Basic & Clinical Pharmacology

Twelfth Edition

Edited by

Bertram G. Katzung, MD, PhD

Professor Emeritus
Department of Cellular & Molecular Pharmacology
University of California, San Francisco

Associate Editors

Susan B. Masters, PhD

Professor of Pharmacology & Academy Chair of Pharmacology Education
Department of Cellular & Molecular Pharmacology
University of California, San Francisco

Anthony J. Trevor, PhD

Professor Emeritus
Department of Cellular & Molecular Pharmacology
University of California, San Francisco

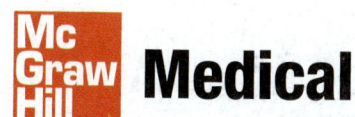

New York   Chicago   San Francisco   Lisbon   London   Madrid   Mexico City
Milan   New Delhi   San Juan   Seoul   Singapore   Sydney   Toronto

The McGraw·Hill Companies

1 2 3 4 5 6 7 8 9 0   DOW/DOW   15 14 13 12 11

ISBN 978-0-07-176401-8
MHID 0-07-176401-1
ISSN 0891-2033

This book was set in Adobe Garamond by Cenveo Publisher Services.
The editors were Michael Weitz and Harriet Lebowitz.
The copyeditors were Donna Frassetto and Rachel D'Annucci Henriquez.
The production supervisor was John Williams.
Project management provided by Rajni Pisharody, Cenveo Publisher Services.
The illustration manager was Armen Ovsepyan; the text designer was Elise Lansdon.
Cover photo: Human insulin, monomeric form; computer-generated model based on Protein Data Bank coordinates. Credit: Scott Camazine/ Photo Researchers, Inc.
The index was prepared by Ann Blum.
RR Donnelley was printer and binder.

This book is printed on acid-free paper.

Contents

Preface

The twelfth edition of *Basic & Clinical Pharmacology* continues the important changes inaugurated in the eleventh edition, with extensive use of full-color illustrations and expanded coverage of transporters, pharmacogenomics, and new drugs. Case studies have been added to several chapters and answers to questions posed in the case studies now appear at the end of each chapter. As in prior editions, the book is designed to provide a comprehensive, authoritative, and readable pharmacology textbook for students in the health sciences. Frequent revision is necessary to keep pace with the rapid changes in pharmacology and therapeutics; the 2–3 year revision cycle of the printed text is among the shortest in the field and the availability of an online version provides even greater currency. In addition to the full-color illustrations, other new features have been introduced. The Case Study Answer section at the end of chapters will make the learning process even more interesting and efficient. The book also offers special features that make it a useful reference for house officers and practicing clinicians.

Information is organized according to the sequence used in many pharmacology courses and in integrated curricula: basic principles; autonomic drugs; cardiovascular-renal drugs; drugs with important actions on smooth muscle; central nervous system drugs; drugs used to treat inflammation, gout, and diseases of the blood; endocrine drugs; chemotherapeutic drugs; toxicology; and special topics. This sequence builds new information on a foundation of information already assimilated. For example, early presentation of autonomic nervous system pharmacology allows students to integrate the physiology and neuroscience they have learned elsewhere with the pharmacology they are learning and prepares them to understand the autonomic effects of other drugs. This is especially important for the cardiovascular and central nervous system drug groups. However, chapters can be used equally well in courses and curricula that present these topics in a different sequence.

Within each chapter, emphasis is placed on discussion of drug groups and prototypes rather than offering repetitive detail about individual drugs. Selection of the subject matter and the order of its presentation are based on the accumulated experience of teaching this material to thousands of medical, pharmacy, dental, podiatry, nursing, and other health science students.

Major features that make this book particularly useful in integrated curricula include sections that specifically address the clinical choice and use of drugs in patients and the monitoring of their effects—in other words, *clinical pharmacology* is an integral part of this text. Lists of the commercial preparations available, including trade and generic names and dosage formulations, are provided at the end of each chapter for easy reference by the house officer or practitioner writing a chart order or prescription.

Significant revisions in this edition include:

- In addition to the Case Studies used to open many chapters, Case Study Answers at the end of these chapters provide an introduction to the clinical applications of the drugs discussed.
- A Drug Summary Table is placed at the conclusion of most chapters; these provide a concise recapitulation of the most important drugs.
- Many new illustrations in full color provide significantly more information about drug mechanisms and effects and help to clarify important concepts.
- Major revisions of the chapters on sympathomimetic, sympathoplegic, antipsychotic, antidepressant, antidiabetic, anti-inflammatory, and antiviral drugs, prostaglandins, nitric oxide, hypothalamic and pituitary hormones, and immunopharmacology.
- Continued expansion of the coverage of general concepts relating to newly discovered receptors, receptor mechanisms, and drug transporters.
- Descriptions of important new drugs released through August 2011.

An important related educational resource is *Katzung & Trevor's Pharmacology: Examination & Board Review*, ninth edition (Trevor AJ, Katzung BG, & Masters SB: McGraw-Hill, 2010). This book provides a succinct review of pharmacology with over one thousand sample examination questions and answers. It is especially helpful to students preparing for board-type examinations. A more highly condensed source of information suitable for review purposes is *USMLE Road Map: Pharmacology*, second edition (Katzung BG, Trevor AJ: McGraw-Hill, 2006).

This edition marks the 30th year of publication of *Basic & Clinical Pharmacology*. The widespread adoption of the first eleven editions indicates that this book fills an important need. We believe that the twelfth edition will satisfy this need even more successfully. Spanish, Portuguese, Italian, French, Indonesian, Japanese, Korean, and Turkish translations are available. Translations into other languages are under way; the publisher may be contacted for further information.

I wish to acknowledge the prior and continuing efforts of my contributing authors and the major contributions of the staff at Lange Medical Publications, Appleton & Lange, and McGraw-Hill, and of our editors for this edition, Donna Frassetto and Rachel D'Annucci Henriquez. I also wish to thank my wife, Alice Camp, for her expert proofreading contributions since the first edition.

This edition is dedicated to the memory of James Ransom, PhD, the long-time Senior Editor at Lange Medical Publications, who provided major inspiration and invaluable guidance through the first eight editions of the book. Without him, this book would not exist.

Suggestions and comments about *Basic & Clinical Pharmacology* are always welcome. They may be sent to me in care of the publisher.

Bertram G. Katzung, MD, PhD
San Francisco
December, 2011

Authors

Emmanuel T. Akporiaye, PhD
Adjunct Professor, Oregon Health Sciences University,
Laboratory Chief, Earle A. Chiles Research Institute,
Providence Cancer Center, Portland

Michael J. Aminoff, MD, DSc, FRCP
Professor, Department of Neurology, University of
California, San Francisco

Allan I. Basbaum, PhD
Professor and Chair, Department of Anatomy and
W.M. Keck Foundation Center for Integrative
Neuroscience, University of California, San Francisco

Neal L. Benowitz, MD
Professor of Medicine and Bioengineering & Therapeutic
Science, University of California, San Francisco,
San Francisco

Italo Biaggioni, MD
Professor of Pharmacology, Vanderbilt University School
of Medicine, Nashville

Daniel D. Bikle, MD, PhD
Professor of Medicine, Department of Medicine, and
Co-Director, Special Diagnostic and Treatment Unit,
University of California, San Francisco, and Veterans
Affairs Medical Center, San Francisco

Homer A. Boushey, MD
Chief, Asthma Clinical Research Center and Division of
Allergy & Immunology; Professor of Medicine,
Department of Medicine, University of California,
San Francisco

Adrienne D. Briggs, MD
Clinical Director, Bone Marrow Transplant Program,
Banner Good Samaritan Hospital, Phoenix

Lundy Campbell, MD
Professor, Department of Anesthesiology and
Perioperative Medicine, University of California
San Francisco, School of Medicine, San Francisco

George P. Chrousos, MD
Professor & Chair, First Department of Pediatrics, Athens
University Medical School, Athens

Edward Chu, MD
Professor of Medicine and Pharmacology & Chemical
Biology; Chief, Division of Hematology-Oncology, Deputy
Director, University of Pittsburgh Cancer Institute,
University of Pittsburgh School of Medicine, Pittsburgh

Robin L. Corelli, PharmD
Clinical Professor, Department of Clinical Pharmacy,
School of Pharmacy, University of California, San
Francisco

Maria Almira Correia, PhD
Professor of Pharmacology, Pharmaceutical Chemistry
and Biopharmaceutical Sciences, Department of Cellular
& Molecular Pharmacology, University of California,
San Francisco

Charles DeBattista, MD
Professor of Psychiatry and Behavioral Sciences, Stanford
University School of Medicine, Stanford

Daniel H. Deck, PharmD
Assistant Clinical Professor, School of Pharmacy,
University of California, San Francisco; Infectious
Diseases Clinical Pharmacist, San Francisco General
Hospital

Cathi E. Dennehy, PharmD
Professor, Department of Clinical Pharmacy, University of
California, San Francisco School of Pharmacy

Betty J. Dong, PharmD, FASHP, FCCP
Professor of Clinical Pharmacy and Clinical Professor of
Family and Community Medicine, Department of Clinical
Pharmacy and Department of Family and Community
Medicine, Schools of Pharmacy and Medicine, University
of California, San Francisco

Kenneth Drasner, MD
Profesor of Anesthesia and Perioperative Care, University
of California, San Francisco

Helge Eilers, MD
Professor of Anesthesia and Perioperative Care, University
of California, San Francisco

Garret A. FitzGerald, MD
Chair, Department of Pharmacology; Director, Institute for Translational Medicine and Therapeutics, Perelman School of Medicine at the University of Pennsylvania, Philadelphia

Daniel E. Furst, MD
Carl M. Pearson Professor of Rheumatology, Director, Rheumatology Clinical Research Center, Department of Rheumatology, University of California, Los Angeles

Augustus O. Grant, MD, PhD
Professor of Medicine, Cardiovascular Division, Duke University Medical Center, Durham

Francis S. Greenspan, MD, FACP
Clinical Professor of Medicine and Radiology and Chief, Thyroid Clinic, Division of Endocrinology, Department of Medicine, University of California, San Francisco

Nicholas H. G. Holford, MB, ChB, FRACP
Professor, Department of Pharmacology and Clinical Pharmacology, University of Auckland Medical School, Auckland

John R. Horn, PharmD, FCCP
Professor of Pharmacy, School of Pharmacy, University of Washington; Associate Director of Pharmacy Services, Department of Medicine, University of Washington Medicine, Seattle

Joseph R. Hume, PhD
Professor and Chairman, Department of Pharmacology; Adjunct Professor, Department of Physiology and Cell Biology, University of Nevada School of Medicine, Reno

Harlan E. Ives, MD, PhD
Professor of Medicine, Department of Medicine, University of California, San Francisco

Samie R. Jaffrey, MD, PhD
Associate Professor of Pharmacology, Department of Pharmacology, Cornell University Weill Medical College, New York City

John P. Kane, MD, PhD
Professor of Medicine, Department of Medicine; Professor of Biochemistry and Biophysics; Associate Director, Cardiovascular Research Institute, University of California, San Francisco

Bertram G. Katzung, MD, PhD
Professor Emeritus, Department of Cellular & Molecular Pharmacology, University of California, San Francisco

Gideon Koren, MD
Professor of Pediatrics, Pharmacology, Pharmacy, Medicine and Medical Genetics; Director, Motherisk Program, University of Toronto

Michael J. Kosnett, MD, MPH
Associate Clinical Professor of Medicine, Division of Clinical Pharmacology and Toxicology, University of Colorado Health Sciences Center, Denver

Marieke Kruidering-Hall, PhD
Associate Professor, Department of Cellular and Molecular Pharmacology, University of California, San Francisco

Douglas F. Lake, PhD
Associate Professor, The Biodesign Institute, Arizona State University, Tempe

Harry W. Lampiris, MD
Associate Professor of Medicine, University of California, San Francisco

Paul W. Lofholm, PharmD
Clinical Professor of Pharmacy, School of Pharmacy, University of California, San Francisco

Christian Lüscher, MD
Departments of Basic and Clincial Neurosciences, Medical Faculty, University Hospital of Geneva, Geneva, Switzerland

Daniel S. Maddix, PharmD
Associate Clinical Professor of Pharmacy, University of California, San Francisco

Howard I. Maibach, MD
Professor of Dermatology, Department of Dermatology, University of California, San Francisco

Mary J. Malloy, MD
Clinical Professor of Pediatrics and Medicine, Departments of Pediatrics and Medicine, Cardiovascular Research Institute, University of California, San Francisco

Susan B. Masters, PhD
Professor of Pharmacology & Academy Chair of Pharmacology Education, Department of Cellular & Molecular Pharmacology, University of California, San Francisco

Kenneth R. McQuaid, MD
Professor of Clinical Medicine, University of California, San Francisco; Chief of Gastroenterology, San Francisco Veterans Affairs Medical Center

Brian S. Meldrum, MB, PhD
Professor Emeritus, GKT School of Medicine, Guy's Campus, London

Herbert Meltzer, MD, PhD
Professor of Psychiatry and Pharmacology, Vanderbilt University, Nashville

Roger A. Nicoll, MD
Professor of Pharmacology and Physiology, Departments of Cellular & Molecular Pharmacology and Physiology, University of California, San Francisco

Martha S. Nolte Kennedy, MD
Clinical Professor, Department of Medicine, University of California, San Francisco

Kent R. Olson, MD
Clinical Professor, Departments of Medicine and Pharmacy, University of California, San Francisco; Medical Director, San Francisco Division, California Poison Control System

Achilles J. Pappano, PhD
Professor Emeritus, Department of Cell Biology and Calhoun Cardiology Center, University of Connecticut Health Center, Farmington

Roger J. Porter, MD
Adjunct Professor of Neurology, University of Pennsylvania, Philadelphia; Adjunct Professor of Pharmacology, Uniformed Services University of the Health Sciences, Bethesda

Shraddha Prakash, MD
Senior Fellow in Rheumatology, David Geffen School of Medicine, University of California, Los Angeles

Ian A. Reid, PhD
Professor Emeritus, Department of Physiology, University of California, San Francisco

David Robertson, MD
Elton Yates Professor of Medicine, Pharmacology and Neurology, Vanderbilt University; Director, Clinical & Translational Research Center, Vanderbilt Institute for Clinical and Translational Research, Nashville

Dirk B. Robertson, MD
Professor of Clinical Dermatology, Department of Dermatology, Emory University School of Medicine, Atlanta

Philip J. Rosenthal, MD
Professor of Medicine, University of California, San Francisco, San Francisco General Hospital

Stephen M. Rosenthal, MD
Professor of Pediatrics, Associate Program Director, Pediatric Endocrinology; Director, Pediatric Endocrine Outpatient Services, University of California, San Francisco

Sharon Safrin, MD
Associate Clinical Professor, Department of Medicine, University of California, San Francisco; President, Safrin Clinical Research

Alan C. Sartorelli, PhD
Alfred Gilman Professor of Pharmacology, Department of Pharmacology, Yale University School of Medicine, New Haven

Mark A. Schumacher, PhD, MD
Associate Professor, Department of Anesthesia and Perioperative Care, University of California, San Francisco

Don Sheppard, MD
Associate Professor, Departments of Microbiology and Immunology and Medicine, McGill University; Program Director, McGill Royal College Training Program in Medical Microbiology and Infectious Diseases, Montreal

Emer M. Smyth, PhD
Assistant Professor, Department of Pharmacology, University of Pennsylvania School of Medicine, Philadelphia

Daniel T. Teitelbaum, MD
Professor, University of Colorado School of Medicine, Aurora, and Colorado School of Mines, Golden

Anthony J. Trevor, PhD
Professor Emeritus, Department of Cellular & Molecular Pharmacology, University of California, San Francisco

Candy Tsourounis, PharmD
Professor of Clinical Pharmacy, Medication Outcomes Center, University of California, San Francisco School of Pharmacy

Robert W. Ulrich, PharmD
Senior Clinical Science Manager, Abbott Laboratories Inc., Covina, California

Mark von Zastrow, MD, PhD
Professor, Departments of Psychiatry and Cellular & Molecular Pharmacology, University of California, San Francisco

Walter L. Way, MD[*]
Professor Emeritus, Departments of Anesthesia and Cellular & Molecular Pharmacology, University of California, San Francisco

Lisa G. Winston, MD
Associate Professor, Department of Medicine, Division of Infectious Diseases, University of California, San Francisco; Hospital Epidemiologist, San Francisco General Hospital

Spencer Yost, MD
Professor, Department of Anesthesia and Perioperative Care, University of California, San Francisco; Medical Director, UCSF-Mt. Zion ICU, Chief of Anesthesia, UCSF-Mt. Zion Hospital

James L. Zehnder, MD
Professor of Pathology and Medicine, Pathology Department, Stanford University School of Medicine, Stanford

*Deceased

Key Features of
Basic & Clinical Pharmacology, 12e

The most comprehensive, authoritative, and engaging pharmacology textbook for students in the health sciences

Key Features

- More than 300 full-color illustrations

- Emphasis is placed on discussion of drug groups and prototypes within each chapter

- NEW case studies open several chapters, adding clinical relevance to the material

- NEW case study answers at the end of the chapters provide an introduction to the clinical application of the drugs discussed

- NEW drug summary tables conclude most chapters, providing a concise summary of the most important drugs

- Expanded coverage of general concepts relating to newly discovered receptors, receptor mechanisms, and drug transporters

- Lists of the commercial preparations available, including trade and generic names and dosage formulations, are provided at the end of each chapter

- Selection of the material and order of presentation is based on the author's years of experience in teaching this material to thousands of students

- Material is organized according to the sequence used in most pharmacology courses

Hundreds of full-color illustrations enrich the text

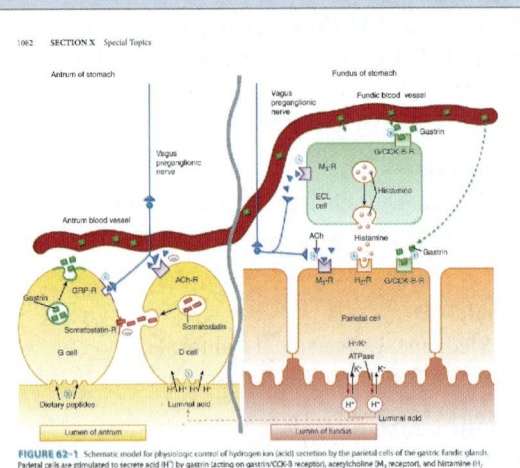

1062   SECTION X   Special Topics

FIGURE 62–1 Schematic model for physiologic control of hydrogen ion (acid) secretion by the parietal cells of the gastric fundic glands. Parietal cells are stimulated to secrete acid (H⁺) by gastrin (acting on gastrin/CCK-B receptor), acetylcholine (M₃ receptor), and histamine (H₂ receptor). Acid is secreted across the parietal cell canalicular membrane by the H⁺/K⁺-ATPase proton pump into the gastric lumen. Gastrin is secreted by antral G cells into blood vessels in response to intraluminal dietary peptides. Within the gastric body, gastrin passes from the blood vessels into the submucosal tissue of the fundic glands, where it binds to gastrin-CCK-B receptors on parietal cells and enterochromaffin-like (ECL) cells. The vagus nerve stimulates postganglionic neurons of the enteric nervous system to release acetylcholine (ACh), which binds to M₃ receptors on parietal cells and ECL cells. Stimulation of ECL cells by gastrin (CCK-B receptor) or acetylcholine (M₃ receptor) stimulates release of histamine. Within the gastric antrum, vagal stimulation of postganglionic enteric neurons enhances gastrin release directly by stimulation of antral G cells (through gastrin-releasing peptide, GRP) and indirectly by inhibition of somatostatin secretion from antral D cells. Acid secretion must eventually be turned off. Antral D cells are stimulated to release somatostatin by the rise in intraluminal H⁺ concentration and by CCK that is released into the bloodstream by duodenal I cells in response to proteins and fats (not shown). Binding of somatostatin to receptors on adjacent antral G cells inhibits further gastrin release. ATPase, H⁺/K⁺-ATPase proton pump; CCK, cholecystokinin; M₃, muscarinic receptors.

In close proximity to the parietal cells are gut endocrine cells called *enterochromaffin-like (ECL) cells*. ECL cells also have receptors for gastrin and acetylcholine, which stimulate histamine release. Histamine binds in the H₂ receptor on the parietal cell, resulting in activation of adenylyl cyclase, which increases intracellular cyclic adenosine monophosphate (cAMP) and activates protein kinases that stimulate acid secretion by the H⁺/K⁺-ATPase. In humans, it is believed that the major effect of gastrin upon acid secretion is mediated indirectly through the release of histamine from ECL cells rather than through direct parietal cell stimulation. In contrast, acetylcholine provides potent direct parietal cell stimulation.

ANTACIDS

Antacids have been used for centuries in the treatment of patients with dyspepsia and acid-peptic disorders. They were the mainstay of treatment for acid-peptic disorders until the advent of H2-receptor antagonists and proton pump inhibitors. They con-

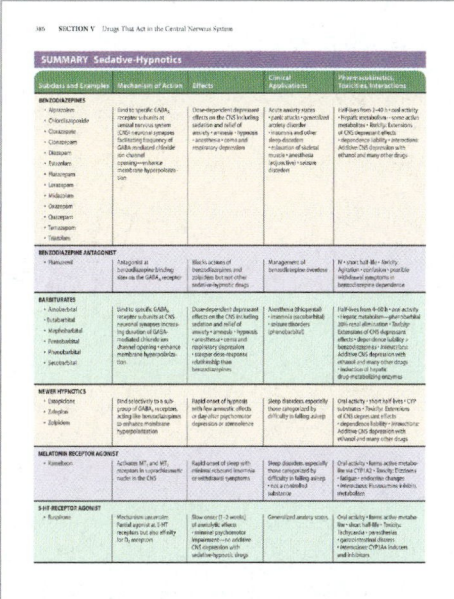

Drug Summary Tables conclude most chapters

Case studies are included in selected chapters

Lists of the commercial preparations available appear at the end of the chapter

C H A P T E R

1

Introduction

Bertram G. Katzung, MD, PhD

C A S E   S T U D Y

A 26-year-old man is brought by friends to the emergency department of the city hospital because he has been behaving strangely for several days. A known user of methamphetamine, he has not eaten or slept in 48 hours. He threatened to shoot one of his friends because he believes this friend is plotting against him. On admission, the man is extremely agitated, appears to be underweight, and is unable to give a coherent history. He has to be restrained to prevent him from walking out of the emergency department and into traffic on the street. His blood pressure is 160/100 mm Hg, heart rate 100, temperature 39°C, and respirations 30/ min. His arms show evidence of numerous intravenous injections. The remainder of his physical examination is unremarkable. After evaluation, the man is given a sedative, fluids, a diuretic, and ammonium chloride parenterally. What is the purpose of the ammonium chloride?

Pharmacology can be defined as the study of substances that interact with living systems through chemical processes, especially by binding to regulatory molecules and activating or inhibiting normal body processes. These substances may be chemicals administered to achieve a beneficial therapeutic effect on some process within the patient or for their toxic effects on regulatory processes in parasites infecting the patient. Such deliberate therapeutic applications may be considered the proper role of **medical pharmacology,** which is often defined as the science of substances used to prevent, diagnose, and treat disease. **Toxicology** is the branch of pharmacology that deals with the undesirable effects of chemicals on living systems, from individual cells to humans to complex ecosystems (Figure 1–1).

THE HISTORY OF PHARMACOLOGY

Prehistoric people undoubtedly recognized the beneficial or toxic effects of many plant and animal materials. Early written records from China and Egypt and the traditions of India list remedies of many types, including a few that are still recognized as useful drugs today. Most, however, were worthless or actually harmful. In the 1500 years or so preceding the present, there were sporadic attempts to introduce rational methods into medicine, but none was successful owing to the dominance of systems of thought that purported to explain all of biology and disease without the need for experimentation and observation. These schools promulgated bizarre notions such as the idea that

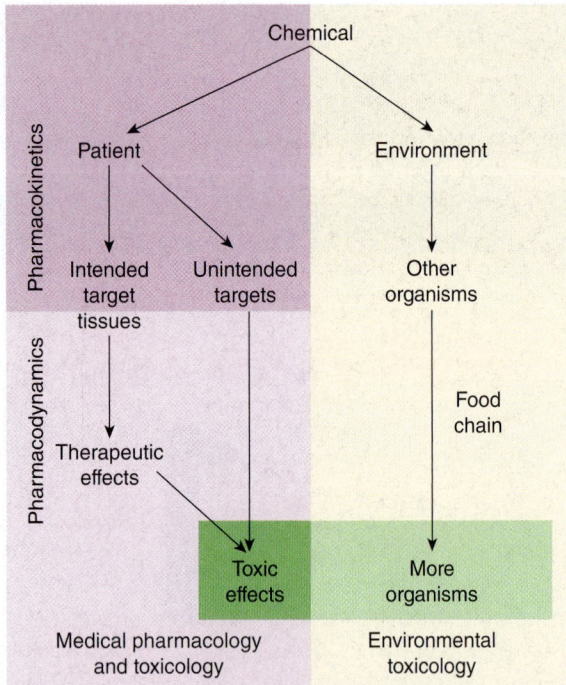

FIGURE 1–1 Major areas of study in pharmacology. The actions of chemicals can be divided into two large domains. The first (*left side*) is that of medical pharmacology and toxicology, which is aimed at understanding the actions of drugs as chemicals on individual organisms, especially humans and domestic animals. Both beneficial and toxic effects are included. Pharmacokinetics deals with the absorption, distribution, and elimination of drugs. Pharmacodynamics concerns the actions of the chemical on the organism. The second domain (*right side*) is that of environmental toxicology, which is concerned with the effects of chemicals on all organisms and their survival in groups and as species.

disease was caused by excesses of bile or blood in the body, that wounds could be healed by applying a salve to the weapon that caused the wound, and so on.

Around the end of the 17th century, and following the example of the physical sciences, reliance on observation and experimentation began to replace theorizing in medicine. As the value of these methods in the study of disease became clear, physicians in Great Britain and on the Continent began to apply them to the effects of traditional drugs used in their own practices. Thus, **materia medica**—the science of drug preparation and the medical use of drugs—began to develop as the precursor to pharmacology. However, any real understanding of the mechanisms of action of drugs was prevented by the absence of methods for purifying active agents from the crude materials that were available and— even more—by the lack of methods for testing hypotheses about the nature of drug actions.

In the late 18th and early 19th centuries, François Magendie, and later his student Claude Bernard, began to develop the methods of **experimental physiology** and **pharmacology.** Advances in chemistry and the further development of physiology in the 18th,

19th, and early 20th centuries laid the foundation needed for understanding how drugs work at the organ and tissue levels. Paradoxically, real advances in basic pharmacology during this time were accompanied by an outburst of unscientific claims by manufacturers and marketers of worthless "patent medicines." Not until the concepts of rational therapeutics, especially that of the **controlled clinical trial,** were reintroduced into medicine— only about 60 years ago—did it become possible to accurately evaluate therapeutic claims.

Around the same time, a major expansion of research efforts in all areas of biology began. As new concepts and new techniques were introduced, information accumulated about drug action and the biologic substrate of that action, the **drug receptor.** During the last half-century, many fundamentally new drug groups and new members of old groups were introduced. The last three decades have seen an even more rapid growth of information and understanding of the molecular basis for drug action. The molecular mechanisms of action of many drugs have now been identified, and numerous receptors have been isolated, structurally characterized, and cloned. In fact, the use of receptor identification methods (described in Chapter 2) has led to the discovery of many orphan receptors—receptors for which no ligand has been discovered and whose function can only be surmised. Studies of the local molecular environment of receptors have shown that receptors and effectors do not function in isolation; they are strongly influenced by other receptors and by companion regulatory proteins.

Pharmacogenomics—the relation of the individual's genetic makeup to his or her response to specific drugs—is close to becoming a practical area of therapy (see Box: Pharmacology & Genetics). Decoding of the genomes of many species—from bacteria to humans—has led to the recognition of unsuspected relationships between receptor families and the ways that receptor proteins have evolved. Discovery that small segments of RNA can interfere with protein synthesis with extreme selectivity has led to investigation of **small interfering RNAs (siRNAs)** and **microRNAs (miRNAs)** as therapeutic agents. Similarly, short nucleotide chains called **antisense oligonucleotides (ANOs)** synthesized to be complementary to natural RNA or DNA can interfere with the readout of genes and the transcription of RNA. These intracellular targets may provide the next major wave of advances in therapeutics.

The extension of scientific principles into everyday therapeutics is still going on, although the medication-consuming public is still exposed to vast amounts of inaccurate, incomplete, or unscientific information regarding the pharmacologic effects of chemicals. This has resulted in the irrational use of innumerable expensive, ineffective, and sometimes harmful remedies and the growth of a huge "alternative health care" industry. Unfortunately, manipulation of the legislative process in the United States has allowed many substances promoted for health—but not promoted specifically as "drugs"—to avoid meeting the Food and Drug Administration (FDA) standards described in Chapter 5. Conversely, lack of understanding of basic scientific principles in biology and statistics and the absence of critical thinking about public health issues have led to rejection of medical

Pharmacology & Genetics

It has been known for centuries that certain diseases are inherited, and we now understand that individuals with such diseases have a heritable abnormality in their DNA. During the last 10 years, the genomes of humans, mice, and many other organisms have been decoded in considerable detail. This has opened the door to a remarkable range of new approaches to research and treatment. It is now possible in the case of some inherited diseases to define exactly which DNA base pairs are anomalous and in which chromosome they appear. In a small number of animal models of such diseases, it has been possible to correct the abnormality by gene therapy, ie, insertion of an appropriate "healthy" gene into somatic cells. Human somatic cell **gene therapy** has been attempted, but the technical difficulties are great.

Studies of a newly discovered receptor or endogenous ligand are often confounded by incomplete knowledge of the exact role of that receptor or ligand. One of the most powerful of the new genetic techniques is the ability to breed animals (usually mice) in which the gene for the receptor or its endogenous ligand has been "knocked out," ie, mutated so that the gene product is absent or nonfunctional. Homozygous **knockout** mice usually have complete suppression of that function, whereas heterozygous animals usually have partial suppression. Observation of the behavior, biochemistry, and physiology of the knockout mice often defines the role of the missing gene product very clearly. When the products of a particular gene are so essential that even heterozygotes do not survive to birth, it is sometimes possible to breed "knockdown" versions with only limited suppression of function. Conversely, "knockin" mice, which overexpress certain proteins of interest, have been bred.

Some patients respond to certain drugs with greater than usual sensitivity to standard doses. It is now clear that such increased sensitivity is often due to a very small genetic modification that results in decreased activity of a particular enzyme responsible for eliminating that drug. (Such variations are discussed in Chapter 4.) **Pharmacogenomics** (or pharmacogenetics) is the study of the genetic variations that cause differences in drug response among individuals or populations. Future clinicians may screen every patient for a variety of such differences before prescribing a drug.

---

science by a segment of the public and to a common tendency to assume that all adverse drug effects are the result of malpractice.

Two general principles that the student should remember are (1) that *all* substances can under certain circumstances be toxic, and the chemicals in botanicals (herbs and plant extracts) are no different from chemicals in manufactured drugs except for the proportion of impurities (greater in botanicals); and, (2) that all dietary supplements and all therapies promoted as health-enhancing should meet the same standards of efficacy and safety as conventional drugs and medical therapies. That is, there should be no artificial separation between scientific medicine and "alternative" or "complementary" medicine.

PHARMACOLOGY & THE PHARMACEUTICAL INDUSTRY

A truly new drug (one that does not simply mimic the structure and action of previously available drugs) requires the discovery of a new drug *target*, ie, the pathophysiologic process or substrate of a disease. Such discoveries are usually made in public sector institutions (universities and research institutes), and the molecules that have beneficial effects on such targets are often discovered in the same laboratories. However, the *development* of new drugs usually takes place in industrial laboratories because optimization of a class of new drugs requires painstaking and expensive chemical, pharmacologic, and toxicologic research. In fact, much of the recent progress in the application of drugs to disease problems can be ascribed to the pharmaceutical industry including "big pharma," the multibillion-dollar corporations that specialize in drug discovery and development. As described in Chapter 5, these companies are uniquely skilled in exploiting discoveries from academic and governmental laboratories and translating these basic findings into commercially successful therapeutic breakthroughs.

Such breakthroughs come at a price, however, and the escalating cost of drugs has become a significant contributor to the inflationary increase in the cost of health care. Development of new drugs is enormously expensive, and to survive and prosper, big pharma must pay the costs of drug development and marketing and return a profit to its shareholders. Today, considerable controversy surrounds drug pricing. Critics claim that the costs of development and marketing are grossly inflated by marketing activities, which may consume as much as 25% or more of a company's budget in advertising and other promotional efforts. Furthermore, profit margins for big pharma have historically exceeded all other industries by a significant factor. Finally, pricing schedules for many drugs vary dramatically from country to country and even within countries, where large organizations can negotiate favorable prices and small ones cannot. Some countries have already addressed these inequities, and it seems likely that all countries will have to do so during the next few decades.

GENERAL PRINCIPLES OF PHARMACOLOGY

THE NATURE OF DRUGS

In the most general sense, a drug may be defined as any substance that brings about a change in biologic function through its chemical actions. In most cases, the drug molecule interacts as an

agonist (activator) or **antagonist** (inhibitor) with a specific molecule in the biologic system that plays a regulatory role. This target molecule is called a **receptor**. The nature of receptors is discussed more fully in Chapter 2. In a very small number of cases, drugs known as **chemical antagonists** may interact directly with other drugs, whereas a few drugs (osmotic agents) interact almost exclusively with water molecules. Drugs may be synthesized within the body (eg, **hormones**) or may be chemicals *not* synthesized in the body (ie, **xenobiotics,** from the Greek *xenos*, meaning "stranger"). **Poisons** are drugs that have almost exclusively harmful effects. However, Paracelsus (1493–1541) famously stated that "the dose makes the poison," meaning that any substance can be harmful if taken in the wrong dosage. **Toxins** are usually defined as poisons of biologic origin, ie, synthesized by plants or animals, in contrast to inorganic poisons such as lead and arsenic.

To interact chemically with its receptor, a drug molecule must have the appropriate size, electrical charge, shape, and atomic composition. Furthermore, a drug is often administered at a location distant from its intended site of action, eg, a pill given orally to relieve a headache. Therefore, a useful drug must have the necessary properties to be transported from its site of administration to its site of action. Finally, a practical drug should be inactivated or excreted from the body at a reasonable rate so that its actions will be of appropriate duration.

The Physical Nature of Drugs

Drugs may be solid at room temperature (eg, aspirin, atropine), liquid (eg, nicotine, ethanol), or gaseous (eg, nitrous oxide). These factors often determine the best route of administration. The most common routes of administration are described in Table 3–3. The various classes of organic compounds—carbohydrates, proteins, lipids, and their constituents—are all represented in pharmacology. As noted above, oligonucleotides, in the form of small segments of RNA, have entered clinical trials and are on the threshold of introduction into therapeutics.

A number of useful or dangerous drugs are inorganic elements, eg, lithium, iron, and heavy metals. Many organic drugs are weak acids or bases. This fact has important implications for the way they are handled by the body, because pH differences in the various compartments of the body may alter the degree of ionization of such drugs (see text that follows).

Drug Size

The molecular size of drugs varies from very small (lithium ion, MW 7) to very large (eg, alteplase [t-PA], a protein of MW 59,050). However, most drugs have molecular weights between 100 and 1000. The lower limit of this narrow range is probably set by the requirements for specificity of action. To have a good "fit" to only one type of receptor, a drug molecule must be sufficiently unique in shape, charge, and other properties, to prevent its binding to other receptors. To achieve such selective binding, it appears that a molecule should in most cases be at least 100 MW units in size. The upper limit in molecular weight is determined primarily by the requirement that drugs must be able to move within the body (eg, from the site of administration to the site of action). Drugs much larger than MW 1000 do not diffuse readily between compartments of the body (see Permeation, in following text). Therefore, very large drugs (usually proteins) must often be administered directly into the compartment where they have their effect. In the case of alteplase, a clot-dissolving enzyme, the drug is administered directly into the vascular compartment by intravenous or intra-arterial infusion.

Drug Reactivity and Drug-Receptor Bonds

Drugs interact with receptors by means of chemical forces or bonds. These are of three major types: **covalent, electrostatic,** and **hydrophobic.** Covalent bonds are very strong and in many cases not reversible under biologic conditions. Thus, the covalent bond formed between the acetyl group of acetylsalicylic acid (aspirin) and cyclooxygenase, its enzyme target in platelets, is not readily broken. The platelet aggregation–blocking effect of aspirin lasts long after free acetylsalicylic acid has disappeared from the bloodstream (about 15 minutes) and is reversed only by the synthesis of new enzyme in new platelets, a process that takes several days. Other examples of highly reactive, covalent bond-forming drugs are the DNA-alkylating agents used in cancer chemotherapy to disrupt cell division in the tumor.

Electrostatic bonding is much more common than covalent bonding in drug-receptor interactions. Electrostatic bonds vary from relatively strong linkages between permanently charged ionic molecules to weaker hydrogen bonds and very weak induced dipole interactions such as van der Waals forces and similar phenomena. Electrostatic bonds are weaker than covalent bonds.

Hydrophobic bonds are usually quite weak and are probably important in the interactions of highly lipid-soluble drugs with the lipids of cell membranes and perhaps in the interaction of drugs with the internal walls of receptor "pockets."

The specific nature of a particular drug-receptor bond is of less practical importance than the fact that drugs that bind through weak bonds to their receptors are generally more selective than drugs that bind by means of very strong bonds. This is because weak bonds require a very precise fit of the drug to its receptor if an interaction is to occur. Only a few receptor types are likely to provide such a precise fit for a particular drug structure. Thus, if we wished to design a highly selective short-acting drug for a particular receptor, we would avoid highly reactive molecules that form covalent bonds and instead choose a molecule that forms weaker bonds.

A few substances that are almost completely inert in the chemical sense nevertheless have significant pharmacologic effects. For example, xenon, an "inert" gas, has anesthetic effects at elevated pressures.

Drug Shape

The shape of a drug molecule must be such as to permit binding to its receptor site via the bonds just described. Optimally, the drug's shape is complementary to that of the receptor site in the same way that a key is complementary to a lock. Furthermore, the phenomenon of **chirality (stereoisomerism)** is so common in biology that more than half of all useful drugs are chiral molecules; that is, they

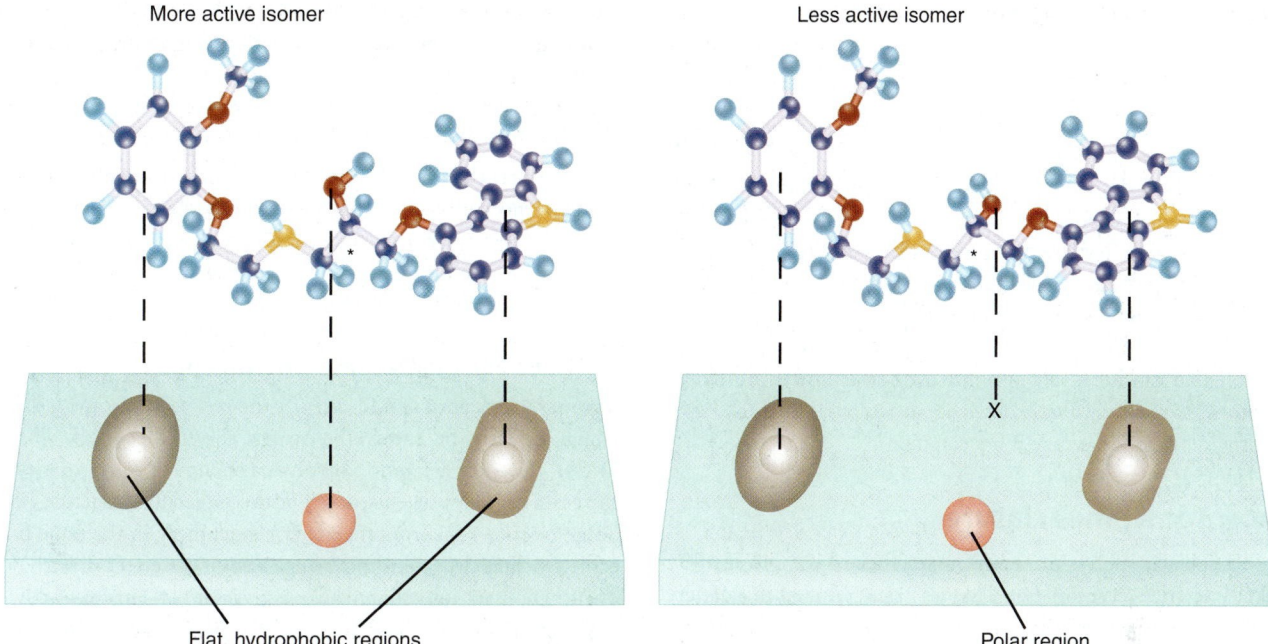

More active isomer

Less active isomer

Flat, hydrophobic regions

Polar region

FIGURE 1–2 Cartoon illustrating the nonsuperimposibility of the two stereoisomers of carvedilol on the β receptor. The "receptor surface" has been grossly oversimplified. The chiral center carbon is denoted with an asterisk. One of the two isomers fits the three-dimensional configuration of binding site of the β-adrenoceptor molecule very well (*left*), and three groups, including an important polar moiety (an hydroxyl group, indicated by the central dashed line), bind to key areas of the surface. The less active isomer cannot orient all three binding areas to the receptor surface (*right*). (Molecule generated by means of Jmol, an open-source Java viewer for chemical structures in 3D [http://jmol.sourceforge.net/] with data from DrugBank [http://www.drugbank.ca].)

can exist as enantiomeric pairs. Drugs with two asymmetric centers have four diastereomers, eg, ephedrine, a sympathomimetic drug. In most cases, one of these enantiomers is much more potent than its mirror image enantiomer, reflecting a better fit to the receptor molecule. If one imagines the receptor site to be like a glove into which the drug molecule must fit to bring about its effect, it is clear why a "left-oriented" drug is more effective in binding to a left-hand receptor than its "right-oriented" enantiomer.

The more active enantiomer at one type of receptor site may not be more active at another receptor type, eg, a type that may be responsible for some other effect. For example, carvedilol, a drug that interacts with adrenoceptors, has a single chiral center and thus two enantiomers (Figure 1–2, Table 1–1). One of these enantiomers, the *(S)(–)* isomer, is a potent β-receptor blocker. The *(R)(+)* isomer is 100-fold weaker at the β receptor. However, the isomers are approximately equipotent as α-receptor blockers. Ketamine is an intravenous anesthetic. The (+) enantiomer is a more potent anesthetic and is less toxic than the (–) enantiomer. Unfortunately, the drug is still used as the racemic mixture.

Finally, because enzymes are usually stereoselective, one drug enantiomer is often more susceptible than the other to drug-metabolizing enzymes. As a result, the duration of action of one enantiomer may be quite different from that of the other. Similarly, drug transporters may be stereoselective.

Unfortunately, most studies of clinical efficacy and drug elimination in humans have been carried out with racemic mixtures of drugs rather than with the separate enantiomers. At present, only a small percentage of the chiral drugs used clinically are marketed as the active isomer—the rest are available only as racemic mixtures. As a result, many patients are receiving drug doses of which 50% is less active, inactive, or actively toxic. Some drugs are currently available in both the racemic and the pure, active isomer forms. Unfortunately, the hope that administration of the pure, active enantiomer would decrease adverse effects relative to those produced by racemic formulations has not been firmly established. However, there is increasing interest at both the scientific and the regulatory levels in making more chiral drugs available as their active enantiomers.

TABLE 1–1 Dissociation constants (K_d) of the enantiomers and racemate of carvedilol.

Form of Carvedilol	α Receptors (K_d, nmol/L[1])	β Receptors (K_d, nmol/L)
R(+) enantiomer	14	45
S(–) enantiomer	16	0.4
R,S(±) enantiomers	11	0.9

[1]The K_d is the concentration for 50% saturation of the receptors and is inversely proportionate to the affinity of the drug for the receptors.

Data from Ruffolo RR et al: The pharmacology of carvedilol. Eur J Pharmacol 1990;38:S82.

Rational Drug Design

Rational design of drugs implies the ability to predict the appropriate molecular structure of a drug on the basis of information about its biologic receptor. Until recently, no receptor was known in sufficient detail to permit such drug design. Instead, drugs were developed through random testing of chemicals or modification of drugs already known to have some effect (see Chapter 5). However, the characterization of many receptors during the past three decades has changed this picture. A few drugs now in use were developed through molecular design based on knowledge of the three-dimensional structure of the receptor site. Computer programs are now available that can iteratively optimize drug structures to fit known receptors. As more becomes known about receptor structure, rational drug design will become more common.

Receptor Nomenclature

The spectacular success of newer, more efficient ways to identify and characterize receptors (see Chapter 2) has resulted in a variety of differing, and sometimes confusing, systems for naming them. This in turn has led to a number of suggestions regarding more rational methods of naming receptors. The interested reader is referred for details to the efforts of the International Union of Pharmacology (IUPHAR) *Committee on Receptor Nomenclature and Drug Classification* (reported in various issues of *Pharmacological Reviews*) and to Alexander SPH, Mathie A, Peters JA: Guide to receptors and channels (GRAC), 4th edition. *Br J Pharmacol* 2009;158(Suppl 1):S1–S254. The chapters in this book mainly use these sources for naming receptors.

DRUG-BODY INTERACTIONS

The interactions between a drug and the body are conveniently divided into two classes. The actions of the drug on the body are termed **pharmacodynamic** processes (Figure 1–1); the principles of pharmacodynamics are presented in greater detail in Chapter 2. These properties determine the group in which the drug is classified, and they play the major role in deciding whether that group is appropriate therapy for a particular symptom or disease. The actions of the body on the drug are called **pharmacokinetic** processes and are described in Chapters 3 and 4. Pharmacokinetic processes govern the absorption, distribution, and elimination of drugs and are of great practical importance in the choice and administration of a particular drug for a particular patient, eg, a patient with impaired renal function. The following paragraphs provide a brief introduction to pharmacodynamics and pharmacokinetics.

Pharmacodynamic Principles

Most drugs must bind to a receptor to bring about an effect. However, at the cellular level, drug binding is only the first in what is often a complex sequence of steps:

- Drug (D) + receptor-effector (R) → drug-receptor-effector complex → effect

- D + R → drug-receptor complex → effector molecule → effect
- D + R → D-R complex → activation of coupling molecule → effector molecule → effect
- Inhibition of metabolism of endogenous activator → increased activator action on an effector molecule → increased effect

Note that the final change in function is accomplished by an **effector** mechanism. The effector may be part of the receptor molecule or may be a separate molecule. A very large number of receptors communicate with their effectors through coupling molecules, as described in Chapter 2.

A. Types of Drug-Receptor Interactions

Agonist drugs bind to and *activate* the receptor in some fashion, which directly or indirectly brings about the effect (Figure 1–3A). Receptor activation involves a change in conformation in the cases that have been studied at the molecular structure level. Some receptors incorporate effector machinery in the same molecule, so that drug binding brings about the effect directly, eg, opening of an ion channel or activation of enzyme activity. Other receptors are linked through one or more intervening coupling molecules to a separate effector molecule. The five major types of drug-receptor-effector coupling systems are discussed in Chapter 2. **Pharmacologic antagonist** drugs, by binding to a receptor, compete with and prevent binding by other molecules. For example, acetylcholine receptor blockers such as atropine are antagonists because they prevent access of acetylcholine and similar agonist drugs to the acetylcholine receptor site and they stabilize the receptor in its inactive state (or some state other than the acetylcholine-activated state). These agents reduce the effects of acetylcholine and similar molecules in the body (Figure 1–3B), but their action can be overcome by increasing the dosage of agonist. Some antagonists bind very tightly to the receptor site in an irreversible or pseudoirreversible fashion and cannot be displaced by increasing the agonist concentration. Drugs that bind to the same receptor molecule but do not prevent binding of the agonist are said to act **allosterically** and may enhance (Figure 1–3C) or inhibit (Figure 1–3D) the action of the agonist molecule. Allosteric inhibition is not overcome by increasing the dose of agonist.

B. Agonists That Inhibit Their Binding Molecules

Some drugs mimic agonist drugs by inhibiting the molecules responsible for terminating the action of an endogenous agonist. For example, acetylcholinesterase *inhibitors*, by slowing the destruction of endogenous acetylcholine, cause cholinomimetic effects that closely resemble the actions of cholinoceptor *agonist* molecules even though cholinesterase inhibitors do not bind or only incidentally bind to cholinoceptors (see Chapter 7). Because they amplify the effects of physiologically released agonist ligands, their effects are sometimes more selective and less toxic than those of exogenous agonists.

C. Agonists, Partial Agonists, and Inverse Agonists

Figure 1–4 describes a useful model of drug-receptor interaction. As indicated, the receptor is postulated to exist in the inactive,

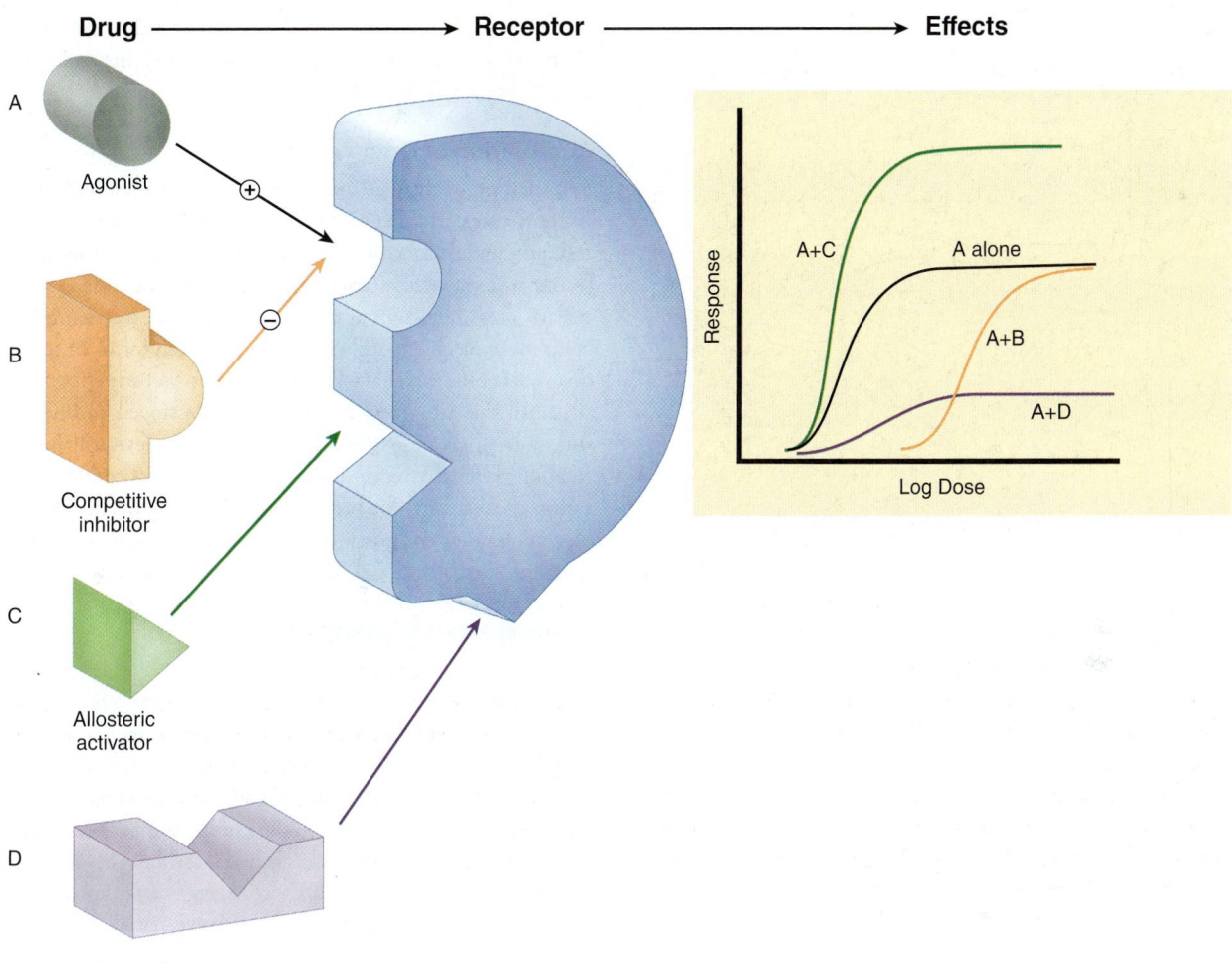

FIGURE 1–3 Drugs may interact with receptors in several ways. The effects resulting from these interactions are diagrammed in the dose-response curves at the right. Drugs that alter the agonist (**A**) response may activate the agonist binding site, compete with the agonist (competitive inhibitors, **B**), or act at separate (allosteric) sites, increasing (**C**) or decreasing (**D**) the response to the agonist. Allosteric activators (**C**) may increase the efficacy of the agonist or its binding affinity. The curve shown reflects an increase in efficacy; an increase in affinity would result in a leftward shift of the curve.

nonfunctional form (R_i) and in the activated form (R_a). Thermodynamic considerations indicate that even in the absence of any agonist, some of the receptor pool must exist in the R_a form some of the time and may produce the same physiologic effect as agonist-induced activity. This effect, occurring in the absence of agonist, is termed **constitutive activity.** Agonists are those drugs that have a much higher affinity for the R_a configuration and stabilize it, so that a large percentage of the total pool resides in the R_a–D fraction and a large effect is produced. The recognition of constitutive activity may depend on the receptor density, the concentration of coupling molecules (if a coupled system), and the number of effectors in the system.

Many agonist drugs, when administered at concentrations sufficient to saturate the receptor pool, can activate their receptor-effector systems to the maximum extent of which the system is capable; that is, they cause a shift of almost all of the receptor pool to the R_a–D pool. Such drugs are termed **full agonists.** Other drugs, called **partial agonists,** bind to the same receptors and activate them in the same way but do not evoke as great a response, no matter how high the concentration. In the model in Figure 1–4, partial agonists do not stabilize the R_a configuration as fully as full agonists, so that a significant fraction of receptors exists in the R_i–D pool. Such drugs are said to have low **intrinsic efficacy.** Thus, pindolol, a β-adrenoceptor partial agonist, may act either as an agonist (if no full agonist is present) or as an antagonist (if a full agonist such as epinephrine is present). (See Chapter 2.) Intrinsic efficacy is independent of affinity (as usually measured) for the receptor.

In the same model, conventional antagonist action can be explained as fixing the fractions of drug-bound R_i and R_a in the same relative amounts as in the absence of any drug. In this situation, no change will be observed, so the drug will appear to be without effect. However, the presence of the antagonist at the receptor site will block access of agonists to the receptor and prevent the usual agonist effect. Such blocking action can be termed **neutral antagonism.**

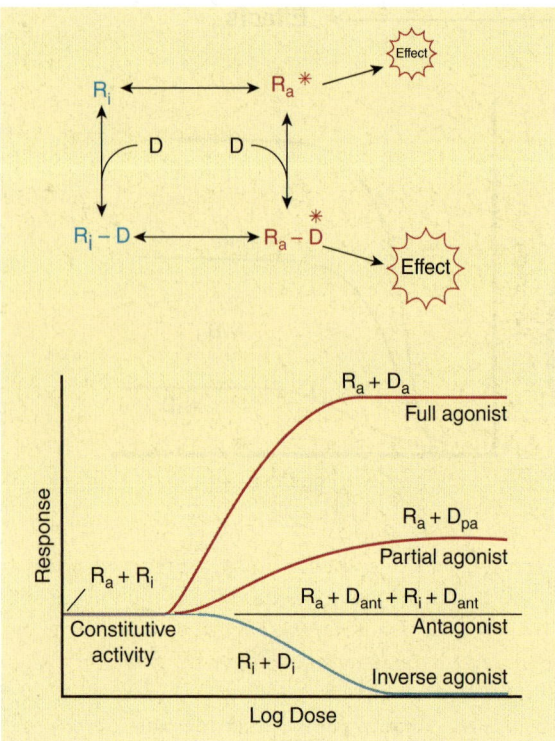

FIGURE 1–4 A model of drug-receptor interaction. The receptor is able to assume two conformations. In the R_i conformation, it is inactive and produces no effect, even when combined with a drug molecule. In the R_a conformation, the receptor can activate downstream mechanisms that produce a small observable effect, even in the absence of drug (constitutive activity). In the absence of drugs, the two isoforms are in equilibrium, and the R_i form is favored. Conventional full agonist drugs have a much higher affinity for the R_a conformation, and mass action thus favors the formation of the R_a–D complex with a much larger observed effect. Partial agonists have an intermediate affinity for both R_i and R_a forms. Conventional antagonists, according to this hypothesis, have equal affinity for both receptor forms and maintain the same level of constitutive activity. Inverse agonists, on the other hand, have a much higher affinity for the R_i form, reduce constitutive activity, and may produce a contrasting physiologic result.

What will happen if a drug has a much stronger affinity for the R_i than for the R_a state and stabilizes a large fraction in the R_i–D pool? In this scenario the drug would reduce any constitutive activity, thus resulting in effects that are the opposite of the effects produced by conventional agonists at that receptor. Such drugs have been termed **inverse agonists** (Figure 1–4). One of the best documented examples of such a system is the γ-aminobutyric acid (GABA$_A$) receptor-effector (a chloride channel) in the nervous system. This receptor is activated by the endogenous transmitter GABA and causes inhibition of postsynaptic cells. Conventional exogenous agonists such as benzodiazepines also facilitate the receptor-effector system and cause GABA-like inhibition with sedation as the therapeutic result. This inhibition can be blocked by conventional neutral antagonists such as flumazenil. In addition, inverse agonists have been found that cause anxiety and

agitation, the inverse of sedation (see Chapter 22). Similar inverse agonists have been found for β-adrenoceptors, histamine H$_1$ and H$_2$ receptors, and several other receptor systems.

D. Duration of Drug Action

Termination of drug action is a result of one of several processes. In some cases, the effect lasts only as long as the drug occupies the receptor, and dissociation of drug from the receptor automatically terminates the effect. In many cases, however, the action may persist after the drug has dissociated because, for example, some coupling molecule is still present in activated form. In the case of drugs that bind covalently to the receptor site, the effect may persist until the drug-receptor complex is destroyed and new receptors or enzymes are synthesized, as described previously for aspirin. In addition, many receptor-effector systems incorporate desensitization mechanisms for preventing excessive activation when agonist molecules continue to be present for long periods. (See Chapter 2 for additional details.)

E. Receptors and Inert Binding Sites

To function as a receptor, an endogenous molecule must first be **selective** in choosing ligands (drug molecules) to bind; and second, it must **change its function** upon binding in such a way that the function of the biologic system (cell, tissue, etc) is altered. The selectivity characteristic is required to avoid constant activation of the receptor by promiscuous binding of many different ligands. The ability to change function is clearly necessary if the ligand is to cause a pharmacologic effect. The body contains a vast array of molecules that are capable of binding drugs, however, and not all of these endogenous molecules are regulatory molecules. Binding of a drug to a nonregulatory molecule such as plasma albumin will result in no detectable change in the function of the biologic system, so this endogenous molecule can be called an **inert binding site.** Such binding is not completely without significance, however, because it affects the distribution of drug within the body and determines the amount of free drug in the circulation. Both of these factors are of pharmacokinetic importance (see also Chapter 3).

Pharmacokinetic Principles

In practical therapeutics, a drug should be able to reach its intended site of action after administration by some convenient route. In many cases, the active drug molecule is sufficiently lipid-soluble and stable to be given as such. In some cases, however, an inactive precursor chemical that is readily absorbed and distributed must be administered and then converted to the active drug by biologic processes—inside the body. Such a precursor chemical is called a **prodrug.**

In only a few situations is it possible to apply a drug directly to its target tissue, eg, by topical application of an anti-inflammatory agent to inflamed skin or mucous membrane. Most often, a drug is administered into one body compartment, eg, the gut, and must move to its site of action in another compartment, eg, the brain in the case of an antiseizure medication. This requires that the drug be **absorbed** into the blood from its site of administration and **distributed** to its site of action, **permeating** through the various

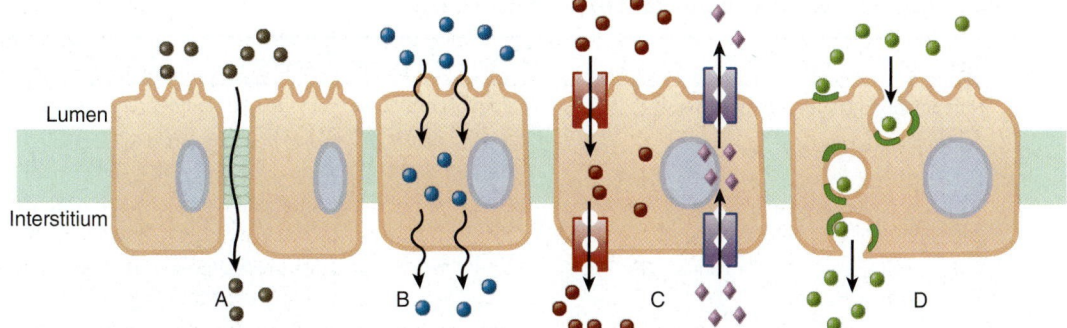

FIGURE 1–5 Mechanisms of drug permeation. Drugs may diffuse passively through aqueous channels in the intercellular junctions (eg, tight junctions, **A**), or through lipid cell membranes (**B**). Drugs with the appropriate characteristics may be transported by carriers into or out of cells (**C**). Very impermeant drugs may also bind to cell surface receptors (dark binding sites), be engulfed by the cell membrane (endocytosis), and then released inside the cell or expelled via the membrane-limited vesicles out of the cell into the extracellular space (exocytosis, **D**).

barriers that separate these compartments. For a drug given orally to produce an effect in the central nervous system, these barriers include the tissues that make up the wall of the intestine, the walls of the capillaries that perfuse the gut, and the blood-brain barrier, the walls of the capillaries that perfuse the brain. Finally, after bringing about its effect, a drug should be **eliminated** at a reasonable rate by metabolic inactivation, by excretion from the body, or by a combination of these processes.

A. Permeation

Drug permeation proceeds by several mechanisms. Passive diffusion in an aqueous or lipid medium is common, but active processes play a role in the movement of many drugs, especially those whose molecules are too large to diffuse readily (Figure 1–5).

1. Aqueous diffusion—Aqueous diffusion occurs within the larger aqueous compartments of the body (interstitial space, cytosol, etc) and across epithelial membrane tight junctions and the endothelial lining of blood vessels through aqueous pores that—in some tissues—permit the passage of molecules as large as MW 20,000–30,000.* See Figure 1–5A.

Aqueous diffusion of drug molecules is usually driven by the concentration gradient of the permeating drug, a downhill movement described by Fick's law (see below). Drug molecules that are bound to large plasma proteins (eg, albumin) do not permeate most vascular aqueous pores. If the drug is charged, its flux is also influenced by electrical fields (eg, the membrane potential and—in parts of the nephron—the transtubular potential).

2. Lipid diffusion—Lipid diffusion is the most important limiting factor for drug permeation because of the large number of lipid barriers that separate the compartments of the body. Because these lipid barriers separate aqueous compartments, the **lipid:aqueous partition coefficient** of a drug determines how readily the molecule moves between aqueous and lipid media. In the case of weak acids and weak bases (which gain or lose electrical charge-bearing protons, depending on the pH), the ability to move from aqueous to lipid or vice versa varies with the pH of the medium, because charged molecules attract water molecules. The ratio of lipid-soluble form to water-soluble form for a weak acid or weak base is expressed by the Henderson-Hasselbalch equation (described in the following text). See Figure 1–5B.

3. Special carriers—Special carrier molecules exist for many substances that are important for cell function and too large or too insoluble in lipid to diffuse passively through membranes, eg, peptides, amino acids, and glucose. These carriers bring about movement by active transport or facilitated diffusion and, unlike passive diffusion, are selective, saturable, and inhibitable. Because many drugs are or resemble such naturally occurring peptides, amino acids, or sugars, they can use these carriers to cross membranes. See Figure 1–5C.

Many cells also contain less selective membrane carriers that are specialized for expelling foreign molecules. One large family of such transporters binds adenosine triphosphate (ATP) and is called the ABC (ATP-binding cassette) family. This family includes the **P-glycoprotein** or **multidrug resistance type 1 (MDR1) transporter** found in the brain, testes, and other tissues, and in some drug-resistant neoplastic cells, Table 1–2. Similar transport molecules from the ABC family, the **multidrug resistance-associated protein (MRP)** transporters, play important roles in the excretion of some drugs or their metabolites into urine and bile and in the resistance of some tumors to chemotherapeutic drugs. Several other transporter families have been identified that do not bind ATP but use ion gradients to drive transport. Some of these (the solute carrier [SLC] family) are particularly important in the uptake of neurotransmitters across nerve-ending membranes. The latter carriers are discussed in more detail in Chapter 6.

4. Endocytosis and exocytosis—A few substances are so large or impermeant that they can enter cells only by endocytosis, the process by which the substance is bound at a cell-surface receptor,

---

*The capillaries of the brain, the testes, and some other tissues are characterized by the absence of pores that permit aqueous diffusion. They may also contain high concentrations of drug export pumps (MDR pumps; see text). These tissues are therefore protected or "sanctuary" sites from many circulating drugs.

TABLE 1–2   Some transport molecules important in pharmacology.

Transporter	Physiologic Function	Pharmacologic Significance
NET	Norepinephrine reuptake from synapse	Target of cocaine and some tricyclic antidepressants
SERT	Serotonin reuptake from synapse	Target of selective serotonin reuptake inhibitors and some tricyclic antidepressants
VMAT	Transport of dopamine and norepinephrine into adrenergic vesicles in nerve endings	Target of reserpine and tetrabenazine
MDR1	Transport of many xenobiotics out of cells	Increased expression confers resistance to certain anticancer drugs; inhibition increases blood levels of digoxin
MRP1	Leukotriene secretion	Confers resistance to certain anticancer and antifungal drugs

MDR1, multidrug resistance protein-1; MRP1, multidrug resistance-associated protein-1; NET, norepinephrine transporter; SERT, serotonin reuptake transporter; VMAT, vesicular monoamine transporter.

engulfed by the cell membrane, and carried into the cell by pinching off of the newly formed vesicle inside the membrane. The substance can then be released inside the cytosol by breakdown of the vesicle membrane, Figure 1–5D. This process is responsible for the transport of vitamin B_{12}, complexed with a binding protein (intrinsic factor) across the wall of the gut into the blood. Similarly, iron is transported into hemoglobin-synthesizing red blood cell precursors in association with the protein transferrin. Specific receptors for the transport proteins must be present for this process to work.

The reverse process (exocytosis) is responsible for the secretion of many substances from cells. For example, many neurotransmitter substances are stored in membrane-bound vesicles in nerve endings to protect them from metabolic destruction in the cytoplasm. Appropriate activation of the nerve ending causes fusion of the storage vesicle with the cell membrane and expulsion of its contents into the extracellular space (see Chapter 6).

B. Fick's Law of Diffusion

The passive flux of molecules down a concentration gradient is given by Fick's law:

$$\text{Flux (molecules per unit time)} = (C_1 - C_2) \times \frac{\text{Area} \times \text{Permeability coefficient}}{\text{Thickness}}$$

where C_1 is the higher concentration, C_2 is the lower concentration, area is the cross-sectional area of the diffusion path, permeability coefficient is a measure of the mobility of the drug molecules in the medium of the diffusion path, and thickness is the thickness (length) of the diffusion path. In the case of lipid diffusion, the lipid:aqueous partition coefficient is a major determinant of mobility of the drug, because it determines how readily the drug enters the lipid membrane from the aqueous medium.

C. Ionization of Weak Acids and Weak Bases; the Henderson-Hasselbalch Equation

The electrostatic charge of an ionized molecule attracts water dipoles and results in a polar, relatively water-soluble and lipid-insoluble complex. Because lipid diffusion depends on relatively high lipid solubility, ionization of drugs may markedly reduce their ability to permeate membranes. A very large percentage of the drugs in use are weak acids or weak bases (Table 1–3). For drugs, a weak acid is best defined as a neutral molecule that can reversibly dissociate into an anion (a negatively charged molecule) and a proton (a hydrogen ion). For example, aspirin dissociates as follows:

$$C_8H_7O_2COOH \rightleftharpoons C_8H_7O_2COO^- + H^+$$

Neutral   Aspirin   Proton
aspirin   anion

A drug that is a weak base can be defined as a neutral molecule that can form a cation (a positively charged molecule) by combining with a proton. For example, pyrimethamine, an antimalarial drug, undergoes the following association-dissociation process:

$$C_{12}H_{11}ClN_3NH_3^+ \rightleftharpoons C_{12}H_{11}ClN_3NH_2 + H^+$$

Pyrimethamine   Neutral   Proton
cation   pyrimethamine

Note that the protonated form of a weak acid is the neutral, more lipid-soluble form, whereas the unprotonated form of a weak base is the neutral form. The law of mass action requires that these reactions move to the left in an acid environment (low pH, excess protons available) and to the right in an alkaline environment. The Henderson-Hasselbalch equation relates the ratio of protonated to unprotonated weak acid or weak base to the molecule's pK_a and the pH of the medium as follows:

$$\log \frac{(\text{Protonated})}{(\text{Unprotonated})} = pK_a - pH$$

This equation applies to both acidic and basic drugs. Inspection confirms that the lower the pH relative to the pK_a, the greater will be the fraction of drug in the protonated form. Because the uncharged form is the more lipid-soluble, more of a weak acid will be in the lipid-soluble form at acid pH, whereas more of a basic drug will be in the lipid-soluble form at alkaline pH.

TABLE 1–3 Ionization constants of some common drugs.

Drug	pKa[1]	Drug	pKa[1]	Drug	pKa[1]
Weak acids		**Weak bases**		**Weak bases (cont'd)**	
Acetaminophen	9.5	Albuterol (salbutamol)	9.3	Isoproterenol	8.6
Acetazolamide	7.2	Allopurinol	9.4, 12.3[2]	Lidocaine	7.9
Ampicillin	2.5	Alprenolol	9.6	Metaraminol	8.6
Aspirin	3.5	Amiloride	8.7	Methadone	8.4
Chlorothiazide	6.8, 9.4[2]	Amiodarone	6.6	Methamphetamine	10.0
Chlorpropamide	5.0	Amphetamine	9.8	Methyldopa	10.6
Ciprofloxacin	6.1, 8.7[2]	Atropine	9.7	Metoprolol	9.8
Cromolyn	2.0	Bupivacaine	8.1	Morphine	7.9
Ethacrynic acid	2.5	Chlordiazepoxide	4.6	Nicotine	7.9, 3.1[2]
Furosemide	3.9	Chloroquine	10.8, 8.4	Norepinephrine	8.6
Ibuprofen	4.4, 5.2[2]	Chlorpheniramine	9.2	Pentazocine	7.9
Levodopa	2.3	Chlorpromazine	9.3	Phenylephrine	9.8
Methotrexate	4.8	Clonidine	8.3	Physostigmine	7.9, 1.8[2]
Methyldopa	2.2, 9.2[2]	Cocaine	8.5	Pilocarpine	6.9, 1.4[2]
Penicillamine	1.8	Codeine	8.2	Pindolol	8.6
Pentobarbital	8.1	Cyclizine	8.2	Procainamide	9.2
Phenobarbital	7.4	Desipramine	10.2	Procaine	9.0
Phenytoin	8.3	Diazepam	3.0	Promethazine	9.1
Propylthiouracil	8.3	Diphenhydramine	8.8	Propranolol	9.4
Salicylic acid	3.0	Diphenoxylate	7.1	Pseudoephedrine	9.8
Sulfadiazine	6.5	Ephedrine	9.6	Pyrimethamine	7.0–7.3[3]
Sulfapyridine	8.4	Epinephrine	8.7	Quinidine	8.5, 4.4[2]
Theophylline	8.8	Ergotamine	6.3	Scopolamine	8.1
Tolbutamide	5.3	Fluphenazine	8.0, 3.9[2]	Strychnine	8.0, 2.3[2]
Warfarin	5.0	Hydralazine	7.1	Terbutaline	10.1
		Imipramine	9.5	Thioridazine	9.5

[1]The pKa is that pH at which the concentrations of the ionized and nonionized forms are equal.
[2]More than one ionizable group.
[3]Isoelectric point.

Application of this principle is made in the manipulation of drug excretion by the kidney. Almost all drugs are filtered at the glomerulus. If a drug is in a lipid-soluble form during its passage down the renal tubule, a significant fraction will be reabsorbed by simple passive diffusion. If the goal is to accelerate excretion of the drug (eg, in a case of drug overdose), it is important to prevent its reabsorption from the tubule. This can often be accomplished by adjusting urine pH to make certain that most of the drug is in the ionized state, as shown in Figure 1–6. As a result of this partitioning effect, the drug is "trapped" in the urine. Thus, weak acids are usually excreted faster in alkaline urine; weak bases are usually excreted faster in acidic urine. Other body fluids in which pH differences from blood pH may cause trapping or reabsorption are the contents of the stomach and small intestine;

breast milk; aqueous humor; and vaginal and prostatic secretions (Table 1–4).

As suggested by Table 1–3, a large number of drugs are weak bases. Most of these bases are amine-containing molecules. The nitrogen of a neutral amine has three atoms associated with it plus a pair of unshared electrons (see the display that follows). The three atoms may consist of one carbon (designated "R") and two hydrogens (a **primary amine**), two carbons and one hydrogen (a **secondary amine**), or three carbon atoms (a **tertiary amine**). Each of these three forms may reversibly bind a proton with the unshared electrons. Some drugs have a fourth carbon-nitrogen bond; these are **quaternary amines**. However, the quaternary amine is permanently charged and has no unshared electrons with which to reversibly bind a proton. Therefore, primary, secondary,

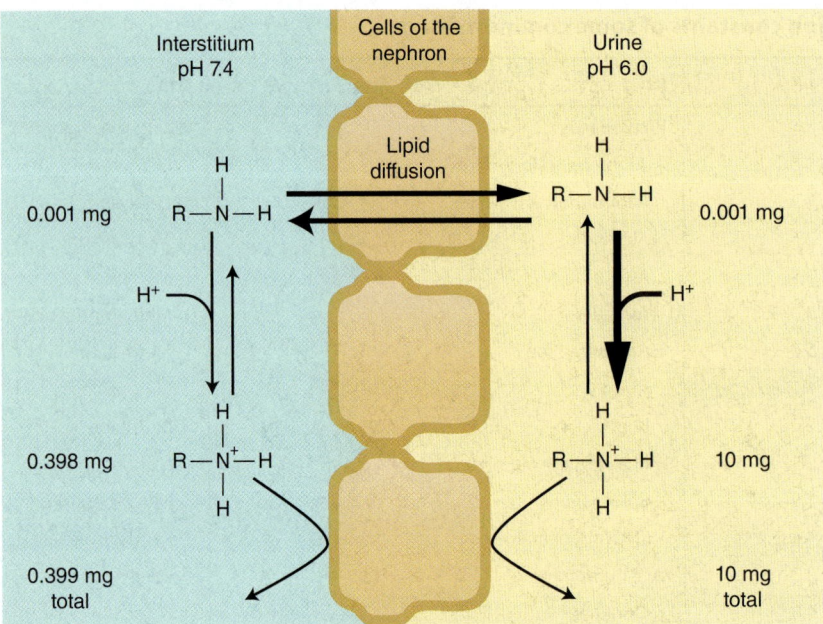

FIGURE 1–6 Trapping of a weak base (methamphetamine) in the urine when the urine is more acidic than the blood. In the hypothetical case illustrated, the diffusible uncharged form of the drug has equilibrated across the membrane, but the total concentration (charged plus uncharged) in the urine (more than 10 mg) is 25 times higher than in the blood (0.4 mg).

and tertiary amines may undergo reversible protonation and vary their lipid solubility with pH, but quaternary amines are always in the poorly lipid-soluble charged form.

Primary	Secondary	Tertiary	Quaternary
H	R	R	R
R:N:	R:N:	R:N:	R:N:R
H	H	R	R

DRUG GROUPS

To learn each pertinent fact about each of the many hundreds of drugs mentioned in this book would be an impractical goal and, fortunately, is unnecessary. Almost all the several thousand drugs currently available can be arranged into about 70 groups. Many of the drugs within each group are very similar in pharmacodynamic actions and in their pharmacokinetic properties as well. For most groups, one or more **prototype drugs** can be identified that typify

TABLE 1–4 Body fluids with potential for drug "trapping" through the pH-partitioning phenomenon.

Body Fluid	Range of pH	Total Fluid: Blood Concentration Ratios for Sulfadiazine (acid, pK$_a$ 6.5)[1]	Total Fluid: Blood Concentration Ratios for Pyrimethamine (base, pK$_a$ 7.0)[1]
Urine	5.0–8.0	0.12–4.65	72.24–0.79
Breast milk	6.4–7.6[2]	0.2–1.77	3.56–0.89
Jejunum, ileum contents	7.5–8.0[3]	1.23–3.54	0.94–0.79
Stomach contents	1.92–2.59[2]	0.11[4]	85,993–18,386
Prostatic secretions	6.45–7.4[2]	0.21	3.25–1.0
Vaginal secretions	3.4–4.2[3]	0.11[4]	2848–452

[1]Body fluid protonated-to-unprotonated drug ratios were calculated using each of the pH extremes cited; a blood pH of 7.4 was used for blood:drug ratio. For example, the steady-state urine:blood ratio for sulfadiazine is 0.12 at a urine pH of 5.0; this ratio is 4.65 at a urine pH of 8.0. Thus, sulfadiazine is much more effectively trapped and excreted in alkaline urine.

[2]Lentner C (editor): *Geigy Scientific Tables,* vol 1, 8th ed. Ciba Geigy, 1981.

[3]Bowman WC, Rand MJ: *Textbook of Pharmacology,* 2nd ed. Blackwell, 1980.

[4]Insignificant change in ratios over the physiologic pH range.

the most important characteristics of the group. This permits classification of other important drugs in the group as variants of the prototype, so that only the prototype must be learned in detail and, for the remaining drugs, only the differences from the prototype.

SOURCES OF INFORMATION

Students who wish to review the field of pharmacology in preparation for an examination are referred to *Pharmacology: Examination and Board Review,* by Trevor, Katzung, and Masters (McGraw-Hill, 2010). This book provides over 1000 questions and explanations in USMLE format. A short study guide is *USMLE Road Map: Pharmacology,* by Katzung and Trevor (McGraw-Hill, 2006). *Road Map* contains numerous tables, figures, mnemonics, and USMLE-type clinical vignettes.

The references at the end of each chapter in this book were selected to provide reviews or classic publications of information specific to those chapters. More detailed questions relating to basic or clinical research are best answered by referring to the journals covering general pharmacology and clinical specialties. For the student and the physician, three periodicals can be recommended as especially useful sources of current information about drugs: *The New England Journal of Medicine,* which publishes much original drug-related clinical research as well as frequent reviews of topics in pharmacology; *The Medical Letter on Drugs and Therapeutics,* which publishes brief critical reviews of new and old therapies, mostly pharmacologic; and *Drugs,* which publishes extensive reviews of drugs and drug groups.

Other sources of information pertinent to the United States should be mentioned as well. The "package insert" is a summary of information that the manufacturer is required to place in the prescription sales package; *Physicians' Desk Reference (PDR)* is a compendium of package inserts published annually with supplements twice a year. It is sold in bookstores and distributed free to licensed physicians. The package insert consists of a brief description of the pharmacology of the product. This brochure contains much practical information, and it is also used as a means of shifting liability for untoward drug reactions from the manufacturer onto the practitioner. Therefore, the manufacturer typically lists every toxic effect ever reported, no matter how rare. *Micromedex* is an extensive subscription website maintained by the Thomson Corporation (http://clinical.thomsonhealthcare.com/products/physicians/). It provides downloads for personal digital assistant devices, online drug dosage and interaction information, and toxicologic information. A useful and objective quarterly handbook that presents information on drug toxicity and interactions is *Drug Interactions: Analysis and Management.* Finally, the FDA maintains an Internet website that carries news regarding recent drug approvals, withdrawals, warnings, etc. It can be accessed at http://www.fda.gov. The MedWatch drug safety program is a free e-mail notification service that provides news of FDA drug warnings and withdrawals. Subscriptions may be obtained at https://service.govdelivery.com/service/user.html?code=USFDA.

REFERENCES

Drug Interactions: Analysis and Management (quarterly). Wolters Kluwer Publications.
Pharmacology: Examination & Board Review, 9th ed. McGraw-Hill Companies, Inc.
Symposium: Allosterism and collateral efficacy. Trends Pharmacol Sci 2007;28(8):entire issue.
USMLE Road Map: Pharmacology, McGraw-Hill Companies, Inc.
The Medical Letter on Drugs and Therapeutics. The Medical Letter, Inc.

CASE STUDY ANSWER

In the case study, the patient intravenously self-administered an overdose of methamphetamine, a weak base. This drug is freely filtered at the glomerulus, but can be rapidly reabsorbed in the renal tubule. Administration of ammonium chloride acidifies the urine, converting a larger fraction of the drug to the protonated, charged form, which is poorly reabsorbed and thus more rapidly eliminated. Note that not all experts recommend forced diuresis and urinary pH manipulation after methamphetamine overdose because of the risk of renal damage (see Figure 1–6).

Drug Receptors & Pharmacodynamics

Mark von Zastrow, MD, PhD[*]

CASE STUDY

A 51-year-old man presents to his medical clinic due to difficulty breathing. The patient is afebrile and normotensive, but tachypneic. Auscultation of the chest reveals diffuse wheezes. The physician provisionally makes the diagnosis of bronchial asthma and administers epinephrine by intramuscular injection, improving the patient's breathing over several minutes. A normal chest X-ray is subsequently obtained, and the medical history is remarkable only for mild hypertension that was recently treated with propranolol. The physician instructs the patient to discontinue use of propranolol, and changes the patient's antihypertensive medication to verapamil. Why is the physician correct to discontinue propranolol? Why is verapamil a better choice for managing hypertension in this patient?

Therapeutic and toxic effects of drugs result from their interactions with molecules in the patient. Most drugs act by associating with specific macromolecules in ways that alter the macromolecules' biochemical or biophysical activities. This idea, more than a century old, is embodied in the term **receptor:** the component of a cell or organism that interacts with a drug and initiates the chain of events leading to the drug's observed effects.

Receptors have become the central focus of investigation of drug effects and their mechanisms of action (pharmacodynamics). The receptor concept, extended to endocrinology, immunology, and molecular biology, has proved essential for explaining many aspects of biologic regulation. Many drug receptors have been isolated and characterized in detail, thus opening the way to precise understanding of the molecular basis of drug action.

The receptor concept has important practical consequences for the development of drugs and for arriving at therapeutic decisions in clinical practice. These consequences form the basis for understanding the actions and clinical uses of drugs described in almost every chapter of this book. They may be briefly summarized as follows:

1. **Receptors largely determine the quantitative relations between dose or concentration of drug and pharmacologic effects.** The receptor's affinity for binding a drug determines the concentration of drug required to form a significant number of drug-receptor complexes, and the total number of receptors may limit the maximal effect a drug may produce.

2. **Receptors are responsible for selectivity of drug action.** The molecular size, shape, and electrical charge of a drug determine whether—and with what affinity—it will bind to a particular receptor among the vast array of chemically different binding sites available in a cell, tissue, or patient. Accordingly, changes in the chemical structure of a drug can dramatically increase or decrease a new drug's affinities for different classes of receptors, with resulting alterations in therapeutic and toxic effects.

3. **Receptors mediate the actions of pharmacologic agonists and antagonists.** Some drugs and many natural ligands, such as hormones and neurotransmitters, regulate the function of receptor macromolecules as **agonists;** this means that they activate the receptor to signal as a direct result of binding to it. Some agonists activate a single kind of receptor to produce all their biologic functions, whereas others selectively promote one receptor function more than another.

Other drugs act as pharmacologic **antagonists;** that is, they bind to receptors but do not activate generation of a signal; consequently, they interfere with the ability of an agonist to activate the receptor. The effect of a so-called "pure" antagonist on a cell or in a patient depends entirely on its preventing the binding of agonist molecules and blocking their biologic actions. Other

---

[*]The author thanks Henry R. Bourne, MD, for major contributions to this chapter.

antagonists, in addition to preventing agonist binding, suppress the basal signaling ("constitutive") activity of receptors. Some of the most useful drugs in clinical medicine are pharmacologic antagonists.

MACROMOLECULAR NATURE OF DRUG RECEPTORS

Most receptors are proteins, presumably because the structures of polypeptides provide both the necessary diversity and the necessary specificity of shape and electrical charge. Receptors vary greatly in structure and can be identified in many ways. Traditionally, drug binding was used to identify or purify receptors from tissue extracts; consequently, receptors were discovered after the drugs that bind to them. However, advances in molecular biology and genome sequencing have effectively reversed this order. Now receptors are being discovered by predicted structure or sequence homology to other (known) receptors, and drugs that bind to them are developed later using chemical screening methods. This effort has revealed, for many known drugs, a larger diversity of receptors than previously anticipated. It has also identified a number of **"orphan" receptors,** so-called because their ligands are presently unknown, which may prove to be useful targets for the development of new drugs.

The best-characterized drug receptors are **regulatory proteins,** which mediate the actions of endogenous chemical signals such as neurotransmitters, autacoids, and hormones. This class of receptors mediates the effects of many of the most useful therapeutic agents. The molecular structures and biochemical mechanisms of these regulatory receptors are described in a later section entitled Signaling Mechanisms & Drug Action.

Other classes of proteins that have been clearly identified as drug receptors include **enzymes,** which may be inhibited (or, less commonly, activated) by binding a drug (eg, dihydrofolate reductase, the receptor for the antineoplastic drug methotrexate); **transport proteins** (eg, Na^+/K^+-ATPase, the membrane receptor for cardioactive digitalis glycosides); and **structural proteins** (eg, tubulin, the receptor for colchicine, an anti-inflammatory agent).

This chapter deals with three aspects of drug receptor function, presented in increasing order of complexity: (1) receptors as determinants of the quantitative relation between the concentration of a drug and the pharmacologic response, (2) receptors as regulatory proteins and components of chemical signaling mechanisms that provide targets for important drugs, and (3) receptors as key determinants of the therapeutic and toxic effects of drugs in patients.

RELATION BETWEEN DRUG CONCENTRATION & RESPONSE

The relation between dose of a drug and the clinically observed response may be complex. In carefully controlled in vitro systems, however, the relation between concentration of a drug and its effect is often simple and can be described with mathematical

precision. This idealized relation underlies the more complex relations between dose and effect that occur when drugs are given to patients.

Concentration-Effect Curves & Receptor Binding of Agonists

Even in intact animals or patients, responses to low doses of a drug usually increase in direct proportion to dose. As doses increase, however, the response increment diminishes; finally, doses may be reached at which no further increase in response can be achieved. In idealized or in vitro systems, the relation between drug concentration and effect is described by a hyperbolic curve (Figure 2–1A) according to the following equation:

$$E = \frac{E_{max} \times C}{C + EC_{50}}$$

where E is the effect observed at concentration C, E_{max} is the maximal response that can be produced by the drug, and EC_{50} is the concentration of drug that produces 50% of maximal effect.

This hyperbolic relation resembles the mass action law, which describes association between two molecules of a given affinity. This resemblance suggests that drug agonists act by binding to ("occupying") a distinct class of biologic molecules with a characteristic affinity for the drug receptor. Radioactive receptor ligands have been used to confirm this occupancy assumption in many drug-receptor systems. In these systems, drug bound to receptors (B) relates to the concentration of free (unbound) drug (C) as depicted in Figure 2–1B and as described by an analogous equation:

$$B = \frac{B_{max} \times C}{C + K_d}$$

in which B_{max} indicates the total concentration of receptor sites (ie, sites bound to the drug at infinitely high concentrations of free drug) and K_d (the equilibrium dissociation constant) represents the concentration of free drug at which half-maximal binding is observed. This constant characterizes the receptor's affinity for binding the drug in a reciprocal fashion: If the K_d is low, binding affinity is high, and vice versa. The EC_{50} and K_d may be identical, but need not be, as discussed below. Dose-response data are often presented as a plot of the drug effect (ordinate) against the *logarithm* of the dose or concentration (abscissa). This mathematical maneuver transforms the hyperbolic curve of Figure 2–1 into a sigmoid curve with a linear midportion (eg, Figure 2–2). This expands the scale of the concentration axis at low concentrations (where the effect is changing rapidly) and compresses it at high concentrations (where the effect is changing slowly), but has no special biologic or pharmacologic significance.

Receptor-Effector Coupling & Spare Receptors

When a receptor is occupied by an agonist, the resulting conformational change is only the first of many steps usually required to

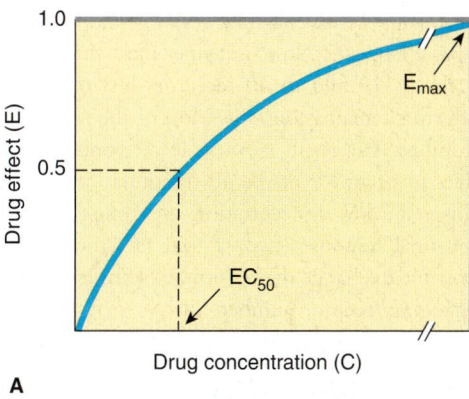
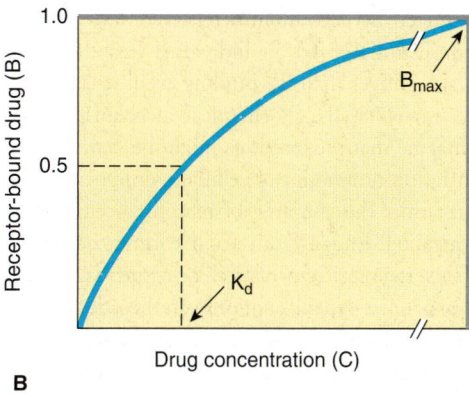

FIGURE 2–1 Relations between drug concentration and drug effect (**A**) or receptor-bound drug (**B**). The drug concentrations at which effect or receptor occupancy is half-maximal are denoted by EC_{50} and K_d, respectively.

produce a pharmacologic response. The transduction process that links drug occupancy of receptors and pharmacologic response is often termed **coupling.** The relative efficiency of occupancy-response coupling is partially determined by the initial conformational change

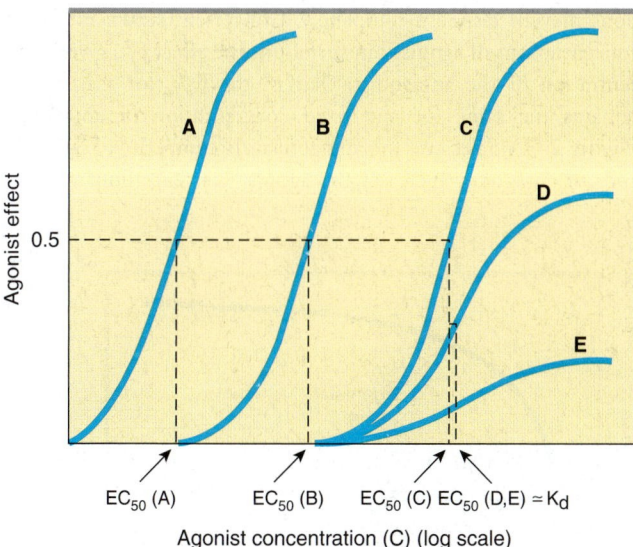

FIGURE 2–2 Logarithmic transformation of the dose axis and experimental demonstration of spare receptors, using different concentrations of an irreversible antagonist. Curve **A** shows agonist response in the absence of antagonist. After treatment with a low concentration of antagonist (curve **B**), the curve is shifted to the right. Maximal responsiveness is preserved, however, because the remaining available receptors are still in excess of the number required. In curve **C,** produced after treatment with a larger concentration of antagonist, the available receptors are no longer "spare"; instead, they are just sufficient to mediate an undiminished maximal response. Still higher concentrations of antagonist (curves **D** and **E**) reduce the number of available receptors to the point that maximal response is diminished. The apparent EC_{50} of the agonist in curves **D** and **E** may approximate the K_d that characterizes the binding affinity of the agonist for the receptor.

in the receptor; thus, the effects of full agonists can be considered more efficiently coupled to receptor occupancy than can the effects of partial agonists (described in text that follows). Coupling efficiency is also determined by the biochemical events that transduce receptor occupancy into cellular response. Sometimes the biologic effect of the drug is linearly related to the number of receptors bound. This is often true for drug-regulated ion channels, eg, in which the ion current produced by the drug is directly proportional to the number of receptors (ion channels) bound. In other cases, the biologic response is a more complex function of drug binding to receptors. This is often true for receptors linked to enzymatic signal transduction cascades, eg, in which the biologic response often increases disproportionately to the number of receptors occupied by drug.

Many factors can contribute to nonlinear occupancy-response coupling, and often these factors are only partially understood. The concept of **"spare" receptors,** regardless of the precise biochemical mechanism involved, can help us to think about these effects. Receptors are said to be "spare" for a given pharmacologic response if it is possible to elicit a maximal biologic response at a concentration of agonist that does not result in occupancy of the full complement of available receptors. Experimentally, spare receptors may be demonstrated by using irreversible antagonists to prevent binding of agonist to a proportion of available receptors and showing that high concentrations of agonist can still produce an undiminished maximal response (Figure 2–2). Thus, the same maximal inotropic response of heart muscle to catecholamines can be elicited even under conditions in which 90% of the β adrenoceptors are occupied by a quasi-irreversible antagonist. Accordingly, myocardial cells are said to contain a large proportion of spare β adrenoceptors.

How can we account for the phenomenon of spare receptors? In the example of the β adrenoceptor, receptor activation promotes binding of guanosine triphosphate (GTP) to an intermediate signaling protein and activation of the signaling intermediate may greatly outlast the agonist-receptor interaction (see the following section on G Proteins & Second Messengers). In such a case, the "spareness" of receptors is *temporal.* Maximal response can be elicited by activation of relatively few receptors because the response initiated by an individual ligand-receptor binding event persists longer than the binding event itself.

In other cases, in which the biochemical mechanism is not understood, we imagine that the receptors might be *spare in number*. If the concentration or amount of cellular components other than the receptors limits the coupling of receptor occupancy to response, then a maximal response can occur without occupancy of all receptors. Thus, the sensitivity of a cell or tissue to a particular concentration of agonist depends not only on the *affinity* of the receptor for binding the agonist (characterized by the K_d) but also on the *degree of spareness*—the total number of receptors present compared with the number actually needed to elicit a maximal biologic response.

The concept of spare receptors is very useful clinically because it allows one to think precisely about the effects of drug dosage without needing to consider biochemical details of the signaling response. The K_d of the agonist-receptor interaction determines what fraction (B/B_{max}) of total receptors will be occupied at a given free concentration (C) of agonist regardless of the receptor concentration:

$$\frac{B}{B_{max}} = \frac{C}{C + K_d}$$

Imagine a responding cell with four receptors and four effectors. Here the number of effectors does not limit the maximal response, and the receptors are *not* spare in number. Consequently, an agonist present at a concentration equal to the K_d will occupy 50% of the receptors, and half of the effectors will be activated,

producing a half-maximal response (ie, two receptors stimulate two effectors). Now imagine that the number of receptors increases 10-fold to 40 receptors but that the total number of effectors remains constant. Most of the receptors are now spare in number. As a result, a much lower concentration of agonist suffices to occupy 2 of the 40 receptors (5% of the receptors), and this same low concentration of agonist is able to elicit a half-maximal response (two of four effectors activated). Thus, it is possible to change the sensitivity of tissues with spare receptors by changing receptor number.

Competitive & Irreversible Antagonists

Receptor antagonists bind to receptors but do not activate them. The primary action of antagonists is to prevent agonists (other drugs or endogenous regulatory molecules) from activating receptors. Some antagonists (so-called "inverse agonists," see Chapter 1), also reduce receptor activity below basal levels observed in the absence of bound ligand. Antagonists are divided into two classes depending on whether or not they *reversibly compete* with agonists for binding to receptors.

In the presence of a fixed concentration of agonist, increasing concentrations of a reversible **competitive antagonist** progressively inhibit the agonist response; high antagonist concentrations prevent response completely. Conversely, sufficiently high concentrations of agonist can surmount the effect of a given concentration of the antagonist; that is, the E_{max} for the agonist remains the same for any fixed concentration of antagonist (Figure 2–3A). Because the antagonism is competitive, the presence of antagonist increases the agonist concentration required

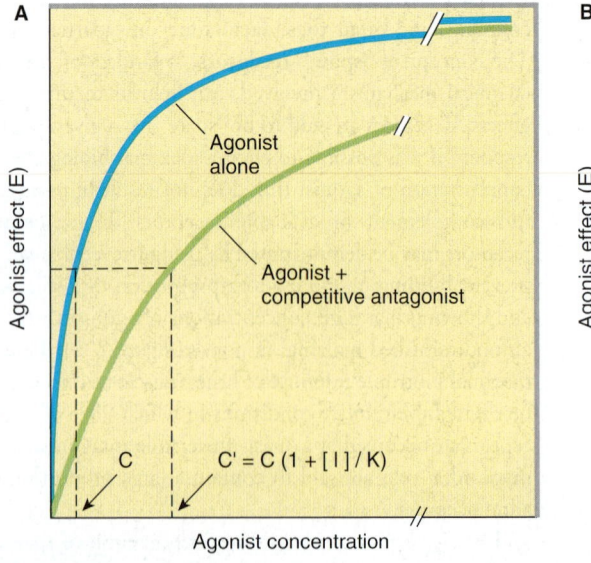
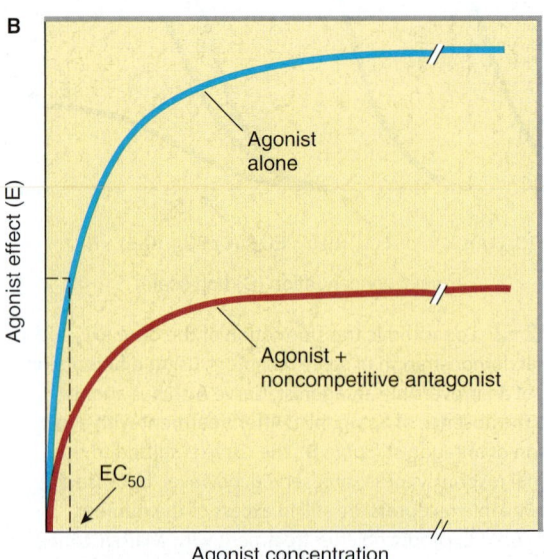

FIGURE 2–3 Changes in agonist concentration-effect curves produced by a competitive antagonist (**A**) or by an irreversible antagonist (**B**). In the presence of a competitive antagonist, higher concentrations of agonist are required to produce a given effect; thus the agonist concentration (C') required for a given effect in the presence of concentration [I] of an antagonist is shifted to the right, as shown. High agonist concentrations can overcome inhibition by a competitive antagonist. This is not the case with an irreversible (or noncompetitive) antagonist, which reduces the maximal effect the agonist can achieve, although it may not change its EC_{50}.

for a given degree of response, and so the agonist concentration-effect curve is shifted to the right.

The concentration (C′) of an agonist required to produce a given effect in the presence of a fixed concentration ([I]) of competitive antagonist is greater than the agonist concentration (C) required to produce the same effect in the absence of the antagonist. The ratio of these two agonist concentrations (dose ratio) is related to the dissociation constant (K_i) of the antagonist by the Schild equation:

$$\frac{C'}{C} = 1 + \frac{[I]}{K_i}$$

Pharmacologists often use this relation to determine the K_i of a competitive antagonist. Even without knowledge of the relation between agonist occupancy of the receptor and response, the K_i can be determined simply and accurately. As shown in Figure 2–3, concentration-response curves are obtained in the presence and in the absence of a fixed concentration of competitive antagonist; comparison of the agonist concentrations required to produce identical degrees of pharmacologic effect in the two situations reveals the antagonist's K_i. If C′ is twice C, for example, then [I] = K_i.

For the clinician, this mathematical relation has two important therapeutic implications:

1. The degree of inhibition produced by a competitive antagonist depends on the concentration of antagonist. The competitive β-adrenoceptor antagonist propranolol provides a useful example. Patients receiving a fixed dose of this drug exhibit a wide range of plasma concentrations, owing to differences among individuals in clearance of propranolol. As a result, inhibitory effects on physiologic responses to norepinephrine and epinephrine (endogenous adrenergic receptor agonists) may vary widely, and the dose of propranolol must be adjusted accordingly.

2. Clinical response to a competitive antagonist also depends on the concentration of agonist that is competing for binding to receptors. Again, propranolol provides a useful example: When this drug is administered at moderate doses sufficient to block the effect of basal levels of the neurotransmitter norepinephrine, resting heart rate is decreased. However, the increase in the release of norepinephrine and epinephrine that occurs with exercise, postural changes, or emotional stress may suffice to overcome this competitive antagonism. Accordingly, the same dose of propranolol may have little effect under these conditions, thereby altering therapeutic response.

Some receptor antagonists bind to the receptor in an **irreversible** or nearly irreversible fashion, either by forming a covalent bond with the receptor or by binding so tightly that, for practical purposes, the receptor is unavailable for binding of agonist. After occupancy of some proportion of receptors by such an antagonist, the number of remaining unoccupied receptors may be too low for the agonist (even at high concentrations) to elicit a response comparable to the previous maximal response (Figure 2–3B). If spare receptors are present, however, a lower dose of an irreversible antagonist may leave enough receptors unoccupied to allow achievement of maximum response to agonist, although a higher agonist concentration will be required (Figure 2–2B and C; see Receptor-Effector Coupling & Spare Receptors).

Therapeutically, irreversible antagonists present distinct advantages and disadvantages. Once the irreversible antagonist has occupied the receptor, it need not be present in unbound form to inhibit agonist responses. Consequently, the duration of action of such an irreversible antagonist is relatively independent of its own rate of elimination and more dependent on the rate of turnover of receptor molecules.

Phenoxybenzamine, an irreversible α-adrenoceptor antagonist, is used to control the hypertension caused by catecholamines released from pheochromocytoma, a tumor of the adrenal medulla. If administration of phenoxybenzamine lowers blood pressure, blockade will be maintained even when the tumor episodically releases very large amounts of catecholamine. In this case, the ability to prevent responses to varying and high concentrations of agonist is a therapeutic advantage. If overdose occurs, however, a real problem may arise. If the α-adrenoceptor blockade cannot be overcome, excess effects of the drug must be antagonized "physiologically," ie, by using a pressor agent that does not act via α receptors.

Antagonists can function noncompetitively in a different way; that is, by binding to a site on the receptor protein separate from the agonist binding site, and thereby modifying receptor activity without blocking agonist binding (see Figure 1–3C and D). Although these drugs act noncompetitively, their actions are reversible if they do not bind covalently. Such drugs are often called *allosteric modulators*. For example, benzodiazepines bind noncompetitively to ion channels activated by the neurotransmitter γ-aminobutyric acid (GABA), enhancing the net activating effect of GABA on channel conductance.

Partial Agonists

Based on the maximal pharmacologic response that occurs when all receptors are occupied, agonists can be divided into two classes: **partial agonists** produce a lower response, at full receptor occupancy, than do **full agonists.** Partial agonists produce concentration-effect curves that resemble those observed with full agonists in the presence of an antagonist that irreversibly blocks some of the receptor sites (compare Figures 2–2 [curve D] and 2–4B). It is important to emphasize that the failure of partial agonists to produce a maximal response is not due to decreased affinity for binding to receptors. Indeed, a partial agonist's inability to cause a maximal pharmacologic response, even when present at high concentrations that saturate binding to all receptors, is indicated by the fact that partial agonists competitively inhibit the responses produced by full agonists (Figure 2–4C). Many drugs used clinically as antagonists are actually weak partial agonists. Partial agonism can be useful in some clinical circumstances. For example, buprenorphine, a partial agonist of μ-opioid receptors, is a generally safer analgesic drug than morphine because it produces less respiratory depression in overdose. Buprenorphine is effectively antianalgesic when administered to

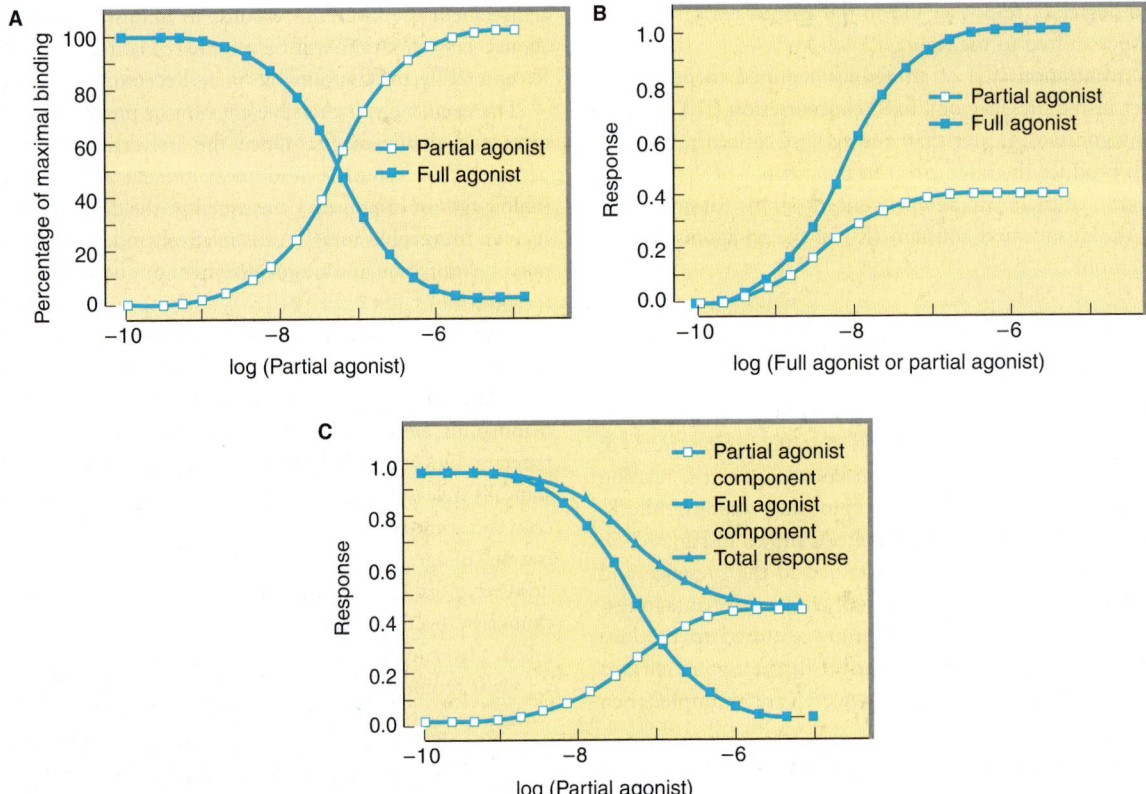

FIGURE 2–4 **A:** The percentage of receptor occupancy resulting from full agonist (present at a single concentration) binding to receptors in the presence of increasing concentrations of a partial agonist. Because the full agonist (filled squares) and the partial agonist (open squares) compete to bind to the same receptor sites, when occupancy by the partial agonist increases, binding of the full agonist decreases. **B:** When each of the two drugs is used alone and response is measured, occupancy of all the receptors by the partial agonist produces a lower maximal response than does similar occupancy by the full agonist. **C:** Simultaneous treatment with a single concentration of full agonist and increasing concentrations of the partial agonist produces the response patterns shown in the bottom panel. The fractional response caused by a single high concentration of the full agonist (filled squares) decreases as increasing concentrations of the partial agonist compete to bind to the receptor with increasing success; at the same time the portion of the response caused by the partial agonist (open squares) increases, while the total response—ie, the sum of responses to the two drugs (filled triangles)—gradually decreases, eventually reaching the value produced by partial agonist alone (compare with B).

morphine-dependent individuals, however, and may precipitate a drug withdrawal syndrome due to competitive inhibition of morphine's agonist action.

Other Mechanisms of Drug Antagonism

Not all the mechanisms of antagonism involve interactions of drugs or endogenous ligands at a single type of receptor, and some types of antagonism do not involve a receptor at all. For example, protamine, a protein that is positively charged at physiologic pH, can be used clinically to counteract the effects of heparin, an anticoagulant that is negatively charged. In this case, one drug acts as a **chemical antagonist** of the other simply by ionic binding that makes the other drug unavailable for interactions with proteins involved in blood clotting.

Another type of antagonism is **physiologic antagonism** between endogenous regulatory pathways mediated by different receptors. For example, several catabolic actions of the glucocorticoid hormones lead to increased blood sugar, an effect that is physiologically opposed by insulin. Although glucocorticoids and insulin act on quite distinct receptor-effector systems, the clinician must sometimes administer insulin to oppose the hyperglycemic effects of a glucocorticoid hormone, whether the latter is elevated by endogenous synthesis (eg, a tumor of the adrenal cortex) or as a result of glucocorticoid therapy.

In general, use of a drug as a physiologic antagonist produces effects that are less specific and less easy to control than are the effects of a receptor-specific antagonist. Thus, for example, to treat bradycardia caused by increased release of acetylcholine from vagus nerve endings, the physician could use isoproterenol, a β-adrenoceptor agonist that increases heart rate by mimicking sympathetic stimulation of the heart. However, use of this physiologic antagonist would be less rational—and potentially more dangerous—than would use of a receptor-specific antagonist such as atropine (a competitive antagonist at the receptors at which acetylcholine slows heart rate).

SIGNALING MECHANISMS & DRUG ACTION

Until now we have considered receptor interactions and drug effects in terms of equations and concentration-effect curves. We must also understand the molecular mechanisms by which a drug acts. Such understanding allows us to ask basic questions with important clinical implications:

- Why do some drugs produce effects that persist for minutes, hours, or even days after the drug is no longer present?
- Why do responses to other drugs diminish rapidly with prolonged or repeated administration?
- How do cellular mechanisms for amplifying external chemical signals explain the phenomenon of spare receptors?
- Why do chemically similar drugs often exhibit extraordinary selectivity in their actions?
- Do these mechanisms provide targets for developing new drugs?

Most transmembrane signaling is accomplished by a small number of different molecular mechanisms. Each type of mechanism has been adapted, through the evolution of distinctive protein families, to transduce many different signals. These protein families include receptors on the cell surface and within the cell, as well as enzymes and other components that generate, amplify, coordinate, and terminate postreceptor signaling by chemical second messengers in the cytoplasm. This section first discusses the mechanisms for carrying chemical information across the plasma membrane and then outlines key features of cytoplasmic second messengers.

Five basic mechanisms of transmembrane signaling are well understood (Figure 2–5). Each uses a different strategy to circumvent the barrier posed by the lipid bilayer of the plasma membrane. These strategies use (1) a lipid-soluble ligand that crosses the membrane and acts on an intracellular receptor; (2) a transmembrane receptor protein whose intracellular enzymatic activity is allosterically regulated by a ligand that binds to a site on the protein's extracellular domain; (3) a transmembrane receptor that binds and stimulates a protein tyrosine kinase; (4) a ligand-gated transmembrane ion channel that can be induced to open or close by the binding of a ligand; or (5) a transmembrane receptor protein that stimulates a GTP-binding signal transducer protein (G protein), which in turn modulates production of an intracellular second messenger.

Although the five established mechanisms do not account for all the chemical signals conveyed across cell membranes, they do transduce many of the most important signals exploited in pharmacotherapy.

Intracellular Receptors for Lipid-Soluble Agents

Several biologic ligands are sufficiently lipid-soluble to cross the plasma membrane and act on intracellular receptors. One class of such ligands includes steroids (corticosteroids, mineralocorticoids, sex steroids, vitamin D), and thyroid hormone, whose receptors stimulate the transcription of genes by binding to specific DNA sequences near the gene whose expression is to be regulated. Many of the target DNA sequences (called **response elements**) have been identified.

These "gene-active" receptors belong to a protein family that evolved from a common precursor. Dissection of the receptors by

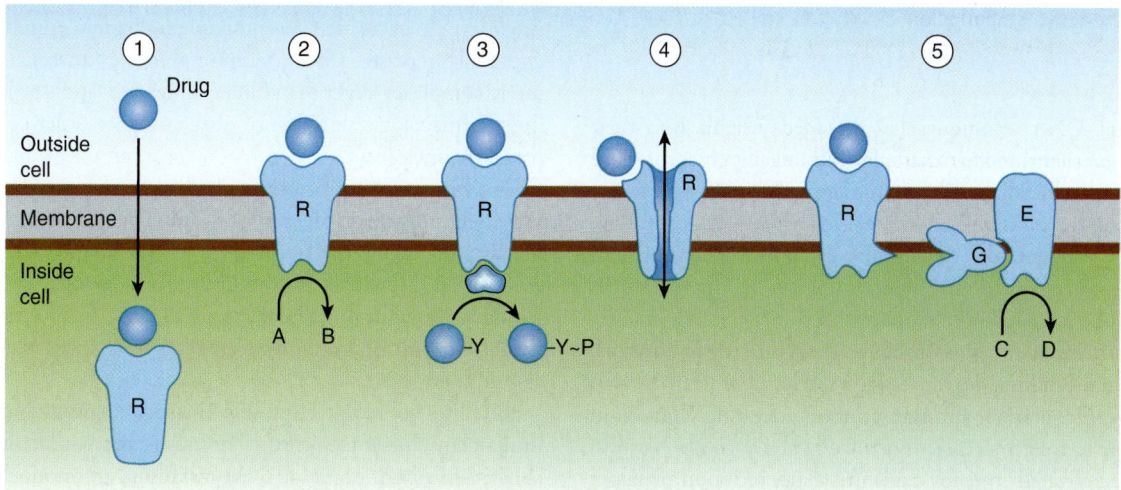

FIGURE 2–5   Known transmembrane signaling mechanisms: **1:** A lipid-soluble chemical signal crosses the plasma membrane and acts on an intracellular receptor (which may be an enzyme or a regulator of gene transcription); **2:** the signal binds to the extracellular domain of a transmembrane protein, thereby activating an enzymatic activity of its cytoplasmic domain; **3:** the signal binds to the extracellular domain of a transmembrane receptor bound to a separate protein tyrosine kinase, which it activates; **4:** the signal binds to and directly regulates the opening of an ion channel; **5:** the signal binds to a cell-surface receptor linked to an effector enzyme by a G protein. (A, C, substrates; B, D, products; R, receptor; G, G protein; E, effector [enzyme or ion channel]; Y, tyrosine; P, phosphate.)

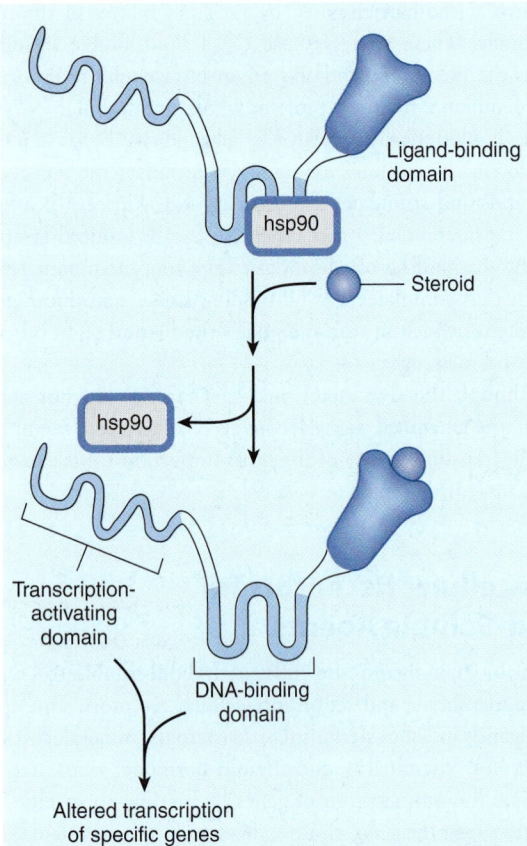

FIGURE 2–6 Mechanism of glucocorticoid action. The glucocorticoid receptor polypeptide is schematically depicted as a protein with three distinct domains. A heat-shock protein, hsp90, binds to the receptor in the absence of hormone and prevents folding into the active conformation of the receptor. Binding of a hormone ligand (steroid) causes dissociation of the hsp90 stabilizer and permits conversion to the active configuration.

recombinant DNA techniques has provided insights into their molecular mechanism. For example, binding of glucocorticoid hormone to its normal receptor protein relieves an inhibitory constraint on the transcription-stimulating activity of the protein. Figure 2–6 schematically depicts the molecular mechanism of glucocorticoid action: In the absence of hormone, the receptor is bound to hsp90, a protein that appears to prevent normal folding of several structural domains of the receptor. Binding of hormone to the ligand-binding domain triggers release of hsp90. This allows the DNA-binding and transcription-activating domains of the receptor to fold into their functionally active conformations, so that the activated receptor can initiate transcription of target genes.

The mechanism used by hormones that act by regulating gene expression has two therapeutically important consequences:

1. All of these hormones produce their effects after a characteristic lag period of 30 minutes to several hours—the time required for the synthesis of new proteins. This means that the gene-active hormones cannot be expected to alter a pathologic state within minutes (eg, glucocorticoids will not immediately relieve the symptoms of acute bronchial asthma).

2. The effects of these agents can persist for hours or days after the agonist concentration has been reduced to zero. The persistence of effect is primarily due to the relatively slow turnover of most enzymes and proteins, which can remain active in cells for hours or days after they have been synthesized. Consequently, it means that the beneficial (or toxic) effects of a gene-active hormone usually decrease slowly when administration of the hormone is stopped.

Ligand-Regulated Transmembrane Enzymes Including Receptor Tyrosine Kinases

This class of receptor molecules mediates the first steps in signaling by insulin, epidermal growth factor (EGF), platelet-derived growth factor (PDGF), atrial natriuretic peptide (ANP), transforming growth factor-β (TGF-β), and many other trophic hormones. These receptors are polypeptides consisting of an extracellular hormone-binding domain and a cytoplasmic enzyme domain, which may be a protein tyrosine kinase, a serine kinase, or a guanylyl cyclase (Figure 2–7). In all these receptors, the two domains are connected by a hydrophobic segment of the polypeptide that crosses the lipid bilayer of the plasma membrane.

The receptor tyrosine kinase signaling pathway begins with binding of ligand, typically a polypeptide hormone or growth factor, to the receptor's extracellular domain. The resulting change in receptor conformation causes two receptor molecules to bind to one another (*dimerize*), which in turn brings together the tyrosine kinase domains, which become enzymatically active, and phosphorylate one another as well as additional downstream signaling proteins. Activated receptors catalyze phosphorylation of tyrosine residues on different target signaling proteins, thereby allowing a single type of activated receptor to modulate a number of biochemical processes. (Some receptor tyrosine kinases form oligomeric complexes larger than dimers upon activation by ligand, but the pharmacologic significance of such higher-order complexes is presently unclear.)

Insulin, for example, uses a single class of receptors to trigger increased uptake of glucose and amino acids and to regulate metabolism of glycogen and triglycerides in the cell. Similarly, each of the growth factors initiates in its specific target cells a complex program of cellular events ranging from altered membrane transport of ions and metabolites to changes in the expression of many genes.

Inhibitors of receptor tyrosine kinases are finding increased use in neoplastic disorders in which excessive growth factor signaling is often involved. Some of these inhibitors are monoclonal antibodies (eg, trastuzumab, cetuximab), which bind to the extracellular domain of a particular receptor and interfere with binding of growth factor. Other inhibitors are membrane-permeant "small molecule" chemicals (eg, gefitinib, erlotinib), which inhibit the receptor's kinase activity in the cytoplasm.

The intensity and duration of action of EGF, PDGF, and other agents that act via receptor tyrosine kinases are limited by a process

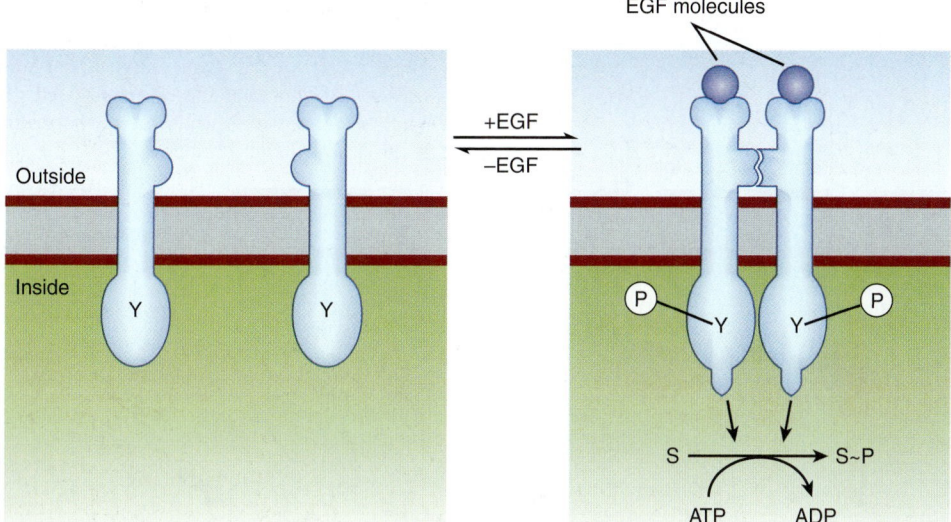

FIGURE 2–7 Mechanism of activation of the epidermal growth factor (EGF) receptor, a representative receptor tyrosine kinase. The receptor polypeptide has extracellular and cytoplasmic domains, depicted above and below the plasma membrane. Upon binding of EGF (circle), the receptor converts from its inactive monomeric state (*left*) to an active dimeric state (*right*), in which two receptor polypeptides bind noncovalently. The cytoplasmic domains become phosphorylated (P) on specific tyrosine residues (Y), and their enzymatic activities are activated, catalyzing phosphorylation of substrate proteins (S).

called receptor **down-regulation.** Ligand binding often induces accelerated endocytosis of receptors from the cell surface, followed by the degradation of those receptors (and their bound ligands). When this process occurs at a rate faster than de novo synthesis of receptors, the total number of cell-surface receptors is reduced (down-regulated), and the cell's responsiveness to ligand is correspondingly diminished. A well-understood example is the EGF receptor tyrosine kinase, which undergoes rapid endocytosis followed by proteolysis in lysosomes after EGF binding; genetic mutations that interfere with this process cause excessive growth factor-induced cell proliferation and are associated with an increased susceptibility to certain types of cancer. Endocytosis of other receptor tyrosine kinases, most notably receptors for nerve growth factor, serves a very different function. Internalized nerve growth factor receptors are not rapidly degraded and are translocated in endocytic vesicles from the distal axon, where receptors are activated by nerve growth factor released from the innervated tissue, to the cell body. In the cell body, the growth factor signal is transduced to transcription factors regulating the expression of genes controlling cell survival. This process effectively transports a critical survival signal from its site of release to its site of signaling effect, and does so over a remarkably long distance—up to 1 meter in certain sensory neurons.

A number of regulators of growth and differentiation, including TGF-β, act on another class of transmembrane receptor enzymes that phosphorylate serine and threonine residues. ANP, an important regulator of blood volume and vascular tone, acts on a transmembrane receptor whose intracellular domain, a guanylyl cyclase, generates cGMP (see below). Receptors in both groups, like the receptor tyrosine kinases, are active in their dimeric forms.

Cytokine Receptors

Cytokine receptors respond to a heterogeneous group of peptide ligands, which include growth hormone, erythropoietin, several kinds of interferon, and other regulators of growth and differentiation. These receptors use a mechanism (Figure 2–8) closely resembling that of receptor tyrosine kinases, except that in this case, the protein tyrosine kinase activity is not intrinsic to the receptor molecule. Instead, a separate protein tyrosine kinase, from the Janus-kinase (JAK) family, binds noncovalently to the receptor. As in the case of the EGF receptor, cytokine receptors dimerize after they bind the activating ligand, allowing the bound JAKs to become activated and to phosphorylate tyrosine residues on the receptor. Phosphorylated tyrosine residues on the receptor's cytoplasmic surface then set in motion a complex signaling dance by binding another set of proteins, called STATs (signal transducers and activators of transcription). The bound STATs are themselves phosphorylated by the JAKs, two STAT molecules dimerize (attaching to one another's tyrosine phosphates), and finally the STAT/STAT dimer dissociates from the receptor and travels to the nucleus, where it regulates transcription of specific genes.

Ligand- and Voltage-Gated Channels

Many of the most useful drugs in clinical medicine act by mimicking or blocking the actions of endogenous ligands that regulate the flow of ions through plasma membrane channels. The natural ligands are acetylcholine, serotonin, GABA, and glutamate. All of these agents are synaptic transmitters.

Each of their receptors transmits its signal across the plasma membrane by increasing transmembrane conductance of the

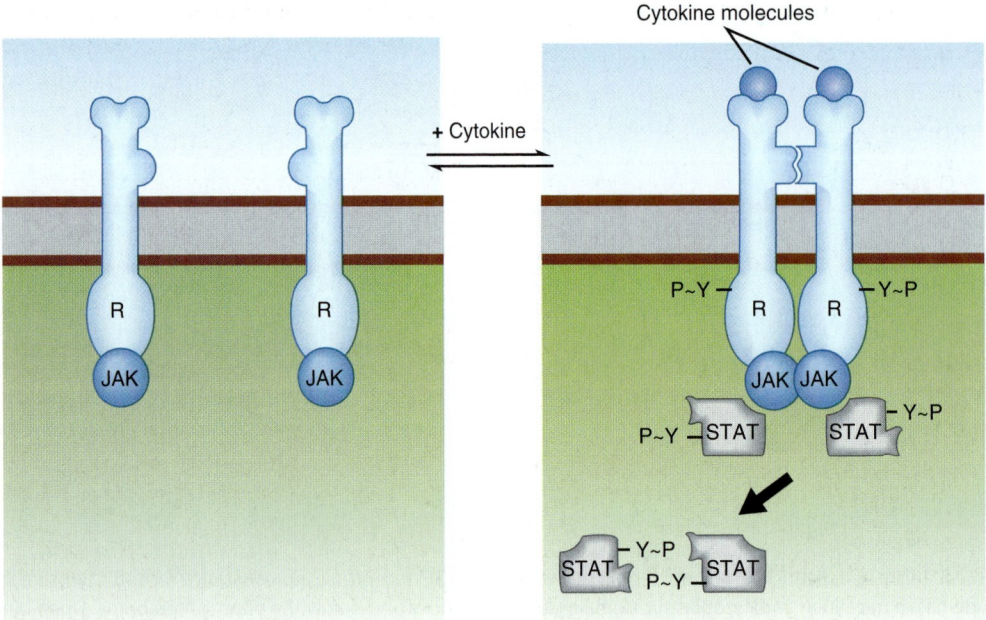

FIGURE 2–8 Cytokine receptors, like receptor tyrosine kinases, have extracellular and intracellular domains and form dimers. However, after activation by an appropriate ligand, separate mobile protein tyrosine kinase molecules (JAK) are activated, resulting in phosphorylation of signal transducers and activation of transcription (STAT) molecules. STAT dimers then travel to the nucleus, where they regulate transcription.

relevant ion and thereby altering the electrical potential across the membrane. For example, acetylcholine causes the opening of the ion channel in the nicotinic acetylcholine receptor (nAChR), which allows Na^+ to flow down its concentration gradient into cells, producing a localized excitatory postsynaptic potential—a depolarization.

The nAChR is one of the best characterized of all cell-surface receptors for hormones or neurotransmitters (Figure 2–9). One form of this receptor is a pentamer made up of four different polypeptide subunits (eg, two α chains plus one β, one γ, and one δ chain, all with molecular weights ranging from 43,000 to 50,000). These polypeptides, each of which crosses the lipid bilayer four times, form a cylindrical structure that is 8 nm in diameter. When acetylcholine binds to sites on the α subunits, a conformational change occurs that results in the transient opening of a central aqueous channel through which sodium ions penetrate from the extracellular fluid into the cell.

The time elapsed between the binding of the agonist to a ligand-gated channel and the cellular response can often be measured in milliseconds. The rapidity of this signaling mechanism is crucially important for moment-to-moment transfer of information across synapses. Ligand-gated ion channels can be regulated by multiple mechanisms, including phosphorylation and endocytosis. In the central nervous system, these mechanisms contribute to synaptic plasticity involved in learning and memory.

Voltage-gated ion channels do not bind neurotransmitters directly but are controlled by membrane potential; such channels are also important drug targets. For example, verapamil inhibits voltage-gated calcium channels that are present in the heart and in

vascular smooth muscle, producing antiarrhythmic effects and reducing blood pressure without mimicking or antagonizing any known endogenous transmitter.

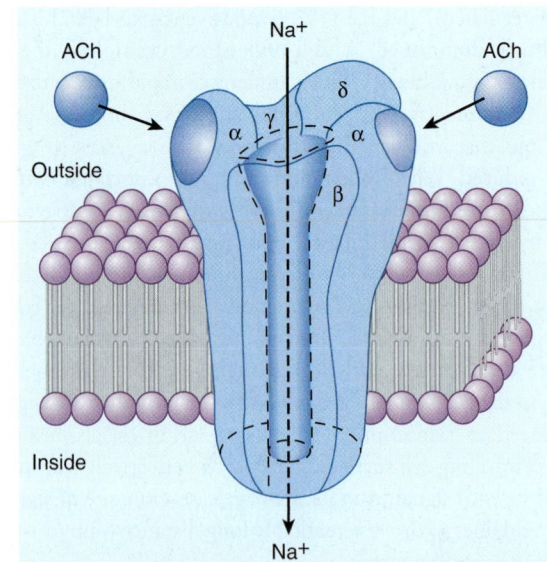

FIGURE 2–9 The nicotinic acetylcholine (ACh) receptor, a ligand-gated ion channel. The receptor molecule is depicted as embedded in a rectangular piece of plasma membrane, with extracellular fluid above and cytoplasm below. Composed of five subunits (two α, one β, one γ, and one δ), the receptor opens a central transmembrane ion channel when ACh binds to sites on the extracellular domain of its α subunits.

G Proteins & Second Messengers

Many extracellular ligands act by increasing the intracellular concentrations of second messengers such as **cyclic adenosine-3′,5′-monophosphate (cAMP), calcium ion,** or the **phosphoinositides** (described below). In most cases, they use a transmembrane signaling system with three separate components. First, the extracellular ligand is selectively detected by a cell-surface receptor. The receptor in turn triggers the activation of a G protein located on the cytoplasmic face of the plasma membrane. The activated G protein then changes the activity of an effector element, usually an enzyme or ion channel. This element then changes the concentration of the intracellular second messenger. For cAMP, the effector enzyme is adenylyl cyclase, a membrane protein that converts intracellular adenosine triphosphate (ATP) to cAMP. The corresponding G protein, G_s, stimulates adenylyl cyclase after being activated by hormones and neurotransmitters that act via specific G_s-coupled receptors. There are many examples of such receptors, including β adrenoceptors, glucagon receptors, thyrotropin receptors, and certain subtypes of dopamine and serotonin receptors.

G_s and other G proteins use a molecular mechanism that involves binding and hydrolysis of GTP (Figure 2–10). This mechanism allows the transduced signal to be amplified. For example, a neurotransmitter such as norepinephrine may encounter its membrane receptor for only a few milliseconds. When the encounter generates a GTP-bound G_s molecule, however, the duration of activation of adenylyl cyclase depends on the longevity of GTP binding to G_s rather than on the receptor's affinity for norepinephrine. Indeed, like other G proteins, GTP-bound G_s may remain active for tens of seconds, enormously amplifying the original signal. This mechanism also helps explain how signaling by G proteins produces the phenomenon of spare receptors. The family of G proteins contains several functionally diverse subfamilies (Table 2–1), each of which mediates effects of a particular set of receptors to a distinctive group of effectors. Note that an endogenous ligand (eg, norepinephrine, acetylcholine, serotonin, many others not listed in Table 2–1) may bind and stimulate receptors that couple to different subsets of G proteins. The apparent promiscuity of such a ligand allows it to elicit different G protein-dependent responses in different cells. For instance, the body responds to danger by using catecholamines (norepinephrine and epinephrine) both to increase heart rate and to induce constriction of blood vessels in the skin, by acting on G_s-coupled β adrenoceptors and G_q-coupled $α_1$ adrenoceptors, respectively. Ligand promiscuity also offers opportunities in drug development (see Receptor Classes & Drug Development in the following text).

Receptors coupled to G proteins are often called "G protein-coupled receptors" **(GPCRs)**, "seven-transmembrane" (7-TM), or "serpentine" receptors. GPCRs make up the largest receptor family and are so-named because the receptor polypeptide chain "snakes" across the plasma membrane seven times (Figure 2–11). Receptors for adrenergic amines, serotonin, acetylcholine (muscarinic but not nicotinic), many peptide hormones, odorants, and even visual receptors (in retinal rod and cone cells) all belong to the GPCR family. All were derived from a common evolutionary precursor. A few GPCRs (eg, $GABA_B$ and metabotropic glutamate receptors) require stable assembly into either *homodimers* (complexes of two identical receptor polypeptides) or *heterodimers* (complexes of different isoforms) for functional activity. However, in contrast to tyrosine kinase and cytokine receptors, most GPCRs are thought to be able to function as monomers.

All GPCRs transduce signals across the plasma membrane in essentially the same way. Often the agonist ligand—eg, a catecholamine or acetylcholine—is bound in a pocket enclosed by the transmembrane regions of the receptor (as in Figure 2–11). The resulting change in conformation of these regions is transmitted to cytoplasmic loops of the receptor, which in turn activate the appropriate G protein by promoting replacement of GDP by GTP, as described above. Amino acids in the third cytoplasmic loop of the GPCR polypeptide are generally thought to play a key role in mediating receptor interaction with G proteins (shown by arrows in Figure 2–11). The structural basis for ligand binding to β adrenoceptors was determined recently using X-ray crystallography.

Receptor Regulation

G protein-mediated responses to drugs and hormonal agonists often attenuate with time (Figure 2–12, top). After reaching an initial high level, the response (eg, cellular cAMP accumulation, Na^+ influx, contractility, etc) diminishes over seconds or minutes, even in the continued presence of the agonist. This **"desensitization"** is often rapidly reversible; a second exposure to agonist, if provided a few minutes after termination of the first exposure, results in a response similar to the initial response.

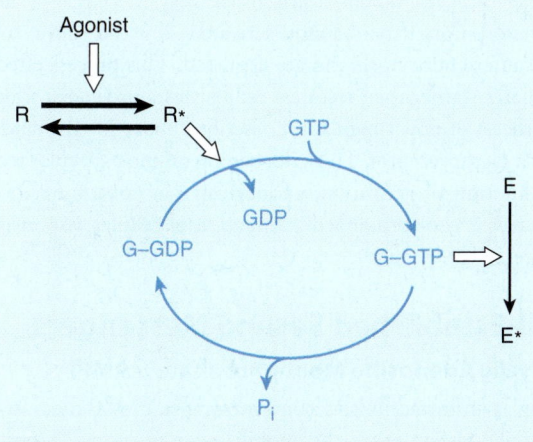

FIGURE 2–10 The guanine nucleotide-dependent activation-inactivation cycle of G proteins. The agonist activates the receptor (R→R*), which promotes release of GDP from the G protein (G), allowing entry of GTP into the nucleotide binding site. In its GTP-bound state (GGTP), the G protein regulates activity of an effector enzyme or ion channel (E→E*). The signal is terminated by hydrolysis of GTP, followed by return of the system to the basal unstimulated state. Open arrows denote regulatory effects. (P_i, inorganic phosphate.)

TABLE 2–1   **G proteins and their receptors and effectors.**

G Protein	Receptors for	Effector/Signaling Pathway
G_s	β-Adrenergic amines, glucagon, histamine, serotonin, and many other hormones	↑ Adenylyl cyclase →↑ cAMP
G_{i1}, G_{i2}, G_{i3}	α_2-Adrenergic amines, acetylcholine (muscarinic), opioids, serotonin, and many others	Several, including: ↓ Adenylyl cyclase →↓ cAMP Open cardiac K^+ channels →↓ heart rate
G_{olf}	Odorants (olfactory epithelium)	↑ Adenylyl cyclase →↑ cAMP
G_o	Neurotransmitters in brain (not yet specifically identified)	Not yet clear
G_q	Acetylcholine (muscarinic), bombesin, serotonin (5-HT_2), and many others	↑ Phospholipase C →↑ IP_3, diacylglycerol, cytoplasmic Ca^{2+}
G_{t1}, G_{t2}	Photons (rhodopsin and color opsins in retinal rod and cone cells)	↑ cGMP phosphodiesterase →↓ cGMP (phototransduction)

cAMP, cyclic adenosine monophosphate; cGMP, cyclic guanosine monophosphate.

Many GPCRs are regulated by phosphorylation, as illustrated by rapid desensitization of the β adrenoceptor. The agonist-induced change in conformation of the receptor causes it to bind, activate, and serve as a substrate for a family of specific receptor kinases, called G protein-coupled receptor kinases (GRKs). The activated GRK then phosphorylates serine residues in the receptor's carboxyl

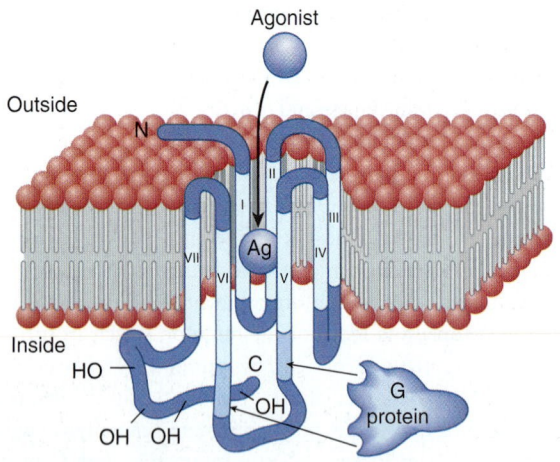

FIGURE 2–11 Transmembrane topology of a typical "serpentine" GPCR. The receptor's amino (N) terminal is extracellular (above the plane of the membrane), and its carboxyl (C) terminal intracellular. The terminals are connected by a polypeptide chain that traverses the plane of the membrane seven times. The hydrophobic transmembrane segments (light color) are designated by Roman numerals (I–VII). The agonist (Ag) approaches the receptor from the extracellular fluid and binds to a site surrounded by the transmembrane regions of the receptor protein. G proteins interact with cytoplasmic regions of the receptor, especially with portions of the third cytoplasmic loop between transmembrane regions V and VI. The receptor's cytoplasmic terminal tail contains numerous serine and threonine residues whose hydroxyl (-OH) groups can be phosphorylated. This phosphorylation may be associated with diminished receptor-G protein interaction.

terminal tail (Figure 2-12, panel B). The presence of phosphoserines increases the receptor's affinity for binding a third protein, β-arrestin. Binding of β-arrestin to cytoplasmic loops of the receptor diminishes the receptor's ability to interact with G_s, thereby reducing the agonist response (ie, stimulation of adenylyl cyclase). Upon removal of agonist, GRK activation is terminated, and the desensitization process can be reversed by cellular phosphatases.

For β adrenoceptors, and many other GPCRs, β-arrestin binding also accelerates endocytosis of receptors from the plasma membrane. Endocytosis of receptors promotes their dephosphorylation by a receptor phosphatase that is present at high concentration on endosome membranes, and receptors then return to the plasma membrane. This helps explain the ability of cells to recover receptor-mediated signaling responsiveness very efficiently after agonist-induced desensitization. Several GPCRs—including β adrenoceptors if persistently activated—instead traffic to lysosomes after endocytosis and are degraded. This process effectively attenuates (rather than restores) cellular responsiveness, similar to the process of down-regulation described above for the epidermal growth factor receptor. Thus, depending on the particular receptor and duration of activation, endocytosis can contribute to either rapid recovery or prolonged attenuation of cellular responsiveness (Figure 2–12).

Well-Established Second Messengers

A. Cyclic Adenosine Monophosphate (cAMP)

Acting as an intracellular second messenger, cAMP mediates such hormonal responses as the mobilization of stored energy (the breakdown of carbohydrates in liver or triglycerides in fat cells stimulated by β-adrenomimetic catecholamines), conservation of water by the kidney (mediated by vasopressin), Ca^{2+} homeostasis (regulated by parathyroid hormone), and increased rate and contractile force of heart muscle (β-adrenomimetic catecholamines). It also regulates the production of adrenal and sex steroids (in response to corticotropin or follicle-stimulating hormone), relaxation of smooth muscle, and many other endocrine and neural processes.

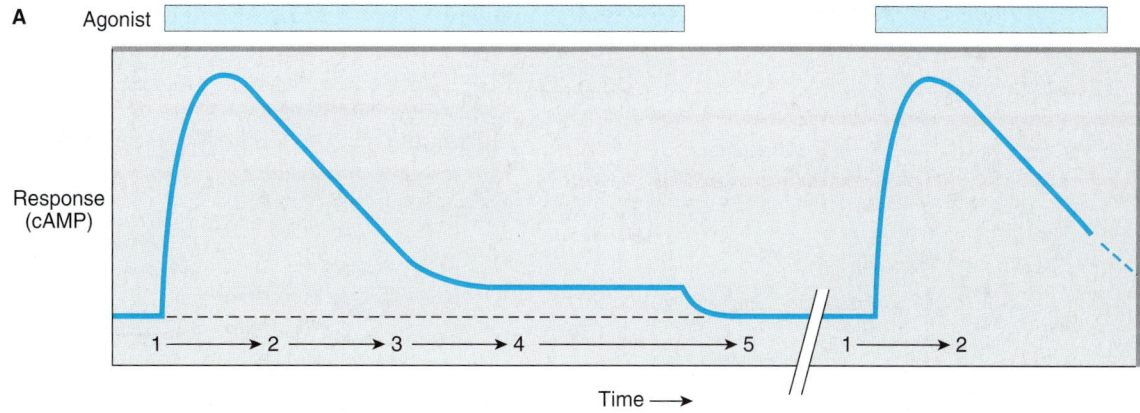

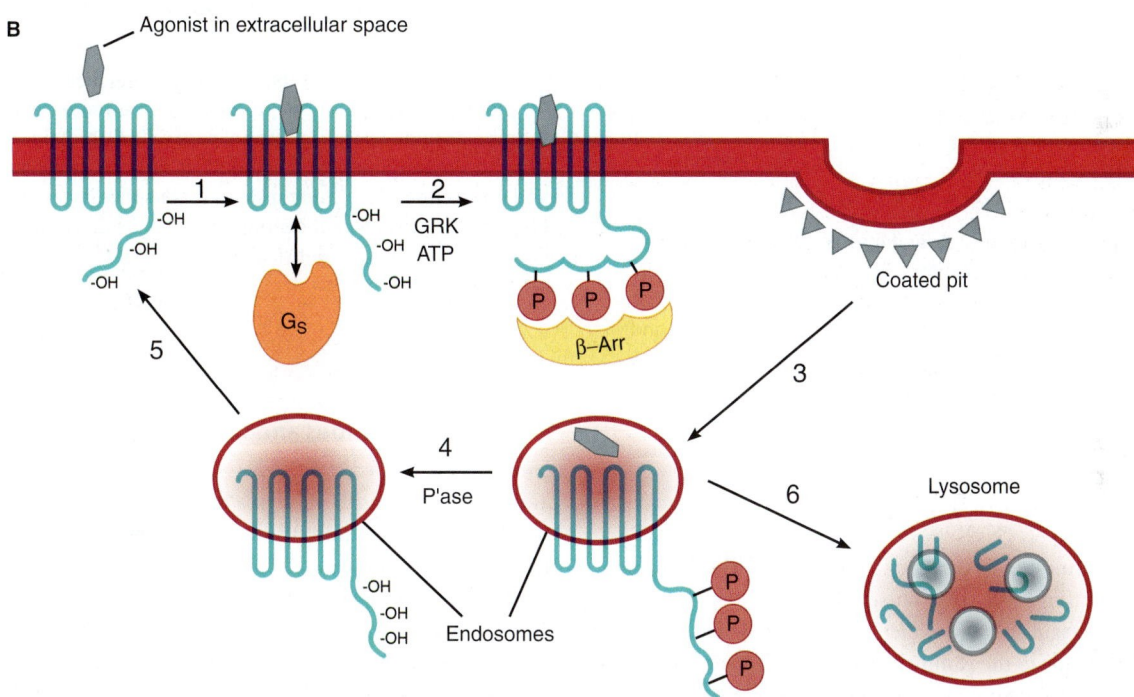

FIGURE 2–12 Rapid desensitization, resensitization, and down-regulation of β adrenoceptors. **A:** Response to a β-adrenoceptor agonist (ordinate) versus time (abscissa). (Numbers refer to the phases of receptor function in B.) Exposure of cells to agonist (indicated by the light-colored bar) produces a cyclic AMP response. A reduced cAMP response is observed in the continued presence of agonist; this "desensitization" typically occurs within a few minutes. If agonist is removed after a short time (typically several to tens of minutes, indicated by broken line on abscissa), cells recover full responsiveness to a subsequent addition of agonist (second light-colored bar). This "resensitization" fails to occur, or occurs incompletely, if cells are exposed to agonist repeatedly or over a more prolonged time period. **B:** Agonist binding to receptors initiates signaling by promoting receptor interaction with G proteins (G$_s$) located in the cytoplasm (step 1 in the diagram). Agonist-activated receptors are phosphorylated by a G protein-coupled receptor kinase (GRK), preventing receptor interaction with G$_s$ and promoting binding of a different protein, β-arrestin (β-Arr), to the receptor (step 2). The receptor-arrestin complex binds to coated pits, promoting receptor internalization (step 3). Dissociation of agonist from internalized receptors reduces β-Arr binding affinity, allowing dephosphorylation of receptors by a phosphatase (P'ase, step 4) and return of receptors to the plasma membrane (step 5); together, these events result in the efficient resensitization of cellular responsiveness. Repeated or prolonged exposure of cells to agonist favors the delivery of internalized receptors to lysosomes (step 6), promoting receptor down-regulation rather than resensitization.

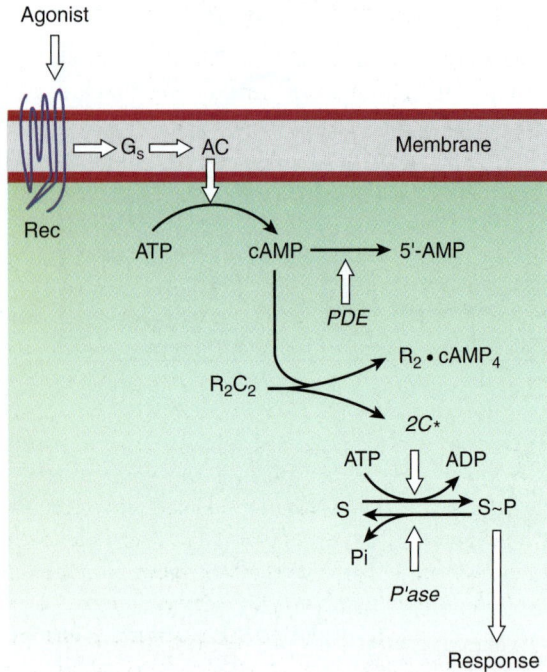

FIGURE 2–13 The cAMP second messenger pathway. Key proteins include hormone receptors (Rec), a stimulatory G protein (G$_s$), catalytic adenylyl cyclase (AC), phosphodiesterases (PDE) that hydrolyze cAMP, cAMP-dependent kinases, with regulatory (R) and catalytic (C) subunits, protein substrates (S) of the kinases, and phosphatases (P'ase), which remove phosphates from substrate proteins. Open arrows denote regulatory effects.

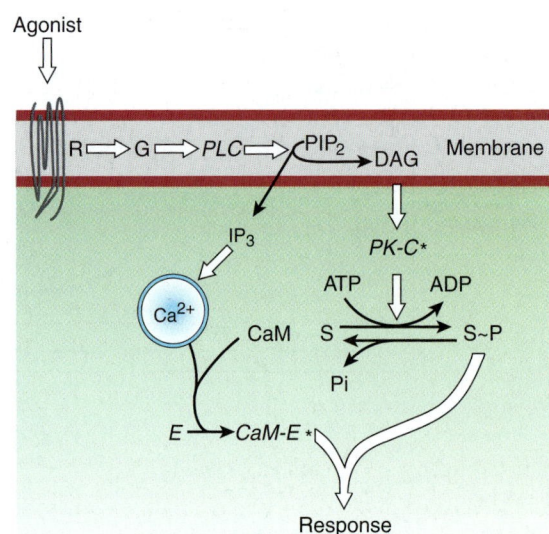

FIGURE 2–14 The Ca^{2+}-phosphoinositide signaling pathway. Key proteins include hormone receptors (R), a G protein (G), a phosphoinositide-specific phospholipase C (PLC), protein kinase C substrates of the kinase (S), calmodulin (CaM), and calmodulin-binding enzymes (E), including kinases, phosphodiesterases, etc. (PIP$_2$, phosphatidylinositol-4,5-bisphosphate; DAG, diacylglycerol; IP$_3$, inositol trisphosphate. Asterisk denotes activated state. Open arrows denote regulatory effects.)

cAMP exerts most of its effects by stimulating cAMP-dependent protein kinases (Figure 2–13). These kinases are composed of a cAMP-binding regulatory (R) dimer and two catalytic (C) chains. When cAMP binds to the R dimer, active C chains are released to diffuse through the cytoplasm and nucleus, where they transfer phosphate from ATP to appropriate substrate proteins, often enzymes. The specificity of the regulatory effects of cAMP resides in the distinct protein substrates of the kinases that are expressed in different cells. For example, liver is rich in phosphorylase kinase and glycogen synthase, enzymes whose reciprocal regulation by cAMP-dependent phosphorylation governs carbohydrate storage and release.

When the hormonal stimulus stops, the intracellular actions of cAMP are terminated by an elaborate series of enzymes. cAMP-stimulated phosphorylation of enzyme substrates is rapidly reversed by a diverse group of specific and nonspecific phosphatases. cAMP itself is degraded to 5′-AMP by several cyclic nucleotide phosphodiesterases (PDE; Figure 2–13). Milrinone, a selective inhibitor of type 3 phosphodiesterases that are expressed in cardiac muscle cells, has been used as an adjunctive agent in treating acute heart failure. Competitive inhibition of cAMP degradation is one way that caffeine, theophylline, and other methylxanthines produce their effects (see Chapter 20).

B. Phosphoinositides and Calcium

Another well-studied second messenger system involves hormonal stimulation of phosphoinositide hydrolysis (Figure 2–14). Some of the hormones, neurotransmitters, and growth factors that trigger this pathway bind to receptors linked to G proteins, whereas others bind to receptor tyrosine kinases. In all cases, the crucial step is stimulation of a membrane enzyme, phospholipase C (PLC), which splits a minor phospholipid component of the plasma membrane, phosphatidylinositol-4,5-bisphosphate (PIP$_2$), into two second messengers, **diacylglycerol (DAG)** and **inositol-1,4,5-trisphosphate (IP$_3$ or InsP$_3$).** Diacylglycerol is confined to the membrane, where it activates a phospholipid- and calcium-sensitive protein kinase called protein kinase C. IP$_3$ is water-soluble and diffuses through the cytoplasm to trigger release of Ca^{2+} by binding to ligand-gated calcium channels in the limiting membranes of internal storage vesicles. Elevated cytoplasmic Ca^{2+} concentration resulting from IP$_3$-promoted opening of these channels promotes the binding of Ca^{2+} to the calcium-binding protein calmodulin, which regulates activities of other enzymes, including calcium-dependent protein kinases.

With its multiple second messengers and protein kinases, the phosphoinositide signaling pathway is much more complex than the cAMP pathway. For example, different cell types may contain one or more specialized calcium- and calmodulin-dependent kinases with limited substrate specificity (eg, myosin light-chain kinase) in addition to a general calcium- and calmodulin-dependent kinase that can phosphorylate a wide variety of protein substrates. Furthermore, at least nine structurally distinct types of protein kinase C have been identified.

As in the cAMP system, multiple mechanisms damp or terminate signaling by this pathway. IP_3 is inactivated by dephosphorylation; diacylglycerol is either phosphorylated to yield phosphatidic acid, which is then converted back into phospholipids, or it is deacylated to yield arachidonic acid; Ca^{2+} is actively removed from the cytoplasm by Ca^{2+} pumps.

These and other nonreceptor elements of the calcium-phosphoinositide signaling pathway are of considerable importance in pharmacotherapy. For example, lithium ion, used in treatment of bipolar (manic-depressive) disorder, affects the cellular metabolism of phosphoinositides (see Chapter 29).

C. Cyclic Guanosine Monophosphate (cGMP)

Unlike cAMP, the ubiquitous and versatile carrier of diverse messages, cGMP has established signaling roles in only a few cell types. In intestinal mucosa and vascular smooth muscle, the cGMP-based signal transduction mechanism closely parallels the cAMP-mediated signaling mechanism. Ligands detected by cell-surface receptors stimulate membrane-bound guanylyl cyclase to produce cGMP, and cGMP acts by stimulating a cGMP-dependent protein kinase. The actions of cGMP in these cells are terminated by enzymatic degradation of the cyclic nucleotide and by dephosphorylation of kinase substrates.

Increased cGMP concentration causes relaxation of vascular smooth muscle by a kinase-mediated mechanism that results in dephosphorylation of myosin light chains (see Figure 12–2). In these smooth muscle cells, cGMP synthesis can be elevated by two transmembrane signaling mechanisms utilizing two different guanylyl cyclases. Atrial natriuretic peptide, a blood-borne peptide hormone, stimulates a transmembrane receptor by binding to its extracellular domain, thereby activating the guanylyl cyclase activity that resides in the receptor's intracellular domain. The other mechanism mediates responses to nitric oxide (NO; see Chapter 19), which is generated in vascular endothelial cells in response to natural vasodilator agents such as acetylcholine and histamine. After entering the target cell, nitric oxide binds to and activates a cytoplasmic guanylyl cyclase (see Figure 19–2). A number of useful vasodilating drugs, such as nitroglycerin and sodium nitroprusside used in treating cardiac ischemia and acute hypertension, act by generating or mimicking nitric oxide. Other drugs produce vasodilation by inhibiting specific phosphodiesterases, thereby interfering with the metabolic breakdown of cGMP. One such drug is sildenafil, used in treating erectile dysfunction and pulmonary hypertension (see Chapter 12).

Interplay among Signaling Mechanisms

The calcium-phosphoinositide and cAMP signaling pathways oppose one another in some cells and are complementary in others. For example, vasopressor agents that contract smooth muscle act by IP_3-mediated mobilization of Ca^{2+}, whereas agents that relax smooth muscle often act by elevation of cAMP. In contrast, cAMP and phosphoinositide second messengers act together to stimulate glucose release from the liver.

Phosphorylation: A Common Theme

Almost all second messenger signaling involves reversible phosphorylation, which performs two principal functions in signaling: amplification and flexible regulation. In **amplification**, rather like GTP bound to a G protein, the attachment of a phosphoryl group to a serine, threonine, or tyrosine residue powerfully amplifies the initial regulatory signal by recording a molecular memory that the pathway has been activated; dephosphorylation erases the memory, taking a longer time to do so than is required for dissociation of an allosteric ligand. In **flexible regulation**, differing substrate specificities of the multiple protein kinases regulated by second messengers provide branch points in signaling pathways that may be independently regulated. In this way, cAMP, Ca^{2+}, or other second messengers can use the presence or absence of particular kinases or kinase substrates to produce quite different effects in different cell types. Inhibitors of protein kinases have great potential as therapeutic agents, particularly in neoplastic diseases. Trastuzumab, an antibody that antagonizes growth factor receptor signaling (discussed earlier), is a useful therapeutic agent for breast cancer. Another example of this general approach is imatinib, a small molecule inhibitor of the cytoplasmic tyrosine kinase Abl, which is activated by growth factor signaling pathways. Imatinib is effective for treating chronic myelogenous leukemia, which is caused by a chromosomal translocation event that produces an active Bcr/Abl fusion protein in hematopoietic cells.

RECEPTOR CLASSES & DRUG DEVELOPMENT

The existence of a specific drug receptor is usually inferred from studying the **structure-activity relationship** of a group of structurally similar congeners of the drug that mimic or antagonize its effects. Thus, if a series of related agonists exhibits identical relative potencies in producing two distinct effects, it is likely that the two effects are mediated by similar or identical receptor molecules. In addition, if identical receptors mediate both effects, a competitive antagonist will inhibit both responses with the same K_i; a second competitive antagonist will inhibit both responses with its own characteristic K_i. Thus, studies of the relation between structure and activity of a series of agonists and antagonists can identify a species of receptor that mediates a set of pharmacologic responses.

Exactly the same experimental procedure can show that observed effects of a drug are mediated by *different* receptors. In this case, effects mediated by different receptors may exhibit different orders of potency among agonists and different K_i values for each competitive antagonist.

Wherever we look, evolution has created many different receptors that function to mediate responses to any individual chemical signal. In some cases, the same chemical acts on completely different structural receptor classes. For example, acetylcholine uses ligand-gated ion channels (nicotinic AChRs) to initiate a fast (in milliseconds) excitatory postsynaptic potential (EPSP) in postganglionic neurons. Acetylcholine also activates a separate class of G protein-coupled receptors (muscarinic AChRs), which mediate slower (seconds to minutes) modulatory effects on the same neurons. In addition, each structural class usually includes multiple subtypes of receptor, often with significantly different signaling or regulatory properties. For example, many biogenic amines (eg, norepinephrine, acetylcholine, and serotonin) activate more than one receptor, each of which may activate a different G protein, as previously described (see also Table 2–1). The existence of many receptor classes and subtypes for the same endogenous ligand has created important opportunities for drug development. For example, propranolol, a selective antagonist of β adrenoceptors, can reduce an accelerated heart rate without preventing the sympathetic nervous system from causing vasoconstriction, an effect mediated by α_1 receptors.

The principle of drug selectivity may even apply to structurally identical receptors expressed in different cells, eg, receptors for steroids such as estrogen (Figure 2–6). Different cell types express different accessory proteins, which interact with steroid receptors and change the functional effects of drug-receptor interaction. For example, tamoxifen acts as an *antagonist* on estrogen receptors expressed in mammary tissue but as an *agonist* on estrogen receptors in bone. Consequently, tamoxifen may be useful not only in the treatment and prophylaxis of breast cancer but also in the prevention of osteoporosis by increasing bone density (see Chapters 40 and 42). Tamoxifen may also create complications in postmenopausal women, however, by exerting an agonist action in the uterus, stimulating endometrial cell proliferation.

New drug development is not confined to agents that act on receptors for extracellular chemical signals. Increasingly, pharmaceutical chemists are determining whether elements of signaling pathways distal to the receptors may also serve as targets of selective and useful drugs. We have already discussed drugs that act on phosphodiesterase and some intracellular kinases. There are several additional kinase inhibitors presently in clinical trials, as well as preclinical efforts directed at developing inhibitors of G proteins.

RELATION BETWEEN DRUG DOSE & CLINICAL RESPONSE

We have dealt with receptors as molecules and shown how receptors can quantitatively account for the relation between dose or concentration of a drug and pharmacologic responses, at least in an idealized system. When faced with a patient who needs treatment, the prescriber must make a choice among a variety of possible drugs and devise a dosage regimen that is likely to produce maximal benefit and minimal toxicity. To make rational therapeutic decisions, the prescriber must understand how drug-receptor interactions underlie the relations between dose and response in patients, the nature and causes of variation in pharmacologic responsiveness, and the clinical implications of selectivity of drug action.

Dose & Response in Patients

A. Graded Dose-Response Relations

To choose among drugs and to determine appropriate doses of a drug, the prescriber must know the relative **pharmacologic**

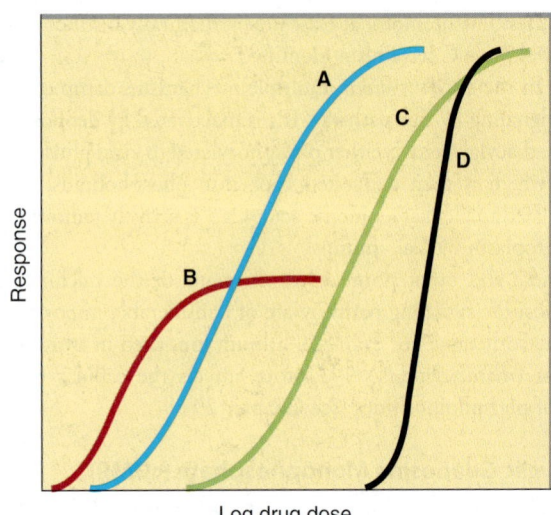

FIGURE 2–15 Graded dose-response curves for four drugs, illustrating different pharmacologic potencies and different maximal efficacies. (See text.)

potency and **maximal efficacy** of the drugs in relation to the desired therapeutic effect. These two important terms, often confusing to students and clinicians, can be explained by referring to Figure 2–15, which depicts graded dose-response curves that relate the dose of four different drugs to the magnitude of a particular therapeutic effect.

1. Potency—Drugs A and B are said to be more potent than drugs C and D because of the relative positions of their dose-response curves along the **dose axis** of Figure 2–15. Potency refers to the concentration (EC_{50}) or dose (ED_{50}) of a drug required to produce 50% of that drug's maximal effect. Thus, the pharmacologic potency of drug A in Figure 2–15 is less than that of drug B, a partial agonist because the EC_{50} of A is greater than the EC_{50} of B. Potency of a drug depends in part on the affinity (K_d) of receptors for binding the drug and in part on the efficiency with which drug-receptor interaction is coupled to response. Note that some doses of drug A can produce larger effects than any dose of drug B, despite the fact that we describe drug B as pharmacologically more potent. The reason for this is that drug A has a larger maximal efficacy (as described below).

For clinical use, it is important to distinguish between a drug's potency and its efficacy. The clinical effectiveness of a drug depends not on its potency (EC_{50}), but on its maximal efficacy (see below) and its ability to reach the relevant receptors. This ability can depend on its route of administration, absorption, distribution through the body, and clearance from the blood or site of action. In deciding which of two drugs to administer to a patient, the prescriber must usually consider their relative effectiveness rather than their relative potency. Pharmacologic potency can largely determine the administered dose of the chosen drug.

For therapeutic purposes, the potency of a drug should be stated in dosage units, usually in terms of a particular therapeutic end point (eg, 50 mg for mild sedation, 1 mcg/kg/min for an increase in heart rate of 25 bpm). Relative potency, the ratio of equi-effective doses (0.2, 10, etc), may be used in comparing one drug with another.

2. Maximal efficacy—This parameter reflects the limit of the dose-response relation on the **response axis.** Drugs A, C, and D in Figure 2–15 have equal maximal efficacy, and all have greater maximal efficacy than drug B. The maximal efficacy (sometimes referred to simply as efficacy) of a drug is obviously crucial for making clinical decisions when a large response is needed. It may be determined by the drug's mode of interactions with receptors (as with partial agonists* or by characteristics of the receptor-effector system involved.

Thus, diuretics that act on one portion of the nephron may produce much greater excretion of fluid and electrolytes than diuretics that act elsewhere. In addition, the *practical* efficacy of a drug for achieving a therapeutic end point (eg, increased cardiac contractility) may be limited by the drug's propensity to cause a toxic effect (eg, fatal cardiac arrhythmia) even if the drug could otherwise produce a greater therapeutic effect.

B. Shape of Dose-Response Curves

Although the responses depicted in curves A, B, and C of Figure 2–15 approximate the shape of a simple Michaelis-Menten relation (transformed to a logarithmic plot), some clinical responses do not. Extremely steep dose-response curves (eg, curve D) may have important clinical consequences if the upper portion of the curve represents an undesirable extent of response (eg, coma caused by a sedative-hypnotic). Steep dose-response curves in patients can result from cooperative interactions of several different actions of a drug (eg, effects on brain, heart, and peripheral vessels, all contributing to lowering of blood pressure).

C. Quantal Dose-Effect Curves

Graded dose-response curves of the sort described above have certain limitations in their application to clinical decision making. For example, such curves may be impossible to construct if the pharmacologic response is an either-or (quantal) event, such as prevention of convulsions, arrhythmia, or death. Furthermore, the clinical relevance of a quantitative dose-response relation in a single patient, no matter how precisely defined, may be limited in application to other patients, owing to the great potential variability among patients in severity of disease and responsiveness to drugs.

---

*Note that "maximal efficacy," used in a therapeutic context, does not have exactly the same meaning that the term denotes in the more specialized context of drug-receptor interactions described earlier in this chapter. In an idealized in vitro system, efficacy denotes the relative maximal efficacy of agonists and partial agonists that act via the same receptor. In therapeutics, efficacy denotes the extent or degree of an effect that can be achieved in the intact patient. Thus, therapeutic efficacy may be affected by the characteristics of a particular drug-receptor interaction, but it also depends on a host of other factors as noted in the text.

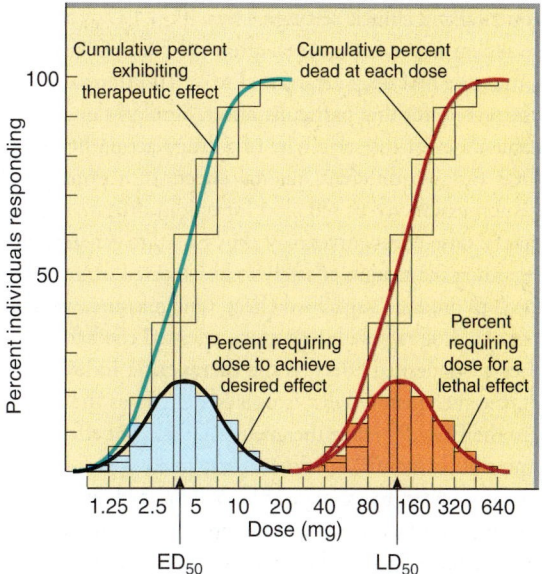

FIGURE 2–16 Quantal dose-effect plots. Shaded boxes (and the accompanying bell-shaped curves) indicate the frequency distribution of doses of drug required to produce a specified effect; that is, the percentage of animals that required a particular dose to exhibit the effect. The open boxes (and the corresponding colored curves) indicate the cumulative frequency distribution of responses, which are lognormally distributed.

Some of these difficulties may be avoided by determining the dose of drug required to produce a specified magnitude of effect in a large number of individual patients or experimental animals and plotting the cumulative frequency distribution of responders versus the log dose (Figure 2–16). The specified quantal effect may be chosen on the basis of clinical relevance (eg, relief of headache) or for preservation of safety of experimental subjects (eg, using low doses of a cardiac stimulant and specifying an increase in heart rate of 20 bpm as the quantal effect), or it may be an inherently quantal event (eg, death of an experimental animal). For most drugs, the doses required to produce a specified quantal effect in individuals are lognormally distributed; that is, a frequency distribution of such responses plotted against the log of the dose produces a gaussian normal curve of variation (colored areas, Figure 2–16). When these responses are summated, the resulting cumulative frequency distribution constitutes a quantal dose-effect curve (or dose-percent curve) of the proportion or percentage of individuals who exhibit the effect plotted as a function of log dose.

The quantal dose-effect curve is often characterized by stating the **median effective dose (ED$_{50}$),** which is the dose at which 50% of individuals exhibit the specified quantal effect. (Note that the abbreviation ED$_{50}$ has a different meaning in this context from its meaning in relation to graded dose-effect curves, described in previous text). Similarly, the dose required to produce a particular toxic effect in 50% of animals is called the **median toxic dose (TD$_{50}$).** If the toxic effect is death of the animal, a **median lethal dose (LD$_{50}$)** may be experimentally defined. Such values provide a convenient way of comparing the potencies of drugs in experimental and clinical settings: Thus, if the ED_{50}s of two drugs for producing a specified quantal effect are 5 and 500 mg, respectively, then the first drug can be said to be 100 times more potent than the second for that particular effect. Similarly, one can obtain a valuable index of the selectivity of a drug's action by comparing its ED_{50}s for two different quantal effects in a population (eg, cough suppression versus sedation for opioid drugs).

Quantal dose-effect curves may also be used to generate information regarding the margin of safety to be expected from a particular drug used to produce a specified effect. One measure, which relates the dose of a drug required to produce a desired effect to that which produces an undesired effect, is the **therapeutic index.** In animal studies, the therapeutic index is usually defined as the ratio of the TD_{50} to the ED_{50} for some therapeutically relevant effect. The precision possible in animal experiments may make it useful to use such a therapeutic index to estimate the potential benefit of a drug in humans. Of course, the therapeutic index of a drug in humans is almost never known with real precision; instead, drug trials and accumulated clinical experience often reveal a range of usually effective doses and a different (but sometimes overlapping) range of possibly toxic doses. The clinically acceptable risk of toxicity depends critically on the severity of the disease being treated. For example, the dose range that provides relief from an ordinary headache in the majority of patients should be very much lower than the dose range that produces serious toxicity, even if the toxicity occurs in a small minority of patients. However, for treatment of a lethal disease such as Hodgkin's lymphoma, the acceptable difference between therapeutic and toxic doses may be smaller.

Finally, note that the quantal dose-effect curve and the graded dose-response curve summarize somewhat different sets of information, although both appear sigmoid in shape on a semilogarithmic plot (compare Figures 2–15 and 2–16). Critical information required for making rational therapeutic decisions can be obtained from each type of curve. Both curves provide information regarding the **potency** and **selectivity** of drugs; the graded dose-response curve indicates the **maximal efficacy** of a drug, and the quantal dose-effect curve indicates the potential **variability** of responsiveness among individuals.

Variation in Drug Responsiveness

Individuals may vary considerably in their response to a drug; indeed, a single individual may respond differently to the same drug at different times during the course of treatment. Occasionally, individuals exhibit an unusual or **idiosyncratic** drug response, one that is infrequently observed in most patients. The idiosyncratic responses are usually caused by genetic differences in metabolism of the drug or by immunologic mechanisms, including allergic reactions.

Quantitative variations in drug response are in general more common and more clinically important. An individual patient is **hyporeactive** or **hyperreactive** to a drug in that the intensity of effect of a given dose of drug is diminished or increased compared with the effect seen in most individuals. (**Note:** The term **hypersensitivity** usually refers to allergic or other immunologic responses to drugs.) With some drugs, the intensity of response to a given dose

may change during the course of therapy; in these cases, responsiveness usually decreases as a consequence of continued drug administration, producing a state of relative **tolerance** to the drug's effects. When responsiveness diminishes rapidly after administration of a drug, the response is said to be subject to **tachyphylaxis.**

Even before administering the first dose of a drug, the prescriber should consider factors that may help in predicting the direction and extent of possible variations in responsiveness. These include the propensity of a particular drug to produce tolerance or tachyphylaxis as well as the effects of age, sex, body size, disease state, genetic factors, and simultaneous administration of other drugs.

Four general mechanisms may contribute to variation in drug responsiveness among patients or within an individual patient at different times.

A. Alteration in Concentration of Drug That Reaches the Receptor

Patients may differ in the rate of absorption of a drug, in distributing it through body compartments, or in clearing the drug from the blood (see Chapter 3). By altering the concentration of drug that reaches relevant receptors, such pharmacokinetic differences may alter the clinical response. Some differences can be predicted on the basis of age, weight, sex, disease state, and liver and kidney function, and by testing specifically for genetic differences that may result from inheritance of a functionally distinctive complement of drug-metabolizing enzymes (see Chapters 3 and 4). Another important mechanism influencing drug availability is active transport of drug from the cytoplasm, mediated by a family of membrane transporters encoded by the so-called multidrug resistance (*MDR*) genes. For example, up-regulation of *MDR* gene-encoded transporter expression is a major mechanism by which tumor cells develop resistance to anticancer drugs.

B. Variation in Concentration of an Endogenous Receptor Ligand

This mechanism contributes greatly to variability in responses to pharmacologic antagonists. Thus, propranolol, a β-adrenoceptor antagonist, markedly slows the heart rate of a patient whose endogenous catecholamines are elevated (as in pheochromocytoma) but does not affect the resting heart rate of a well-trained marathon runner. A partial agonist may exhibit even more dramatically different responses: Saralasin, a weak partial agonist at angiotensin II receptors, lowers blood pressure in patients with hypertension caused by increased angiotensin II production and raises blood pressure in patients who produce normal amounts of angiotensin.

C. Alterations in Number or Function of Receptors

Experimental studies have documented changes in drug response caused by increases or decreases in the number of receptor sites or by alterations in the efficiency of coupling of receptors to distal effector mechanisms. In some cases, the change in receptor number is caused by other hormones; for example, thyroid hormones increase both the number of β receptors in rat heart muscle and cardiac sensitivity to catecholamines. Similar changes probably contribute to the tachycardia of thyrotoxicosis in patients and may account for the usefulness of propranolol, a β-adrenoceptor antagonist, in ameliorating symptoms of this disease.

In other cases, the agonist ligand itself induces a decrease in the number (eg, down-regulation) or coupling efficiency (eg, desensitization) of its receptors. These mechanisms (discussed previously under Signaling Mechanisms & Drug Actions) may contribute to two clinically important phenomena: first, tachyphylaxis or tolerance to the effects of some drugs (eg, biogenic amines and their congeners), and second, the "overshoot" phenomena that follow withdrawal of certain drugs. These phenomena can occur with either agonists or antagonists. An antagonist may increase the number of receptors in a critical cell or tissue by preventing down-regulation caused by an endogenous agonist. When the antagonist is withdrawn, the elevated number of receptors can produce an exaggerated response to physiologic concentrations of agonist. Potentially disastrous withdrawal symptoms can result for the opposite reason when administration of an agonist drug is discontinued. In this situation, the number of receptors, which has been decreased by drug-induced down-regulation, is too low for endogenous agonist to produce effective stimulation. For example, the withdrawal of clonidine (a drug whose α_2-adrenoceptor agonist activity reduces blood pressure) can produce hypertensive crisis, probably because the drug down-regulates α_2 adrenoceptors (see Chapter 11).

Genetic factors also can play an important role in altering the number or function of specific receptors. For example, a specific genetic variant of the α_{2C} adrenoceptor—when inherited together with a specific variant of the α_1 adrenoceptor—confers increased risk for developing heart failure, which may be reduced by early intervention using antagonist drugs. The identification of such genetic factors, part of the rapidly developing field of pharmacogenetics, holds promise for clinical diagnosis and in the future may help physicians design the most appropriate pharmacologic therapy for individual patients.

Another interesting example of genetic determination of effects on drug response is seen in the treatment of cancers involving excessive growth factor signaling. Somatic mutations affecting the tyrosine kinase domain of the epidermal growth factor receptor confer enhanced sensitivity to kinase inhibitors such as gefitinib in certain lung cancers. This effect enhances the antineoplastic effect of the drug and, because the somatic mutation is specific to the tumor and not present in the host, the therapeutic index of these drugs can be significantly enhanced in patients whose tumors harbor such mutations.

D. Changes in Components of Response Distal to the Receptor

Although a drug initiates its actions by binding to receptors, the response observed in a patient depends on the functional integrity of biochemical processes in the responding cell and physiologic regulation by interacting organ systems. Clinically, changes in these postreceptor processes represent the largest and most important class of mechanisms that cause variation in responsiveness to drug therapy.

Before initiating therapy with a drug, the prescriber should be aware of patient characteristics that may limit the clinical response. These characteristics include the age and general health of the patient and—most importantly—the severity and pathophysiologic mechanism of the disease. The most important potential cause of failure to achieve a satisfactory response is that the diagnosis is wrong or physiologically incomplete. Drug therapy is always most successful when it is accurately directed at the pathophysiologic mechanism responsible for the disease.

When the diagnosis is correct and the drug is appropriate, an unsatisfactory therapeutic response can often be traced to compensatory mechanisms in the patient that respond to and oppose the beneficial effects of the drug. Compensatory increases in sympathetic nervous tone and fluid retention by the kidney, for example, can contribute to tolerance to antihypertensive effects of a vasodilator drug. In such cases, additional drugs may be required to achieve a useful therapeutic result.

Clinical Selectivity: Beneficial versus Toxic Effects of Drugs

Although we classify drugs according to their principal actions, it is clear that *no drug causes only a single, specific effect*. Why is this so? It is exceedingly unlikely that any kind of drug molecule will bind to only a single type of receptor molecule, if only because the number of potential receptors in every patient is astronomically large. Even if the chemical structure of a drug allowed it to bind to only one kind of receptor, the biochemical processes controlled by such receptors would take place in many cell types and would be coupled to many other biochemical functions; as a result, the patient and the prescriber would probably perceive more than one drug effect. Accordingly, drugs are only *selective*—rather than specific—in their actions, because they bind to one or a few types of receptor more tightly than to others and because these receptors control discrete processes that result in distinct effects.

It is only because of their selectivity that drugs are useful in clinical medicine. Selectivity can be measured by comparing binding affinities of a drug to different receptors or by comparing ED_{50}s for different effects of a drug in vivo. In drug development and in clinical medicine, selectivity is usually considered by separating effects into two categories: **beneficial** or **therapeutic effects** versus **toxic** or **adverse effects.** Pharmaceutical advertisements and prescribers occasionally use the term **side effect,** implying that the effect in question is insignificant or occurs via a pathway that is to one side of the principal action of the drug; such implications are frequently erroneous.

A. Beneficial and Toxic Effects Mediated by the Same Receptor-Effector Mechanism

Much of the serious drug toxicity in clinical practice represents a direct pharmacologic extension of the therapeutic actions of the drug. In some of these cases (eg, bleeding caused by anticoagulant therapy; hypoglycemic coma due to insulin), toxicity may be avoided by judicious management of the dose of drug administered, guided by careful monitoring of effect (measurements of blood coagulation or serum glucose) and aided by ancillary measures (avoiding tissue trauma that may lead to hemorrhage; regulation of carbohydrate intake). In still other cases, the toxicity may be avoided by not administering the drug at all, if the therapeutic indication is weak or if other therapy is available.

In certain situations, a drug is clearly necessary and beneficial but produces unacceptable toxicity when given in doses that produce optimal benefit. In such situations, it may be necessary to add another drug to the treatment regimen. In treating hypertension, for example, administration of a second drug often allows the prescriber to reduce the dose and toxicity of the first drug (see Chapter 11).

B. Beneficial and Toxic Effects Mediated by Identical Receptors but in Different Tissues or by Different Effector Pathways

Many drugs produce both their desired effects and adverse effects by acting on a single receptor type in different tissues. Examples discussed in this book include: digitalis glycosides, which act by inhibiting Na^+/K^+-ATPase in cell membranes; methotrexate, which inhibits the enzyme dihydrofolate reductase; and glucocorticoid hormones.

Three therapeutic strategies are used to avoid or mitigate this sort of toxicity. First, the drug should always be administered at the lowest dose that produces acceptable benefit. Second, adjunctive drugs that act through different receptor mechanisms and produce different toxicities may allow lowering the dose of the first drug, thus limiting its toxicity (eg, use of other immunosuppressive agents added to glucocorticoids in treating inflammatory disorders). Third, selectivity of the drug's actions may be increased by manipulating the concentrations of drug available to receptors in different parts of the body, for example, by aerosol administration of a glucocorticoid to the bronchi in asthma.

C. Beneficial and Toxic Effects Mediated by Different Types of Receptors

Therapeutic advantages resulting from new chemical entities with improved receptor selectivity were mentioned earlier in this chapter and are described in detail in later chapters. Such drugs include α- and β-selective adrenoceptor agonists and antagonists, H_1 and H_2 antihistamines, nicotinic and muscarinic blocking agents, and receptor-selective steroid hormones. All these receptors are grouped in functional families, each responsive to a small class of endogenous agonists. The receptors and their associated therapeutic uses were discovered by analyzing effects of the physiologic chemical signals—catecholamines, histamine, acetylcholine, and corticosteroids.

Several other drugs were discovered by exploiting therapeutic or toxic effects of chemically similar agents observed in a clinical context. Examples include quinidine, the sulfonylureas, thiazide diuretics, tricyclic antidepressants, opioid drugs, and phenothiazine antipsychotics. Often the new agents turn out to interact with receptors for endogenous substances (eg, opioids and phenothiazines for endogenous opioid and dopamine receptors, respectively). It is likely that other new drugs will be found to do so in the future, perhaps leading to the discovery of new classes of receptors and endogenous ligands for future drug development.

Thus, the propensity of drugs to bind to different classes of receptor sites is not only a potentially vexing problem in treating patients, it also presents a continuing challenge to pharmacology and an opportunity for developing new and more useful drugs.

REFERENCES

Berridge MJ: Unlocking the secrets of cell signaling. Ann Rev Physiol 2005;67:1.

Cabrera-Vera TM et al: Insights into G protein structure, function, and regulation. Endocr Rev 2003;24:765.

Civelli O et al: Orphan GPCRs and their ligands. Pharmacol Ther 2006;110:525.

Davies MA, Samuels Y: Analysis of the genome to personalize therapy for melanoma. Oncogene 2010;29:5545.

Feng XH, Derynck R: Specificity and versatility in TGF-beta signaling through Smads. Annu Rev Cell Dev Biol 2005;21:659.

Galandrin S, Oligny-Longpre G, Bouvier M: The evasive nature of drug efficacy: Implications for drug discovery. Trends Pharmacol Sci 2007;28:423.

Ginty DD, Segal RA: Retrograde neurotrophin signaling: Trk-ing along the axon. Curr Opin Neurobiol 2002;12:268.

Gouaux E, MacKinnon R: Principles of selective ion transport in channels and pumps. Science 2005;310:1461.

Hermiston ML et al: Reciprocal regulation of lymphocyte activation by tyrosine kinases and phosphatases. J Clin Invest 2002;109:9.

Kenakin T: Principles: Receptor theory in molecular pharmacology. Trends Pharmacol Sci 2004;25:186.

Mosesson Y, Yarden Y: Oncogenic growth factor receptors: Implications for signal transduction therapy. Semin Cancer Biol 2004;14:262.

Pawson T: Dynamic control of signaling by modular adaptor proteins. Curr Opin Cell Biol 2007;19:112.

Rajagopal S, Rajagopal K, Lefkowitz RJ: Teaching old receptors new tricks- biasing seven-transmembrane receptors. Nat Rev Drug Discov 2010;9:373.

Roden DM, George AL Jr: The genetic basis of variability in drug responses. Nat Rev Drug Discov 2002;1:37.

Rosenbaum DM, Rasmussen SG, Kobilka BK: The structure and function of G-protein-coupled receptors. Nature 2009;459:356.

Rotella DP: Phosphodiesterase 5 inhibitors: Current status and potential applications. Nat Rev Drug Discov 2002;1:674.

Small KM, McGraw DW, Liggett SB: Pharmacology and physiology of human adrenergic receptor polymorphisms. Ann Rev Pharmacol Toxicol 2003;43:381.

Sorkin A, von Zastrow M: Endocytosis and signaling: Intertwining molecular networks. Nat Rev Mol Cell Biol 2009;10:609.

Yu FH et al: Overview of molecular relationships in the voltage-gated ion channel superfamily. Pharmacol Rev 2005;57:387.

Yuan TL, Cantley LC: PI3K pathway alterations in cancer: Variations on a theme. Oncogene 2008;27:5497.

CASE STUDY ANSWER

Propranolol, a nonselective β-adrenoceptor blocker, is a useful antihypertensive agent because it reduces cardiac output and probably vascular resistance as well. However, it also prevents β₂-receptor-induced bronchodilation and may precipitate bronchoconstriction in susceptible individuals. Calcium channel blockers such as verapamil also reduce blood pressure but do not cause bronchoconstriction or prevent bronchodilation. Selection of the most appropriate drug or drug group for one condition requires awareness of the other conditions a patient may have and the receptor selectivity of the drug groups available.

Pharmacokinetics & Pharmacodynamics: Rational Dosing & the Time Course of Drug Action

Nicholas H. G. Holford, MB, ChB, FRACP

CASE STUDY

An 85-year-old, 60-kg woman with a serum creatinine of 1.8 mg/dL has atrial fibrillation. A decision has been made to use digoxin to control the rapid heart rate. The target concentration of digoxin for the treatment of atrial fibrillation is 2 ng/mL. Tablets of digoxin contain 62.5 micrograms and 250 micrograms (mcg). What maintenance dose would you recommend?

The goal of therapeutics is to achieve a desired beneficial effect with minimal adverse effects. When a medicine has been selected for a patient, the clinician must determine the dose that most closely achieves this goal. A rational approach to this objective combines the principles of pharmacokinetics with pharmacodynamics to clarify the dose-effect relationship (Figure 3–1). Pharmacodynamics governs the concentration-effect part of the interaction, whereas pharmacokinetics deals with the dose-concentration part (Holford & Sheiner, 1981). The pharmacokinetic processes of absorption, distribution, and elimination determine how rapidly and for how long the drug will appear at the target organ. The pharmacodynamic concepts of maximum response and sensitivity determine the magnitude of the effect at a particular concentration (see E_{max} and C_{50}, Chapter 2; C_{50} is also known as EC_{50}).

Figure 3–1 illustrates a fundamental hypothesis of pharmacology, namely, that a relationship exists between a beneficial or toxic effect of a drug and the concentration of the drug. This hypothesis has been documented for many drugs, as indicated by the Target

Concentrations and Toxic Concentrations columns in Table 3–1. The apparent lack of such a relationship for some drugs does not weaken the basic hypothesis but points to the need to consider the time course of concentration at the actual site of pharmacologic effect (see below).

Knowing the relationship between dose, drug concentration, and effects allows the clinician to take into account the various pathologic and physiologic features of a particular patient that make him or her different from the average individual in responding to a drug. The importance of pharmacokinetics and pharmacodynamics in patient care thus rests upon the improvement in therapeutic benefit and reduction in toxicity that can be achieved by application of these principles.

PHARMACOKINETICS

The "standard" dose of a drug is based on trials in healthy volunteers and patients with average ability to absorb, distribute, and eliminate

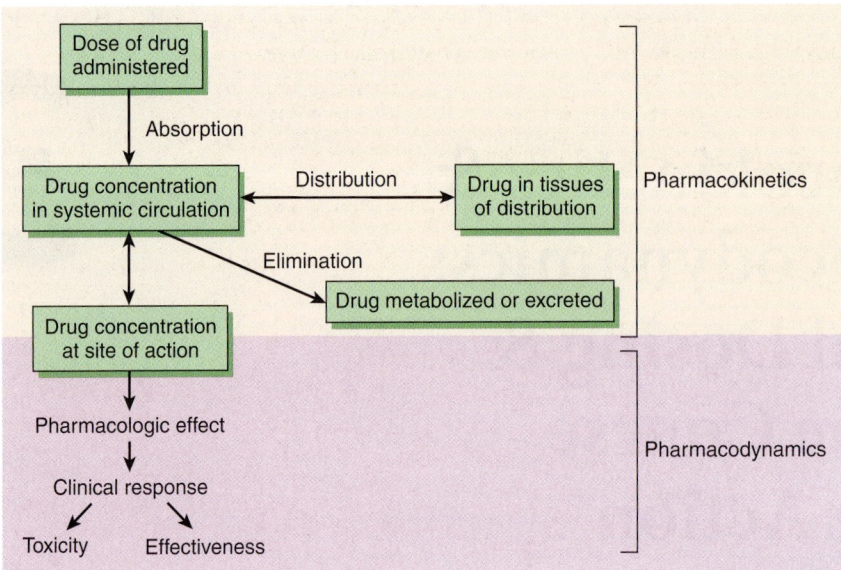

FIGURE 3–1   The relationship between dose and effect can be separated into pharmacokinetic (dose-concentration) and pharmacodynamic (concentration-effect) components. Concentration provides the link between pharmacokinetics and pharmacodynamics and is the focus of the target concentration approach to rational dosing. The three primary processes of pharmacokinetics are absorption, distribution, and elimination.

the drug (see Clinical Trials: The IND and NDA in Chapter 5). This dose will not be suitable for every patient. Several physiologic processes (eg, maturation of organ function in infants) and pathologic processes (eg, heart failure, renal failure) dictate dosage adjustment in individual patients. These processes modify specific pharmacokinetic parameters. The two basic parameters are **clearance,** the measure of the ability of the body to eliminate the drug; and **volume of distribution,** the measure of the apparent space in the body available to contain the drug. These parameters are illustrated schematically in Figure 3–2 where the volume of the beakers into which the drugs diffuse represents the volume of distribution and the size of the outflow "drain" in Figures 3–2B and 3–2D represents the clearance.

Volume of Distribution

Volume of distribution (V) relates the amount of drug in the body to the concentration of drug (C) in blood or plasma:

$$V = \frac{\text{Amount of drug in body}}{C} \qquad (1)$$

The volume of distribution may be defined with respect to blood, plasma, or water (unbound drug), depending on the concentration used in equation (1) ($C = C_b$, C_p, or C_u).

That the V calculated from equation (1) is an *apparent* volume may be appreciated by comparing the volumes of distribution of drugs such as digoxin or chloroquine (Table 3–1) with some of the physical volumes of the body (Table 3–2). Volume of distribution can vastly exceed any physical volume in the body because

it is the volume *apparently* necessary to contain the amount of drug *homogeneously* at the concentration found in the blood, plasma, or water. Drugs with very high volumes of distribution have much higher concentrations in extravascular tissue than in the vascular compartment, ie, they are *not* homogeneously distributed. Drugs that are completely retained within the vascular compartment, on the other hand, have a minimum possible volume of distribution equal to the blood component in which they are distributed, eg, 0.04 L/kg body weight or 2.8 L/70 kg (Table 3–2) for a drug that is restricted to the plasma compartment.

Clearance

Drug clearance principles are similar to the clearance concepts of renal physiology. Clearance of a drug is the factor that predicts the rate of elimination in relation to the drug concentration:

$$CL = \frac{\text{Rate of elimination}}{C} \qquad (2)$$

Clearance, like volume of distribution, may be defined with respect to blood (CL_b), plasma (CL_p), or unbound in water (CL_u), depending on the concentration measured.

It is important to note the additive character of clearance. Elimination of drug from the body may involve processes occurring in the kidney, the lung, the liver, and other organs. Dividing the rate of elimination at each organ by the concentration of drug presented to it yields the respective clearance at that organ.

TABLE 3–1 Pharmacokinetic and pharmacodynamic parameters for selected drugs. (See Speight & Holford, 1997, for a more comprehensive listing.)

Drug	Oral Availability (F) (%)	Urinary Excretion (%)[1]	Bound in Plasma (%)	Clearance (L/h/70 kg)[2]	Volume of Distribution (L/70 kg)	Half-Life (h)	Target Concentration	Toxic Concentration
Acetaminophen	88	3	0	21	67	2	15 mg/L	> 300 mg/L
Acyclovir	23	75	15	19.8	48	2.4	...	...
Amikacin	...	98	4	5.46	19	2.3	10 mg/L[3]...	...
Amoxicillin	93	86	18	10.8	15	1.7	...	...
Amphotericin	...	4	90	1.92	53	18	...	...
Ampicillin	62	82	18	16.2	20	1.3	...	...
Aspirin	68	1	49	39	11	0.25	...	...
Atenolol	56	94	5	10.2	67	6.1	1 mg/L	...
Atropine	50	57	18	24.6	120	4.3	...	...
Captopril	65	38	30	50.4	57	2.2	50 ng/mL	...
Carbamazepine	70	1	74	5.34	98	15	6 mg/L	> 9 mg/L
Cephalexin	90	91	14	18	18	0.9	...	...
Cephalothin	...	52	71	28.2	18	0.57	...	...
Chloramphenicol	80	25	53	10.2	66	2.7	...	...
Chlordiazepoxide	100	1	97	2.28	21	10	1 mg/L	...
Chloroquine	89	61	61	45	13,000	214	20 ng/mL	250 ng/mL
Chlorpropamide	90	20	96	0.126	6.8	33	...	...
Cimetidine	62	62	19	32.4	70	1.9	0.8 mg/L	...
Ciprofloxacin	60	65	40	25.2	130	4.1	...	...
Clonidine	95	62	20	12.6	150	12	1 ng/mL	...
Cyclosporine	30	1	98	23.9	244	15	200 ng/mL	> 400 ng/mL
Diazepam	100	1	99	1.62	77	43	300 ng/mL	...
Digoxin	70	67	25	9	500	39	1 ng/mL	> 2 ng/mL
Diltiazem	44	4	78	50.4	220	3.7	...	...
Disopyramide	83	55	2	5.04	41	6	3 mg/mL	> 8 mg/mL
Enalapril	95	90	55	9	40	3	> 0.5 ng/mL	...
Erythromycin	35	12	84	38.4	55	1.6	...	...
Ethambutol	77	79	5	36	110	3.1	...	> 10 mg/L
Fluoxetine	60	3	94	40.2	2500	53	...	...
Furosemide	61	66	99	8.4	7.7	1.5	...	> 25 mg/L
Gentamicin	...	76	10	4.7	20	3	3 mg/L[3]	...
Hydralazine	40	10	87	234	105	1	100 ng/mL	...
Imipramine	40	2	90	63	1600	18	200 ng/mL	> 1 mg/L
Indomethacin	98	15	90	8.4	18	2.4	1 mg/L	> 5 mg/L
Labetalol	18	5	50	105	660	4.9	0.1 mg/L	...
Lidocaine	35	2	70	38.4	77	1.8	3 mg/L	> 6 mg/L
Lithium	100	95	0	1.5	55	22	0.7 mEq/L	> 2 mEq/L

(continued)

TABLE 3–1 Pharmacokinetic and pharmacodynamic parameters for selected drugs. (Continued)

Drug	Oral Availability (F) (%)	Urinary Excretion (%)[1]	Bound in Plasma (%)	Clearance (L/h/70 kg)[2]	Volume of Distribution (L/70 kg)	Half-Life (h)	Target Concentration	Toxic Concentration
Meperidine	52	12	58	72	310	3.2	0.5 mg/L	...
Methotrexate	70	48	34	9	39	7.2	750 µM-h[4,5]	> 950 µM-h
Metoprolol	38	10	11	63	290	3.2	25 ng/mL	...
Metronidazole	99	10	10	5.4	52	8.5	4 mg/L	...
Midazolam	44	56	95	27.6	77	1.9	...	...
Morphine	24	8	35	60	230	1.9	15 ng/mL	...
Nifedipine	50	0	96	29.4	55	1.8	50 ng/mL	...
Nortriptyline	51	2	92	30	1300	31	100 ng/mL	> 500 ng/mL
Phenobarbital	100	24	51	0.258	38	98	15 mg/L	> 30 mg/L
Phenytoin	90	2	89	Conc dependent[5]	45	Conc dependent[6]	10 mg/L	> 20 mg/L
Prazosin	68	1	95	12.6	42	2.9	...	...
Procainamide	83	67	16	36	130	3	5 mg/L	> 14 mg/L
Propranolol	26	1	87	50.4	270	3.9	20 ng/mL	...
Pyridostigmine	14	85	...	36	77	1.9	75 ng/mL	...
Quinidine	80	18	87	19.8	190	6.2	3 mg/L	> 8 mg/L
Ranitidine	52	69	15	43.8	91	2.1	100 ng/mL	...
Rifampin	?	7	89	14.4	68	3.5	...	...
Salicylic acid	100	15	85	0.84	12	13	200 mg/L	> 200 mg/L
Sulfamethoxazole	100	14	62	1.32	15	10	...	...
Terbutaline	14	56	20	14.4	125	14	2 ng/mL	...
Tetracycline	77	58	65	7.2	105	11	...	...
Theophylline	96	18	56	2.8	35	8.1	10 mg/L	> 20 mg/L
Tobramycin	...	90	10	4.62	18	2.2	...	...
Tocainide	89	38	10	10.8	210	14	10 mg/L	...
Tolbutamide	93	0	96	1.02	7	5.9	100 mg/L	...
Trimethoprim	100	69	44	9	130	11	...	...
Tubocurarine	...	63	50	8.1	27	2	0.6 mg/L	...
Valproic acid	100	2	93	0.462	9.1	14	75 mg/L	> 150 mg/L
Vancomycin	...	79	30	5.88	27	5.6	20 mg/L[3]	...
Verapamil	22	3	90	63	350	4	...	...
Warfarin	93	3	99	0.192	9.8	37	...	...
Zidovudine	63	18	25	61.8	98	1.1	...	...

[1] Assuming creatinine clearance 100 mL/min/70 kg.

[2] Convert to mL/min by multiplying the number given by 16.6.

[3] Average steady-state concentration.

[4] Target area under the concentration-time curve after a single dose.

[5] Can be estimated from measured C using $CL = V_{max}/(K_m + C)$; $V_{max} = 415$ mg/d, $K_m = 5$ mg/L. See text.

[6] Varies because of concentration-dependent clearance.

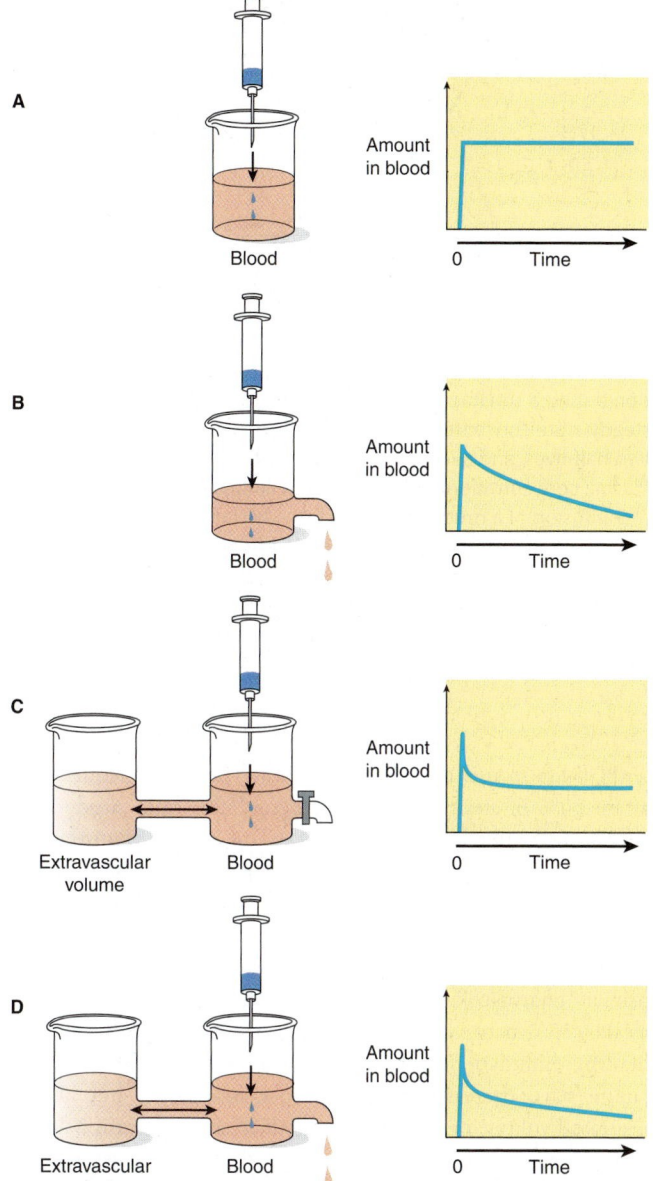

FIGURE 3–2 Models of drug distribution and elimination. The effect of adding drug to the blood by rapid intravenous injection is represented by expelling a known amount of the agent into a beaker. The time course of the amount of drug in the beaker is shown in the graphs at the right. In the first example (**A**), there is no movement of drug out of the beaker, so the graph shows only a steep rise to maximum followed by a plateau. In the second example (**B**), a route of elimination is present, and the graph shows a slow decay after a sharp rise to a maximum. Because the level of material in the beaker falls, the "pressure" driving the elimination process also falls, and the slope of the curve decreases. This is an exponential decay curve. In the third model (**C**), drug placed in the first compartment ("blood") equilibrates rapidly with the second compartment ("extravascular volume") and the amount of drug in "blood" declines exponentially to a new steady state. The fourth model (**D**) illustrates a more realistic combination of elimination mechanism and extravascular equilibration. The resulting graph shows an early distribution phase followed by the slower elimination phase.

TABLE 3–2 **Physical volumes (in L/kg body weight) of some body compartments into which drugs may be distributed.**

Compartment and Volume	Examples of Drugs
Water	
Total body water (0.6 L/kg[1])	Small water-soluble molecules: eg, ethanol
Extracellular water (0.2 L/kg)	Larger water-soluble molecules: eg, gentamicin
Blood (0.08 L/kg); plasma (0.04 L/kg)	Strongly plasma protein-bound molecules and very large molecules: eg, heparin
Fat (0.2-0.35 L/kg)	Highly lipid-soluble molecules: eg, DDT
Bone (0.07 L/kg)	Certain ions: eg, lead, fluoride

[1]An average figure. Total body water in a young lean man might be 0.7 L/kg; in an obese woman, 0.5 L/kg.

Added together, these separate clearances equal total systemic clearance:

$$CL_{kidney} = \frac{Rate\ of\ elimination_{kidney}}{C} \qquad (3a)$$

$$CL_{liver} = \frac{Rate\ of\ elimination_{liver}}{C} \qquad (3b)$$

$$CL_{other} = \frac{Rate\ of\ elimination_{other}}{C} \qquad (3c)$$

$$CL_{systemic} = CL_{kidney} + CL_{liver} + CL_{other} \qquad (3d)$$

"Other" tissues of elimination could include the lungs and additional sites of metabolism, eg, blood or muscle.

The two major sites of drug elimination are the kidneys and the liver. Clearance of unchanged drug in the urine represents renal clearance. Within the liver, drug elimination occurs via biotransformation of parent drug to one or more metabolites, or excretion of unchanged drug into the bile, or both. The pathways of biotransformation are discussed in Chapter 4. For most drugs, clearance is constant over the concentration range encountered in clinical settings, ie, elimination is not saturable, and the rate of drug elimination is directly proportional to concentration (rearranging equation [2]):

$$Rate\ of\ elimination = CL \times C \qquad (4)$$

This is usually referred to as first-order elimination. When clearance is first-order, it can be estimated by calculating the **area under the curve (AUC)** of the time-concentration profile after a dose. Clearance is calculated from the dose divided by the AUC.

A. Capacity-Limited Elimination

For drugs that exhibit capacity-limited elimination (eg, phenytoin, ethanol), clearance will vary depending on the concentration of drug that is achieved (Table 3–1). Capacity-limited elimination is also known as mixed-order, saturable, dose- or concentration-dependent, nonlinear, and Michaelis-Menten elimination.

Most drug elimination pathways will become saturated if the dose and therefore the concentration are high enough. When blood flow to an organ does not limit elimination (see below), the relation between elimination rate and concentration (C) is expressed mathematically in equation (5):

$$\text{Rate of elimination} = \frac{V_{max} \times C}{K_m + C} \qquad (5)$$

The maximum elimination capacity is V_{max}, and K_m is the drug concentration at which the rate of elimination is 50% of V_{max}. At concentrations that are high relative to the K_m, the elimination rate is almost independent of concentration—a state of "pseudo-zero order" elimination. If dosing rate exceeds elimination capacity, steady state cannot be achieved: The concentration will keep on rising as long as dosing continues. This pattern of capacity-limited elimination is important for three drugs in common use: ethanol, phenytoin, and aspirin. Clearance has no real meaning for drugs with capacity-limited elimination, and AUC should not be used to describe the elimination of such drugs.

B. Flow-Dependent Elimination

In contrast to capacity-limited drug elimination, some drugs are cleared very readily by the organ of elimination, so that at any clinically realistic concentration of the drug, most of the drug in the blood perfusing the organ is eliminated on the first pass of the drug through it. The elimination of these drugs will thus depend primarily on the rate of drug delivery to the organ of elimination. Such drugs (see Table 4–7) can be called "high-extraction" drugs since they are almost completely extracted from the blood by the organ. Blood flow to the organ is the main determinant of drug delivery, but plasma protein binding and blood cell partitioning may also be important for extensively bound drugs that are highly extracted.

Half-Life

Half-life ($t_{1/2}$) is the time required to change the amount of drug in the body by one-half during elimination (or during a constant infusion). In the simplest case—and the most useful in designing drug dosage regimens—the body may be considered as a single compartment (as illustrated in Figure 3–2B) of a size equal to the volume of distribution (V). The time course of drug in the body will depend on both the volume of distribution and the clearance:

$$t_{1/2} = \frac{0.7 \times V}{CL} \qquad (6)$$

Because drug elimination can be described by an exponential process, the time taken for a twofold decrease can be shown to be proportional to the natural logarithm of 2. The constant 0.7 in equation (6) is an approximation to the natural logarithm of 2.

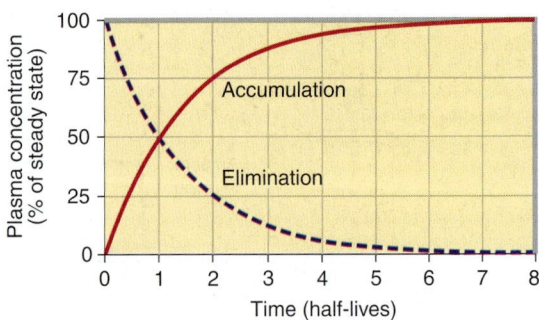

FIGURE 3–3 The time course of drug accumulation and elimination. **Solid line:** Plasma concentrations reflecting drug accumulation during a constant-rate infusion of a drug. Fifty percent of the steady-state concentration is reached after one half-life, 75% after two half-lives, and over 90% after four half-lives. **Dashed line:** Plasma concentrations reflecting drug elimination after a constant-rate infusion of a drug had reached steady state. Fifty percent of the drug is lost after one half-life, 75% after two half-lives, etc. The "rule of thumb" that four half-lives must elapse after starting a drug-dosing regimen before full effects will be seen is based on the approach of the accumulation curve to over 90% of the final steady-state concentration.

Half-life is useful because it indicates the time required to attain 50% of steady state—or to decay 50% from steady-state conditions—after a change in the rate of drug administration. Figure 3–3 shows the time course of drug accumulation during a constant-rate drug infusion and the time course of drug elimination after stopping an infusion that has reached steady state.

Disease states can affect both of the physiologically related primary pharmacokinetic parameters: volume of distribution and clearance. A change in half-life will not necessarily reflect a change in drug elimination. For example, patients with chronic renal failure have decreased renal clearance of digoxin but also a decreased volume of distribution; the increase in digoxin half-life is not as great as might be expected based on the change in renal function. The decrease in volume of distribution is due to the decreased renal and skeletal muscle mass and consequent decreased tissue binding of digoxin to Na^+/K^+-ATPase.

Many drugs will exhibit multicompartment pharmacokinetics (as illustrated in Figures 3–2C and 3–2D). Under these conditions, the "true" terminal half-life, as given in Table 3–1, will be greater than that calculated from equation (6).

Drug Accumulation

Whenever drug doses are repeated, the drug will accumulate in the body until dosing stops. This is because it takes an infinite time (in theory) to eliminate all of a given dose. In practical terms, this means that if the dosing interval is shorter than four half-lives, accumulation will be detectable.

Accumulation is inversely proportional to the fraction of the dose lost in each dosing interval. The fraction lost is 1 minus the fraction remaining just before the next dose. The fraction remaining can be predicted from the dosing interval and the half-life. A convenient index of accumulation is the **accumulation factor:**

$$\text{Accumulation factor} = \frac{1}{\text{Fraction lost in one dosing interval}}$$

$$= \frac{1}{1 - \text{Fraction remaining}} \qquad (7)$$

For a drug given once every half-life, the accumulation factor is 1/0.5, or 2. The accumulation factor predicts the ratio of the steady-state concentration to that seen at the same time following the first dose. Thus, the peak concentrations after intermittent doses at steady state will be equal to the peak concentration after the first dose multiplied by the accumulation factor.

Bioavailability

Bioavailability is defined as the fraction of unchanged drug reaching the systemic circulation following administration by any route (Table 3–3). The area under the blood concentration-time curve (AUC) is proportional to the extent of bioavailability for a drug if its elimination is first-order (Figure 3–4). For an intravenous dose of the drug, bioavailability is assumed to be equal to unity. For a drug administered orally, bioavailability may be less than 100% for two main reasons—incomplete extent of absorption across the gut wall and first-pass elimination by the liver (see below).

A. Extent of Absorption

After oral administration, a drug may be incompletely absorbed, eg, only 70% of a dose of digoxin reaches the systemic circulation. This is mainly due to lack of absorption from the gut. Other drugs are either too hydrophilic (eg, atenolol) or too lipophilic (eg, acy-

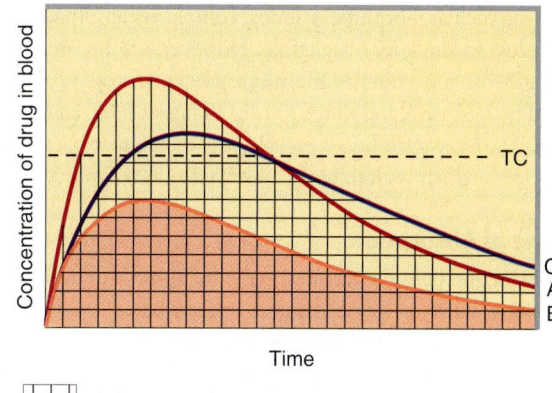

A: Drug rapidly and completely available

B: Only half of availability of A but rate equal to A

C: Drug completely available but rate only half of A

FIGURE 3-4 Blood concentration-time curves, illustrating how changes in the rate of absorption and extent of bioavailability can influence both the duration of action and the effectiveness of the same total dose of a drug administered in three different formulations. The dashed line indicates the target concentration (TC) of the drug in the blood.

clovir) to be absorbed easily, and their low bioavailability is also due to incomplete absorption. If too hydrophilic, the drug cannot cross the lipid cell membrane; if too lipophilic, the drug is not soluble enough to cross the water layer adjacent to the cell. Drugs may not be absorbed because of a reverse transporter associated with P-glycoprotein. This process actively pumps drug out of gut wall cells back into the gut lumen. Inhibition of P-glycoprotein and gut wall metabolism, eg, by grapefruit juice, may be associated with substantially increased drug absorption.

B. First-Pass Elimination

Following absorption across the gut wall, the portal blood delivers the drug to the liver prior to entry into the systemic circulation. A drug can be metabolized in the gut wall (eg, by the CYP3A4 enzyme system) or even in the portal blood, but most commonly it is the liver that is responsible for metabolism before the drug reaches the systemic circulation. In addition, the liver can excrete the drug into the bile. Any of these sites can contribute to this reduction in bioavailability, and the overall process is known as first-pass elimination. The effect of first-pass hepatic elimination on bioavailability is expressed as the extraction ratio (ER):

$$\text{ER} = \frac{CL_{liver}}{Q} \qquad (8a)$$

where Q is hepatic blood flow, normally about 90 L/h in a person weighing 70 kg.

The systemic bioavailability of the drug (F) can be predicted from the extent of absorption (f) and the extraction ratio (ER):

$$F = f \times (1 - \text{ER}) \qquad (8b)$$

TABLE 3–3 Routes of administration, bioavailability, and general characteristics.

Route	Bioavailability (%)	Characteristics
Intravenous (IV)	100 (by definition)	Most rapid onset
Intramuscular (IM)	75 to ≤ 100	Large volumes often feasible; may be painful
Subcutaneous (SC)	75 to ≤100	Smaller volumes than IM; may be painful
Oral (PO)	5 to < 100	Most convenient; first-pass effect may be significant
Rectal (PR)	30 to < 100	Less first-pass effect than oral
Inhalation	5 to < 100	Often very rapid onset
Transdermal	80 to ≤ 100	Usually very slow absorption; used for lack of first-pass effect; prolonged duration of action

A drug such as morphine is almost completely absorbed (f = 1), so that loss in the gut is negligible. However, the hepatic extraction ratio for morphine is morphine clearance (60 L/h/70 kg) divided by hepatic blood flow (90 L/h/70 kg) or 0.67, so (1 − ER) is 0.33. The bioavailability of morphine is therefore expected to be about 33%, which is close to the observed value (Table 3–1).

C. Rate of Absorption

The distinction between rate and extent of absorption is shown in Figure 3–4. The rate of absorption is determined by the site of administration and the drug formulation. Both the rate of absorption and the extent of input can influence the clinical effectiveness of a drug. For the three different dosage forms depicted in Figure 3–4, there would be significant differences in the intensity of clinical effect. Dosage form B would require twice the dose to attain blood concentrations equivalent to those of dosage form A. Differences in rate of absorption may become important for drugs given as a single dose, such as a hypnotic used to induce sleep. In this case, drug from dosage form A would reach its target concentration earlier than drug from dosage form C; concentrations from A would also reach a higher level and remain above the target concentration for a longer period. In a multiple dosing regimen, dosage forms A and C would yield the same average blood level concentrations, although dosage form A would show somewhat greater maximum and lower minimum concentrations.

The mechanism of drug absorption is said to be zero-order when the rate is independent of the amount of drug remaining in the gut, eg, when it is determined by the rate of gastric emptying or by a controlled-release drug formulation. In contrast, when the dose is dissolved in gastrointestinal fluids, the rate of absorption is usually proportional to the gastrointestinal concentration and is said to be first-order.

Extraction Ratio & the First-Pass Effect

Systemic clearance is not affected by bioavailability. However, clearance can markedly affect the extent of availability because it determines the extraction ratio (equation [8a]). Of course, therapeutic blood concentrations may still be reached by the oral route of administration if larger doses are given. However, in this case, the concentrations of the drug *metabolites* will be increased significantly over those that would occur following intravenous administration. Lidocaine and verapamil are both used to treat cardiac arrhythmias and have bioavailability less than 40%, but lidocaine is never given orally because its metabolites are believed to contribute to central nervous system toxicity. Other drugs that are highly extracted by the liver include isoniazid, morphine, propranolol, and several tricyclic antidepressants (Table 3–1).

Drugs with high extraction ratios will show marked variations in bioavailability between subjects because of differences in hepatic function and blood flow. These differences can explain the marked variation in drug concentrations that occurs among individuals given similar doses of highly extracted drugs. For drugs that are highly extracted by the liver, bypassing hepatic sites of elimination (eg, in hepatic cirrhosis with portosystemic shunting) will result in substantial increases in drug availability, whereas for drugs that are poorly extracted by the liver (for which the difference between entering and exiting drug concentration is small), shunting of blood past the liver will cause little change in availability. Drugs in Table 3–1 that are poorly extracted by the liver include chlorpropamide, diazepam, phenytoin, theophylline, tolbutamide, and warfarin.

Alternative Routes of Administration & the First-Pass Effect

There are several reasons for different routes of administration used in clinical medicine (Table 3–3)—for convenience (eg, oral), to maximize concentration at the site of action and minimize it elsewhere (eg, topical), to prolong the duration of drug absorption (eg, transdermal), or to avoid the first-pass effect.

The hepatic first-pass effect can be avoided to a great extent by use of sublingual tablets and transdermal preparations and to a lesser extent by use of rectal suppositories. Sublingual absorption provides direct access to systemic—not portal—veins. The transdermal route offers the same advantage. Drugs absorbed from suppositories in the lower rectum enter vessels that drain into the inferior vena cava, thus bypassing the liver. However, suppositories tend to move upward in the rectum into a region where veins that lead to the liver predominate. Thus, only about 50% of a rectal dose can be assumed to bypass the liver.

Although drugs administered by inhalation bypass the hepatic first-pass effect, the lung may also serve as a site of first-pass loss by excretion and possibly metabolism for drugs administered by nongastrointestinal ("parenteral") routes.

THE TIME COURSE OF DRUG EFFECT

The principles of pharmacokinetics (discussed in this chapter) and those of pharmacodynamics (discussed in Chapter 2 and Holford & Sheiner, 1981) provide a framework for understanding the time course of drug effect.

Immediate Effects

In the simplest case, drug effects are directly related to plasma concentrations, but this does not necessarily mean that effects simply parallel the time course of concentrations. Because the relationship between drug concentration and effect is not linear (recall the E_{max} model described in Chapter 2), the effect will not usually be linearly proportional to the concentration.

Consider the effect of an angiotensin-converting enzyme (ACE) inhibitor, such as enalapril, on plasma ACE. The half-life of enalapril is about 3 hours. After an oral dose of 10 mg, the peak plasma concentration at 3 hours is about 64 ng/mL. Enalapril is usually given once a day, so seven half-lives will elapse from the time of peak concentration to the end of the dosing interval. The concentration of enalapril after each half-life and the corresponding extent of ACE inhibition are shown in Figure 3–5. The extent of inhibition of ACE is calculated using the E_{max} model, where E_{max}, the maximum extent of inhibition, is 100% and the C_{50}, the

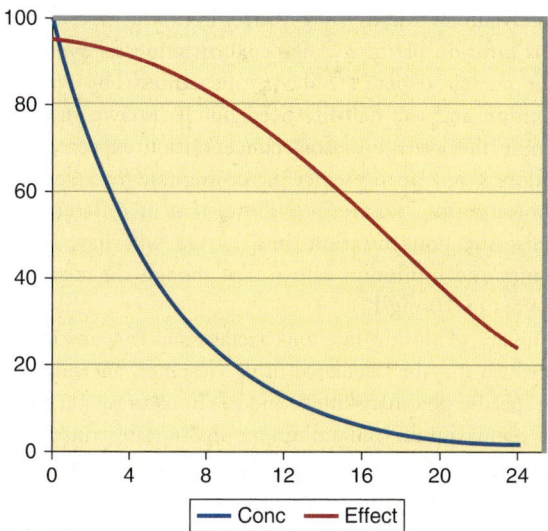

FIGURE 3–5 Time course of angiotensin-converting enzyme (ACE) inhibitor concentrations and effects. The blue line shows the plasma enalapril concentrations in nanograms per milliliter after a single oral dose. The red line indicates the percentage inhibition of its target, ACE. Note the different shapes of the concentration-time course (exponentially decreasing) and the effect-time course (linearly decreasing in its central portion).

concentration of the drug that produces 50% of maximum effect, is about 1 ng/mL.

Note that plasma concentrations of enalapril change by a factor of 16 over the first 12 hours (four half-lives) after the peak, but ACE inhibition has only decreased by 20%. Because the concentrations over this time are so high in relation to the C_{50}, the effect on ACE is almost constant. After 24 hours, ACE is still 33% inhibited. This explains why a drug with a short half-life can be given once a day and still maintain its effect throughout the day. The key factor is a high initial concentration in relation to the C_{50}. Even though the plasma concentration at 24 hours is less than 1% of its peak, this low concentration is still half the C_{50}. This is very common for drugs that act on enzymes (eg, ACE inhibitors) or compete at receptors (eg, propranolol).

When concentrations are in the range between four times and one fourth of the C_{50}, the time course of effect is essentially a linear function of time. It takes four half-lives for concentrations to drop from an effect of 80% to 20% of E_{max}—15% of the effect is lost every half-life over this concentration range. At concentrations below one fourth the C_{50}, the effect becomes almost directly proportional to concentration and the time course of drug effect will follow the exponential decline of concentration. It is only when the concentration is low in relation to the C_{50} that the concept of a "half-life of drug effect" has any meaning.

Delayed Effects

Changes in drug effects are often delayed in relation to changes in plasma concentration. This delay may reflect the time required for the drug to distribute from plasma to the site of action. This will be the case for almost all drugs. The delay due to distribution is a

pharmacokinetic phenomenon that can account for delays of a few minutes. This distributional delay can account for the lag of effects after rapid intravenous injection of central nervous system (CNS)–active agents such as thiopental.

A common reason for more delayed drug effects—especially those that take many hours or even days to occur—is the slow turnover of a physiologic substance that is involved in the expression of the drug effect. For example, warfarin works as an anticoagulant by inhibiting vitamin K epoxidase in the liver. This action of warfarin occurs rapidly, and inhibition of the enzyme is closely related to plasma concentrations of warfarin. The *clinical effect* of warfarin, eg, on the International Normalized Ratio (INR), reflects a decrease in the concentration of the prothrombin complex of clotting factors. Inhibition of vitamin K epoxidase decreases the synthesis of these clotting factors, but the complex has a long half-life (about 14 hours), and it is this half-life that determines how long it takes for the concentration of clotting factors to reach a new steady state and for a drug effect to reflect the average warfarin plasma concentration.

Cumulative Effects

Some drug effects are more obviously related to a cumulative action than to a rapidly reversible one. The renal toxicity of aminoglycoside antibiotics (eg, gentamicin) is greater when administered as a constant infusion than with intermittent dosing. It is the accumulation of aminoglycoside in the renal cortex that is thought to cause renal damage. Even though both dosing schemes produce the same average steady-state concentration, the intermittent dosing scheme produces much higher peak concentrations, which saturate an uptake mechanism into the cortex; thus, total aminoglycoside accumulation is less. The difference in toxicity is a predictable consequence of the different patterns of concentration and the saturable uptake mechanism.

The effect of many drugs used to treat cancer also reflects a cumulative action—eg, the extent of binding of a drug to DNA is proportional to drug concentration and is usually irreversible. The effect on tumor growth is therefore a consequence of cumulative exposure to the drug. Measures of cumulative exposure, such as AUC, provide a means to individualize treatment.

THE TARGET CONCENTRATION APPROACH TO DESIGNING A RATIONAL DOSAGE REGIMEN

A rational dosage regimen is based on the assumption that there is a **target concentration** that will produce the desired therapeutic effect. By considering the pharmacokinetic factors that determine the dose-concentration relationship, it is possible to individualize the dose regimen to achieve the target concentration. The effective concentration ranges shown in Table 3–1 are a guide to the concentrations measured when patients are being effectively treated. The initial target concentration should usually be chosen from the lower end of this range. In some cases, the target concentration will also depend on the specific therapeutic objective—eg, the control of atrial fibrillation by digoxin often requires a target concentration of 2 ng/mL, while heart failure is usually adequately managed with a target concentration of 1 ng/mL.

Maintenance Dose

In most clinical situations, drugs are administered in such a way as to maintain a steady state of drug in the body, ie, just enough drug is given in each dose to replace the drug eliminated since the preceding dose. Thus, calculation of the appropriate maintenance dose is a primary goal. Clearance is the most important pharmacokinetic term to be considered in defining a rational steady-state drug dosage regimen. At steady state, the dosing rate ("rate in") must equal the rate of elimination ("rate out"). Substitution of the target concentration (TC) for concentration (C) in equation (4) predicts the maintenance dosing rate:

$$Dosing\ rate_{ss} = Rate\ of\ elimination_{ss}$$
$$= CL \times TC \qquad (9)$$

Thus, if the desired target concentration is known, the clearance in that patient will determine the dosing rate. If the drug is given by a route that has a bioavailability less than 100%, then the dosing rate predicted by equation (9) must be modified. For oral dosing:

$$Dosing\ rate_{oral} = \frac{Dosing\ rate}{F_{oral}} \qquad (10)$$

If intermittent doses are given, the maintenance dose is calculated from:

$$Maintenance\ dose = Dosing\ rate \times Dosing\ interval \qquad (11)$$

(See Box: Example: Maintenance Dose Calculations.)

Note that the steady-state concentration achieved by continuous infusion or the average concentration following intermittent dosing depends only on clearance. The volume of distribution and the half-life need not be known in order to determine the average plasma concentration expected from a given dosing rate or to predict the dosing rate for a desired target concentration. Figure 3–6 shows that at different dosing intervals, the concentration-time curves will have different maximum and minimum values even though the average level will always be 10 mg/L.

Estimates of dosing rate and average steady-state concentrations, which may be calculated using clearance, are independent of any specific pharmacokinetic model. In contrast, the determination of maximum and minimum steady-state concentrations requires further assumptions about the pharmacokinetic model. The accumulation factor (equation [7]) assumes that the drug follows a one-compartment body model (Figure 3–2B), and the peak concentration prediction assumes that the absorption rate is much faster than the elimination rate. For the calculation of estimated maximum and minimum concentrations in a clinical situation, these assumptions are usually reasonable.

Loading Dose

When the time to reach steady state is appreciable, as it is for drugs with long half-lives, it may be desirable to administer a loading dose that promptly raises the concentration of drug in plasma to the target concentration. In theory, only the amount of the loading dose need be computed—not the rate of its administration—and, to a first approximation, this is so. The volume of distribution is the proportionality factor that relates the total amount of drug in the body to the concentration; if a loading dose is to achieve the target concentration, then from equation (1):

Example: Maintenance Dose Calculations

A target plasma theophylline concentration of 10 mg/L is desired to relieve acute bronchial asthma in a patient. If the patient is a nonsmoker and otherwise normal except for asthma, we may use the mean clearance given in Table 3–1, ie, 2.8 L/h/70 kg. Since the drug will be given as an intravenous infusion, F = 1.

$$Dosing\ rate = CL \times TC$$
$$= 2.8\ L\,/\,h\,/\,70\ kg \times 10\ mg\,/\,L$$
$$= 28\ mg\,/\,h\,/\,70\ kg$$

Therefore, in this patient, the proper infusion rate would be 28 mg/h/70 kg.

If the asthma attack is relieved, the clinician might want to maintain this plasma level using oral theophylline, which might be given every 12 hours using an extended-release formulation to approximate a continuous intravenous infusion. According to

Table 3–1, F_{oral} is 0.96. When the dosing interval is 12 hours, the size of each maintenance dose would be:

$$\underset{dose}{Maintenance} = \frac{Dosing\ rate}{F} \times Dosing\ interval$$
$$= \frac{28\ mg\,/\,h}{0.96} \times 12\ hours$$
$$= 350\ mg$$

A tablet or capsule size close to the ideal dose of 350 mg would then be prescribed at 12-hourly intervals. If an 8-hour dosing interval was used, the ideal dose would be 233 mg; and if the drug was given once a day, the dose would be 700 mg. In practice, F could be omitted from the calculation since it is so close to 1.

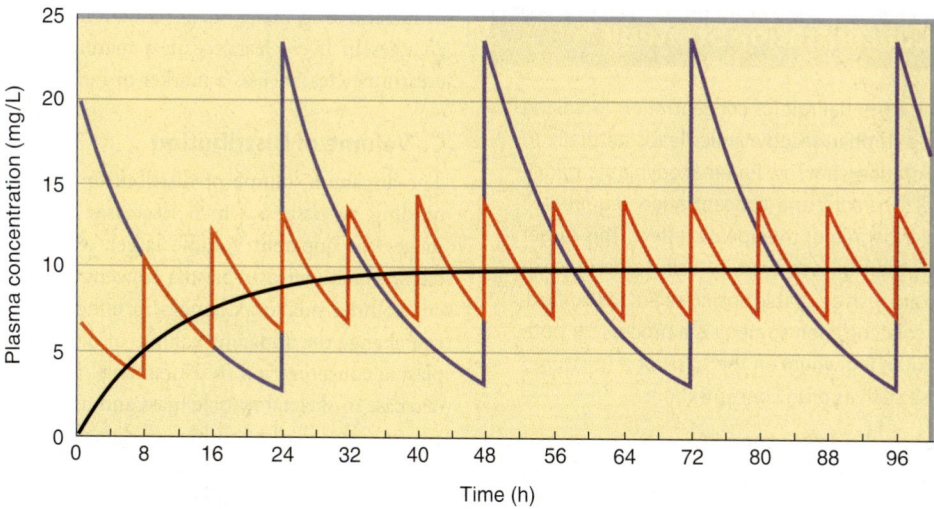

FIGURE 3–6 Relationship between frequency of dosing and maximum and minimum plasma concentrations when a steady-state theophylline plasma level of 10 mg/L is desired. The smoothly rising black line shows the plasma concentration achieved with an intravenous infusion of 28 mg/h. The doses for 8-hourly administration (orange line) are 224 mg; for 24-hourly administration (blue line), 672 mg. In each of the three cases, the mean steady-state plasma concentration is 10 mg/L.

$$\text{Loading dose} = \begin{array}{c}\text{Amount in the body} \\ \text{immediately following} \\ \text{the loading dose}\end{array}$$

$$= V \times TC \qquad (12)$$

For the theophylline example given in the Box, Example: Maintenance Dose Calculations, the loading dose would be 350 mg (35 L × 10 mg/L) for a 70-kg person. For most drugs, the loading dose can be given as a single dose by the chosen route of administration.

Up to this point, we have ignored the fact that some drugs follow more complex multicompartment pharmacokinetics, eg, the distribution process illustrated by the two-compartment model in Figure 3–2. This is justified in the great majority of cases. However, in some cases the distribution phase may not be ignored, particularly in connection with the calculation of loading doses. If the rate of absorption is rapid relative to distribution (this is always true for rapid intravenous administration), the concentration of drug in plasma that results from an appropriate loading dose—calculated using the apparent volume of distribution—can initially be considerably higher than desired. Severe toxicity may occur, albeit transiently. This may be particularly important, eg, in the administration of antiarrhythmic drugs such as lidocaine, where an almost immediate toxic response may occur. Thus, while the estimation of the *amount* of a loading dose may be quite correct, the *rate of administration* can sometimes be crucial in preventing excessive drug concentrations, and slow administration of an intravenous drug (over minutes rather than seconds) is almost always prudent practice.

When intermittent doses are given, the loading dose calculated from equation (12) will only reach the average steady-state concentration and will not match the peak steady-state concentration (Figure 3–6). To match the peak steady-state concentration, the loading dose can be calculated from equation (13):

$$\text{Loading dose} = \text{Maintenance dose} \times \text{Accumulation factor} \qquad (13)$$

TARGET CONCENTRATION INTERVENTION: APPLICATION OF PHARMACOKINETICS & PHARMACODYNAMICS TO DOSE INDIVIDUALIZATION

The basic principles outlined above can be applied to the interpretation of clinical drug concentration measurements on the basis of three major pharmacokinetic variables: absorption, clearance, and volume of distribution (and the derived variable, half-life). In addition, it may be necessary to consider two pharmacodynamic variables: maximum effect attainable in the target tissue and the sensitivity of the tissue to the drug. Diseases may modify all of these parameters, and the ability to predict the effect of disease states on pharmacokinetic parameters is important in properly adjusting dosage in such cases. (See Box: The Target Concentration Strategy.)

Pharmacokinetic Variables

A. Absorption

The amount of drug that enters the body depends on the patient's adherence to the prescribed regimen and on the rate and extent of transfer from the site of administration to the blood.

The Target Concentration Strategy

Recognition of the essential role of concentration in linking pharmacokinetics and pharmacodynamics leads naturally to the target concentration strategy. Pharmacodynamic principles can be used to predict the concentration required to achieve a particular degree of therapeutic effect. This target concentration can then be achieved by using pharmacokinetic principles to arrive at a suitable dosing regimen (Holford, 1999). The target concentration strategy is a process for optimizing the dose in an individual on the basis of a measured surrogate response such as drug concentration:

1. Choose the target concentration, TC.
2. Predict volume of distribution (V) and clearance (CL) based on standard population values (eg, Table 3–1) with adjustments for factors such as weight and renal function.
3. Give a loading dose or maintenance dose calculated from TC, V, and CL.
4. Measure the patient's response and drug concentration.
5. Revise V and/or CL based on the measured concentration.
6. Repeat steps 3–5, adjusting the predicted dose to achieve TC.

Overdosage and underdosage relative to the prescribed dosage—both aspects of failure of adherence—can frequently be detected by concentration measurements when gross deviations from expected values are obtained. If adherence is found to be adequate, absorption abnormalities in the small bowel may be the cause of abnormally low concentrations. Variations in the extent of bioavailability are rarely caused by irregularities in the manufacture of the particular drug formulation. More commonly, variations in bioavailability are due to metabolism during absorption.

B. Clearance

Abnormal clearance may be anticipated when there is major impairment of the function of the kidney, liver, or heart. Creatinine clearance is a useful quantitative indicator of renal function. Conversely, drug clearance may be a useful indicator of the functional consequences of heart, kidney, or liver failure, often with greater precision than clinical findings or other laboratory tests. For example, when renal function is changing rapidly, estimation of the clearance of aminoglycoside antibiotics may be a more accurate indicator of glomerular filtration than serum creatinine.

Hepatic disease has been shown to reduce the clearance and prolong the half-life of many drugs. However, for many other drugs known to be eliminated by hepatic processes, no changes in clearance or half-life have been noted with similar hepatic disease. This reflects the fact that hepatic disease does not always affect the hepatic intrinsic clearance. At present, there is no reliable marker of hepatic drug-metabolizing function that can be used to predict changes in liver clearance in a manner analogous to the use of creatinine clearance as a marker of renal drug clearance.

C. Volume of Distribution

The apparent volume of distribution reflects a balance between binding to tissues, which decreases plasma concentration and makes the apparent volume larger, and binding to plasma proteins, which increases plasma concentration and makes the apparent volume smaller. Changes in either tissue or plasma binding can change the apparent volume of distribution determined from plasma concentration measurements. Older people have a relative decrease in skeletal muscle mass and tend to have a smaller apparent volume of distribution of digoxin (which binds to muscle proteins). The volume of distribution may be overestimated in obese patients if based on body weight and the drug does not enter fatty tissues well, as is the case with digoxin. In contrast, theophylline has a volume of distribution similar to that of total body water. Adipose tissue has almost as much water in it as other tissues, so that the apparent total volume of distribution of theophylline is proportional to body weight even in obese patients.

Abnormal accumulation of fluid—edema, ascites, pleural effusion—can markedly increase the volume of distribution of drugs such as gentamicin that are hydrophilic and have small volumes of distribution.

D. Half-Life

The differences between clearance and half-life are important in defining the underlying mechanisms for the effect of a disease state on drug disposition. For example, the half-life of diazepam increases with patient age. When clearance is related to age, it is found that clearance of this drug does not change with age. The increasing half-life for diazepam actually results from changes in the volume of distribution with age; the metabolic processes responsible for eliminating the drug are fairly constant.

Pharmacodynamic Variables

A. Maximum Effect

All pharmacologic responses must have a maximum effect (E_{max}). No matter how high the drug concentration goes, a point will be reached beyond which no further increment in response is achieved.

If increasing the dose in a particular patient does not lead to a further clinical response, it is possible that the maximum effect has been reached. Recognition of maximum effect is helpful in avoiding ineffectual increases of dose with the attendant risk of toxicity.

B. Sensitivity

The sensitivity of the target organ to drug concentration is reflected by the concentration required to produce 50% of maximum effect, the C_{50}. Diminished sensitivity to the drug can be detected by measuring drug concentrations that are usually associated with therapeutic response in a patient who has not responded. This may be a result of abnormal physiology—eg, hyperkalemia diminishes responsiveness to digoxin—or drug antagonism—eg, calcium channel blockers impair the inotropic response to digoxin.

Increased sensitivity to a drug is usually signaled by exaggerated responses to small or moderate doses. The pharmacodynamic nature of this sensitivity can be confirmed by measuring drug concentrations that are low in relation to the observed effect.

INTERPRETATION OF DRUG CONCENTRATION MEASUREMENTS

Clearance

Clearance is the single most important factor determining drug concentrations. The interpretation of measurements of drug concentrations depends on a clear understanding of three factors that may influence clearance: the dose, the organ blood flow, and the intrinsic function of the liver or kidneys. Each of these factors should be considered when interpreting clearance estimated from a drug concentration measurement. It must also be recognized that changes in protein binding may lead the unwary to believe there is a change in clearance when in fact drug elimination is not altered (see Box: Plasma Protein Binding: Is It Important?). Factors affecting protein binding include the following:

1. **Albumin concentration:** Drugs such as phenytoin, salicylates, and disopyramide are extensively bound to plasma albumin. Albumin levels are low in many disease states, resulting in lower total drug concentrations.

2. **Alpha$_1$-acid glycoprotein concentration:** α_1-Acid glycoprotein is an important binding protein with binding sites for drugs such as quinidine, lidocaine, and propranolol. It is increased in acute inflammatory disorders and causes major changes in total plasma concentration of these drugs even though drug elimination is unchanged.

3. **Capacity-limited protein binding:** The binding of drugs to plasma proteins is capacity-limited. Therapeutic concentrations of salicylates and prednisolone show concentration-dependent protein binding. Because unbound drug concentration is determined by dosing rate and clearance—which is not altered, in the case of these low-extraction-ratio drugs, by protein binding—increases in dosing rate will cause corresponding changes in the pharmacodynamically important unbound concentration. In contrast, total drug concentration will increase less rapidly than the dosing rate would suggest as protein binding approaches saturation at higher concentrations.

Dosing History

An accurate dosing history is essential if one is to obtain maximum value from a drug concentration measurement. In fact, if the dosing history is unknown or incomplete, a drug concentration measurement loses all predictive value.

Timing of Samples for Concentration Measurement

Information about the rate and extent of drug absorption in a particular patient is rarely of great clinical importance. However, absorption usually occurs during the first 2 hours after a drug dose and varies according to food intake, posture, and activity. Therefore, it is important to avoid drawing blood until absorption is complete (about 2 hours after an oral dose). Attempts to measure peak concentrations early after oral dosing are usually unsuccessful and compromise the validity of the measurement, because one cannot be certain that absorption is complete.

Some drugs such as digoxin and lithium take several hours to distribute to tissues. Digoxin samples should be taken at least 6 hours after the last dose and lithium just before the next dose (usually 24 hours after the last dose). Aminoglycosides distribute

---

Plasma Protein Binding: Is It Important?

Plasma protein binding is often mentioned as a factor playing a role in pharmacokinetics, pharmacodynamics, and drug interactions. However, there are no clinically relevant examples of changes in drug disposition or effects that can be clearly ascribed to changes in plasma protein binding (Benet & Hoener, 2002). The idea that if a drug is displaced from plasma proteins it would increase the unbound drug concentration and increase the drug effect and, perhaps, produce toxicity seems a simple and obvious mechanism. Unfortunately, this simple theory, which is appropriate for a test tube, does not work in the body, which is an open system capable of eliminating unbound drug.

First, a seemingly dramatic change in the unbound fraction from 1% to 10% releases less than 5% of the total amount of drug in the body into the unbound pool because less than one third of the drug in the body is bound to plasma proteins even in the most extreme cases, eg, warfarin. Drug displaced from plasma protein will of course distribute throughout the volume of distribution, so that a 5% increase in the amount of unbound drug in the body produces at most a 5% increase in pharmacologically active unbound drug at the site of action.

Second, when the amount of unbound drug in plasma increases, the rate of elimination will increase (if unbound clearance is unchanged), and after four half-lives the unbound concentration will return to its previous steady-state value. When drug interactions associated with protein binding displacement and clinically important effects have been studied, it has been found that the displacing drug is also an inhibitor of clearance, and it is the change in *clearance* of the *unbound* drug that is the relevant mechanism explaining the interaction.

The clinical importance of plasma protein binding is only to help interpretation of measured drug concentrations. When plasma proteins are lower than normal, then total drug concentrations will be lower but unbound concentrations will not be affected.

quite rapidly, but it is still prudent to wait 1 hour after giving the dose before taking a sample.

Clearance is readily estimated from the dosing rate and mean steady-state concentration. Blood samples should be appropriately timed to estimate steady-state concentration. Provided steady state has been approached (at least three half-lives of constant dosing), a sample obtained near the midpoint of the dosing interval will usually be close to the mean steady-state concentration.

Initial Predictions of Volume of Distribution & Clearance

A. Volume of Distribution

Volume of distribution is commonly calculated for a particular patient using body weight (70-kg body weight is assumed for the values in Table 3–1). If a patient is obese, drugs that do not readily penetrate fat (eg, gentamicin and digoxin) should have their volumes calculated from fat-free mass (FFM) as shown below. Total body weight (WT) is in kilograms and height (HTM) is in meters:

$$\text{For women: FFM (kg)} = \frac{37.99 \times HTM^2 \times WT}{35.98 \times HTM^2 + WT} \quad (14a)$$

$$\text{For men: FFM (kg)} = \frac{42.92 \times HTM^2 \times WT}{30.93 \times HTM^2 + WT} \quad (14b)$$

Patients with edema, ascites, or pleural effusions offer a larger volume of distribution to the aminoglycoside antibiotics (eg, gentamicin) than is predicted by body weight. In such patients, the weight should be corrected as follows: Subtract an estimate of the weight of the excess fluid accumulation from the measured weight. Use the resultant "normal" body weight to calculate the normal volume of distribution. Finally, this normal volume should be increased by 1 L for each estimated kilogram of excess fluid. This correction is important because of the relatively small volumes of distribution of these water-soluble drugs.

B. Clearance

Drugs cleared by the renal route often require adjustment of clearance in proportion to renal function. This can be conveniently estimated from the creatinine clearance, calculated from a single serum creatinine measurement and the predicted creatinine production rate.

The predicted creatinine production rate in women is 85% of the calculated value, because they have a smaller muscle mass per kilogram and it is muscle mass that determines creatinine production. Muscle mass as a fraction of body weight decreases with age, which is why age appears in the Cockcroft-Gault equation.[*]

The decrease of renal function with age is independent of the decrease in creatinine production. Because of the difficulty of obtaining complete urine collections, creatinine clearance calculated in this way is at least as reliable as estimates based on urine collections. The fat-free mass (equation [14]) should be considered rather than total body weight for obese patients, and correction should be made for muscle wasting in severely ill patients.

Revising Individual Estimates of Volume of Distribution & Clearance

The commonsense approach to the interpretation of drug concentrations compares predictions of pharmacokinetic parameters and expected concentrations to measured values. If measured concentrations differ by more than 20% from predicted values, revised estimates of V or CL for that patient should be calculated using equation (1) or equation (2). If the change calculated is more than a 100% increase or 50% decrease in either V or CL, the assumptions made about the timing of the sample and the dosing history should be critically examined.

For example, if a patient is taking 0.25 mg of digoxin a day, a clinician may expect the digoxin concentration to be about 1 ng/mL. This is based on typical values for bioavailability of 70% and total clearance of about 7 L/h (CL_{renal} 4 L/h, $CL_{nonrenal}$ 3 L/h). If the patient has heart failure, the nonrenal (hepatic) clearance might be halved because of hepatic congestion and hypoxia, so the expected clearance would become 5.5 L/h. The concentration is then expected to be about 1.3 ng/mL. Suppose that the concentration actually measured is 2 ng/mL. Common sense would suggest halving the daily dose to achieve a target concentration of 1 ng/mL. This approach implies a revised clearance of 3.5 L/h. The smaller clearance compared with the expected value of 5.5 L/h may reflect additional renal functional impairment due to heart failure.

This technique will often be misleading if steady state has not been reached. At least a week of regular dosing (three to four half-lives) must elapse before the implicit method will be reliable.

REFERENCES

Benet LZ, Hoener B: Changes in plasma protein binding have little clinical relevance. Clin Pharmacol Ther 2002;71:115.

Holford NHG: Pharmacokinetic and pharmacodynamic principles. 2011; http://www.fmhs.auckland.ac.nz/sms/pharmacology/holford/teaching/medsci722

Holford NHG: Target concentration intervention: Beyond Y2K. Br J Clin Pharmacol 1999;48:9.

Holford NHG, Sheiner LB: Understanding the dose-effect relationship. Clin Pharmacokinet 1981;6:429.

Speight T, Holford NHG: *Avery's Drug Treatment*, 4th ed. Adis International, 1997.

---

[*] The Cockcroft-Gault equation is given in Chapter 60.

CASE STUDY ANSWER

Sixty seven percent of total standard digoxin clearance is renal, so the standard renal clearance is 0.67×9 L/h = 6 L/h/70 kg with creatinine clearance of 100 mL/min and nonrenal clearance is $(1 - 0.67) \times 9$ L/h = 3 L/h/70 kg (see Table 3–1 for standard pharmacokinetic parameters). Her predicted creatinine clearance is 22 mL/min (Cockcroft & Gault), so for digoxin, her renal clearance is $6 \times 22/100 \times$ 60/70 = 1.1 L/h, nonrenal clearance $2.7 \times 60/70 = 2.6$ L/h, and total clearance 3.7 L/h. The parenteral maintenance dose rate is 2 mcg/L $\times$ 3.7 L/h = 7.4 mcg/h. Once-a-day oral dosing with bioavailability of 0.7 would require a daily maintenance dose of $7.4/0.7 \times 24 = 254$ mcg/day. A practical dose would be one 250 mcg tablet per day.

Drug Biotransformation

Maria Almira Correia, PhD

Humans are exposed daily to a wide variety of foreign compounds called **xenobiotics**—substances absorbed across the lungs or skin or, more commonly, ingested either unintentionally as compounds present in food and drink or deliberately as drugs for therapeutic or "recreational" purposes. Exposure to environmental xenobiotics may be inadvertent and accidental or—when they are present as components of air, water, and food—inescapable. Some xenobiotics are innocuous, but many can provoke biologic responses. Such biologic responses often depend on conversion of the absorbed substance into an active metabolite. The discussion that follows is applicable to xenobiotics in general (including drugs) and to some extent to endogenous compounds.

WHY IS DRUG BIOTRANSFORMATION NECESSARY?

Renal excretion plays a pivotal role in terminating the biologic activity of some drugs, particularly those that have small molecular volumes or possess polar characteristics, such as functional groups that are fully ionized at physiologic pH. However, many drugs do not possess such physicochemical properties. Pharmacologically active organic molecules tend to be lipophilic and remain unionized or only partially ionized at physiologic pH; these are readily reabsorbed from the glomerular filtrate in the nephron. Certain lipophilic compounds are often strongly bound to plasma proteins and may not be readily filtered at the glomerulus. Consequently, most drugs would have a prolonged duration of action if termination of their action depended solely on renal excretion.

An alternative process that can lead to the termination or alteration of biologic activity is metabolism. In general, lipophilic xenobiotics are transformed to more polar and hence more readily excreted products. The role that metabolism plays in the inactivation of lipid-soluble drugs can be quite dramatic. For example, lipophilic barbiturates such as thiopental and pentobarbital would have extremely long half-lives if it were not for their metabolic conversion to more water-soluble compounds.

Metabolic products are often less pharmacodynamically active than the parent drug and may even be inactive. However, some biotransformation products have *enhanced* activity or toxic properties. It is noteworthy that the synthesis of endogenous substrates such as steroid hormones, cholesterol, active vitamin D congeners, and bile acids involves many pathways catalyzed by enzymes associated with the metabolism of xenobiotics. Finally, drug-metabolizing enzymes have been exploited in the design of pharmacologically inactive prodrugs that are converted to active molecules in the body.

THE ROLE OF BIOTRANSFORMATION IN DRUG DISPOSITION

Most metabolic biotransformations occur at some point between absorption of the drug into the general circulation and its renal elimination. A few transformations occur in the intestinal lumen or intestinal wall. In general, all of these reactions can be assigned to one of two major categories called **phase I** and **phase II reactions** (Figure 4–1).

Phase I reactions usually convert the parent drug to a more polar metabolite by introducing or unmasking a functional group (–OH, –NH₂, –SH). Often these metabolites are inactive, although in some instances activity is only modified or even enhanced.

If phase I metabolites are sufficiently polar, they may be readily excreted. However, many phase I products are not eliminated rapidly and undergo a subsequent reaction in which an endogenous substrate such as glucuronic acid, sulfuric acid, acetic acid, or an amino acid combines with the newly incorporated functional group to form a highly polar conjugate. Such conjugation or synthetic reactions are the hallmarks of phase II metabolism. A great variety of drugs undergo these sequential biotransformation reactions, although in some instances the parent drug may already possess a functional group that may form a conjugate directly. For example, the hydrazide moiety of isoniazid is known to form an *N*-acetyl conjugate in a phase II reaction. This conjugate is then a

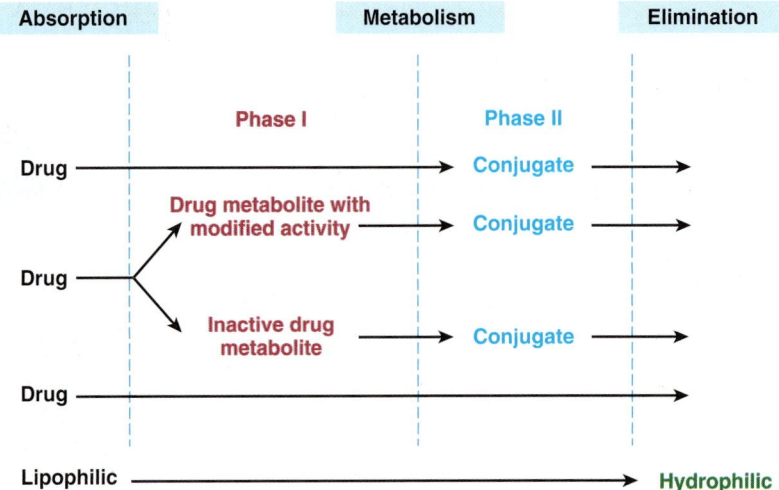

FIGURE 4–1 Phase I and phase II reactions, and direct elimination, in drug biodisposition. Phase II reactions may also precede phase I reactions.

substrate for a phase I type reaction, namely, hydrolysis to isonicotinic acid (Figure 4–2). Thus, phase II reactions may actually precede phase I reactions.

WHERE DO DRUG BIOTRANSFORMATIONS OCCUR?

Although every tissue has some ability to metabolize drugs, the liver is the principal organ of drug metabolism. Other tissues that display considerable activity include the gastrointestinal tract, the lungs, the skin, the kidneys, and the brain. After oral administration, many drugs (eg, isoproterenol, meperidine, pentazocine,

morphine) are absorbed intact from the small intestine and transported first via the portal system to the liver, where they undergo extensive metabolism. This process is called the **first-pass effect** (see Chapter 3). Some orally administered drugs (eg, clonazepam, chlorpromazine, cyclosporine) are more extensively metabolized in the intestine than in the liver, while others (eg, midazolam) undergo significant ($\approx 50\%$) intestinal metabolism. Thus, intestinal metabolism can contribute to the overall first-pass effect, and individuals with compromised liver function may rely increasingly on such intestinal metabolism for drug elimination. Compromise of intestinal metabolism of certain drugs (eg, felodipine, cyclosporine A) can also result in significant elevation of their plasma levels and clinically relevant drug-drug interactions (DDIs, see below). First-pass effects may so greatly limit the bioavailability of orally administered drugs (eg, lidocaine) that alternative routes of administration must be used to achieve therapeutically effective blood levels. Furthermore, the lower gut harbors intestinal microorganisms that are capable of many biotransformation reactions. In addition, drugs may be metabolized by gastric acid (eg, penicillin), by digestive enzymes (eg, polypeptides such as insulin), or by enzymes in the wall of the intestine (eg, sympathomimetic catecholamines).

Although drug biotransformation in vivo can occur by spontaneous, noncatalyzed chemical reactions, most transformations are catalyzed by specific cellular enzymes. At the subcellular level, these enzymes may be located in the endoplasmic reticulum (ER), mitochondria, cytosol, lysosomes, or even the nuclear envelope or plasma membrane.

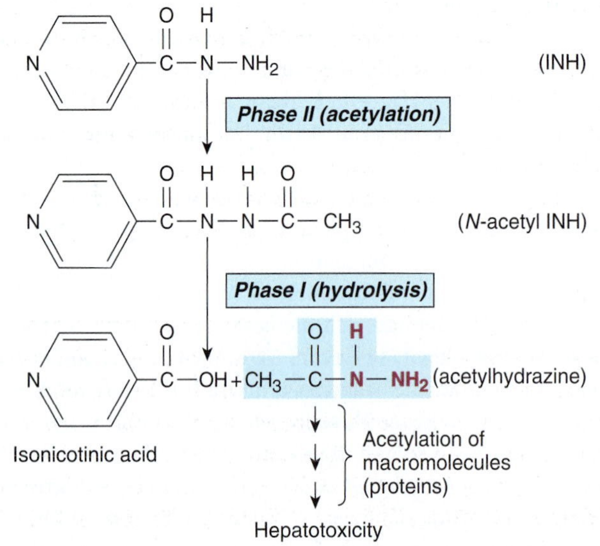

FIGURE 4–2 Phase II activation of isoniazid (INH) to a hepatotoxic metabolite.

MICROSOMAL MIXED FUNCTION OXIDASE SYSTEM & PHASE I REACTIONS

Many drug-metabolizing enzymes are located in the lipophilic endoplasmic reticulum membranes of the liver and other tissues.

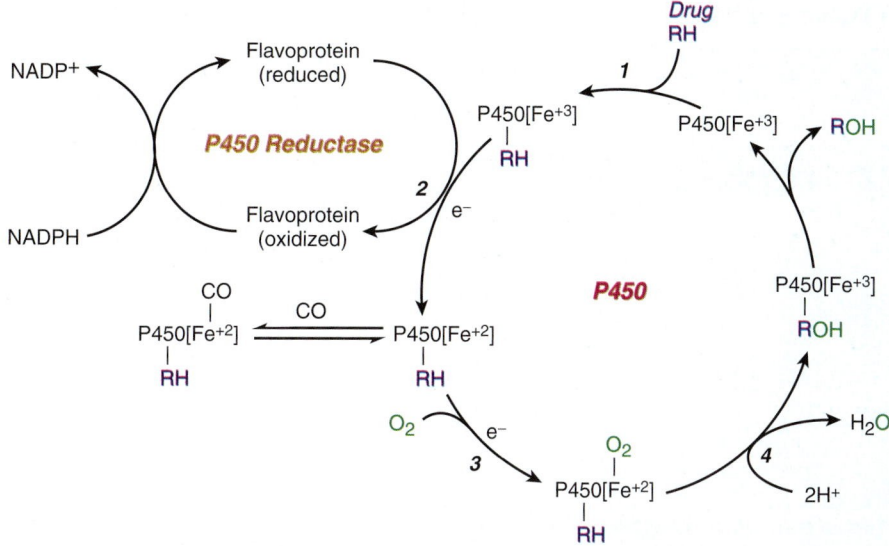

FIGURE 4–3 Cytochrome P450 cycle in drug oxidations. RH, parent drug; ROH, oxidized metabolite; e⁻, electron.

When these lamellar membranes are isolated by homogenization and fractionation of the cell, they re-form into vesicles called **microsomes.** Microsomes retain most of the morphologic and functional characteristics of the intact membranes, including the rough and smooth surface features of the rough (ribosome-studded) and smooth (no ribosomes) endoplasmic reticulum. Whereas the rough microsomes tend to be dedicated to protein synthesis, the smooth microsomes are relatively rich in enzymes responsible for oxidative drug metabolism. In particular, they contain the important class of enzymes known as the **mixed function oxidases** (MFOs), or **monooxygenases.** The activity of these enzymes requires both a reducing agent (nicotinamide adenine dinucleotide phosphate [NADPH]) and molecular oxygen; in a typical reaction, one molecule of oxygen is consumed (reduced) per substrate molecule, with one oxygen atom appearing in the product and the other in the form of water.

In this oxidation-reduction process, two microsomal enzymes play a key role. The first of these is a flavoprotein, **NADPH-cytochrome P450 oxidoreductase** (POR). One mole of this enzyme contains 1 mol each of flavin mononucleotide (FMN) and flavin adenine dinucleotide (FAD). The second microsomal enzyme is a hemoprotein called **cytochrome P450,** which serves as the terminal oxidase. In fact, the microsomal membrane harbors multiple forms of this hemoprotein, and this multiplicity is increased by repeated administration of or exposure to exogenous chemicals (see text that follows). The name cytochrome P450 (abbreviated as **P450** or **CYP**) is derived from the spectral properties of this hemoprotein. In its reduced (ferrous) form, it binds carbon monoxide to give a complex that absorbs light maximally at 450 nm. The relative abundance of P450s, compared with that of the reductase in the liver, contributes to making P450 heme reduction a rate-limiting step in hepatic drug oxidations.

Microsomal drug oxidations require P450, P450 reductase, NADPH, and molecular oxygen. A simplified scheme of the oxidative cycle is presented in Figure 4–3. Briefly, oxidized (Fe^{3+}) P450 combines with a drug substrate to form a binary complex (step 1). NADPH donates an electron to the flavoprotein P450 reductase, which in turn reduces the oxidized P450-drug complex (step 2). A second electron is introduced from NADPH via the same P450 reductase, which serves to reduce molecular oxygen and to form an "activated oxygen"-P450-substrate complex (step 3). This complex in turn transfers activated oxygen to the drug substrate to form the oxidized product (step 4).

The potent oxidizing properties of this activated oxygen permit oxidation of a large number of substrates. Substrate specificity is very low for this enzyme complex. High lipid solubility is the only common structural feature of the wide variety of structurally unrelated drugs and chemicals that serve as substrates in this system (Table 4–1). However, compared with many other enzymes including phase II enzymes, P450s are remarkably sluggish catalysts, and their drug biotransformation reactions are slow.

HUMAN LIVER P450 ENZYMES

Gene arrays combined with immunoblotting analyses of microsomal preparations, as well as the use of relatively selective functional markers and selective P450 inhibitors, have identified numerous P450 isoforms (CYP: 1A2, 2A6, 2B6, 2C8, 2C9, 2C18, 2C19, 2D6, 2E1, 3A4, 3A5, 4A11, and 7) in the human liver. Of these, **CYP1A2, CYP2A6, CYP2B6, CYP2C9, CYP2D6, CYP2E1,** and **CYP3A4** appear to be the most important forms, accounting for approximately 15%, 4%, 1%, 20%, 5%, 10%, and 30%, respectively, of the total human liver P450 content. Together, they

TABLE 4–1 Phase I reactions.

Reaction Class	Structural Change	Drug Substrates
Oxidations		
Cytochrome P450-dependent oxidations:		
Aromatic hydroxylations		Acetanilide, propranolol, phenobarbital, phenytoin, phenylbutazone, amphetamine, warfarin, 17α-ethinyl estradiol, naphthalene, benzpyrene
Aliphatic hydroxylations	$RCH_2CH_3 \longrightarrow RCH_2CH_2OH$ $RCH_2CH_3 \longrightarrow RCHCH_3$ $\qquad\qquad\qquad\quad OH$	Amobarbital, pentobarbital, secobarbital, chlorpropamide, ibuprofen, meprobamate, glutethimide, phenylbutazone, digitoxin
Epoxidation	$RCH{=}CHR \longrightarrow R{-}\underset{H}{C}{-}\overset{O}{\underset{H}{C}}{-}R$	Aldrin
Oxidative dealkylation		
N-Dealkylation	$RNHCH_3 \longrightarrow RNH_2 + CH_2O$	Morphine, ethylmorphine, benzphetamine, aminopyrine, caffeine, theophylline
O-Dealkylation	$ROCH_3 \longrightarrow ROH + CH_2O$	Codeine, *p*-nitroanisole
S-Dealkylation	$RSCH_3 \longrightarrow RSH + CH_2O$	6-Methylthiopurine, methitural
***N*-Oxidation**		
Primary amines	$RNH_2 \longrightarrow RNHOH$	Aniline, chlorphentermine
Secondary amines	$\underset{R_2}{\overset{R_1}{NH}} \longrightarrow \underset{R_2}{\overset{R_1}{N}}{-}OH$	2-Acetylaminofluorene, acetaminophen
Tertiary amines	$\underset{R_3}{\overset{R_1}{R_2{-}N}} \longrightarrow \underset{R_3}{\overset{R_1}{R_2{-}N}}{\to}O$	Nicotine, methaqualone
***S*-Oxidation**	$\underset{R_2}{\overset{R_1}{S}} \longrightarrow \underset{R_2}{\overset{R_1}{S}}{=}O$	Thioridazine, cimetidine, chlorpromazine
Deamination	$\underset{NH_2}{RCHCH_3} \longrightarrow R{-}\underset{NH_2}{\overset{OH}{C}}{-}CH_3 \longrightarrow R{-}\underset{O}{CCH_3} + NH_3$	Amphetamine, diazepam
Desulfuration	$\underset{R_2}{\overset{R_1}{C}}{=}S \longrightarrow \underset{R_2}{\overset{R_1}{C}}{=}O$	Thiopental

(*continued*)

TABLE 4–1 Phase I reactions. (Continued)

Reaction Class	Structural Change	Drug Substrates
Cytochrome P450- dependent oxidations: (continued)		
	R_1 R_1 P=S $\longrightarrow$ P=O R_2 R_2	Parathion
Dechlorination	$CCl_4 \longrightarrow [CCl_3^\cdot] \longrightarrow CHCl_3$	Carbon tetrachloride
Cytochrome P450-independent oxidations:		
Flavin monooxygenase (Ziegler's enzyme)	$R_3N \longrightarrow R_3N^+ \to O^- \overset{H^+}{\longrightarrow} R_3N^+OH$	Chlorpromazine, amitriptyline, benzphetamine
	$RCH_2N-CH_2R \longrightarrow RCH_2-N-CH_2R \longrightarrow$ $\quad\quad$ | $\quad\quad\quad\quad\quad\quad\quad\quad$ | $\quad\quad$ H $\quad\quad\quad\quad\quad\quad\quad\quad$ OH $RCH=N-CH_2R$ $\quad\quad\quad$ | $\quad\quad\quad$ O^-	Desipramine, nortriptyline
	$-N$ $\quad\quad$ $-N$ $\quad\quad$ $-N$ $\quad\quad$ \ $\quad\quad\quad\quad$ \ $\quad\quad\quad\quad$ \ $\quad\quad$ C—SH $\longrightarrow$ C—SOH $\longrightarrow$ C—SO$_2$H $\quad\quad$ / $\quad\quad\quad\quad$ / $\quad\quad\quad\quad$ / $-N$ $\quad\quad$ $-N$ $\quad\quad$ $-N$	Methimazole, propylthiouracil
Amine oxidases	$RCH_2NH_2 \longrightarrow RCHO + NH_3$	Phenylethylamine, epinephrine
Dehydrogenations	$RCH_2OH \longrightarrow RCHO$	Ethanol
Reductions		
Azo reductions	$RN=NR_1 \longrightarrow RNH-NHR_1 \longrightarrow RNH_2 + R_1NH_2$	Prontosil, tartrazine
Nitro reductions	$RNO_2 \longrightarrow RNO \longrightarrow RNHOH \longrightarrow RNH_2$	Nitrobenzene, chloramphenicol, clonazepam, dantrolene
Carbonyl reductions	$RCR' \longrightarrow RCHR'$ $\;$ || $\quad\quad\quad$ | $\;$ O $\quad\quad\quad$ OH	Metyrapone, methadone, naloxone
Hydrolyses		
Esters	$R_1COOR_2 \longrightarrow R_1COOH + R_2OH$	Procaine, succinylcholine, aspirin, clofibrate, methylphenidate
Amides	$RCONHR_1 \longrightarrow RCOOH + R_1NH_2$	Procainamide, lidocaine, indomethacin

are responsible for catalyzing the bulk of the hepatic drug and xenobiotic metabolism (Table 4–2, Figure 4–4).

It is noteworthy that CYP3A4 alone is responsible for the metabolism of over 50% of the prescription drugs metabolized by the liver. The involvement of individual P450s in the metabolism of a given drug may be screened in vitro by means of selective functional markers, selective chemical P450 inhibitors, and P450 antibodies. In vivo, such screening may be accomplished by means of relatively selective noninvasive markers, which include breath tests or urinary analyses of specific metabolites after administration of a P450-selective substrate probe.

Enzyme Induction

Some of the chemically dissimilar P450 substrate drugs, on repeated administration, *induce* P450 expression by enhancing the

TABLE 4–2 Human liver P450s (CYPs), and some of the drugs metabolized (substrates), inducers, and selective inhibitors.

CYP	Substrates	Inducers	Inhibitors
1A2	Acetaminophen, antipyrine, caffeine, clomipramine, phenacetin, tacrine, tamoxifen, theophylline, warfarin	Smoking, charcoal-broiled foods, cruciferous vegetables, omeprazole	Galangin, furafylline, fluvoxamine
2A6	Coumarin, tobacco nitrosamines, nicotine (to cotinine and 2′-hydroxynicotine)	Rifampin, phenobarbital	Tranylcypromine, menthofuran, methoxsalen
2B6	Artemisinin, bupropion, cyclophosphamide, efavirenz, ifosfamide, ketamine, S-mephobarbital, S-mephenytoin (N-demethylation to nirvanol), methadone, nevirapine, propofol, selegiline, sertraline, ticlopidine	Phenobarbital, cyclophosphamide	Ticlopidine, clopidogrel
2C8	Taxol, all-trans-retinoic acid	Rifampin, barbiturates	Trimethoprim
2C9	Celecoxib, flurbiprofen, hexobarbital, ibuprofen, losartan, phenytoin, tolbutamide, trimethadione, sulfaphenazole, S-warfarin, ticrynafen	Barbiturates, rifampin	Tienilic acid, sulfaphenazole
2C18	Tolbutamide, phenytoin	Phenobarbital	
2C19	Diazepam, S-mephenytoin, naproxen, nirvanol, omeprazole, propranolol	Barbiturates, rifampin	N3-benzylnirvanol, N3-benzylphenobarbital, fluconazole
2D6	Bufuralol, bupranolol, clomipramine, clozapine, codeine, debrisoquin, dextromethorphan, encainide, flecainide, fluoxetine, guanoxan, haloperidol, hydrocodone, 4-methoxy-amphetamine, metoprolol, mexiletine, oxycodone, paroxetine, phenformin, propafenone, propoxyphene, risperidone, selegiline (deprenyl), sparteine, tamoxifen, thioridazine, timolol, tricyclic antidepressants	Unknown	Quinidine, paroxetine
2E1	Acetaminophen, chlorzoxazone, enflurane, halothane, ethanol (a minor pathway)	Ethanol, isoniazid	4-Methylpyrazole, disulfiram
3A4[1]	Acetaminophen, alfentanil, amiodarone, astemizole, cisapride, cocaine, cortisol, cyclosporine, dapsone, diazepam, dihydroergot-amine, dihydropyridines, diltiazem, erythromycin, ethinyl estradiol, gestodene, indinavir, lidocaine, lovastatin, macrolides, methadone, miconazole, midazolam, mifepristone, nifedipine, paclitaxel, proges-terone, quinidine, rapamycin, ritonavir, saquinavir, spironolactone, sulfamethoxazole, sufentanil, tacrolimus, tamoxifen, terfenadine, testosterone, tetrahydrocannabinol, triazolam, troleandomycin, verapamil	Barbiturates, carbamazepine, glucocorticoids, pioglitazone, phenytoin, rifampin, St. John's wort	Azamulin, clarithromycin, diltiazem, erythromycin, fluconazole, grapefruit juice (furanocoumarins), itraconazole, ketoconazole, ritonavir, troleandomycin

[1]CYP3A5 has similar substrate and inhibitor profiles, but except for a few drugs is generally less active than CYP3A4.

rate of its synthesis or reducing its rate of degradation (Table 4–2). Induction results in accelerated substrate metabolism and usually in a decrease in the pharmacologic action of the inducer and also of co-administered drugs. However, in the case of drugs meta-bolically transformed to reactive metabolites, enzyme induction may exacerbate metabolite-mediated toxicity.

Various substrates induce P450 isoforms having different molecular masses and exhibiting different substrate specificities and immunochemical and spectral characteristics.

Environmental chemicals and pollutants are also capable of inducing P450 enzymes. As previously noted, exposure to benzo[a]pyrene and other polycyclic aromatic hydrocarbons, which are present in tobacco smoke, charcoal-broiled meat, and other organic pyrolysis products, is known to induce CYP1A enzymes and to alter the rates of drug metabolism. Other environ-mental chemicals known to induce specific P450s include the polychlorinated biphenyls (PCBs), which were once used widely in

industry as insulating materials and plasticizers, and 2,3,7,8-tetrachlorodibenzo-p-dioxin (dioxin, TCDD), a trace byproduct of the chemical synthesis of the defoliant 2,4,5-T (see Chapter 56).

Increased P450 synthesis requires enhanced transcription and translation along with increased synthesis of heme, its prosthetic cofactor. A cytoplasmic receptor (termed AhR) for polycyclic aro-matic hydrocarbons (eg, benzo[a]pyrene, dioxin) has been identi-fied. The translocation of the inducer-receptor complex into the nucleus, followed by ligand-induced dimerization with Arnt, a closely related nuclear protein, leads to subsequent activation of regulatory elements of CYP1A genes, resulting in their induction. This is also the mechanism of CYP1A induction by cruciferous vegetables, and the proton pump inhibitor, omeprazole. A preg-nane X receptor (PXR), a member of the steroid-retinoid-thyroid hormone receptor family, has recently been shown to mediate CYP3A induction by various chemicals (dexamethasone, rifampin, mifepristone, phenobarbital, atorvastatin, and hyperforin,

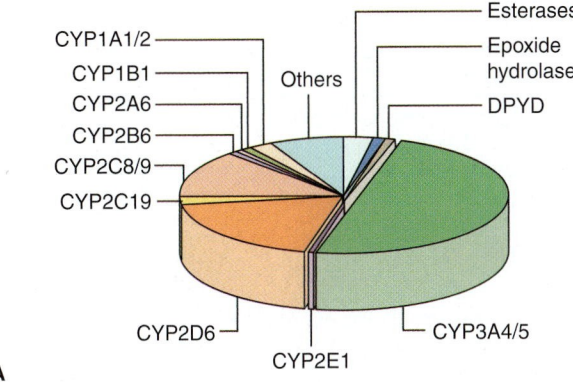

A

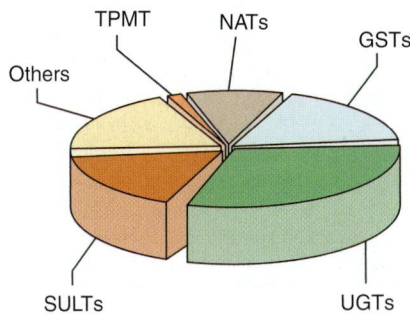

B

FIGURE 4–4 Relative contributions of various cytochrome P450 isoforms (**A**) and different phase II pathways (**B**) to metabolism of drugs in clinical use. Many drugs are metabolized by two or more of these pathways. Note that two pathways, CYP3A4/5 and UGT, are involved in the metabolism of more than 75% of drugs in use. DPYD, dihydropyrimidine dehydrogenase; GST, glutathione-*S*-transferase; NAT, *N*-acetyltransferase; SULT, sulfotransferase; TPMT, thiopurine methyltransferase; UGT, UDP-glucuronosyltransferase. (Reproduced, with permission, from Brunton LL, Lazo JS, Parker KL: *Goodman & Gilman's The Pharmacological Basis of Therapeutics*, 11th ed. McGraw-Hill Medical, 2006.)

a constituent of St. John's wort) in the liver and intestinal mucosa. A similar receptor, the constitutive androstane receptor (CAR), has been identified for the relatively large and structurally diverse phenobarbital class of inducers of CYP2B6, CYP2C9, and CYP3A4. Peroxisome proliferator receptor α (PPAR-α) is yet another nuclear receptor highly expressed in liver and kidneys, which uses lipid-lowering drugs (eg, fenofibrate and gemfibrozil) as ligands. Consistent with its major role in the regulation of fatty acid metabolism, PPAR-α mediates the induction of CYP4A enzymes, responsible for the metabolism of fatty acids such as arachidonic acid and its physiologically relevant derivatives. It is noteworthy that on binding of its particular ligand, PXR, CAR, and PPAR-α each form heterodimers with another nuclear receptor, the retinoid X-receptor (RXR). This heterodimer in turn binds to response elements within the promoter regions of specific *P450* genes to induce gene expression.

P450 enzymes may also be induced by **substrate stabilization,** eg, decreased degradation, as is the case with troleandomycin- or clotrimazole-mediated induction of CYP3A enzymes, the ethanol-mediated induction of CYP2E1, and the isosafrole-mediated induction of CYP1A2.

Enzyme Inhibition

Certain drug substrates inhibit cytochrome P450 enzyme activity (Table 4–2). Imidazole-containing drugs such as cimetidine and ketoconazole bind tightly to the P450 heme iron and effectively reduce the metabolism of endogenous substrates (eg, testosterone) or other co-administered drugs through competitive inhibition. Macrolide antibiotics such as troleandomycin, erythromycin, and erythromycin derivatives are metabolized, apparently by CYP3A, to metabolites that complex the cytochrome P450 heme iron and render it catalytically inactive. Another compound that acts through this mechanism is the inhibitor proadifen (SKF-525-A, used in research), which binds tightly to the heme iron and quasi-irreversibly inactivates the enzyme, thereby inhibiting the metabolism of potential substrates.

Some substrates irreversibly inhibit P450s via covalent interaction of a metabolically generated reactive intermediate that may react with the P450 apoprotein or heme moiety or even cause the heme to fragment and irreversibly modify the apoprotein. The antibiotic chloramphenicol is metabolized by CYP2B1 to a species that modifies the P450 protein and thus also inactivates the enzyme. A growing list of such **suicide inhibitors**—inactivators that attack the heme or the protein moiety—includes certain steroids (ethinyl estradiol, norethindrone, and spironolactone); fluroxene; allobarbital; the analgesic sedatives allylisopropylacetylurea, diethylpentenamide, and ethchlorvynol; carbon disulfide; grapefruit furanocoumarins; selegiline; phencyclidine; ticlopidine and clopidogrel; ritonavir; and propylthiouracil. On the other hand, the barbiturate secobarbital is found to inactivate CYP2B1 by modification of *both* its heme and protein moieties. Other metabolically activated drugs whose P450 inactivation mechanism is not fully elucidated are mifepristone, troglitazone, raloxifene, and tamoxifen.

PHASE II REACTIONS

Parent drugs or their phase I metabolites that contain suitable chemical groups often undergo coupling or conjugation reactions with an endogenous substance to yield **drug conjugates** (Table 4–3). In general, conjugates are polar molecules that are readily excreted and often inactive. Conjugate formation involves high-energy intermediates and specific transfer enzymes. Such enzymes (**transferases**) may be located in microsomes or in the cytosol. Of these, uridine 5′-diphosphate (UDP)-glucuronosyl transferases (**UGTs**) are the most dominant enzymes (Figure 4–4). These microsomal enzymes catalyze the coupling of an activated endogenous substance (such as the UDP derivative of glucuronic acid) with a drug (or endogenous compound such as bilirubin, the end product of heme metabolism). Nineteen *UGT* genes (*UGTA1*

TABLE 4–3 Phase II reactions.

Type of Conjugation	Endogenous Reactant	Transferase (Location)	Types of Substrates	Examples
Glucuronidation	UDP glucuronic acid	UDP glucuronosyltransferase (microsomes)	Phenols, alcohols, carboxylic acids, hydroxylamines, sulfonamides	Nitrophenol, morphine, acetaminophen, diazepam, N-hydroxydapsone, sulfathiazole, meprobamate, digitoxin, digoxin
Acetylation	Acetyl-CoA	N–Acetyltransferase (cytosol)	Amines	Sulfonamides, isoniazid, clonazepam, dapsone, mescaline
Glutathione conjugation	Glutathione (GSH)	GSH-S-transferase (cytosol, microsomes)	Epoxides, arene oxides, nitro groups, hydroxylamines	Acetaminophen, ethacrynic acid, bromobenzene
Glycine conjugation	Glycine	Acyl-CoA glycinetransferase (mitochondria)	Acyl-CoA derivatives of carboxylic acids	Salicylic acid, benzoic acid, nicotinic acid, cinnamic acid, cholic acid, deoxycholic acid
Sulfation	Phosphoadenosyl phosphosulfate	Sulfotransferase (cytosol)	Phenols, alcohols, aromatic amines	Estrone, aniline, phenol, 3-hydroxycoumarin, acetaminophen, methyldopa
Methylation	S-Adenosylmethionine	Transmethylases (cytosol)	Catecholamines, phenols, amines	Dopamine, epinephrine, pyridine, histamine, thiouracil
Water conjugation	Water	Epoxide hydrolase (microsomes)	Arene oxides, cis-disubstituted and monosubstituted oxiranes	Benzopyrene 7,8-epoxide, styrene 1,2-oxide, carbamazepine epoxide
		(cytosol)	Alkene oxides, fatty acid epoxides	Leukotriene A_4

and *UGT2*) encode UGT proteins involved in the metabolism of drugs and xenobiotics. Similarly, 11 human sulfotransferases (**SULTs**) catalyze the sulfation of substrates using 3′-phosphoadenosine 5′-phosphosulfate (**PAPS**) as the endogenous sulfate donor. Cytosolic and microsomal glutathione (**GSH**) transferases (**GSTs**) are also engaged in the metabolism of drugs and xenobiotics, and in that of leukotrienes and prostaglandins, respectively. Chemicals containing an aromatic amine or a hydrazine moiety (eg, isoniazid) are substrates of cytosolic *N*-acetyltransferases (**NATs**), encoded by *NAT1* and *NAT2* genes, which utilize **acetyl-CoA** as the endogenous cofactor.

S-Adenosyl-L-methionine (**SAMe**; AdoMet)-mediated *O*-, *N*-, and *S*-methylation of drugs and xenobiotics by methyltransferases (**MTs**) also occurs. Finally, endobiotic, drug, and xenobiotic epoxides generated via P450-catalyzed oxidations can also be hydrolyzed by microsomal or cytosolic epoxide hydrolases (**EHs**). Conjugation of an activated drug such as the *S*-CoA derivative of benzoic acid, with an endogenous substrate, such as glycine, also occurs. Because the endogenous substrates originate in the diet, nutrition plays a critical role in the regulation of drug conjugations.

Phase II reactions are relatively faster than P450-catalyzed reactions, thus effectively accelerating drug biotransformation.

Drug conjugations were once believed to represent terminal inactivation events and as such have been viewed as "true detoxification" reactions. However, this concept must be modified, because it is now known that certain conjugation reactions (acyl glucuronidation of nonsteroidal anti-inflammatory drugs, *O*-sulfation of *N*-hydroxyacetylaminofluorene, and *N*-acetylation

of isoniazid) may lead to the formation of reactive species responsible for the toxicity of the drugs. Furthermore, sulfation is known to activate the orally active prodrug minoxidil into a very efficacious vasodilator, and morphine-6-glucuronide is more potent than morphine itself.

METABOLISM OF DRUGS TO TOXIC PRODUCTS

Metabolism of drugs and other foreign chemicals may not always be an innocuous biochemical event leading to detoxification and elimination of the compound. Indeed, as previously noted, several compounds have been shown to be metabolically transformed to reactive intermediates that are toxic to various organs. Such toxic reactions may not be apparent at low levels of exposure to parent compounds when alternative detoxification mechanisms are not yet overwhelmed or compromised and when the availability of endogenous detoxifying cosubstrates (GSH, glucuronic acid, sulfate) is not limited. However, when these resources are exhausted, the toxic pathway may prevail, resulting in overt organ toxicity or carcinogenesis. The number of specific examples of such drug-induced toxicity is expanding rapidly. An example is acetaminophen (paracetamol)-induced hepatotoxicity (Figure 4–5). Acetaminophen, an analgesic antipyretic drug, is quite safe in therapeutic doses (1.2 g/d for an adult). It normally undergoes glucuronidation and sulfation to the corresponding conjugates, which together make up 95% of the total excreted metabolites. The alternative P450-dependent GSH conjugation pathway

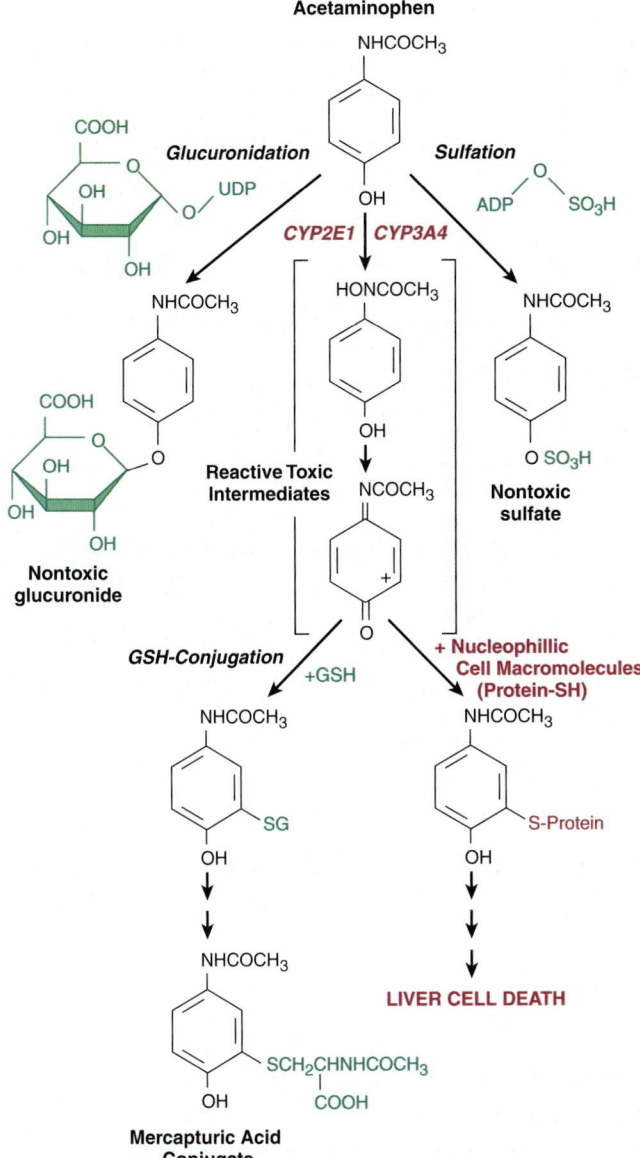

FIGURE 4–5 Metabolism of acetaminophen (top center) to hepatotoxic metabolites. GSH, glutathione; SG, glutathione moiety.

accounts for the remaining 5%. When acetaminophen intake far exceeds therapeutic doses, the glucuronidation and sulfation pathways are saturated, and the P450-dependent pathway becomes increasingly important. Little or no hepatotoxicity results as long as hepatic GSH is available for conjugation. However, with time, hepatic GSH is depleted faster than it can be regenerated, and a reactive, toxic metabolite accumulates. In the absence of intracellular nucleophiles such as GSH, this reactive metabolite (*N*-acetylbenzoiminoquinone) reacts with nucleophilic groups of cellular proteins, resulting in hepatotoxicity.

The chemical and toxicologic characterization of the electrophilic nature of the reactive acetaminophen metabolite has led to the development of effective antidotes—cysteamine and *N*-acetylcysteine. Administration of *N*-acetylcysteine (the safer of

the two) within 8–16 hours after acetaminophen overdosage has been shown to protect victims from fulminant hepatotoxicity and death (see Chapter 58). Administration of GSH is not effective because it does not cross cell membranes readily.

CLINICAL RELEVANCE OF DRUG METABOLISM

The dose and frequency of administration required to achieve effective therapeutic blood and tissue levels vary in different patients because of individual differences in drug distribution and rates of drug metabolism and elimination. These differences are determined by genetic factors and nongenetic variables, such as age, sex, liver size, liver function, circadian rhythm, body temperature, and nutritional and environmental factors such as concomitant exposure to inducers or inhibitors of drug metabolism. The discussion that follows summarizes the most important of these variables.

Individual Differences

Individual differences in metabolic rate depend on the nature of the drug itself. Thus, within the same population, steady-state plasma levels may reflect a 30-fold variation in the metabolism of one drug and only a two-fold variation in the metabolism of another.

Genetic Factors

Genetic factors that influence enzyme levels account for some of these differences, giving rise to "genetic polymorphisms" in drug metabolism. The first examples of drugs found to be subject to genetic polymorphisms were the muscle relaxant succinylcholine, the anti-tuberculosis drug isoniazid, and the anticoagulant warfarin. A true genetic polymorphism is defined as the occurrence of a variant allele of a gene at a population frequency of ≥ 1%, resulting in altered expression or functional activity of the gene product, or both. Well-defined and clinically relevant genetic polymorphisms in both phase I and phase II drug-metabolizing enzymes exist that result in altered efficacy of drug therapy or adverse drug reactions (**ADRs**). The latter frequently necessitate dose adjustment (Table 4–4), a consideration particularly crucial for drugs with low therapeutic indices.

A. Phase I Enzyme Polymorphisms

Genetically determined defects in the phase I oxidative metabolism of several drugs have been reported (Table 4–4). These defects are often transmitted as autosomal recessive traits and may be expressed at any one of the multiple metabolic transformations that a chemical might undergo. Human liver P450s 3A4, 2C9, 2D6, 2C19, 1A2, and 2B6 are responsible for about 75% of all clinically relevant phase I drug metabolism (Figure 4–4), and thus for about 60% of all physiologic drug biotransformation and elimination. Thus, genetic polymorphisms of these enzymes, by significantly influencing phase I drug metabolism, can alter their

TABLE 4–4 Some examples of genetic polymorphisms in phase I and phase II drug metabolism.

Enzyme Involved	Defect	Genotype	Drug and Therapeutic Use	Clinical Consequences[1]
CYP1A2	N-Demethylation	EM	Caffeine (CNS stimulant)	Reduced CNS stimulation due to increased gene inducibility and thus increased metabolism/clearance in cigarette smokers and frequent ingesters of omeprazole.
	N-Demethylation	PM	Caffeine (CNS stimulant)	Enhanced CNS stimulation.
CYP2A6	Oxidation	PM	Nicotine (cholinoceptor stimulant)	Nicotine toxicity. Lesser craving for frequent cigarette smoking.
	Oxidation	EM	Nicotine (cholinoceptor stimulant)	Increased nicotine metabolism. Greater craving for frequent cigarette smoking.
	Oxidation	PM	Coumarin (anticoagulant)	Increased risk of bleeding.
	Oxidation	EM	Coumarin (anticoagulant)	Increased clearance. Greater risk of platelet aggregation and thrombosis.
CYP2B6	Oxidation, N-Dechloroethylation	PM	Cyclophosphamide, ifosfamide (anticancer)	Reduced clearance. Increased risk of ADRs.
	Oxidation	PM	Efavirenz (anti-HIV)	Reduced clearance. Increased risk of ADRs.
CYP2C8	Hydroxylation	PM	Repaglinide, rosiglitazone, pioglitazone (antidiabetic)	Reduced clearance. Increased risk of ADRs.
	Hydroxylation	PM	Paclitaxel (anticancer)	Reduced clearance. Increased risk of ADRs (myelosuppression).
	N-Deethylation/N-Dealkylation	PM	Amodiaquine, chloroquine (antimalarial)	Reduced clearance. Increased risk of ADRs.
	N-Deethylation	PM	Amiodarone (antiarrhythmic)	Reduced clearance. Increased risk of ADRs.
CYP2C9	Hydroxylation	PM	Celecoxib, diclofenac, flurbiprofen, S-ibuprofen (NSAIDs)	Reduced clearance. Increased risk of ADRs.
	Hydroxylation	PM	S-Warfarin, S-acenocoumarol (anticoagulants)	Enhanced bleeding risk. Clinically highly relevant. Dose adjustment required.
	Hydroxylation	PM	Tolbutamide (antidiabetic)	Cardiotoxicity.
	Hydroxylation	PM	Phenytoin (antiepileptic)	Nystagmus, diplopia, and ataxia.
CYP2C19	N-Demethylation	PM	Amitriptyline, clomipramine (antidepressants)	Reduced clearance. Increased risk of ADRs. Dose adjustment required.
	Oxidation	PM	Moclobemide (MAOI)	
	N-Demethylation	PM	Citalopram (SSRI)	Increased risk of gastrointestinal side effects.
	O-Demethylation	PM	Omeprazole (PPI)	Increased therapeutic efficacy.
	Hydroxylation	PM	Mephenytoin (antiepileptic)	Overdose toxicity.
	N-Demethylation	EM	Escitalopram (antidepressants)	Increased gene transcription resulting in increased activity and thus reduced therapeutic efficacy.
	O-Demethylation	EM	Omeprazole (PPI)	Reduced therapeutic efficacy.
	Hydroxylation	EM	Tamoxifen (anticancer)	Increased metabolic activation, increased therapeutic efficacy; reduced risk of relapse. Dose adjustment required.
	Oxidative cyclization	EM	Chlorproguanil (antimalarial)	Increased metabolic activation, increased therapeutic efficacy. Dose adjustment required.
	Oxidation	EM	Clopidogrel (antiplatelet)	Increased metabolic activation, increased therapeutic efficacy. Dose adjustment required.
CYP2D6	Oxidation	PM	Bufuralol (β-adrenoceptor blocker)	Exacerbation of β blockade, nausea.
	O-Demethylation	PM	Codeine (analgesic)	Reduced metabolic activation to morphine and thus reduced analgesia.
	Oxidation	PM	Debrisoquin (antihypertensive)	Orthostatic hypotension.

(continued)

TABLE 4–4 **Some examples of genetic polymorphisms in phase I and phase II drug metabolism. (Continued)**

Enzyme Involved	Defect	Genotype	Drug and Therapeutic Use	Clinical Consequences[1]
	N-Demethylation	PM	Nortriptyline (antidepressant)	Reduced clearance. Increased risk of ADRs.
	Oxidation	PM	Sparteine	Oxytocic symptoms.
	O-Demethylation	PM	Dextromethorphan (antitussive)	Reduced clearance. Increased risk of ADRs.
	O-Demethylation	PM	Tramadol (analgesic)	Increased risk of seizures.
	Hydroxylation	PM	Tamoxifen (anticancer)	Reduced metabolic activation to the therapeutically active endoxifen and thus reduced therapeutic efficacy.
	O-Demethylation	UM	Codeine (analgesic)	Increased metabolic activation to morphine and thus increased risk of respiratory depression.
	N-Demethylation	UM	Nortriptyline (antidepressant)	Reduced therapeutic efficacy due to increased clearance.
	O-Demethylation	UM	Tramadol (analgesic)	Reduced therapeutic efficacy due to increased clearance.
CYP3A4		PM?	All drugs metabolized by this enzyme would be potentially affected	Reduced clearance. Dose adjustment may be required to avoid drug-drug interactions.
CYP3A5		PM?	Saquinavir, and other CYP3A substrates	Usually less catalytically active than CYP3A4. A higher frequency of a functional CYP3A5∗1 allele is seen in Africans than in Caucasians; the latter most often carry the defective CYP3A5∗3 allele. This may significantly affect therapeutics of CYP3A substrates in CYP3A5∗1 or CYP3A5∗3 homozygous individuals.
ALDH	Aldehyde dehydrogenation	PM	Ethanol (recreational drug)	Facial flushing, hypotension, tachycardia, nausea, vomiting.
BCHE	Ester hydrolysis	PM	Succinylcholine (muscle relaxant) Mivacurium (neuromuscular blocker)	Prolonged apnea. Prolonged muscle paralysis.
			Cocaine (CNS stimulant)	Increased blood pressure, tachycardia, ventricular arrhythmias.
GST	GSH-conjugation	PM	Acetaminophen (analgesic), Busulfan (anticancer)	Impaired GSH conjugation due to gene deletion.
NAT2	N-Acetylation	PM	Hydralazine (antihypertensive)	Lupus erythematosus-like syndrome.
	N-Acetylation	PM	Isoniazid (antitubercular)	Peripheral neuropathy.
TPMT	S-Methylation	PM	6-Thiopurines (anticancer)	Myelotoxicity.
UGT1A1	Glucuronidation	PM	Bilirubin (heme metabolite)	Hyperbilirubinemia.
			Irinotecan (anticancer)	Reduced clearance. Dose adjustment may be required to avoid toxicity (GI dysfunction, immunosuppression).

[1]Observed or predictable.

ADR, adverse drug reaction; EM, extensive metabolizer; PM, poor metabolizer; UM, ultrarapid metabolizer.

pharmacokinetics and the magnitude or the duration of drug response and associated events.

Three P450 genetic polymorphisms have been particularly well characterized, affording some insight into possible underlying molecular mechanisms, and are clinically noteworthy, as they require therapeutic dosage adjustment. The first is the **debrisoquin-sparteine oxidation** type of polymorphism, which apparently occurs in 3–10% of Caucasians and is inherited as an autosomal recessive trait. In affected individuals, the **CYP2D6**-dependent oxidations of debrisoquin and other drugs (Table 4–2; Figure 4–6) are impaired. These defects in oxidative drug metabolism are probably co-inherited. The precise molecular basis for the defect appears to be faulty expression of the P450 protein due to either defective mRNA splicing or protein folding, resulting in little or no isoform-catalyzed drug metabolism and thereby conferring a **poor metabolizer (PM)** phenotype. This PM phenotype correlates with a higher risk of relapse in patients with breast cancer treated with tamoxifen, an anti-cancer drug that relies on its CYP2D6-dependent metabolic activation to endoxifen for its efficacy. More recently, however, another polymorphic genotype has been reported that results in **ultrarapid metabolism** of relevant drugs due to the presence of CYP2D6 allelic variants with

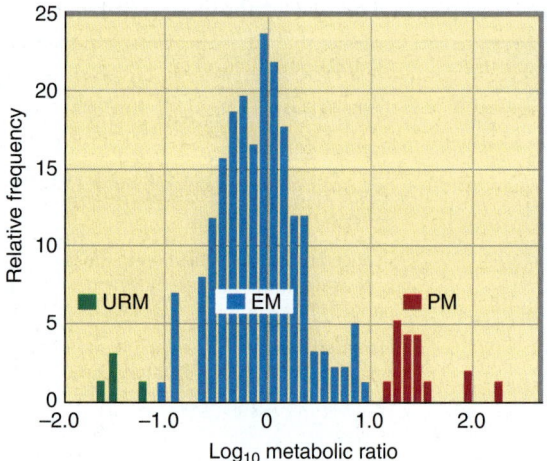

FIGURE 4–6 Genetic polymorphism in debrisoquin 4-hydroxylation by CYP2D6 in a Caucasian population. The semilog frequency distribution histogram of the metabolic ratio (MR; defined as percent of dose excreted as unchanged debrisoquin divided by the percent of dose excreted as 4-hydroxydebrisoquin metabolite) in the 8-hour urine collected after oral ingestion of 12.8 mg debrisoquin sulfate (equivalent to 10 mg free debrisoquin base). Individuals with MR values > 12.6 were phenotyped as poor metabolizers (PM, *red bars*), and those with MR values < 12.6 but > 0.2 were designated as extensive metabolizers (EM, *blue bars*). Those with MR values < 0.2 were designated as ultrarapid metabolizers (URM, *green bars*) based on the MR values (0.01–0.1) of individuals with documented multiple copies of CYP2D6 allelic variants resulting from inherited amplification of this gene. (Data from Woolhouse et al: Debrisoquin hydroxylation polymorphism among Ghanians and Caucasians. Clin Pharmacol Ther 1979;26:584.)

up to 13 gene copies in tandem. This ultrarapid metabolizer (**UM**) genotype is most common in Ethiopians and Saudi Arabians, populations that display it in up to one third of individuals. As a result, these subjects require two-fold to three-fold higher daily doses of nortriptyline (an antidepressant and a CYP2D6 substrate) to achieve therapeutic plasma levels. The poor responsiveness to antidepressant therapy of the UM phenotype also clinically correlates with a higher incidence of suicides relative to that of deaths due to natural causes in this patient population. Conversely, in these UM populations the prodrug codeine (another CYP2D6 substrate) is metabolized much faster to morphine, often resulting in undesirable adverse effects of morphine, such as abdominal pain. Indeed, intake of high doses of codeine by a mother of the ultrarapid metabolizer type was held responsible for the morphine-induced death of her breast-fed infant.

The second well-studied genetic drug polymorphism involves the stereoselective **aromatic (4)-hydroxylation** of the anticonvulsant mephenytoin, catalyzed by **CYP2C19.** This polymorphism, which is also inherited as an autosomal recessive trait, occurs in 3–5% of Caucasians and 18–23% of Japanese populations. It is genetically independent of the debrisoquin-sparteine polymorphism. In normal "**extensive metabolizers**" (EMs) (*S*)-mephenytoin is extensively hydroxylated by CYP2C19 at the 4 position of the phenyl ring before its glucuronidation and rapid

excretion in the urine, whereas (*R*)-mephenytoin is slowly *N*-demethylated to nirvanol, an active metabolite. PMs however, appear to totally lack the stereospecific (*S*)-mephenytoin hydroxylase activity, so both (*S*)- and (*R*)-mephenytoin enantiomers are *N*-demethylated to nirvanol, which accumulates in much higher concentrations. Thus, PMs of mephenytoin show signs of profound sedation and ataxia after doses of the drug that are well tolerated by normal metabolizers. Two defective CYP2C19 variant alleles (CYP2C19*2 and CYP2C19*3), the latter predominant in Asians, are responsible for the PM genotype. The molecular bases include splicing defects resulting in a truncated, nonfunctional protein. CYP2C19 is responsible for the metabolism of various clinically relevant drugs (Table 4–4). Thus, it is clinically important to recognize that the safety of each of these drugs may be severely reduced in persons with the PM phenotype. On the other hand, the PM phenotype can notably increase the therapeutic efficacy of omeprazole, a proton-pump inhibitor, in gastric ulcer and gastroesophageal reflux diseases.

Another CYP2C19 variant allele (CYP2C19*17) exists that is associated with increased transcription and thus higher CYP2C19 expression and even higher functional activity than that of the wild type CYP2C19-carrying EMs. Individuals carrying this CYP2C19*17 allele exhibit higher metabolic activation of prodrugs such as the breast cancer drug tamoxifen, the antimalarial chlorproguanil, and the antiplatelet drug clopidogrel. The former event is associated with a lower risk of breast cancer relapse, and the latter event with an increased risk of bleeding. Carriers of the CYP2C19*17 allele are also known to enhance the metabolism and thus the elimination of drugs such as the antidepressants escitalopram and imipramine, as well as the antifungal voriconazole. This consequently impairs the therapeutic efficacy of these drugs, thus requiring clinical dosage adjustments.

The third relatively well-characterized genetic polymorphism is that of **CYP2C9.** Two well-characterized variants of this enzyme exist, each with amino acid mutations that result in altered metabolism. The CYP2C9*2 allele encodes an Arg144Cys mutation, exhibiting impaired functional interactions with **POR.** The other allelic variant, CYP2C9*3, encodes an enzyme with an Ile359Leu mutation that has lowered affinity for many substrates. For example, individuals displaying the CYP2C9*3 phenotype have greatly reduced tolerance for the anticoagulant warfarin. The warfarin clearance in CYP2C9*3-homozygous individuals is about 10% of normal values, and these people have a much lower tolerance for the drug than those who are homozygous for the normal wild type allele. These individuals also have a much higher risk of adverse effects with warfarin (eg, bleeding) and with other CYP2C9 substrates such as phenytoin, losartan, tolbutamide, and some nonsteroidal anti-inflammatory drugs (Table 4–4).

Allelic variants of CYP3A4 have also been reported, but their contribution to its well-known interindividual variability in drug metabolism apparently is limited. On the other hand, the expression of **CYP3A5,** another human liver isoform, is markedly polymorphic, ranging from 0% to 100% of the total hepatic CYP3A content. This CYP3A5 protein polymorphism is now known to result from a single nucleotide polymorphism (**SNP**) within intron 3, which enables normally spliced CYP3A5 transcripts in

5% of Caucasians, 29% of Japanese, 27% of Chinese, 30% of Koreans, and 73% of African Americans. Thus, it can significantly contribute to interindividual differences in the metabolism of preferential CYP3A5 substrates such as midazolam. Two other CYP3A5 allelic variants that result in a PM phenotype are also known.

Polymorphisms in the *CYP2A6* gene have also been recently characterized, and their prevalence is apparently racially linked. CYP2A6 is responsible for nicotine oxidation, and tobacco smokers with low CYP2A6 activity consume less and have a lower incidence of lung cancer. CYP2A6 1B allelic variants associated with faster rates of nicotine metabolism have been recently discovered. It remains to be determined whether patients with these faster variants will fall into the converse paradigm of increased smoking behavior and lung cancer incidence.

Additional genetic polymorphisms in drug metabolism (eg, **CYP2B6**) that are inherited independently from those already described are being discovered. For instance, a 20- to 250-fold variation in interindividual CYP2B6 expression partly due to genetic polymorphisms has been reported. This may have a significant impact on the metabolism of several clinically relevant drugs such as cyclophosphamide, methadone, efavirenz, selegiline, and propofol. Studies of theophylline metabolism in monozygotic and dizygotic twins that included pedigree analysis of various families have revealed that a distinct polymorphism may exist for this drug and may be inherited as a recessive genetic trait. Genetic drug metabolism polymorphisms also appear to occur for aminopyrine and carbocysteine oxidations. Regularly updated information on human P450 polymorphisms is available at http://www.imm.ki.se/CYPalleles/.

Although genetic polymorphisms in drug oxidations often involve specific P450 enzymes, such genetic variations can also occur in other enzymes. Recently, genetic polymorphisms in POR, the essential P450 electron donor, have been reported. In particular, an allelic variant (at a 28% frequency) encoding a POR A503V mutation has been reported to result in impaired CYP17-dependent sex steroid synthesis and impaired CYP3A4- and CYP2D6-dependent drug metabolism in vitro. Its involvement in clinically relevant drug metabolism, while predictable, remains to be established. Descriptions of a polymorphism in the oxidation of trimethylamine, believed to be metabolized largely by the **flavin monooxygenase (Ziegler's enzyme),** result in the "fish-odor syndrome" in slow metabolizers, thus suggesting that genetic variants of other non–P450-dependent oxidative enzymes may also contribute to such polymorphisms.

B. Phase II Enzyme Polymorphisms

Succinylcholine is metabolized only half as rapidly in persons with genetically determined deficiency in pseudocholinesterase (now generally referred to as butyrylcholinesterase [**BCHE**]) as in persons with normally functioning enzyme. Different mutations, inherited as autosomal recessive traits, account for the enzyme deficiency. Deficient individuals treated with succinylcholine as a surgical muscle relaxant may become susceptible to prolonged respiratory paralysis (succinylcholine apnea). Similar pharmacogenetic differences are seen in the acetylation of isoniazid. The defect

in slow acetylators (of isoniazid and similar amines) appears to be caused by the synthesis of less of the NAT2 enzyme rather than of an abnormal form of it. Inherited as an autosomal recessive trait, the **slow acetylator phenotype** occurs in about 50% of blacks and whites in the USA, more frequently in Europeans living in high northern latitudes, and much less commonly in Asians and Inuits (Eskimos). The slow acetylator phenotype is also associated with a higher incidence of isoniazid-induced peripheral neuritis, drug-induced autoimmune disorders, and bicyclic aromatic amine-induced bladder cancer.

A clinically important polymorphism of the *TPMT* (thiopurine *S*-methyltransferase) gene is encountered in Europeans (frequency, 1:300), resulting in a rapidly degraded mutant enzyme and consequently deficient *S*-methylation of aromatic and heterocyclic sulfhydryl compounds including the anti-cancer thiopurine drugs 6-mercaptopurine, thioguanine, and azathioprine, required for their detoxification. Patients inheriting this polymorphism as an autosomal recessive trait are at high risk of thiopurine drug-induced fatal hematopoietic toxicity.

Genetic polymorphisms in the expression of other phase II enzymes (UGTs and GSTs) also occur. Thus, UGT polymorphisms (*UGT1A1*28*) are associated with hyperbilirubinemic diseases (Gilbert's syndrome) as well as toxic side effects due to impaired drug conjugation and/or elimination (eg, the anticancer drug irinotecan). Similarly, genetic polymorphisms (*GSTM1*) in GST (mu1 isoform) expression can lead to significant adverse effects and toxicities of drugs dependent on its GSH conjugation for elimination.

C. The Role of Pharmacogenetic Testing in Clinically Safe & Effective Drug Therapy

Despite our improved understanding of the molecular basis of pharmacogenetic defects in drug-metabolizing enzymes, their impact on drug therapy and ADRs, and the availability of validated pharmacogenetic biomarkers to identify patients at risk, this clinically relevant information has not been effectively translated to patient care. Thus, the much-heralded potential for personalized medicine, except in a few instances of drugs with a relatively low therapeutic index (eg, warfarin), has remained largely unrealized. This is so even though 98% of US physicians are apparently aware that such genetic information may significantly influence therapy. This is partly due to the lack of adequate training in translating this knowledge to medical practice, and partly due to the logistics of genetic testing and the issue of cost-effectiveness. Severe ADRs are known to contribute to 100,000 annual US deaths, about 7% of all hospital admissions, and an increased average length of hospital stay. Genotype information could greatly enhance safe and efficacious clinical therapy through dose adjustment or alternative drug therapy, thereby curbing much of the rising ADR incidence and its associated costs.

Diet & Environmental Factors

Diet and environmental factors contribute to individual variations in drug metabolism. Charcoal-broiled foods and cruciferous vegetables are known to induce CYP1A enzymes, whereas grapefruit juice is known to inhibit the CYP3A metabolism of co-administered drug substrates (Table 4–2). Cigarette smokers metabolize some drugs more rapidly than nonsmokers because of enzyme induction (see previous section). Industrial workers exposed to some pesticides metabolize certain drugs more rapidly than unexposed individuals. Such differences make it difficult to determine effective and safe doses of drugs that have narrow therapeutic indices.

Age & Sex

Increased susceptibility to the pharmacologic or toxic activity of drugs has been reported in very young and very old patients compared with young adults (see Chapters 59 and 60). Although this may reflect differences in absorption, distribution, and elimination, differences in drug metabolism also play a role. Slower metabolism could be due to reduced activity of metabolic enzymes or reduced availability of essential endogenous cofactors.

Sex-dependent variations in drug metabolism have been well documented in rats but not in other rodents. Young adult male rats metabolize drugs much faster than mature female rats or prepubertal male rats. These differences in drug metabolism have been clearly associated with androgenic hormones. Clinical reports suggest that similar sex-dependent differences in drug metabolism also exist in humans for ethanol, propranolol, some benzodiazepines, estrogens, and salicylates.

Drug-Drug Interactions during Metabolism

Many substrates, by virtue of their relatively high lipophilicity, are not only retained at the active site of the enzyme but remain non-specifically bound to the lipid endoplasmic reticulum membrane. In this state, they may induce microsomal enzymes, particularly after repeated use. Acutely, depending on the residual drug levels at the active site, they also may competitively inhibit metabolism of a simultaneously administered drug.

Enzyme-inducing drugs include various sedative-hypnotics, antipsychotics, anticonvulsants, the antitubercular drug rifampin, and insecticides (Table 4–5). Patients who routinely ingest barbiturates, other sedative-hypnotics, or certain antipsychotic drugs may require considerably higher doses of warfarin to maintain a therapeutic effect. On the other hand, discontinuance of the sedative inducer may result in reduced metabolism of the anticoagulant and bleeding—a toxic effect of the ensuing enhanced plasma levels of the anticoagulant. Similar interactions have been observed in individuals receiving various combinations of drug regimens such as rifampin, antipsychotics, or sedatives with contraceptive agents, sedatives with anticonvulsant drugs, and even alcohol with hypoglycemic drugs (tolbutamide).

It must also be noted that an inducer may enhance not only the metabolism of other drugs but also its own metabolism. Thus, continued use of some drugs may result in a pharmacokinetic type of **tolerance**—progressively reduced therapeutic effectiveness due to enhancement of their own metabolism.

TABLE 4–5 Partial list of drugs that enhance drug metabolism in humans.

Inducer	Drugs Whose Metabolism Is Enhanced
Benzo[a]pyrene	Theophylline
Carbamazepine	Carbamazepine, clonazepam, itraconazole
Chlorcyclizine	Steroid hormones
Ethchlorvynol	Warfarin
Glutethimide	Antipyrine, glutethimide, warfarin
Griseofulvin	Warfarin
Phenobarbital and other barbiturates[1]	Barbiturates, chloramphenicol, chlorpromazine, cortisol, coumarin anticoagulants, desmethylimipramine, digitoxin, doxorubicin, estradiol, itraconazole, phenylbutazone, phenytoin, quinine, testosterone
Phenylbutazone	Aminopyrine, cortisol, digitoxin
Phenytoin	Cortisol, dexamethasone, digitoxin, itraconazole, theophylline
Rifampin	Coumarin anticoagulants, digitoxin, glucocorticoids, itraconazole, methadone, metoprolol, oral contraceptives, prednisone, propranolol, quinidine, saquinavir
Ritonavir[2]	Midazolam
St. John's wort	Alprazolam, cyclosporine, digoxin, indinavir, oral contraceptives, ritonavir, simvastatin, tacrolimus, warfarin

[1]Secobarbital is an exception. See Table 4–6 and text.

[2]With chronic (repeated) administration; acutely, ritonavir is a potent CYP3A4 inhibitor/inactivator.

Conversely, simultaneous administration of two or more drugs may result in impaired elimination of the more slowly metabolized drug and prolongation or potentiation of its pharmacologic effects (Table 4–6). Both competitive substrate inhibition and irreversible substrate-mediated enzyme inactivation may augment plasma drug levels and lead to toxic effects from drugs with narrow therapeutic indices. Indeed, such acute interactions of terfenadine (a second-generation antihistamine) with a CYP3A4 substrate-inhibitor (ketoconazole, erythromycin, or grapefruit juice) resulted in fatal cardiac arrhythmias (torsades de pointe) requiring its withdrawal from the market. Similar drug-drug interactions with CYP3A4 substrate-inhibitors (such as the antibiotics erythromycin and clarithromycin, the antidepressant nefazodone, the antifungals itraconazole and ketoconazole, and the HIV protease inhibitors indinavir and ritonavir), and consequent cardiotoxicity led to withdrawal or restricted use of the 5-HT$_4$ agonist, cisapride. Similarly, allopurinol both prolongs the duration and enhances the chemotherapeutic and toxic actions of mercaptopurine by competitive inhibition of xanthine oxidase. Consequently, to avoid bone marrow toxicity, the dose of mercaptopurine must be reduced in patients receiving allopurinol. Cimetidine, a drug used in the treatment of peptic ulcer, has been shown to potentiate the pharmacologic actions of anticoagulants and sedatives. The metabolism of the sedative chlordiazepoxide has been shown to be

TABLE 4–6 Partial list of drugs that inhibit drug metabolism in humans.

Inhibitor[1]	Drug Whose Metabolism Is Inhibited
Allopurinol, chloramphenicol, isoniazid	Antipyrine, dicumarol, probenecid, tolbutamide
Chlorpromazine	Propranolol
Cimetidine	Chlordiazepoxide, diazepam, warfarin, others
Dicumarol	Phenytoin
Diethylpentenamide	Diethylpentenamide
Disulfiram	Antipyrine, ethanol, phenytoin, warfarin
Ethanol	Chlordiazepoxide (?), diazepam (?), methanol
Grapefruit juice[2]	Alprazolam, atorvastatin, cisapride, cyclosporine, midazolam, triazolam
Itraconazole	Alfentanil, alprazolam, astemizole, atorvastatin, buspirone, cisapride, cyclosporine, delavirdine, diazepam, digoxin, felodipine, indinavir, loratadine, lovastatin, midazolam, nisoldipine, phenytoin, quinidine, ritonavir, saquinavir, sildenafil, simvastatin, sirolimus, tacrolimus, triazolam, verapamil, warfarin
Ketoconazole	Astemizole, cyclosporine, terfenadine
Nortriptyline	Antipyrine
Oral contraceptives	Antipyrine
Phenylbutazone	Phenytoin, tolbutamide
Ritonavir	Amiodarone, cisapride, itraconazole, midazolam, triazolam
Saquinavir	Cisapride, ergot derivatives, midazolam, triazolam
Secobarbital	Secobarbital
Spironolactone	Digoxin
Troleandomycin	Theophylline, methylprednisolone

[1]While some inhibitors are selective for a given P450 enzyme, others are more general and can inhibit several P450s concurrently.

[2]Active components in grapefruit juice include furanocoumarins such as 6′, 7′-dihydroxybergamottin (which inactivates both intestinal and liver CYP3A4) as well as other unknown components that inhibit P-glycoprotein-mediated intestinal drug efflux and consequently further enhance the bioavailability of certain drugs such as cyclosporine.

inhibited by 63% after a single dose of cimetidine; such effects are reversed within 48 hours after withdrawal of cimetidine.

Impaired metabolism may also result if a simultaneously administered drug irreversibly inactivates a common metabolizing enzyme. These inhibitors, in the course of their metabolism by cytochrome P450, inactivate the enzyme and result in impairment of their own metabolism and that of other cosubstrates. This is indeed the case of the furanocoumarins in grapefruit juice that inactivate CYP3A4 in the intestinal mucosa and consequently

enhance its proteolytic degradation. This impairment of their intestinal first-pass CYP3A4-dependent metabolism significantly enhances the bioavailability of drugs, such as felodipine, nifedipine, terfenadine, verapamil, ethinylestradiol, saquinavir, and cyclosporine A, and is associated with clinically relevant drug-drug and food-drug interactions.

Recovery from these interactions is dependent on CYP3A4 resynthesis and thus may be slow.

Interactions between Drugs & Endogenous Compounds

Some drugs require conjugation with endogenous substrates such as GSH, glucuronic acid, or sulfate for their inactivation. Consequently, different drugs may compete for the same endogenous substrates, and the faster-reacting drug may effectively deplete endogenous substrate levels and impair the metabolism of the slower-reacting drug. If the latter has a steep dose-response curve or a narrow margin of safety, potentiation of its therapeutic and toxic effects may result.

Diseases Affecting Drug Metabolism

Acute or chronic diseases that affect liver architecture or function markedly affect hepatic metabolism of some drugs. Such conditions include alcoholic hepatitis, active or inactive alcoholic cirrhosis, hemochromatosis, chronic active hepatitis, biliary cirrhosis, and acute viral or drug-induced hepatitis. Depending on their severity, these conditions may significantly impair hepatic drug-metabolizing enzymes, particularly microsomal oxidases, and thereby markedly affect drug elimination. For example, the half-lives of chlordiazepoxide and diazepam in patients with liver cirrhosis or acute viral hepatitis are greatly increased, with a corresponding increase in their effects. Consequently, these drugs may cause coma in patients with liver disease when given in ordinary doses.

Some drugs are metabolized so readily that even marked reduction in liver function does not significantly prolong their action. However, cardiac disease, by limiting blood flow to the liver, may impair disposition of those drugs whose metabolism is flow-limited (Table 4–7). These drugs are so readily metabolized by the liver that hepatic clearance is essentially equal to liver blood

TABLE 4–7 Rapidly metabolized drugs whose hepatic clearance is blood flow-limited.

Alprenolol	Lidocaine
Amitriptyline	Meperidine
Clomethiazole	Morphine
Desipramine	Pentazocine
Imipramine	Propoxyphene
Isoniazid	Propranolol
Labetalol	Verapamil

flow. Pulmonary disease may also affect drug metabolism, as indicated by the impaired hydrolysis of procainamide and procaine in patients with chronic respiratory insufficiency and the increased half-life of antipyrine (a P450 functional probe) in patients with lung cancer. The impaired enzyme activity or defective formation of enzymes associated with heavy metal poisoning or porphyria also results in reduced hepatic drug metabolism.

Although the effects of endocrine dysfunction on drug metabolism have been well explored in experimental animal models, corresponding data for humans with endocrine disorders are scanty. Thyroid dysfunction has been associated with altered metabolism of some drugs and of some endogenous compounds as well. Hypothyroidism increases the half-life of antipyrine, digoxin, methimazole, and some β blockers, whereas hyperthyroidism has the opposite effect. A few clinical studies in diabetic patients indicate no apparent impairment of drug metabolism, although impairment has been noted in diabetic rats. Malfunctions of the pituitary, adrenal cortex, and gonads markedly reduce hepatic drug metabolism in rats. On the basis of these findings, it may be supposed that such disorders could significantly affect drug metabolism in humans. However, until sufficient evidence is obtained from clinical studies in patients, such extrapolations must be considered tentative.

Finally, the release of inflammatory mediators, cytokines, and nitric oxide associated with bacterial or viral infections, cancer, or inflammation are known to impair drug metabolism by inactivating P450s and enhancing their degradation.

REFERENCES

Benowitz NL: Pharmacology of nicotine: Addiction, smoking-induced disease, and therapeutics. Annu Rev Pharmacol Toxicol 2009;49:57.

Correia MA: Human and rat liver cytochromes P450: Functional markers, diagnostic inhibitor probes and parameters frequently used in P450 studies. In: Ortiz de Montellano P (editor). *Cytochrome P450: Structure, Mechanism and Biochemistry*, 3rd ed. Kluwer-Academic/Plenum Press, 2005.

Correia MA, Ortiz de Montellano P: Inhibitors of cytochrome P-450 and possibilities for their therapeutic application. In: Ruckpaul K (editor): *Frontiers in Biotransformation*, vol 8. Taylor & Francis, 1993.

Correia MA, Ortiz de Montellano P: Inhibition of cytochrome P450 enzymes. In: Ortiz de Montellano P (editor). Cytochrome P450: Structure, *Mechanism and Biochemistry*, 3rd ed. KluwerAcademic/Plenum Press, 2005.

Daly AK: Pharmacogenetics and human genetic polymorphisms. Biochem J 2010;429:435.

Guengerich FP: Human cytochrome P450 enzymes. In: Ortiz de Montellano P (editor). *Cytochrome P450: Structure, Mechanism and Biochemistry*, 3rd ed. Kluwer-Academic/Plenum Press, 2005.

Guengerich FP: Role of cytochrome P450 enzymes in drug-drug interactions. Adv Pharmacol 1997;43:7.

Hustert E et al: The genetic determinants of the CYP3A5 polymorphism. Pharmacogenetics 2001;11:773.

Ingelman-Sundberg M et al: Influence of cytochrome P450 polymorphisms on drug therapies: Pharmacogenetic, pharmacoepigenetic and clinical aspects. Pharmacol Ther 2007;116:496.

Ingelman-Sundberg M, Sim SC: Pharmacogenetic biomarkers as tools for improved drug therapy; emphasis on the cytochrome P450 system. Biochem Biophys Res Commun 2010;396:90.

Ingelman-Sundberg M: Pharmacogenetics: An opportunity for a safer and more efficient pharmacotherapy. J Intern Med 2001;250:186.

Kroemer HK, Klotz U: Glucuronidation of drugs: A reevaluation of the pharmacological significance of the conjugates and modulating factors. Clin Pharmacokinet 1992;23:292.

Kuehl P et al: Sequence diversity in CYP3A promoters and characterization of the genetic basis of polymorphic CYP3A5 expression. Nat Genet 2001;27:383.

Lown KS et al: Grapefruit juice increases felodipine oral availability in humans by decreasing intestinal CYP3A protein expression. J Clin Invest 1997;99:2545.

Meyer UA: Pharmacogenetics—Five decades of therapeutic lessons from genetic diversity. Nat Rev Genet 2004;5:669.

Morgan ET et al: Regulation of drug-metabolizing enzymes and transporters in infection, inflammation, and cancer. Drug Metab Dispos 2008;36:205.

Nelson DR et al: The P450 superfamily: Update on new sequences, gene mapping, accession numbers, and nomenclature. Pharmacogenetics 1996;6:1.

Nelson DR et al: Updated human P450 sequences available at http://drnelson.utmem.edu/human.P450.seqs.html.

Sueyoshi T, Negishi M: Phenobarbital response elements of cytochrome P450 genes and nuclear receptors. Annu Rev Pharmacol Toxicol 2001;41:123.

Thummel KE, Wilkinson GR: In vitro and in vivo drug interactions involving human CYP3A. Annu Rev Pharmacol Toxicol 1998;38:389.

Wang L, McLeod HL, Weinshilboum RM: Genomics and drug response. N Engl J Med 2011;364:1144.

Williams SN et al: Induction of cytochrome P450 enzymes. In: Ortiz de Montellano PR (editor). *Cytochrome P450. Structure, Mechanism, and Biochemistry.* Plenum Press, 2005; *and references therein.*

Willson TM, Kliewer SA: PXR, CAR and drug metabolism. Nat Rev Drug Discov 2002;1:259.

Xu C et al: CYP2A6 genetic variation and potential consequences. Adv Drug Delivery Rev 2002;54:1245.

Development & Regulation of Drugs

Bertram G. Katzung, MD, PhD[*]

A few useful drugs have been known since humans first began ingesting or injecting substances and recording the results (see The History of Pharmacology in Chapter 1), but the majority of agents in current use have been developed during the last 100 years using a variety of pharmacologic and toxicologic techniques. These new chemicals and the efforts to market them have in turn led to a variety of methods of legal regulation. This chapter describes the methods of new drug development and some aspects of drug regulation in the United States.

The most common first steps in the development of a new drug are the discovery or synthesis of a potential new drug compound or the elucidation of a new drug target. When a new drug molecule is synthesized or discovered, subsequent steps seek an understanding of the drug's interactions with its biologic targets. Repeated application of this approach leads to compounds with increased efficacy, potency, and selectivity (Figure 5–1). In the United States, the safety and efficacy of drugs must be defined before marketing can be legally carried out. In addition to in vitro studies, relevant biologic effects, drug metabolism, pharmacokinetic profiles, and particularly an assessment of the relative safety of the drug must be characterized in vivo in animals before human drug trials can be started. With regulatory approval, human testing may then go forward (usually in three phases) before the drug is considered for approval for general use. A fourth phase of data gathering and safety monitoring is becoming increasingly important and follows after approval for marketing. Once approved, the great majority of drugs become available for use by any appropriately licensed practitioner. Highly toxic drugs that are nevertheless considered valuable in lethal diseases may be approved for restricted use by practitioners who have undergone special training in their use and who maintain detailed records.

THE PHARMACEUTICAL INDUSTRY

Careful analysis indicates that a majority of new drugs *originate* in research carried out in public sector institutions (universities, research institutes). However, because of the economic investment required and the need to efficiently access and integrate multiple technologies, most new drugs are then *developed* in pharmaceutical companies. Enormous and increasing costs, with estimates from $150 million to several billion, are involved in the development of a single new drug that reaches the marketplace. Only 2 of 10 marketed drugs return their research and development (R&D) investments, thus providing considerable motivation to develop "blockbuster drugs." Thousands of compounds may be synthesized and hundreds of thousands tested from libraries of compounds for each successful new drug lead, which then frequently needs to be further optimized for reasons of potency, selectivity, drug metabolism, and dosing convenience before each drug reaches the market. Increasing regulatory challenges and litigation resulting from real or suspected drug toxicity after approval further increase the cost of developing new drugs. Unfortunately, only 10–15% of the new drugs that achieve marketing approval represent significant advances in safety and effectiveness; the remainder are merely molecular variants ("me-too drugs") on true breakthrough drugs.

In spite of the cost of development, the financial rewards in drug development can be enormous. The global market for pharmaceuticals in 2007 was estimated to be $712 billion and the return on investment in the pharmaceutical industry is among the highest of all industries. This is ensured by setting the price of a new, important drug very high and lowering the price only when competition forces it down; for example, when me-too variants or generic versions of the original molecule become available. Even in Europe, where drug prices are lower than in the USA, industry profits are comparable. The 2007 worldwide sales of the top-selling drug (Lipitor) exceeded $12 billion. In the USA, approximately 10–12% of the health care dollar is presently spent on prescription drugs. At the same time, the investment in drugs can have

[*]The author thanks Barry A. Berkowitz, PhD, a previous author of this chapter, for his contributions.

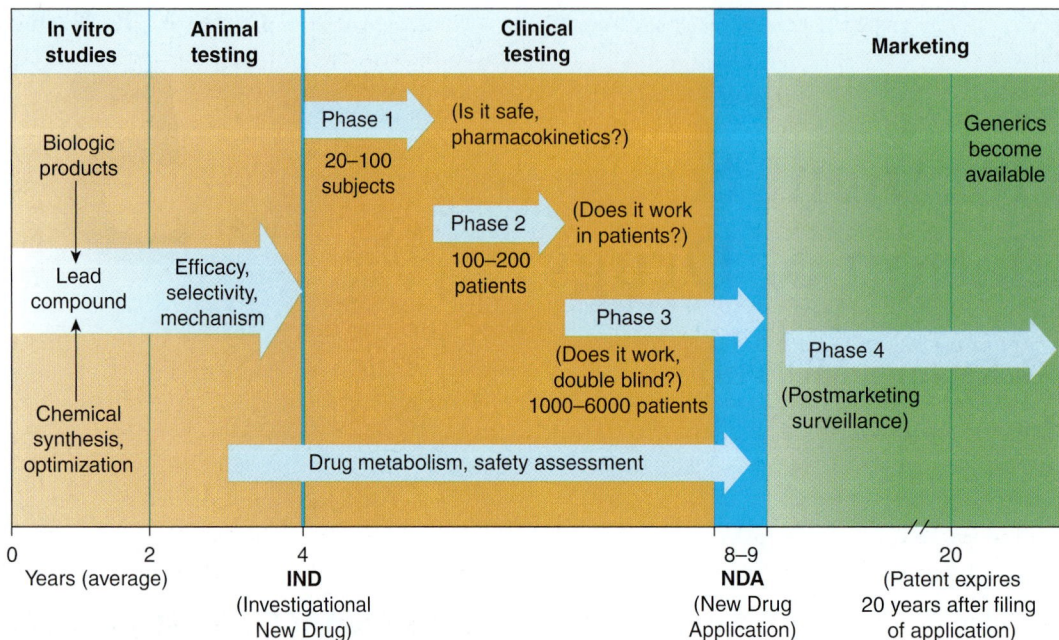

FIGURE 5–1 The development and testing process required to bring a drug to market in the USA. Some of the requirements may be different for drugs used in life-threatening diseases (see text).

enormous health benefits—new drugs can reduce suffering and save lives.

DRUG DISCOVERY

Most new drugs or drug products are discovered or developed through the following approaches: (1) identification or elucidation of a new drug target; (2) rational design of a new molecule based on an understanding of biologic mechanisms and drug receptor structure; (3) screening for biologic activity of large numbers of natural products, banks of previously discovered chemical entities, or large libraries of peptides, nucleic acids, and other organic molecules; and (4) chemical modification of a known active molecule, resulting in a me-too analog. Steps (1) and (2) are often carried out in academic research laboratories, but the costs of steps (3) and (4) usually ensure that industry carries them out.

Once a new drug target or promising molecule has been identified, the process of moving from the basic science laboratory to the clinic begins. This **translational research** involves the preclinical and clinical steps described next.

Drug Screening

Regardless of the source or the key idea leading to a drug candidate molecule, testing it involves a sequence of experimentation and characterization called drug screening. A variety of assays at the molecular, cellular, organ system, and whole animal levels are used to define the activity and selectivity of the drug. The type and number of initial screening tests depend on the pharmacologic and therapeutic goal. For example, anti-infective drugs may be tested against a variety of infectious organisms, some of which are

resistant to standard agents; hypoglycemic drugs may be tested for their ability to lower blood sugar, etc.

The molecule will also be studied for a broad array of other actions to determine the mechanism of action and selectivity of the drug. This can reveal both expected and unexpected toxic effects. Occasionally, an unexpected therapeutic action is serendipitously discovered by a careful observer. The selection of compounds for development is most efficiently conducted in animal models of human disease. Where good predictive preclinical models exist (eg, antibacterials, hypertension, or thrombotic disease), we generally have good or excellent drugs. Good drugs or breakthrough improvements are conspicuously lacking and slow for diseases for which preclinical models are poor or not yet available, eg, autism and Alzheimer's disease.

Studies are performed during drug screening to define the **pharmacologic profile** of the drug at the molecular, cellular, organ, system, and organism levels. The value of these tests is highly dependent on the reproducibility and reliability of the assays. For example, a broad range of tests would be performed on a drug designed to act as an antagonist for a new vascular target for the treatment of hypertension.

At the molecular level, the compound would be screened for activity on the target, for example, receptor binding affinity to cell membranes containing the homologous animal receptors (or if possible, on the cloned human receptors). Early studies would be done to predict effects that might later cause undesired drug metabolism or toxicologic complications. For example, studies on liver cytochrome P450 enzymes would be performed to determine whether the molecule of interest is likely to be a substrate or inhibitor of these enzymes or to interfere with the metabolism of other drugs. Effects on cardiac ion channels such as the hERG

potassium channel, possibly predictive of life-threatening arrhythmias, are considered.

Effects on cell function determine whether the drug is an agonist, partial agonist, inverse agonist, or antagonist at the relevant receptors. Isolated tissues, especially vascular smooth muscle, would be used to characterize the pharmacologic activity and selectivity of the new compound in comparison with reference compounds. Comparison with other drugs would also be undertaken in other in vitro preparations such as gastrointestinal and bronchial smooth muscle. At each step in this process, the compound would have to meet specific performance and selectivity criteria to be carried further.

Whole animal studies are generally necessary to determine the effect of the drug on organ systems and disease models. Cardiovascular and renal function studies of new drugs are generally first performed in normal animals. Studies on disease models, if available, are then performed. For a candidate antihypertensive drug, animals with hypertension would be treated to see whether blood pressure was lowered in a dose-related manner and to characterize other effects of the compound. Evidence would be collected on duration of action and efficacy after oral and parenteral administration. If the agent possessed useful activity, it would be further studied for possible adverse effects on other major organs, including the respiratory, gastrointestinal, endocrine, and central nervous systems.

These studies might suggest the need for further chemical modification (compound optimization) to achieve more desirable pharmacokinetic or pharmacodynamic properties. For example, oral administration studies might show that the drug was poorly absorbed or rapidly metabolized in the liver; modification to improve bioavailability might be indicated. If the drug was to be administered long term, an assessment of tolerance development would be made. For drugs related to or having mechanisms of action similar to those known to cause physical or psychological dependence, abuse potential would also be studied. Drug interactions would be examined.

The desired result of this screening procedure (which may have to be repeated several times with analogs or congeners of the original molecule) is a **lead compound**, ie, a leading candidate for a successful new drug. A patent application would be filed for a novel compound (a composition of matter patent) that is efficacious, or for a new and nonobvious therapeutic use (a use patent) for a previously known chemical entity.

PRECLINICAL SAFETY & TOXICITY TESTING

All drugs are toxic in some individuals at some dose. Seeking to correctly define the limiting toxicities of drugs and the therapeutic index comparing benefits and risks of a new drug is an essential part of the new drug development process. Most drug candidates fail to reach the market, but the art of drug development consists of effective assessment and management of risk versus benefit and not total risk avoidance.

Candidate drugs that survive the initial screening procedures must be carefully evaluated for potential risks before and during clinical testing. Depending on the proposed use of the drug, preclinical toxicity testing includes most or all of the procedures shown in Table 5–1. Although no chemical can be certified as completely "safe" (free of risk), the objective is to estimate the risk associated with exposure to the drug candidate and to consider this in the context of therapeutic needs and likely duration of drug use.

The goals of preclinical toxicity studies include identifying potential human toxicities, designing tests to further define the toxic mechanisms, and predicting the most relevant toxicities to be monitored in clinical trials. In addition to the studies shown in Table 5–1, several quantitative estimates are desirable. These include the **no-effect dose**—the maximum dose at which a specified toxic effect is not seen; the **minimum lethal dose**—the smallest dose that is observed to kill any experimental animal; and, if necessary, the **median lethal dose (LD_{50})**—the dose that kills

TABLE 5–1 Safety tests.

Type of Test	Approach and Goals
Acute toxicity	Usually two species, two routes. Determine the no-effect dose and the maximum tolerated dose. In some cases, determine the acute dose that is lethal in approximately 50% of animals.
Subacute or subchronic toxicity	Three doses, two species. Two weeks to 3 months of testing may be required before clinical trials. The longer the duration of expected clinical use, the longer the subacute test. Determine biochemical, physiologic effects.
Chronic toxicity	Rodent and at least one nonrodent species for ≥ 6 months. Required when drug is intended to be used in humans for prolonged periods. Usually run concurrently with clinical trials. Determine same end points as subacute toxicity tests.
Effect on reproductive performance	Two species, usually one rodent and rabbits. Test effects on animal mating behavior, reproduction, parturition, progeny, birth defects, postnatal development.
Carcinogenic potential	Two years, two species. Required when drug is intended to be used in humans for prolonged periods. Determine gross and histologic pathology.
Mutagenic potential	Test effects on genetic stability and mutations in bacteria (Ames test) or mammalian cells in culture; dominant lethal test and clastogenicity in mice.

approximately 50% of the animals. Presently, the LD$_{50}$ is estimated from the smallest number of animals possible. These doses are used to calculate the initial dose to be tried in humans, usually taken as one hundredth to one tenth of the no-effect dose in animals.

It is important to recognize the limitations of preclinical testing. These include the following:

1. Toxicity testing is time-consuming and expensive. Two to 6 years may be required to collect and analyze data on toxicity before the drug can be considered ready for testing in humans.

2. Large numbers of animals may be needed to obtain valid preclinical data. Scientists are properly concerned about this situation, and progress has been made toward reducing the numbers required while still obtaining valid data. Cell and tissue culture in vitro methods and computer modeling are increasingly being used, but their predictive value is still limited. Nevertheless, some segments of the public attempt to halt all animal testing in the unfounded belief that it has become unnecessary.

3. Extrapolations of therapeutic index and toxicity data from animals to humans are reasonably predictive for many but not for all toxicities. Seeking an improved process, a Predictive Safety Testing Consortium of five of America's largest pharmaceutical companies with an advisory role by the Food and Drug Administration (FDA) has been formed to share internally developed laboratory methods to predict the safety of new treatments before they are tested in humans. In 2007, this group presented to the FDA a list of biomarkers for early kidney damage.

4. For statistical reasons, rare adverse effects are unlikely to be detected in preclinical testing.

EVALUATION IN HUMANS

Less than one third of the drugs tested in clinical trials reach the marketplace. Federal law in the USA and ethical considerations require that the study of new drugs in humans be conducted in accordance with stringent guidelines. Scientifically valid results are not guaranteed simply by conforming to government regulations, however, and the design and execution of a good clinical trial require interdisciplinary personnel including basic scientists, clinical pharmacologists, clinician specialists, statisticians, and others. The need for careful design and execution is based on three major confounding factors inherent in the study of any drug in humans.

Confounding Factors in Clinical Trials

A. The Variable Natural History of Most Diseases

Many diseases tend to wax and wane in severity; some disappear spontaneously, even, on occasion, cancer. A good experimental design takes into account the natural history of the disease by evaluating a large enough population of subjects over a sufficient period of time. Further protection against errors of interpretation caused by disease fluctuations is sometimes provided by using a **crossover design,** which consists of alternating periods of administration of test drug, placebo preparation (the control), and the standard treatment (positive control), if any, in each subject. These sequences are systematically varied, so that different subsets of patients receive each of the possible sequences of treatment.

B. The Presence of Other Diseases and Risk Factors

Known and unknown diseases and risk factors (including lifestyles of subjects) may influence the results of a clinical study. For example, some diseases alter the pharmacokinetics of drugs (see Chapters 3 and 4). Other drugs and some foods alter the pharmacokinetics of many drugs. Concentrations of blood or tissue components being monitored as a measure of the effect of the new agent may be influenced by other diseases or other drugs. Attempts to avoid this hazard usually involve the crossover technique (when feasible) and proper selection and assignment of patients to each of the study groups. This requires obtaining accurate diagnostic tests, medical and pharmacologic histories (including use of recreational drugs), and the use of statistically valid methods of randomization in assigning subjects to particular study groups. There is growing interest in analyzing genetic variations as part of the trial that may influence whether a person responds to a particular drug. It has been shown that age, gender, and pregnancy influence the pharmacokinetics of some drugs, but these factors have not been adequately studied because of legal restrictions and reluctance to expose these populations to unknown risks.

C. Subject and Observer Bias and Other Factors

Most patients tend to respond in a positive way to any therapeutic intervention by interested, caring, and enthusiastic medical personnel. The manifestation of this phenomenon in the subject is the **placebo response** (Latin, "I shall please") and may involve objective physiologic and biochemical changes as well as changes in subjective complaints associated with the disease. The placebo response is usually quantitated by administration of an inert material with exactly the same physical appearance, odor, consistency, etc, as the active dosage form. The magnitude of the response varies considerably from patient to patient and may also be influenced by the duration of the study. In some conditions, a positive response may be noted in as many as 30–40% of subjects given placebo. Placebo adverse effects and "toxicity" also occur but usually involve subjective effects: stomach upset, insomnia, sedation, and so on.

Subject bias effects can be quantitated—and minimized relative to the response measured during active therapy—by the **single-blind** design. This involves use of a placebo as described above, administered to the same subjects in a crossover design, if possible, or to a separate control group of well-matched subjects. Observer bias can be taken into account by disguising the identity of the medication being used—placebo or active form—from both the subjects and the personnel evaluating the subjects' responses (**double-blind** design). In this design, a third party holds the code identifying each medication packet, and the code is not broken until all the clinical data have been collected.

Drug effects seen in clinical trials are obviously affected by the patient taking the drugs at the dose and frequency prescribed. In a recent phase 2 study, one third of the patients who said they were taking the drug were found by blood analysis to have not taken the

Drug Studies—The Types of Evidence[*]

As described in this chapter, drugs are studied in a variety of ways, from 30-minute test tube experiments with isolated enzymes and receptors to decades-long observations of populations of patients. The conclusions that can be drawn from such different types of studies can be summarized as follows.

Basic research is designed to answer specific, usually single, questions under tightly controlled laboratory conditions, eg, does drug *x* inhibit enzyme *y*? The basic question may then be extended, eg, if drug *x* inhibits enzyme *y*, what is the concentration-response relationship? Such experiments are usually reproducible and often lead to reliable insights into the mechanism of the drug's action.

First-in-human studies include phase 1–3 trials. Once a drug receives FDA approval for use in humans, *case reports* and *case series* consist of observations by clinicians of the effects of drug (or other) treatments in one or more patients. These results often reveal unpredictable benefits and toxicities but do not generally test a prespecified hypothesis and cannot prove cause and effect. *Analytic epidemiologic studies* consist of observations designed to test a specified hypothesis, eg, that thiazolidinedione antidiabetic drugs are associated with adverse cardiovascular events. *Cohort* epidemiologic studies utilize populations of patients that have (exposed group) and have not (control group) been exposed to the agents under study and ask whether the exposed groups show a higher or lower incidence of the effect. *Case control* epidemiologic studies utilize populations of patients that have displayed the end point under study and ask whether they have been exposed or not exposed to the drugs in question. Such epidemiologic studies add weight to conjectures but cannot control all confounding variables and therefore cannot conclusively prove cause and effect.

Meta-analyses utilize rigorous evaluation and grouping of similar studies to increase the number of subjects studied and hence the statistical power of results obtained in multiple published studies. While the numbers may be dramatically increased by meta-analysis, the individual studies still suffer from their varying methods and end points and a meta-analysis cannot prove cause and effect. *Large randomized controlled trials* are designed to answer specific questions about the effects of medications on clinical end points or important surrogate end points, using large enough samples of patients and allocating them to control and experimental treatments using rigorous randomization methods. Randomization is the best method for distributing all foreseen confounding factors, as well as unknown confounders, equally between the experimental and control groups. When properly carried out, such studies are rarely invalidated and can be very convincing.

[*]I thank Ralph Gonzales, MD, for helpful comments.

---

drug. Confirmation of **compliance** with protocols (also known as **adherence**) is a necessary element to consider.

The various types of studies and the conclusions that may be drawn from them are described in the accompanying text box. (See Box: Drug Studies—The Types of Evidence.)

The Food & Drug Administration

The FDA is the administrative body that oversees the drug evaluation process in the USA and grants approval for marketing of new drug products. To receive FDA approval for marketing, the originating institution or company (almost always the latter) must submit evidence of safety and effectiveness. Outside the USA, the regulatory and drug approval process is generally similar to that in the USA.

As its name suggests, the FDA is also responsible for certain aspects of food safety, a role it shares with the US Department of Agriculture (USDA). Shared responsibility results in complications when questions arise regarding the use of drugs, eg, antibiotics, in food animals. A different type of problem arises when so-called food supplements are found to contain active drugs, eg, sildenafil analogs in "energy food" supplements.

The FDA's authority to regulate drugs derives from specific legislation (Table 5–2). If a drug has not been shown through adequately controlled testing to be "safe and effective" for a specific use, it cannot be marketed in interstate commerce for this use.[*]

Unfortunately, "safe" can mean different things to the patient, the physician, and society. Complete absence of risk is impossible to demonstrate, but this fact may not be understood by the public, who frequently assume that any medication sold with the approval of the FDA should be free of serious "side effects." This confusion is a major factor in litigation and dissatisfaction with aspects of drugs and medical care.

The history of drug regulation (Table 5–2) reflects several health events that precipitated major shifts in public opinion. The Pure Food and Drug Act of 1906 became law in response to revelations of unsanitary and unethical practices in the meat-packing industry. The Federal Food, Drug, and Cosmetic Act of 1938 was largely a reaction to deaths associated with the use of a preparation of sulfanilamide marketed before it and its vehicle were adequately

---

[*]Although the FDA does not directly control drug commerce within states, a variety of state and federal laws control interstate production and marketing of drugs.

TABLE 5–2 Some major legislation pertaining to drugs in the United States.

Law	Purpose and Effect
Pure Food and Drug Act of 1906	Prohibited mislabeling and adulteration of drugs.
Opium Exclusion Act of 1909	Prohibited importation of opium.
Amendment (1912) to the Pure Food and Drug Act	Prohibited false or fraudulent advertising claims.
Harrison Narcotic Act of 1914	Established regulations for use of opium, opiates, and cocaine (marijuana added in 1937).
Food, Drug, and Cosmetic Act of 1938	Required that new drugs be safe as well as pure (but did not require proof of efficacy). Enforcement by FDA.
Durham-Humphrey Act of 1952	Vested in the FDA the power to determine which products could be sold without prescription.
Kefauver-Harris Amendments (1962) to the Food, Drug, and Cosmetic Act	Required proof of efficacy as well as safety for new drugs and for drugs released since 1938; established guidelines for reporting of information about adverse reactions, clinical testing, and advertising of new drugs.
Comprehensive Drug Abuse Prevention and Control Act (1970)	Outlined strict controls in the manufacture, distribution, and prescribing of habit-forming drugs; established drug schedules and programs to prevent and treat drug addiction.
Orphan Drug Amendments of 1983	Provided incentives for development of drugs that treat diseases with less than 200,000 patients in USA.
Drug Price Competition and Patent Restoration Act of 1984	Abbreviated new drug applications for generic drugs. Required bioequivalence data. Patent life extended by amount of time drug delayed by FDA review process. Cannot exceed 5 extra years or extend to more than 14 years post-NDA approval.
Prescription Drug User Fee Act (1992, reauthorized 2007)	Manufacturers pay user fees for certain new drug applications.
Dietary Supplement Health and Education Act (1994)	Established standards with respect to dietary supplements but prohibited full FDA review of supplements and botanicals as drugs. Required the establishment of specific ingredient and nutrition information labeling that defines dietary supplements and classifies them as part of the food supply but allows unregulated advertising.
Bioterrorism Act of 2002	Enhanced controls on dangerous biologic agents and toxins. Seeks to protect safety of food, water, and drug supply.
Food and Drug Administration Amendments Act of 2007	Granted FDA greater authority over drug marketing, labeling, and direct-to-consumer advertising; required post-approval studies, established active surveillance systems, made clinical trial operations and results more visible to the public.

tested. The Kefauver-Harris amendments of 1962 were, in part, the result of a teratogenic drug disaster involving thalidomide. This agent was introduced in Europe in 1957–1958 and, based on animal tests then commonly used, was marketed as a "nontoxic" hypnotic and promoted as being especially useful during pregnancy. In 1961, reports were published suggesting that thalidomide was responsible for a dramatic increase in the incidence of a rare birth defect called phocomelia, a condition involving shortening or complete absence of the arms and legs. Epidemiologic studies provided strong evidence for the association of this defect with thalidomide use by women during the first trimester of pregnancy, and the drug was withdrawn from sale worldwide. An estimated 10,000 children were born with birth defects because of maternal exposure to this one agent. The tragedy led to the requirement for more extensive testing of new drugs for teratogenic effects and stimulated passage of the Kefauver-Harris Amendments of 1962, even though the drug was not then approved for use in the USA. In spite of its disastrous fetal toxicity and effects in pregnancy, thalidomide is a relatively safe drug for humans other than the fetus. Even the most serious risk of toxicities may be avoided or managed if understood, and despite its toxicity, thalidomide is

now approved by the FDA for limited use as a potent immunoregulatory agent and to treat certain forms of leprosy.

Clinical Trials: The IND & NDA

Once a new drug is judged ready to be studied in humans, a Notice of Claimed Investigational Exemption for a New Drug (IND) must be filed with the FDA (Figure 5–1). The IND includes (1) information on the composition and source of the drug, (2) chemical and manufacturing information, (3) all data from animal studies, (4) proposed plans for clinical trials, (5) the names and credentials of physicians who will conduct the clinical trials, and (6) a compilation of the key data relevant to study of the drug in humans that has been made available to investigators and their institutional review boards.

It often requires 4–6 years of clinical testing to accumulate and analyze all required data. Testing in humans is begun only after sufficient acute and subacute animal toxicity studies have been completed. Chronic safety testing in animals, including carcinogenicity studies, is usually done concurrently with clinical trials. In each of the three formal phases of clinical trials, volunteers or patients must be informed of the investigational status of the drug as well as the possible risks and must be allowed to decline or to consent to participate and receive the drug. These regulations are based on the ethical principles set forth in the Declaration of Helsinki (1966). In addition to the approval of the sponsoring organization and the FDA, an interdisciplinary institutional review board (IRB) at the facility where the clinical drug trial will be conducted must review and approve the scientific and ethical plans for testing in humans.

In **phase 1**, the effects of the drug as a function of dosage are established in a small number (20–100) of healthy volunteers. Although a goal is to find the maximum tolerated dose, the study is designed to prevent severe toxicity. If the drug is expected to have significant toxicity, as may be the case in cancer and AIDS therapy, volunteer patients with the disease are used in phase 1 rather than normal volunteers. Phase 1 trials are done to determine the probable limits of the safe clinical dosage range. These trials may be nonblind or "open"; that is, both the investigators and the subjects know what is being given. Alternatively, they may be "blinded" and placebo controlled. The choice of design depends on the drug, disease, goals of investigators, and ethical considerations. Many predictable toxicities are detected in this phase. Pharmacokinetic measurements of absorption, half-life, and metabolism are often done. Phase 1 studies are usually performed in research centers by specially trained clinical pharmacologists.

In **phase 2**, the drug is studied in patients with the target disease to determine its efficacy ("proof of concept"), and the doses to be used in any follow-on trials. A modest number of patients (100–200) are studied in detail. A single-blind design may be used, with an inert placebo medication and an established active drug (positive control) in addition to the investigational agent. Phase 2 trials are usually done in special clinical centers (eg, university hospitals). A broader range of toxicities may be detected in this phase. Phase 2 trials have the highest rate of drug failures, and only 25% of innovative drugs move on to phase 3.

In **phase 3**, the drug is evaluated in much larger numbers of patients with the target disease—usually thousands—to further establish and confirm safety and efficacy. Using information gathered in phases 1 and 2, phase 3 trials are designed to minimize errors caused by placebo effects, variable course of the disease, etc. Therefore, double-blind and crossover techniques are often used. Phase 3 trials are usually performed in settings similar to those anticipated for the ultimate use of the drug. Phase 3 studies can be difficult to design and execute and are usually expensive because of the large numbers of patients involved and the masses of data that must be collected and analyzed. The drug is formulated as intended for the market. The investigators are usually specialists in the disease being treated. Certain toxic effects, especially those caused by immunologic processes, may first become apparent in phase 3.

If phase 3 results meet expectations, application is made for permission to market the new agent. Marketing approval requires submission of a New Drug Application (NDA)—or for biologicals, a Biological License Application—to the FDA. The application contains, often in hundreds of volumes, full reports of all preclinical and clinical data pertaining to the drug under review. The number of subjects studied in support of the new drug application

has been increasing and currently averages more than 5000 patients for new drugs of novel structure (new molecular entities). The duration of the FDA review leading to approval (or denial) of the new drug application may vary from months to years. Priority approvals are designated for products that represent significant improvements compared with marketed products; in 2007, the median priority approval time was 6 months. Standard approvals, which take longer, are designated for products judged similar to those on the market—in 2007, the median standard approval time was 10.2 months. If problems arise, eg, unexpected but possibly serious toxicities, additional studies may be required and the approval process may extend to several years.

In cases in which an urgent need is perceived (eg, cancer chemotherapy), the process of preclinical and clinical testing and FDA review may be accelerated. For serious diseases, the FDA may permit extensive but controlled marketing of a new drug before phase 3 studies are completed; for life-threatening diseases, it may permit controlled marketing even before phase 2 studies have been completed. Roughly 50% of drugs in phase 3 trials involve early, controlled marketing. Such "accelerated approval" is usually granted with the requirement that careful monitoring of the effectiveness and toxicity of the drug be carried out and reported to the FDA. Unfortunately, FDA enforcement of this requirement has not always been adequate.

Once approval to market a drug has been obtained, **phase 4** begins. This constitutes monitoring the safety of the new drug under actual conditions of use in large numbers of patients. The importance of careful and complete reporting of toxicity by physicians after marketing begins can be appreciated by noting that many important drug-induced effects have an incidence of 1 in 10,000 or less and that some adverse effects may become apparent only after chronic dosing. The sample size required to disclose drug-induced events or toxicities is very large for such rare events. For example, several hundred thousand patients may have to be exposed before the first case is observed of a toxicity that occurs with an average incidence of 1 in 10,000. Therefore, low-incidence drug effects are not generally detected before phase 4 no matter how carefully the studies are executed. Phase 4 has no fixed duration. As with monitoring of drugs granted accelerated approval, phase 4 monitoring has often been lax.

The time from the filing of a patent application to approval for marketing of a new drug may be 5 years or considerably longer. Since the lifetime of a patent is 20 years in the USA, the owner of the patent (usually a pharmaceutical company) has exclusive rights for marketing the product for only a limited time after approval of the new drug application. Because the FDA review process can be lengthy, the time consumed by the review is sometimes added to the patent life. However, the extension (up to 5 years) cannot increase the total life of the patent to more than 14 years after approval of a new drug application. As of 2005, the average effective patent life for major pharmaceuticals was 11 years. After expiration of the patent, any company may produce the drug, file an abbreviated new drug application (ANDA), demonstrate required equivalence, and, with FDA approval, market the drug as a **generic** product without paying license fees to the original patent owner. Currently, 67% of prescriptions in the USA are for generic drugs. Even biotechnology-based drugs such as antibodies and other proteins are now qualifying for generic designation, and this has fueled regulatory concerns.

A **trademark** is the drug's proprietary trade name and is usually registered; this registered name may be legally protected as long as it is used. A generically equivalent product, unless specially licensed, cannot be sold under the trademark name and is often designated by the official generic name. Generic prescribing is described in Chapter 65.

The FDA drug approval process is one of the rate-limiting factors in the time it takes for a drug to be marketed and to reach patients. The Prescription Drug User Fee Act (PDUFA) of 1992, reauthorized in 2007, attempts to make more FDA resources available to the drug approval process and increase efficiency through use of fees collected from the drug companies that produce certain human drugs and biologic products. In 2009, the FDA approved 19 new molecular entity drug applications for new nonbiologic entities and six biological license applications, one more than in 2008. The traditional sequential and linear drug development process previously described is being increasingly modified in an attempt to safely accelerate clinical trials that provide "proof of mechanism" of action and "proof of concept" that the drug does work in the target disease. In these newer approaches, certain development activities such as full dose-response studies, final drug formulation work, and long-term toxicology studies may be deferred. It is hoped that this approach will focus resources on drugs more likely to succeed and minimize later-stage failures. In one example, a phase 0 (phase zero) clinical trial is designed to study the pharmacodynamic, pharmacokinetic properties of a drug and its links to useful biomarkers and measures of mechanism. Unlike a phase 1 trial with dose-response studies, in a phase 0 trial, a limited number of low doses are administered. These trials are not designed to be therapeutic.

Conflicts of Interest

Several factors in the development and marketing of drugs result in conflicts of interest. Use of pharmaceutical industry funding to support FDA approval processes raises the possibility of conflicts of interest within the FDA. Supporters of this policy point out that chronic FDA underfunding by the government allows for few alternatives. Another important source of conflicts of interest is the dependence of the FDA on outside panels of experts that are recruited from the scientific and clinical community to advise the government agency on questions regarding drug approval or withdrawal. Such experts are often recipients of grants from the companies producing the drugs in question. The need for favorable data in the new drug application leads to phase 2 and 3 trials in which the new agent is compared only to placebo, not to older, effective drugs. As a result, data regarding the efficacy and toxicity of the new drug *relative to a known effective agent* may not be available when the new drug is first marketed.

Manufacturers promoting a new agent may pay physicians to use it in preference to older drugs with which they are more familiar. Manufacturers sponsor small and often poorly designed clinical studies after marketing approval and aid in the publication of favorable results but may retard publication of unfavorable results. The need for physicians to meet continuing medical education (CME) requirements in order to maintain their licenses encourages manufacturers to sponsor conferences and courses, often in highly attractive vacation sites, and new drugs are often featured in such courses. Recognition of the obvious conflicts of interest is leading some clinical specialty organizations to reject industry support of such conferences. Finally, the common practice of distributing free samples of new drugs to practicing physicians has both positive and negative effects. The samples allow physicians to try out new drugs without incurring any cost to the patient. On the other hand, new drugs are usually much more expensive than older agents and when the free samples run out, the patient (or insurance carrier) may be forced to pay much more for treatment than if the older, cheaper, and possibly equally effective drug were used. Finally, when the patent for a drug is nearing expiration, the patent-holding manufacturer may try to extend its exclusive marketing privilege by paying generic manufacturers to *not* introduce a generic version ("pay to delay").

Translational Research

Unfortunately, the rate of introduction of new drugs has fallen during the last two decades. This has raised concerns about our ability to deal with the increasing prevalence of resistant microorganisms, and the problems of degenerative diseases in an aging population. In an effort to facilitate this process, the National Institutes of Health are currently (2011) considering the establishment of a new institute specializing in translational research.

Adverse Drug Reactions

An adverse drug event (ADE) or reaction to a drug (ADR) is a harmful or unintended response. Adverse drug reactions are claimed to be the fourth leading cause of death, higher than pulmonary disease, AIDS, accidents, and automobile deaths. The FDA has further estimated that 300,000 preventable adverse events occur in hospitals, many as a result of confusing medical information or lack of information (for example, regarding drug incompatibilities). Some adverse reactions, such as overdose, excessive effects, and drug interactions, may occur in anyone. Adverse reactions occurring only in susceptible patients include intolerance, idiosyncrasy (frequently genetic in origin), and allergy (usually immunologically mediated). During IND studies and clinical trials before FDA approval, all adverse events (serious, life-threatening, disabling, reasonably drug related, or unexpected) must be reported. After FDA approval to market a drug, surveillance, evaluation, and reporting must continue for any adverse events that are related to use of the drug, including overdose, accident, failure of expected action, events occurring from drug withdrawal, and unexpected events not listed in labeling. Events that are both serious and unexpected must be reported to the FDA within 15 days. In 2008, the FDA began publishing quarterly a list of drugs being investigated for potential safety risks. The ability to predict and avoid adverse drug reactions and optimize a drug's therapeutic index is an increasing focus of pharmacogenetic and personalized medicine.

It is hoped that greater use of electronic health records will reduce some of these risks (see Chapter 65).

Orphan Drugs & Treatment of Rare Diseases

Drugs for rare diseases—so-called orphan drugs—can be difficult to research, develop, and market. Proof of drug safety and efficacy in small populations must be established, but doing so is a complex process. Furthermore, because basic research in the pathophysiology and mechanisms of rare diseases receives relatively little attention or funding in both academic and industrial settings, recognized rational targets for drug action may be few. In addition, the cost of developing a drug can greatly influence priorities when the target population is relatively small. Funding for development of drugs for rare diseases or ignored diseases that do not receive priority attention from the traditional industry has received increasing support via philanthropy or similar funding from not-for-profit foundations such as the Cystic Fibrosis Foundation, the Huntington's Disease Society of America, and the Gates Foundation.

The Orphan Drug Amendments of 1983 provides incentives for the development of drugs for treatment of a rare disease or condition defined as "any disease or condition which (a) affects less than 200,000 persons in the U.S. or (b) affects more than 200,000 persons in the U.S. but for which there is no reasonable expectation that the cost of developing and making available in the U.S. a drug for such disease or condition will be recovered from sales in the U.S. of such drug." Since 1983, the FDA has approved for marketing more than 300 orphan drugs to treat more than 82 rare diseases.

REFERENCES

Avorn J: Debate about funding comparative effectiveness research. N Engl J Med 2009;360:1927.

Avorn J: *Powerful Medicines: The Benefits and Risks and Costs of Prescription Drugs.* Alfred A. Knopf, 2004.

Boutron I et al: Reporting and interpretation of randomized controlled trials with statistically nonsignificant results for primary outcomes. JAMA 2010;303:2058.

Brown WA: The placebo effect. Sci Am 1998;1:91.

DiMasi JA: Rising research and development costs for new drugs in a cost containment environment. J Health Econ 2003;22:151.

Editor's Page: Code of Ethics of the World Medical Association: Declaration of Helsinki. Clin Res 1966;14:193.

Evans RP: *Drug and Biological Development: From Molecule to Product and Beyond.* Springer, 2007.

FDA website: http://www.fda.gov

Ferrara N et al: Discovery and development of bevacizumab, an anti-VEGF antibody for treating cancer. Nat Rev Drug Discov 2004;3(5):391.

Grabowski H, Vernon J, DiMasi J: Returns on research and development for 1990s new drug introductions. Pharmacoeconomics 2002;20(Suppl 3):11.

Hennekens CH, DeMets D: Statistical association and causation. Contributions of different types of evidence. JAMA 2011;305:1134.

Hoffman GA, Harrington A, Fields, HK: Pain and the placebo response: What have we learned. Perspect Biol Med 2005;48:248.

Holaday JW, Berkowitz BA: Antiangiogenic drugs: Insights into drug development from endostatin, Avastin, and thalidomide. Mol Interv 2009;9:157.

Huang S-M, Temple R: Is this the drug or dose for you? Impact and consideration of ethnic factors in global drug development, regulatory review, and clinical practice. Clin Pharmacol Ther 2008;84:287; or http://www.fda.gov/cder/genomics/publications.htm

Hughes B: 2009 FDA drug approvals. Nat Rev Drug Discov 2010;9:89

Kesselheim AS et al: Whistle-blowers experiences in fraud litigation against pharmaceutical companies. N Engl J Med 2010;362:1832.

Lee C-J et al: *Clinical Trials of Drugs and Biopharmaceuticals.* CRC Publishing, 2005.

Lesko LJ: The critical path of warfarin dosing: Finding an optimal dosing strategy using pharmacogenetics. Clin Pharmacol Ther 2008;84:301; http://www.fda.gov/cder/genomics/publications.htm

Light DW: Global drug discovery: Europe is ahead. Health Affairs 2009;28:969.

Mogolian E, Mrydral P: What's the difference between brand-name and generic prescription drugs? Sci Am 2004;Dec 13; http://www.sciam.com/article.cfm?id=whats-the-difference-betw-2004-12-13

Ng R: *Drugs from Discovery to Approval.* Wiley-Blackwell, 2008.

Pharmaceutical Research and Manufacturers of America website: http://www.phrma.org

Rockey SJ, Collins FS: Managing financial conflict of interest in biomedical research. JAMA 2010;303:2400

Scheindlin S: Demystifying the new drug application. Molec Interventions 2004;4:188.

Sistare FD, DeGeorge JJ: Preclinical predictors of clinical safety: Opportunities for improvement. Clin Pharmacol Ther 2007;82(2):210.

Stevens AJ et al: The role of public sector research in the discovery of drugs and vaccines. N Engl J Med 2011;364:535.

CHAPTER

6

Introduction to Autonomic Pharmacology

Bertram G. Katzung, MD, PhD

CASE STUDY

A teenage boy is seen at the office of a dental surgeon for extraction of an impacted wisdom tooth. He is so nervous that the dentist decides to administer a sedative to calm the boy. After intravenous administration of the sedative (promethazine), the boy relaxes and the extraction is accomplished with no complications. However, when the boy stands up from the dental chair, he turns very pale and faints. Lying on the floor, he rapidly regains consciousness, but has a rapid heart rate of 120 bpm and a blood pressure of only 110/70 mm Hg. When he sits up, his heart rate increases to 140 bpm, his pressure drops to 80/40 mm Hg, and he complains of faintness. He is helped to a couch in the reception area, where he rests for 30 minutes. At the end of this time the boy is able to sit up without symptoms and, after an additional 15 minutes, is able to stand without difficulty. What autonomic effects might promethazine have that would explain the patient's signs and symptoms? Why did his heart rate increase when his blood pressure dropped?

The nervous system is conventionally divided into the central nervous system (CNS; the brain and spinal cord) and the peripheral nervous system (PNS; neuronal tissues outside the CNS). The motor (efferent) portion of the nervous system can be divided into two major subdivisions: autonomic and somatic. The **autonomic nervous system (ANS)** is largely independent (autonomous) in that its activities are not under direct conscious control. It is concerned primarily with visceral functions such as cardiac output, blood flow to various organs, and digestion, which are necessary for life. Evidence is accumulating that the ANS, especially the vagus nerve, also influences immune function and some CNS functions such as seizure discharge. The **somatic** subdivision is largely concerned with consciously controlled functions such as movement, respiration, and posture. Both systems have important afferent (sensory) inputs that provide information regarding the internal and external environments and modify motor output through reflex arcs of varying size and complexity.

The nervous system has several properties in common with the endocrine system, which is the other major system for control of body function. These include high-level integration in the brain, the ability to influence processes in distant regions of the body, and extensive use of negative feedback. Both systems use chemicals for the transmission of information. In the nervous system, chemical transmission occurs between nerve cells and between nerve cells and their effector cells. Chemical transmission takes place through the release of small amounts of transmitter substances from the nerve terminals into the synaptic cleft. The transmitter crosses the cleft by diffusion and activates or inhibits the postsynaptic cell by binding to a specialized receptor molecule. In a few cases, *retrograde* transmission may occur from the postsynaptic cell to the presynaptic neuron terminal and modify its subsequent activity.

By using drugs that mimic or block the actions of chemical transmitters, we can selectively modify many autonomic functions.

These functions involve a variety of effector tissues, including cardiac muscle, smooth muscle, vascular endothelium, exocrine glands, and presynaptic nerve terminals. Autonomic drugs are useful in many clinical conditions. Unfortunately, a very large number of drugs used for other purposes have unwanted effects on autonomic function (see Case Study).

ANATOMY OF THE AUTONOMIC NERVOUS SYSTEM

The ANS lends itself to division on anatomic grounds into two major portions: the **sympathetic (thoracolumbar)** division and the **parasympathetic (craniosacral)** division (Figure 6–1). Neurons in both divisions originate in nuclei within the CNS and give rise to preganglionic efferent fibers that exit from the brain stem or spinal cord and terminate in motor ganglia. The sympathetic preganglionic

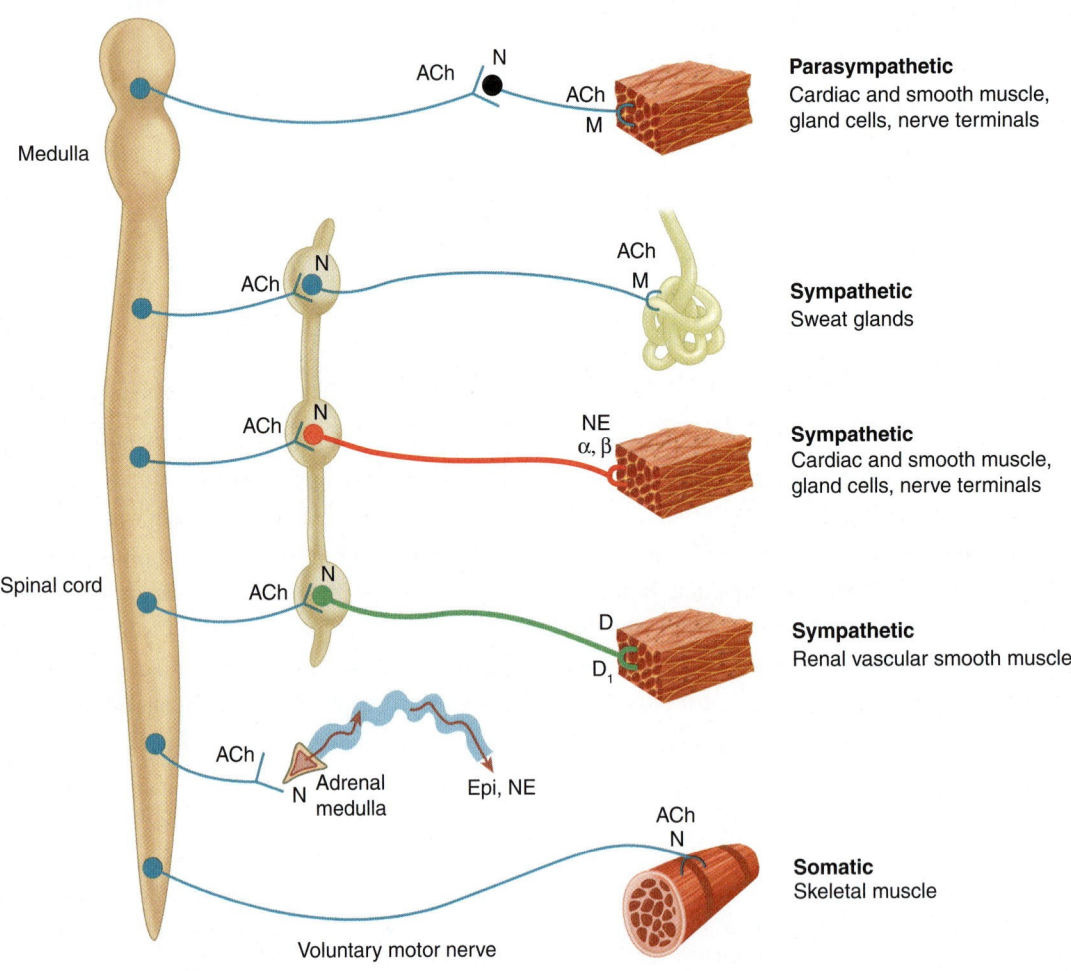

FIGURE 6–1 Schematic diagram comparing some anatomic and neurotransmitter features of autonomic and somatic motor nerves. Only the primary transmitter substances are shown. Parasympathetic ganglia are not shown because most are in or near the wall of the organ innervated. Cholinergic nerves are shown in blue; noradrenergic in red; and dopaminergic in green. Note that some sympathetic postganglionic fibers release acetylcholine or dopamine rather than norepinephrine. The adrenal medulla, a modified sympathetic ganglion, receives sympathetic preganglionic fibers and releases epinephrine and norepinephrine into the blood. ACh, acetylcholine; D, dopamine; Epi, epinephrine; M, muscarinic receptors; N, nicotinic receptors; NE, norepinephrine.

fibers leave the CNS through the thoracic and lumbar spinal nerves. The parasympathetic preganglionic fibers leave the CNS through the cranial nerves (especially the third, seventh, ninth, and tenth) and the third and fourth sacral spinal nerve roots.

Most sympathetic preganglionic fibers are short and terminate in ganglia located in the **paravertebral** chains that lie on either side of the spinal column. The remaining sympathetic preganglionic fibers are somewhat longer and terminate in **prevertebral ganglia,** which lie in front of the vertebrae, usually on the ventral surface of the aorta. From the ganglia, postganglionic sympathetic fibers run to the tissues innervated. Some preganglionic parasympathetic fibers terminate in parasympathetic ganglia located outside the organs innervated: the **ciliary, pterygopalatine, submandibular, otic,** and several **pelvic ganglia.** However, the majority of parasympathetic preganglionic fibers terminate on ganglion cells distributed diffusely or in networks in the walls of the innervated

organs. Note that the terms "sympathetic" and "parasympathetic" are anatomic designations and do not depend on the type of transmitter chemical released from the nerve endings nor on the kind of effect—excitatory or inhibitory—evoked by nerve activity.

In addition to these clearly defined peripheral motor portions of the ANS, large numbers of afferent fibers run from the periphery to integrating centers, including the enteric plexuses in the gut, the autonomic ganglia, and the CNS. Many of the sensory pathways that end in the CNS terminate in the integrating centers of the hypothalamus and medulla and evoke reflex motor activity that is carried to the effector cells by the efferent fibers described previously. There is increasing evidence that some of these sensory fibers also have peripheral motor functions.

The **enteric nervous system (ENS)** is a large and highly organized collection of neurons located in the walls of the gastrointestinal (GI) system (Figure 6–2). It is sometimes considered a third

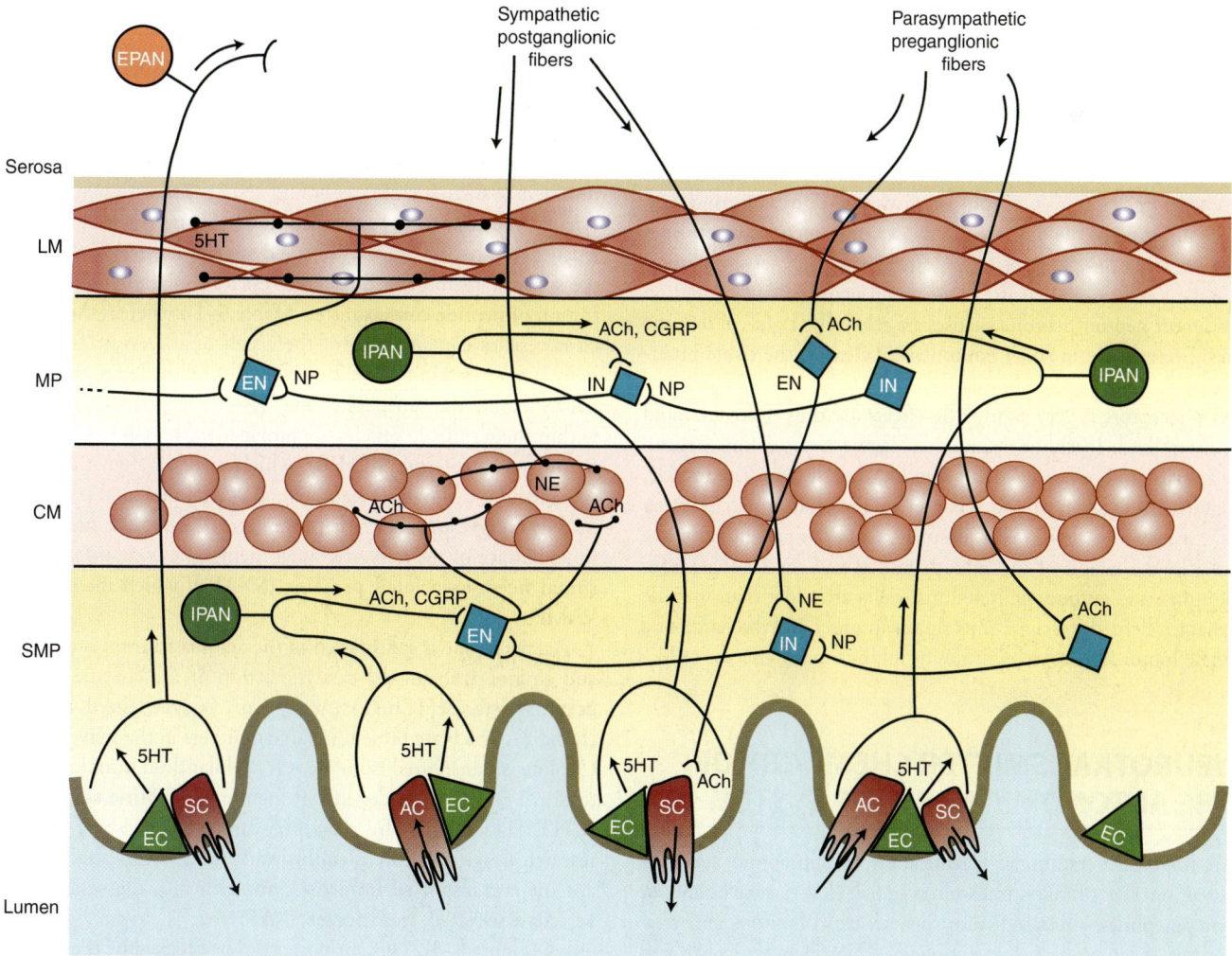

FIGURE 6–2 A highly simplified diagram of the intestinal wall and some of the circuitry of the enteric nervous system (ENS). The ENS receives input from both the sympathetic and the parasympathetic systems and sends afferent impulses to sympathetic ganglia and to the central nervous system. Many transmitter or neuromodulator substances have been identified in the ENS; see Table 6–1. ACh, acetylcholine; AC, absorptive cell; CM, circular muscle layer; EC, enterochromaffin cell; EN, excitatory neuron; EPAN, extrinsic primary afferent neuron; 5HT, serotonin; IN, inhibitory neuron; IPAN, intrinsic primary afferent neuron; LM, longitudinal muscle layer; MP, myenteric plexus; NE, norepinephrine; NP, neuropeptides; SC, secretory cell; SMP, submucosal plexus.

division of the ANS. It is found in the wall of the GI tract from the esophagus to the distal colon and is involved in both motor and secretory activities of the gut. It is particularly critical in the motor activity of the colon. The ENS includes the **myenteric plexus** (the plexus of Auerbach) and the **submucous plexus** (the plexus of Meissner). These neuronal networks receive preganglionic fibers from the parasympathetic system and postganglionic sympathetic axons. They also receive sensory input from within the wall of the gut. Fibers from the neuronal cell bodies in these plexuses travel forward, backward, and in a circular direction to the smooth muscle of the gut to control motility and to secretory cells in the mucosa. Sensory fibers transmit chemical and mechanical information from the mucosa and from stretch receptors to motor neurons in the plexuses and to postganglionic neurons in the sympathetic ganglia. The parasympathetic and sympathetic fibers that synapse on enteric plexus neurons appear to play a modulatory role, as indicated by the observation that deprivation of input from both ANS divisions does not abolish GI activity. In fact, selective denervation may result in greatly enhanced motor activity.

The ENS functions in a semiautonomous manner, utilizing input from the motor outflow of the ANS for modulation of GI activity and sending sensory information back to the CNS. The ENS also provides the necessary synchronization of impulses that, for example, ensures forward, not backward, propulsion of gut contents and relaxation of sphincters when the gut wall contracts.

The anatomy of autonomic synapses and junctions determines the localization of transmitter effects around nerve endings. Classic synapses such as the mammalian neuromuscular junction and most neuron-neuron synapses are relatively "tight" in that the nerve terminates in small boutons very close to the tissue innervated, so that the diffusion path from nerve terminal to postsynaptic receptors is very short. The effects are thus relatively rapid and localized. In contrast, junctions between autonomic neuron terminals and effector cells (smooth muscle, cardiac muscle, glands) differ from classic synapses in that transmitter is often released from a chain of varicosities in the postganglionic nerve fiber in the region of the smooth muscle cells rather than from boutons, and autonomic junctional clefts are wider than somatic synaptic clefts. Effects are thus slower in onset and discharge of a single motor fiber often activates or inhibits many effector cells.

NEUROTRANSMITTER CHEMISTRY OF THE AUTONOMIC NERVOUS SYSTEM

An important traditional classification of autonomic nerves is based on the primary transmitter molecules—acetylcholine or norepinephrine—released from their terminal boutons and varicosities. A large number of peripheral ANS fibers synthesize and release acetylcholine; they are **cholinergic** fibers; that is, they work by releasing acetylcholine. As shown in Figure 6–1, these include all preganglionic efferent autonomic fibers and the somatic (nonautonomic) motor fibers to skeletal muscle as well. Thus, almost all efferent fibers leaving the CNS are cholinergic. In addition, most parasympathetic postganglionic and a few sympathetic

postganglionic fibers are cholinergic. A significant number of parasympathetic postganglionic neurons utilize nitric oxide or peptides as the primary transmitter or cotransmitters.

Most postganglionic sympathetic fibers release norepinephrine (also known as noradrenaline); they are **noradrenergic** (often called simply "adrenergic") fibers; that is, they work by releasing norepinephrine (noradrenaline). These transmitter characteristics are presented schematically in Figure 6–1. As noted, some sympathetic fibers release acetylcholine. Dopamine is a very important transmitter in the CNS, and there is evidence that it may be released by some peripheral sympathetic fibers. Adrenal medullary cells, which are embryologically analogous to postganglionic sympathetic neurons, release a mixture of epinephrine and norepinephrine. Finally, most autonomic nerves also release several **cotransmitter** substances (described in the text that follows), in addition to the primary transmitters just described.

Five key features of neurotransmitter function provide potential targets for pharmacologic therapy: **synthesis, storage, release,** and **termination of action** of the transmitter, and **receptor effects.** These processes are discussed next.

Cholinergic Transmission

The terminals and varicosities of cholinergic neurons contain large numbers of small membrane-bound vesicles concentrated near the synaptic portion of the cell membrane (Figure 6–3) as well as a smaller number of large dense-cored vesicles located farther from the synaptic membrane. The large vesicles contain a high concentration of peptide cotransmitters (Table 6–1), whereas the smaller clear vesicles contain most of the acetylcholine. Vesicles are initially synthesized in the neuron cell body and carried to the terminal by axonal transport. They may also be recycled several times within the terminal. Vesicles are provided with **vesicle-associated membrane proteins (VAMPs),** which serve to align them with release sites on the inner neuronal cell membrane and participate in triggering the release of transmitter. The release site on the inner surface of the nerve terminal membrane contains **synaptosomal nerve-associated proteins (SNAPs),** which interact with VAMPs.

Acetylcholine is synthesized in the cytoplasm from acetyl-CoA and choline through the catalytic action of the enzyme **choline acetyltransferase (ChAT).** Acetyl-CoA is synthesized in mitochondria, which are present in large numbers in the nerve ending. Choline is transported from the extracellular fluid into the neuron terminal by a sodium-dependent membrane **choline transporter (CHT;** Figure 6–3). This symporter can be blocked by a group of research drugs called **hemicholiniums.** Once synthesized, acetylcholine is transported from the cytoplasm into the vesicles by a **vesicle-associated transporter (VAT)** that is driven by proton efflux (Figure 6–3). This antiporter can be blocked by the research drug **vesamicol.** Acetylcholine synthesis is a rapid process capable of supporting a very high rate of transmitter release. Storage of acetylcholine is accomplished by the packaging of "quanta" of acetylcholine molecules (usually 1000 to 50,000 molecules in each vesicle). Most of the vesicular acetylcholine (ACh) is bound to negatively charged **vesicular proteoglycan (VPG).**

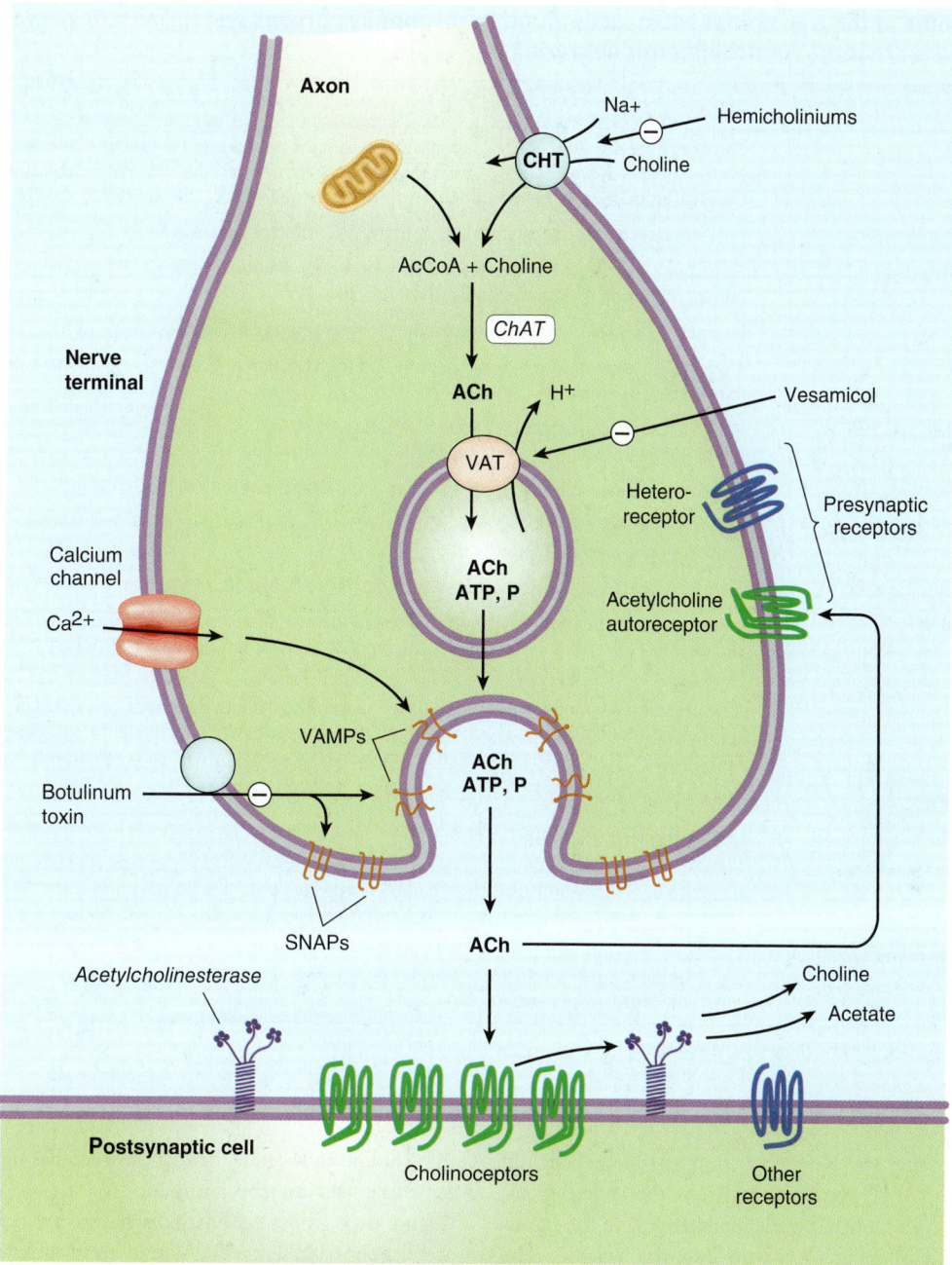

FIGURE 6–3 Schematic illustration of a generalized cholinergic junction (not to scale). Choline is transported into the presynaptic nerve terminal by a sodium-dependent choline transporter (CHT). This transporter can be inhibited by hemicholinium drugs. In the cytoplasm, acetylcholine is synthesized from choline and acetyl-CoA (AcCoA) by the enzyme choline acetyltransferase (ChAT). Acetylcholine is then transported into the storage vesicle by a second carrier, the vesicle-associated transporter (VAT), which can be inhibited by vesamicol. Peptides (P), adenosine triphosphate (ATP), and proteoglycan are also stored in the vesicle. Release of transmitter occurs when voltage-sensitive calcium channels in the terminal membrane are opened, allowing an influx of calcium. The resulting increase in intracellular calcium causes fusion of vesicles with the surface membrane and exocytotic expulsion of acetylcholine and cotransmitters into the junctional cleft (see text). This step can be blocked by botulinum toxin. Acetylcholine's action is terminated by metabolism by the enzyme acetylcholinesterase. Receptors on the presynaptic nerve ending modulate transmitter release. SNAPs, synaptosome-associated proteins; VAMPs, vesicle-associated membrane proteins.

Vesicles are concentrated on the inner surface of the nerve terminal facing the synapse through the interaction of so-called SNARE proteins on the vesicle (a subgroup of VAMPs called v-SNAREs, especially **synaptobrevin**) and on the inside of the terminal cell membrane (SNAPs called t-SNAREs, especially **syntaxin** and **SNAP-25**). Physiologic release of transmitter from the vesicles is dependent on extracellular calcium and occurs when an action potential reaches the terminal and triggers sufficient

TABLE 6–1 Some of the transmitter substances found in autonomic nervous system, enteric nervous system, and nonadrenergic, noncholinergic neurons.[1]

Substance	Probable Roles
Acetylcholine (ACh)	The primary transmitter at ANS ganglia, at the somatic neuromuscular junction, and at parasympathetic postganglionic nerve endings. A primary excitatory transmitter to smooth muscle and secretory cells in the ENS. Probably also the major neuron-to-neuron ("ganglionic") transmitter in the ENS.
Adenosine triphosphate (ATP)	Acts as a transmitter or cotransmitter at many ANS-effector synapses.
Calcitonin gene-related peptide (CGRP)	Found with substance P in cardiovascular sensory nerve fibers. Present in some secretomotor ENS neurons and interneurons. A cardiac stimulant.
Cholecystokinin (CCK)	May act as a cotransmitter in some excitatory neuromuscular ENS neurons.
Dopamine	A modulatory transmitter in some ganglia and the ENS. Probably a postganglionic sympathetic transmitter in renal blood vessels.
Enkephalin and related opioid peptides	Present in some secretomotor and interneurons in the ENS. Appear to inhibit ACh release and thereby inhibit peristalsis. May *stimulate* secretion.
Galanin	Present in secretomotor neurons; may play a role in appetite-satiety mechanisms.
GABA (γ-aminobutyric acid)	May have presynaptic effects on excitatory ENS nerve terminals. Has some relaxant effect on the gut. Probably not a major transmitter in the ENS.
Gastrin-releasing peptide (GRP)	Extremely potent excitatory transmitter to gastrin cells. Also known as mammalian bombesin.
Neuropeptide Y (NPY)	Found in many noradrenergic neurons. Present in some secretomotor neurons in the ENS and may inhibit secretion of water and electrolytes by the gut. Causes long-lasting vasoconstriction. It is also a cotransmitter in some parasympathetic postganglionic neurons.
Nitric oxide (NO)	A cotransmitter at inhibitory ENS and other neuromuscular junctions; may be especially important at sphincters. Cholinergic nerves innervating blood vessels appear to activate the synthesis of NO by vascular endothelium. NO is synthesized on demand by nitric oxide synthase, NOS, not stored; see Chapter 19.
Norepinephrine (NE)	The primary transmitter at most sympathetic postganglionic nerve endings.
Serotonin (5-HT)	An important transmitter or cotransmitter at excitatory neuron-to-neuron junctions in the ENS.
Substance P, related tachykinins	Substance P is an important sensory neuron transmitter in the ENS and elsewhere. Tachykinins appear to be excitatory cotransmitters with ACh at ENS neuromuscular junctions. Found with CGRP in cardiovascular sensory neurons. Substance P is a vasodilator (probably via release of nitric oxide).
Vasoactive intestinal peptide (VIP)	Excitatory secretomotor transmitter in the ENS; may also be an inhibitory ENS neuromuscular cotransmitter. A probable cotransmitter in many cholinergic neurons. A vasodilator (found in many perivascular neurons) and cardiac stimulant.

[1]See Chapter 21 for transmitters found in the central nervous system.

influx of calcium ions via N-type calcium channels. Calcium interacts with the VAMP **synaptotagmin** on the vesicle membrane and triggers fusion of the vesicle membrane with the terminal membrane and opening of a pore into the synapse. The opening of the pore and inrush of cations results in release of the acetylcholine from the proteoglycan and exocytotic expulsion into the synaptic cleft. One depolarization of a somatic motor nerve may release several hundred quanta into the synaptic cleft. One depolarization of an autonomic postganglionic nerve varicosity or terminal probably releases less and releases it over a larger area. In addition to acetylcholine, several cotransmitters are released at the same time (Table 6–1). The acetylcholine vesicle release process is blocked by **botulinum toxin** through the enzymatic removal of two amino acids from one or more of the fusion proteins.

After release from the presynaptic terminal, acetylcholine molecules may bind to and activate an acetylcholine receptor (**cholinoceptor**). Eventually (and usually very rapidly), all of the acetylcholine released diffuses within range of an **acetylcholinesterase (AChE)** molecule. AChE very efficiently splits acetylcholine

into choline and acetate, neither of which has significant transmitter effect, and thereby terminates the action of the transmitter (Figure 6–3). Most cholinergic synapses are richly supplied with acetylcholinesterase; the half-life of acetylcholine molecules in the synapse is therefore very short (a fraction of a second). Acetylcholinesterase is also found in other tissues, eg, red blood cells. (Other cholinesterases with a lower specificity for acetylcholine, including butyrylcholinesterase [pseudocholinesterase], are found in blood plasma, liver, glia, and many other tissues.)

Adrenergic Transmission

Adrenergic neurons (Figure 6–4) transport a precursor amino acid (tyrosine) into the nerve ending, then synthesize the catecholamine transmitter (Figure 6–5), and finally store it in membrane-bound vesicles. In most sympathetic postganglionic neurons, norepinephrine is the final product. In the adrenal medulla and certain areas of the brain, some norepinephrine is further converted to epinephrine. In dopaminergic neurons, synthesis terminates with

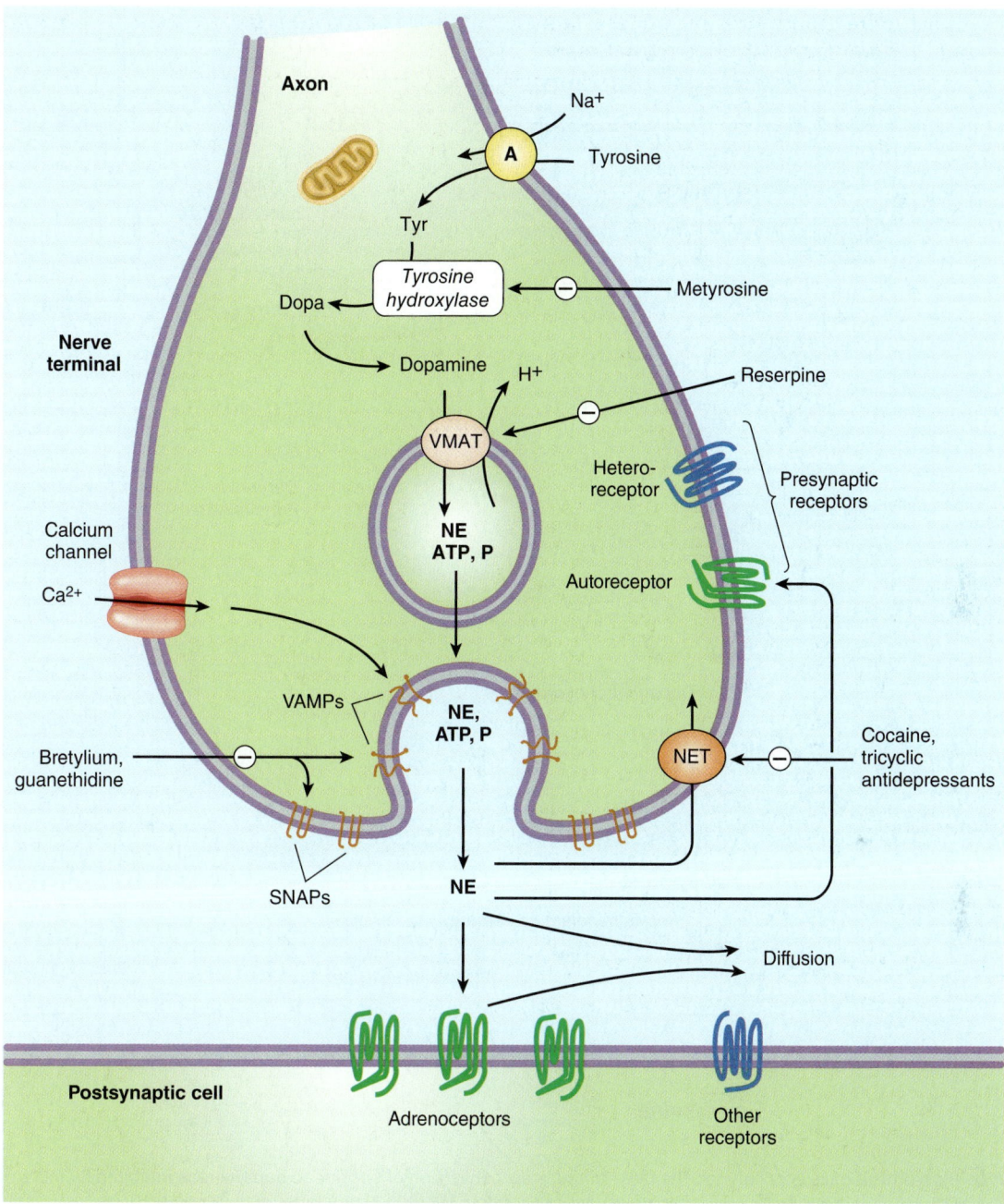

FIGURE 6–4 Schematic diagram of a generalized noradrenergic junction (not to scale). Tyrosine is transported into the noradrenergic ending or varicosity by a sodium-dependent carrier (A). Tyrosine is converted to dopamine (see Figure 6–5 for details), and transported into the vesicle by the vesicular monoamine transporter (VMAT), which can be blocked by reserpine. The same carrier transports norepinephrine (NE) and several other amines into these granules. Dopamine is converted to NE in the vesicle by dopamine-β-hydroxylase. Physiologic release of transmitter occurs when an action potential opens voltage-sensitive calcium channels and increases intracellular calcium. Fusion of vesicles with the surface membrane results in expulsion of norepinephrine, cotransmitters, and dopamine-β-hydroxylase. Release can be blocked by drugs such as guanethidine and bretylium. After release, norepinephrine diffuses out of the cleft or is transported into the cytoplasm of the terminal by the norepinephrine transporter (NET), which can be blocked by cocaine and tricyclic antidepressants, or into postjunctional or perijunctional cells. Regulatory receptors are present on the presynaptic terminal. SNAPs, synaptosome-associated proteins; VAMPs, vesicle-associated membrane proteins.

dopamine. Several processes in these nerve terminals are potential sites of drug action. One of these, the conversion of tyrosine to dopa, is the rate-limiting step in catecholamine transmitter synthesis. It can be inhibited by the tyrosine analog **metyrosine.** A high-affinity antiporter for catecholamines located in the wall of

the storage vesicle (**vesicular monoamine transporter, VMAT**) can be inhibited by the **reserpine** alkaloids. Reserpine causes depletion of transmitter stores. Another transporter (**norepinephrine transporter, NET**) carries norepinephrine and similar molecules back into the cell cytoplasm from the synaptic cleft

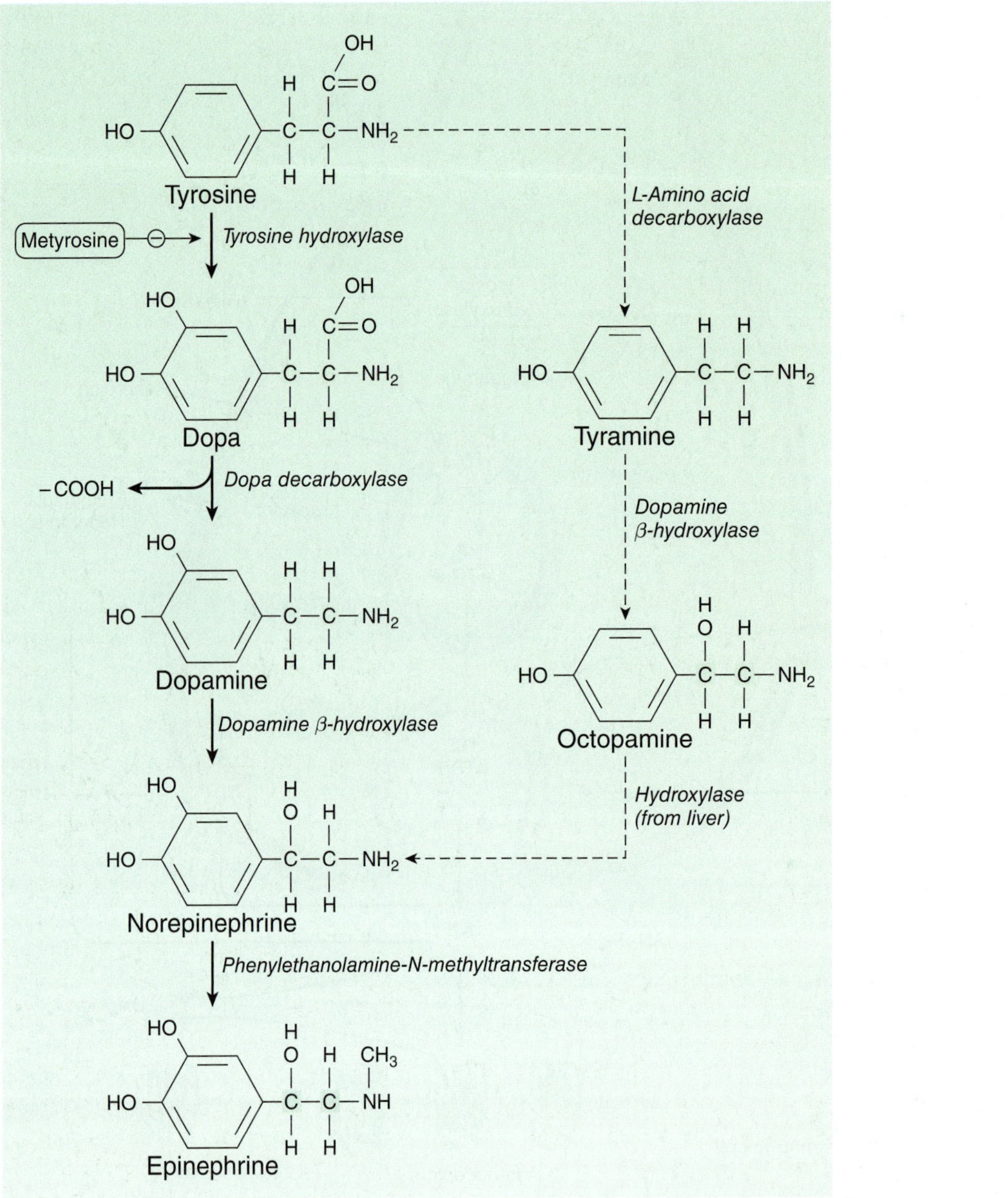

FIGURE 6–5 Biosynthesis of catecholamines. The rate-limiting step, conversion of tyrosine to dopa, can be inhibited by metyrosine (α-methyltyrosine). The alternative pathway shown by the dashed arrows has not been found to be of physiologic significance in humans. However, tyramine and octopamine may accumulate in patients treated with monoamine oxidase inhibitors. (Reproduced, with permission, from Greenspan FS, Gardner DG [editors]: *Basic and Clinical Endocrinology,* 7th ed. McGraw-Hill, 2003.)

(Figure 6–4; NET). NET is also commonly called uptake 1 or reuptake 1 and is partially responsible for the termination of synaptic activity. NET can be inhibited by **cocaine** and **tricyclic antidepressant** drugs, resulting in an increase of transmitter activity in the synaptic cleft (see Box: Neurotransmitter Uptake Carriers).

Release of the vesicular transmitter store from noradrenergic nerve endings is similar to the calcium-dependent process previously described for cholinergic terminals. In addition to the primary transmitter (norepinephrine), adenosine triphosphate (ATP), dopamine-β-hydroxylase, and peptide cotransmitters are also released into the synaptic cleft. Indirectly acting and mixed sympathomimetics, eg, **tyramine, amphetamines,** and **ephedrine,** are capable of releasing stored transmitter from noradrenergic nerve endings by a calcium-independent process. These drugs are poor agonists (some are inactive) at adrenoceptors, but they are excellent substrates for monoamine transporters. As a result, they are avidly taken up into noradrenergic nerve endings by NET. In the nerve ending, they are then transported by VMAT into the vesicles, displacing norepinephrine, which is subsequently expelled into the synaptic space by reverse transport via NET. Amphetamines

Neurotransmitter Uptake Carriers

As noted in Chapter 1, several large families of transport proteins have been identified. The most important of these are the ABC (ATP-Binding Cassette) and SLC (SoLute Carrier) transporter families. As indicated by the name, the ABC carriers utilize ATP for transport. The SLC proteins are cotransporters and in most cases, use the movement of sodium down its concentration gradient as the energy source. Under some circumstances, they also transport transmitters in the reverse direction in a sodium-independent fashion.

NET, SLC6A2, the norepinephrine transporter, is a member of the SLC family, as are similar transporters responsible for the reuptake of dopamine (**DAT,** SLC6A3) and 5-HT (serotonin, **SERT,** SLC6A4) into the neurons that release these transmitters. These transport proteins are found in peripheral tissues and in the CNS wherever neurons utilizing these transmitters are located.

NET is important in the peripheral actions of cocaine and the amphetamines. In the CNS, NET and SERT are important targets of several antidepressant drug classes (see Chapter 30). The most important inhibitory transmitter in the CNS, γ-aminobutyric acid (GABA), is the substrate for at least three SLC transporters: GAT1, GAT2, and GAT3. GAT1 is the target of an antiseizure medication (see Chapter 24). Other SLC proteins transport glutamate, the major excitatory CNS transmitter.

---

also inhibit monoamine oxidase and have other effects that result in increased norepinephrine activity in the synapse. Their action does not require vesicle exocytosis.

Norepinephrine and epinephrine can be metabolized by several enzymes, as shown in Figure 6–6. Because of the high activity of monoamine oxidase in the mitochondria of the nerve terminal, there is significant turnover of norepinephrine even in the resting terminal. Since the metabolic products are excreted in the urine, an estimate of catecholamine turnover can be obtained from laboratory analysis of total metabolites (sometimes referred to as "VMA and metanephrines") in a 24-hour urine sample. However, metabolism is not the primary mechanism for termination of action of norepinephrine physiologically released from noradrenergic nerves. Termination of noradrenergic transmission results from two processes: simple diffusion away from the receptor site (with eventual metabolism in the plasma or liver) and reuptake into the nerve terminal by NET (Figure 6–4) or into perisynaptic glia or other cells.

Cotransmitters in Cholinergic & Adrenergic Nerves

As previously noted, the vesicles of both cholinergic and adrenergic nerves contain other substances in addition to the primary transmitter, sometimes in the same vesicles and sometimes in a

separate vesicle population. Some of the substances identified to date are listed in Table 6–1. Many of these substances are also *primary* transmitters in the nonadrenergic, noncholinergic nerves described in the text that follows. They appear to play several roles in the function of nerves that release acetylcholine or norepinephrine. In some cases, they provide a faster or slower action to supplement or modulate the effects of the primary transmitter. They also participate in feedback inhibition of the same and nearby nerve terminals.

AUTONOMIC RECEPTORS

Historically, structure-activity analyses, with careful comparisons of the potency of series of autonomic agonist and antagonist analogs, led to the definition of different autonomic receptor subtypes, including muscarinic and nicotinic cholinoceptors, and α, β, and dopamine adrenoceptors (Table 6–2). Subsequently, binding of isotope-labeled ligands permitted the purification and characterization of several of the receptor molecules. Molecular biology now provides techniques for the discovery and expression of genes that code for related receptors within these groups (see Chapter 2).

The primary acetylcholine receptor subtypes were named after the alkaloids originally used in their identification: muscarine and nicotine, thus **muscarinic** and **nicotinic receptors.** In the case of receptors associated with noradrenergic nerves, the use of the names of the agonists (noradrenaline, phenylephrine, isoproterenol, and others) was not practicable. Therefore, the term **adrenoceptor** is widely used to describe receptors that respond to catecholamines such as norepinephrine. By analogy, the term **cholinoceptor** denotes receptors (both muscarinic and nicotinic) that respond to acetylcholine. In North America, receptors were colloquially named after the nerves that usually innervate them; thus, **adrenergic** (or noradrenergic) **receptors** and **cholinergic receptors.** The general class of adrenoceptors can be further subdivided into **α-adrenoceptor, β-adrenoceptor,** and **dopaminereceptor** types on the basis of both agonist and antagonist selectivity and on genomic grounds. Development of more selective blocking drugs has led to the naming of subclasses within these major types; for example, within the α-adrenoceptor class, α_1 and α_2 receptors differ in both agonist and antagonist selectivity. Specific examples of such selective drugs are given in the chapters that follow.

NONADRENERGIC, NONCHOLINERGIC (NANC) NEURONS

It has been known for many years that autonomic effector tissues (eg, gut, airways, bladder) contain nerve fibers that do not show the histochemical characteristics of either cholinergic or adrenergic fibers. Both motor and sensory NANC fibers are present. Although peptides are the most common transmitter substances found in these nerve endings, other substances, eg, nitric oxide synthase and purines, are also present in many nerve terminals (Table 6–1). Capsaicin, a neurotoxin derived from chili peppers, can cause the

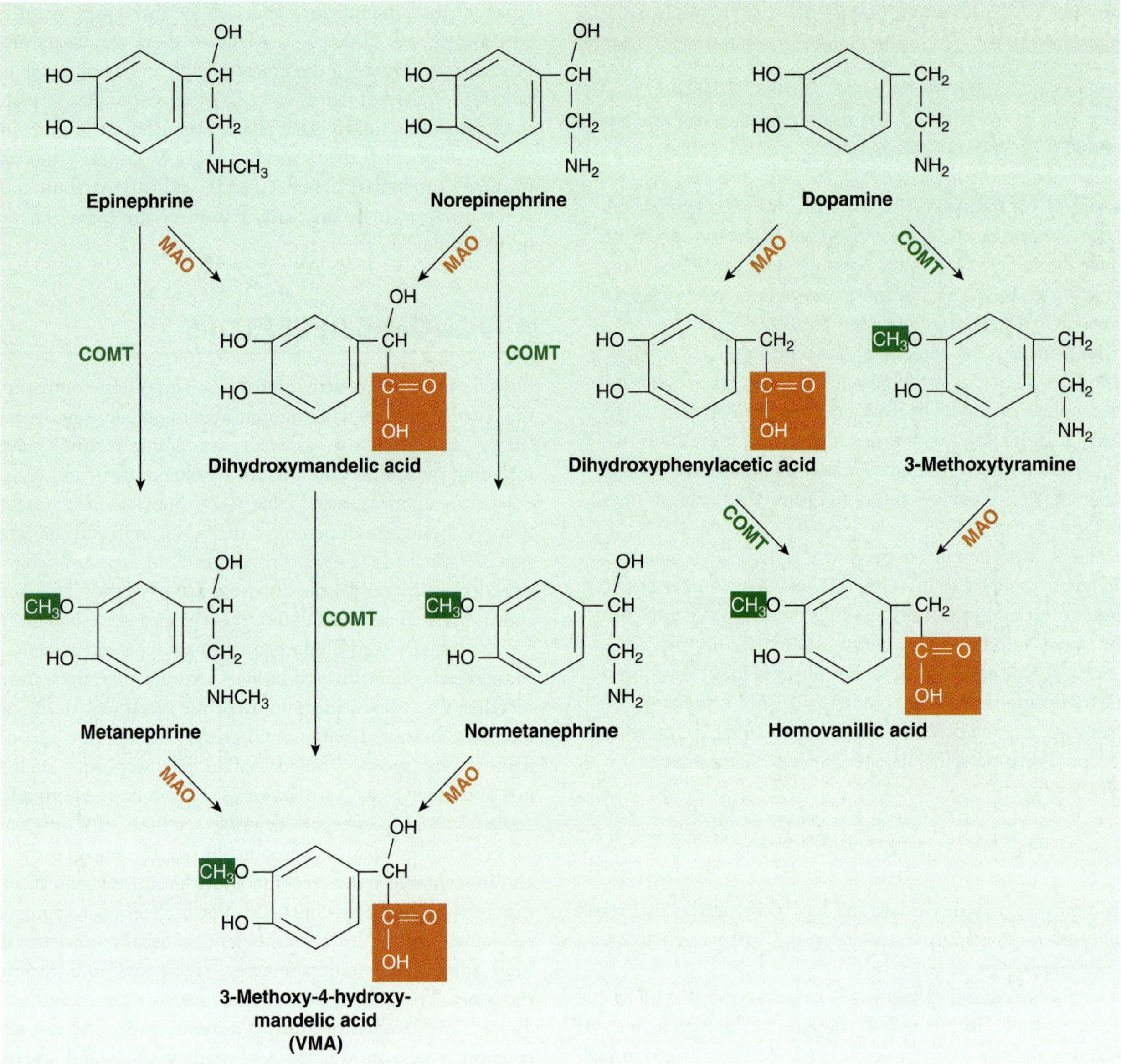

FIGURE 6–6 Metabolism of catecholamines by catechol-*O*-methyltransferase (COMT) and monoamine oxidase (MAO). (Modified and reproduced, with permission, from Greenspan FS, Gardner DG [editors]: *Basic and Clinical Endocrinology,* 7th ed. McGraw-Hill, 2003.)

release of transmitter (especially substance P) from such neurons and, if given in high doses, destruction of the neuron.

The enteric system in the gut wall (Figure 6–2) is the most extensively studied system containing NANC neurons in addition to cholinergic and adrenergic fibers. In the small intestine, for example, these neurons contain one or more of the following: nitric oxide synthase (which produces nitric oxide; NO), calcitonin gene-related peptide, cholecystokinin, dynorphin, enkephalins, gastrin-releasing peptide, 5-hydroxytryptamine (serotonin), neuropeptide Y, somatostatin, substance P, and vasoactive intestinal peptide (VIP). Some neurons contain as many as five different transmitters.

The sensory fibers in the nonadrenergic, noncholinergic systems are probably better termed "sensory-efferent" or "sensory-local effector" fibers because, when activated by a sensory input,

they are capable of releasing transmitter peptides from the sensory ending itself, from local axon branches, and from collaterals that terminate in the autonomic ganglia. These peptides are potent agonists in many autonomic effector tissues.

FUNCTIONAL ORGANIZATION OF AUTONOMIC ACTIVITY

Autonomic function is integrated and regulated at many levels, from the CNS to the effector cells. Most regulation uses negative feedback, but several other mechanisms have been identified. Negative feedback is particularly important in the responses of the ANS to the administration of autonomic drugs.

TABLE 6–2 Major autonomic receptor types.

Receptor Name	Typical Locations	Result of Ligand Binding
Cholinoceptors		
Muscarinic M_1	CNS neurons, sympathetic postganglionic neurons, some presynaptic sites	Formation of IP_3 and DAG, increased intracellular calcium
Muscarinic M_2	Myocardium, smooth muscle, some presynaptic sites; CNS neurons	Opening of potassium channels, inhibition of adenylyl cyclase
Muscarinic M_3	Exocrine glands, vessels (smooth muscle and endothelium); CNS neurons	Like M_1 receptor-ligand binding
Muscarinic M_4	CNS neurons; possibly vagal nerve endings	Like M_2 receptor-ligand binding
Muscarinic M_5	Vascular endothelium, especially cerebral vessels; CNS neurons	Like M_1 receptor-ligand binding
Nicotinic N_N	Postganglionic neurons, some presynaptic cholinergic terminals; receptors typically contain two $\alpha3$ and one $\beta4$ type subunits in addition to γ and δ subunits	Opening of Na^+, K^+ channels, depolarization
Nicotinic N_M	Skeletal muscle neuromuscular end plates; receptors typically contain two $\alpha1$ and $\beta1$ type subunits in addition to γ and δ subunits	Opening of Na^+, K^+ channels, depolarization
Adrenoceptors		
Alpha$_1$	Postsynaptic effector cells, especially smooth muscle	Formation of IP_3 and DAG, increased intracellular calcium
Alpha$_2$	Presynaptic adrenergic nerve terminals, platelets, lipocytes, smooth muscle	Inhibition of adenylyl cyclase, decreased cAMP
Beta$_1$	Postsynaptic effector cells, especially heart, lipocytes, brain; presynaptic adrenergic and cholinergic nerve terminals, juxtaglomerular apparatus of renal tubules, ciliary body epithelium	Stimulation of adenylyl cyclase, increased cAMP
Beta$_2$	Postsynaptic effector cells, especially smooth muscle and cardiac muscle	Stimulation of adenylyl cyclase and increased cAMP. Activates cardiac G_i under some conditions.
Beta$_3$	Postsynaptic effector cells, especially lipocytes; heart	Stimulation of adenylyl cyclase and increased cAMP[1]
Dopamine receptors		
D_1 (DA$_1$), D_5	Brain; effector tissues, especially smooth muscle of the renal vascular bed	Stimulation of adenylyl cyclase and increased cAMP
D_2 (DA$_2$)	Brain; effector tissues, especially smooth muscle; presynaptic nerve terminals	Inhibition of adenylyl cyclase; increased potassium conductance
D_3	Brain	Inhibition of adenylyl cyclase
D_4	Brain, cardiovascular system	Inhibition of adenylyl cyclase

[1]Cardiac β_3-receptor function is poorly understood, but activation does *not* appear to result in stimulation of rate or force.

Central Integration

At the highest level—midbrain and medulla—the two divisions of the ANS and the endocrine system are integrated with each other, with sensory input, and with information from higher CNS centers, including the cerebral cortex. These interactions are such that early investigators called the parasympathetic system a **trophotropic** one (ie, leading to growth) used to "rest and digest" and the sympathetic system an **ergotropic** one (ie, leading to energy expenditure), which is activated for "fight or flight." Although such terms offer little insight into the mechanisms involved, they do provide simple descriptions applicable to many of the actions of the systems (Table 6–3). For example, slowing of the heart and stimulation of digestive activity are typical energy-conserving and storing actions of the parasympathetic system. In contrast, cardiac stimulation, increased blood sugar, and cutaneous vasoconstriction are responses produced by sympathetic discharge that are suited to fighting or surviving attack.

At a more subtle level of interactions in the brain stem, medulla, and spinal cord, there are important cooperative interactions between the parasympathetic and sympathetic systems. For some organs, sensory fibers associated with the parasympathetic system exert reflex control over motor outflow in the sympathetic system. Thus, the sensory carotid sinus baroreceptor fibers in the glossopharyngeal nerve have a major influence on sympathetic outflow from the vasomotor center. This example is described in greater detail in the following text. Similarly, parasympathetic sensory fibers in the wall of the urinary bladder significantly influence sympathetic inhibitory outflow to that organ. Within the ENS, sensory fibers from the wall of the gut synapse on both preganglionic and postganglionic motor cells that control intestinal smooth muscle and secretory cells (Figure 6–2).

Integration of Cardiovascular Function

Autonomic reflexes are particularly important in understanding cardiovascular responses to autonomic drugs. As indicated in Figure 6–7, the primary controlled variable in cardiovascular function is **mean arterial pressure.** Changes in any variable contributing to mean arterial pressure (eg, a drug-induced increase in peripheral vascular resistance) evoke powerful **homeostatic** secondary responses that tend to compensate for the directly evoked

TABLE 6–3 Direct effects of autonomic *nerve* activity on some organ systems. Autonomic *drug* effects are similar but not identical (see text).

Organ	Effect of			
	Sympathetic Activity		**Parasympathetic Activity**	
	Action[1]	**Receptor**[2]	**Action**	**Receptor**[2]
Eye				
Iris radial muscle	Contracts	α_1	...	...
Iris circular muscle	...	...	Contracts	M_3
Ciliary muscle	[Relaxes]	β	Contracts	M_3
Heart				
Sinoatrial node	Accelerates	β_1, β_2	Decelerates	M_2
Ectopic pacemakers	Accelerates	β_1, β_2	...	...
Contractility	Increases	β_1, β_2	Decreases (atria)	M_2
Blood vessels				
Skin, splanchnic vessels	Contracts	α	...	...
Skeletal muscle vessels	Relaxes	β_2	...	...
	[Contracts]	α	...	...
	Relaxes[3]	M_3	...	...
Endothelium of vessels in heart, brain, viscera	...	...	Synthesizes and releases EDRF[4]	M_3, M_5[5]
Bronchiolar smooth muscle	Relaxes	β_2	Contracts	M_3
Gastrointestinal tract				
Smooth muscle				
Walls	Relaxes	$\alpha_2,$ [6]β_2	Contracts	M_3
Sphincters	Contracts	α_1	Relaxes	M_3
Secretion	...	...	Increases	M_3
Genitourinary smooth muscle				
Bladder wall	Relaxes	β_2	Contracts	M_3
Sphincter	Contracts	α_1	Relaxes	M_3
Uterus, pregnant	Relaxes	β_2	...	...
	Contracts	α	Contracts	M_3
Penis, seminal vesicles	Ejaculation	α	Erection	M
Skin				
Pilomotor smooth muscle	Contracts	α	...	...
Sweat glands			...	...
Eccrine	Increases	M	...	...
Apocrine (stress)	Increases	α	...	...
Metabolic functions				
Liver	Gluconeogenesis	β_2, α	...	...
Liver	Glycogenolysis	β_2, α	...	...
Fat cells	Lipolysis	β_3	...	...
Kidney	Renin release	β_1	...	...

[1]Less important actions are shown in brackets.

[2]Specific receptor type: α, alpha; β, beta; M, muscarinic.

[3]Vascular smooth muscle in skeletal muscle has sympathetic cholinergic dilator fibers.

[4]The endothelium of most blood vessels releases EDRF (endothelium-derived relaxing factor), which causes marked vasodilation, in response to muscarinic stimuli. Parasympathetic fibers innervate muscarinic receptors in vessels in the viscera and brain, and sympathetic cholinergic fibers innervate skeletal muscle blood vessels. The muscarinic receptors in the other vessels of the peripheral circulation are not innervated and respond only to circulating muscarinic agonists.

[5]Cerebral blood vessels dilate in response to M_5 receptor activation.

[6]Probably through presynaptic inhibition of parasympathetic activity.

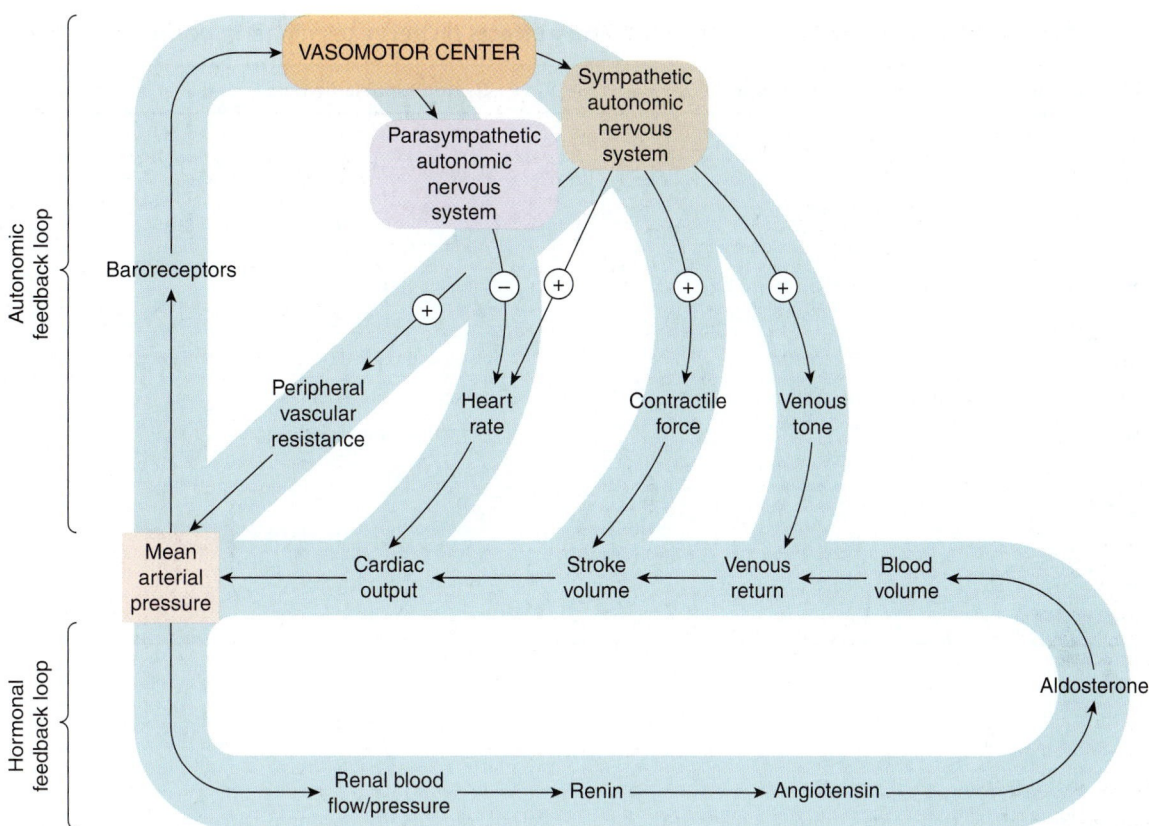

FIGURE 6–7 Autonomic and hormonal control of cardiovascular function. Note that two feedback loops are present: the autonomic nervous system loop and the hormonal loop. The sympathetic nervous system directly influences four major variables: peripheral vascular resistance, heart rate, force, and venous tone. It also directly modulates renin production (not shown). The parasympathetic nervous system directly influences heart rate. In addition to its role in stimulating aldosterone secretion, angiotensin II directly increases peripheral vascular resistance and facilitates sympathetic effects (not shown). The net feedback effect of each loop is to compensate for changes in arterial blood pressure. Thus, decreased blood pressure due to blood loss would evoke increased sympathetic outflow and renin release. Conversely, elevated pressure due to the administration of a vasoconstrictor drug would cause reduced sympathetic outflow, reduced renin release, and increased parasympathetic (vagal) outflow.

change. The homeostatic response may be sufficient to reduce the change in mean arterial pressure and to reverse the drug's effects on heart rate. A slow infusion of norepinephrine provides a useful example. This agent produces direct effects on both vascular and cardiac muscle. It is a powerful vasoconstrictor and, by increasing peripheral vascular resistance, increases mean arterial pressure. In the absence of reflex control—in a patient who has had a heart transplant, for example—the drug's effect on the heart is also stimulatory; that is, it increases heart rate and contractile force. However, in a subject with intact reflexes, the negative feedback response to increased mean arterial pressure causes decreased sympathetic outflow to the heart and a powerful increase in parasympathetic (vagus nerve) discharge at the cardiac pacemaker. This response is mediated by increased firing by the baroreceptor nerves of the carotid sinus and the aortic arch. Increased baroreceptor activity causes the changes mentioned in central sympathetic and vagal outflow. As a result, the *net* effect of ordinary pressor doses of norepinephrine in a normal subject is to produce a marked increase in peripheral vascular resistance, an increase in mean arterial pressure, and a consistent *slowing*

of heart rate. Bradycardia, the reflex compensatory response elicited by this agent, is the *exact opposite* of the drug's direct action; yet it is completely predictable if the integration of cardiovascular function by the ANS is understood.

Presynaptic Regulation

The principle of negative feedback control is also found at the presynaptic level of autonomic function. Important presynaptic feedback inhibitory control mechanisms have been shown to exist at most nerve endings. A well-documented mechanism involves the α_2 receptor located on noradrenergic nerve terminals. This receptor is activated by norepinephrine and similar molecules; activation diminishes further release of norepinephrine from these nerve endings (Table 6–4). The mechanism of this G protein-mediated effect involves inhibition of the inward calcium current that causes vesicular fusion and transmitter release. Conversely, a presynaptic β receptor appears to facilitate the release of norepinephrine from some adrenergic neurons. Presynaptic receptors

TABLE 6–4 Autoreceptor, heteroreceptor, and modulatory effects on nerve terminals in peripheral synapses.[1]

Transmitter/Modulator	Receptor Type	Neuron Terminals Where Found
Inhibitory effects		
Acetylcholine	M_2, M_1	Adrenergic, enteric nervous system
Norepinephrine	Alpha$_2$	Adrenergic
Dopamine	D_2; less evidence for D_1	Adrenergic
Serotonin (5-HT)	5-HT$_1$, 5-HT$_2$, 5-HT$_3$	Cholinergic preganglionic
ATP and adenosine	P_2 (ATP), P_1 (adenosine)	Adrenergic autonomic and ENS cholinergic neurons
Histamine	H_3, possibly H_2	H_3 type identified on CNS adrenergic and serotonergic neurons
Enkephalin	Delta (also mu, kappa)	Adrenergic, ENS cholinergic
Neuropeptide Y	Y_1, Y_2 (NPY)	Adrenergic, some cholinergic
Prostaglandin E$_1$, E$_2$	EP$_3$	Adrenergic
Excitatory effects		
Epinephrine	Beta$_2$	Adrenergic, somatic motor cholinergic
Acetylcholine	N_M	Somatic motor cholinergic
Angiotensin II	AT$_1$	Adrenergic

[1]A provisional list. The number of transmitters and locations will undoubtedly increase with additional research.

that respond to the primary transmitter substance released by the nerve ending are called **autoreceptors.** Autoreceptors are usually inhibitory, but in addition to the excitatory β receptors on noradrenergic fibers, many cholinergic fibers, especially somatic motor fibers, have excitatory nicotinic autoreceptors.

Control of transmitter release is not limited to modulation by the transmitter itself. Nerve terminals also carry regulatory receptors that respond to many other substances. Such **heteroreceptors** may be activated by substances released from other nerve terminals that synapse with the nerve ending. For example, some vagal fibers in the myocardium synapse on sympathetic noradrenergic nerve terminals and inhibit norepinephrine release. Alternatively, the ligands for these receptors may diffuse to the receptors from the blood or from nearby tissues. Some of the transmitters and receptors identified to date are listed in Table 6–4. Presynaptic regulation by a variety of endogenous chemicals probably occurs in all nerve fibers.

Postsynaptic Regulation

Postsynaptic regulation can be considered from two perspectives: modulation by previous activity at the primary receptor (which may up- or down-regulate receptor number or desensitize receptors; see Chapter 2), and modulation by other simultaneous events.

The first mechanism has been well documented in several receptor-effector systems. Up-regulation and down-regulation are known to occur in response to decreased or increased activation, respectively, of the receptors. An extreme form of up-regulation occurs after denervation of some tissues, resulting in **denervation supersensitivity** of the tissue to activators of that receptor type. In

skeletal muscle, for example, nicotinic receptors are normally restricted to the end-plate regions underlying somatic motor nerve terminals. Surgical denervation results in marked proliferation of nicotinic cholinoceptors over all parts of the fiber, including areas not previously associated with any motor nerve junctions. A pharmacologic supersensitivity related to denervation supersensitivity occurs in autonomic effector tissues after administration of drugs that deplete transmitter stores and prevent activation of the postsynaptic receptors for a sufficient period of time. For example, prolonged administration of large doses of reserpine, a norepinephrine depleter, can cause increased sensitivity of the smooth muscle and cardiac muscle effector cells served by the depleted sympathetic fibers.

The second mechanism involves modulation of the primary transmitter-receptor event by events evoked by the same or other transmitters acting on different postsynaptic receptors. Ganglionic transmission is a good example of this phenomenon (Figure 6–8). The postganglionic cells are activated (depolarized) as a result of binding of an appropriate ligand to a neuronal nicotinic (N_N) acetylcholine receptor. The resulting fast **excitatory postsynaptic potential (EPSP)** evokes a propagated action potential if threshold is reached. This event is often followed by a small and slowly developing but longer-lasting hyperpolarizing afterpotential—a slow **inhibitory postsynaptic potential (IPSP).** This hyperpolarization involves opening of potassium channels by M_2 cholinoceptors. The IPSP is followed by a small, slow excitatory postsynaptic potential caused by closure of potassium channels linked to M_1 cholinoceptors. Finally, a late, very slow EPSP may be evoked by peptides released from other fibers. These slow potentials serve to modulate the responsiveness of the postsynaptic cell to subsequent primary

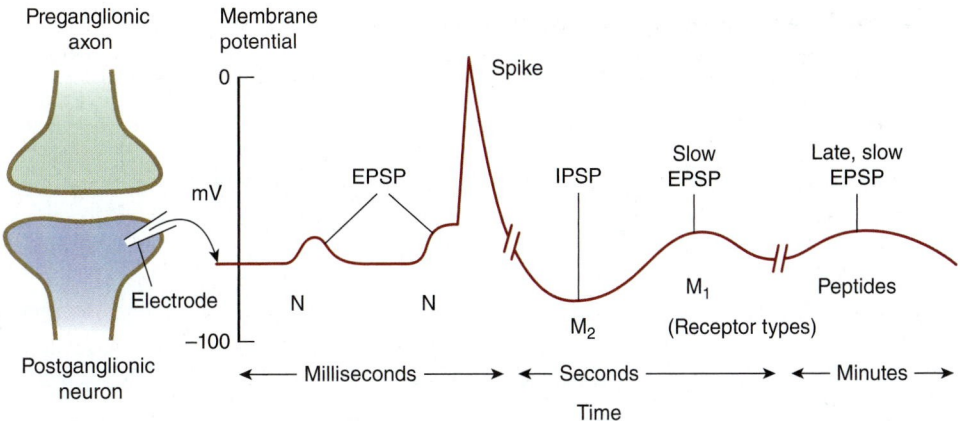

FIGURE 6–8 Excitatory and inhibitory postsynaptic potentials (EPSP and IPSP) in an autonomic ganglion cell. The postganglionic neuron shown at the left with a recording electrode might undergo the membrane potential changes shown schematically in the recording. The response begins with two EPSP responses to nicotinic (N) receptor activation, the first not reaching threshold. The second, suprathreshold, EPSP evokes an action potential, which is followed by an IPSP, probably evoked by M_2 receptor activation (with possible participation from dopamine receptor activation). The IPSP is, in turn, followed by a slower, M_1-dependent EPSP, and this is sometimes followed by a still slower peptide-induced excitatory postsynaptic potential.

excitatory presynaptic nerve activity. (See Chapter 21 for additional examples.)

PHARMACOLOGIC MODIFICATION OF AUTONOMIC FUNCTION

Because transmission involves different mechanisms in different segments of the ANS, some drugs produce highly specific effects, whereas others are much less selective in their actions.

A summary of the steps in transmission of impulses, from the CNS to the autonomic effector cells, is presented in Table 6–5. Drugs that block action potential propagation (local anesthetics and some natural toxins) are very nonselective in their action, since they act on a process that is common to all neurons. On the other hand, drugs that act on the biochemical processes involved in transmitter synthesis and storage are more selective, since the biochemistry of each transmitter differs, eg, norepinephrine synthesis is very different from acetylcholine synthesis. Activation or blockade of effector cell receptors offers maximum

Pharmacology of the Eye

The eye is a good example of an organ with multiple autonomic functions, controlled by several autonomic receptors. As shown in Figure 6–9, the anterior chamber is the site of several autonomic effector tissues. These tissues include three muscles (pupillary dilator and constrictor muscles in the iris and the ciliary muscle) and the secretory epithelium of the ciliary body.

Parasympathetic nerve activity and muscarinic cholinomimetics mediate contraction of the circular pupillary constrictor muscle and of the ciliary muscle. Contraction of the pupillary constrictor muscle causes miosis, a reduction in pupil size. Miosis is usually present in patients exposed to large systemic or small topical doses of cholinomimetics, especially organophosphate cholinesterase inhibitors. Ciliary muscle contraction causes accommodation of focus for near vision. Marked contraction of the ciliary muscle, which often occurs with cholinesterase inhibitor

intoxication, is called *cyclospasm*. Ciliary muscle contraction also puts tension on the trabecular meshwork, opening its pores and facilitating outflow of the aqueous humor into the canal of Schlemm. Increased outflow reduces intraocular pressure, a very useful result in patients with glaucoma. All of these effects are prevented or reversed by muscarinic blocking drugs such as atropine.

Alpha adrenoceptors mediate contraction of the radially oriented pupillary dilator muscle fibers in the iris and result in mydriasis. This occurs during sympathetic discharge and when α-agonist drugs such as phenylephrine are placed in the conjunctival sac. Beta adrenoceptors on the ciliary epithelium facilitate the secretion of aqueous humor. Blocking these receptors (with β-blocking drugs) reduces the secretory activity and reduces intraocular pressure, providing another therapy for glaucoma.

TABLE 6–5 Steps in autonomic transmission: Effects of drugs.

Process Affected	Drug Example	Site	Action
Action potential propagation	Local anesthetics, tetrodotoxin,[1] saxitoxin[2]	Nerve axons	Block voltage-gated sodium channels; block conduction
Transmitter synthesis	Hemicholiniums	Cholinergic nerve terminals: membrane	Block uptake of choline and slow synthesis
	α-Methyltyrosine (metyrosine)	Adrenergic nerve terminals and adrenal medulla: cytoplasm	Inhibits tyrosine hydroxylase and blocks synthesis of catecholamines
Transmitter storage	Vesamicol	Cholinergic terminals: VAT on vesicles	Prevents storage, depletes
	Reserpine	Adrenergic terminals: VMAT on vesicles	Prevents storage, depletes
Transmitter release	Many[3]	Nerve terminal membrane receptors	Modulate release
	ω-Conotoxin GVIA[4]	Nerve terminal calcium channels	Reduces transmitter release
	Botulinum toxin	Cholinergic vesicles	Prevents release
	α-Latrotoxin[5]	Cholinergic and adrenergic vesicles	Causes explosive transmitter release
	Tyramine, amphetamine	Adrenergic nerve terminals	Promote transmitter release
Transmitter reuptake after release	Cocaine, tricyclic antidepressants	Adrenergic nerve terminals, NET	Inhibit uptake; increase transmitter effect on postsynaptic receptors
Receptor activation or blockade	Norepinephrine	Receptors at adrenergic junctions	Binds α receptors; causes contraction
	Phentolamine	Receptors at adrenergic junctions	Binds α receptors; prevents activation
	Isoproterenol	Receptors at adrenergic junctions	Binds β receptors; activates adenylyl cyclase
	Propranolol	Receptors at adrenergic junctions	Binds β receptors; prevents activation
	Nicotine	Receptors at nicotinic cholinergic junctions (autonomic ganglia, neuromuscular end plates)	Binds nicotinic receptors; opens ion channel in postsynaptic membrane
	Tubocurarine	Neuromuscular end plates	Prevents activation
	Bethanechol	Receptors, parasympathetic effector cells (smooth muscle, glands)	Binds and activates muscarinic receptors
	Atropine	Receptors, parasympathetic effector cells	Binds muscarinic receptors; prevents activation
Enzymatic inactivation of transmitter	Neostigmine	Cholinergic synapses (acetylcholinesterase)	Inhibits enzyme; prolongs and intensifies transmitter action
	Tranylcypromine	Adrenergic nerve terminals (monoamine oxidase)	Inhibits enzyme; increases stored transmitter pool

[1]Toxin of puffer fish, California newt.

[2]Toxin of *Gonyaulax* (red tide organism).

[3]Norepinephrine, dopamine, acetylcholine, angiotensin II, various prostaglandins, etc.

[4]Toxin of marine snails of the genus *Conus*.

[5]Black widow spider venom.

VAT, vesicle-associated transporter; VMAT, vesicular monoamine transporter; NET, norepinephrine transporter.

flexibility and selectivity of effect attainable with currently available drugs: adrenoceptors are easily distinguished from cholinoceptors. Furthermore, individual receptor subgroups can often be selectively activated or blocked within each major type. Some examples are given in the Box: Pharmacology of the Eye. Even greater selectivity may be attainable in the future using drugs that target post-traditional receptor processes, eg, receptors for second messengers.

The next four chapters provide many more examples of this useful diversity of autonomic control processes.

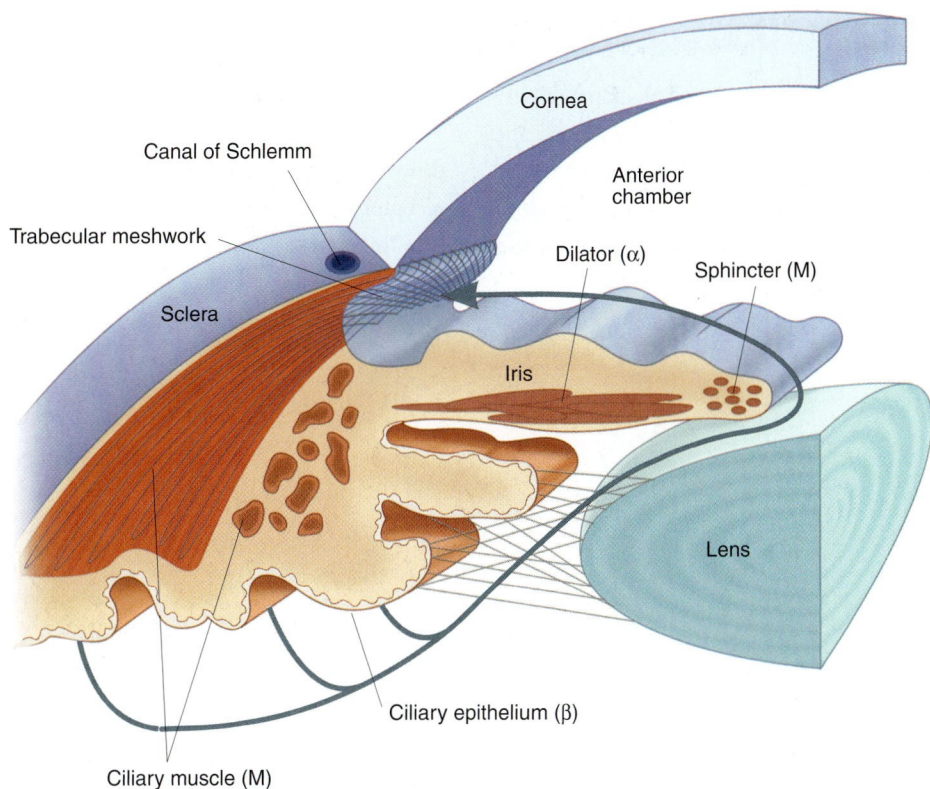

FIGURE 6–9 Structures of the anterior chamber of the eye. Tissues with significant autonomic functions and the associated ANS receptors are shown in this schematic diagram. Aqueous humor is secreted by the epithelium of the ciliary body, flows into the space in front of the iris, flows through the trabecular meshwork, and exits via the canal of Schlemm (*arrow*). Blockade of the β adrenoceptors associated with the ciliary epithelium causes decreased secretion of aqueous. Blood vessels (not shown) in the sclera are also under autonomic control and influence aqueous drainage.

REFERENCES

Andersson K-E, Wein AJ: Pharmacology of the lower urinary tract: Basis for current and future treatments of urinary incontinence. Pharmacol Rev 2004;56:581.

Bengel FM et al: Clinical determinants of ventricular sympathetic reinnervation after orthotopic heart transplantation. Circulation 2002;106:831.

Birdsall NJM: Class A GPCR heterodimers: Evidence from binding studies. Trends Pharmacol Sci 2010;31:499.

Boehm S, Kubista H: Fine tuning of sympathetic transmitter release via ionotropic and metabotropic presynaptic receptors. Pharmacol Rev 2002;54:43.

Broten TP et al: Role of endothelium-derived relaxing factor in parasympathetic coronary vasodilation. Am J Physiol 1992;262:H1579.

Burnstock G: Non-synaptic transmission at autonomic neuroeffector junctions. Neurochem Int 2008;52:14.

Fagerlund MJ, Eriksson LI: Current concepts in neuromuscular transmission. Br J Anaesthesia 2009;103:108.

Freeman R: Neurogenic orthostatic hypotension. N Engl J Med 2008;358:615.

Furchgott RF: Role of endothelium in responses of vascular smooth muscle to drugs. Annu Rev Pharmacol Toxicol 1984;24:175.

Galligan JJ: Ligand-gated ion channels in the enteric nervous system. Neurogastroenterol Motil 2002;14:611.

Gershon MD, Tack J: The serotonin signaling system: From basic understanding to drug development for functional GI disorders. Gastroenterology 2007;132:397.

Goldstein DS et al: Dysautonomias: Clinical disorders of the autonomic nervous system. Ann Intern Med 2002;137:753.

Johnston GR, Webster NR: Cytokines and the immunomodulatory function of the vagus nerve. Br J Anaesthesiol 2009;102:453.

Kirstein SL, Insel PA: Autonomic nervous system pharmacogenomics: A progress report. Pharmacol Rev 2004;56:31.

Langer SZ: Presynaptic receptors regulating transmitter release. Neurochem Int 2008;52:26.

Mikoshiba K: IP$_3$ receptor/Ca^{2+} channel: From discovery to new signaling concepts. J Neurochem 2007;102:1426.

Shibasaki M, Crandall CG: Mechanisms and controllers of eccrine sweating in humans. Front Biosci (Schol Ed) 2011;2:685.

Symposium: Gastrointestinal Reviews. Curr Opin Pharmacol 2007;7:555.

Tobin G, Giglio D, Lundgren O: Muscarinic receptor subtypes in the alimentary tract. J Physiol Pharmacol 2009;60:3.

Toda N, Herman AG: Gastrointestinal function regulation by nitrergic efferent nerves. Pharmacol Rev 2005;57:315.

Vernino S, Hopkins S, Wang Z: Autonomic ganglia, acetylcholine antibodies, and autoimmune gangliopathy. Auton Neurosci 2009;146:3.

Verrier RL, Tan A: Heart rate, autonomic markers, and cardiac mortality. Heart Rhythm 2009;6 (Suppl 11):S68.

Westfall DP, Todorov LD, Mihaylova-Todorova ST: ATP as a cotransmitter in sympathetic nerves and its inactivation by releasable enzymes. J Pharmacol Exp Ther 2002;303:439.

Whittaker VP: Some currently neglected aspects of cholinergic function. J Mol Neurosci 2010;40:7

CASE STUDY ANSWER

Promethazine has potent α-adrenoceptor blocking activity in addition to its sedative, antianxiety effect. As a result, the normal autonomic response to postural change (sympathetic vasoconstriction upon standing up) was temporarily lost in the patient in this case. Marked orthostatic hypotension and syncope resulted with transient recovery upon lying down. The heart rate increased when the baroreceptors detected the drop in blood pressure because promethazine blocks α receptors (dominant in the vessels) but not β receptors (dominant in the heart).

Cholinoceptor-Activating & Cholinesterase-Inhibiting Drugs

Achilles J. Pappano, PhD

CASE STUDY

In mid-afternoon, a coworker brings 43-year-old JM to the emergency department because he is unable to continue picking vegetables. His gait is unsteady and he walks with support from his colleague. JM has difficulty speaking and swallowing, his vision is blurred, and his eyes are filled with tears. His coworker notes that JM was working in a field that had been sprayed early in the morning with a material that had the odor of sulfur. Within 3 hours after starting his work, JM complained of tightness in his chest that made breathing difficult, and he called for help before becoming disoriented.

How would you proceed to evaluate and treat JM? What should be done for his coworker?

Acetylcholine-receptor stimulants and cholinesterase inhibitors make up a large group of drugs that mimic acetylcholine (cholinomimetic agents) (Figure 7–1). Cholinoceptor stimulants are classified pharmacologically by their spectrum of action, depending on the type of receptor—muscarinic or nicotinic—that is activated. Cholinomimetics are also classified by their mechanism of action because some bind directly to (and activate) cholinoceptors whereas others act indirectly by inhibiting the hydrolysis of endogenous acetylcholine.

SPECTRUM OF ACTION OF CHOLINOMIMETIC DRUGS

Early studies of the parasympathetic nervous system showed that the alkaloid **muscarine** mimicked the effects of parasympathetic nerve discharge; that is, the effects were **parasympathomimetic.** Application of muscarine to ganglia and to autonomic effector tissues (smooth muscle, heart, exocrine glands) showed that the parasympathomimetic action of the alkaloid occurred through an action on receptors at effector cells, not those in ganglia. The effects of acetylcholine itself and of other cholinomimetic drugs at autonomic neuroeffector junctions are called *parasympathomimetic effects* and are mediated by **muscarinic receptors.** In contrast, low concentrations of the alkaloid **nicotine** stimulated autonomic ganglia and skeletal muscle neuromuscular junctions but not autonomic effector cells. The ganglion and skeletal muscle receptors were therefore labeled nicotinic. When acetylcholine was later identified as the physiologic transmitter at both muscarinic and **nicotinic receptors,** both receptors were recognized as cholinoceptor subtypes.

Cholinoceptors are members of either G protein–linked (muscarinic) or ion channel (nicotinic) families on the basis of their transmembrane signaling mechanisms. Muscarinic receptors contain seven transmembrane domains whose third cytoplasmic loop is coupled to G proteins that function as transducers (see Figure 2–11). These receptors regulate the production of intracellular second messengers and modulate certain ion channels via their G proteins. Agonist selectivity is determined by the subtypes of muscarinic receptors and G proteins that are present in a given cell (Table 7–1). When expressed in cells, muscarinic receptors form dimers or oligomers that are thought to function in receptor movement between the endoplasmic reticulum and plasma membrane. Conceivably, agonist or antagonist ligands could signal by changing the ratio of monomeric to oligomeric receptors. Muscarinic receptors are located on plasma membranes of cells in the central nervous system, in organs innervated by parasympathetic

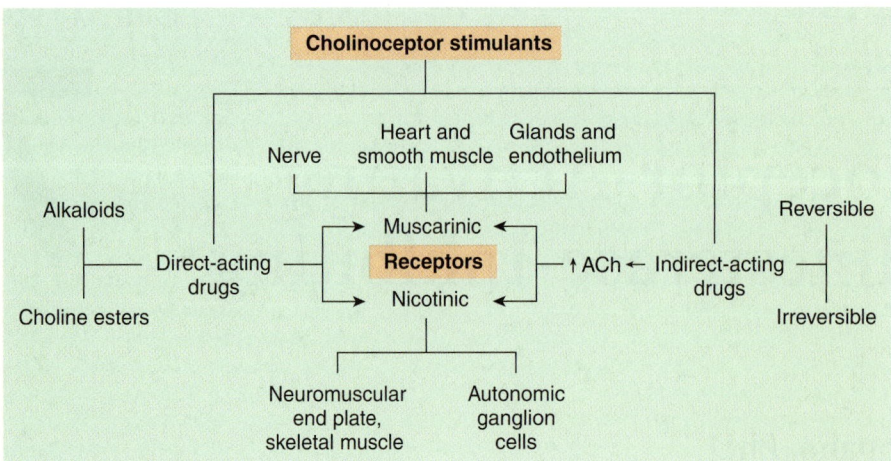

FIGURE 7–1 The major groups of cholinoceptor-activating drugs, receptors, and target tissues. ACh, acetylcholine.

nerves as well as on some tissues that are not innervated by these nerves, eg, endothelial cells (Table 7–1), and on those tissues innervated by postganglionic sympathetic cholinergic nerves.

Nicotinic receptors are part of a transmembrane polypeptide whose subunits form cation-selective ion channels (see Figure 2–9). These receptors are located on plasma membranes of postganglionic cells in all autonomic ganglia, of muscles innervated by somatic motor fibers, and of some central nervous system neurons (see Figure 6–1).

Nonselective cholinoceptor stimulants in sufficient dosage can produce very diffuse and marked alterations in organ system function because acetylcholine has multiple sites of action where it initiates both excitatory and inhibitory effects. Fortunately, drugs are available that have a degree of selectivity, so that desired effects can often be achieved while avoiding or minimizing adverse effects.

Selectivity of action is based on several factors. Some drugs stimulate either muscarinic receptors or nicotinic receptors selectively. Some agents stimulate nicotinic receptors at neuromuscular junctions preferentially and have less effect on nicotinic receptors in ganglia. Organ selectivity can also be achieved by using appropriate routes of administration ("pharmacokinetic selectivity"). For example, muscarinic stimulants can be administered topically to the surface of the eye to modify ocular function while minimizing systemic effects.

TABLE 7–1 Subtypes and characteristics of cholinoceptors.

Receptor Type	Other Names	Location	Structural Features	Postreceptor Mechanism
M_1		Nerves	Seven transmembrane segments, $G_{q/11}$ protein-linked	IP_3, DAG cascade
M_2	Cardiac M_2	Heart, nerves, smooth muscle	Seven transmembrane segments, $G_{i/o}$ protein-linked	Inhibition of cAMP production, activation of K^+ channels
M_3		Glands, smooth muscle, endothelium	Seven transmembrane segments, $G_{q/11}$ protein-linked	IP_3, DAG cascade
M_4		CNS	Seven transmembrane segments, $G_{i/o}$ protein-linked	Inhibition of cAMP production
M_5		CNS	Seven transmembrane segments, $G_{q/11}$ protein-linked	IP_3, DAG cascade
N_M	Muscle type, end plate receptor	Skeletal muscle neuromuscular junction	Pentamer[1] $[(\alpha 1)_2 \beta 1 \delta \gamma)]$	Na^+, K^+ depolarizing ion channel
N_N	Neuronal type, ganglion receptor	CNS, postganglionic cell body, dendrites	Pentamer[1] with α and β subunits only, eg, $(\alpha 4)_2(\beta 2)_3$ (CNS) or $\alpha 3 \alpha 5 (\beta 2)_3$ (ganglia)	Na^+, K^+ depolarizing ion channel

[1]Pentameric structure in *Torpedo* electric organ and fetal mammalian muscle has two $\alpha 1$ subunits and one each of $\beta 1$, δ, and γ subunits. The stoichiometry is indicated by subscripts, eg, $[(\alpha 1)_2 \beta 1 \delta \gamma]$. In adult muscle, the γ subunit is replaced by an ε subunit. There are twelve neuronal nicotinic receptors with nine α ($\alpha 2$–$\alpha 10$) subunits and three ($\beta 2$–$\beta 4$) subunits. The subunit composition varies among different mammalian tissues.

DAG, diacylglycerol; IP_3, inositol trisphosphate.

Data from Millar NS: Assembly and subunit diversity of nicotinic acetylcholine receptors. Biochem Soc Trans 2003;31:869.

MODE OF ACTION OF CHOLINOMIMETIC DRUGS

Direct-acting cholinomimetic agents bind to and activate muscarinic or nicotinic receptors (Figure 7–1). Indirect-acting agents produce their primary effects by inhibiting acetylcholinesterase, which hydrolyzes acetylcholine to choline and acetic acid (see Figure 6–3). By inhibiting acetylcholinesterase, the indirect-acting drugs increase the endogenous acetylcholine concentration in synaptic clefts and neuroeffector junctions. The excess acetylcholine, in turn, stimulates cholinoceptors to evoke increased responses. These drugs act primarily where acetylcholine is physiologically released and are thus *amplifiers* of endogenous acetylcholine.

Some cholinesterase inhibitors also inhibit butyrylcholinesterase (pseudocholinesterase). However, inhibition of butyrylcholinesterase plays little role in the action of indirect-acting cholinomimetic drugs because this enzyme is not important in the physiologic termination of synaptic acetylcholine action. Some quaternary cholinesterase inhibitors also have a modest direct action as well, eg, neostigmine, which activates neuromuscular nicotinic cholinoceptors directly in addition to blocking cholinesterase.

■ BASIC PHARMACOLOGY OF THE DIRECT-ACTING CHOLINOCEPTOR STIMULANTS

The direct-acting cholinomimetic drugs can be divided on the basis of chemical structure into esters of choline (including acetylcholine) and alkaloids (such as muscarine and nicotine). Many of these drugs have effects on both receptors; acetylcholine is typical. A few of them are highly selective for the muscarinic or for the nicotinic receptor. However, none of the clinically useful drugs is selective for receptor subtypes in either class.

Chemistry & Pharmacokinetics

A. Structure

Four important choline esters that have been studied extensively are shown in Figure 7–2. Their permanently charged quaternary ammonium group renders them relatively insoluble in lipids. Many naturally occurring and synthetic cholinomimetic drugs that are not choline esters have been identified; a few of these are shown in Figure 7–3. The muscarinic receptor is strongly stereoselective: *(S)*-bethanechol is almost 1000 times more potent than *(R)*-bethanechol.

B. Absorption, Distribution, and Metabolism

Choline esters are poorly absorbed and poorly distributed into the central nervous system because they are hydrophilic. Although all are hydrolyzed in the gastrointestinal tract (and less active by the oral route), they differ markedly in their susceptibility to hydrolysis by cholinesterase. Acetylcholine is very rapidly hydrolyzed (see Chapter 6); large amounts must be infused intravenously to achieve concentrations sufficient to produce detectable effects. A

large intravenous bolus injection has a brief effect, typically 5–20 seconds, whereas intramuscular and subcutaneous injections produce only local effects. Methacholine is more resistant to hydrolysis, and the carbamic acid esters carbachol and bethanechol are still more resistant to hydrolysis by cholinesterase and have correspondingly longer durations of action. The β-methyl group (methacholine, bethanechol) reduces the potency of these drugs at nicotinic receptors (Table 7–2).

The tertiary natural cholinomimetic alkaloids (pilocarpine, nicotine, lobeline; Figure 7–3) are well absorbed from most sites of administration. Nicotine, a liquid, is sufficiently lipid-soluble to be absorbed across the skin. Muscarine, a quaternary amine, is less completely absorbed from the gastrointestinal tract than the tertiary amines but is nevertheless toxic when ingested—eg, in certain mushrooms—and it even enters the brain. Lobeline is a plant derivative similar to nicotine. These amines are excreted chiefly by the kidneys. Acidification of the urine accelerates clearance of the tertiary amines (see Chapter 1).

Pharmacodynamics

A. Mechanism of Action

Activation of the parasympathetic nervous system modifies organ function by two major mechanisms. First, acetylcholine released

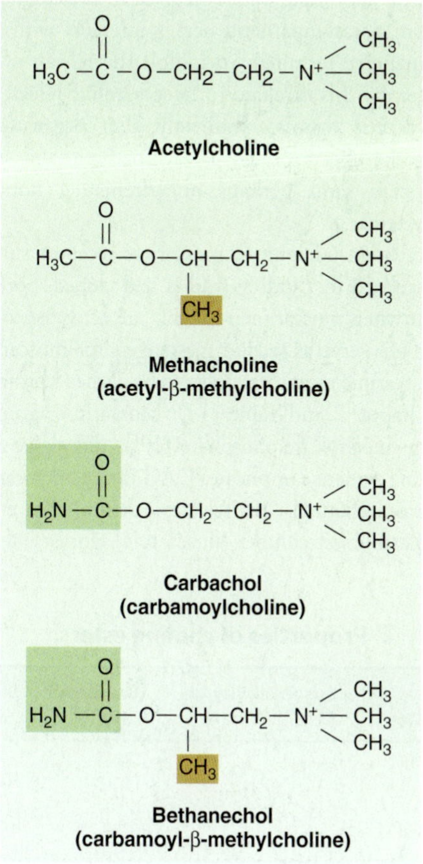

FIGURE 7–2 Molecular structures of four choline esters. Acetylcholine and methacholine are acetic acid esters of choline and β-methylcholine, respectively. Carbachol and bethanechol are carbamic acid esters of the same alcohols.

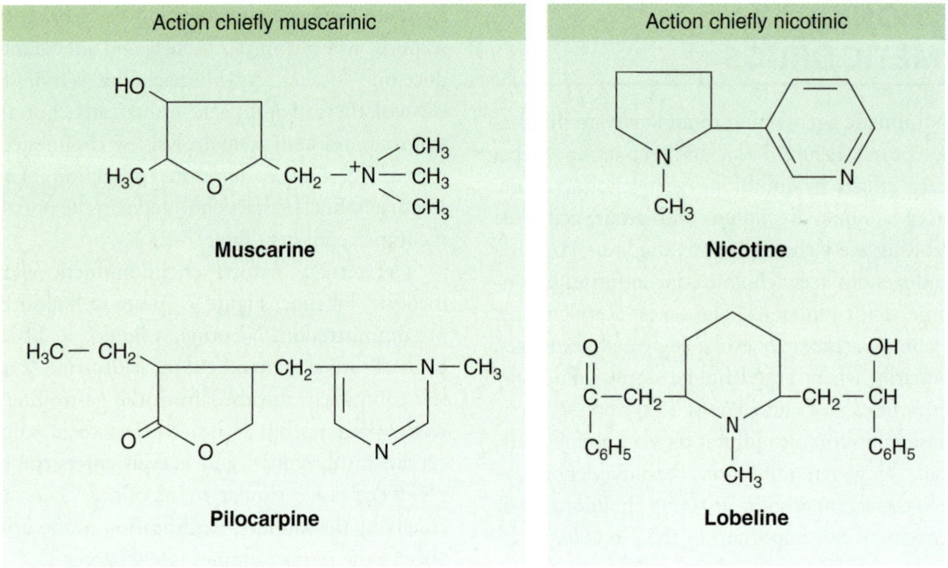

FIGURE 7–3 Structures of some cholinomimetic alkaloids.

from parasympathetic nerves activates muscarinic receptors on effector cells to alter organ function directly. Second, acetylcholine released from parasympathetic nerves interacts with muscarinic receptors on nerve terminals to inhibit the release of their neurotransmitter. By this mechanism, acetylcholine release and circulating muscarinic agonists indirectly alter organ function by modulating the effects of the parasympathetic and sympathetic nervous systems and perhaps nonadrenergic, noncholinergic (NANC) systems.

As indicated in Chapter 6, muscarinic receptor subtypes have been characterized by binding studies and cloned. Several cellular events occur when muscarinic receptors are activated, one or more of which might serve as second messengers for muscarinic activation. All muscarinic receptors appear to be of the G protein-coupled type (see Chapter 2 and Table 7–1). Muscarinic agonist binding activates the inositol trisphosphate (IP_3), diacylglycerol (DAG) cascade. Some evidence implicates DAG in the opening of smooth muscle calcium channels; IP_3 releases calcium from endoplasmic and sarcoplasmic reticulum. Muscarinic agonists also increase

cellular cGMP concentrations. Activation of muscarinic receptors also increases potassium flux across cardiac cell membranes (Figure 7–4A) and decreases it in ganglion and smooth muscle cells. This effect is mediated by the binding of an activated G protein βγ subunit directly to the channel. Finally, muscarinic receptor activation in some tissues (eg, heart, intestine) inhibits adenylyl cyclase activity. Moreover, muscarinic agonists attenuate the activation of adenylyl cyclase and modulate the increase in cAMP levels induced by hormones such as catecholamines. These muscarinic effects on cAMP generation reduce the physiologic response of the organ to stimulatory hormones.

The mechanism of nicotinic receptor activation has been studied in great detail, taking advantage of three factors: (1) the receptor is present in extremely high concentration in the membranes of the electric organs of electric fish; (2) α-bungarotoxin, a component of certain snake venoms, binds tightly to the receptors and is readily labeled as a marker for isolation procedures; and (3) receptor activation results in easily measured electrical and ionic changes in the cells involved. The nicotinic receptor in muscle tissues is a pentamer of four types of glycoprotein subunits (one monomer occurs twice) with a total molecular weight of about 250,000 (Figure 7–4B). The neuronal nicotinic receptor consists of α and β subunits only (Table 7–1). Each subunit has four transmembrane segments. The nicotinic receptor has two agonist binding sites at the interfaces formed by the two α subunits and two adjacent subunits (β, γ, ε). Agonist binding to the receptor sites causes a conformational change in the protein (channel opening) that allows sodium and potassium ions to diffuse rapidly down their concentration gradients (calcium ions may also carry charge through the nicotinic receptor ion channel). Binding of an agonist molecule by one of the two receptor sites only modestly increases the probability of channel opening; simultaneous binding of agonist by both of the receptor sites

TABLE 7–2 Properties of choline esters.

Choline Ester	Susceptibility to Cholinesterase	Muscarinic Action	Nicotinic Action
Acetylcholine chloride	++++	+++	+++
Methacholine chloride	+	++++	None
Carbachol chloride	Negligible	++	+++
Bethanechol chloride	Negligible	++	None

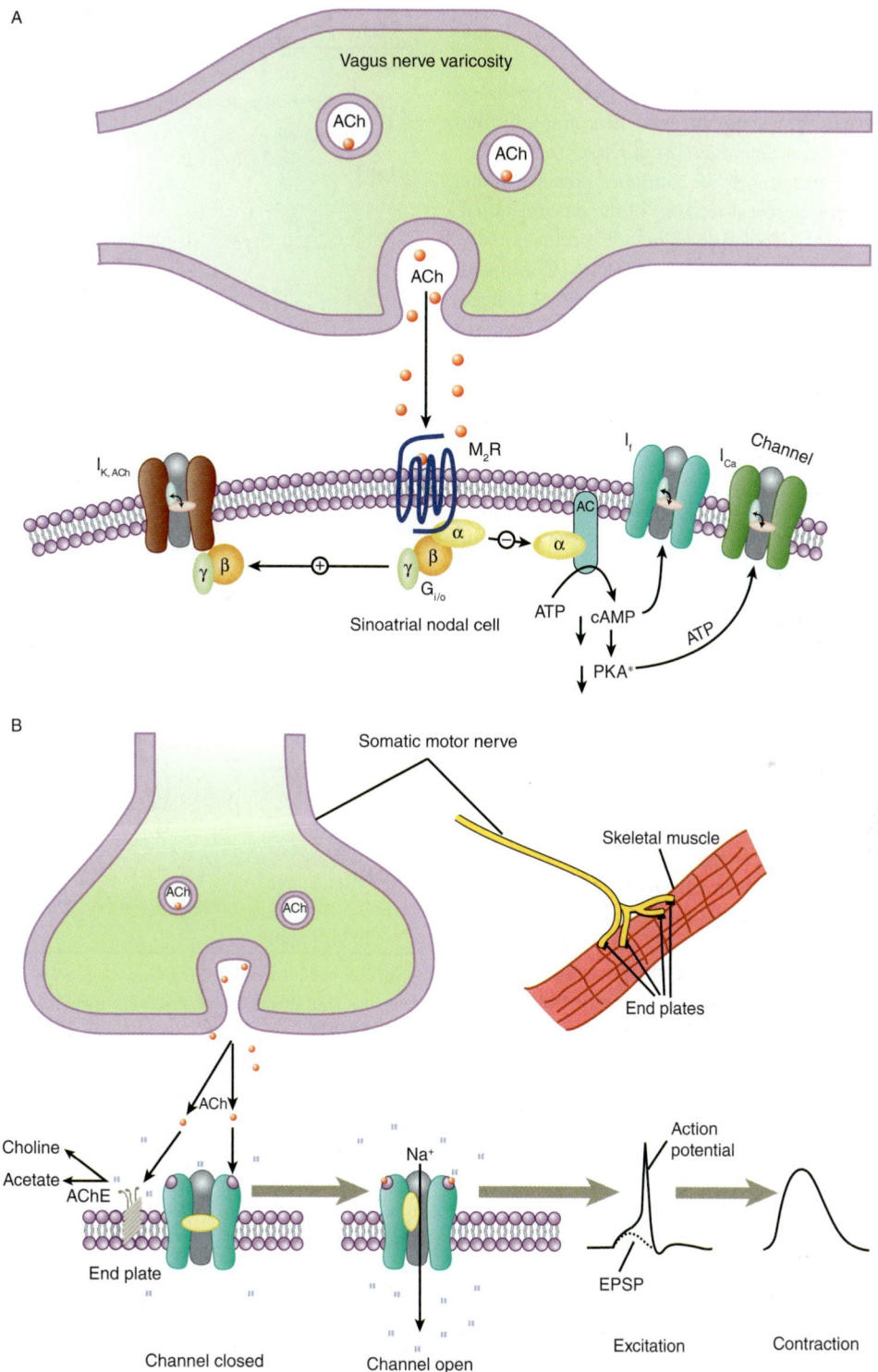

FIGURE 7–4 Muscarinic and nicotinic signaling. **A:** Muscarinic transmission to the sinoatrial node in heart. Acetylcholine (ACh) released from a varicosity of a postganglionic cholinergic axon interacts with a muscarinic receptor (M_2R) linked via $G_{i/o}$ to K^+ channel opening, which causes hyperpolarization, and to inhibition of cAMP synthesis. Reduced cAMP causes voltage-dependent opening of pacemaker channels (I_f) to shift to more negative potentials, and reduces the phosphorylation and availability of L-type Ca^{2+} channels (I_{Ca}). **B:** Nicotinic transmission at the skeletal neuromuscular junction. ACh released from the motor nerve terminal interacts with subunits of the pentameric nicotinic receptor to open it, allowing Na^+ influx to produce an excitatory postsynaptic potential (EPSP). The EPSP depolarizes the muscle membrane, generating an action potential, and triggering contraction. Acetylcholinesterase (AChE) in the extracellular matrix hydrolyzes ACh.

greatly enhances opening probability. Nicotinic receptor activation causes depolarization of the nerve cell or neuromuscular end plate membrane. In skeletal muscle, the depolarization initiates an action potential that propagates across the muscle membrane and causes contraction (Figure 7–4B).

Prolonged agonist occupancy of the nicotinic receptor abolishes the effector response; that is, the postganglionic neuron stops firing (ganglionic effect), and the skeletal muscle cell relaxes (neuromuscular end plate effect). Furthermore, the continued presence of the nicotinic agonist prevents electrical recovery of the postjunctional membrane. Thus, a state of "depolarizing blockade" occurs initially during persistent agonist occupancy of the receptor. Continued agonist occupancy is associated with return of membrane voltage to the resting level. The receptor becomes desensitized to agonist, and this state is refractory to reversal by other agonists. As described in Chapter 27, this effect can be exploited for producing muscle paralysis.

B. Organ System Effects

Most of the direct organ system effects of muscarinic cholinoceptor stimulants are readily predicted from knowledge of the effects of parasympathetic nerve stimulation (see Table 6–3) and the distribution of muscarinic receptors. Effects of a typical agent such as acetylcholine are listed in Table 7–3. The effects of nicotinic agonists are similarly predictable from knowledge of the physiology of the autonomic ganglia and skeletal muscle motor end plate.

1. Eye—Muscarinic agonists instilled into the conjunctival sac cause contraction of the smooth muscle of the iris sphincter (resulting in miosis) and of the ciliary muscle (resulting in accommodation). As a result, the iris is pulled away from the angle of the anterior chamber, and the trabecular meshwork at the base of the ciliary muscle is opened. Both effects facilitate aqueous humor outflow into the canal of Schlemm, which drains the anterior chamber.

2. Cardiovascular system—The primary cardiovascular effects of muscarinic agonists are reduction in peripheral vascular resistance and changes in heart rate. The direct effects listed in Table 7–3 are modified by important homeostatic reflexes, as described in Chapter 6 and depicted in Figure 6–7. Intravenous infusions of minimally effective doses of acetylcholine in humans (eg, 20–50 mcg/min) cause vasodilation, resulting in a reduction in blood pressure, often accompanied by a reflex increase in heart rate. Larger doses of acetylcholine produce bradycardia and decrease atrioventricular node conduction velocity in addition to hypotension.

The direct cardiac actions of muscarinic stimulants include the following: (1) an increase in a potassium current ($I_{K(ACh)}$) in the cells of the sinoatrial and atrioventricular nodes, in Purkinje cells, and also in atrial and ventricular muscle cells; (2) a decrease in the slow inward calcium current (I_{Ca}) in heart cells; and (3) a reduction in the hyperpolarization-activated current (I_f) that underlies diastolic depolarization (Figure 7–4A). All these actions are mediated by M_2 receptors and contribute to slowing the pacemaker rate. Effects (1) and (2) cause hyperpolarization, reduce action potential duration, and decrease the contractility of atrial and

TABLE 7–3 Effects of direct-acting cholinoceptor stimulants.*

Organ	Response
Eye	
Sphincter muscle of iris	Contraction (miosis)
Ciliary muscle	Contraction for near vision
Heart	
Sinoatrial node	Decrease in rate (negative chronotropy)
Atria	Decrease in contractile strength (negative inotropy). Decrease in refractory period
Atrioventricular node	Decrease in conduction velocity (negative dromotropy). Increase in refractory period
Ventricles	Small decrease in contractile strength
Blood vessels	
Arteries, veins	Dilation (via EDRF). Constriction (high-dose direct effect)
Lung	
Bronchial muscle	Contraction (bronchoconstriction)
Bronchial glands	Stimulation
Gastrointestinal tract	
Motility	Increase
Sphincters	Relaxation
Secretion	Stimulation
Urinary bladder	
Detrusor	Contraction
Trigone and sphincter	Relaxation
Glands	
Sweat, salivary, lacrimal, nasopharyngeal	Secretion

EDRF, endothelium-derived relaxing factor.

*Only the direct effects are indicated; homeostatic responses to these direct actions may be important (see text).

ventricular cells. Predictably, knockout of M_2 receptors eliminates the bradycardic effect of vagal stimulation and the negative chronotropic effect of carbachol on sinoatrial rate.

The direct slowing of sinoatrial rate and atrioventricular conduction that is produced by muscarinic agonists is often opposed by reflex sympathetic discharge, elicited by the decrease in blood pressure (see Figure 6–7). The resultant sympathetic-parasympathetic interaction is complex because muscarinic modulation of sympathetic influences occurs by inhibition of norepinephrine release and by postjunctional cellular effects. Muscarinic receptors that are present on postganglionic parasympathetic nerve terminals allow neurally released acetylcholine to inhibit its own secretion. The neuronal muscarinic receptors need not be the same subtype as found on effector cells. Therefore, the net effect on heart rate depends on local concentrations of the agonist in the heart and in the vessels and on the level of reflex responsiveness.

Parasympathetic innervation of the ventricles is much less extensive than that of the atria; activation of ventricular muscarinic receptors causes much less physiologic effect than that seen in atria. However, the effects of muscarinic agonists on ventricular function are clearly evident during sympathetic nerve stimulation because of muscarinic modulation of sympathetic effects ("accentuated antagonism").

In the intact organism, intravascular injection of muscarinic agonists produces marked vasodilation. However, earlier studies of isolated blood vessels often showed a contractile response to these agents. It is now known that acetylcholine-induced vasodilation arises from activation of M_3 receptors and requires the presence of intact endothelium (Figure 7–5). Muscarinic agonists release endothelium-derived relaxing factor (EDRF), identified as nitric oxide (NO), from the endothelial cells. The NO diffuses to adjacent vascular smooth muscle, where it activates guanylyl cyclase and increases cGMP, resulting in relaxation (see Figure 12–2). Isolated vessels prepared with the endothelium preserved consistently reproduce the vasodilation seen in the intact organism. The relaxing effect of acetylcholine was maximal at 3×10^{-7} M (Figure 7–5). This effect was eliminated in the absence of endothelium, and acetylcholine, at concentrations greater than 10^{-7} M, then caused contraction. This results from a direct effect of acetylcholine on vascular smooth muscle in which activation of M_3 receptors stimulates IP_3 production and releases intracellular calcium.

Parasympathetic nerves can regulate arteriolar tone in vascular beds in thoracic and abdominal visceral organs. Acetylcholine released from postganglionic parasympathetic nerves relaxes coronary arteriolar smooth muscle via the NO/cGMP pathway in humans as described above. Damage to the endothelium, as occurs with atherosclerosis, eliminates this action, and acetylcholine is then able to contract arterial smooth muscle and produce vasoconstriction. Parasympathetic nerve stimulation also causes vasodilation in cerebral blood vessels; however, the effect often appears as a result of NO released either from NANC (nitrergic) neurons or as a cotransmitter from cholinergic nerves. The relative contributions of cholinergic and NANC neurons to the vascular effects of parasympathetic nerve stimulation are not known for most viscera. Skeletal muscle receives sympathetic cholinergic vasodilator nerves, but the view that acetylcholine causes vasodilation in this vascular bed has not been verified experimentally. Nitric oxide, rather than acetylcholine, may be released from these neurons. However, this vascular bed responds to exogenous choline esters because of the presence of M_3 receptors on endothelial and smooth muscle cells.

The cardiovascular effects of all the choline esters are similar to those of acetylcholine—the main difference being in their potency and duration of action. Because of the resistance of methacholine, carbachol, and bethanechol to acetylcholinesterase, lower doses given intravenously are sufficient to produce effects similar to those of acetylcholine, and the duration of action of these synthetic choline esters is longer. The cardiovascular effects of most of the cholinomimetic natural alkaloids and the synthetic analogs are also generally similar to those of acetylcholine.

Pilocarpine is an interesting exception to the above statement. If given intravenously (an experimental exercise), it may produce hypertension after a brief initial hypotensive response. The longer-lasting hypertensive effect can be traced to sympathetic ganglionic discharge caused by activation of postganglionic cell membrane M_1 receptors, which close K^+ channels and elicit slow excitatory (depolarizing) postsynaptic potentials. This effect, like the hypotensive effect, can be blocked by atropine, an antimuscarinic drug.

3. Respiratory system—Muscarinic stimulants contract the smooth muscle of the bronchial tree. In addition, the glands of the tracheobronchial mucosa are stimulated to secrete. This combination of effects can occasionally cause symptoms, especially in individuals with asthma. The bronchoconstriction caused by muscarinic agonists is eliminated in knockout animals in which the M_3 receptor has been mutated.

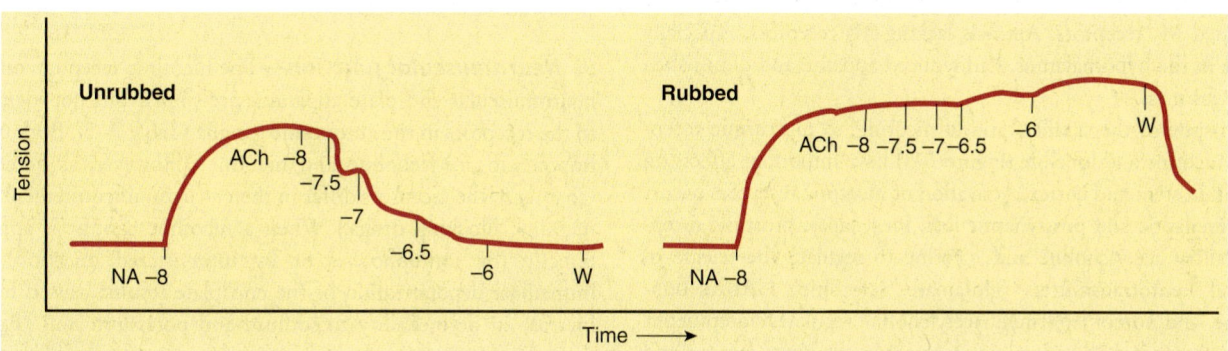

FIGURE 7–5 Activation of endothelial cell muscarinic receptors by acetylcholine (Ach) releases endothelium-derived relaxing factor (nitric oxide), which causes relaxation of vascular smooth muscle precontracted with norepinephrine, 10^{-8} M. Removal of the endothelium by rubbing eliminates the relaxant effect and reveals contraction caused by direct action of Ach on vascular smooth muscle. (NA, noradrenaline [norepinephrine]. Numbers indicate the log concentration applied at the time indicated.) (Modified and reproduced, with permission, from Furchgott RF, Zawadzki JV: The obligatory role of endothelial cells in the relaxation of arterial smooth muscle by acetylcholine. Nature 1980;288:373.)

4. Gastrointestinal tract—Administration of muscarinic agonists, as in parasympathetic nervous system stimulation, increases the secretory and motor activity of the gut. The salivary and gastric glands are strongly stimulated; the pancreas and small intestinal glands are stimulated less so. Peristaltic activity is increased throughout the gut, and most sphincters are relaxed. Stimulation of contraction in this organ system involves depolarization of the smooth muscle cell membrane and increased calcium influx. Muscarinic agonists do not cause contraction of the ileum in mutant mice lacking M_2 and M_3 receptors. The M_3 receptor is required for direct activation of smooth muscle contraction, whereas the M_2 receptor reduces cAMP formation and relaxation caused by sympathomimetic drugs.

5. Genitourinary tract—Muscarinic agonists stimulate the detrusor muscle and relax the trigone and sphincter muscles of the bladder, thus promoting voiding. The function of M_2 and M_3 receptors in the urinary bladder appears to be the same as in intestinal smooth muscle. The human uterus is not notably sensitive to muscarinic agonists.

6. Miscellaneous secretory glands—Muscarinic agonists stimulate secretion by thermoregulatory sweat, lacrimal, and nasopharyngeal glands.

7. Central nervous system—The central nervous system contains both muscarinic and nicotinic receptors, the brain being relatively richer in muscarinic sites and the spinal cord containing a preponderance of nicotinic sites. The physiologic roles of these receptors are discussed in Chapter 21.

All five muscarinic receptor subtypes have been detected in the central nervous system. The roles of M_1 through M_3 have been analyzed by means of experiments in knockout mice. The M_1 subtype is richly expressed in brain areas involved in cognition. Knockout of M_1 receptors was associated with impaired neuronal plasticity in the forebrain, and pilocarpine did not induce seizures in M_1 mutant mice. The central nervous system effects of the synthetic muscarinic agonist oxotremorine (tremor, hypothermia, and antinociception) were lacking in mice with homozygously mutated M_2 receptors. Animals lacking M_3 receptors, especially those in the hypothalamus, had reduced appetite and diminished body fat mass.

In spite of the smaller ratio of nicotinic to muscarinic receptors, nicotine and lobeline (Figure 7–3) have important effects on the brain stem and cortex. Activation of nicotinic receptors occurs at presynaptic and postsynaptic loci. Presynaptic nicotinic receptors allow acetylcholine and nicotine to regulate the release of several neurotransmitters (glutamate, serotonin, GABA, dopamine, and norepinephrine). Acetylcholine regulates norepinephrine release via $\alpha3\beta4$ nicotinic receptors in the hippocampus and inhibits acetylcholine release from neurons in the hippocampus and cortex. The $\alpha4\beta2$ oligomer is the most abundant nicotinic receptor in the brain. Chronic exposure to nicotine has a dual effect at nicotinic receptors: activation (depolarization) followed by desensitization. The former effect is associated with greater

release of dopamine in the mesolimbic system. This effect is thought to contribute to the mild alerting action and the addictive property of nicotine absorbed from tobacco. When the $\beta2$ subunits are deleted in reconstitution experiments, acetylcholine binding is reduced, as is the release of dopamine. The later desensitization of the nicotinic receptor is accompanied by increased high-affinity agonist binding and an upregulation of nicotinic binding sites, especially those of the $\alpha4\beta2$ oligomer. Sustained desensitization may contribute to the benefits of nicotine replacement therapy in smoking cessation regimens. In high concentrations, nicotine induces tremor, emesis, and stimulation of the respiratory center. At still higher levels, nicotine causes convulsions, which may terminate in fatal coma. The lethal effects on the central nervous system and the fact that nicotine is readily absorbed form the basis for the use of nicotine as an insecticide.

8. Peripheral nervous system—Autonomic ganglia are important sites of nicotinic synaptic action. The nicotinic agents shown in Figure 7–3 cause marked activation of these nicotinic receptors and initiate action potentials in postganglionic neurons (see Figure 6–8). Nicotine itself has a somewhat greater affinity for neuronal than for skeletal muscle nicotinic receptors. The action is the same on both parasympathetic and sympathetic ganglia. The initial response therefore often resembles simultaneous discharge of both the parasympathetic and the sympathetic nervous systems. In the case of the cardiovascular system, the effects of nicotine are chiefly sympathomimetic. Dramatic hypertension is produced by parenteral injection of nicotine; sympathetic tachycardia may alternate with a bradycardia mediated by vagal discharge. In the gastrointestinal and urinary tracts, the effects are largely parasympathomimetic: nausea, vomiting, diarrhea, and voiding of urine are commonly observed. Prolonged exposure may result in depolarizing blockade of the ganglia.

Neuronal nicotinic receptors are present on sensory nerve endings—especially afferent nerves in coronary arteries and the carotid and aortic bodies as well as on the glomus cells of the latter. Activation of these receptors by nicotinic stimulants and of muscarinic receptors on glomus cells by muscarinic stimulants elicits complex medullary responses, including respiratory alterations and vagal discharge.

9. Neuromuscular junction—The nicotinic receptors on the neuromuscular end plate apparatus are similar but not identical to the receptors in the autonomic ganglia (Table 7–1). Both types respond to acetylcholine and nicotine. (However, as noted in Chapter 8, the receptors differ in their structural requirements for nicotinic blocking drugs.) When a nicotinic agonist is applied directly (by iontophoresis or by intra-arterial injection), an immediate depolarization of the end plate results, caused by an increase in permeability to sodium and potassium ions (Figure 7–4). The contractile response varies from disorganized fasciculations of independent motor units to a strong contraction of the entire muscle depending on the synchronization of depolarization of end plates throughout the muscle. Depolarizing nicotinic agents that are not rapidly hydrolyzed (like nicotine itself) cause rapid development of depolarization blockade; transmission blockade persists even when the membrane has repolarized (discussed further in Chapters 8 and 27). This latter phase of block is manifested as flaccid paralysis in the case of skeletal muscle.

■ BASIC PHARMACOLOGY OF THE INDIRECT-ACTING CHOLINOMIMETICS

The actions of acetylcholine released from autonomic and somatic motor nerves are terminated by enzymatic hydrolysis of the molecule. Hydrolysis is accomplished by the action of acetylcholinesterase, which is present in high concentrations in cholinergic synapses. The indirect-acting cholinomimetics have their primary effect at the active site of this enzyme, although some also have direct actions at nicotinic receptors. The chief differences between members of the group are chemical and pharmacokinetic—their pharmacodynamic properties are almost identical.

Chemistry & Pharmacokinetics

A. Structure

There are three chemical groups of cholinesterase inhibitors: (1) simple alcohols bearing a quaternary ammonium group, eg, edrophonium; (2) carbamic acid esters of alcohols having quaternary or tertiary ammonium groups (carbamates, eg, neostigmine); and (3) organic derivatives of phosphoric acid (organophosphates, eg, echothiophate). Examples of the first two groups are shown in Figure 7–6. Edrophonium, neostigmine, and pyridostigmine are synthetic quaternary ammonium agents used in medicine. Physostigmine (eserine) is a naturally occurring tertiary amine of

greater lipid solubility that is also used in therapeutics. Carbaryl (carbaril) is typical of a large group of carbamate insecticides designed for very high lipid solubility, so that absorption into the insect and distribution to its central nervous system are very rapid.

A few of the estimated 50,000 organophosphates are shown in Figure 7–7. Many of the organophosphates (echothiophate is an exception) are highly lipid-soluble liquids. Echothiophate, a thiocholine derivative, is of clinical value because it retains the very long duration of action of other organophosphates but is more stable in aqueous solution. Soman is an extremely potent "nerve gas." Parathion and malathion are thiophosphate (sulfur-containing phosphate) prodrugs that are inactive as such; they are converted to the phosphate derivatives in animals and plants and are used as insecticides.

B. Absorption, Distribution, and Metabolism

Absorption of the quaternary carbamates from the conjunctiva, skin, gut and lungs is predictably poor, since their permanent charge renders them relatively insoluble in lipids. Thus, much larger doses are required for oral administration than for parenteral injection. Distribution into the central nervous system is negligible. Physostigmine, in contrast, is well absorbed from all sites and can be used topically in the eye (Table 7–4). It is distributed into the central nervous system and is more toxic than the more polar quaternary carbamates. The carbamates are relatively stable in aqueous solution but can be metabolized by nonspecific esterases in the body as well as by cholinesterase. However, the duration of their effect is determined chiefly by the stability of the inhibitor-enzyme complex (see Mechanism of Action, below), not by metabolism or excretion.

The organophosphate cholinesterase inhibitors (except for echothiophate) are well absorbed from the skin, lung, gut, and

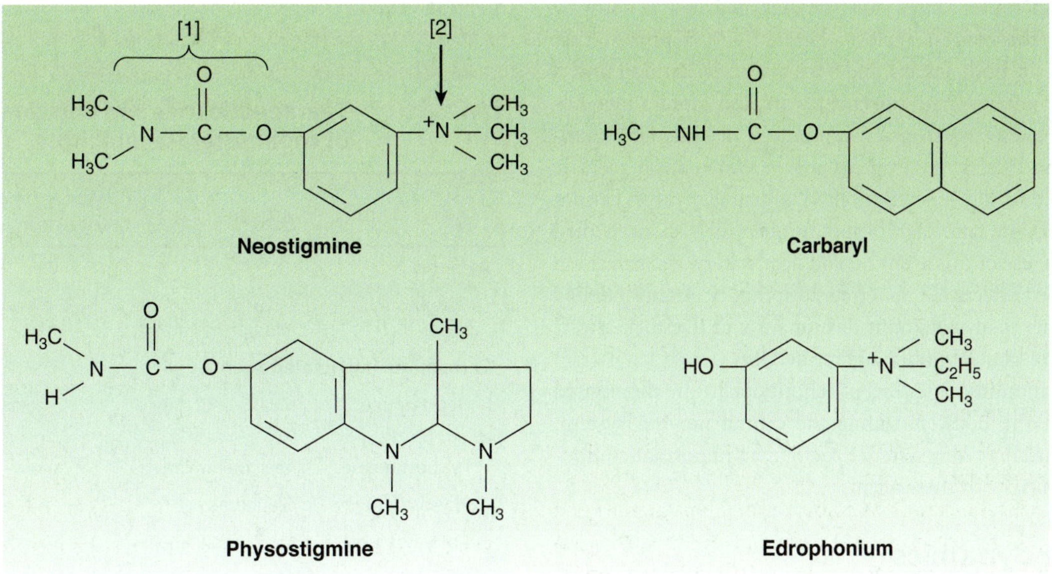

FIGURE 7–6 Cholinesterase inhibitors. Neostigmine exemplifies the typical ester composed of carbamic acid ([1]) and a phenol bearing a quaternary ammonium group ([2]). Physostigmine, a naturally occurring carbamate, is a tertiary amine. Edrophonium is not an ester but binds to the active site of the enzyme. Carbaryl is used as an insecticide.

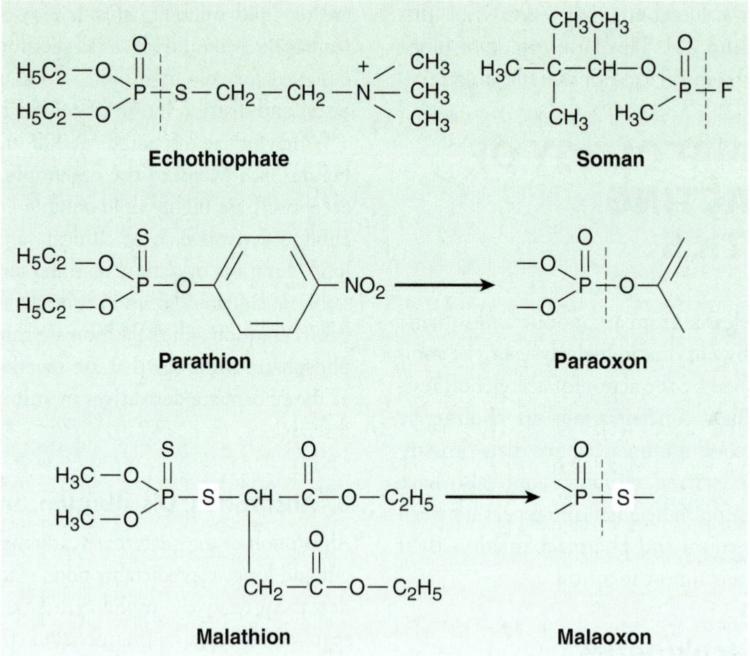

FIGURE 7–7 Structures of some organophosphate cholinesterase inhibitors. The dashed lines indicate the bond that is hydrolyzed in binding to the enzyme. The shaded ester bonds in malathion represent the points of detoxification of the molecule in mammals and birds.

conjunctiva—thereby making them dangerous to humans and highly effective as insecticides. They are relatively less stable than the carbamates when dissolved in water and thus have a limited half-life in the environment (compared with another major class of insecticides, the halogenated hydrocarbons, eg, DDT). Echothiophate is highly polar and more stable than most other organophosphates. When prepared in aqueous solution for ophthalmic use, it retains activity for weeks.

The thiophosphate insecticides (parathion, malathion, and related compounds) are quite lipid-soluble and are rapidly absorbed by all routes. They must be activated in the body by conversion to the oxygen analogs (Figure 7–7), a process that occurs rapidly in both insects and vertebrates. Malathion and a few other organophosphate insecticides are also rapidly metabolized by other pathways to inactive products in birds and mammals but not in insects; these agents are therefore considered safe enough for sale to the general public. Unfortunately, fish cannot detoxify malathion, and significant numbers of fish have died from the heavy use of this agent on and near waterways. Parathion is not detoxified effectively in vertebrates; thus, it is considerably more dangerous than malathion to humans and livestock and is not available for general public use in the USA.

All the organophosphates except echothiophate are distributed to all parts of the body, including the central nervous system. Therefore, central nervous system toxicity is an important component of poisoning with these agents.

Pharmacodynamics

A. Mechanism of Action

Acetylcholinesterase is the primary target of these drugs, but butyrylcholinesterase is also inhibited. Acetylcholinesterase is an extremely active enzyme. In the initial catalytic step, acetylcholine binds to the enzyme's active site and is hydrolyzed, yielding free choline and the acetylated enzyme. In the second step, the covalent acetyl-enzyme bond is split, with the addition of water (hydration). The entire process occurs in approximately 150 microseconds.

All the cholinesterase inhibitors increase the concentration of endogenous acetylcholine at cholinoceptors by inhibiting acetylcholinesterase. However, the molecular details of their interaction with the enzyme vary according to the three chemical subgroups mentioned above.

TABLE 7–4 Therapeutic uses and durations of action of cholinesterase inhibitors.

	Uses	Approximate Duration of Action
Alcohols		
Edrophonium	Myasthenia gravis, ileus, arrhythmias	5–15 minutes
Carbamates and related agents		
Neostigmine	Myasthenia gravis, ileus	0.5–2 hours
Pyridostigmine	Myasthenia gravis	3–6 hours
Physostigmine	Glaucoma	0.5–2 hours
Ambenonium	Myasthenia gravis	4–8 hours
Demecarium	Glaucoma	4–6 hours
Organophosphates		
Echothiophate	Glaucoma	100 hours

The first group, of which edrophonium is the example, consists of quaternary alcohols. These agents reversibly bind electrostatically and by hydrogen bonds to the active site, thus preventing access of acetylcholine. The enzyme-inhibitor complex does not involve a covalent bond and is correspondingly short-lived (on the order of 2–10 minutes). The second group consists of carbamate esters, eg, neostigmine and physostigmine. These agents undergo a two-step hydrolysis sequence analogous to that described for acetylcholine. However, the covalent bond of the *carbamoylated* enzyme is considerably more resistant to the second (hydration) process, and this step is correspondingly prolonged (on the order of 30 minutes to 6 hours). The third group consists of the organophosphates. These agents also undergo initial binding and hydrolysis by the enzyme, resulting in a *phosphorylated* active site. The covalent phosphorus-enzyme bond is extremely stable and hydrolyzes in water at a very slow rate (hundreds of hours). After the initial binding-hydrolysis step, the phosphorylated enzyme complex may undergo a process called **aging.** This process apparently involves the breaking of one of the oxygen-phosphorus bonds of the inhibitor and further strengthens the phosphorus-enzyme bond. The rate of aging varies with the particular organophosphate compound. For example, aging occurs within 10 minutes with the chemical warfare agent soman, but as much as 48 hours later with the drug VX. If given before aging has occurred, strong nucleophiles like pralidoxime are able to break the phosphorus-enzyme bond and can be used as "cholinesterase regenerator" drugs for organophosphate insecticide poisoning (see Chapter 8). Once aging has occurred, the enzyme-inhibitor complex is even more stable and is more difficult to break, even with oxime regenerator compounds.

The organophosphate inhibitors are sometimes referred to as "irreversible" cholinesterase inhibitors, and edrophonium and the carbamates are considered "reversible" inhibitors because of the marked differences in duration of action. However, the molecular mechanisms of action of the three groups do not support this simplistic description.

B. Organ System Effects

The most prominent pharmacologic effects of cholinesterase inhibitors are on the cardiovascular and gastrointestinal systems, the eye, and the skeletal muscle neuromuscular junction (as described in the Case Study). Because the primary action is to amplify the actions of endogenous acetylcholine, the effects are similar (but not always identical) to the effects of the direct-acting cholinomimetic agonists.

1. Central nervous system—In low concentrations, the lipid-soluble cholinesterase inhibitors cause diffuse activation on the electroencephalogram and a subjective alerting response. In higher concentrations, they cause generalized convulsions, which may be followed by coma and respiratory arrest.

2. Eye, respiratory tract, gastrointestinal tract, urinary tract—The effects of the cholinesterase inhibitors on these organ systems, all of which are well innervated by the parasympathetic nervous system, are qualitatively quite similar to the effects of the direct-acting cholinomimetics (Table 7–3).

3. Cardiovascular system—The cholinesterase inhibitors can increase activity in both sympathetic and parasympathetic ganglia supplying the heart and at the acetylcholine receptors on neuro-effector cells (cardiac and vascular smooth muscles) that receive cholinergic innervation.

In the heart, the effects on the parasympathetic limb predominate. Thus, cholinesterase inhibitors such as edrophonium, physostigmine, or neostigmine mimic the effects of vagal nerve activation on the heart. Negative chronotropic, dromotropic, and inotropic effects are produced, and cardiac output falls. The fall in cardiac output is attributable to bradycardia, decreased atrial contractility, and some reduction in ventricular contractility. The latter effect occurs as a result of prejunctional inhibition of norepinephrine release as well as inhibition of postjunctional cellular sympathetic effects.

Cholinesterase inhibitors have minimal effects by direct action on vascular smooth muscle because most vascular beds lack cholinergic innervation (coronary vasculature is an exception). At moderate doses, cholinesterase inhibitors cause an increase in systemic vascular resistance and blood pressure that is initiated at sympathetic ganglia in the case of quaternary nitrogen compounds and also at central sympathetic centers in the case of lipid-soluble agents. Atropine, acting in the central and peripheral nervous systems, can prevent the increase of blood pressure and the increased plasma norepinephrine.

The *net* cardiovascular effects of moderate doses of cholinesterase inhibitors therefore consist of modest bradycardia, a fall in cardiac output, and an increased vascular resistance that results in a rise in blood pressure. (Thus, in patients with Alzheimer's disease who have hypertension, treatment with cholinesterase inhibitors requires that blood pressure be monitored to adjust antihypertensive therapy.) At high (toxic) doses of cholinesterase inhibitors, marked bradycardia occurs, cardiac output decreases significantly, and hypotension supervenes.

4. Neuromuscular junction—The cholinesterase inhibitors have important therapeutic and toxic effects at the skeletal muscle neuromuscular junction. Low (therapeutic) concentrations moderately prolong and intensify the actions of physiologically released acetylcholine. This increases the strength of contraction, especially in muscles weakened by curare-like neuromuscular blocking agents or by myasthenia gravis. At higher concentrations, the accumulation of acetylcholine may result in fibrillation of muscle fibers. Antidromic firing of the motor neuron may also occur, resulting in fasciculations that involve an entire motor unit. With marked inhibition of acetylcholinesterase, depolarizing neuromuscular blockade occurs and that may be followed by a phase of nondepolarizing blockade as seen with succinylcholine (see Table 27–2 and Figure 27–7).

Some quaternary carbamate cholinesterase inhibitors, eg, neostigmine, have an additional *direct* nicotinic agonist effect at the neuromuscular junction. This may contribute to the effectiveness of these agents as therapy for myasthenia.

■ CLINICAL PHARMACOLOGY OF THE CHOLINOMIMETICS

The major therapeutic uses of the cholinomimetics are to treat diseases of the eye (glaucoma, accommodative esotropia), the gastrointestinal and urinary tracts (postoperative atony, neurogenic bladder), and the neuromuscular junction (myasthenia gravis, curare-induced neuromuscular paralysis), and to treat patients with Alzheimer's disease. Cholinesterase inhibitors are occasionally used in the treatment of atropine overdosage and, very rarely, in the therapy of certain atrial arrhythmias.

Clinical Uses

A. The Eye

Glaucoma is a disease characterized by increased intraocular pressure. Muscarinic stimulants and cholinesterase inhibitors reduce intraocular pressure by causing contraction of the ciliary body so as to facilitate outflow of aqueous humor and perhaps also by diminishing the rate of its secretion (see Figure 6–9). In the past, glaucoma was treated with either direct agonists (pilocarpine, methacholine, carbachol) or cholinesterase inhibitors (physostigmine, demecarium, echothiophate, isoflurophate). For chronic glaucoma, these drugs have been largely replaced by topical β blockers and prostaglandin derivatives.

Acute angle-closure glaucoma is a medical emergency that is frequently treated initially with drugs but usually requires surgery for permanent correction. Initial therapy often consists of a combination of a direct muscarinic agonist and a cholinesterase inhibitor (eg, pilocarpine plus physostigmine) as well as other drugs. Once the intraocular pressure is controlled and the danger of vision loss is diminished, the patient can be prepared for corrective surgery (iridectomy). Open-angle glaucoma and some cases of secondary glaucoma are chronic diseases that are not amenable to traditional surgical correction, although newer laser techniques appear to be useful. Other treatments for glaucoma are described in the Box, Treatment of Glaucoma in Chapter 10.

Accommodative esotropia (strabismus caused by hypermetropic accommodative error) in young children is sometimes diagnosed and treated with cholinomimetic agonists. Dosage is similar to or higher than that used for glaucoma.

B. Gastrointestinal and Urinary Tracts

In clinical disorders that involve depression of smooth muscle activity without obstruction, cholinomimetic drugs with direct or indirect muscarinic effects may be helpful. These disorders include postoperative ileus (atony or paralysis of the stomach or bowel following surgical manipulation) and congenital megacolon. Urinary retention may occur postoperatively or postpartum or may be secondary to spinal cord injury or disease (neurogenic bladder). Cholinomimetics are also sometimes used to increase the tone of the lower esophageal sphincter in patients with reflux esophagitis. Of the choline esters, bethanechol is the most widely used for these disorders. For gastrointestinal problems, it is usually administered orally in a dose of 10–25 mg three or four times

daily. In patients with urinary retention, bethanechol can be given subcutaneously in a dose of 5 mg and repeated in 30 minutes if necessary. Of the cholinesterase inhibitors, neostigmine is the most widely used for these applications. For paralytic ileus or atony of the urinary bladder, neostigmine can be given subcutaneously in a dose of 0.5–1 mg. If patients are able to take the drug by mouth, neostigmine can be given orally in a dose of 15 mg. In all of these situations, the clinician must be certain that there is no mechanical obstruction to outflow before using the cholinomimetic. Otherwise, the drug may exacerbate the problem and may even cause perforation as a result of increased pressure.

Pilocarpine has long been used to increase salivary secretion. Cevimeline, a quinuclidine derivative of acetylcholine, is a new direct-acting muscarinic agonist used for the treatment of dry mouth associated with Sjögren's syndrome and that caused by radiation damage of the salivary glands.

C. Neuromuscular Junction

Myasthenia gravis is an autoimmune disease affecting skeletal muscle neuromuscular junctions. In this disease, antibodies are produced against the main immunogenic region found on $\alpha 1$ subunits of the nicotinic receptor-channel complex. Antibodies are detected in 85% of myasthenic patients. The antibodies reduce nicotinic receptor function by (1) cross-linking receptors, a process that stimulates their internalization and degradation; (2) causing lysis of the postsynaptic membrane; and (3) binding to the nicotinic receptor and inhibiting function. Frequent findings are ptosis, diplopia, difficulty in speaking and swallowing, and extremity weakness. Severe disease may affect all the muscles, including those necessary for respiration. The disease resembles the neuromuscular paralysis produced by *d*-tubocurarine and similar nondepolarizing neuromuscular blocking drugs (see Chapter 27). Patients with myasthenia are exquisitely sensitive to the action of curariform drugs and other drugs that interfere with neuromuscular transmission, eg, aminoglycoside antibiotics.

Cholinesterase inhibitors—but not direct-acting acetylcholine receptor agonists—are extremely valuable as therapy for myasthenia. Patients with ocular myasthenia may be treated with cholinesterase inhibitors alone (Figure 7–4B). Patients having more widespread muscle weakness are also treated with immunosuppressant drugs (steroids, cyclosporine, and azathioprine). In some patients, the thymus gland is removed; very severely affected patients may benefit from administration of immunoglobulins and from plasmapheresis.

Edrophonium is sometimes used as a diagnostic test for myasthenia. A 2 mg dose is injected intravenously after baseline muscle strength has been measured. If no reaction occurs after 45 seconds, an additional 8 mg may be injected. If the patient has myasthenia gravis, an improvement in muscle strength that lasts about 5 minutes can usually be observed.

Clinical situations in which severe myasthenia (myasthenic crisis) must be distinguished from excessive drug therapy (cholinergic crisis) usually occur in very ill myasthenic patients and must be managed in hospital with adequate emergency support systems (eg, mechanical ventilators) available. Edrophonium can be used to assess the adequacy of treatment with the longer-acting cholinesterase inhibitors usually prescribed in patients with myasthenia gravis. If excessive amounts of cholinesterase inhibitor have been used, patients may become paradoxically weak because of nicotinic depolarizing blockade of the motor end plate. These patients may also exhibit symptoms of excessive stimulation of muscarinic receptors (abdominal cramps, diarrhea, increased salivation, excessive bronchial secretions, miosis, bradycardia). Small doses of edrophonium (1–2 mg intravenously) will produce no relief or even worsen weakness if the patient is receiving excessive cholinesterase inhibitor therapy. On the other hand, if the patient improves with edrophonium, an increase in cholinesterase inhibitor dosage may be indicated.

Long-term therapy for myasthenia gravis is usually accomplished with pyridostigmine; neostigmine or ambenonium are alternatives. The doses are titrated to optimum levels based on changes in muscle strength. These drugs are relatively short-acting and therefore require frequent dosing (every 6 hours for pyridostigmine and ambenonium and every 4 hours for neostigmine; Table 7–4). Sustained-release preparations are available but should be used only at night and if needed. Longer-acting cholinesterase inhibitors such as the organophosphate agents are not used, because the dose requirement in this disease changes too rapidly to permit smooth control of symptoms with long-acting drugs.

If muscarinic effects of such therapy are prominent, they can be controlled by the administration of antimuscarinic drugs such as atropine. Frequently, tolerance to the muscarinic effects of the cholinesterase inhibitors develops, so atropine treatment is not required.

Neuromuscular blockade is frequently produced as an adjunct to surgical anesthesia, using nondepolarizing neuromuscular relaxants such as pancuronium and newer agents (see Chapter 27). After surgery, it is usually desirable to reverse this pharmacologic paralysis promptly. This can be easily accomplished with cholinesterase inhibitors; neostigmine and edrophonium are the drugs of choice. They are given intravenously or intramuscularly for prompt effect.

D. Heart

The short-acting cholinesterase inhibitor edrophonium was used to treat supraventricular tachyarrhythmias, particularly paroxysmal supraventricular tachycardia. In this application, edrophonium has been replaced by newer drugs with different mechanisms (adenosine and the calcium channel blockers verapamil and diltiazem, see Chapter 14).

E. Antimuscarinic Drug Intoxication

Atropine intoxication is potentially lethal in children (see Chapter 8) and may cause prolonged severe behavioral disturbances and arrhythmias in adults. The tricyclic antidepressants, when taken in overdosage (often with suicidal intent), also cause severe muscarinic blockade (see Chapter 30). The muscarinic receptor blockade produced by all these agents is competitive in nature and can be overcome by increasing the amount of endogenous acetylcholine at the neuroeffector junctions. Theoretically, a cholinesterase inhibitor could be used to reverse these effects. Physostigmine has been used for this application because it enters the central nervous system and reverses the central as well as the peripheral signs of

muscarinic blockade. However, as described below, physostigmine itself can produce dangerous central nervous system effects, and such therapy is therefore used only in patients with dangerous elevation of body temperature or very rapid supraventricular tachycardia (see also Chapter 58).

F. Central Nervous System

Tacrine is a drug with anticholinesterase and other cholinomimetic actions that has been used for the treatment of mild to moderate Alzheimer's disease. Tacrine's efficacy is modest, and hepatic toxicity is significant. Donepezil, galantamine, and rivastigmine are newer, more selective acetylcholinesterase inhibitors that appear to have the same modest clinical benefit as tacrine in treatment of cognitive dysfunction in Alzheimer's patients. Donepezil may be given once daily because of its long half-life, and it lacks the hepatotoxic effect of tacrine. However, no trials comparing these newer drugs with tacrine have been reported. These drugs are discussed in Chapter 60.

Toxicity

The toxic potential of the cholinoceptor stimulants varies markedly depending on their absorption, access to the central nervous system, and metabolism.

A. Direct-Acting Muscarinic Stimulants

Drugs such as pilocarpine and the choline esters cause predictable signs of muscarinic excess when given in overdosage. These effects include nausea, vomiting, diarrhea, urinary urgency, salivation, sweating, cutaneous vasodilation, and bronchial constriction. The effects are all blocked competitively by atropine and its congeners.

Certain mushrooms, especially those of the genus *Inocybe*, contain muscarinic alkaloids. Ingestion of these mushrooms causes typical signs of muscarinic excess within 15–30 minutes. These effects can be very uncomfortable but are rarely fatal. Treatment is with atropine, 1–2 mg parenterally. (*Amanita muscaria*, the first source of muscarine, contains very low concentrations of the alkaloid.)

B. Direct-Acting Nicotinic Stimulants

Nicotine itself is the only common cause of this type of poisoning. (Varenicline toxicity is discussed elsewhere in this chapter.) The acute toxicity of the alkaloid is well defined but much less important than the chronic effects associated with smoking. In addition to tobacco products, nicotine is also used in insecticides.

1. Acute toxicity—The fatal dose of nicotine is approximately 40 mg, or 1 drop of the pure liquid. This is the amount of nicotine in two regular cigarettes. Fortunately, most of the nicotine in cigarettes is destroyed by burning or escapes via the "sidestream" smoke. Ingestion of nicotine insecticides or of tobacco by infants and children is usually followed by vomiting, limiting the amount of the alkaloid absorbed.

The toxic effects of a large dose of nicotine are simple extensions of the effects described previously. The most dangerous are (1) central stimulant actions, which cause convulsions and may progress to coma and respiratory arrest; (2) skeletal muscle end plate depolarization, which may lead to depolarization blockade and respiratory paralysis; and (3) hypertension and cardiac arrhythmias.

Treatment of acute nicotine poisoning is largely symptom-directed. Muscarinic excess resulting from parasympathetic ganglion stimulation can be controlled with atropine. Central stimulation is usually treated with parenteral anticonvulsants such as diazepam. Neuromuscular blockade is not responsive to pharmacologic treatment and may require mechanical ventilation.

Fortunately, nicotine is metabolized and excreted relatively rapidly. Patients who survive the first 4 hours usually recover completely if hypoxia and brain damage have not occurred.

2. Chronic nicotine toxicity—The health costs of tobacco smoking to the smoker and its socioeconomic costs to the general public are still incompletely understood. However, the 1979 *Surgeon General's Report on Health Promotion and Disease Prevention* stated that "cigarette smoking is clearly the largest single preventable cause of illness and premature death in the United States." This statement has been supported by numerous subsequent studies. Unfortunately, the fact that the most important of the tobacco-associated diseases are delayed in onset reduces the health incentive to stop smoking.

Clearly, the addictive power of cigarettes is directly related to their nicotine content. It is not known to what extent nicotine per se contributes to the other well-documented adverse effects of chronic tobacco use. It appears highly probable that nicotine contributes to the increased risk of vascular disease and sudden coronary death associated with smoking. Also, nicotine probably contributes to the high incidence of ulcer recurrences in smokers with peptic ulcer.

There are several approaches to help patients stop smoking. One approach is replacement therapy with nicotine in the form of gum, transdermal patch, nasal spray, or inhaler. All these forms have low abuse potential and are effective in patients motivated to stop smoking. Their action derives from slow absorption of nicotine that occupies $\alpha4\beta2$ receptors in the central nervous system and reduces the desire to smoke and the pleasurable feelings of smoking.

Another quite effective agent for smoking cessation is **varenicline**, a synthetic drug with partial agonist action at $\alpha4\beta2$ nicotinic receptors. Varenicline also has antagonist properties that persist because of its long half-life; this prevents the stimulant effect of nicotine at presynaptic $\alpha4\beta2$ receptors that causes release of dopamine. However, its use is limited by nausea and insomnia and also by exacerbation of psychiatric illnesses, including anxiety and depression. Suicidal ideation has also been reported in some patients; this is currently being evaluated. The efficacy of varenicline is superior to that of bupropion, an antidepressant (see Chapter 30). Some of bupropion's efficacy in smoking cessation therapy stems from its noncompetitive antagonism (see Chapter 2) of nicotinic receptors where it displays some selectivity among neuronal subtypes.

C. Cholinesterase Inhibitors

The acute toxic effects of the cholinesterase inhibitors, like those of the direct-acting agents, are direct extensions of their pharmacologic actions. The major source of such intoxications is pesticide use in agriculture and in the home. Approximately 100 organophosphate and 20 carbamate cholinesterase inhibitors are available in pesticides and veterinary vermifuges used in the USA. Cholinesterase inhibitors used in agriculture can cause slowly or rapidly developing symptoms, as described in the Case Study, which persist for days. The cholinesterase inhibitors used as chemical warfare agents (soman, sarin, VX) induce effects rapidly because of the large concentrations present.

Acute intoxication must be recognized and treated promptly in patients with heavy exposure. The dominant initial signs are those of muscarinic excess: miosis, salivation, sweating, bronchial constriction, vomiting, and diarrhea. Central nervous system involvement (cognitive disturbances, convulsions, and coma) usually follows rapidly, accompanied by peripheral nicotinic effects, especially depolarizing neuromuscular blockade. Therapy always includes (1) maintenance of vital signs—respiration in particular may be impaired; (2) decontamination to prevent further absorption—this may require removal of all clothing and washing of the skin in cases of exposure to dusts and sprays; and (3) atropine parenterally in large doses, given as often as required to control signs of muscarinic excess. Therapy often also includes treatment with pralidoxime, as described in Chapter 8, and administration of benzodiazepines for seizures.

Preventive therapy for cholinesterase inhibitors used as chemical warfare agents has been developed to protect soldiers and civilians. Personnel are given autoinjection syringes containing a carbamate, pyridostigmine, and atropine. Protection is provided by pyridostigmine, which, by prior binding to the enzyme, impedes binding of organophosphate agents and thereby prevents prolonged inhibition of cholinesterase. The protection is limited to the peripheral nervous system because pyridostigmine does not readily enter the central nervous system. Enzyme inhibition by pyridostigmine dissipates within hours (Table 7–4), a duration of time that allows clearance of the organophosphate agent from the body.

Chronic exposure to certain organophosphate compounds, including some organophosphate cholinesterase inhibitors, causes delayed neuropathy associated with demyelination of axons. **Triorthocresyl phosphate,** an additive in lubricating oils, is the prototype agent of this class. The effects are not caused by cholinesterase inhibition but rather by neuropathy target esterase (NTE) inhibition whose symptoms (weakness of upper and lower extremities, unsteady gait) appear 1–2 weeks after exposure. Another nerve toxicity called intermediate syndrome occurs 1–4 days after exposure to organophosphate insecticides. This syndrome is also characterized by muscle weakness; its origin is not known but it appears to be related to cholinesterase inhibition.

SUMMARY Drugs Used for Cholinomimetic Effects

Subclass	Mechanism of Action	Effects	Clinical Applications	Pharmacokinetics, Toxicities, Interactions
DIRECT-ACTING CHOLINE ESTERS				
• Bethanechol	Muscarinic agonist • negligible effect at nicotinic receptors	Activates M_1 through M_3 receptors in all peripheral tissues • causes increased secretion, smooth muscle contraction (except vascular smooth muscle relaxes), and changes in heart rate	Postoperative and neurogenic ileus and urinary retention	Oral and parenteral, duration ~ 30 min • does not enter central nervous system (CNS) • *Toxicity:* Excessive parasympathomimetic effects, especially bronchospasm in asthmatics • *Interactions:* Additive with other parasympathomimetics
• *Carbachol: Nonselective muscarinic and nicotinic agonist; otherwise similar to bethanechol; used topically almost exclusively for glaucoma*				
DIRECT-ACTING MUSCARINIC ALKALOIDS OR SYNTHETICS				
• Pilocarpine	Like bethanechol, partial agonist	Like bethanechol	Glaucoma; Sjögren's syndrome	Oral lozenge and topical • *Toxicity & interactions:* Like bethanechol
• *Cevimeline: Synthetic M_3-selective; similar to pilocarpine*				
DIRECT-ACTING NICOTINIC AGONISTS				
• Nicotine	Agonist at both N_N and N_M receptors	Activates autonomic postganglionic neurons (both sympathetic and parasympathetic) and skeletal muscle neuromuscular end plates • enters CNS and activates N_N receptors	Medical use in smoking cessation • nonmedical use in smoking and in insecticides	Oral gum, patch for smoking cessation • *Toxicity:* Increased gastrointestinal (GI) activity, nausea, vomiting, diarrhea acutely • increased blood pressure • high doses cause seizures • long-term GI and cardiovascular risk factor • *Interactions:* Additive with CNS stimulants
• *Varenicline: Selective partial agonist at α4β2 nicotinic receptors; used exclusively for smoking cessation*				
SHORT-ACTING CHOLINESTERASE INHIBITOR (ALCOHOL)				
• Edrophonium	Alcohol, binds briefly to active site of acetylcholinesterase (AChE) and prevents access of acetylcholine (ACh)	Amplifies all actions of ACh • increases parasympathetic activity and somatic neuromuscular transmission	Diagnosis and acute treatment of myasthenia gravis	Parenteral • quaternary amine • does not enter CNS • *Toxicity:* Parasympathomimetic excess • *Interactions:* Additive with parasympathomimetics
INTERMEDIATE-ACTING CHOLINESTERASE INHIBITORS (CARBAMATES)				
• Neostigmine	Forms covalent bond with AChE, but hydrolyzed and released	Like edrophonium, but longer-acting	Myasthenia gravis • postoperative and neurogenic ileus and urinary retention	Oral and parenteral; quaternary amine, does not enter CNS. Duration 2–4 h • *Toxicity & interactions:* Like edrophonium
• *Pyridostigmine: Like neostigmine, but longer-acting (4–6 h); used in myasthenia*				
• *Physostigmine: Like neostigmine, but natural alkaloid tertiary amine; enters CNS*				
LONG-ACTING CHOLINESTERASE INHIBITORS (ORGANOPHOSPHATES)				
• Echothiophate	Like neostigmine, but released more slowly	Like neostigmine, but longer-acting	Obsolete • was used in glaucoma	Topical only • *Toxicity:* Brow ache, uveitis, blurred vision
• *Malathion: Insecticide, relatively safe for mammals and birds because metabolized by other enzymes to inactive products; some medical use as ectoparasiticide*				
• *Parathion, others: Insecticide, dangerous for all animals; toxicity important because of agricultural use and exposure of farm workers (see text)*				
• *Sarin, others: "Nerve gas," used exclusively in warfare and terrorism*				

PREPARATIONS AVAILABLE

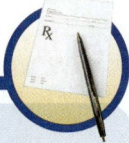

DIRECT-ACTING CHOLINOMIMETICS

Acetylcholine (Miochol-E)
Ophthalmic: 1% intraocular solution

Bethanechol (generic, Urecholine)
Oral: 5, 10, 25, 50 mg tablets
Parenteral: 5 mg/mL for SC injection

Carbachol
Ophthalmic (topical, Isopto Carbachol, Carboptic): 0.75, 1.5, 2.25, 3% solution
Ophthalmic (intraocular, Miostat, Carbastat): 0.01% solution

Cevimeline (Evoxac)
Oral: 30 mg capsules

Nicotine
Transdermal: 5-21 mg/day absorbed/patch
Inhalation: 0.5-4 mg/dose
Gum: 2-4 mg/dose

Pilocarpine (generic, Isopto Carpine)
Ophthalmic (topical): 0.5, 1, 2, 3, 4, 6, 8, 10% solutions, 4% gel
Ophthalmic sustained-release inserts (Ocusert Pilo-20, Ocusert Pilo-40): release 20 and 40 mcg pilocarpine per hour for 1 week, respectively
Oral (Salagen): 5 mg tablets

Varenicline (Chantix)
Oral: 0.5, 1 mg tablets

CHOLINESTERASE INHIBITORS

Ambenonium (Mytelase)
Oral: 10 mg tablets

Demecarium (Humorsol)
Ophthalmic: 0.125, 0.25% solution

Donepezil (Aricept)
Oral: 5, 10, 23 mg tablets

Echothiophate (Phospholine)
Ophthalmic: 1.5 mg powder to reconstitute for 0.03, 0.06, 0.125% solution

Edrophonium (generic, Tensilon)
Parenteral: 10 mg/mL for IM or IV injection

Galantamine (Reminyl, Razadyne)
Oral: 4, 8, 12 mg tablets; 8, 16, 24 mg extended-release capsules; 4 mg/mL solution

Neostigmine (generic, Prostigmin)
Oral: 15 mg tablets
Parenteral: 0.2, 0.5, 1, 2.5 mg/mL solution

Physostigmine (generic, Eserine)
Ophthalmic: 0.25% ointment; 0.25, 0.5% solution
Parenteral: 1 mg/mL for IM or slow IV injection

Pyridostigmine (Mestinon, Regonol)
Oral: 30, 60 mg tablets; 180 mg sustained-release tablets; 12 mg/mL syrup
Parenteral: 5 mg/mL for IM or slow IV injection

Rivastigmine (Exelon)
Oral: 1.5, 3, 4.5, 6 mg tablets; 2 mg/mL solution; transdermal patch 4.6 or 9.5 mg/24 h

Tacrine (Cognex)
Oral: 10, 20, 30, 40 mg tablets

REFERENCES

Aaron CK: Organophosphates and carbamates. In: Shannon MW, Borron SW, Burns MJ (editors): *Haddad and Winchester's Clinical Management of Poisoning and Drug Overdose,* 4th ed. Philadelphia: Saunders, 2007:1171.

Benowitz N: Nicotine addiction. N Engl J Med 2010;362:2295.

Celie PH et al: Nicotine and carbamylcholine binding to nicotinic acetylcholine receptors as studied in AChBP crystal structures. Neuron 2004;41:907.

Chen L: In pursuit of the high-resolution structure of nicotinic acetylcholine receptors. J Physiol 2004;588:557.

Conti-Fine B, Milani M, Kaminski HJ: Myasthenia gravis: past, present, and future. J Clin Invest 2006;116:2843.

Ehlert FJ: Contractile role of M2 and M3 muscarinic receptors in gastrointestinal, airway and urinary bladder smooth muscle. Life Sci 2003;74:355.

Gerthoffer WT: Signal-transduction pathways that regulate visceral smooth muscle function. III. Coupling of muscarinic receptors to signaling kinases and effector proteins in gastrointestinal smooth muscles. Am J Physiol 2005;288:G849.

Giacobini E (editor): *Cholinesterases and Cholinesterase Inhibitors.* London: Martin Dunitz, 2000.

Harvey RD, Belevych AE: Muscarinic regulation of cardiac ion channels. Br J Pharmacol 2003;139:1074.

Hern JA et al: Formation and dissociation of M_1 muscarinic receptor dimers seen by total internal reflection fluorescence imaging of single molecules. Proc Natl Acad Sci USA 2010;107:2693.

Lamping KG et al: Muscarinic (M) receptors in coronary circulation. Arterioscler Thromb Vasc Biol 2004;24:1253.

Lazartigues E et al: Spontaneously hypertensive rats cholinergic hyper-responsiveness: Central and peripheral pharmacological mechanisms. Br J Pharmacol 1999;127:1657.

Matsui M et al: Increased relaxant action of forskolin and isoproterenol against muscarinic agonist-induced contractions in smooth muscle from M_2 receptor knockout mice. J Pharmacol Exp Ther 2003;305:106.

Mavragani CP, Moutsopoulos HM: Conventional therapy of Sjögren's syndrome. Clin Rev Allergy Immunol 2007;32:284.

Millar NS: Assembly and subunit diversity of nicotinic acetylcholine receptors. Biochem Soc Trans 2003;31:869.

Molitor H: A comparative study of the effects of five choline compounds used in therapeutics: Acetylcholine chloride, acetyl-beta-methylcholine chloride, carbaminoyl choline, ethyl ether beta-methylcholine chloride, carbaminoyl beta-methylcholine chloride. J Pharmacol Exp Ther 1936;58:337.

Okamoto H et al: Muscarinic agonist potencies at three different effector systems linked to the M(2) or M(3) receptor in longitudinal smooth muscle of guinea-pig small intestine. Br J Pharmacol 2002;135:1765.

Picciotto MR et al: It is not "either/or": Activation and desensitization of nicotinic acetylcholine receptors both contribute to behaviors related to nicotine addiction and mood. Prog Neurobiol 2008;84:329.

The Surgeon General: *Smoking and Health.* US Department of Health and Human Services, 1979.

Wess J et al: Muscarinic acetylcholine receptors: Mutant mice provide new insights for drug development. Nat Rev Drug Discov 2007;6:721.

CASE STUDY ANSWER

The patient's presentation is characteristic of poisoning by organophosphate cholinesterase inhibitors. Ask the coworker if he can identify the agent used. Decontaminate the patient by removal of clothing and washing affected areas. Ensure an open airway and ventilate with oxygen. For muscarinic excess, administer atropine (0.5–5 mg) intravenously until signs of muscarinic excess (dyspnea, lacrimation, confusion) subside. To treat nicotinic excess, infuse 2-PAM (initially a 1–2% solution in 15–30 minutes) followed by infusion of 1% solution (200–500 mg/h) until muscle fasciculations cease. If needed, decontaminate the coworker and isolate all contaminated clothing.

Cholinoceptor-Blocking Drugs

8

Achilles J. Pappano, PhD

CASE STUDY

JH, a 63-year-old architect, complains of urinary symptoms to his family physician. He has hypertension, and during the last 8 years, he has been adequately managed with a thiazide diuretic and an angiotensin-converting enzyme inhibitor. During the same period, JH developed the signs of benign prostatic hypertrophy, which eventually required prostatectomy to relieve symptoms. He now complains that he has an increased urge to urinate as well as urinary frequency, and this has disrupted the pattern of his daily life. What do you suspect is the cause of JH's problem? What information would you gather to confirm your diagnosis? What treatment steps would you initiate?

Cholinoceptor antagonists, like agonists, are divided into muscarinic and nicotinic subgroups on the basis of their specific receptor affinities. Ganglion blockers and neuromuscular junction blockers make up the antinicotinic drugs. The ganglion-blocking drugs have little clinical use and are discussed at the end of this chapter. Neuromuscular blockers are discussed in Chapter 27. This chapter emphasizes drugs that block muscarinic cholinoceptors.

Five subtypes of muscarinic receptors have been identified, primarily on the basis of data from ligand-binding and cDNA-cloning experiments (see Chapters 6 and 7). A standard terminology (M_1 through M_5) for these subtypes is now in common use, and evidence—based mostly on selective agonists and antagonists—indicates that functional differences exist between several of these subtypes.

The M_1 receptor subtype is located on central nervous system (CNS) neurons, sympathetic postganglionic cell bodies, and many presynaptic sites. M_2 receptors are located in the myocardium, smooth muscle organs, and some neuronal sites. M_3 receptors are most common on effector cell membranes, especially glandular and smooth muscle cells. M_4 and M_5 receptors are less prominent and appear to play a greater role in the CNS than in the periphery.

■ BASIC PHARMACOLOGY OF THE MUSCARINIC RECEPTOR-BLOCKING DRUGS

Muscarinic antagonists are sometimes called parasympatholytic because they block the effects of parasympathetic autonomic discharge. However, they do not "lyse" parasympathetic nerves, and they have some effects that are not predictable from block of the parasympathetic nervous system. For these reasons, the term "antimuscarinic" is preferable.

Naturally occurring compounds with antimuscarinic effects have been known and used for millennia as medicines, poisons, and cosmetics. **Atropine** is the prototype of these drugs. Many similar plant alkaloids are known, and hundreds of synthetic antimuscarinic compounds have been prepared.

Chemistry & Pharmacokinetics

A. Source and Chemistry

Atropine and its naturally occurring congeners are tertiary amine alkaloid esters of tropic acid (Figure 8–1). Atropine (hyoscyamine) is found in the plant *Atropa belladonna*, or deadly nightshade, and

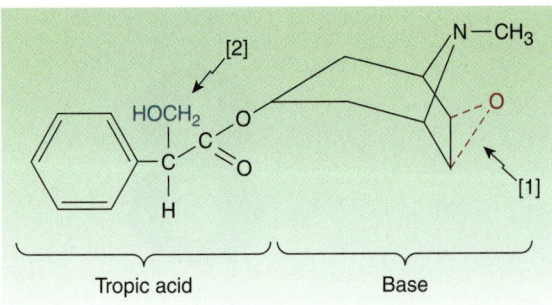

FIGURE 8–1 The structure of atropine (oxygen [red] at [1] is missing) or scopolamine (oxygen present). In homatropine, the hydroxymethyl at [2] is replaced by a hydroxyl group, and the oxygen at [1] is absent.

in *Datura stramonium*, also known as jimson-weed (Jamestown weed), sacred Datura, or thorn apple. **Scopolamine** (hyoscine) occurs in *Hyoscyamus niger*, or henbane, as the *l*(–) stereoisomer. Naturally occurring atropine is *l*(–)-hyoscyamine, but the compound readily racemizes, so the commercial material is racemic *d,l*-hyoscyamine. The *l*(–) isomers of both alkaloids are at least 100 times more potent than the *d*(+) isomers.

A variety of semisynthetic and fully synthetic molecules have antimuscarinic effects. The tertiary members of these classes (Figure 8–2) are often used for their effects on the eye or the CNS. Many antihistaminic (see Chapter 16), antipsychotic (see Chapter 29), and antidepressant (see Chapter 30) drugs have similar structures and, predictably, significant antimuscarinic effects.

Quaternary amine antimuscarinic agents (Figure 8–2) have been developed to produce more peripheral effects and reduced CNS effects.

B. Absorption

Natural alkaloids and most tertiary antimuscarinic drugs are well absorbed from the gut and conjunctival membranes. When applied in a suitable vehicle, some (eg, scopolamine) are even absorbed across the skin (transdermal route). In contrast, only 10–30% of a dose of a quaternary antimuscarinic drug is absorbed after oral administration, reflecting the decreased lipid solubility of the charged molecule.

C. Distribution

Atropine and the other tertiary agents are widely distributed in the body. Significant levels are achieved in the CNS within 30 minutes to 1 hour, and this can limit the dose tolerated when the drug is taken for its peripheral effects. Scopolamine is rapidly and fully distributed into the CNS where it has greater effects than most other antimuscarinic drugs. In contrast, the quaternary derivatives are poorly taken up by the brain and therefore are relatively free—at low doses—of CNS effects.

D. Metabolism and Excretion

After administration, the elimination of atropine from the blood occurs in two phases: the $t_{1/2}$ of the rapid phase is 2 hours and that of the slow phase is approximately 13 hours. About 50% of the dose is excreted unchanged in the urine. Most of the rest appears in the urine as hydrolysis and conjugation products. The drug's effect on parasympathetic function declines rapidly in all organs except the eye. Effects on the iris and ciliary muscle persist for ≥ 72 hours.

Pharmacodynamics

A. Mechanism of Action

Atropine causes reversible (surmountable) blockade (see Chapter 2) of cholinomimetic actions at muscarinic receptors; that is, blockade by a small dose of atropine can be overcome by a larger concentration of acetylcholine or equivalent muscarinic agonist. Mutation experiments suggest that aspartate in the third transmembrane segment of the heptahelical receptor forms an ionic bond with the nitrogen atom of acetylcholine; this amino acid is also required for binding of antimuscarinic drugs. When atropine binds to the muscarinic receptor, it prevents actions such as the release of inositol trisphosphate (IP₃) and the inhibition of adenylyl cyclase that are caused by muscarinic agonists (see Chapter 7). Muscarinic antagonists were traditionally viewed as neutral compounds that occupied the receptor and prevented agonist binding. Recent evidence indicates that muscarinic receptors are constitutively active, and most drugs that block the actions of acetylcholine are inverse agonists (see Chapter 1) that shift the equilibrium to the inactive state of the receptor. Muscarinic blocking drugs that are inverse agonists include atropine, pirenzepine, trihexyphenidyl, AF-DX 116, 4-DAMP, ipratropium, glycopyrrolate, and a methyl derivative of scopolamine (Table 8–1).

The effectiveness of antimuscarinic drugs varies with the tissue and with the source of agonist. Tissues most sensitive to atropine are the salivary, bronchial, and sweat glands. Secretion of acid by the gastric parietal cells is the least sensitive. In most tissues, antimuscarinic agents block exogenously administered cholinoceptor agonists more effectively than endogenously released acetylcholine.

Atropine is highly selective for muscarinic receptors. Its potency at nicotinic receptors is much lower, and actions at nonmuscarinic receptors are generally undetectable clinically.

Atropine does not distinguish among the M_1, M_2, and M_3 subgroups of muscarinic receptors. In contrast, other antimuscarinic drugs are moderately selective for one or another of these subgroups (Table 8–1). Most synthetic antimuscarinic drugs are considerably less selective than atropine in interactions with nonmuscarinic receptors. For example, some quaternary amine antimuscarinic agents have significant ganglion-blocking actions, and others are potent histamine receptor blockers. The antimuscarinic effects of other agents, eg, antipsychotic and antidepressant drugs, have been mentioned. Their relative selectivity for muscarinic receptor subtypes has not been defined.

B. Organ System Effects

1. Central nervous system—In the doses usually used, atropine has minimal stimulant effects on the CNS, especially the parasympathetic medullary centers, and a slower, longer-lasting sedative effect on the brain. Scopolamine has more marked central effects, producing

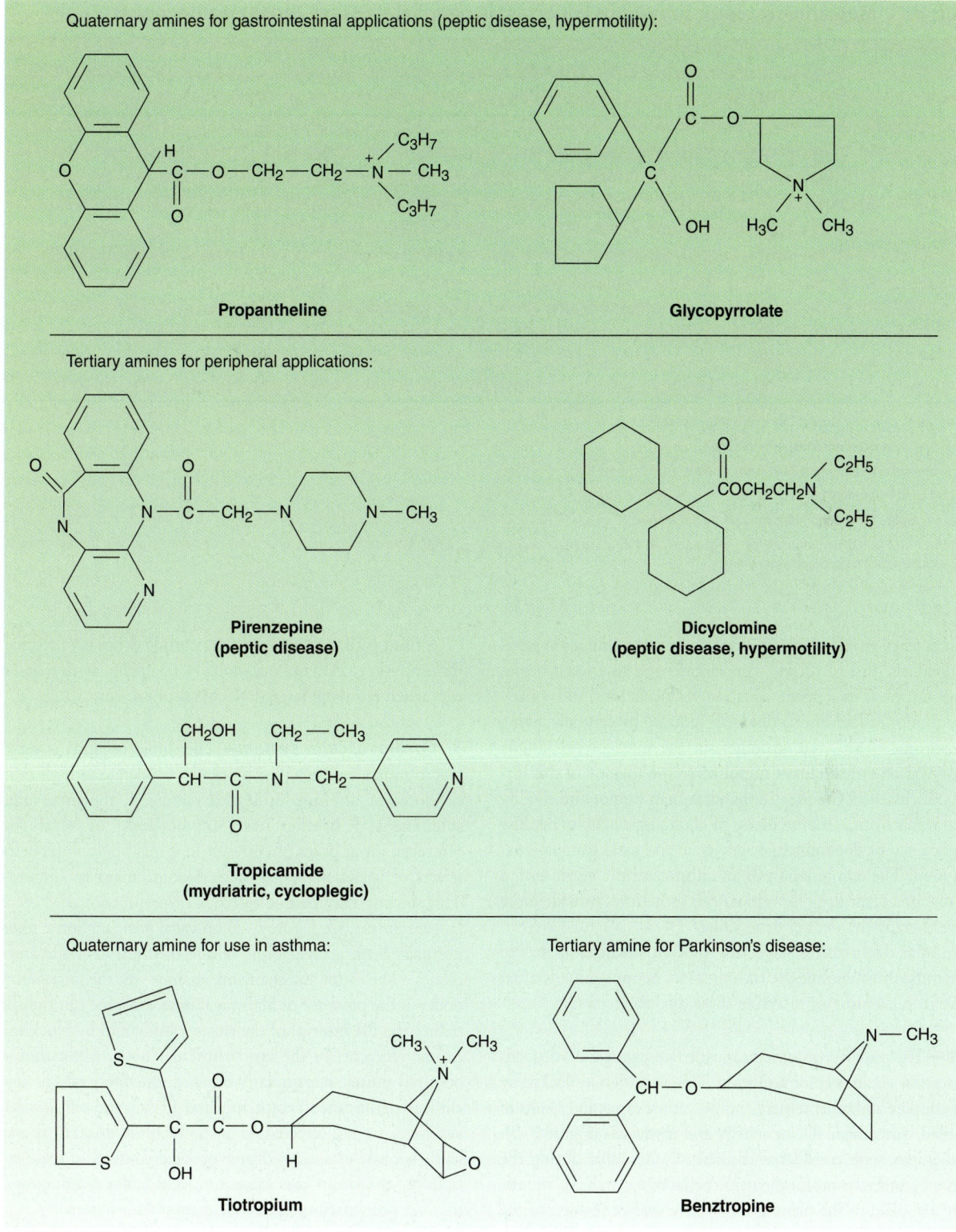

FIGURE 8–2 Structures of some semisynthetic and synthetic antimuscarinic drugs.

TABLE 8–1 Muscarinic receptor subgroups important in peripheral tissues and their antagonists.

Property	Subgroup		
	M$_1$	M$_2$	M$_3$
Primary locations	Nerves	Heart, nerves, smooth muscle	Glands, smooth muscle, endothelium
Dominant effector system	↑ IP$_3$, ↑ DAG	↓ cAMP, ↑ K$^+$ channel current	↑ IP$_3$, ↑ DAG
Antagonists	Pirenzepine, telenzepine, dicyclomine,[2] trihexyphenidyl[3]	Gallamine,[1] methoctramine, AF-DX 116[4]	4-DAMP, darifenacin, solifenacin, oxybutynin, tolterodine
Approximate dissociation constant[5]			
Atropine	1	1	1
Pirenzepine	25	300	500
AF-DX 116	2000	65	4000
Darifenacin	70	55	8

[1]In clinical use as a neuromuscular blocking agent (obsolete).

[2]In clinical use as an intestinal antispasmodic agent.

[3]In clinical use in the treatment of Parkinson's disease.

[4]Compound used in research only.

[5]Relative to atropine. Smaller numbers indicate higher affinity.

AF-DX 116, 11-({2-[(diethylamino)methyl]-1-piperidinyl}acetyl)-5,11-dihydro-6H-pyrido-[2,3-b](1,4)benzodiazepine-6-one; DAG, diacylglycerol; IP$_3$, inositol trisphosphate; 4-DAMP, 4-diphenylacetoxy-N-methylpiperidine.

drowsiness when given in recommended dosages and amnesia in sensitive individuals. In toxic doses, scopolamine, and to a lesser degree atropine, can cause excitement, agitation, hallucinations, and coma.

The tremor of Parkinson's disease is reduced by centrally acting antimuscarinic drugs, and atropine—in the form of belladonna extract—was one of the first drugs used in the therapy of this disease. As discussed in Chapter 28, parkinsonian tremor and rigidity seem to result from a *relative* excess of cholinergic activity because of a deficiency of dopaminergic activity in the basal ganglia-striatum system. The combination of an antimuscarinic agent with a dopamine precursor drug (levodopa) can sometimes provide more effective therapy than either drug alone.

Vestibular disturbances, especially motion sickness, appear to involve muscarinic cholinergic transmission. Scopolamine is often effective in preventing or reversing these disturbances.

2. Eye—The pupillary constrictor muscle (see Figure 6–9) depends on muscarinic cholinoceptor activation. This activation is blocked by topical atropine and other tertiary antimuscarinic drugs and results in unopposed sympathetic dilator activity and **mydriasis** (Figure 8–3). Dilated pupils were considered cosmetically desirable during the Renaissance and account for the name belladonna (Italian, "beautiful lady") applied to the plant and its active extract because of the use of the extract as eye drops during that time.

The second important ocular effect of antimuscarinic drugs is to weaken contraction of the ciliary muscle, or **cycloplegia.** Cycloplegia results in loss of the ability to accommodate; the fully atropinized eye cannot focus for near vision (Figure 8–3).

Both mydriasis and cycloplegia are useful in ophthalmology. They are also potentially hazardous, since acute glaucoma may be induced in patients with a narrow anterior chamber angle.

A third ocular effect of antimuscarinic drugs is to reduce lacrimal secretion. Patients occasionally complain of dry or "sandy" eyes when receiving large doses of antimuscarinic drugs.

3. Cardiovascular system—The sinoatrial node is very sensitive to muscarinic receptor blockade. Moderate to high therapeutic doses of atropine cause tachycardia in the innervated and spontaneously beating heart by blockade of vagal slowing. However, lower doses often result in initial bradycardia before the effects of peripheral vagal block become manifest (Figure 8–4). This slowing may be due to block of prejunctional M$_1$ receptors (autoreceptors, see Figure 6–3) on vagal postganglionic fibers that normally limit acetylcholine release in the sinus node and other tissues. The same mechanisms operate in the atrioventricular node; in the presence of high vagal tone, atropine can significantly reduce the PR interval of the electrocardiogram by blocking muscarinic receptors in the atrioventricular node. Muscarinic effects on atrial muscle are similarly blocked, but these effects are of no clinical significance except in atrial flutter and fibrillation. The ventricles are less affected by antimuscarinic drugs at therapeutic levels because of a lesser degree of vagal control. In toxic concentrations, the drugs can cause intraventricular conduction block that has been attributed to a local anesthetic action.

Most blood vessels, except those in thoracic and abdominal viscera, receive no direct innervation from the parasympathetic system. However, parasympathetic nerve stimulation dilates coronary arteries, and sympathetic cholinergic nerves cause vasodilation in the skeletal muscle vascular bed (see Chapter 6). Atropine can block this vasodilation. Furthermore, almost all vessels contain endothelial muscarinic receptors that mediate vasodilation (see Chapter 7). These receptors are readily blocked by antimuscarinic

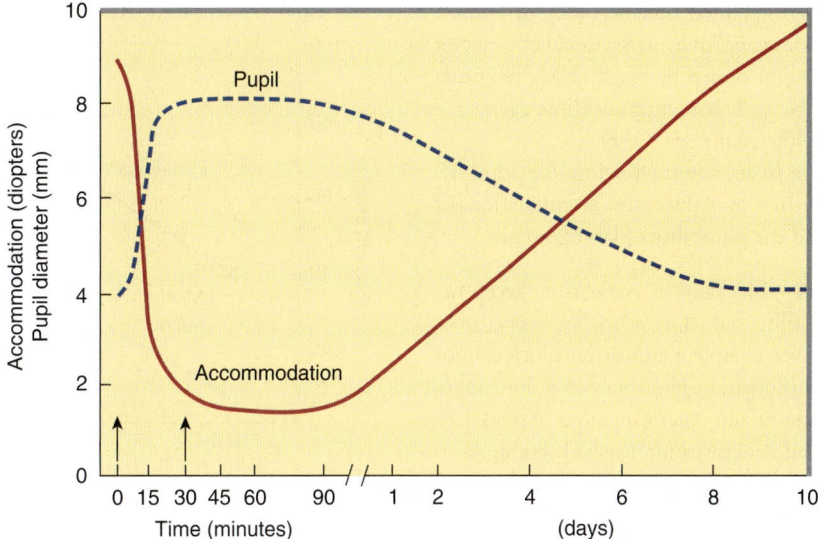

FIGURE 8–3 Effects of topical scopolamine drops on pupil diameter (mm) and accommodation (diopters) in the normal human eye. One drop of 0.5% solution of drug was applied at zero time, and a second drop was administered at 30 minutes (*arrows*). The responses of 42 eyes were averaged. Note the extremely slow recovery. (Redrawn from Marron J: Cycloplegia and mydriasis by use of atropine, scopolamine, and homatropine-paredrine. Arch Ophthalmol 1940;23:340.)

drugs. At toxic doses, and in some individuals at normal doses, antimuscarinic agents cause cutaneous vasodilation, especially in the upper portion of the body. The mechanism is unknown.

The net cardiovascular effects of atropine in patients with normal hemodynamics are not dramatic: tachycardia may occur, but there is little effect on blood pressure. However, the cardiovascular effects of administered direct-acting muscarinic agonists are easily prevented.

4. Respiratory system—Both smooth muscle and secretory glands of the airway receive vagal innervation and contain muscarinic receptors. Even in normal individuals, administration of atropine can cause some bronchodilation and reduce secretion. The effect is more significant in patients with airway disease, although the antimuscarinic drugs are not as useful as the β-adrenoceptor stimulants in the treatment of asthma (see Chapter 20). The effectiveness of nonselective antimuscarinic drugs in treating chronic obstructive

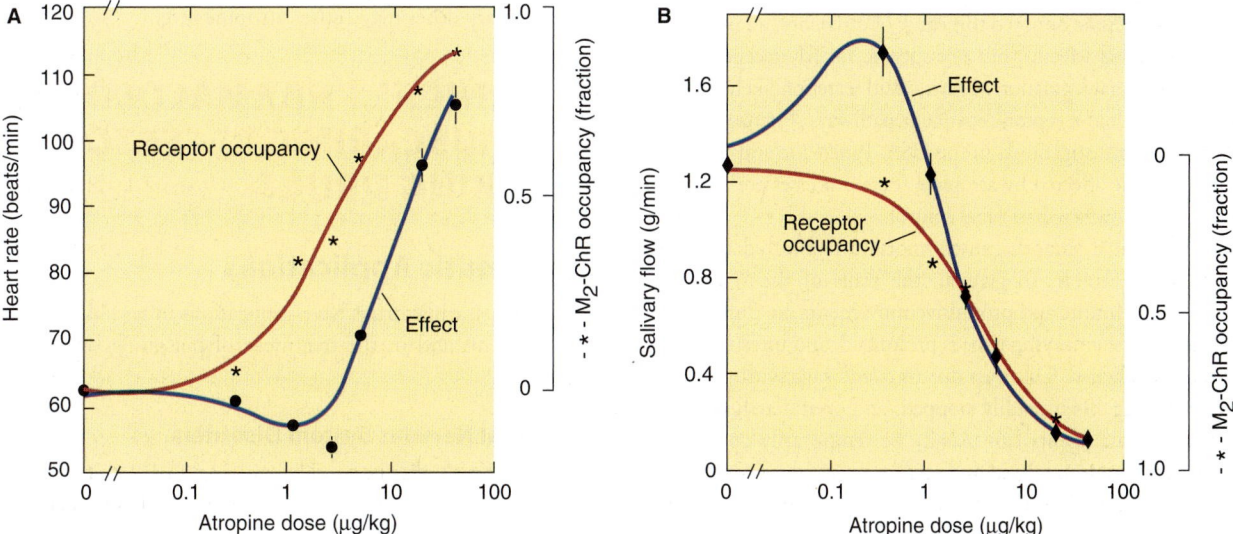

FIGURE 8–4 Effects of increasing doses of atropine on heart rate (**A**) and salivary flow (**B**) compared with muscarinic receptor occupancy in humans. The parasympathomimetic effect of low-dose atropine is attributed to blockade of prejunctional muscarinic receptors that suppress acetylcholine release. (Modified and reproduced, with permission, from Wellstein A, Pitschner HF: Complex dose-response curves of atropine in man explained by different functions of M_1 and M_2 cholinoceptors. Naunyn Schmiedebergs Arch Pharmacol 1988;338:19.)

pulmonary disease (COPD) is limited because block of autoinhibitory M_2 receptors on postganglionic parasympathetic nerves can oppose the bronchodilation caused by block of M_3 receptors on airway smooth muscle. Nevertheless, antimuscarinic agents are valuable in some patients with asthma or COPD.

Antimuscarinic drugs are frequently used before the administration of inhalant anesthetics to reduce the accumulation of secretions in the trachea and the possibility of laryngospasm.

5. Gastrointestinal tract—Blockade of muscarinic receptors has dramatic effects on motility and some of the secretory functions of the gut. However, even complete muscarinic block cannot totally abolish activity in this organ system, since local hormones and noncholinergic neurons in the enteric nervous system (see Chapters 6 and 62) also modulate gastrointestinal function. As in other tissues, exogenously administered muscarinic stimulants are more effectively blocked than are the effects of parasympathetic (vagal) nerve activity. The removal of autoinhibition, a negative feedback mechanism by which neural acetylcholine suppresses its own release, might explain the lower efficacy of antimuscarinic drugs against the effects of endogenous acetylcholine.

Antimuscarinic drugs have marked effects on salivary secretion; dry mouth occurs frequently in patients taking antimuscarinic drugs for Parkinson's disease or urinary conditions (Figure 8–5). Gastric secretion is blocked less effectively: the volume and amount of acid, pepsin, and mucin are all reduced, but large doses of atropine may be required. Basal secretion is blocked more effectively than that stimulated by food, nicotine, or alcohol. Pirenzepine and a more potent analog, telenzepine, reduce gastric acid secretion with fewer adverse effects than atropine and other less selective agents. This was thought to result from a selective blockade of excitatory M_1 muscarinic receptors on vagal ganglion cells innervating the stomach, as suggested by their high ratio of M_1 to M_3 affinity (Table 8–1). However, carbachol was found to stimulate gastric acid secretion in animals with M_1 receptors knocked out; M_3 receptors were implicated and pirenzepine opposed this effect of carbachol, an indication that pirenzepine is selective but not specific for M_1 receptors. The mechanism of vagal regulation of gastric acid secretion likely involves multiple muscarinic receptor-dependent pathways. Pirenzepine and telenzepine are investigational in the USA. Pancreatic and intestinal secretion are little affected by atropine; these processes are primarily under hormonal rather than vagal control.

Gastrointestinal smooth muscle motility is affected from the stomach to the colon. In general, the walls of the viscera are relaxed, and both tone and propulsive movements are diminished. Therefore, gastric emptying time is prolonged, and intestinal transit time is lengthened. Diarrhea due to overdosage with parasympathomimetic agents is readily stopped, and even diarrhea caused by nonautonomic agents can usually be temporarily controlled. However, intestinal "paralysis" induced by antimuscarinic drugs is temporary; local mechanisms within the enteric nervous system usually reestablish at least some peristalsis after 1–3 days of antimuscarinic drug therapy.

6. Genitourinary tract—The antimuscarinic action of atropine and its analogs relaxes smooth muscle of the ureters and bladder

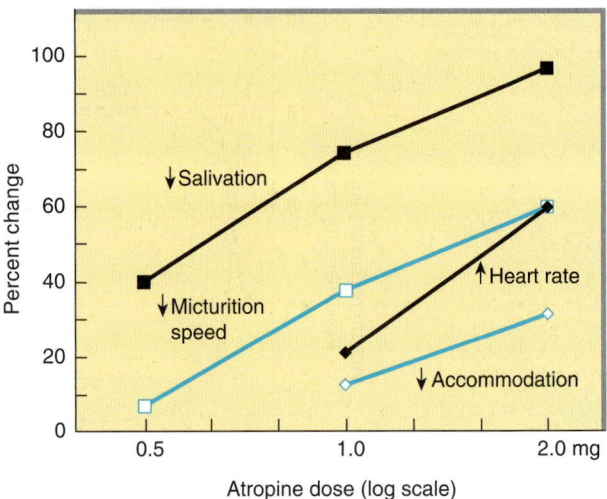

FIGURE 8–5 Effects of subcutaneous injection of atropine on salivation, speed of micturition (voiding), heart rate, and accommodation in normal adults. Note that salivation is the most sensitive of these variables, accommodation the least. (Data from Herxheimer A: Br J Pharmacol 1958;13:184.)

wall and slows voiding (Figure 8–5). This action is useful in the treatment of spasm induced by mild inflammation, surgery, and certain neurologic conditions, but it can precipitate urinary retention in men who have prostatic hyperplasia (see following section, Clinical Pharmacology of the Muscarinic Receptor-Blocking Drugs). The antimuscarinic drugs have no significant effect on the uterus.

7. Sweat glands—Atropine suppresses thermoregulatory sweating. Sympathetic cholinergic fibers innervate eccrine sweat glands, and their muscarinic receptors are readily accessible to antimuscarinic drugs. In adults, body temperature is elevated by this effect only if large doses are administered, but in infants and children even ordinary doses may cause "atropine fever."

■ CLINICAL PHARMACOLOGY OF THE MUSCARINIC RECEPTOR-BLOCKING DRUGS

Therapeutic Applications

The antimuscarinic drugs have applications in several of the major organ systems and in the treatment of poisoning by muscarinic agonists.

A. Central Nervous System Disorders

1. Parkinson's disease—The treatment of Parkinson's disease is often an exercise in polypharmacy, since no single agent is fully effective over the course of the disease. Most antimuscarinic drugs promoted for this application (see Table 28–1) were developed before levodopa became available. Their use is accompanied by all of the adverse effects described below, but the drugs remain useful as adjunctive therapy in some patients.

2. Motion sickness—Certain vestibular disorders respond to antimuscarinic drugs (and to antihistaminic agents with antimuscarinic effects). Scopolamine is one of the oldest remedies for seasickness and is as effective as any more recently introduced agent. It can be given by injection or by mouth or as a transdermal patch. The patch formulation produces significant blood levels over 48–72 hours. Useful doses by any route usually cause significant sedation and dry mouth.

B. Ophthalmologic Disorders

Accurate measurement of refractive error in uncooperative patients, eg, young children, requires ciliary paralysis. Also, ophthalmoscopic examination of the retina is greatly facilitated by mydriasis. Therefore, antimuscarinic agents, administered topically as eye drops or ointment, are very helpful in doing a complete examination. For adults and older children, the shorter-acting drugs are preferred (Table 8–2). For younger children, the greater efficacy of atropine is sometimes necessary, but the possibility of antimuscarinic poisoning is correspondingly increased. Drug loss from the conjunctival sac via the nasolacrimal duct into the nasopharynx can be diminished by the use of the ointment form rather than drops. Formerly, ophthalmic antimuscarinic drugs were selected from the tertiary amine subgroup to ensure good penetration after conjunctival application. Recent experiments in animals, however, suggest that glycopyrrolate, a quaternary agent, is as rapid in onset and as long-lasting as atropine.

Antimuscarinic drugs should never be used for mydriasis unless cycloplegia or prolonged action is required. Alpha-adrenoceptor stimulant drugs, eg, phenylephrine, produce a short-lasting mydriasis that is usually sufficient for funduscopic examination (see Chapter 9).

A second ophthalmologic use is to prevent synechia (adhesion) formation in uveitis and iritis. The longer-lasting preparations, especially homatropine, are valuable for this indication.

C. Respiratory Disorders

The use of atropine became part of routine preoperative medication when anesthetics such as ether were used, because these irritant anesthetics markedly increased airway secretions and were associated with frequent episodes of laryngospasm. Preanesthetic injection of atropine or scopolamine could prevent these hazardous effects. Scopolamine also produces significant amnesia for the events associated with surgery and obstetric delivery, a side effect that was considered desirable. On the other hand, urinary retention and intestinal hypomotility following surgery were often exacerbated by antimuscarinic drugs. Newer inhalational anesthetics are far less irritating to the airways.

Patients with **COPD,** a condition that occurs more frequently in older patients, particularly chronic smokers, benefit from bronchodilators, especially antimuscarinic agents. **Ipratropium** and **tiotropium** (see Figure 8–2), synthetic analogs of atropine, are used as inhalational drugs in COPD. The aerosol route of administration has the advantage of maximal concentration at the bronchial target tissue with reduced systemic effects. This application is discussed in greater detail in Chapter 20. Tiotropium has a longer bronchodilator action than ipratropium and can be given once daily because it dissociates slowly from M_3 receptors. It has a terminal elimination $t_{1/2}$ of 5–6 days; steady-state plasma levels are achieved in about 25 days with single daily administration. Tiotropium reduces the incidence of COPD exacerbations and is a useful adjunct to pulmonary rehabilitation in increasing exercise tolerance. The hyperactive neural bronchoconstrictor reflex present in most individuals with **asthma** is mediated by the vagus, acting on muscarinic receptors on bronchial smooth muscle cells. Ipratropium and tiotropium are also used as inhalational drugs in asthma.

D. Cardiovascular Disorders

Marked reflex vagal discharge sometimes accompanies the pain of myocardial infarction (eg, vasovagal attack) and may depress sinoatrial or atrioventricular node function sufficiently to impair cardiac output. Parenteral atropine or a similar antimuscarinic drug is appropriate therapy in this situation. Rare individuals without other detectable cardiac disease have hyperactive carotid sinus reflexes and may experience faintness or even syncope as a result of vagal discharge in response to pressure on the neck, eg, from a tight collar. Such individuals may benefit from the judicious use of atropine or a related antimuscarinic agent.

Pathophysiology can influence muscarinic activity in other ways as well. Circulating autoantibodies against the second extracellular loop of cardiac M_2 muscarinic receptors have been detected in some patients with idiopathic dilated cardiomyopathy and those afflicted with Chagas' disease caused by the protozoan *Trypanosoma cruzi*. Patients with Graves' disease (hyperthyroidism) also have such autoantibodies that may facilitate the development of atrial fibrillation. These antibodies exert parasympathomimetic actions on the heart that are prevented by atropine. In animals immunized with a peptide from the second extracellular loop of the M_2 receptor, the antibody is an allosteric modulator of the receptor. Although their role in the pathology of heart diseases is unknown, these antibodies should provide clues to the molecular basis of receptor activation because their site of action differs from the orthosteric site where acetylcholine binds (see Chapter 2).

E. Gastrointestinal Disorders

Antimuscarinic agents are now rarely used for peptic ulcer disease in the USA (see Chapter 62). Antimuscarinic agents can provide some relief in the treatment of common traveler's diarrhea and other mild or self-limited conditions of hypermotility. They are

TABLE 8–2 Antimuscarinic drugs used in ophthalmology.

Drug	Duration of Effect (days)	Usual Concentration (%)
Atropine	7–10	0.5–1
Scopolamine	3–7	0.25
Homatropine	1–3	2–5
Cyclopentolate	1	0.5–2
Tropicamide	0.25	0.5–1

often combined with an opioid antidiarrheal drug, an extremely effective therapy. In this combination, however, the very low dosage of the antimuscarinic drug functions primarily to discourage abuse of the opioid agent. The classic combination of atropine with diphenoxylate, a nonanalgesic congener of meperidine, is available under many names (eg, Lomotil) in both tablet and liquid form (see Chapter 62).

F. Urinary Disorders

Atropine and other antimuscarinic drugs have been used to provide symptomatic relief in the treatment of urinary urgency caused by minor inflammatory bladder disorders (Table 8–3). However, specific antimicrobial therapy is essential in bacterial cystitis. In the human urinary bladder, M_2 and M_3 receptors are expressed predominantly with the M_3 subtype mediating direct activation of contraction. As in intestinal smooth muscle, the M_2 subtype appears to act indirectly by inhibiting relaxation by norepinephrine and epinephrine.

Receptors for acetylcholine on the urothelium (the epithelial lining of the urinary tract) and on afferent nerves as well as the detrusor muscle provide a broad basis for the action of antimuscarinic drugs in the treatment of overactive bladder. **Oxybutynin,**

TABLE 8–3 Antimuscarinic drugs used in gastrointestinal and genitourinary conditions.

Drug	Usual Dosage
Quaternary amines	
Anisotropine	50 mg tid
Clidinium	2.5 mg tid–qid
Glycopyrrolate	1 mg bid–tid
Isopropamide	5 mg bid
Mepenzolate	25–50 mg qid
Methantheline	50–100 mg qid
Methscopolamine	2.5 mg qid
Oxyphenonium	5–10 mg qid
Propantheline	15 mg qid
Tridihexethyl	25–50 mg tid–qid
Trospium	20 mg bid
Tertiary amines	
Atropine	0.4 mg tid–qid
Darifenacin	7.5 mg qd
Dicyclomine	10–20 mg qid
Oxybutynin	5 mg tid
Oxyphencyclimine	10 mg bid
Propiverine	15 mg bid–tid
Scopolamine	0.4 mg tid
Solifenacin	5 mg qd
Tolterodine	2 mg bid

which is somewhat selective for M_3 receptors, is used to relieve bladder spasm after urologic surgery, eg, prostatectomy. It is also valuable in reducing involuntary voiding in patients with neurologic disease, eg, children with meningomyelocele. Oral oxybutynin or instillation of the drug by catheter into the bladder in such patients appears to improve bladder capacity and continence and to reduce infection and renal damage. Transdermally applied oxybutynin or its oral extended-release formulation reduces the need for multiple daily doses. **Trospium,** a nonselective antagonist, has been approved and is comparable in efficacy and side effects to oxybutynin. **Darifenacin** and **solifenacin** are recently approved antagonists that have greater selectivity for M_3 receptors than oxybutynin or trospium. Darifenacin and solifenacin have the advantage of once-daily dosing because of their long half-lives. **Tolterodine** and **fesoterodine,** M_3-selective antimuscarinics, are available for use in adults with urinary incontinence. They have many of the qualities of darifenacin and solifenacin and are available in extended-release tablets. The convenience of the newer and longer-acting drugs has not been accompanied by improvements in overall efficacy or by reductions in side effects such as dry mouth. An alternative treatment for urinary incontinence refractory to antimuscarinic drugs is intrabladder injection of botulinum toxin A. Botulinum toxin is reported to reduce urinary incontinence for several months after a single treatment by interfering with the co-release of ATP with neuronal acetylcholine (see Figure 6–3). Blockade of the activation of sensory nerves in the urothelium by ATP may account for a large part of this effect of botulinum toxin. This approach is not an FDA-approved indication at present.

Imipramine, a tricyclic antidepressant drug with strong antimuscarinic actions, has long been used to reduce incontinence in institutionalized elderly patients. It is moderately effective but causes significant CNS toxicity. **Propiverine,** a newer antimuscarinic agent, has been approved for this purpose.

Antimuscarinic agents have also been used in urolithiasis to relieve the painful ureteral smooth muscle spasm caused by passage of the stone. However, their usefulness in this condition is debatable.

G. Cholinergic Poisoning

Severe cholinergic excess is a medical emergency, especially in rural communities where cholinesterase inhibitor insecticides are commonly used and in cultures where wild mushrooms are frequently eaten. The potential use of cholinesterase inhibitors as chemical warfare "nerve gases" also requires an awareness of the methods for treating acute poisoning (see Chapter 58).

1. Antimuscarinic therapy—

Both the nicotinic and the muscarinic effects of the cholinesterase inhibitors can be life-threatening. Unfortunately, there is no effective method for directly blocking the nicotinic effects of cholinesterase inhibition, because nicotinic agonists *and* antagonists cause blockade of transmission (see Chapter 27). To reverse the muscarinic effects, a tertiary (not quaternary) amine drug must be used (preferably atropine) to treat the CNS effects as well as the peripheral effects of the organophosphate inhibitors. Large doses of atropine may be needed to oppose the muscarinic effects of extremely potent agents like parathion and chemical warfare nerve gases: 1–2 mg of atropine sulfate may be given intravenously every 5–15 minutes until signs of effect (dry mouth, reversal of miosis) appear. The drug may have to be given many times, since the acute effects of the cholinesterase inhibitor may last 24–48 hours or longer. In this life-threatening situation, as much as 1 g of atropine per day may be required for as long as 1 month for full control of muscarinic excess.

2. Cholinesterase regenerator compounds—A second class of compounds, composed of substituted oximes capable of regenerating active enzyme from the organophosphorus-cholinesterase complex, is also available to treat organophosphorus poisoning. These oxime agents include pralidoxime (PAM), diacetylmonoxime (DAM), obidoxime, and others.

Pralidoxime   **Diacetylmonoxime**

Organophosphates cause phosphorylation of the serine OH group at the active site of cholinesterase. The oxime group (=NOH) has a very high affinity for the phosphorus atom, for which it competes with serine OH. These oximes can hydrolyze the phosphorylated enzyme and regenerate active enzyme from the organophosphorus-cholinesterase complex if the complex has not "aged" (see Chapter 7). Pralidoxime is the most extensively studied—in humans—of the agents shown and the only one available for clinical use in the USA. It is most effective in regenerating the cholinesterase associated with skeletal muscle neuromuscular junctions. Pralidoxime and obidoxime are ineffective in reversing the central effects of organophosphate poisoning because each has positively charged quaternary ammonium groups that prevent entry into the CNS. Diacetylmonoxime, on the other hand, crosses the blood-brain barrier and, in experimental animals, can regenerate some of the CNS cholinesterase.

Pralidoxime is administered by intravenous infusion, 1–2 g given over 15–30 minutes. In spite of the likelihood of aging of the phosphate-enzyme complex, recent reports suggest that administration of multiple doses of pralidoxime over several days may be useful in severe poisoning. In excessive doses, pralidoxime can induce neuromuscular weakness and other adverse effects. Pralidoxime is *not* recommended for the reversal of inhibition of acetylcholinesterase by carbamate inhibitors. Further details of treatment of anticholinesterase toxicity are given in Chapter 58.

A third approach to protection against excessive acetylcholinesterase inhibition is *pretreatment* with reversible enzyme inhibitors to prevent binding of the irreversible organophosphate inhibitor. This prophylaxis can be achieved with pyridostigmine but is reserved for situations in which possibly lethal poisoning is anticipated, eg, chemical warfare (see Chapter 7). Simultaneous use of atropine is required to control muscarinic excess.

Mushroom poisoning has traditionally been divided into rapid-onset and delayed-onset types. The rapid-onset type is usually apparent within 30 minutes to 2 hours after ingestion of the mushrooms, and can be caused by a variety of toxins. Some of these produce simple upset stomach; others can have disulfiram-like effects; some cause hallucinations; and a few mushrooms (eg, Inocybe species) can produce signs of muscarinic excess: nausea, vomiting, diarrhea, urinary urgency, sweating, salivation, and sometimes bronchoconstriction. Parenteral atropine, 1–2 mg, is effective treatment in such intoxications. Despite its name, *Amanita muscaria* contains not only muscarine (the alkaloid was named after the mushroom), but also numerous other alkaloids, including antimuscarinic agents, and ingestion of *A muscaria* often causes signs of atropine poisoning, not muscarine excess.

Delayed-onset mushroom poisoning, usually caused by *Amanita phalloides, A virosa, Galerina autumnalis,* or *G marginata,* manifests its first symptoms 6–12 hours after ingestion. Although the initial symptoms usually include nausea and vomiting, the major toxicity involves hepatic and renal cellular injury by amatoxins that inhibit RNA polymerase. Atropine is of no value in this form of mushroom poisoning (see Chapter 58).

H. Other Applications

Hyperhidrosis (excessive sweating) is sometimes reduced by antimuscarinic agents. However, relief is incomplete at best, probably because apocrine rather than eccrine glands are usually involved.

Adverse Effects

Treatment with atropine or its congeners directed at one organ system almost always induces undesirable effects in other organ systems. Thus, mydriasis and cycloplegia are adverse effects when an antimuscarinic agent is used to reduce gastrointestinal secretion or motility, even though they are therapeutic effects when the drug is used in ophthalmology.

At higher concentrations, atropine causes block of all parasympathetic functions. However, atropine is a remarkably safe drug *in adults.* Atropine poisoning has occurred as a result of attempted suicide, but most cases are due to attempts to induce hallucinations. Poisoned individuals manifest dry mouth, mydriasis, tachycardia, hot and flushed skin, agitation, and delirium for as long as 1 week. Body temperature is frequently elevated. These effects are memorialized in the adage, "dry as a bone, blind as a bat, red as a beet, mad as a hatter."

Unfortunately, children, especially infants, are very sensitive to the hyperthermic effects of atropine. Although accidental administration of over 400 mg has been followed by recovery, deaths have followed doses as small as 2 mg. Therefore, atropine should be considered a highly dangerous drug when overdose occurs in infants or children.

Overdoses of atropine or its congeners are generally treated symptomatically (see Chapter 58). Poison control experts discourage the use of physostigmine or another cholinesterase inhibitor to reverse the effects of atropine overdose because symptomatic management is more effective and less dangerous. When physostigmine is deemed necessary, *small* doses are given *slowly* intravenously

(1–4 mg in adults, 0.5–1 mg in children). Symptomatic treatment may require temperature control with cooling blankets and seizure control with diazepam.

Poisoning caused by high doses of quaternary antimuscarinic drugs is associated with all of the peripheral signs of parasympathetic blockade but few or none of the CNS effects of atropine. These more polar drugs may cause significant ganglionic blockade, however, with marked orthostatic hypotension (see below). Treatment of the antimuscarinic effects, if required, can be carried out with a quaternary cholinesterase inhibitor such as neostigmine. Control of hypotension may require the administration of a sympathomimetic drug such as phenylephrine.

Recent evidence indicates that some centrally acting drugs (tricyclic antidepressants, selective serotonin reuptake inhibitors, anti-anxiety agents) with antimuscarinic actions impair memory and cognition in older patients.

Contraindications

Contraindications to the use of antimuscarinic drugs are relative, not absolute. Obvious muscarinic excess, especially that caused by cholinesterase inhibitors, can always be treated with atropine.

Antimuscarinic drugs are contraindicated in patients with glaucoma, especially angle-closure glaucoma. Even systemic use of moderate doses may precipitate angle closure (and acute glaucoma) in patients with shallow anterior chambers.

In elderly men, antimuscarinic drugs should always be used with caution and should be avoided in those with a history of prostatic hyperplasia.

Because the antimuscarinic drugs slow gastric emptying, they may *increase* symptoms in patients with gastric ulcer. Nonselective antimuscarinic agents should never be used to treat acid-peptic disease (see Chapter 62).

■ BASIC & CLINICAL PHARMACOLOGY OF THE GANGLION-BLOCKING DRUGS

Ganglion-blocking agents competitively block the action of acetylcholine and similar agonists at nicotinic receptors of both parasympathetic and sympathetic autonomic ganglia. Some members of the group also block the ion channel that is gated by the nicotinic cholinoceptor. The ganglion-blocking drugs are important and used in pharmacologic and physiologic research because they can block all autonomic outflow. However, their lack of selectivity confers such a broad range of undesirable effects that they have limited clinical use.

Chemistry & Pharmacokinetics

All ganglion-blocking drugs of interest are synthetic amines. **Tetraethylammonium (TEA),** the first to be recognized as having this action, has a very short duration of action. **Hexamethonium ("C6")** was developed and was introduced clinically as the first drug effective for management of hypertension. As shown in

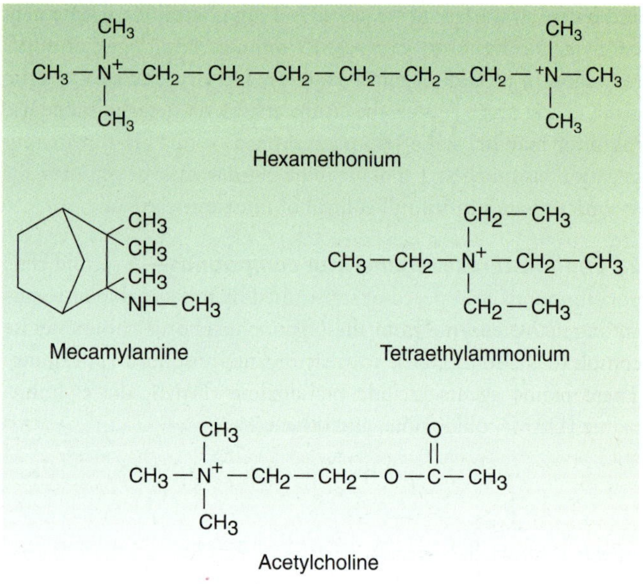

FIGURE 8–6 Some ganglion-blocking drugs. Acetylcholine is shown for reference.

Figure 8–6, there is an obvious relationship between the structures of the agonist acetylcholine and the nicotinic antagonists tetraethylammonium and hexamethonium. Decamethonium, the "C10" analog of hexamethonium, is a depolarizing neuromuscular blocking agent.

Mecamylamine, a secondary amine, was developed to improve the degree and extent of absorption from the gastrointestinal tract because the quaternary amine ganglion-blocking compounds were poorly and erratically absorbed after oral administration. **Trimethaphan,** a short-acting ganglion blocker, is inactive orally and is given by intravenous infusion.

Pharmacodynamics

A. Mechanism of Action

Ganglionic nicotinic receptors, like those of the skeletal muscle neuromuscular junction, are subject to both depolarizing and nondepolarizing blockade (see Chapters 7 and 27). Nicotine itself, carbamoylcholine, and even acetylcholine (if amplified with a cholinesterase inhibitor) can produce depolarizing ganglion block.

Drugs now used as ganglion blockers are classified as nondepolarizing competitive antagonists. However, hexamethonium actually produces most of its blockade by occupying sites in or on the nicotinic ion channel, not by occupying the cholinoceptor itself. In contrast, trimethaphan appears to block the nicotinic receptor, not the channel pore. Blockade can be surmounted by increasing the concentration of an agonist, eg, acetylcholine.

B. Organ System Effects

1. Central nervous system—Mecamylamine, unlike the quaternary amine agents and trimethaphan, crosses the blood-brain barrier and readily enters the CNS. Sedation, tremor, choreiform movements, and mental aberrations have been reported as effects of mecamylamine.

2. Eye—The ganglion-blocking drugs cause a predictable cycloplegia with loss of accommodation because the ciliary muscle receives innervation primarily from the parasympathetic nervous system. The effect on the pupil is not so easily predicted, since the iris receives both sympathetic innervation (mediating pupillary dilation) and parasympathetic innervation (mediating pupillary constriction). Ganglionic blockade often causes moderate dilation of the pupil because parasympathetic tone usually dominates this tissue.

3. Cardiovascular system—Blood vessels receive chiefly vasoconstrictor fibers from the sympathetic nervous system; therefore, ganglionic blockade causes a marked decrease in arteriolar and venomotor tone. The blood pressure may fall precipitously because both peripheral vascular resistance and venous return are decreased (see Figure 6–7). Hypotension is especially marked in the upright position (orthostatic or postural hypotension), because postural reflexes that normally prevent venous pooling are blocked.

Cardiac effects include diminished contractility and, because the sinoatrial node is usually dominated by the parasympathetic nervous system, a moderate tachycardia.

4. Gastrointestinal tract—Secretion is reduced, although not enough to effectively treat peptic disease. Motility is profoundly inhibited, and constipation can be marked.

5. Other systems—Genitourinary smooth muscle is partially dependent on autonomic innervation for normal function. Therefore, ganglionic blockade causes hesitancy in urination and may precipitate urinary retention in men with prostatic hyperplasia.

Sexual function is impaired in that both erection and ejaculation may be prevented by moderate doses.

Thermoregulatory sweating is reduced by the ganglion-blocking drugs. However, hyperthermia is not a problem except in very warm environments, because cutaneous vasodilation is usually sufficient to maintain a normal body temperature.

6. Response to autonomic drugs—Patients receiving ganglion-blocking drugs are fully responsive to autonomic drugs acting on muscarinic, α-, and β-adrenergic receptors because these effector cell receptors are not blocked. In fact, responses may be exaggerated or even reversed (eg, intravenously administered norepinephrine may cause tachycardia rather than bradycardia), because homeostatic reflexes, which normally moderate autonomic responses, are absent.

Clinical Applications & Toxicity

Ganglion blockers are used infrequently because more selective autonomic blocking agents are available. Mecamylamine blocks central nicotinic receptors and has been advocated as a possible adjunct with the transdermal nicotine patch to reduce nicotine craving in patients attempting to quit smoking. Trimethaphan is occasionally used in the treatment of hypertensive emergencies and dissecting aortic aneurysm; in producing hypotension, which can be of value in neurosurgery to reduce bleeding in the operative field; and in the treatment of patients undergoing electroconvulsive therapy. The toxicity of the ganglion-blocking drugs is limited to the autonomic effects already described. For most patients, these effects are intolerable except for acute use.

SUMMARY Drugs with Anticholinergic Actions

Subclass	Mechanism of Action	Effects	Clinical Applications	Pharmacokinetics, Toxicities, Interactions
MOTION SICKNESS DRUGS				
• Scopolamine	Unknown mechanism in CNS	Reduces vertigo, postoperative nausea	Prevention of motion sickness and postoperative nausea and vomiting	Transdermal patch used for motion sickness • IM injection for postoperative use • *Toxicity:* Tachycardia, blurred vision, xerostomia, delirium • *Interactions:* With other antimuscarinics
GASTROINTESTINAL DISORDERS				
• Dicyclomine	Competitive antagonism at M_3 receptors	Reduces smooth muscle and secretory activity of gut	Irritable bowel syndrome, minor diarrhea	Available in oral and parenteral forms • short $t_{1/2}$ but action lasts up to 6 hours • *Toxicity:* Tachycardia, confusion, urinary retention, increased intraocular pressure • *Interactions:* With other antimuscarinics
• *Hyoscyamine: Longer duration of action*				
• *Glycopyrrolate: Similar to dicyclomine*				
OPHTHALMOLOGY				
• Atropine	Competitive antagonism at all M receptors	Causes mydriasis and cycloplegia	Retinal examination; prevention of synechiae after surgery	Used as drops • long (5–6 days) action • *Toxicity:* Increased intraocular pressure in closed-angle glaucoma • *Interactions:* With other antimuscarinics
• *Scopolamine: Faster onset of action than atropine*				
• *Homatropine: Shorter duration of action (12–24 h)*				
• *Cyclopentolate: Shorter duration of action (3–6 h)*				
• *Tropicamide: Shortest duration of action (15–60 min)*				
RESPIRATORY (ASTHMA, COPD)				
• Ipratropium	Competitive, nonselective antagonist at M receptors	Reduces or prevents bronchospasm	Prevention and relief of acute episodes of bronchospasm	Aerosol canister, up to qid • *Toxicity:* Xerostomia, cough • *Interactions:* With other antimuscarinics
• *Tiotropium: Longer duration of action; used qd*				
URINARY				
• Oxybutynin	Slightly M_3-selective muscarinic antagonist	Reduces detrusor smooth muscle tone, spasms	Urge incontinence; postoperative spasms	Oral, IV, patch formulations • *Toxicity:* Tachycardia, constipation, increased intraocular pressure, xerostomia • Patch: Pruritus • *Interactions:* With other antimuscarinics
• *Darifenacin, solifenacin, and tolterodine: Tertiary amines with somewhat greater selectivity for M_3 receptors*				
• *Trospium: Quaternary amine with less CNS effect*				
CHOLINERGIC POISONING				
• Atropine	Nonselective competitive antagonist at all muscarinic receptors in CNS and periphery	Blocks muscarinic excess at exocrine glands, heart, smooth muscle	Mandatory antidote for severe cholinesterase inhibitor poisoning	Intravenous infusion until antimuscarinic signs appear • continue as long as necessary • *Toxicity:* Insignificant as long as AChE inhibition continues
• Pralidoxime	Very high affinity for phosphorus atom but does not enter CNS	Regenerates active AChE; can relieve skeletal muscle end plate block	Usual antidote for early-stage (48 h) cholinesterase inhibitor poisoning	Intravenous every 4–6 h • *Toxicity:* Can cause muscle weakness in overdose

AChE, acetylcholinesterase; CNS, central nervous system; COPD, chronic obstructive pulmonary disease.

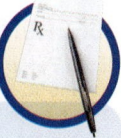

P R E P A R A T I O N S   A V A I L A B L E

ANTIMUSCARINIC ANTICHOLINERGIC DRUGS*

Atropine (generic)
Oral: 0.4, 0.6 mg tablets
Parenteral: 0.05, 0.1, 0.4, 0.5, 1 mg/mL for injection; Atropen: 0.25, 0.5, 2 mg pen injectors
Ophthalmic (generic, Isopto Atropine): 0.5, 1, 2% drops; 0.5, 1% ointments

Belladonna alkaloids, extract or tincture (generic)
Oral: 0.27–0.33 mg/mL liquid

Clidinium (generic, Quarzan, others)
Oral: 2.5, 5 mg capsules

Cyclopentolate (generic, Cyclogyl, others)
Ophthalmic: 0.5, 1, 2% solution

Darifenacin (Enablex)
Oral: 7.5, 15 mg tablets (extended release)

Dicyclomine (generic, Bentyl, others)
Oral: 10, 20 mg capsules; 20 mg tablets; 10 mg/5 mL syrup
Parenteral: 10 mg/mL for intramuscular injection

Fesoterodine (Toviaz)
Oral: 4, 8 mg extended-release tablets

Flavoxate (Urispas)
Oral: 100 mg tablets

Glycopyrrolate (generic, Robinul)
Oral: 1, 2 mg tablets
Parenteral: 0.2 mg/mL for injection

Homatropine (generic, Isopto Homatropine, others)
Ophthalmic: 2, 5% solution

l-Hyoscyamine (Anaspaz, Cystospaz-M, Levsin, others)
Oral: 0.125, 0.25 mg tablets; 0.375, 0.75 mg timed-release capsules; 0.125 mg/5 mL oral elixir and solution
Parenteral: 0.5 mg/mL for injection

Ipratropium (generic, Atrovent)
Aerosol: 200 dose metered-dose inhaler (0.17 mg/dose)
Solution for nebulizer: 0.02%
Nasal spray: 0.03, 0.06%

Mepenzolate (Cantil)
Oral: 25 mg tablets

Methantheline (Banthine)
Oral: 50 mg tablets

Methscopolamine (generic, Pamine)
Oral: 2.5, 5 mg tablets

Oxybutynin (generic, Ditropan)
Oral: 5 mg tablets; 5, 10 mg extended-release tablets; patch (3.9 mg/day); 5 mg/5 mL syrup
Topical: 10% gel

Propantheline (generic, Pro-Banthine, others)
Oral: 7.5, 15 mg tablets

Scopolamine (generic)
Oral: 0.4 mg tablets
Parenteral: 0.4 mg/mL for injection
Ophthalmic (Isopto Hyoscine): 0.25% solution
Transdermal (Transderm Scop): 1.5 mg (delivers 0.5 mg/24 h)patch; extended-release patch (delivers 0.33 mg/24 h)

Solifenacin (Vesicare)
Oral: 5, 10 mg tablets

Tiotropium (Spiriva)
Aerosol: 18 mcg tablet for inhaler

Tolterodine (Detrol)
Oral: 1, 2 mg tablets; 2, 4 mg extended-release capsules

Tridihexethyl (Pathilon)
Oral: 25 mg tablets

Tropicamide (generic, Mydriacyl Ophthalmic, others)
Ophthalmic: 0.5, 1% drops

Trospium (Spasmex, Sanctura)
Oral: 20 mg tablets; 60 mg extended-release capsule
Suppository: 0.75, 1.0 mg
Parenteral: 0.6 mg/mL

GANGLION BLOCKERS

Mecamylamine (Inversine)
Oral: 2.5, 10 mg tablets

Trimethaphan (Arfonad)
Parenteral: 50 mg/mL

CHOLINESTERASE REGENERATOR

Pralidoxime (generic, Protopam)
Parenteral: 1 g vial with 20 mL diluent for IV administration; 600 mg in 2 mL autoinjector

*Antimuscarinic drugs used in parkinsonism are listed in Chapter 28.

REFERENCES

Aihaara T et al: Cholinergically stimulated gastric acid secretion is mediated by M_3 and M_5 but not M_1 muscarinic acetylcholine receptors in mice. Am J Physiol 2005;288:G1199.

Andersson KE: Antimuscarinics for treatment of overactive bladder. Lancet Neurol 2004;3:46.

Brodde OE et al: Presence, distribution and physiological function of adrenergic and muscarinic receptor subtypes in the human heart. Basic Res Cardiol 2001;96:528.

Carrière I et al: Drugs with anticholinergic properties, cognitive decline, and dementia in an elderly general population. Arch Intern Med 2009;169:1317.

Casaburi R et al: Improvement in exercise tolerance with the combination of tiotropium and pulmonary rehabilitation in patients with COPD. Chest 2005;127:809.

Casarosa P et al: The constitutive activity of the human muscarinic M3 receptor unmasks differences in the pharmacology of anticholinergics. J Pharmacol Exp Ther 2010;333:201.

Chapple CR et al: A comparison of the efficacy and tolerability of solifenacin succinate and extended release tolterodine at treating overactive bladder syndrome: Results of the STAR trial. Eur Urol 2005;48:464.

Fowler CJ et al: The neural control of micturition. Nat Rev Neurosci 2008:9:453.

Fukusaki M et al: Effects of controlled hypotension with sevoflurane anesthesia on hepatic function of surgical patients. Eur J Anaesthesiol 1999;16:111.

Hegde SS: Muscarinic receptors in the bladder: From basic research to therapeutics. Br J Pharmacol 2006;147:S80.

Kranke P et al: The efficacy and safety of transdermal scopolamine for the prevention of postoperative nausea and vomiting: A quantitative systematic review. Anesth Analg 2002;95:133.

Lawrence GW et al: Excitatory cholinergic and purinergic signaling in bladder are equally susceptible to botulinum neurotoxin A consistent with co-release of transmitters from efferent fibers. J Pharmacol Exp Ther 2010;334:1080.

Moreland RB et al: Emerging pharmacologic approaches for the treatment of lower urinary tract disorders. J Pharm Exp Ther 2004;308:797.

Olson K: Mushrooms. In: Olson K (editor). *Poisoning & Drug Overdose,* 5th ed. McGraw-Hill, 2007.

Petrides G et al: Trimethaphan (Arfonad) control of hypertension and tachycardia during electroconvulsive therapy: A double-blind study. J Clin Anesth 1996;8:104.

Profita M et al: Smoke, choline acetyltransferase, muscarinic receptors, and fibroblast proliferation in chronic obstructive pulmonary disease. J Pharmacol Exp Ther 2009;329:753.

Stavrakis S et al: Activating autoantibodies to the beta-1 adrenergic and m2 muscarinic receptors facilitate atrial fibrillation in patients with Graves' hyperthyroidism. J Am Coll Cardiol 2009;54:1309.

Xie G et al: Cholinergic agonist-induced pepsinogen secretion from murine gastric chief cells is mediated by M_1 and M_3 muscarinic receptors. Am J Physiol 2005;289:G521.

Young JM et al: Mecamylamine: New therapeutic uses and toxicity/risk profile. Clin Ther 2001;23:532.

Zhang L et al: A missense mutation in the CHRM2 gene is associated with familial dilated cardiomyopathy. Circ Res 2008;102:1426.

Treatment of Anticholinesterase Poisoning

Jokanovic M: Medical treatment of acute poisoning with organophosphorus and carbamate pesticides. Toxicol Lett 2009;190:107.

Newmark J: Nerve agents: Pathophysiology and treatment of poisoning. Semin Neurol 2004:24:185.

Thiermann H et al: Pharmacokinetics of obidoxime in patients poisoned with organophosphorus compounds. Toxicol Lett 2010;197:236.

Weinbroum AA: Pathophysiological and clinical aspects of combat anticholinesterase poisoning. Br Med Bull 2005;72:119.

Worek R et al: Recent advances in evaluation of oxime efficacy in nerve agent poisoning by in vitro analysis. Toxicol Appl Pharmacol 2007;219:226.

CASE STUDY ANSWER

JH's symptoms are often displayed by patients following prostatectomy to relieve significant obstruction of bladder outflow. Urge incontinence can occur in patients whose prostatic hypertrophy caused instability of the detrusor muscle. He should be advised that urinary incontinence and urinary frequency can diminish with time after prostatectomy as detrusor muscle instability subsides. JH can be helped by daily administration of a single tablet of extended-release tolterodine (4 mg/day) or oxybutynin (5–10 mg/day). A transdermal patch containing oxybutynin (3.9 mg/day) is also available.

Adrenoceptor Agonists & Sympathomimetic Drugs

Italo Biaggioni, MD, & David Robertson, MD[*]

CASE STUDY

A 68-year-old man presents with a complaint of light-headedness on standing that is worse after meals and in hot environments. Symptoms started about 4 years ago and have slowly progressed to the point that he is disabled. He has fainted several times, but always recovers consciousness almost as soon as he falls. Review of symptoms reveals slight worsening of constipation, urinary retention out of proportion to prostate size, and decreased sweating. He is otherwise healthy with no history of hypertension, diabetes, or Parkinson's disease. Because of his urinary retention, he was placed on the α_1 antagonist tamsulosin but he could not tolerate it because of worsening of orthostatic hypotension. Physical examination revealed a blood pressure of 167/84 mm Hg supine and 106/55 mm Hg standing. There was an inadequate compensatory increase in heart rate (from 84 to 88 bpm), considering the degree of orthostatic hypotension. Physical examination is otherwise unremarkable with no evidence of peripheral neuropathy or parkinsonian features. Laboratory examinations are negative except for plasma norepinephrine, which is low at 98 pg/mL (normal is 250–400 pg/mL for his age). A diagnosis of pure autonomic failure is made, based on the clinical picture and the absence of drugs that could induce orthostatic hypotension and diseases commonly associated with autonomic neuropathy (eg, diabetes, Parkinson's disease). What precautions should this patient observe in using sympathomimetic drugs? Can such drugs be used in his treatment?

The sympathetic nervous system is an important regulator of virtually all organ systems. This is particularly evident in the regulation of blood pressure. As illustrated in the case study, the autonomic nervous system is crucial for the maintenance of blood pressure even under relatively minor situations of stress (eg, the gravitational stress of standing).

The ultimate effects of sympathetic stimulation are mediated by release of norepinephrine from nerve terminals, which then activates adrenoceptors on postsynaptic sites (see Chapter 6). Also, in response to a variety of stimuli such as stress, the adrenal medulla releases epinephrine, which is transported in the blood to target tissues. In other words, epinephrine acts as a hormone, whereas norepinephrine acts as a neurotransmitter.

Drugs that mimic the actions of epinephrine or norepinephrine have traditionally been termed **sympathomimetic drugs.** The sympathomimetics can be grouped by mode of action and by the spectrum of receptors that they activate. Some of these drugs (eg, norepinephrine and epinephrine) are *direct* agonists; that is, they directly interact with and activate adrenoceptors. Others are *indirect* agonists because their actions are dependent on their ability to enhance the actions of endogenous catecholamines. These indirect agents may have either of two different mechanisms: (1) they may displace stored catecholamines from the adrenergic nerve ending (eg, the mechanism of action of tyramine), or they may decrease the clearance of released norepinephrine either by (2a) inhibiting reuptake of catecholamines already released (eg, the mechanism of action of cocaine and tricyclic antidepressants) or (2b) preventing the enzymatic metabolism of norepinephrine (monoamine oxidase and catechol-*O*-methyltransferase inhibitors). Some drugs have both direct and indirect actions. Both

[*]The authors thank Drs. Vsevolod Gurevich and Randy Blakely for helpful comments.

types of sympathomimetics, direct and indirect, ultimately cause activation of adrenoceptors, leading to some or all of the characteristic effects of endogenous catecholamines.

The pharmacologic effects of direct agonists depend on the route of administration, their relative affinity for adrenoreceptor subtypes, and the relative expression of these receptor subtypes in target tissues. The pharmacologic effects of indirect sympathomimetics are greater under conditions of increased sympathetic activity and norepinephrine storage and release.

MOLECULAR PHARMACOLOGY UNDERLYING THE ACTIONS OF SYMPATHOMIMETIC DRUGS

The effects of catecholamines are mediated by cell-surface receptors. Adrenoceptors are typical G protein-coupled receptors (GPCRs; see Chapter 2). The receptor protein has an extracellular N-terminus, traverses the membrane seven times (transmembrane domains) forming three extracellular and three intracellular loops, and has an intracellular C-terminus (Figure 9–1). G protein-coupled receptors are coupled by G proteins to the various effector proteins whose activities are regulated by those receptors. Each

G protein is a heterotrimer consisting of α, β, and γ subunits. G proteins are classified on the basis of their distinctive α subunits. G proteins of particular importance for adrenoceptor function include G_s, the stimulatory G protein of adenylyl cyclase; G_i and G_o, the inhibitory G proteins of adenylyl cyclase; and G_q and G_{11}, the G proteins coupling α receptors to phospholipase C. The activation of G protein-coupled receptors by catecholamines promotes the dissociation of guanosine diphosphate (GDP) from the α subunit of the appropriate G protein. Guanosine triphosphate (GTP) then binds to this G protein, and the α subunit dissociates from the β-γ unit. The activated GTP-bound α subunit then regulates the activity of its effector. Effectors of adrenoceptor-activated α subunits include adenylyl cyclase, cGMP phosphodiesterase, phospholipase C, and ion channels. The α subunit is inactivated by hydrolysis of the bound GTP to GDP and phosphate, and the subsequent reassociation of the α subunit with the β-γ subunit. The β-γ subunits have additional independent effects, acting on a variety of effectors such as ion channels and enzymes.

Adrenoreceptors were initially characterized pharmacologically, with α receptors having the comparative potencies epinephrine ≥ norepinephrine >> isoproterenol, and β receptors having the comparative potencies isoproterenol > epinephrine ≥ norepinephrine. The development of selective antagonists revealed the presence of subtypes of these receptors, which were finally characterized by

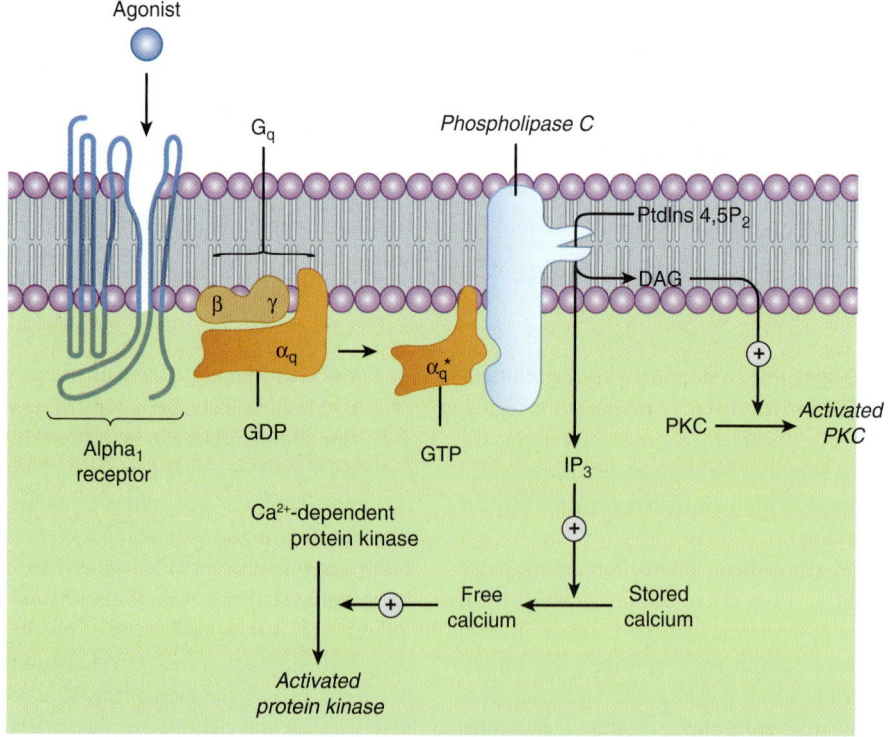

FIGURE 9–1 Activation of α_1 responses. Stimulation of α_1 receptors by catecholamines leads to the activation of a G_q-coupling protein. The activated α subunit (α_q*) of this G protein activates the effector, phospholipase C, which leads to the release of IP_3 (inositol 1,4,5-trisphosphate) and DAG (diacylglycerol) from phosphatidylinositol 4,5-bisphosphate ($PtdIns\ 4,5P_2$). IP_3 stimulates the release of sequestered stores of calcium, leading to an increased concentration of cytoplasmic Ca^{2+}. Ca^{2+} may then activate Ca^{2+}-dependent protein kinases, which in turn phosphorylate their substrates. DAG activates protein kinase C (PKC). GTP, guanosine triphosphate; GDP, guanosine diphosphate. See text for additional effects of α_1-receptor activation.

TABLE 9–1 Adrenoceptor types and subtypes.

Receptor	Agonist	Antagonist	G Protein	Effects	Gene on Chromosome
α_1 type	Phenylephrine	Prazosin	G_q	↑ IP3, DAG common to all	
α_{1A}					C8
α_{1B}					C5
α_{1D}					C20
α_2 type	Clonidine	Yohimbine	G_i	↓ cAMP common to all	
α_{2A}	Oxymetazoline				C10
α_{2B}		Prazosin			C2
α_{2C}		Prazosin			C4
β type	Isoproterenol	Propranolol	G_s	↑ cAMP common to all	
β_1	Dobutamine	Betaxolol			C10
β_2	Albuterol	Butoxamine			C5
β_3					C8
Dopamine type	Dopamine				
D_1	Fenoldopam		G_s	↑ cAMP	C5
D_2	Bromocriptine		G_i	↓ cAMP	C11
D_3			G_i	↓ cAMP	C3
D_4		Clozapine	G_i	↓ cAMP	C11
D_5			G_s	↑ cAMP	C4

molecular cloning. We now know that unique genes encode the receptor subtypes listed in Table 9–1.

Likewise, the endogenous catecholamine dopamine produces a variety of biologic effects that are mediated by interactions with specific dopamine receptors (Table 9–1). These receptors are distinct from α and β receptors and are particularly important in the brain (see Chapters 21 and 29) and in the splanchnic and renal vasculature. Molecular cloning has identified several distinct genes encoding five receptor subtypes, two D_1-like receptors (D_1 and D_5) and three D_2-like (D_2, D_3, and D_4). Further complexity occurs because of the presence of introns within the coding region of the D_2-like receptor genes, which allows for alternative splicing of the exons in this major subtype. There is extensive polymorphic variation in the D_4 human receptor gene. These subtypes may have importance for understanding the efficacy and adverse effects of novel antipsychotic drugs (see Chapter 29).

Receptor Types

A. Alpha Receptors

Alpha$_1$ receptors are coupled via G proteins in the G_q family to phospholipase C. This enzyme hydrolyzes polyphosphoinositides, leading to the formation of **inositol 1,4,5-trisphosphate (IP$_3$)** and **diacylglycerol (DAG)** (Table 9–1, Figure 9–1). IP$_3$ promotes the release of sequestered Ca^{2+} from intracellular stores, which increases the cytoplasmic concentration of free Ca^{2+} and the activation of various calcium-dependent protein kinases. Activation of these receptors may also increase influx of calcium across the cell's plasma

membrane. IP$_3$ is sequentially dephosphorylated, which ultimately leads to the formation of free inositol. DAG activates protein kinase C, which modulates activity of many signaling pathways. In addition, α_1 receptors activate signal transduction pathways that were originally described for peptide growth factor receptors that activate tyrosine kinases. For example, α_1 receptors have been found to activate mitogen-activated kinases (MAP kinases) and polyphospho-inositol-3-kinase (PI-3-kinase). These pathways may have importance for the α_1-receptor–mediated stimulation of cell growth and proliferation through the regulation of gene expression.

Alpha$_2$ receptors inhibit adenylyl cyclase activity and cause intracellular cyclic adenosine monophosphate (cAMP) levels to decrease. Alpha$_2$-receptor–mediated inhibition of adenylyl cyclase activity is transduced by the inhibitory regulatory protein, G_i (Figure 9–2). It is likely that not only α, but also the β-γ subunits of G_i contribute to inhibition of adenylyl cyclase. Alpha$_2$ receptors use other signaling pathways, including regulation of ion channel activities and the activities of important enzymes involved in signal transduction. Indeed, some of the effects of α_2 adrenoceptors are independent of their ability to inhibit adenylyl cyclase; for example, α_2-receptor agonists cause platelet aggregation and a decrease in platelet cAMP levels, but it is not clear whether aggregation is the result of the decrease in cAMP or other mechanisms involving G_i-regulated effectors.

B. Beta Receptors

Activation of all three receptor subtypes (β_1, β_2, and β_3) results in stimulation of adenylyl cyclase and increased conversion of

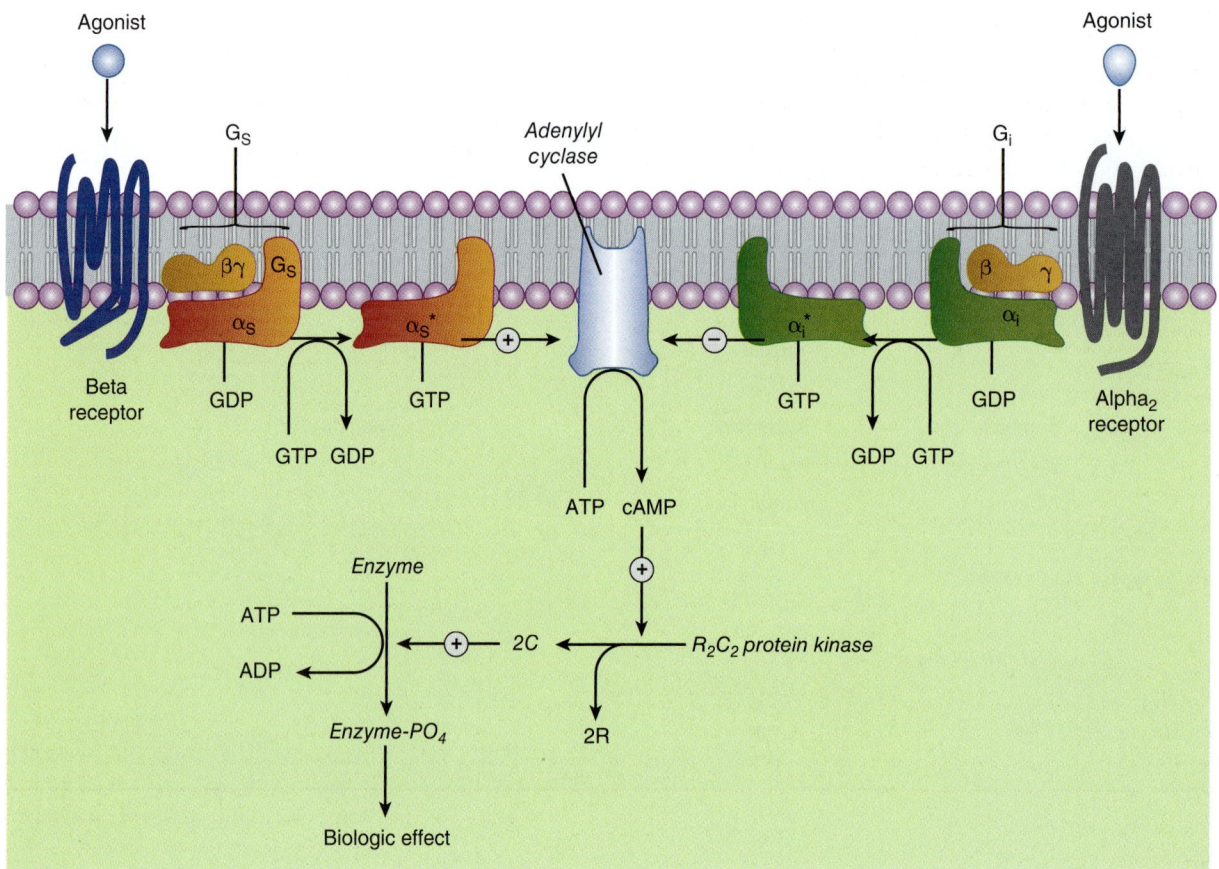

FIGURE 9–2 Activation and inhibition of adenylyl cyclase by agonists that bind to catecholamine receptors. Binding to β adrenoceptors stimulates adenylyl cyclase by activating the stimulatory G protein, G_s, which leads to the dissociation of its α subunit charged with GTP. This activated α_s subunit directly activates adenylyl cyclase, resulting in an increased rate of synthesis of cAMP. Alpha$_2$-adrenoceptor ligands inhibit adenylyl cyclase by causing dissociation of the inhibitory G protein, G_i, into its subunits; ie, an activated α_i subunit charged with GTP and a β-γ unit. The mechanism by which these subunits inhibit adenylyl cyclase is uncertain. cAMP binds to the regulatory subunit (R) of cAMP-dependent protein kinase, leading to the liberation of active catalytic subunits (C) that phosphorylate specific protein substrates and modify their activity. These catalytic units also phosphorylate the cAMP response element binding protein (CREB), which modifies gene expression. See text for other actions of β and α_2 adrenoceptors.

adenosine triphosphate (ATP) to cAMP (Table 9–1, Figure 9–2). Activation of the cyclase enzyme is mediated by the stimulatory coupling protein G_s. Cyclic AMP is the major second messenger of β-receptor activation. For example, in the liver of many species, β-receptor–activated cAMP synthesis leads to a cascade of events culminating in the activation of glycogen phosphorylase. In the heart, β-receptor–activated cAMP synthesis increases the influx of calcium across the cell membrane and its sequestration inside the cell. Beta-receptor activation also promotes the relaxation of smooth muscle. Although the mechanism of the smooth muscle effect is uncertain, it may involve the phosphorylation of myosin light-chain kinase to an inactive form (see Figure 12–1). Beta adrenoceptors may activate voltage-sensitive calcium channels in the heart via G_s-mediated enhancement independently of changes in cAMP concentration. Under certain circumstances, β_2 receptors may couple to G_q proteins. These receptors have been demonstrated to activate additional kinases, such as MAP kinases, by

forming multi-subunit complexes within cells, which contain multiple signaling molecules.

The β_3 adrenoreceptor is a lower affinity receptor compared with β_1 and β_2 receptors but is more resistant to desensitization. It is found in several tissues, but its physiologic or pathologic role in humans is not clear. Selective agonists and antagonists have been developed but are not clinically available.

C. Dopamine Receptors

The D_1 receptor is typically associated with the stimulation of adenylyl cyclase (Table 9–1); for example, D_1-receptor–induced smooth muscle relaxation is presumably due to cAMP accumulation in the smooth muscle of those vascular beds in which dopamine is a vasodilator. D_2 receptors have been found to inhibit adenylyl cyclase activity, open potassium channels, and decrease calcium influx.

Receptor Selectivity

Many clinically available adrenergic agonists have selectivity for the major (α_1 and α_2 versus β) adrenoreceptor types, but not for the subtypes of these major groups. Examples of clinically useful sympathomimetic agonists that are relatively selective for α_1-, α_2-, and β-adrenoceptor subgroups are compared with some nonselective agents in Table 9–2. Selectivity means that a drug may preferentially bind to one subgroup of receptors at concentrations too low to interact extensively with another subgroup. However, selectivity is not usually absolute (nearly absolute selectivity has been termed "specificity"), and at higher concentrations, a drug may also interact with related classes of receptors. The effects of a given drug may depend not only on its selectivity to adrenoreceptor types, but also to the relative expression of receptor subtypes in a given tissue. (see Box: Receptor Selectivity and Physiologic Functions of Adrenoceptor Subtypes).

Receptor Regulation

Responses mediated by adrenoceptors are not fixed and static. The number and function of adrenoceptors on the cell surface and their responses may be regulated by catecholamines themselves, other hormones and drugs, age, and a number of disease states (see Chapter 2). These changes may modify the magnitude of a tissue's physiologic response to catecholamines and can be important clinically during the course of treatment. One of the best-studied examples of receptor regulation is the **desensitization** of adrenoceptors that may occur after exposure to catecholamines and other sympathomimetic drugs. After a cell or tissue has been exposed for a period of time to an agonist, that tissue often becomes less responsive to further stimulation by that agent (see Figure 2–12).

> ### Receptor Selectivity and Physiologic Functions of Adrenoceptor Subtypes: Lessons from Knockout Mice
>
> Since pharmacologic tools used to evaluate the function of adrenoceptor subtypes have some limitations, a number of knockout mice have been developed with one or more adrenoceptor genes subjected to loss of function mutations, as described in Chapter 1 (see Box: Pharmacology & Genetics). These models have their own complexities, and extrapolations from mice to humans may be uncertain. Nonetheless, these studies have yielded some novel insights. For example, α-adrenoceptor subtypes play an important role in cardiac responses, the α_{2A}-adrenoceptor subtype is critical in transducing the effects of α_2 agonists on blood pressure control, and β_1 receptors play a predominant role in directly increasing heart rate in the mouse heart.

Other terms such as tolerance, refractoriness, and tachyphylaxis have also been used to denote desensitization. This process has potential clinical significance because it may limit the therapeutic response to sympathomimetic agents.

Many mechanisms have been found to contribute to desensitization. Some mechanisms function relatively slowly, over the course of hours or days, and these typically involve transcriptional or translational changes in the receptor protein level, or its migration to the cell surface. Other mechanisms of desensitization occur quickly, within minutes. Rapid modulation of receptor function in desensitized cells may involve critical covalent modification of the receptor, especially by phosphorylation on specific amino acid residues, association of these receptors with other proteins, or changes in their subcellular location.

There are two major categories of desensitization of responses mediated by G protein-coupled receptors. **Homologous** desensitization refers to loss of responsiveness exclusively of the receptors that have been exposed to repeated or sustained activation by an agonist. **Heterologous** desensitization refers to the process by which desensitization of one receptor by its agonists also results in desensitization of another receptor that has not been directly activated by the agonist in question.

A major mechanism of desensitization that occurs rapidly involves phosphorylation of receptors by members of the **G protein-coupled receptor kinase (GRK)** family, of which there are seven members. Specific adrenoceptors become substrates for these kinases only when they are bound to an agonist. This mechanism is an example of homologous desensitization because it specifically involves only agonist-occupied receptors.

Phosphorylation of these receptors enhances their affinity for **arrestins,** a family of four widely expressed proteins. Upon binding of arrestin, the capacity of the receptor to activate G proteins is blunted, presumably as a result of steric hindrance

TABLE 9–2 Relative receptor affinities.

	Relative Receptor Affinities
Alpha agonists	
Phenylephrine, methoxamine	$\alpha_1 > \alpha_2 >>>>> \beta$
Clonidine, methylnorepinephrine	$\alpha_2 > \alpha_1 >>>>> \beta$
Mixed alpha and beta agonists	
Norepinephrine	$\alpha_1 = \alpha_2; \beta_1 >> \beta_2$
Epinephrine	$\alpha_1 = \alpha_2; \beta_1 = \beta_2$
Beta agonists	
Dobutamine[1]	$\beta_1 > \beta_2 >>>> \alpha$
Isoproterenol	$\beta_1 = \beta_2 >>>> \alpha$
Albuterol, terbutaline, metaproterenol, ritodrine	$\beta_2 >> \beta_1 >>>> \alpha$
Dopamine agonists	
Dopamine	$D_1 = D_2 >> \beta >> \alpha$
Fenoldopam	$D_1 >> D_2$

[1]See text.

(see Figure 2–12). Arrestin then interacts with clathrin and clathrin adaptor AP2, leading to endocytosis of the receptor. In addition to blunting responses requiring the presence of the receptor on the cell surface, these regulatory processes may also contribute to novel mechanisms of receptor signaling via intracellular pathways.

Receptor desensitization may also be mediated by second-messenger feedback. For example, β adrenoceptors stimulate cAMP accumulation, which leads to activation of protein kinase A; protein kinase A can phosphorylate residues on β receptors, resulting in inhibition of receptor function. For the β_2 receptor, phosphorylation occurs on serine residues both in the third cytoplasmic loop and in the carboxyl terminal tail of the receptor. Similarly, activation of protein kinase C by G_q-coupled receptors may lead to phosphorylation of this class of G protein-coupled receptors. This second-messenger feedback mechanism has been termed heterologous desensitization because activated protein kinase A or protein kinase C may phosphorylate any structurally similar receptor with the appropriate consensus sites for phosphorylation by these enzymes.

Adrenoceptor Polymorphisms

Since elucidation of the sequences of the genes encoding the α_1, α_2, and β subtypes of adrenoceptors, it has become clear that there are relatively common genetic polymorphisms for many of these receptor subtypes in humans. Some of these may lead to changes in critical amino acid sequences that have pharmacologic importance. Often, distinct polymorphisms occur in specific combinations termed **haplotypes.** Some polymorphisms have been shown to alter susceptibility to diseases such as heart failure, others to alter the propensity of a receptor to desensitize, and still others to alter therapeutic responses to drugs in diseases such as asthma. This remains an area of active research because studies have reported inconsistent results as to the pathophysiologic importance of some polymorphisms.

The Norepinephrine Transporter

When norepinephrine is released into the synaptic cleft, it binds to postsynaptic adrenoceptors to elicit the expected physiologic effect. However, just as the release of neurotransmitters is a tightly regulated process, the mechanisms for removal of neurotransmitter must also be highly effective. The norepinephrine transporter (NET) is the principal route by which this occurs. It is particularly efficient in the synapses of the heart, where up to 90% of released norepinephrine is removed by the NET. Remaining synaptic norepinephrine may escape into the extrasynaptic space and enter the bloodstream or be taken up into extraneuronal cells and metabolized by catecholamine-*N*-methyltransferase. In other sites such as the vasculature, where synaptic structures are less well developed, removal may still be 60% or more by NET. The NET, often situated on the presynaptic neuronal membrane, pumps the synaptic norepinephrine back into the neuron cell cytoplasm. In the cell, this norepinephrine may reenter the vesicles or undergo metabolism through monoamine oxidase to dihydroxyphenylglycol

(DHPG). Elsewhere in the body similar transporters remove dopamine (dopamine transporter, DAT), serotonin (serotonin transporter, SERT), and other neurotransmitters. The NET, surprisingly, has equivalent affinity for dopamine as for norepinephrine, and it can sometimes clear dopamine in brain areas where DAT is low, like the cortex.

Blockade of the NET, eg, by the nonselective psychostimulant cocaine or the NET selective agents atomoxetine or reboxetine, impairs this primary site of norepinephrine removal and thus synaptic norepinephrine levels rise, leading to greater stimulation of α and β adrenoceptors. In the periphery this effect may produce a clinical picture of sympathetic activation, but it is often counterbalanced by concomitant stimulation of α_2 adrenoceptors in the brainstem that reduces sympathetic activation.

However, the function of the norepinephrine and dopamine transporters is complex, and drugs can interact with the NET to actually reverse the direction of transport and induce the release of intraneuronal neurotransmitter. This is illustrated in Figure 9–3. Under normal circumstances (panel A), presynaptic NET (red) inactivates and recycles norepinephrine (NE, red) released by vesicular fusion. In panel B, amphetamine (black) acts as both an NET substrate and a reuptake blocker, eliciting reverse transport and blocking normal uptake, thereby increasing NE levels in and beyond the synaptic cleft. In panel C, agents such as methylphenidate and cocaine (hexagons) block NET-mediated NE reuptake and enhance NE signaling.

■ MEDICINAL CHEMISTRY OF SYMPATHOMIMETIC DRUGS

Phenylethylamine may be considered the parent compound from which sympathomimetic drugs are derived (Figure 9–4). This compound consists of a benzene ring with an ethylamine side chain. Substitutions may be made on (1) the benzene ring, (2) the terminal amino group, and (3) the α or β carbons of the ethylamino chain. Substitution by –OH groups at the 3 and 4 positions yields sympathomimetic drugs collectively known as catecholamines. The effects of modification of phenylethylamine are to change the affinity of the drugs for α and β receptors, spanning the range from almost pure α activity (methoxamine) to almost pure β activity (isoproterenol), as well as to influence the intrinsic ability to activate the receptors.

In addition to determining relative affinity to receptor subtype, chemical structure also determines the pharmacokinetic properties and bioavailability of these molecules.

A. Substitution on the Benzene Ring

Maximal α and β activity is found with catecholamines, ie, drugs having –OH groups at the 3 and 4 positions on the benzene ring. The absence of one or the other of these groups, particularly the hydroxyl at C_3, without other substitutions on the ring may dramatically reduce the potency of the drug. For example, phenylephrine (Figure 9–5) is much less potent than epinephrine;

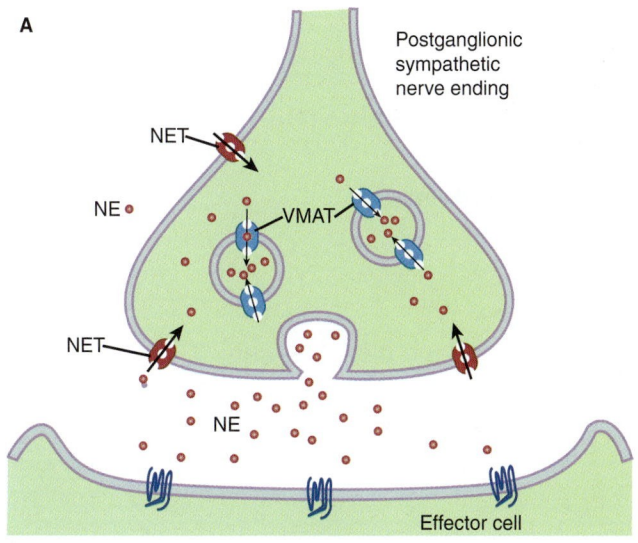

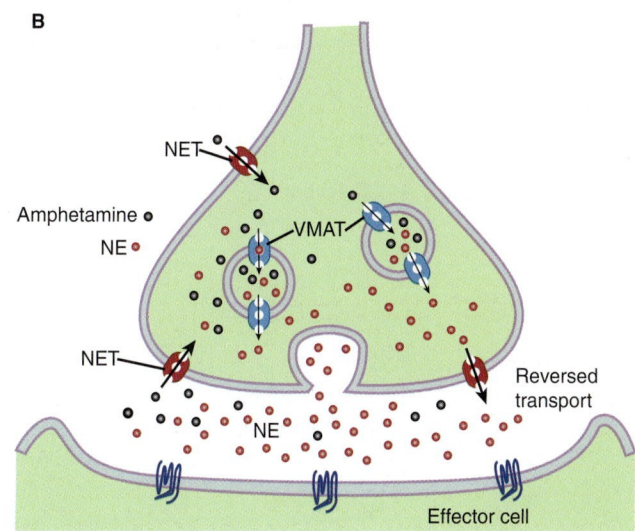

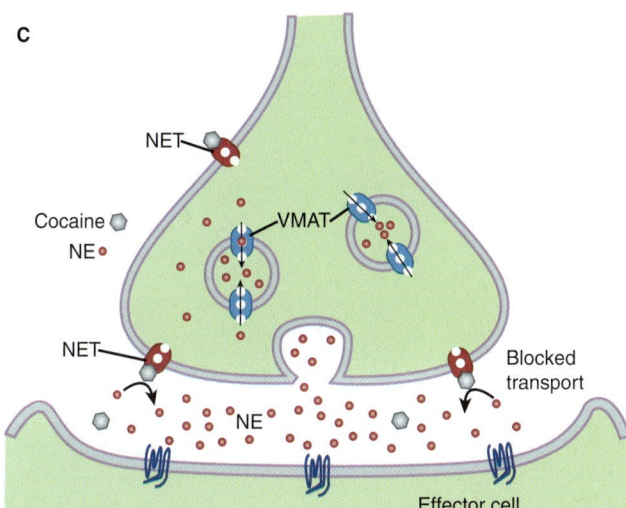

FIGURE 9–3 Pharmacologic targeting of monoamine transporters. Commonly used drugs such as antidepressants, amphetamines, and cocaine target monoamine (norepinephrine, dopamine, and serotonin) transporters with different potencies. **A** shows the mechanism of reuptake of norepinephrine (NE) back into the noradrenergic neuron via the norepinephrine transporter (NET), where a proportion is sequestered in presynaptic vesicles through the vesicular monoamine transporter (VMAT). **B** and **C** show the effects of amphetamine and cocaine on these pathways. See text for details.

indeed, α-receptor affinity is decreased about 100-fold and β activity is almost negligible except at very high concentrations. On the other hand, catecholamines are subject to inactivation by catechol-*O*-methyltransferase (COMT), and because this enzyme is found in the gut and liver, catecholamines are not active orally (see Chapter 6). Absence of one or both –OH groups on the phenyl ring increases the bioavailability after oral administration and prolongs the duration of action. Furthermore, absence of ring –OH groups tends to increase the distribution of the molecule to the central nervous system. For example, ephedrine and amphetamine (Figure 9–5) are orally active, have a prolonged duration of action, and produce central nervous system effects not typically observed with the catecholamines.

B. Substitution on the Amino Group

Increasing the size of alkyl substituents on the amino group tends to increase β-receptor activity. For example, methyl substitution on norepinephrine, yielding epinephrine, enhances activity at β2 receptors. Beta activity is further enhanced with isopropyl substitution at the amino group (isoproterenol). Beta2-selective agonists generally require a large amino substituent group. The larger the substituent on the amino group, the lower the activity at α receptors; for example, isoproterenol is very weak at α receptors.

C. Substitution on the Alpha Carbon

Substitutions at the α carbon block oxidation by monoamine oxidase (MAO) and prolong the action of such drugs, particularly the

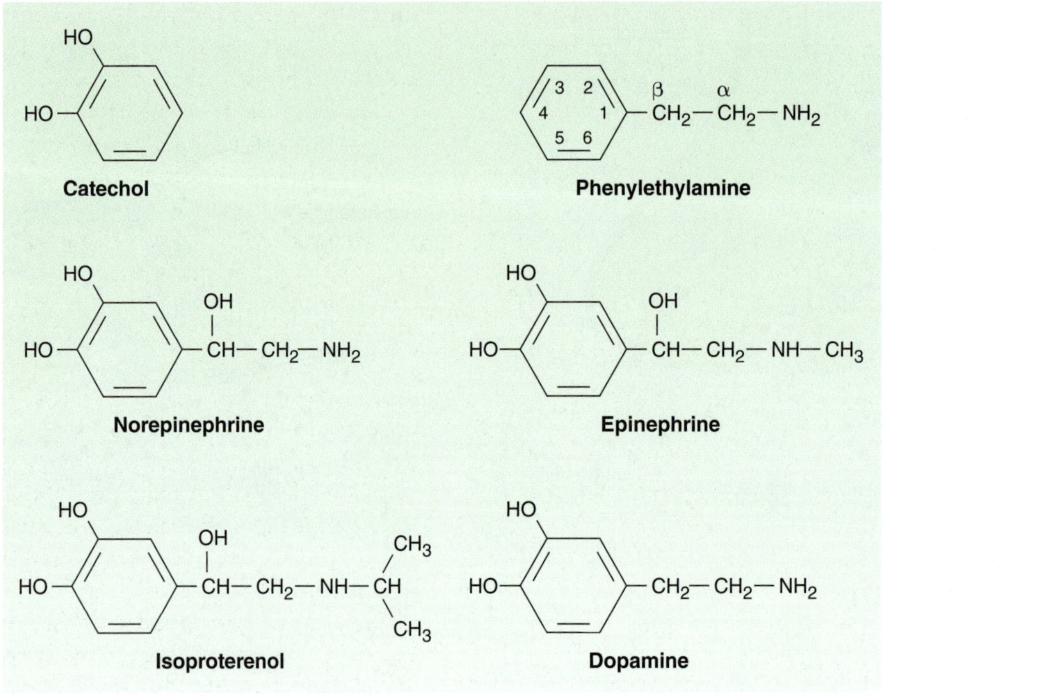

Catechol

Phenylethylamine

Norepinephrine

Epinephrine

Isoproterenol

Dopamine

FIGURE 9–4 Phenylethylamine and some important catecholamines. Catechol is shown for reference.

noncatecholamines. Ephedrine and amphetamine are examples of α-substituted compounds (Figure 9–5). Alpha-methyl compounds are also called phenylisopropylamines. In addition to their resistance to oxidation by MAO, some phenylisopropylamines have an enhanced ability to displace catecholamines from storage sites in noradrenergic nerves (see Chapter 6). Therefore, a portion of their activity is dependent on the presence of normal norepinephrine stores in the body; they are indirectly acting sympathomimetics.

D. Substitution on the Beta Carbon

Direct-acting agonists typically have a β-hydroxyl group, although dopamine does not. In addition to facilitating activation of adrenoceptors, this hydroxyl group may be important for storage of sympathomimetic amines in neural vesicles.

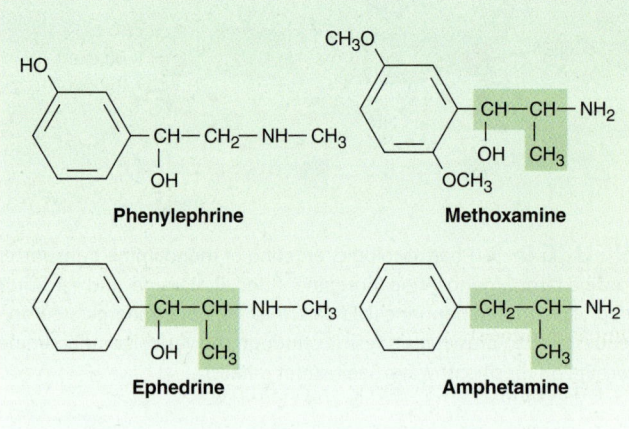

Phenylephrine

Methoxamine

Ephedrine

Amphetamine

FIGURE 9–5 Some examples of noncatecholamine sympathomimetic drugs. The isopropyl group is highlighted in color.

ORGAN SYSTEM EFFECTS OF SYMPATHOMIMETIC DRUGS

Cardiovascular System

General outlines of the cellular actions of sympathomimetics are presented in Tables 6–3 and 9–3. Sympathomimetics have prominent cardiovascular effects because of widespread distribution of α and β adrenoceptors in the heart, blood vessels, and neural and hormonal systems involved in blood pressure regulation. The net effect of a given sympathomimetic in the intact organism depends

not only on its relative selectivity for α or β adrenoceptors and its pharmacologic action at those receptors; any effect these agents have on blood pressure is counteracted by compensatory baroreflex mechanisms aimed at restoring homeostasis.

The effects of sympathomimetic drugs on blood pressure can be explained on the basis of their effects on heart rate, myocardial function, peripheral vascular resistance, and venous return (see Figure 6–7 and Table 9–4). The endogenous catecholamines, norepinephrine and epinephrine, have complex cardiovascular effects

TABLE 9–3 Distribution of adrenoceptor subtypes.

Type	Tissue	Actions
α_1	Most vascular smooth muscle (innervated)	Contraction
	Pupillary dilator muscle	Contraction (dilates pupil)
	Pilomotor smooth muscle	Erects hair
	Prostate	Contraction
	Heart	Increases force of contraction
α_2	Postsynaptic CNS neurons	Probably multiple
	Platelets	Aggregation
	Adrenergic and cholinergic nerve terminals	Inhibits transmitter release
	Some vascular smooth muscle	Contraction
	Fat cells	Inhibits lipolysis
β_1	Heart, juxtaglomerular cells	Increases force and rate of contraction; increases renin release
β_2	Respiratory, uterine, and vascular smooth muscle	Promotes smooth muscle relaxation
	Skeletal muscle	Promotes potassium uptake
	Human liver	Activates glycogenolysis
β_3	Fat cells	Activates lipolysis
D_1	Smooth muscle	Dilates renal blood vessels
D_2	Nerve endings	Modulates transmitter release

because they activate both α and β receptors. It is easier to understand these actions by first describing the cardiovascular effect of sympathomimetics that are selective for a given adrenoreceptor.

A. Effects of Alpha₁-Receptor Activation

Alpha₁ receptors are widely expressed in vascular beds, and their activation leads to arterial and venous vasoconstriction. Their direct effect on cardiac function is of relatively less importance. A relatively pure α agonist such as phenylephrine increases peripheral arterial resistance and decreases venous capacitance. The enhanced arterial resistance usually leads to a dose-dependent rise in blood pressure (Figure 9–6). In the presence of normal cardiovascular reflexes, the rise in blood pressure elicits a baroreceptor-mediated increase in vagal tone with slowing of the heart rate, which may be quite marked (Figure 9–7). However, cardiac output may not diminish in proportion to this reduction in rate, since increased venous return may increase stroke volume. Furthermore, direct α-adrenoceptor stimulation of the heart may have a modest positive inotropic action. The magnitude of the restraining effect of the baroreflex is quite dramatic. If baroreflex function is

removed by pretreatment with the ganglionic blocker trimethaphan, the pressor effect of phenylephrine is increased approximately tenfold, and bradycardia is no longer observed (Figure 9–7), confirming that the decrease in heart rate associated with the increase in blood pressure induced by phenylephrine was reflex in nature rather than a direct effect of α_1-receptor activation.

Patients who have an impairment of autonomic function (due to pure autonomic failure as in the case study or to more common conditions such as diabetic autonomic neuropathy) exhibit this extreme hypersensitivity to most pressor and depressor stimuli, including medications. This is to a large extent due to failure of baroreflex buffering. Such patients may have exaggerated increases in heart rate or blood pressure when taking sympathomimetics with β- and α-adrenergic activity, respectively. This, however, can be used as an advantage in their treatment. The α agonist midodrine is commonly used to ameliorate orthostatic hypotension in these patients.

There are major differences in receptor types predominantly expressed in the various vascular beds (Table 9–4). The skin vessels have predominantly α receptors and constrict in response to epinephrine and norepinephrine, as do the splanchnic vessels. Vessels in skeletal muscle may constrict or dilate depending on whether α or β receptors are activated. The blood vessels of the nasal mucosa express α receptors, and local vasoconstriction induced by sympathomimetics explains their decongestant action (see Therapeutic Uses of Sympathomimetic Drugs).

B. Effects of Alpha₂-Receptor Activation

Alpha₂ adrenoceptors are present in the vasculature, and their activation leads to vasoconstriction. This effect, however, is observed only when α_2 agonists are given locally, by rapid intravenous injection or in very high oral doses. When given systemically, these vascular effects are obscured by the central effects of α_2 receptors, which lead to inhibition of sympathetic tone and blood pressure. Hence, α_2 agonists are used as *sympatholytics* in the treatment of hypertension (see Chapter 11). In patients with pure autonomic failure, characterized by neural degeneration of postganglionic noradrenergic fibers, clonidine may increase blood pressure because the central sympatholytic effects of clonidine become irrelevant, whereas the peripheral vasoconstriction remains intact.

C. Effects of Beta-Receptor Activation

The blood pressure response to a β-adrenoceptor agonist depends on its contrasting effects on the heart and the vasculature. Stimulation of β receptors in the heart increases cardiac output by increasing contractility and by direct activation of the sinus node to increase heart rate. Beta agonists also decrease peripheral resistance by activating β_2 receptors, leading to vasodilation in certain vascular beds (Table 9–4). Isoproterenol is a nonselective β agonist; it activates both β_1 and β_2 receptors. The net effect is to maintain or slightly increase systolic pressure and to lower diastolic pressure, so that mean blood pressure is decreased (Figure 9–6).

Direct effects on the heart are determined largely by β_1 receptors, although β_2 and to a lesser extent α receptors are also involved, especially in heart failure. Beta-receptor activation results in increased calcium influx in cardiac cells. This has both

TABLE 9–4 Cardiovascular responses to sympathomimetic amines.

	Phenylephrine	Epinephrine	Isoproterenol
Vascular resistance (tone)			
Cutaneous, mucous membranes (α)	↑↑	↑↑	0
Skeletal muscle (β_2, α)	↑	↓ or ↑	↓↓
Renal (α, D_1)	↑	↑	↓
Splanchnic (α, β)	↑↑	↓ or ↑[1]	↓
Total peripheral resistance	↑↑↑	↓ or ↑[1]	↓↓
Venous tone (α, β)	↑	↑	↓
Cardiac			
Contractility (β_1)	0 or ↑	↑↑↑	↑↑↑
Heart rate (predominantly β_1)	↓↓ (vagal reflex)	↑ or ↓	↑↑↑
Stroke volume	0, ↓, ↑	↑	↑
Cardiac output	↓	↑	↑↑
Blood pressure			
Mean	↑↑	↑	↓
Diastolic	↑↑	↓ or ↑[1]	↓↓
Systolic	↑↑	↑↑	0 or ↓
Pulse pressure	0	↑↑	↑↑

[1]Small doses decrease, large doses increase.

↑ = increase; ↓ = decrease; 0 = no change.

electrical and mechanical consequences. Pacemaker activity—both normal (sinoatrial node) and abnormal (eg, Purkinje fibers)—is increased (**positive chronotropic** effect). Conduction velocity in the atrioventricular node is increased (**positive dromotropic** effect), and the refractory period is decreased. Intrinsic contractility is increased (**positive inotropic** effect), and relaxation is accelerated. As a result, the twitch response of isolated cardiac muscle is increased in tension but abbreviated in duration. In the intact heart, intraventricular pressure rises and falls more rapidly, and ejection time is decreased. These direct effects are easily demonstrated in the absence of reflexes evoked by changes in blood pressure, eg, in isolated myocardial preparations and in patients with ganglionic blockade. In the presence of normal reflex activity, the direct effects on heart rate may be dominated by a reflex response to blood pressure changes. Physiologic stimulation of the heart by catecholamines tends to increase coronary blood flow. Expression of β_3 adrenoreceptors has been detected in the human heart and may be upregulated in disease states, but its relevance to human disease is unclear.

D. Effects of Dopamine-Receptor Activation

Intravenous administration of dopamine promotes vasodilation of renal, splanchnic, coronary, cerebral, and perhaps other resistance vessels, via activation of D_1 receptors. Activation of the D_1 receptors in the renal vasculature may also induce natriuresis. The renal effects of dopamine have been used clinically to improve perfusion to the kidney in situations of oliguria (abnormally low urinary output). The activation of presynaptic D_2 receptors suppresses

norepinephrine release, but it is unclear if this contributes to cardiovascular effects of dopamine. In addition, dopamine activates β_1 receptors in the heart. At low doses, peripheral resistance may decrease. At higher rates of infusion, dopamine activates vascular α receptors, leading to vasoconstriction, including in the renal vascular bed. Consequently, high rates of infusion of dopamine may mimic the actions of epinephrine.

Noncardiac Effects of Sympathomimetics

Adrenoceptors are distributed in virtually all organ systems. This section focuses on the activation of adrenoceptors that are responsible for the therapeutic effects of sympathomimetics or that explain their adverse effects. A more detailed description of the therapeutic use of sympathomimetics is given later in this chapter.

Activation of β_2 receptors in **bronchial smooth muscle** leads to bronchodilation, and β_2 agonists are important in the treatment of asthma (see Chapter 20 and Table 9–3).

In the **eye,** the radial pupillary dilator muscle of the iris contains α receptors; activation by drugs such as phenylephrine causes mydriasis (see Figure 6–9). Alpha stimulants also have important effects on intraocular pressure. Alpha agonists increase the outflow of aqueous humor from the eye and can be used clinically to reduce intraocular pressure. In contrast, β agonists have little effect, but β *antagonists* decrease the production of aqueous humor. These effects are important in the treatment of glaucoma (see Chapter 10), a leading cause of blindness.

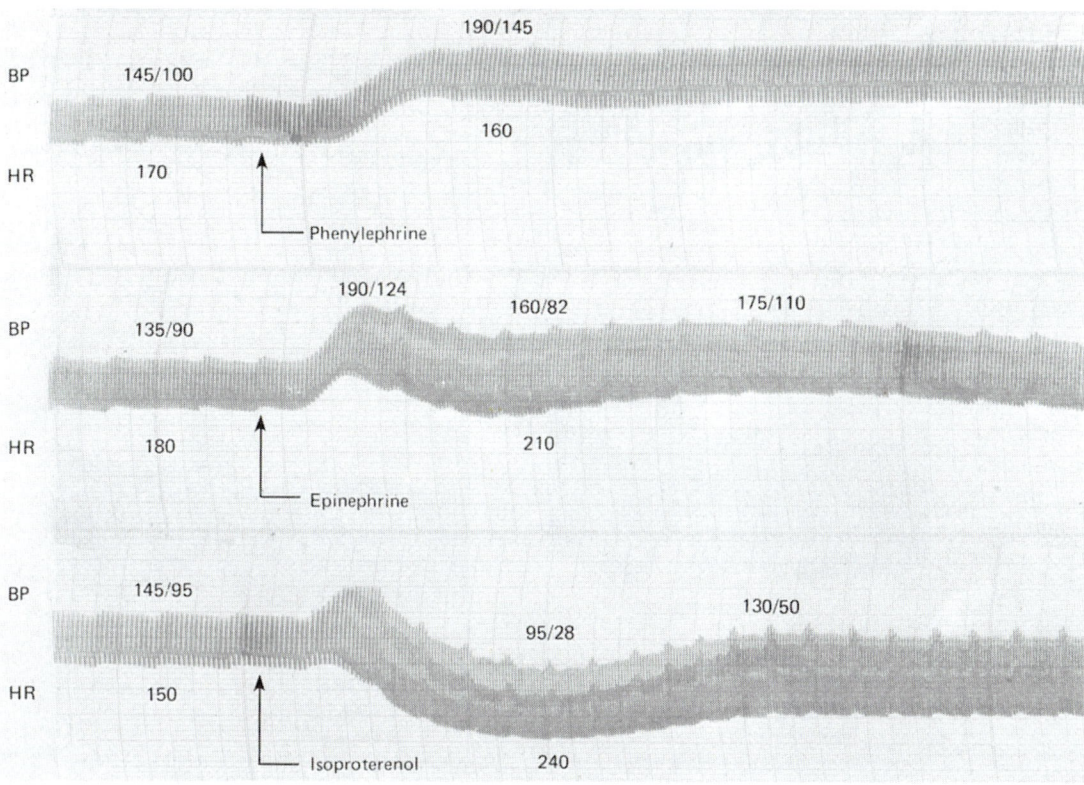

FIGURE 9–6 Effects of an α-selective (phenylephrine), β-selective (isoproterenol), and nonselective (epinephrine) sympathomimetic, given as an intravenous bolus injection to a dog. Reflexes are blunted but not eliminated in this anesthetized animal. BP, blood pressure; HR, heart rate.

In **genitourinary** organs, the bladder base, urethral sphincter, and prostate contain α receptors that mediate contraction and therefore promote urinary continence. The specific subtype of α_1 receptor involved in mediating constriction of the bladder base and prostate is uncertain, but α_{1A} receptors probably play an important role. This effect explains why urinary retention is a potential adverse effect of administration of the α_1 agonist midodrine.

Alpha-receptor activation in the ductus deferens, seminal vesicles, and prostate plays a role in normal ejaculation. The detumescence of erectile tissue that normally follows ejaculation is also brought about by norepinephrine (and possibly neuropeptide Y) released from sympathetic nerves. Alpha activation appears to have a similar detumescent effect on erectile tissue in female animals.

The **salivary glands** contain adrenoceptors that regulate the secretion of amylase and water. However, certain sympathomimetic drugs, eg, clonidine, produce symptoms of dry mouth. The mechanism of this effect is uncertain; it is likely that central nervous system effects are responsible, although peripheral effects may contribute.

The **apocrine sweat glands,** located on the palms of the hands and a few other areas, respond to adrenoceptor stimulants with increased sweat production. These are the apocrine nonthermoregulatory glands usually associated with psychological stress. (The diffusely distributed thermoregulatory eccrine sweat glands are regulated by *sympathetic cholinergic* postganglionic nerves that activate muscarinic cholinoceptors; see Chapter 6.)

Sympathomimetic drugs have important effects on intermediary **metabolism.** Activation of β adrenoceptors in fat cells leads to increased lipolysis with enhanced release of free fatty acids and glycerol into the blood. Beta$_3$ adrenoceptors play a role in mediating this response in animals, but their role in humans is probably minor. Human fat cells also contain α_2 receptors that inhibit lipolysis by decreasing intracellular cAMP. Sympathomimetic drugs enhance glycogenolysis in the liver, which leads to increased glucose release into the circulation. In the human liver, the effects of catecholamines are probably mediated mainly by β receptors, though α_1 receptors may also play a role. Catecholamines in high concentration may also cause metabolic acidosis. Activation of β_2 adrenoceptors by endogenous epinephrine or by sympathomimetic drugs promotes the uptake of potassium into cells, leading to a fall in extracellular potassium. This may result in a fall in the plasma potassium concentration during stress or protect against a rise in plasma potassium during exercise. Blockade of these receptors may accentuate the rise in plasma potassium that occurs during exercise. On the other hand, epinephrine has been used to treat hyperkalemia in certain conditions, but other alternatives are more commonly used. Beta receptors and α_2 receptors that are expressed in pancreatic islets tend to increase and decrease insulin secretion, respectively, although the major regulator of insulin release is the plasma concentration of glucose.

Catecholamines are important endogenous regulators of **hormone secretion** from a number of glands. As mentioned above,

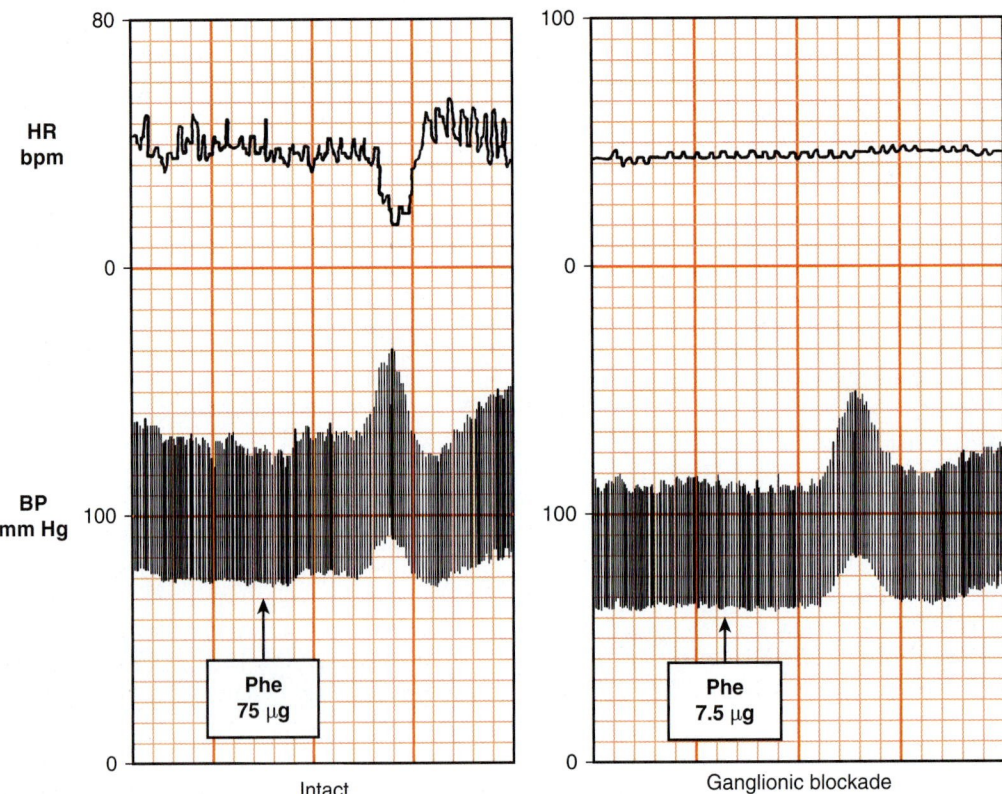

FIGURE 9–7 Effects of ganglionic blockade on the response to phenylephrine (Phe) in a human subject. **Left:** The cardiovascular effect of the selective α agonist phenylephrine when given as an intravenous bolus to a subject with intact autonomic baroreflex function. Note that the increase in blood pressure (BP) is associated with a baroreflex-mediated compensatory decrease in heart rate (HR). **Right:** The response in the same subject after autonomic reflexes were abolished by the ganglionic blocker trimethaphan. Note that resting blood pressure is decreased and heart rate is increased by trimethaphan because of sympathetic and parasympathetic withdrawal (HR scale is different). In the absence of baroreflex buffering, approximately a tenfold lower dose of phenylephrine is required to produce a similar increase in blood pressure. Note also the lack of compensatory decrease in heart rate.

insulin secretion is stimulated by β receptors and inhibited by α_2 receptors. Similarly, renin secretion is stimulated by β_1 and inhibited by α_2 receptors; indeed, β-receptor antagonist drugs may lower blood pressure in patients with hypertension at least in part by lowering plasma renin. Adrenoceptors also modulate the secretion of parathyroid hormone, calcitonin, thyroxine, and gastrin; however, the physiologic significance of these control mechanisms is probably limited. In high concentrations, epinephrine and related agents cause leukocytosis, in part by promoting demargination of sequestered white blood cells back into the general circulation.

The action of sympathomimetics on the **central nervous system** varies dramatically, depending on their ability to cross the blood-brain barrier. The catecholamines are almost completely excluded by this barrier, and subjective CNS effects are noted only at the highest rates of infusion. These effects have been described as ranging from "nervousness" to "an adrenaline rush" or "a feeling of impending disaster." Furthermore, peripheral effects of β-adrenoceptor agonists such as tachycardia and tremor are similar to the somatic manifestations of anxiety. In contrast, noncatecholamines with indirect actions, such as amphetamines, which readily enter the central nervous system from the circulation,

produce qualitatively very different CNS effects. These actions vary from mild alerting, with improved attention to boring tasks; through elevation of mood, insomnia, euphoria, and anorexia; to full-blown psychotic behavior. These effects are not readily assigned to either α- or β-mediated actions and may represent enhancement of dopamine-mediated processes or other effects of these drugs in the CNS.

SPECIFIC SYMPATHOMIMETIC DRUGS

Endogenous Catecholamines

Epinephrine (adrenaline) is an agonist at both α and β receptors. It is therefore a very potent vasoconstrictor and cardiac stimulant. The rise in systolic blood pressure that occurs after epinephrine release or administration is caused by its positive inotropic and chronotropic actions on the heart (predominantly β_1 receptors) and the vasoconstriction induced in many vascular beds (α receptors). Epinephrine also activates β_2 receptors in some vessels (eg, skeletal muscle blood vessels), leading to their dilation. Consequently, total peripheral resistance may actually fall, explaining the fall in diastolic pressure that is sometimes seen with epinephrine injection (Figure 9–6; Table 9–4). Activation of β_2 receptors in skeletal muscle contributes to increased blood flow during exercise. Under physiologic conditions, epinephrine functions largely as a hormone; after release from the adrenal medulla into the blood, it acts on distant cells.

Norepinephrine (levarterenol, noradrenaline) is an agonist at both α_1 and α_2 receptors. Norepinephrine also activates β_1 receptors with similar potency as epinephrine, but has relatively little effect on β_2 receptors. Consequently, norepinephrine increases peripheral resistance and both diastolic and systolic blood pressure. Compensatory baroreflex activation tends to overcome the direct positive chronotropic effects of norepinephrine; however, the positive inotropic effects on the heart are maintained.

Dopamine is the immediate precursor in the synthesis of norepinephrine (see Figure 6–5). Its cardiovascular effects were described above. Endogenous dopamine may have more important effects in regulating sodium excretion and renal function. It is an important neurotransmitter in the central nervous system and is involved in the reward stimulus relevant to addiction. Its deficiency in the basal ganglia leads to Parkinson's disease, which is treated with its precursor levodopa. Dopamine receptors are also targets for antipsychotic drugs.

Direct-Acting Sympathomimetics

Phenylephrine was discussed previously when describing the actions of a relatively pure α_1 agonist (Table 9–2). Because it is not a catechol derivative (Figure 9–4), it is not inactivated by COMT and has a longer duration of action than the catecholamines. It is an effective mydriatic and decongestant and can be used to raise the blood pressure (Figure 9–6).

Midodrine is a prodrug that is enzymatically hydrolyzed to desglymidodrine, a selective α_1-receptor agonist. The peak concentration of desglymidodrine is achieved about 1 hour after midodrine is administered. The primary indication for midodrine is the treatment of orthostatic hypotension, typically due to impaired autonomic nervous system function. Although the drug has efficacy in diminishing the fall of blood pressure when the patient is standing, it may cause hypertension when the subject is supine. The Food and Drug Administration considered withdrawing approval of this drug in 2010 because required postapproval studies that verify the clinical benefit of the drug had not been done. Action was suspended in response to prescriber and patient requests.

Methoxamine acts pharmacologically like phenylephrine, since it is predominantly a direct-acting α_1-receptor agonist. It may cause a prolonged increase in blood pressure due to vasoconstriction; it also causes a vagally mediated bradycardia. Methoxamine is available for parenteral use, but clinical applications are rare and limited to hypotensive states.

Alpha$_2$-selective agonists have an important ability to decrease blood pressure through actions in the central nervous system even though direct application to a blood vessel may cause vasoconstriction. Such drugs (eg, **clonidine, methyldopa, guanfacine, guanabenz**) are useful in the treatment of hypertension (and some other conditions) and are discussed in Chapter 11. Sedation is a recognized side effect of these drugs, and newer α_2-agonists (with activity also at imidazoline receptors) with fewer central nervous system side effects are available outside the USA for the treatment of hypertension (**moxonidine,** rilmenidine). On the other hand, the primary indication of **dexmedetomidine** is for sedation of initially intubated and mechanically ventilated patients during treatment in an intensive care setting. It also reduces the requirements for opioids in pain control. Finally, **tizanidine** is used as a central muscle relaxant.

Xylometazoline and **oxymetazoline** are direct-acting α agonists. These drugs have been used as topical decongestants because of their ability to promote constriction of the nasal mucosa. When taken in large doses, oxymetazoline may cause hypotension, presumably because of a central clonidine-like effect (see Chapter 11). Oxymetazoline has significant affinity for α_{2A} receptors.

Isoproterenol (isoprenaline) is a very potent β-receptor agonist and has little effect on α receptors. The drug has positive chronotropic and inotropic actions; because isoproterenol activates β receptors almost exclusively, it is a potent vasodilator. These actions lead to a marked increase in cardiac output associated with a fall in diastolic and mean arterial pressure and a lesser decrease or a slight increase in systolic pressure (Table 9–4; Figure 9–6).

Beta-selective agonists are very important because the separation of β_1 and β_2 effects (Table 9–2), although incomplete, is sufficient to reduce adverse effects in several clinical applications.

Beta$_1$-selective agents include **dobutamine** and a partial agonist, **prenalterol** (Figure 9–8). Because they are less effective in activating vasodilator β_2 receptors, they may increase cardiac output with less reflex tachycardia than occurs with nonselective β agonists such as isoproterenol. **Dobutamine** was initially considered a relatively β_1-selective agonist, but its actions are more complex. Its chemical structure resembles dopamine, but its actions are mediated mostly by activation of α and β receptors. Clinical preparations of dobutamine are a racemic mixture of (−) and (+) isomers, each with contrasting activity at α_1 and α_2 receptors. The (+) isomer is a potent β_1 agonist and an α_1-receptor antagonist. The (−) isomer is a potent α_1 agonist, which is capable of causing significant vasoconstriction when given alone. The resultant cardiovascular effects of dobutamine reflect this complex pharmacology. Dobutamine has a positive inotropic action caused by the isomer with predominantly β-receptor activity. It has relatively greater inotropic than chronotropic effect compared with isoproterenol. Activation of α_1 receptors probably explains why peripheral resistance does not decrease significantly.

Beta$_2$-selective agents have achieved an important place in the treatment of asthma and are discussed in Chapter 20. An additional application is to achieve uterine relaxation in premature labor (ritodrine; see below). Some examples of β_2-selective drugs currently in use are shown in Figures 9–8 and 20–4; many more are available or under investigation.

Mixed-Acting Sympathomimetics

Ephedrine occurs in various plants and has been used in China for over 2000 years; it was introduced into Western medicine in 1924 as the first orally active sympathomimetic drug. It is found

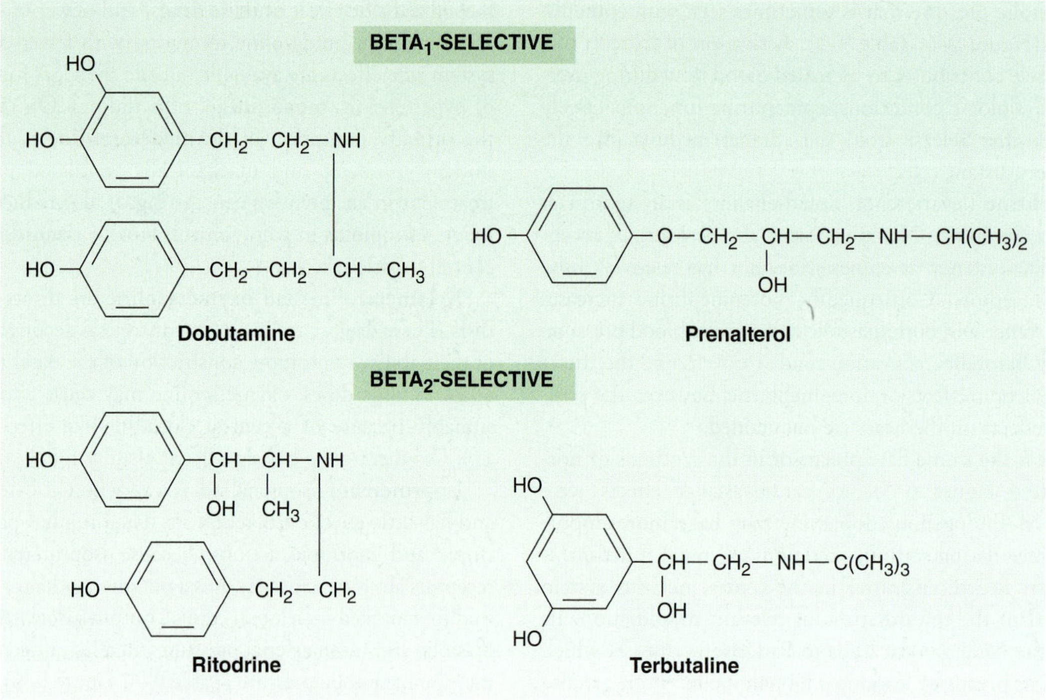

FIGURE 9–8 Examples of β_1- and β_2-selective agonists.

in ma huang, a popular herbal medication (see Chapter 64). Ma huang contains multiple ephedrine-like alkaloids in addition to ephedrine. Because ephedrine is a noncatechol phenylisopropylamine (Figure 9–5), it has high bioavailability and a relatively long duration of action—hours rather than minutes. As with many other phenylisopropylamines, a significant fraction of the drug is excreted unchanged in the urine. Since it is a weak base, its excretion can be accelerated by acidification of the urine.

Ephedrine has not been extensively studied in humans despite its long history of use. Its ability to activate β receptors probably accounted for its earlier use in asthma. Because it gains access to the central nervous system, it is a mild stimulant. Ingestion of ephedrine alkaloids contained in ma huang has raised important safety concerns. **Pseudoephedrine,** one of four ephedrine enantiomers, has been available over the counter as a component of many decongestant mixtures. However, the use of pseudoephedrine as a precursor in the illicit manufacture of methamphetamine has led to restrictions on its sale.

Phenylpropanolamine was a common component in over-the-counter appetite suppressants. It was removed from the market because its use was associated with hemorrhagic strokes in young women. The mechanism of this potential adverse effect is unknown, but the drug can increase blood pressure in patients with impaired autonomic reflexes.

Indirect-Acting Sympathomimetics

As noted previously, indirect-acting sympathomimetics can have one of two different mechanisms (Figure 9–3). First, they may enter the sympathetic nerve ending and displace stored catecholamine transmitter. Such drugs have been called amphetamine-like or "displacers." Second, they may inhibit the reuptake of released transmitter by interfering with the action of the norepinephrine transporter, NET.

A. Amphetamine-Like

Amphetamine is a racemic mixture of phenylisopropylamine (Figure 9–5) that is important chiefly because of its use and misuse as a central nervous system stimulant (see Chapter 32). Pharmacokinetically, it is similar to ephedrine; however, amphetamine even more readily enters the central nervous system, where it has marked stimulant effects on mood and alertness and a depressant effect on appetite. Its D-isomer is more potent than the L-isomer. Amphetamine's actions are mediated through the release of norepinephrine and, to some extent, dopamine.

Methamphetamine (*N*-methylamphetamine) is very similar to amphetamine with an even higher ratio of central to peripheral actions. **Phenmetrazine** is a variant phenylisopropylamine with amphetamine-like effects. It has been promoted as an anorexiant and is also a popular drug of abuse. **Methylphenidate** is an amphetamine variant whose major pharmacologic effects and abuse potential are similar to those of amphetamine. Methylphenidate may be effective in some children with attention deficit hyperactivity disorder (see Therapeutic Uses of Sympathomimetic Drugs). **Modafinil** is a psychostimulant that differs from amphetamine in structure, neurochemical profile, and behavioral effects. Its mechanism of action is not fully known. It inhibits both norepinephrine and dopamine transporters, and it increases synaptic concentrations not only of norepinephrine and dopamine, but also of serotonin and glutamate, while decreasing GABA levels. It is used primarily to improve wakefulness in narcolepsy and some other conditions. It is often associated with increases in blood pressure and heart rate, though these are usually mild (see Therapeutic Uses of Sympathomimetic Drugs).

Tyramine (see Figure 6–5) is a normal by product of tyrosine metabolism in the body and can be produced in high concentrations in protein-rich foods by decarboxylation of tyrosine during fermentation (Table 9–5). It is readily metabolized by MAO in the liver and is normally inactive when taken orally because of a very high first-pass effect, ie, low bioavailability. If administered parenterally, it has an indirect sympathomimetic action caused by the release of stored catecholamines. Consequently, tyramine's spectrum of action is similar to that of norepinephrine. In patients treated with MAO inhibitors—particularly inhibitors of the MAO-A isoform—this effect of tyramine may be greatly intensified, leading to marked increases in blood pressure. This occurs because of increased bioavailability of tyramine and increased neuronal stores of catecholamines. Patients taking MAO inhibitors must be very careful to avoid tyramine-containing foods. There are differences in the effects of various MAO inhibitors on tyramine bioavailability, and isoform-specific or reversible enzyme antagonists may be safer (see Chapters 28 and 30).

TABLE 9–5 Foods reputed to have a high content of tyramine or other sympathomimetic agents.

Food	Tyramine Content of an Average Serving
Beer	4–45 mg
Broad beans, fava beans	Negligible (but contains dopamine)
Cheese, natural or aged	Nil to 130 mg (cheddar, Gruyère, and Stilton especially high)
Chicken liver	Nil to 9 mg
Chocolate	Negligible (but contains phenylethylamine)
Sausage, fermented (eg, salami, pepperoni, summer sausage)	Nil to 74 mg
Smoked or pickled fish (eg, pickled herring)	Nil to 198 mg
Snails	(No data found)
Wine (red)	Nil to 3 mg
Yeast (eg, dietary brewer's yeast supplements)	2–68 mg

Note: In a patient taking an irreversible monoamine oxidase (MAO) inhibitor drug, 20–50 mg of tyramine in a meal may increase the blood pressure significantly (see also Chapter 30: Antidepressant Agents). Note that only cheese, sausage, pickled fish, and yeast supplements contain sufficient tyramine to be consistently dangerous. This does not rule out the possibility that some preparations of other foods might contain significantly greater than average amounts of tyramine. Amounts in mg as per regular food portion.

B. Catecholamine Reuptake Inhibitors

Many inhibitors of the amine transporters for norepinephrine, dopamine, and serotonin are used clinically. Although specificity is not absolute, some are highly selective for one of the transporters. Many antidepressants, particularly the older tricyclic antidepressants, can inhibit norepinephrine and serotonin reuptake to different degrees. This may lead to orthostatic tachycardia as a side effect. Some antidepressants of this class, particularly imipramine, can induce orthostatic hypotension presumably by their clonidine-like effect or by blocking α_1 receptors, but the mechanism remains unclear.

Atomoxetine is a selective inhibitor of the norepinephrine reuptake transporter. Its actions, therefore, are mediated by potentiation of norepinephrine levels in noradrenergic synapses. It is used in the treatment of attention deficit disorders (see below). Atomoxetine has surprisingly little cardiovascular effect because it has a clonidine-like effect in the central nervous system to decrease sympathetic outflow while at the same time potentiating the effects of norepinephrine in the periphery. However, it may increase blood pressure in some patients. Norepinephrine reuptake is particularly important in the heart, especially during sympathetic stimulation, and this explains why atomoxetine and other norepinephrine reuptake inhibitors frequently cause orthostatic tachycardia. **Reboxetine** has similar characteristics as atomoxetine. **Sibutramine** is a serotonin and norepinephrine reuptake inhibitor and was initially approved by the FDA as an appetite suppressant for long-term treatment of obesity. It has been taken off the market in the United States and several other countries because it has been associated with a small increase in cardiovascular events including strokes in patients with a history of cardiovascular disease, which outweighed the benefits gained by modest weight reduction. **Duloxetine** is a widely used antidepressant with balanced serotonin and norepinephrine reuptake inhibitory effects (see Chapter 30). Increased cardiovascular risk has not been reported with duloxetine. Duloxetine and **milnacipran,** another serotonin and norepinephrine transporter blocker, are approved for the treatment of pain in fibromyalgia (see Chapter 30).

Cocaine is a local anesthetic with a peripheral sympathomimetic action that results from inhibition of transmitter reuptake at noradrenergic synapses (Figure 9-3). It readily enters the central nervous system and produces an amphetamine-like psychological effect that is shorter lasting and more intense than amphetamine. The major action of cocaine in the central nervous system is to inhibit dopamine reuptake into neurons in the "pleasure centers" of the brain. These properties and the fact that a rapid onset of action can be obtained when smoked, snorted into the nose, or injected, has made cocaine a heavily abused drug (see Chapter 32). It is interesting that dopamine-transporter knockout mice still self-administer cocaine, suggesting that cocaine may have additional pharmacologic targets.

Dopamine Agonists

Levodopa, which is converted to dopamine in the body, and **dopamine agonists** with central actions are of considerable value in the treatment of Parkinson's disease and prolactinemia. These agents are discussed in Chapters 28 and 37.

Fenoldopam is a D_1-receptor agonist that selectively leads to peripheral vasodilation in some vascular beds. The primary indication for fenoldopam is in the intravenous treatment of severe hypertension (see Chapter 11).

THERAPEUTIC USES OF SYMPATHOMIMETIC DRUGS

Cardiovascular Applications

In keeping with the critical role of the sympathetic nervous system in the control of blood pressure, a major area of application of the sympathomimetics is in cardiovascular conditions.

A. Treatment of Acute Hypotension

Acute hypotension may occur in a variety of settings such as severe hemorrhage, decreased blood volume, cardiac arrhythmias, neurologic disease or accidents, adverse reactions or overdose of medications such as antihypertensive drugs, and infection. If cerebral, renal, and cardiac perfusion is maintained, hypotension itself does not usually require vigorous direct treatment. Rather, placing the patient in the recumbent position and ensuring adequate fluid volume while the primary problem is determined and treated is usually the correct course of action. The use of sympathomimetic drugs merely to elevate a blood pressure that is not an immediate threat to the patient may increase morbidity. Sympathomimetic drugs may be used in a hypotensive emergency to preserve cerebral and coronary blood flow. The treatment is usually of short duration while the appropriate intravenous fluid or blood is being administered. Direct-acting α agonists such as **norepinephrine, phenylephrine,** and **methoxamine** have been used in this setting when vasoconstriction is desired.

Shock is a complex acute cardiovascular syndrome that results in a critical reduction in perfusion of vital tissues and a wide range of systemic effects. Shock is usually associated with hypotension, an altered mental state, oliguria, and metabolic acidosis. If untreated, shock usually progresses to a refractory deteriorating state and death. The three major mechanisms responsible for shock are hypovolemia, cardiac insufficiency, and altered vascular resistance. Volume replacement and treatment of the underlying disease are the mainstays of the treatment of shock. Although sympathomimetic drugs have been used in the treatment of virtually all forms of shock, their efficacy is unclear.

In most forms of shock, intense vasoconstriction, mediated by reflex sympathetic nervous system activation, is present. Indeed, efforts aimed at reducing rather than increasing peripheral resistance may be more fruitful to improve cerebral, coronary, and renal perfusion. A decision to use vasoconstrictors or vasodilators is best made on the basis of information about the underlying cause. Their use may require invasive monitoring.

Cardiogenic shock and acute heart failure, usually due to massive myocardial infarction, has a poor prognosis. Mechanically assisted perfusion and emergency cardiac surgery have been utilized in some settings. Optimal fluid replacement requires monitoring of pulmonary capillary wedge pressure and other parameters of cardiac function. Positive inotropic agents such as dopamine or dobutamine may provide short-term relief of heart failure symptoms in patients with advanced ventricular dysfunction. In low to moderate doses, these drugs may increase cardiac output and, compared with norepinephrine, cause relatively little peripheral vasoconstriction. Isoproterenol increases heart rate and work more than either dopamine or dobutamine. See Chapter 13 for a discussion of shock associated with myocardial infarction.

Unfortunately, the patient with shock may not respond to any of these therapeutic maneuvers; the temptation is then to use vasoconstrictors to maintain blood pressure. Coronary perfusion may be improved, but this gain may be offset by increased myocardial oxygen demands as well as more severe vasoconstriction in blood vessels to the abdominal viscera. Therefore, the goal of therapy in shock should be to optimize tissue perfusion, not blood pressure.

B. Chronic Orthostatic Hypotension

On standing, gravitational forces induce venous pooling, resulting in decreased venous return. Normally, a decrease in blood pressure is prevented by reflex sympathetic activation with increased heart rate, and peripheral arterial and venous vasoconstriction. Impairment of autonomic reflexes that regulate blood pressure can lead to chronic orthostatic hypotension. This is more often due to medications that can interfere with autonomic function (eg, imipramine and other tricyclic antidepressants, α blockers for the treatment of urinary retention, and diuretics) diabetes, and other diseases causing peripheral autonomic neuropathies, and less commonly, primary degenerative disorders of the autonomic nervous system, as in the case study described at the beginning of the chapter.

Increasing peripheral resistance is one of the strategies to treat chronic orthostatic hypotension, and drugs activating α receptors can be used for this purpose. Midodrine, an orally active α_1 agonist, is frequently used for this indication. Other sympathomimetics, such as oral ephedrine or phenylephrine, can be tried.

C. Cardiac Applications

Catecholamines such as isoproterenol and epinephrine have been used in the temporary emergency management of complete heart block and cardiac arrest. Epinephrine may be useful in cardiac arrest in part by redistributing blood flow during cardiopulmonary resuscitation to coronaries and to the brain. However, electronic pacemakers are both safer and more effective in heart block and should be inserted as soon as possible if there is any indication of continued high-degree block.

Dobutamine injection is used as a pharmacologic **cardiac stress test.** Dobutamine augments myocardial contractility and promotes coronary and systemic vasodilation. These actions lead to increased heart rate and increased myocardial work and can reveal areas of ischemia in the myocardium that are detected by echocardiogram or nuclear medicine techniques. Dobutamine is often used in patients unable to exercise during the stress test.

D. Inducing Local Vasoconstriction

Reduction of local or regional blood flow is desirable for achieving hemostasis in surgery, for reducing diffusion of local anesthetics away from the site of administration, and for reducing mucous membrane congestion. In each instance, α-receptor activation is desired, and the choice of agent depends on the maximal efficacy required, the desired duration of action, and the route of administration.

Effective pharmacologic hemostasis, often necessary for facial, oral, and nasopharyngeal surgery, requires drugs of high efficacy that can be administered in high concentration by local application. Epinephrine is usually applied topically in nasal packs (for epistaxis) or in a gingival string (for gingivectomy). Cocaine is still sometimes used for nasopharyngeal surgery because it combines a hemostatic effect with local anesthesia. Occasionally, cocaine is mixed with epinephrine for maximum hemostasis and local anesthesia.

Combining α agonists with some local anesthetics greatly prolongs the duration of infiltration nerve block; the total dose of local anesthetic (and the probability of toxicity) can therefore be reduced. Epinephrine, 1:200,000, is the favored agent for this application, but norepinephrine, phenylephrine, and other α agonists have also been used. Systemic effects on the heart and peripheral vasculature may occur even with local drug administration but are usually minimal. Use of epinephrine with local anesthesia of acral vascular beds (digits, nose, and ears) has not been advised because of fear of ischemic necrosis. Recent studies suggest that it can be used (with caution) for this indication.

Mucous membrane decongestants are α agonists that reduce the discomfort of hay fever and, to a lesser extent, the common cold by decreasing the volume of the nasal mucosa. These effects are probably mediated by α_1 receptors. Unfortunately, rebound hyperemia may follow the use of these agents, and repeated topical use of high drug concentrations may result in ischemic changes in the mucous membranes, probably as a result of vasoconstriction of nutrient arteries. Constriction of these vessels may involve activation of α_2 receptors, and phenylephrine is often used in nasal decongestant sprays. A longer duration of action—at the cost of much lower local concentrations and greater potential for cardiac and central nervous system effects—can be achieved by the oral administration of agents such as ephedrine or one of its isomers, pseudoephedrine. Long-acting topical decongestants include xylometazoline and oxymetazoline. Most of these mucous membrane decongestants are available as over-the-counter products.

Pulmonary Applications

One of the most important uses of sympathomimetic drugs is in the therapy of bronchial asthma. Beta$_2$-selective drugs (albuterol, metaproterenol, terbutaline) are used for this purpose. Short-acting preparations can be used only transiently for acute treatment of asthma symptoms. For chronic asthma treatment in adults, long-acting β_2 agonists should only be used as an addition to steroids because they may increase morbidity if used alone. There is less agreement about their benefit in children. Long-acting β_2 agonists are also used in patients with chronic obstructive pulmonary disease (COPD). Nonselective drugs are now rarely used because they are likely to have more adverse effects than the selective drugs. The use of β agonists for the management of asthma is discussed in Chapter 20.

Anaphylaxis

Anaphylactic shock and related immediate (type I) IgE-mediated reactions affect both the respiratory and the cardiovascular systems. The syndrome of bronchospasm, mucous membrane congestion, angioedema, and severe hypotension usually responds rapidly to the parenteral administration of **epinephrine,** 0.3–0.5 mg (0.3–0.5 mL of a 1:1000 epinephrine solution). Intramuscular injection may be the preferred route of administration, since skin blood flow (and hence systemic drug absorption from subcutaneous injection) is unpredictable in hypotensive patients. In some patients with impaired cardiovascular function, intravenous injection of epinephrine may be required. Glucocorticoids and antihistamines (both H$_1$- and H$_2$-receptor antagonists) may be useful as secondary therapy in anaphylaxis. The use of these agents precedes the era of controlled clinical trials, but extensive experimental and clinical experience supports the use of epinephrine as the agent of choice in anaphylaxis, presumably because epinephrine activates α, β$_1$, and β$_2$ receptors, all of which may be important in reversing the pathophysiologic processes underlying anaphylaxis. It is recommended that patients at risk for insect sting hypersensitivity, severe food allergies, or other types of anaphylaxis carry epinephrine in an autoinjector (EpiPen) for self-administration.

Ophthalmic Applications

Phenylephrine is an effective mydriatic agent frequently used to facilitate examination of the retina. It is also a useful decongestant for minor allergic hyperemia and itching of the conjunctival membranes. Sympathomimetics administered as ophthalmic drops are also useful in localizing the lesion in Horner's syndrome. (See Box: An Application of Basic Pharmacology to a Clinical Problem.)

Glaucoma responds to a variety of sympathomimetic and sympathoplegic drugs. (See Box, The Treatment of Glaucoma, in Chapter 10.) Epinephrine and its prodrug dipivefrin are now rarely used, but β-blocking agents are among the most important therapies. **Apraclonidine** and **brimonidine** are α$_2$-selective agonists that also lower intraocular pressure and are approved for use in glaucoma. The mechanism of action of these drugs in treating glaucoma is still uncertain; direct neuroprotective effects may be involved in addition to the benefits of lowering intraocular pressure.

Genitourinary Applications

As noted above, β$_2$-selective agents relax the pregnant uterus. **Ritodrine, terbutaline,** and similar drugs have been used to suppress premature labor. The goal is to defer labor long enough to ensure adequate maturation of the fetus. These drugs may delay labor for several days. This may afford time to administer corticosteroid drugs, which decrease the incidence of neonatal respiratory distress syndrome. However, meta-analysis of older trials and a randomized study suggest that β-agonist therapy may have no significant benefit on perinatal infant mortality and may increase maternal morbidity.

Oral sympathomimetic therapy is occasionally useful in the treatment of stress incontinence. Ephedrine or pseudoephedrine may be tried.

An Application of Basic Pharmacology to a Clinical Problem

Horner's syndrome is a condition—usually unilateral—that results from interruption of the sympathetic nerves to the face. The effects include vasodilation, ptosis, miosis, and loss of sweating on the affected side. The syndrome can be caused by either a preganglionic or a postganglionic lesion, such as a tumor. Knowledge of the location of the lesion (preganglionic or postganglionic) helps determine the optimal therapy.

A localized lesion in a nerve causes degeneration of the distal portion of that fiber and loss of transmitter contents from the degenerated nerve ending—without affecting neurons innervated by the fiber. Therefore, a preganglionic lesion leaves the postganglionic adrenergic neuron intact, whereas a postganglionic lesion results in degeneration of the adrenergic nerve endings and loss of stored catecholamines from them. Because indirectly acting sympathomimetics require normal stores of catecholamines, such drugs can be used to test for the presence of normal adrenergic nerve endings. The iris, because it is easily visible and responsive to topical sympathomimetics, is a convenient assay tissue in the patient.

If the lesion of Horner's syndrome is postganglionic, indirectly acting sympathomimetics (eg, cocaine, hydroxyamphetamine) will not dilate the abnormally constricted pupil because catecholamines have been lost from the nerve endings in the iris. In contrast, the pupil dilates in response to phenylephrine, which acts directly on the α receptors on the smooth muscle of the iris. A patient with a preganglionic lesion, on the other hand, shows a normal response to both drugs, since the postganglionic fibers and their catecholamine stores remain intact in this situation.

Central Nervous System Applications

The amphetamines have a mood-elevating (euphoriant) effect; this effect is the basis for the widespread abuse of this drug group (see Chapter 32). The amphetamines also have an alerting, sleep-deferring action that is manifested by improved attention to repetitive tasks and by acceleration and desynchronization of the electroencephalogram. A therapeutic application of this effect is in the treatment of narcolepsy. **Modafinil,** a new amphetamine substitute, is approved for use in narcolepsy and is claimed to have fewer disadvantages (excessive mood changes, insomnia, and abuse potential) than amphetamine in this condition. The appetite-suppressing effect of these agents is easily demonstrated in experimental animals. In obese humans, an encouraging initial response may be observed, but there is no evidence that long-term improvement in weight control can be achieved with amphetamines alone, especially when administered for a relatively short course. A final application of the central nervous system-active sympathomimetics is in the attention deficit hyperactivity disorder (ADHD), a behavioral syndrome consisting of short attention span, hyperkinetic physical behavior, and learning problems. Some patients with this syndrome respond well to low doses of **methylphenidate** and related agents. Extended-release formulations of methylphenidate may simplify dosing regimens and increase adherence to therapy, especially in school-age children. Slow or continuous-release preparations of the α_2 agonists clonidine and guanfacine are also effective in children with ADHD. Clinical trials suggest that modafinil may also be useful in ADHD, but because the safety profile in children has not been defined, it has not gained approval by the FDA for this indication.

Additional Therapeutic Uses

Although the primary use of the α_2 agonist **clonidine** is in the treatment of hypertension (see Chapter 11), the drug has been found to have efficacy in the treatment of diarrhea in diabetics with autonomic neuropathy, perhaps because of its ability to enhance salt and water absorption from the intestine. In addition, clonidine has efficacy in diminishing craving for narcotics and alcohol during withdrawal and may facilitate cessation of cigarette smoking. Clonidine has also been used to diminish menopausal hot flushes and is being used experimentally to reduce hemodynamic instability during general anesthesia. **Dexmedetomidine** is an α_2 agonist used for sedation under intensive care circumstances and during anesthesia (see Chapter 25). It blunts the sympathetic response to surgery, which may be beneficial in some situations. It lowers opioid requirements for pain control and does not depress ventilation. Clonidine is also sometimes used as a premedication before anesthesia. **Tizanidine** is an α_2 agonist that is used as a muscle relaxant (see Chapter 27).

SUMMARY Sympathomimetic Drugs

Subclass	Mechanism of Action	Effects	Clinical Applications	Pharmacokinetics, Toxicities, Interactions
α₁ AGONISTS				
• Midodrine	Activates phospholipase C, resulting in increased intracellular calcium and vasoconstriction	Vascular smooth muscle contraction increasing blood pressure (BP)	Orthostatic hypotension	Oral • prodrug converted to active drug with a 1-h peak effect • *Toxicity:* Supine hypertension, piloerection (goose bumps), and urinary retention
• *Phenylephrine: Can be used IV for short-term maintenance of BP in acute hypotension and intranasally to produce local vasoconstriction as a decongestant*				
α₂ AGONISTS				
• Clonidine	Inhibits adenylyl cyclase and interacts with other intracellular pathways	Vasoconstriction is masked by central sympatholytic effect, which lowers BP	Hypertension	Oral • transdermal • peak effect 1–3 h • half-life of oral drug ~12 h • produces dry mouth and sedation
• *α-Methyldopa, guanfacine, and guanabenz: Also used as central sympatholytics*				
• *Dexmedetomidine: Prominent sedative effects and used in anesthesia*				
• *Tizanidine: Used as a muscle relaxant*				
• *Apraclonidine and brimonidine: Used in glaucoma to reduce intraocular pressure*				
β₁ AGONISTS				
• Dobutamine[1]	Activates adenylyl cyclase, increasing myocardial contractility	Positive inotropic effect	Cardiogenic shock, acute heart failure	IV • requires dose titration to desired effect
B₂ AGONISTS				
• Albuterol	Activates adenylyl cyclase	Bronchial smooth muscle dilation	Asthma	Inhalation • duration 4–6 h • *Toxicity:* Tremor, tachycardia
• *See other β₂ agonists in Chapter 20*				
DOPAMINE				
D₁ Agonists				
• Fenoldopam	Activates adenylyl cyclase	Vascular smooth muscle relaxation	Hypertension	Requires dose titration to desired effect
D₂ Agonists				
• Bromocriptine	Inhibits adenylyl cyclase and interacts with other intracellular pathways	Mimics dopamine actions in the central nervous system	Parkinson's disease, prolactinemia	Oral • *Toxicity:* Nausea, headache, orthostatic hypotension
• *See other D₂ agonists in Chapters 28 and 37*				

[1]*Dobutamine has other actions in addition to β₁-agonist effect. See text for details.*

PREPARATIONS AVAILABLE[1]

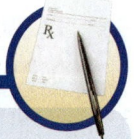

Amphetamine, racemic mixture (generic)
(attention deficit hyperactivity disorder [ADHD], narcolepsy)
Oral: 5, 10 mg tablets
Oral (Adderall): 1:1:1:1 mixtures of amphetamine sulfate, amphetamine aspartate, dextroamphetamine sulfate, and dextroamphetamine saccharate, formulated to contain a total of 5, 7.5, 10, 12.5, 15, 20, or 30 mg in tablets; or 10, 20, or 30 mg in capsules

Apraclonidine (Iopidine)
(glaucoma)
Topical: 0.5, 1% ophthalmic solutions

Armodafinil (Nuvigil)
(narcolepsy)
Oral: 50, 150, 250 mg tablets

Brimonidine (Alphagan)
(glaucoma)
Topical: 0.15, 0.2% ophthalmic solution

Dexmedetomidine (Precedex)
(sedation)
Parenteral: 100 mcg/mL

Dexmethylphenidate (Focalin)
(ADHD)
Oral: 2.5, 5, 10 mg tablets
Oral sustained release: 5, 10, 15, 20, 30 mg capsules

Dextroamphetamine (generic, Dexedrine)
(ADHD, narcolepsy)
Oral: 5, 10 mg tablets
Oral sustained release: 5, 10, 15 mg capsules
Oral mixtures with amphetamine: see Amphetamine (Adderall)

Dobutamine (generic, Dobutrex)
(hypotension)
Parenteral: 12.5 mg/mL in 20 mL vials for injection

Dopamine (generic, Intropin)
(hypotension)
Parenteral: 40, 80, 160 mg/mL for injection; 80, 160, 320 mg/100 mL in 5% D/W for injection

Ephedrine (generic)
(hypotension, asthma)
Oral: 25 mg capsules
Parenteral: 50 mg/mL for injection

Epinephrine (generic, Adrenalin Chloride, others)
(anaphylaxis, hypotension, asthma)
Parenteral: 1:1000 (1 mg/mL), 1:2000 (0.5 mg/mL), 1:10,000 (0.1 mg/mL), 1:100,000 (0.01 mg/mL) for injection
Parenteral autoinjector (EpiPen): 1:1000 (1 mg/mL), 1:2000 (0.5 mg/mL)
Ophthalmic: 0.1, 0.5, 1, 2% drops
Nasal: 0.1% drops and spray
Aerosol for bronchospasm (Primatene Mist, Bronkaid Mist): 0.22 mg/spray
Solution for nebulizer aerosol: 1:100

Fenoldopam (Corlopam)
(hypertension)
Parenteral: 10 mg/mL for IV infusion

Hydroxyamphetamine (Paremyd)
(mydriatic)
Ophthalmic: 1% drops (includes 0.25% tropicamide)

Isoproterenol (generic, Isuprel)
(bradycardia)
Parenteral: 1:5000 (0.2 mg/mL), 1:50,000 (0.02 mg/mL) for injection

Metaraminol (Aramine)
(hypotension)
Parenteral: 10 mg/mL for injection

Methamphetamine (Desoxyn)
(ADHD)
Oral: 5 mg tablets

Methylphenidate (generic, Ritalin, Ritalin-SR)
(ADHD, narcolepsy)
Oral: 5, 10, 20 mg tablets
Oral sustained release: 10, 18, 20, 27, 36, 54 mg tablets; 20, 30, 40 mg capsules

Midodrine (ProAmatine)
(hypotension)
Oral: 2.5, 5, 10 mg tablets

Modafinil (Provigil)
(narcolepsy)
Oral: 100, 200 mg tablets

Naphazoline (generic, Privine)
(decongestant)
Nasal: 0.05% drops and spray
Ophthalmic: 0.012, 0.02, 0.03, 0.1% drops

Norepinephrine (generic, Levophed)
(hypotension)
Parenteral: 1 mg/mL for injection

Oxymetazoline (generic, Afrin, Neo-Synephrine 12 Hour, Visine LR)
(decongestant)
Nasal: 0.05% spray
Ophthalmic: 0.025% drops

Phenylephrine (generic, Neo-Synephrine)
(hypotension, decongestant)
Oral: 10 mg chewable tablets
Parenteral: 10 mg/mL for injection
Nasal: 0.125, 0.16, 0.25, 0.5, 1% drops and spray
Ophthalmic: 0.12, 2.5, 10% solution

Pseudoephedrine (generic, Sudafed)
(decongestant)
Oral: 30, 60 mg tablets; 30, 60 mg capsules; 15, 30 mg/5 mL syrups; 7.5 mg/0.8 mL drops
Oral extended release: 120, 240 mg tablets, capsules

Tetrahydrozoline (generic, Visine)
(decongestant)
Nasal: 0.05, 0.1% drops
Ophthalmic: 0.05% drops

Tizanidine (Zanaflex)
(muscle relaxant)
Oral: 2, 4, 6 mg capsules; 2, 4 mg tablets

Xylometazoline (generic, Otrivin)
(decongestant)
Nasal: 0.05, 0.1% drops

---

[1]Primary clinical indications are given in parentheses. α_2 agonists used in hypertension are listed in Chapter 11. β_2 Agonists used in asthma are listed in Chapter 20. Norepinephrine transporter inhibitors are listed in Chapter 30. The primary clinical indications are given in parentheses.

REFERENCES

Brown SG: Cardiovascular aspects of anaphylaxis: Implications for treatment and diagnosis. Curr Opin Allergy Clin Immunol 2005;5:359.

Evans WE, McLeod HL: Pharmacogenomics—drug disposition, drug targets, and side effects. N Engl J Med 2003;348:538.

Gainetdinov RR et al: Desensitization of G protein-coupled receptors and neuronal functions. Annu Rev Neurosci 2004;27:107.

Hawrylyshyn KA et al: Update on human alpha1-adrenoceptor subtype signaling and genomic organization. Trends Pharmacol Sci 2004;25:449.

Holmes A, Lachowicz JE, Sibley DR: Phenotypic analysis of dopamine receptor knockout mice: Recent insights into the functional specificity of dopamine receptor subtypes. Neuropharmacology 2004;47:1117.

Johnson M: Molecular mechanisms of β_2-adrenergic receptor function, response, and regulation. J Allergy Clin Immunol 2006;117:18.

Kaufmann H, Biaggioni I: Orthostatic hypotension. In Shapira AHV (editor): *Neurology and Clinical Neurosciences.* Mosby Elsevier, 2007:354-361.

Koch WJ: Genetic and phenotypic targeting of beta-adrenergic signaling in heart failure. Mol Cell Biochem 2004;263:5.

Koshimizu T et al: Recent progress in alpha1-adrenoceptor pharmacology. Biol Pharm Bull 2002;25:401.

Lefkowitz RJ, Shenoy SK: Transduction of receptor signals by beta-arrestins. Science 2005;308:512.

Minzenberg MJ, Carter CS: Modafinil: A review of neurochemical actions and effects on cognition. Neuropsychopharmacol 2008;33:1477.

Mitler MM, Hayduk R: Benefits and risks of pharmacotherapy for narcolepsy. Drug Saf 2002;25:791.

Oldenburg O et al: Treatment of orthostatic hypotension. Curr Opin Pharmacol 2002;2:740.

Philipp M, Hein L: Adrenergic receptor knockout mice: Distinct functions of 9 receptor subtypes. Pharmacol Ther 2004;101:65.

Rockman HA, Koch WJ, Lefkowitz RJ: Seven-transmembrane-spanning receptors and heart function. Nature 2002;415:206.

Sandilands AJ, O'Shaughnessy KM: The functional significance of genetic variation within the beta-adrenoceptor. Br J Clin Pharmacol 2005;60:235.

Sicherer SH, Simons FE: Self-injectable epinephrine for first-aid management of anaphylaxis. Pediatrics 2007;119:638.

Simons FE: Anaphylaxis. J Allergy Clin Immunol 2008;121:S402.

Small KM, McGraw DW, Liggett SB: Pharmacology and physiology of human adrenergic receptor polymorphisms. Ann Rev Pharmacol Toxicol 2003;43:381.

Wechsler ME, Israel E: How pharmacogenomics will play a role in the management of asthma. Am J Respir Crit Care Med 2005;172:12.

Wechsler ME et al: Beta-adrenergic receptor polymorphisms and response to salmeterol. Am J Respir Crit Care Med 2006;173:519.

CASE STUDY ANSWER

The clinical picture is that of autonomic failure. The best indicator of this is the profound drop in orthostatic blood pressure without an adequate compensatory increase in heart rate. Pure autonomic failure is a neurodegenerative disorder selectively affecting peripheral autonomic fibers. Patients' blood pressure is critically dependent on whatever residual sympathetic tone they have, hence the symptomatic worsening of orthostatic hypotension that occurred when this patient was given the α blocker tamsulosin. Conversely, these patients are hypersensitive to the pressor effects of α agonists and other sympathomimetics. For example, the α agonist midodrine can increase blood pressure significantly at doses that have no effect in normal subjects and can be used to treat their orthostatic hypotension. Caution should be observed in the use of sympathomimetics (including over-the-counter agents) and sympatholytic drugs.

10

Adrenoceptor Antagonist Drugs

David Robertson, MD, & Italo Biaggioni, MD[*]

A 46-year-old woman sees her physician because of palpitations and headaches. She enjoyed good health until 1 year ago when spells of rapid heartbeat began. These became more severe and were eventually accompanied by throbbing headaches and drenching sweats. Physical examination revealed a blood pressure of 150/90 mm Hg and heart rate of 88 bpm. During the physical examination, palpation of the abdomen elicited a sudden and typical episode, with a rise in blood pressure to 210/120 mm Hg, heart rate to 122 bpm, profuse sweating, and facial pallor. This was accompanied by severe headache. What is the likely cause of her episodes? What caused the blood pressure and heart rate to rise so high during the examination? What treatments might help this patient?

Catecholamines play a role in many physiologic and pathophysiologic responses as described in Chapter 9. Drugs that block their receptors therefore have important effects, some of which are of great clinical value. These effects vary dramatically according to the drug's selectivity for α and β receptors. The classification of adrenoceptors into α_1, α_2, and β subtypes and the effects of activating these receptors are discussed in Chapters 6 and 9. Blockade of peripheral dopamine receptors is of minor clinical importance at present. In contrast, blockade of central nervous system dopamine receptors is very important; drugs that act on these receptors are discussed in Chapters 21 and 29. This chapter deals with pharmacologic antagonist drugs whose major effect is to occupy α_1, α_2, or β receptors outside the central nervous system and prevent their activation by catecholamines and related agonists.

For pharmacologic research, α_1- and α_2-adrenoceptor antagonist drugs have been very useful in the experimental exploration of autonomic nervous system function. In clinical therapeutics, nonselective α antagonists are used in the treatment of pheochromocytoma (tumors that secrete catecholamines), and α_1-selective antagonists are used in primary hypertension and benign prostatic hyperplasia. Beta-receptor antagonist drugs are useful in a much wider variety of clinical conditions and are firmly established in the treatment of hypertension, ischemic heart disease, arrhythmias, endocrinologic and neurologic disorders, glaucoma, and other conditions.

■ BASIC PHARMACOLOGY OF THE ALPHA-RECEPTOR ANTAGONIST DRUGS

Mechanism of Action

Alpha-receptor antagonists may be reversible or irreversible in their interaction with these receptors. Reversible antagonists dissociate from receptors, and the block can be surmounted with sufficiently high concentrations of agonists; irreversible drugs do not dissociate and cannot be surmounted. Phentolamine and prazosin (Figure 10–1) are examples of reversible antagonists. These drugs and labetalol—drugs used primarily for their antihypertensive effects—as well as several ergot derivatives (see Chapter 16) are also reversible α-adrenoceptor antagonists or partial agonists. Phenoxybenzamine, an agent related to the nitrogen mustards,

[*]The authors thank Dr Randy Blakely for helpful comments, Dr Brett English for improving tables, and our students at Vanderbilt for advice on conceptual clarity.

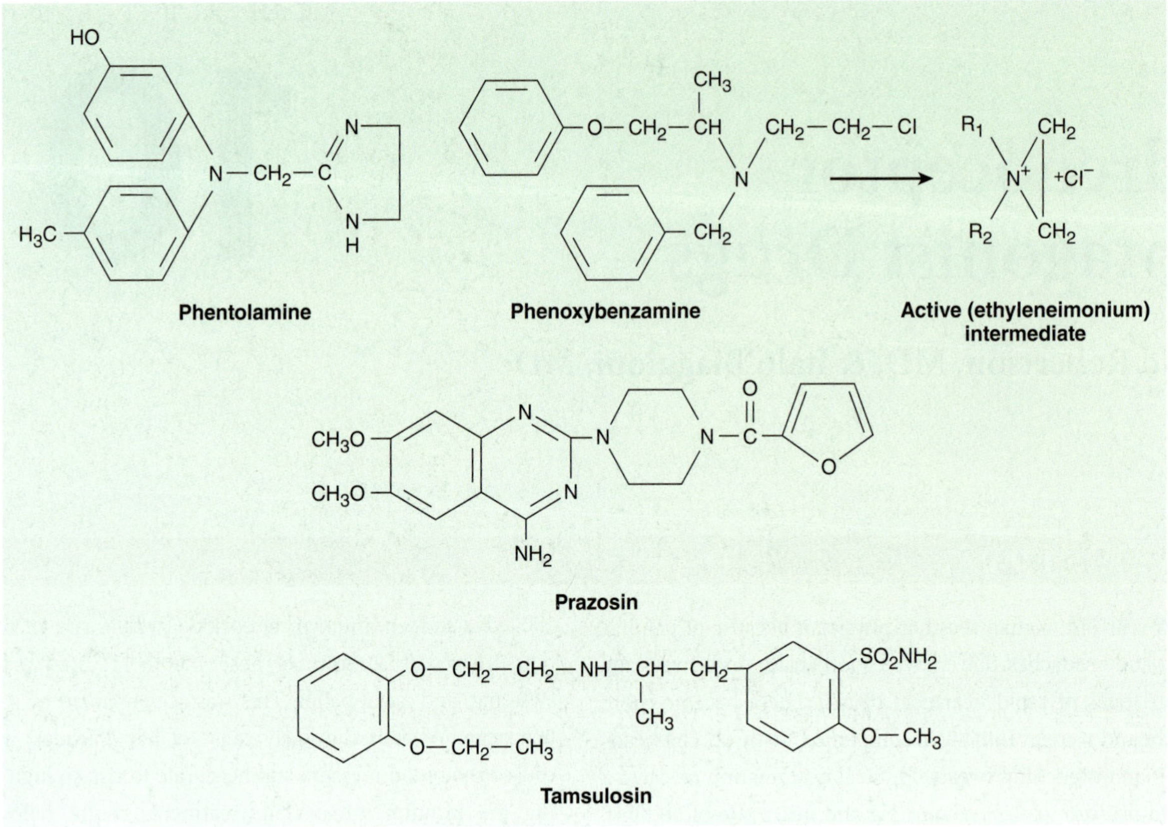

FIGURE 10–1   Structure of several α-receptor–blocking drugs.

forms a reactive ethyleneimonium intermediate (Figure 10–1) that covalently binds to α receptors, resulting in irreversible blockade. Figure 10–2 illustrates the effects of a reversible drug in comparison with those of an irreversible agent.

As discussed in Chapters 1 and 2, the duration of action of a reversible antagonist is largely dependent on the half-life of the drug in the body and the rate at which it dissociates from its receptor: The shorter the half-life of the drug in the body, the less time it takes for the effects of the drug to dissipate. In contrast, the effects of an irreversible antagonist may persist long after the drug has been cleared from the plasma. In the case of phenoxybenzamine, the restoration of tissue responsiveness after extensive α-receptor blockade is dependent on synthesis of new receptors, which may take several days. The rate of return of α_1-adrenoceptor responsiveness may be particularly important in patients having a sudden cardiovascular event or who become candidates for urgent surgery.

Pharmacologic Effects

A. Cardiovascular Effects

Because arteriolar and venous tone are determined to a large extent by α receptors on vascular smooth muscle, α-receptor antagonist drugs cause a lowering of peripheral vascular resistance and blood pressure (Figure 10–3). These drugs can prevent the pressor effects of usual doses of α agonists; indeed, in the case of agonists with both α and β_2 effects (eg, epinephrine), selective α-receptor antagonism may convert a pressor to a depressor response (Figure 10–3). This change in response is called **epinephrine reversal;** it illustrates how the activation of both α and β receptors in the vasculature may lead to opposite responses. Alpha-receptor antagonists often cause orthostatic hypotension and reflex tachycardia; nonselective ($\alpha_1 = \alpha_2$, Table 10–1) blockers usually cause significant tachycardia if blood pressure is lowered below normal. Orthostatic hypotension is due to antagonism of sympathetic nervous system stimulation of α_1 receptors in vascular smooth muscle; contraction of veins is an important component of the normal capacity to maintain blood pressure in the upright position since it decreases venous pooling in the periphery. Constriction of arterioles in the legs also contributes to the normal orthostatic response. Tachycardia may be more marked with agents that block α_2-presynaptic receptors in the heart, since the augmented release of norepinephrine will further stimulate β receptors in the heart.

B. Other Effects

Blockade of α receptors in other tissues elicits miosis (small pupils) and nasal stuffiness. Alpha$_1$ receptors are expressed in the base of the bladder and the prostate, and their blockade decreases resistance to the flow of urine. Alpha blockers, therefore, are used

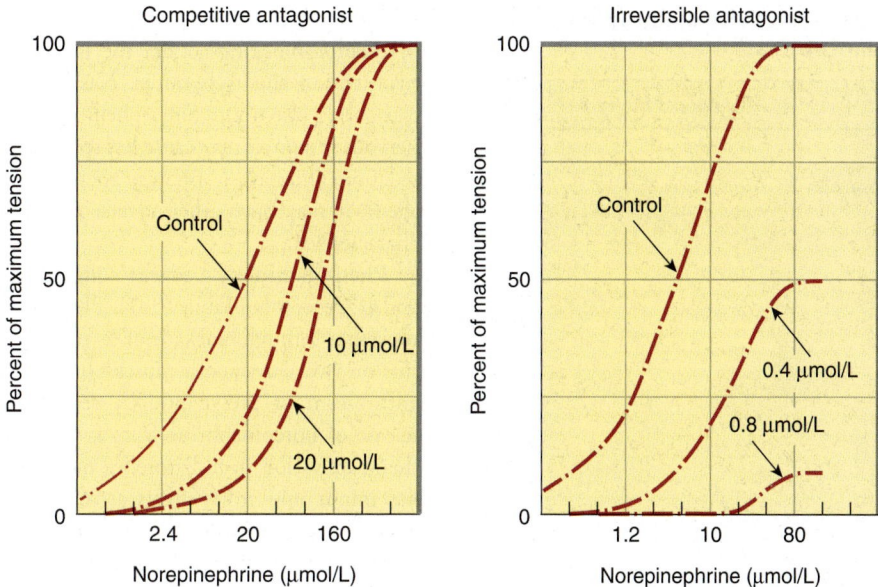

FIGURE 10–2 Dose-response curves to norepinephrine in the presence of two different α-adrenoceptor–blocking drugs. The tension produced in isolated strips of cat spleen, a tissue rich in α receptors, was measured in response to graded doses of norepinephrine. **Left:** Tolazoline, a reversible blocker, shifted the curve to the right without decreasing the maximum response when present at concentrations of 10 and 20 μmol/L. **Right:** Dibenamine, an analog of phenoxybenzamine and irreversible in its action, reduced the maximum response attainable at both concentrations tested. (Modified and reproduced, with permission, from Bickerton RK: The response of isolated strips of cat spleen to sympathomimetic drugs and their antagonists. J Pharmacol Exp Ther 1963;142:99.)

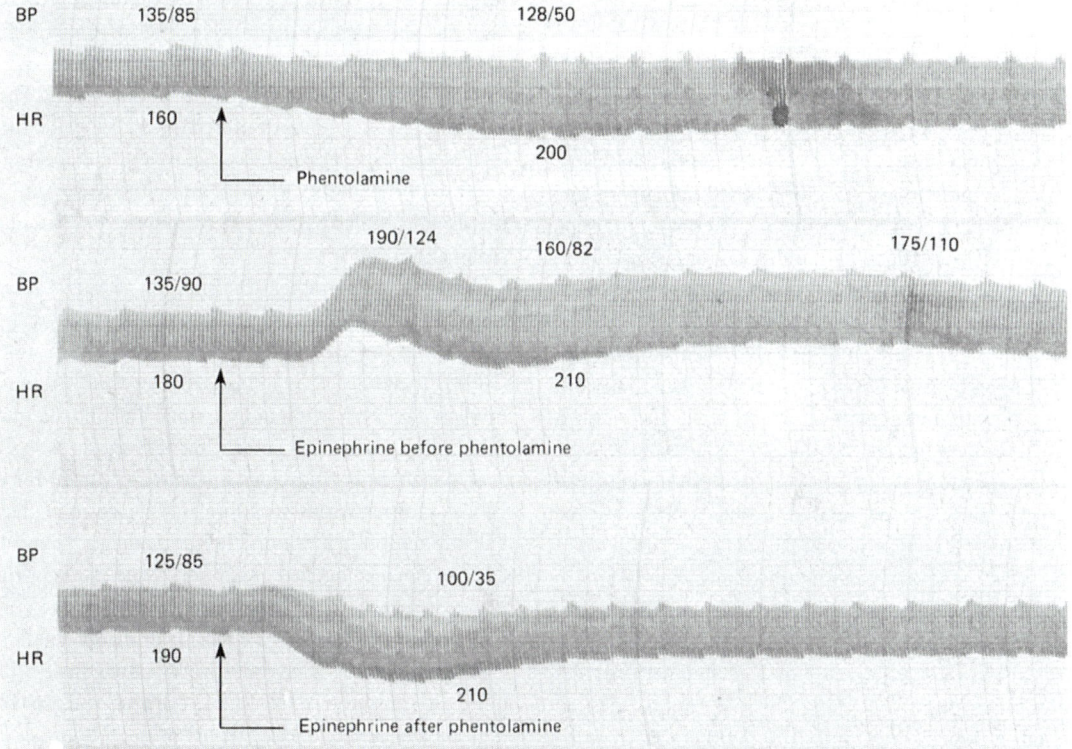

FIGURE 10–3 **Top:** Effects of phentolamine, an α-receptor–blocking drug, on blood pressure in an anesthetized dog. Epinephrine reversal is demonstrated by tracings showing the response to epinephrine before **(middle)** and after **(bottom)** phentolamine. All drugs given intravenously. BP, blood pressure; HR, heart rate.

TABLE 10–1 Relative selectivity of antagonists for adrenoceptors.

	Receptor Affinity
Alpha antagonists	
Prazosin, terazosin, doxazosin	$\alpha_1 >>>> \alpha_2$
Phenoxybenzamine	$\alpha_1 > \alpha_2$
Phentolamine	$\alpha_1 = \alpha_2$
Yohimbine, tolazoline	$\alpha_2 >> \alpha_1$
Mixed antagonists	
Labetalol, carvedilol	$\beta_1 = \beta_2 \geq \alpha_1 > \alpha_2$
Beta antagonists	
Metoprolol, acebutolol, alprenolol, atenolol, betaxolol, celiprolol, esmolol, nebivolol	$\beta_1 >>> \beta_2$
Propranolol, carteolol, penbutolol, pindolol, timolol	$\beta_1 = \beta_2$
Butoxamine	$\beta_2 >>> \beta_1$

therapeutically for the treatment of urinary retention due to prostatic hyperplasia (see below). Individual agents may have other important effects in addition to α-receptor antagonism (see below).

SPECIFIC AGENTS

Phenoxybenzamine binds covalently to α receptors, causing irreversible blockade of long duration (14–48 hours or longer). It is somewhat selective for α_1 receptors but less so than prazosin (Table 10–1). The drug also inhibits reuptake of released norepinephrine by presynaptic adrenergic nerve terminals. Phenoxybenzamine blocks histamine (H_1), acetylcholine, and serotonin receptors as well as α receptors (see Chapter 16).

The pharmacologic actions of phenoxybenzamine are primarily related to antagonism of α-receptor–mediated events. The most significant effect is attenuation of catecholamine-induced vasoconstriction. While phenoxybenzamine causes relatively little fall in blood pressure in normal supine individuals, it reduces blood pressure when sympathetic tone is high, eg, as a result of upright posture or because of reduced blood volume. Cardiac output may be increased because of reflex effects and because of some blockade of presynaptic α_2 receptors in cardiac sympathetic nerves.

Phenoxybenzamine is absorbed after oral administration, although bioavailability is low and its kinetic properties are not well known. The drug is usually given orally, starting with dosages of 10 mg/d and progressively increasing the dose until the desired effect is achieved. A dosage of less than 100 mg/d is usually sufficient to achieve adequate α-receptor blockade. The major use of phenoxybenzamine is in the treatment of pheochromocytoma (see below).

Most adverse effects of phenoxybenzamine derive from its α-receptor–blocking action; the most important are orthostatic hypotension and tachycardia. Nasal stuffiness and inhibition of ejaculation also occur. Since phenoxybenzamine enters the central nervous system, it may cause less specific effects, including fatigue, sedation, and nausea. Because phenoxybenzamine is an alkylating agent, it may have other adverse effects that have not yet been characterized.

Phentolamine is a potent competitive antagonist at both α_1 and α_2 receptors (Table 10–1). Phentolamine reduces peripheral resistance through blockade of α_1 receptors and possibly α_2 receptors on vascular smooth muscle. Its cardiac stimulation is due to antagonism of presynaptic α_2 receptors (leading to enhanced release of norepinephrine from sympathetic nerves) and sympathetic activation from baroreflex mechanisms. Phentolamine also has minor inhibitory effects at serotonin receptors and agonist effects at muscarinic and H_1 and H_2 histamine receptors. Phentolamine's principal adverse effects are related to cardiac stimulation, which may cause severe tachycardia, arrhythmias, and myocardial ischemia. Phentolamine has been used in the treatment of pheochromocytoma. In addition it is sometimes used to reverse local anesthesia in soft tissue sites; local anesthetics are often given with vasoconstrictors that slow their removal. Local phentolamine permits reversal at the end of the procedure. Unfortunately oral and intravenous formulations of phentolamine are no longer consistently available in the United States.

Prazosin is a piperazinyl quinazoline effective in the management of hypertension (see Chapter 11). It is highly selective for α_1 receptors and typically 1000-fold less potent at α_2 receptors. This may partially explain the relative absence of tachycardia seen with prazosin compared with that of phentolamine and phenoxybenzamine. Prazosin relaxes both arterial and venous vascular smooth muscle, as well as smooth muscle in the prostate, due to blockade of α_1 receptors. Prazosin is extensively metabolized in humans; because of metabolic degradation by the liver, only about 50% of the drug is available after oral administration. The half-life is normally about 3 hours.

Terazosin is another reversible α_1-selective antagonist that is effective in hypertension (see Chapter 11); it is also approved for use in men with urinary symptoms due to benign prostatic hyperplasia (BPH). Terazosin has high bioavailability but is extensively metabolized in the liver, with only a small fraction of unchanged drug excreted in the urine. The half-life of terazosin is 9–12 hours.

Doxazosin is efficacious in the treatment of hypertension and BPH. It differs from prazosin and terazosin in having a longer half-life of about 22 hours. It has moderate bioavailability and is extensively metabolized, with very little parent drug excreted in urine or feces. Doxazosin has active metabolites, although their contribution to the drug's effects is probably small.

Tamsulosin is a competitive α_1 antagonist with a structure quite different from that of most other α_1-receptor blockers. It has high bioavailability and a half-life of 9–15 hours. It is metabolized extensively in the liver. Tamsulosin has higher affinity for α_{1A} and α_{1D} receptors than for the α_{1B} subtype. Evidence suggests that tamsulosin has relatively greater potency in inhibiting contraction in *prostate* smooth muscle versus *vascular* smooth muscle compared with other α_1-selective antagonists. The drug's efficacy in BPH suggests that the α_{1A} subtype may be the most important α subtype mediating prostate smooth muscle contraction. Furthermore, compared with other antagonists, tamsulosin has less effect on standing blood pressure in patients. Nevertheless, caution is appropriate in using any α antagonist in patients with diminished sympathetic nervous system function. Patients receiving oral tamsulosin and undergoing cataract surgery are at increased risk of the intraoperative floppy iris syndrome (IFIS), characterized by the billowing of a flaccid iris, propensity for iris prolapse, and progressive intraoperative pupillary constriction. These effects increase the risk of cataract surgery, and complications are more likely in the ensuing 14 days if patients are taking these agents.

OTHER ALPHA-ADRENOCEPTOR ANTAGONISTS

Alfuzosin is an α_1-selective quinazoline derivative that is approved for use in BPH. It has a bioavailability of about 60%, is extensively metabolized, and has an elimination half-life of about 5 hours. It may increase risk of QT prolongation in susceptible individuals. **Silodosin** resembles tamsulosin in blocking the α_{1A} receptor and is used in treatment of BPH. **Indoramin** is another α_1-selective antagonist that also has efficacy as an antihypertensive. It is not available in the USA. **Urapidil** is an α_1 antagonist (its primary effect) that also has weak α_2-agonist and 5-HT$_{1A}$-agonist actions and weak antagonist action at β_1 receptors. It is used in Europe as an antihypertensive agent and for benign prostatic hyperplasia. **Labetalol** has both α_1-selective and β-antagonistic effects; it is discussed below. Neuroleptic drugs such as **chlorpromazine** and **haloperidol** are potent dopamine receptor antagonists but are also antagonists at α receptors. Their antagonism of α receptors probably contributes to some of their adverse effects, particularly hypotension. Similarly, the antidepressant **trazodone** has the capacity to block α_1 receptors. Ergot derivatives, eg, **ergotamine** and **dihydroergotamine,** cause reversible α-receptor blockade, probably via a partial agonist action (see Chapter 16).

Yohimbine, an indole alkaloid, is an α_2-selective antagonist. It is sometimes used in the treatment of orthostatic hypotension because it promotes norepinephrine release through blockade of α_2 receptors in both the central nervous system and the periphery. This increases central sympathetic activation and also promotes increased norepinephrine release in the periphery. It was once widely used to treat male erectile dysfunction but has been superseded by phosphodiesterase-5 inhibitors like sildenafil (see Chapter 12). Yohimbine can greatly elevate blood pressure if administered to patients receiving norepinephrine transport blocking drugs. Yohimbine reverses the antihypertensive effects of α_2-adrenoceptor agonists such as clonidine. It is used in veterinary medicine to reverse anesthesia produced by xylazine, an α_2 agonist used to calm animals. Although yohimbine has been taken off the market in the USA solely for financial reasons, it is available as a "nutritional" supplement.

■ CLINICAL PHARMACOLOGY OF THE ALPHA-RECEPTOR–BLOCKING DRUGS

Pheochromocytoma

Pheochromocytoma is a tumor of the adrenal medulla or sympathetic ganglion cells. The tumor secretes catecholamines, especially norepinephrine and epinephrine. The patient in the case study at the beginning of this chapter had a left adrenal pheochromocytoma that was identified by imaging. In addition, she had elevated plasma and urinary norepinephrine, epinephrine, and their metabolites, normetanephrine and metanephrine.

The diagnosis of pheochromocytoma is confirmed on the basis of elevated plasma or urinary levels of catecholamines, metanephrine, and normetanephrine (see Chapter 6). Once diagnosed biochemically, techniques to localize a pheochromocytoma include computed tomography and magnetic resonance imaging scans and scanning with radiomarkers such as ^{131}I-meta-iodobenzylguanidine (MIBG), a norepinephrine transporter substrate that is taken up by tumor cells.

The major clinical use of phenoxybenzamine is in the management of pheochromocytoma. Patients have many symptoms and signs of catecholamine excess, including intermittent or sustained hypertension, headaches, palpitations, and increased sweating.

Release of stored catecholamines from pheochromocytomas may occur in response to physical pressure, chemical stimulation, or spontaneously. When it occurs during operative manipulation of pheochromocytoma, the resulting hypertension may be controlled with α-receptor blockade or nitroprusside. Nitroprusside is preferred because its effects can be more readily titrated and it has a shorter duration of action.

Alpha-receptor antagonists are most useful in the preoperative management of patients with pheochromocytoma (Figure 10–4). Administration of phenoxybenzamine in the preoperative period helps to control hypertension and tends to reverse chronic changes resulting from excessive catecholamine secretion such as plasma volume contraction, if present. Furthermore, the patient's operative course may be simplified. Oral doses of 10 mg/d can be increased at intervals of several days until hypertension is controlled. Some physicians give phenoxybenzamine to patients with pheochromocytoma for 1–3 weeks before surgery. Other surgeons prefer to operate on patients in the absence of treatment with phenoxybenzamine, counting on modern anesthetic techniques to control blood pressure and heart rate during surgery. Phenoxybenzamine can be very useful in the chronic treatment of inoperable or metastatic pheochromocytoma. Although there is less experience with alternative drugs, hypertension in patients with pheochromocytoma may also respond to reversible α_1-selective antagonists or to conventional calcium channel antagonists. Beta-receptor antagonists may be required after α-receptor blockade has been instituted to reverse the cardiac effects of excessive catecholamines. Beta antagonists should not be used prior to establishing effective α-receptor blockade, since unopposed

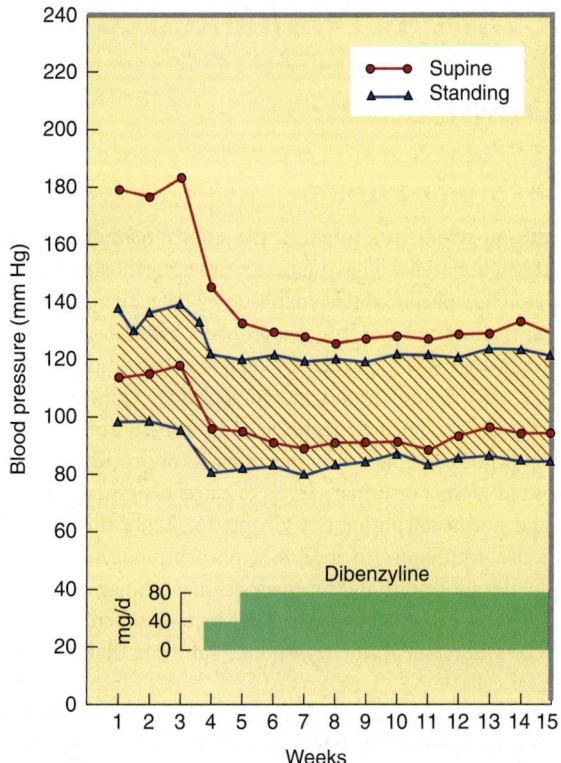

FIGURE 10–4 Effects of phenoxybenzamine (Dibenzyline) on blood pressure in a patient with pheochromocytoma. Dosage of the drug was begun in the fourth week as shown by the shaded bar. Supine systolic and diastolic pressures are indicated by the circles, and the standing pressures by triangles and the hatched area. Note that the α-blocking drug dramatically reduced blood pressure. The reduction in orthostatic hypotension, which was marked before treatment, is probably due to normalization of blood volume, a variable that is sometimes markedly reduced in patients with longstanding pheochromocytoma-induced hypertension. (Redrawn and reproduced, with permission, from Engelman E, Sjoerdsma A: Chronic medical therapy for pheochromocytoma. Ann Intern Med 1961;61:229.)

β-receptor blockade could theoretically cause blood pressure elevation from increased vasoconstriction.

Pheochromocytoma is sometimes treated with **metyrosine** (α-methyltyrosine), the α-methyl analog of tyrosine. This agent is a competitive inhibitor of tyrosine hydroxylase, the rate-limiting step in the synthesis of dopamine, norepinephrine, and epinephrine (see Figure 6–5). Metyrosine is especially useful in symptomatic patients with inoperable or metastatic pheochromocytoma. Because it has access to the central nervous system, metyrosine can cause extrapyramidal effects due to reduced dopamine levels.

Hypertensive Emergencies

The α-adrenoceptor antagonist drugs have limited application in the management of hypertensive emergencies, but labetalol has been used in this setting (see Chapter 11). In theory, α-adrenoceptor antagonists are most useful when increased blood pressure reflects excess circulating concentrations of α agonists, eg, in pheochromocytoma, overdosage of sympathomimetic drugs, or clonidine withdrawal. However, other drugs are generally preferable, since

considerable experience is necessary to use α-adrenoceptor antagonist drugs safely in these settings.

Chronic Hypertension

Members of the prazosin family of α_1-selective antagonists are efficacious drugs in the treatment of mild to moderate systemic hypertension (see Chapter 11). They are generally well tolerated, but they are not usually recommended as monotherapy for hypertension because other classes of antihypertensives are more effective in preventing heart failure. Their major adverse effect is orthostatic hypotension, which may be severe after the first few doses but is otherwise uncommon. Nonselective α antagonists are not used in primary systemic hypertension. Prazosin and related drugs may also be associated with dizziness. Orthostatic changes in blood pressure should be checked routinely in any patient being treated for hypertension.

It is interesting that the use of α-adrenoceptor antagonists such as prazosin has been found to be associated with either no changes in plasma lipids or increased concentrations of high-density lipoproteins (HDL), which could be a favorable alteration. The mechanism for this effect is not known.

Peripheral Vascular Disease

Alpha-receptor–blocking drugs do not seem to be effective in the treatment of peripheral vascular occlusive disease characterized by morphologic changes that limit flow in the vessels. Occasionally, individuals with Raynaud's phenomenon and other conditions involving excessive reversible vasospasm in the peripheral circulation do benefit from prazosin or phenoxybenzamine, although calcium channel blockers may be preferable for most patients.

Urinary Obstruction

Benign prostatic hyperplasia is common in elderly men. Various surgical treatments are effective in relieving the urinary symptoms of BPH; however, drug therapy is efficacious in many patients. The mechanism of action in improving urine flow involves partial reversal of smooth muscle contraction in the enlarged prostate and in the bladder base. It has been suggested that some α_1-receptor antagonists may have additional effects on cells in the prostate that help improve symptoms.

Prazosin, doxazosin, and terazosin are all efficacious in patients with BPH. These drugs are particularly useful in patients who also have hypertension. Considerable interest has focused on which α_1-receptor subtype is most important for smooth muscle contraction in the prostate: *subtype-selective* α_{1A}-receptor antagonists may have improved efficacy and safety in treating this disease. As indicated above, tamsulosin is also efficacious in BPH and has relatively minor effects on blood pressure at a low dose. This drug may be preferred in patients who have experienced orthostatic hypotension with other α_1-receptor antagonists.

Erectile Dysfunction

A combination of phentolamine with the nonspecific smooth muscle relaxant papaverine, when injected directly into the penis, may cause erections in men with sexual dysfunction. Long-term administration may result in fibrotic reactions. Systemic absorption may lead to orthostatic hypotension; priapism may require direct treatment with an α-adrenoceptor agonist such as phenylephrine. Alternative therapies for erectile dysfunction include prostaglandins (see Chapter 18), sildenafil and other cGMP phosphodiesterase inhibitors (see Chapter 12), and apomorphine.

Applications of Alpha$_2$ Antagonists

Alpha$_2$ antagonists have relatively little clinical usefulness. They have limited benefit in male erectile dysfunction. There has been experimental interest in the development of highly selective antagonists for treatment of type 2 diabetes (α$_2$ receptors inhibit insulin secretion), and for treatment of psychiatric depression. It is likely that better understanding of the subtypes of α$_2$ receptors will lead to development of clinically useful subtype-selective new drugs.

■ BASIC PHARMACOLOGY OF THE BETA-RECEPTOR ANTAGONIST DRUGS

Beta-receptor antagonists share the common feature of antagonizing the effects of catecholamines at β adrenoceptors. Beta-blocking drugs occupy β receptors and competitively reduce receptor occupancy by catecholamines and other β agonists. (A few members of this group, used only for experimental purposes, bind irreversibly to β receptors.) Most β-blocking drugs in clinical use are pure antagonists; that is, the occupancy of a β receptor by such a drug causes no activation of the receptor. However, some are partial agonists; that is, they cause partial activation of the receptor, albeit less than that caused by the full agonists epinephrine and isoproterenol. As described in Chapter 2, partial agonists inhibit the activation of β receptors in the presence of high catecholamine concentrations but moderately activate the receptors in the absence of endogenous agonists. Finally, evidence suggests that some β blockers (eg, betaxolol, metoprolol) are *inverse agonists*— drugs that reduce constitutive activity of β receptors—in some tissues. The clinical significance of this property is not known.

The β-receptor–blocking drugs differ in their relative affinities for β$_1$ and β$_2$ receptors (Table 10–1). Some have a higher affinity for β$_1$ than for β$_2$ receptors, and this selectivity may have important clinical implications. Since none of the clinically available β-receptor antagonists are absolutely specific for β$_1$ receptors, the selectivity is dose-related; it tends to diminish at higher drug concentrations. Other major differences among β antagonists relate to their pharmacokinetic characteristics and local anesthetic membrane-stabilizing effects.

Chemically, most β-receptor antagonist drugs (Figure 10–5) resemble isoproterenol to some degree (see Figure 9–4).

Pharmacokinetic Properties of the Beta-Receptor Antagonists

A. Absorption

Most of the drugs in this class are well absorbed after oral administration; peak concentrations occur 1–3 hours after ingestion.

Sustained-release preparations of propranolol and metoprolol are available.

B. Bioavailability

Propranolol undergoes extensive hepatic (first-pass) metabolism; its bioavailability is relatively low (Table 10–2). The proportion of drug reaching the systemic circulation increases as the dose is increased, suggesting that hepatic extraction mechanisms may become saturated. A major consequence of the low bioavailability of propranolol is that oral administration of the drug leads to much lower drug concentrations than are achieved after intravenous injection of the same dose. Because the first-pass effect varies among individuals, there is great individual variability in the plasma concentrations achieved after oral propranolol. For the same reason, bioavailability is limited to varying degrees for most β antagonists with the exception of betaxolol, penbutolol, pindolol, and sotalol.

C. Distribution and Clearance

The β antagonists are rapidly distributed and have large volumes of distribution. Propranolol and penbutolol are quite lipophilic and readily cross the blood-brain barrier (Table 10–2). Most β antagonists have half-lives in the range of 3–10 hours. A major exception is esmolol, which is rapidly hydrolyzed and has a half-life of approximately 10 minutes. Propranolol and metoprolol are extensively metabolized in the liver, with little unchanged drug appearing in the urine. The cytochrome P450 2D6 (CYP2D6) genotype is a major determinant of interindividual differences in metoprolol plasma clearance (see Chapter 4). Poor metabolizers exhibit threefold to tenfold higher plasma concentrations after administration of metoprolol than extensive metabolizers. Atenolol, celiprolol, and pindolol are less completely metabolized. Nadolol is excreted unchanged in the urine and has the longest half-life of any available β antagonist (up to 24 hours). The half-life of nadolol is prolonged in renal failure. The elimination of drugs such as propranolol may be prolonged in the presence of liver disease, diminished hepatic blood flow, or hepatic enzyme inhibition. It is notable that the pharmacodynamic effects of these drugs are sometimes prolonged well beyond the time predicted from half-life data.

Pharmacodynamics of the Beta-Receptor Antagonist Drugs

Most of the effects of these drugs are due to occupation and blockade of β receptors. However, some actions may be due to other effects, including partial agonist activity at β receptors and local anesthetic action, which differ among the β blockers (Table 10–2).

A. Effects on the Cardiovascular System

Beta-blocking drugs given chronically lower blood pressure in patients with hypertension (see Chapter 11). The mechanisms involved are not fully understood but probably include suppression of renin release and effects in the central nervous system. These drugs do *not* usually cause hypotension in healthy individuals with normal blood pressure.

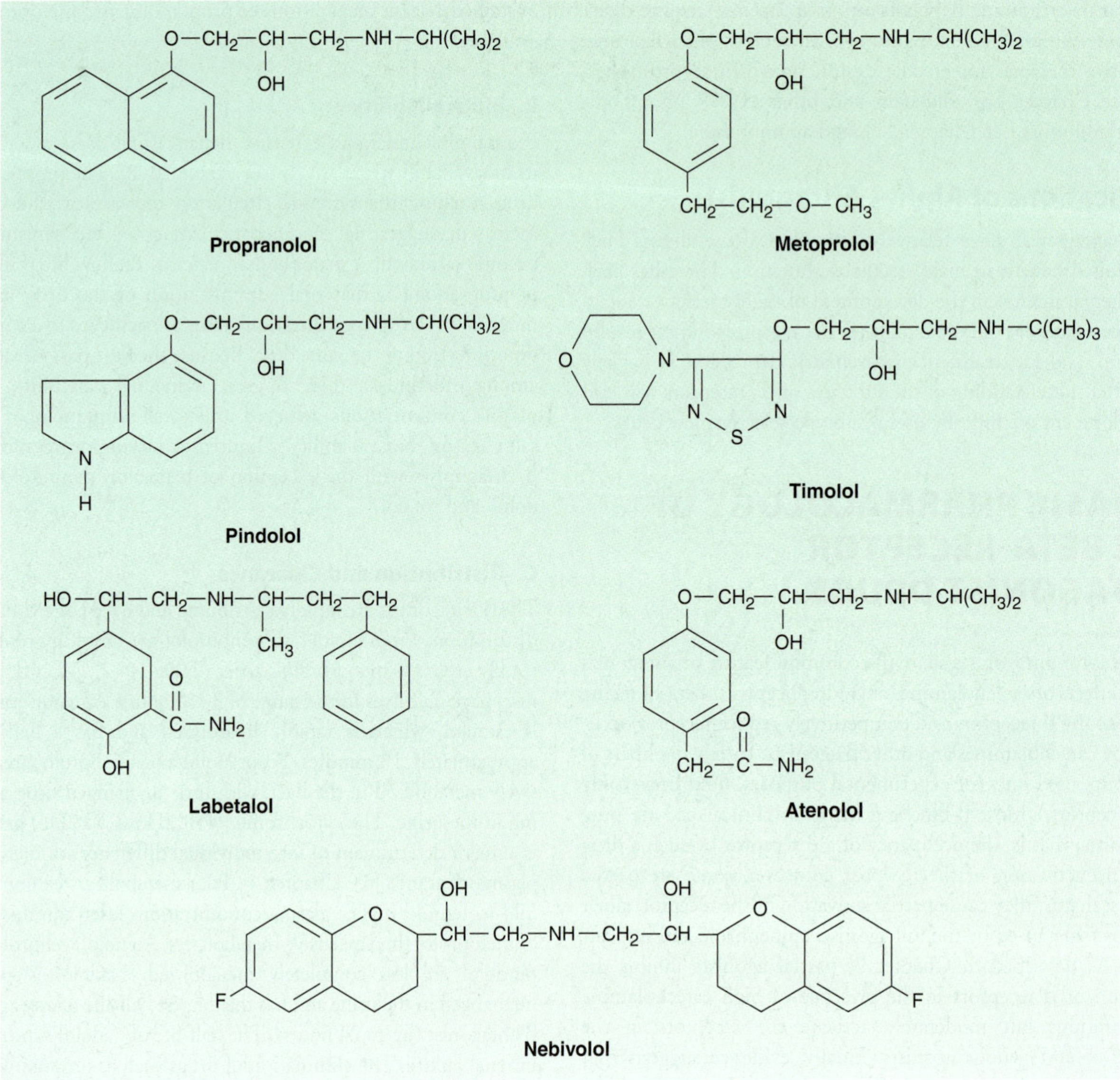

FIGURE 10–5 Structures of some β-receptor antagonists.

Beta-receptor antagonists have prominent effects on the heart (Figure 10–6) and are very valuable in the treatment of angina (see Chapter 12) and chronic heart failure (see Chapter 13) and following myocardial infarction (see Chapter 14). The negative inotropic and chronotropic effects reflect the role of adrenoceptors in regulating these functions. Slowed atrioventricular conduction with an increased PR interval is a related result of adrenoceptor blockade in the atrioventricular node. In the vascular system, β-receptor blockade opposes β_2-mediated vasodilation. This may acutely lead to a rise in peripheral resistance from unopposed α-receptor–mediated effects as the sympathetic nervous system discharges in response to lowered blood pressure due to the fall in cardiac output. Nonselective and β_1-blocking drugs antagonize the release of renin caused by the sympathetic nervous system.

Overall, although the acute effects of these drugs may include a rise in peripheral resistance, chronic drug administration leads to a fall in peripheral resistance in patients with hypertension.

B. Effects on the Respiratory Tract

Blockade of the β_2 receptors in bronchial smooth muscle may lead to an increase in airway resistance, particularly in patients with asthma. Beta$_1$-receptor antagonists such as metoprolol and atenolol may have some advantage over nonselective β antagonists when blockade of β_1 receptors in the heart is desired and β_2-receptor blockade is undesirable. However, no currently available β_1-selective antagonist is sufficiently specific to *completely* avoid interactions with β_2 adrenoceptors. Consequently, these drugs should generally be avoided in patients with asthma. On the other

TABLE 10–2 Properties of several beta-receptor–blocking drugs.

	Selectivity	Partial Agonist Activity	Local Anesthetic Action	Lipid Solubility	Elimination Half-life	Approximate Bioavailability
Acebutolol	β_1	Yes	Yes	Low	3–4 hours	50
Atenolol	β_1	No	No	Low	6–9 hours	40
Betaxolol	β_1	No	Slight	Low	14–22 hours	90
Bisoprolol	β_1	No	No	Low	9–12 hours	80
Carteolol	None	Yes	No	Low	6 hours	85
Carvedilol[1]	None	No	No	Moderate	7–10 hours	25–35
Celiprolol	β_1	Yes	No	Low	4–5 hours	70
Esmolol	β_1	No	No	Low	10 minutes	0
Labetalol[1]	None	Yes	Yes	Low	5 hours	30
Metoprolol	β_1	No	Yes	Moderate	3–4 hours	50
Nadolol	None	No	No	Low	14–24 hours	33
Nebivolol	β_1	?[2]	No	Low	11–30 hours	12–96
Penbutolol	None	Yes	No	High	5 hours	>90
Pindolol	None	Yes	Yes	Moderate	3–4 hours	90
Propranolol	None	No	Yes	High	3.5–6 hours	30[3]
Sotalol	None	No	No	Low	12 hours	90
Timolol	None	No	No	Moderate	4–5 hours	50

[1]Carvedilol and labetalol also cause α_1-adrenoceptor blockade.

[2]β_3 agonist.

[3]Bioavailability is dose-dependent.

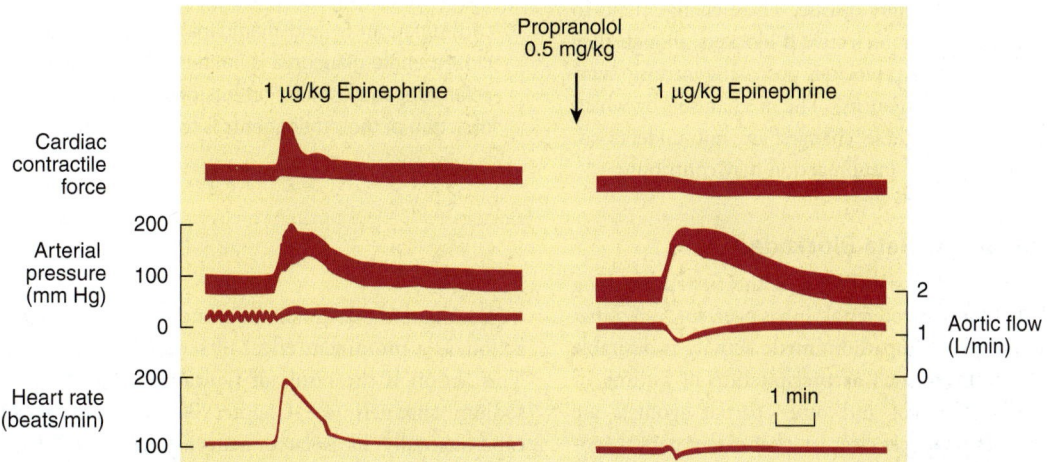

FIGURE 10–6 The effect in an anesthetized dog of the injection of epinephrine before and after propranolol. In the presence of a β-receptor–blocking agent, epinephrine no longer augments the force of contraction (measured by a strain gauge attached to the ventricular wall) nor increases cardiac rate. Blood pressure is still elevated by epinephrine because vasoconstriction is not blocked. (Reproduced, with permission, from Shanks RG: The pharmacology of β sympathetic blockade. Am J Cardiol 1966;18:312.)

hand, many patients with chronic obstructive pulmonary disease (COPD) may tolerate these drugs quite well and the benefits, for example in patients with concomitant ischemic heart disease, may outweigh the risks.

C. Effects on the Eye

Beta-blocking agents reduce intraocular pressure, especially in glaucoma. The mechanism usually reported is decreased aqueous humor production. (See Clinical Pharmacology and Box: The Treatment of Glaucoma.)

D. Metabolic and Endocrine Effects

Beta-receptor antagonists such as propranolol inhibit sympathetic nervous system stimulation of lipolysis. The effects on carbohydrate metabolism are less clear, though glycogenolysis in the human liver is at least partially inhibited after β_2-receptor blockade. Glucagon is the primary hormone used to combat hypoglycemia; it is unclear to what extent β antagonists impair recovery from hypoglycemia, but they should be used with caution in insulin-dependent diabetic patients. This may be particularly important in diabetic patients with inadequate glucagon reserve and in pancreatectomized patients since catecholamines may be the major factors in stimulating glucose release from the liver in response to hypoglycemia. Beta$_1$-receptor–selective drugs may be less prone to inhibit recovery from hypoglycemia. Beta-receptor antagonists are much safer in those type 2 diabetic patients who do not have hypoglycemic episodes.

The chronic use of β-adrenoceptor antagonists has been associated with increased plasma concentrations of very-low-density lipoproteins (VLDL) and decreased concentrations of HDL cholesterol. Both of these changes are potentially unfavorable in terms of risk of cardiovascular disease. Although low-density lipoprotein (LDL) concentrations generally do not change, there is a variable decline in the HDL cholesterol/LDL cholesterol ratio that may increase the risk of coronary artery disease. These changes tend to occur with both selective and nonselective β blockers, though they may be less likely to occur with β blockers possessing intrinsic sympathomimetic activity (partial agonists). The mechanisms by which β-receptor antagonists cause these changes are not understood, though changes in sensitivity to insulin action may contribute.

E. Effects Not Related to Beta-Blockade

Partial β-agonist activity was significant in the first β-blocking drug synthesized, dichloroisoproterenol. It has been suggested that retention of some intrinsic sympathomimetic activity is desirable to prevent untoward effects such as precipitation of asthma or excessive bradycardia. Pindolol and other partial agonists are noted in Table 10–2. It is not yet clear to what extent partial agonism is clinically valuable. Furthermore, these drugs may not be as effective as the pure antagonists in secondary prevention of myocardial infarction. However, they may be useful in patients who develop symptomatic bradycardia or bronchoconstriction in response to pure antagonist β-adrenoceptor drugs, but only if they are strongly indicated for a particular clinical indication.

The Treatment of Glaucoma

Glaucoma is a major cause of blindness and of great pharmacologic interest because the chronic form often responds to drug therapy. The primary manifestation is increased intraocular pressure not initially associated with symptoms. Without treatment, increased intraocular pressure results in damage to the retina and optic nerve, with restriction of visual fields and, eventually, blindness. Intraocular pressure is easily measured as part of the routine ophthalmologic examination. Two major types of glaucoma are recognized: open-angle and closed-angle (also called narrow-angle). The closed-angle form is associated with a shallow anterior chamber, in which a dilated iris can occlude the outflow drainage pathway at the angle between the cornea and the ciliary body (see Figure 6–9). This form is associated with acute and painful increases of pressure, which must be controlled on an emergency basis with drugs or prevented by surgical removal of part of the iris (iridectomy). The open-angle form of glaucoma is a chronic condition, and treatment is largely pharmacologic. Because intraocular pressure is a function of the balance between fluid input and drainage out of the globe, the strategies for the treatment of open-angle glaucoma fall into two classes: reduction of aqueous humor secretion and enhancement of aqueous outflow. Five general groups of drugs—cholinomimetics, α agonists, β blockers, prostaglandin $F_{2\alpha}$ analogs, and diuretics—have been found to be useful in reducing intraocular pressure and can be related to these strategies as shown in Table 10–3. Of the five drug groups listed in Table 10–3, the prostaglandin analogs and the β blockers are the most popular. This popularity results from convenience (once- or twice-daily dosing) and relative lack of adverse effects (except, in the case of β blockers, in patients with asthma or cardiac pacemaker or conduction pathway disease). Other drugs that have been reported to reduce intraocular pressure include prostaglandin E_2 and marijuana. The use of drugs in acute closed-angle glaucoma is limited to cholinomimetics, acetazolamide, and osmotic agents preceding surgery. The onset of action of the other agents is too slow in this situation.

Local anesthetic action, also known as "membrane-stabilizing" action, is a prominent effect of several β blockers (Table 10–2). This action is the result of typical local anesthetic blockade of sodium channels (see Chapter 26) and can be demonstrated experimentally in isolated neurons, heart muscle, and skeletal muscle membrane. However, it is unlikely that this effect is important after systemic administration of these drugs, since the concentration in plasma usually achieved by these routes is too low for the anesthetic effects to be evident. The membrane-stabilizing β blockers are not used topically on the eye, because local anesthesia of the cornea would be highly undesirable. Sotalol

TABLE 10–3 Drugs used in open-angle glaucoma.

	Mechanism	Methods of Administration
Cholinomimetics		
Pilocarpine, carbachol, physostigmine, echothiophate, demecarium	Ciliary muscle contraction, opening of trabecular meshwork; increased outflow	Topical drops or gel; plastic film slow-release insert
Alpha agonists		
Nonselective	Increased outflow	Topical drops
Epinephrine, dipivefrin		
Alpha$_2$-selective	Decreased aqueous secretion	
Apraclonidine		Topical, postlaser only
Brimonidine		Topical
Beta blockers		
Timolol, betaxolol, carteolol, levobunolol, metipranolol	Decreased aqueous secretion from the ciliary epithelium	Topical drops
Carbonic anhydrase inhibitors		
Dorzolamide, brinzolamide	Decreased aqueous secretion due to lack of HCO_3^-	Topical
Acetazolamide, dichlorphenamide, methazolamide		Oral
Prostaglandins		
Latanoprost, bimatoprost, travoprost, unoprostone	Increased outflow	Topical

is a nonselective β-receptor antagonist that lacks local anesthetic action but has marked class III antiarrhythmic effects, reflecting potassium channel blockade (see Chapter 14).

SPECIFIC AGENTS (SEE TABLE 10–2)

Propranolol is the prototypical β-blocking drug. As noted above, it has low and dose-dependent bioavailability. A long-acting form of propranolol is available; prolonged absorption of the drug may occur over a 24-hour period. The drug has negligible effects at α and muscarinic receptors; however, it may block some serotonin receptors in the brain, though the clinical significance is unclear. It has no detectable partial agonist action at β receptors.

Metoprolol, atenolol, and several other drugs (Table 10–2) are members of the β$_1$-selective group. These agents may be safer in patients who experience bronchoconstriction in response to propranolol. Since their β$_1$ selectivity is rather modest, they should be used with great caution, if at all, in patients with a history of asthma. However, in selected patients with COPD the benefits may exceed the risks, eg, in patients with myocardial infarction. Beta$_1$-selective antagonists may be preferable in patients with diabetes or peripheral vascular disease when therapy with a β blocker is required, since β$_2$ receptors are probably important in liver (recovery from hypoglycemia) and blood vessels (vasodilation).

Nebivolol is the most highly selective β$_1$-adrenergic receptor blocker, though some of its metabolites do not have this level of specificity. Nebivolol has the additional quality of eliciting vasodilation. This is due to an action of the drug on endothelial nitric

oxide production. Nebivolol may increase insulin sensitivity and does not adversely affect lipid profile.

Nadolol is noteworthy for its very long duration of action; its spectrum of action is similar to that of timolol. **Timolol** is a nonselective agent with no local anesthetic activity. It has excellent ocular hypotensive effects when administered topically in the eye. **Levobunolol** (nonselective) and **betaxolol** (β$_1$-selective) are also used for topical ophthalmic application in glaucoma; the latter drug may be less likely to induce bronchoconstriction than nonselective antagonists. **Carteolol** is a nonselective β-receptor antagonist.

Pindolol, acebutolol, carteolol, bopindolol,[*] **oxprenolol,**[*] **celiprolol,**[*] and **penbutolol** are of interest because they have partial β-agonist activity. They are effective in the major cardiovascular applications of the β-blocking group (hypertension and angina). Although these partial agonists may be less likely to cause bradycardia and abnormalities in plasma lipids than are antagonists, the overall clinical significance of intrinsic sympathomimetic activity remains uncertain. Pindolol, perhaps as a result of actions on serotonin signaling, may potentiate the action of traditional antidepressant medications. Celiprolol is a β$_1$-selective antagonist with a modest capacity to activate β$_2$ receptors.

There is limited evidence suggesting that celiprolol may have less adverse bronchoconstrictor effect in asthma and may even promote bronchodilation. Acebutolol is also a β$_1$-selective antagonist.

[*]Not available in the USA

Labetalol is a reversible adrenoceptor antagonist available as a racemic mixture of two pairs of chiral isomers (the molecule has two centers of asymmetry). The (S,S)- and (R,S)-isomers are nearly inactive, the (S,R)-isomer is a potent α blocker, and the (R,R)-isomer is a potent β blocker. Labetalol's affinity for α receptors is less than that of phentolamine, but labetalol is α_1-selective. Its β-blocking potency is somewhat lower than that of propranolol. Hypotension induced by labetalol is accompanied by less tachycardia than occurs with phentolamine and similar α blockers.

Carvedilol, medroxalol,[*] and **bucindolol**[*] are nonselective β-receptor antagonists with some capacity to block α_1-adrenergic receptors. Carvedilol antagonizes the actions of catecholamines more potently at β receptors than at α_1 receptors. The drug has a half-life of 6–8 hours. It is extensively metabolized in the liver, and stereoselective metabolism of its two isomers is observed. Since metabolism of (R)-carvedilol is influenced by polymorphisms in CYP2D6 activity and by drugs that inhibit this enzyme's activity (such as quinidine and fluoxetine, see Chapter 4), drug interactions may occur. Carvedilol also appears to attenuate oxygen free radical–initiated lipid peroxidation and to inhibit vascular smooth muscle mitogenesis independently of adrenoceptor blockade. These effects may contribute to the clinical benefits of the drug in chronic heart failure (see Chapter 13).

Esmolol is an ultra-short–acting β_1-selective adrenoceptor antagonist. The structure of esmolol contains an ester linkage; esterases in red blood cells rapidly metabolize esmolol to a metabolite that has a low affinity for β receptors. Consequently, esmolol has a short half-life (about 10 minutes). Therefore, during continuous infusions of esmolol, steady-state concentrations are achieved quickly, and the therapeutic actions of the drug are terminated rapidly when its infusion is discontinued. Esmolol may be safer to use than longer-acting antagonists in critically ill patients who require a β-adrenoceptor antagonist. Esmolol is useful in controlling supraventricular arrhythmias, arrhythmias associated with thyrotoxicosis, perioperative hypertension, and myocardial ischemia in acutely ill patients.

Butoxamine is a research drug selective for β_2 receptors. Selective β_2-blocking drugs have not been actively sought because there is no obvious clinical application for them; none is available for clinical use.

■ CLINICAL PHARMACOLOGY OF THE BETA-RECEPTOR–BLOCKING DRUGS

Hypertension

The β-adrenoceptor–blocking drugs have proved to be effective and well tolerated in hypertension. Although many hypertensive patients respond to a β blocker used alone, the drug is often used with either a diuretic or a vasodilator. In spite of the short half-life of many β antagonists, these drugs may be administered once or twice daily and still have an adequate therapeutic effect. Labetalol, a competitive α and β antagonist, is effective in hypertension, though its ultimate role is yet to be determined. Use of these agents is discussed in greater detail in Chapter 11. There is some evidence that drugs in this class may be less effective in the elderly and in individuals of African ancestry. However, these differences are relatively small and may not apply to an individual patient. Indeed, since effects on blood pressure are easily measured, the therapeutic outcome for this indication can be readily detected in any patient.

Ischemic Heart Disease

Beta-adrenoceptor blockers reduce the frequency of anginal episodes and improve exercise tolerance in many patients with angina (see Chapter 12). These actions relate to the blockade of cardiac β receptors, resulting in decreased cardiac work and reduction in oxygen demand. Slowing and regularization of the heart rate may contribute to clinical benefits (Figure 10–7). Multiple large-scale prospective studies indicate that the long-term use of **timolol, propranolol,** or **metoprolol** in patients who have had a myocardial infarction prolongs survival (Figure 10–8). At the present time, data are less compelling for the use of other than the three mentioned β-adrenoceptor antagonists for this indication. It is significant that surveys in many populations have indicated that β-receptor antagonists are underused, leading to unnecessary morbidity and mortality. In addition, β-adrenoceptor antagonists are strongly indicated in the acute phase of a myocardial infarction. In this setting, relative contraindications include bradycardia, hypotension, moderate or severe left ventricular failure, shock, heart block, and active airways disease. It has been suggested that certain polymorphisms in β_2-adrenoceptor genes may influence survival among patients receiving antagonists after acute coronary syndromes.

Cardiac Arrhythmias

Beta antagonists are often effective in the treatment of both supraventricular and ventricular arrhythmias (see Chapter 14). It has been suggested that the improved survival following myocardial infarction in patients using β antagonists (Figure 10–8) is due to suppression of arrhythmias, but this has not been proved. By increasing the atrioventricular nodal refractory period, β antagonists slow ventricular response rates in atrial flutter and fibrillation. These drugs can also reduce ventricular ectopic beats, particularly if the ectopic activity has been precipitated by catecholamines. Sotalol has antiarrhythmic effects involving ion channel blockade in addition to its β-blocking action; these are discussed in Chapter 14.

Heart Failure

Clinical trials have demonstrated that at least three β antagonists—metoprolol, bisoprolol, and carvedilol—are effective in reducing mortality in selected patients with chronic heart failure. Although administration of these drugs may worsen acute congestive heart failure, cautious long-term use with gradual dose increments in patients who tolerate them may prolong life. Although mechanisms are uncertain, there appear to be beneficial effects on

---

[*]Not available in the USA.

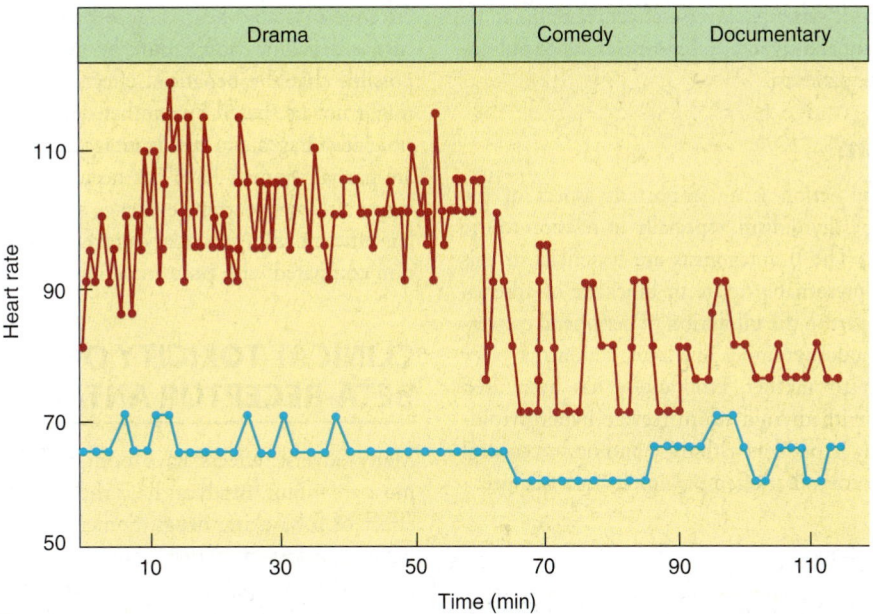

FIGURE 10–7 Heart rate in a patient with ischemic heart disease measured by telemetry while watching television. Measurements were begun 1 hour after receiving placebo (*upper line, red*) or 40 mg of oxprenolol (*lower line, blue*), a nonselective β antagonist with partial agonist activity. Not only was the heart rate decreased by the drug under the conditions of this experiment, it also varied much less in response to stimuli. (Modified and reproduced, with permission, from Taylor SH: Oxprenolol in clinical practice. Am J Cardiol 1983;52:34D.)

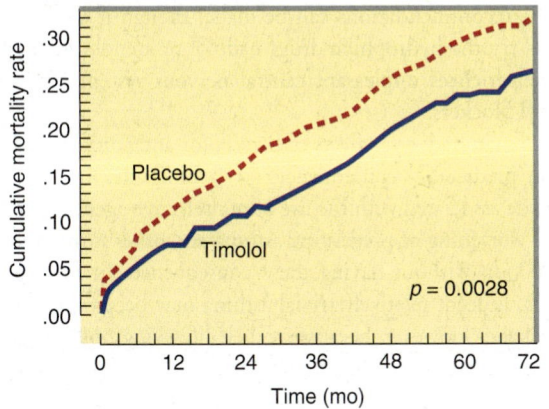

FIGURE 10–8 Effects of β-blocker therapy on life-table cumulated rates of mortality from all causes over 6 years among 1884 patients surviving myocardial infarctions. Patients were randomly assigned to treatment with placebo (*dashed red line*) or timolol (*solid blue line*). (Reproduced, with permission, from Pederson TR: Six-year follow-up of the Norwegian multicenter study on timolol after acute myocardial infarction. N Engl J Med 1985;313:1055.)

myocardial remodeling and in decreasing the risk of sudden death (see Chapter 13).

Other Cardiovascular Disorders

Beta-receptor antagonists have been found to increase stroke volume in some patients with obstructive cardiomyopathy. This beneficial effect is thought to result from the slowing of ventricular ejection and decreased outflow resistance. Beta antagonists are useful in dissecting aortic aneurysm to decrease the rate of development of systolic pressure. Beta antagonists are also useful in selected at-risk patients in the prevention of adverse cardiovascular outcomes resulting from noncardiac surgery.

Glaucoma (See Box: The Treatment of Glaucoma)

Systemic administration of β-blocking drugs for other indications was found serendipitously to reduce intraocular pressure in patients with glaucoma. Subsequently, it was found that topical administration also reduces intraocular pressure. The mechanism appears to involve reduced production of aqueous humor by the ciliary body, which is physiologically activated by cAMP. Timolol and related β antagonists are suitable for local use in the eye because they lack local anesthetic properties. Beta antagonists appear to have an efficacy comparable to that of epinephrine or pilocarpine in open-angle glaucoma and are far better tolerated by most patients. While the maximal daily dose applied locally (1 mg) is small compared with the systemic doses commonly used in the treatment of hypertension or angina (10–60 mg), sufficient timolol may be absorbed from the eye to cause serious adverse effects on the heart and airways in susceptible individuals. Topical timolol may interact with orally administered verapamil and increase the risk of heart block.

Betaxolol, carteolol, levobunolol, and metipranolol are also approved for the treatment of glaucoma. Betaxolol has the potential advantage of being β_1-selective; to what extent this potential advantage might diminish systemic adverse effects remains to be determined. The drug apparently has caused worsening of pulmonary symptoms in some patients.

Hyperthyroidism

Excessive catecholamine action is an important aspect of the pathophysiology of hyperthyroidism, especially in relation to the heart (see Chapter 38). The β antagonists are beneficial in this condition. The effects presumably relate to blockade of adrenoceptors and perhaps in part to the inhibition of peripheral conversion of thyroxine to triiodothyronine. The latter action may vary from one β antagonist to another. Propranolol has been used extensively in patients with thyroid storm (severe hyperthyroidism); it is used cautiously in patients with this condition to control supraventricular tachycardias that often precipitate heart failure.

Neurologic Diseases

Propranolol reduces the frequency and intensity of **migraine headache**. Other β-receptor antagonists with preventive efficacy include metoprolol and probably also atenolol, timolol, and nadolol. The mechanism is not known. Since sympathetic activity may enhance skeletal muscle tremor, it is not surprising that β antagonists have been found to reduce certain **tremors** (see Chapter 28). The somatic manifestations of anxiety may respond dramatically to low doses of propranolol, particularly when taken prophylactically. For example, benefit has been found in musicians with **performance anxiety ("stage fright")**. Propranolol may contribute to the symptomatic treatment of alcohol withdrawal in some patients.

Miscellaneous

Beta-receptor antagonists have been found to diminish portal vein pressure in patients with cirrhosis. There is evidence that both propranolol and nadolol decrease the incidence of the first episode of bleeding from esophageal varices and decrease the mortality rate associated with bleeding in patients with cirrhosis. Nadolol in combination with isosorbide mononitrate appears to be more efficacious than sclerotherapy in preventing rebleeding in patients who have previously bled from esophageal varices. Variceal band ligation in combination with a β antagonist may be more efficacious.

CHOICE OF A BETA-ADRENOCEPTOR ANTAGONIST DRUG

Propranolol is the standard against which newer β antagonists developed for systemic use have been compared. In many years of very wide use, propranolol has been found to be a safe and effective drug for many indications. Since it is possible that some actions of a β-receptor antagonist may relate to some other effect of the drug, these drugs should not be considered interchangeable for all applications. For example, only β antagonists known to be effective in stable heart failure or in prophylactic therapy after myocardial infarction should be used for those indications. It is possible that the beneficial effects of one drug in these settings might not be shared by another drug in the same class. The possible advantages and disadvantages of β-receptor antagonists that are partial agonists have not been clearly defined in clinical settings, although current evidence suggests that they are probably less efficacious in secondary prevention after a myocardial infarction compared with pure antagonists.

CLINICAL TOXICITY OF THE BETA-RECEPTOR ANTAGONIST DRUGS

Many adverse effects have been reported for propranolol but most are minor. Bradycardia is the most common adverse cardiac effect of β-blocking drugs. Sometimes patients note coolness of hands and feet in winter. Central nervous system effects include mild sedation, vivid dreams, and rarely, depression. Discontinuing the use of β blockers in any patient who develops psychiatric depression should be seriously considered if clinically feasible. It has been claimed that β-receptor antagonist drugs with low lipid solubility are associated with a lower incidence of central nervous system adverse effects than compounds with higher lipid solubility (Table 10–2). Further studies designed to compare the central nervous system adverse effects of various drugs are required before specific recommendations can be made, though it seems reasonable to try the hydrophilic drugs nadolol or atenolol in a patient who experiences unpleasant central nervous system effects with other β blockers.

The major adverse effects of β-receptor antagonist drugs relate to the predictable consequences of β blockade. Beta$_2$-receptor blockade associated with the use of nonselective agents commonly causes worsening of preexisting asthma and other forms of airway obstruction without having these consequences in normal individuals. Indeed, relatively trivial asthma may become severe after β blockade. However, because of their lifesaving potential in cardiovascular disease, strong consideration should be given to individualized therapeutic trials in some classes of patients, eg, those with chronic obstructive pulmonary disease who have appropriate indications for β blockers. While β$_1$-selective drugs may have less effect on airways than nonselective β antagonists, they must be used very cautiously in patients with reactive airway disease. Beta$_1$-selective antagonists are generally well tolerated in patients with mild to moderate peripheral vascular disease, but caution is required in patients with severe peripheral vascular disease or vasospastic disorders.

Beta-receptor blockade depresses myocardial contractility and excitability. In patients with abnormal myocardial function, cardiac output may be dependent on sympathetic drive. If this stimulus is removed by β blockade, cardiac decompensation may ensue. Thus, caution must be exercised in starting a β-receptor antagonist in patients with compensated heart failure even though long-term use of these drugs in these patients may prolong life. A life-threatening adverse cardiac effect of a β antagonist may be overcome directly with isoproterenol or with glucagon (glucagon stimulates the heart via glucagon receptors, which are not blocked by β antagonists), but neither of these methods is without hazard. A very small dose of a β antagonist (eg, 10 mg of propranolol) may provoke severe cardiac failure in a susceptible individual. Beta blockers may interact with the calcium antagonist verapamil; severe hypotension, bradycardia, heart failure, and cardiac conduction abnormalities have all been described. These adverse effects may even arise in susceptible patients taking a topical (ophthalmic) β blocker and oral verapamil.

Patients with ischemic heart disease or renovascular hypertension may be at increased risk if β blockade is suddenly interrupted. The mechanism of this effect might involve up-regulation of the number of β receptors. Until better evidence is available regarding the magnitude of the risk, prudence dictates the gradual tapering rather than abrupt cessation of dosage when these drugs are discontinued, especially drugs with short half-lives, such as propranolol and metoprolol.

The incidence of hypoglycemic episodes exacerbated by β-blocking agents in diabetics is unknown. Nevertheless, it is inadvisable to use β antagonists in insulin-dependent diabetic patients who are subject to frequent hypoglycemic reactions if alternative therapies are available. Beta$_1$-selective antagonists offer some advantage in these patients, since the rate of recovery from hypoglycemia may be faster compared with that in diabetics receiving nonselective β-adrenoceptor antagonists. There is considerable potential benefit from these drugs in diabetics after a myocardial infarction, so the balance of risk versus benefit must be evaluated in individual patients.

SUMMARY Sympathetic Antagonists

Subclass	Mechanism of Action	Effects	Clinical Applications	Pharmacokinetics, Toxicities, Interactions
ALPHA-ADRENOCEPTOR ANTAGONISTS				
• Phenoxybenzamine	Irreversibly blocks α_1 and α_2• indirect baroreflex activation	Lowers blood pressure (BP) • heart rate (HR) rises due to baroreflex activation	Pheochromocytoma • high catecholamine states	Irreversible blocker • duration > 1 day • *Toxicity:* Orthostatic hypotension • tachycardia • myocardial ischemia
• Phentolamine	Reversibly blocks α_1 and α_2	Blocks α-mediated vasoconstriction, lowers BP, increases HR (baroreflex)	Pheochromocytoma	Half-life ~45 min after IV injection
• Prazosin • Doxazosin • Terazosin	Block α_1, but not α_2	Lower BP	Hypertension • benign prostatic hyperplasia	Larger depressor effect with first dose may cause orthostatic hypotension
• Tamsulosin	Tamsulosin is slightly selective for α_{1A}	α_{1A} Blockade may relax prostatic smooth muscles more than vascular smooth muscle	Benign prostatic hyperplasia	Orthostatic hypotension may be less common with this subtype
• Yohimbine	Blocks α_2• elicits increased central sympathetic activity • increased norepinephrine release	Raises BP and HR	Male erectile dysfunction • hypotension	May cause anxiety • excess pressor effect if norepinephrine transporter is blocked
• Labetalol (see carvedilol section below)	$\beta > \alpha_1$ block	Lowers BP with limited HR increase	Hypertension	Oral, parenteral • *Toxicity:* Less tachycardia than other α_1 agents
BETA-ADRENOCEPTOR ANTAGONISTS				
• Propranolol • Nadolol • Timolol	Block β_1 and β_2	Lower HR and BP • reduce renin	Hypertension • angina pectoris • arrhythmias • migraine • hyperthyroidism	Oral, parenteral • *Toxicity:* Bradycardia • worsened asthma • fatigue • vivid dreams • cold hands
• Metoprolol • Atenolol • Alprenolol • Betaxolol • Nebivolol	Block $\beta_1 > \beta_2$	Lower HR and BP • reduce renin • may be safer in asthma	Angina pectoris • hypertension • arrhythmias	*Toxicity:* Bradycardia • fatigue • vivid dreams • cold hands

(continued)

Subclass	Mechanism of Action	Effects	Clinical Applications	Pharmacokinetics, Toxicities, Interactions
• Butoxamine[1]	Blocks $\beta_2 > \beta_1$	Increases peripheral resistance	No clinical indication	*Toxicity:* Asthma provocation
• Pindolol • Acebutolol • Carteolol • Bopindolol[1] • Oxprenolol[1] • Celiprolol[1] • Penbutolol	β_1, β_2, with intrinsic sympathomimetic (partial agonist) effect	Lowers BP • modestly lower HR	Hypertension • arrhythmias • migraine • may avoid worsening of bradycardia	Oral • *Toxicity:* Fatigue • vivid dreams • cold hands
• Carvedilol • Medroxalol[1] • Bucindolol[1] (see labetalol above)	$\beta > \alpha_1$ block		Heart failure	Oral, long half-life • *Toxicity:* Fatigue
• Esmolol	$\beta_1 > \beta_2$	Very brief cardiac β blockade	Rapid control of BP and arrhythmias, thyrotoxicosis and myocardial ischemia intraoperatively	Parenteral only • half-life ~ 10 min • *Toxicity:* Bradycardia • hypotension
TYROSINE HYDROXYLASE INHIBITOR				
• Metyrosine	Blocks tyrosine hydroxylase • reduces synthesis of dopamine, norepinephrine, and epinephrine	Lowers BP • in central nervous system may elicit extrapyramidal effects (due to low dopamine)	Pheochromocytoma	*Toxicity:* Extrapyramidal symptoms • orthostatic hypotension • crystalluria

[1]Not available in the USA.

PREPARATIONS AVAILABLE*

ALPHA BLOCKERS

Alfuzosin (Uroxatral)
   Oral: 10 mg tablets (extended release)
Doxazosin (generic, Cardura)
   Oral: 1, 2, 4, 8 mg tablets; 4, 8 mg extended-release tablets
Phenoxybenzamine (Dibenzyline)
   Oral: 10 mg capsules
Phentolamine (generic)
   Parenteral: 5 mg/vial for injection
Prazosin (generic, Minipress)
   Oral: 1, 2, 5 mg capsules
Silodosin (Rapaflow)
   Oral: 4, 8 mg capsules
Tamsulosin (Flomax)
   Oral: 0.4 mg capsule
Terazosin (generic, Hytrin)
   Oral: 1, 2, 5, 10 mg tablets, capsules
Tolazoline (Priscoline)
   Parenteral: 25 mg/mL for injection

BETA BLOCKERS

Acebutolol (generic, Sectral)
   Oral: 200, 400 mg capsules
Atenolol (generic, Tenormin)
   Oral: 25, 50, 100 mg tablets
   Parenteral: 0.5 mg/mL for IV injection
Betaxolol
   Oral (Kerlone): 10, 20 mg tablets
   Ophthalmic (generic, Betoptic): 0.25%, 0.5% drops
Bisoprolol (generic, Zebeta)
   Oral: 5, 10 mg tablets
Carteolol
   Oral (Cartrol): 2.5, 5 mg tablets
   Ophthalmic (generic, Ocupress): 1% drops
Carvedilol (Coreg)
   Oral: 3.125, 6.25, 12.5, 25 mg tablets; 10, 20, 40, 80 mg extended-release capsules
Esmolol (Brevibloc)
   Parenteral: 10 mg/mL for IV injection; 250 mg/mL for IV infusion

*In the USA

Labetalol (generic, Normodyne, Trandate)
Oral: 100, 200, 300 mg tablets
Parenteral: 5 mg/mL for injection

Levobunolol (Betagan Liquifilm, others)
Ophthalmic: 0.25, 0.5% drops

Metipranolol (Optipranolol)
Ophthalmic: 0.3% drops

Metoprolol (generic, Lopressor, Toprol)
Oral: 50, 100 mg tablets
Oral sustained release: 25, 50, 100, 200 mg tablets
Parenteral: 1 mg/mL for injection

Nadolol (generic, Corgard)
Oral: 20, 40, 80, 120, 160 mg tablets

Nebivolol (Bystolic)
Oral: 2.5, 5, 10 mg tablets

Penbutolol (Levatol)
Oral: 20 mg tablets

Pindolol (generic, Visken)
Oral: 5, 10 mg tablets

Propranolol (generic, Inderal)
Oral: 10, 20, 40, 60, 80, 90 mg tablets; 4, 8, 80 mg/mL solutions
Oral sustained release: 60, 80, 120, 160 mg capsules
Parenteral: 1 mg/mL for injection

Sotalol (generic, Betapace)
Oral: 80, 120, 160, 240 mg tablets

Timolol
Oral (generic, Blocadren): 5, 10, 20 mg tablets
Ophthalmic (generic, Timoptic): 0.25, 0.5% drops, gel

TYROSINE HYDROXYLASE INHIBITOR

Metyrosine (Demser)
Oral: 250 mg capsules

REFERENCES

Ambrosio G et al: β-Blockade with nebivolol for prevention of acute ischaemic events in elderly patients with heart failure. Heart 2011;97:209.

Bell CM et al. Association between tamsulosin and serious ophthalmic adverse events in older men following cataract surgery. JAMA 2009;301:1991.

Blakely RD, DeFelice LJ: All aglow about presynaptic receptor regulation of neurotransmitter transporters. Mol Pharmacol 2007;71:1206.

Blaufarb I, Pfeifer TM, Frishman WH: Beta-blockers: Drug interactions of clinical significance. Drug Saf 1995;13:359.

Boyer TD: Primary prophylaxis for variceal bleeding: Are we there yet? Gastroenterology 2005;128:1120.

Berruezo A, Brugada J: Beta blockers: Is the reduction of sudden death related to pure electrophysiologic effects? Cardiovasc Drug Ther 2008;22:163.

Brantigan CO, Brantigan TA, Joseph N: Effect of beta blockade and beta stimulation on stage fright. Am J Med 1982;72:88.

Bristow M: Antiadrenergic therapy of chronic heart failure: Surprises and new opportunities. Circulation 2003;107:1100.

Cheng J, Kamiya K, Kodama I: Carvedilol: Molecular and cellular basis for its multifaceted therapeutic potential. Cardiovasc Drug Rev 2001;19:152.

Cleland JG: Beta-blockers for heart failure: Why, which, when, and where. Med Clin North Am 2003;87:339.

Eisenhofer G et al: Current progress and future challenges in the biochemical diagnosis and treatment of pheochromocytomas and paragangliomas. Horm Metab Res 2008;40:329.

Ellison KE, Gandhi G: Optimising the use of beta-adrenoceptor antagonists in coronary artery disease. Drugs 2005;65:787.

Fitzgerald JD: Do partial agonist beta-blockers have improved clinical utility? Cardiovasc Drugs Ther 1993;7:303.

Freemantle N et al: Beta blockade after myocardial infarction: Systematic review and meta regression analysis. BMJ 1999;318:1730.

Kamp O et al: Nebivolol: Haemodynamic effects and clinical significance of combined β-blockade and nitric oxide release. Drugs 2010;70:41.

Kaplan SA et al: Combination therapy using oral β-blockers and intracavernosal injection in men with erectile dysfunction. Urology 1998;52:739.

Kyprianou N: Doxazosin and terazosin suppress prostate growth by inducing apoptosis: Clinical significance. J Urol 2003;169:1520.

Lanfear et al: β₂-Adrenergic receptor genotype and survival among patients receiving β-blocker therapy after an acute coronary syndrome. JAMA 2005;294:1526.

Lepor H et al: The efficacy of terazosin, finasteride, or both in benign prostate hyperplasia. N Engl J Med 1996;335:533.

Maggio PM, Taheri PA: Perioperative issues: Myocardial ischemia and protection–beta-blockade. Surg Clin North Am 2005;85:1091.

Marquis RE, Whitson JT: Management of glaucoma: Focus on pharmacological therapy. Drugs Aging 2005;22:1.

McVary KT: Alfuzosin for symptomatic benign prostatic hyperplasia: Long-term experience. J Urol 2006;175:35.

Nickerson M: The pharmacology of adrenergic blockade. Pharmacol Rev 1949;1:27.

Nickel JC, Sander S, Moon TD: A meta-analysis of the vascular-related safety profile and efficacy of alpha-adrenergic blockers for symptoms related to benign prostatic hyperplasia. Int J Clin Pract 2008;62:1547.

Perez DM: Structure-function of alpha₁-adrenergic receptors. Biochem Pharmacol 2007;73:1051.

Pojoga L et al: Beta-2 adrenergic receptor diplotype defines a subset of salt-sensitive hypertension. Hypertension 2006;48:892.

Roehrborn CG, Schwinn DA: Alpha₁-adrenergic receptors and their inhibitors in lower urinary tract symptoms and benign prostatic hyperplasia. J Urol 2004;171:1029.

Schwinn DA, Roehrborn CG. Alpha1-adrenoceptor subtypes and lower urinary tract symptoms. Int J Urol 2008;15:193.

Tank J et al: Yohimbine attenuates baroreflex-mediated bradycardia in humans. Hypertension 2007:50:899.

Wespes E: Intracavernous injection as an option for aging men with erectile dysfunction. Aging Male 2002;5:177.

Wilt TJ, MacDonald R, Rutks I: Tamsulosin for benign prostatic hyperplasia. Cochrane Database Syst Rev 2003;(1):CD002081.

CASE STUDY ANSWER

The patient had a pheochromocytoma. The tumor secretes catecholamines, especially norepinephrine and epinephrine, resulting in increases in blood pressure (via α_1 receptors) and heart rate (via β_1 receptors). The pheochromocytoma was in the left adrenal gland and was identified by MIBG imaging, which labels tissues that have norepinephrine transporters on their cell surface (see text). In addition, she had elevated plasma and urinary norepinephrine, epinephrine, and their metabolites, normetanephrine and metanephrine. The catecholamines made the blood pressure surge and the heart rate increase, producing a typical episode during her examination, perhaps set off in this case by external pressure as the physician palpated the abdomen. Her profuse sweating was typical and partly due to α_1 receptors, though the large magnitude of drenching sweats in pheochromocytoma has never been fully explained. Treatment would consist of preoperative control of blood pressure and normalization of blood volume if reduced, followed by surgical resection of the tumor. Control of blood pressure extremes might be necessary during surgery, probably with nitroprusside.

SECTION III CARDIOVASCULAR-RENAL DRUGS

CHAPTER

11

Antihypertensive Agents

Neal L. Benowitz, MD

CASE STUDY

A 35-year-old man presents with a blood pressure of 150/95 mm Hg. He has been generally healthy, is sedentary, drinks several cocktails per day, and does not smoke cigarettes. He has a family history of hypertension, and his father died of a myocardial infarction at age 55. Physical examination is remarkable only for moderate obesity. Total cholesterol is 220, and high-density lipoprotein (HDL) cholesterol level is 40 mg/dL. Fasting glucose is 105 mg/dL. Chest x-ray is normal. Electrocardiogram shows left ventricular enlargement. How would you treat this patient?

Hypertension is the most common cardiovascular disease. In a survey carried out in 2007/2008, hypertension was found in 29% of American adults. The prevalence varies with age, race, education, and many other variables. According to some studies, 60–80% of both men and women will develop hypertension by age 80. Sustained arterial hypertension damages blood vessels in kidney, heart, and brain and leads to an increased incidence of renal failure, coronary disease, heart failure, stroke, and dementia. Effective pharmacologic lowering of blood pressure has been shown to prevent damage to blood vessels and to substantially reduce morbidity and mortality rates. Unfortunately, several surveys indicate that only one third to one half of Americans with hypertension have adequate blood pressure control. Many effective drugs are available. Knowledge of their antihypertensive mechanisms and sites of action allows accurate prediction of efficacy and toxicity. As a result, rational use of these agents, alone or in combination, can lower blood pressure with minimal risk of serious toxicity in most patients.

HYPERTENSION & REGULATION OF BLOOD PRESSURE

Diagnosis

The diagnosis of hypertension is based on repeated, reproducible measurements of elevated blood pressure (Table 11–1). The diagnosis serves primarily as a prediction of consequences for the patient; it seldom includes a statement about the cause of hypertension.

Epidemiologic studies indicate that the risks of damage to kidney, heart, and brain are directly related to the extent of blood pressure elevation. Even mild hypertension (blood pressure

TABLE 11–1 Classification of hypertension on the basis of blood pressure.

Systolic/Diastolic Pressure (mm Hg)	Category
< 120/80	Normal
120–135/80–89	Prehypertension
≥ 140/90	Hypertension
140–159/90–99	Stage 1
≥ 160/100	Stage 2

From the Joint National Committee on prevention, detection, evaluation, and treatment of high blood pressure. JAMA 2003;289:2560.

140/90 mm Hg) increases the risk of eventual end-organ damage. Starting at 115/75 mm Hg, cardiovascular disease risk doubles with each increment of 20/10 mm Hg throughout the blood pressure range. Both systolic hypertension and diastolic hypertension are associated with end-organ damage; so-called isolated systolic hypertension is not benign. The risks—and therefore the urgency of instituting therapy—increase in proportion to the magnitude of blood pressure elevation. The risk of end-organ damage at any level of blood pressure or age is greater in African Americans and relatively less in premenopausal women than in men. Other positive risk factors include smoking; metabolic syndrome, including obesity, dyslipidemia, and diabetes; manifestations of end-organ damage at the time of diagnosis; and a family history of cardiovascular disease.

It should be noted that the diagnosis of hypertension depends on measurement of blood pressure and not on symptoms reported by the patient. In fact, hypertension is usually asymptomatic until overt end-organ damage is imminent or has already occurred.

Etiology of Hypertension

A specific cause of hypertension can be established in only 10–15% of patients. Patients in whom no specific cause of hypertension can be found are said to have *essential* or *primary hypertension*. Patients with a specific etiology are said to have *secondary hypertension*. It is important to consider specific causes in each case, however, because some of them are amenable to definitive surgical treatment: renal artery constriction, coarctation of the aorta, pheochromocytoma, Cushing's disease, and primary aldosteronism.

In most cases, elevated blood pressure is associated with an overall increase in resistance to flow of blood through arterioles, whereas cardiac output is usually normal. Meticulous investigation of autonomic nervous system function, baroreceptor reflexes, the renin-angiotensin-aldosterone system, and the kidney has failed to identify a single abnormality as the cause of increased peripheral vascular resistance in essential hypertension. It appears, therefore, that elevated blood pressure is usually caused by a combination of several (multifactorial) abnormalities. Epidemiologic evidence points to genetic factors, psychological stress, and environmental and dietary factors (increased salt and decreased potassium or calcium intake) as

contributing to the development of hypertension. Increase in blood pressure with aging does not occur in populations with low daily sodium intake. Patients with labile hypertension appear more likely than normal controls to have blood pressure elevations after salt loading.

The heritability of essential hypertension is estimated to be about 30%. Mutations in several genes have been linked to various rare causes of hypertension. Functional variations of the genes for angiotensinogen, angiotensin-converting enzyme (ACE), the β_2 adrenoceptor, and α adducin (a cytoskeletal protein) appear to contribute to some cases of essential hypertension.

Normal Regulation of Blood Pressure

According to the hydraulic equation, arterial blood pressure (BP) is directly proportionate to the product of the blood flow (cardiac output, CO) and the resistance to passage of blood through precapillary arterioles (peripheral vascular resistance, PVR):

$$BP = CO \times PVR$$

Physiologically, in both normal and hypertensive individuals, blood pressure is maintained by moment-to-moment regulation of cardiac output and peripheral vascular resistance, exerted at three anatomic sites (Figure 11–1): arterioles, postcapillary venules (capacitance vessels), and heart. A fourth anatomic control site, the kidney, contributes to maintenance of blood pressure by regulating the volume of intravascular fluid. Baroreflexes, mediated by autonomic nerves, act in combination with humoral mechanisms, including the renin-angiotensin-aldosterone system, to coordinate function at these four control sites and to maintain normal blood pressure. Finally, local release of vasoactive substances from vascular endothelium may also be involved in the regulation of vascular

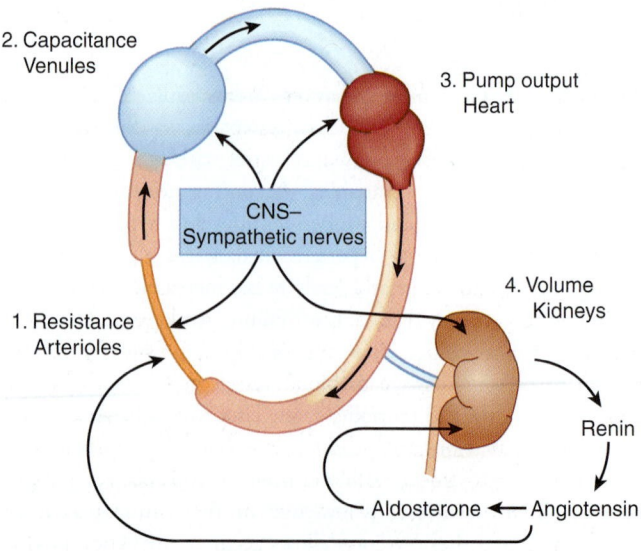

FIGURE 11–1 Anatomic sites of blood pressure control.

resistance. For example, endothelin-1 (see Chapter 17) constricts and nitric oxide (see Chapter 19) dilates blood vessels.

Blood pressure in a hypertensive patient is controlled by the same mechanisms that are operative in normotensive subjects. Regulation of blood pressure in hypertensive patients differs from healthy patients in that the baroreceptors and the renal blood volume-pressure control systems appear to be "set" at a higher level of blood pressure. All antihypertensive drugs act by interfering with these normal mechanisms, which are reviewed below.

A. Postural Baroreflex

Baroreflexes are responsible for rapid, moment-to-moment adjustments in blood pressure, such as in transition from a reclining to an upright posture (Figure 11–2). Central sympathetic neurons arising from the vasomotor area of the medulla are tonically active. Carotid baroreceptors are stimulated by the stretch of the vessel walls brought about by the internal pressure (arterial blood pressure). Baroreceptor activation inhibits central sympathetic discharge. Conversely, reduction in stretch results in a reduction in baroreceptor activity. Thus, in the case of a transition to upright posture, baroreceptors sense the reduction in arterial pressure that results from pooling of blood in the veins below the level of the heart as reduced wall stretch, and sympathetic discharge is disinhibited. The reflex increase in sympathetic outflow acts through nerve endings to increase peripheral vascular resistance (constriction of arterioles) and cardiac output (direct stimulation of the heart and constriction of capacitance vessels, which increases venous return to the heart), thereby restoring normal blood pressure. The same baroreflex acts in response to any event that lowers arterial pressure, including a primary reduction in peripheral vascular resistance (eg, caused by a vasodilating agent) or a reduction in intravascular volume (eg, due to hemorrhage or to loss of salt and water via the kidney).

B. Renal Response to Decreased Blood Pressure

By controlling blood volume, the kidney is primarily responsible for long-term blood pressure control. A reduction in renal perfusion pressure causes intrarenal redistribution of blood flow and increased reabsorption of salt and water. In addition, decreased pressure in renal arterioles as well as sympathetic neural activity (via β adrenoceptors) stimulates production of renin, which increases production of angiotensin II (see Figure 11–1 and Chapter 17). Angiotensin II causes (1) direct constriction of resistance vessels and (2) stimulation of aldosterone synthesis in the adrenal cortex, which increases renal sodium absorption and intravascular blood volume. Vasopressin released from the posterior pituitary gland also plays a role in maintenance of blood pressure through its ability to regulate water reabsorption by the kidney (see Chapters 15 and 17).

■ BASIC PHARMACOLOGY OF ANTIHYPERTENSIVE AGENTS

All antihypertensive agents act at one or more of the four anatomic control sites depicted in Figure 11–1 and produce their effects by interfering with normal mechanisms of blood pressure regulation. A useful classification of these agents categorizes them according to the principal regulatory site or mechanism on which they act (Figure 11–3). Because of their common mechanisms of action, drugs within each category tend to produce a similar spectrum of toxicities. The categories include the following:

1. **Diuretics,** which lower blood pressure by depleting the body of sodium and reducing blood volume and perhaps by other mechanisms.

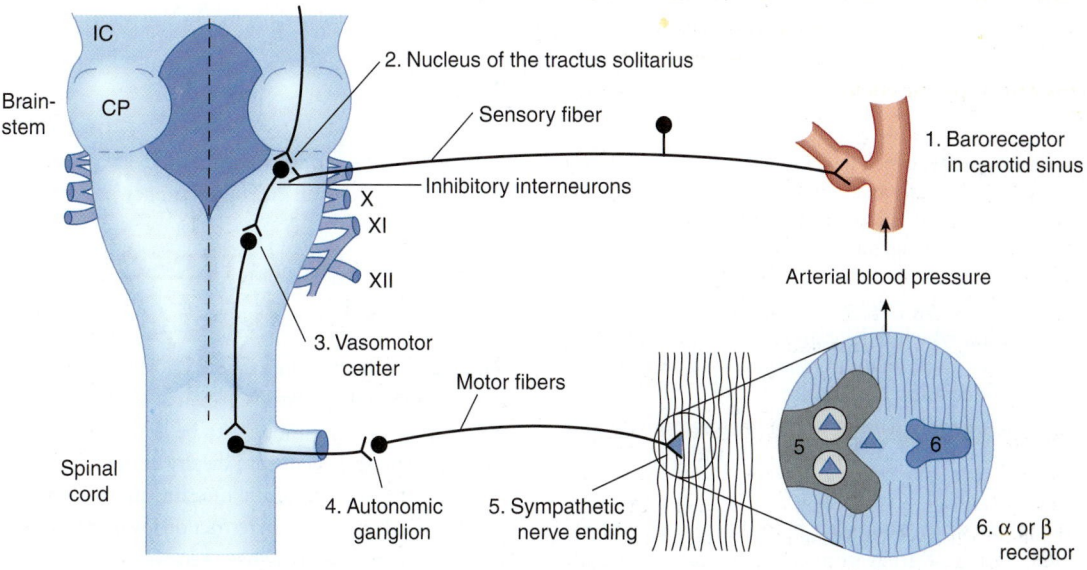

FIGURE 11–2 Baroreceptor reflex arc.

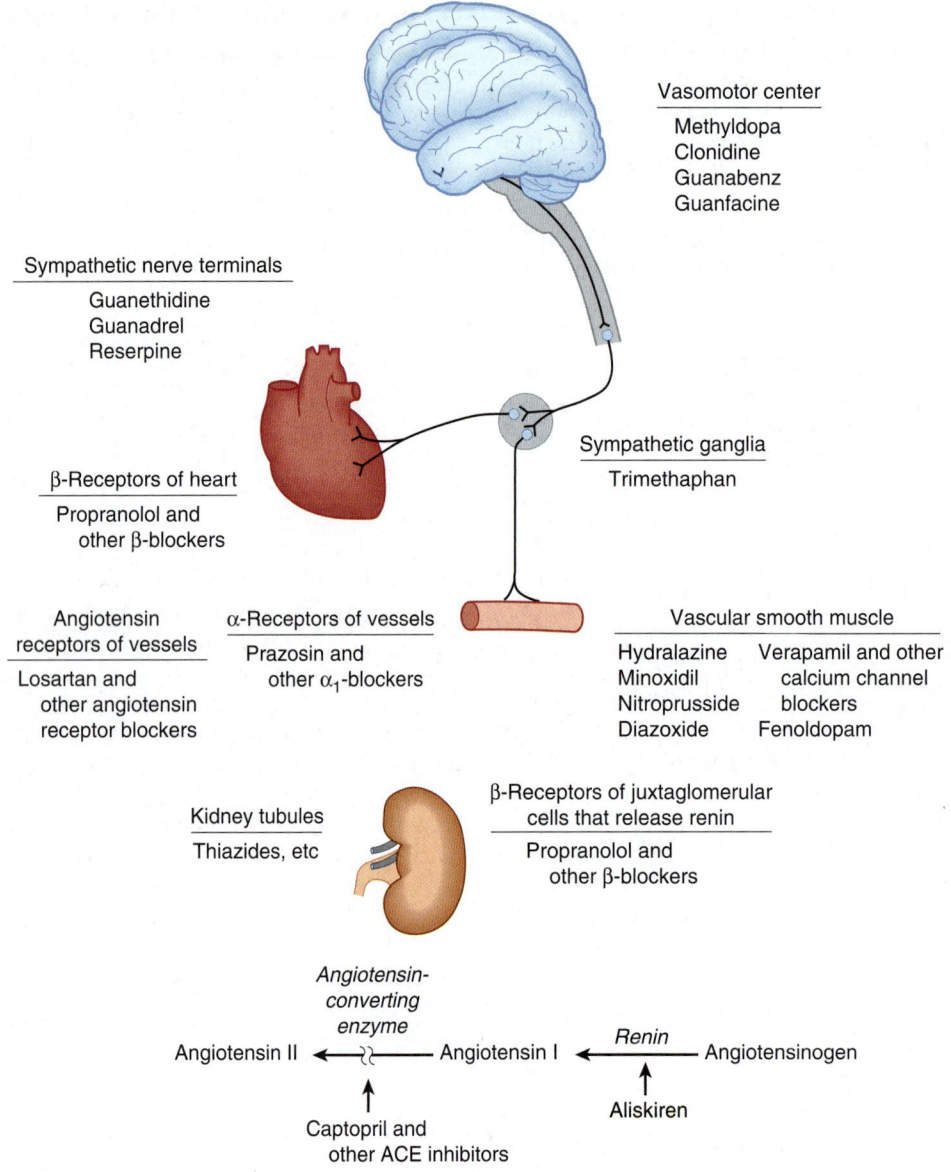

FIGURE 11–3 Sites of action of the major classes of antihypertensive drugs.

2. **Sympathoplegic agents,** which lower blood pressure by reducing peripheral vascular resistance, inhibiting cardiac function, and increasing venous pooling in capacitance vessels. (The latter two effects reduce cardiac output.) These agents are further subdivided according to their putative sites of action in the sympathetic reflex arc (see below).

3. **Direct vasodilators,** which reduce pressure by relaxing vascular smooth muscle, thus dilating resistance vessels and—to varying degrees—increasing capacitance as well.

4. **Agents that block production or action of angiotensin** and thereby reduce peripheral vascular resistance and (potentially) blood volume.

The fact that these drug groups act by different mechanisms permits the combination of drugs from two or more groups with increased efficacy and, in some cases, decreased toxicity. (See Box: Resistant Hypertension & Polypharmacy.)

DRUGS THAT ALTER SODIUM & WATER BALANCE

Dietary sodium restriction has been known for many years to decrease blood pressure in hypertensive patients. With the advent of diuretics, sodium restriction was thought to be less important. However, there is now general agreement that dietary control of blood pressure is a relatively nontoxic therapeutic measure and may even be preventive. Even modest dietary sodium restriction lowers blood pressure (though to varying extents) in many hypertensive persons.

Resistant Hypertension & Polypharmacy

Monotherapy of hypertension (treatment with a single drug) is desirable because compliance is likely to be better and cost is lower, and because in some cases adverse effects are fewer. However, most patients with hypertension require two or more drugs, preferably acting by different mechanisms (polypharmacy). According to some estimates, up to 40% of patients may respond inadequately even to two agents and are considered to have "resistant hypertension." Some of these patients have treatable secondary hypertension that has been missed, but most do not and three or more drugs are required.

One rationale for polypharmacy in hypertension is that most drugs evoke compensatory regulatory mechanisms for maintaining blood pressure (see Figures 6–7 and 11–1), which may markedly limit their effect. For example, vasodilators such as hydralazine cause a significant decrease in peripheral vascular resistance, but evoke a strong compensatory tachycardia and salt and water retention (Figure 11–4) that is capable of almost completely reversing their effect. The addition of a β blocker prevents the tachycardia; addition of a diuretic (eg, hydrochlorothiazide) prevents the salt and water retention. In effect, all three drugs increase the sensitivity of the cardiovascular system to each other's actions.

A second reason is that some drugs have only modest maximum efficacy but reduction of long-term morbidity mandates their use. Many studies of angiotensin-converting enzyme (ACE) inhibitors report a maximal lowering of blood pressure of less than 10 mm Hg. In patients with stage 2 hypertension (pressure > 160/100 mm Hg), this is inadequate to prevent all the sequelae of hypertension, but ACE inhibitors have important long-term benefits in preventing or reducing renal disease in diabetic persons, and reduction of heart failure.

Finally, the toxicity of some effective drugs prevents their use at maximally effective dosage. The widespread indiscriminate use of β blockers has been criticized because several large clinical trials indicate that some members of the group, eg, metoprolol and carvedilol, have a greater benefit than others, eg, atenolol. However, all β blockers appear to have similar benefits in reducing mortality after myocardial infarction, so these drugs are particularly indicated in patients with an infarct and hypertension.

In practice, when hypertension does not respond adequately to a regimen of one drug, a second drug from a different class with a different mechanism of action and different pattern of toxicity is added. If the response is still inadequate and compliance is known to be good, a third drug should be added. If three drugs (usually including a diuretic) are inadequate, dietary sodium restriction and an additional drug may be necessary.

Mechanisms of Action & Hemodynamic Effects of Diuretics

Diuretics lower blood pressure primarily by depleting body sodium stores. Initially, diuretics reduce blood pressure by reducing blood volume and cardiac output; peripheral vascular resistance may increase. After 6–8 weeks, cardiac output returns toward normal while peripheral vascular resistance declines. Sodium is believed to contribute to vascular resistance by increasing vessel stiffness and neural reactivity, possibly related to altered sodium-calcium exchange with a resultant increase in intracellular calcium. These effects are reversed by diuretics or sodium restriction.

Diuretics are effective in lowering blood pressure by 10–15 mm Hg in most patients, and diuretics alone often provide adequate treatment for mild or moderate essential hypertension. In more severe hypertension, diuretics are used in combination with sympathoplegic and vasodilator drugs to control the tendency toward sodium retention caused by these agents. Vascular responsiveness—ie, the ability to either constrict or dilate—is diminished by sympathoplegic and vasodilator drugs, so that the vasculature behaves like an inflexible tube. As a consequence, blood pressure becomes exquisitely sensitive to blood volume. Thus, in severe hypertension, when multiple drugs are used, blood pressure may be well controlled when blood volume is 95% of normal but much too high when blood volume is 105% of normal.

Use of Diuretics

The sites of action within the kidney and the pharmacokinetics of various diuretic drugs are discussed in Chapter 15. Thiazide diuretics are appropriate for most patients with mild or moderate hypertension and normal renal and cardiac function. More powerful diuretics (eg, those acting on the loop of Henle) such as furosemide are necessary in severe hypertension, when multiple drugs with sodium-retaining properties are used; in renal insufficiency, when glomerular filtration rate is less than 30 or 40 mL/min; and in cardiac failure or cirrhosis, in which sodium retention is marked.

Potassium-sparing diuretics are useful both to avoid excessive potassium depletion and to enhance the natriuretic effects of other diuretics. Aldosterone receptor antagonists in particular also have a favorable effect on cardiac function in people with heart failure.

Some pharmacokinetic characteristics and the initial and usual maintenance dosages of hydrochlorothiazide are listed in Table 11–2. Although thiazide diuretics are more natriuretic at higher

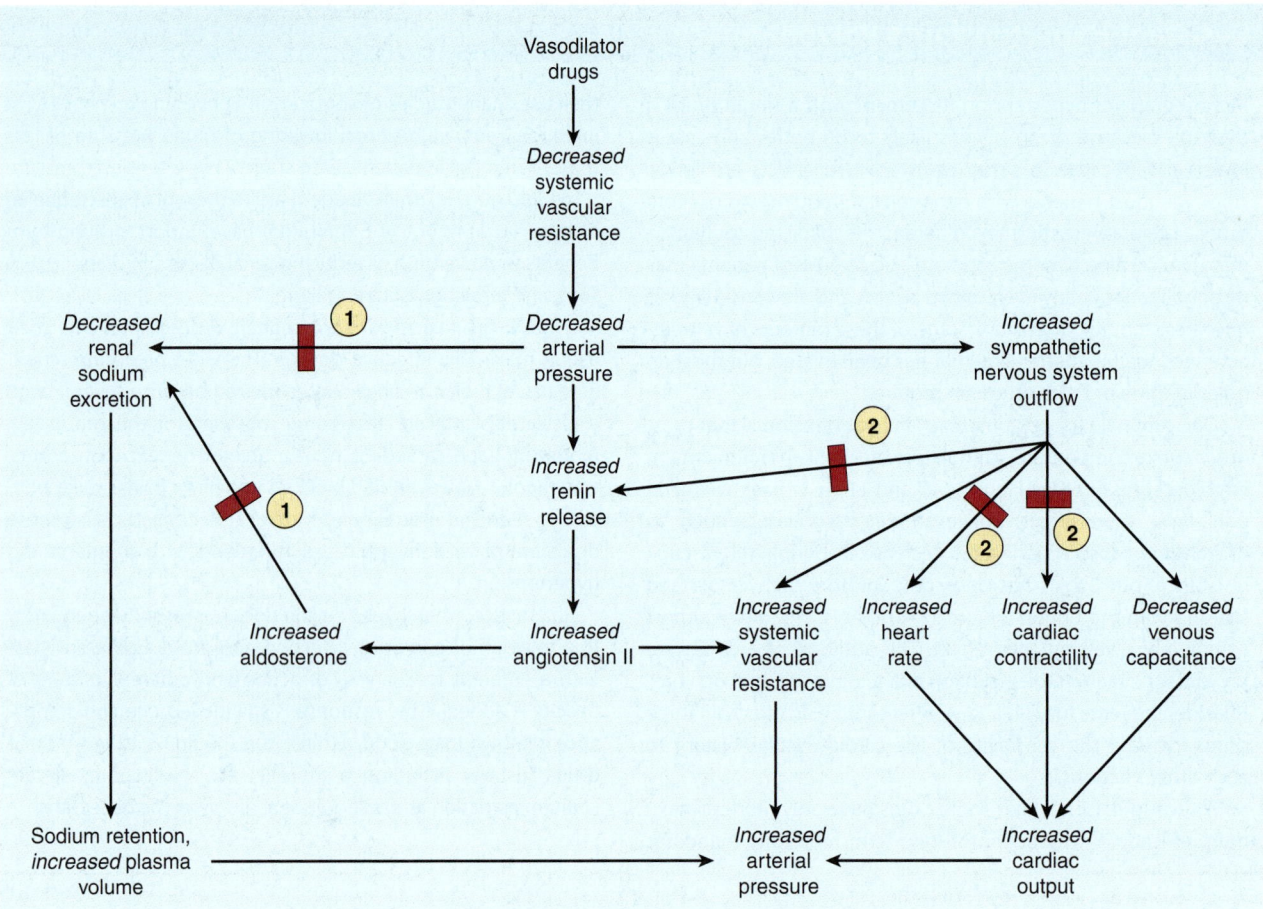

FIGURE 11–4 Compensatory responses to vasodilators; basis for combination therapy with β blockers and diuretics. ① Effect blocked by diuretics. ② Effect blocked by β blockers.

doses (up to 100–200 mg of hydrochlorothiazide), when used as a single agent, lower doses (25–50 mg) exert as much anti-hypertensive effect as do higher doses. In contrast to thiazides, the blood pressure response to loop diuretics continues to increase at doses many times greater than the usual therapeutic dose.

Toxicity of Diuretics

In the treatment of hypertension, the most common adverse effect of diuretics (except for potassium-sparing diuretics) is potassium depletion. Although mild degrees of hypokalemia are tolerated well by many patients, hypokalemia may be hazardous in persons taking digitalis, those who have chronic arrhythmias, or those with acute myocardial infarction or left ventricular dysfunction. Potassium loss is coupled to reabsorption of sodium, and restriction of dietary sodium intake therefore minimizes potassium loss. Diuretics may also cause magnesium depletion, impair glucose tolerance, and increase serum lipid concentrations. Diuretics increase uric acid concentrations and may precipitate gout. The use of low doses minimizes these adverse metabolic effects without impairing the antihypertensive action. Potassium-sparing diuretics may produce hyperkalemia, particularly in patients with renal insufficiency and those taking ACE inhibitors or angiotensin receptor blockers; spironolactone (a steroid) is associated with gynecomastia.

DRUGS THAT ALTER SYMPATHETIC NERVOUS SYSTEM FUNCTION

In many patients, hypertension is initiated and sustained at least in part by sympathetic neural activation. In patients with moderate to severe hypertension, most effective drug regimens include an agent that inhibits function of the sympathetic nervous system. Drugs in this group are classified according to the site at which they impair the sympathetic reflex arc (Figure 11–2). This neuro-anatomic classification explains prominent differences in cardiovascular effects of drugs and allows the clinician to predict interactions of these drugs with one another and with other drugs.

The subclasses of sympathoplegic drugs exhibit different patterns of potential toxicity. Drugs that lower blood pressure by actions on the central nervous system tend to cause sedation and mental depression and may produce disturbances of sleep, including nightmares. Drugs that act by inhibiting transmission through

TABLE 11–2 Pharmacokinetic characteristics and dosage of selected oral antihypertensive drugs.

Drug	Half-life (h)	Bioavailability (percent)	Suggested Initial Dose	Usual Maintenance Dose Range	Reduction of Dosage Required in Moderate Renal Insufficiency[1]
Amlodipine	35	65	2.5 mg/d	5–10 mg/d	No
Atenolol	6	60	50 mg/d	50–100 mg/d	Yes
Benazepril	0.6[2]	35	5–10 mg/d	20–40 mg/d	Yes
Captopril	2.2	65	50–75 mg/d	75–150 mg/d	Yes
Clonidine	8–12	95	0.2 mg/d	0.2–1.2 mg/d	Yes
Diltiazem	3.5	40	120–140 mg/d	240–360 mg/d	No
Guanethidine	120	3–50	10 mg/d	25–50 mg/d	Possible
Hydralazine	1.5–3	25	40 mg/d	40–200 mg/d	No
Hydrochlorothiazide	12	70	25 mg/d	25–50 mg/d	No
Lisinopril	12	25	10 mg/d	10–80 mg/d	Yes
Losartan	1–2[3]	36	50 mg/d	25–100 mg/d	No
Methyldopa	2	25	1 g/d	1–2 g/d	No
Metoprolol	3–7	40	50–100 mg/d	200–400 mg/d	No
Minoxidil	4	90	5–10 mg/d	40 mg/d	No
Nebivolol	12	Nd[4]	5 mg/d	10–40 mg/d	No
Nifedipine	2	50	30 mg/d	30–60 mg/d	No
Prazosin	3–4	70	3 mg/d	10–30 mg/d	No
Propranolol	3–5	25	80 mg/d	80–480 mg/d	No
Reserpine	24–48	50	0.25 mg/d	0.25 mg/d	No
Verapamil	4–6	22	180 mg/d	240–480 mg/d	No

[1]Creatinine clearance ≥ 30 mL/min. Many of these drugs do require dosage adjustment if creatinine clearance falls below 30 mL/min.

[2]The active metabolite of benazepril has a half-life of 10 hours.

[3]The active metabolite of losartan has a half-life of 3–4 hours.

[4]Nd, not determined.

autonomic ganglia (ganglion blockers) produce toxicity from inhibition of parasympathetic regulation, in addition to profound sympathetic blockade and are no longer used. Drugs that act chiefly by reducing release of norepinephrine from sympathetic nerve endings cause effects that are similar to those of surgical sympathectomy, including inhibition of ejaculation, and hypotension that is increased by upright posture and after exercise. Drugs that block postsynaptic adrenoceptors produce a more selective spectrum of effects depending on the class of receptor to which they bind. Although not discussed in this chapter, it should be noted that renal sympathetic denervation is effective in lowering blood pressure in patients with hypertension resistant to antihypertensive drugs.

Finally, one should note that *all* of the agents that lower blood pressure by altering sympathetic function can elicit compensatory effects through mechanisms that are not dependent on adrenergic nerves. Thus, the antihypertensive effect of any of these agents used alone may be limited by retention of sodium by the kidney and expansion of blood volume. For this reason, sympathoplegic antihypertensive drugs are most effective when used concomitantly with a diuretic.

CENTRALLY ACTING SYMPATHOPLEGIC DRUGS

Centrally acting sympathoplegic drugs were once widely used in the treatment of hypertension. With the exception of clonidine, these drugs are rarely used today.

Mechanisms & Sites of Action

These agents reduce sympathetic outflow from vasomotor centers in the brainstem but allow these centers to retain or even increase their sensitivity to baroreceptor control. Accordingly, the antihypertensive and toxic actions of these drugs are generally less dependent on posture than are the effects of drugs that act directly on peripheral sympathetic neurons.

Methyldopa (L-α-methyl-3,4-dihydroxyphenylalanine) is an analog of L-dopa and is converted to α-methyldopamine and α-methylnorepinephrine; this pathway directly parallels the synthesis of norepinephrine from dopa illustrated in Figure 6–5. Alpha-methylnorepinephrine is stored in adrenergic nerve vesicles, where it stoichiometrically replaces norepinephrine, and is released by nerve stimulation to interact with postsynaptic adrenoceptors. However, this replacement of norepinephrine by a false transmitter in peripheral neurons is *not* responsible for methyldopa's antihypertensive effect, because the α-methylnorepinephrine released is an effective agonist at the α adrenoceptors that mediate peripheral sympathetic constriction of arterioles and venules. In fact, methyldopa's antihypertensive action appears to be due to stimulation of *central* α adrenoceptors by α-methylnorepinephrine or α-methyldopamine.

The antihypertensive action of **clonidine,** a 2-imidazoline derivative, was discovered in the course of testing the drug for use as a nasal decongestant.

After intravenous injection, clonidine produces a brief rise in blood pressure followed by more prolonged hypotension. The pressor response is due to direct stimulation of α adrenoceptors in arterioles. The drug is classified as a partial agonist at α receptors because it also inhibits pressor effects of other α agonists.

Considerable evidence indicates that the hypotensive effect of clonidine is exerted at α adrenoceptors in the medulla of the brain. In animals, the hypotensive effect of clonidine is prevented by central administration of α antagonists. Clonidine reduces sympathetic and increases parasympathetic tone, resulting in blood pressure lowering and bradycardia. The reduction in pressure is accompanied by a decrease in circulating catecholamine levels. These observations suggest that clonidine sensitizes brainstem vasomotor centers to inhibition by baroreflexes.

Thus, studies of clonidine and methyldopa suggest that normal regulation of blood pressure involves central adrenergic neurons that modulate baroreceptor reflexes. Clonidine and α-methylnorepinephrine bind more tightly to α_2 than to α_1 adrenoceptors. As noted in Chapter 6, α_2 receptors are located on presynaptic adrenergic neurons as well as some postsynaptic sites. It is possible that clonidine and α-methylnorepinephrine act in the brain to reduce norepinephrine release onto relevant receptor sites. Alternatively, these drugs may act on postsynaptic α_2 adrenoceptors to inhibit activity of appropriate neurons. Finally, clonidine also binds to a nonadrenoceptor site, the **imidazoline receptor,** which may also mediate antihypertensive effects.

Methyldopa and clonidine produce slightly different hemodynamic effects: clonidine lowers heart rate and cardiac output more than does methyldopa. This difference suggests that these two drugs do not have identical sites of action. They may act primarily on different populations of neurons in the vasomotor centers of the brainstem.

Guanabenz and **guanfacine** are centrally active antihypertensive drugs that share the central α-adrenoceptor–stimulating effects of clonidine. They do not appear to offer any advantages over clonidine and are rarely used.

METHYLDOPA

Methyldopa was widely used in the past but is now used primarily for hypertension during pregnancy. It lowers blood pressure chiefly by reducing peripheral vascular resistance, with a variable reduction in heart rate and cardiac output.

Most cardiovascular reflexes remain intact after administration of methyldopa, and blood pressure reduction is not markedly dependent on posture. Postural (orthostatic) hypotension sometimes occurs, particularly in volume-depleted patients. One potential advantage of methyldopa is that it causes reduction in renal vascular resistance.

α-Methyldopa
(α-methyl group in color)

Pharmacokinetics & Dosage

Pharmacokinetic characteristics of methyldopa are listed in Table 11–2. Methyldopa enters the brain via an aromatic amino acid transporter. The usual oral dose of methyldopa produces its maximal antihypertensive effect in 4–6 hours, and the effect can persist for up to 24 hours. Because the effect depends on accumulation and storage of a metabolite (α-methylnorepinephrine) in the vesicles of nerve endings, the action persists after the parent drug has disappeared from the circulation.

Toxicity

The most common undesirable effect of methyldopa is sedation, particularly at the onset of treatment. With long-term therapy, patients may complain of persistent mental lassitude and impaired mental concentration. Nightmares, mental depression, vertigo, and extrapyramidal signs may occur but are relatively infrequent. Lactation, associated with increased prolactin secretion, can occur both in men and in women treated with methyldopa. This toxicity is probably mediated by inhibition of dopaminergic mechanisms in the hypothalamus.

Other important adverse effects of methyldopa are development of a positive Coombs test (occurring in 10–20% of patients undergoing therapy for longer than 12 months), which sometimes makes cross-matching blood for transfusion difficult and rarely is associated with hemolytic anemia, as well as hepatitis and drug fever. Discontinuation of the drug usually results in prompt reversal of these abnormalities.

CLONIDINE

Blood pressure lowering by clonidine results from reduction of cardiac output due to decreased heart rate and relaxation of capacitance vessels, as well as a reduction in peripheral vascular resistance.

Clonidine

Reduction in arterial blood pressure by clonidine is accompanied by decreased renal vascular resistance and maintenance of renal blood flow. As with methyldopa, clonidine reduces blood pressure in the supine position and only rarely causes postural hypotension. Pressor effects of clonidine are not observed after ingestion of therapeutic doses of clonidine, but severe hypertension can complicate a massive overdose.

Pharmacokinetics & Dosage

Typical pharmacokinetic characteristics are listed in Table 11–2.

Clonidine is lipid-soluble and rapidly enters the brain from the circulation. Because of its relatively short half-life and the fact that its antihypertensive effect is directly related to blood concentration, oral clonidine must be given twice a day (or as a patch, below) to maintain smooth blood pressure control. However, as is not the case with methyldopa, the dose-response curve of clonidine is such that increasing doses are more effective (but also more toxic).

A transdermal preparation of clonidine that reduces blood pressure for 7 days after a single application is also available. This preparation appears to produce less sedation than clonidine tablets but is often associated with local skin reactions.

Toxicity

Dry mouth and sedation are common. Both effects are centrally mediated and dose-dependent and coincide temporally with the drug's antihypertensive effect.

Clonidine should not be given to patients who are at risk for mental depression and should be withdrawn if depression occurs during therapy. Concomitant treatment with tricyclic antidepressants may block the antihypertensive effect of clonidine. The interaction is believed to be due to α-adrenoceptor–blocking actions of the tricyclics.

Withdrawal of clonidine after protracted use, particularly with high dosages (more than 1 mg/d), can result in life-threatening hypertensive crisis mediated by increased sympathetic nervous activity. Patients exhibit nervousness, tachycardia, headache, and sweating after omitting one or two doses of the drug. Because of the risk of severe hypertensive crisis when clonidine is suddenly withdrawn, all patients who take clonidine should be warned of the possibility. If the drug must be stopped, it should be done gradually while other antihypertensive agents are being substituted. Treatment of the hypertensive crisis consists of reinstitution of clonidine therapy or administration of α- and β-adrenoceptor–blocking agents.

GANGLION-BLOCKING AGENTS

Historically, drugs that block activation of postganglionic autonomic neurons by acetylcholine were among the first agents used in the treatment of hypertension. Most such drugs are no longer available clinically because of intolerable toxicities related to their primary action (see below).

Ganglion blockers competitively block nicotinic cholinoceptors on postganglionic neurons in both sympathetic and parasympathetic ganglia. In addition, these drugs may directly block the nicotinic acetylcholine channel, in the same fashion as neuromuscular nicotinic blockers (see Figure 27–6).

The adverse effects of ganglion blockers are direct extensions of their pharmacologic effects. These effects include both sympathoplegia (excessive orthostatic hypotension and sexual dysfunction) and parasympathoplegia (constipation, urinary retention, precipitation of glaucoma, blurred vision, dry mouth, etc). These severe toxicities are the major reason for the abandonment of ganglion blockers for the therapy of hypertension.

ADRENERGIC NEURON-BLOCKING AGENTS

These drugs lower blood pressure by preventing normal physiologic release of norepinephrine from postganglionic sympathetic neurons.

Guanethidine

In high enough doses, guanethidine can produce profound sympathoplegia. The resulting high maximal efficacy of this agent made it the mainstay of outpatient therapy of severe hypertension for many years. For the same reason, guanethidine can produce all of the toxicities expected from "pharmacologic sympathectomy," including marked postural hypotension, diarrhea, and impaired ejaculation. Because of these adverse effects, guanethidine is now rarely used.

Guanethidine is too polar to enter the central nervous system. As a result, this drug has none of the central effects seen with many of the other antihypertensive agents described in this chapter.

Guanadrel is a guanethidine-like drug that is available in the USA. **Bethanidine** and **debrisoquin**, antihypertensive agents not available for clinical use in the USA, are similar.

A. Mechanism and Sites of Action

Guanethidine inhibits the release of norepinephrine from sympathetic nerve endings (see Figure 6–4). This effect is probably responsible for most of the sympathoplegia that occurs in patients. Guanethidine is transported across the sympathetic nerve membrane by the same mechanism that transports norepinephrine itself (NET, uptake 1), and uptake is essential for the drug's action. Once guanethidine has entered the nerve, it is concentrated in transmitter vesicles, where it replaces norepinephrine. Because it replaces norepinephrine, the drug causes a gradual depletion of norepinephrine stores in the nerve ending.

Because neuronal uptake is necessary for the hypotensive activity of guanethidine, drugs that block the catecholamine uptake process or displace amines from the nerve terminal (see Chapter 6) block its effects. These include cocaine, amphetamine, tricyclic antidepressants, phenothiazines, and phenoxybenzamine.

B. Pharmacokinetics and Dosage

Because of guanethidine's long half-life (5 days), the onset of sympathoplegia is gradual (maximal effect in 1–2 weeks), and sympathoplegia persists for a comparable period after cessation of therapy. The dose should not ordinarily be increased at intervals shorter than 2 weeks.

C. Toxicity

Therapeutic use of guanethidine is often associated with symptomatic postural hypotension and hypotension following exercise, particularly when the drug is given in high doses. Guanethidine-induced sympathoplegia in men may be associated with delayed or retrograde ejaculation (into the bladder). Guanethidine commonly causes diarrhea, which results from increased gastrointestinal motility due to parasympathetic predominance in controlling the activity of intestinal smooth muscle.

Interactions with other drugs may complicate guanethidine therapy. Sympathomimetic agents, at doses available in over-the-counter cold preparations, can produce hypertension in patients taking guanethidine. Similarly, guanethidine can produce hypertensive crisis by releasing catecholamines in patients with pheochromocytoma. When tricyclic antidepressants are administered to patients taking guanethidine, the drug's antihypertensive effect is attenuated, and severe hypertension may follow.

Reserpine

Reserpine, an alkaloid extracted from the roots of an Indian plant, *Rauwolfia serpentina,* was one of the first effective drugs used on a large scale in the treatment of hypertension. At present, it is rarely used owing to its adverse effects.

A. Mechanism and Sites of Action

Reserpine blocks the ability of aminergic transmitter vesicles to take up and store biogenic amines, probably by interfering with the vesicular membrane-associated transporter (VMAT, see Figure 6–4). This effect occurs throughout the body, resulting in depletion of norepinephrine, dopamine, and serotonin in both central and peripheral neurons. Chromaffin granules of the adrenal medulla are also depleted of catecholamines, although to a lesser extent than are the vesicles of neurons. Reserpine's effects on adrenergic vesicles appear irreversible; trace amounts of the drug remain bound to vesicular membranes for many days.

Depletion of peripheral amines probably accounts for much of the beneficial antihypertensive effect of reserpine, but a central component cannot be ruled out. Reserpine readily enters the brain, and depletion of cerebral amine stores causes sedation, mental depression, and parkinsonism symptoms.

At lower doses used for treatment of mild hypertension, reserpine lowers blood pressure by a combination of decreased cardiac output and decreased peripheral vascular resistance.

B. Pharmacokinetics and Dosage

See Table 11–2.

C. Toxicity

At the low doses usually administered, reserpine produces little postural hypotension. Most of the unwanted effects of reserpine result from actions on the brain or gastrointestinal tract.

High doses of reserpine characteristically produce sedation, lassitude, nightmares, and severe mental depression; occasionally, these occur even in patients receiving low doses (0.25 mg/d). Much less frequently, ordinary low doses of reserpine produce extrapyramidal effects resembling Parkinson's disease, probably as a result of dopamine depletion in the corpus striatum. Although these central effects are uncommon, it should be stressed that they may occur at any time, even after months of uneventful treatment. Patients with a history of mental depression should not receive reserpine, and the drug should be stopped if depression appears.

Reserpine rather often produces mild diarrhea and gastrointestinal cramps and increases gastric acid secretion. The drug should not be given to patients with a history of peptic ulcer.

ADRENOCEPTOR ANTAGONISTS

The detailed pharmacology of α- and β-adrenoceptor blockers is presented in Chapter 10.

BETA-ADRENOCEPTOR–BLOCKING AGENTS

Of the large number of β blockers tested, most have been shown to be effective in lowering blood pressure. The pharmacologic properties of several of these agents differ in ways that may confer therapeutic benefits in certain clinical situations.

Propranolol

Propranolol was the first β blocker shown to be effective in hypertension and ischemic heart disease. Propranolol has now been largely replaced by cardioselective β blockers such as metoprolol and atenolol. All β-adrenoceptor–blocking agents are useful for lowering blood pressure in mild to moderate hypertension. In severe hypertension, β blockers are especially useful in preventing the reflex tachycardia that often results from treatment with direct vasodilators. Beta blockers have been shown to reduce mortality after a myocardial infarction and some also reduce mortality in patients with heart failure; they are particularly advantageous for treating hypertension in patients with these conditions (see Chapter 13).

A. Mechanism and Sites of Action

Propranolol's efficacy in treating hypertension as well as most of its toxic effects result from nonselective β blockade. Propranolol decreases blood pressure primarily as a result of a decrease in cardiac output. Other β blockers may decrease cardiac output or decrease peripheral vascular resistance to various degrees, depending on cardioselectivity and partial agonist activities.

Propranolol inhibits the stimulation of renin production by catecholamines (mediated by β_1 receptors). It is likely that propranolol's effect is due in part to depression of the renin-angiotensin-aldosterone system. Although most effective in patients with high plasma renin activity, propranolol also reduces blood pressure in hypertensive patients with normal or even low renin activity. Beta blockers might also act on peripheral presynaptic β adrenoceptors to reduce sympathetic vasoconstrictor nerve activity.

In mild to moderate hypertension, propranolol produces a significant reduction in blood pressure without prominent postural hypotension.

B. Pharmacokinetics and Dosage

See Table 11–2. Resting bradycardia and a reduction in the heart rate during exercise are indicators of propranolol's β-blocking effect, and changes in these parameters may be used as guides for regulating dosage. Propranolol can be administered twice daily, and slow-release preparations are available.

C. Toxicity

The principal toxicities of propranolol result from blockade of cardiac, vascular, or bronchial β receptors and are described in more detail in Chapter 10. The most important of these predictable extensions of the β-blocking action occur in patients with bradycardia or cardiac conduction disease, asthma, peripheral vascular insufficiency, and diabetes.

When propranolol is discontinued after prolonged regular use, some patients experience a withdrawal syndrome, manifested by nervousness, tachycardia, increased intensity of angina, and increase of blood pressure. Myocardial infarction has been reported in a few patients. Although the incidence of these complications is probably low, propranolol should not be discontinued abruptly. The withdrawal syndrome may involve up-regulation or supersensitivity of β adrenoceptors.

Metoprolol & Atenolol

Metoprolol and atenolol, which are cardioselective, are the most widely used β blockers in the treatment of hypertension. Metoprolol is approximately equipotent to propranolol in inhibiting stimulation of β₁ adrenoceptors such as those in the heart but 50- to 100-fold less potent than propranolol in blocking β₂ receptors. Relative cardioselectivity may be advantageous in treating hypertensive patients who also suffer from asthma, diabetes, or peripheral vascular disease. Although cardioselectivity is not complete, metoprolol causes less bronchial constriction than propranolol at doses that produce equal inhibition of β₁-adrenoceptor responses. Metoprolol is extensively metabolized by CYP2D6 with high first-pass metabolism. The drug has a relatively short half-life of 4–6 hours, but the extended-release preparation can be dosed once daily (Table 11–2). Sustained-release metoprolol is effective in reducing mortality from heart failure and is particularly useful in patients with hypertension and heart failure.

Atenolol is not extensively metabolized and is excreted primarily in the urine with a half-life of 6 hours; it is usually dosed once daily. Recent studies have found atenolol less effective than metoprolol in preventing the complications of hypertension. A possible reason for this difference is that once-daily dosing does not maintain adequate blood levels of atenolol. The usual dosage is 50–100 mg/d. Patients with reduced renal function should receive lower doses.

Nadolol, Carteolol, Betaxolol, & Bisoprolol

Nadolol and carteolol, nonselective β-receptor antagonists, are not appreciably metabolized and are excreted to a considerable extent in the urine. Betaxolol and bisoprolol are β₁-selective blockers that are primarily metabolized in the liver but have long half-lives. Because of these relatively long half-lives, these drugs can be administered once daily. Nadolol is usually begun at a dosage of 40 mg/d, carteolol at 2.5 mg/d, betaxolol at 10 mg/d, and bisoprolol at 5 mg/d. Increases in dosage to obtain a satisfactory therapeutic effect should take place no more often than every 4 or 5 days. Patients with reduced renal function should receive correspondingly reduced doses of nadolol and carteolol.

Pindolol, Acebutolol, & Penbutolol

Pindolol, acebutolol, and penbutolol are partial agonists, ie, β blockers with some intrinsic sympathomimetic activity. They lower blood pressure by decreasing vascular resistance and appear to depress cardiac output or heart rate less than other β blockers, perhaps because of significantly greater agonist than antagonist effects at β₂ receptors. This may be particularly beneficial for patients with bradyarrhythmias or peripheral vascular disease. Daily doses of pindolol start at 10 mg; of acebutolol, at 400 mg; and of penbutolol, at 20 mg.

Labetalol, Carvedilol, & Nebivolol

These drugs have both β-blocking and vasodilating effects. Labetalol is formulated as a racemic mixture of four isomers (it has two centers of asymmetry). Two of these isomers—the (S,S)- and (R,S)-isomers—are relatively inactive, a third (S,R)- is a potent α blocker, and the last (R,R)- is a potent β blocker. Labetalol has a 3:1 ratio of β:α antagonism after oral dosing. Blood pressure is lowered by reduction of systemic vascular resistance (via α blockade) without significant alteration in heart rate or cardiac output. Because of its combined α- and β-blocking activity, labetalol is useful in treating the hypertension of pheochromocytoma and hypertensive emergencies. Oral daily doses of labetalol range from 200 to 2400 mg/d. Labetalol is given as repeated intravenous bolus injections of 20–80 mg to treat hypertensive emergencies.

Carvedilol, like labetalol, is administered as a racemic mixture. The S(−) isomer is a nonselective β-adrenoceptor blocker, but both S(−) and R(+) isomers have approximately equal α-blocking potency. The isomers are stereoselectively metabolized in the liver, which means that their elimination half-lives may differ. The average half-life is 7–10 hours. The usual starting dosage of carvedilol for ordinary hypertension is 6.25 mg twice daily. Carvedilol reduces mortality in patients with heart failure and is therefore particularly useful in patients with both heart failure and hypertension.

Nebivolol is a β₁-selective blocker with vasodilating properties that are *not* mediated by α blockade. D-Nebivolol has highly selective β₁ blocking effects, while the L-isomer causes vasodilation; the drug is marketed as a racemic mixture. The vasodilating effect may be due to an increase in endothelial release of nitric oxide via induction of endothelial nitric oxide synthase. The hemodynamic effects of nebivolol therefore differ from those of pure β blockers in that peripheral vascular resistance is acutely lowered (by nebivolol) as opposed to increased acutely (by the older agents). Nebivolol is extensively metabolized and has active metabolites. The half-life is 10–12 hours, but the drug can be given once daily. Dosing is generally started at 5 mg/d, with dose escalation as high as 40 mg, if necessary. The efficacy of nebivolol is similar to that of other antihypertensive agents, but several studies report fewer adverse effects.

Esmolol

Esmolol is a β1-selective blocker that is rapidly metabolized via hydrolysis by red blood cell esterases. It has a short half-life (9–10 minutes) and is administered by constant intravenous infusion. Esmolol is generally administered as a loading dose (0.5–1 mg/kg), followed by a constant infusion. The infusion is typically started at 50–150 mcg/kg/min, and the dose increased every 5 minutes, up to 300 mcg/kg/min, as needed to achieve the desired therapeutic effect. Esmolol is used for management of intraoperative and postoperative hypertension, and sometimes for hypertensive emergencies, particularly when hypertension is associated with tachycardia.

PRAZOSIN & OTHER ALPHA₁ BLOCKERS

Mechanism & Sites of Action

Prazosin, terazosin, and doxazosin produce most of their antihypertensive effects by selectively blocking α1 receptors in arterioles and venules. These agents produce less reflex tachycardia when lowering blood pressure than do nonselective α antagonists such as phentolamine. Alpha1-receptor selectivity allows norepinephrine to exert unopposed negative feedback (mediated by presynaptic α2 receptors) on its own release (see Chapter 6); in contrast, phentolamine blocks both presynaptic and postsynaptic α receptors, with the result that reflex activation of sympathetic neurons by phentolamine's effects produces greater release of transmitter onto β receptors and correspondingly greater cardioacceleration.

Alpha blockers reduce arterial pressure by dilating both resistance and capacitance vessels. As expected, blood pressure is reduced more in the upright than in the supine position. Retention of salt and water occurs when these drugs are administered without a diuretic. The drugs are more effective when used in combination with other agents, such as a β blocker and a diuretic, than when used alone. Owing to their beneficial effects in men with prostatic hyperplasia and bladder obstruction symptoms, these drugs are used primarily in men with concurrent hypertension and benign prostatic hyperplasia.

Pharmacokinetics & Dosage

Pharmacokinetic characteristics of prazosin are listed in Table 11–2. Terazosin is also extensively metabolized but undergoes very little

first-pass metabolism and has a half-life of 12 hours. Doxazosin has an intermediate bioavailability and a half-life of 22 hours.

Terazosin can often be given once daily, with doses of 5–20 mg/d. Doxazosin is usually given once daily starting at 1 mg/d and progressing to 4 mg/d or more as needed. Although long-term treatment with these α blockers causes relatively little postural hypotension, a precipitous drop in standing blood pressure develops in some patients shortly after the first dose is absorbed. For this reason, the first dose should be small and should be administered at bedtime. Although the mechanism of this first-dose phenomenon is not clear, it occurs more commonly in patients who are salt- and volume-depleted.

Aside from the first-dose phenomenon, the reported toxicities of the α1 blockers are relatively infrequent and mild. These include dizziness, palpitations, headache, and lassitude. Some patients develop a positive test for antinuclear factor in serum while on prazosin therapy, but this has not been associated with rheumatic symptoms. The α1 blockers do not adversely and may even beneficially affect plasma lipid profiles, but this action has not been shown to confer any benefit on clinical outcomes.

OTHER ALPHA-ADRENOCEPTOR–BLOCKING AGENTS

The nonselective agents, **phentolamine** and **phenoxybenzamine,** are useful in diagnosis and treatment of pheochromocytoma and in other clinical situations associated with exaggerated release of catecholamines (eg, phentolamine may be combined with propranolol to treat the clonidine withdrawal syndrome, described previously). Their pharmacology is described in Chapter 10.

VASODILATORS

Mechanism & Sites of Action

This class of drugs includes the oral vasodilators, hydralazine and minoxidil, which are used for long-term outpatient therapy of hypertension; the parenteral vasodilators, nitroprusside, diazoxide, and fenoldopam, which are used to treat hypertensive emergencies; the calcium channel blockers, which are used in both circumstances; and the nitrates, which are used mainly in angina (Table 11–3).

Chapter 12 contains additional discussion of vasodilators. All the vasodilators that are useful in hypertension relax smooth muscle of arterioles, thereby decreasing systemic vascular resistance. Sodium nitroprusside and the nitrates also relax veins. Decreased arterial resistance and decreased mean arterial blood pressure elicit compensatory responses, mediated by baroreceptors and the sympathetic nervous system (Figure 11–4), as well as renin, angiotensin, and aldosterone. Because sympathetic reflexes are intact, vasodilator therapy does not cause orthostatic hypotension or sexual dysfunction.

Vasodilators work best in combination with other antihypertensive drugs that oppose the compensatory cardiovascular responses. (See Box: Resistant Hypertension & Polypharmacy.)

TABLE 11–3 Mechanisms of action of vasodilators.

Mechanism	Examples
Release of nitric oxide from drug or endothelium	Nitroprusside, hydralazine, nitrates,[1] histamine, acetylcholine
Reduction of calcium influx	Verapamil, diltiazem, nifedipine
Hyperpolarization of smooth muscle membrane through opening of potassium channels	Minoxidil, diazoxide
Activation of dopamine receptors	Fenoldopam

[1]See Chapter 12.

HYDRALAZINE

Hydralazine, a hydrazine derivative, dilates arterioles but not veins. It has been available for many years, although it was initially thought not to be particularly effective because tachyphylaxis to its antihypertensive effects developed rapidly. The benefits of combination therapy are now recognized, and hydralazine may be used more effectively, particularly in severe hypertension. The combination of hydralazine with nitrates is effective in heart failure and should be considered in patients with both hypertension and heart failure, especially in African-American patients.

Pharmacokinetics & Dosage

Hydralazine is well absorbed and rapidly metabolized by the liver during the first pass, so that bioavailability is low (averaging 25%) and variable among individuals. It is metabolized in part by acetylation at a rate that appears to be bimodally distributed in the population (see Chapter 4). As a consequence, rapid acetylators have greater first-pass metabolism, lower blood levels, and less antihypertensive benefit from a given dose than do slow acetylators. The half-life of hydralazine ranges from 1.5 to 3 hours, but vascular effects persist longer than do blood concentrations, possibly due to avid binding to vascular tissue.

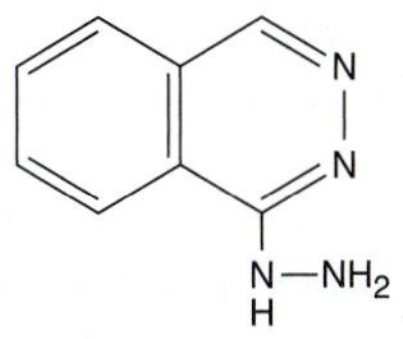

Hydralazine

Usual dosage ranges from 40 mg/d to 200 mg/d. The higher dosage was selected as the dose at which there is a small possibility of developing the lupus erythematosus-like syndrome described in the next section. However, higher dosages result in greater vasodilation and may be used if necessary. Dosing two or three times daily provides smooth control of blood pressure.

Toxicity

The most common adverse effects of hydralazine are headache, nausea, anorexia, palpitations, sweating, and flushing. In patients with ischemic heart disease, reflex tachycardia and sympathetic stimulation may provoke angina or ischemic arrhythmias. With dosages of 400 mg/d or more, there is a 10–20% incidence—chiefly in persons who slowly acetylate the drug—of a syndrome characterized by arthralgia, myalgia, skin rashes, and fever that resembles lupus erythematosus. The syndrome is not associated with renal damage and is reversed by discontinuance of hydralazine. Peripheral neuropathy and drug fever are other serious but uncommon adverse effects.

MINOXIDIL

Minoxidil is a very efficacious orally active vasodilator. The effect results from the opening of potassium channels in smooth muscle membranes by minoxidil sulfate, the active metabolite. Increased potassium permeability stabilizes the membrane at its resting potential and makes contraction less likely. Like hydralazine, minoxidil dilates arterioles but not veins. Because of its greater potential antihypertensive effect, minoxidil should replace hydralazine when maximal doses of the latter are not effective or in patients with renal failure and severe hypertension, who do not respond well to hydralazine.

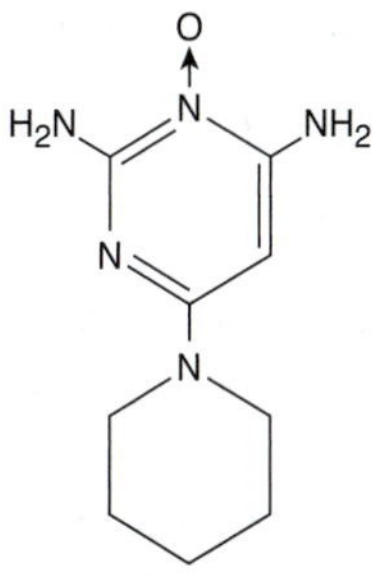

Minoxidil

Pharmacokinetics & Dosage

Pharmacokinetic parameters of minoxidil are listed in Table 11–2. Even more than with hydralazine, the use of minoxidil is associated with reflex sympathetic stimulation and sodium and fluid retention. Minoxidil must be used in combination with a β blocker and a loop diuretic.

Toxicity

Tachycardia, palpitations, angina, and edema are observed when doses of β blockers and diuretics are inadequate. Headache, sweating, and hypertrichosis, which is particularly bothersome in women, are relatively common. Minoxidil illustrates how one person's toxicity may become another person's therapy. Topical minoxidil (as Rogaine) is used as a stimulant to hair growth for correction of baldness.

SODIUM NITROPRUSSIDE

Sodium nitroprusside is a powerful parenterally administered vasodilator that is used in treating hypertensive emergencies as well as severe heart failure. Nitroprusside dilates both arterial and venous vessels, resulting in reduced peripheral vascular resistance and venous return. The action occurs as a result of activation of guanylyl cyclase, either via release of nitric oxide or by direct stimulation of the enzyme. The result is increased intracellular cGMP, which relaxes vascular smooth muscle (Figure 12–2).

In the absence of heart failure, blood pressure decreases, owing to decreased vascular resistance, whereas cardiac output does not change or decreases slightly. In patients with heart failure and low cardiac output, output often increases owing to afterload reduction.

Nitroprusside

Pharmacokinetics & Dosage

Nitroprusside is a complex of iron, cyanide groups, and a nitroso moiety. It is rapidly metabolized by uptake into red blood cells with liberation of cyanide. Cyanide in turn is metabolized by the mitochondrial enzyme rhodanase, in the presence of a sulfur donor, to the less toxic thiocyanate. Thiocyanate is distributed in extracellular fluid and slowly eliminated by the kidney.

Nitroprusside rapidly lowers blood pressure, and its effects disappear within 1–10 minutes after discontinuation. The drug is given by intravenous infusion. Sodium nitroprusside in aqueous solution is sensitive to light and must therefore be made up fresh before each administration and covered with opaque foil. Infusion solutions should be changed after several hours. Dosage typically begins at 0.5 mcg/kg/min and may be increased up to 10 mcg/kg/min as necessary to control blood pressure. Higher rates of infusion, if continued for more than an hour, may result in toxicity. Because of its efficacy and rapid onset of effect, nitroprusside should be administered by infusion pump and arterial blood pressure continuously monitored via intra-arterial recording.

Toxicity

Other than excessive blood pressure lowering, the most serious toxicity is related to accumulation of cyanide; metabolic acidosis, arrhythmias, excessive hypotension, and death have resulted. In a few cases, toxicity after relatively low doses of nitroprusside suggested

a defect in cyanide metabolism. Administration of sodium thiosulfate as a sulfur donor facilitates metabolism of cyanide. Hydroxocobalamin combines with cyanide to form the nontoxic cyanocobalamin. Both have been advocated for prophylaxis or treatment of cyanide poisoning during nitroprusside infusion. Thiocyanate may accumulate over the course of prolonged administration, usually several days or more, particularly in patients with renal insufficiency who do not excrete thiocyanate at a normal rate. Thiocyanate toxicity is manifested as weakness, disorientation, psychosis, muscle spasms, and convulsions, and the diagnosis is confirmed by finding serum concentrations greater than 10 mg/dL. Rarely, delayed hypothyroidism occurs, owing to thiocyanate inhibition of iodide uptake by the thyroid. Methemoglobinemia during infusion of nitroprusside has also been reported.

DIAZOXIDE

Diazoxide is an effective and relatively long-acting parenterally administered arteriolar dilator that is occasionally used to treat hypertensive emergencies. Diminishing usage suggests that it may be withdrawn. Injection of diazoxide results in a rapid fall in systemic vascular resistance and mean arterial blood pressure. Studies of its mechanism suggest that it prevents vascular smooth muscle contraction by opening potassium channels and stabilizing the membrane potential at the resting level.

Diazoxide

Pharmacokinetics & Dosage

Diazoxide is similar chemically to the thiazide diuretics but has no diuretic activity. It is bound extensively to serum albumin and to vascular tissue. Diazoxide is partially metabolized; its metabolic pathways are not well characterized. The remainder is excreted unchanged. Its half-life is approximately 24 hours, but the relationship between blood concentration and hypotensive action is not well established. The blood pressure-lowering effect after a rapid injection is established within 5 minutes and lasts for 4–12 hours.

When diazoxide was first marketed, a dose of 300 mg by rapid injection was recommended. It appears, however, that excessive hypotension can be avoided by beginning with smaller doses (50–150 mg). If necessary, doses of 150 mg may be repeated every 5 to 15 minutes until blood pressure is lowered satisfactorily. Nearly all patients respond to a maximum of three or four doses. Alternatively, diazoxide may be administered by intravenous infusion at rates of 15–30 mg/min. Because of reduced protein binding, hypotension occurs after smaller doses in persons with chronic renal failure, and smaller doses should be administered to these patients. The hypotensive effects of diazoxide are also greater when patients are pretreated with β blockers to prevent the reflex tachycardia and associated increase in cardiac output.

Toxicity

The most significant toxicity from diazoxide has been excessive hypotension, resulting from the recommendation to use a fixed dose of 300 mg in all patients. Such hypotension has resulted in stroke and myocardial infarction. The reflex sympathetic response can provoke angina, electrocardiographic evidence of ischemia, and cardiac failure in patients with ischemic heart disease, and diazoxide should be avoided in this situation.

Diazoxide inhibits insulin release from the pancreas (probably by opening potassium channels in the beta cell membrane) and is used to treat hypoglycemia secondary to insulinoma. Occasionally, hyperglycemia complicates diazoxide use, particularly in persons with renal insufficiency.

In contrast to the structurally related thiazide diuretics, diazoxide causes renal salt and water *retention*. However, because the drug is used for short periods only, this is rarely a problem.

FENOLDOPAM

Fenoldopam is a peripheral arteriolar dilator used for hypertensive emergencies and postoperative hypertension. It acts primarily as an agonist of dopamine D_1 receptors, resulting in dilation of peripheral arteries and natriuresis. The commercial product is a racemic mixture with the (R)-isomer mediating the pharmacologic activity.

Fenoldopam is rapidly metabolized, primarily by conjugation. Its half-life is 10 minutes. The drug is administered by continuous intravenous infusion. Fenoldopam is initiated at a low dosage (0.1 mcg/kg/min), and the dose is then titrated upward every 15 or 20 minutes to a maximum dose of 1.6 mcg/kg/min or until the desired blood pressure reduction is achieved.

As with other direct vasodilators, the major toxicities are reflex tachycardia, headache, and flushing. Fenoldopam also increases intraocular pressure and should be avoided in patients with glaucoma.

CALCIUM CHANNEL BLOCKERS

In addition to their antianginal (see Chapter 12) and antiarrhythmic effects (see Chapter 14), calcium channel blockers also reduce peripheral resistance and blood pressure. The mechanism of action in hypertension (and, in part, in angina) is inhibition of calcium influx into arterial smooth muscle cells.

Verapamil, diltiazem, and the **dihydropyridine** family (**amlodipine, felodipine, isradipine, nicardipine, nifedipine,** and **nisoldipine**) are all equally effective in lowering blood pressure, and many formulations are currently approved for this use in the USA. **Clevidipine** is a newer member of this group that is formulated for intravenous use only.

Hemodynamic differences among calcium channel blockers may influence the choice of a particular agent. Nifedipine and the other dihydropyridine agents are more selective as vasodilators and have less cardiac depressant effect than verapamil and diltiazem. Reflex sympathetic activation with slight tachycardia maintains or increases cardiac output in most patients given dihydropyridines. Verapamil has the greatest depressant effect on the heart and may decrease heart rate and cardiac output. Diltiazem has intermediate actions. The pharmacology and toxicity of these drugs is discussed in more detail in Chapter 12. Doses of calcium channel blockers used in treating hypertension are similar to those used in treating angina. Some epidemiologic studies reported an increased risk of myocardial infarction or mortality in patients receiving short-acting nifedipine for hypertension. It is therefore recommended that short-acting oral dihydropyridines not be used for hypertension. Sustained-release calcium blockers or calcium blockers with long half-lives provide smoother blood pressure control and are more appropriate for treatment of chronic hypertension. Intravenous nicardipine and clevidipine are available for the treatment of hypertension when oral therapy is not feasible; parenteral verapamil and diltiazem can also be used for the same indication. Nicardipine is typically infused at rates of 2–15 mg/h. Clevidipine is infused starting at 1–2 mg/h and progressing to 4–6 mg/h. It has a rapid onset of action and has been used in acute hypertension occurring during surgery. Oral short-acting nifedipine has been used in emergency management of severe hypertension.

■ INHIBITORS OF ANGIOTENSIN

Renin, angiotensin, and aldosterone play important roles in at least some people with essential hypertension. Approximately 20% of patients with essential hypertension have inappropriately low and 20% have inappropriately high plasma renin activity. Blood pressure of patients with high-renin hypertension responds well to drugs that interfere with the system, supporting a role for excess renin and angiotensin in this population.

Mechanism & Sites of Action

Renin release from the kidney cortex is stimulated by reduced renal arterial pressure, sympathetic neural stimulation, and reduced sodium delivery or increased sodium concentration at the distal renal tubule (see Chapter 17). Renin acts upon angiotensinogen to split off the inactive precursor decapeptide angiotensin I. Angiotensin I is then converted, primarily by endothelial ACE, to the arterial vasoconstrictor octapeptide angiotensin II (Figure 11–5), which is in turn converted in the adrenal gland to angiotensin III. Angiotensin II has vasoconstrictor and sodium-retaining activity. Angiotensin II and III both stimulate aldosterone release. Angiotensin may contribute to maintaining high vascular resistance in hypertensive states associated with high plasma renin activity, such as renal arterial stenosis, some types of intrinsic renal disease, and malignant hypertension, as well as in essential hypertension after treatment with sodium restriction, diuretics, or vasodilators. However, even in low-renin hypertensive states, these drugs can lower blood pressure (see below).

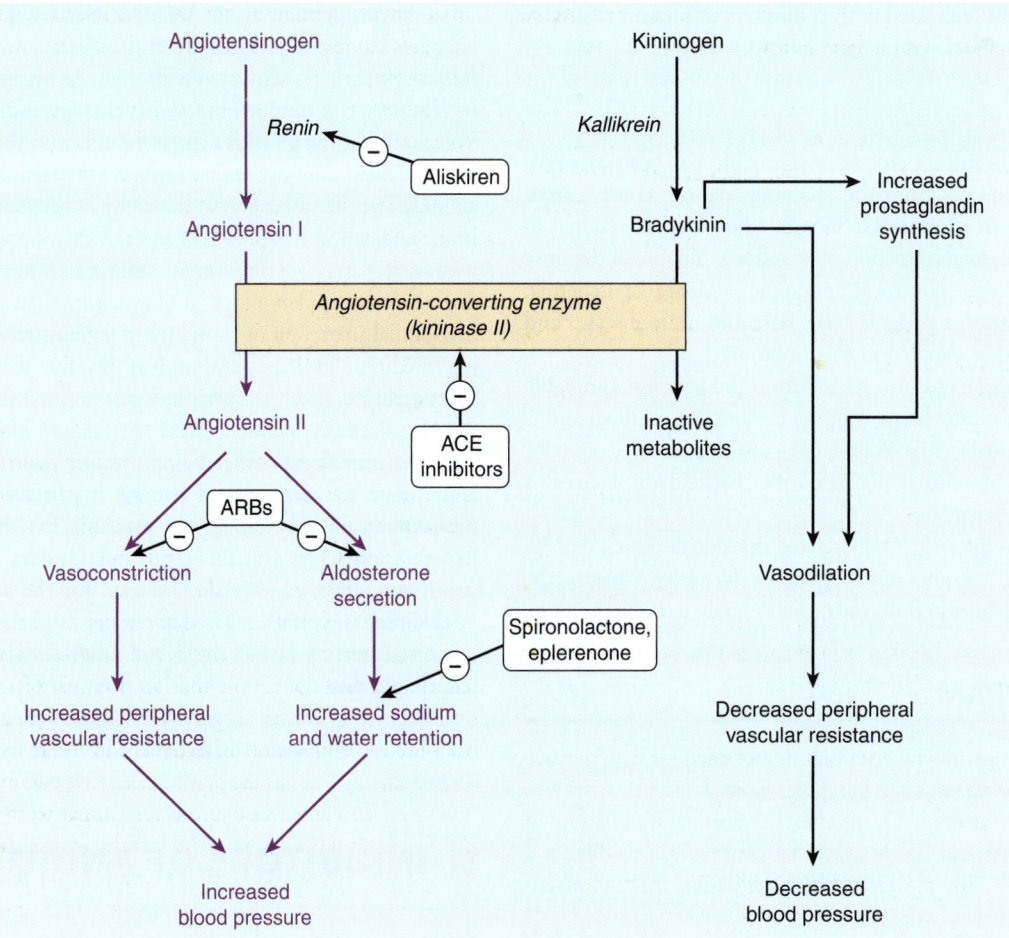

FIGURE 11–5 Sites of action of drugs that interfere with the renin-angiotensin-aldosterone system. ACE, angiotensin-converting enzyme; ARBs, angiotensin receptor blockers.

A parallel system for angiotensin generation exists in several other tissues (eg, heart) and may be responsible for trophic changes such as cardiac hypertrophy. The converting enzyme involved in tissue angiotensin II synthesis is also inhibited by ACE inhibitors.

Three classes of drugs act specifically on the renin-angiotensin system: ACE inhibitors; the competitive inhibitors of angiotensin at its receptors, including losartan and other nonpeptide antagonists; and aliskiren, an orally active renin antagonist (see Chapter 17). A fourth group of drugs, the aldosterone receptor inhibitors (eg, spironolactone, eplerenone) are discussed with the diuretics. In addition, β blockers, as noted earlier, can reduce renin secretion.

ANGIOTENSIN-CONVERTING ENZYME (ACE) INHIBITORS

Captopril and other drugs in this class inhibit the converting enzyme peptidyl dipeptidase that hydrolyzes angiotensin I to angiotensin II and (under the name plasma kininase) inactivates

bradykinin, a potent vasodilator, which works at least in part by stimulating release of nitric oxide and prostacyclin. The hypotensive activity of captopril results both from an inhibitory action on the renin-angiotensin system and a stimulating action on the kallikrein-kinin system (Figure 11–5). The latter mechanism has been demonstrated by showing that a bradykinin receptor antagonist, **icatibant** (see Chapter 17), blunts the blood pressure-lowering effect of captopril.

Enalapril is an oral prodrug that is converted by hydrolysis to a converting enzyme inhibitor, enalaprilat, with effects similar to those of captopril. Enalaprilat itself is available only for intravenous use, primarily for hypertensive emergencies. Lisinopril is a lysine derivative of enalaprilat. **Benazepril, fosinopril, moexipril, perindopril, quinapril, ramipril,** and **trandolapril** are other long-acting members of the class. All are prodrugs, like enalapril, and are converted to the active agents by hydrolysis, primarily in the liver.

Angiotensin II inhibitors lower blood pressure principally by decreasing peripheral vascular resistance. Cardiac output and heart rate are not significantly changed. Unlike direct vasodilators, these agents do not result in reflex sympathetic activation and can be used safely in persons with ischemic heart disease. The absence of reflex tachycardia may be due to downward resetting of the baroreceptors or to enhanced parasympathetic activity.

Although converting enzyme inhibitors are most effective in conditions associated with high plasma renin activity, there is no good correlation among subjects between plasma renin activity and antihypertensive response. Accordingly, renin profiling is unnecessary.

ACE inhibitors have a particularly useful role in treating patients with chronic kidney disease because they diminish proteinuria and stabilize renal function (even in the absence of lowering of blood pressure). This effect is particularly valuable in diabetes, and these drugs are now recommended in diabetes even in the absence of hypertension. These benefits probably result from improved intrarenal hemodynamics, with decreased glomerular efferent arteriolar resistance and a resulting reduction of intraglomerular capillary pressure. ACE inhibitors have also proved to be extremely useful in the treatment of heart failure, and after myocardial infarction, and there is recent evidence that ACE inhibitors reduce the incidence of diabetes in patients with high cardiovascular risk (see Chapter 13).

Pharmacokinetics & Dosage

Captopril's pharmacokinetic parameters and dosing recommendations are set forth in Table 11–2. Peak concentrations of enalaprilat, the active metabolite of enalapril, occur 3–4 hours after dosing with enalapril. The half-life of enalaprilat is about 11 hours. Typical doses of enalapril are 10–20 mg once or twice daily. Lisinopril has a half-life of 12 hours. Doses of 10–80 mg once daily are effective in most patients. All of the ACE inhibitors except fosinopril and moexipril are eliminated primarily by the kidneys; doses of these drugs should be reduced in patients with renal insufficiency.

Toxicity

Severe hypotension can occur after initial doses of any ACE inhibitor in patients who are hypovolemic as a result of diuretics, salt restriction, or gastrointestinal fluid loss. Other adverse effects common to all ACE inhibitors include acute renal failure (particularly in patients with bilateral renal artery stenosis or stenosis of the renal artery of a solitary kidney), hyperkalemia, dry cough sometimes accompanied by wheezing, and angioedema. Hyperkalemia is more likely to occur in patients with renal insufficiency or diabetes. Bradykinin and substance P seem to be responsible for the cough and angioedema seen with ACE inhibition.

ACE inhibitors are contraindicated during the second and third trimesters of pregnancy because of the risk of fetal hypotension, anuria, and renal failure, sometimes associated with fetal malformations or death. Recent evidence also implicates first-trimester exposure to ACE inhibitors in increased teratogenic risk. Captopril, particularly when given in high doses to patients with renal insufficiency, may cause neutropenia or proteinuria. Minor toxic effects seen more typically include altered sense of taste, allergic skin rashes, and drug fever, which may occur in up to 10% of patients.

Important drug interactions include those with potassium supplements or potassium-sparing diuretics, which can result in hyperkalemia. Nonsteroidal anti-inflammatory drugs may impair the hypotensive effects of ACE inhibitors by blocking bradykinin-mediated vasodilation, which is at least in part, prostaglandin mediated.

ANGIOTENSIN RECEPTOR-BLOCKING AGENTS

Losartan and **valsartan** were the first marketed blockers of the angiotensin II type 1 (AT_1) receptor. **Candesartan, eprosartan, irbesartan, telmisartan,** and **olmesartan** are also available. They have no effect on bradykinin metabolism and are therefore more selective blockers of angiotensin effects than ACE inhibitors. They also have the potential for more complete inhibition of angiotensin action compared with ACE inhibitors because there are enzymes other than ACE that are capable of generating angiotensin II. Angiotensin receptor blockers provide benefits similar to those of ACE inhibitors in patients with heart failure and chronic kidney disease. Losartan's pharmacokinetic parameters are listed in Table 11–2. The adverse effects are similar to those described for ACE inhibitors, including the hazard of use during pregnancy. Cough and angioedema can occur but are less common with angiotensin receptor blockers than with ACE inhibitors.

■ CLINICAL PHARMACOLOGY OF ANTIHYPERTENSIVE AGENTS

Hypertension presents a unique problem in therapeutics. It is usually a lifelong disease that causes few symptoms until the advanced stage. For effective treatment, medicines that may be expensive and sometimes produce adverse effects must be consumed daily. Thus, the physician must establish with certainty that hypertension is persistent and requires treatment and must exclude secondary causes of hypertension that might be treated by definitive surgical procedures. Persistence of hypertension, particularly in persons with mild elevation of blood pressure, should be established by finding an elevated blood pressure on at least three different office visits. Ambulatory blood pressure monitoring may be the best predictor of risk and therefore of need for therapy in mild hypertension. Isolated systolic hypertension and hypertension in the elderly also benefit from therapy.

Once the presence of hypertension is established, the question of whether to treat and which drugs to use must be considered. The level of blood pressure, the age of the patient, the severity of organ damage (if any) due to high blood pressure, and the presence of cardiovascular risk factors all must be considered. Assessment of renal function and the presence of proteinuria are useful in antihypertensive drug selection. At this stage, the patient must be educated about the nature of hypertension and the importance of treatment so that he or she can make an informed decision regarding therapy.

Once the decision is made to treat, a therapeutic regimen must be developed. Selection of drugs is dictated by the level of blood pressure, the presence and severity of end organ damage, and the presence of other diseases. Severe high blood pressure with life-threatening complications requires more rapid treatment with more efficacious drugs. Most patients with essential hypertension, however, have had elevated blood pressure for months or years, and therapy is best initiated in a gradual fashion.

Education about the natural history of hypertension and the importance of treatment compliance as well as potential adverse effects of drugs is essential. Obesity should be treated and drugs that increase blood pressure (sympathomimetic decongestants, nonsteroidal anti-inflammatory drugs, oral contraceptives, and some herbal medications) should be eliminated if possible. Follow-up visits should be frequent enough to convince the patient that the physician thinks the illness is serious. With each follow-up visit, the importance of treatment should be reinforced and questions concerning dosing or side effects of medication encouraged. Other factors that may improve compliance are simplifying dosing regimens and having the patient monitor blood pressure at home.

OUTPATIENT THERAPY OF HYPERTENSION

The initial step in treating hypertension may be nonpharmacologic. As discussed previously, sodium restriction may be effective treatment for many patients with mild hypertension. The average American diet contains about 200 mEq of sodium per day. A reasonable dietary goal in treating hypertension is 70–100 mEq of sodium per day, which can be achieved by not salting food during or after cooking and by avoiding processed foods that contain large amounts of sodium. Eating a diet rich in fruits, vegetables, and low-fat dairy products with a reduced content of saturated and total fat, and moderation of alcohol intake (no more than two drinks per day) also lower blood pressure.

Weight reduction even without sodium restriction has been shown to normalize blood pressure in up to 75% of overweight patients with mild to moderate hypertension. Regular exercise has been shown in some but not all studies to lower blood pressure in hypertensive patients.

For pharmacologic management of mild hypertension, blood pressure can be normalized in many patients with a single drug. However, most patients with hypertension require two or more antihypertensive medications (see Box: Resistant Hypertension & Polypharmacy). Thiazide diuretics, β blockers, ACE inhibitors, angiotensin receptor blockers, and calcium channel blockers have all been shown to reduce complications of hypertension and may be used for initial drug therapy. There has been concern that diuretics, by adversely affecting the serum lipid profile or impairing

glucose tolerance, may add to the risk of coronary disease, thereby offsetting the benefit of blood pressure reduction. However, a recent large clinical trial comparing different classes of antihypertensive mediations for initial therapy found that chlorthalidone (a thiazide diuretic) was as effective as other agents in reducing coronary heart disease death and nonfatal myocardial infarction, and was superior to amlodipine in preventing heart failure and superior to lisinopril in preventing stroke.

The presence of concomitant disease should influence selection of antihypertensive drugs because two diseases may benefit from a single drug. For example, drugs that inhibit the renin-angiotensin system are particularly useful in patients with diabetes or evidence of chronic kidney disease with proteinuria. Beta blockers or calcium channel blockers are useful in patients who also have angina; diuretics, ACE inhibitors, angiotensin receptor blockers, β blockers or hydralazine combined with nitrates in patients who also have heart failure; and α_1 blockers in men who have benign prostatic hyperplasia. Race may also affect drug selection: African Americans respond better on average to diuretics and calcium channel blockers than to β blockers and ACE inhibitors. Ethnic Chinese patients are more sensitive to the effects of β blockers and may require lower doses.

If a single drug does not adequately control blood pressure, drugs with different sites of action can be combined to effectively lower blood pressure while minimizing toxicity ("stepped care"). If a diuretic is not used initially, it is often selected as the second drug. If three drugs are required, combining a diuretic, a sympathoplegic agent or an ACE inhibitor, and a direct vasodilator (eg, hydralazine or a calcium channel blocker) is often effective. In the USA, fixed-dose drug combinations containing a β blocker, an ACE inhibitor, or an angiotensin receptor blocker plus a thiazide, and a calcium channel blocker plus an ACE inhibitor are available. Fixed-dose combinations have the drawback of not allowing for titration of individual drug doses but have the advantage of allowing fewer pills to be taken, potentially enhancing compliance.

Assessment of blood pressure during office visits should include measurement of recumbent, sitting, and standing pressures. An attempt should be made to normalize blood pressure in the posture or activity level that is customary for the patient. The large Hypertension Optimal Treatment study suggests that the optimal blood pressure end point is 138/83 mm Hg. Lowering blood pressure below this level produces no further benefit. In diabetic patients, however, there is a continued reduction of event rates with progressively lower blood pressures. Systolic hypertension (> 140 mm Hg in the presence of normal diastolic blood pressure) is a strong cardiovascular risk factor in people older than 50 years of age and should be treated.

In addition to noncompliance with medication, causes of failure to respond to drug therapy include excessive sodium intake and inadequate diuretic therapy with excessive blood volume, and drugs such as tricyclic antidepressants, nonsteroidal anti-inflammatory drugs, over-the-counter sympathomimetics, abuse of stimulants (amphetamine or cocaine), or excessive doses of caffeine and oral contraceptives that can interfere with actions of some antihypertensive drugs or directly raise blood pressure.

MANAGEMENT OF HYPERTENSIVE EMERGENCIES

Despite the large number of patients with chronic hypertension, hypertensive emergencies are relatively rare. Marked or sudden elevation of blood pressure may be a serious threat to life, however, and prompt control of blood pressure is indicated. Most frequently, hypertensive emergencies occur in patients whose hypertension is severe and poorly controlled and in those who suddenly discontinue antihypertensive medications.

Clinical Presentation & Pathophysiology

Hypertensive emergencies include hypertension associated with vascular damage (termed malignant hypertension) and hypertension associated with hemodynamic complications such as heart failure, stroke, or dissecting aortic aneurysm. The underlying pathologic process in malignant hypertension is a progressive arteriopathy with inflammation and necrosis of arterioles. Vascular lesions occur in the kidney, which releases renin, which in turn stimulates production of angiotensin and aldosterone, which further increase blood pressure.

Hypertensive encephalopathy is a classic feature of malignant hypertension. Its clinical presentation consists of severe headache, mental confusion, and apprehension. Blurred vision, nausea and vomiting, and focal neurologic deficits are common. If untreated, the syndrome may progress over a period of 12–48 hours to convulsions, stupor, coma, and even death.

Treatment of Hypertensive Emergencies

The general management of hypertensive emergencies requires monitoring the patient in an intensive care unit with continuous recording of arterial blood pressure. Fluid intake and output must be monitored carefully and body weight measured daily as an indicator of total body fluid volume during the course of therapy.

Parenteral antihypertensive medications are used to lower blood pressure rapidly (within a few hours); as soon as reasonable blood pressure control is achieved, oral antihypertensive therapy should be substituted because this allows smoother long-term management of hypertension. The goal of treatment in the first few hours or days is not complete normalization of blood pressure because chronic hypertension is associated with autoregulatory changes in cerebral blood flow. Thus, rapid normalization of blood pressure may lead to cerebral hypoperfusion and brain injury. Rather, blood pressure should be lowered by about 25%, maintaining diastolic blood pressure at no less than 100–110 mm Hg. Subsequently, blood pressure can be reduced to normal levels using oral medications over several weeks. The drug most commonly used to treat hypertensive emergencies is the vasodilator sodium nitroprusside. Other parenteral drugs that may be effective include fenoldopam, nitroglycerin, labetalol, calcium channel blockers, diazoxide, and hydralazine. Esmolol is often used to manage intraoperative and postoperative hypertension. Diuretics such as furosemide are administered to prevent the volume expansion that typically occurs during administration of powerful vasodilators.

SUMMARY Drugs Used in Hypertension

Subclass	Mechanism of Action	Effects	Clinical Applications	Pharmacokinetics, Toxicities, Interactions
DIURETICS				
• Thiazides: Hydrochlorothiazide	Block Na/Cl transporter in renal distal convoluted tubule	Reduce blood volume and poorly understood vascular effects	Hypertension, mild heart failure	
• Loop diuretics: Furosemide	Block Na/K/2Cl transporter in renal loop of Henle	Like thiazides • greater efficacy	Severe hypertension, heart failure	See Chapter 15
• Spironolactone	Block aldosterone receptor in renal collecting tubule	Increase Na and decrease K excretion • poorly understood reduction in heart failure mortality	Aldosteronism, heart failure, hypertension	
• Eplerenone				
SYMPATHOPLEGICS, CENTRALLY ACTING				
• Clonidine, methyl dopa	Activate α_2 adrenoceptors	Reduce central sympathetic outflow • reduce norepinephrine release from noradrenergic nerve endings	Hypertension • clonidine also used in withdrawal from abused drugs	Oral • clonidine also patch • Toxicity: sedation • methyldopa hemolytic anemia
SYMPATHETIC NERVE TERMINAL BLOCKERS				
• Reserpine	Blocks vesicular amine transporter in noradrenergic nerves and depletes transmitter stores	Reduce all sympathetic effects, especially cardiovascular, and reduce blood pressure	Hypertension but rarely used	Oral • long duration (days) • Toxicity: Reserpine: psychiatric depression, gastrointestinal disturbances
• Guanethidine	Interferes with amine release and replaces norepinephrine in vesicles	Same as reserpine	Same as reserpine	Guanethidine: Severe orthostatic hypotension • sexual dysfunction

(continued)

Subclass	Mechanism of Action	Effects	Clinical Applications	Pharmacokinetics, Toxicities, Interactions
α BLOCKERS				
• Prazosin • Terazosin • Doxazosin	Selectively block α_1 adrenoceptors	Prevent sympathetic vasoconstriction • reduce prostatic smooth muscle tone	Hypertension • benign prostatic hyperplasia	Oral • *Toxicity:* Orthostatic hypotension
β BLOCKERS				
• Metoprolol, others • Carvedilol	Block β_1 receptors; carvedilol also blocks α receptors	Prevent sympathetic cardiac stimulation • reduce renin secretion	Hypertension • heart failure	See Chapter 10
• *Propranolol: Nonselective prototype β blocker* • *Atenolol: Very widely used β_1-selective blocker*				
VASODILATORS				
• Verapamil • Diltiazem	Nonselective block of L-type calcium channels	Reduce cardiac rate and output • reduce vascular resistance	Hypertension, angina, arrhythmias	See Chapter 12
• Nifedipine, amlodipine, other dihydropyridines	Block vascular calcium channels > cardiac calcium channels	Reduce vascular resistance	Hypertension, angina	See Chapter 12
• Hydralazine	Causes nitric oxide release	Vasodilation • reduce vascular resistance • arterioles more sensitive than veins • reflex tachycardia	Hypertension • minoxidil also used to treat hair loss	Oral • *Toxicity:* Angina, tachycardia • Hydralazine: Lupus-like syndrome
• Minoxidil	Metabolite opens K channels in vascular smooth muscle			Minoxidil: Hypertrichosis
PARENTERAL AGENTS				
• Nitroprusside • Fenoldopam • Diazoxide • Labetalol	Releases nitric oxide Activates D_1 receptors Opens K channels α, β blocker	Powerful vasodilation	Hypertensive emergencies	Parenteral • short duration • *Toxicity:* Excessive hypotension, shock
ANGIOTENSIN-CONVERTING ENZYME (ACE) INHIBITORS				
• Captopril, many others	Inhibit angiotensin-converting enzyme	Reduce angiotensin II levels • reduce vasoconstriction and aldosterone secretion • increase bradykinin	Hypertension • heart failure, diabetes	Oral • *Toxicity:* Cough, angioedema • hyperkalemia • renal impairment • teratogenic
ANGIOTENSIN RECEPTOR BLOCKERS (ARBs)				
• Losartan, many others	Block AT_1 angiotensin receptors	Same as ACE inhibitors but no increase in bradykinin	Hypertension • heart failure	Oral • *Toxicity:* Same as ACE inhibitors but less cough
RENIN INHIBITOR				
• Aliskiren	Inhibits enzyme activity of renin	Reduces angiotensin I and II and aldosterone	Hypertension	Oral • *Toxicity:* Hyperkalemia, renal impairment • potential teratogen

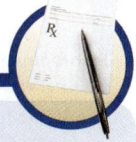

PREPARATIONS AVAILABLE

BETA-ADRENOCEPTOR BLOCKERS

Acebutolol (generic, Sectral)
Oral: 200, 400 mg capsules

Atenolol (generic, Tenormin)
Oral: 25, 50, 100 mg tablets
Parenteral: 0.5 mg/mL for injection

Betaxolol (Kerlone)
Oral: 10, 20 mg tablets

Bisoprolol (Zebeta)
Oral: 5, 10 mg tablets

Carteolol (Cartrol)
Oral: 2.5, 5 mg tablets

Carvedilol (Coreg)
Oral: 3.125, 6.25, 12.5, 25 mg tablets; 10, 20, 40, 80 mg extended-release capsules

Esmolol (BreviBloc)
Parenteral: 10, 250 mg/mL for injection

Labetalol (generic, Normodyne, Trandate)
Oral: 100, 200, 300 mg tablets
Parenteral: 5 mg/mL for injection

Metoprolol (generic, Lopressor)
Oral: 50, 100 mg tablets
Oral extended-release (Toprol-XL): 25, 50, 100, 200 mg tablets
Parenteral: 1 mg/mL for injection

Nadolol (generic, Corgard)
Oral: 20, 40, 80, 120, 160 mg tablets

Nebivolol (Bystolic)
Oral: 2.5, 5, 10 mg tablets

Penbutolol (Levatol)
Oral: 20 mg tablets

Pindolol (generic, Visken)
Oral: 5, 10 mg tablets

Propranolol (generic, Inderal)
Oral: 10, 20, 40, 60, 80, 90 mg tablets; 4, 8 mg/mL oral solution; Intensol, 80 mg/mL solution
Oral sustained-release (generic, Inderal LA): 60, 80, 120, 160 mg capsules
Parenteral: 1 mg/mL for injection

Timolol (generic, Blocadren)
Oral: 5, 10, 20 mg tablets

CENTRALLY ACTING SYMPATHOPLEGIC DRUGS

Clonidine (generic, Catapres)
Oral: 0.1, 0.2, 0.3 mg tablets
Transdermal (Catapres-TTS): patches that release 0.1, 0.2, 0.3 mg/24 h

Guanabenz (generic, Wytensin)
Oral: 4, 8 mg tablets

Guanfacine (Tenex)
Oral: 1, 2 mg tablets

Methyldopa (generic)
Oral: 250, 500 mg tablets
Parenteral (Methyldopate HCl): 50 mg/mL for injection

POSTGANGLIONIC SYMPATHETIC NERVE TERMINAL BLOCKERS

Guanadrel (Hylorel)
Oral: 10, 25 mg tablets

Guanethidine (Ismelin)
Oral: 10, 25 mg tablets

Reserpine (generic)
Oral: 0.1, 0.25 mg tablets

ALPHA$_1$-SELECTIVE ADRENOCEPTOR BLOCKERS

Doxazosin (generic, Cardura)
Oral: 1, 2, 4, 8 mg tablets

Prazosin (generic, Minipress)
Oral: 1, 2, 5 mg capsules

Terazosin (generic, Hytrin)
Oral: 1, 2, 5, 10 mg capsules and tablets

GANGLION-BLOCKING AGENTS

Mecamylamine (Inversine)
Oral: 2.5 mg tablets

VASODILATORS USED IN HYPERTENSION

Diazoxide (Hyperstat IV)
Parenteral: 15 mg/mL ampule
Oral (Proglycem): 50 mg capsule; 50 mg/mL oral suspension (for insulinoma)

Fenoldopam (generic, Corlopam)
Parenteral: 10 mg/mL for IV infusion

Hydralazine (generic, Apresoline)
Oral: 10, 25, 50, 100 mg tablets
Parenteral: 20 mg/mL for injection

Minoxidil (generic, Loniten)
Oral: 2.5, 10 mg tablets
Topical (generic, Rogaine): 2% lotion

Nitroprusside (generic, Nitropress)
Parenteral: 50 mg/vial

CALCIUM CHANNEL BLOCKERS

Amlodipine (generic, Norvasc)
Oral 2.5, 5, 10 mg tablets

Clevidipine (Cleviprex)
Parenteral: 0.5 mg/mL emulsion for injection

Diltiazem (generic, Cardizem)
Oral: 30, 60, 90, 120 mg tablets (unlabeled in hypertension)
Oral sustained-release (Cardizem CD, Cardizem SR, Dilacor XL): 60, 90, 120, 180, 240, 300, 360, 420 mg capsules
Parenteral: 5 mg/mL for injection

Felodipine (generic, Plendil)
Oral extended-release: 2.5, 5, 10 mg tablets

Isradipine (generic, DynaCirc)
Oral: 2.5, 5 mg capsules; 5, 10 mg controlled-release tablets

Nicardipine (generic, Cardene)
Oral: 20, 30 mg capsules
Oral sustained-release (Cardene SR): 30, 45, 60 mg capsules
Parenteral (Cardene I.V.): 0.1, 2.5 mg/mL for injection

Nifedipine (generic, Adalat, Procardia)
Oral: 10, 20 mg capsules (off-label use in hypertension)

Oral extended-release (Adalat CC, Procardia-XL): 30, 60, 90 mg tablets

Nisoldipine (Sular)
Oral extended-release: 8.5, 17, 25.5, 34 mg tablets

Verapamil (generic, Calan, Isoptin)
Oral: 40, 80, 120 mg tablets
Oral sustained-release (generic, Calan SR, Verelan): 120, 180, 240 mg tablets; 100, 120, 180, 200, 240, 300, 360 mg capsules
Parenteral: 2.5 mg/mL for injection

ANGIOTENSIN-CONVERTING ENZYME INHIBITORS

Benazepril (generic, Lotensin)
Oral: 5, 10, 20, 40 mg tablets

Captopril (generic, Capoten)
Oral: 12.5, 25, 50, 100 mg tablets

Enalapril (generic, Vasotec)
Oral: 2.5, 5, 10, 20 mg tablets
Parenteral (Enalaprilat): 1.25 mg/mL for injection

Fosinopril (generic, Monopril)
Oral: 10, 20, 40 mg tablets

Lisinopril (generic, Prinivil, Zestril)
Oral: 2.5, 5, 10, 20, 40 mg tablets

Moexipril (generic, Univasc)
Oral: 7.5, 15 mg tablets

Perindopril (Aceon)
Oral: 2, 4, 8 mg tablets

Quinapril (Accupril)
Oral: 5, 10, 20, 40 mg tablets

Ramipril (Altace)
Oral: 1.25, 2.5, 5, 10 mg capsules

Trandolapril (Mavik)
Oral: 1, 2, 4 mg tablets

ANGIOTENSIN RECEPTOR BLOCKERS

Azilsartan (Edarbi)
Oral: 40, 80 mg tablets

Candesartan (Atacand)
Oral: 4, 8, 16, 32 mg tablets

Eprosartan (Teveten)
Oral: 600 mg tablets

Irbesartan (Avapro)
Oral: 75, 150, 300 mg tablets

Losartan (Cozaar)
Oral: 25, 50, 100 mg tablets

Olmesartan (Benicar)
Oral: 5, 20, 40 mg tablets

Telmisartan (Micardis)
Oral: 20, 40, 80 mg tablets

Valsartan (Diovan)
Oral: 40, 80, 160, 320 mg tablet

RENIN INHIBITOR

Aliskiren (Tekturna)
Oral: 150, 300 mg tablets

REFERENCES

ACE Inhibitors in Diabetic Nephropathy Trialist Group: Should all patients with type 1 diabetes mellitus and microalbuminuria receive angiotensin-converting enzyme inhibitors? A meta-analysis of individual patient data. Ann Intern Med 2001;134:370.

ALLHAT Officers and Coordinators for the ALLHAT Collaborative Research Group: Major outcomes of high-risk hypertensive patients randomized to angiotensin-converting enzyme inhibitor or calcium channel blockers vs diuretic: The antihypertensive and lipid-lowering treatment to prevent heart attack trial. JAMA 2002;288:2981.

Appel LJ et al: The importance of population-wide sodium reduction as a means to prevent cardiovascular disease and stroke: A call to action from the American Heart Association. Circulation 2011;123:1138.

Appel LJ et al: Intensive blood-pressure control in hypertensive chronic kidney disease. N Engl J Med 2010;363:918.

Appel LJ et al: Effects of comprehensive lifestyle modification on blood pressure control: Main results of the PREMIER clinical trial. JAMA 2003;289:2083.

Aronow WS et al: ACCF/AHA 2011 Expert consensus document on hypertension in the elderly: A report of the American College of Cardiology Foundation Task Force on Clinical Expert Consensus Documents. Circulation 2011; 123:2434.

Aronson S et al: The ECLIPSE trials: Comparative studies of clevidipine to nitroglycerin, sodium nitroprusside, and nicardipine for acute hypertension in cardiac surgery patients. Anesth Alang 2008;107:1110.

August P: Initial treatment of hypertension. N Engl J Med 2003;348:610.

Bangalore S et al: Beta-blockers for primary prevention of heart failure in patients with hypertension: Insights from a meta-analysis. J Am Coll Cardiol 2008;52:1062.

Calhoun DA et al: Resistant hypertension: Diagnosis, evaluation, and treatment: A scientific statement from the American Heart Association Professional Education Committee of the Council for High Blood Pressure Research. Circulation 2008;117:e510.

Chobanian AV et al: The Seventh report of the Joint National Committee on Prevention, Detection, Evaluation, and Treatment of High Blood Pressure. JAMA 2003;289:2560.

Egan BM et al: US trends in prevalence, awareness, treatment, and control of hypertension, 1988-2008. JAMA 2010;303:2043.

Esler MD et al: Renal sympathetic denervation in patients with treatment-resistant hypertension (The Symplicity HTN-2 Trial): A randomised controlled trial. Lancet 2010;376:1903.

Garg J, Messerli AW, Bakris GL: Evaluation and treatment of patients with systemic hypertension. Circulation 2002;105:2458.

Hajjar I et al: Hypertension, white matter hyperintensities, and concurrent impairments in mobility, cognition, and mood: The Cardiovascular Health Study. Circulation 2011;123:858.

Heran BS et al: Blood pressure lowering efficacy of angiotensin converting enzyme (ACE) inhibitors for primary hypertension. Cochrane Database Syst Rev 2008;(4):CD003823.

Jamerson K et al: Benazepril plus amlodipine or hydrochlorothiazide for hypertension in high-risk patients. N Engl J Med 2008;359:2417.

Khan NA et al: The 2008 Canadian Hypertension Education Program recommendations for the management of hypertension: Part 2—therapy. Can J Cardiol 2008;24:465.

Krum H et al: Device-based antihypertensive therapy: Therapeutic modulation of the autonomic nervous system. Circulation 2011;123:209.

Mark PE, Varon J: Hypertensive crisis. Challenges and management. Chest 2007;131:1949.

Mauer M et al: Renal and retinal effects of enalapril and losartan in type 1 diabetes. N Engl J Med 2009;361:40.

Moser M, Setaro JF: Resistant or difficult-to-control hypertension. N Engl J Med 2006;355:385.

Psaty BM et al: Health outcomes associated with various antihypertensive therapies used as first-line agents: A network meta-analysis. JAMA 2003;289:2534.

Ram CV: Angiotensin receptor blockers: Current status and future prospects. Am J Med 2008;121:656.

Sacks FM, Campos H: Dietary therapy in hypertension. N Engl J Med 2010;362:2102.

Thompson AM et al: Antihypertensive treatment and secondary prevention of cardiovascular disease events among persons without hypertension: A meta-analysis. JAMA 2011;305:913.

Verdecchia P et al: Angiotensin-converting enzyme inhibitors and calcium channel blockers for coronary heart disease and stroke prevention. Hypertension 2005;46:386.

Vermes E et al: Enalapril reduces the incidence of diabetes in patients with chronic heart failure: Insight from the Studies of Left Ventricular Dysfunction (SOLVD). Circulation 2003;107:1291.

Wang TJ, Ramachandran SV: Epidemiology of uncontrolled hypertension in the United States. Circulation 2005;112:1651.

Wing LMH et al: A comparison of outcomes with angiotensin-converting-enzyme inhibitors and diuretics for hypertension in the elderly. N Engl J Med 2003;348:583.

CASE STUDY ANSWER

The patient has JNC stage 1 hypertension (see Table 11-1). The first question in management is how urgent is it to treat the hypertension. Cardiovascular risk factors in this man include family history of early coronary disease and elevated cholesterol. Evidence of end-organ impact includes left ventricular enlargement on EKG. The strong family history suggests that this patient has essential hypertension. However, the patient should undergo the usual screening tests including renal function, thyroid function, and serum electrolyte measurements. An echocardiogram should also be considered to determine whether the patient has left ventricular hypertrophy secondary to valvular or other structural heart disease as opposed to hypertension.

Initial management in this patient can be behavioral, including dietary changes and aerobic exercise. However, most patients like this will require medication. Thiazide diuretics in low doses are inexpensive, have relatively few side effects, and are effective in many patients with mild hypertension. Other first-line agents include angiotensin-converting enzyme inhibitors and calcium channel blockers. Beta blockers might be considered if the patient had coronary disease or had labile hypertension. A single agent should be prescribed and the patient reassessed in a month. If a second agent is needed, one of the two agents should be a thiazide diuretic. Once blood pressure is controlled, patients should be followed periodically to reinforce the need for compliance with both lifestyle changes and medications.

12

Vasodilators & the Treatment of Angina Pectoris

Bertram G. Katzung, MD, PhD[*]

CASE STUDY

A 74-year-old man presents with a history of anterior chest pressure whenever he walks more than one block. The chest discomfort is diffuse, and he cannot localize it; sometimes it radiates to his lower jaw. The discomfort is more severe when he walks after meals but is relieved within 5–10 minutes when he stops walking. Assuming that a diagnosis of stable effort angina is correct, what medical treatments should be implemented to reduce the acute pain of an attack and to prevent future attacks?

Ischemic heart disease is one of the most common cardiovascular disease in developed countries, and angina pectoris is the most common condition involving tissue ischemia in which vasodilator drugs are used. The name *angina pectoris* denotes chest pain caused by accumulation of metabolites resulting from myocardial ischemia. The organic nitrates, eg, **nitroglycerin,** are the mainstay of therapy for the immediate relief of angina. Another group of vasodilators, the **calcium channel blockers,** is also important, especially for prophylaxis, and β **blockers,** which are *not* vasodilators, are also useful in prophylaxis. Several newer groups of drugs are under investigation, including drugs that alter myocardial metabolism and selective cardiac rate inhibitors.

By far the most common cause of angina is atheromatous obstruction of the large coronary vessels (coronary artery disease, CAD). Inadequate blood flow in the presence of CAD results in **effort angina,** also known as **classic angina.** However, transient spasm of localized portions of these vessels, which is usually associated with underlying atheromas, can also cause significant myocardial ischemia and pain (**vasospastic** or **variant angina**). Variant angina is also called **Prinzmetal** angina.

The primary cause of angina pectoris is an imbalance between the oxygen requirement of the heart and the oxygen supplied to it via the coronary vessels. In effort angina, the imbalance occurs when the myocardial oxygen requirement increases, especially during exercise, and coronary blood flow does not increase proportionately. The resulting ischemia usually leads to pain. In fact, coronary flow reserve is frequently impaired in such patients because of endothelial dysfunction, which is associated with impaired vasodilation. As a result, ischemia may occur at a lower level of myocardial oxygen demand. In some individuals, the ischemia is not always accompanied by pain, resulting in "silent" or "ambulatory" ischemia. In variant angina, oxygen delivery decreases as a result of reversible coronary vasospasm.

Unstable angina, an **acute coronary syndrome,** is said to be present when episodes of angina occur at rest and when there is an increase in the severity, frequency, and duration of chest pain in patients with previously stable angina. Unstable angina is caused by episodes of increased epicardial coronary artery resistance or small platelet clots occurring in the vicinity of an atherosclerotic plaque. In most cases, formation of labile partially occlusive thrombi at the site of a fissured or ulcerated plaque is the mechanism for reduction in flow. The course and the prognosis of unstable angina are variable, but this subset of acute coronary syndrome is associated with a high risk of myocardial infarction and death and is considered a medical emergency.

---

[*]The author thanks Dr. Kanu Chatterjee, MB, FRCP, who was coauthor of this chapter in prior editions.

In theory, the imbalance between oxygen delivery and myocardial oxygen demand can be corrected by **decreasing oxygen demand** or by **increasing delivery** (by increasing coronary flow). In effort angina, oxygen demand can be reduced by decreasing cardiac work or, according to some studies, by shifting myocardial metabolism to substrates that require less oxygen per unit of adenosine triphosphate (ATP) produced. In variant angina, on the other hand, spasm of coronary vessels can be reversed by nitrate or calcium channel-blocking vasodilators. Lipid-lowering drugs, especially the "statins," have become extremely important in the long-term treatment of atherosclerotic disease (see Chapter 35). In unstable angina, vigorous measures are taken to achieve both—increase oxygen delivery and decrease oxygen demand.

PATHOPHYSIOLOGY OF ANGINA

Determinants of Myocardial Oxygen Demand

The major determinants of myocardial oxygen requirement are set forth in Table 12–1. The effect of arterial blood pressure is mediated through its effect on wall stress. As a consequence of its continuous activity, the heart's oxygen needs are relatively high, and it extracts approximately 75% of the available oxygen even in the absence of stress. The myocardial oxygen requirement increases when there is an increase in heart rate, contractility, arterial pressure, or ventricular volume. These hemodynamic alterations frequently occur during physical exercise and sympathetic discharge, which often precipitate angina in patients with obstructive coronary artery disease.

Drugs that reduce cardiac size, rate, or force reduce cardiac oxygen demand. Thus, vasodilators, β blockers, and calcium blockers have predictable benefits in angina. A small, late component of sodium current helps to maintain the long plateau and prolong the calcium current of myocardial action potentials. Drugs that block this late sodium current can indirectly reduce calcium influx and consequently reduce cardiac contractile force. The heart favors fatty acids as a substrate for energy production. However, oxidation of fatty acids requires more oxygen per unit of ATP generated than oxidation of carbohydrates. Therefore, drugs that shift myocardial metabolism toward greater use of glucose (fatty acid oxidation inhibitors) have the potential, at least in theory, to reduce the oxygen demand without altering hemodynamics.

TABLE 12–1   Determinants of myocardial oxygen consumption.

Wall stress
Intraventricular pressure
Ventricular radius (volume)
Wall thickness
Heart rate
Contractility

Determinants of Coronary Blood Flow & Myocardial Oxygen Supply

Increased demand for oxygen in the normal heart is met by augmenting coronary blood flow. Coronary blood flow is directly related to the perfusion pressure (aortic diastolic pressure) and the duration of diastole. Because coronary flow drops to negligible values during systole, the duration of diastole becomes a limiting factor for myocardial perfusion during tachycardia. Coronary blood flow is inversely proportional to coronary vascular resistance. Resistance is determined mainly by intrinsic factors—including metabolic products and autonomic activity—and by various pharmacologic agents. Damage to the endothelium of coronary vessels has been shown to alter their ability to dilate and to increase coronary vascular resistance.

Determinants of Vascular Tone

Peripheral arteriolar and venous tone (smooth muscle tension) both play a role in determining myocardial wall stress (Table 12–1). Arteriolar tone directly controls peripheral vascular resistance and thus arterial blood pressure. In systole, intraventricular pressure must exceed aortic pressure to eject blood; arterial blood pressure thus determines the *systolic* wall stress in an important way. Venous tone determines the capacity of the venous circulation and controls the amount of blood sequestered in the venous system versus the amount returned to the heart. Venous tone thereby determines the *diastolic* wall stress.

The regulation of smooth muscle contraction and relaxation is shown schematically in Figure 12–1. The mechanisms of action of the major types of vasodilators are listed in Table 11–2. As shown in Figures 12–1 and 12–2, drugs may relax vascular smooth muscle in several ways:

1. **Increasing cGMP:** As indicated in Figures 12–1 and 12–2, cGMP facilitates the dephosphorylation of myosin light chains, preventing the interaction of myosin with actin. **Nitric oxide** is an effective activator of soluble guanylyl cyclase and acts mainly through this mechanism. Important molecular donors of nitric oxide include **nitroprusside** (see Chapters 11 and 19) and the organic **nitrates** used in angina.

2. **Decreasing intracellular Ca^{2+}: Calcium channel blockers** predictably cause vasodilation because they reduce intracellular Ca^{2+}, a major modulator of the activation of myosin light chain kinase (Figure 12–1). **Beta blockers** and **calcium channel blockers** also reduce Ca^{2+} influx in cardiac muscle fibers, thereby reducing rate, contractility, and oxygen requirement under most circumstances.

3. **Stabilizing or preventing depolarization of the vascular smooth muscle cell membrane:** The membrane potential of excitable cells is stabilized near the resting potential by increasing potassium permeability. Potassium channel openers, such as minoxidil sulfate (see Chapter 11) increase the permeability of K^+ channels, probably ATP-dependent K^+ channels. Certain newer agents under investigation for use in angina (eg, **nicorandil**) may act, in part, by this mechanism.

4. **Increasing cAMP in vascular smooth muscle cells:** As shown in Figure 12–1, an increase in cAMP increases the rate of inactivation of myosin light chain kinase, the enzyme responsible

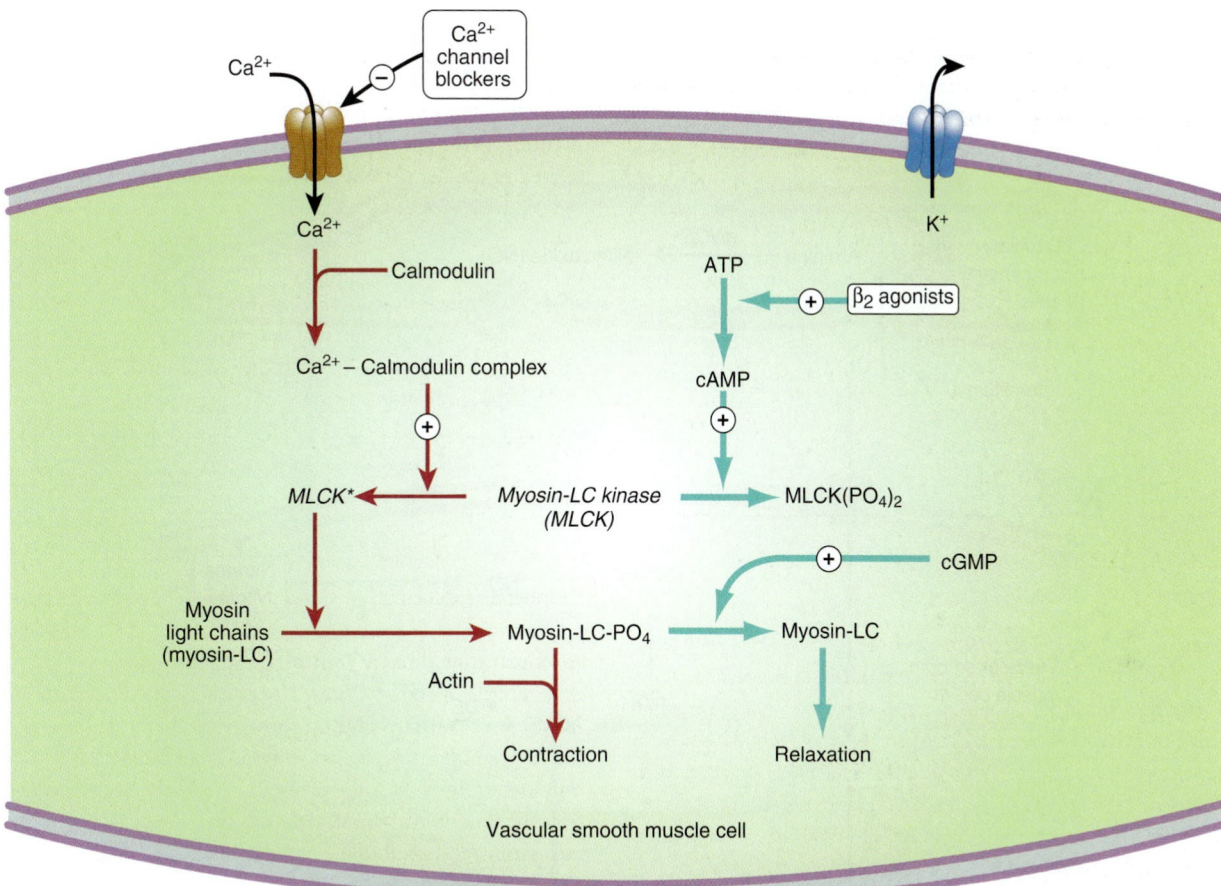

FIGURE 12–1 Control of smooth muscle contraction and site of action of calcium channel-blocking drugs. Contraction is triggered (red arrows) by influx of calcium (which can be blocked by calcium channel blockers) through transmembrane calcium channels. The calcium combines with calmodulin to form a complex that converts the enzyme myosin light-chain kinase to its active form (*MLCK**). The latter phosphorylates the myosin light chains, thereby initiating the interaction of myosin with actin. Other proteins, calponin and caldesmon (not shown), inhibit the ATPase activity of myosin during the relaxation of smooth muscle. Interaction with the Ca^{2+}-calmodulin complex reduces their interaction with myosin during the contraction cycle. Beta$_2$ agonists (and other substances that increase cAMP) may cause relaxation in smooth muscle (blue arrows) by accelerating the inactivation of MLCK and by facilitating the expulsion of calcium from the cell (not shown). cGMP facilitates relaxation by the mechanism shown in Figure 12–2.

for triggering the interaction of actin with myosin in these cells. This appears to be the mechanism of vasodilation caused by β$_2$ agonists, drugs that are *not* used in angina (because they cause too much cardiac stimulation), and by fenoldopam, a D$_1$ agonist used in hypertensive emergencies.

BASIC PHARMACOLOGY OF DRUGS USED TO TREAT ANGINA

Drug Action in Angina

The three drug groups traditionally used in angina (organic nitrates, calcium channel blockers, and β blockers) *decrease myocardial oxygen requirement* by decreasing the determinants of oxygen demand (heart rate, ventricular volume, blood pressure, and contractility). In some patients, the nitrates and the calcium channel blockers may cause a redistribution of coronary flow and *increase oxygen delivery*

to ischemic tissue. In variant angina, these two drug groups also increase myocardial oxygen delivery by reversing coronary artery spasm. The newer drugs, represented by ranolazine and ivabradine, are discussed later.

NITRATES & NITRITES

Chemistry

These agents are simple nitric and nitrous acid esters of polyalcohols. **Nitroglycerin** may be considered the prototype of the group. Although nitroglycerin is used in the manufacture of dynamite, the systemic formulations used in medicine are not explosive. The conventional sublingual tablet form of nitroglycerin may lose potency when stored as a result of volatilization and adsorption to plastic surfaces. Therefore, it should be kept in tightly closed glass containers. Nitroglycerin is not sensitive to light.

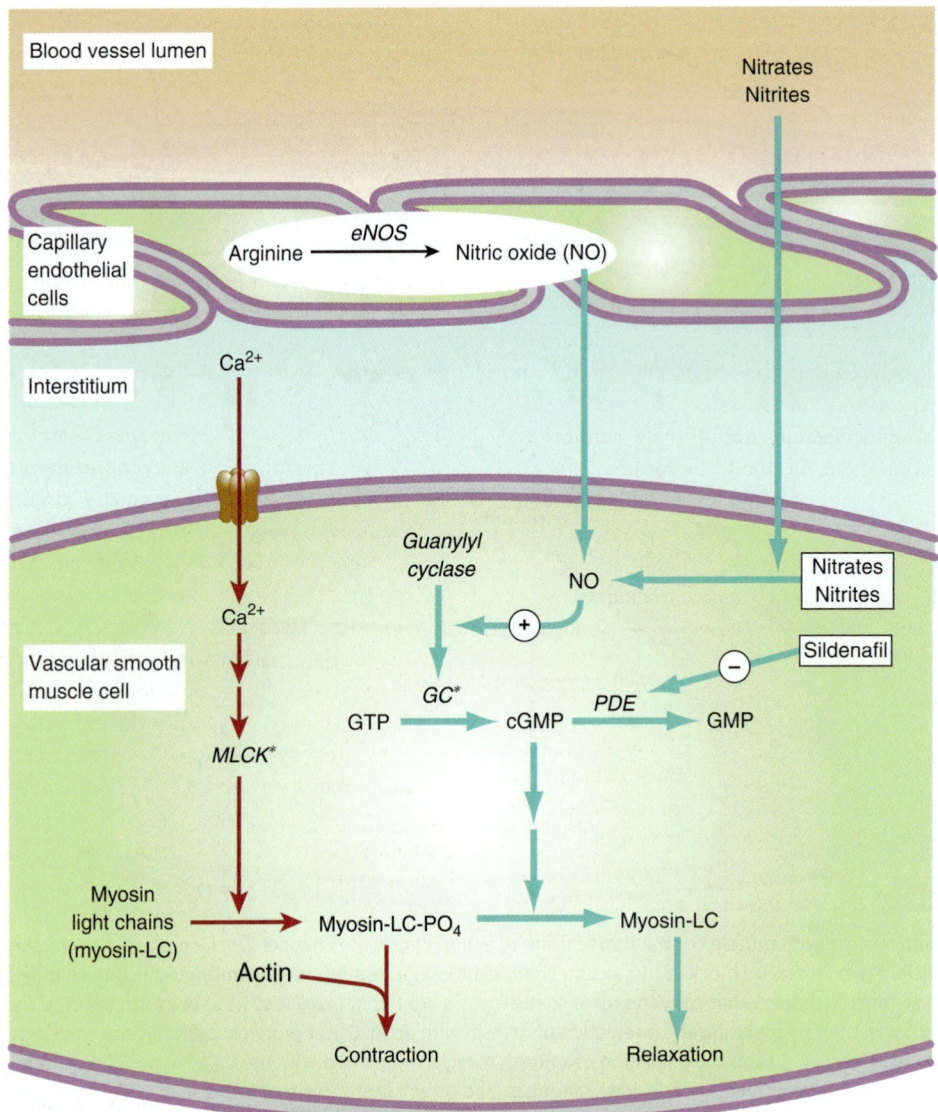

FIGURE 12–2 Mechanism of action of nitrates, nitrites, and other substances that increase the concentration of nitric oxide (NO) in vascular smooth muscle cells. Steps leading to relaxation are shown with blue arrows. MLCK*, activated myosin light-chain kinase (see Figure 12–1). GC*, activated guanylyl cyclase; PDE, phosphodiesterase; eNOS, endothelial nitric oxide synthase.

All therapeutically active agents in the nitrate group appear to have identical mechanisms of action and similar toxicities, although susceptibility to tolerance may vary. Therefore, pharmacokinetic factors govern the choice of agent and mode of therapy when using the nitrates.

$$H_2C - O - NO_2$$
$$HC - O - NO_2$$
$$H_2C - O - NO_2$$

Nitroglycerin
(glyceryl trinitrate)

Pharmacokinetics

The liver contains a high-capacity organic nitrate reductase that removes nitrate groups in a stepwise fashion from the parent molecule and ultimately inactivates the drug. Therefore, oral bioavailability of the traditional organic nitrates (eg, nitroglycerin and **isosorbide dinitrate**) is low (typically < 10–20%). For this reason, the sublingual route, which avoids the first-pass effect, is preferred for achieving a therapeutic blood level rapidly. Nitroglycerin and isosorbide dinitrate both are absorbed efficiently by this route and reach therapeutic blood levels within a few minutes. However, the total dose administered by this route must be limited to avoid excessive effect; therefore, the total duration of effect is brief (15–30 minutes). When much longer duration of action is needed, oral preparations can be given that contain an amount of drug sufficient to result in sustained systemic blood levels of the parent drug plus active metabolites. Other routes of administration available for nitroglycerin include transdermal and buccal absorption from slow-release preparations (described below).

Amyl nitrite and related nitrites are highly volatile liquids. Amyl nitrite is available in fragile glass ampules packaged in a protective cloth covering. The ampule can be crushed with the fingers, resulting in rapid release of vapors inhalable through the cloth covering. The inhalation route provides very rapid absorption and, like the sublingual route, avoids the hepatic first-pass effect. Because of its unpleasant odor and short duration of action, amyl nitrite is now obsolete for angina.

Once absorbed, the unchanged nitrate compounds have half-lives of only 2–8 minutes. The partially denitrated metabolites have much longer half-lives (up to 3 hours). Of the nitroglycerin metabolites (two dinitroglycerins and two mononitro forms), the 1,2-dinitro derivative has significant vasodilator efficacy and probably provides most of the therapeutic effect of orally administered nitroglycerin. The 5-mononitrate metabolite of isosorbide dinitrate is an active metabolite of the latter drug and is available for oral use as **isosorbide mononitrate**. It has a bioavailability of 100%.

Excretion, primarily in the form of glucuronide derivatives of the denitrated metabolites, is largely by way of the kidney.

Pharmacodynamics

A. Mechanism of Action in Smooth Muscle

After more than a century of study, the mechanism of action of nitroglycerin is still not fully understood. There is general agreement that the drug must be bioactivated with the release of nitric oxide. Unlike nitroprusside and some other direct nitric oxide donors, nitroglycerin activation requires enzymatic action. Nitroglycerin can be denitrated by glutathione S-transferase in smooth muscle and other cells. A mitochondrial enzyme, aldehyde dehydrogenase isoform 2 (ALDH2) and possibly isoform 3, ALDH3, is also capable of activating nitroglycerin and releasing nitric oxide. The differential selectivity of glutathione S-transferase and ALDH2 for different organic nitrates suggests that the ALDH2 may be the more important enzyme for nitroglycerin bioactivation. Free nitrite ion is released, which is then converted to **nitric oxide** (see Chapter 19). Nitric oxide (probably complexed with cysteine) combines with the heme group of soluble guanylyl cyclase, activating that enzyme and causing an increase in cGMP. As shown in Figure 12–2, formation of cGMP represents a first step toward smooth muscle relaxation. The production of prostaglandin E or prostacyclin (PGI$_2$) and membrane hyperpolarization may also be involved. There is no evidence that autonomic receptors are involved in the primary nitrate response. However, autonomic *reflex* responses, evoked when hypotensive doses are given, are common.

As described in the following text, tolerance is an important consideration in the use of nitrates. Although tolerance may be caused in part by a decrease in tissue sulfhydryl groups, eg, on cysteine, it can be only partially prevented or reversed with a sulfhydryl-regenerating agent. Increased generation of oxygen free radicals during nitrate therapy may be another important mechanism of tolerance. Recent evidence suggests that diminished availability of calcitonin gene-related peptide (CGRP, a potent vasodilator) is also associated with nitrate tolerance.

Nicorandil and several other investigational antianginal agents appear to combine the activity of nitric oxide release with potassium channel-opening action, thus providing an additional mechanism for causing vasodilation. Nitroglycerin has not been reported to open potassium channels.

B. Organ System Effects

Nitroglycerin relaxes all types of smooth muscle regardless of the cause of the preexisting muscle tone (Figure 12–3). It has practically no direct effect on cardiac or skeletal muscle.

1. Vascular smooth muscle—All segments of the vascular system from large arteries through large veins relax in response to nitroglycerin. Most evidence suggests a gradient of response, with veins responding at the lowest concentrations, arteries at slightly higher ones. The epicardial coronary arteries are sensitive, but concentric atheromas can prevent significant dilation. On the other hand, eccentric lesions permit an increase in flow when nitrates relax the smooth muscle on the side away from the lesion. Arterioles and precapillary sphincters are dilated least, partly because of reflex responses and partly because different vessels vary in their ability to release nitric oxide from the drug.

A primary direct result of an effective dose of nitroglycerin is marked relaxation of veins with increased venous capacitance and decreased ventricular preload. Pulmonary vascular pressures and heart size are significantly reduced. In the absence of heart failure, cardiac output is reduced. Because venous capacitance is increased, orthostatic hypotension may be marked and syncope can result. Dilation of large epicardial coronary arteries may improve oxygen delivery in the presence of eccentric atheromas. Temporal artery pulsations and a throbbing headache associated with meningeal artery pulsations are common effects of nitroglycerin and amyl nitrite. In heart failure, preload is often abnormally high; the nitrates and other vasodilators, by reducing preload, may have a beneficial effect on cardiac output in this condition (see Chapter 13).

The indirect effects of nitroglycerin consist of those compensatory responses evoked by baroreceptors and hormonal mechanisms responding to decreased arterial pressure (see Figure 6–7); this often results in tachycardia and increased cardiac contractility. Retention of salt and water may also be significant, especially with intermediate- and long-acting nitrates. These compensatory responses contribute to the development of tolerance.

In normal subjects without coronary disease, nitroglycerin can induce a significant, if transient, increase in total coronary blood flow. In contrast, there is no evidence that total coronary flow is increased in patients with angina due to atherosclerotic obstructive coronary artery disease. However, some studies suggest that *redistribution* of coronary flow from normal to ischemic regions may play a role in nitroglycerin's therapeutic effect. Nitroglycerin also exerts a weak negative inotropic effect on the heart via nitric oxide.

2. Other smooth muscle organs—Relaxation of smooth muscle of the bronchi, gastrointestinal tract (including biliary system), and genitourinary tract has been demonstrated experimentally. Because of their brief duration, these actions of the

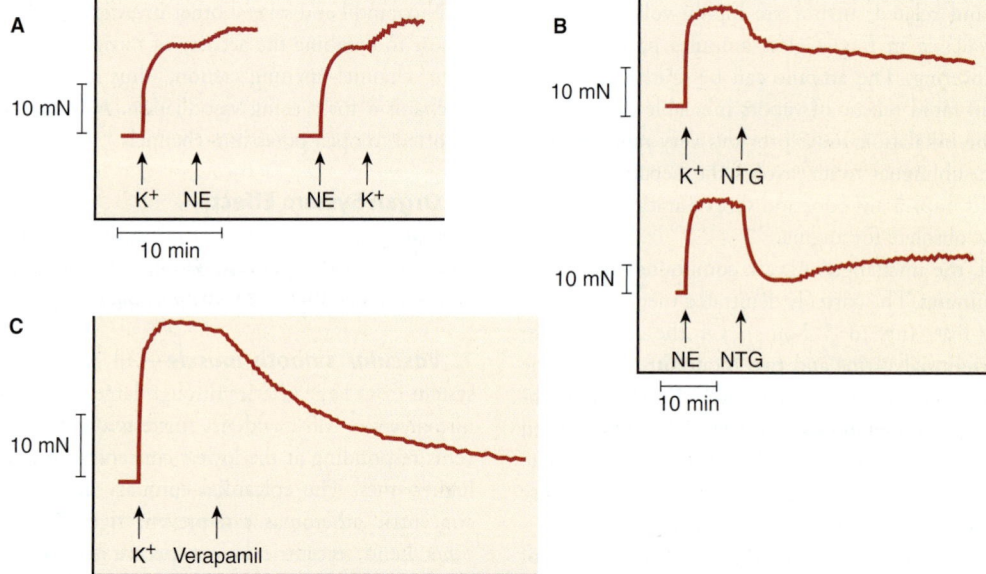

FIGURE 12–3 Effects of vasodilators on contractions of human vein segments studied in vitro. **A** shows contractions induced by two vaso-constrictor agents, norepinephrine (NE) and potassium (K⁺). **B** shows the relaxation induced by nitroglycerin (NTG), 4 μmol/L. The relaxation is prompt. **C** shows the relaxation induced by verapamil, 2.2 μmol/L. The relaxation is slower but more sustained. (Modified and reproduced, with permission, from Mikkelsen E, Andersson KE, Bengtsson B: Effects of verapamil and nitroglycerin on contractile responses to potassium and noradrenaline in isolated human peripheral veins. Acta Pharmacol Toxicol 1978;42:14.)

nitrates are rarely of any clinical value. During recent decades, the use of amyl nitrite and isobutyl nitrite (not nitrates) by inhalation as recreational (sex-enhancing) drugs has become popular with some segments of the population. Nitrites readily release nitric oxide in erectile tissue as well as vascular smooth muscle and activate guanylyl cyclase. The resulting increase in cGMP causes dephosphorylation of myosin light chains and relaxation (Figure 12–2), which enhances erection. The pharmacologic approach to erectile dysfunction is are discussed in the Box: Drugs Used in the Treatment of Erectile Dysfunction.

3. Action on platelets—Nitric oxide released from nitroglycerin stimulates guanylyl cyclase in platelets as in smooth muscle. The increase in cGMP that results is responsible for a decrease in platelet aggregation. Unfortunately, recent prospective trials have established no survival benefit when nitroglycerin is used in acute myocardial infarction. In contrast, intravenous nitroglycerin may be of value in unstable angina, in part through its action on platelets.

4. Other effects—Nitrite ion reacts with hemoglobin (which contains ferrous iron) to produce methemoglobin (which contains ferric iron). Because methemoglobin has a very low affinity for oxygen, large doses of nitrites can result in pseudocyanosis, tissue hypoxia, and death. Fortunately, the plasma level of nitrite resulting from even large doses of organic and inorganic nitrates is too low to cause significant methemoglobinemia in adults. In nursing infants, the intestinal flora is capable of converting significant amounts of inorganic nitrate, eg, from well water, to nitrite ion. In addition, sodium nitrite is used as a curing agent for meats, eg,

corned beef. Thus, inadvertent exposure to large amounts of nitrite ion can occur and may produce serious toxicity.

One therapeutic application of this otherwise toxic effect of nitrite has been discovered. Cyanide poisoning results from complexing of cytochrome iron by the CN^- ion. Methemoglobin iron has a very high affinity for CN^-; thus, administration of sodium nitrite ($NaNO_2$) soon after cyanide exposure regenerates active cytochrome. The cyanmethemoglobin produced can be further detoxified by the intravenous administration of sodium thiosulfate ($Na_2S_2O_3$); this results in formation of thiocyanate ion (SCN^-), a less toxic ion that is readily excreted. Methemoglobinemia, if excessive, can be treated by giving methylene blue intravenously. This antidotal procedure is now being replaced by hydroxocobalamin, a form of vitamin B_{12}, which also has a very high affinity for cyanide and converts it to another form of vitamin B_{12}.

Toxicity & Tolerance

A. Acute Adverse Effects

The major acute toxicities of organic nitrates are direct extensions of therapeutic vasodilation: orthostatic hypotension, tachycardia, and throbbing headache. Glaucoma, once thought to be a contraindication, does not worsen, and nitrates can be used safely in the presence of increased intraocular pressure. Nitrates are contraindicated, however, if intracranial pressure is elevated. Rarely, transdermal nitroglycerin patches have ignited when external defibrillator electroshock was applied to the chest of patients in ventricular fibrillation. Such patches should be removed before use of external defibrillators to prevent superficial burns.

Drugs Used in the Treatment of Erectile Dysfunction

Erectile dysfunction in men has long been the subject of research (by both amateur and professional scientists). Among the substances used in the past and generally discredited are "Spanish Fly" (a bladder and urethral irritant), yohimbine (an α_2 antagonist; see Chapter 10), nutmeg, and mixtures containing lead, arsenic, or strychnine. Substances currently favored by practitioners of herbal medicine but of dubious value include ginseng and kava.

Scientific studies of the process have shown that erection requires *relaxation* of the nonvascular smooth muscle of the corpora cavernosa. This relaxation permits inflow of blood at nearly arterial pressure into the sinuses of the cavernosa, and it is the pressure of the blood that causes erection. (With regard to other aspects of male sexual function, ejaculation requires intact sympathetic motor function, while orgasm involves independent superficial and deep sensory nerves.) Physiologic erection occurs in response to the release of nitric oxide from nonadrenergic-noncholinergic nerves (see Chapter 6) associated with parasympathetic discharge. Thus, parasympathetic motor innervation must be intact and nitric oxide synthesis must be active. (It appears that a similar process occurs in female erectile tissues.) Certain other smooth muscle relaxants—eg, PGE_1 analogs or α antagonists—if present in high enough concentration, can independently cause sufficient cavernosal relaxation to result in erection. As noted in the text, nitric oxide activates guanylyl cyclase, which increases the concentration of cGMP, and the latter second messenger stimulates the dephosphorylation of myosin light chains (Figure 12–2) and relaxation of the smooth muscle. Thus, any drug that increases cGMP might be of value in erectile dysfunction if normal innervation is present. **Sildenafil** (Viagra) acts to increase cGMP by inhibiting its breakdown by phosphodiesterase isoform 5 (PDE-5). The drug has been very successful in the marketplace because it can be taken orally. However, sildenafil is of little or no value in men with loss of potency due to cord injury or other damage to innervation and in men lacking libido. Furthermore, sildenafil potentiates the action of nitrates used for angina, and severe hypotension and a few myocardial infarctions have been reported in men taking both drugs. It is recommended that at least 6 hours pass between use of a nitrate and the ingestion of sildenafil. Sildenafil also has effects on color vision, causing difficulty in blue-green discrimination. Two similar PDE-5 inhibitors, **tadalafil** and **vardenafil**, are available. It is important to be aware that numerous nonprescription mail-order products that contain sildenafil analogs such as hydroxythiohomosildenafil and sulfoaildenafil have been marketed as "male enhancement" agents. These products are not approved by the FDA and incur the same risk of dangerous interactions with nitrates as the approved agents.

PDE-5 inhibitors have also been studied for possible use in other conditions. Clinical studies show distinct benefit in some patients with pulmonary arterial hypertension but not in patients with advanced idiopathic pulmonary fibrosis. The drugs have possible benefit in systemic hypertension, cystic fibrosis, and benign prostatic hyperplasia. Both sildenafil and tadalafil are currently approved for pulmonary hypertension. Preclinical studies suggest that sildenafil may be useful in preventing apoptosis and cardiac remodeling after ischemia and reperfusion.

The drug most commonly used in patients who do not respond to sildenafil is **alprostadil**, a PGE_1 analog (see Chapter 18) that can be injected directly into the cavernosa or placed in the urethra as a minisuppository, from which it diffuses into the cavernosal tissue. Phentolamine can be used by injection into the cavernosa. These drugs will cause erection in most men who do not respond to sildenafil.

B. Tolerance

With continuous exposure to nitrates, isolated smooth muscle may develop complete tolerance (tachyphylaxis), and the intact human becomes progressively more tolerant when long-acting preparations (oral, transdermal) or continuous intravenous infusions are used for more than a few hours without interruption. The mechanisms by which tolerance develops are not completely understood. As previously noted, diminished release of nitric oxide resulting from reduced bioactivation may be partly responsible for tolerance to nitroglycerin. Systemic compensation also plays a role in tolerance in the intact human. Initially, significant sympathetic discharge occurs, and after one or more days of therapy with long-acting nitrates, retention of salt and water may reverse the favorable hemodynamic changes normally caused by nitroglycerin.

Tolerance does not occur equally with all nitric oxide donors. Nitroprusside, for example, retains activity over long periods. Other organic nitrates appear to be less susceptible than nitroglycerin to the development of tolerance. In cell-free systems, soluble guanylate cyclase is inhibited, possibly by nitrosylation of the enzyme, only after prolonged exposure to exceedingly high nitroglycerin concentrations. In contrast, treatment with antioxidants that protect ALDH2 and similar enzymes appears to prevent or reduce tolerance. This suggests that tolerance is a function of diminished bioactivation of organic nitrates and to a lesser degree, a loss of soluble guanylate cyclase responsiveness to nitric oxide.

Continuous exposure to high levels of nitrates can occur in the chemical industry, especially where explosives are manufactured. When contamination of the workplace with volatile organic nitrate compounds is severe, workers find that upon starting their work week (Monday), they suffer headache and transient dizziness ("Monday disease"). After a day or so, these symptoms disappear owing to the development of tolerance. Over the weekend, when exposure to the chemicals is reduced, tolerance disappears, so symptoms recur each Monday. Other hazards of industrial exposure, including dependence, have been reported. There is no evidence that physical dependence develops as a result of the *therapeutic* use of short-acting nitrates for angina, even in large doses.

C. Carcinogenicity of Nitrate and Nitrite Derivatives

Nitrosamines are small molecules with the structure R_2–N–NO formed from the combination of nitrates and nitrites with amines. Some nitrosamines are powerful carcinogens in animals, apparently through conversion to reactive derivatives. Although there is no direct proof that these agents cause cancer in humans, there is a strong epidemiologic correlation between the incidence of esophageal and gastric carcinoma and the nitrate content of food in certain cultures. Nitrosamines are also found in tobacco and in cigarette smoke. There is no evidence that the small doses of nitrates used in the treatment of angina result in significant body levels of nitrosamines.

Mechanisms of Clinical Effect

The beneficial and deleterious effects of nitrate-induced vasodilation are summarized in Table 12–2.

A. Nitrate Effects in Angina of Effort

Decreased venous return to the heart and the resulting reduction of intracardiac volume are important beneficial hemodynamic effects of nitrates. Arterial pressure also decreases. Decreased

intraventricular pressure and left ventricular volume are associated with decreased wall tension (Laplace relation) and decreased myocardial oxygen requirement. In rare instances, a paradoxical *increase* in myocardial oxygen demand may occur as a result of excessive reflex tachycardia and increased contractility.

Intracoronary, intravenous, or sublingual nitrate administration consistently increases the caliber of the large epicardial coronary arteries except where blocked by concentric atheromas. Coronary arteriolar resistance tends to decrease, though to a lesser extent. However, nitrates administered by the usual systemic routes may *decrease* overall coronary blood flow (and myocardial oxygen consumption) if cardiac output is reduced due to decreased venous return. The reduction in oxygen consumption is the major mechanism for the relief of effort angina.

B. Nitrate Effects in Variant Angina

Nitrates benefit patients with variant angina by relaxing the smooth muscle of the epicardial coronary arteries and relieving coronary artery spasm.

C. Nitrate Effects in Unstable Angina

Nitrates are also useful in the treatment of the acute coronary syndrome of unstable angina, but the precise mechanism for their beneficial effects is not clear. Because both increased coronary vascular tone and increased myocardial oxygen demand can precipitate rest angina in these patients, nitrates may exert their beneficial effects both by dilating the epicardial coronary arteries and by simultaneously reducing myocardial oxygen demand. As previously noted, nitroglycerin also decreases platelet aggregation, and this effect may be of importance in unstable angina.

Clinical Use of Nitrates

Some of the forms of nitroglycerin and its congeners are listed in Table 12–3. Because of its rapid onset of action (1–3 minutes), sublingual nitroglycerin is the most frequently used agent for the immediate treatment of angina. Because its duration of action is short (not exceeding 20–30 minutes), it is not suitable for maintenance therapy. The onset of action of intravenous nitroglycerin is also rapid (minutes), but its hemodynamic effects are quickly reversed when the infusion is stopped. Clinical use of intravenous nitroglycerin is therefore restricted to the treatment of severe, recurrent rest angina. Slowly absorbed preparations of nitroglycerin include a buccal form, oral preparations, and several transdermal forms. These formulations have been shown to provide blood concentrations for long periods but, as noted above, this leads to the development of tolerance.

The hemodynamic effects of sublingual or chewable isosorbide dinitrate and the oral organic nitrates are similar to those of nitroglycerin given by the same route. The recommended dosage schedules for commonly used long-acting nitrate preparations, along with their durations of action, are listed in Table 12–3. Although transdermal administration may provide blood levels of nitroglycerin for 24 hours or longer, the full hemodynamic effects usually do not persist for more than 6–8 hours. The clinical efficacy of

TABLE 12–2 Beneficial and deleterious effects of nitrates in the treatment of angina.

Effect	Result
Potential beneficial effects	
Decreased ventricular volume	Decreased myocardial oxygen requirement
Decreased arterial pressure	
Decreased ejection time	
Vasodilation of epicardial coronary arteries	Relief of coronary artery spasm
Increased collateral flow	Improved perfusion to ischemic myocardium
Decreased left ventricular diastolic pressure	Improved subendocardial perfusion
Potential deleterious effects	
Reflex tachycardia	Increased myocardial oxygen requirement
Reflex increase in contractility	Increased myocardial oxygen requirement
Decreased diastolic perfusion time due to tachycardia	Decreased coronary perfusion

TABLE 12–3 Nitrate and nitrite drugs used in the treatment of angina.

Drug	Dose	Duration of Action
Short-acting		
Nitroglycerin, sublingual	0.15–1.2 mg	10–30 minutes
Isosorbide dinitrate, sublingual	2.5–5 mg	10–60 minutes
Amyl nitrite, inhalant	0.18–0.3 mL	3–5 minutes
Long-acting		
Nitroglycerin, oral sustained-action	6.5–13 mg per 6–8 hours	6–8 hours
Nitroglycerin, 2% ointment, transdermal	1–1.5 inches per 4 hours	3–6 hours
Nitroglycerin, slow-release, buccal	1–2 mg per 4 hours	3–6 hours
Nitroglycerin, slow-release patch, transdermal	10–25 mg per 24 hours (one patch per day)	8–10 hours
Isosorbide dinitrate, sublingual	2.5–10 mg per 2 hours	1.5–2 hours
Isosorbide dinitrate, oral	10–60 mg per 4–6 hours	4–6 hours
Isosorbide dinitrate, chewable oral	5–10 mg per 2–4 hours	2–3 hours
Isosorbide mononitrate, oral	20 mg per 12 hours	6–10 hours

slow-release forms of nitroglycerin in maintenance therapy of angina is thus limited by the development of significant tolerance. Therefore, a nitrate-free period of at least 8 hours between doses should be observed to reduce or prevent tolerance.

OTHER NITRO-VASODILATORS

Nicorandil is a nicotinamide nitrate ester that has vasodilating properties in normal coronary arteries but more complex effects in patients with angina. Clinical studies suggest that it reduces both preload and afterload. It also provides some myocardial protection via preconditioning by activation of cardiac K_{ATP} channels. One large trial showed a significant reduction in relative risk of fatal and nonfatal coronary events in patients receiving the drug. Nicorandil is currently approved for use in the treatment of angina in Europe and Japan and has been submitted for approval in the USA.

CALCIUM CHANNEL-BLOCKING DRUGS

It has been known since the late 1800s that transmembrane calcium influx is necessary for the contraction of smooth and cardiac muscle. The discovery of a calcium channel in cardiac muscle was followed by the finding of several different types of calcium channels in different tissues (Table 12–4). The discovery of these channels made possible the measurement of the calcium current, I_{Ca}, and subsequently, the development of clinically useful blocking

TABLE 12–4 Properties of several recognized voltage-activated calcium channels.

Type	Channel Name	Where Found	Properties of the Calcium Current	Blocked By
L	$Ca_V1.1$–$Ca_V1.4$	Cardiac, skeletal, smooth muscle, neurons ($Ca_V1.4$ is found in retina), endocrine cells, bone	Long, large, high threshold	Verapamil, DHPs, Cd^{2+}, ω-aga-IIIA
T	$Ca_V3.1$–$Ca_V3.3$	Heart, neurons	Short, small, low threshold	sFTX, flunarizine, Ni^{2+} ($Ca_V3.2$ only), mibefradil[1]
N	$Ca_V2.2$	Neurons, sperm[2]	Short, high threshold	Ziconotide,[3] gabapentin,[4] ω-CTXGVIA, ω-aga-IIIA, Cd^{2+}
P/Q	$Ca_V2.1$	Neurons	Long, high threshold	ω-CTX-MVIIC, ω-aga-IVA
R	$Ca_V2.3$	Neurons, sperm[2]	Pacemaking	SNX-482, ω-aga-IIIA

[1]Antianginal drug withdrawn from market.

[2]Channel types associated with sperm flagellar activity may be of the Catsper1–4 variety.

[3]Synthetic snail peptide analgesic (see Chapter 31).

[4]Antiseizure agent (see Chapter 24).

DHPs, dihydropyridines (eg, nifedipine); sFTX, synthetic funnel web spider toxin; ω-CTX, conotoxins extracted from several marine snails of the genus *Conus;* ω-aga-IIIA and ω-aga-IVA, toxins of the funnel web spider, *Agelenopsis aperta;* SNX-482, a toxin of the African tarantula, *Hysterocrates gigas.*

TABLE 12–5 Clinical pharmacology of some calcium channel-blocking drugs.

Drug	Oral Bioavailability (%)	Half-life (hours)	Indication	Dosage
Dihydropyridines				
Amlodipine	65–90	30–50	Angina, hypertension	5–10 mg orally once daily
Felodipine	15–20	11–16	Hypertension, Raynaud's phenomenon	5–10 mg orally once daily
Isradipine	15–25	8	Hypertension	2.5–10 mg orally twice daily
Nicardipine	35	2–4	Angina, hypertension	20–40 mg orally every 8 hours
Nifedipine	45–70	4	Angina, hypertension, Raynaud's phenomenon	3–10 mcg/kg IV; 20–40 mg orally every 8 hours
Nisoldipine	< 10	6–12	Hypertension	20–40 mg orally once daily
Nitrendipine	10–30	5–12	Investigational	20 mg orally once or twice daily
Miscellaneous				
Diltiazem	40–65	3–4	Angina, hypertension, Raynaud's phenomenon	75–150 mcg/kg IV; 30–80 mg orally every 6 hours
Verapamil	20–35	6	Angina, hypertension, arrhythmias, migraine	75–150 mcg/kg IV; 80–160 mg orally every 8 hours

drugs. Although the blockers currently available for clinical use in cardiovascular conditions are exclusively L-type calcium channel blockers, selective blockers of other types of calcium channels are under intensive investigation. Certain antiseizure drugs are thought to act, at least in part, through calcium channel (especially T-type) blockade in neurons (see Chapter 24).

Chemistry & Pharmacokinetics

Verapamil, the first clinically useful member of this group, was the result of attempts to synthesize more active analogs of papaverine, a vasodilator alkaloid found in the opium poppy. Since then, dozens of agents of varying structure have been found to have the same fundamental pharmacologic action (Table 12–5). Three chemically dissimilar calcium channel blockers are shown in Figure 12–4. Nifedipine is the prototype of the dihydropyridine family of calcium channel blockers; dozens of molecules in this family have been investigated, and several are currently approved in the USA for angina and other indications. Nifedipine is the most extensively studied of this group, but the properties of the other dihydropyridines can be assumed to be similar to it unless otherwise noted.

The calcium channel blockers are orally active agents and are characterized by high first-pass effect, high plasma protein binding, and extensive metabolism. Verapamil and diltiazem are also used by the intravenous route.

Pharmacodynamics

A. Mechanism of Action

The voltage-gated L-type calcium channel is the dominant type in cardiac and smooth muscle and is known to contain several drug receptors. It consists of $\alpha 1$ (the larger, pore-forming subunit), $\alpha 2$, β, γ, and δ subunits. Four variant $\alpha 1$ subunits have

been recognized. Nifedipine and other dihydropyridines have been demonstrated to bind to one site on the $\alpha 1$ subunit, whereas verapamil and diltiazem appear to bind to closely related but not identical receptors in another region of the same subunit. Binding of a drug to the verapamil or diltiazem receptors allosterically affects dihydropyridine binding. These receptor regions are stereoselective, since marked differences in both stereoisomer-binding affinity and pharmacologic potency are observed for enantiomers of verapamil, diltiazem, and optically active nifedipine congeners.

Blockade of calcium channels by these drugs resembles that of sodium channel blockade by local anesthetics (see Chapters 14 and 26). The drugs act from the inner side of the membrane and bind more effectively to open channels and inactivated channels. Binding of the drug reduces the frequency of opening in response to depolarization. The result is a marked decrease in transmembrane calcium current, which in smooth muscle results in long-lasting relaxation (Figure 12–3) and in cardiac muscle results in reduction in contractility throughout the heart and decreases in sinus node pacemaker rate and atrioventricular node conduction velocity.[*] Although some neuronal cells harbor L-type calcium channels, their sensitivity to these drugs is lower because the channels in these cells spend less time in the open and inactivated states.

Smooth muscle responses to calcium influx through *ligand-gated* calcium channels are also reduced by these drugs but not as markedly. The block can be partially reversed by elevating the concentration of calcium, although the levels of calcium required are not easily attainable in patients. Block can also be partially

---

[*] At very low doses and under certain circumstances, some dihydropyridines increase calcium influx. Some special dihydropyridines, eg, Bay K 8644, actually increase calcium influx over most of their dose range.

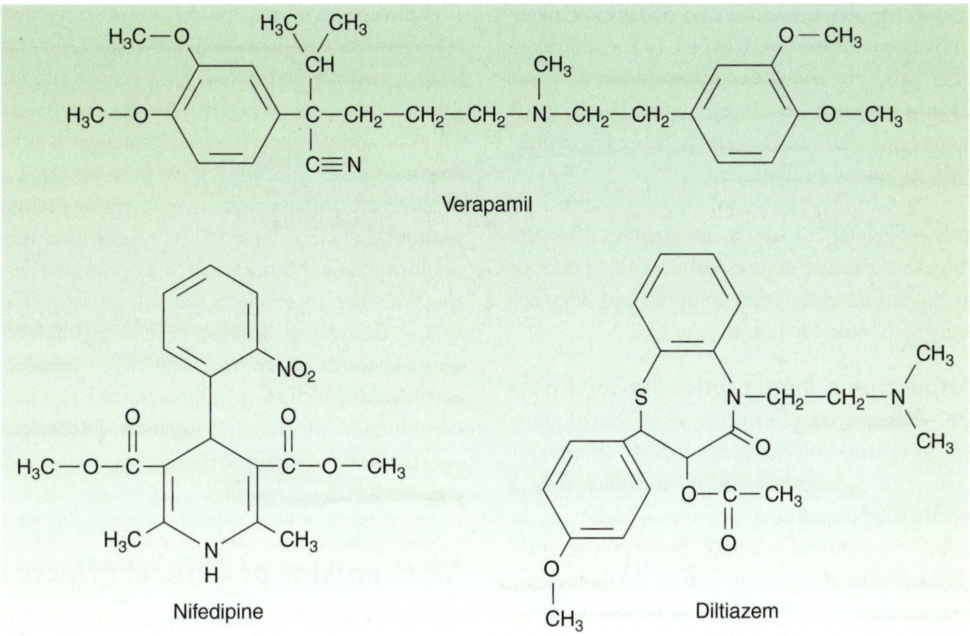

FIGURE 12-4 Chemical structures of several calcium channel-blocking drugs.

reversed by the use of drugs that increase the transmembrane flux of calcium, such as sympathomimetics.

Other types of calcium channels are less sensitive to blockade by these calcium channel blockers (Table 12–4). Therefore, tissues in which these other channel types play a major role—neurons and most secretory glands—are much less affected by these drugs than are cardiac and smooth muscle. **Mibefradil** is a selective T-type calcium channel blocker that was introduced for antiarrhythmic use but has been withdrawn. Ion channels other than calcium channels are much less sensitive to these drugs. Potassium channels in vascular smooth muscle are inhibited by verapamil, thus limiting the vasodilation produced by this drug. Sodium channels as well as calcium channels are blocked by **bepridil**, an obsolete antiarrhythmic drug.

B. Organ System Effects

1. Smooth muscle—Most types of smooth muscle are dependent on transmembrane calcium influx for normal resting tone and contractile responses. These cells are relaxed by the calcium channel blockers (Figure 12–3). Vascular smooth muscle appears to be the most sensitive, but similar relaxation can be shown for bronchiolar, gastrointestinal, and uterine smooth muscle. In the vascular system, arterioles appear to be more sensitive than veins; orthostatic hypotension is not a common adverse effect. Blood pressure is reduced with all calcium channel blockers (see Chapter 11). Women may be more sensitive than men to the hypotensive action of diltiazem. The reduction in peripheral vascular resistance is one mechanism by which these agents may benefit the patient with angina of effort. Reduction of coronary artery spasm has been demonstrated in patients with variant angina.

Important differences in vascular selectivity exist among the calcium channel blockers. In general, the dihydropyridines have a greater ratio of vascular smooth muscle effects relative to cardiac effects than do diltiazem and verapamil. The relatively smaller effect of verapamil on vasodilation may be the result of simultaneous blockade of vascular smooth muscle potassium channels described earlier. Furthermore, the dihydropyridines may differ in their potency in different vascular beds. For example, **nimodipine** is claimed to be particularly selective for cerebral blood vessels. Splice variants in the structure of the $\alpha 1$ channel subunit appear to account for these differences.

2. Cardiac muscle—Cardiac muscle is highly dependent on calcium influx during each action potential for normal function. Impulse generation in the sinoatrial node and conduction in the atrioventricular node—so-called slow-response, or calcium-dependent, action potentials—may be reduced or blocked by all of the calcium channel blockers. Excitation-contraction coupling in all cardiac cells requires calcium influx, so these drugs reduce cardiac contractility in a dose-dependent fashion. In some cases, cardiac output may also decrease. This reduction in cardiac mechanical function is another mechanism by which the calcium channel blockers can reduce the oxygen requirement in patients with angina.

Important differences between the available calcium channel blockers arise from the details of their interactions with cardiac ion channels and, as noted above, differences in their relative smooth muscle versus cardiac effects. Sodium channel block is modest with verapamil, and still less marked with diltiazem. It is negligible with nifedipine and other dihydropyridines. Verapamil and diltiazem interact kinetically with the calcium channel receptor in a different manner than the dihydropyridines; they block tachycardias in calcium-dependent cells, eg, the atrioventricular node, more selectively than do the dihydropyridines. (See Chapter 14 for additional details.) On the other hand, the dihydropyridines appear to block smooth muscle calcium channels at concentrations below those required for significant cardiac effects; they are therefore less depressant on the heart than verapamil or diltiazem.

3. Skeletal muscle—Skeletal muscle is not depressed by the calcium channel blockers because it uses intracellular pools of calcium to support excitation-contraction coupling and does not require as much transmembrane calcium influx.

4. Cerebral vasospasm and infarct following subarachnoid hemorrhage—Nimodipine, a member of the dihydropyridine group of calcium channel blockers, has a high affinity for cerebral blood vessels and appears to reduce morbidity after a subarachnoid hemorrhage. Nimodipine was approved for use in patients who have had a hemorrhagic stroke, but it has recently been withdrawn. **Nicardipine** has similar effects and is used by intravenous and intracerebral arterial infusion to prevent cerebral vasospasm associated with stroke. Verapamil as well, despite its lack of vasoselectivity, is used by the intra-arterial route in stroke. Some evidence suggests that calcium channel blockers may also reduce cerebral damage after thromboembolic stroke.

5. Other effects—Calcium channel blockers minimally interfere with stimulus-secretion coupling in glands and nerve endings because of differences between calcium channel type and sensitivity in different tissues. Verapamil has been shown to inhibit insulin release in humans, but the dosages required are greater than those used in management of angina and other cardiovascular conditions.

A significant body of evidence suggests that the calcium channel blockers may interfere with platelet aggregation in vitro and prevent or attenuate the development of atheromatous lesions in animals. However, clinical studies have not established their role in human blood clotting and atherosclerosis.

Verapamil has been shown to block the P-glycoprotein responsible for the transport of many foreign drugs out of cancer (and other) cells (see Chapter 1); other calcium channel blockers appear to have a similar effect. This action is not stereospecific. Verapamil has been shown to partially reverse the resistance of cancer cells to many chemotherapeutic drugs in vitro. Some clinical results suggest similar effects in patients (see Chapter 54). Animal research suggests possible future roles of calcium blockers in the treatment of osteoporosis, fertility disorders and male contraception, immune modulation, and even schistosomiasis. Verapamil does not appear to block transmembrane divalent metal ion transporters such as DMT1.

Toxicity

The most important toxic effects reported for calcium channel blockers are direct extensions of their therapeutic action. Excessive inhibition of calcium influx can cause serious cardiac depression, including bradycardia, atrioventricular block, cardiac arrest, and heart failure. These effects have been rare in clinical use.

Retrospective case-control studies reported that immediate-acting nifedipine increased the risk of myocardial infarction in patients with hypertension. Slow-release and long-acting dihydropyridine calcium channel blockers are usually well tolerated. However, dihydropyridines, compared with angiotensin-converting enzyme (ACE) inhibitors, have been reported to increase the risk of adverse cardiac events in patients with hypertension with or without diabetes. These results suggest that relatively short-acting calcium channel blockers such as prompt-release nifedipine have the potential to enhance the risk of adverse cardiac events and should be avoided. Patients receiving β-blocking drugs are more sensitive to the cardiodepressant effects of calcium channel blockers. Minor toxicities (troublesome but not usually requiring discontinuance of therapy) include flushing, dizziness, nausea, constipation, and peripheral edema. Constipation is particularly common with verapamil.

Mechanisms of Clinical Effects

Calcium channel blockers decrease myocardial contractile force, which reduces myocardial oxygen requirements. Calcium channel block in arterial smooth muscle decreases arterial and intraventricular pressure. Some of these drugs (eg, verapamil, diltiazem) also possess a nonspecific antiadrenergic effect, which may contribute to peripheral vasodilation. As a result of all of these effects, left ventricular wall stress declines, which reduces myocardial oxygen requirements. Decreased heart rate with the use of verapamil or diltiazem causes a further decrease in myocardial oxygen demand. Calcium channel-blocking agents also relieve and prevent focal coronary artery spasm in variant angina. Use of these agents has thus emerged as the most effective prophylactic treatment for this form of angina pectoris.

Sinoatrial and atrioventricular nodal tissues, which are mainly composed of calcium-dependent, slow-response cells, are affected markedly by verapamil, moderately by diltiazem, and much less by dihydropyridines. Thus, verapamil and diltiazem decrease atrioventricular nodal conduction and are often effective in the management of supraventricular reentry tachycardia and in decreasing ventricular responses in atrial fibrillation or flutter. Nifedipine does not affect atrioventricular conduction. Nonspecific sympathetic antagonism is most marked with diltiazem and much less with verapamil. Nifedipine does not appear to have this effect. Significant reflex tachycardia in response to hypotension occurs most frequently with nifedipine and less so with diltiazem and verapamil. These differences in pharmacologic effects should be considered in selecting calcium channel-blocking agents for the management of angina.

Clinical Uses of Calcium Channel-Blocking Drugs

In addition to angina, calcium channel blockers have well-documented efficacy in hypertension (see Chapter 11) and supraventricular tachyarrhythmias (see Chapter 14). They also show moderate efficacy in a variety of other conditions, including hypertrophic cardiomyopathy, migraine, and Raynaud's phenomenon. Nifedipine has some efficacy in preterm labor but is more toxic and not as effective as **atosiban,** an investigational oxytocin antagonist (see Chapter 17).

The pharmacokinetic properties of these drugs are set forth in Table 12–5. The choice of a particular calcium channel-blocking agent should be made with knowledge of its specific potential adverse effects as well as its pharmacologic properties. Nifedipine does not decrease atrioventricular conduction and therefore can be used more safely than verapamil or diltiazem in the presence of atrioventricular conduction abnormalities. A combination of verapamil or diltiazem with β blockers may produce atrioventricular block and depression of ventricular function. In the presence of overt heart failure, all calcium channel blockers can cause further worsening of failure as a result of their negative inotropic effect. **Amlodipine,** however, does not increase mortality in patients with heart failure due to nonischemic left ventricular systolic dysfunction and can be used safely in these patients.

In patients with relatively low blood pressure, dihydropyridines can cause further deleterious lowering of pressure. Verapamil and diltiazem appear to produce less hypotension and may be better tolerated in these circumstances. In patients with a history of atrial tachycardia, flutter, and fibrillation, verapamil and diltiazem provide a distinct advantage because of their antiarrhythmic effects. In the patient receiving digitalis, verapamil should be used with caution, because it may increase digoxin blood levels through a pharmacokinetic interaction. Although increases in digoxin blood level have also been demonstrated with diltiazem and nifedipine, such interactions are less consistent than with verapamil.

In patients with unstable angina, immediate-release short-acting calcium channel blockers can increase the risk of adverse cardiac events and therefore are contraindicated (see Toxicity, above). However, in patients with non–Q-wave myocardial infarction, diltiazem can decrease the frequency of postinfarction angina and may be used.

BETA-BLOCKING DRUGS

Although they are not vasodilators (with the exception of carvedilol and nebivolol), β-blocking drugs (see Chapter 10) are extremely useful in the management of effort angina. The beneficial effects of β-blocking agents are related to their hemodynamic effects—decreased heart rate, blood pressure, and contractility—which decrease myocardial oxygen requirements at rest and during exercise. Lower heart rate is also associated with an increase in diastolic perfusion time that may increase coronary perfusion. However, reduction of heart rate and blood pressure, and consequently decreased myocardial oxygen consumption, appear to be the most important mechanisms for relief of angina and improved exercise tolerance. Beta blockers may also be valuable in treating silent or ambulatory ischemia. Because this condition causes no pain, it is usually detected by the appearance of typical electrocardiographic signs of ischemia. The total amount of "ischemic time" per day is reduced by long-term therapy with a β blocker. Beta-blocking

agents decrease mortality of patients with recent myocardial infarction and improve survival and prevent stroke in patients with hypertension. Randomized trials in patients with stable angina have shown better outcome and symptomatic improvement with β blockers compared with calcium channel blockers.

Undesirable effects of β-blocking agents in angina include an increase in end-diastolic volume and an increase in ejection time, both of which tend to increase myocardial oxygen requirement. These deleterious effects of β-blocking agents can be balanced by the concomitant use of nitrates as described below.

Contraindications to the use of β blockers are asthma and other bronchospastic conditions, severe bradycardia, atrioventricular blockade, bradycardia-tachycardia syndrome, and severe unstable left ventricular failure. Potential complications include fatigue, impaired exercise tolerance, insomnia, unpleasant dreams, worsening of claudication, and erectile dysfunction.

NEWER ANTIANGINAL DRUGS

Because of the high prevalence of angina, new drugs are actively sought for its treatment. Some of the drugs or drug groups currently under investigation are listed in Table 12–6.

Ranolazine is a newer antianginal drug that appears to act by reducing a late sodium current (I_{Na}) that facilitates calcium entry via the sodium-calcium exchanger (see Chapter 13). The resulting reduction in intracellular calcium concentration reduces cardiac contractility and work. Ranolazine is approved for use in angina in the USA.

Certain metabolic modulators (eg, **trimetazidine**) are known as **pFOX inhibitors** because they partially inhibit the fatty acid oxidation pathway in myocardium. Because metabolism shifts to oxidation of fatty acids in ischemic myocardium, the oxygen requirement per unit of ATP produced increases. Partial inhibition of the enzyme

TABLE 12–6 New drugs or drug groups under investigation for use in angina.

Drugs
Amiloride
Capsaicin
Direct bradycardic agents, eg, ivabradine
Inhibitors of slowly inactivating sodium current, eg, ranolazine
Metabolic modulators, eg, trimetazidine
Nitric oxide donors, eg, L-arginine
Potassium channel activators, eg, nicorandil
Protein kinase G facilitators, eg, detanonoate
Rho-kinase inhibitors, eg, fasudil
Sulfonylureas, eg, glibenclamide
Thiazolidinediones
Vasopeptidase inhibitors
Xanthine oxidase inhibitors, eg, allopurinol

required for fatty acid oxidation (long-chain 3-ketoacyl thiolase, LC-3KAT) appears to improve the metabolic status of ischemic tissue. (Ranolazine was initially assigned to this group of agents.). Trimetazidine is not approved for use in angina in the USA. A much older drug, **allopurinol,** represents another type of metabolic modifier. Allopurinol inhibits xanthine oxidase (see Chapter 36), an enzyme that contributes to oxidative stress and endothelial dysfunction. A recent study suggests that high-dose allopurinol prolongs exercise time in patients with atherosclerotic angina.

So-called *bradycardic* drugs, relatively selective I_f sodium channel blockers (eg, **ivabradine**), reduce cardiac rate by inhibiting the hyperpolarization-activated sodium channel in the sinoatrial node. No other significant hemodynamic effects have been reported. Ivabradine appears to reduce anginal attacks with an efficacy similar to that of calcium channel blockers and β blockers. The lack of effect on gastrointestinal and bronchial smooth muscle is an advantage of ivabradine, and Food and Drug Administration approval is expected.

The Rho kinases comprise a family of enzymes that inhibit vascular relaxation and diverse functions of several other cell types. Excessive activity of these enzymes has been implicated in coronary spasm, pulmonary hypertension, apoptosis, and other conditions. Drugs targeting the enzyme have therefore been sought for possible clinical applications. **Fasudil** is an inhibitor of smooth muscle Rho kinase and reduces coronary vasospasm in experimental animals. In clinical trials in patients with CAD, it has improved performance in stress tests.

■ CLINICAL PHARMACOLOGY OF DRUGS USED TO TREAT ANGINA

Because the most common cause of angina is atherosclerotic disease of the coronaries (CAD), therapy must address the underlying causes of CAD as well as the immediate symptoms of angina. In addition to reducing the need for antianginal therapy, such primary management has been shown to reduce major cardiac events such as myocardial infarction.

First-line therapy of CAD depends on modification of risk factors such as smoking, hypertension (see Chapter 11), hyperlipidemia (see Chapter 35), obesity, and clinical depression. In addition, antiplatelet drugs (see Chapter 34) are very important.

Specific pharmacologic therapy to prevent myocardial infarction and death consists of antiplatelet agents (aspirin, ADP receptor blockers, Chapter 34) and lipid-lowering agents, especially statins (Chapter 35). Aggressive therapy with statins has been shown to reduce the incidence and severity of ischemia in patients during exercise testing and the incidence of cardiac events (including infarction and death) in clinical trials. ACE inhibitors also reduce the risk of adverse cardiac events in patients at high risk for CAD, although they have not been consistently shown to exert antianginal effects. In patients with unstable angina and non-ST-segment elevation myocardial infarction, aggressive therapy consisting of coronary stenting, antilipid drugs, heparin, and antiplatelet agents is recommended.

The treatment of established angina and other manifestations of myocardial ischemia includes the corrective measures previously described as well as treatment to prevent or relieve symptoms. Treatment of symptoms is based on reduction of myocardial oxygen demand and increase of coronary blood flow to the potentially ischemic myocardium to restore the balance between myocardial oxygen supply and demand.

Angina of Effort

Many studies have demonstrated that nitrates, calcium channel blockers, and β blockers increase time to onset of angina and ST depression during treadmill tests in patients with angina of effort (Figure 12–5). Although exercise tolerance increases, there is usually no change in the angina threshold, ie, the rate-pressure product at which symptoms occur.

For maintenance therapy of chronic stable angina, long-acting nitrates, calcium channel-blocking agents, or β blockers may be chosen; the drug of choice depends on the individual patient's response. In hypertensive patients, monotherapy with either slow-release or long-acting calcium channel blockers or β blockers may be adequate. In normotensive patients, long-acting nitrates may be suitable. The combination of a β blocker with a calcium channel blocker (eg, propranolol with nifedipine) or two different calcium channel blockers (eg, nifedipine and verapamil) has been shown to be more effective than individual drugs used alone. If response to a single drug is inadequate, a drug from a different class should be added to maximize the beneficial reduction of cardiac work while minimizing undesirable effects (Table 12–7). Some patients may require therapy with all three drug groups.

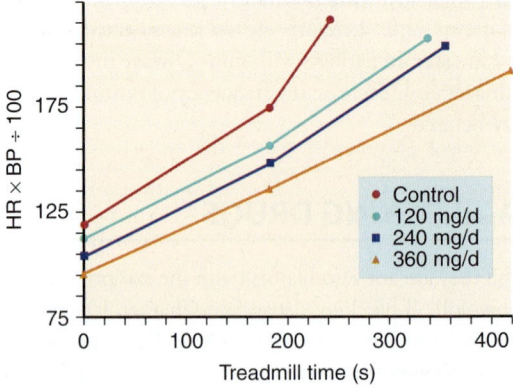

FIGURE 12–5 Effects of diltiazem on the double product (heart rate × systolic blood pressure) in a group of 20 patients with angina of effort. In a double-blind study using a standard protocol, patients were tested on a treadmill during treatment with placebo and three doses of the drug. Heart rate (HR) and systolic blood pressure (BP) were recorded at 180 seconds of exercise (midpoints of lines) and at the time of onset of anginal symptoms (rightmost points). Note that the drug treatment decreased the double product at all times during exercise and prolonged the time to appearance of symptoms. (Data from Lindenberg BS et al: Efficacy and safety of incremental doses of diltiazem for the treatment of angina. J Am Coll Cardiol 1983;2:1129. Used with permission of the American College of Cardiology.)

TABLE 12–7 Effects of nitrates alone and with β blockers or calcium channel blockers in angina pectoris.

	Nitrates Alone	Beta Blockers or Calcium Channel Blockers	Combined Nitrates with Beta Blockers or Calcium Channel Blockers
Heart rate	Reflex[1] increase	Decrease	Decrease
Arterial pressure	Decrease	Decrease	Decrease
End-diastolic volume	Decrease	Increase	None or decrease
Contractility	Reflex[1] increase	Decrease	None
Ejection time	Decrease[1]	Increase	None

[1]Baroreceptor reflex.

Note: Undesirable effects are shown in italics.

Surgical revascularization (ie, coronary artery bypass grafting [CABG]) and catheter-based revascularization (ie, percutaneous coronary intervention [PCI]) are the primary methods for promptly restoring coronary blood flow and increasing oxygen supply in unstable or medically refractory angina.

Vasospastic Angina

Nitrates and the calcium channel blockers are effective drugs for relieving and preventing ischemic episodes in patients with variant angina. In approximately 70% of patients treated with nitrates plus calcium channel blockers, angina attacks are completely abolished; in another 20%, marked reduction of frequency of anginal episodes is observed. Prevention of coronary artery spasm (with or without fixed atherosclerotic coronary artery lesions) is the principal mechanism for this beneficial response. All presently available calcium channel blockers appear to be equally effective, and the choice of a particular drug should depend on the patient. Surgical revascularization and angioplasty are not indicated in patients with variant angina.

Unstable Angina & Acute Coronary Syndromes

In patients with unstable angina with recurrent ischemic episodes at rest, recurrent platelet-rich nonocclusive thrombus formation is the principal mechanism. Aggressive antiplatelet therapy with a combination of aspirin and clopidogrel is indicated. Intravenous heparin or subcutaneous low-molecular-weight heparin is also indicated in most patients. If percutaneous coronary intervention with stenting is required, glycoprotein IIb/IIIa inhibitors such as abciximab should be added. In addition, therapy with nitroglycerin and β blockers should be considered; calcium channel blockers should be added in refractory cases for relief of myocardial

ischemia. Primary lipid-lowering and ACE-inhibitor therapy should also be initiated.

TREATMENT OF PERIPHERAL ARTERY DISEASE (PAD) & INTERMITTENT CLAUDICATION

Atherosclerosis can result in ischemia of peripheral muscles just as coronary artery disease causes cardiac ischemia. Pain (claudication) occurs in skeletal muscles, especially in the legs, during exercise and disappears with rest. Although claudication is not immediately life-threatening, peripheral artery disease is associated with increased mortality, can severely limit exercise tolerance, and may be associated with chronic ischemic ulcers and susceptibility to infection.

Intermittent claudication results from obstruction of blood flow by atheromas in large and medium arteries. Treatment is primarily directed at reversal or control of atherosclerosis and requires measurement and control of hyperlipidemia (see Chapter 35), hypertension (see Chapter 11), and obesity; cessation of smoking; and control of diabetes, if present. Physical therapy and exercise training is of proven benefit. Conventional vasodilators are of no benefit because vessels distal to the obstructive lesions are usually already dilated at rest. Antiplatelet drugs such as aspirin or clopidogrel are often used to prevent clotting in the region of plaques. Two drugs are used almost exclusively for peripheral artery disease. **Pentoxifylline,** a xanthine derivative, is thought to act by reducing the viscosity of blood, allowing it to flow more easily through partially obstructed areas. **Cilostazol,** a phosphodiesterase type 3 (PDE3) inhibitor, is poorly understood, but may have selective antiplatelet and vasodilating effects. Both drugs have been shown to increase exercise tolerance in patients with severe claudication. Percutaneous angioplasty with stenting is often effective in patients with medically intractable signs and symptoms of ischemia.

SUMMARY Drugs Used in Angina Pectoris

Subclass	Mechanism of Action	Effects	Clinical Applications	Pharmacokinetics, Toxicities, Interactions
NITRATES				
• Nitroglycerin	Releases nitric oxide in smooth muscle, which activates guanylyl cyclase and increases cGMP	Smooth muscle relaxation, especially in vessels • other smooth muscle is relaxed but not as markedly • vasodilation decreases venous return and heart size • may increase coronary flow in some areas and in variant angina	Angina: Sublingual form for acute episodes • oral and transdermal forms for prophylaxis • IV form for acute coronary syndrome	High first-pass effect, so sublingual dose is much smaller than oral • high lipid solubility ensures rapid absorption • *Toxicity:* Orthostatic hypotension, tachycardia, headache • *Interactions:* Synergistic hypotension with phosphodiesterase type 5 inhibitors (sildenafil, etc)
• *Isosorbide dinitrate: Very similar to nitroglycerin, slightly longer duration of action*				
• *Isosorbide mononitrate: Active metabolite of the dinitrate; used orally for prophylaxis*				
BETA BLOCKERS				
• Propranolol	Nonselective competitive antagonist at β adrenoceptors	Decreased heart rate, cardiac output, and blood pressure • decreases myocardial oxygen demand	Prophylaxis of angina • for other applications, see Chapters 10, 11, and 13	Oral and parenteral, 4–6 h duration of action • *Toxicity:* Asthma, atrioventricular block, acute heart failure, sedation • *Interactions:* Additive with all cardiac depressants
• *Atenolol, metoprolol, others: β₁-Selective blockers, less risk of bronchospasm, but still significant*				
• *See Chapters 10 and 11 for other β blockers and their applications*				
CALCIUM CHANNEL BLOCKERS				
• Verapamil, diltiazem	Nonselective block of L-type calcium channels in vessels and heart	Reduced vascular resistance, cardiac rate, and cardiac force results in decreased oxygen demand	Prophylaxis of angina, hypertension, others	Oral, IV, duration 4–8 h • *Toxicity:* Atrioventricular block, acute heart failure; constipation, edema • *Interactions:* Additive with other cardiac depressants and hypotensive drugs
• Nifedipine (a dihydropyridine)	Block of vascular L-type calcium channels > cardiac channels	Like verapamil and diltiazem; less cardiac effect	Prophylaxis of angina, hypertension	Oral, duration 4–6 h • *Toxicity:* Excessive hypotension, baroreceptor reflex tachycardia • *Interactions:* Additive with other vasodilators
• *Other dihydropyridines: Like nifedipine but slower onset and longer duration (up to 12 h or longer)*				
MISCELLANEOUS				
• Ranolazine	Inhibits late sodium current in heart • also may modify fatty acid oxidation	Reduces cardiac oxygen demand • fatty acid oxidation modification may improve efficiency of cardiac oxygen utilization	Prophylaxis of angina	Oral, duration 6–8 h • *Toxicity:* QT interval prolongation, nausea, constipation, dizziness • *Interactions:* Inhibitors of CYP3A increase ranolazine concentration and duration of action
• *Ivabradine: Investigational inhibitor of sinoatrial pacemaker; reduction of heart rate reduces oxygen demand*				

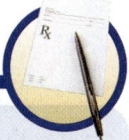

P R E P A R A T I O N S   A V A I L A B L E

NITRATES & NITRITES

Amyl nitrite (generic)
Inhalant: 0.3 mL capsules

Isosorbide dinitrate (generic, Isordil)
Oral: 5, 10, 20, 30, 40 mg tablets; 5, 10 mg chewable tablets
Oral sustained-release (Isochron, Dilatrate SR): 40 mg tablets and capsules
Sublingual: 2.5, 5 mg sublingual tablets

Isosorbide mononitrate (Ismo, others)
Oral: 10, 20 mg tablets; extended-release: 30, 60, 120 mg tablets

Nitroglycerin
Sublingual or buccal: 0.3, 0.4, 0.6 mg tablets; 0.4 mg/metered dose aerosol spray
Oral sustained-release (generic, Nitro-Time): 2.5, 6.5, 9 mg capsules
Parenteral (generic): 5 mg/mL for IV administration; 100, 200, 400 mcg/mL in dextrose for IV infusion
Transdermal patches (generic, Nitrek, Nitro-Dur, Transderm-Nitro): to release at rates of 0.1, 0.2, 0.3, 0.4, 0.6, or 0.8 mg/h
Topical ointment (generic, Nitro-Bid): 20 mg/mL ointment (1 inch, or 25 mm, of ointment contains about 15 mg nitroglycerin)

CALCIUM CHANNEL BLOCKERS

Amlodipine (generic, Norvasc, AmVaz)
Oral: 2.5, 5, 10 mg tablets

Clevidipine (Cleviprex) (approved only for use in hypertensive emergencies)
Parenteral: 0.5 mg/mL for IV infusion

Diltiazem (Cardizem, generic)
Oral: 30, 60, 90, 120 mg tablets
Oral sustained-release (Cardizem SR, Dilacor XL, others): 60, 90, 120, 180, 240, 300, 360, 420 mg capsules, tablets
Parenteral: 5 mg/mL for injection

Felodipine (generic, Plendil)
Oral extended-release: 2.5, 5, 10 mg tablets

Isradipine (DynaCirc)
Oral: 2.5, 5 mg capsules
Oral controlled-release: 5, 10 mg tablets

Nicardipine (Cardene, others)
Oral: 20, 30 mg capsules
Oral sustained-release (Cardene SR): 30, 45, 60 mg capsules
Parenteral (Cardene I.V.): 2.5 mg/mL

Nifedipine (Adalat, Procardia, others)
Oral: 10, 20 mg capsules
Oral extended-release (Procardia XL, Adalat CC): 30, 60, 90 mg tablets

Nisoldipine (Sular)
Oral extended-release: 8.5, 17, 25.5, 34 mg tablets

Verapamil (generic, Calan, Isoptin)
Oral: 40, 80, 120 mg tablets
Oral sustained-release: 100, 120, 180, 240 mg tablets or capsules
Parenteral: 2.5 mg/mL for injection

BETA BLOCKERS

See Chapter 10.

SODIUM CHANNEL BLOCKERS

Ranolazine (Ranexa)
Oral: 500, 1000 mg extended-release tablets

DRUGS FOR ERECTILE DYSFUNCTION

Sildenafil (Viagra, Revatio)
Oral: 20 (approved for use in pulmonary arterial hypertension), 25, 50, 100 mg tablets

Tadalafil (Cialis, Adcirca)
Oral: 2.5, 5, 10, 20 mg tablets (20 mg approved for use in pulmonary hypertension)

Vardenafil (Levitra)
Oral: 2.5, 5, 10, 20 mg tablets

DRUGS FOR PERIPHERAL ARTERY DISEASE

Cilostazol (generic, Pletal)
Oral: 50, 100 mg tablets

Pentoxifylline (generic, Trental)
Oral: 400 mg controlled-release, extended-release tablets

REFERENCES

Borer JS: Clinical effect of 'pure' heart rate slowing with a prototype If inhibitor: placebo-controlled experience with ivabradine. Adv Cardiol 2006;43:54.

Carmichael P, Lieben J: Sudden death in explosives workers. Arch Environ Health 1963;7:50.

Chaitman BR: Efficacy and safety of a metabolic modulator drug in chronic stable angina: Review of evidence from clinical trials. J Cardiovasc Pharmacol Ther 2004;9(Suppl 1):S47.

Chaitman BR et al: Effects of ranolazine, with atenolol, amlodipine, or diltiazem on exercise tolerance and angina frequency in patients with severe chronic angina. A randomized controlled trial. JAMA 2004;291:309.

Chen Z, Zhang J, Stamler JS: Identification of the enzymatic mechanism of nitroglycerin bioactivation. Proc Nat Acad Sci 2002;99:8306.

DeWitt CR, Waksman JC: Pharmacology, pathophysiology and management of calcium channel blocker and beta-blocker toxicity. Toxicol Rev 2004;23:223.

Fraker TD Jr, Fihn SD: 2007 Chronic angina focused update of the ACC/AHA 2002 guidelines for the management of patients with chronic stable angina. J Am Coll Cardiol 2007;50:2264.

Ignarro LJ et al: Mechanism of vascular smooth muscle relaxation by organic nitrates, nitrites, nitroprusside, and nitric oxide: Evidence for the involvement of S-nitrosothiols as active intermediates. J Pharmacol Exp Ther 1981;218:739.

Kannam JP, Aroesty JM, Gersh BJ: Overview of the management of stable angina pectoris. UpToDate, 2010. http://www.uptodate.com.

Kast R et al: Cardiovascular effects of a novel potent and highly selective asaindole-based inhibitor of Rho-kinase. Br J Pharmacol 2007;152:1070.

Lacinova L: Voltage-dependent calcium channels. Gen Physiol Biophys 2005;24(Suppl 1):1.

Mayer B, Beretta M: The enigma of nitroglycerin bioactivation and nitrate tolerance: News, views and troubles. Br J Pharmacol 2008;155:170.

McLaughlin VV et al: Expert consensus document on pulmonary hypertension. J Am Coll Cardiol 2009;53:1573.

Peng J, Li Y-J: New insights into nitroglycerin effects and tolerance: Role of calcitonin gene-related peptide. Eur J Pharmacol 2008; 586:9.

Pollack CV, Braunwald E: 2007 Update to the ACC/AHA guidelines for the management of patients with unstable angina and non-ST-segment elevation myocardial infarction: Implications for emergency department practice. Ann Emerg Med 2008;51:591.

Saint DA: The cardiac persistent sodium current: An appealing therapeutic target? Br J Pharmacol 2008;153:1133.

Simmons M, Laham RJ: New therapies for angina pectoris. UpToDate, 2010. http://www.uptodate.com

Stone GW et al: A prospective natural-history study of coronary atherosclerosis. N Eng J Med 2011;364:226.

Triggle DJ: Calcium channel antagonists: clinical uses—past, present and future. Biochem Pharmacol 2007;74:1.

CASE STUDY ANSWER

The case described is typical of stable atherosclerotic angina. Treatment of acute episodes should include sublingual tablets or sprayed nitroglycerin, 0.4–0.6 mg. Relief of discomfort within 2–4 minutes can be expected. If anginal episodes are frequent, or to prevent episodes of angina, a β blocker such as metoprolol should be tried first. If contraindications to the use of a β blocker are present, a medium- to long-acting calcium channel blocker such as verapamil, diltiazem, or amlodipine is likely to be effective.

13

Drugs Used in Heart Failure

Bertram G. Katzung, MD, PhD[*]

A 65-year-old man has developed shortness of breath with exertion several weeks after experiencing a viral illness. This is accompanied by swelling of the feet and ankles and increasing fatigue. On physical examination he is found to be mildly short of breath lying down, but feels better sitting upright. Pulse is 105 and regular, and blood pressure is 90/60 mm Hg. His lungs show crackles at both bases, and his jugular venous pressure is elevated. The liver is enlarged, and there is 3+ edema of the ankles and feet. An echocardiogram shows a dilated, poorly contracting heart with a left ventricular ejection fraction of about 20% (normal: 60%). The presumptive diagnosis is dilated cardiomyopathy secondary to a viral infection with stage C, class III heart failure. What treatment is indicated?

Heart failure occurs when cardiac output is inadequate to provide the oxygen needed by the body. It is a highly lethal condition, with a 5-year mortality rate conventionally said to be about 50%. The most common cause of heart failure in the USA is coronary artery disease, with hypertension also an important factor. Two major types of failure may be distinguished. Approximately 50% of younger patients have **systolic failure,** with reduced mechanical pumping action (contractility) and reduced ejection fraction. The remaining group has **diastolic failure,** with stiffening and loss of adequate relaxation playing a major role in reducing filling and cardiac output; ejection fraction may be normal even though stroke volume is significantly reduced. The proportion of patients with diastolic failure increases with age. Because other cardiovascular conditions (especially myocardial infarction) are now being treated more effectively, more patients are surviving long enough for heart failure to develop, making heart failure one of the cardiovascular conditions that is actually increasing in prevalence.

Heart failure is a progressive disease that is characterized by a gradual reduction in cardiac performance, punctuated in many cases by episodes of acute decompensation, often requiring hospitalization.

Treatment is therefore directed at two somewhat different goals: (1) reducing symptoms and slowing progression as much as possible during relatively stable periods and (2) managing acute episodes of decompensated failure. These factors are discussed in Clinical Pharmacology of Drugs Used in Heart Failure.

Although it is believed that the primary defect in early systolic heart failure resides in the excitation-contraction coupling machinery of the heart, the clinical condition also involves many other processes and organs, including the baroreceptor reflex, the sympathetic nervous system, the kidneys, angiotensin II and other peptides, aldosterone, and apoptosis of cardiac cells. Recognition of these factors has resulted in evolution of a variety of drug treatment strategies (Table 13–1).

Large clinical trials have shown that therapy directed at noncardiac targets is more valuable in the long-term treatment of heart failure than traditional positive inotropic agents (cardiac glycosides [digitalis]). Extensive trials have shown that ACE inhibitors, angiotensin receptor blockers, certain β blockers, aldosterone receptor antagonists, and combined hydralazine-nitrate therapy are the only agents in current use that actually prolong life in patients with chronic heart failure. These strategies are useful in both systolic and diastolic failure. Positive inotropic drugs, on the other hand, are helpful mainly in acute systolic failure. Cardiac glycosides also reduce symptoms in chronic systolic

---

[*]The author thanks Dr. William W. Parmley, MD, who was coauthor of this chapter in prior editions.

TABLE 13–1 Drug groups used in heart failure.

Chronic heart failure	Acute heart failure
Diuretics	Diuretics
Aldosterone receptor antagonists	Vasodilators
Angiotensin-converting enzyme inhibitors	Beta agonists
Angiotensin receptor blockers	Bipyridines
Beta blockers	Natriuretic peptide
Cardiac glycosides	
Vasodilators	

heart failure. Other positive inotropic drugs have consistently *reduced* survival in chronic failure, and their use is discouraged.

Control of Normal Cardiac Contractility

The vigor of contraction of heart muscle is determined by several processes that lead to the movement of actin and myosin filaments in the cardiac sarcomere (Figure 13–1). Ultimately, contraction results from the interaction of *activator* calcium (during systole) with the actin-troponin-tropomyosin system, thereby releasing the actin-myosin interaction. This activator calcium is released from the sarcoplasmic reticulum (SR). The amount released depends on the amount stored in the SR and on the amount of *trigger* calcium that enters the cell during the plateau of the action potential.

A. Sensitivity of the Contractile Proteins to Calcium and Other Contractile Protein Modifications

The determinants of calcium sensitivity, ie, the curve relating the shortening of cardiac myofibrils to the cytoplasmic calcium concentration, are incompletely understood, but several types of drugs can be shown to affect calcium sensitivity in vitro. **Levosimendan** is the most recent example of a drug that increases calcium sensitivity (it may also inhibit phosphodiesterase) and reduces symptoms in models of heart failure.

A recent report suggests that an experimental drug, **omecantiv mecarbil** (CK-1827452), alters the rate of transition of myosin from a low-actin-binding state to a strongly actin-bound force-generating state. Preliminary studies in experimental animal models of heart failure indicate that this agent may provide a new approach to the treatment of heart failure in humans. Clinical trials are underway.

B. Amount of Calcium Released from the Sarcoplasmic Reticulum

A small rise in free cytoplasmic calcium, brought about by calcium influx during the action potential, triggers the opening of calcium-gated, ryanodine-sensitive calcium channels (RyR2) in the membrane of the cardiac SR and the rapid release of a large amount of the ion into the cytoplasm in the vicinity of the actin-troponin-tropomyosin complex. The amount released is proportional to the amount stored in the SR and the amount of trigger calcium that

enters the cell through the cell membrane. (Ryanodine is a potent negative inotropic plant alkaloid that interferes with the release of calcium through cardiac SR channels.)

C. Amount of Calcium Stored in the Sarcoplasmic Reticulum

The SR membrane contains a very efficient calcium uptake transporter known as the sarcoplasmic endoplasmic reticulum Ca^{2+}-ATPase (SERCA). This pump maintains free cytoplasmic calcium at very low levels during diastole by pumping calcium into the SR. SERCA is normally inhibited by phospholamban; phosphorylation of phospholamban by protein kinase A (eg, by β agonists) removes this inhibition. The amount of calcium sequestered in the SR is thus determined, in part, by the amount accessible to this transporter and the activity of the sympathetic nervous system. This in turn is dependent on the balance of calcium influx (primarily through the voltage-gated membrane L-type calcium channels) and calcium efflux, the amount removed from the cell (primarily via the sodium-calcium exchanger, a transporter in the cell membrane). The amount of Ca^{2+} released from the SR depends on the response of the RyR channels to trigger Ca^{2+}.

D. Amount of Trigger Calcium

The amount of trigger calcium that enters the cell depends on the availability of membrane calcium channels and the duration of their opening. As described in Chapters 6 and 9, sympathomimetics cause an increase in calcium influx through an action on these channels. Conversely, the calcium channel blockers (see Chapter 12) reduce this influx and depress contractility.

E. Activity of the Sodium-Calcium Exchanger

This antiporter (NCX) uses the sodium gradient to move calcium against its concentration gradient from the cytoplasm to the extracellular space. Extracellular concentrations of these ions are much less labile than intracellular concentrations under physiologic conditions. The sodium-calcium exchanger's ability to carry out this transport is thus strongly dependent on the intracellular concentrations of both ions, especially sodium.

F. Intracellular Sodium Concentration and Activity of Na^+/K^+-ATPase

Na^+/K^+-ATPase, by removing intracellular sodium, is the major determinant of sodium concentration in the cell. The sodium influx through voltage-gated channels, which occurs as a normal part of almost all cardiac action potentials, is another determinant, although the amount of sodium that enters with each action potential is much less than 1% of the total intracellular sodium. Na^+/K^+-ATPase appears to be the primary target of **digoxin** and other cardiac glycosides.

Pathophysiology of Heart Failure

Heart failure is a syndrome with many causes that may involve one or both ventricles. Cardiac output is usually below the normal range ("low-output" failure). Systolic dysfunction, with reduced

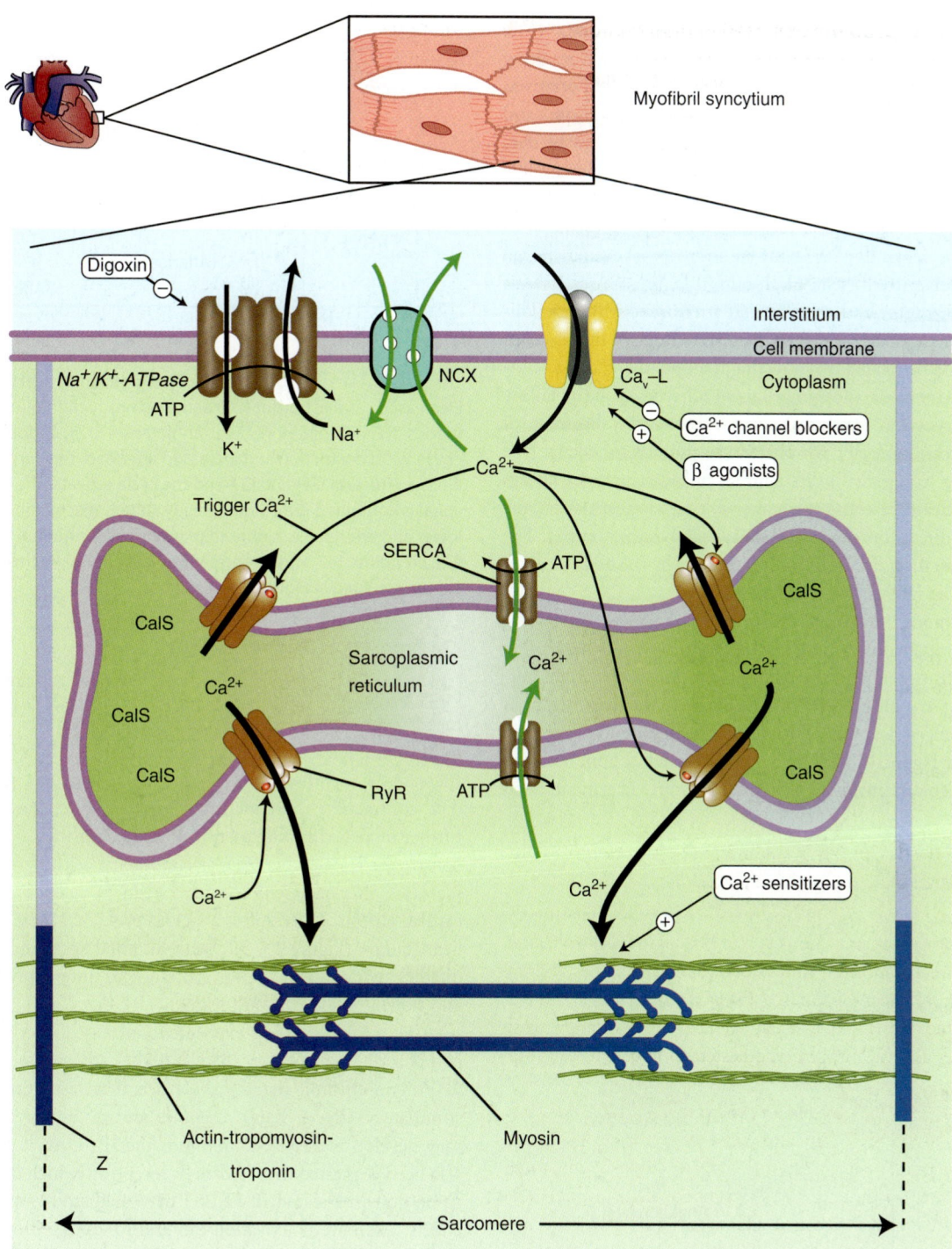

FIGURE 13–1 Schematic diagram of a cardiac muscle sarcomere, with sites of action of several drugs that alter contractility. Na$^+$/K$^+$-ATPase, the sodium pump, is the site of action of cardiac glycosides. NCX is the sodium-calcium exchanger. Ca$_v$-L is the voltage-gated, L-type calcium channel. SERCA (sarcoplasmic endoplasmic reticulum Ca^{2+}-ATPase) is a calcium transporter ATPase that pumps calcium into the sarcoplasmic reticulum (SR). CalS is calcium bound to calsequestrin, a high-capacity Ca^{2+}-binding protein. RyR (ryanodine RyR2 receptor) is a calcium-activated calcium channel in the membrane of the SR that is triggered to release stored calcium. Calcium sensitizers act at the actin-troponin-tropomyosin complex where activator calcium brings about the contractile interaction of actin and myosin. Black arrows represent processes that initiate contraction or support basal tone. Green arrows represent processes that promote relaxation.

cardiac output and significantly reduced ejection fraction (< 45%; normal > 60%), is typical of acute failure, especially that resulting from myocardial infarction. Diastolic dysfunction often occurs as a result of hypertrophy and stiffening of the myocardium, and although cardiac output is reduced, ejection fraction may be normal. Heart failure due to diastolic dysfunction does not usually respond optimally to positive inotropic drugs.

"High-output" failure is a rare form of heart failure. In this condition, the demands of the body are so great that even increased cardiac output is insufficient. High-output failure can result from hyperthyroidism, beriberi, anemia, and arteriovenous shunts. This form of failure responds poorly to the drugs discussed in this chapter and should be treated by correcting the underlying cause.

The primary signs and symptoms of all types of heart failure include tachycardia, decreased exercise tolerance, shortness of breath, and cardiomegaly. Peripheral and pulmonary edema (the congestion of congestive heart failure) are often but not always present. Decreased exercise tolerance with rapid muscular fatigue is the major direct consequence of diminished cardiac output. The other manifestations result from the attempts by the body to compensate for the intrinsic cardiac defect.

Neurohumoral (extrinsic) compensation involves two major mechanisms (previously presented in Figure 6–7)—the sympathetic nervous system and the renin-angiotensin-aldosterone hormonal response—plus several others. Some of the detrimental as well as beneficial features of these compensatory responses are illustrated in Figure 13–2. The baroreceptor reflex appears to be reset, with a lower sensitivity to arterial pressure, in patients with

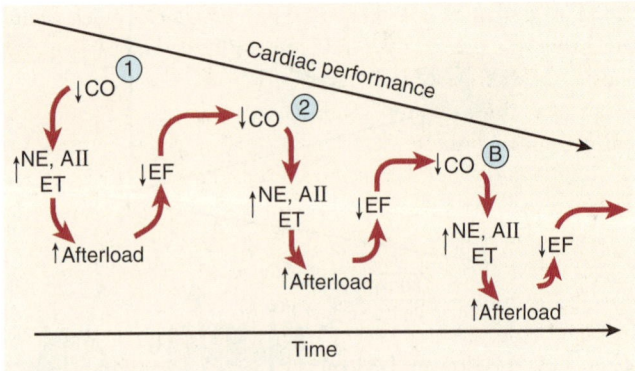

FIGURE 13–3 Vicious spiral of progression of heart failure. Decreased cardiac output (CO) activates production of neurohormones (NE, norepinephrine; AII, angiotensin II; ET, endothelin), which cause vasoconstriction and increased afterload. This further reduces ejection fraction (EF) and CO, and the cycle repeats. The downward spiral is continued until a new steady state is reached in which CO is lower and afterload is higher than is optimal for normal activity. Circled points 1, 2, and B represent points on the ventricular function curves depicted in Figure 13–4.

heart failure. As a result, baroreceptor sensory input to the vasomotor center is reduced even at normal pressures; sympathetic outflow is increased, and parasympathetic outflow is decreased. Increased sympathetic outflow causes tachycardia, increased cardiac contractility, and increased vascular tone. Vascular tone is further increased by angiotensin II and endothelin, a potent vasoconstrictor released by vascular endothelial cells. Vasoconstriction increases afterload, which further reduces ejection fraction and cardiac output. The result is a vicious cycle that is characteristic of heart failure (Figure 13–3). Neurohumoral antagonists and vasodilators reduce heart failure mortality by interrupting the cycle and slowing the downward spiral.

After a relatively short exposure to increased sympathetic drive, complex down-regulatory changes in the cardiac β_1-adrenoceptor–G protein-effector system take place that result in diminished stimulatory effects. Beta$_2$ receptors are *not* down-regulated and may develop increased coupling to the IP$_3$-DAG cascade. It has also been suggested that cardiac β_3 receptors (which do not appear to be down-regulated in failure) may mediate *negative* inotropic effects. Excessive β activation can lead to leakage of calcium from the SR via RyR channels and contributes to stiffening of the ventricles and arrhythmias. Prolonged β activation also increases caspases, the enzymes responsible for apoptosis. Increased angiotensin II production leads to increased aldosterone secretion (with sodium and water retention), to increased afterload, and to remodeling of both heart and vessels (discussed below). Other hormones are released, including natriuretic peptide, endothelin, and vasopressin (see Chapter 17). Within the heart, failure-induced changes have been documented in calcium handling in the SR by SERCA and phospholamban; in transcription factors that lead to hypertrophy and fibrosis; in mitochondrial function, which is critical for energy production in the overworked heart;

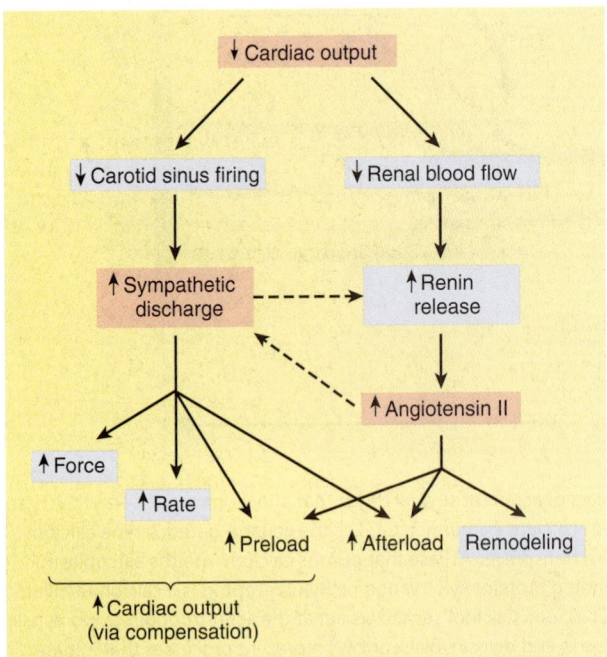

FIGURE 13–2 Some compensatory responses that occur during congestive heart failure. In addition to the effects shown, sympathetic discharge facilitates renin release, and angiotensin II increases norepinephrine release by sympathetic nerve endings (*dashed arrows*).

and in ion channels, especially potassium channels, which facilitate arrhythmogenesis, a primary cause of death in heart failure. Phosphorylation of RyR channels in the sarcoplasmic reticulum enhances and dephosphorylation reduces Ca^{2+} release; studies in animal models indicate that the enzyme primarily responsible for RyR dephosphorylation, protein phosphatase 1 (PP1), is up-regulated in heart failure. These cellular changes provide many potential targets for future drugs.

The most important intrinsic compensatory mechanism is **myocardial hypertrophy.** This increase in muscle mass helps maintain cardiac performance. However, after an initial beneficial effect, hypertrophy can lead to ischemic changes, impairment of diastolic filling, and alterations in ventricular geometry. **Remodeling** is the term applied to dilation (other than that due to passive stretch) and other slow structural changes that occur in the stressed myocardium. It may include proliferation of connective tissue cells as well as abnormal myocardial cells with some biochemical characteristics of fetal myocytes. Ultimately, myocytes in the failing heart die at an accelerated rate through apoptosis, leaving the remaining myocytes subject to even greater stress.

Pathophysiology of Cardiac Performance

Cardiac performance is a function of four primary factors:

1. **Preload:** When some measure of left ventricular performance such as stroke volume or stroke work is plotted as a function of left ventricular filling pressure or end-diastolic fiber length, the resulting curve is termed the left ventricular function curve (Figure 13–4). The ascending limb (< 15 mm Hg filling pressure) represents the classic Frank-Starling relation described in physiology texts. Beyond approximately 15 mm Hg, there is a plateau of performance. Preloads greater than 20–25 mm Hg result in pulmonary congestion. As noted above, preload is usually increased in heart failure because of increased blood volume and venous tone. Because the function curve of the failing heart is lower, the plateau is reached at much lower values of stroke work or output. Increased fiber length or filling pressure increases oxygen demand in the myocardium, as described in Chapter 12. Reduction of high filling pressure is the goal of salt restriction and diuretic therapy in heart failure. Venodilator drugs (eg, nitroglycerin) also reduce preload by redistributing blood away from the chest into peripheral veins.

2. **Afterload:** Afterload is the resistance against which the heart must pump blood and is represented by aortic impedance and systemic vascular resistance. As noted in Figure 13–2, as cardiac output falls in chronic failure, a reflex increase in systemic vascular resistance occurs, mediated in part by increased sympathetic outflow and circulating catecholamines and in part by activation of the renin-angiotensin system. Endothelin, a potent vasoconstrictor peptide, is also involved. This sets the stage for the use of drugs that reduce arteriolar tone in heart failure.

3. **Contractility:** Heart muscle obtained by biopsy from patients with chronic low-output failure demonstrates a reduction in intrinsic contractility. As contractility decreases in the patient, there is a reduction in the velocity of muscle shortening, the rate of intraventricular pressure development (dP/dt), and the stroke output achieved (Figure 13–4). However, the heart is usually still capable of some increase in all of these measures of contractility in response to inotropic drugs.

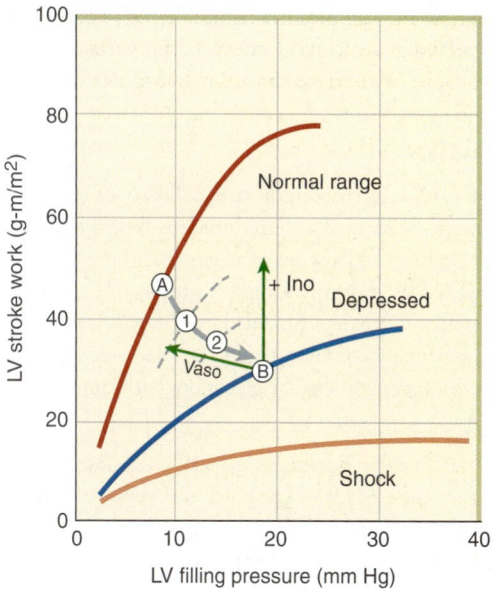

FIGURE 13–4 Relation of left ventricular (LV) performance to filling pressure in patients with acute myocardial infarction, an important cause of heart failure. The upper line indicates the range for normal, healthy individuals. At a given level of exercise, the heart operates at a stable point, eg, point A. In heart failure, function is shifted down and to the right, through points 1 and 2, finally reaching point B. A "pure" positive inotropic drug (+ Ino) would move the operating point upward by increasing cardiac stroke work. A vasodilator (Vaso) would move the point leftward by reducing filling pressure. Successful therapy usually results in both effects. (Modified and reproduced with permission, from Swan HJC, Parmley WW: Congestive heart failure. In: Sodeman WA Jr, Sodeman TM [editors]: *Pathologic Physiology*. Saunders, 1979.)

4. **Heart rate:** The heart rate is a major determinant of cardiac output. As the intrinsic function of the heart decreases in failure and stroke volume diminishes, an increase in heart rate—through sympathetic activation of β adrenoceptors—is the first compensatory mechanism that comes into play to maintain cardiac output.

■ BASIC PHARMACOLOGY OF DRUGS USED IN HEART FAILURE

Although digitalis is not the first drug and never the only drug used in heart failure, we begin our discussion with this group because other drugs are discussed in more detail in other chapters.

DIGITALIS

Digitalis is the genus name for the family of plants that provide most of the medically useful **cardiac glycosides,** eg, digoxin. Such plants have been known for thousands of years but were used erratically and with variable success until 1785, when William

Withering, an English physician and botanist, published a monograph describing the clinical effects of an extract of the purple foxglove plant (*Digitalis purpurea*, a major source of these agents).

Chemistry

All of the cardiac glycosides, or cardenolides—of which **digoxin** is the prototype—combine a steroid nucleus linked to a lactone ring at the 17 position and a series of sugars at carbon 3 of the nucleus. Because they lack an easily ionizable group, their solubility is not pH-dependent. Digoxin is obtained from *Digitalis lanata*, the white foxglove, but many common plants (eg, oleander, lily of the valley, and milkweed) contain cardiac glycosides with similar properties.

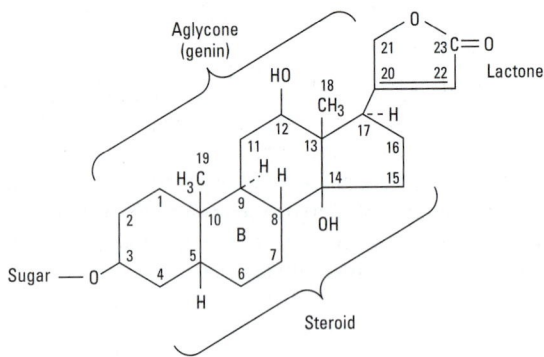

Pharmacokinetics

Digoxin, the only cardiac glycoside used in the USA, is 65–80% absorbed after oral administration. Absorption of other glycosides varies from zero to nearly 100%. Once present in the blood, all cardiac glycosides are widely distributed to tissues, including the central nervous system.

Digoxin is not extensively metabolized in humans; almost two thirds is excreted unchanged by the kidneys. Its renal clearance is proportional to creatinine clearance, and the half-life is 36–40 hours in patients with normal renal function. Equations and nomograms are available for adjusting digoxin dosage in patients with renal impairment.

Pharmacodynamics

Digoxin has multiple direct and indirect cardiovascular effects, with both therapeutic and toxic consequences. In addition, it has undesirable effects on the central nervous system and gut.

At the molecular level, all therapeutically useful cardiac glycosides **inhibit Na$^+$/K$^+$-ATPase,** the membrane-bound transporter often called the **sodium pump** (Figure 13–1). Although several isoforms of this ATPase occur and have varying sensitivity to cardiac glycosides, they are highly conserved in evolution. Inhibition of this transporter over most of the dose range has been extensively documented in all tissues studied. It is probable that this inhibitory action is largely responsible for the therapeutic effect (positive inotropy) as well as a major portion of the toxicity of digitalis. Other molecular-level effects of digitalis have been studied in the

heart and are discussed below. The fact that a receptor for cardiac glycosides exists on the sodium pump has prompted some investigators to propose that an endogenous digitalis-like steroid, possibly **ouabain** or **marinobufagenin,** must exist. Furthermore, additional functions of Na$^+$/K$^+$-ATPase have been postulated, involving apoptosis, cell growth and differentiation, immunity, and carbohydrate metabolism.

A. Cardiac Effects

1. Mechanical effects—Cardiac glycosides increase contraction of the cardiac sarcomere by increasing the free calcium concentration in the vicinity of the contractile proteins during systole. The increase in calcium concentration is the result of a two-step process: first, an **increase of intracellular sodium** concentration because of Na$^+$/K$^+$-ATPase inhibition; and second, a relative **reduction of calcium expulsion** from the cell by the sodium-calcium exchanger (NCX in Figure 13–1) caused by the increase in intracellular sodium. The increased cytoplasmic calcium is sequestered by SERCA in the SR for later release. Other mechanisms have been proposed but are not well supported.

The net result of the action of therapeutic concentrations of a cardiac glycoside is a distinctive increase in cardiac contractility (Figure 13–5, bottom trace, panels A and B). In isolated myocardial preparations, the rate of development of tension and of relaxation are both increased, with little or no change in time to peak tension. This effect occurs in both normal and failing myocardium, but in the intact patient the responses are modified by cardiovascular reflexes and the pathophysiology of heart failure.

2. Electrical effects—The effects of digitalis on the electrical properties of the heart are a mixture of direct and autonomic actions. Direct actions on the membranes of cardiac cells follow a well-defined progression: an early, brief prolongation of the action potential, followed by shortening (especially the plateau phase). The decrease in action potential duration is probably the result of increased potassium conductance that is caused by increased intracellular calcium (see Chapter 14). All these effects can be observed at therapeutic concentrations in the absence of overt toxicity (Table 13–2).

At higher concentrations, resting membrane potential is reduced (made less negative) as a result of inhibition of the sodium pump and reduced intracellular potassium. As toxicity progresses, oscillatory depolarizing afterpotentials appear following normally evoked action potentials (Figure 13–5, panel C). The afterpotentials (also known as **delayed after-depolarizations,** DADs) are associated with overloading of the intracellular calcium stores and oscillations in the free intracellular calcium ion concentration. When afterpotentials reach threshold, they elicit action potentials (**premature depolarizations,** ectopic "beats") that are coupled to the preceding normal action potentials. If afterpotentials in the Purkinje conducting system regularly reach threshold in this way, bigeminy will be recorded on the electrocardiogram (Figure 13–6). With further intoxication, each afterpotential-evoked action potential will itself elicit a suprathreshold after-potential, and a self-sustaining tachycardia will

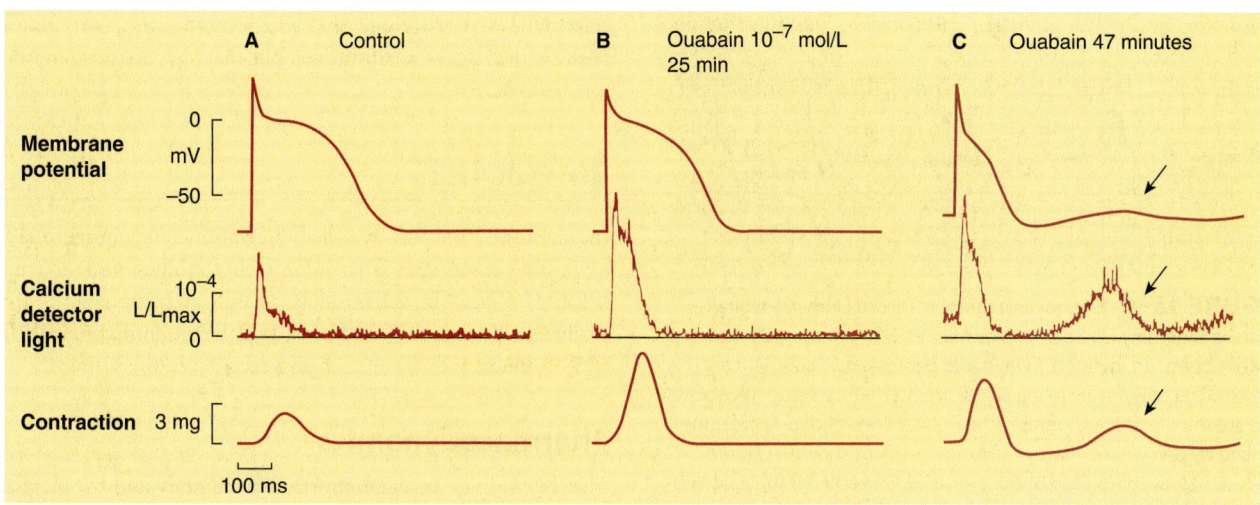

FIGURE 13–5 Effects of a cardiac glycoside, ouabain, on isolated cardiac tissue. The top tracing shows action potentials evoked during the control period (panel **A**), early in the "therapeutic" phase (**B**), and later, when toxicity is present (**C**). The middle tracing shows the light (L) emitted by the calcium-detecting protein aequorin (relative to the maximum possible, L_{max}) and is roughly proportional to the free intracellular calcium concentration. The bottom tracing records the tension elicited by the action potentials. The early phase of ouabain action (panel **B**) shows a slight shortening of action potential and a marked increase in free intracellular calcium concentration and contractile tension. The toxic phase (panel **C**) is associated with depolarization of the resting potential, a marked shortening of the action potential, and the appearance of an oscillatory depolarization, calcium increment, and contraction (*arrows*). (Unpublished data kindly provided by P Hess and H Gil Wier.)

be established. If allowed to progress, such a tachycardia may deteriorate into fibrillation; in the case of ventricular fibrillation, the arrhythmia will be rapidly fatal unless corrected.

Autonomic actions of cardiac glycosides on the heart involve both the parasympathetic and the sympathetic systems. In the lower portion of the dose range, cardioselective parasympathomimetic effects predominate. In fact, these atropine-blockable effects account for a significant portion of the early electrical effects of digitalis (Table 13–2). This action involves sensitization of the baroreceptors, central vagal stimulation, and facilitation of muscarinic transmission at the cardiac muscle cell. Because cholinergic innervation is much richer in the atria, these actions affect atrial and atrioventricular nodal function more than Purkinje or ventricular function. Some of the cholinomimetic effects are useful in the treatment of certain arrhythmias. At toxic levels, sympathetic outflow is increased by digitalis. This effect is not essential for typical digitalis toxicity but sensitizes the myocardium and exaggerates all the toxic effects of the drug.

The most common cardiac manifestations of digitalis toxicity include atrioventricular junctional rhythm, premature ventricular depolarizations, bigeminal rhythm, and second-degree atrioventricular blockade. However, it is claimed that digitalis can cause virtually any arrhythmia.

B. Effects on Other Organs

Cardiac glycosides affect all excitable tissues, including smooth muscle and the central nervous system. The gastrointestinal tract is the most common site of digitalis toxicity outside the heart. The effects include anorexia, nausea, vomiting, and diarrhea. This toxicity is caused in part by direct effects on the gastrointestinal tract and in part by central nervous system actions.

Central nervous system effects include vagal and chemoreceptor trigger zone stimulation. Less often, disorientation and hallucinations—especially in the elderly—and visual disturbances are noted. The latter effect may include aberrations of color perception. Gynecomastia is a rare effect reported in men taking digitalis.

TABLE 13–2 Effects of digoxin on electrical properties of cardiac tissues.

Tissue or Variable	Effects at Therapeutic Dosage	Effects at Toxic Dosage
Sinus node	↓ Rate	↓ Rate
Atrial muscle	↓ Refractory period	↓ Refractory period, arrhythmias
Atrioventricular node	↓ Conduction velocity, ↑ refractory period	↓ Refractory period, arrhythmias
Purkinje system, ventricular muscle	Slight ↓ refractory period	Extrasystoles, tachycardia, fibrillation
Electrocardiogram	↑ PR interval, ↓ QT interval	Tachycardia, fibrillation, arrest at extremely high dosage

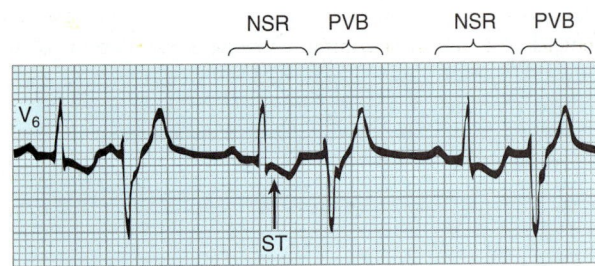

FIGURE 13–6 Electrocardiographic record showing digitalis-induced bigeminy. The complexes marked NSR are normal sinus rhythm beats; an inverted T wave and depressed ST segment are present. The complexes marked PVB are premature ventricular beats and are the electrocardiographic manifestations of depolarizations evoked by delayed oscillatory afterpotentials as shown in Figure 13–5. (Modified and reproduced, with permission, from Goldman MJ: *Principles of Clinical Electrocardiography*, 12th ed. Lange, 1986.)

C. Interactions with Potassium, Calcium, and Magnesium

Potassium and digitalis interact in two ways. First, they inhibit each other's binding to Na^+/K^+-ATPase; therefore, hyperkalemia reduces the enzyme-inhibiting actions of cardiac glycosides, whereas hypokalemia facilitates these actions. Second, abnormal cardiac automaticity is inhibited by hyperkalemia (see Chapter 14). Moderately increased extracellular K^+ therefore reduces the effects of digitalis, especially the toxic effects.

Calcium ion facilitates the toxic actions of cardiac glycosides by accelerating the overloading of intracellular calcium stores that appears to be responsible for digitalis-induced abnormal automaticity. Hypercalcemia therefore increases the risk of a digitalis-induced arrhythmia. The effects of magnesium ion are opposite to those of calcium. These interactions mandate careful evaluation of serum electrolytes in patients with digitalis-induced arrhythmias.

OTHER POSITIVE INOTROPIC DRUGS USED IN HEART FAILURE

Istaroxime is an investigational steroid derivative that increases contractility by inhibiting Na^+/K^+-ATPase (like cardiac glycosides) but in addition facilitates sequestration of Ca^{2+} by the SR. The latter action may render the drug less arrhythmogenic than digoxin. Istaroxime is in phase 2 clinical trials.

Drugs that inhibit **phosphodiesterases**, the family of enzymes that inactivate cAMP and cGMP, have long been used in therapy of heart failure. Although they have positive inotropic effects, most of their benefits appear to derive from vasodilation, as discussed below. The bipyridines **inamrinone** and **milrinone** are the most successful of these agents found to date, but their usefulness is limited. **Levosimendan,** a drug that sensitizes the troponin system to calcium, also appears to inhibit phosphodiesterase and to cause some vasodilation in addition to its inotropic effects. Some clinical trials suggest that this drug may be useful in patients with heart failure, and the drug has been approved in some countries

(not the USA). A group of β-adrenoceptor stimulants has also been used as digitalis substitutes, but they may increase mortality (see below).

BIPYRIDINES

Inamrinone (previously called amrinone) and **milrinone** are bipyridine compounds that inhibit phosphodiesterase isozyme 3 (PDE-3). They are active orally as well as parenterally but are available only in parenteral forms. They have elimination half-lives of 3–6 hours, with 10–40% being excreted in the urine.

Pharmacodynamics

The bipyridines increase myocardial contractility by increasing inward calcium flux in the heart during the action potential; they may also alter the intracellular movements of calcium by influencing the sarcoplasmic reticulum. They also have an important vasodilating effect. Inhibition of phosphodiesterase results in an increase in cAMP and the increase in contractility and vasodilation.

The toxicity of inamrinone includes nausea and vomiting; arrhythmias, thrombocytopenia, and liver enzyme changes have also been reported in a significant number of patients. This drug has been withdrawn in some countries. Milrinone appears less likely to cause bone marrow and liver toxicity than inamrinone, but it does cause arrhythmias. Inamrinone and milrinone are now used only intravenously and only for acute heart failure or severe exacerbation of chronic heart failure.

BETA-ADRENOCEPTOR AGONISTS

The general pharmacology of these agents is discussed in Chapter 9. The selective β_1 agonist that has been most widely used in patients with heart failure is **dobutamine.** This parenteral drug produces an increase in cardiac output together with a decrease in ventricular filling pressure. Some tachycardia and an increase in myocardial oxygen consumption have been reported. Therefore, the potential for producing angina or arrhythmias in patients with coronary artery disease is significant, as is the tachyphylaxis that accompanies the use of any β stimulant. Intermittent dobutamine infusion may benefit some patients with chronic heart failure.

Dopamine has also been used in acute heart failure and may be particularly helpful if there is a need to raise blood pressure.

DRUGS WITHOUT POSITIVE INOTROPIC EFFECTS USED IN HEART FAILURE

These agents—not positive inotropic drugs—are the first-line therapies for chronic heart failure. The drugs most commonly used are diuretics, ACE inhibitors, angiotensin receptor antagonists, aldosterone antagonists, and β blockers (Table 13–1). In acute failure, diuretics and vasodilators play important roles.

DIURETICS

Diuretics, especially furosemide, are drugs of choice in heart failure and are discussed in detail in Chapter 15. They have no direct effect on cardiac contractility; their major mechanism of action in heart failure is to reduce venous pressure and ventricular preload. This results in reduction of salt and water retention and edema and its symptoms. The reduction of cardiac size, which leads to improved pump efficiency, is of major importance in systolic failure. **Spironolactone and eplerenone,** the aldosterone antagonist diuretics (see Chapter 15), have the additional benefit of decreasing morbidity and mortality in patients with severe heart failure who are also receiving ACE inhibitors and other standard therapy. One possible mechanism for this benefit lies in accumulating evidence that aldosterone may also cause myocardial and vascular fibrosis and baroreceptor dysfunction in addition to its renal effects.

ANGIOTENSIN-CONVERTING ENZYME INHIBITORS, ANGIOTENSIN RECEPTOR BLOCKERS, & RELATED AGENTS

ACE inhibitors such as **captopril** are introduced in Chapter 11 and discussed again in Chapter 17. These versatile drugs reduce peripheral resistance and thereby reduce afterload; they also reduce salt and water retention (by reducing aldosterone secretion) and in that way reduce preload. The reduction in tissue angiotensin levels also reduces sympathetic activity through diminution of angiotensin's presynaptic effects on norepinephrine release. Finally, these drugs reduce the long-term remodeling of the heart and vessels, an effect that may be responsible for the observed reduction in mortality and morbidity (see Clinical Pharmacology).

Angiotensin AT_1 receptor blockers such as **losartan** (see Chapters 11 and 17) appear to have similar but more limited beneficial effects. Angiotensin receptor blockers should be considered in patients intolerant of ACE inhibitors because of incessant cough. In some trials, **candesartan** was beneficial when *added* to an ACE inhibitor.

Aliskiren, a renin inhibitor recently approved for hypertension, is in clinical trials for heart failure. Preliminary results suggest an efficacy similar to that of ACE inhibitors.

VASODILATORS

Vasodilators are effective in acute heart failure because they provide a reduction in preload (through venodilation), or reduction in afterload (through arteriolar dilation), or both. Some evidence suggests that long-term use of hydralazine and isosorbide dinitrate can also reduce damaging remodeling of the heart.

A synthetic form of the endogenous peptide brain natriuretic peptide (BNP) is approved for use in acute (not chronic) cardiac failure as **nesiritide.** This recombinant product increases cGMP in smooth muscle cells and reduces venous and arteriolar tone in experimental preparations. It also causes diuresis. The peptide has a short half-life of about 18 minutes and is administered as a bolus intravenous dose followed by continuous infusion. Excessive hypotension is the most common adverse effect. Reports of significant renal damage and deaths have resulted in extra warnings regarding this agent, and it should be used with great caution.

Plasma concentrations of *endogenous* BNP rise in most patients with heart failure and are correlated with severity. Measurement of plasma BNP has become a useful diagnostic or prognostic test in some centers.

Related peptides include atrial natriuretic peptide (ANP) and urodilatin, a similar peptide produced in the kidney. **Carperitide** and **ularitide,** respectively, are investigational synthetic analogs of these endogenous peptides and are in clinical trials (see Chapter 15).

Bosentan and **tezosentan,** orally active competitive inhibitors of endothelin (see Chapter 17), have been shown to have some benefits in experimental animal models with heart failure, but results in human trials have been disappointing. Bosentan is approved for use in pulmonary hypertension (see Chapter 11). It has significant teratogenic and hepatotoxic effects.

BETA-ADRENOCEPTOR BLOCKERS

Most patients with chronic heart failure respond favorably to certain β blockers in spite of the fact that these drugs can precipitate acute decompensation of cardiac function (see Chapter 10). Studies with **bisoprolol, carvedilol, metoprolol,** and **nebivolol** showed a reduction in mortality in patients with stable severe heart failure, but this effect was not observed with another β blocker, bucindolol. A full understanding of the beneficial action of β blockade is lacking, but suggested mechanisms include attenuation of the adverse effects of high concentrations of catecholamines (including apoptosis), up-regulation of β receptors, decreased heart rate, and reduced remodeling through inhibition of the mitogenic activity of catecholamines.

■ CLINICAL PHARMACOLOGY OF DRUGS USED IN HEART FAILURE

The American College of Cardiology/American Heart Association (ACC/AHA) guidelines for management of chronic heart failure specify four stages in the development of heart failure (Table 13–3). Patients in stage A are at high risk because of other disease but have no signs or symptoms of heart failure. Stage B patients have evidence of structural heart disease but no symptoms of heart failure. Stage C patients have structural heart disease and symptoms of failure, and symptoms are responsive to ordinary therapy. Stage D patients have heart failure refractory to ordinary therapy, and special interventions (resynchronization therapy, transplant) are required.

Once stage C is reached, the severity of heart failure is usually described according to a scale devised by the New York Heart Association. Class I failure is associated with no limitations on ordinary activities, and symptoms that occur only with greater than ordinary exercise. Class II is characterized by slight limitation of activities, and results in fatigue and palpitations with ordinary

TABLE 13–3 Classification and treatment of chronic heart failure.

ACC/AHA Stage[1]	NYHA Class[2]	Description	Management
A	Prefailure	No symptoms but risk factors present[3]	Treat obesity, hypertension, diabetes, hyperlipidemia, etc
B	I	Symptoms with severe exercise	ACEI/ARB, β blocker, diuretic
C	II/III	Symptoms with marked (class II) or mild (class III) exercise	Add aldosterone antagonist, digoxin; CRT, hydralazine/nitrate[4]
D	IV	Severe symptoms at rest	Transplant, LVAD

[1]American College of Cardiology/American Heart Association classification.

[2]New York Heart Association classification.

[3]Risk factors include hypertension, myocardial infarct, diabetes.

[4]For selected populations, eg, African American.

ACEI, angiotensin-converting enzyme inhibitor; ARB, angiotensin receptor blocker; CRT, cardiac resynchronization therapy; LVAD, left ventricular assist device.

physical activity. Class III failure results in no symptoms at rest, but fatigue, shortness of breath, and tachycardia occur with less than ordinary physical activity. Class IV is associated with symptoms even when the patient is at rest.

MANAGEMENT OF CHRONIC HEART FAILURE

The major steps in the management of patients with chronic heart failure are outlined in Table 13–3. The 2009 update to the ACC/AHA 2005 guidelines suggests that treatment of patients at high risk (stages A and B) should be focused on control of hypertension, hyperlipidemia, and diabetes, if present. Once symptoms and signs of failure are present, stage C has been entered, and active treatment of failure must be initiated.

SODIUM REMOVAL

Sodium removal—by dietary salt restriction and a diuretic—is the mainstay in management of symptomatic heart failure, especially if edema is present. In very mild failure a **thiazide** diuretic may be tried, but a loop agent such as **furosemide** is usually required. Sodium loss causes secondary loss of potassium, which is particularly hazardous if the patient is to be given digitalis. Hypokalemia can be treated with potassium supplementation or through the addition of an ACE inhibitor or a potassium-sparing diuretic such as spironolactone. Spironolactone or eplerenone should probably be considered in all patients with moderate or severe heart failure, since both appear to reduce both morbidity and mortality.

ACE INHIBITORS & ANGIOTENSIN RECEPTOR BLOCKERS

In patients with left ventricular dysfunction but no edema, an ACE inhibitor should be the first drug used. Several large studies have showed clearly that ACE inhibitors are superior to both placebo and to vasodilators and must be considered, along with diuretics, as first-line therapy for chronic heart failure. However, ACE inhibitors cannot replace digoxin in patients already receiving the glycoside because patients withdrawn from digoxin deteriorate while on ACE inhibitor therapy.

By reducing preload and afterload in asymptomatic patients, ACE inhibitors (eg, **enalapril**) slow the progress of ventricular dilation and thus slow the downward spiral of heart failure. Consequently, ACE inhibitors are beneficial in all subsets of patients—from those who are asymptomatic to those in severe chronic failure. This benefit appears to be a class effect; that is, all ACE inhibitors appear to be effective.

The angiotensin II AT_1 receptor blockers (ARBs, eg, **losartan**) produce beneficial hemodynamic effects similar to those of ACE inhibitors. However, large clinical trials suggest that angiotensin receptor blockers are best reserved for patients who cannot tolerate ACE inhibitors (usually because of cough).

VASODILATORS

Vasodilator drugs can be divided into selective arteriolar dilators, venous dilators, and drugs with nonselective vasodilating effects. The choice of agent should be based on the patient's signs and symptoms and hemodynamic measurements. Thus, in patients with high filling pressures in whom the principal symptom is dyspnea, venous dilators such as long-acting **nitrates** will be most helpful in reducing filling pressures and the symptoms of pulmonary congestion. In patients in whom fatigue due to low left ventricular output is a primary symptom, an arteriolar dilator such as **hydralazine** may be helpful in increasing forward cardiac output. In most patients with severe chronic failure that responds poorly to other therapy, the problem usually involves both elevated filling pressures and reduced cardiac output. In these circumstances, dilation of both arterioles and veins is required. In a trial in African-American patients already receiving ACE inhibitors, addition of hydralazine and isosorbide dinitrate reduced mortality. As a result, a fixed combination of these two agents has been made available as isosorbide dinitrate/hydralazine (**BiDil**), and this is currently approved for use only in African Americans.

BETA BLOCKERS & ION CHANNEL BLOCKERS

Trials of β-blocker therapy in patients with heart failure are based on the hypothesis that excessive tachycardia and adverse effects of high catecholamine levels on the heart contribute to the downward course of heart failure. The results clearly indicate that such therapy is beneficial if initiated cautiously at low doses, even though acutely blocking the supportive effects of catecholamines can worsen heart failure. Several months of therapy may be required before improvement is noted; this usually consists of a slight rise in ejection fraction, slower heart rate, and reduction in symptoms. As noted above, not all β blockers have proved useful, but **bisoprolol, carvedilol, metoprolol,** and **nebivolol** have been shown to reduce mortality.

In contrast, the calcium-blocking drugs appear to have no role in the treatment of patients with heart failure. Their depressant effects on the heart may worsen heart failure. On the other hand, slowing of heart rate with **ivabradine** (an I_f blocker, see Chapter 12) appears to be of benefit.

Digitalis

Digoxin is indicated in patients with heart failure and atrial fibrillation. It is usually given only when diuretics and ACE inhibitors have failed to control symptoms. Only about 50% of patients with normal sinus rhythm (usually those with documented systolic dysfunction) will have relief of heart failure from digitalis. Better results are obtained in patients with atrial fibrillation. If the decision is made to use a cardiac glycoside, digoxin is the one chosen in most cases (and the only one available in the USA). When symptoms are mild, slow loading (digitalization) with 0.125–0.25 mg per day is safer and just as effective as the rapid method (0.5–0.75 mg every 8 hours for three doses, followed by 0.125–0.25 mg per day).

Determining the optimal level of digitalis effect may be difficult. Unfortunately, toxic effects may occur before the therapeutic end point is detected. Measurement of plasma digoxin levels is useful in patients who appear unusually resistant or sensitive; a level of 1 ng/mL or less is appropriate.

Because it has a moderate but persistent positive inotropic effect, digitalis can, in theory, reverse all the signs and symptoms of heart failure. Although the net effect of the drug on mortality is mixed, it reduces hospitalization and deaths from progressive heart failure at the expense of an increase in sudden death. It is important to note that the mortality rate is reduced in patients with serum digoxin concentrations of less than 0.9 ng/mL but increased in those with digoxin levels greater than 1.5 ng/mL.

Other Clinical Uses of Digitalis

Digitalis is useful in the management of atrial arrhythmias because of its cardioselective parasympathomimetic effects. In atrial flutter and fibrillation, the depressant effect of the drug on atrioventricular conduction helps control an excessively high ventricular rate. Digitalis has also been used in the control of paroxysmal atrial and atrioventricular nodal tachycardia. At present, calcium channel blockers and adenosine are preferred for this application. Digoxin is explicitly contraindicated in patients with Wolff-Parkinson-White syndrome and atrial fibrillation (see Chapter 14).

Toxicity

In spite of its limited benefits and recognized hazards, digitalis is still heavily used and toxicity is common. Therapy for toxicity manifested as visual changes or gastrointestinal disturbances generally requires no more than reducing the dose of the drug. If cardiac arrhythmia is present and can be ascribed to digitalis, more vigorous therapy may be necessary. Serum digitalis and potassium levels and the electrocardiogram should always be monitored during therapy of significant digitalis toxicity. Electrolyte status should be corrected if abnormal (see above). Monitoring of potassium levels is particularly important in patients on renal dialysis.

In severe digitalis intoxication, serum potassium will already be elevated at the time of diagnosis (because of potassium loss from the intracellular compartment of skeletal muscle and other tissues). Furthermore, automaticity is usually depressed, and antiarrhythmic agents administered in this setting may lead to cardiac arrest. Such patients are best treated with prompt insertion of a temporary cardiac pacemaker catheter and administration of digitalis antibodies (**digoxin immune fab**). These antibodies recognize digitoxin and cardiac glycosides from many other plants in addition to digoxin. They are extremely useful in reversing severe intoxication with most glycosides.

Digitalis-induced arrhythmias are frequently made worse by cardioversion; this therapy should be reserved for ventricular fibrillation if the arrhythmia is glycoside-induced.

CARDIAC RESYNCHRONIZATION THERAPY

Patients with normal sinus rhythm and a wide QRS interval, eg, greater than 120 ms, have impaired synchronization of right and left ventricular contraction. Poor synchronization of ventricular contraction results in diminished cardiac output. Resynchronization, with left ventricular or biventricular pacing, has been shown to reduce mortality in patients with chronic heart failure who were already receiving optimal medical therapy.

MANAGEMENT OF DIASTOLIC HEART FAILURE

Most clinical trials have been carried out in patients with systolic dysfunction, so the evidence regarding the superiority or inferiority of drugs in heart failure with preserved ejection fraction is meager. Most authorities support the use of the drug groups described above, and the SENIORS 2009 study suggests that nebivolol is effective in both systolic and diastolic failure. Control of hypertension is particularly important, and revascularization should be considered if coronary artery disease is present.

Tachycardia limits filling time; therefore, bradycardic drugs may be particularly useful, at least in theory.

MANAGEMENT OF ACUTE HEART FAILURE

Acute heart failure occurs frequently in patients with chronic failure. Such episodes are usually associated with increased exertion, emotion, excess salt intake, nonadherence to medical therapy, or increased metabolic demand occasioned by fever, anemia, etc. A particularly common and important cause of acute failure—with or without chronic failure—is acute myocardial infarction.

Patients with acute myocardial infarction are best treated with emergency revascularization using either coronary angioplasty and a stent, or a thrombolytic agent. Even with revascularization, acute failure may develop in such patients. Many of the signs and symptoms of acute and chronic failure are identical, but their therapies diverge because of the need for more rapid response and the relatively greater frequency and severity of pulmonary vascular congestion in the acute form.

Measurements of arterial pressure, cardiac output, stroke work index, and pulmonary capillary wedge pressure are particularly useful in patients with acute myocardial infarction and acute heart failure. Such patients can be usefully characterized on the basis of three hemodynamic measurements: arterial pressure, left ventricular filling pressure, and cardiac index. When filling pressure is greater than 15 mm Hg and stroke work index is less than 20 g-m/m^2, the mortality rate is high. Intermediate levels of these two variables imply a much better prognosis.

Intravenous treatment is the rule in acute heart failure. Among diuretics, **furosemide** is the most commonly used. **Dopamine** or **dobutamine** are positive inotropic drugs with prompt onset and short durations of action; they are most useful in patients with severe hypotension. **Levosimendan** has been approved for use in acute failure in Europe, and noninferiority has been demonstrated against dobutamine. Vasodilators in use in patients with acute decompensation include **nitroprusside, nitroglycerine,** and **nesiritide.** Reduction in afterload often improves ejection fraction, but improved survival has not been documented. A small subset of patients in acute heart failure will have hyponatremia, presumably due to increased vasopressin activity. A V_{1a} and V_2 receptor antagonist, **conivaptan,** is approved for parenteral treatment of euvolemic hyponatremia. Several clinical trials have indicated that this drug and related V_2 antagonists (**tolvaptan**) may have a beneficial effect in some patients with acute heart failure and hyponatremia. Thus far, vasopressin antagonists do not seem to reduce mortality.

SUMMARY Drugs Used in Heart Failure

Subclass	Mechanism of Action	Effects	Clinical Applications	Pharmacokinetics, Toxicities, Interactions
DIURETICS				
• Furosemide	Loop diuretic: Decreases NaCl and KCl reabsorption in thick ascending limb of the loop of Henle in the nephron (see Chapter 15)	Increased excretion of salt and water • reduces cardiac preload and afterload • reduces pulmonary and peripheral edema	Acute and chronic heart failure • severe hypertension • edematous conditions	Oral and IV • duration 2–4 h • *Toxicity:* Hypovolemia, hypokalemia, orthostatic hypotension, ototoxicity, sulfonamide allergy
• Hydrochlorothiazide	Decreases NaCl reabsorption in the distal convoluted tubule	Same as furosemide, but less efficacious	Mild chronic failure • mild-moderate hypertension • hypercalciuria • has not been shown to reduce mortality	Oral only • duration 10–12 h • *Toxicity:* Hyponatremia, hypokalemia, hyperglycemia, hyperuricemia, hyperlipidemia, sulfonamide allergy

• *Three other loop diuretics: Bumetanide and torsemide similar to furosemide; ethacrynic acid not a sulfonamide*
• *Many other thiazides: All basically similar to hydrochlorothiazide, differing only in pharmacokinetics*

ALDOSTERONE ANTAGONISTS				
• Spironolactone	Blocks cytoplasmic aldosterone receptors in collecting tubules of nephron • possible membrane effect	Increased salt and water excretion • reduces remodeling • reduces mortality	Chronic heart failure • aldosteronism (cirrhosis, adrenal tumor) • hypertension • has been shown to reduce mortality	Oral • duration 24–72 h (slow onset and offset) • *Toxicity:* Hyperkalemia, antiandrogen actions

• *Eplerenone: Similar to spironolactone; more selective antialdosterone effect; no significant antiandrogen action; has been shown to reduce mortality*

(continued)

Subclass	Mechanism of Action	Effects	Clinical Applications	Pharmacokinetics, Toxicities, Interactions
ANGIOTENSIN ANTAGONISTS				
Angiotensin-converting enzyme (ACE) inhibitors: • Captopril	Inhibits ACE • reduces AII formation by inhibiting conversion of AI to AII	Arteriolar and venous dilation • reduces aldosterone secretion • reduces cardiac remodeling	Chronic heart failure • hypertension • diabetic renal disease • has been shown to reduce mortality	Oral • half-life 2–4 h but given in large doses so duration 12–24 h • *Toxicity:* Cough, hyperkalemia, angioneurotic edema • *Interactions:* Additive with other angiotensin antagonists
Angiotensin receptor blockers (ARBs): • Losartan	Antagonize AII effects at AT_1 receptors	Like ACE inhibitors	Like ACE inhibitors • used in patients intolerant to ACE inhibitors • has been shown to reduce mortality	Oral • duration 6–8 h • *Toxicity:* Hyperkalemia; angioneurotic edema • *Interactions:* Additive with other angiotensin antagonists
• *Enalapril, many other ACE inhibitors: Like captopril*				
• *Candesartan, many other ARBs: Like losartan*				
BETA BLOCKERS				
• Carvedilol	Competitively blocks β_1 receptors (see Chapter 10)	Slows heart rate • reduces blood pressure • poorly understood effects • reduces heart failure mortality	Chronic heart failure: To slow progression • reduce mortality in moderate and severe heart failure • many other indications in Chapter 10	Oral • duration 10–12 h • *Toxicity:* Bronchospasm, bradycardia, atrioventricular block, acute cardiac decompensation • see Chapter 10 for other toxicities and interactions
• *Metoprolol, bisoprolol, nebivolol: Select group of β blockers that have been shown to reduce heart failure mortality*				
CARDIAC GLYCOSIDE				
• Digoxin	Na^+/K^+-ATPase inhibition results in reduced Ca^{2+} expulsion and increased Ca^{2+} stored in sarcoplasmic reticulum	Increases cardiac contractility • cardiac parasympathomimetic effect (slowed sinus heart rate, slowed atrioventricular conduction)	Chronic symptomatic heart failure • rapid ventricular rate in atrial fibrillation • has not been definitively shown to reduce mortality	Oral, parenteral • duration 36–40 h • *Toxicity:* Nausea, vomiting, diarrhea • cardiac arrhythmias
VASODILATORS				
Venodilators: • Isosorbide dinitrate	Releases nitric oxide (NO) • activates guanylyl cyclase (see Chapter 12)	Venodilation • reduces preload and ventricular stretch	Acute and chronic heart failure • angina	Oral • 4–6 h duration • *Toxicity:* Postural hypotension, tachycardia, headache • *Interactions:* Additive with other vasodilators and synergistic with phosphodiesterase type 5 inhibitors
Arteriolar dilators: • Hydralazine	Probably increases NO synthesis in endothelium (see Chapter 11)	Reduces blood pressure and afterload • results in increased cardiac output	Hydralazine plus nitrates have reduced mortality	Oral • 8–12 h duration • *Toxicity:* Tachycardia, fluid retention, lupus-like syndrome
Combined arteriolar and venodilator: • Nitroprusside	Releases NO spontaneously • activates guanylyl cyclase	Marked vasodilation • reduces preload and afterload	Acute cardiac decompensation • hypertensive emergencies (malignant hypertension)	IV only • duration 1–2 min • *Toxicity:* Excessive hypotension, thiocyanate and cyanide toxicity • *Interactions:* Additive with other vasodilators
BETA-ADRENOCEPTOR AGONISTS				
• Dobutamine	$Beta_1$-selective agonist • increases cAMP synthesis	Increases cardiac contractility, output	Acute decompensated heart failure • intermittent therapy in chronic failure reduces symptoms	IV only • duration a few minutes • *Toxicity:* Arrhythmias • *Interactions:* Additive with other sympathomimetics
• Dopamine	Dopamine receptor agonist • higher doses activate β and α adrenoceptors	Increases renal blood flow • higher doses increase cardiac force and blood pressure	Acute decompensated heart failure • shock	IV only • duration a few minutes • *Toxicity:* Arrhythmias • *Interactions:* Additive with sympathomimetics

(continued)

Subclass	Mechanism of Action	Effects	Clinical Applications	Pharmacokinetics, Toxicities, Interactions
BIPYRIDINES				
• Inamrinone, milrinone	Phosphodiesterase type 3 inhibitors • decrease cAMP breakdown	Vasodilators; lower peripheral vascular resistance • also increase cardiac contractility	Acute decompensated heart failure • increase mortality in chronic failure	IV only • duration 3–6 h • *Toxicity:* Arrhythmias • *Interactions:* Additive with other arrhythmogenic agents
NATRIURETIC PEPTIDE				
• Nesiritide	Activates BNP receptors, increases cGMP	Vasodilation • diuresis	Acute decompensated failure • has not been shown to reduce mortality	IV only • duration 18 minutes • *Toxicity:* Renal damage, hypotension, may increase mortality

P R E P A R A T I O N S   A V A I L A B L E

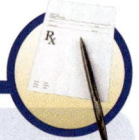

DIURETICS

See Chapter 15.

DIGITALIS

Digoxin (generic, Lanoxicaps, Lanoxin)
　Oral: 0.125, 0.25 mg tablets; 0.05, 0.1, 0.2 mg capsules[*]; 0.05 mg/mL elixir
　Parenteral: 0.1, 0.25 mg/mL for injection

DIGITALIS ANTIBODY

Digoxin immune fab (ovine) (Digibind, DigiFab)
　Parenteral: 38 or 40 mg per vial with 75 mg sorbitol lyophilized powder to reconstitute for IV injection. Each vial will bind approximately 0.5 mg digoxin or digitoxin.

SYMPATHOMIMETICS MOST COMMONLY USED IN CONGESTIVE HEART FAILURE

Dobutamine (generic)
　Parenteral: 12.5 mg/mL for IV infusion

Dopamine (generic, Intropin)
　Parenteral: 40, 80, 160 mg/mL for IV injection; 80, 160, 320 mg/dL in 5% dextrose for IV infusion

ANGIOTENSIN-CONVERTING ENZYME INHIBITORS

Benazepril (generic, Lotensin)
　Oral: 5, 10, 20, 40 mg tablets

Captopril (generic, Capoten)
　Oral: 12.5, 25, 50, 100 mg tablets

Enalapril (generic, Vasotec, Vasotec I.V.)
　Oral: 2.5, 5, 10, 20 mg tablets
　Parenteral: 1.25 mg enalaprilat/mL

Fosinopril (generic, Monopril)
　Oral: 10, 20, 40 mg tablets

Lisinopril (generic, Prinivil, Zestril)
　Oral: 2.5, 5, 10, 20, 30, 40 mg tablets

Moexipril (generic, Univasc)
　Oral: 7.5, 15 mg tablets

Perindopril (Aceon)
　Oral: 2, 4, 8 mg tablets

Quinapril (generic, Accupril)
　Oral: 5, 10, 20, 40 mg tablets

Ramipril (Altace)
　Oral: 1.25, 2.5, 5, 10 mg capsules

Trandolapril (Mavik)
　Oral: 1, 2, 4 mg tablets

ANGIOTENSIN RECEPTOR BLOCKERS

Candesartan (Atacand)
　Oral: 4, 8, 16, 32 mg tablets

Eprosartan (Teveten)
　Oral: 600 mg tablets

Irbesartan (Avapro)
　Oral: 75, 150, 300 mg tablets

Losartan (Cozaar)
　Oral: 25, 50, 100 mg tablets

Olmesartan (Benicar)
　Oral: 5, 20, 40 mg tablets

Telmisartan (Micardis)
　Oral: 20, 40, 80 mg tablets

Valsartan (Diovan)
　Oral: 40, 80, 160, 320 mg tablets

BETA BLOCKERS THAT HAVE REDUCED MORTALITY IN HEART FAILURE

Bisoprolol (generic, Zebeta, off-label use)
　Oral: 5, 10 mg tablets

Carvedilol (Coreg)
Oral: 3.125, 6.25, 12.5, 25 mg tablets; 10, 20, 40, 80 mg extended-release capsules

Metoprolol (Lopressor, Toprol XL)
Oral: 50, 100 mg tablets; 25, 50, 100, 200 mg extended-release tablets
Parenteral: 1 mg/mL for IV injection

Nebivolol (Bystolic)
Oral: 2.5, 5, 10 mg tablets

ALDOSTERONE ANTAGONISTS

Spironolactone (generic, Aldactone)
Oral: 25, 50 mg tablets

Eplerenone (Inspra)
Oral: 25, 50 mg tablets

OTHER DRUGS

Hydralazine (generic) (see Chapter 11)

Isosorbide dinitrate (see Chapter 12)

Nitroglycerine (see Chapter 12)

Hydralazine plus isosorbide dinitrate fixed dose (BiDil)
Oral: 37.5 mg hydralazine + 20 mg isosorbide dinitrate tablets

Inamrinone (generic)
Parenteral: 5 mg/mL for IV injection

Milrinone (generic, Primacor)
Parenteral: 1 mg/mL for IV injection

Nesiritide (Natrecor)
Parenteral: 1.58 mg powder to reconstitute for IV injection

Bosentan (Tracleer)
Oral: 62.5, 125 mg tablets

*Digoxin capsules (Lanoxicaps) have greater bioavailability than digoxin tablets.

REFERENCES

Abraham WT, Greenberg BH, Yancy CW: Pharmacologic therapies across the continuum of left ventricular dysfunction. Am J Cardiol 2008;102 (Suppl):21G.

Ahmed A et al: Effectiveness of digoxin in reducing one-year mortality in chronic heart failure in the Digitalis Investigation Group trial. Am J Cardiol 2009;103:82.

Arnold JM et al: Canadian Cardiovascular Society Consensus Conference Recommendations on Heart Failure. Can J Cardiol 2006;22:23.

Bagrov AY, Shapiro JI, Federova OV: Endogenous cardiotonic steroids: Physiology, pharmacology, and novel therapeutic targets. Pharmacol Rev 2009;61:9.

Cleland JCF et al: The effect of cardiac resynchronization on morbidity and mortality in heart failure. N Engl J Med 2005;352:1539.

Colucci WS: Overview of the therapy of heart failure due to systolic dysfunction. UpToDate, 2010. http://www.UpToDate.com.

CONSENSUS Trial Study Group: Effects of enalapril on mortality in severe congestive heart failure. N Engl J Med 1987;316:1429.

DeLuca L et al: Overview of emerging pharmacologic agents for acute heart failure syndromes. Eur J Heart Fail 2008;10:201.

Elkayam U et al: Vasodilators in the management of acute heart failure. Crit Care Med 2008;36:S95.

Ikeda Y, Hoshijima M, Chien KR: Toward biologically targeted therapy of calcium cycling defects in heart failure. Physiology 2008;28:6.

Jessup M et al: 2009 Focused update incorporated into the ACC/AHA 2005 guidelines for the diagnosis and management of heart failure in adults. J Am Coll Cardiol 2009;53:e1.

Klapholtz M: β-Blocker use for the stages of heart failure. Mayo Clin Proc 2009;84:718.

Lingrel JB: The physiological significance of the cardiotonic steroid/ouabain-binding site of the Na,K-ATPase. Annu Rev Physiol 2010;72:395.

Malik FI et al: Cardiac myosin activation: A potential therapeutic approach for systolic heart failure. Science 2011;331:1439.

Post SR, Hammond HK, Insel PA: β-Adrenergic receptors and receptor signaling in heart failure. Annu Rev Pharmacol Toxicol 1999;39:343.

Ramani GV, Ur PA, Mehra MR: Chronic heart failure: Contemporary diagnosis and management. Mayo Clin Proc 2010;85:180.

Rathbone SS et al: Association of serum digoxin concentration and outcomes in patients with heart failure. JAMA 2003;289:871.

Seed A et al: Neurohumoral effects of the new orally active renin inhibitor, aliskiren, in chronic heart failure. Eur J Heart Fail 2007;9:1120.

Shekelle PG et al: Efficacy of angiotensin-converting enzyme inhibitors and beta blockers in the management of left ventricular systolic dysfunction according to race, gender, and diabetic status: A meta-analysis of major clinical trials. J Am Coll Cardiol 2003;41:1529.

Taur Y, Frishman WH: The cardiac ryanodine receptor (RyR2) and its role in heart disease. Cardiol Rev 2005;13:142.

Taylor AL et al: Combination of isosorbide dinitrate and hydralazine in blacks with heart failure. N Engl J Med 2004;351:2049.

Topalian S, Ginsberg F, Parrillo JE: Cardiogenic shock. Crit Care Med 2008;36:S66.

van Veldhuisen DJ et al: Beta-blockade with nebivolol in elderly heart failure patients with impaired and preserved left ventricular ejection fraction. Data from SENIORS (Study of Effects of Nebivolol Intervention on Outcomes and Rehospitalization in Seniors with Heart Failure). J Am Coll Cardiol 2009;53:2150.

CASE STUDY ANSWER

The patient has a low ejection fraction with systolic heart failure. He was placed on a low-sodium diet and treated with a diuretic (furosemide 40 mg twice daily). On this therapy, he was less short of breath on exertion and could also lie flat without dyspnea. An angiotensin-converting enzyme (ACE) inhibitor was added (enalapril 20 mg twice daily), and over the next few weeks, he continued to feel better. Because of continued shortness of breath on exercise, digoxin 0.25 mg/d was added with a further improvement in exercise tolerance. Addition of a β blocker and eplerenone is being considered.

Agents Used in Cardiac Arrhythmias

Joseph R. Hume, PhD, &
Augustus O. Grant, MD, PhD

CASE STUDY

A 69-year-old retired teacher presents with a 1-month history of palpitations, intermittent shortness of breath, and fatigue. She has a history of hypertension. An ECG shows atrial fibrillation with a ventricular response of 122 bpm and signs of left ventricular hypertrophy. She is anticoagulated with warfarin and started on sustained-release metoprolol 50 mg/d. After 7 days, her rhythm reverts to normal sinus spontaneously. However, over the ensuing month, she continues to have intermittent palpitations and fatigue. Continuous ECG recording over a 48-hour period documents paroxysms of atrial fibrillation with heart rates of 88–114 bpm. An echocardiogram shows a left ventricular ejection fraction of 38% with no localized wall motion abnormality. At this stage, would you initiate treatment with an antiarrhythmic drug to maintain normal sinus rhythm, and if so, what drug would you choose?

Cardiac arrhythmias are a common problem in clinical practice, occurring in up to 25% of patients treated with digitalis, 50% of anesthetized patients, and over 80% of patients with acute myocardial infarction. Arrhythmias may require treatment because rhythms that are too rapid, too slow, or asynchronous can reduce cardiac output. Some arrhythmias can precipitate more serious or even lethal rhythm disturbances; for example, early premature ventricular depolarizations can precipitate ventricular fibrillation. In such patients, antiarrhythmic drugs may be lifesaving. On the other hand, the hazards of antiarrhythmic drugs—and in particular the fact that they can *precipitate* lethal arrhythmias in some patients—has led to a reevaluation of their relative risks and benefits. In general, treatment of asymptomatic or minimally symptomatic arrhythmias should be avoided for this reason.

Arrhythmias can be treated with the drugs discussed in this chapter and with nonpharmacologic therapies such as pacemakers, cardioversion, catheter ablation, and surgery. This chapter describes the pharmacology of drugs that suppress arrhythmias by a direct action on the cardiac cell membrane. Other modes of therapy are discussed briefly (see Box: The Nonpharmacologic Therapy of Cardiac Arrhythmias).

ELECTROPHYSIOLOGY OF NORMAL CARDIAC RHYTHM

The electrical impulse that triggers a normal cardiac contraction originates at regular intervals in the sinoatrial (SA) node (Figure 14–1), usually at a frequency of 60–100 bpm. This impulse spreads rapidly through the atria and enters the atrioventricular (AV) node, which is normally the only conduction pathway between the atria and ventricles. Conduction through the AV node is slow, requiring about 0.15 seconds. (This delay provides time for atrial contraction to propel blood into the ventricles.) The impulse then propagates over the His-Purkinje system and invades all parts of the ventricles, beginning with the endocardial surface near the apex and ending with the epicardial surface at the base of the heart. Ventricular activation is complete in less than 0.1 seconds; therefore, contraction of all of the ventricular muscle is normally synchronous and hemodynamically effective.

Arrhythmias consist of cardiac depolarizations that deviate from the above description in one or more aspects: there is an abnormality in the site of origin of the impulse, its rate or regularity, or its conduction.

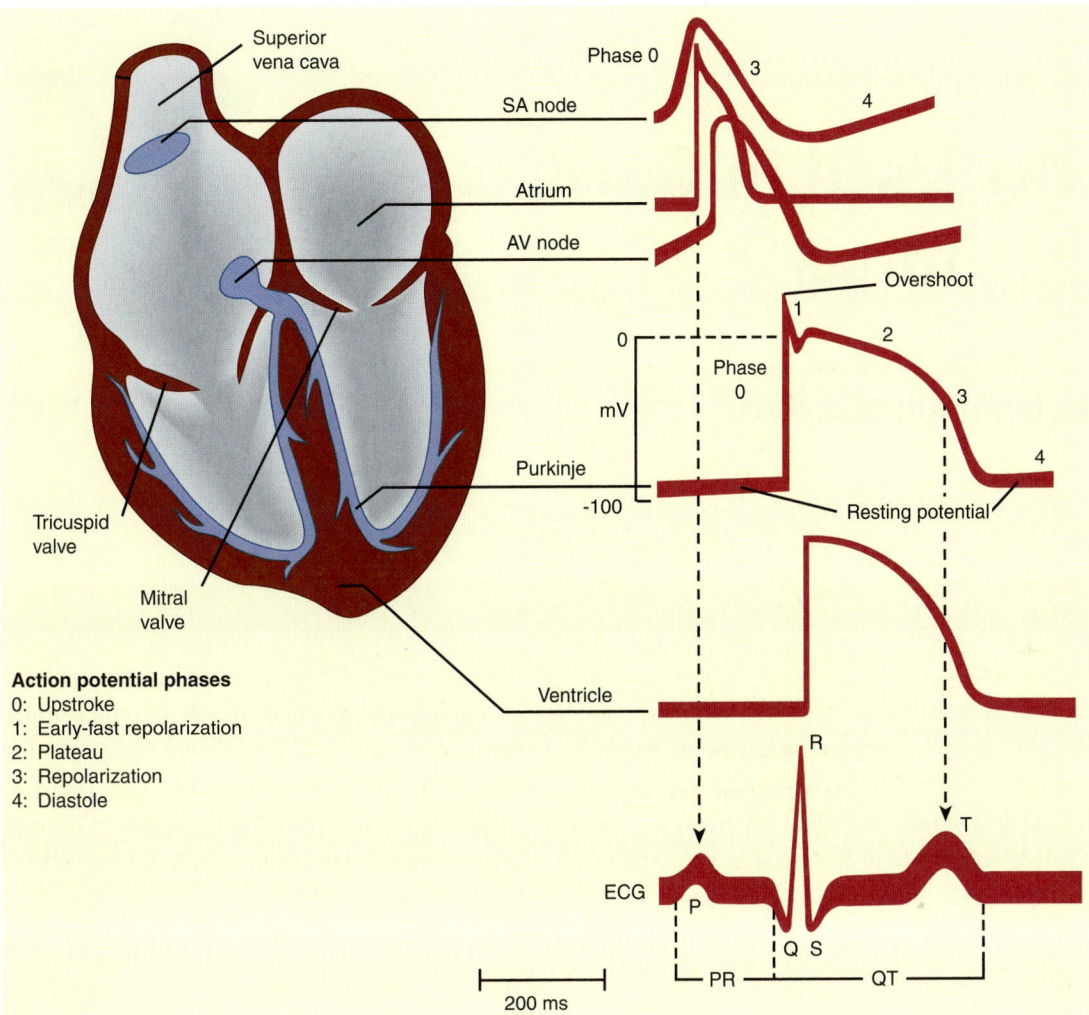

FIGURE 14–1 Schematic representation of the heart and normal cardiac electrical activity (intracellular recordings from areas indicated and ECG). Sinoatrial (SA) node, atrioventricular (AV) node, and Purkinje cells display pacemaker activity (phase 4 depolarization). The ECG is the body surface manifestation of the depolarization and repolarization waves of the heart. The P wave is generated by atrial depolarization, the QRS by ventricular muscle depolarization, and the T wave by ventricular repolarization. Thus, the PR interval is a measure of conduction time from atrium to ventricle, and the QRS duration indicates the time required for all of the ventricular cells to be activated (ie, the intraventricular conduction time). The QT interval reflects the duration of the ventricular action potential.

Ionic Basis of Membrane Electrical Activity

The transmembrane potential of cardiac cells is determined by the concentrations of several ions—chiefly sodium (Na^+), potassium (K^+), calcium (Ca^{2+}), and chloride (Cl^-)—on either side of the membrane and the permeability of the membrane to each ion. These water-soluble ions are unable to freely diffuse across the lipid cell membrane in response to their electrical and concentration gradients; they require aqueous channels (specific pore-forming proteins) for such diffusion. Thus, ions move across cell membranes in response to their gradients only at specific times during the cardiac cycle when these ion channels are open. The movements of the ions produce currents that form the basis of the cardiac action potential. Individual channels are relatively ion-specific, and the flux of ions through them is controlled by "gates" (flexible portions of the

peptide chains that make up the channel proteins). Each type of channel has its own type of gate (sodium, calcium, and some potassium channels are each thought to have two types of gates). The channels primarily responsible for the cardiac action potential (sodium, calcium, and several potassium) are opened and closed ("gated") by voltage changes across the cell membrane; that is, they are voltage-sensitive. Most are also modulated by ion concentrations and metabolic conditions, and some potassium channels are primarily ligand- rather than voltage-gated.

All the ionic currents that are currently thought to contribute to the cardiac action potential are illustrated in Figure 14–2. At rest, most cells are not significantly permeable to sodium, but at the start of each action potential, they become quite permeable (see below). In electrophysiologic terms, the conductance of the fast sodium

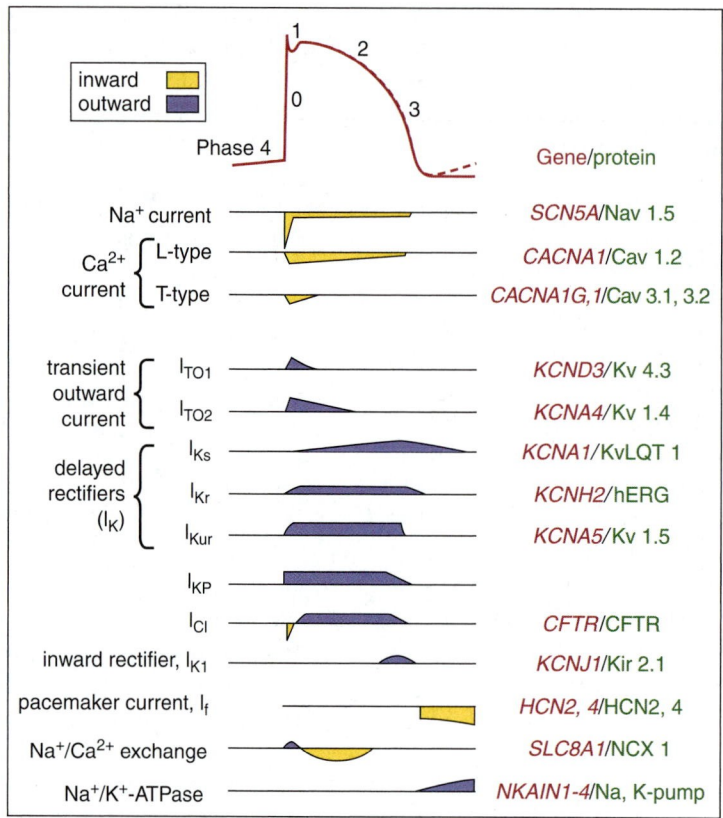

FIGURE 14–2 Schematic diagram of the ion permeability changes and transport processes that occur during an action potential and the diastolic period following it. Yellow indicates inward (depolarizing) membrane currents; blue indicates outward (repolarizing) membrane currents. Multiple subtypes of potassium and calcium currents, with different sensitivities to blocking drugs, have been identified. The right side of the figure lists the genes and proteins responsible for each type of channel or transporter.

channel suddenly increases in response to a depolarizing stimulus. Similarly, calcium enters and potassium leaves the cell with each action potential. Therefore, in addition to ion channels, the cell must have mechanisms to maintain stable transmembrane ionic conditions by establishing and maintaining ion gradients. The most important of these active mechanisms is the sodium pump, Na^+/K^+-ATPase, described in Chapter 13. This pump and other active ion carriers contribute indirectly to the transmembrane potential by maintaining the gradients necessary for diffusion through channels. In addition, some pumps and exchangers produce net current flow (eg, by exchanging three Na^+ for two K^+ ions) and hence are termed "electrogenic."

When the cardiac cell membrane becomes permeable to a specific ion (ie, when the channels selective for that ion are open), movement of that ion across the cell membrane is determined by Ohm's law: current = voltage ÷ resistance, or current = voltage × conductance. Conductance is determined by the properties of the individual ion channel protein. The voltage term is the difference between the actual membrane potential and the reversal potential for that ion (the membrane potential at which no current would flow even if channels were open). For example, in the case of sodium in a cardiac cell at rest, there is a substantial concentration gradient (140 mmol/L Na^+ outside; 10–15 mmol/L Na^+ inside) and an electrical gradient (0 mV outside; −90 mV inside) that

would drive Na^+ into cells. Sodium does not enter the cell at rest because sodium channels are closed; when sodium channels open, the very large influx of Na^+ accounts for phase 0 depolarization of the action potential. The situation for K^+ in the resting cardiac cell is quite different. Here, the concentration gradient (140 mmol/L inside; 4 mmol/L outside) would drive the ion out of the cell, but the electrical gradient would drive it in; that is, the inward gradient is in equilibrium with the outward gradient. In fact, certain potassium channels ("inward rectifier" channels) are open in the resting cell, but little current flows through them because of this balance. The equilibrium, or **reversal potential,** for ions is determined by the **Nernst equation:**

$$E_{ion} = 61 \times \log\left(\frac{C_e}{C_i}\right)$$

where C_e and C_i are the extracellular and intracellular concentrations, respectively, multiplied by their activity coefficients. Note that raising extracellular potassium makes E_K less negative. When this occurs, the membrane depolarizes until the new E_K is reached. Thus, extracellular potassium concentration and inward rectifier channel function are the major factors determining the membrane potential of the resting cardiac cell. The conditions required for application of the Nernst equation are approximated at the peak of

the overshoot (using sodium concentrations) and during rest (using potassium concentrations) in most nonpacemaker cardiac cells. If the permeability is significant for both potassium and sodium, the Nernst equation is not a good predictor of membrane potential, but the **Goldman-Hodgkin-Katz equation** may be used:

$$E_{mem} = 61 \times \log \left(\frac{P_K \times K_e + P_{Na} \times Na_e}{P_K \times K_i + P_{Na} \times Na_i} \right)$$

In pacemaker cells (whether normal or ectopic), spontaneous depolarization (the pacemaker potential) occurs during diastole (phase 4, Figure 14–1). This depolarization results from a gradual increase of depolarizing current through special hyperpolarization-activated ion channels (I_f, also called I_h) in pacemaker cells. The effect of changing extracellular potassium is more complex in a pacemaker cell than it is in a nonpacemaker cell because the effect on permeability to potassium is much more important in a pacemaker (see Box: Effects of Potassium). In a pacemaker—especially an ectopic one—the end result of an increase in extracellular potassium is usually to slow or stop the pacemaker. Conversely, hypokalemia often facilitates ectopic pacemakers.

The Active Cell Membrane

In normal atrial, Purkinje, and ventricular cells, the action potential upstroke (phase 0) is dependent on sodium current. From a functional point of view, it is convenient to describe the behavior of the sodium current in terms of three channel states (Figure 14–3). The cardiac sodium channel protein has been

Effects of Potassium

The effects of changes in serum potassium on cardiac action potential duration, pacemaker rate, and arrhythmias can appear somewhat paradoxical if changes are predicted based solely on a consideration of changes in the potassium *electrochemical gradient*. In the heart, however, changes in serum potassium concentration have the additional effect of altering potassium *conductance* (increased extracellular potassium increases potassium conductance) independent of simple changes in electrochemical driving force, and this effect often predominates. As a result, the actual observed effects of **hyperkalemia** include reduced action potential duration, slowed conduction, decreased pacemaker rate, and decreased pacemaker arrhythmogenesis. Conversely, the actual observed effects of **hypokalemia** include prolonged action potential duration, increased pacemaker rate, and increased pacemaker arrhythmogenesis. Furthermore, pacemaker rate and arrhythmias involving ectopic pacemaker cells appear to be more sensitive to changes in serum potassium concentration, compared with cells of the sinoatrial node. These effects of serum potassium on the heart probably contribute to the observed increased sensitivity to potassium channel-blocking antiarrhythmic agents (quinidine or sotalol) during hypokalemia, eg, accentuated action potential prolongation and tendency to cause torsades de pointes.

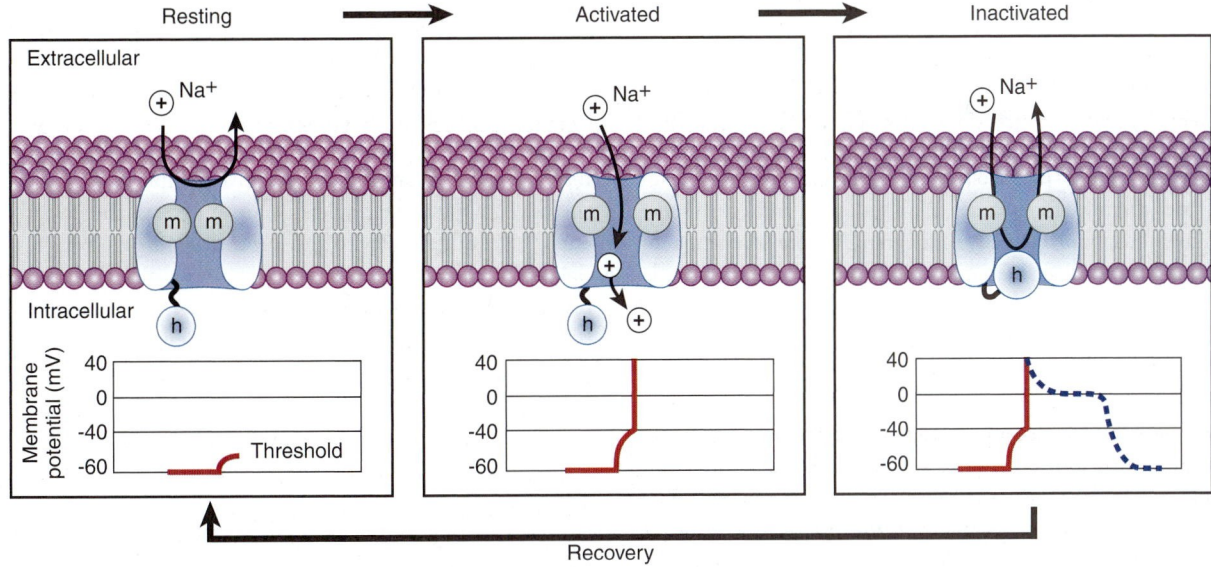

FIGURE 14–3 A schematic representation of Na⁺ channels cycling through different conformational states during the cardiac action potential. Transitions between resting, activated, and inactivated states are dependent on membrane potential and time. The activation gate is shown as *m* and the inactivation gate as *h*. Potentials typical for each state are shown under each channel schematic as a function of time. The dashed line indicates that part of the action potential during which most Na⁺ channels are completely or partially inactivated and unavailable for reactivation.

cloned, and it is now recognized that these channel states actually represent different protein conformations. In addition, regions of the protein that confer specific behaviors, such as voltage sensing, pore formation, and inactivation, are now being identified. The gates described below and in Figure 14–3 represent such regions.

Depolarization to the threshold voltage results in opening of the activation (*m*) gates of sodium channels (Figure 14–3, middle). If the inactivation (*h*) gates of these channels have not already closed, the channels are now open or activated, and sodium permeability is markedly increased, greatly exceeding the permeability for any other ion. Extracellular sodium therefore diffuses down its electrochemical gradient into the cell, and the membrane potential very rapidly approaches the sodium equilibrium potential, E_{Na} (about +70 mV when Na_e = 140 mmol/L and Na_i = 10 mmol/L). This intense sodium current is very brief because opening of the *m* gates upon depolarization is promptly followed by closure of the *h* gates and inactivation of the sodium channels (Figure 14–3, right).

Most calcium channels become activated and inactivated in what appears to be the same way as sodium channels, but in the case of the most common type of cardiac calcium channel (the "L" type), the transitions occur more slowly and at more positive potentials. The action potential plateau (phases 1 and 2) reflects the turning off of most of the sodium current, the waxing and waning of calcium current, and the slow development of a repolarizing potassium current.

Final repolarization (phase 3) of the action potential results from completion of sodium and calcium channel inactivation and the growth of potassium permeability, so that the membrane potential once again approaches the potassium equilibrium potential. The major potassium currents involved in phase 3 repolarization include a rapidly activating potassium current (I_{Kr}) and a slowly activating potassium current (I_{Ks}). These two potassium currents are sometimes discussed together as "I_K." It is noteworthy that a different potassium current, distinct from I_{Kr} and I_{Ks}, may control repolarization in SA nodal cells. This explains why some drugs that block either I_{Kr} or I_{Ks} may prolong repolarization in Purkinje and ventricular cells, but have little effect on SA nodal repolarization (see Box: Molecular & Genetic Basis of Cardiac Arrhythmias).

The Effect of Resting Potential on Action Potentials

A key factor in the pathophysiology of arrhythmias and the actions of antiarrhythmic drugs is the relation between the resting potential of a cell and the action potentials that can be evoked in it (Figure 14–4, left panel). Because the inactivation gates of sodium channels in the resting membrane close over the potential range –75 to –55 mV, fewer sodium channels are "available" for diffusion of sodium ions when an action potential is evoked from a resting potential of –60 mV than when it is evoked from a resting potential of –80 mV. Important consequences of the reduction in peak sodium permeability include reduced maximum upstroke

velocity (called $\dot{V}_{max}$, for maximum rate of change of membrane voltage), reduced action potential amplitude, reduced excitability, and reduced conduction velocity.

During the plateau of the action potential, most sodium channels are inactivated. Upon repolarization, recovery from inactivation takes place (in the terminology of Figure 14–3, the *h* gates reopen), making the channels again available for excitation. The time between phase 0 and sufficient recovery of sodium channels in phase 3 to permit a new propagated response to an external stimulus is the **refractory period.** Changes in refractoriness (determined by either altered recovery from inactivation or altered action potential duration) can be important in the genesis or suppression of certain arrhythmias. Another important effect of less negative resting potential is prolongation of this recovery time, as shown in Figure 14–4 (right panel). The prolongation of recovery time is reflected in an increase in the effective refractory period.

A brief, sudden, depolarizing stimulus, whether caused by a propagating action potential or by an external electrode arrangement, causes the opening of large numbers of activation gates before a significant number of inactivation gates can close. In contrast, slow reduction (depolarization) of the resting potential, whether brought about by hyperkalemia, sodium pump blockade, or ischemic cell damage, results in depressed sodium currents during the upstrokes of action potentials. Depolarization of the resting potential to levels positive to –55 mV abolishes sodium currents, since all sodium channels are inactivated. However, such severely depolarized cells have been found to support special action potentials under circumstances that increase calcium permeability or decrease potassium permeability. These "slow responses"—slow upstroke velocity and slow conduction— depend on a calcium inward current and constitute the normal electrical activity in the SA and AV nodes, since these tissues have a normal resting potential in the range of –50 to –70 mV. Slow responses may also be important for certain arrhythmias.

Modern techniques of molecular biology and electrophysiology can identify multiple subtypes of calcium and potassium channels. One way in which such subtypes may differ is in sensitivity to drug effects, so drugs targeting specific channel subtypes may be developed in the future.

MECHANISMS OF ARRHYTHMIAS

Many factors can precipitate or exacerbate arrhythmias: ischemia, hypoxia, acidosis or alkalosis, electrolyte abnormalities, excessive catecholamine exposure, autonomic influences, drug toxicity (eg, digitalis or antiarrhythmic drugs), overstretching of cardiac fibers, and the presence of scarred or otherwise diseased tissue. However, all arrhythmias result from (1) disturbances in impulse formation, (2) disturbances in impulse conduction, or (3) both.

Disturbances of Impulse Formation

The interval between depolarizations of a pacemaker cell is the sum of the duration of the action potential and the duration of the diastolic interval. Shortening of either duration results in an

Molecular & Genetic Basis of Cardiac Arrhythmias

It is now possible to define the molecular basis of several congenital and acquired cardiac arrhythmias. The best example is the polymorphic ventricular tachycardia known as torsades de pointes (shown in Figure 14–8), which is associated with prolongation of the QT interval (especially at the onset of the tachycardia), syncope, and sudden death. This must represent prolongation of the action potential of at least some ventricular cells (Figure 14–1). The effect can, in theory, be attributed to either increased inward current (gain of function) or decreased outward current (loss of function) during the plateau of the action potential. In fact, recent molecular genetic studies have identified up to 300 different mutations in at least eight ion channel genes that produce the congenital long QT (LQT) syndrome (Table 14–1), and different mutations may have different clinical implications. Loss-of-function mutations in potassium channel genes produce decreases in outward repolarizing current and are responsible for LQT subtypes 1, 2, 5, 6, and 7. HERG and KCNE2 (MiRP1) genes encode subunits of the rapid delayed rectifier potassium current (I_{Kr}), whereas KCNQ1 and KCNE1 (minK) encode subunits of the slow delayed rectifier potassium current (I_{Ks}). KCNJ2 encodes an inwardly rectifying potassium current (I_{Kir}). In contrast, gain-of-function mutations in the sodium channel gene (SCN5A) or calcium channel gene (CACNA1c) cause increases in inward plateau current and are responsible for LQT subtypes 3 and 8, respectively.

Molecular genetic studies have identified the reason why congenital and acquired cases of torsades de pointes can be so strikingly similar. The potassium channel I_{Kr} (encoded by HERG) is blocked or modified by many drugs (eg, quinidine, sotalol) or electrolyte abnormalities (hypokalemia, hypomagnesemia, hypocalcemia) that also produce torsades de pointes. Thus, the identification of the precise molecular mechanisms underlying various forms of

the LQT syndromes now raises the possibility that specific therapies may be developed for individuals with defined molecular abnormalities. Indeed, preliminary reports suggest that the sodium channel blocker mexiletine can correct the clinical manifestations of congenital LQT subtype 3 syndrome. It is likely that torsades de pointes originates from triggered upstrokes arising from early afterdepolarizations (Figure 14–5). Thus, therapy is directed at correcting hypokalemia, eliminating triggered upstrokes (eg, by using β blockers or magnesium), or shortening the action potential (eg, by increasing heart rate with isoproterenol or pacing)—or all of these.

The molecular basis of several other congenital cardiac arrhythmias associated with sudden death has also recently been identified. Three forms of short QT syndrome have been identified that are linked to gain-of-function mutations in three different potassium channel genes (KCNH2, KCNQ1, and KCNJ2). Catecholaminergic polymorphic ventricular tachycardia, a disease that is characterized by stress- or emotion-induced syncope, can be caused by genetic mutations in two different proteins in the sarcoplasmic reticulum that control intracellular calcium homeostasis. Mutations in two different ion channel genes (HCN4 and SCN5A) have been linked to congenital forms of sick sinus syndrome. The Brugada syndrome, which is characterized by ventricular fibrillation associated with persistent ST-segment elevation, and progressive cardiac conduction disorder (PCCD), characterized by impaired conduction in the His-Purkinje system and right or left bundle block leading to complete atrioventricular block, have both been linked to several loss-of-function mutations in the sodium channel gene, SCN5A. At least one form of familial atrial fibrillation is caused by a gain-of-function mutation in the potassium channel gene, KCNQ1.

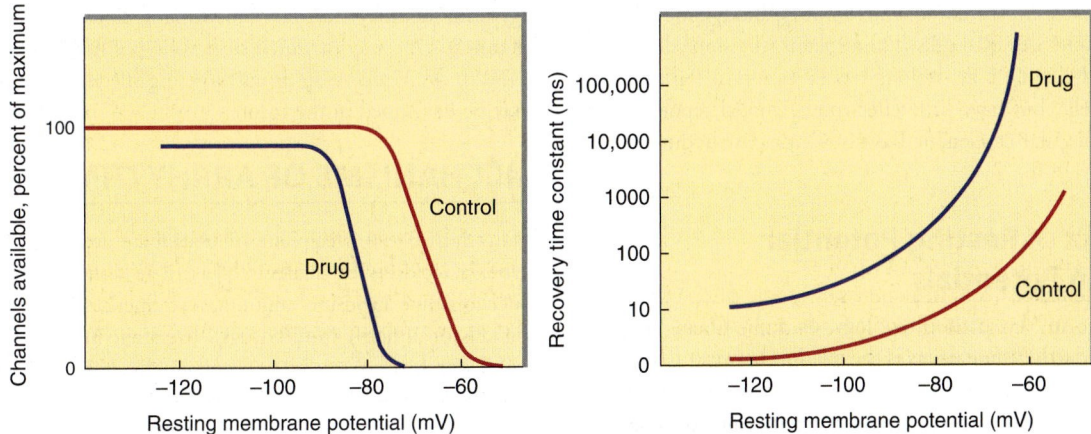

FIGURE 14–4 Dependence of sodium channel function on the membrane potential preceding the stimulus. **Left:** The fraction of sodium channels available for opening in response to a stimulus is determined by the membrane potential immediately preceding the stimulus. The decrease in the fraction available when the resting potential is depolarized in the absence of a drug (control curve) results from the voltage-dependent closure of h gates in the channels. The curve labeled Drug illustrates the effect of a typical local anesthetic antiarrhythmic drug. Most sodium channels are inactivated during the plateau of the action potential. **Right:** The time constant for recovery from inactivation after repolarization also depends on the resting potential. In the absence of drug, recovery occurs in less than 10 ms at normal resting potentials (−85 to −95 mV). Depolarized cells recover more slowly (note logarithmic scale). In the presence of a sodium channel-blocking drug, the time constant of recovery is increased, but the increase is far greater at depolarized potentials than at more negative ones.

TABLE 14–1 Molecular and genetic basis of some cardiac arrhythmias.

Type	Chromosome Involved	Defective Gene	Ion Channel or Proteins Affected	Result
LQT-1	11	KCNQ1	I_{Ks}	LF
LQT-2	7	KCNH2 (HERG)	I_{Kr}	LF
LQT-3	3	SCN5A	I_{Na}	GF
LQT-4	4	Ankyrin-B[1]		LF
LQT-5	21	KCNE1 (minK)	I_{Ks}	LF
LQT-6	21	KCNE2 (MiRP1)	I_{Kr}	LF
LQT-7[2]	17	KCNJ2	I_{Kir}	LF
LQT-8[3]	12	CACNA1c	I_{Ca}	GF
SQT-1	7	KCNH2	I_{Kr}	GF
SQT-2	11	KCNQ1	I_{Ks}	GF
SQT-3	17	KCNJ2	I_{Kir}	GF
CPVT-1[4]	1	hRyR2	Ryanodine receptor	GF
CPVT-2	1	CASQ2	Calsequestrin	LF
Sick sinus syndrome	15 or 3	HCN4 or SCN5A[5]		LF
Brugada syndrome	3	SCN5A	I_{Na}	LF
PCCD	3	SCN5A	I_{Na}	LF
Familial atrial fibrillation	11	KCNQ1	I_{Ks}	GF

[1]Ankyrins are intracellular proteins that associate with a variety of transport proteins including Na^+ channels, Na^+/K^+-ATPase, Na^+, Ca^{2+} exchange, and Ca^{2+} release channels.

[2]Also known as Andersen syndrome.

[3]Also known as Timothy syndrome; multiple organ dysfunction, including autism.

[4]CPVT, catecholaminergic polymorphic ventricular tachycardia; mutations in intracellular ryanodine Ca^{2+} release channel or the Ca^{2+} buffer protein, calsequestrin, may result in enhanced sarcoplasmic reticulum Ca^{2+} leakage or enhanced Ca^{2+} release during adrenergic stimulation, causing triggered arrhythmogenesis.

[5]HCN4 encodes a pacemaker current in sinoatrial nodal cells; mutations in sodium channel gene (SCN5A) cause conduction defects.

GF, gain of function; LF, loss of function; LQT, long QT syndrome; PCCD, progressive cardiac conduction disorder; SQT, short QT syndrome.

increase in pacemaker rate. The more important of the two, diastolic interval, is determined primarily by the slope of phase 4 depolarization (pacemaker potential). Vagal discharge and β-receptor–blocking drugs slow normal pacemaker rate by reducing the phase 4 slope (acetylcholine also makes the maximum diastolic potential more negative). Acceleration of pacemaker discharge is often brought about by increased phase 4 depolarization slope, which can be caused by hypokalemia, β-adrenoceptor stimulation, positive chronotropic drugs, fiber stretch, acidosis, and partial depolarization by currents of injury.

Latent pacemakers (cells that show slow phase 4 depolarization even under normal conditions, eg, some Purkinje fibers) are particularly prone to acceleration by the above mechanisms. However, all cardiac cells, including normally quiescent atrial and ventricular cells, may show repetitive pacemaker activity when depolarized under appropriate conditions, especially if hypokalemia is also present.

Afterdepolarizations (Figure 14–5) are transient depolarizations that interrupt phase 3 (**early afterdepolarizations, EADs**) or phase 4 (**delayed afterdepolarizations, DADs**). EADs are usually exacerbated at *slow* heart rates and are thought to contribute to the development of long QT-related arrhythmias (see Box: Molecular & Genetic Basis of Cardiac Arrhythmias). DADs, on the other hand, often occur when intracellular calcium is increased (see Chapter 13). They are exacerbated by *fast* heart rates and are thought to be responsible for some arrhythmias related to digitalis excess, to catecholamines, and to myocardial ischemia.

Disturbances of Impulse Conduction

Severely depressed conduction may result in simple **block,** eg, AV nodal block or bundle branch block. Because parasympathetic control of AV conduction is significant, partial AV block is sometimes relieved by atropine. Another common abnormality of conduction is **reentry** (also known as "circus movement"), in which one impulse reenters and excites areas of the heart more than once (Figure 14–6).

The path of the reentering impulse may be confined to very small areas, eg, within or near the AV node, or it may involve large portions of the atrial or ventricular walls. Some forms of reentry are strictly anatomically determined; for example, in Wolff-Parkinson-White syndrome, the reentry circuit consists of atrial tissue, the AV node, ventricular tissue, and an accessory AV connection (bundle of Kent, a bypass tract). In other cases (eg, atrial or ventricular fibrillation),

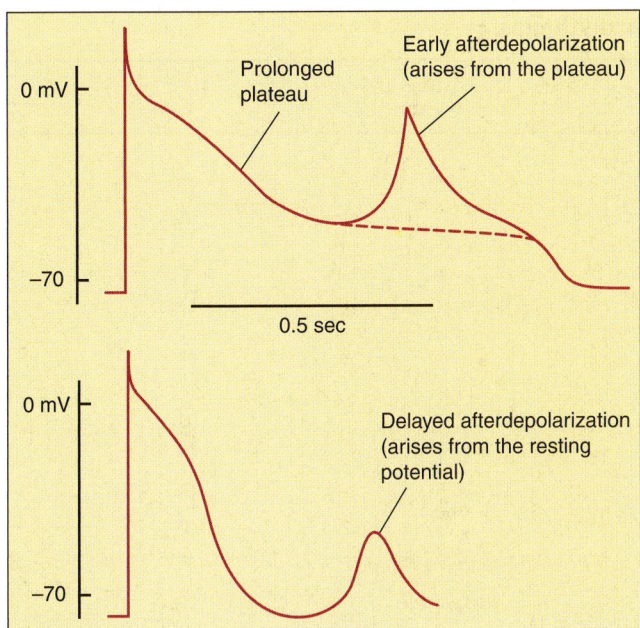

FIGURE 14–5 Two forms of abnormal activity, early (**top**) and delayed afterdepolarizations (**bottom**). In both cases, abnormal depolarizations arise during or after a normally evoked action potential. They are therefore often referred to as "triggered" automaticity; that is, they require a normal action potential for their initiation.

multiple reentry circuits, determined by the varying properties of the cardiac tissue, may meander through the heart in apparently random paths. The circulating impulse often gives off "daughter impulses" that can spread to the rest of the heart. Depending on how many

round trips through the pathway the reentrant impulse makes before dying out, the arrhythmia may be manifest as one or a few extra beats or as a sustained tachycardia.

For reentry to occur, three conditions must coexist, as indicated in Figure 14–6. (1) There must be an obstacle (anatomic or physiologic) to homogeneous conduction, thus establishing a circuit around which the reentrant wavefront can propagate. (2) There must be unidirectional block at some point in the circuit; that is, conduction must die out in one direction but continue in the opposite direction (as shown in Figure 14–6, the impulse can gradually decrease as it invades progressively more depolarized tissue until it finally blocks—a process known as decremental conduction). (3) Conduction time around the circuit must be long enough that the retrograde impulse does not enter refractory tissue as it travels around the obstacle; that is, the conduction time must exceed the effective refractory period. It is important to note that reentry depends on conduction that has been depressed by some critical amount, usually as a result of injury or ischemia. If conduction velocity is too slow, bidirectional block rather than unidirectional block occurs; if the reentering impulse is too weak, conduction may fail, or the impulse may arrive so late that it collides with the next regular impulse. On the other hand, if conduction is too rapid—ie, almost normal—bidirectional conduction rather than unidirectional block will occur. Even in the presence of unidirectional block, if the impulse travels around the obstacle too rapidly, it will reach tissue that is still refractory. Representative electrocardiograms of important arrhythmias are shown in Figures 14–7 and 14–8.

Slowing of conduction may be due to depression of sodium current, depression of calcium current (the latter especially in the AV node), or both. Drugs that abolish reentry usually work by

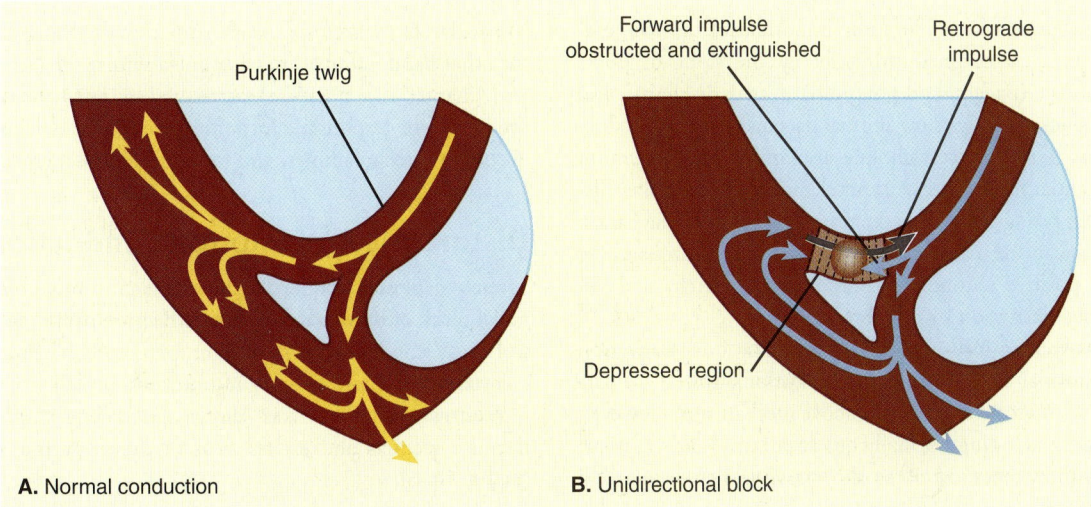

FIGURE 14–6 Schematic diagram of a reentry circuit that might occur in small bifurcating branches of the Purkinje system where they enter the ventricular wall. **A:** Normally, electrical excitation branches around the circuit, is transmitted to the ventricular branches, and becomes extinguished at the other end of the circuit due to collision of impulses. **B:** An area of unidirectional block develops in one of the branches, preventing anterograde impulse transmission at the site of block, but the retrograde impulse may be propagated through the site of block if the impulse finds excitable tissue; that is, the refractory period is shorter than the conduction time. This impulse then reexcites tissue it had previously passed through, and a reentry arrhythmia is established.

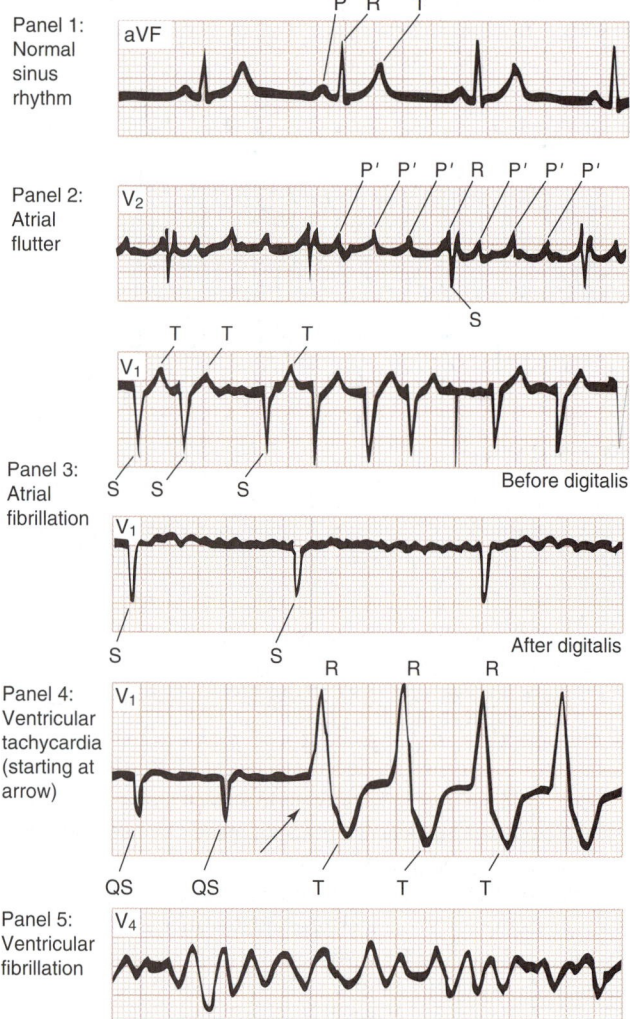

Panel 1:
Normal sinus rhythm

aVF

P R T

Panel 2:
Atrial flutter

V₂

P' P' P' R P' P' P'

S

Panel 3:
Atrial fibrillation

V₁

T T T

S S S

Before digitalis

V₁

After digitalis

S S

Panel 4:
Ventricular tachycardia (starting at arrow)

V₁

R R R

QS QS T T T

Panel 5:
Ventricular fibrillation

V₄

FIGURE 14–7 Electrocardiograms of normal sinus rhythm and some common arrhythmias. Major deflections (P, Q, R, S, and T) are labeled in each electrocardiographic record except in panel 5, in which electrical activity is completely disorganized and none of these deflections is recognizable. (Modified and reproduced, with permission, from Goldman MJ: *Principles of Clinical Electrocardiography*, 11th ed. McGraw-Hill, 1982.)

BASIC PHARMACOLOGY OF THE ANTIARRHYTHMIC AGENTS

Mechanisms of Action

Arrhythmias are caused by abnormal pacemaker activity or abnormal impulse propagation. Thus, the aim of therapy of the arrhythmias is to reduce ectopic pacemaker activity and modify conduction or refractoriness in reentry circuits to disable circus movement. The major pharmacologic mechanisms currently available for accomplishing these goals are (1) sodium channel blockade, (2) blockade of sympathetic autonomic effects in the heart, (3) prolongation of the effective refractory period, and (4) calcium channel blockade.

Antiarrhythmic drugs decrease the automaticity of ectopic pacemakers more than that of the SA node. They also reduce conduction and excitability and increase the refractory period to a greater extent in depolarized tissue than in normally polarized tissue. This is accomplished chiefly by selectively blocking the sodium or calcium channels of depolarized cells (Figure 14–9). Therapeutically useful channel-blocking drugs bind readily to activated channels (ie, during phase 0) or inactivated channels (ie, during phase 2) but bind poorly or not at all to rested channels. Therefore, these drugs block electrical activity when there is a fast tachycardia (many channel activations and inactivations per unit time) or when there is significant loss of resting potential (many inactivated channels during rest). This type of drug action is often described as **use-dependent** or **state-dependent;** that is, channels that are being used frequently, or in an inactivated state, are more susceptible to block. Channels in normal cells that become blocked by a drug during normal activation-inactivation cycles will rapidly lose the drug from the receptors during the resting portion of the cycle (Figure 14–9). Channels in myocardium that is chronically depolarized (ie, has a resting potential more positive than –75 mV) recover from block very slowly if at all (see also right panel, Figure 14–4).

In cells with abnormal automaticity, most of these drugs reduce the phase 4 slope by blocking either sodium or calcium channels, thereby reducing the ratio of sodium (or calcium) permeability to potassium permeability. As a result, the membrane potential during phase 4 stabilizes closer to the potassium equilibrium potential. In addition, some agents may increase the threshold (make it more positive). β-Adrenoceptor–blocking drugs indirectly reduce the phase 4 slope by blocking the positive chronotropic action of norepinephrine in the heart.

In reentry arrhythmias, which depend on critically depressed conduction, most antiarrhythmic agents slow conduction further by one or both of two mechanisms: (1) steady-state reduction in the number of available unblocked channels, which reduces the excitatory currents to a level below that required for propagation (Figure 14–4, left); and (2) prolongation of recovery time of the channels still able to reach the rested and available state, which increases the effective refractory period (Figure 14–4, right). As a result, early extrasystoles are unable to propagate at all; later impulses propagate more slowly and are subject to bidirectional conduction block.

further slowing depressed conduction (by blocking the sodium or calcium current) and causing bidirectional block. In theory, accelerating conduction (by increasing sodium or calcium current) would also be effective, but only under unusual circumstances does this mechanism explain the action of any available drug.

Lengthening (or shortening) of the refractory period may also make reentry less likely. The longer the refractory period in tissue near the site of block, the greater the chance that the tissue will still be refractory when reentry is attempted. (Alternatively, the shorter the refractory period in the depressed region, the less likely it is that unidirectional block will occur.) Thus, increased dispersion of refractoriness is one contributor to reentry, and drugs may suppress arrhythmias by reducing such dispersion.

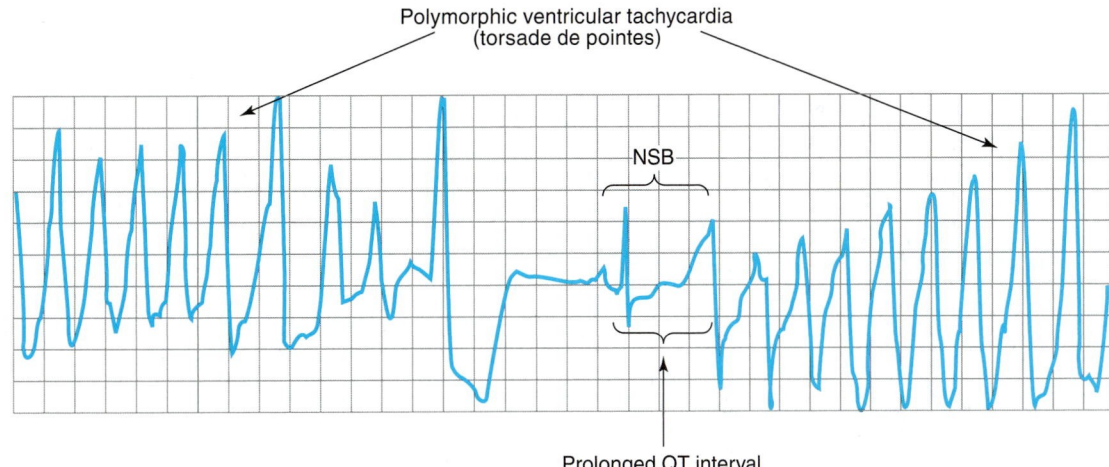

Polymorphic ventricular tachycardia
(torsade de pointes)

NSB

Prolonged QT interval

FIGURE 14–8 Electrocardiogram from a patient with the long QT syndrome during two episodes of torsades de pointes. The polymorphic ventricular tachycardia is seen at the start of this tracing and spontaneously halts at the middle of the panel. A single normal sinus beat (NSB) with an extremely prolonged QT interval follows, succeeded immediately by another episode of ventricular tachycardia of the torsades type. The usual symptoms include dizziness or transient loss of consciousness. (Reproduced, with permission, from *Basic and Clinical Pharmacology*, 10th edition, McGraw-Hill, 2007.)

By these mechanisms, antiarrhythmic drugs can suppress ectopic automaticity and abnormal conduction occurring in depolarized cells—rendering them electrically silent—while minimally affecting the electrical activity in normally polarized parts of the heart. However, as dosage is increased, these agents also depress conduction in normal tissue, eventually resulting in *drug-induced* arrhythmias. Furthermore, a drug concentration that is therapeutic (antiarrhythmic) under the initial circumstances of treatment may become "proarrhythmic" (arrhythmogenic) during fast heart rates (more development of block), acidosis (slower recovery from block for most drugs), hyperkalemia, or ischemia.

■ SPECIFIC ANTIARRHYTHMIC AGENTS

The most widely used scheme for the classification of antiarrhythmic drug actions recognizes four classes:

1. Class 1 action is sodium channel blockade. Subclasses of this action reflect effects on the action potential duration (APD) and the kinetics of sodium channel blockade. Drugs with class 1A action prolong the APD and dissociate from the channel with intermediate kinetics; drugs with class 1B action shorten the APD in some tissues of the heart and dissociate from the channel with rapid kinetics; and drugs with class 1C action have minimal effects on the APD and dissociate from the channel with slow kinetics.

2. Class 2 action is sympatholytic. Drugs with this action reduce β-adrenergic activity in the heart.

3. Class 3 action manifests as prolongation of the APD. Most drugs with this action block the rapid component of the delayed rectifier potassium current, I_{Kr}.

4. Class 4 action is blockade of the cardiac calcium current. This action slows conduction in regions where the action potential upstroke is calcium dependent, eg, the SA and AV nodes.

A given drug may have multiple classes of action as indicated by its membrane and electrocardiographic (ECG) effects (Tables 14–2 and 14–3). For example, amiodarone shares all four classes of action. Drugs are usually discussed according to the predominant class of action. Certain antiarrhythmic agents, eg, adenosine and magnesium, do not fit readily into this scheme and are described separately.

SODIUM CHANNEL-BLOCKING DRUGS (CLASS 1)

Drugs with local anesthetic action block sodium channels and reduce the sodium current, I_{Na}. They are the oldest group of antiarrhythmic drugs and are still widely used.

PROCAINAMIDE (SUBGROUP 1A)

Cardiac Effects

By blocking sodium channels, procainamide slows the upstroke of the action potential, slows conduction, and prolongs the QRS duration of the ECG. The drug also prolongs the APD (a class 3 action) by nonspecific blockade of potassium channels. The drug may be somewhat less effective than quinidine (see below) in suppressing abnormal ectopic pacemaker activity but more effective in blocking sodium channels in depolarized cells.

Procainamide

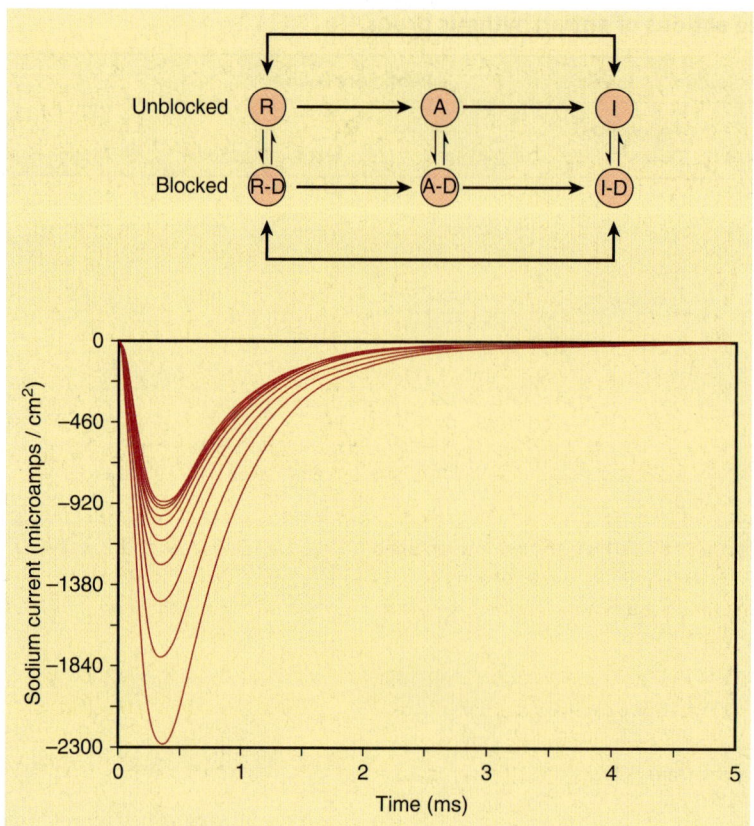

FIGURE 14–9 State- and frequency-dependent block of sodium channels by antiarrhythmic drugs. **Top:** Diagram of a mechanism for the selective depressant action of antiarrhythmic drugs on sodium channels. The upper portion of the figure shows the population of channels moving through a cycle of activity during an action potential in the absence of drugs: R (rested) → A (activated) → I (inactivated). Recovery takes place via the I → R pathway. Antiarrhythmic drugs (D) that act by blocking sodium channels can bind to their receptors in the channels, as shown by the vertical arrows, to form drug-channel complexes, indicated as R-D, A-D, and I-D. Binding of the drugs to the receptor varies with the state of the channel. Most sodium channel blockers bind to the active and inactivated channel receptor much more strongly than to the rested channel. Furthermore, recovery from the I-D state to the R-D state is much slower than from I to R. As a result, rapid activity (more activations and inactivations) and depolarization of the resting potential (more channels in the I state) will favor blockade of the channels and selectively suppress arrhythmic cells. **Bottom:** Progressive reduction of inward sodium current (downward deflections) in the presence of a lidocaine derivative. The largest curve is the initial sodium current elicited by a depolarizing voltage step; subsequent sodium current amplitudes are progressively reduced owing to prior accumulated block and block during each depolarization. (Adapted, with permission, from Starmer FC, Grant AO, Strauss HC: Mechanisms of use-dependent block of sodium channels in excitable membranes by local anesthetics. Biophys J 1984;46:15.)

Procainamide has direct depressant actions on SA and AV nodes, and these actions are only slightly counterbalanced by drug-induced vagal block.

Extracardiac Effects

Procainamide has ganglion-blocking properties. This action reduces peripheral vascular resistance and can cause hypotension, particularly with intravenous use. However, in therapeutic concentrations, its peripheral vascular effects are less prominent than those of quinidine. Hypotension is usually associated with excessively rapid procainamide infusion or the presence of severe underlying left ventricular dysfunction.

Toxicity

Procainamide's cardiotoxic effects include excessive action potential prolongation, QT-interval prolongation, and induction of torsades de pointes arrhythmia and syncope. Excessive slowing of conduction can also occur. New arrhythmias can be precipitated.

A troublesome adverse effect of long-term procainamide therapy is a syndrome resembling lupus erythematosus and usually consisting of arthralgia and arthritis. In some patients, pleuritis, pericarditis, or parenchymal pulmonary disease also occurs. Renal lupus is rarely induced by procainamide. During long-term therapy, serologic abnormalities (eg, increased antinuclear antibody titer) occur in nearly all patients, and in the absence of symptoms, these are not an indication to stop drug therapy. Approximately one third of patients receiving long-term procainamide therapy develop these reversible lupus-related symptoms.

Other adverse effects include nausea and diarrhea (in about 10% of cases), rash, fever, hepatitis (< 5%), and agranulocytosis (approximately 0.2%).

TABLE 14–2 Membrane actions of antiarrhythmic drugs.

| Drug | Block of Sodium Channels | | Refractory Period | | Calcium Channel Blockade | Effect on Pacemaker Activity | Sympatholytic Action |
	Normal Cells	Depolarized Cells	Normal Cells	Depolarized Cells			
Adenosine	0	0	0	0	+	0	+
Amiodarone	+	+++	↑↑	↑↑	+	↓↓	+
Diltiazem	0	0	0	0	+++	↓↓	0
Disopyramide	+	+++	↑	↑↑	+	↓	0
Dofetilide	0	0	↑	?	0	0	0
Dronedarone	+	+	na	na	+	na	+
Esmolol	0	+	0	na	0	↓↓	+++
Flecainide	+	+++	0	↑	0	↓↓	0
Ibutilide	0	0	↑	?	0	0	0
Lidocaine	0	+++	↓	↑↑	0	↓↓	0
Mexiletine	0	+++	0	↑↑	0	↓↓	0
Procainamide	+	+++	↑	↑↑↑	0	↓	+
Propafenone	+	++	↑	↑↑	+	↓↓	+
Propranolol	0	+	↓	↑↑	0	↓↓	+++
Quinidine	+	++	↑	↑↑	0	↓↓	+
Sotalol	0	0	↑↑	↑↑↑	0	↓↓	++
Verapamil	0	+	0	↑	+++	↓↓	+
Vernakalant	+	+	+	+	na	0	na

na, data not available.

Pharmacokinetics & Dosage

Procainamide can be administered safely by intravenous and intramuscular routes and is well absorbed orally. A metabolite (N-acetylprocainamide, NAPA) has class 3 activity. Excessive accumulation of NAPA has been implicated in torsades de pointes during procainamide therapy, especially in patients with renal failure. Some individuals rapidly acetylate procainamide and develop high levels of NAPA. The lupus syndrome appears to be less common in these patients.

Procainamide is eliminated by hepatic metabolism to NAPA and by renal elimination. Its half-life is only 3–4 hours, which necessitates frequent dosing or use of a slow-release formulation (the usual practice). NAPA is eliminated by the kidneys. Thus, procainamide dosage must be reduced in patients with renal failure. The reduced volume of distribution and renal clearance associated with heart failure also require reduction in dosage. The half-life of NAPA is considerably longer than that of procainamide, and it therefore accumulates more slowly. Thus, it is important to measure plasma levels of both procainamide and NAPA, especially in patients with circulatory or renal impairment.

If a rapid procainamide effect is needed, an intravenous loading dose of up to 12 mg/kg can be given at a rate of 0.3 mg/kg/min or less rapidly. This dose is followed by a maintenance dosage of 2–5 mg/min, with careful monitoring of plasma levels. The risk of gastrointestinal (GI) or cardiac toxicity rises at plasma concentrations greater than 8 mcg/mL or NAPA concentrations greater than 20 mcg/mL.

To control ventricular arrhythmias, a total procainamide dosage of 2–5 g/d is usually required. In an occasional patient who accumulates high levels of NAPA, less frequent dosing may be possible. This is also possible in renal disease, where procainamide elimination is slowed.

Therapeutic Use

Procainamide is effective against most atrial and ventricular arrhythmias. However, many clinicians attempt to avoid long-term therapy because of the requirement for frequent dosing and the common occurrence of lupus-related effects. Procainamide is the drug of second or third choice (after lidocaine or amiodarone) in most coronary care units for the treatment of sustained ventricular arrhythmias associated with acute myocardial infarction.

QUINIDINE (SUBGROUP 1A)

Cardiac Effects

Quinidine has actions similar to those of procainamide: it slows the upstroke of the action potential, slows conduction, and prolongs

TABLE 14–3 Clinical pharmacologic properties of antiarrhythmic drugs.

Drug	Effect on SA Nodal Rate	Effect on AV Nodal Refractory Period	PR Interval	QRS Duration	QT Interval	Usefulness in Arrhythmias		Half-Life
						Supra-ventricular	Ventricular	
Adenosine	↓↑	↑↑↑	↑↑↑	0	0	++++	?	< 10 s
Amiodarone	↓↓[1]	↑↑	Variable	↑	↑↑↑↑	+++	+++	(weeks)
Diltiazem	↑↓	↑↑	↑	0	0	+++	–	4–8 h
Disopyramide	↑↓[1,2]	↑↓[2]	↑↓[2]	↑↑	↑↑	+	+++	7–8 h
Dofetilide	↓(?)	0	0	0	↑↑	++	None	7 h
Dronedarone					↑	+++	–	24 h
Esmolol	↓↓	↑↑	↑↑	0	0	+	+	10 min
Flecainide	None,↓	↑	↑	↑↑↑	0	+[3]	++++	20 h
Ibutilide	↓ (?)	0	0	0	↑↑	++	?	6 h
Lidocaine	None[1]	None	0	0	0	None[4]	+++	1–2 h
Mexiletine	None[1]	None	0	0	0	None	+++	12 h
Procainamide	↓[1]	↑↓[2]	↑↓[2]	↑↑	↑↑	+	+++	3–4 h
Propafenone	0, ↓	↑	↑	↑↑↑	0	+	+++	5–7 h
Propranolol	↓↓	↑↑	↑↑	0	0	+	+	5 h
Quinidine	↑↓[1,2]	↑↓[2]	↑↓[2]	↑↑	↑↑	+	+++	6 h
Sotalol	↓↓	↑↑	↑↑	0	↑↑↑	+++	+++	7 h
Verapamil	↓↓	↑↑	↑↑	0	0	+++	–	7 h
Vernakalant		↑	↑			+++	–	2 h

[1]May suppress diseased sinus nodes.

[2]Anticholinergic effect and direct depressant action.

[3]Especially in Wolff-Parkinson-White syndrome.

[4]May be effective in atrial arrhythmias caused by digitalis.

[5]Half-life of active metabolites much longer.

the QRS duration of the ECG, by blockade of sodium channels. The drug also prolongs the action potential duration by blockade of several potassium channels. Its toxic cardiac effects include excessive QT-interval prolongation and induction of torsades de pointes arrhythmia. Toxic concentrations of quinidine also produce excessive sodium channel blockade with slowed conduction throughout the heart.

Quinidine

Extracardiac Effects

Adverse GI effects of diarrhea, nausea, and vomiting are observed in one third to one half of patients. A syndrome of headache, dizziness, and tinnitus (**cinchonism**) is observed at toxic drug concentrations. Idiosyncratic or immunologic reactions, including thrombocytopenia, hepatitis, angioneurotic edema, and fever, are observed rarely.

Pharmacokinetics & Therapeutic Use

Quinidine is readily absorbed from the GI tract and eliminated by hepatic metabolism. It is rarely used because of cardiac and extracardiac adverse effects and the availability of better-tolerated antiarrhythmic drugs.

DISOPYRAMIDE (SUBGROUP 1A)

Cardiac Effects

The effects of disopyramide are very similar to those of procainamide and quinidine. Its cardiac antimuscarinic effects are even more marked than those of quinidine. Therefore, a drug that slows AV conduction should be administered with disopyramide when treating atrial flutter or fibrillation.

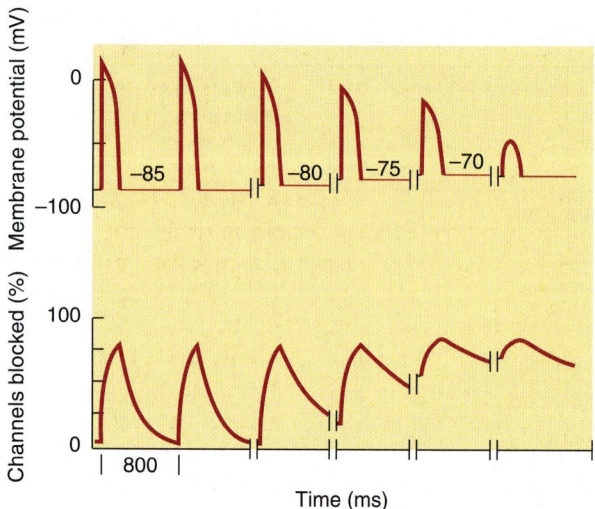

Disopyramide

Toxicity

Toxic concentrations of disopyramide can precipitate all of the electrophysiologic disturbances described under quinidine. As a result of its negative inotropic effect, disopyramide may precipitate heart failure de novo or in patients with preexisting depression of left ventricular function. Because of this effect, disopyramide is not used as a first-line antiarrhythmic agent in the USA. It should not be used in patients with heart failure.

Disopyramide's atropine-like activity accounts for most of its symptomatic adverse effects: urinary retention (most often, but not exclusively, in male patients with prostatic hyperplasia), dry mouth, blurred vision, constipation, and worsening of preexisting glaucoma. These effects may require discontinuation of the drug.

Pharmacokinetics & Dosage

In the USA, disopyramide is only available for oral use. The typical oral dosage of disopyramide is 150 mg three times a day, but up to 1 g/d has been used. In patients with renal impairment, dosage must be reduced. Because of the danger of precipitating heart failure, loading doses are not recommended.

Therapeutic Use

Although disopyramide has been shown to be effective in a variety of supraventricular arrhythmias, in the USA it is approved only for the treatment of ventricular arrhythmias.

LIDOCAINE (SUBGROUP 1B)

Lidocaine has a low incidence of toxicity and a high degree of effectiveness in arrhythmias associated with acute myocardial infarction. It is used only by the intravenous route.

Lidocaine

Cardiac Effects

Lidocaine blocks activated and inactivated sodium channels with rapid kinetics (Figure 14–10); the inactivated state block ensures

FIGURE 14–10 Computer simulation of the effect of resting membrane potential on the blocking and unblocking of sodium channels by lidocaine as the membrane depolarizes. **Upper tracing:** Action potentials in a ventricular muscle cell. **Lower tracing:** Percentage of channels blocked by the drug. An 800 ms time segment is shown. Extra passage of time is indicated by breaks in the traces. **Left side:** At the normal resting potential of –85 mV, the drug combines with open (activated) and inactivated channels during each action potential, but block is rapidly reversed during diastole because the affinity of the drug for its receptor is so low when the channel recovers to the resting state at –85 mV. **Middle:** Metabolic injury is simulated, eg, ischemia due to coronary occlusion, that causes gradual depolarization over time. With subsequent action potentials arising from more depolarized potentials, the fraction of channels blocked increases because more channels remain in the inactivated state at less negative potentials (Figure 14–4, left), and the time constant for unblocking during diastole rapidly increases at less negative resting potentials (Figure 14–4, right). **Right:** Because of marked drug binding, conduction block and loss of excitability in this tissue result; that is, the "sick" (depolarized) tissue is selectively suppressed.

greater effects on cells with long action potentials such as Purkinje and ventricular cells, compared with atrial cells. The rapid kinetics at normal resting potentials result in recovery from block between action potentials and no effect on conduction. The increased inactivation and slower unbinding kinetics result in the selective depression of conduction in depolarized cells. Little effect is seen on the ECG in normal sinus rhythm.

Toxicity

Lidocaine is one of the least cardiotoxic of the currently used sodium channel blockers. Proarrhythmic effects, including SA node arrest, worsening of impaired conduction, and ventricular arrhythmias, are uncommon with lidocaine use. In large doses, especially in patients with preexisting heart failure, lidocaine may cause hypotension—partly by depressing myocardial contractility.

Lidocaine's most common adverse effects—like those of other local anesthetics—are neurologic: paresthesias, tremor, nausea of central origin, lightheadedness, hearing disturbances, slurred speech, and convulsions. These occur most commonly in elderly or otherwise vulnerable patients or when a bolus of the drug is given too rapidly. The effects are dose-related and usually short-lived; seizures respond to intravenous diazepam. In general, if plasma levels above 9 mcg/mL are avoided, lidocaine is well tolerated.

Pharmacokinetics & Dosage

Because of its extensive first-pass hepatic metabolism, only 3% of orally administered lidocaine appears in the plasma. Thus, lidocaine must be given parenterally. Lidocaine has a half-life of 1–2 hours. In adults, a loading dose of 150–200 mg administered over about 15 minutes (as a single infusion or as a series of slow boluses) should be followed by a maintenance infusion of 2–4 mg/min to achieve a therapeutic plasma level of 2–6 mcg/mL. Determination of lidocaine plasma levels is of great value in adjusting the infusion rate. Occasional patients with myocardial infarction or other acute illness require (and tolerate) higher concentrations. This may be due to increased plasma α_1-acid glycoprotein, an acute-phase reactant protein that binds lidocaine, making less free drug available to exert its pharmacologic effects.

In patients with heart failure, lidocaine's volume of distribution and total body clearance may both be decreased. Therefore, both loading and maintenance doses should be decreased. Since these effects counterbalance each other, the half-life may not be increased as much as predicted from clearance changes alone. In patients with liver disease, plasma clearance is markedly reduced and the volume of distribution is often increased; the elimination half-life in such cases may be increased threefold or more. In liver disease, the maintenance dose should be decreased, but usual loading doses can be given. Elimination half-life determines the time to steady state. Although steady-state concentrations may be achieved in 8–10 hours in normal patients and patients with heart failure, 24–36 hours may be required in those with liver disease. Drugs that decrease liver blood flow (eg, propranolol, cimetidine) reduce lidocaine clearance and so increase the risk of toxicity unless infusion rates are decreased. With infusions lasting more than 24 hours, clearance falls and plasma concentrations rise. Renal disease has no major effect on lidocaine disposition.

Therapeutic Use

Lidocaine is the agent of choice for termination of ventricular tachycardia and prevention of ventricular fibrillation after cardioversion in the setting of acute ischemia. However, routine *prophylactic* use of lidocaine in this setting may actually increase total mortality, possibly by increasing the incidence of asystole, and is not the standard of care. Most physicians administer IV lidocaine only to patients with arrhythmias.

MEXILETINE (SUBGROUP 1B)

Mexiletine is an orally active congener of lidocaine. Its electrophysiologic and antiarrhythmic actions are similar to those of lidocaine. (The anticonvulsant phenytoin [see Chapter 24] also exerts similar electrophysiologic effects and has been used as an antiarrhythmic.) Mexiletine is used in the treatment of ventricular

arrhythmias. The elimination half-life is 8–20 hours and permits administration two or three times per day. The usual daily dosage of mexiletine is 600–1200 mg/d. Dose-related adverse effects are seen frequently at therapeutic dosage. These are predominantly neurologic, including tremor, blurred vision, and lethargy. Nausea is also a common effect.

Mexiletine

Mexiletine has also shown significant efficacy in relieving chronic pain, especially pain due to diabetic neuropathy and nerve injury. The usual dosage is 450–750 mg/d orally. This application is off label.

FLECAINIDE (SUBGROUP 1C)

Flecainide is a potent blocker of sodium and potassium channels with slow unblocking kinetics. (Note that although it does block certain potassium channels, it does not prolong the action potential or the QT interval.) It is currently used for patients with otherwise normal hearts who have supraventricular arrhythmias. It has no antimuscarinic effects.

Flecainide

Flecainide is very effective in suppressing premature ventricular contractions. However, it may cause severe exacerbation of arrhythmia even when normal doses are administered to patients with preexisting ventricular tachyarrhythmias and those with a previous myocardial infarction and ventricular ectopy. This was dramatically demonstrated in the Cardiac Arrhythmia Suppression Trial (CAST), which was terminated prematurely because of a two and one-half-fold increase in mortality rate in the patients receiving flecainide and similar group 1C drugs. Flecainide is well absorbed and has a half-life of approximately 20 hours. Elimination is both by hepatic metabolism and by the kidney. The usual dosage of flecainide is 100–200 mg twice a day.

PROPAFENONE (SUBGROUP 1C)

Propafenone has some structural similarities to propranolol and possesses weak β-blocking activity. Its spectrum of action is very similar to that of quinidine, but it does not prolong the action potential. Its sodium channel-blocking kinetics are similar to that of flecainide. Propafenone is metabolized in the liver, with an average half-life of 5–7 hours. The usual daily dosage of propafenone is 450–900 mg in three divided doses. The drug is used primarily for supraventricular arrhythmias. The most common adverse effects are a metallic taste and constipation; arrhythmia exacerbation can also occur.

MORICIZINE (SUBGROUP 1C)

Moricizine is an antiarrhythmic phenothiazine derivative that was used for treatment of ventricular arrhythmias. It is a relatively potent sodium channel blocker that does not prolong action potential duration. Moricizine has been withdrawn from the US market.

BETA-ADRENOCEPTOR–BLOCKING DRUGS (CLASS 2)

Cardiac Effects

Propranolol and similar drugs have antiarrhythmic properties by virtue of their β-receptor–blocking action and direct membrane effects. As described in Chapter 10, some of these drugs have selectivity for cardiac β_1 receptors, some have intrinsic sympathomimetic activity, some have marked direct membrane effects, and some prolong the cardiac action potential. The relative contributions of the β-blocking and direct membrane effects to the antiarrhythmic effects of these drugs are not fully known. Although β blockers are fairly well tolerated, their efficacy for suppression of ventricular ectopic depolarizations is lower than that of sodium channel blockers. However, there is good evidence that these agents can prevent recurrent infarction and sudden death in patients recovering from acute myocardial infarction (see Chapter 10).

Esmolol is a short-acting β blocker used primarily as an antiarrhythmic drug for intraoperative and other acute arrhythmias. See Chapter 10 for more information. **Sotalol** is a nonselective β-blocking drug that prolongs the action potential (class 3 action).

DRUGS THAT PROLONG EFFECTIVE REFRACTORY PERIOD BY PROLONGING THE ACTION POTENTIAL (CLASS 3)

These drugs prolong action potentials, usually by blocking potassium channels in cardiac muscle or by enhancing inward current, eg, through sodium channels. Action potential prolongation by most of these drugs often exhibits the undesirable property of "reverse use-dependence": action potential prolongation is least marked at fast rates (where it is desirable) and most marked at slow rates, where it can contribute to the risk of torsades de pointes.

Although most drugs in the class evoke QT prolongation, there is considerable variability among drugs in their proarrhythmic tendency to cause torsades de pointes despite significant QT-interval prolongation. Recent studies suggest that excessive QT prolongation alone may not be the best predictor of drug-induced torsades de pointes. Other important factors in addition to QT prolongation

include action potential stability and development of a triangular shape (triangulation), reverse use-dependence, and dispersion of repolarization.

AMIODARONE

In the USA, amiodarone is approved for oral and intravenous use to treat serious ventricular arrhythmias. However, the drug is also highly effective for the treatment of supraventricular arrhythmias such as atrial fibrillation. As a result of its broad spectrum of antiarrhythmic action, it is very extensively used for a wide variety of arrhythmias. Amiodarone has unusual pharmacokinetics and important extracardiac adverse effects. **Dronedarone,** an analog that lacks iodine atoms, recently received Food and Drug Administration approval for the treatment of atrial flutter and fibrillation. **Celivarone** is another noniodinated benzofuran derivative similar to dronedarone that is currently undergoing clinical trials for the prevention of ventricular tachycardia recurrence.

Amiodarone

Cardiac Effects

Amiodarone markedly prolongs the action potential duration (and the QT interval on the ECG) by blockade of I_{Kr}. During chronic administration, I_{Ks} is also blocked. The action potential duration is prolonged uniformly over a wide range of heart rates; that is, the drug does not have reverse use-dependent action. In spite of its present classification as a class 3 agent, amiodarone also significantly blocks inactivated sodium channels. Its action potential-prolonging action reinforces this effect. Amiodarone also has weak adrenergic and calcium channel-blocking actions. Consequences of these actions include slowing of the heart rate and AV node conduction. The broad spectrum of actions may account for its relatively high efficacy and its low incidence of torsades de pointes despite significant QT-interval prolongation.

Extracardiac Effects

Amiodarone causes peripheral vasodilation. This action is prominent after intravenous administration and may be related to the action of the vehicle.

Toxicity

Amiodarone may produce symptomatic bradycardia and heart block in patients with preexisting sinus or AV node disease. The drug accumulates in many tissues, including the heart (10–50 times more so than in plasma), lung, liver, and skin, and is concentrated in tears. Dose-related pulmonary toxicity is the most important adverse effect. Even on a low dose of 200 mg/d or less, fatal pulmonary fibrosis may be observed in 1% of patients.

Abnormal liver function tests and hypersensitivity hepatitis may develop during amiodarone treatment and liver function tests should be monitored regularly. The skin deposits result in a photodermatitis and a gray-blue skin discoloration in sun-exposed areas, eg, the malar regions. After a few weeks of treatment, asymptomatic corneal microdeposits are present in virtually all patients treated with amiodarone. Halos develop in the peripheral visual fields of some patients. Drug discontinuation is usually not required. Rarely, an optic neuritis may progress to blindness.

Amiodarone blocks the peripheral conversion of thyroxine (T_4) to triiodothyronine (T_3). It is also a potential source of large amounts of inorganic iodine. Amiodarone may result in hypothyroidism or hyperthyroidism. Thyroid function should be evaluated before initiating treatment and should be monitored periodically. Because effects have been described in virtually every organ system, amiodarone treatment should be reevaluated whenever new symptoms develop in a patient, including arrhythmia aggravation.

Pharmacokinetics

Amiodarone is variably absorbed with a bioavailability of 35–65%. It undergoes hepatic metabolism, and the major metabolite, desethylamiodarone, is bioactive. The elimination half-life is complex, with a rapid component of 3–10 days (50% of the drug) and a slower component of several weeks. After discontinuation of the drug, effects are maintained for 1–3 months. Measurable tissue levels may be observed up to 1 year after discontinuation. A total loading dose of 10 g is usually achieved with 0.8–1.2 g daily doses. The maintenance dose is 200–400 mg daily. Pharmacologic effects may be achieved rapidly by intravenous loading. QT-prolonging effect is modest with this route of administration, whereas bradycardia and AV block may be significant.

Amiodarone has many important drug interactions, and all medications should be reviewed when the drug is initiated and when the dose is adjusted. Amiodarone is a substrate for liver cytochrome CYP3A4, and its levels are increased by drugs that inhibit this enzyme, eg, the histamine H_2 blocker cimetidine. Drugs that induce CYP3A4, eg, rifampin, decrease amiodarone concentration when coadministered. Amiodarone inhibits several cytochrome P450 enzymes and may result in high levels of many drugs, including statins, digoxin, and warfarin. The dose of warfarin should be reduced by one third to one half following initiation of amiodarone, and prothrombin times should be closely monitored.

Therapeutic Use

Low doses (100–200 mg/d) of amiodarone are effective in maintaining normal sinus rhythm in patients with atrial fibrillation. The drug is effective in the prevention of recurrent ventricular tachycardia. It is not associated with an increase in mortality in patients with coronary artery disease or heart failure. In many centers, the implanted cardioverter-defibrillator (ICD) has succeeded drug therapy as the primary treatment modality for ventricular tachycardia, but amiodarone may be used for ventricular tachycardia as adjuvant therapy to decrease the frequency of uncomfortable cardioverter defibrillator discharges. The drug increases the pacing and defibrillation threshold and these devices require retesting after a maintenance dose has been achieved.

DRONEDARONE

Dronedarone is a structural analog of amiodarone in which the iodine atoms have been removed from the phenyl ring and a methanesulfonyl group added to the benzofuran ring. The design was intended to eliminate action of the parent drug on thyroxine metabolism and to modify the half-life of the drug. No thyroid dysfunction or pulmonary toxicity has been reported in short-term studies. However, liver toxicity, including two severe cases requiring liver transplantation, has been reported. Like amiodarone, dronedarone has multichannel actions, including blocking I_{Kr}, I_{Ks}, I_{Ca}, and I_{Na}. It also has β-adrenergic–blocking action. The drug has a half-life of 24 hours and can be administered twice daily at a fixed dose of 400 mg. Dronedarone absorption increases twofold to threefold when taken with food, and this information should be communicated to patients as a part of the dosing instructions. Dronedarone elimination is primarily non-renal. However, it inhibits tubular secretion of creatinine, resulting in a 10–20% increase in serum creatinine. However, because glomerular filtration rate is unchanged, no adjustments are required. Dronedarone is both a substrate and an inhibitor of CY3A4 and should not be co-administered with potent inhibitors of this enzyme, such as the azole and similar antifungal agents, and protease inhibitors.

Dronedarone restores sinus rhythm in a small percentage of patients (< 15%) with atrial fibrillation. It produces a 10- to 15-bpm reduction of the ventricular rate compared to placebo. Dronedarone doubled the interval between episodes of atrial fibrillation recurrence in patients with paroxysmal atrial fibrillation. Initial studies suggested a reduction in mortality or hospitalization in patients with atrial fibrillation. However, a study of dronedarone's effects in permanent atrial fibrillation was terminated in 2011 because of increased risk of death, stroke, and heart failure. Similarly, a trial of dronedarone in advanced heart failure was terminated prematurely because of an increase in mortality. The drug carries a "black box" warning against its use in acute decompensated or advanced (class IV) heart failure.

VERNAKALANT

The limited success of highly specific drugs that target single ion channels and the efficacy of multi-ion channel blockers such as amiodarone have shifted the emphasis in antiarrhythmic drug development to the latter class of drugs. Vernakalant is a multi-ion channel blocker that was developed for the treatment of atrial fibrillation.

Vernakalant prolongs the atrial effective refractory period and slows conduction over the AV node. Ventricular effective refractory period is unchanged. In the maximal clinical dose of 1800 mg/day, vernakalant does not change the QT interval on the ECG. Vernakalant blocks I_{Kur}, I_{ACh}, and I_{to}. These currents play key roles in atrial repolarization and their block accounts for the prolongation of the atrial effective refractory period. The drug is a less potent blocker of I_{Kr} and, as a result, produces less APD prolongation in the ventricle; that is, the APD-prolonging effect is relatively atrium specific. Vernakalant also produces use-dependent block of the sodium channel. Recovery from block is fast, such that significant blockade is observed only at fast rates or at low membrane potentials. In the therapeutic concentration range, vernakalant has no effect on heart rate.

Toxicity

Adverse effects of vernakalant include dysgeusia (disturbance of taste), sneezing, paresthesia, cough, and hypotension.

Pharmacokinetics & Therapeutic Uses

Pharmacokinetic data for vernakalant are limited. After IV administration, the drug is metabolized in the liver by CYP2D6 with a half-life of 2 hours. However, on an oral regimen of 900 mg twice daily, a sustained blood concentration was observed over a 12-hour interval. Clinical trials with the oral drug have used a twice-daily dosing regimen.

Intravenous vernakalant is effective in converting recent-onset atrial fibrillation to normal sinus rhythm in 50% of patients. Final approval for this purpose is pending. The drug is undergoing clinical trials for maintenance of normal sinus rhythm in patients with paroxysmal or persistent atrial fibrillation.

SOTALOL

Sotalol has both β-adrenergic receptor-blocking (class 2) and action potential-prolonging (class 3) actions. The drug is formulated as a racemic mixture of D- and L-sotalol. All the β-adrenergic–blocking activity resides in the L-isomer; the D- and L-isomers share action potential prolonging actions. Beta-adrenergic–blocking action is not cardioselective and is maximal at doses below those required for action potential prolongation.

$$CH_3SO_2NH \text{—} \bigcirc \text{—} \overset{\overset{\displaystyle OH}{|}}{CHCH_2NHCH(CH_3)_2}$$

Sotalol

Sotalol is well absorbed orally with bioavailability of approximately 100%. It is not metabolized in the liver and is not bound to plasma proteins. Excretion is predominantly by the kidneys in the unchanged form with a half-life of approximately 12 hours. Because of its relatively simple pharmacokinetics, solatol exhibits few direct drug interactions. Its most significant cardiac adverse effect is an extension of its pharmacologic action: a dose-related incidence of torsades de pointes that approaches 6% at the highest recommended daily dose. Patients with overt heart failure may experience further depression of left ventricular function during treatment with sotalol.

Sotalol is approved for the treatment of life-threatening ventricular arrhythmias and the maintenance of sinus rhythm in patients with atrial fibrillation. It is also approved for treatment of supraventricular and ventricular arrhythmias in the pediatric age group. Sotalol decreases the threshold for cardiac defibrillation.

DOFETILIDE

Dofetilide has class 3 action potential prolonging action. This action is effected by a dose-dependent blockade of the rapid component of the delayed rectifier potassium current (I_{Kr}) and the blockade of I_{Kr} increases in hypokalemia. Dofetilide produces no relevant blockade of the other potassium channels or the sodium channel. Because of the slow rate of recovery from blockade, the extent of blockade shows little dependence on stimulation frequency. However, dofetilide does show less action potential prolongation at rapid rates because of the increased importance of other potassium channels such as I_{Ks} at higher frequencies.

Dofetilide is 100% bioavailable. Verapamil increases peak plasma dofetilide concentration by increasing intestinal blood flow. Eighty percent of an oral dose is eliminated unchanged by the kidneys; the remainder is eliminated in the urine as inactive metabolites. Inhibitors of the renal cation secretion mechanism, eg, cimetidine, prolong the half-life of dofetilide. Since the QT-prolonging effects and risks of ventricular proarrhythmia are directly related to plasma concentration, dofetilide dosage must be based on the estimated creatinine clearance. Treatment with dofetilide should be initiated in hospital after baseline measurement of the rate-corrected QT interval (QT_c) and serum electrolytes. A baseline QT_c of > 450 ms (500 ms in the presence of an intraventricular conduction delay), bradycardia of < 50 bpm, and hypokalemia are relative contraindications to its use.

Dofetilide is approved for the maintenance of normal sinus rhythm in patients with atrial fibrillation. It is also effective in restoring normal sinus rhythm in patients with atrial fibrillation.

IBUTILIDE

Ibutilide, like dofetilide, slows cardiac depolarization by blockade of the rapid component (I_{Kr}) of the delayed rectifier potassium current. Activation of slow inward sodium current has also been suggested as an additional mechanism of action potential prolongation. After intravenous administration, ibutilide is rapidly cleared by hepatic metabolism. The metabolites are excreted by the kidney. The elimination half-life averages 6 hours.

Intravenous ibutilide is used for the acute conversion of atrial flutter and atrial fibrillation to normal sinus rhythm. The drug is more effective in atrial flutter than atrial fibrillation, with a mean time to termination of 20 minutes. The most important adverse effect is excessive QT-interval prolongation and torsades de pointes. Patients require continuous ECG monitoring for 4 hours after ibutilide infusion or until QT_c returns to baseline.

CALCIUM CHANNEL-BLOCKING DRUGS (CLASS 4)

These drugs, of which verapamil is the prototype, were first introduced as antianginal agents and are discussed in greater detail in Chapter 12. Verapamil and diltiazem also have antiarrhythmic effects. The dihydropyridines (eg, nifedipine) do not share antiarrhythmic efficacy and may *precipitate* arrhythmias.

VERAPAMIL

Cardiac Effects

Verapamil blocks both activated and inactivated L-type calcium channels. Thus, its effect is more marked in tissues that fire frequently, those that are less completely polarized at rest, and those in which activation depends exclusively on the calcium current, such as the SA and AV nodes. AV nodal conduction time and effective refractory period are consistently prolonged by therapeutic concentrations. Verapamil usually slows the SA node by its direct action, but its hypotensive action may occasionally result in a small reflex increase of SA rate.

Verapamil can suppress both early and delayed afterdepolarizations and may antagonize slow responses arising in severely depolarized tissue.

Extracardiac Effects

Verapamil causes peripheral vasodilation, which may be beneficial in hypertension and peripheral vasospastic disorders. Its effects on smooth muscle produce a number of extracardiac effects (see Chapter 12).

Toxicity

Verapamil's cardiotoxic effects are dose-related and usually avoidable. A common error has been to administer intravenous verapamil to a patient with ventricular tachycardia misdiagnosed as supraventricular tachycardia. In this setting, hypotension and ventricular fibrillation can occur. Verapamil's negative inotropic effects may limit its clinical usefulness in diseased hearts (see Chapter 12). Verapamil can induce AV block when used in large doses or in patients with AV nodal disease. This block can be treated with atropine and β-receptor stimulants.

Adverse extracardiac effects include constipation, lassitude, nervousness, and peripheral edema.

Pharmacokinetics & Dosage

The half-life of verapamil is approximately 7 hours. It is extensively metabolized by the liver; after oral administration, its bioavailability is only about 20%. Therefore, verapamil must be administered with caution in patients with hepatic dysfunction or impaired hepatic perfusion.

In adult patients without heart failure or SA or AV nodal disease, parenteral verapamil can be used to terminate supraventricular tachycardia, although adenosine is the agent of first choice. Verapamil dosage is an initial bolus of 5 mg administered over 2–5 minutes, followed a few minutes later by a second 5 mg bolus if needed. Thereafter, doses of 5–10 mg can be administered every 4–6 hours, or a constant infusion of 0.4 mcg/kg/min may be used.

Effective oral dosages are higher than intravenous dosage because of first-pass metabolism and range from 120 mg to 640 mg daily, divided into three or four doses.

Therapeutic Use

Supraventricular tachycardia is the major arrhythmia indication for verapamil. Adenosine or verapamil are preferred over older treatments (propranolol, digoxin, edrophonium, and vasoconstrictor agents) and cardioversion for termination. Verapamil can also reduce the ventricular rate in atrial fibrillation and flutter. It only rarely converts atrial flutter and fibrillation to sinus rhythm. Verapamil is occasionally useful in ventricular arrhythmias. However, intravenous verapamil in a patient with sustained ventricular tachycardia can cause hemodynamic collapse.

DILTIAZEM

Diltiazem appears to be similar in efficacy to verapamil in the management of supraventricular arrhythmias, including rate control in atrial fibrillation. An intravenous form of diltiazem is available for the latter indication and causes hypotension or bradyarrhythmias relatively infrequently.

MISCELLANEOUS ANTIARRHYTHMIC AGENTS

Certain agents used for the treatment of arrhythmias do not fit the conventional class 1–4 organization. These include digitalis (discussed in Chapter 13), adenosine, magnesium, and potassium. It is also becoming clear that certain nonantiarrhythmic drugs, such as drugs acting on the renin-angiotensin-aldosterone system, fish oil, and statins, can reduce recurrence of tachycardias and fibrillation in patients with coronary heart disease or congestive heart failure.

ADENOSINE

Mechanism & Clinical Use

Adenosine is a nucleoside that occurs naturally throughout the body. Its half-life in the blood is less than 10 seconds. Its mechanism of action involves activation of an inward rectifier K^+ current and inhibition of calcium current. The results of these actions are marked hyperpolarization and suppression of calcium-dependent action potentials. When given as a bolus dose, adenosine directly inhibits AV nodal conduction and increases the AV nodal refractory period but has lesser effects on the SA node. Adenosine is currently the drug of choice for prompt conversion of paroxysmal supraventricular tachycardia to sinus rhythm because of its high efficacy (90–95%) and very short duration of action. It is usually given in a bolus dose of 6 mg followed, if necessary, by a dose of 12 mg. An uncommon variant of ventricular tachycardia is adenosine-sensitive. The drug is less effective in the presence of adenosine receptor blockers such as theophylline or caffeine, and its effects are potentiated by adenosine uptake inhibitors such as dipyridamole.

The Nonpharmacologic Therapy of Cardiac Arrhythmias

It was recognized over 100 years ago that reentry in simple in vitro models (eg, rings of conducting tissues) was permanently interrupted by transecting the reentry circuit. This concept is now applied in cardiac arrhythmias with defined anatomic pathways—eg, atrioventricular reentry using accessory pathways, atrioventricular node reentry, atrial flutter, and some forms of ventricular tachycardia—by treatment with **radiofrequency catheter ablation** or extreme cold, **cryoablation.** Mapping of reentrant pathways and ablation can be carried out by means of catheters threaded into the heart from peripheral arteries and veins. Recent studies have shown that paroxysmal and persistent atrial fibrillation may arise from one of the pulmonary veins. Both forms of atrial fibrillation can be cured by electrically isolating the pulmonary

veins by radiofrequency catheter ablation or during concomitant cardiac surgery.

Another form of nonpharmacologic therapy is the **implantable cardioverter-defibrillator (ICD),** a device that can automatically detect and treat potentially fatal arrhythmias such as ventricular fibrillation. ICDs are now widely used in patients who have been resuscitated from such arrhythmias, and several trials have shown that ICD treatment reduces mortality in patients with coronary artery disease who have an ejection fraction $\leq 30\%$ and in patients with class II or III heart failure and no prior history of arrhythmias. The increasing use of nonpharmacologic antiarrhythmic therapies reflects both advances in the relevant technologies and an increasing appreciation of the dangers of long-term therapy with currently available drugs.

Toxicity

Adenosine causes flushing in about 20% of patients and shortness of breath or chest burning (perhaps related to bronchospasm) in over 10%. Induction of high-grade AV block may occur but is very short-lived. Atrial fibrillation may occur. Less common toxicities include headache, hypotension, nausea, and paresthesias.

MAGNESIUM

Originally used for patients with digitalis-induced arrhythmias who were hypomagnesemic, magnesium infusion has been found to have antiarrhythmic effects in some patients with normal serum magnesium levels. The mechanisms of these effects are not known, but magnesium is recognized to influence Na^+/K^+-ATPase, sodium channels, certain potassium channels, and calcium channels. Magnesium therapy appears to be indicated in patients with digitalis-induced arrhythmias if hypomagnesemia is present; it is also indicated in some patients with torsades de pointes even if serum magnesium is normal. The usual dosage is 1 g (as sulfate) given intravenously over 20 minutes and repeated once if necessary. A full understanding of the action and indications for the use of magnesium as an antiarrhythmic drug awaits further investigation.

POTASSIUM

The significance of the potassium ion concentrations inside and outside the cardiac cell membrane was discussed earlier in this chapter. The effects of increasing serum K^+ can be summarized as (1) a resting potential depolarizing action and (2) a membrane potential stabilizing action, the latter caused by increased potassium permeability. Hypokalemia results in an increased risk of early and delayed afterdepolarizations, and ectopic pacemaker activity, especially in the presence of digitalis. Hyperkalemia depresses ectopic pacemakers (severe hyperkalemia is required to suppress the SA node) and slows conduction. Because both insufficient and excess potassium is potentially arrhythmogenic, potassium therapy is directed toward normalizing potassium gradients and pools in the body.

■ PRINCIPLES IN THE CLINICAL USE OF ANTIARRHYTHMIC AGENTS

The margin between efficacy and toxicity is particularly narrow for antiarrhythmic drugs. Risks and benefits must be carefully considered (see Box: Antiarrhythmic Drug-Use Principles Applied to Atrial Fibrillation).

Pretreatment Evaluation

Several important steps must be taken before initiation of any antiarrhythmic therapy:

1. **Eliminate the cause.** Precipitating factors must be recognized and eliminated if possible. These include not only abnormalities of internal homeostasis, such as hypoxia or electrolyte abnormalities (especially hypokalemia or hypomagnesemia), but also drug therapy and underlying disease states such as hyperthyroidism or cardiac disease. It is important to separate this abnormal substrate from triggering factors, such as myocardial ischemia or acute cardiac dilation, which may be treatable and reversible by different means.

2. **Make a firm diagnosis.** A firm arrhythmia diagnosis should be established. For example, the misuse of verapamil in patients with ventricular tachycardia mistakenly diagnosed as supraventricular tachycardia can lead to catastrophic hypotension and cardiac arrest. As increasingly sophisticated methods to characterize underlying arrhythmia mechanisms become available and are validated, it may be possible to direct certain drugs toward specific arrhythmia mechanisms.

3. **Determine the baseline condition.** Underlying heart disease is a critical determinant of drug selection for a particular arrhythmia in a particular patient. A key question is whether the heart is structurally abnormal. Few antiarrhythmic drugs have documented safety in patients with congestive heart failure or ischemic heart disease. In fact, some drugs pose a documented proarrhythmic risk in certain disease states, eg, class 1C drugs in patients with ischemic heart disease. A reliable baseline should be established against which to judge the efficacy of any

Antiarrhythmic Drug-Use Principles Applied to Atrial Fibrillation

Atrial fibrillation is the most common sustained arrhythmia observed clinically. Its prevalence increases from ~ 0.5% in individuals younger than 65 years of age to 10% in individuals older than 80. Diagnosis is usually straightforward by means of an ECG. The ECG may also enable the identification of a prior myocardial infarction, left ventricular hypertrophy, and ventricular pre-excitation. Hyperthyroidism is an important treatable cause of atrial fibrillation, and a thyroid panel should be obtained at the time of diagnosis to exclude this possibility. With the clinical history and physical examination as a guide, the presence and extent of the underlying heart disease should be evaluated, preferably using noninvasive techniques such as echocardiography.

Treatment of atrial fibrillation is initiated to relieve patient symptoms and prevent the complications of thromboembolism and tachycardia-induced heart failure, the result of prolonged uncontrolled heart rates. The initial treatment objective is control of the ventricular rate. This is usually achieved by use of a calcium channel-blocking drug alone or in combination with a β-adrenergic blocker. Digoxin may be of value in the presence of heart failure. A second objective is a restoration and maintenance of normal sinus rhythm. Several studies show that rate control (maintenance of ventricular rate in the range of 60–80 bpm) has a better benefit-to-risk outcome than rhythm control (conversion to normal sinus rhythm) in the long-term health of patients with atrial fibrillation. If rhythm control is deemed desirable, sinus rhythm is usually restored by DC cardioversion in the USA; in some countries, a class 1 antiarrhythmic drug is used initially. For patients with paroxysmal atrial fibrillation, normal sinus rhythm may be restored with a single large oral dose of propafenone or flecainide, provided that safety is initially documented in a monitored setting. Intravenous ibutilide can restore sinus rhythm promptly. For restoration of sinus rhythm in an emergency, eg, atrial fibrillation associated with hypotension or angina, DC cardioversion is the preferred modality. A class 1 or class 3 antiarrhythmic drug is then used to maintain normal sinus rhythm.

subsequent antiarrhythmic intervention. Several methods are now available for such baseline quantification. These include prolonged ambulatory monitoring, electrophysiologic studies that reproduce a target arrhythmia, reproduction of a target arrhythmia by treadmill exercise, or the use of transtelephonic monitoring for recording of sporadic but symptomatic arrhythmias.

4. **Question the need for therapy.** The mere identification of an abnormality of cardiac rhythm does not necessarily require that the arrhythmia be treated. An excellent justification for conservative treatment was provided by the Cardiac Arrhythmia Suppression Trial (CAST) referred to earlier.

Benefits & Risks

The benefits of antiarrhythmic therapy are actually relatively difficult to establish. Two types of benefits can be envisioned: reduction of arrhythmia-related symptoms, such as palpitations, syncope, or cardiac arrest; and reduction in long-term mortality in asymptomatic patients. Among drugs discussed here, only β blockers have been definitely associated with reduction of mortality in relatively asymptomatic patients, and the mechanism underlying this effect is not established (see Chapter 10).

Antiarrhythmic therapy carries with it a number of risks. In some cases, the risk of an adverse reaction is clearly related to high dosages or plasma concentrations. Examples include lidocaine-induced tremor or quinidine-induced cinchonism. In other cases, adverse reactions are unrelated to high plasma concentrations (eg, procainamide-induced agranulocytosis). For many serious adverse reactions to antiarrhythmic drugs, the *combination* of drug therapy and the underlying heart disease appears important.

Several specific syndromes of arrhythmia provocation by antiarrhythmic drugs have also been identified, each with its underlying pathophysiologic mechanism and risk factors. Drugs such as quinidine, sotalol, ibutilide, and dofetilide, which act—at least in part—by slowing repolarization and prolonging cardiac action potentials, can result in marked QT prolongation and torsades de pointes. Treatment for torsades requires recognition of the arrhythmia, withdrawal of any offending agent, correction of hypokalemia, and treatment with maneuvers to increase heart rate (pacing or isoproterenol); intravenous magnesium also appears effective, even in patients with normal magnesium levels.

Drugs that markedly slow conduction, such as flecainide, or high concentrations of quinidine, can result in an increased frequency of reentry arrhythmias, notably ventricular tachycardia in patients with prior myocardial infarction in whom a potential reentry circuit may be present. Treatment here consists of recognition, withdrawal of the offending agent, and intravenous sodium.

Conduct of Antiarrhythmic Therapy

The urgency of the clinical situation determines the route and rate of drug initiation. When immediate drug action is required, the intravenous route is preferred. Therapeutic drug levels can be achieved by administration of multiple *slow* intravenous boluses. Drug therapy can be considered effective when the target arrhythmia is suppressed (according to the measure used to quantify it at baseline) and toxicities are absent. Conversely, drug therapy should not be considered ineffective unless toxicities occur at a time when arrhythmias are not suppressed.

Monitoring plasma drug concentrations can be a useful adjunct to managing antiarrhythmic therapy. Plasma drug concentrations are also important in establishing compliance during long-term therapy as well as in detecting drug interactions that may result in very high concentrations at low drug dosages or very low concentrations at high dosages.

SUMMARY Antiarrhythmic Drugs

Subclass	Mechanism of Action	Effects	Clinical Applications	Pharmacokinetics, Toxicities, Interactions
CLASS 1A				
• Procainamide	I_{Na} (primary) and I_{Kr} (secondary) blockade	Slows conduction velocity and pacemaker rate • prolongs action potential duration and dissociates from I_{Na} channel with intermediate kinetics • direct depressant effects on sinoatrial (SA) and atrioventricular (AV) nodes	Most atrial and ventricular arrhythmias • drug of second choice for most sustained ventricular arrhythmias associated with acute myocardial infarction	Oral, IV, IM • eliminated by hepatic metabolism to N-acetylprocainamide (NAPA; see text) and renal elimination • NAPA implicated in torsades de pointes in patients with renal failure • *Toxicity:* Hypotension • long-term therapy produces reversible lupus-related symptoms
• Quinidine: Similar to procainamide but more toxic (cinchonism, torsades); rarely used in arrhythmias; see Chapter 52 for malaria				
• Disopyramide: Similar to procainamide but significant antimuscarinic effects; may precipitate heart failure; not commonly used				
CLASS 1B				
• Lidocaine	Sodium channel (I_{Na}) blockade	Blocks activated and inactivated channels with fast kinetics • does not prolong and may shorten action potential	Terminate ventricular tachycardias and prevent ventricular fibrillation after cardioversion	IV • first-pass hepatic metabolism • reduce dose in patients with heart failure or liver disease • *Toxicity:* Neurologic symptoms
• Mexiletine: Orally active congener of lidocaine; used in ventricular arrhythmias, chronic pain syndromes				
CLASS 1C				
• Flecainide	Sodium channel (I_{Na}) blockade	Dissociates from channel with slow kinetics • no change in action potential duration	Supraventricular arrhythmias in patients with normal heart • do not use in ischemic conditions (post-myocardial infarction)	Oral • hepatic and kidney metabolism • half life ~ 20 h • *Toxicity:* Proarrhythmic
• Propafenone: Orally active, weak β-blocking activity; supraventricular arrhythmias; hepatic metabolism				
• Moricizine: Phenothiazine derivative, orally active; ventricular arrhythmias, proarrhythmic. Withdrawn in USA.				
CLASS 2				
• Propranolol	β-Adrenoceptor blockade	Direct membrane effects (sodium channel block) and prolongation of action potential duration • slows SA node automaticity and AV nodal conduction velocity	Atrial arrhythmias and prevention of recurrent infarction and sudden death	Oral, parenteral • duration 4–6 h • *Toxicity:* Asthma, AV blockade, acute heart failure • *Interactions:* With other cardiac depressants and hypotensive drugs
• Esmolol: Short-acting, IV only; used for intraoperative and other acute arrhythmias				
CLASS 3				
• Amiodarone	Blocks I_{Kr}, I_{Na}, I_{Ca-L} channels, β adrenoceptors	Prolongs action potential duration and QT interval • slows heart rate and AV node conduction • low incidence of torsades de pointes	Serious ventricular arrhythmias and supraventricular arrhythmias	Oral, IV • variable absorption and tissue accumulation • hepatic metabolism, elimination complex and slow • *Toxicity:* Bradycardia and heart block in diseased heart, peripheral vasodilation, pulmonary and hepatic toxicity • hyper- or hypothyroidism. *Interactions:* Many, based on CYP metabolism
• Dofetilide	I_{Kr} block	Prolongs action potential, effective refractory period	Maintenance or restoration of sinus rhythm in atrial fibrillation	Oral • renal excretion • *Toxicity:* Torsades de pointes (initiate in hospital) • *Interactions:* Additive with other QT-prolonging drugs
• Sotalol: β-Adrenergic and I_{Kr} blocker, direct action potential prolongation properties, use for ventricular arrhythmias, atrial fibrillation				
• Ibutilide: Potassium channel blocker, may activate inward current; IV use for conversion in atrial flutter and fibrillation				
• Dronedarone: Amiodarone derivative; multichannel actions, reduces mortality in patients with atrial fibrillation				
• Vernakalant: Investigational, multichannel actions in atria, prolongs atrial refractoriness, effective in atrial fibrillation				

(continued)

Subclass	Mechanism of Action	Effects	Clinical Applications	Pharmacokinetics, Toxicities, Interactions
CLASS 4				
• Verapamil	Calcium channel (I_{Ca-L} type) blockade	Slows SA node automaticity and AV nodal conduction velocity • decreases cardiac contractility • reduces blood pressure	Supraventricular tachycardias, hypertension, angina	Oral, IV • hepatic metabolism • caution in patients with hepatic dysfunction • *Toxicity & Interactions*: See Chapter 12
• *Diltiazem: Equivalent to verapamil*				
MISCELLANEOUS				
• Adenosine	Activates inward rectifier I_K • blocks I_{Ca}	Very brief, usually complete AV blockade	Paroxysmal supraventricular tachycardias	IV only • duration 10–15 seconds• *Toxicity*: Flushing, chest tightness, dizziness • *Interactions*: Minimal
• Magnesium	Poorly understood • interacts with Na^+/K^+-ATPase, K^+, and Ca^{2+} channels	Normalizes or increases plasma Mg^{2+}	Torsades de pointes • digitalis-induced arrhythmias	IV • duration dependent on dosage • *Toxicity*: Muscle weakness in overdose
• Potassium	Increases K^+ permeability, K^+ currents	Slows ectopic pacemakers • slows conduction velocity in heart	Digitalis-induced arrhythmias • arrhythmias associated with hypokalemia	Oral, IV • *Toxicity*: Reentrant arrhythmias, fibrillation or arrest in overdose

PREPARATIONS AVAILABLE

SODIUM CHANNEL BLOCKERS

Disopyramide (generic, Norpace)
Oral: 100, 150 mg capsules
Oral controlled-release (generic, Norpace CR): 100, 150 capsules

Flecainide (generic, Tambocor)
Oral: 50, 100, 150 mg tablets

Lidocaine (generic, Xylocaine)
Parenteral: 100 mg/mL for IM injection; 10, 20 mg/mL for IV injection; 40, 100, 200 mg/mL for IV admixtures; 2, 4, 8 mg/mL premixed IV (5% D/W) solution

Mexiletine (Mexitil)
Oral: 150, 200, 250 mg capsules

Procainamide (generic, Pronestyl, others)
Oral: 250, 375, 500 mg tablets and capsules
Oral sustained-release (generic, Procan-SR): 250, 500, 750, 1000 mg tablets
Parenteral: 500 mg/mL for injection

Propafenone (generic, Rythmol)
Oral: 150, 225, 300 mg tablets, capsules

Quinidine sulfate [83% quinidine base] (generic)
Oral: 200, 300 mg tablets
Oral sustained-release (Quinidex Extentabs): 300 mg tablets

Quinidine gluconate [62% quinidine base] (generic)
Oral sustained-release: 324 mg tablets
Parenteral: 80 mg/mL for injection

Quinidine polygalacturonate [60% quinidine base] (Cardioquin)
Oral: 275 mg tablets

BETA BLOCKERS LABELED FOR USE AS ANTIARRHYTHMICS

Acebutolol (generic, Sectral)
Oral: 200, 400 mg capsules

Esmolol (Brevibloc)
Parenteral: 10 mg/mL, 250 mg/mL for IV injection

Propranolol (generic, Inderal)
Oral: 10, 20, 40, 60, 80, 90 mg tablets
Oral sustained-release: 60, 80, 120, 160 mg capsules
Oral solution: 4, 8 mg/mL
Parenteral: 1 mg/mL for injection

ACTION POTENTIAL-PROLONGING AGENTS

Amiodarone (generic, Cordarone)
Oral: 100, 200, 400 mg tablets
Parenteral: 150 mg/3 mL for IV infusion

Dofetilide (Tikosyn)
Oral: 125, 250, 500 mcg capsules

Dronedarone (Multac)
Oral: 400 mg tablets

Ibutilide (Corvert)
Parenteral: 0.1 g/mL solution for IV infusion

Sotalol (generic, Betapace)
Oral: 80, 120, 160, 240 mg capsules

CALCIUM CHANNEL BLOCKERS

Diltiazem (generic, Cardizem, Dilacor)
Oral: 30, 60, 90, 120 mg tablets; 60, 90, 120, 180, 240, 300, 340, 420 mg extended- or sustained-release capsules (*not labeled for use in arrhythmias*)
Parenteral: 5 mg/mL for IV injection

Verapamil (generic, Calan, Isoptin)
Oral: 40, 80, 120 mg tablets
Oral sustained-release (Calan SR, Isoptin SR): 100, 120, 180, 240 mg capsules
Parenteral: 5 mg/2 mL for injection

MISCELLANEOUS

Adenosine (generic, Adenocard)
Parenteral: 3 mg/mL for injection

Magnesium sulfate
Parenteral: 125, 500 mg/mL for IV infusion

REFERENCES

Antzelevitch C, Shimizu W: Cellular mechanisms underlying the long QT syndrome. Curr Opin Cardiol 2002;17:43.

Chen YH et al: KCNQ1 gain-of-function mutation in familial atrial fibrillation. Science 2003;299:251.

Cho HC, Marban E: Biological therapies for cardiac arrhythmias-can genes and cells replace drugs and devices? Circ Res 2010;106:674.

Cho H-S, Takano M, Noma A: The electrophysiological properties of spontaneously beating pacemaker cells isolated from mouse sinoatrial node. J Physiol 2003;550:169.

Das MK, Zipes DP: Antiarrhythmic and nonantiarrhythmic drugs for sudden cardiac death prevention. J Cardiovasc Pharmacol 2010;55(5):438.

Duan D et al: Functional role of anion channels in cardiac diseases. Acta Pharmacol Sin 2005;26:265.

Dumaine R, Antzelevitch C: Molecular mechanisms underlying the long QT syndrome. Curr Opin Cardiol 2002;17:36.

Echt DS et al for the CAST Investigators: Mortality and morbidity in patients receiving encainide, flecainide, or placebo. The Cardiac Arrhythmia Suppression Trial. N Engl J Med 1991;324:781.

Fedida D: Vernakalant (RSD1235): A novel, atrial-selective antifibrillatory agent. Expert Opin Investig Drugs 2007;16:519.

Fuster V et al: ACC/AHA/ESC Guidelines for the management of patients with atrial fibrillation. Circulation 2006;114:700.

Grant AO: Recent advances in the treatment of arrhythmias. Circ J 2003;67:651.

Grant AO: Cardiac ion channels. Circ Arrhythmia Electrophysiol 2009;2:185.

Hondeghem LM: Relative contributions of TRIaD and QT to proarrhythmia. J Cardiovasc Electrophysiol 2007;18:655.

IRCCS Fondazione Salvatore Maugeri: Genetic mutations and inherited arrhythmias. http://www.fsm.it/cardmoc.

Keating MT, Sanguinetti MC: Molecular and cellular mechanisms of cardiac arrhythmias. Cell 2001;104:569.

Khan IA: Clinical and therapeutic aspects of congenital and acquired long QT syndrome. Am J Med 2002;112:58.

Marrus SB, Nerbonne JM: Mechanisms linking short- and long-term electrical remodeling in the heart. . .is it a stretch? Channels 2008;2(2):117.

Mohler PJ, Gramolini AO, Bennett V: Ankyrins. J Cell Biol 2002;115:1565.

Morady F: Catheter ablation of supraventricular arrhythmias: State of the art. J Cardiovasc Electrophysiol 2004;15:124.

Splawski I, et al: Severe arrhythmia disorder caused by cardiac L-type calcium channel mutations. Proc Natl Acad Sci USA 2005;102:8089.

Srivatsa U, Wadhani N, Singh AB: Mechanisms of antiarrhythmic drug actions and their clinical relevance for controlling disorders of cardiac rhythm. Curr Cardiol Rep 2002;4:401.

Starmer FC, Grant AO, Strauss HC: Mechanisms of use-dependent block of sodium channels in excitable membranes by local anesthetics. Biophys J 1984;46:15.

Subbiah RN, Campbell TJ, Vandenberg JI: Inherited cardiac arrhythmia syndromes: What have they taught us about arrhythmias and anti-arrhythmic therapy? Clin Exp Pharmacol Physiol 2004;31:906.

van Gelder I et al: A comparison of rate control and rhythm control in patients with recurrent persistent atrial fibrillation. N Engl J Med 2002;347:1834.

Wehrens XHT, Lehnart SE, Marks AR: Ryanodine receptor-targeted anti-arrhythmic therapy. NY Acad Sci 2005;1047:366.

Wolbrette D et al: Dronedarone for the treatment of atrial fibrillation and atrial flutter: Approval and efficacy. Vasc Health Risk Manag 2010;6:517.

Wyse DG et al: A comparison of rate control and rhythm control in patients with atrial fibrillation. N Engl J Med 2002;347:1825.

CASE STUDY ANSWER

The patient has significant symptoms during recurrent episodes of atrial fibrillation. The peak heart rate is not particularly high. Maintenance of sinus rhythm appears to be important in this patient. The echocardiogram demonstrates impairment of left ventricular function. Selection of a drug that is tolerated in heart failure and has documented ability to convert or prevent atrial fibrillation, eg, dofetilide or amiodarone, would be appropriate.

Diuretic Agents

Harlan E. Ives, MD, PhD

CASE STUDY

A 65-year-old man comes to the emergency department with severe shortness of breath. His wife reports that he has long known that he is hypertensive but never had symptoms, so he refused to take antihypertensive medications. During the last month, he has noted increasing ankle edema, reduced exercise tolerance, and difficulty sleeping lying down, but he reports no episodes of chest pain or discomfort. He now has pitting edema to the knees and is acutely uncomfortable lying down. Vital signs include blood pressure 190/140 mm Hg, pulse 120 bpm, and respiratory rate 20/min. Chest auscultation reveals loud rhonchi, but an electrocardiogram is negative except for evidence of left ventricular hypertrophy. He is given a diuretic intravenously and admitted to intensive care. What diuretic would be most appropriate for this man's case of acute pulmonary edema associated with heart failure? What are the possible toxicities of this therapy?

Abnormalities in fluid volume and electrolyte composition are common and important clinical disorders. Drugs that block specific transport functions of the renal tubules are valuable clinical tools in the treatment of these disorders. Although various agents that increase urine volume (diuretics) have been described since antiquity, it was not until 1937 that carbonic anhydrase inhibitors were first described and not until 1957 that a much more useful and powerful diuretic agent (chlorothiazide) became available.

Technically, a "diuretic" is an agent that increases urine volume, whereas a "natriuretic" causes an increase in renal sodium excretion and an "aquaretic" increases excretion of solute-free water. Because natriuretics almost always also increase water excretion, they are usually called diuretics. Osmotic diuretics and antidiuretic hormone antagonists (see Agents That Alter Water Excretion) are aquaretics that are not directly natriuretic.

This chapter is divided into three sections. The first section covers major renal tubule transport mechanisms. The nephron is divided structurally and functionally into several segments (Figure 15–1, Table 15–1). Several autacoids, which exert multiple, complex events on renal physiologic processes (adenosine, prostaglandins, and urodilatin, a renal autacoid closely related to atrial natriuretic peptide), are also discussed. The second section describes the pharmacology of diuretic agents. Many diuretics exert their effects on specific membrane transport proteins in renal tubular epithelial cells. Other diuretics exert osmotic effects that prevent water reabsorption (mannitol), inhibit enzymes (acetazolamide), or interfere with hormone receptors in renal epithelial cells (vaptans, or vasopressin antagonists). The physiology of each nephron segment is closely linked to the basic pharmacology of the drugs acting there, which is discussed in the second section. The third section of the chapter describes the clinical applications of diuretics.

■ RENAL TUBULE TRANSPORT MECHANISMS

PROXIMAL TUBULE

Sodium bicarbonate ($NaHCO_3$), sodium chloride (NaCl), glucose, amino acids, and other organic solutes are reabsorbed via specific transport systems in the early proximal tubule (proximal convoluted tubule, PCT). Potassium ions (K^+) are reabsorbed via the paracellular pathway. Water is reabsorbed passively, maintaining the osmolality of proximal tubular fluid at a nearly constant level. As tubule fluid is processed along the length of the proximal tubule, the luminal concentrations of these solutes decrease relative to the concentration of inulin, an experimental marker that is filtered but neither secreted nor absorbed by renal tubules. Approximately 66% of filtered sodium ions (Na^+), 85% of the $NaHCO_3$, 65% of the K^+, 60% of the water, and virtually all of the filtered glucose and amino acids are reabsorbed in the proximal tubule.

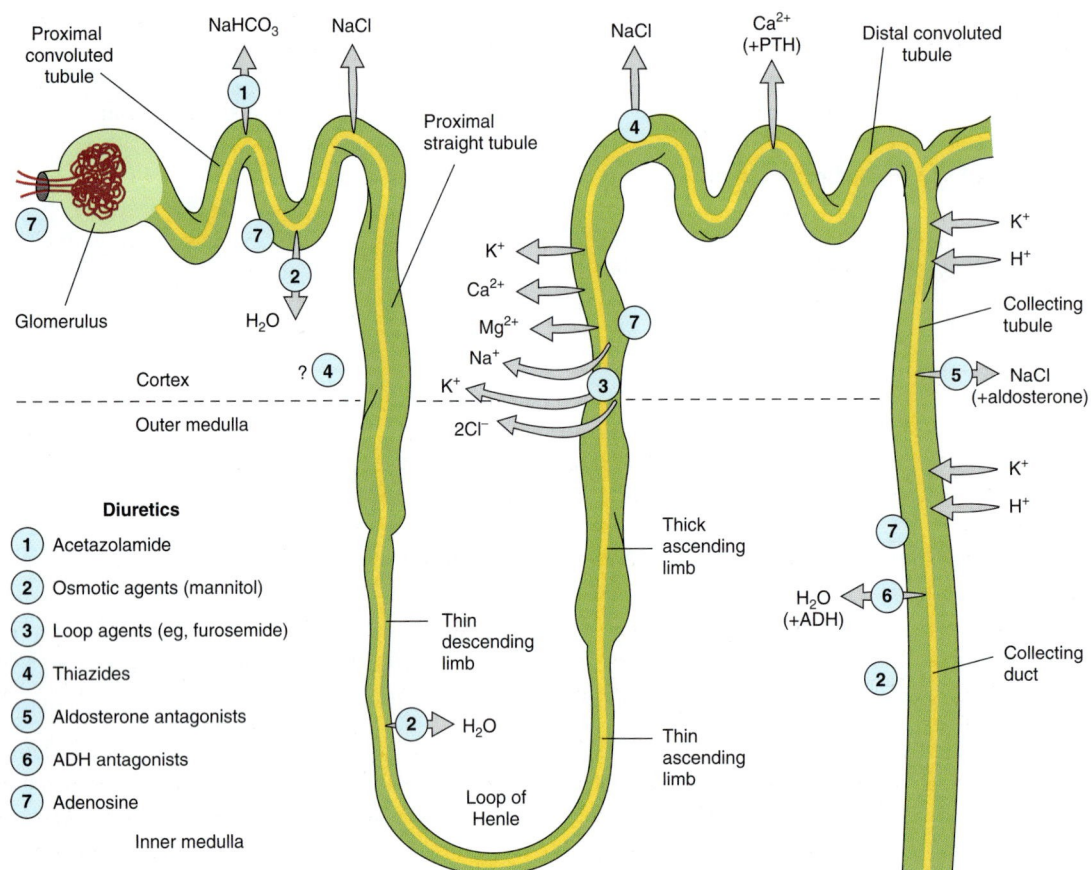

FIGURE 15–1 Tubule transport systems and sites of action of diuretics. ADH, antidiuretic hormone; PTH, parathyroid hormone.

TABLE 15–1 Major segments of the nephron and their functions.

Segment	Functions	Water Permeability	Primary Transporters and Drug Targets at Apical Membrane	Diuretic with Major Action
Glomerulus	Formation of glomerular filtrate	Extremely high	None	None
Proximal convoluted tubule (PCT)	Reabsorption of 65% of filtered Na^+/K^+, CA^{2+}, and Mg^{2+}; 85% of $NaHCO_3$, and nearly 100% of glucose and amino acids. Isosmotic reabsorption of water.	Very high	Na/H[1] (NHE3), carbonic anhydrase	Carbonic anhydrase inhibitors Adenosine antagonists (under investigation)
Proximal tubule, straight segments	Secretion and reabsorption of organic acids and bases, including uric acid and most diuretics	Very high	Acid (eg, uric acid) and base transporters	None
Thin descending limb of Henle's loop	Passive reabsorption of water	High	Aquaporins	None
Thick ascending limb of Henle's loop (TAL)	Active reabsorption of 15–25% of filtered $Na^+/K^+/Cl^-$; secondary reabsorption of Ca^{2+} and Mg^{2+}	Very low	Na/K/2Cl (NKCC2)	Loop diuretics
Distal convoluted tubule (DCT)	Active reabsorption of 4–8% of filtered Na^+ and Cl^-; Ca^{2+} reabsorption under parathyroid hormone control	Very low	Na/Cl (NCC)	Thiazides
Cortical collecting tubule (CCT)	Na^+ reabsorption (2–5%) coupled to K^+ and H^+ secretion	Variable[2]	Na channels (ENaC), K channels,[1] H[+] transporter,[1] aquaporins	K^+-sparing diuretics Adenosine antagonists (under investigation)
Medullary collecting duct	Water reabsorption under vasopressin control	Variable[2]	Aquaporins	Vasopressin antagonists

[1]Not a target of currently available drugs.
[2]Controlled by vasopressin activity.

Of the various solutes reabsorbed in the proximal tubule, the most relevant to diuretic action are NaHCO₃ and NaCl. Of the currently available diuretics, only one group (carbonic anhydrase inhibitors, which block NaHCO₃ reabsorption) acts predominantly in the PCT. In view of the large quantity of NaCl absorbed in this segment, a drug that specifically blocked proximal tubular absorption of NaCl could be a particularly powerful diuretic. Adenosine receptor antagonists, which are currently under intense clinical investigation, act mainly in the PCT and appear to induce a NaCl, rather than a NaHCO₃ diuresis. Sodium bicarbonate reabsorption by the PCT is initiated by the action of a Na⁺/H⁺ exchanger (NHE3) located in the luminal membrane of the proximal tubule epithelial cell (Figure 15–2). This transport system allows Na⁺ to enter the cell from the tubular lumen in exchange for a proton (H⁺) from inside the cell. As in all portions of the nephron, Na⁺/K⁺-ATPase in the basolateral membrane pumps the reabsorbed Na⁺ into the interstitium so as to maintain a low intracellular Na⁺ concentration. The H⁺ secreted into the lumen combines with bicarbonate (HCO₃⁻) to form H₂CO₃ (carbonic acid), which is rapidly dehydrated to CO₂ and H₂O by carbonic anhydrase. Carbon dioxide produced by dehydration of H₂CO₃ enters the proximal tubule cell by simple diffusion where it is then rehydrated back to H₂CO₃, also facilitated by intracellular carbonic anhydrase. After dissociation of H₂CO₃, the H⁺ is available for transport by the Na⁺/H⁺ exchanger, and the HCO₃⁻ is transported out of the cell by a basolateral membrane transporter (Figure 15–2). Bicarbonate reabsorption by the proximal tubule is thus dependent on carbonic anhydrase activity. This enzyme can be inhibited by acetazolamide and other carbonic anhydrase inhibitors.

Adenosine, which is released as a result of hypoxia and ATP consumption, is a molecule with four different receptors and complex effects on Na⁺ transport in several segments of the nephron. Although it reduces glomerular filtration rate (GFR) to decrease energy consumption by the kidney, adenosine actually increases proximal reabsorption of Na⁺ via stimulation of NHE3 activity. A new class of drugs, the adenosine A₁-receptor antagonists, have recently been found to significantly blunt both proximal tubule NHE3 activity and collecting duct NaCl reabsorption, and to have potent vasomotor effects in the renal microvasculature (see below, under Autacoids, Pharmacology of Diuretic Agents, and under Heart Failure).

Because HCO₃⁻ and organic solutes have been largely removed from the tubular fluid in the late proximal tubule, the residual luminal fluid contains predominantly NaCl. Under these conditions, Na⁺ reabsorption continues, but the H⁺ secreted by the Na⁺/H⁺ exchanger can no longer bind to HCO₃⁻. Free H⁺ causes luminal pH to fall, activating a poorly defined Cl⁻/base exchanger (Figure 15–2). The net effect of parallel Na⁺/H⁺ exchange and Cl⁻/base exchange is NaCl reabsorption. As yet, there are no diuretic agents that are known to act on this conjoint process.

Water is reabsorbed in the PCT in response to osmotic forces, so luminal fluid osmolality remains nearly constant along its length, and an impermeant solute like inulin rises in concentration as water is reabsorbed. If large amounts of an impermeant solute such as mannitol (an osmotic diuretic) are present in the tubular fluid, water reabsorption causes the concentration of the solute to rise, so that as salt concentrations become diminished further, water reabsorption is prevented.

Organic acid secretory systems are located in the middle third of the straight part of the proximal tubule (S₂ segment). These systems secrete a variety of organic acids (uric acid, nonsteroidal anti-inflammatory drugs [NSAIDs], diuretics, antibiotics, etc) into the luminal fluid from the blood. These systems thus help deliver diuretics to the luminal side of the tubule, where most of them act. Organic base secretory systems (creatinine, choline, etc) are also present, in the early (S₁) and middle (S₂) segments of the proximal tubule.

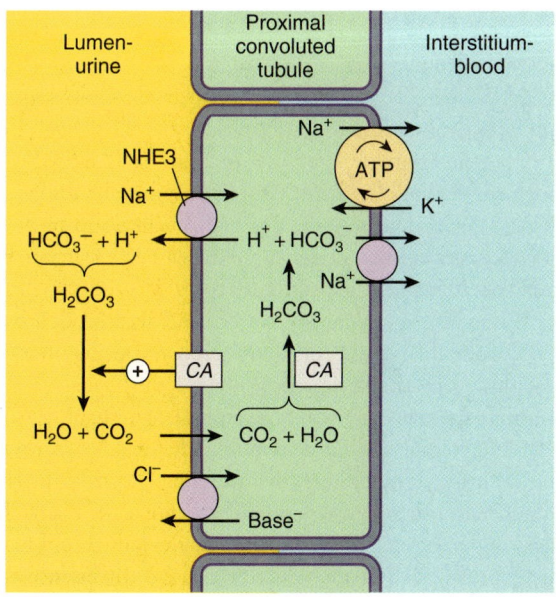

FIGURE 15–2 Apical membrane Na⁺/H⁺ exchange (via NHE3) and bicarbonate reabsorption in the proximal convoluted tubule cell. Na⁺/K⁺-ATPase is present in the basolateral membrane to maintain intracellular sodium and potassium levels within the normal range. Because of rapid equilibration, concentrations of the solutes are approximately equal in the interstitial fluid and the blood. Carbonic anhydrase (CA) is found in other locations in addition to the brush border of the luminal membrane.

LOOP OF HENLE

At the boundary between the inner and outer stripes of the outer medulla, the proximal tubule empties into the thin descending limb of Henle's loop. Water is extracted from the descending limb of this loop by osmotic forces found in the hypertonic medullary interstitium. As in the proximal tubule, impermeant luminal solutes such as mannitol oppose this water extraction and thus have aquaretic activity. The thin *ascending* limb is relatively water-impermeable but is permeable to some solutes.

The thick ascending limb (TAL), which follows the thin limb of Henle's loop, actively reabsorbs NaCl from the lumen (about 25% of the filtered sodium), but unlike the proximal tubule and the thin descending limb of Henle's loop, it is nearly impermeable to water.

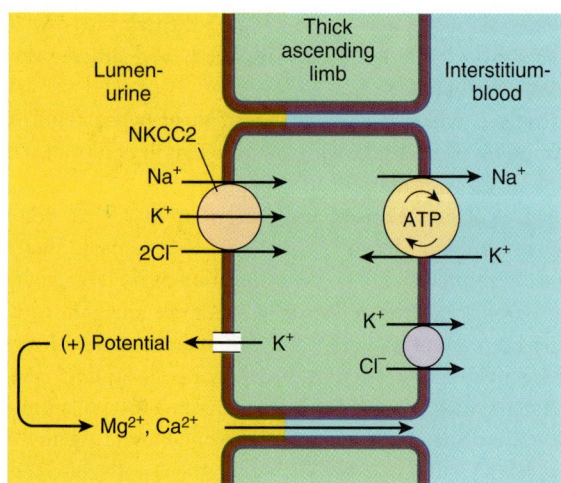

FIGURE 15–3 Ion transport pathways across the luminal and basolateral membranes of the thick ascending limb cell. The lumen positive electrical potential created by K⁺ back diffusion drives divalent (and monovalent) cation reabsorption via the paracellular pathway. NKCC2 is the primary transporter in the luminal membrane.

Salt reabsorption in the TAL therefore dilutes the tubular fluid, and it is called a *diluting segment*. Medullary portions of the TAL contribute to medullary hypertonicity and thereby also play an important role in concentration of urine by the collecting duct.

The NaCl transport system in the luminal membrane of the TAL is a Na⁺/K⁺/2Cl⁻ cotransporter (called NKCC2 or NK2CL) (Figure 15–3). This transporter is selectively blocked by diuretic agents known as "loop" diuretics (see later in chapter). Although the Na⁺/K⁺/2Cl⁻ transporter is itself electrically neutral (two cations and two anions are cotransported), the action of the transporter contributes to excess K⁺ accumulation within the cell. Back diffusion of this K⁺ into the tubular lumen causes a lumen-positive electrical potential that provides the driving force for reabsorption of cations—including magnesium and calcium—via the paracellular pathway. Thus, inhibition of salt transport in the TAL by loop diuretics, which reduces the lumen-positive potential, causes an increase in urinary excretion of divalent cations in addition to NaCl.

DISTAL CONVOLUTED TUBULE

Only about 10% of the filtered NaCl is reabsorbed in the distal convoluted tubule (DCT). Like the TAL of Henle's loop, this segment is relatively impermeable to water, and NaCl reabsorption further dilutes the tubular fluid. The mechanism of NaCl transport in the DCT is an electrically neutral thiazide-sensitive Na⁺ and Cl⁻ cotransporter (NCC, Figure 15–4).

Because K⁺ does not recycle across the apical membrane of the DCT as it does in the TAL, there is no lumen-positive potential in this segment, and Ca²⁺ and Mg²⁺ are not driven out of the tubular lumen by electrical forces. Instead, Ca²⁺ is actively reabsorbed by the DCT epithelial cell via an apical Ca²⁺ channel and basolateral Na⁺/Ca²⁺ exchanger (Figure 15–4). This process is regulated by parathyroid hormone.

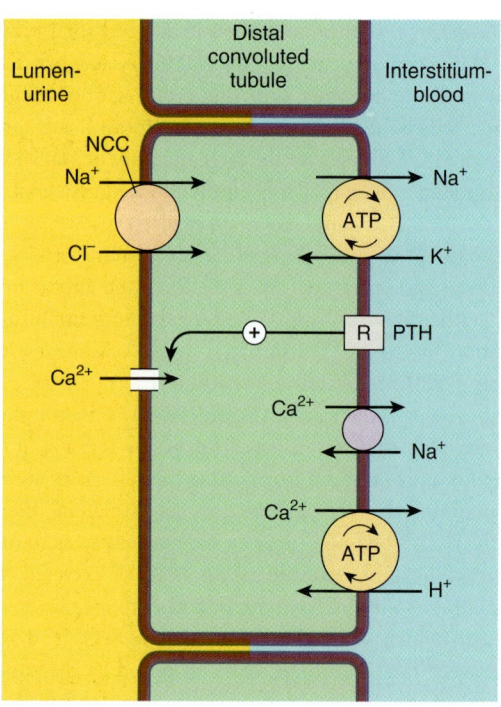

FIGURE 15–4 Ion transport pathways across the luminal and basolateral membranes of the distal convoluted tubule cell. As in all tubular cells, Na⁺/K⁺ ATPase is present in the basolateral membrane. NCC is the primary sodium and chloride transporter in the luminal membrane. (R, parathyroid hormone [PTH] receptor.)

COLLECTING TUBULE SYSTEM

The collecting tubule system that connects the DCT to the renal pelvis and the ureter consists of several sequential tubular segments: the connecting tubule, the collecting tubule, and the collecting duct (formed by the connection of two or more collecting tubules). Although these tubule segments may be anatomically distinct, the physiologic gradations are more gradual, and in terms of diuretic activity it is easier to think of this complex as a single segment of the nephron containing several distinct cell types. The collecting tubule system is responsible for only 2–5% of NaCl reabsorption by the kidney. Despite this small contribution, it plays an important role in renal physiology and in diuretic action. As the final site of NaCl reabsorption, the collecting system is responsible for tight regulation of body fluid volume and for determining the final Na⁺ concentration of the urine. Furthermore, the collecting system is the site at which mineralocorticoids exert a significant influence. Lastly, this is the most important site of K⁺ secretion by the kidney and the site at which virtually all diuretic-induced changes in K⁺ balance occur.

The mechanism of NaCl reabsorption in the collecting tubule system is distinct from the mechanisms found in other tubule segments. The **principal cells** are the major sites of Na⁺, K⁺, and water transport (Figures 15–5 and 15–6), and the **intercalated cells** (α, β) are the primary sites of H⁺ (α cells) or bicarbonate (β cells) secretion. The α and β intercalated cells are very similar, except that the membrane locations of the H⁺-ATPase and Cl/HCO₃⁻ exchanger are reversed. Principal cells do not contain apical

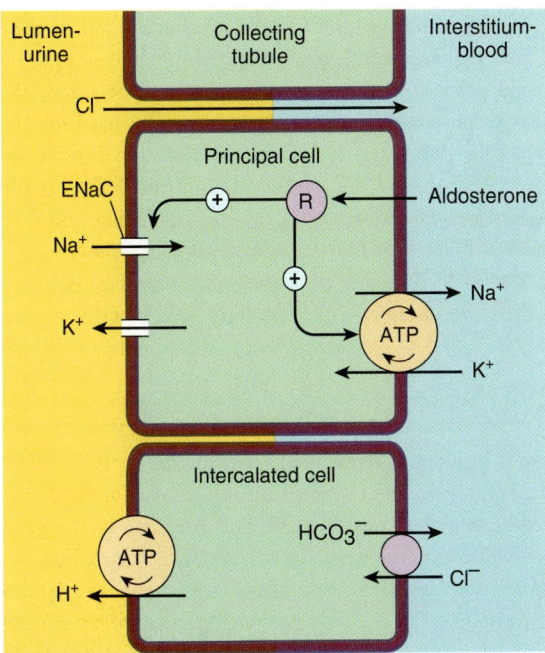

FIGURE 15–5 Ion transport pathways across the luminal and basolateral membranes of collecting tubule and collecting duct cells. Inward diffusion of Na^+ via the epithelial sodium channel (ENaC) leaves a lumen-negative potential, which drives reabsorption of Cl^- and efflux of K^+. (R, aldosterone receptor.)

increase in the transepithelial electrical potential and a dramatic increase in both Na^+ reabsorption and K^+ secretion.

The collecting tubule system is also the site at which the final urine concentration is determined. In addition to their role in control of Na^+ absorption and K^+ secretion (Figure 15–5), principal cells also contain a regulated system of water channels (Figure 15–6). Antidiuretic hormone (ADH, also called arginine vasopressin, AVP) controls the permeability of these cells to water by regulating the insertion of pre-formed water channels (aquaporin-2, AQP2) into the apical membrane. Vasopressin receptors in the vasculature and central nervous system (CNS) are V_1 receptors, and those in the kidney are V_2 receptors. V_2 receptors act via a G protein-coupled, cAMP-mediated process. In the absence of ADH, the collecting tubule (and duct) is impermeable to water, and dilute urine is produced. ADH markedly increases water permeability, and this leads to the formation of a more concentrated final urine. ADH also stimulates the insertion of urea transporter UT1 molecules into the apical membranes of collecting duct cells in the medulla.

Urea concentration in the medulla plays an important role maintaining the high osmolarity of the medulla and in the concentration of urine. ADH secretion is regulated by serum osmolality and by volume status. A new class of drugs, the vaptans (see under Agents That Alter Water Excretion), are ADH antagonists.

cotransport systems for Na^+ and other ions, unlike cells in other nephron segments. Principal cell membranes exhibit separate ion channels for Na^+ and K^+. Since these channels exclude anions, transport of Na^+ or K^+ leads to a net movement of charge across the membrane. Because Na^+ entry into the principal cell predominates over K^+ secretion into the lumen, a 10–50 mV lumen-negative electrical potential develops. Sodium that enters the principal cell from the tubular fluid is then transported back to the blood via the basolateral Na^+/K^+-ATPase (Figure 15–5). The 10–50 mV lumen-negative electrical potential drives the transport of Cl^- back to the blood via the paracellular pathway and draws K^+ out of cells through the apical membrane K^+ channel. Thus, there is an important relationship between Na^+ delivery to the collecting tubule system and the resulting secretion of K^+. Upstream diuretics increase Na^+ delivery to this site and enhance K^+ secretion. If Na^+ is delivered to the collecting system with an anion that cannot be reabsorbed as readily as Cl^- (eg, HCO_3^-), the lumen-negative potential is increased, and K^+ secretion is enhanced. This mechanism, combined with enhanced aldosterone secretion due to volume depletion, is the basis for most diuretic-induced K^+ wasting. Adenosine antagonists, which act upstream at the proximal tubule, but also at the collecting duct, are perhaps the only diuretics that violate this principle (see below). Reabsorption of Na^+ via the epithelial Na channel (ENaC) and its coupled secretion of K^+ is regulated by aldosterone. This steroid hormone, through its actions on gene transcription, increases the activity of both apical membrane channels and the basolateral Na^+/K^+-ATPase. This leads to an

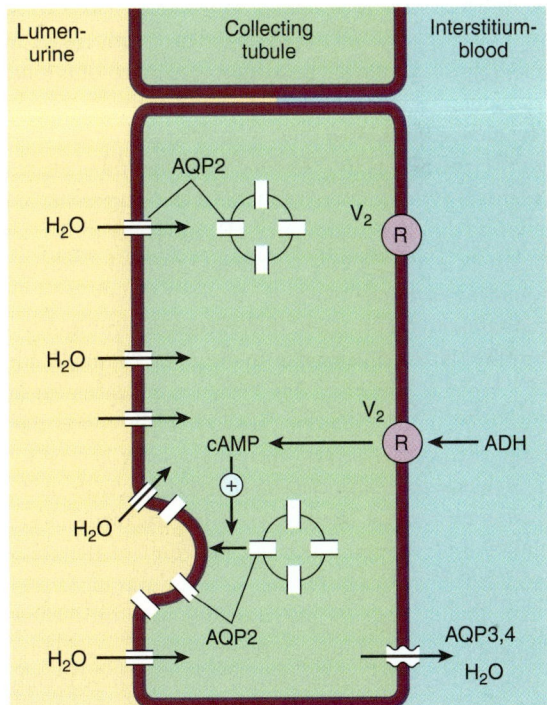

FIGURE 15–6 Water transport across the luminal and basolateral membranes of collecting duct cells. Above, low water permeability exists in the absence of antidiuretic hormone (ADH). Below, in the presence of ADH, aquaporins are inserted into the apical membrane, greatly increasing water permeability. (AQP2, apical aquaporin water channels; AQP3,4, basolateral aquaporin water channels; V_2, vasopressin V_2 receptor.)

RENAL AUTACOIDS

A number of locally produced compounds exhibit physiologic effects within the kidney and are therefore referred to as *autacoids*, or *paracrine factors*. Several of these autacoids (adenosine, the prostaglandins, and urodilatin) appear to have important effects on the pharmacology of diuretics. Since these effects are complex, they will be treated independently of the individual tubule segments discussed above.

ADENOSINE

Adenosine is an unphosphorylated ribonucleoside whose actions in the kidney have been intensively studied. As in all tissues, renal adenosine concentrations rise in response to hypoxia and ATP consumption. In most tissues, hypoxia results in compensatory vasodilation and, if cardiac output is sufficient, increased blood flow. The kidney has different requirements because increased blood flow leads to an increase in GFR and greater solute delivery to the tubules. This increased delivery would increase tubule work and ATP consumption. In contrast, in the hypoxic kidney, adenosine actually decreases blood flow and GFR. Because the medulla is always more hypoxic than the cortex, adenosine increases Na^+ reabsorption from the reduced flow in the cortex, so that delivery to medullary segments will be even further reduced.

There are four distinct adenosine receptors (A_1, A_{2a}, A_{2b}, and A_3), all of which have been found in the kidney. However, probably only one of these (A_1) is of importance with regard to the pharmacology of diuretics. The adenosine A_1 receptor is found on the pre-glomerular afferent arteriole, as well as the PCT and most other tubule segments. Adenosine is known to affect ion transport in the PCT, the medullary TAL, and collecting tubules. In addition, adenosine (via A_1 receptors on the afferent arteriole) reduces blood flow to the glomerulus (and GFR) and is also the key signaling molecule in the process of tubuloglomerular feedback (see below, under Heart Failure).

In addition to its effects on GFR, adenosine significantly alters Na^+ transport in several segments. In the proximal tubule, adenosine has a biphasic effect on NHE3 activity: enhancement at low concentrations and inhibition at very high concentrations. However, adenosine receptor antagonists have generally been found to block the enhancement of NHE3 activity and thus exhibit diuretic activity (see below). It is particularly interesting that unlike other diuretics that act upstream of the collecting tubules, adenosine antagonists do not cause wasting of K. This important finding suggests that in addition to their effects on NHE3, adenosine antagonists must also blunt K^+ secretion in the cortical collecting tubule. Adenosine A_1 receptors have been found in the collecting tubule, but the precise mechanism by which adenosine blunts K^+ secretion is not well understood.

PROSTAGLANDINS

Prostaglandins are autacoids that contribute importantly to renal physiology, and to the function of many other organs (see Chapter 18). Five prostaglandin subtypes (PGE_2, PGI_2, PGD_2,

$PGF_{2\alpha}$, and thromboxane [TXA_2] are synthesized in the kidney and have receptors in this organ. The role of some of these receptors in renal physiology is not yet completely understood. However, PGE_2 (acting on EP_1, EP_3, and possibly EP_2) has been shown to play a role in the activity of certain diuretics. Among its many actions, PGE_2 blunts Na^+ reabsorption in the TAL of Henle's loop and ADH-mediated water transport in collecting tubules. These actions of PGE_2 contribute significantly to the diuretic efficacy of loop diuretics. Blockade of prostaglandin synthesis with NSAIDs can therefore interfere with loop diuretic activity.

PEPTIDES

There is growing interest in the natriuretic peptides (ANP, BNP, and CNP, see Chapter 17), which induce natriuresis through several different mechanisms. ANP and BNP are synthesized in the heart, while CNP comes primarily from the CNS. Some of these peptides exert both vascular effects (see Chapter 17) and sodium transport effects in the kidney, which participate in causing natriuresis. A fourth natriuretic peptide, urodilatin, is structurally very similar to ANP but is synthesized and functions only in the kidney. Urodilatin is made in distal tubule epithelial cells and blunts Na^+ reabsorption through effects on Na^+ uptake channels and Na^+/K^+-ATPase at the downstream collecting tubule system. In addition, through effects on vascular smooth muscle, it reduces glomerular afferent and increases glomerular efferent vasomotor tone. These effects cause an increase in GFR, which adds to the natriuretic activity. Ularitide is a recombinant peptide that mimics the activity of urodilatin. It is currently under intense investigation and may become available for clinical use in the near future.

The cardiac peptides ANP and BNP have pronounced systemic vascular effects. The receptors ANP_A and ANP_B, also known as NPR_A and NPR_B, are transmembrane molecules with guanylyl cyclase catalytic activity at the cytoplasmic domains. Of interest, both peptides increase GFR through effects on glomerular arteriolar vasomotor tone and also exhibit diuretic activity. CNP has very little diuretic activity. Three agents in this group are in clinical use or under investigation: nesiritide (BNP), carperitide (ANP, available only in Japan), and ularitide (urodilatin, under investigation). Intravenous ularitide has been studied extensively for use in acute heart failure. It can dramatically improve cardiovascular parameters and promote diuresis without reducing creatinine clearance. There is also evidence that nesiritide (simulating BNP) may enhance the activity of other diuretics while helping to maintain stable renal function.

■ BASIC PHARMACOLOGY OF DIURETIC AGENTS

CARBONIC ANHYDRASE INHIBITORS

Carbonic anhydrase is present in many nephron sites, but the predominant location of this enzyme is the epithelial cells of the PCT (Figure 15–2), where it catalyzes the dehydration of H_2CO_3

to CO_2 at the luminal membrane and rehydration of CO_2 to H_2CO_3 in the cytoplasm as previously described. By blocking carbonic anhydrase, inhibitors blunt $NaHCO_3$ reabsorption and cause diuresis.

Carbonic anhydrase inhibitors were the forerunners of modern diuretics. They were discovered in 1937 when it was found that bacteriostatic sulfonamides caused an alkaline diuresis and hyperchloremic metabolic acidosis. With the development of newer agents, carbonic anhydrase inhibitors are now rarely used as diuretics, but they still have several specific applications that are discussed below. The prototypical carbonic anhydrase inhibitor is **acetazolamide**.

Pharmacokinetics

The carbonic anhydrase inhibitors are well absorbed after oral administration. An increase in urine pH from the HCO_3^- diuresis is apparent within 30 minutes, is maximal at 2 hours, and persists for 12 hours after a single dose. Excretion of the drug is by secretion in the proximal tubule S_2 segment. Therefore, dosing must be reduced in renal insufficiency.

Pharmacodynamics

Inhibition of carbonic anhydrase activity profoundly depresses HCO_3^- reabsorption in the PCT. At its maximal safe dosage, 85% of the HCO_3^- reabsorptive capacity of the superficial PCT is inhibited. Some HCO_3^- can still be absorbed at other nephron sites by carbonic anhydrase–independent mechanisms, so the overall effect of maximal acetazolamide dosage is only about 45% inhibition of whole kidney HCO_3^- reabsorption. Nevertheless, carbonic anhydrase inhibition causes significant HCO_3^- losses and hyperchloremic metabolic acidosis (Table 15–2). Because of reduced HCO_3^- in the glomerular filtrate and the fact that HCO_3^- depletion leads to enhanced NaCl reabsorption by the remainder of the nephron, the diuretic efficacy of acetazolamide decreases significantly with use over several days.

At present, the major clinical applications of acetazolamide involve carbonic anhydrase–dependent HCO_3^- and fluid transport at

TABLE 15–2 Changes in urinary electrolyte patterns and body pH in response to diuretic drugs.

| Group | Urinary Electrolytes | | | |
	NaCl	NaHCO₃	K⁺	Body pH
Carbonic anhydrase inhibitors	+	+++	+	↓
Loop agents	++++	0	+	↑
Thiazides	++	+	+	↑
Loop agents plus thiazides	++++	+	++	↑
K⁺-sparing agents	+	(+)	−	↓

+, increase; −, decrease; 0, no change; ↓, acidosis; ↑, alkalosis.

TABLE 15–3 Carbonic anhydrase inhibitors used orally in the treatment of glaucoma.

Drug	Usual Oral Dosage
Dichlorphenamide	50 mg 1–3 times daily
Methazolamide	50–100 mg 2–3 times daily

sites other than the kidney. The ciliary body of the eye secretes HCO_3^- from the blood into the aqueous humor. Likewise, formation of cerebrospinal fluid by the choroid plexus involves HCO_3^- secretion. Although these processes remove HCO_3^- from the blood (the direction opposite of that in the proximal tubule), they are similarly inhibited by carbonic anhydrase inhibitors.

Clinical Indications & Dosage (Table 15–3)

A. Glaucoma

The reduction of aqueous humor formation by carbonic anhydrase inhibitors decreases the intraocular pressure. This effect is valuable in the management of glaucoma, making it the most common indication for use of carbonic anhydrase inhibitors. Topically active agents, which reduce intraocular pressure without producing renal or systemic effects, are available (dorzolamide, brinzolamide).

B. Urinary Alkalinization

Uric acid and cystine are relatively insoluble and may form stones in acidic urine. Therefore, in cystinuria, a disorder of cystine reabsorption, solubility of cystine can be enhanced by increasing urinary pH from 7.0 to 7.5 with carbonic anhydrase inhibitors. In the case of uric acid, pH needs to be raised only to 6.0 or 6.5. In the absence of HCO_3^- administration, these effects of acetazolamide last only 2–3 days, so prolonged therapy requires oral HCO_3^-. Excessive urinary alkalinization can lead to stone formation from calcium salts (see below), so urine pH should be followed during treatment with acetazolamide.

C. Metabolic Alkalosis

Metabolic alkalosis is generally treated by correction of abnormalities in total body K^+, intravascular volume, or mineralocorticoid levels. However, when the alkalosis is due to excessive use of diuretics in patients with severe heart failure, replacement of intravascular volume may be contraindicated. In these cases, acetazolamide can be useful in correcting the alkalosis as well as producing a small additional diuresis for correction of volume overload. Acetazolamide can also be used to rapidly correct the metabolic alkalosis that may appear following the correction of respiratory acidosis.

D. Acute Mountain Sickness

Weakness, dizziness, insomnia, headache, and nausea can occur in mountain travelers who rapidly ascend above 3000 m. The symptoms are usually mild and last for a few days. In more serious cases, rapidly progressing pulmonary or cerebral edema can be life-threatening. By decreasing cerebrospinal fluid formation and by decreasing the pH of the cerebrospinal fluid and brain, acetazolamide can increase ventilation and diminish symptoms of mountain sickness. This mild metabolic central and cerebrospinal fluid (CSF) acidosis is also useful in the treatment of sleep apnea.

E. Other Uses

Carbonic anhydrase inhibitors have been used as adjuvants in the treatment of epilepsy and in some forms of hypokalemic periodic paralysis. They are also useful in treating patients with CSF leakage (usually caused by tumor or head trauma, but often idiopathic). By reducing the rate of CSF formation and intracranial pressure, carbonic anhydrase inhibitors can significantly slow the rate of CSF leakage. Finally, they also increase urinary phosphate excretion during severe hyperphosphatemia.

Toxicity

A. Hyperchloremic Metabolic Acidosis

Acidosis predictably results from chronic reduction of body HCO_3^- stores by carbonic anhydrase inhibitors (Table 15–2) and limits the diuretic efficacy of these drugs to 2 or 3 days. Unlike the diuretic effect, acidosis persists as long as the drug is continued.

B. Renal Stones

Phosphaturia and hypercalciuria occur during the bicarbonaturic response to inhibitors of carbonic anhydrase. Renal excretion of solubilizing factors (eg, citrate) may also decline with chronic use. Calcium salts are relatively insoluble at alkaline pH, which means that the potential for renal stone formation from these salts is enhanced.

C. Renal Potassium Wasting

Potassium (K^+) wasting can occur because the increased Na^+ presented to the collecting tubule (with HCO_3^-) is partially reabsorbed, increasing the lumen-negative electrical potential in that segment and enhancing K^+ secretion. This effect can be counteracted by simultaneous administration of potassium chloride or a K^+-sparing diuretic. Potassium wasting is theoretically a problem with any diuretic that presents increased Na^+ delivery to the collecting tubule. However, the new adenosine A_1-receptor antagonists (see below) appear to avoid this toxicity by blunting Na^+ reabsorption in the collecting tubules as well as the proximal tubules.

D. Other Toxicities

Drowsiness and paresthesias are common following large doses of acetazolamide. Carbonic anhydrase inhibitors may accumulate in patients with renal failure, leading to nervous system toxicity. Hypersensitivity reactions (fever, rashes, bone marrow suppression, and interstitial nephritis) may also occur.

Contraindications

Carbonic anhydrase inhibitor–induced alkalinization of the urine decreases urinary excretion of NH_4^+ (by converting it to rapidly reabsorbed NH_3) and may contribute to the development of **hyperammonemia** and **hepatic encephalopathy** in patients with cirrhosis.

ADENOSINE A₁-RECEPTOR ANTAGONISTS

In addition to their potentially beneficial effect in preventing tubuloglomerular feedback (see below, under Heart Failure), adenosine receptor antagonists interfere with the activation of NHE3 in the PCT and the adenosine-mediated enhancement of collecting tubule K^+ secretion. Thus, adenosine receptor antagonists should be very useful diuretics.

Caffeine and theophylline have long been known to be weak diuretics because of their modest and nonspecific inhibition of adenosine receptors. A more selective A_1 antagonist, rolofylline, was recently withdrawn from study because of CNS toxicity and unexpected negative effects on GFR. However, newer adenosine inhibitors that are much more potent and more specific have been synthesized. Several of these (Aventri [BG9928], SLV320, and BG9719) are under study and if found to be less toxic than rolofylline, may become available as diuretics that avoid the diuretic effects of K^+ wasting and decreased GFR resulting from tubuloglomerular feedback.

LOOP DIURETICS

Loop diuretics selectively inhibit NaCl reabsorption in the TAL. Because of the large NaCl absorptive capacity of this segment and the fact that the diuretic action of these drugs is not limited by development of acidosis, as is the case with the carbonic anhydrase inhibitors, loop diuretics are the most efficacious diuretic agents currently available.

Chemistry

The two prototypical drugs of this group are **furosemide** and **ethacrynic acid.** The structures of these diuretics are shown in Figure 15–7. In addition to furosemide, **bumetanide** and **torsemide** are sulfonamide loop diuretics.

Ethacrynic acid—not a sulfonamide derivative—is a phenoxyacetic acid derivative containing an adjacent ketone and methylene group (Figure 15–7). The methylene group (shaded in figure) forms an adduct with the free sulfhydryl group of cysteine. The cysteine adduct appears to be an active form of the drug.

Organic **mercurial diuretics** also inhibit salt transport in the TAL but are no longer used because of their toxicity.

Pharmacokinetics

The loop diuretics are rapidly absorbed. They are eliminated by the kidney by glomerular filtration and tubular secretion. Absorption of oral torsemide is more rapid (1 hour) than that of furosemide (2–3 hours) and is nearly as complete as with intravenous administration. The duration of effect for furosemide is usually 2–3 hours. The effect of torsemide lasts 4–6 hours. Half-life

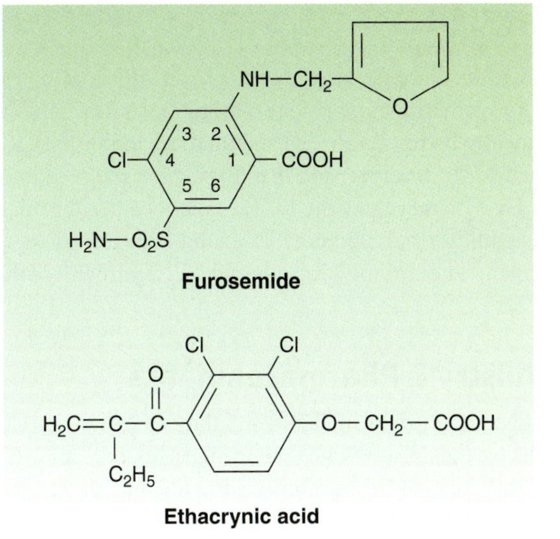

Furosemide

Ethacrynic acid

FIGURE 15–7 Two loop diuretics. The shaded methylene group on ethacrynic acid is reactive and may combine with free sulfhydryl groups.

TABLE 15–4 Typical dosages of loop diuretics.

Drug	Total Daily Oral Dose[1]
Bumetanide	0.5–2 mg
Ethacrynic acid	50–200 mg
Furosemide	20–80 mg
Torsemide	5–20 mg

[1]As single dose or in two divided doses.

depends on renal function. Since loop agents act on the luminal side of the tubule, their diuretic activity correlates with their secretion by the proximal tubule. Reduction in the secretion of loop diuretics may result from simultaneous administration of agents such as NSAIDs or probenecid, which compete for weak acid secretion in the proximal tubule. Metabolites of ethacrynic acid and furosemide have been identified, but it is not known if they have any diuretic activity. Torsemide has at least one active metabolite with a half-life considerably longer than that of the parent compound.

Pharmacodynamics

Loop diuretics inhibit NKCC2, the luminal $Na^+/K^+/2Cl^-$ transporter in the TAL of Henle's loop. By inhibiting this transporter, the loop diuretics reduce the reabsorption of NaCl and also diminish the lumen-positive potential that comes from K^+ recycling (Figure 15–3). This positive potential normally drives divalent cation reabsorption in the TAL (Figure 15–3), and by reducing this potential, loop diuretics cause an increase in Mg^{2+} and Ca^{2+} excretion. Prolonged use can cause significant hypomagnesemia in some patients. Since vitamin D–induced intestinal absorption and parathyroid hormone-induced renal reabsorption of Ca^{2+} can be increased, loop diuretics do not generally cause *hypocalcemia*. However, in disorders that cause hypercalcemia, Ca^{2+} excretion can be usefully enhanced by treatment with loop diuretics combined with saline infusions.

Loop diuretics have also been shown to induce expression of one of the cyclooxygenases (COX-2), which participates in the synthesis of prostaglandins from arachidonic acid. At least one of these prostaglandins, PGE_2, inhibits salt transport in the TAL and thus participates in the renal actions of loop diuretics. NSAIDs (eg, indomethacin), which blunt cyclooxygenase activity, can interfere with the actions of loop diuretics by reducing prostaglandin

synthesis in the kidney. This interference is minimal in otherwise normal subjects but may be significant in patients with nephrotic syndrome or hepatic cirrhosis.

Loop agents have direct effects on blood flow through several vascular beds. Furosemide increases renal blood flow via prostaglandin actions on kidney vasculature. Both furosemide and ethacrynic acid have also been shown to reduce pulmonary congestion and left ventricular filling pressures in heart failure before a measurable increase in urinary output occurs. These effects on peripheral vascular tone are also due to release of renal prostaglandins that were induced by the diuretics.

Clinical Indications & Dosage (Table 15–4)

The most important indications for the use of the loop diuretics include **acute pulmonary edema, other edematous conditions,** and **acute hypercalcemia.** The use of loop diuretics in these conditions is discussed below in Clinical Pharmacology. Other indications for loop diuretics include hyperkalemia, acute renal failure, and anion overdose.

A. Hyperkalemia

In mild hyperkalemia—or after acute management of severe hyperkalemia by other measures—loop diuretics can significantly enhance urinary excretion of K^+. This response is enhanced by simultaneous NaCl and water administration.

B. Acute Renal Failure

Loop agents can increase the rate of urine flow and enhance K^+ excretion in acute renal failure. However, they cannot prevent or shorten the duration of renal failure. If a large pigment load has precipitated acute renal failure (or threatens to), loop agents may help flush out intratubular casts and ameliorate intratubular obstruction. On the other hand, loop agents can actually worsen cast formation in myeloma and light chain nephropathy because increased distal Cl^- concentration enhances secretion of Tamm-Horsfall protein, which then aggregates with myeloma Bence Jones proteins.

C. Anion Overdose

Loop diuretics are useful in treating toxic ingestions of bromide, fluoride, and iodide, which are reabsorbed in the TAL. Saline solution must be administered to replace urinary losses of Na^+ and to provide Cl^-, so as to avoid extracellular fluid volume depletion.

Toxicity

A. Hypokalemic Metabolic Alkalosis

By inhibiting salt reabsorption in the TAL, loop diuretics increase Na^+ delivery to the collecting duct. Increased delivery leads to increased secretion of K^+ and H^+ by the duct, causing hypokalemic metabolic alkalosis (Table 15–2). This toxicity is a function of the magnitude of the diuresis and can be reversed by K^+ replacement and correction of hypovolemia.

B. Ototoxicity

Loop diuretics occasionally cause dose-related hearing loss that is usually reversible. It is most common in patients who have diminished renal function or who are also receiving other ototoxic agents such as aminoglycoside antibiotics.

C. Hyperuricemia

Loop diuretics can cause hyperuricemia and precipitate attacks of gout. This is caused by hypovolemia-associated enhancement of uric acid reabsorption in the proximal tubule. It may be prevented by using lower doses to avoid development of hypovolemia.

D. Hypomagnesemia

Magnesium depletion is a predictable consequence of the chronic use of loop agents and occurs most often in patients with dietary magnesium deficiency. It can be reversed by administration of oral magnesium preparations.

E. Allergic and Other Reactions

All loop diuretics, with the exception of ethacrynic acid, are sulfonamides. Therefore, skin rash, eosinophilia, and less often, interstitial nephritis are occasional adverse effects of these drugs. This toxicity usually resolves rapidly after drug withdrawal. Allergic reactions are much less common with ethacrynic acid.

Because Henle's loop is indirectly responsible for water reabsorption by the downstream collecting duct, loop diuretics can cause severe dehydration. Hyponatremia is less common than with the thiazides (see below), but patients who increase water intake in response to hypovolemia-induced thirst can become severely hyponatremic with loop agents. Loop agents can cause hypercalciuria, which can lead to mild hypocalcemia and secondary hyperparathyroidism. On the other hand, loop agents can have the opposite effect (hypercalcemia) in volume-depleted patients who have another—previously occult—cause for hypercalcemia, such as metastatic breast or squamous cell lung carcinoma.

Contraindications

Furosemide, bumetanide, and torsemide may exhibit allergic cross-reactivity in patients who are sensitive to other sulfonamides, but this appears to be very rare. Overzealous use of any diuretic is dangerous in hepatic cirrhosis, borderline renal failure, or heart failure.

THIAZIDES

The thiazide diuretics were discovered in 1957, as a result of efforts to synthesize more potent carbonic anhydrase inhibitors. It subsequently became clear that the thiazides inhibit NaCl, rather than $NaHCO_3^-$ transport and that their action was predominantly in the DCT, rather than the PCT. Some members of this group retain significant carbonic anhydrase inhibitory activity (eg, chlorthalidone). The prototypical thiazide is **hydrochlorothiazide (HCTZ).**

Chemistry & Pharmacokinetics

Like carbonic anhydrase inhibitors and three loop diuretics, all of the thiazides have an unsubstituted sulfonamide group (Figure 15–8).

All thiazides can be administered orally, but there are differences in their metabolism. Chlorothiazide, the parent of the group, is not very lipid-soluble and must be given in relatively large doses. It is the only thiazide available for parenteral administration. HCTZ is considerably more potent and should be used in much lower doses (Table 15–5). Chlorthalidone is slowly absorbed and has a longer duration of action. Although indapamide is excreted primarily by the biliary system, enough of the active form is cleared by the kidney to exert its diuretic effect in the DCT.

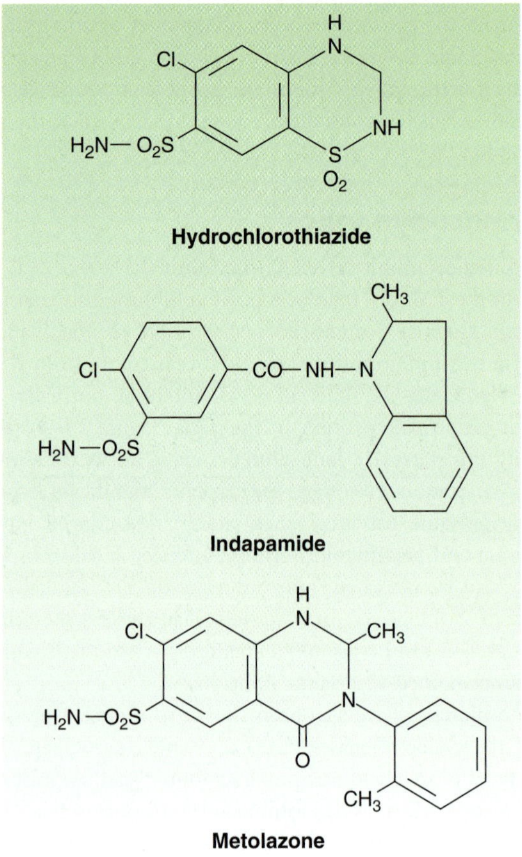

FIGURE 15–8 Hydrochlorothiazide and related agents.

All thiazides are secreted by the organic acid secretory system in the proximal tubule and compete with the secretion of uric acid by that system. As a result, thiazide use may blunt uric acid secretion and elevate serum uric acid level.

Pharmacodynamics

Thiazides inhibit NaCl reabsorption from the luminal side of epithelial cells in the DCT by blocking the Na^+/Cl^- transporter (NCC). In contrast to the situation in the TAL, in which loop diuretics inhibit Ca^{2+} reabsorption, thiazides actually enhance Ca^{2+} reabsorption. This enhancement has been postulated to result from effects in both the proximal and distal convoluted tubules. In the proximal tubule, thiazide-induced volume depletion leads to enhanced Na^+ and passive Ca^{2+} reabsorption. In the DCT, lowering of intracellular Na^+ by thiazide-induced blockade of Na^+ entry enhances Na^+/Ca^{2+} exchange in the basolateral membrane (Figure 15–4), and increases overall reabsorption of Ca^{2+}. Although thiazides rarely cause hypercalcemia as the result of this enhanced reabsorption, they can unmask hypercalcemia due to other causes (eg, hyperparathyroidism, carcinoma, sarcoidosis). Thiazides are useful in the treatment of kidney stones caused by hypercalciuria.

The action of thiazides depends in part on renal prostaglandin production. As described for loop diuretics, the actions of thiazides can also be inhibited by NSAIDs under certain conditions.

Clinical Indications & Dosage (Table 15–5)

The major indications for thiazide diuretics are (1) hypertension, (2) heart failure, (3) nephrolithiasis due to idiopathic hypercalciuria, and (4) nephrogenic diabetes insipidus. Use of the thiazides in each of these conditions is described below in Clinical Pharmacology of Diuretic Agents.

TABLE 15–5 Thiazides and related diuretics.

Drug	Total Daily Oral Dose	Frequency of Daily Administration
Bendroflumethiazide	2.5–10 mg	Single dose
Chlorothiazide	0.5–2 g	Two divided doses
Chlorthalidone[1]	25–50 mg	Single dose
Hydrochlorothiazide	25–100 mg	Single dose
Hydroflumethiazide	12.5–50 mg	Two divided doses
Indapamide[1]	2.5–10 mg	Single dose
Methyclothiazide	2.5–10 mg	Single dose
Metolazone[1]	2.5–10 mg	Single dose
Polythiazide	1–4 mg	Single dose
Quinethazone[1]	25–100 mg	Single dose
Trichlormethiazide	1–4 mg	Single dose

[1]Not a thiazide but a sulfonamide qualitatively similar to the thiazides.

Toxicity

A. Hypokalemic Metabolic Alkalosis and Hyperuricemia

These toxicities are similar to those observed with loop diuretics (see previous text and Table 15–2).

B. Impaired Carbohydrate Tolerance

Hyperglycemia may occur in patients who are overtly diabetic or who have even mildly abnormal glucose tolerance tests. The effect is due to both impaired pancreatic release of insulin and diminished tissue utilization of glucose. Hyperglycemia may be partially reversible with correction of hypokalemia.

C. Hyperlipidemia

Thiazides cause a 5–15% increase in total serum cholesterol and low-density lipoproteins (LDLs). These levels may return toward baseline after prolonged use.

D. Hyponatremia

Hyponatremia is an important adverse effect of thiazide diuretics. It is caused by a combination of hypovolemia-induced elevation of ADH, reduction in the diluting capacity of the kidney, and increased thirst. It can be prevented by reducing the dose of the drug or limiting water intake.

E. Allergic Reactions

The thiazides are sulfonamides and share cross-reactivity with other members of this chemical group. Photosensitivity or generalized dermatitis occurs rarely. Serious allergic reactions are extremely rare but do include hemolytic anemia, thrombocytopenia, and acute necrotizing pancreatitis.

F. Other Toxicities

Weakness, fatigability, and paresthesias similar to those of carbonic anhydrase inhibitors may occur. Impotence has been reported but is probably related to volume depletion.

Contraindications

Excessive use of any diuretic is dangerous in patients with hepatic cirrhosis, borderline renal failure, or heart failure (see text that follows).

POTASSIUM-SPARING DIURETICS

Potassium-sparing diuretics prevent K^+ secretion by antagonizing the effects of aldosterone in collecting tubules. Inhibition may occur by direct pharmacologic antagonism of mineralocorticoid receptors (**spironolactone, eplerenone**) or by inhibition of Na^+ influx through ion channels in the luminal membrane (**amiloride, triamterene**). This latter property appears to be shared by adenosine antagonists, which primarily blunt Na^+ reabsorption in the PCT, but also blunt Na^+ reabsorption and K^+ secretion in collecting tubules. Finally, ularitide (recombinant urodilatin), which is currently still under investigation, blunts Na^+ uptake and Na^+/K^+-ATPase in collecting tubules and increases GFR through its vascular effects. Nesiritide, which is now commercially available for intravenous use only, increases GFR and blunts Na^+ reabsorption in both proximal and collecting tubules.

Chemistry & Pharmacokinetics

The structures of spironolactone and amiloride are shown in Figure 15–9.

Spironolactone is a synthetic steroid that acts as a competitive antagonist to aldosterone. Onset and duration of its action are determined by the kinetics of the aldosterone response in the target tissue. Substantial inactivation of spironolactone occurs in the liver. Overall, spironolactone has a rather slow onset of action, requiring several days before full therapeutic effect is achieved. Eplerenone is a spironolactone analog with much greater selectivity for the mineralocorticoid receptor. It is several hundredfold less active on androgen and progesterone receptors than spironolactone, and therefore, eplerenone has considerably fewer adverse effects.

Amiloride and triamterene are direct inhibitors of Na^+ influx in the CCT (cortical collecting tubule). Triamterene is metabolized in the liver, but renal excretion is a major route of elimination for the active form and the metabolites. Because triamterene is extensively metabolized, it has a shorter half-life and must be given more frequently than amiloride (which is not metabolized).

Pharmacodynamics

Potassium-sparing diuretics reduce Na^+ absorption in the collecting tubules and ducts. Potassium absorption (and K^+ secretion) at this site is regulated by aldosterone, as described above. Aldosterone antagonists interfere with this process. Similar effects are observed with respect to H^+ handling by the intercalated cells of the collecting tubule, in part explaining the metabolic acidosis seen with aldosterone antagonists (Table 15–2).

Spironolactone and eplerenone bind to mineralocorticoid receptors and blunt aldosterone activity. Amiloride and triamterene do not block aldosterone, but instead directly interfere with Na^+ entry through the epithelial Na^+ channels (ENaC, Figure 15–5), in the apical membrane of the collecting tubule. Since K^+ secretion is coupled with Na^+ entry in this segment, these agents are also effective K^+-sparing diuretics.

The actions of the aldosterone antagonists depend on renal prostaglandin production. The actions of K^+-sparing diuretics can be inhibited by NSAIDs under certain conditions.

Clinical Indications & Dosage (Table 15–6)

Potassium-sparing diuretics are most useful in states of mineralocorticoid excess or hyperaldosteronism (also called aldosteronism), due either to primary hypersecretion (Conn's syndrome, ectopic adrenocorticotropic hormone production) or secondary hyperaldosteronism (evoked by heart failure, hepatic cirrhosis, nephrotic syndrome, or other conditions associated with diminished effective intravascular volume). Use of diuretics such as thiazides or loop agents can cause or exacerbate volume contraction and may cause secondary hyperaldosteronism. In the setting of enhanced mineralocorticoid secretion and excessive delivery of Na^+ to distal nephron sites, renal K^+ wasting occurs. Potassium-sparing diuretics of either type may be used in this setting to blunt the K^+ secretory response.

It has also been found that low doses of eplerenone (25–50 mg/d) may interfere with some of the fibrotic and inflammatory effects of aldosterone. By doing so, it can slow the progression of albuminuria in diabetic patients. More important is that eplerenone has been found to reduce myocardial perfusion defects after myocardial infarction. In one clinical study, eplerenone reduced

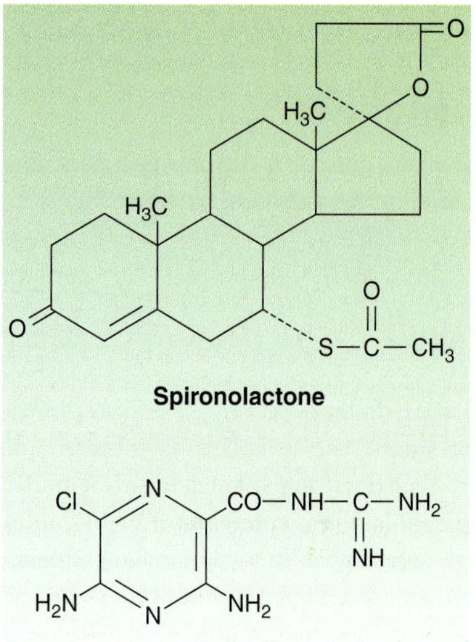

FIGURE 15–9 Potassium-sparing diuretics.

TABLE 15–6 Potassium-sparing diuretics and combination preparations.

Trade Name	Potassium-Sparing Agent	Hydrochlorothiazide
Aldactazide	Spironolactone 25 mg	50 mg
Aldactone	Spironolactone 25, 50, or 100 mg	...
Dyazide	Triamterene 37.5 mg	25 mg
Dyrenium	Triamterene 50 or 100 mg	...
Inspra[1]	Eplerenone 25, 50, or 100 mg	...
Maxzide	Triamterene 75 mg	50 mg
Maxzide-25 mg	Triamterene 37.5 mg	25 mg
Midamor	Amiloride 5 mg	...
Moduretic	Amiloride 5 mg	50 mg

[1]Eplerenone is currently approved for use only in hypertension.

mortality rate by 15% (compared with placebo) in patients with mild to moderate heart failure after myocardial infarction.

Toxicity

A. Hyperkalemia

Unlike most other diuretics, K^+-sparing diuretics reduce urinary excretion of K^+ (Table 15–2) and can cause mild, moderate, or even life-threatening hyperkalemia. The risk of this complication is greatly increased by renal disease (in which maximal K^+ excretion may be reduced) or by the use of other drugs that reduce or inhibit renin (β blockers, NSAIDs, aliskiren) or angiotensin II activity (angiotensin-converting enzyme inhibitors, angiotensin receptor inhibitors). Since most other diuretic agents lead to K^+ losses, hyperkalemia is more common when K^+-sparing diuretics are used as the sole diuretic agent, especially in patients with renal insufficiency. With fixed-dosage combinations of K^+-sparing and thiazide diuretics, the thiazide-induced hypokalemia and metabolic alkalosis are ameliorated. However, because of variations in the bioavailability of the components of fixed-dosage forms, the thiazide-associated adverse effects often predominate. Therefore, it is generally preferable to adjust the doses of the two drugs separately.

B. Hyperchloremic Metabolic Acidosis

By inhibiting H^+ secretion in parallel with K^+ secretion, the K^+-sparing diuretics can cause acidosis similar to that seen with type IV renal tubular acidosis.

C. Gynecomastia

Synthetic steroids may cause endocrine abnormalities by actions on other steroid receptors. Gynecomastia, impotence, and benign prostatic hyperplasia (very rare) all have been reported with spironolactone. Such effects have not been reported with eplerenone, presumably because it is much more selective than spironolactone for the mineralocorticoid receptor and virtually inactive on androgen or progesterone receptors.

D. Acute Renal Failure

The combination of triamterene with indomethacin has been reported to cause acute renal failure. This has not been reported with other K^+-sparing diuretics.

E. Kidney Stones

Triamterene is only slightly soluble and may precipitate in the urine, causing kidney stones.

Contraindications

Potassium-sparing agents can cause severe, even fatal, hyperkalemia in susceptible patients. Patients with chronic renal insufficiency are especially vulnerable and should rarely be treated with these diuretics. Oral K^+ administration should be discontinued if K^+-sparing diuretics are administered. Concomitant use of other agents that blunt the renin-angiotensin system (β blockers, ACE inhibitors, ARBs) increases the likelihood of hyperkalemia. Patients with liver disease may have impaired metabolism of triamterene and spironolactone, so dosing must be carefully adjusted. Strong CYP3A4 inhibitors (eg, erythromycin, fluconazole, diltiazem, and grapefruit juice) can markedly increase blood levels of eplerenone, but not spironolactone.

AGENTS THAT ALTER WATER EXCRETION (AQUARETICS)

OSMOTIC DIURETICS

The proximal tubule and descending limb of Henle's loop are freely permeable to water (Table 15–1). Any osmotically active agent that is filtered by the glomerulus but not reabsorbed causes water to be retained in these segments and promotes a water diuresis. Such agents can be used to reduce intracranial pressure and to promote prompt removal of renal toxins. The prototypic osmotic diuretic is **mannitol**. Glucose is not used clinically as a diuretic but frequently causes osmotic diuresis (glycosuria) in patients with hyperglycemia.

Pharmacokinetics

Mannitol is poorly absorbed by the GI tract, and when administered orally, it causes osmotic diarrhea rather than diuresis. For systemic effect, mannitol must be given intravenously. Mannitol is not metabolized and is excreted by glomerular filtration within 30–60 minutes, without any important tubular reabsorption or secretion. It must be used cautiously in patients with even mild renal insufficiency (see below).

Pharmacodynamics

Osmotic diuretics have their major effect in the proximal tubule and the descending limb of Henle's loop. Through osmotic effects, they also oppose the action of ADH in the collecting tubule. The presence of a nonreabsorbable solute such as mannitol prevents the normal absorption of water by interposing a countervailing osmotic force. As a result, urine volume increases. The increase in urine flow rate decreases the contact time between fluid and the tubular epithelium, thus reducing Na^+ as well as water reabsorption. The resulting natriuresis is of lesser magnitude than the water diuresis, leading eventually to excessive water loss and hypernatremia.

Clinical Indications & Dosage

A. Increase of Urine Volume

Osmotic diuretics are used to increase water excretion in preference to sodium excretion. This effect can be useful when avid Na^+ retention limits the response to conventional agents. It can be used to maintain urine volume and to prevent anuria that might otherwise result from presentation of large pigment loads to the kidney (eg, from hemolysis or rhabdomyolysis). Some oliguric patients do not respond to osmotic diuretics. Therefore, a test dose of mannitol

(12.5 g intravenously) should be given before starting a continuous infusion. Mannitol should not be continued unless there is an increase in urine flow rate to more than 50 mL/h during the 3 hours after the test dose. Mannitol (12.5–25 g intravenously) can be repeated every 1–2 hours to maintain urine flow rate greater than 100 mL/h. Prolonged use of mannitol is not advised.

B. Reduction of Intracranial and Intraocular Pressure

Osmotic diuretics alter Starling forces so that water leaves cells and reduces intracellular volume. This effect is used to reduce intracranial pressure in neurologic conditions and to reduce intraocular pressure before ophthalmologic procedures. A dose of 1–2 g/kg mannitol is administered intravenously. Intracranial pressure, which must be monitored, should fall in 60–90 minutes.

Toxicity

A. Extracellular Volume Expansion

Mannitol is rapidly distributed in the extracellular compartment and extracts water from cells. Prior to the diuresis, this leads to expansion of the extracellular volume and hyponatremia. This effect can complicate heart failure and may produce florid pulmonary edema. Headache, nausea, and vomiting are commonly observed in patients treated with osmotic diuretics.

B. Dehydration, Hyperkalemia, and Hypernatremia

Excessive use of mannitol without adequate water replacement can ultimately lead to severe dehydration, free water losses, and hypernatremia. As water is extracted from cells, intracellular K^+ concentration rises, leading to cellular losses and hyperkalemia. These complications can be avoided by careful attention to serum ion composition and fluid balance.

C. Hyponatremia

When used in patients with severe renal impairment, parenterally administered mannitol cannot be excreted and is retained intravenously. This causes osmotic extraction of water from cells, leading to hyponatremia.

ANTIDIURETIC HORMONE (ADH, VASOPRESSIN) AGONISTS

Vasopressin and **desmopressin** are used in the treatment of central diabetes insipidus. They are discussed in Chapter 37. Their renal action appears to be mediated primarily via V_2 ADH receptors, although V_{1a} receptors may also be involved.

ANTIDIURETIC HORMONE ANTAGONISTS

A variety of medical conditions, including congestive heart failure (CHF) and the syndrome of inappropriate ADH secretion (SIADH), cause water retention as a result of excessive ADH secretion. Patients with CHF who are on diuretics frequently develop hyponatremia secondary to excessive ADH secretion. Dangerous hyponatremia can result.

Until recently, two nonselective agents, lithium (discussed in Chapter 29) and demeclocycline (a tetracycline antimicrobial drug discussed in Chapter 44), were used for their well-known interference with ADH activity. The mechanism for this interference has not been completely determined for either of these agents. Demeclocycline is used more often than lithium because of the many side effects of lithium administration. However, demeclocycline is now being rapidly replaced by several specific ADH receptor antagonists (vaptans), which have yielded encouraging clinical results.

There are three known vasopressin receptors, V_{1a}, V_{1b}, and V_2. V_1 receptors are expressed in the vasculature and CNS, while V_2 receptors are expressed specifically in the kidney. **Conivaptan** (currently available only for intravenous use) exhibits activity against both V_{1a} and V_2 receptors (see below). The oral agents **tolvaptan**, lixivaptan, and satavaptan are selectively active against the V_2 receptor. Lixivaptan and satavaptan are still under clinical investigation, but tolvaptan, which recently received Food and Drug Administration approval, is very effective in treatment of hyponatremia and as an adjunct to standard diuretic therapy in patients with CHF.

Pharmacokinetics

The half-life of conivaptan and demeclocycline is 5–10 hours, while that of tolvaptan is 12–24 hours.

Pharmacodynamics

Antidiuretic hormone antagonists inhibit the effects of ADH in the collecting tubule. Conivaptan and tolvaptan are direct ADH receptor antagonists, while both lithium and demeclocycline reduce ADH-induced cAMP by mechanisms that are not yet completely clarified.

Clinical Indications & Dosage

A. Syndrome of Inappropriate ADH Secretion

Antidiuretic hormone antagonists are used to manage SIADH when water restriction has failed to correct the abnormality. This generally occurs in the outpatient setting, where water restriction cannot be enforced, but can occur in the hospital when large quantities of intravenous fluid are needed for other purposes. Demeclocycline (600–1200 mg/d) or tolvaptan (15–60 mg/d) can be used for SIADH. Appropriate plasma levels of demeclocycline (2 mcg/mL) should be maintained by monitoring, but tolvaptan levels are not routinely monitored. Unlike demeclocycline or tolvaptan, conivaptan is administered intravenously and is not suitable for chronic use in outpatients. Lixivaptan and satavaptan may also soon be available for oral use.

B. Other Causes of Elevated Antidiuretic Hormone

Antidiuretic hormone is also elevated in response to diminished effective circulating blood volume, as often occurs in heart failure. When treatment by volume replacement is not desirable, hyponatremia may result. As for SIADH, water restriction is often the treatment of choice. In patients with heart failure, this approach is often unsuccessful in view of increased thirst and the large number of oral medications being used. For patients with heart failure, intravenous conivaptan may be particularly useful because it has been found that the blockade of V_{1a} receptors by this drug leads to decreased peripheral vascular resistance and increased cardiac output.

Toxicity

A. Nephrogenic Diabetes Insipidus

If serum Na^+ is not monitored closely, any ADH antagonist can cause severe hypernatremia and nephrogenic diabetes insipidus. If lithium is being used for a psychiatric disorder, nephrogenic diabetes insipidus can be treated with a thiazide diuretic or amiloride (see Diabetes Insipidus, below).

B. Renal Failure

Both lithium and demeclocycline have been reported to cause acute renal failure. Long-term lithium therapy may also cause chronic interstitial nephritis.

C. Other

Dry mouth and thirst are common with many of these drugs. Tolvaptan may cause hypotension. Multiple adverse effects associated with lithium therapy have been found and are discussed in Chapter 29. Demeclocycline should be avoided in patients with liver disease (see Chapter 44) and in children younger than 12 years.

DIURETIC COMBINATIONS

LOOP AGENTS & THIAZIDES

Some patients are refractory to the usual dose of loop diuretics or become refractory after an initial response. Since these agents have a short half-life (2–6 hours), refractoriness may be due to an excessive interval between doses. Renal Na^+ retention may be greatly increased during the time period when the drug is no longer active. After the dosing interval for loop agents is minimized or the dose is maximized, the use of two drugs acting at different nephron sites may exhibit dramatic synergy. Loop agents and thiazides in combination often produce diuresis when neither agent acting alone is even minimally effective. There are several reasons for this phenomenon.

First, salt reabsorption in either the TAL or the DCT can increase when the other is blocked. Inhibition of both can therefore produce more than an additive diuretic response. Second, thiazide diuretics often produce a mild natriuresis in the proximal tubule that is usually masked by increased reabsorption in the TAL. The combination of loop diuretics and thiazides can therefore block Na^+ reabsorption, to some extent, from all three segments.

Metolazone is the thiazide-like drug usually used in patients refractory to loop agents alone, but it is likely that other thiazides would be as effective. Moreover, metolazone is available only in an oral preparation, whereas chlorothiazide can be given parenterally.

The combination of loop diuretics and thiazides can mobilize large amounts of fluid, even in patients who have not responded to single agents. Therefore, close hemodynamic monitoring is essential. Routine outpatient use is not recommended. Furthermore, K^+ wasting is extremely common and may require parenteral K^+ administration with careful monitoring of fluid and electrolyte status.

POTASSIUM-SPARING DIURETICS & PROXIMAL TUBULE DIURETICS, LOOP AGENTS, OR THIAZIDES

Hypokalemia often develops in patients taking carbonic anhydrase inhibitors, loop diuretics, or thiazides. This can usually be managed by dietary NaCl restriction or by taking dietary KCl supplements. When hypokalemia cannot be managed in this way, the addition of a K^+-sparing diuretic can significantly lower K^+ excretion. Although this approach is generally safe, it should be avoided in patients with renal insufficiency and in those receiving angiotensin antagonists such as ACE inhibitors, in whom life-threatening hyperkalemia can develop in response to K^+-sparing diuretics. It is not yet known whether adenosine receptor antagonists, which are K^+-sparing diuretics (but which act primarily in the proximal tubule), will cause hyperkalemia.

■ CLINICAL PHARMACOLOGY OF DIURETIC AGENTS

A summary of the effects of diuretics on urinary electrolyte excretion is shown in Table 15–2.

EDEMATOUS STATES

A common reason for diuretic use is for reduction of peripheral or pulmonary edema that has accumulated as a result of cardiac, renal, or vascular diseases that reduce blood flow to the kidney. This reduction is sensed as insufficient effective arterial blood volume and leads to salt and water retention, which expands blood volume and eventually causes edema formation. Judicious use of diuretics can mobilize this interstitial edema without significant reductions in plasma volume. However, excessive diuretic therapy may compromise the effective arterial blood volume and reduce the perfusion of vital organs. Therefore, the use of diuretics to mobilize edema requires careful monitoring of the patient's hemodynamic status and an understanding of the pathophysiology of the underlying illness.

HEART FAILURE

When cardiac output is reduced by heart failure, the resultant changes in blood pressure and blood flow to the kidney are sensed as hypovolemia and lead to renal retention of salt and water. This physiologic response initially increases intravascular volume and venous return to the heart and may partially restore the cardiac output toward normal (see Chapter 13).

If the underlying disease causes cardiac output to deteriorate despite expansion of plasma volume, the kidney continues to retain salt and water, which then leaks from the vasculature and becomes interstitial or pulmonary edema. At this point, diuretic use becomes necessary to reduce the accumulation of edema, particularly in the lungs. Reduction of pulmonary vascular congestion with diuretics may actually improve oxygenation and thereby improve myocardial function. Reduction of preload can reduce the size of the heart, allowing it to work at a more efficient fiber length. Edema associated with heart failure is generally managed with loop diuretics. In some instances, salt and water retention may become so severe that a combination of thiazides and loop diuretics is necessary.

In treating the heart failure patient with diuretics, it must always be remembered that cardiac output in these patients is being maintained in part by high filling pressures. Therefore, excessive use of diuretics may diminish venous return and further impair cardiac output. This is especially critical in right ventricular heart failure. Systemic, rather than pulmonary vascular, congestion is the hallmark of this disorder. Diuretic-induced volume contraction predictably reduces venous return and can severely compromise cardiac output if left ventricular filling pressure is reduced below 15 mm Hg (see Chapter 13). Reduction in cardiac output, resulting from either left or right ventricular dysfunction, also eventually leads to renal dysfunction resulting from reduced perfusion pressures.

Increased delivery of salt to the TAL leads to activation of the macula densa and a reduction in GFR by tubuloglomerular feedback. The mechanism of this feedback is secretion of adenosine by macula densa cells, which causes afferent arteriolar vasoconstriction through activation of A_1 adenosine receptors on the afferent arteriole. This vasoconstriction reduces GFR. Tubuloglomerular feedback–mediated reduction in GFR exacerbates the reduction that was initially caused by decreased cardiac output. Recent work with adenosine receptor antagonists has shown that it may soon be possible to circumvent this complication of diuretic therapy in heart failure patients by blunting tubuloglomerular feedback.

Diuretic-induced metabolic alkalosis, exacerbated by hypokalemia, is another adverse effect that may further compromise cardiac function. This complication can be treated with replacement of K^+ and restoration of intravascular volume with saline; however, severe heart failure may preclude the use of saline even in patients who have received excessive diuretic therapy. In these cases, adjunctive use of acetazolamide helps to correct the alkalosis.

Another serious toxicity of diuretic use in the cardiac patient is hypokalemia. Hypokalemia can exacerbate underlying cardiac arrhythmias and contribute to digitalis toxicity. This can usually be avoided by having the patient reduce Na^+ intake while taking diuretics, thus decreasing Na^+ delivery to the K^+-secreting collecting tubule. Patients who are noncompliant with a low Na^+ diet must take oral KCl supplements or a K^+-sparing diuretic.

KIDNEY DISEASE AND RENAL FAILURE

A variety of diseases interfere with the kidney's critical role in volume homeostasis. Although some renal disorders cause salt wasting, most cause retention of salt and water. When renal failure is severe (GFR < 5 mL/min), diuretic agents are of little benefit, because glomerular filtration is insufficient to generate or sustain a natriuretic response. However, a large number of patients, and even dialysis patients, with milder degrees of renal insufficiency (GFR of 5–15 mL/min), can be treated with diuretics when they retain excessive volumes of fluid between dialysis treatments.

There is still interest in the question as to whether diuretic therapy can alter the severity or the outcome of acute renal failure. This is because "nonoliguric" forms of acute renal insufficiency have better outcomes than "oliguric" (< 400–500 mL/24 h urine output) acute renal failure. Almost all studies of this question have shown that diuretic therapy helps in the short-term fluid management of these patients with acute renal failure, but that it has no impact on the long-term outcome.

Many glomerular diseases, such as those associated with diabetes mellitus or systemic lupus erythematosus, exhibit renal retention of salt and water. The cause of this sodium retention is not precisely known, but it probably involves disordered regulation of the renal microcirculation and tubular function through release of vasoconstrictors, prostaglandins, cytokines, and other mediators. When edema or hypertension develops in these patients, diuretic therapy can be very effective.

Certain forms of renal disease, particularly diabetic nephropathy, are frequently associated with development of hyperkalemia at a relatively early stage of renal failure. In these cases, a thiazide or loop diuretic will enhance K^+ excretion by increasing delivery of salt to the K^+-secreting collecting tubule.

Patients with renal diseases leading to the nephrotic syndrome often present complex problems in volume management. These patients may exhibit fluid retention in the form of ascites or edema but have reduced plasma volume due to reduced plasma oncotic pressures. This is very often the case in patients with "minimal change" nephropathy. In these patients, diuretic use may cause further reductions in plasma volume that can impair GFR and may lead to orthostatic hypotension. Most other causes of nephrotic syndrome are associated with primary retention of salt and water by the kidney, leading to expanded plasma volume and hypertension despite the low plasma oncotic pressure. In these cases, diuretic therapy may be beneficial in controlling the volume-dependent component of hypertension.

In choosing a diuretic for the patient with kidney disease, there are a number of important limitations. Acetazolamide must usually be avoided because it causes $NaHCO_3$ excretion and can exacerbate acidosis. Potassium-sparing diuretics may cause hyperkalemia. Thiazide diuretics were previously thought to be ineffective when GFR falls below 30 mL/min. More recently, it has been found that thiazides, which are of little benefit when used alone, can be used to significantly reduce the dose of loop diuretics needed to promote diuresis in a patient with GFR of 5–15 mL/min. Thus, high-dose loop diuretics (up to

500 mg of furosemide/d) or a combination of metolazone (5–10 mg/d) and much smaller doses of furosemide (40–80 mg/d) may be useful in treating volume overload in dialysis or predialysis patients. There has been some interest in the use of osmotic diuretics such as mannitol, because this drug can shrink swollen epithelial cells and may theoretically reduce tubular obstruction. Unfortunately, there is no evidence that mannitol can prevent ischemic or toxic acute renal failure. Mannitol may be useful in the management of hemoglobinuria or myoglobinuria. Lastly, although excessive use of diuretics can impair renal function in all patients, the consequences are obviously more serious in patients with underlying renal disease.

HEPATIC CIRRHOSIS

Liver disease is often associated with edema and ascites in conjunction with elevated portal hydrostatic pressures and reduced plasma oncotic pressures. Mechanisms for retention of Na^+ by the kidney in this setting include diminished renal perfusion (from systemic vascular alterations), diminished plasma volume (due to ascites formation), and diminished oncotic pressure (hypoalbuminemia). In addition, there may be primary Na^+ retention due to elevated plasma aldosterone levels.

When ascites and edema become severe, diuretic therapy can be very useful. However, cirrhotic patients are often resistant to loop diuretics because of decreased secretion of the drug into the tubular fluid and because of high aldosterone levels. In contrast, cirrhotic edema is unusually responsive to spironolactone and eplerenone. The combination of loop diuretics and an aldosterone receptor antagonist may be useful in some patients. However, considerable caution is necessary in the use of aldosterone antagonists in cirrhotic patients with even mild renal insufficiency because of the potential for causing serious hyperkalemia.

It is important to note that, even more than in heart failure, overly aggressive use of diuretics in this setting can be disastrous. Vigorous diuretic therapy can cause marked depletion of intravascular volume, hypokalemia, and metabolic alkalosis. Hepatorenal syndrome and hepatic encephalopathy are the unfortunate consequences of excessive diuretic use in the cirrhotic patient.

IDIOPATHIC EDEMA

Idiopathic edema (fluctuating salt retention and edema) is a syndrome found most often in 20–30 year-old women. Despite intensive study, the pathophysiology remains obscure. Some studies suggest that surreptitious, intermittent diuretic use may actually contribute to the syndrome and should be ruled out before additional therapy is pursued. While spironolactone has been used for idiopathic edema, it should probably be managed with moderate salt restriction alone if possible. Compression stockings have also been used but appear to be of variable benefit.

NONEDEMATOUS STATES

HYPERTENSION

The diuretic and mild vasodilator actions of the thiazides are useful in treating virtually all patients with essential hypertension and may be sufficient in many. Although hydrochlorothiazide is the most widely used diuretic for hypertension, chlorthalidone may be more effective because of its much longer half-life. Loop diuretics are usually reserved for patients with mild renal insufficiency (GFR < 30–40 mL/min) or heart failure. Moderate restriction of dietary Na^+ intake (60–100 mEq/d) has been shown to potentiate the effects of diuretics in essential hypertension and to lessen renal K^+ wasting. A K^+-sparing diuretic can be added to reduce K^+ wasting.

There has been debate about whether thiazides should be used as the initial therapy in treatment of hypertension. Their relatively mild efficacy sometimes limits their use as monotherapy. However, a very large study of over 30,000 participants has shown that inexpensive diuretics like thiazides result in outcomes that are similar or superior to those found with ACE inhibitor or calcium channel-blocker therapy. This important result reinforces the importance of thiazide therapy in hypertension.

Although diuretics are often successful as monotherapy, they also play an important role in patients who require multiple drugs to control blood pressure. Diuretics enhance the efficacy of many agents, particularly ACE inhibitors. Patients being treated with powerful vasodilators such as hydralazine or minoxidil usually require simultaneous diuretics because the vasodilators cause significant salt and water retention.

NEPHROLITHIASIS

Approximately two thirds of kidney stones contain Ca^{2+} phosphate or Ca^{2+} oxalate. While there are numerous medical conditions (hyperparathyroidism, hypervitaminosis D, sarcoidosis, malignancies, etc) that cause hypercalciuria, many patients with such stones exhibit a defect in proximal tubular Ca^{2+} reabsorption. This can be treated with thiazide diuretics, which enhance Ca^{2+} reabsorption in the DCT and thus reduce the urinary Ca^{2+} concentration. Fluid intake should be increased, but salt intake must be reduced, since excess dietary NaCl will overwhelm the hypocalciuric effect of thiazides. Dietary Ca^{2+} should not be restricted, as this can lead to negative total body Ca^{2+} balance. Calcium stones may also be caused by increased intestinal absorption of Ca^{2+}, or they may be idiopathic. In these situations, thiazides are also effective but should be used as adjunctive therapy with other measures.

HYPERCALCEMIA

Hypercalcemia can be a medical emergency (see Chapter 42). Because loop diuretics reduce Ca^{2+} reabsorption significantly, they can be quite effective in promoting Ca^{2+} diuresis. However, loop diuretics alone can cause marked volume contraction. If this occurs, loop diuretics are ineffective (and potentially counterproductive) because Ca^{2+} reabsorption in the proximal tubule would be enhanced. Thus, saline must be administered simultaneously with loop diuretics if an effective Ca^{2+} diuresis is to be maintained. The usual approach is to infuse normal saline and furosemide (80–120 mg) intravenously. Once the diuresis begins, the rate of saline infusion can be matched with the urine flow rate to avoid volume depletion. Potassium chloride may be added to the saline infusion as needed.

DIABETES INSIPIDUS

Diabetes insipidus is due to either deficient production of ADH (neurogenic or central diabetes insipidus) or inadequate responsiveness to ADH (nephrogenic diabetes insipidus [NDI]). Administration of supplementary ADH or one of its analogs is effective only in central diabetes insipidus. Thiazide diuretics can reduce polyuria and polydipsia in both types of diabetes insipidus. Lithium, used in the treatment of manic-depressive disorder, is a common cause of NDI, and thiazide diuretics have been found to be very helpful in treating it. This seemingly paradoxic beneficial effect of thiazides was previously thought to be mediated through plasma volume reduction, with an associated fall in GFR, leading to enhanced proximal reabsorption of NaCl and water and decreased delivery of fluid to the downstream diluting segments. However, in the case of Li^+-induced NDI, it is now known that HCTZ causes increased osmolality in the inner medulla (papilla) and a partial correction of the Li^+-induced reduction in aquaporin-2 expression. HCTZ also leads to increased expression of Na^+ transporters in the DCT and CCT segments of the nephron. Thus, the maximum volume of dilute urine that can be produced is significantly reduced in NDI. Dietary sodium restriction can potentiate the beneficial effects of thiazides on urine volume in this setting. Serum Li^+ levels must be carefully monitored in these patients, because diuretics may reduce renal clearance of Li^+ and raise plasma Li^+ levels into the toxic range (see Chapter 29). Lithium-induced polyuria can also be partially reversed by amiloride, which blocks Li^+ entry into collecting duct cells, much as it blocks Na^+ entry. As mentioned above, thiazides are also beneficial in other forms of nephrogenic diabetes insipidus. It is not yet clear whether this is via the same mechanism that has been found in Li^+-induced NDI.

SUMMARY Diuretic Agents

Subclass	Mechanism of Action	Effects	Clinical Applications	Pharmacokinetics, Toxicities, Interactions
CARBONIC ANHYDRASE INHIBITORS				
• Acetazolamide, others	Inhibition of the enzyme prevents dehydration of H_2CO_3 and hydration of CO_2 in the proximal convoluted tubule	Reduces reabsorption of HCO_3^-, causing self-limited diuresis • hyperchloremic metabolic acidosis reduces body pH, reduces intraocular pressure	Glaucoma, mountain sickness, edema with alkalosis	Oral and topical preparations available • duration of action ~ 8–12 h • *Toxicity:* Metabolic acidosis, renal stones, hyperammonemia in cirrhotics
• Brinzolamide, dorzolamide: Topical for glaucoma				
LOOP DIURETICS				
• Furosemide	Inhibition of the Na/K/2Cl transporter in the ascending limb of Henle's loop	Marked increase in NaCl excretion, some K wasting, hypokalemic metabolic alkalosis, increased urine Ca and Mg	Pulmonary edema, peripheral edema, hypertension, acute hypercalcemia or hyperkalemia, acute renal failure, anion overdose	Oral and parenteral preparations • duration of action 2–4 h • *Toxicity:* Ototoxicity, hypovolemia, K wasting, hyperuricemia, hypomagnesemia
• Bumetanide, torsemide: Sulfonamide loop agents like furosemide				
• Ethacrynic acid: Not a sulfonamide but has typical loop activity and some uricosuric action				
THIAZIDES				
• Hydrochlorothiazide	Inhibition of the Na/Cl transporter in the distal convoluted tubule	Modest increase in NaCl excretion • some K wasting • hypokalemic metabolic alkalosis • decreased urine Ca	Hypertension, mild heart failure, nephrolithiasis, nephrogenic diabetes insipidus	Oral • duration 8–12 h • *Toxicity:* Hypokalemic metabolic alkalosis, hyperuricemia, hyperglycemia, hyponatremia
• Metolazone: Popular for use with loop agents for synergistic effects				
• Chlorothiazide: Only parenteral thiazide available (IV)				
• Chlorthalidone: Long half-life (50–60 h) due to binding to red blood cells				

(continued)

Subclass	Mechanism of Action	Effects	Clinical Applications	Pharmacokinetics, Toxicities, Interactions
POTASSIUM-SPARING DIURETICS				
• Spironolactone	Pharmacologic antagonist of aldosterone in collecting tubules • weak antagonism of androgen receptors	Reduces Na retention and K wasting in kidney • poorly understood antagonism of aldosterone in heart and vessels	Aldosteronism from any cause • hypokalemia due to other diuretics • postmyocardial infarction	Slow onset and offset of effect • duration 24–48 h • *Toxicity:* Hyperkalemia, gynecomastia (spironolactone, not eplerenone) • additive interaction with other K-retaining drugs
• Amiloride	Blocks epithelial sodium channels in collecting tubules	Reduces Na retention and K wasting • increases lithium clearance	Hypokalemia from other diuretics • reduces lithium-induced polyuria	Orally active • duration 24 h • *Toxicity:* Hyperkalemic metabolic acidosis
• *Eplerenone: Like spironolactone, more selective for aldosterone receptor*				
• *Triamterene: Mechanism like amiloride, much less potent, more toxic*				
OSMOTIC DIURETICS				
• Mannitol	Physical osmotic effect on tissue water distribution because it is retained in the vascular compartment	Marked increase in urine flow, reduced brain volume, decreased intraocular pressure, initial hyponatremia, then hypernatremia	Renal failure due to increased solute load (rhabdomyolysis, chemotherapy), increased intracranial pressure, glaucoma	IV administration • *Toxicity:* Nausea, vomiting, headache
VASOPRESSIN (ADH) ANTAGONISTS				
• Conivaptan	Antagonist at V_{1a} and V_2 ADH receptors	Reduces water reabsorption, increases plasma Na concentration, vasodilation	Hyponatremia, congestive heart failure	IV only, usually continuous • *Toxicity:* Infusion site reactions, thirst, polyuria, hypernatremia
• Tolvaptan	Selective antagonist at V_2 ADH receptors	Reduces water reabsorption, increases plasma Na concentration	Hyponatremia, SIADH	Oral • duration 12–24 h • *Toxicity:* Polyuria (frequency), thirst, hypernatremia

PREPARATIONS AVAILABLE

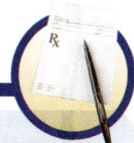

Acetazolamide (generic, Diamox)
Oral: 125, 250 mg tablets
Oral sustained-release: 500 mg capsules
Parenteral: 500 mg powder for injection

Amiloride (generic, Midamor, combination drugs[1])
Oral: 5 mg tablets

Bendroflumethiazide (Naturetin, combination drugs[1])
Oral: 5, 10 mg tablets

Brinzolamide (Azopt) (For ocular conditions)
Ophthalmic: 1% suspension

Bumetanide (generic, Bumex)
Oral: 0.5, 1, 2 mg tablets
Parenteral: 0.5 mg/2 mL ampule for IV or IM injection

Chlorothiazide (generic, Diuril)
Oral: 250, 500 mg tablets; 250 mg/5 mL oral suspension
Parenteral: 500 mg for injection

Chlorthalidone (generic, Hygroton, Thalitone, combination drugs[1])
Oral: 25, 50, 100 mg tablets

Conivaptan (Vaprisol)
Parenteral: 5 mg/mL; 20 mg/100 mL D5W for IV injection

Demeclocycline (Declomycin)
Oral: 150 mg tablets and capsules; 300 mg tablets

Dichlorphenamide (Daranide)
Oral: 50 mg tablets

Dorzolamide (Trusopt) (For ocular conditions)
Ophthalmic: 2% solution

Eplerenone (Inspra)
Oral: 25, 50 mg tablets

Ethacrynic acid (Edecrin)
Oral: 25, 50 mg tablets
Parenteral: 50 mg IV injection

Furosemide (generic, Lasix, others)
Oral: 20, 40, 80 mg tablets; 8, 10 mg/mL oral solutions
Parenteral: 10 mg/mL for IM or IV injection

Hydrochlorothiazide (generic, Esidrix, Hydro-DIURIL, combination drugs[1])
Oral: 12.5 mg capsules; 25, 50, 100 mg tablets; 10, 100 mg/mL solution

Hydroflumethiazide (generic, Saluron)
Oral: 50 mg tablets

Indapamide (generic, Lozol)
Oral: 1.25, 2.5 mg tablets

Mannitol (generic, Osmitrol)
Parenteral: 5, 10, 15, 20% solution, for injection

Methazolamide (generic, Neptazane) (For ocular conditions)
Oral: 25, 50 mg tablets

Methyclothiazide (generic, Aquatensen, Enduron)
Oral: 2.5, 5 mg tablets

Metolazone (Mykrox, Zaroxolyn) (Note: Bioavailability of Mykrox is greater than that of Zaroxolyn.)
Oral: 0.5 (Mykrox); 2.5, 5, 10 mg (Zaroxolyn) tablets

Nesiritide (Natrecor)
Parenteral: 1.5 mg vial for dilution into 250 mL IV solution (6 mcg/mL)

Polythiazide (Renese, combination drugs[1])
Oral: 1, 2, 4 mg tablets

Quinethazone (Hydromox)
Oral: 50 mg tablets

Spironolactone (generic, Aldactone , combination drugs[1])
Oral: 25, 50, 100 mg tablets

Tolvaptan (Samsca)
Oral: 15, 30 mg tablets

Torsemide (Demadex)
Oral: 5, 10, 20, 100 mg tablets
Parenteral: 10 mg/mL for injection

Triamterene (Dyrenium)
Oral: 50, 100 mg capsules

Trichlormethiazide (generic, Diurese, Naqua, others)
Oral: 2, 4 mg tablets

[1]Combination drugs: see Table 15-6

REFERENCES

ALLHAT Officers and Coordinators for the ALLHAT Collaborative Research Group: Major outcomes in high-risk hypertensive patients randomized to angiotensin-converting enzyme inhibitor or calcium channel blocker vs diuretic: The Antihypertensive and Lipid-Lowering Treatment to Prevent Heart Attack Trial (ALLHAT). JAMA 2002;288:2981.

Berl T et al: Oral Tolvaptan is safe and effective in chronic hyponatremia. J Am Soc Nephrol 2010;21:705.

BMJ group: Eplerenone after myocardial infarction? Drug Ther Bull 2008;46(1):1.

Brenner BM (editor): *Brenner & Rector's The Kidney*, 8th ed. Saunders, 2008.

Chow T et al: *Ginkgo biloba* and acetazolamide prophylaxis for acute mountain sickness. Arch Intern Med 2005;165:296.

Cooper BE: Diuresis in renal failure: Treat the patient, not the urine output. Crit Care Med 2009;37:761.

Costello-Boerrigter LC, Boerrigter G, Burnett JC Jr: Revisiting salt and water retention: New diuretics, aquaretics, and natriuretics. Med Clin North Am 2003;87:475.

Ely JW et al: Approach to leg edema of unclear etiology. J Am Board Family Med 2006;19:148.

Ernst ME, Moser M: Use of diuretics in patients with hypertension. N Engl J Med 2009;361:2153.

Forssmann W-G, Meyer M, Forssmann K: The renal urodilatin system: Clinical implications. Cardiovasc Res 2001;51(3):450.

Ginès P, Schrier RW: Renal failure in cirrhosis. N Engl J Med 2009;361:1279.

Gross P: Treatment of hyponatremia. Intern Med 2008;47:885.

Hall PM: Nephrolithiasis: Treatment, causes, and prevention. Cleveland Clinic J Med 2009;76:583.

Hao C-M, Breyer MD: Physiological regulation of prostaglandins in the kidney. Annu Rev Physiol 2008;70:357.

Hays RM: Vasopressin antagonists: Progress and promise. N Engl J Med 2006;355:146.

Hill JA, Yancy CW, Abraham WT: Beyond diuretics: Management of volume overload in acute heart failure syndromes. Am J Med 2006; 119:S37.

Hocher B: Adenosine A1 receptor antagonists in clinical research and development. Kidney Int 2010;78(5):438.

Kaplan NM: The place of diuretics in preventing cardiovascular events. J Hum Hypertens 2004;18:S29.

Kim G-H et al: Antidiuretic effect of hydrochlorothiazide in lithium-induced nephrogenic diabetes insipidus is associated with upregulation of aquaporin-2, Na-Cl co-transporter, and epithelial sodium channel. J Am Soc Nephrol 2004;15:2836.

Lee C, Burnett J: Natriuretic peptides and therapeutic applications. Heart Failure Rev 2007;12:131.

Lüss H et al: Renal effects of ularitide in patients with decompensated heart failure. Am Heart J 2008;155:1012.

Mitrovic V et al: Cardio-renal effects of the A1 adenosine receptor antagonist SLV320 in patients with heart failure. Circ Heart Fail 2009;2:523.

Na KY et al: Upregulation of Na$^+$ transporter abundance in response to chronic thiazide or loop diuretic treatment in rats. Am J Physiol 2003;284:F133.

Nijenhuis T et al: Enhanced passive Ca^{2+} reabsorption and reduced Mg^{2+} channel abundance explains thiazide-induced hypocalciuria and hypomagnesemia. J Clin Invest 2005;115:1651.

Rejnmark L et al: Effects of long-term treatment with loop diuretics on bone mineral density, calciotropic hormones and bone turnover. J Intern Med 2005;257:176.

Shlipak MG, Massie BM: The clinical challenge of cardiorenal syndrome. Circulation 2004;110:1514.

Sica DA, Gehr TWB: Diuretic use in stage 5 chronic kidney disease and end-stage renal disease. Curr Opin Nephrol Hypertens 2003;12:483.

Smyth EM et al: Prostanoids in health and disease. J Lipid Res 2009;50:S423.

Tavares M et al: New pharmacologic therapies in acute heart failure. Crit Care Med 2008;36:S112.

Tovar-Palacio C et al: Ion and diuretic specificity of chimeric proteins between apical Na$^+$-K$^+$-2Cl$^-$and Na$^+$-Cl$^-$ cotransporters. Am J Physiol 2004;287:F570.

Vallon V et al: Adenosine and kidney function. Physiol Rev 2006;86:901.

Vallon V et al: Adenosine and kidney function: Potential implications in patients with heart failure. Eur J Heart Failure 2008;10:176.

Vigen R, Weideman RA, Reilly RF: Thiazides diuretics in the treatment of neph-rolithiasis; are we using them in an evidence-based fashion? Int Urol Nephrol 2010;Epub Aug 25.

Wakai, R, Roberts IG, Schierhout G: Mannitol for acute traumatic brain injury. Cochrane Library (online publication) Issue 4, 2008.

Wilcox C: New insights into diuretic use in patients with chronic renal disease. J Am Soc Nephrol 2002;13:798.

CASE STUDY ANSWER

The diuretic most commonly used for congestive heart failure is a loop diuretic like furosemide, which is administered IV, in a dosage of 40 mg, followed if necessary by oral administration, 20–80 mg/24 h. For this patient, furosemide would probably be needed chronically, since it blunts the symptoms of congestive heart failure but does not reverse the ventricular damage that caused the symptoms. A common problem when beginning effective diuretic treatment is a reduction of glomerular filtration rate. Other adverse effects of loop diuretics include hypokalemia, metabolic alkalosis, ototoxicity, hyperuricemia, hypomagnesemia, and allergic reactions.

SECTION IV DRUGS WITH IMPORTANT ACTIONS ON SMOOTH MUSCLE

CHAPTER

16

Histamine, Serotonin, & the Ergot Alkaloids

Bertram G. Katzung, MD, PhD

CASE STUDY

A 35-year-old man visits his family practitioner with a complaint of red, raised, itchy wheals on his arms and legs. Two days earlier, he had eaten a spicy meal at a restaurant he had not previously visited. The following morning, he woke up with the palms of his hands and the soles of his feet red and itchy. During the day, similar raised, itchy lesions appeared on his arms and legs, and some are now appearing on his trunk. He reports a similar, milder episode 2 years ago, from which he recovered without treatment. Physical examination reveals no respiratory symptoms and no evidence of pharyngeal edema. The practitioner makes a diagnosis of urticaria (hives) caused by food allergy and suggests that the patient take an over-the-counter antihistamine. The following day the patient calls saying that the antihistamine has reduced the itching slightly, but the wheals are still present and new ones are appearing. What other therapeutic measures are appropriate?

It has long been known that many tissues contain substances that, when released by various stimuli, cause physiologic effects such as reddening of the skin, pain or itching, and bronchospasm. Later, it was discovered that many of these substances are also present in nervous tissue and have multiple functions. Histamine and serotonin (5-hydroxytryptamine, 5-HT) are biologically active amines that function as neurotransmitters and are found in non-neural tissues, have complex physiologic and pathologic effects through multiple receptor subtypes, and are often released locally. Together with endogenous peptides (see Chapter 17), prostaglandins and leukotrienes (see Chapter 18), and cytokines (see Chapter 55), they constitute the **autacoid group** of drugs.

Because of their broad and largely undesirable peripheral effects, neither histamine nor serotonin has any clinical application in the treatment of disease. However, compounds that *selectively* activate certain receptor subtypes or selectively antagonize the actions of these amines are of considerable clinical usefulness. This chapter therefore emphasizes the basic pharmacology of the agonist amines and the clinical pharmacology of the more selective agonist and antagonist drugs. The ergot alkaloids, compounds with partial agonist activity at serotonin and several other receptors, are discussed at the end of the chapter.

■ HISTAMINE

Histamine was synthesized in 1907 and later isolated from mammalian tissues. Early hypotheses concerning the possible physiologic roles of tissue histamine were based on similarities between the effects of intravenously administered histamine and the symptoms of anaphylactic shock and tissue injury. Marked species variation is observed, but in humans histamine is an important mediator of immediate allergic (such as urticaria) and inflammatory reactions, although it plays only a modest role in anaphylaxis. Histamine plays an important role in gastric acid secretion (see Chapter 62) and functions as a neurotransmitter and neuromodulator (see Chapters 6 and 21). Newer evidence indicates that histamine also plays a role in immune functions and chemotaxis of white blood cells.

BASIC PHARMACOLOGY OF HISTAMINE

Chemistry & Pharmacokinetics

Histamine occurs in plants as well as in animal tissues and is a component of some venoms and stinging secretions.

Histamine is formed by decarboxylation of the amino acid L-histidine, a reaction catalyzed in mammalian tissues by the enzyme histidine decarboxylase. Once formed, histamine is either stored or rapidly inactivated. Very little histamine is excreted unchanged. The major metabolic pathways involve conversion to N-methylhistamine, methylimidazoleacetic acid, and imidazoleacetic acid (IAA). Certain neoplasms (systemic mastocytosis, urticaria pigmentosa, gastric carcinoid, and occasionally myelogenous leukemia) are associated with increased numbers of mast cells or basophils and with increased excretion of histamine and its metabolites.

$$\text{HN} \diagdown \text{N} \diagup \text{---} \text{CH}_2 \text{---} \text{CH}_2 \text{---} \text{NH}_2$$

Histamine

Most tissue histamine is sequestered and bound in granules (vesicles) in mast cells or basophils; the histamine content of many tissues is directly related to their mast cell content. The bound form of histamine is biologically inactive, but as noted below, many stimuli can trigger the release of mast cell histamine, allowing the free amine to exert its actions on surrounding tissues. Mast cells are especially rich at sites of potential tissue injury—nose, mouth, and feet; internal body surfaces; and blood vessels, particularly at pressure points and bifurcations.

Non-mast cell histamine is found in several tissues, including the brain, where it functions as a neurotransmitter. Strong evidence implicates endogenous neurotransmitter histamine in many brain functions such as neuroendocrine control, cardiovascular regulation, thermal and body weight regulation, and sleep and arousal (see Chapters 21 and 37).

A second important nonneuronal site of histamine storage and release is the enterochromaffin-like (ECL) cells of the fundus of the stomach. ECL cells release histamine, one of the primary gastric acid secretagogues, to activate the acid-producing parietal cells of the mucosa (see Chapter 62).

Storage & Release of Histamine

The stores of histamine in mast cells can be released through several mechanisms.

A. Immunologic Release

Immunologic processes account for the most important pathophysiologic mechanism of mast cell and basophil histamine release. These cells, if sensitized by IgE antibodies attached to their surface membranes, degranulate explosively when exposed to the appropriate antigen (see Figure 55–5, effector phase). This type of release also requires energy and calcium. Degranulation leads to the simultaneous release of histamine, adenosine triphosphate (ATP), and other mediators that are stored together in the granules. Histamine released by this mechanism is a mediator in immediate (type I) allergic reactions, such as hay fever and acute urticaria. Substances released during IgG- or IgM-mediated immune reactions that activate the complement cascade also release histamine from mast cells and basophils.

By a negative feedback control mechanism mediated by H_2 receptors, histamine appears to modulate its own release and that of other mediators from sensitized mast cells in some tissues. In humans, mast cells in skin and basophils show this negative feedback mechanism; lung mast cells do not. Thus, histamine may act to limit the intensity of the allergic reaction in the skin and blood.

Endogenous histamine has a modulating role in a variety of inflammatory and immune responses. Upon injury to a tissue, released histamine causes local vasodilation and leakage of plasma-containing mediators of acute inflammation (complement, C-reactive protein) and antibodies. Histamine has an active chemotactic attraction for inflammatory cells (neutrophils, eosinophils, basophils, monocytes, and lymphocytes). Histamine inhibits the release of lysosome contents and several T- and B-lymphocyte functions. Most of these actions are mediated by H_2 or H_4 receptors. Release of peptides from nerves in response to inflammation is also probably modulated by histamine, in this case acting through presynaptic H_3 receptors.

B. Chemical and Mechanical Release

Certain amines, including drugs such as morphine and tubocurarine, can displace histamine from its bound form within cells. This type of release does not require energy and is not associated with mast cell injury or degranulation. Loss of granules from the mast cell also releases histamine, since sodium ions in the extracellular fluid rapidly displace the amine from the complex. Chemical and mechanical mast cell injury causes degranulation and histamine

release. **Compound 48/80,** an experimental drug, selectively releases histamine from tissue mast cells by an exocytotic degranulation process requiring energy and calcium.

Pharmacodynamics

A. Mechanism of Action

Histamine exerts its biologic actions by combining with specific cellular receptors located on the surface membrane. Four different histamine receptors have been characterized and are designated H_1–H_4; they are described in Table 16–1. Unlike the other amine transmitter receptors discussed previously, no subfamilies have been found within these major types, although different splice variants of several receptor types have been described.

All four receptor types have been cloned and belong to the large superfamily of receptors having seven membrane-spanning regions and coupled with G proteins (GPCR). The structures of the H_1 and H_2 receptors differ significantly and appear to be more closely related to muscarinic and 5-HT_1 receptors, respectively, than to each other. The H_4 receptor has about 40% homology with the H_3 receptor but does not seem to be closely related to any other histamine receptor. All four histamine receptors have been shown to have constitutive activity in some systems; thus, some antihistamines previously considered to be traditional pharmacologic antagonists must now be considered to be inverse agonists (see Chapters 1 and 2). Indeed, many first- and second-generation H_1 blockers (see below) function as inverse agonists. Furthermore, a single molecule may be an agonist at one histamine receptor and an antagonist or inverse agonist at another. For example, clobenpropit, an agonist at H_4 receptors, is an antagonist or inverse agonist at H_3 receptors (Table 16–1).

In the brain, H_1 and H_2 receptors are located on postsynaptic membranes, whereas H_3 receptors are predominantly presynaptic. Activation of H_1 receptors, which are present in endothelium, smooth muscle cells, and nerve endings, usually elicits an increase in phosphoinositol hydrolysis and an increase in inositol trisphosphate (IP_3) and intracellular calcium. Activation of H_2 receptors, present in gastric mucosa, cardiac muscle cells, and some immune cells, increases intracellular cyclic adenosine monophosphate (cAMP) via G_s. Like the β_2 adrenoceptor, under certain circumstances the H_2 receptor may couple to G_q, activating the IP_3-DAG (inositol 1,4,5-trisphosphate-diacylglycerol) cascade. Activation of H_3 receptors decreases transmitter release from histaminergic and other neurons,

probably mediated by a decrease in calcium influx through N-type calcium channels in nerve endings. H_4 receptors are found mainly on leukocytes in the bone marrow and circulating blood. H_4 receptors appear to have very important chemotactic effects on eosinophils and mast cells. In this role, they seem to play a part in inflammation and allergy. They may also modulate production of these cell types and they may mediate, in part, the previously recognized effects of histamine on cytokine production.

B. Tissue and Organ System Effects of Histamine

Histamine exerts powerful effects on smooth and cardiac muscle, on certain endothelial and nerve cells, on the secretory cells of the stomach, and on inflammatory cells. However, sensitivity to histamine varies greatly among species. Guinea pigs are exquisitely sensitive; humans, dogs, and cats somewhat less so; and mice and rats very much less so.

1. Nervous system—Histamine is a powerful stimulant of sensory nerve endings, especially those mediating pain and itching. This H_1-mediated effect is an important component of the urticarial response and reactions to insect and nettle stings. Some evidence suggests that local high concentrations can also depolarize efferent (axonal) nerve endings (see Triple Response, item 8 in this list). In the mouse, and probably in humans, respiratory neurons signaling inspiration and expiration are modulated by H_1 receptors. H_1 and H_3 receptors play important roles in appetite and satiety; antipsychotic drugs that block these receptors cause significant weight gain (see Chapter 29). Presynaptic H_3 receptors play important roles in modulating release of several transmitters in the nervous system. H_3 agonists reduce the release of acetylcholine, amine, and peptide transmitters in various areas of the brain and in peripheral nerves.

2. Cardiovascular system—In humans, injection or infusion of histamine causes a decrease in systolic and diastolic blood pressure and an increase in heart rate. The blood pressure changes are caused by the direct vasodilator action of histamine on arterioles and precapillary sphincters; the increase in heart rate involves both stimulatory actions of histamine on the heart and a reflex tachycardia. Flushing, a sense of warmth, and headache may also occur during histamine administration, consistent with the vasodilation.

TABLE 16–1 Histamine receptor subtypes.

Receptor Subtype	Distribution	Postreceptor Mechanism	Partially Selective Agonists	Partially Selective Antagonists or Inverse Agonists
H_1	Smooth muscle, endothelium, brain	G_q, $\uparrow IP_3$, DAG	Histaprodifen	Mepyramine,[1] triprolidine, cetirizine
H_2	Gastric mucosa, cardiac muscle, mast cells, brain	G_s, $\uparrow$ cAMP	Amthamine	Cimetidine,[1] ranitidine,[1] tiotidine
H_3	Presynaptic autoreceptors and heteroreceptors: brain, myenteric plexus, other neurons	G_i, $\downarrow$ cAMP	R-α-Methylhistamine, imetit, immepip	Thioperamide,[1] iodophenpropit, clobenpropit,[1] tiprolisant[1]
H_4	Eosinophils, neutrophils, CD4 T cells	G_i, $\downarrow$ cAMP	Clobenpropit, imetit, clozapine	Thioperamide[1]

[1]Inverse agonist.

cAMP, cyclic adenosine monophosphate; DAG, diacylglycerol; IP_3, inositol trisphosphate.

Vasodilation elicited by small doses of histamine is caused by H_1-receptor activation and is mediated mainly by release of nitric oxide from the endothelium (see Chapter 19). The decrease in blood pressure is usually accompanied by a reflex tachycardia. Higher doses of histamine activate the H_2-mediated cAMP process of vasodilation and direct cardiac stimulation. In humans, the cardiovascular effects of small doses of histamine can usually be antagonized by H_1-receptor antagonists alone.

Histamine-induced edema results from the action of the amine on H_1 receptors in the vessels of the microcirculation, especially the postcapillary vessels. The effect is associated with the separation of the endothelial cells, which permits the transudation of fluid and molecules as large as small proteins into the perivascular tissue. This effect is responsible for urticaria (hives), which signals the release of histamine in the skin. Studies of endothelial cells suggest that actin and myosin within these cells cause contraction, resulting in separation of the endothelial cells and increased permeability.

Direct cardiac effects of histamine include both increased contractility and increased pacemaker rate. These effects are mediated chiefly by H_2 receptors. In human atrial muscle, histamine can also decrease contractility; this effect is mediated by H_1 receptors. The physiologic significance of these cardiac actions is not clear. Some of the cardiovascular signs and symptoms of anaphylaxis are due to released histamine, although several other mediators are involved and appear to be more important than histamine in humans.

3. Bronchiolar smooth muscle—In both humans and guinea pigs, histamine causes bronchoconstriction mediated by H_1 receptors. In the guinea pig, this effect is the cause of death from histamine toxicity, but in humans with normal airways, bronchoconstriction following small doses of histamine is not marked. However, patients with asthma are very sensitive to histamine. The bronchoconstriction induced in these patients probably represents a hyperactive neural response, since such patients also respond excessively to many other stimuli, and the response to histamine can be blocked by autonomic blocking drugs such as ganglion blocking agents as well as by H_1-receptor antagonists (see Chapter 20). Although methacholine provocation is more commonly used, tests using small doses of inhaled histamine have been used in the diagnosis of bronchial hyperreactivity in patients with suspected asthma or cystic fibrosis. Such individuals may be 100 to 1000 times more sensitive to histamine (and methacholine) than are normal subjects. Curiously, a few species (eg, rabbit) respond to histamine with broncho*dilation*, reflecting the dominance of the H_2 receptor in their airways.

4. Gastrointestinal tract smooth muscle—Histamine causes contraction of intestinal smooth muscle, and histamine-induced contraction of guinea pig ileum is a standard bioassay for this amine. The human gut is not as sensitive as that of the guinea pig, but large doses of histamine may cause diarrhea, partly as a result of this effect. This action of histamine is mediated by H_1 receptors.

5. Other smooth muscle organs—In humans, histamine generally has insignificant effects on the smooth muscle of the eye and genitourinary tract. However, pregnant women suffering anaphylactic reactions may abort as a result of histamine-induced contractions, and in some species the sensitivity of the uterus is sufficient to form the basis for a bioassay.

6. Secretory tissue—Histamine has long been recognized as a powerful stimulant of gastric acid secretion and, to a lesser extent, of gastric pepsin and intrinsic factor production. The effect is caused by activation of H_2 receptors on gastric parietal cells and is associated with increased adenylyl cyclase activity, cAMP concentration, and intracellular Ca^{2+} concentration. Other stimulants of gastric acid secretion such as acetylcholine and gastrin do not increase cAMP even though their maximal effects on acid output can be reduced—but not abolished—by H_2-receptor antagonists. These actions are discussed in more detail in Chapter 62. Histamine also stimulates secretion in the small and large intestine. In contrast, H_3-selective histamine agonists *inhibit* acid secretion stimulated by food or pentagastrin in several species.

Histamine has much smaller effects on the activity of other glandular tissue at ordinary concentrations. Very high concentrations can cause adrenal medullary discharge.

7. Metabolic effects—Recent studies of H_3-receptor knockout mice demonstrate that absence of this receptor results in animals with increased food intake, decreased energy expenditure, and obesity. They also show insulin resistance and increased blood levels of leptin and insulin. It is not yet known whether the H_3 receptor has a similar role in humans, but intensive research is underway to determine whether H_3 agonists are useful in the treatment of obesity.

8. The "triple response"—Intradermal injection of histamine causes a characteristic red spot, edema, and flare response that was first described many years ago. The effect involves three separate cell types: smooth muscle in the microcirculation, capillary or venular endothelium, and sensory nerve endings. At the site of injection, a reddening appears owing to dilation of small vessels, followed soon by an edematous wheal at the injection site and a red irregular flare surrounding the wheal. The flare is said to be caused by an axon reflex. A sensation of itching may accompany these effects.

Similar local effects may be produced by injecting histamine liberators (compound 48/80, morphine, etc) intradermally or by applying the appropriate antigens to the skin of a sensitized person. Although most of these local effects can be prevented by adequate doses of an H_1-receptor–blocking agent, H_2 and H_3 receptors may also be involved.

9. Other effects possibly mediated by histamine receptors—In addition to the local stimulation of peripheral pain nerve endings via H_3 and H_1 receptors, histamine may play a role in nociception in the central nervous system. **Burimamide,** an early candidate for H_2-blocking action, and newer analogs with no effect on H_1, H_2, or H_3 receptors, have been shown to have significant analgesic action in rodents when administered into the central nervous system. The analgesia is said to be comparable to that produced by opioids, but tolerance, respiratory depression,

and constipation have not been reported. Although the mechanism of this action is not known, these compounds may represent an important new class of analgesics.

Other Histamine Agonists

Small substitutions on the imidazole ring of histamine significantly modify the selectivity of the compounds for the histamine receptor subtypes. Some of these are listed in Table 16–1.

CLINICAL PHARMACOLOGY OF HISTAMINE

Clinical Uses

In pulmonary function laboratories, histamine aerosol has been used as a **provocative test** of bronchial hyperreactivity. Histamine has no other current clinical applications.

Toxicity & Contraindications

Adverse effects of histamine release, like those following administration of histamine, are dose related. Flushing, hypotension, tachycardia, headache, wheals, bronchoconstriction, and gastrointestinal upset are noted. These effects are also observed after the ingestion of spoiled fish (scombroid fish poisoning), and there is evidence that histamine produced by bacterial action in the flesh of the fish is the major causative agent.

Histamine should not be given to patients with asthma (except as part of a carefully monitored test of pulmonary function) or to patients with active ulcer disease or gastrointestinal bleeding.

HISTAMINE ANTAGONISTS

The effects of histamine released in the body can be reduced in several ways. **Physiologic antagonists,** especially epinephrine, have smooth muscle actions opposite to those of histamine, but they act at different receptors. This is important clinically because injection of epinephrine can be lifesaving in systemic **anaphylaxis** and in other conditions in which massive release of histamine—and other more important mediators—occurs.

Release inhibitors reduce the degranulation of mast cells that results from immunologic triggering by antigen-IgE interaction. **Cromolyn** and **nedocromil** appear to have this effect (see Chapter 20) and have been used in the treatment of asthma, although the molecular mechanism underlying their action is not fully understood. Beta$_2$-adrenoceptor agonists also appear capable of reducing histamine release.

Histamine **receptor antagonists** represent a third approach to the reduction of histamine-mediated responses. For over 60 years, compounds have been available that competitively antagonize many of the actions of histamine on smooth muscle. However, not until the H$_2$-receptor antagonist burimamide was described in 1972 was it possible to antagonize the gastric acid-stimulating activity of histamine. The development of selective H$_2$-receptor antagonists has led to more effective therapy for peptic disease (see Chapter 62).

Selective H$_3$ and H$_4$ antagonists are not yet available for clinical use. However, potent and partially selective experimental H$_3$-receptor antagonists, thioperamide and clobenpropit, have been developed.

■ HISTAMINE RECEPTOR ANTAGONISTS

H$_1$-RECEPTOR ANTAGONISTS

Compounds that competitively block histamine or act as inverse agonists at H$_1$ receptors have been used in the treatment of allergic conditions for many years, and in the discussion that follows are referred to as antagonists. Many H$_1$ antagonists are currently marketed in the USA. A large number are available without prescription, both alone and in combination formulations such as "cold pills" and "sleep aids" (see Chapter 63).

BASIC PHARMACOLOGY OF H$_1$-RECEPTOR ANTAGONISTS

Chemistry & Pharmacokinetics

The H$_1$ antagonists are conveniently divided into first-generation and second-generation agents. These groups are distinguished by the relatively strong sedative effects of most of the first-generation drugs. The first-generation agents are also more likely to block autonomic receptors. Second-generation H$_1$ blockers are less sedating, owing in part to their less complete distribution into the central nervous system. All the H$_1$ antagonists are stable amines with the general structure illustrated in Figure 16–1. Doses of some of these drugs are given in Table 16–2.

These agents are rapidly absorbed after oral administration, with peak blood concentrations occurring in 1–2 hours. They are widely distributed throughout the body, and the first-generation drugs enter the central nervous system readily. Some of them are extensively metabolized, primarily by microsomal systems in the liver. Several of the second-generation agents are metabolized by the CYP3A4 system and thus are subject to important interactions when other drugs (such as ketoconazole) inhibit this subtype of P450 enzymes. Most of the drugs have an effective duration of action of 4–6 hours following a single dose, but meclizine and several second-generation agents are longer-acting, with a duration of action of 12–24 hours. The newer agents are considerably less lipid-soluble than the first-generation drugs and are substrates of the P-glycoprotein transporter in the blood-brain barrier; as a result they enter the central nervous system with difficulty or not at all. Many H$_1$ antagonists have active metabolites. The active metabolites of hydroxyzine, terfenadine, and loratadine are available as drugs (cetirizine, fexofenadine, and desloratadine, respectively).

Pharmacodynamics

Both neutral H$_1$ antagonists and inverse H$_1$ agonists reduce or block the actions of histamine by reversible competitive binding

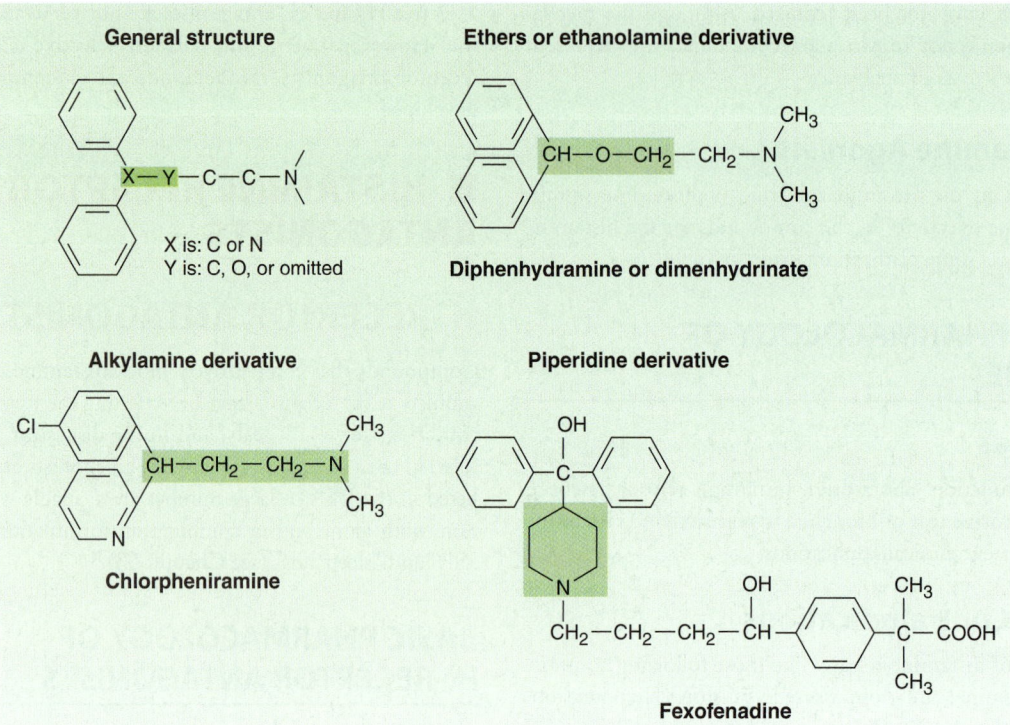

FIGURE 16–1 General structure of H_1-antagonist drugs and examples of the major subgroups. Chemical subgroups are indicated by shading.

to the H_1 receptor. Several have been clearly shown to be inverse agonists, and it is possible that all act by this mechanism. They have negligible potency at the H_2 receptor and little at the H_3 receptor. For example, histamine-induced contraction of bronchiolar or gastrointestinal smooth muscle can be completely blocked by these agents, but the effects on gastric acid secretion and the heart are unmodified.

The first-generation H_1-receptor antagonists have many actions in addition to blockade of the actions of histamine. The large number of these actions probably results from the similarity of the general structure (Figure 16–1) to the structure of drugs that have effects at muscarinic cholinoceptor, α adrenoceptor, serotonin, and local anesthetic receptor sites. Some of these actions are of therapeutic value and some are undesirable.

1. Sedation—A common effect of first-generation H_1 antagonists is sedation, but the intensity of this effect varies among chemical subgroups (Table 16–2) and among patients as well. The effect is sufficiently prominent with some agents to make them useful as "sleep aids" (see Chapter 63) and unsuitable for daytime use. The effect resembles that of some antimuscarinic drugs and is considered very different from the disinhibited sedation produced by sedative-hypnotic drugs. Compulsive use has not been reported. At ordinary dosages, children occasionally (and adults rarely) manifest excitation rather than sedation. At very high toxic dose levels, marked stimulation, agitation, and even convulsions may precede coma. Second-generation H_1 antagonists have little or no sedative or stimulant actions. These drugs (or their active metabolites) also have far fewer autonomic effects than the first-generation antihistamines.

2. Antinausea and antiemetic actions—Several first-generation H_1 antagonists have significant activity in preventing motion sickness (Table 16–2). They are less effective against an episode of motion sickness already present. Certain H_1 antagonists, notably doxylamine (in Bendectin), were used widely in the past in the treatment of nausea and vomiting of pregnancy (see below).

3. Antiparkinsonism effects—Some of the H_1 antagonists, especially **diphenhydramine,** have significant acute suppressant effects on the extrapyramidal symptoms associated with certain antipsychotic drugs. This drug is given parenterally for acute dystonic reactions to antipsychotics.

4. Anticholinoceptor actions—Many first-generation agents, especially those of the ethanolamine and ethylenediamine subgroups, have significant atropine-like effects on peripheral muscarinic receptors. This action may be responsible for some of the (uncertain) benefits reported for nonallergic rhinorrhea but may also cause urinary retention and blurred vision.

5. Adrenoceptor-blocking actions—Alpha-receptor blocking effects can be demonstrated for many H_1 antagonists, especially those in the phenothiazine subgroup, eg, **promethazine.** This action may cause orthostatic hypotension in susceptible individuals. Beta-receptor blockade is not observed.

6. Serotonin-blocking action—Strong blocking effects at serotonin receptors have been demonstrated for some first-generation

TABLE 16–2 Some H$_1$ antihistaminic drugs in clinical use.

Drugs	Usual Adult Dose	Anticholinergic Activity	Comments
FIRST-GENERATION ANTIHISTAMINES			
Ethanolamines			
Carbinoxamine (Clistin)	4–8 mg	+++	Slight to moderate sedation
Dimenhydrinate (salt of diphenhydramine) (Dramamine)	50 mg	+++	Marked sedation; anti-motion sickness activity
Diphenhydramine (Benadryl, etc)	25–50 mg	+++	Marked sedation; anti-motion sickness activity
Piperazine derivatives			
Hydroxyzine (Atarax, etc)	15–100 mg	nd	Marked sedation
Cyclizine (Marezine)	25–50 mg	–	Slight sedation; anti-motion sickness activity
Meclizine (Bonine, etc)	25–50 mg	–	Slight sedation; anti-motion sickness activity
Alkylamines			
Brompheniramine (Dimetane, etc)	4–8 mg	+	Slight sedation
Chlorpheniramine (Chlor-Trimeton, etc)	4–8 mg	+	Slight sedation; common component of OTC "cold" medication
Phenothiazine derivative			
Promethazine (Phenergan, etc)	10–25 mg	+++	Marked sedation; antiemetic; α block
Miscellaneous			
Cyproheptadine (Periactin, etc)	4 mg	+	Moderate sedation; significant antiserotonin activity
SECOND-GENERATION ANTIHISTAMINES			
Piperidine			
Fexofenadine (Allegra)	60 mg	–	
Miscellaneous			
Loratadine (Claritin), desloratadine (Clarinex)	10 mg (desloratadine, 5 mg)	–	Longer action; used at 5 mg dosage
Cetirizine (Zyrtec)	5–10 mg	–	

nd, no data found.

H$_1$ antagonists, notably **cyproheptadine**. This drug is promoted as an antiserotonin agent and is discussed with that drug group. Nevertheless, its structure resembles that of the phenothiazine antihistamines, and it is a potent H$_1$-blocking agent.

7. *Local anesthesia*—Several first-generation H$_1$ antagonists are potent local anesthetics. They block sodium channels in excitable membranes in the same fashion as procaine and lidocaine. Diphenhydramine and promethazine are actually more potent than procaine as local anesthetics. They are occasionally used to produce local anesthesia in patients allergic to conventional local anesthetic drugs. A small number of these agents also block potassium channels; this action is discussed below (see Toxicity).

8. *Other actions*—Certain H$_1$ antagonists, eg, cetirizine, inhibit mast cell release of histamine and some other mediators of inflammation. This action is not due to H$_1$-receptor blockade and may reflect an H$_4$-receptor effect (see below). The mechanism is not fully understood but could play a role in the beneficial effects of these drugs in the treatment of allergies such as rhinitis. A few

H$_1$ antagonists (eg, terfenadine, acrivastine) have been shown to inhibit the P-glycoprotein transporter found in cancer cells, the epithelium of the gut, and the capillaries of the brain. The significance of this effect is not known.

CLINICAL PHARMACOLOGY OF H$_1$-RECEPTOR ANTAGONISTS

Clinical Uses

First-generation H$_1$-receptor blockers are among the most extensively promoted and used over-the-counter drugs. The prevalence of allergic conditions and the *relative* safety of the drugs contribute to this heavy use. The fact that they do cause sedation contributes to heavy prescribing and over-the-counter use of second-generation antihistamines.

A. Allergic Reactions

The H$_1$ antihistaminic agents are often the first drugs used to prevent or treat the symptoms of allergic reactions. In allergic rhinitis (hay fever), the H$_1$ antagonists are second-line drugs after glucocorticoids administered by nasal spray. In urticaria, in which histamine is the primary mediator, the H_1 antagonists are the drugs of choice and are often quite effective if given before exposure. However, in bronchial asthma, which involves several mediators, the H_1 antagonists are largely ineffective.

Angioedema may be precipitated by histamine release but appears to be maintained by peptide kinins that are not affected by antihistaminic agents. For atopic dermatitis, antihistaminic drugs such as diphenhydramine are used mostly for their sedative side effect, which reduces awareness of itching.

The H_1 antihistamines used for treating allergic conditions such as hay fever are usually selected with the goal of minimizing sedative effects; in the USA, the drugs in widest use are the alkylamines and the second-generation nonsedating agents. However, the sedative effect and the therapeutic efficacy of different agents vary widely among individuals. In addition, the clinical effectiveness of one group may diminish with continued use, and switching to another group may restore drug effectiveness for as yet unexplained reasons.

The second-generation H_1 antagonists are used mainly for the treatment of allergic rhinitis and chronic urticaria. Several double-blind comparisons with older agents (eg, chlorpheniramine) indicated about equal therapeutic efficacy. However, sedation and interference with safe operation of machinery, which occur in about 50% of subjects taking first-generation antihistamines, occurred in only about 7% of subjects taking second-generation agents. The newer drugs are much more expensive, even in over-the-counter generic formulations.

B. Motion Sickness and Vestibular Disturbances

Scopolamine (see Chapter 8) and certain first-generation H_1 antagonists are the most effective agents available for the prevention of motion sickness. The antihistaminic drugs with the greatest effectiveness in this application are diphenhydramine and promethazine. Dimenhydrinate, which is promoted almost exclusively for the treatment of motion sickness, is a salt of diphenhydramine and has similar efficacy. The piperazines (cyclizine and meclizine) also have significant activity in preventing motion sickness and are less sedating than diphenhydramine in most patients. Dosage is the same as that recommended for allergic disorders (Table 16–2). Both scopolamine and the H_1 antagonists are more effective in preventing motion sickness when combined with ephedrine or amphetamine.

It has been claimed that the antihistaminic agents effective in prophylaxis of motion sickness are also useful in Ménière's syndrome, but efficacy in the latter application is not established.

C. Nausea and Vomiting of Pregnancy

Several H_1-antagonist drugs have been studied for possible use in treating "morning sickness." The piperazine derivatives were withdrawn from such use when it was demonstrated that they have teratogenic effects in rodents. Doxylamine, an ethanolamine H_1 antagonist, was promoted for this application as a component of Bendectin, a prescription medication that also contained pyridoxine. Possible teratogenic effects of doxylamine were widely publicized

in the lay press after 1978 as a result of a few case reports of fetal malformation that occurred after maternal ingestion of Bendectin. However, several large prospective studies involving over 60,000 pregnancies, of which more than 3000 involved maternal Bendectin ingestion, disclosed no increase in the incidence of birth defects. Nonetheless, because of the continuing controversy, adverse publicity, and lawsuits, the manufacturer of Bendectin withdrew the product from the market.

Toxicity

The wide spectrum of nonantihistaminic effects of the H_1 antihistamines is described above. Several of these effects (sedation, antimuscarinic action) have been used for therapeutic purposes, especially in over-the-counter remedies (see Chapter 63). Nevertheless, these two effects constitute the most common undesirable actions when these drugs are used to block histamine receptors.

Less common toxic effects of systemic use include excitation and convulsions in children, postural hypotension, and allergic responses. Drug allergy is relatively common after topical use of H_1 antagonists. The effects of severe systemic overdosage of the older agents resemble those of atropine overdosage and are treated in the same way (see Chapters 8 and 58). Overdosage of astemizole or terfenadine may induce cardiac arrhythmias; the same effect may be caused at normal dosage by interaction with enzyme inhibitors (see Drug Interactions). These drugs are no longer marketed in the USA.

Drug Interactions

Lethal ventricular arrhythmias occurred in several patients taking either of the early second-generation agents, terfenadine or astemizole, in combination with ketoconazole, itraconazole, or macrolide antibiotics such as erythromycin. These antimicrobial drugs inhibit the metabolism of many drugs by CYP3A4 and cause significant increases in blood concentrations of the antihistamines. The mechanism of this toxicity involves blockade of the HERG (I_{Kr}) potassium channels in the heart that contribute to repolarization of the action potential (see Chapter 14). The result is prolongation and a change in shape of the action potential, and these changes lead to arrhythmias. Both terfenadine and astemizole were withdrawn from the US market in recognition of these problems. Where still available, terfenadine and astemizole should be considered to be contraindicated in patients taking ketoconazole, itraconazole, or macrolides and in patients with liver disease. Grapefruit juice also inhibits CYP3A4 and has been shown to increase blood levels of terfenadine significantly.

For those H_1 antagonists that cause significant sedation, concurrent use of other drugs that cause central nervous system depression produces additive effects and is contraindicated while driving or operating machinery. Similarly, the autonomic blocking effects of older antihistamines are additive with those of antimuscarinic and α-blocking drugs.

H₂-RECEPTOR ANTAGONISTS

The development of H_2-receptor antagonists was based on the observation that H_1 antagonists had no effect on histamine-induced acid secretion in the stomach. Molecular manipulation of the histamine molecule resulted in drugs that blocked acid secretion and had no H_1 agonist or antagonist effects. Like the other histamine receptors, the H_2 receptor displays constitutive activity, and some H_2 blockers are inverse agonists.

The high prevalence of peptic ulcer disease created great interest in the therapeutic potential of the H_2-receptor antagonists when first discovered. Although these agents are not the most efficacious available, their ability to reduce gastric acid secretion with very low toxicity has made them extremely popular as over-the-counter preparations. These drugs are discussed in more detail in Chapter 62.

H_3- & H_4-RECEPTOR ANTAGONISTS

Although no selective H_3 or H_4 ligands are presently available for general clinical use, there is great interest in their therapeutic potential. H_3-selective ligands may be of value in sleep disorders, narcolepsy, obesity, and cognitive and psychiatric disorders. Tiprolisant, an inverse H_3-receptor agonist, has been shown to reduce sleep cycles in mutant mice and in humans with narcolepsy. Increased obesity has been demonstrated in both H_1- and H_3-receptor knockout mice. As noted in Chapter 29, several newer antipsychotic drugs have significant affinity for H_3 receptors.

Because of the homology between the H_3 and H_4 receptors, many H_3 ligands also have affinity for the H_4 receptor. H_4 blockers have potential in chronic inflammatory conditions such as asthma, in which eosinophils and mast cells play a prominent role. No selective H_4 ligand is available for use in humans, but in addition to research agents listed in Table 16–1, many H_1-selective blockers (eg, diphenhydramine, cetirizine, loratadine) show some affinity for this receptor. Several studies have suggested that H_4-receptor antagonists may be useful in pruritus, asthma, allergic rhinitis, and pain conditions.

■ SEROTONIN (5-HYDROXYTRYPTAMINE)

Before the identification of 5-hydroxytryptamine (5-HT), it was known that when blood is allowed to clot, a vasoconstrictor (tonic) substance is released from the clot into the serum. This substance was called serotonin. Independent studies established the existence of a smooth muscle stimulant in intestinal mucosa. This was called enteramine. The synthesis of 5-hydroxytryptamine in 1951 led to the identification of serotonin and enteramine as the same metabolite of 5-hydroxytryptophan.

Serotonin is an important neurotransmitter, a local hormone in the gut, a component of the platelet clotting process, and is thought to play a role in migraine headache and several other clinical conditions, including carcinoid syndrome. This syndrome is an unusual manifestation of carcinoid tumor, a neoplasm of enterochromaffin cells. In patients whose tumor is not surgically resectable, a serotonin antagonist may constitute a useful treatment.

BASIC PHARMACOLOGY OF SEROTONIN

Chemistry & Pharmacokinetics

Like histamine, serotonin is widely distributed in nature, being found in plant and animal tissues, venoms, and stings. It is synthesized in biologic systems from the amino acid L-tryptophan by hydroxylation of the indole ring followed by decarboxylation of the amino acid (Figure 16–2). Hydroxylation at C5 by tryptophan hydroxylase-1 is the rate-limiting step and can be blocked by *p*-chlorophenylalanine (PCPA; fenclonine) and by *p*-chloroamphetamine. These agents have been used experimentally to reduce serotonin synthesis in carcinoid syndrome but are too toxic for general clinical use.

After synthesis, the free amine is stored or is rapidly inactivated, usually by oxidation by monoamine oxidase (MAO). In the pineal gland, serotonin serves as a precursor of melatonin, a melanocyte-stimulating hormone. In mammals (including humans), over 90% of the serotonin in the body is found in enterochromaffin cells in the gastrointestinal tract. In the blood, serotonin is found in platelets, which are able to concentrate the amine by means of an active serotonin transporter mechanism (SERT) similar to that in the membrane of serotonergic nerve endings. Once transported into the platelet or nerve ending, 5-HT is concentrated in vesicles by a vesicle-associated transporter (VAT) that is blocked by reserpine. Serotonin is also found in the raphe nuclei of the brainstem, which contain cell bodies of serotonergic

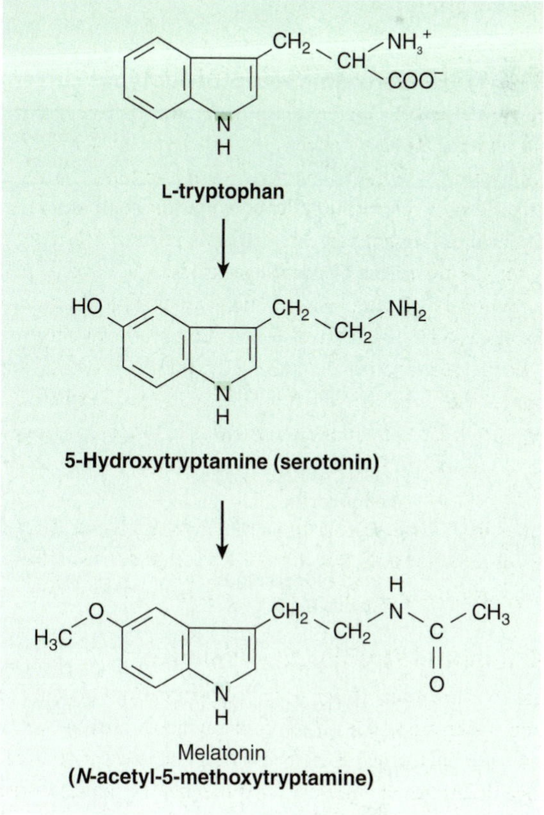

FIGURE 16–2 Synthesis of serotonin and melatonin from L-tryptophan.

neurons that synthesize, store, and release serotonin as a transmitter. Stored serotonin can be depleted by reserpine in much the same manner as this drug depletes catecholamines from vesicles in adrenergic nerves and the adrenal medulla (see Chapter 6).

Brain serotonergic neurons are involved in numerous diffuse functions such as mood, sleep, appetite, and temperature regulation, as well as the perception of pain, the regulation of blood pressure, and vomiting (see Chapter 21). Serotonin also appears to be involved in clinical conditions such as depression, anxiety, and migraine. Serotonergic neurons are also found in the enteric nervous system of the gastrointestinal tract and around blood vessels. In rodents (but not in humans), serotonin is found in mast cells.

The function of serotonin in enterochromaffin cells is not fully understood. These cells synthesize serotonin, store the amine in a complex with adenosine triphosphate (ATP) and other substances in granules, and release serotonin in response to mechanical and neuronal stimuli. This serotonin interacts in a paracrine fashion with several different 5-HT receptors in the gut. Some of the released serotonin diffuses into blood vessels and is taken up and stored in platelets.

Serotonin is metabolized by MAO, and the intermediate product, 5-hydroxyindoleacetaldehyde, is further oxidized by aldehyde dehydrogenase to 5-hydroxyindoleacetic acid (5-HIAA). In humans consuming a normal diet, the excretion of 5-HIAA is a measure of serotonin synthesis. Therefore, the 24-hour excretion of 5-HIAA can be used as a diagnostic test for tumors that synthesize excessive quantities of serotonin, especially carcinoid tumor. A few foods (eg, bananas) contain large amounts of serotonin or its precursors and must be prohibited during such diagnostic tests.

Pharmacodynamics

A. Mechanisms of Action

Serotonin exerts many actions and, like histamine, displays many species differences, making generalizations difficult. The actions of serotonin are mediated through a remarkably large number of cell membrane receptors. The serotonin receptors that have been characterized thus far are listed in Table 16–3. Seven families of 5-HT-receptor subtypes (those given numeric subscripts 1 through 7) have been identified, six involving G protein-coupled receptors of the usual 7-transmembrane serpentine type and one a ligand-gated ion channel. The latter (5-HT_3) receptor is a member of the nicotinic/$GABA_A$ family of Na^+/K^+ channel proteins.

B. Tissue and Organ System Effects

1. Nervous system—Serotonin is present in a variety of sites in the brain. Its role as a neurotransmitter and its relation to the actions of drugs acting in the central nervous system are discussed in Chapters 21 and 30. Serotonin is also a precursor of melatonin in the pineal gland (Figure 16–2; see Box: Melatonin Pharmacology). **Repinotan**, a 5-HT_{1A} agonist currently in clinical trials, appears to have some antinociceptive action at higher doses while reversing opioid-induced respiratory depression.

TABLE 16–3 Serotonin receptor subtypes currently recognized. (See also Chapter 21.)

Receptor Subtype	Distribution	Postreceptor Mechanism	Partially Selective Agonists	Partially Selective Antagonists
5-HT_{1A}	Raphe nuclei, hippocampus	G_i, ↓ cAMP	8-OH-DPAT,[1] repinotan	WAY100635[1]
5-HT_{1B}	Substantia nigra, globus pallidus, basal ganglia	G_i, ↓ cAMP	Sumatriptan, L694247[1]	
5-HT_{1D}	Brain	G_i, ↓ cAMP	Sumatriptan, eletriptan	
5-HT_{1E}	Cortex, putamen	G_i, ↓ cAMP		
5-HT_{1F}	Cortex, hippocampus	G_i, ↓ cAMP	LY3344864[1]	
5-HT_{1P}	Enteric nervous system	G_o, slow EPSP	5-Hydroxyindalpine	Renzapride
5-HT_{2A}	Platelets, smooth muscle, cerebral cortex	G_q, ↑ IP_3	α-Methyl-5-HT, DOI[1]	Ketanserin
5-HT_{2B}	Stomach fundus	G_q, ↑ IP_3	α-Methyl-5-HT, DOI[1]	RS127445[1]
5-HT_{2C}	Choroid, hippocampus, substantia nigra	G_q, ↑ IP_3	α-Methyl-5-HT, DOI,[1] lorcaserin	Mesulergine
5-HT_3	Area postrema, sensory and enteric nerves	Receptor is a Na^+/K^+ ion channel	2-Methyl-5-HT, *m*-chlorophenylbiguanide	Granisetron, ondansetron, others
5-HT_4	CNS and myenteric neurons, smooth muscle	G_s, ↑ cAMP	BIMU8,[1] renzapride, metoclopramide	GR113808[1]
$5\text{-HT}_{5A,B}$	Brain	↓ cAMP		
$5\text{-HT}_{6,7}$	Brain	G_s, ↑ cAMP		Clozapine (5-HT_7)

[1]Research agents; for chemical names see Alexander SPH, Mathie A, Peters JA: Guide to receptors and channels (GRAC). Br J Pharmacol 2009;158 (Suppl 1):S12.

cAMP, cyclic adenosine monophosphate; EPSP, excitatory postsynaptic potential; IP_3, inositol trisphosphate.

Melatonin Pharmacology

Melatonin is N-acetyl-5-methoxytryptamine (Figure 16–2), a simple methoxylated and N-acetylated product of serotonin found in the pineal gland. It is produced and released primarily at night and has long been suspected of playing a role in diurnal cycles of animals and the sleep-wake behavior of humans. Melatonin receptors have been characterized in the central nervous system and several peripheral tissues. In the brain, MT_1 and MT_2 receptors are found in membranes of neurons in the suprachiasmatic nucleus of the hypothalamus, an area associated—from lesioning experiments—with circadian rhythm. MT_1 and MT_2 are seven-transmembrane G_i protein-coupled receptors. The result of receptor binding is inhibition of adenylyl cyclase. A third receptor, MT_3, is an enzyme; binding to this site has a poorly defined physiologic role, possibly related to intraocular pressure. Activation of the MT_1 receptor results in sleepiness, whereas the MT_2 receptor may be related to the light-dark synchronization of the biologic circadian clock. Melatonin has also been implicated in energy metabolism and obesity, and administration of the agent reduces body weight in certain animal models. However, its role in these processes is poorly understood and there is no evidence that melatonin itself is of any value in obesity in humans. Other studies suggest that melatonin has antiapoptotic effects in experimental models. Recent research implicates melatonin receptors in depressive disorders.

Melatonin is promoted commercially as a sleep aid by the food supplement industry (see Chapter 64). There is an extensive literature supporting its use in ameliorating jet lag. It is used in oral doses of 0.5–5 mg, usually administered at the destination bedtime. **Ramelteon** is a selective MT_1 and MT_2 agonist that is approved for the medical treatment of insomnia. This drug has no addiction liability (it is not a controlled substance), and it appears to be distinctly more efficacious than melatonin (but less efficacious than benzodiazepines) as a hypnotic. It is metabolized by P450 enzymes and should not be used in individuals taking CYP1A2 inhibitors. It has a half-life of 1–3 hours and an active metabolite with a half-life of up to 5 hours. The toxicity of ramelteon is as yet poorly defined, but prolactin levels were elevated in one clinical trial. **Agomelatine**, an MT_1 and MT_2 agonist and a 5-HT_{2C} antagonist, has recently been approved in Europe for use in major depressive disorder.

5-HT_3 receptors in the gastrointestinal tract and in the vomiting center of the medulla participate in the vomiting reflex (see Chapter 62). They are particularly important in vomiting caused by chemical triggers such as cancer chemotherapy drugs. 5-HT_{1P} and 5-HT_4 receptors also play important roles in enteric nervous system function.

Like histamine, serotonin is a potent stimulant of pain and itch sensory nerve endings and is responsible for some of the symptoms caused by insect and plant stings. In addition, serotonin is a powerful activator of chemosensitive endings located in the coronary vascular bed. Activation of 5-HT_3 receptors on these afferent vagal nerve endings is associated with the **chemoreceptor reflex** (also known as the Bezold-Jarisch reflex). The reflex response consists of marked bradycardia and hypotension, and its physiologic role is uncertain. The bradycardia is mediated by vagal outflow to the heart and can be blocked by atropine. The hypotension is a consequence of the decrease in cardiac output that results from bradycardia. A variety of other agents can activate the chemoreceptor reflex. These include nicotinic cholinoceptor agonists and some cardiac glycosides, eg, ouabain.

2. Respiratory system—Serotonin has a small direct stimulant effect on bronchiolar smooth muscle in normal humans, probably via 5-HT_{2A} receptors. It also appears to facilitate acetylcholine release from bronchial vagal nerve endings. In patients with carcinoid syndrome, episodes of bronchoconstriction occur in response to elevated levels of the amine or peptides released from the tumor. Serotonin may also cause hyperventilation as a result of the chemoreceptor reflex or stimulation of bronchial sensory nerve endings.

3. Cardiovascular system—Serotonin directly causes the contraction of vascular smooth muscle, mainly through 5-HT_2 receptors. In humans, serotonin is a powerful vasoconstrictor except in skeletal muscle and the heart, where it dilates blood vessels. At least part of this 5-HT-induced vasodilation requires the presence of vascular endothelial cells. When the endothelium is damaged, coronary vessels are constricted by 5-HT. As noted previously, serotonin can also elicit reflex bradycardia by activation of 5-HT_3 receptors on chemoreceptor nerve endings. A triphasic blood pressure response is often seen following injection of serotonin in experimental animals. Initially, there is a decrease in heart rate, cardiac output, and blood pressure caused by the chemoreceptor response. After this decrease, blood pressure increases as a result of vasoconstriction. The third phase is again a decrease in blood pressure attributed to vasodilation in vessels supplying skeletal muscle. Pulmonary and renal vessels seem especially sensitive to the vasoconstrictor action of serotonin.

Studies in knockout mice suggest that 5-HT, acting on 5-HT_{1A}, 5-HT_2, and 5-HT_4 receptors, is needed for normal cardiac development in the fetus. On the other hand, chronic exposure of adults to 5-HT_{2B} agonists is associated with valvulopathy and adult mice lacking the 5-HT_{2B} receptor gene are protected from cardiac hypertrophy. Preliminary studies suggest that 5-HT_{2B} antagonists can prevent development of pulmonary hypertension in animal models.

Serotonin also constricts veins, and venoconstriction with increased capillary filling appears to be responsible for the flush that is observed after serotonin administration or release from a carcinoid tumor. Serotonin has small direct positive chronotropic and inotropic effects on the heart, which are probably of no clinical

Serotonin Syndrome and Similar Syndromes

Excess synaptic serotonin causes a serious, potentially fatal syndrome that is diagnosed on the basis of a history of administration of a serotonergic drug within recent weeks and physical findings (Table 16–4). It has some characteristics in common with neuroleptic malignant syndrome (NMS) and malignant hyperthermia (MH), but its pathophysiology and management are quite different.

As suggested by the drugs that precipitate it, serotonin syndrome occurs when overdose with a single drug, or concurrent use of several drugs, results in excess serotonergic activity in the central nervous system. It is predictable and not idiosyncratic, but milder forms may easily be misdiagnosed. In experimental animal models, many of the signs of the syndrome can be reversed by administration of 5-HT$_2$ antagonists; however, other 5-HT receptors may be involved as well. Dantrolene is of no value, unlike the treatment of MH.

NMS is idiosyncratic rather than predictable and appears to be associated with hypersensitivity to the parkinsonism-inducing effects of D$_2$-blocking antipsychotics in certain individuals. MH is associated with a genetic defect in the RyR1 calcium channel of skeletal muscle sarcoplasmic reticulum that permits uncontrolled calcium release from the sarcoplasmic reticulum when precipitating drugs are given (see Chapter 27).

significance. However, prolonged elevation of the blood level of serotonin (which occurs in carcinoid syndrome) is associated with pathologic alterations in the endocardium (subendocardial fibroplasia), which may result in valvular or electrical malfunction.

Serotonin causes blood platelets to aggregate by activating 5-HT$_2$ receptors. This response, in contrast to aggregation induced during normal clot formation, is not accompanied by the release of serotonin stored in the platelets. The physiologic role of this effect is unclear.

4. Gastrointestinal tract—Serotonin is a powerful stimulant of gastrointestinal smooth muscle, increasing tone and facilitating peristalsis. This action is caused by the direct action of serotonin on 5-HT$_2$ smooth muscle receptors plus a stimulating action on ganglion cells located in the enteric nervous system (see Chapter 6). 5-HT$_{1A}$ and 5-HT$_7$ receptors may also be involved in this complex action. Activation of 5-HT$_4$ receptors in the enteric nervous system causes increased acetylcholine release and thereby mediates a motility-enhancing or "prokinetic" effect of selective serotonin agonists such as cisapride. These agents are useful in several gastrointestinal disorders (see Chapter 62). Overproduction of serotonin (and other substances) in carcinoid tumor is associated with severe diarrhea. Serotonin has little effect on gastrointestinal secretions, and what effects it has are generally inhibitory.

5. Skeletal muscle and the eye—5-HT$_2$ receptors are present on skeletal muscle membranes, but their physiologic role is not understood. **Serotonin syndrome** is a condition associated with skeletal muscle contractions and precipitated when MAO inhibitors are given with serotonin agonists, especially antidepressants of the selective serotonin reuptake inhibitor class (SSRIs; see Chapter 30). Although the hyperthermia of serotonin syndrome results from excessive muscle contraction, serotonin syndrome is probably caused by a central nervous system effect of these drugs (Table 16–4 and Box: Serotonin Syndrome and Similar Syndromes).

Studies in animal models of glaucoma indicate that 5-HT$_{2A}$ agonists reduce intraocular pressure. This action can be blocked by ketanserin and similar 5-HT$_2$ antagonists.

CLINICAL PHARMACOLOGY OF SEROTONIN

Serotonin Agonists

Serotonin has no clinical applications as a drug. However, several receptor subtype-selective agonists have proved to be of value. **Buspirone,** a 5-HT$_{1A}$ agonist, has received wide attention for its usefulness as an effective nonbenzodiazepine anxiolytic (see

TABLE 16–4 Characteristics of serotonin syndrome and other hyperthermic syndromes.

Syndrome	Precipitating Drugs	Clinical Presentation	Therapy[1]
Serotonin syndrome	SSRIs, second-generation antidepressants, MAOIs, linezolid, tramadol, meperidine, fentanyl, ondansetron, sumatriptan, MDMA, LSD, St. John's wort, ginseng	Hypertension, hyperreflexia, tremor, clonus, hyperthermia, hyperactive bowel sounds, diarrhea, mydriasis, agitation, coma; onset within hours	**Sedation (benzodiazepines), paralysis, intubation, and ventilation;** consider 5-HT$_2$ block with cyproheptadine or chlorpromazine
Neuroleptic malignant syndrome	D$_2$-blocking antipsychotics	Acute severe parkinsonism; hypertension, hyperthermia, normal or reduced bowel sounds, onset over 1–3 days	**Diphenhydramine** (parenteral), cooling if temperature is very high, sedation with benzodiazepines
Malignant hyperthermia	Volatile anesthetics, succinylcholine	Hyperthermia, muscle rigidity, hypertension, tachycardia; onset within minutes	**Dantrolene,** cooling

[1]Precipitating drugs should be discontinued immediately. First-line therapy is in **bold** font.

MAOIs, monoamine oxidase inhibitors; MDMA, methylenedioxy-methamphetamine (ecstasy); SSRIs, selective serotonin reuptake inhibitors.

Chapter 22). **Dexfenfluramine,** another selective 5-HT agonist, was widely used as an appetite suppressant but was withdrawn because of cardiac valve toxicity. Appetite suppression appears to be associated with agonist action at 5-HT$_{2C}$ receptors in the central nervous system.

5-HT$_{1D/1B}$ Agonists & Migraine Headache

The 5-HT$_{1D/1B}$ agonists (**triptans, eg, sumatriptan**) are used almost exclusively for migraine headache. Migraine in its "classic" form is characterized by an aura of variable duration that may involve nausea, vomiting, visual scotomas or even hemianopsia, and speech abnormalities; the aura is followed by a severe throbbing unilateral headache that lasts for a few hours to 1–2 days. "Common" migraine lacks the aura phase, but the headache is similar. After a century of intense study, the pathophysiology of migraine is still poorly understood and controversial. Although the symptom pattern and duration of prodrome and headache vary markedly among patients, the severity of migraine headache justifies vigorous therapy in the great majority of cases.

Migraine involves the trigeminal nerve distribution to intracranial (and possibly extracranial) arteries. These nerves release peptide neurotransmitters, especially **calcitonin gene-related peptide** (CGRP; see Chapter 17), an extremely powerful vasodilator. Substance P and neurokinin A may also be involved. Extravasation of plasma and plasma proteins into the perivascular space appears to be a common feature of animal migraine models and is found in biopsy specimens from migraine patients. This effect probably reflects the action of the neuropeptides on the vessels. The mechanical stretching caused by this perivascular edema may be the immediate cause of activation of pain nerve endings in the dura. The onset of headache is sometimes associated with a marked increase in amplitude of temporal artery pulsations, and relief of pain by administration of effective therapy is sometimes accompanied by diminution of the arterial pulsations.

The mechanisms of action of drugs used in migraine are poorly understood, in part because they include such a wide variety of drug groups and actions. In addition to the triptans, these include ergot alkaloids, nonsteroidal anti-inflammatory analgesic agents, β-adrenoceptor blockers, calcium channel blockers, tricyclic antidepressants and SSRIs, and several antiseizure agents. Furthermore, some of these drug groups are effective only for prophylaxis and not for the acute attack.

Two primary hypotheses have been proposed to explain the actions of these drugs. First, the triptans, the ergot alkaloids, and antidepressants may activate 5-HT$_{1D/1B}$ receptors on presynaptic trigeminal nerve endings to inhibit the release of vasodilating peptides, and antiseizure agents may suppress excessive firing of these nerve endings. Second, the vasoconstrictor actions of direct 5-HT agonists (the triptans and ergot) may prevent vasodilation and stretching of the pain endings. It is possible that both mechanisms contribute in the case of some drugs. Sumatriptan and its congeners are currently first-line therapy for acute severe migraine attacks in most patients (Figure 16–3). However, they should not be used in patients at risk for coronary artery disease. Anti-inflammatory analgesics such as aspirin and ibuprofen are often helpful in

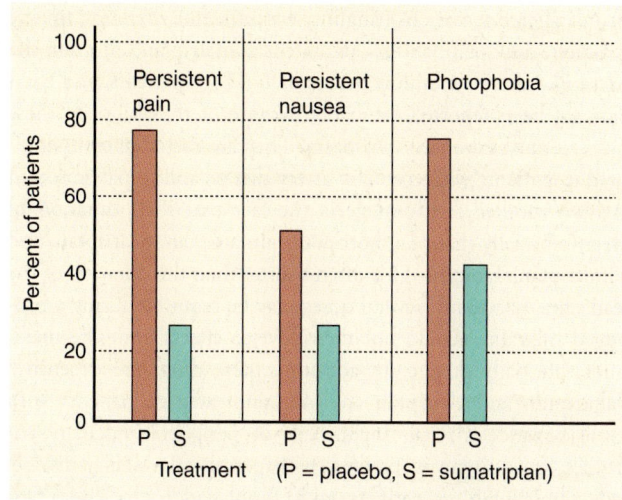

FIGURE 16–3 Effects of sumatriptan (734 patients) or placebo (370 patients) on symptoms of acute migraine headache 60 minutes after injection of 6 mg subcutaneously. All differences between placebo and sumatriptan were statistically significant. (Data from Cady RK et al: Treatment of acute migraine with subcutaneous sumatriptan. JAMA 1991;265:2831.)

controlling the pain of migraine. Rarely, parenteral opioids may be needed in refractory cases. For patients with very severe nausea and vomiting, parenteral metoclopramide may be helpful.

Propranolol, amitriptyline, and some calcium channel blockers have been found to be effective for the prophylaxis of migraine in some patients. They are of no value in the treatment of acute migraine. The anticonvulsants **valproic acid** and **topiramate** (see Chapter 24) have also been found to have prophylactic efficacy in many migraine patients. **Flunarizine,** a calcium channel blocker used in Europe, has been reported in clinical trials to effectively reduce the severity of the acute attack and to prevent recurrences. **Verapamil** appears to have modest efficacy as prophylaxis against migraine.

Sumatriptan and the other triptans are selective agonists for 5-HT$_{1D}$ and 5-HT$_{1B}$ receptors; the similarity of the triptan structure to that of the 5-HT nucleus can be seen in the structure below. These receptor types are found in cerebral and meningeal vessels and mediate vasoconstriction. They are also found on neurons and probably function as presynaptic inhibitory receptors.

Sumatriptan

The efficacies of all the triptan 5-HT$_1$ agonists in migraine are equal to each other and equivalent to or greater than those of other acute drug treatments, eg, parenteral, oral, and rectal ergot alkaloids. The pharmacokinetics of the triptans differ significantly and are set forth in Table 16–5. Most adverse effects are mild and include altered sensations (tingling, warmth, etc), dizziness, muscle weakness, neck pain, and for parenteral sumatriptan, injection site reactions. Chest discomfort occurs in 1–5% of patients, and chest pain has been reported, probably because of the ability of these drugs to cause coronary vasospasm. They are therefore contraindicated in patients with coronary artery disease and in patients with angina. Another disadvantage is the fact that their duration of effect (especially that of almotriptan, sumatriptan, rizatriptan, and zolmitriptan, Table 16–5) is often shorter than the duration of the headache. As a result, several doses may be required during a prolonged migraine attack, but their adverse effects limit the maximum safe daily dosage. In addition, these drugs are expensive. Naratriptan and eletriptan are contraindicated in patients with severe hepatic or renal impairment or peripheral vascular syndromes; frovatriptan in patients with peripheral vascular disease; and zolmitriptan in patients with Wolff-Parkinson-White syndrome. The brand name triptans are extremely expensive; thus generic sumatriptan should be used whenever possible.

Other Serotonin Agonists in Clinical Use

Cisapride, a 5-HT$_4$ agonist, was used in the treatment of gastroesophageal reflux and motility disorders. Because of toxicity, it is now available only for compassionate use in the USA. **Tegaserod**, a 5-HT$_4$ partial agonist, is used for irritable bowel syndrome with constipation. These drugs are discussed in Chapter 62.

Compounds such as **fluoxetine** and other SSRIs, which modulate serotonergic transmission by blocking reuptake of the transmitter, are among the most widely prescribed drugs for the management of depression and similar disorders. These drugs are discussed in Chapter 30.

SEROTONIN ANTAGONISTS

The actions of serotonin, like those of histamine, can be antagonized in several ways. Such antagonism is clearly desirable in those rare patients who have carcinoid tumor and may also be valuable in certain other conditions.

As noted, serotonin synthesis can be inhibited by *p*-chlorophenylalanine and *p*-chloroamphetamine. However, these agents are too toxic for general use. Storage of serotonin can be inhibited by the use of reserpine, but the sympatholytic effects of this drug (see Chapter 11) and the high levels of circulating serotonin that result from release prevent its use in carcinoid. Therefore, receptor blockade is the major therapeutic approach to conditions of serotonin excess.

SEROTONIN-RECEPTOR ANTAGONISTS

A wide variety of drugs with actions at other receptors (eg, α adrenoceptors, H$_1$-histamine receptors) also have serotonin receptor-blocking effects. **Phenoxybenzamine** (see Chapter 10) has a long-lasting blocking action at 5-HT$_2$ receptors. In addition, the ergot alkaloids discussed in the last portion of this chapter are partial agonists at serotonin receptors.

Cyproheptadine resembles the phenothiazine antihistaminic agents in chemical structure and has potent H$_1$-receptor–blocking as well as 5-HT$_2$–blocking actions. The actions of cyproheptadine are predictable from its H$_1$ histamine and 5-HT receptor affinities. It prevents the smooth muscle effects of both amines but has no effect on the gastric secretion stimulated by histamine. It also has significant antimuscarinic effects and causes sedation.

The major clinical applications of cyproheptadine are in the treatment of the smooth muscle manifestations of carcinoid tumor and in cold-induced urticaria. The usual dosage in adults is 12–16 mg/d in three or four divided doses. It is of some value in serotonin syndrome, but because it is available only in tablet form, cyproheptadine must be crushed and administered by stomach tube in unconscious patients.

Ketanserin blocks 5-HT$_2$ receptors on smooth muscle and other tissues and has little or no reported antagonist activity at other 5-HT or H$_1$ receptors. However, this drug potently blocks vascular α$_1$ adrenoceptors. The drug blocks 5-HT$_2$ receptors on platelets and antagonizes platelet aggregation promoted by serotonin. The mechanism involved in ketanserin's hypotensive action probably involves α$_1$ adrenoceptor blockade more than 5-HT$_2$ receptor blockade. Ketanserin is available in Europe for the treatment of hypertension and vasospastic conditions but has not been approved in the USA. **Ritanserin**, another 5-HT$_2$ antagonist, has little or no α-blocking

TABLE 16–5 Pharmacokinetics of triptans.

Drug	Routes	Time to Onset (h)	Single Dose (mg)	Maximum Dose per Day (mg)	Half-Life (h)
Almotriptan	Oral	2.6	6.25–12.5	25	3.3
Eletriptan	Oral	2	20–40	80	4
Frovatriptan	Oral	3	2.5	7.5	27
Naratriptan	Oral	2	1–2.5	5	5.5
Rizatriptan	Oral	1–2.5	5–10	30	2
Sumatriptan	Oral, nasal, subcutaneous, rectal	1.5 (0.2 for subcutaneous)	25–100 (PO), 20 nasal, 6 subcutaneous, 25 rectal	200	2
Zolmitriptan	Oral, nasal	1.5–3	2.5–5	10	2.8

Ergot Poisoning: Not Just an Ancient Disease

As noted in the text, epidemics of ergotism, or poisoning by ergot-contaminated grain, are known to have occurred sporadically in ancient times and through the Middle Ages. It is easy to imagine the social chaos that might result if fiery pain, gangrene, hallucinations, convulsions, and abortions occurred simultaneously throughout a community in which all or most of the people believed in witchcraft, demonic possession, and the visitation of supernatural punishments upon humans for their misdeeds. Fortunately, such beliefs are uncommon today. However, ergotism has not disappeared. A most convincing demonstration of

ergotism occurred in the small French village of Pont-Saint-Esprit in 1951. It was described in the *British Medical Journal* in 1951 (Gabbai et al, 1951) and in a later book-length narrative account (Fuller, 1968). Several hundred individuals suffered symptoms of hallucinations, convulsions, and ischemia—and several died—after eating bread made from contaminated flour. Similar events have occurred even more recently when poverty, famine, or incompetence resulted in the consumption of contaminated grain. Ergot toxicity caused by excessive self-medication with pharmaceutical ergot preparations is still occasionally reported.

action. It has been reported to alter bleeding time and to reduce thromboxane formation, presumably by altering platelet function.

Ondansetron is the prototypical 5-HT$_3$ antagonist. This drug and its analogs are very important in the prevention of nausea and vomiting associated with surgery and cancer chemotherapy. They are discussed in Chapter 62.

Considering the diverse effects attributed to serotonin and the heterogeneous nature of 5-HT receptors, other selective 5-HT antagonists may prove to be clinically useful.

■ THE ERGOT ALKALOIDS

Ergot alkaloids are produced by *Claviceps purpurea,* a fungus that infects grasses and grains—especially rye—under damp growing or storage conditions. This fungus synthesizes histamine, acetylcholine, tyramine, and other biologically active products in addition to a score or more of unique ergot alkaloids. These alkaloids affect α adrenoceptors, dopamine receptors, 5-HT receptors, and perhaps other receptor types. Similar alkaloids are produced by fungi parasitic to a number of other grass-like plants.

The accidental ingestion of ergot alkaloids in contaminated grain can be traced back more than 2000 years from descriptions of epidemics of ergot poisoning (**ergotism**). The most dramatic effects of poisoning are dementia with florid hallucinations; prolonged vasospasm, which may result in gangrene; and stimulation of uterine smooth muscle, which in pregnancy may result in abortion. In medieval times, ergot poisoning was called **St. Anthony's fire** after the saint whose help was sought in relieving the burning pain of vasospastic ischemia. Identifiable epidemics have occurred sporadically up to modern times (see Box: Ergot Poisoning: Not Just an Ancient Disease) and mandate continuous surveillance of all grains used for food. Poisoning of grazing animals is common in many areas because the fungi may grow on pasture grasses.

In addition to the effects noted above, the ergot alkaloids produce a variety of other central nervous system and peripheral effects. Detailed structure-activity analysis and appropriate semisynthetic modifications have yielded a large number of agents of experimental and clinical interest.

BASIC PHARMACOLOGY OF ERGOT ALKALOIDS

Chemistry & Pharmacokinetics

Two major families of compounds that incorporate the tetracyclic **ergoline** nucleus may be identified; the amine alkaloids and the peptide alkaloids (Table 16–6). Drugs of therapeutic and toxicologic importance are found in both groups.

The ergot alkaloids are variably absorbed from the gastrointestinal tract. The oral dose of ergotamine is about 10 times larger than the intramuscular dose, but the speed of absorption and peak blood levels after oral administration can be improved by administration with caffeine (see below). The amine alkaloids are also absorbed from the rectum and the buccal cavity and after administration by aerosol inhaler. Absorption after intramuscular injection is slow but usually reliable. Semisynthetic analogs such as bromocriptine and cabergoline are well absorbed from the gastrointestinal tract.

The ergot alkaloids are extensively metabolized in the body. The primary metabolites are hydroxylated in the A ring, and peptide alkaloids are also modified in the peptide moiety.

Pharmacodynamics

A. Mechanism of Action

The ergot alkaloids act on several types of receptors. As shown by the color outlines in Table 16–6, the nuclei of both catecholamines (phenylethylamine, *left panel*) and 5-HT (indole, *right panel*) can be discerned in the ergoline nucleus. Their effects include agonist, partial agonist, and antagonist actions at α adrenoceptors and serotonin receptors (especially 5-HT$_{1A}$ and 5-HT$_{1D}$; less for 5-HT$_2$ and 5-HT$_3$); and agonist or partial agonist actions at central nervous system dopamine receptors (Table 16–7). Furthermore, some members of the ergot family have a high affinity for presynaptic receptors, whereas others are more selective for postjunctional receptors. There is a powerful stimulant effect on the uterus that seems to be most closely associated with agonist or partial agonist effects at 5-HT$_2$ receptors. Structural variations increase the selectivity of certain members of the family for specific receptor types.

TABLE 16–6 Major ergoline derivatives (ergot alkaloids).

	R_1	R_8
6-Methylergoline	—H	—H
Lysergic acid	—H	—COOH
Lysergic acid diethylamide (LSD)	—H	O ∥ —C—N(CH₂—CH₃)₂
Ergonovine (ergometrine)	—H	O CH₂OH ∥ | —C—NHCHCH₃

	R_2	R_2'	R_5'
Ergotamine[1]	—H	—CH₃	—CH₂— (phenyl)
α-Ergocryptine	—H	—CH(CH₃)₂	—CH₂—CH(CH₃)₂
Bromocriptine	—Br	—CH(CH₃)₂	—CH₂—CH(CH₃)₂

[1]Dihydroergotamine lacks the double bond between carbons 9 and 10.

B. Organ System Effects

1. Central nervous system—As indicated by traditional descriptions of ergotism, certain of the naturally occurring alkaloids are powerful hallucinogens. Lysergic acid diethylamide (LSD; "acid") is a synthetic ergot compound that clearly demonstrates this action. The drug has been used in the laboratory as a potent peripheral 5-HT₂ *antagonist*, but good evidence suggests that its behavioral effects are mediated by *agonist* effects at prejunctional or postjunctional 5-HT₂ receptors in the central nervous system. In spite of extensive research, no clinical value has been discovered for LSD's dramatic central nervous system effects.

Abuse of this drug has waxed and waned but is still widespread. It is discussed in Chapter 32.

Dopamine receptors in the central nervous system play important roles in extrapyramidal motor control and the regulation of pituitary prolactin release. The actions of the peptide ergoline **bromocriptine** on the extrapyramidal system are discussed in Chapter 28. Of all the currently available ergot derivatives, bromocriptine, **cabergoline**, and **pergolide** have the highest selectivity for the pituitary dopamine receptors. These drugs directly suppress prolactin secretion from pituitary cells by activating regulatory dopamine receptors (see Chapter 37). They compete for

TABLE 16–7 Effects of ergot alkaloids at several receptors.[1]

Ergot Alkaloid	α Adrenoceptor	Dopamine Receptor	Serotonin Receptor (5-HT₂)	Uterine Smooth Muscle Stimulation
Bromocriptine	–	+++	–	0
Ergonovine	++	– (PA)	+++	
Ergotamine	– – (PA)	0	+ (PA)	+++
Lysergic acid diethylamide (LSD)	0	+++	– – (++ in CNS)	+
Methysergide	+/0	+/0	– – – (PA)	+/0

[1]Agonist effects are indicated by +, antagonist by –, no effect by 0. Relative affinity for the receptor is indicated by the number of + or – signs. PA means partial agonist (both agonist and antagonist effects can be detected).

binding to these sites with dopamine itself and with other dopamine agonists such as apomorphine. They bind with high affinity and dissociate slowly.

2. Vascular smooth muscle—The action of ergot alkaloids on vascular smooth muscle is drug, species, and vessel dependent, so few generalizations are possible. In humans, ergotamine and similar compounds constrict most vessels in nanomolar concentrations (Figure 16–4). The vasospasm is prolonged. This response is partially blocked by conventional α-blocking agents. However, ergotamine's effect is also associated with "epinephrine reversal" (see Chapter 10) and with *blockade* of the response to other α agonists. This dual effect reflects the drug's partial agonist action (Table 16–7). Because ergotamine dissociates very slowly from the α receptor, it produces very long-lasting agonist and antagonist effects at this receptor. There is little or no effect at β adrenoceptors.

Although much of the vasoconstriction elicited by ergot alkaloids can be ascribed to partial agonist effects at α adrenoceptors, some may be the result of effects at 5-HT receptors. Ergotamine, ergonovine, and methysergide all have partial agonist effects at 5-HT$_2$ vascular receptors. The remarkably specific antimigraine action of the ergot derivatives was originally thought to be related to their actions on vascular serotonin receptors. Current hypotheses, however, emphasize their action on prejunctional neuronal 5-HT receptors.

After overdosage with ergotamine and similar agents, vasospasm is severe and prolonged (see Toxicity, below). This vasospasm is not easily reversed by α antagonists, serotonin antagonists, or combinations of both.

Ergotamine is typical of the ergot alkaloids that have a strong vasoconstrictor spectrum of action. The hydrogenation of ergot alkaloids at the 9 and 10 positions (Table 16–6) yields dihydro derivatives that have reduced serotonin partial agonist and vasoconstrictor effects and increased selective α-receptor–blocking actions.

3. Uterine smooth muscle—The stimulant action of ergot alkaloids on the uterus, as on vascular smooth muscle, appears to combine α agonist, serotonin agonist, and other effects. Furthermore, the sensitivity of the uterus to the stimulant effects of ergot increases dramatically during pregnancy, perhaps because of increasing dominance of α$_1$ receptors as pregnancy progresses. As a result, the uterus at term is more sensitive to ergot than earlier in pregnancy and far more sensitive than the nonpregnant organ.

In very small doses, ergot preparations can evoke rhythmic contraction and relaxation of the uterus. At higher concentrations, these drugs induce powerful and prolonged contracture. Ergonovine is more selective than other ergot alkaloids in affecting the uterus and is the agent of choice in obstetric applications of the ergot drugs although oxytocin, the peptide hormone, is preferred in most cases.

4. Other smooth muscle organs—In most patients, the ergot alkaloids have little or no significant effect on bronchiolar or urinary smooth muscle. The gastrointestinal tract, on the other hand, is quite sensitive. Nausea, vomiting, and diarrhea may be induced even by low doses in some patients. The effect is consistent with action on the central nervous system emetic center and on gastrointestinal serotonin receptors.

CLINICAL PHARMACOLOGY OF ERGOT ALKALOIDS

Clinical Uses

In spite of their significant toxicities, ergot alkaloids are still widely used in patients with migraine headache or pituitary dysfunction, but only occasionally in the postpartum patient.

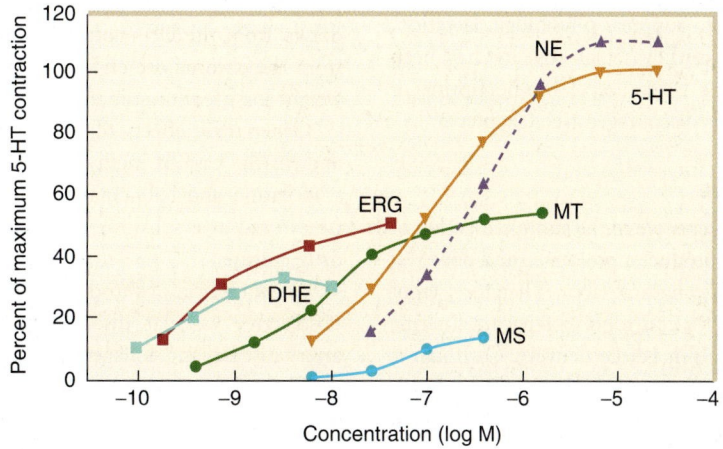

FIGURE 16–4 Effects of ergot derivatives on contraction of isolated segments of human basilar artery strips removed at surgery. All of the ergot derivatives are partial agonists, and all are more potent than the full agonists, norepinephrine and serotonin. DHE, dihydroergotamine; ERG, ergotamine; 5-HT, serotonin; MS, methysergide; MT, methylergometrine; NE, norepinephrine. (Modified and reproduced, with permission, from Müller-Schweinitzer E. In: *5-Hydroxytryptamine Mechanisms in Primary Headaches.* Oleson J, Saxena PR [editors]. Raven Press, 1992.)

A. Migraine

Ergot derivatives are highly specific for migraine pain; they are not analgesic for any other condition. Although the triptan drugs discussed above are preferred by most clinicians and patients, traditional therapy with ergotamine can also be effective when given during the prodrome of an attack; it becomes progressively less effective if delayed. Ergotamine tartrate is available for oral, sublingual, rectal suppository, and inhaler use. It is often combined with caffeine (100 mg caffeine for each 1 mg ergotamine tartrate) to facilitate absorption of the ergot alkaloid.

The vasoconstriction induced by ergotamine is long-lasting and cumulative when the drug is taken repeatedly, as in a severe migraine attack. Therefore, patients must be carefully informed that no more than 6 mg of the oral preparation may be taken for each attack and no more than 10 mg per week. For very severe attacks, ergotamine tartrate, 0.25–0.5 mg, may be given intravenously or intramuscularly. Dihydroergotamine, 0.5–1 mg intravenously, is favored by some clinicians for treatment of intractable migraine. Intranasal dihydroergotamine may also be effective. Methysergide, which was used for migraine prophylaxis in the past, was withdrawn because of toxicity, see below.

B. Hyperprolactinemia

Increased serum levels of the anterior pituitary hormone prolactin are associated with secreting tumors of the gland and also with the use of centrally acting dopamine antagonists, especially the D_2-blocking antipsychotic drugs. Because of negative feedback effects, hyperprolactinemia is associated with amenorrhea and infertility in women as well as galactorrhea in both sexes. Rarely, the prolactin surge that occurs around the end of term pregnancy may be associated with heart failure; cabergoline has been used to treat this cardiac condition successfully.

Bromocriptine is extremely effective in reducing the high levels of prolactin that result from pituitary tumors and has even been associated with regression of the tumor in some cases. The usual dosage of bromocriptine is 2.5 mg two or three times daily. Cabergoline is similar but more potent. Bromocriptine has also been used in the same dosage to suppress physiologic lactation. However, serious postpartum cardiovascular toxicity has been reported in association with the latter use of bromocriptine or pergolide, and this application is discouraged (see Chapter 37).

C. Postpartum Hemorrhage

The uterus at term is extremely sensitive to the stimulant action of ergot, and even moderate doses produce a prolonged and powerful spasm of the muscle quite unlike natural labor. Therefore, ergot derivatives should be used only for control of postpartum uterine bleeding and should never be given before delivery. Oxytocin is the preferred agent for control of postpartum hemorrhage, but if this peptide agent is ineffective, ergonovine maleate, 0.2 mg given intramuscularly, can be tried. It is usually effective within 1–5 minutes and is less toxic than other ergot derivatives for this application. It is given at the time of delivery of the placenta or immediately afterward if bleeding is significant.

D. Diagnosis of Variant Angina

Ergonovine given intravenously produces prompt vasoconstriction during coronary angiography to diagnose variant angina if reactive segments of the coronary arteries are present. In Europe, methylergometrine has been used for this purpose.

E. Senile Cerebral Insufficiency

Dihydroergotoxine, a mixture of dihydro-α-ergocryptine and three similar dihydrogenated peptide ergot alkaloids (ergoloid mesylates), has been promoted for many years for the relief of senility and more recently for the treatment of Alzheimer's dementia. There is no useful evidence that this drug has significant benefit.

Toxicity & Contraindications

The most common toxic effects of the ergot derivatives are gastrointestinal disturbances, including diarrhea, nausea, and vomiting. Activation of the medullary vomiting center and of the gastrointestinal serotonin receptors is involved. Since migraine attacks are often associated with these symptoms before therapy is begun, these adverse effects are rarely contraindications to the use of ergot.

A more dangerous toxic effect—usually associated with overdosage—of agents like ergotamine and ergonovine is prolonged vasospasm. This sign of vascular smooth muscle stimulation may result in gangrene and may require amputation. Bowel infarction has also been reported and may require resection. Peripheral vascular vasospasm caused by ergot is refractory to most vasodilators, but infusion of large doses of nitroprusside or nitroglycerin has been successful in some cases.

Chronic therapy with methysergide was associated with connective tissue proliferation in the retroperitoneal space, the pleural cavity, and the endocardial tissue of the heart. These changes occurred insidiously over months and presented as hydronephrosis (from obstruction of the ureters) or a cardiac murmur (from distortion of the valves of the heart). In some cases, valve damage required surgical replacement. As a result, this drug was withdrawn from the US market. Similar fibrotic change has resulted from the chronic use of 5-HT agonists promoted in the past for weight loss (fenfluramine, dexfenfluramine).

Other toxic effects of the ergot alkaloids include drowsiness and, in the case of methysergide, occasional instances of central stimulation and hallucinations. In fact, methysergide was sometimes used as a substitute for LSD by members of the so-called drug culture.

Contraindications to the use of ergot derivatives consist of the obstructive vascular diseases, especially symptomatic coronary artery disease, and collagen diseases.

There is no evidence that ordinary use of ergotamine for migraine is hazardous in pregnancy. However, most clinicians counsel restraint in the use of the ergot derivatives by pregnant patients. Use to deliberately cause abortion is contraindicated because the high doses required often cause dangerous vasoconstriction.

SUMMARY Drugs with Actions on Histamine and Serotonin Receptors; Ergot Alkaloids

Subclass	Mechanism of Action	Effects	Clinical Applications	Pharmacokinetics, Toxicities, Interactions
H₁ ANTIHISTAMINES **First generation:** • Diphenhydramine	Competitive antagonism/inverse agonism at H₁ receptors	Reduces or prevents histamine effects on smooth muscle, immune cells • also blocks muscarinic and α adrenoceptors • highly sedative	IgE immediate allergies, especially hay fever, urticaria • often used as a sedative, antiemetic, and anti-motion sickness drug	Oral and parenteral • duration 4–6 h • *Toxicity:* Sedation when used in hay fever, muscarinic blockade symptoms, orthostatic hypotension • *Interactions:* Additive sedation with other sedatives, including alcohol • some inhibition of CYP2D6, may prolong action of some β blockers
Second generation: • Cetirizine	Competitive antagonism/inverse agonism at H₁ receptors	Reduces or prevents histamine effects on smooth muscle, immune cells	IgE immediate allergies, especially hay fever, urticaria	Oral • duration 12–24 h • *Toxicity:* Sedation and arrhythmias in overdose • *Interactions:* Minimal

• *Other first-generation H₁ blockers: Chlorpheniramine is a less sedating H₁ blocker with fewer autonomic effects*
• *Other second-generation H₁ blockers: Loratadine, desloratadine, and fexofenadine are very similar to cetirizine*

H₂ ANTIHISTAMINES
• Cimetidine (see Chapter 62)

SEROTONIN AGONISTS **5-HT₁ᵦ/₁ᴅ:** • Sumatriptan	Partial agonist at 5-HT₁ᵦ/₁ᴅ receptors	Effects not fully understood • may reduce release of calcitonin gene-related peptide and perivascular edema in cerebral circulation	Migraine and cluster headache	Oral, nasal, parenteral • duration 2 h • *Toxicity:* Paresthesias, dizziness, coronary vasoconstriction • *Interactions:* Additive with other vasoconstrictors

• *Other triptans: Similar to sumatriptan except for pharmacokinetics (2–6 h duration of action); much more expensive than generic sumatriptan*

5-HT₄:
• Tegaserod (see Chapter 62)

SEROTONIN BLOCKERS **5-HT₂:** • Ketanserin (not available in USA)	Competitive blockade at 5-HT₂ receptors	Prevents vasoconstriction and bronchospasm of carcinoid syndrome	Hypertension • carcinoid syndrome associated with carcinoid tumor	Oral • duration 12–24 h • *Toxicity:* Hypotension

5-HT₃:
• Ondansetron (see Chapter 62)

ERGOT ALKALOIDS **Vasoselective:** • Ergotamine	Mixed partial agonist effects at 5-HT₂ and α adrenoceptors	Causes marked smooth muscle contraction but blocks α-agonist vasoconstriction	Migraine and cluster headache	Oral, parenteral • duration 12–24 h • *Toxicity:* Prolonged vasospasm causing angina, gangrene; uterine spasm
Uteroselective: • Ergonovine	Mixed partial agonist effects at 5-HT₂ and α adrenoceptors	Same as ergotamine • some selectivity for uterine smooth muscle	Postpartum bleeding • migraine headache	Oral, parenteral (methylergonovine) • duration 2–4 h • *Toxicity:* Same as ergotamine
CNS selective: • Lysergic acid diethylamide	Central nervous system (CNS) 5-HT₂ and dopamine agonist • 5-HT₂ antagonist in periphery	Hallucinations • psychotomimetic	None • widely abused	Oral • duration several hours • *Toxicity:* Prolonged psychotic state, flashbacks

• *Bromocriptine, pergolide: Ergot derivatives used in Parkinson's disease (see Chapter 28) and prolactinoma (see Chapter 37)*

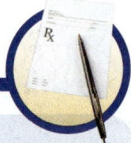

PREPARATIONS AVAILABLE

ANTIHISTAMINES (H₁ BLOCKERS)*

Azelastine
Nasal (Astelin): 137 mcg/puff nasal spray
Ophthalmic (Optivar): 0.5 mg/mL solution

Brompheniramine (generic, Brovex)
Oral: 6, 12 mg extended-release tablets; 12 mg chewable tablets;
2, 8, 12 mg/5 mL suspension

Buclizine (Bucladin-S Softabs)
Oral: 50 mg tablets

Carbinoxamine (generic, Histex)
Oral: 4 mg tablets; 8, 10 mg extended-release capsules; 1.5, 3.6,
4 mg/5 mL liquid

Cetirizine (generic, Zyrtec)
Oral: 5, 10 mg tablets; 5, 10 mg chewable tablets; 5 mg/5 mL syrup

Chlorpheniramine (generic, Chlor-Trimeton)
Oral: 2 mg chewable tablets; 4 mg tablets; 2 mg/5 mL syrup
Oral sustained-release: 8, 12, 16 mg tablets; 8, 12 mg capsules

Clemastine (generic, Tavist)
Oral: 1.34, 2.68 mg tablets; 0.67 mg/5 mL syrup

Cyclizine (Marezine)
Oral: 50 mg tablets

Cyproheptadine (generic)
Oral: 4 mg tablets; 2 mg/5 mL syrup

Desloratadine (Clarinex)
Oral: 5 mg tablets; 2.5, 5 mg rapidly disintegrating tablets;
2.5 mg/5 mL syrup

Dimenhydrinate (Dramamine, others)†
Oral: 50 mg tablets; 50 mg chewable tablets; 12.5/5 mL,
12.5 mg/4 mL, 15.62 mg/5 mL liquid
Parenteral: 50 mg/mL for IM or IV injection

Diphenhydramine (generic, Benadryl)
Oral: 12.5, 25 mg chewable tablets; 25, 50 mg tablets, capsules
12.5 mg orally disintegrating tablets; 12.5, 25 mg/5 mL elixir
and syrup
Parenteral: 50 mg/mL for injection

Epinastine (Elestat)
Ophthalmic: 0.05% solution

Fexofenadine (generic, Allegra)
Oral: 30, 60, 180 mg tablets; 30 mg rapidly disintegrating tablets;
6 mg/mL suspension

Hydroxyzine (generic, Vistaril)
Oral: 10, 25, 50 mg tablets; 25, 50, 100 mg capsules; 10 mg/5 mL
syrup; 25 mg/5 mL suspension
Parenteral: 25, 50 mg/mL for injection

Ketotifen (Zaditor)
Ophthalmic: 0.025% solution

Levocabastine (Livostin)
Ophthalmic: 0.05% solution

Levocetirizine (Xyzal)
Oral: 5 mg tablets

Loratadine (generic, Claritin, Tavist)
Oral: 10 mg tablets; 5 mg chewable tablets; 10 mg rapidly
disintegrating tablets; 1 mg/mL syrup

Meclizine (generic, Antivert)
Oral: 12.5, 25, 50 mg tablets; 25 mg capsules;
25 mg chewable tablets

Olopatadine (Patanol)
Ophthalmic: 0.1% solution

Phenindamine (Nolahist)
Oral: 25 mg tablets

Promethazine (generic, Phenergan)
Oral: 12.5, 25, 50 mg tablets; 6.25 mg/5 mL syrups
Parenteral: 25, 50 mg/mL for injection
Rectal: 12.5, 25, 50 mg suppositories

Triprolidine (Zymine)
Oral: 1.25 mg/5 mL liquid

H₂ BLOCKERS

See Chapter 62.

5-HT AGONISTS

Almotriptan (Axert)
Oral: 6.25, 12.5 mg tablets

Eletriptan (Relpax)
Oral: 24.2, 48.5 mg tablets (equivalent to 20, 40 mg base)

Frovatriptan (Frova)
Oral: 2.5 mg tablets

Naratriptan (Amerge)
Oral: 1, 2.5 mg tablets

Rizatriptan
Oral: 5, 10 mg tablets (Maxalt); 5, 10 mg orally disintegrating
tablets (Maxalt-MLT)

Sumatriptan (generic, Imitrex)
Oral: 25, 50, 100 mg tablets; generic formulation available
Nasal: 5, 20 mg unit dose spray devices
Parenteral: 4, 6 mg/0.5 mL in SELFdose autoinjection units for
subcutaneous injection

Zolmitriptan (Zomig)
Oral: 2.5, 5 mg tablets; 2.5 mg orally disintegrating tablets
Nasal: 5 mg

5-HT ANTAGONISTS

See Chapter 62.

MELATONIN RECEPTOR AGONISTS

Ramelteon (Rozarem)
Oral: 8 mg tablets

ERGOT ALKALOIDS

Dihydroergotamine
Nasal (Migranal): 4 mg/mL nasal spray
Parenteral (D.H.E. 45): 1 mg/mL for injection

Ergonovine (Ergotrate)
Oral: 0.2 mg tablets

Ergotamine mixtures (generic, Cafergot)
Oral: 1 mg ergotamine/100 mg caffeine tablets
Rectal: 2 mg ergotamine/100 mg caffeine suppositories

Ergotamine tartrate (Ergomar)
Sublingual: 2 mg sublingual tablets

Methylergonovine (Methergine)
Oral: 0.2 mg tablets
Parenteral: 0.2 mg/mL for injection

---

*Several other antihistamines are available only in combination products with, for example, phenylephrine.
†Dimenhydrinate is the chlorotheophylline salt of diphenhydramine.

REFERENCES

Histamine

Arrang J-M, Morisset S, Gbahou F: Constitutive activity of the histamine H_3 receptor. Trends Pharmacol Sci 2007;28:350.

Barnes PJ: Histamine and serotonin. Pulm Pharmacol Ther 2001;14:329.

Bond RA, IJzerman AP: Recent developments in constitutive receptor activity and inverse agonism, and their potential for GPCR drug discovery. Trend Pharmacol Sci 2006;27:92.

deShazo RD, Kemp SF: Pharmacotherapy of allergic rhinitis. www.UpToDate.com, 2010.

Gemkow MJ et al: The histamine H_3 receptor as a therapeutic drug target for CNS disorders. Drug Discov Today 2009;14:509.

Lieberman P: Anaphylaxis. Med Clin North Am 2006;90:77.

Lin J-S et al: An inverse agonist of the histamine H_3 receptor improves wakefulness in narcolepsy: Studies in orexin$^{-/-}$ mice and patients. Neurobiol Dis 2008;30:74.

Preuss H et al: Constitutive activity and ligand selectivity of human, guinea pig, rat, and canine histamine H_2 receptors. J Pharmacol Exp Therap 2007;321:983.

Smits RA, Leurs R, deEdech JP: Major advances in the development of histamine H_4 receptor ligands. Drug Discov Today 2009;14:745.

Thurmond RL, Gelfand EW, Dunford PJ: The role of histamine H_1 and H_4 receptors in allergic inflammation: The search for new antihistamines. Nat Rev Drug Dis 2008;7:41.

Tokita S, Takahashi K, Kotani H: Recent advances in molecular pharmacology of the histamine systems: Physiology and pharmacology of histamine H_3 receptor: Roles in feeding regulation and therapeutic potential for metabolic disorders. J Pharmacol Sci 2006;101:12.

Serotonin

Bajwa ZH, Sabahat A: Acute treatment of migraine in adults. www.UpToDate.com, 2010.

Barrenetxe J, Delagrange P, Martinez JA: Physiologic and metabolic functions of melatonin. J Physiol Biochem 2004;60:61.

Boyer EW, Shannon M: The serotonin syndrome. N Engl J Med 2005;352:1112.

Elangbam CS: Drug-induced valvulopathy: An update. Toxicol Path 2010;38:837.

Frank C: Recognition and treatment of serotonin syndrome. Can Fam Physician 2008;54:988.

Isbister GK, Buckley NA, Whyte IM: Serotonin toxicity: A practical approach to diagnosis and treatment. Med J Aust 2007;187:361.

Loder E: Triptan therapy in migraine. N Engl J Med 2010;363:63.

Porvasnik SL et al: PRX-08066, a novel 5-hydroxytryptamine receptor 2B antagonist, reduces monocrotaline-induced pulmonary hypertension and right ventricular hypertrophy in rats. J Pharmacol Exp Ther 2010;334:364.

Prunet-Marcassus B et al: Melatonin reduces body weight gain in Sprague-Dawley rats with diet-induced obesity. Endocrinology 2003;144:5347.

Raymond JR et al: Multiplicity of mechanisms of serotonin receptor signal transduction. Pharmacol Ther 2001;92:179.

Sack RL: Jet lag. N Engl J Med 2010;362:440.

Ergot Alkaloids: Historical

Fuller JG: *The Day of St. Anthony's Fire.* Macmillan, 1968; Signet, 1969.

Gabbai Dr, Lisbonne Dr, Pourquier Dr: Ergot poisoning at Pont St. Esprit. Br Med J 1951;Sept 15:650.

Ergot Alkaloids: Pharmacology

Dierckx RA et al: Intraarterial sodium nitroprusside infusion in the treatment of severe ergotism. Clin Neuropharmacol 1986;9:542.

Dildy GA: Postpartum hemorrhage: New management options. Clin Obstet Gynecol 2002;45:330.

Mantegani S, Brambilla E, Varasi M: Ergoline derivatives: Receptor affinity and selectivity. Farmaco 1999;54:288.

Porter JK, Thompson FN Jr: Effects of fescue toxicosis on reproduction in livestock. J Animal Sci 1992;70:1594.

Snow V et al: Pharmacologic management of acute attacks of migraine and prevention of migraine headache. Ann Intern Med 2002;137:840.

CASE STUDY ANSWER

The patient demonstrates typical symptoms, signs, and course of urticaria due to food allergy. The failure of the antihistamine to control fully the signs and symptoms is also common. In such cases, addition of oral corticosteroids is often the most effective measure. Because the condition is self-limiting (assuming the patient does not repeat the allergen challenge), a tapering high-dose regimen, using prednisone, is relatively safe and effective. This consists of 50–100 mg prednisone on days 1 and 2, 30–75 mg on days 3 and 4, 15–40 mg on days 5 and 6, 5–10 mg on days 7, 8, and 9, and none thereafter if symptoms do not recur.

Vasoactive Peptides

Ian A. Reid, PhD

CASE STUDY

During a routine check, a 45-year-old man was found to have high blood pressure (165/100 mm Hg). Blood pressure remained high on two follow-up visits. His physician initially prescribed hydrochlorothiazide, a diuretic commonly used to treat hypertension. Although his blood pressure was reduced by hydrochlorothiazide, it remained at a hypertensive level (145/95 mm Hg), and he was referred to the university hypertension clinic. Your evaluation reveals that the patient has elevated plasma renin activity and aldosterone concentration. Hydrochlorothiazide is therefore replaced with enalapril, an angiotensin-converting enzyme inhibitor. Enalapril lowers the blood pressure to almost normotensive levels. However, after several weeks on the new drug, the patient returns complaining of a persistent cough. In addition, some signs of angioedema are detected. How does enalapril lower blood pressure? Why does it occasionally cause coughing and angioedema? What other drugs could be used to inhibit renin secretion or suppress the renin-angiotensin system, and decrease blood pressure, without the adverse effects of enalapril?

Peptides are used by most tissues for cell-to-cell communication. As noted in Chapters 6 and 21, they play important roles as transmitters in the autonomic and central nervous systems. Several peptides exert important direct effects on vascular and other smooth muscles. These peptides include vasoconstrictors (**angiotensin II, vasopressin, endothelins, neuropeptide Y**, and **urotensin**) and vasodilators (**bradykinin** and related **kinins, natriuretic peptides, vasoactive intestinal peptide, substance P, neurotensin, calcitonin gene-related peptide**, and **adrenomedullin**). This chapter focuses on the smooth muscle actions of the peptides.

■ ANGIOTENSIN

BIOSYNTHESIS OF ANGIOTENSIN

The pathway for the formation and metabolism of angiotensin II (ANG II) is summarized in Figure 17–1. The principal steps include enzymatic cleavage of angiotensin I (ANG I) from angiotensinogen by renin, conversion of ANG I to ANG II by converting enzyme, and degradation of ANG II by several peptidases.

Renin

Renin is an aspartyl protease enzyme that specifically catalyzes the hydrolytic release of the decapeptide ANG I from angiotensinogen. It is synthesized as a prepromolecule that is processed to prorenin, which has poorly understood actions (see below), and then to active renin, a glycoprotein consisting of 340 amino acids.

Renin in the circulation originates in the kidneys. Enzymes with renin-like activity are present in several extrarenal tissues, including blood vessels, uterus, salivary glands, and adrenal cortex, but no physiologic role for these enzymes has been established. Within the kidney, renin is synthesized and stored in the juxtaglomerular apparatus of the nephron. Specialized granular cells called juxtaglomerular cells are the site of synthesis, storage, and release of renin. The macula densa is a specialized segment of the nephron that is closely associated with the vascular components of the juxtaglomerular apparatus. The vascular and tubular components of the juxtaglomerular apparatus, including the juxtaglomerular cells, are innervated by noradrenergic neurons.

Control of Renin Release

The rate at which renin is released by the kidney is the primary determinant of activity of the renin-angiotensin system. Active

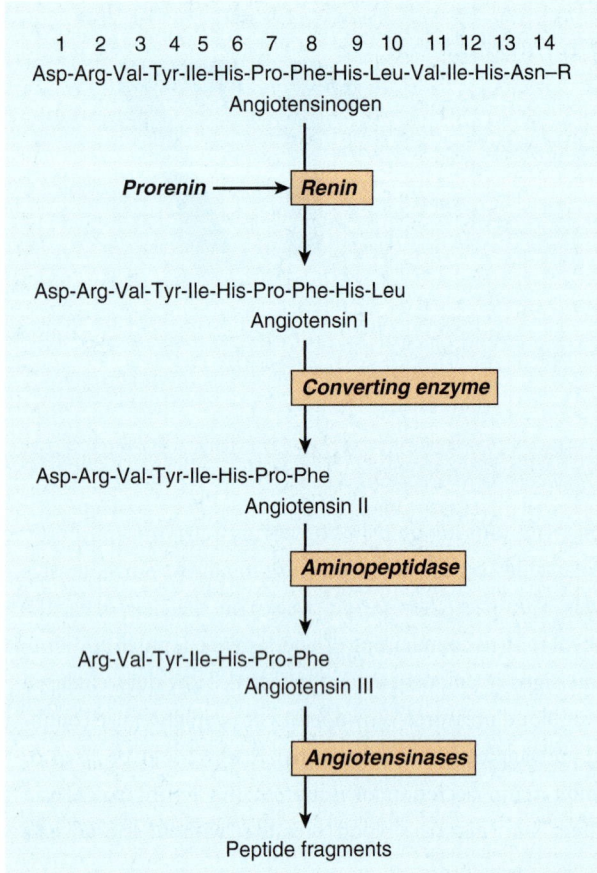

FIGURE 17–1 Chemistry of the renin-angiotensin system. The amino acid sequence of the amino terminal of human angiotensinogen is shown. R denotes the remainder of the protein molecule. See text for additional steps in the formation and metabolism of angiotensin peptides.

renin is released by exocytosis immediately upon stimulation of the juxtaglomerular apparatus. Prorenin is released constitutively, usually at a rate higher than that of active renin, thus accounting for the fact that prorenin can constitute 80–90% of the total renin in the circulation. The significance of circulating prorenin is discussed at the end of this section. Active renin release is controlled by a variety of factors, including a renal vascular receptor, the macula densa, the sympathetic nervous system, and ANG II.

A. Macula Densa

Renin release is controlled in part by the macula densa, a structure that has a close anatomic association with the afferent arteriole. The initial step involves the detection of some function of NaCl concentration in, or delivery to, the distal tubule, possibly by the $Na^+/K^+/2Cl^-$ cotransporter. The macula densa then signals changes in renin release by the juxtaglomerular cells such that there is an inverse relationship between NaCl delivery or concentration and renin release. Potential candidates for signal transmission include prostaglandin E_2 (PGE_2) and nitric oxide, which stimulate renin release, and adenosine, which inhibits it.

B. Renal Baroreceptor

The renal baroreceptor mediates an inverse relationship between renal artery pressure and renin release. The mechanism is not completely understood but it appears that the juxtaglomerular cells are sensitive to stretch and that increased stretch results in decreased renin release. The decrease may result from influx of calcium which, somewhat paradoxically, inhibits renin release. The paracrine factors PGE_2, nitric oxide, and adenosine have also been implicated in the baroreceptor control of renin release.

C. Sympathetic Nervous System

Norepinephrine released from renal sympathetic nerves stimulates renin release indirectly by α-adrenergic activation of the renal baroreceptor and macula densa mechanisms, and directly by an action on the juxtaglomerular cells. In humans, the direct effect is mediated by β_1 adrenoceptors. Through this mechanism, reflex activation of the sympathetic nervous system by hypotension or hypovolemia leads to activation of the renin-angiotensin system.

D. Angiotensin

Angiotensin II inhibits renin release. The inhibition results from increased blood pressure acting by way of the renal baroreceptor and macula densa mechanisms, and from a direct action of the peptide on the juxtaglomerular cells. The direct inhibition is mediated by increased intracellular Ca^{2+} concentration and forms the basis of a short-loop negative feedback mechanism controlling renin release. Interruption of this feedback with drugs that inhibit the renin-angiotensin system (see below) results in stimulation of renin release.

E. Intracellular Signaling Pathways

The release of renin by the juxtaglomerular cells is controlled by interplay among three intracellular messengers: cAMP, cyclic guanosine monophosphate (cGMP), and free cytosolic Ca^{2+} concentration (Figure 17–2). cAMP plays a major role; maneuvers that increase cAMP levels, including activation of adenylyl cyclase, inhibition of cAMP phosphodiesterases, and administration of cAMP analogs, increase renin release. Increases in Ca^{2+} can result from increased entry of extracellular Ca^{2+} or mobilization of Ca^{2+} from intracellular stores, while increases in cGMP levels can result from activation of soluble or particulate guanylyl cyclase. Ca^{2+} and cGMP appear to alter renin release indirectly, primarily by changing cAMP levels.

F. Pharmacologic Alteration of Renin Release

The release of renin is altered by a wide variety of pharmacologic agents. Renin release is stimulated by vasodilators (hydralazine, minoxidil, nitroprusside), β-adrenoceptor agonists, α-adrenoceptor antagonists, phosphodiesterase inhibitors (eg, theophylline, milrinone, rolipram), and most diuretics and anesthetics. This stimulation can be accounted for by the control mechanisms just described. Drugs that inhibit renin release are discussed below.

Many of the peptides reviewed in this chapter also alter renin release. Release is stimulated by adrenomedullin, bradykinin, and

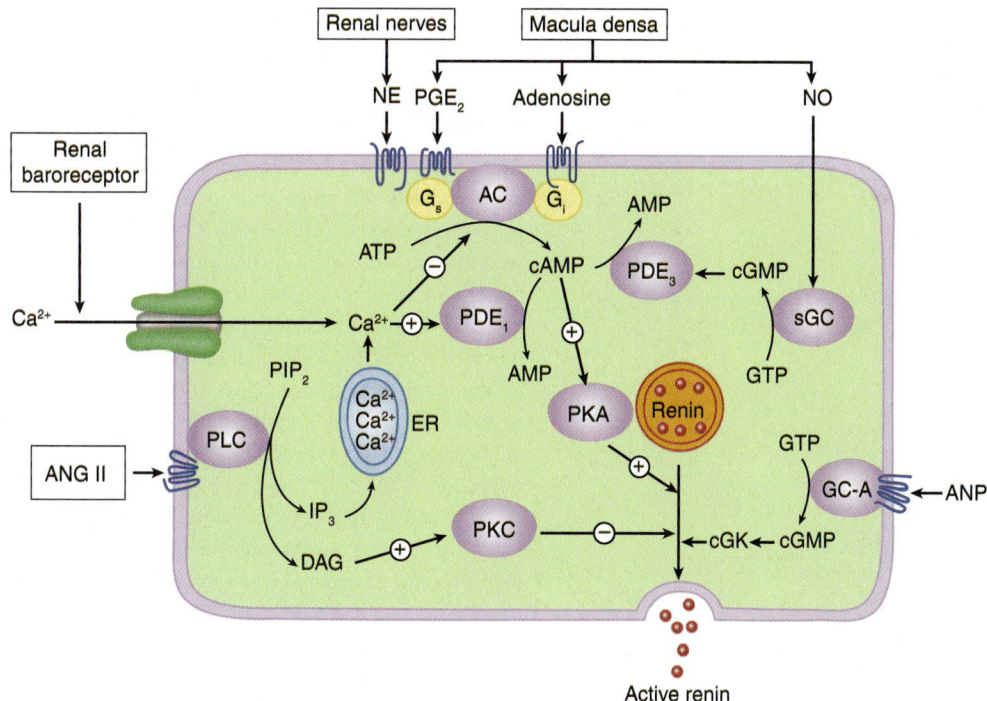

FIGURE 17–2 Major physiologic inputs to renin release and proposed integration with signaling pathways in the juxtaglomerular cell. AC, adenylyl cyclase; ANG II, angiotensin II; ANP, atrial natriuretic peptide; cGK, protein kinase G; DAG, diacylglycerol; GC-A, particulate guanylyl cyclase; ER, endoplasmic reticulum; IP_3, inositol trisphosphate; NE, norepinephrine; NO, nitric oxide; PDE, phosphodiesterase; PKA, protein kinase A; PLC, phospholipase C; sGC, soluble guanylyl cyclase. (Redrawn, with permission, from Castrop H et al: Physiology of kidney renin. Physiol Rev 2010;90:607.)

calcitonin gene-related peptide, and inhibited by atrial natriuretic peptide, endothelin, substance P, and vasopressin.

Angiotensinogen

Angiotensinogen is the circulating protein substrate from which renin cleaves ANG I. It is synthesized in the liver. Human angiotensinogen is a glycoprotein with a molecular weight of approximately 57,000. The 14 amino acids at the amino terminal of the molecule are shown in Figure 17–1. In humans, the concentration of angiotensinogen in the circulation is less than the K_m of the renin-angiotensinogen reaction and is therefore an important determinant of the rate of formation of angiotensin.

The production of angiotensinogen is increased by corticosteroids, estrogens, thyroid hormones, and ANG II. It is also elevated during pregnancy and in women taking estrogen-containing oral contraceptives. The increased plasma angiotensinogen concentration is thought to contribute to the hypertension that may occur in these situations.

Angiotensin I

Although ANG I contains the peptide sequences necessary for all of the actions of the renin-angiotensin system, it has little or no biologic activity. Instead, it must be converted to ANG II by converting enzyme (Figure 17–1). ANG I may also be acted on by plasma or tissue aminopeptidases to form [des-Asp^1]angiotensin I;

this in turn is converted to [des-Asp^1]angiotensin II (commonly known as angiotensin III) by converting enzyme.

Converting Enzyme (ACE, Peptidyl Dipeptidase, Kininase II)

Converting enzyme is a dipeptidyl carboxypeptidase with two active sites that catalyzes the cleavage of dipeptides from the carboxyl terminal of certain peptides. Its most important substrates are ANG I, which it converts to ANG II, and bradykinin, which it inactivates (see Kinins, below). It also cleaves enkephalins and substance P, but the physiologic significance of these effects has not been established. The action of converting enzyme is prevented by a penultimate prolyl residue in the substrate, and ANG II is therefore not hydrolyzed by converting enzyme. Converting enzyme is distributed widely in the body. In most tissues, converting enzyme is located on the luminal surface of vascular endothelial cells and is thus in close contact with the circulation.

A homolog of converting enzyme known as ACE2 was recently found to be highly expressed in vascular endothelial cells of the kidneys, heart, and testes. Unlike converting enzyme, ACE2 has only one active site and functions as a carboxypeptidase rather than a dipeptidyl carboxypeptidase. It removes a single amino acid from the C-terminal of ANG I forming ANG 1-9 (Figure 17–3), which is inactive but is converted to ANG 1-7 by ACE. ACE2 also converts ANG

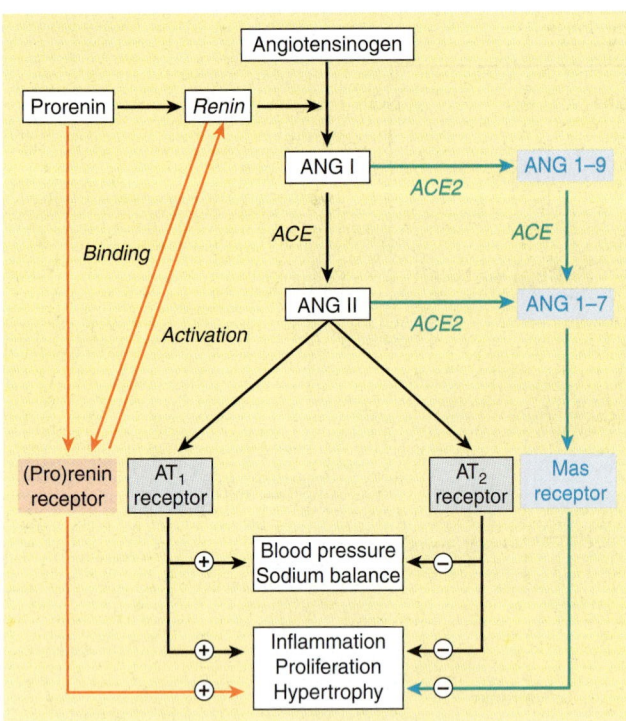

FIGURE 17–3 The renin-angiotensin system showing the established system (black) and recently discovered pathways involving the (pro)renin receptor (red) and ANG 1-7 (blue). (Redrawn, with permission, from Castrop H et al: Physiology of kidney renin. Physiol Rev 2010;90:607.)

II to ANG 1-7. ANG 1-7 has vasodilator activity, apparently mediated by the orphan heterotrimeric guanine nucleotide-binding protein-coupled receptor (Mas receptor). This vasodilation may serve to counteract the vasoconstrictor activity of ANG II. ACE2 also differs from ACE in that it does not hydrolyze bradykinin and is not inhibited by converting enzyme inhibitors (see below). Thus, the enzyme more closely resembles an angiotensinase than a converting enzyme.

Angiotensinase

Angiotensin II, which has a plasma half-life of 15–60 seconds, is removed rapidly from the circulation by a variety of peptidases collectively referred to as angiotensinase. It is metabolized during passage through most vascular beds (a notable exception being the lung). Most metabolites of ANG II are biologically inactive, but the initial product of aminopeptidase action—[des-Asp^1]angiotensin II—retains considerable biologic activity.

ACTIONS OF ANGIOTENSIN II

Angiotensin II exerts important actions at vascular smooth muscle, adrenal cortex, kidney, heart, and brain via the receptors described below. Through these actions, the renin-angiotensin system plays a key role in the regulation of fluid and electrolyte balance and arterial blood pressure. Excessive activity of the renin-angiotensin system can result in hypertension and disorders of fluid and electrolyte homeostasis.

Blood Pressure

Angiotensin II is a very potent pressor agent—on a molar basis, approximately 40 times more potent than norepinephrine. The pressor response to intravenous ANG II is rapid in onset (10–15 seconds) and sustained during long-term infusions. A large component of the pressor response is due to direct contraction of vascular—especially arteriolar—smooth muscle. In addition, however, ANG II can also increase blood pressure through actions on the brain and autonomic nervous system. The pressor response to ANG II is usually accompanied by little or no reflex bradycardia because the peptide acts on the brain to reset the baroreceptor reflex control of heart rate to a higher pressure.

Angiotensin II also interacts with the autonomic nervous system. It stimulates autonomic ganglia, increases the release of epinephrine and norepinephrine from the adrenal medulla, and most important, facilitates sympathetic transmission by an action at adrenergic nerve terminals. The latter effect involves both increased release and reduced reuptake of norepinephrine. Angiotensin II also has a less important direct positive inotropic action on the heart.

Adrenal Cortex & Kidney

Angiotensin II acts directly on the zona glomerulosa of the adrenal cortex to stimulate aldosterone synthesis and release. At higher concentrations, ANG II also stimulates glucocorticoid synthesis. Angiotensin II acts on the kidney to cause renal vasoconstriction, increase proximal tubular sodium reabsorption, and inhibit the release of renin.

Central Nervous System

In addition to its central effects on blood pressure, ANG II acts on the central nervous system to stimulate drinking (dipsogenic effect) and increase the secretion of vasopressin and adrenocorticotropic hormone (ACTH). The physiologic significance of the effects of ANG II on drinking and pituitary hormone secretion is not known.

Cell Growth

Angiotensin II is mitogenic for vascular and cardiac muscle cells and may contribute to the development of cardiovascular hypertrophy. It also exerts a variety of important effects on the vascular endothelium. Indeed, overactivity of the renin-angiotensin system has been implicated as one of the most significant factors in the development of hypertensive vascular disease. Considerable evidence now indicates that ACE inhibitors and ANG II receptor antagonists (see below) slow or prevent morphologic changes (remodeling) following myocardial infarction that would otherwise lead to heart failure. The stimulation of vascular and cardiac growth by ANG II is mediated by other pathways, probably receptor and nonreceptor tyrosine kinases such as the Janus tyrosine kinase Jak2, and by increased transcription of specific genes (see Chapter 2).

ANGIOTENSIN RECEPTORS & MECHANISM OF ACTION

Angiotensin II receptors are widely distributed in the body. Like the receptors for other peptide hormones, ANG II receptors are G protein-coupled and located on the plasma membrane of target cells, and this permits rapid onset of the various actions of ANG II. Two distinct subtypes of ANG II receptors, termed **AT$_1$** and **AT$_2$,** have been identified on the basis of their differential affinity for antagonists and their sensitivity to sulfhydryl-reducing agents. AT$_1$ receptors have a high affinity for the inhibitor losartan and a low affinity for PD 123177 (an experimental nonpeptide antagonist), whereas AT$_2$ receptors have a high affinity for PD 123177 and a low affinity for losartan. Angiotensin II and saralasin (see below) bind equally to both subtypes. The relative proportion of the two subtypes varies from tissue to tissue: AT$_1$ receptors predominate in vascular smooth muscle. Most of the known actions of ANG II are mediated by the AT$_1$ receptor, a G$_q$ protein-coupled receptor. Binding of ANG II to AT$_1$ receptors in vascular smooth muscle results in activation of phospholipase C and generation of inositol trisphosphate and diacylglycerol (see Chapter 2). These events, which occur within seconds, result in smooth muscle contraction.

The AT$_2$ receptor has a structure and affinity for ANG II similar to those of the AT$_1$ receptor. In contrast, however, stimulation of AT$_2$ receptors causes vasodilation that may serve to counteract the vasoconstriction resulting from AT$_1$ receptor stimulation. AT$_2$ receptor-mediated vasodilation appears to be nitric oxide-dependent and may involve the bradykinin B$_2$ receptor-nitric oxide-cGMP pathway. AT$_2$ receptors are present at high density in all tissues during fetal development, but they are much less abundant in the adult where they are expressed at high concentration only in the adrenal medulla, reproductive tissues, vascular endothelium, and parts of the brain. AT$_2$ receptors are up-regulated in pathologic conditions including heart failure and myocardial infarction. The functions of the AT$_2$ receptor appear to include fetal tissue development, inhibition of growth and proliferation, cell differentiation, apoptosis, and vasodilation.

INHIBITION OF THE RENIN-ANGIOTENSIN SYSTEM

In view of the importance of the renin-angiotensin system in cardiovascular disease, considerable effort has been directed to developing drugs that inhibit the system. A wide variety of agents that block the formation or action of ANG II is now available. Some of these drugs block renin release, but most inhibit the conversion of ANG I to ANG II, block angiotensin AT$_1$ receptors, or inhibit the enzymatic action of renin.

Drugs That Block Renin Release

Several drugs that interfere with the sympathetic nervous system inhibit the release of renin. Examples are clonidine and propranolol. Clonidine inhibits renin release by causing a centrally mediated reduction in renal sympathetic nerve activity, and it may also exert a direct intrarenal action. Propranolol and other β-adrenoceptor–blocking drugs act by blocking the intrarenal and extrarenal β receptors involved in the neural control of renin release.

Angiotensin-Converting Enzyme Inhibitors

An important class of orally active ACE inhibitors, directed against the active site of ACE, is now extensively used. **Captopril** and **enalapril** are examples of the many potent ACE inhibitors that are available. These drugs differ in their structure and pharmacokinetics, but they are interchangeable in clinical use. ACE inhibitors decrease systemic vascular resistance without increasing heart rate, and they promote natriuresis. As described in Chapters 11 and 13, they are effective in the treatment of hypertension, decrease morbidity and mortality in heart failure and left ventricular dysfunction after myocardial infarction, and delay the progression of diabetic nephropathy.

ACE inhibitors not only block the conversion of ANG I to ANG II but also inhibit the degradation of other substances, including bradykinin, substance P, and enkephalins. The action of ACE inhibitors to inhibit bradykinin metabolism contributes significantly to their hypotensive action (see Figure 11–5) and is apparently responsible for some adverse side effects, including cough and angioedema. These drugs are contraindicated in pregnancy because they cause fetal kidney damage.

Angiotensin Receptor Blockers

Potent peptide antagonists of the action of ANG II are available for research use. The best-known of these is the partial agonist, **saralasin**. Saralasin lowers blood pressure in hypertensive patients but may elicit pressor responses, particularly when circulating ANG II levels are low. Because it must be administered intravenously, saralasin is used only for investigation of renin-dependent hypertension and other hyperreninemic states.

The *non*peptide ANG II receptor blockers (ARBs) are of much greater interest. **Losartan, valsartan, eprosartan, irbesartan, candesartan, olmesartan,** and **telmisartan** are orally active, potent, and specific competitive antagonists of angiotensin AT$_1$ receptors. The efficacy of these drugs in hypertension is similar to that of ACE inhibitors, but they are associated with a lower incidence of cough. Like ACE inhibitors, ARBs slow the progression of diabetic nephropathy and valsartan has been reported to decrease the incidence of diabetes in patients with impaired glucose tolerance. The antagonists are also effective in the treatment of heart failure and provide a useful alternative when ACE inhibitors are not well tolerated. ARBs are generally well tolerated but should not be used by patients with nondiabetic renal disease or in pregnancy.

Marfan syndrome is a connective tissue disorder associated with aortic disease and other abnormalities involving increased transforming growth factor (TGF)-β signaling. Since ANG II increases TGF-β levels, it was reasoned that blockade of the renin-angiotensin system might be beneficial in Marfan syndrome. Promising initial results have been obtained with losartan, and clinical trials are underway.

The currently available ARBs are selective for the AT_1 receptor. Since prolonged treatment with the drugs disinhibits renin release and increases circulating ANG II levels, there may be increased stimulation of AT_2 receptors. This may be significant in view of the evidence that activation of the AT_2 receptor causes vasodilation and other beneficial effects. AT_2 receptor antagonists such as PD 123177 are available for research but have no clinical applications at this time. However, a selective AT_2 *agonist*, compound 21, lowers blood pressure in hypertensive animals and may be beneficial in human hypertension. The clinical benefits of ARBs are similar to those of ACE inhibitors, and it is not clear if one group of drugs has significant advantages over the other. Combination therapy with an ACE inhibitor plus an ARB has a number of potential advantages and is currently being investigated.

Renin Inhibitors

Cleavage of angiotensinogen by renin (Figures 17–1 and 17–3) is the rate-limiting step in the formation of ANG II and thus represents a logical target for inhibition of the renin-angiotensin system. Drugs that inhibit renin have been available for many years but have been limited by low potency, poor bioavailability, and short duration of action. However, a new class of nonpeptide, low-molecular-weight, orally active inhibitors has recently been developed. Aliskiren is the most advanced of these and the first to be approved for the treatment of hypertension. In healthy subjects, aliskiren produces a dose-dependent reduction in plasma renin activity and ANG I and II and aldosterone concentrations. In patients with hypertension, many of whom have elevated plasma renin levels, aliskiren suppresses plasma renin activity and causes dose-related reductions in blood pressure similar to those produced by ACE inhibitors and ARBs. The safety and tolerability of aliskiren appear to be comparable to angiotensin antagonists and placebo. Aliskiren is contraindicated in pregnancy.

Inhibition of the renin-angiotensin system with ACE inhibitors or ARBs may be incomplete because the drugs disrupt the negative feedback action of ANG II on renin release and thereby increase plasma renin activity. Other antihypertensive drugs, notably hydrochlorothiazide and other diuretics, also increase plasma renin activity. Aliskiren not only decreases baseline plasma renin activity in hypertensive subjects but also eliminates the rise produced by ACE inhibitors, ARBs, and diuretics and thereby results in a greater antihypertensive effect. Renin inhibition has thus proved to be an important new approach to the treatment of hypertension.

Prorenin Receptors

For many years, prorenin was considered to be an inactive precursor of renin, with no function of its own. Thus the observation noted above in the section on renin that prorenin circulates at high levels was surprising. Recently, however, a receptor that preferentially binds prorenin has been identified. Since it also binds active renin, the receptor is referred to as the (pro)renin receptor.

The receptor is a 350-amino acid protein with a single transmembrane domain. When prorenin binds to the (pro)renin receptor, it undergoes a conformational change and becomes fully active. The catalytic activity of active renin also increases further when it binds to the receptor. The activated prorenin and renin interact with circulating angiotensinogen to form angiotensin (Figure 17–3). However, binding of prorenin to the receptor also activates intracellular signaling pathways that differ depending on the cell type. For example, in mesangial and vascular smooth muscle cells, prorenin binding activates MAP kinases and expression of profibrotic molecules. Thus, elevated prorenin levels (as occur, for example, in diabetes mellitus) could produce a variety of adverse effects via both angiotensin-dependent and independent pathways. Recent research indicates that the (pro)renin receptor is functionally linked to the vacuolar proton-ATPase (ATP6ap2) and is necessary for Wnt signaling pathways involved (independently of renin) in stem cell biology, embryology, and cancer.

A synthetic peptide named handle region peptide (HRP), which consists of the amino acid sequence corresponding to the "handle" region of the prorenin prosegment, has been synthesized and shown to competitively inhibit binding of prorenin to the (pro)renin receptor. HRP has beneficial effects in the kidneys of diabetic rats and there is considerable interest in developing noncompetitive antagonists of the (pro)renin receptor.

This novel receptor could be important in cardiovascular and other diseases, but at the present time its role in human pathology is far from clear.

■ KININS

BIOSYNTHESIS OF KININS

Kinins are potent vasodilator peptides formed enzymatically by the action of enzymes known as kallikreins or kininogenases acting on protein substrates called kininogens. The kallikrein-kinin system has several features in common with the renin-angiotensin system.

Kallikreins

Kallikreins are present in plasma and in several organs and tissues, including the kidneys, pancreas, intestine, sweat glands, and salivary glands. Plasma prekallikrein can be activated to kallikrein by trypsin, Hageman factor, and possibly kallikrein itself. In general, the biochemical properties of tissue kallikreins are different from those of plasma kallikreins. Kallikreins can convert prorenin to active renin, but the physiologic significance of this action has not been established.

Kininogens

Kininogens—the precursors of kinins and substrates of kallikreins—are present in plasma, lymph, and interstitial fluid. Two kininogens are known to be present in plasma: a low-molecular-weight form (LMW kininogen) and a high-molecular-weight form (HMW kininogen). About 15–20% of the total plasma kininogen is in the HMW form. It is thought that LMW kininogen crosses capillary walls and serves as the substrate for tissue kallikreins, whereas HMW kininogen is confined to the bloodstream and serves as the substrate for plasma kallikrein.

FORMATION OF KININS IN PLASMA & TISSUES

The pathway for the formation and metabolism of kinins is shown in Figure 17–4. Three kinins have been identified in mammals: **bradykinin, lysylbradykinin** (also known as **kallidin**), and **methionyllysylbradykinin.** Each contains bradykinin in its structure.

Each kinin is formed from a kininogen by the action of a different enzyme. Bradykinin is released by plasma kallikrein, lysylbradykinin by tissue kallikrein, and methionyllysylbradykinin by pepsin and pepsin-like enzymes. The three kinins have been found in plasma and urine. Bradykinin is the predominant kinin in plasma, whereas lysylbradykinin is the major urinary form.

PHYSIOLOGIC & PATHOLOGIC EFFECTS OF KININS

Effects on the Cardiovascular System

Kinins produce marked arteriolar dilation in several vascular beds, including the heart, skeletal muscle, kidney, liver, and intestine. In this respect, kinins are approximately 10 times more potent on a molar basis than histamine. The vasodilation may result from a direct inhibitory effect of kinins on arteriolar smooth muscle or may be mediated by the release of nitric oxide or vasodilator prostaglandins such as PGE_2 and PGI_2. In contrast, the predominant effect of kinins on veins is contraction; again, this may result from direct stimulation of venous smooth muscle or from the release of venoconstrictor prostaglandins such as $PGF_{2\alpha}$. Kinins also produce contraction of most visceral smooth muscle.

When injected intravenously, kinins produce a rapid but brief fall in blood pressure that is due to their arteriolar vasodilator action. Intravenous infusions of the peptide fail to produce a sustained decrease in blood pressure; prolonged hypotension can only be produced by progressively increasing the rate of infusion. The rapid reversibility of the hypotensive response to kinins is due primarily to reflex increases in heart rate, myocardial contractility, and cardiac output. In some species, bradykinin produces a biphasic change in blood pressure—an initial hypotensive response followed by an increase above the preinjection level. The increase in blood pressure may be due to a reflex activation of the sympathetic nervous system, but under some conditions, bradykinin can directly release catecholamines from the adrenal medulla and stimulate sympathetic ganglia. Bradykinin also increases blood pressure when injected into the central nervous system, but the physiologic significance of this effect is not clear, since it is unlikely that kinins cross the blood-brain barrier. (Note, however, that bradykinin can increase the permeability of the blood-brain barrier to some other substances.) Kinins have no consistent effect on sympathetic or parasympathetic nerve endings.

The arteriolar dilation produced by kinins causes an increase in pressure and flow in the capillary bed, thus favoring efflux of fluid from blood to tissues. This effect may be facilitated by increased capillary permeability resulting from contraction of endothelial cells and widening of intercellular junctions, and by increased venous pressure secondary to constriction of veins. As a result of these changes, water and solutes pass from the blood to the extracellular fluid, lymph flow increases, and edema may result.

The role that endogenous kinins play in the regulation of blood pressure is not clear. They do not appear to participate in the control of blood pressure under resting conditions but may play a role in postexercise hypotension.

Effects on Endocrine & Exocrine Glands

As noted earlier, prekallikreins and kallikreins are present in several glands, including the pancreas, kidney, intestine, salivary glands, and sweat glands, and they can be released into the secretory fluids of these glands. The function of the enzymes in these tissues is not known. Since kinins have such marked effects on smooth muscle, they may modulate the tone of salivary and pancreatic ducts, help regulate gastrointestinal motility, and act as local modulators of blood flow. Kinins also influence the transepithelial transport of water, electrolytes, glucose, and amino acids, and may regulate the transport of these substances in the gastrointestinal tract and kidney. Finally, kallikreins may play a role in the physiologic activation of various prohormones, including proinsulin and prorenin.

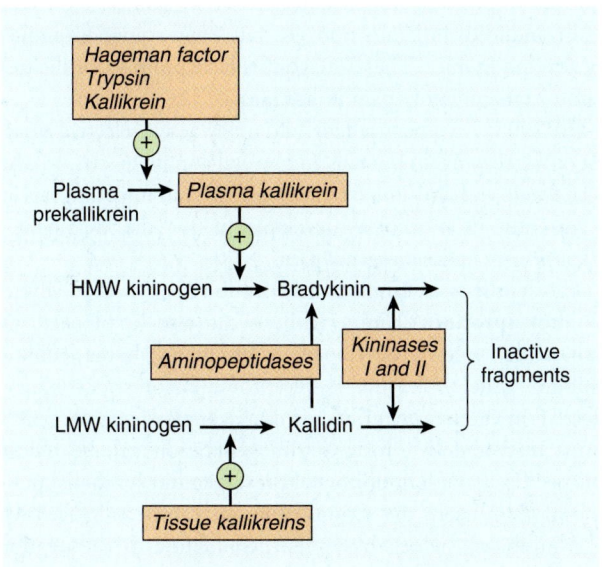

FIGURE 17–4 The kallikrein-kinin system. Kininase II is identical to converting enzyme peptidyl dipeptidase (ACE).

Role in Inflammation & Pain

Bradykinin has long been known to produce the four classic symptoms of inflammation—redness, local heat, swelling, and pain. Kinins are rapidly generated after tissue injury and play a pivotal role in the development and maintenance of these inflammatory processes.

Kinins are potent pain-producing substances when applied to a blister base or injected intradermally. They elicit pain by stimulating nociceptive afferents in the skin and viscera.

Other Effects

There is evidence that bradykinin may play a beneficial, protective role in certain cardiovascular diseases and ischemic stroke-induced brain injury. On the other hand, it has been implicated in cancer and some central nervous system diseases.

KININ RECEPTORS & MECHANISMS OF ACTION

The biologic actions of kinins are mediated by specific receptors located on the membranes of the target tissues. Two types of kinin receptors, termed B_1 and B_2, have been defined based on the rank orders of agonist potencies; both are G protein-coupled receptors. (Note that B here stands for bradykinin, not for β adrenoceptor.) Bradykinin displays the highest affinity in most B_2 receptor systems, followed by lys-bradykinin and then by met-lys-bradykinin. One exception is the B_2 receptor that mediates contraction of venous smooth muscle; this appears to be most sensitive to lys-bradykinin. Recent evidence suggests the existence of two B_2-receptor subtypes, which have been termed B_{2A} and B_{2B}.

B_1 receptors appear to have a very limited distribution in mammalian tissues and have few known functional roles. Studies with knockout mice that lack functional B_1 receptors suggest that these receptors participate in the inflammatory response and may also be important in long-lasting kinin effects such as collagen synthesis and cell multiplication. By contrast, B_2 receptors have a widespread distribution that is consistent with the multitude of biologic effects that are mediated by this receptor type. Agonist binding to B_2 receptors sets in motion multiple signal transduction events, including calcium mobilization, chloride transport, formation of nitric oxide, and activation of phospholipase C, phospholipase A_2, and adenylyl cyclase.

METABOLISM OF KININS

Kinins are metabolized rapidly (half-life < 15 seconds) by nonspecific exopeptidases or endopeptidases, commonly referred to as kininases. Two plasma kininases have been well characterized. Kininase I, apparently synthesized in the liver, is a carboxypeptidase that releases the carboxyl terminal arginine residue. Kininase II is present in plasma and vascular endothelial cells throughout the body. It is identical to angiotensin-converting enzyme (ACE, peptidyl dipeptidase), discussed above. Kininase II inactivates kinins by cleaving the carboxyl terminal dipeptide phenylalanyl-arginine. Like angiotensin I, bradykinin is almost completely hydrolyzed during a single passage through the pulmonary vascular bed.

DRUGS AFFECTING THE KALLIKREIN-KININ SYSTEM

Drugs that modify the activity of the kallikrein-kinin system are available, though none are in wide clinical use. Considerable effort has been directed toward developing kinin receptor antagonists, since such drugs have considerable therapeutic potential as anti-inflammatory and antinociceptive agents. Competitive antagonists of both B_1 and B_2 receptors are available for research use. Examples of B_1 receptor antagonists are the peptides [Leu$_8$-des-Arg$_9$]bradykinin and Lys[Leu$_8$-des-Arg$_9$]bradykinin. The first B_2 receptor antagonists to be discovered were also peptide derivatives of bradykinin. These first-generation antagonists were used extensively in animal studies of kinin receptor pharmacology. However, their half-life is short, and they are almost inactive on the human B_2 receptor.

Icatibant is a second-generation B_2 receptor antagonist. It is a decapeptide with an affinity for the B_2 receptor similar to that of bradykinin and is absorbed rapidly after subcutaneous administration. Icatibant has been shown to be effective in the treatment of hereditary angioedema, an autosomal dominant disorder characterized by recurrent episodes of bradykinin-mediated angioedema of the airways, gastrointestinal tract, extremities, and genitalia. It may also be useful in other conditions including drug-induced angioedema, airway disease, thermal injury, ascites, and pancreatitis.

Recently, a third generation of B_2-receptor antagonists was developed; examples are FR 173657, FR 172357, and NPC 18884. These antagonists block both human and animal B_2 receptors and are orally active. They have been reported to inhibit bradykinin-induced bronchoconstriction in guinea pigs, carrageenin-induced inflammation in rats, and capsaicin-induced nociception in mice. These antagonists have promise for the treatment of inflammatory pain in humans.

SSR240612 is a new, potent, and orally active selective antagonist of B_1 receptors in humans and several animal species. It exhibits analgesic and anti-inflammatory activities in mice and rats and is currently in preclinical development for the treatment of inflammatory and neurogenic pain.

The synthesis of kinins can be inhibited with the kallikrein inhibitor **aprotinin**. Kinin synthesis can also be blocked with **ecallantide,** a newly developed recombinant plasma kallikrein inhibitor which, like the B_2-receptor antagonist icatibant, is effective in the treatment of hereditary angioedema. Actions of kinins mediated by prostaglandin generation can be blocked nonspecifically with inhibitors of prostaglandin synthesis such as aspirin. Conversely, the actions of kinins can be enhanced with ACE inhibitors, which block the degradation of the peptides. Indeed, as noted above, inhibition of bradykinin metabolism by ACE inhibitors contributes significantly to their antihypertensive action.

Selective B2 agonists are under study and have been shown to be effective in some animal models of human cardiovascular disease. These drugs have potential for the treatment of hypertension, myocardial hypertrophy, and other diseases.

VASOPRESSIN

Vasopressin (**arginine vasopressin, AVP; antidiuretic hormone, ADH**) plays an important role in the long-term control of blood pressure through its action on the kidney to increase water reabsorption. This and other aspects of the physiology of AVP are discussed in Chapters 15 and 37 and will not be reviewed here.

AVP also plays an important role in the short-term regulation of arterial pressure by its vasoconstrictor action. It increases total peripheral resistance when infused in doses less than those required to produce maximum urine concentration. Such doses do not normally increase arterial pressure because the vasopressor activity of the peptide is buffered by a reflex decrease in cardiac output. When the influence of this reflex is removed, eg, in shock, pressor sensitivity to AVP is greatly increased. Pressor sensitivity to AVP is also enhanced in patients with idiopathic orthostatic hypotension. Higher doses of AVP increase blood pressure even when baroreceptor reflexes are intact.

VASOPRESSIN RECEPTORS & ANTAGONISTS

Three subtypes of AVP receptors have been identified; all are G protein-coupled. **V1a receptors** mediate the vasoconstrictor action of AVP; **V1b receptors** mediate release of ACTH by pituitary corticotropes; and **V2 receptors** mediate the antidiuretic action. V1a effects are mediated by Gq activation of phospholipase C, formation of inositol trisphosphate, and increased intracellular calcium concentration. V2 effects are mediated by Gs activation of adenylyl cyclase.

AVP analogs selective for vasoconstrictor or antidiuretic activity have been synthesized. The most specific V1 vasoconstrictor agonist synthesized to date is [Phe^2, Ile^3, Orn^8]vasotocin. Selective V2 antidiuretic analogs include 1-deamino[D-Arg^8]arginine vasopressin (dDAVP) and 1-deamino[Val^4,D-Arg^8]arginine vasopressin (dVDAVP).

AVP has proved beneficial in the treatment of vasodilatory shock states, at least in part by virtue of its V1a agonist activity. **Terlipressin** (triglycyl lysine vasopressin), a synthetic vasopressin analog that is converted to lysine vasopressin in the body, is also effective. It may have advantages over AVP because it is more selective for V1 receptors and has a longer half-life.

Antagonists of the vasoconstrictor action of AVP are also available. The peptide antagonist d(CH2)5[Tyr(Me)^2]AVP also has antioxytocic activity but does not antagonize the antidiuretic action of AVP. A related antagonist d(CH2)5[Tyr(Me)^2,Dab^5]AVP lacks oxytocin antagonism but has less anti-V1 activity. Recently, nonpeptide, orally active V1a-receptor antagonists have been discovered, examples being **relcovaptan** and **SRX251.**

The V1a antagonists have been particularly useful in revealing the important role that AVP plays in blood pressure regulation in situations such as dehydration and hemorrhage. They have potential as therapeutic agents for the treatment of such diverse diseases and conditions as Raynaud's disease, hypertension, heart failure, brain edema, motion sickness, cancer, preterm labor, and anger reduction. To date, most studies have focused on heart failure; promising results have been obtained with V2 antagonists such as **tolvaptan**, which is, however, currently approved only for use in hyponatremia. V1a antagonists also have potential, and **conivaptan** (YM087), a drug with both V1a and V2 antagonist activity, has also been approved for treatment of hyponatremia (see Chapter 15).

NATRIURETIC PEPTIDES

Synthesis & Structure

The atria and other tissues of mammals contain a family of peptides with natriuretic, diuretic, vasorelaxant, and other properties. The family includes atrial natriuretic peptide (ANP), brain natriuretic peptide (BNP), and C-type natriuretic peptide (CNP). The peptides share a common 17-amino-acid disulfide ring with variable C- and N-terminals (Figure 17–5). A fourth peptide, urodilatin, has the same structure as ANP with an extension of four amino acids at the N-terminal. The renal effects of these peptides are discussed in Chapter 15.

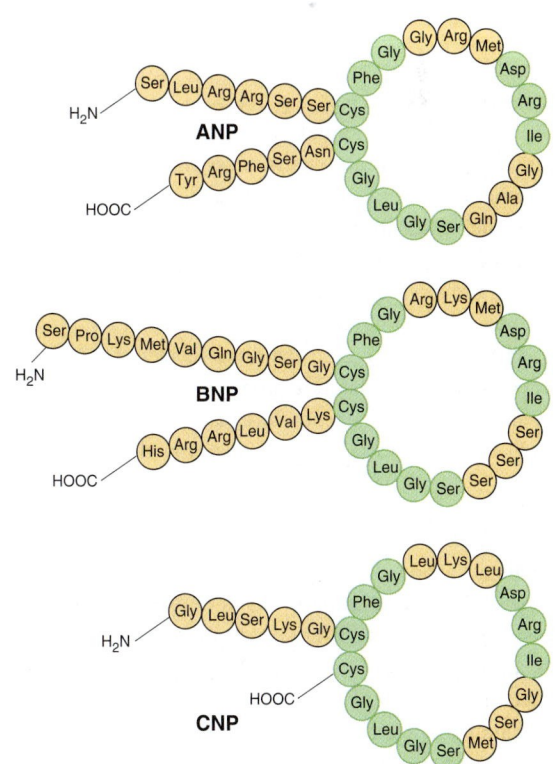

FIGURE 17–5 Structures of atrial natriuretic peptide (ANP), brain natriuretic peptide (BNP), and C-type natriuretic peptide (CNP). Sequences common to the peptides are indicated in green.

ANP is derived from the carboxyl terminal end of a common precursor termed preproANP. ANP is synthesized primarily in cardiac atrial cells, but it is also synthesized in ventricular myocardium, by neurons in the central and peripheral nervous systems, and in the lungs.

The most important stimulus to the release of ANP from the heart is atrial stretch via mechanosensitive ion channels. ANP release is also increased by volume expansion, changing from the standing to the supine position, and exercise. ANP release can also be increased by sympathetic stimulation via α_{1A} adrenoceptors, endothelins via the ET_A-receptor subtype (see below), glucocorticoids, and AVP. Plasma ANP concentration increases in several pathologic states, including heart failure, primary aldosteronism, chronic renal failure, and inappropriate ADH secretion syndrome.

Administration of ANP produces prompt and marked increases in sodium excretion and urine flow. Glomerular filtration rate increases, with little or no change in renal blood flow, so that the filtration fraction increases. The ANP-induced natriuresis is due to both the increase in glomerular filtration rate and a decrease in proximal tubular sodium reabsorption. ANP also inhibits the release of renin, aldosterone, and AVP; these changes may also increase sodium and water excretion. Finally, ANP causes vasodilation and decreases arterial blood pressure. Suppression of ANP production or blockade of its action impairs the natriuretic response to volume expansion, and increases blood pressure.

BNP was originally isolated from porcine brain but, like ANP, it is synthesized primarily in the heart. It exists in two forms, having either 26 or 32 amino acids (Figure 17–5). Like ANP, the release of BNP appears to be volume related; indeed, the two peptides may be co-secreted. BNP exhibits natriuretic, diuretic, and hypotensive activities similar to those of ANP but circulates at a lower concentration.

CNP consists of 22 amino acids (Figure 17–5). It is located predominantly in the central nervous system but is also present in several other tissues including the vascular endothelium, kidneys, and intestine. It has not been found in significant concentrations in the circulation. CNP has less natriuretic and diuretic activity than ANP and BNP but is a potent vasodilator and may play a role in the regulation of peripheral resistance.

Urodilatin is synthesized in the distal tubules of the kidneys by alternative processing of the ANP precursor. It elicits potent natriuresis and diuresis, and thus functions as a paracrine regulator of sodium and water excretion. It also relaxes vascular smooth muscle.

Pharmacodynamics & Pharmacokinetics

The biologic actions of the natriuretic peptides are mediated through association with specific high-affinity receptors located on the surface of the target cells. Three receptor subtypes termed ANP_A, ANP_B, and ANP_C (also known as NPR_1, NPR_2, and NPR_3) have been identified. The ANP_A receptor consists of a 120 kDa membrane-spanning protein with enzymatic activity associated with its intracellular domain. Its primary ligands are ANP and BNP. The ANP_B receptor is similar in structure to the ANP_A receptor, but its primary ligand appears to be CNP. The ANP_A and ANP_B receptors, but not the ANP_C receptor, are guanylyl cyclase enzymes.

The natriuretic peptides have a short half-life in the circulation. They are metabolized in the kidneys, liver, and lungs by the neutral endopeptidase NEP 24.11. Inhibition of this endopeptidase results in increases in circulating levels of the natriuretic peptides, natriuresis, and diuresis. The peptides are also removed from the circulation by binding to ANP_C receptors in the vascular endothelium. This receptor binds the natriuretic peptides with equal affinity. The receptor and bound peptide are internalized, the peptide is degraded enzymatically, and the receptor is returned to the cell surface. Patients with heart failure have high plasma levels of ANP and BNP; the latter has emerged as a diagnostic and prognostic marker in this condition.

■ VASOPEPTIDASE INHIBITORS

Vasopeptidase inhibitors constitute a new class of cardiovascular drugs that inhibit two metalloprotease enzymes, NEP 24.11 and ACE. They thus simultaneously increase the levels of natriuretic peptides and decrease the formation of ANG II. As a result, they enhance vasodilation, reduce vasoconstriction, and increase sodium excretion, in turn reducing peripheral vascular resistance and blood pressure.

Recently developed vasopeptidase inhibitors include **omapatrilat, sampatrilat,** and **fasidotrilat.** Omapatrilat, which has received the most attention, lowers blood pressure in animal models of hypertension as well as in hypertensive patients, and improves cardiac function in patients with heart failure. Unfortunately, omapatrilat causes a significant incidence of angioedema in addition to cough and dizziness and has not been approved for clinical use.

■ ENDOTHELINS

The endothelium is the source of a variety of substances with vasodilator (PGI_2 and nitric oxide) and vasoconstrictor activities. The latter include the endothelin family, potent vasoconstrictor peptides that were first isolated from aortic endothelial cells.

Biosynthesis, Structure, & Clearance

Three isoforms of endothelin have been identified: the originally described endothelin, **ET-1,** and two similar peptides, **ET-2** and **ET-3.** Each isoform is a product of a different gene and is synthesized as a prepro form that is processed to a propeptide and then to the mature peptide. Processing to the mature peptides occurs through the action of endothelin-converting enzyme. Each endothelin is a 21-amino-acid peptide containing two disulfide bridges. The structure of ET-1 is shown in Figure 17–6.

Endothelins are widely distributed in the body. ET-1 is the predominant endothelin secreted by the vascular endothelium. It is also produced by neurons and astrocytes in the central nervous system and in endometrial, renal mesangial, Sertoli, breast epithelial, and other cells. ET-2 is produced predominantly in the kidneys and intestine, whereas ET-3 is found in highest concentration

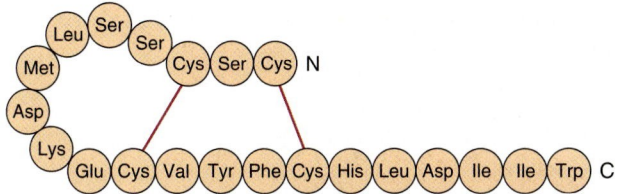

FIGURE 17–6 Structure of human endothelin-1.

in the brain but is also present in the gastrointestinal tract, lungs, and kidneys. Endothelins are present in the blood but in low concentration; they apparently act locally in a paracrine or autocrine fashion rather than as circulating hormones.

The expression of the ET-1 gene is increased by growth factors and cytokines, including transforming growth factor-β (TGF-β) and interleukin 1 (IL-1), vasoactive substances including ANG II and AVP, and mechanical stress. Expression is inhibited by nitric oxide, prostacyclin, and ANP.

Clearance of endothelins from the circulation is rapid and involves both enzymatic degradation by NEP 24.11 and clearance by the ET_B receptor.

Actions

Endothelins exert widespread actions in the body. In particular, they cause potent dose-dependent vasoconstriction in most vascular beds. Intravenous administration of ET-1 causes a rapid and transient decrease in arterial blood pressure followed by a sustained increase. The depressor response results from release of prostacyclin and nitric oxide from the vascular endothelium, whereas the pressor response is due to direct contraction of vascular smooth muscle. Endothelins also exert direct positive inotropic and chronotropic actions on the heart and are potent coronary vasoconstrictors. They act on the kidneys to cause vasoconstriction and decrease glomerular filtration rate and sodium and water excretion. In the respiratory system, they cause potent contraction of tracheal and bronchial smooth muscle. Endothelins interact with several endocrine systems, increasing the secretion of renin, aldosterone, AVP, and ANP. They exert a variety of actions on the central and peripheral nervous systems, the gastrointestinal system, the liver, the urinary tract, the male and female reproductive systems, the eye, the skeletal system, and the skin. Finally, ET-1 is a potent mitogen for vascular smooth muscle cells, cardiac myocytes, and glomerular mesangial cells.

Endothelin receptors are widespread in the body. Two endothelin receptor subtypes, termed ET_A and ET_B, have been cloned and sequenced. ET_A receptors have a high affinity for ET-1 and a low affinity for ET-3 and are located on smooth muscle cells, where they mediate vasoconstriction (Figure 17–7). ET_B receptors have approximately equal affinities for ET-1 and ET-3 and are primarily located on vascular endothelial cells, where they mediate release of PGI_2 and nitric oxide. Some ET_B receptors are also present on smooth muscle cells and mediate vasoconstriction. Both receptor subtypes belong to the G protein-coupled seven-transmembrane domain family of receptors.

The signal transduction mechanisms triggered by binding of ET-1 to its vascular receptors include stimulation of phospholipase C, formation of inositol trisphosphate, and release of calcium from the endoplasmic reticulum, which results in vasoconstriction. Conversely, stimulation of PGI_2 and nitric oxide synthesis results in decreased intracellular calcium concentration and vasodilation.

INHIBITORS OF ENDOTHELIN SYNTHESIS & ACTION

The endothelin system can be blocked with receptor antagonists and drugs that block endothelin-converting enzyme. Endothelin ET_A or ET_B receptors can be blocked selectively, or both can be blocked with nonselective ET_A-ET_B antagonists.

Bosentan is a nonselective receptor blocker. It is active orally, and blocks both the initial transient depressor (ET_B) and the prolonged pressor (ET_A) responses to intravenous endothelin. Many orally active endothelin receptor antagonists with increased selectivity have been developed and are available for research use. Examples include the selective ET_A antagonists **ambrisentan,** which has been approved by the Food and Drug Administration to treat pulmonary artery hypertension, and **sitaxsentan.**

Bosentan

The formation of endothelins can be blocked by inhibiting endothelin-converting enzyme with phosphoramidon. Phosphoramidon is not specific for endothelin-converting enzyme, but more selective inhibitors including CGS35066 are now available for research. Although the therapeutic potential of these drugs appeared similar to that of the endothelin receptor antagonists (see below), their use has been eclipsed by endothelin antagonists.

Physiologic & Pathologic Roles of Endothelin: Effects of Endothelin Antagonists

Systemic administration of endothelin receptor antagonists or endothelin-converting enzyme inhibitors causes vasodilation and decreases arterial pressure in humans and experimental animals. Intra-arterial administration of the drugs also causes slow-onset forearm vasodilation in humans. These observations provide evidence that the endothelin system participates in the regulation of vascular tone, even under resting conditions. The activity of the

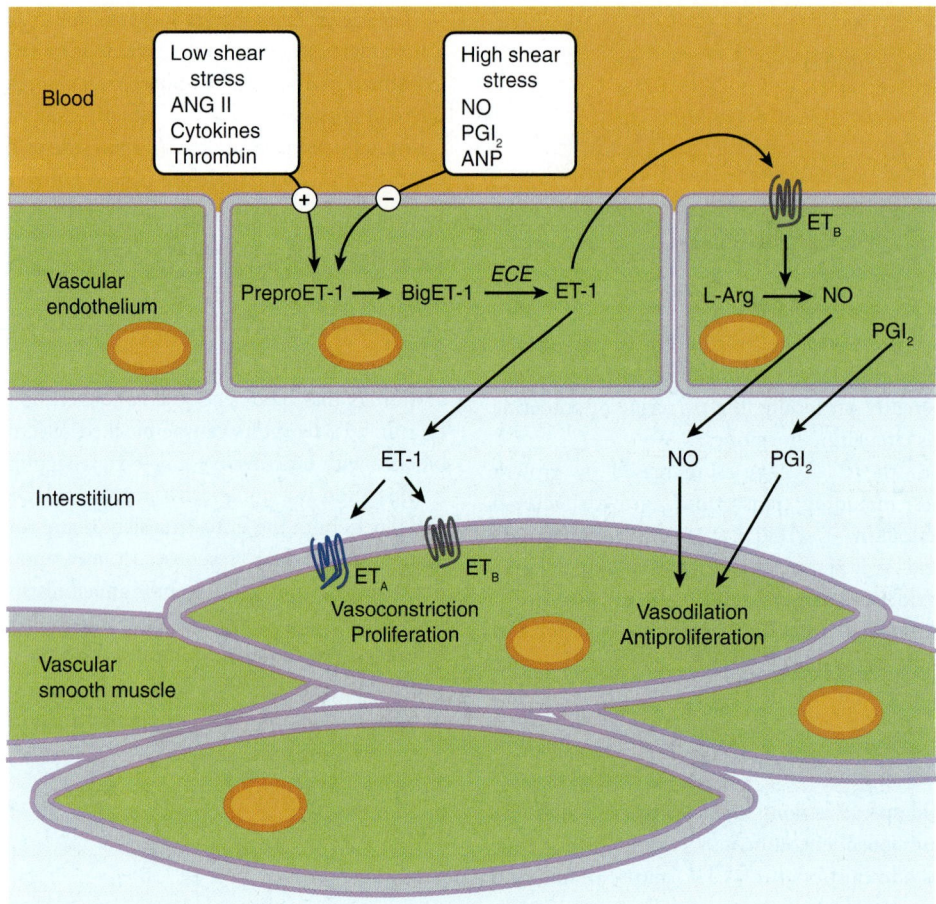

FIGURE 17–7 Generation of endothelin-1 (ET-1) in the vascular endothelium, and its direct and indirect effects on smooth muscle cells mediated by ET_A and ET_B receptors. ANG II, angiotensin II; ANP, atrial natriuretic peptide; ECE, endothelial-converting enzyme; NO, nitric oxide; PGI_2, prostaglandin I_2.

system is higher in males than in females. It increases with age, an effect that can be counteracted by regular aerobic exercise.

Increased production of ET-1 has been implicated in a variety of cardiovascular diseases, including hypertension, cardiac hypertrophy, heart failure, atherosclerosis, coronary artery disease, and myocardial infarction. ET-1 also participates in pulmonary diseases, including asthma and pulmonary hypertension; renal diseases; and several malignancies, including ovarian cancer.

Endothelin antagonists have considerable potential for the treatment of these diseases. Indeed, endothelin antagonism with bosentan, sitaxsentan, and ambrisentan has proved to be a moderately effective and generally well-tolerated treatment for patients with pulmonary arterial hypertension, an important condition with few effective treatments. Other promising targets for these drugs are resistant hypertension, chronic renal disease, connective tissue disease, and subarachnoid hemorrhage. On the other hand, clinical trials of the drugs in the treatment of congestive heart failure have been disappointing.

Endothelin antagonists occasionally cause systemic hypotension, increased heart rate, facial flushing or edema, and headaches. Potential gastrointestinal effects include nausea, vomiting, and constipation. Because of their teratogenic effects, endothelin antagonists are contraindicated in pregnancy. Bosentan has been associated with fatal hepatotoxicity, and patients taking this drug must have monthly liver function tests. Negative pregnancy test results are required for women of child-bearing age to take this drug.

■ VASOACTIVE INTESTINAL PEPTIDE

Vasoactive intestinal peptide (VIP) is a 28-amino-acid peptide that belongs to the glucagon-secretin family of peptides. VIP is widely distributed in the central and peripheral nervous systems, where it functions as one of the major peptide neurotransmitters. It is present in cholinergic presynaptic neurons in the central nervous system, and in peripheral peptidergic neurons innervating diverse tissues including the heart, lungs, gastrointestinal and urogenital tracts, skin, eyes, ovaries, and thyroid gland. Many blood vessels are innervated by VIP neurons. VIP is also present in key organs of the immune system including the thymus, spleen, and lymph nodes. Although VIP is present in blood, where it undergoes rapid degradation, it does not appear to function as a hormone. VIP participates in a wide variety of biologic functions including metabolic processes, secretion of endocrine and exocrine glands, cell differentiation, smooth muscle relaxation, and the immune response.

VIP exerts significant effects on the cardiovascular system. It produces marked vasodilation in most vascular beds and in this regard is more potent on a molar basis than acetylcholine. In the heart, VIP causes coronary vasodilation and exerts positive inotropic and chronotropic effects. It may thus participate in the regulation of coronary blood flow, cardiac contraction, and heart rate.

The effects of VIP are mediated by G protein-coupled receptors; two subtypes, **VPAC1** and **VPAC2,** have been cloned from human tissues. Both subtypes are widely distributed in the central nervous system and in the heart, blood vessels, and other tissues. VIP has a high affinity for both receptor subtypes. Binding of VIP to its receptors results in activation of adenylyl cyclase and formation of cAMP, which is responsible for the vasodilation and many other effects of the peptide. Other actions may be mediated by inositol trisphosphate synthesis and calcium mobilization. VIP can also bind with low affinity to the VIP-like peptide pituitary adenylyl cyclase-activating peptide receptor, PAC1.

VIP analogs with longer half-lives than the native peptide are now available for research use. An example is stearyl-Nle^{17}-VIP. These drugs have potential as therapeutic agents for cardiovascular, pulmonary, gastrointestinal, and nervous system diseases. They may also be effective in treating various inflammatory diseases and diabetes. Indeed, some VIP derivatives are currently undergoing preclinical and clinical testing for the treatment of type 2 diabetes and chronic obstructive pulmonary disease. Unfortunately, their use is currently limited by several issues including poor oral availability, rapid metabolism in the blood, and hypotension. VIP receptor antagonists are also being developed.

■ SUBSTANCE P

Substance P belongs to the **tachykinin** family of peptides, which share the common carboxyl terminal sequence Phe-Gly-Leu-Met. Other members of this family are **neurokinin A** and **neurokinin B.** Substance P is an undecapeptide, while neurokinins A and B are decapeptides.

Substance P is present in the central nervous system, where it is a neurotransmitter (see Chapter 21), and in the gastrointestinal tract, where it may play a role as a transmitter in the enteric nervous system and as a local hormone (see Chapter 6).

Substance P is the most important member of the tachykinin family. It exerts a variety of incompletely understood central actions that implicate the peptide in behavior, anxiety, depression, nausea, and emesis. It is a potent arteriolar vasodilator, producing marked hypotension in humans and several animal species. The vasodilation is mediated by release of nitric oxide from the endothelium. Conversely, substance P causes contraction of venous, intestinal, and bronchial smooth muscle. It also stimulates secretion by the salivary glands and causes diuresis and natriuresis by the kidneys.

The actions of substance P and neurokinins A and B are mediated by three G_q protein-coupled tachykinin receptors designated **NK$_1$, NK$_2$,** and **NK$_3$.** Substance P is the preferred ligand for the NK$_1$ receptor, the predominant tachykinin receptor in the human brain. However, neurokinins A and B also possess considerable affinity for this receptor. In humans, most of the central and peripheral effects of substance P are mediated by NK$_1$ receptors. All three receptor subtypes are coupled to inositol trisphosphate synthesis and calcium mobilization.

Several nonpeptide NK$_1$ receptor antagonists have been developed. These compounds are highly selective and orally active, and enter the brain. Recent clinical trials have shown that these antagonists may be useful in treating depression and other disorders and in preventing chemotherapy-induced emesis. The first of these to be approved for the prevention of chemotherapy-induced and postoperative nausea and vomiting is **aprepitant** (see Chapter 62). **Fosaprepitant** is a prodrug that is converted to aprepitant after intravenous administration and may be a useful parenteral alternative to oral aprepitant.

■ NEUROTENSIN

Neurotensin (NT) is a tridecapeptide that was first isolated from the central nervous system but subsequently was found to be present in the gastrointestinal tract and in the circulation. It is synthesized as part of a larger precursor that also contains **neuromedin N,** a six-amino-acid NT-like peptide.

In the brain, processing of the precursor leads primarily to the formation of NT and neuromedin N; these are released together from nerve endings. In the gut, processing leads mainly to the formation of NT and a larger peptide that contains the neuromedin N sequence at the carboxyl terminal. Both peptides are secreted into the circulation after ingestion of food. Most of the activity of NT is mediated by the last six amino acids, NT(8-13).

Like many other neuropeptides, NT serves a dual function as a neurotransmitter or neuromodulator in the central nervous system and as a local hormone in the periphery. When administered centrally, NT exerts potent effects including hypothermia, antinociception, and modulation of dopamine and glutamate neurotransmission. When administered into the peripheral circulation, it causes vasodilation, hypotension, increased vascular permeability, increased secretion of several anterior pituitary hormones, hyperglycemia, inhibition of gastric acid and pepsin secretion, and inhibition of gastric motility. It also exerts effects on the immune system.

In the central nervous system, there are close associations between NT and dopamine systems, and NT may be involved in clinical disorders involving dopamine pathways such as schizophrenia, Parkinson's disease, and drug abuse. Consistent with this, it has been shown that central administration of NT produces effects in rodents similar to those produced by antipsychotic drugs.

The effects of NT are mediated by three subtypes of NT receptors, designated **NTR$_1$, NTR$_2$,** and **NTR$_3$,** also known as **NTS$_1$, NTS$_2$,** and **NTS$_3$.** NTR$_1$ and NTR$_2$ receptors belong to the G_q protein-coupled superfamily with seven transmembrane domains;

the NTR$_3$ receptor is a single transmembrane domain protein that belongs to a family of sorting proteins.

NT receptor agonists that cross the blood-brain barrier, all peptide analogs of NT(8-13), have been developed. Conversely, NT receptors can be blocked with the nonpeptide antagonists SR142948A and meclinertant (SR48692). SR142948A is a potent antagonist of the hypothermia and analgesia produced by centrally administered NT. It also blocks the cardiovascular effects of systemic NT. The development of drugs that selectively target or block NT receptors has resulted in potential therapeutic agents for the treatment of schizophrenia and Parkinson's disease, as well as drug abuse.

CALCITONIN GENE-RELATED PEPTIDE

Calcitonin gene-related peptide (**CGRP**) is a member of the calcitonin family of peptides, which also includes calcitonin, adrenomedullin (see below), and amylin. CGRP consists of 37 amino acids. Like calcitonin, CGRP is present in large quantities in the C cells of the thyroid gland. It is also distributed widely in the central and peripheral nervous systems, cardiovascular and respiratory systems, and gastrointestinal tract. In the cardiovascular system CGRP-containing fibers are more abundant around arteries than around veins, and in atria than in ventricles. CGRP fibers are associated with most smooth muscles of the gastrointestinal tract. CGRP is found with substance P (see above) in some of these regions and with acetylcholine in others.

When CGRP is injected into the central nervous system, it produces a variety of effects, including hypertension and suppression of feeding. When injected into the systemic circulation, the peptide causes hypotension and tachycardia. The hypotensive action of CGRP results from the potent vasodilator action of the peptide; indeed, CGRP is the most potent vasodilator yet discovered. It dilates multiple vascular beds, but the coronary circulation is particularly sensitive. The vasodilation is mediated via a nonendothelial mechanism through activation of adenylyl cyclase.

Although CGRP receptors have traditionally been divided into two classes, CGRP$_1$ and CGRP$_2$, it now seems likely that the actions of CGRP are mediated by a single receptor. Specifically, the seven-transmembrane G protein-coupled calcitonin-like protein receptor (CLR) co-assembles with the receptor activity-modifying protein RAMP1 to form a functional single CGRP receptor that can activate both G$_s$ and G$_q$. Peptide and nonpeptide antagonists of the receptor have been developed. CGRP$_{8-37}$ has been used extensively to investigate the actions of CGRP but displays affinity for related receptors including those for adrenomedullin (see below). Nonpeptide CGRP receptor antagonists target the interface between CLR and RAMP1 and thereby make them more selective for the CGRP receptor. These antagonists display species selectivity and are more selective for human than rodent receptors. Examples are **olcegepant** and **telcagepant.**

Evidence is accumulating that release of CGRP from trigeminal nerves plays a central role in the pathophysiology of migraine. The peptide is released during migraine attacks, and successful treatment of migraine with a selective serotonin agonist normalizes cranial CGRP levels. Clinical trials with olcegepant and telcagepant have demonstrated that CGRP antagonism is an effective, well-tolerated treatment for migraine.

ADRENOMEDULLIN

Adrenomedullin (AM) was first discovered in human adrenal medullary pheochromocytoma tissue. It is a 52-amino-acid peptide with a six-amino-acid ring and a C-terminal amidation sequence. Like CGRP, AM is a member of the calcitonin family of peptides. A related peptide termed adrenomedullin 2, also called intermedin, has been identified in humans and other mammals.

AM is widely distributed in the body. The highest concentrations are found in the adrenal glands, hypothalamus, and anterior pituitary, but high levels are also present in the kidneys, lungs, cardiovascular system, and gastrointestinal tract. AM in plasma apparently originates in the heart and vasculature.

In animals, AM dilates resistance vessels in the kidney, brain, lung, hind limbs, and mesentery, resulting in a marked, long-lasting hypotension. The hypotension in turn causes reflex increases in heart rate and cardiac output. These responses also occur during intravenous infusion of the peptide in healthy human subjects. AM also acts on the kidneys to increase sodium excretion and renin release, and it exerts other endocrine effects including inhibition of aldosterone and insulin secretion. It acts on the central nervous system to increase sympathetic outflow.

The diverse actions of AM are mediated by a receptor closely related to the CGRP receptor (see above). CLR co-assembles with RAMP subtypes 2 and 3, thus forming a receptor-coreceptor system. Binding of AM to CLR activates G$_s$ and triggers cAMP formation in vascular smooth muscle cells, and increases nitric oxide production in endothelial cells. Other signaling pathways are also involved.

Circulating AM levels increase during intense exercise. They also increase in a number of pathologic states, including essential hypertension, cardiac and renal failure, and septic shock. The roles of AM in these states remain to be defined, but it is currently thought that the peptide functions as a physiologic antagonist of the actions of vasoconstrictors including ET-1 and ANG II. By virtue of these actions, AM may protect against cardiovascular overload and injury, and AM may be beneficial in the treatment of some cardiovascular diseases.

NEUROPEPTIDE Y

Neuropeptide Y (NPY) is a member of the family that also includes peptide YY and pancreatic polypeptide. Each of these peptides consists of 36 amino acids.

NPY is one of the most abundant neuropeptides in both the central and peripheral nervous systems. In the sympathetic nervous system, NPY is frequently localized in noradrenergic neurons and apparently functions both as a vasoconstrictor and as a cotransmitter with norepinephrine. Peptide YY and pancreatic polypeptide are both gut endocrine peptides.

NPY produces a variety of central nervous system effects, including increased feeding (it is one of the most potent orexigenic molecules in the brain), hypotension, hypothermia, respiratory depression, and activation of the hypothalamic-pituitary-adrenal axis. Other effects include vasoconstriction of cerebral blood vessels, positive chronotropic and inotropic actions on the heart, and hypertension. The peptide is a potent renal vasoconstrictor and suppresses renin secretion, but can cause diuresis and natriuresis. Prejunctional neuronal actions include inhibition of transmitter release from sympathetic and parasympathetic nerves. Vascular actions include direct vasoconstriction, potentiation of the action of vasoconstrictors, and inhibition of the action of vasodilators.

These diverse effects are mediated by four subtypes of NPY receptors designated Y_1, Y_2, Y_4, and Y_5. The receptors have been cloned and shown to be G_i protein-coupled receptors linked to mobilization of Ca^{2+} and inhibition of adenylyl cyclase. Y_1 and Y_2 receptors are of major importance in the cardiovascular and other peripheral effects of the peptide. Y_4 receptors have a high affinity for pancreatic polypeptide and may be a receptor for the pancreatic peptide rather than for NPY. Y_5 receptors are found mainly in the central nervous system and may be involved in the control of food intake. They also mediate the activation of the hypothalamic-pituitary-adrenal axis by NPY.

Selective nonpeptide NPY receptor antagonists are now available for research. The first nonpeptide Y_1 receptor antagonist, BIBP3226, is also the most thoroughly studied. It has a short half-life in vivo. In animal models, it blocks the vasoconstrictor and pressor responses to NPY. Structurally related Y_1 antagonists include BIB03304 and H409/22; the latter has been tested in humans. SR120107A and SR120819A are orally active Y_1 antagonists and have a long duration of action. BIIE0246 is the first nonpeptide antagonist selective for the Y_2 receptor; it does not cross the blood-brain barrier. Useful Y_4 antagonists are not available. The Y_5 antagonists MK-0557 and S-2367 have been tested in clinical trials for obesity.

These drugs have been useful in analyzing the role of NPY in cardiovascular regulation. It now appears that the peptide is not important in the regulation of hemodynamics under normal resting conditions but may be of increased importance in cardiovascular disorders including hypertension and heart failure. Other studies have implicated NPY in feeding disorders, obesity, alcoholism, anxiety, depression, epilepsy, pain, cancer, and bone physiology. Y_1 and particularly Y_5 receptor antagonists have potential as antiobesity agents.

■ UROTENSIN

Urotensin II (UII) was originally identified in fish, but isoforms are now known to be present in the human and other mammalian species. Human UII is an 11-amino acid peptide. Major sites of UII expression in humans include the brain, spinal cord, and kidneys. UII is also present in plasma, and potential sources of this circulating peptide include the heart, lungs, liver, and kidneys. The stimulus to UII release has not been identified but increased blood pressure has been implicated in some studies.

In vitro, UII is a potent constrictor of vascular smooth muscle; its activity depends on the type of blood vessel and the species from which it was obtained. Vasoconstriction occurs primarily in arterial vessels, where UII can be more potent than ET-1, making it the most potent known vasoconstrictor. However, under some conditions, UII may cause vasodilation. In vivo, UII has complex hemodynamic effects, the most prominent being regional vasoconstriction and cardiac depression. In some ways, these effects resemble those produced by ET-1. Nevertheless, the role of the peptide in the normal regulation of vascular tone and blood pressure in humans appears to be minor.

The actions of UII are mediated by a G_q protein-coupled receptor referred to as the UT receptor. UT receptors are widely distributed in the brain, spinal cord, heart, vascular smooth muscle, skeletal muscle, and pancreas. Some effects of the peptide including vasoconstriction are mediated by the phospholipase C, inositol trisphosphate-diacylglycerol signal transduction pathway.

Urantide ("urotensin antagonist peptide"), a penicillamine-substituted derivative of UII, is a UII receptor antagonist. A nonpeptide antagonist, **palosuran,** has also been developed and used in clinical studies.

Although UII appears to play only a minor role in health, evidence is accumulating that it is involved in cardiovascular and other diseases. In particular, it has been reported that plasma UII levels are increased in hypertension, heart failure, atherosclerosis, diabetes mellitus, and renal failure, and palosuran may benefit diabetic patients with renal disease. Nevertheless, the role of UII in disease is poorly understood. Indeed it is possible that rather than contributing to these diseases, UII may actually play a protective role.

SUMMARY Drugs That Interact with Vasoactive Peptide Systems

Subclass	Mechanism of Action	Effects	Clinical Applications
ANGIOTENSIN RECEPTOR ANTAGONISTS			
• Valsartan	Selective competitive antagonist of angiotensin AT_1 receptors	Arteriolar dilation • decreased aldosterone secretion • increased sodium and water excretion	Hypertension
• *Eprosartan, irbesartan, candesartan, olmesartan, telmisartan: Similar to valsartan*			
CONVERTING ENZYME INHIBITORS			
• Enalapril	Inhibits conversion of angiotensin I to angiotensin II	Arteriolar dilation • decreased aldosterone secretion • increased sodium and water excretion	Hypertension • heart failure
• *Captopril and many others: Similar to enalapril*			
RENIN INHIBITORS			
• Aliskiren	Inhibits catalytic activity of renin	Arteriolar dilation • decreased aldosterone secretion • increased sodium and water excretion	Hypertension
KININ INHIBITORS			
• Icatibant	Selective antagonist of kinin B_2 receptors	Blocks effects of kinins on pain, hyperalgesia, and inflammation	Hereditary angioedema
• *Ecallantide: Plasma kallikrein inhibitor*			
VASOPRESSIN AGONISTS			
• Arginine vasopressin	Agonist of vasopressin V_1 (and V_2) receptors	Vasoconstriction	Vasodilatory shock
• *Terlipressin: More selective for V_1 receptor*			
VASOPRESSIN ANTAGONISTS			
• Conivaptan	Antagonist of vasopressin V_1 (and V_2) receptors	Vasodilation	Potential use in hypertension and heart failure • hyponatremia
• *Relcovaptan: Increased selectivity for V_1 receptor*			
NATRIURETIC PEPTIDES			
• Nesiritide	Agonist of natriuretic peptide receptors	Increased sodium and water excretion • vasodilation	Heart failure
• *Uralitide: Synthetic form of urodilatin*			
VASOPEPTIDASE INHIBITORS			
• Omapatrilat	Decreases metabolism of natriuretic peptides and formation of angiotensin II	Vasodilation • increased sodium and water excretion	Hypertension • heart failure[1]
ENDOTHELIN ANTAGONISTS			
• Bosentan	Nonselective antagonist of endothelin ET_A and ET_B receptors	Vasodilation	Pulmonary arterial hypertension
• *Sitaxsentan, ambrisentan: Selective for ET_A receptors*			
VASOACTIVE INTESTINAL PEPTIDE AGONISTS			
• Stearyl-Nle[17]-VIP	Agonist of VPAC1 and VPAC2 receptors	Vasodilation • multiple metabolic, endocrine, and other effects	Type 2 diabetes • chronic obstructive pulmonary disease[1]

(continued)

Subclass	Mechanism of Action	Effects	Clinical Applications
SUBSTANCE P ANTAGONISTS			
• Aprepitant	Selective antagonist of tachykinin NK_1 receptors	Blocks several central nervous system effects of substance P	Prevention of chemotherapy-induced nausea and vomiting
• *Fosaprepitant: Prodrug that is converted to aprepitant*			
NEUROTENSIN AGONISTS			
• PD149163	Agonist of central neurotensin receptors	Interacts with central dopamine systems	Potential for treatment of schizophrenia and Parkinson's disease
NEUROTENSIN ANTAGONISTS			
• Meclinertant	Antagonist of central and peripheral neurotensin receptors	Blocks some central and peripheral (vasodilator) actions of neurotensin	None identified
CALCITONIN GENE-RELATED PEPTIDE ANTAGONISTS			
• Telcagepant, *olcegepant*	Antagonists of the calcitonin gene-related peptide (CGRP) receptor	Blocks some central and peripheral (vasodilator) actions of CGRP	Migraine[1]
NEUROPEPTIDE Y ANTAGONISTS			
• BIBP3226	Selective antagonist of neuropeptide Y_1 receptors	Blocks vasoconstrictor response to neurotensin	Potential antiobesity agent
• *BIIE0246: Selective for Y_2 receptor*			
• *MK-0557: Selective for Y_5 receptor*			
UROTENSIN ANTAGONISTS			
• Palosuran	Antagonist of urotensin receptors	Blocks vasoconstrictor action of urotensin	Diabetic renal failure[1]

[1]Undergoing preclinical or clinical evaluation.

REFERENCES

Angiotensin

Balakumar P, Jagadeesh G: Cardiovascular and renal pathologic implications of pro-renin, renin, and the (pro)renin receptor: Promising young players from the old renin-angiotensin-aldosterone system. J Cardiovasc Pharmacol 2010;56:570.

Beierwaltes WH: The role of calcium in the regulation of renin secretion. Am J Physiol Renal Physiol 2010;298:F1.

Castrop H et al: Physiology of kidney renin. Physiol Rev 2010;90:607.

Ichihara A et al: New approaches to blockade of the renin-angiotensin-aldosterone system: Characteristics and usefulness of the direct renin inhibitor aliskiren. J Pharmacol Sci 2009;113:296.

Ichihara A et al: Renin, prorenin and the kidney: A new chapter in an old saga. J Nephrol 2009;22:306.

Kurtz A: Renin release: Sites, mechanisms, and control. Annu Rev Physiol 2011;73:377.

Matt P et al: Recent advances in understanding Marfan syndrome: Should we now treat surgical patients with losartan? J Thorac Cardiovasc Surg 2008;135:389.

McMurray JJ et al: Effect of valsartan on the incidence of diabetes and cardiovascular events. N Engl J Med 2010;362:1477.

Nguyen G: Renin, (pro)renin and receptor: An update. Clin Sci (Lond) 2011;120:169.

Sihn G et al: Physiology of the (pro)renin receptor: Wnt of change? Kidney Int 2010;78:246.

Uresin Y et al: Efficacy and safety of the direct renin inhibitor aliskiren and ramipril alone or in combination in patients with diabetes and hypertension. J Renin Angiotensin Aldosterone Syst 2007;8:190.

Varagic J et al: New angiotensins. J Mol Med 2008;86:663.

Zheng Z et al: A systematic review and meta-analysis of aliskiren and angiotensin receptor blockers in the management of essential hypertension. J Renin Angiotensin Aldosterone Syst 2011;12:102

Kinins

Cicardi M et al: Ecallantide for the treatment of acute attacks in hereditary angioedema. N Engl J Med 2010;363:523.

Cicardi M et al: Icatibant, a new bradykinin-receptor antagonist, in hereditary angioedema. N Engl J Med 2010;363:532.

Costa-Neto CM et al: Participation of kallikrein-kinin system in different pathologies. Int Immunopharmacol 2008;8:135.

Leeb-Lundberg LM et al: International union of pharmacology. XLV. Classification of the kinin receptor family: From molecular mechanisms to pathophysiological consequences. Pharmacol Rev 2005;57:27.

Longhurst HJ: Management of acute attacks of hereditary angioedema: Potential role of icatibant. Vasc Health Risk Manag 2010;6:795.

Vasopressin

Lange M, Ertmer C, Westphal M: Vasopressin vs. terlipressin in the treatment of cardiovascular failure in sepsis. Intensive Care Med 2008;34:821.

Manning M et al: Peptide and non-peptide agonists and antagonists for the vasopressin and oxytocin V1a, V1b, V2 and OT receptors: Research tools and potential therapeutic agents. Prog Brain Res 2008;170:473.

Maybauer MO et al: Physiology of the vasopressin receptors. Best Pract Res Clin Anaesthesiol 2008;22:253.

Natriuretic Peptides

Federico C: Natriuretic peptide system and cardiovascular disease. Heart Views 2010;11:1.

Luss H et al: Renal effects of ularitide in patients with decompensated heart failure. Am Heart J 2008;155:1012.

Saito Y: Roles of atrial natriuretic peptide and its therapeutic use. J Cardiol 2010;56:262.

Vogel MW, Chen HH: Novel natriuretic peptides: New compounds and new approaches. Curr Heart Fail Rep 2011;8:22.

Endothelins

Cartin-Ceba R et al: Safety and efficacy of ambrisentan for the therapy of portopulmonary hypertension. Chest 2011;139:109.

Kasimay O et al: Diet-supported aerobic exercise reduces blood endothelin-1 and nitric oxide levels in individuals with impaired glucose tolerance. J Clin Lipidol 2010;4:427.

Kawanabe Y, Nauli SM: Endothelin. Cell Mol Life Sci 2011;68:195.

Tostes RC et al: Endothelin, sex and hypertension. Clin Sci (Lond) 2008;114:85.

Vasoactive Intestinal Peptide

Onoue S, Misaka S, Yamada S: Structure-activity relationship of vasoactive intestinal peptide (VIP): Potent agonists and potential clinical applications. Naunyn Schmiedebergs Arch Pharmacol 2008;377:579.

White CM et al: Therapeutic potential of vasoactive intestinal peptide and its receptors in neurological disorders. CNS Neurol Disord Drug Targets 2010;9:661.

Substance P

Curran MP, Robinson DM: Aprepitant: A review of its use in the prevention of nausea and vomiting. Drugs 2009;69:1853.

Hokfelt T, Pernow B, Wahren J: Substance P: A pioneer amongst neuropeptides. J Intern Med 2001;249:27.

Mizuta K et al: Expression and coupling of neurokinin receptor subtypes to inositol phosphate and calcium signaling pathways in human airway smooth muscle cells. Am J Physiol Lung Cell Mol Physiol 2008;294:L523.

Navari RM: Fosaprepitant: A neurokinin-1 receptor antagonist for the prevention of chemotherapy-induced nausea and vomiting. Expert Rev Anticancer Ther 2008;8:1733.

Neurotensin

Boules M et al: Neurotensin agonists: Potential in the treatment of schizophrenia. CNS Drugs 2007;21:13.

Ferraro L et al: Emerging evidence for neurotensin receptor 1 antagonists as novel pharmaceutics in neurodegenerative disorders. Mini Rev Med Chem 2009;9:1429.

Hwang JI et al: Phylogenetic history, pharmacological features, and signal transduction of neurotensin receptors in vertebrates. Ann N Y Acad Sci 2009;1163:169.

Katsanos GS et al: Biology of neurotensin: Revisited study. Int J Immunopathol Pharmacol 2008;21:255.

Calcitonin Gene-Related Peptide

Edvinsson L, Ho TW: CGRP receptor antagonism and migraine. Neurotherapeutics 2010;7:164.

Villalon CM, Olesen J: The role of CGRP in the pathophysiology of migraine and efficacy of CGRP receptor antagonists as acute antimigraine drugs. Pharmacol Ther 2009;124:309.

Walker CS et al: Regulation of signal transduction by calcitonin gene-related peptide receptors. Trends Pharmacol Sci 2010;31:476.

Adrenomedullin

Bell D, McDermott BJ: Intermedin (adrenomedullin-2): A novel counter-regulatory peptide in the cardiovascular and renal systems. Br J Pharmacol 2008;153(Suppl 1):S247.

Yanagawa B, Nagaya N: Adrenomedullin: Molecular mechanisms and its role in cardiac disease. Amino Acids 2007;32:157.

Neuropeptide Y

Brothers SP, Wahlestedt C: Therapeutic potential of neuropeptide Y (NPY) receptor ligands. EMBO Mol Med 2010;2:429.

Parker SL, Balasubramaniam A: Neuropeptide Y Y2 receptor in health and disease. Br J Pharmacol 2008;153:420.

Thorsell A: Brain neuropeptide Y and corticotropin-releasing hormone in mediating stress and anxiety. Exp Biol Med 2010;235:1163.

Urotensin

Cheriyan J et al: The effects of urotensin II and urantide on forearm blood flow and systemic haemodynamics in humans. Br J Clin Pharmacol 2009;68:518.

McDonald J, Batuwangala M, Lambert DG: Role of urotensin II and its receptor in health and disease. J Anesth 2007;21:378.

Russell FD: Urotensin II in cardiovascular regulation. Vasc Health Risk Manag 2008;4:775.

General

Paulis L, Unger T: Novel therapeutic targets for hypertension. Nat Rev Cardiol 2010;7:431.

Takahashi K et al: The renin-angiotensin system, adrenomedullins and urotensin II in the kidney: Possible renoprotection via the kidney peptide systems. Peptides 2009;30:1575.

CASE STUDY ANSWER

Enalapril lowers blood pressure by blocking the conversion of angiotensin I to angiotensin II (ANG II). Since converting enzyme also inactivates bradykinin, enalapril increases bradykinin levels, and this is responsible for adverse side effects such as cough and angioedema. This problem could be avoided by using a renin inhibitor, eg, aliskiren, or an ANG II receptor antagonist, eg, losartan, instead of an ACE inhibitor, to block the renin-angiotensin system.

The Eicosanoids: Prostaglandins, Thromboxanes, Leukotrienes, & Related Compounds

Emer M. Smyth, PhD, & Garret A. FitzGerald, MD

The eicosanoids are oxygenation products of polyunsaturated long-chain fatty acids. They are ubiquitous in the animal kingdom and are also found—together with their precursors—in a variety of plants. They constitute a very large family of compounds that are highly potent and display an extraordinarily wide spectrum of biologic activity. Because of their biologic activity, the eicosanoids, their specific receptor antagonists and enzyme inhibitors, and their plant and fish oil precursors have great therapeutic potential.

ARACHIDONIC ACID & OTHER POLYUNSATURATED PRECURSORS

Arachidonic acid (AA), or 5,8,11,14-eicosatetraenoic acid, the most abundant of the eicosanoid precursors, is a 20-carbon (C20) fatty acid containing four double bonds (designated C20:4–6). AA must first be released or mobilized from the sn-2 position of membrane phospholipids by one or more lipases of the phospholipase A_2 (PLA_2) type (Figure 18–1) for eicosanoid synthesis to occur. At least three classes of phospholipases mediate arachidonate release from membrane lipids: cytosolic (c) PLA_2, secretory (s) PLA_2, and calcium-independent (i) PLA_2. Chemical and physical stimuli activate the Ca^{2+}-dependent translocation of group IVA $cPLA_2$, which has high affinity for AA, to the membrane, where it releases arachidonate. Multiple additional PLA_2 isoforms (group VI $iPLA_2$ and $sPLA_2$ from groups IIA, V, and X) have been characterized. Under nonstimulated conditions, AA liberated by $iPLA_2$ is reincorporated into cell membranes, so there is negligible eicosanoid biosynthesis. While $cPLA_2$ dominates in

the acute release of AA, inducible $sPLA_2$ contributes under conditions of sustained or intense stimulation of AA production. AA can also be released by a combination of phospholipase C and diglyceride lipase.

Following mobilization, AA is oxygenated by four separate routes: the cyclooxygenase (COX), lipoxygenase, P450 epoxygenase, and isoeicosanoid pathways (Figure 18–1). Among factors determining the type of eicosanoid synthesized are (1) the substrate lipid species, (2) the type of cell, and (3) the manner in which the cell is stimulated. Distinct but related products can be

ACRONYMS

AA	Arachidonic acid
COX	Cyclooxygenase
DHET	Dihydroxyeicosatrienoic acid
EET	Epoxyeicosatrienoic acid
HETE	Hydroxyeicosatetraenoic acid
HPETE	Hydroxyperoxyeicosatetraenoic acid
LTB, LTC	Leukotriene B, C, etc
LOX	Lipoxygenase
LXA, LXB	Lipoxin A, B
NSAID	Nonsteroidal anti-inflammatory drug
PGE, PGF	Prostaglandin E, F, etc
PLA, PLC	Phospholipase A, C
TXA, TXB	Thromboxane A, B

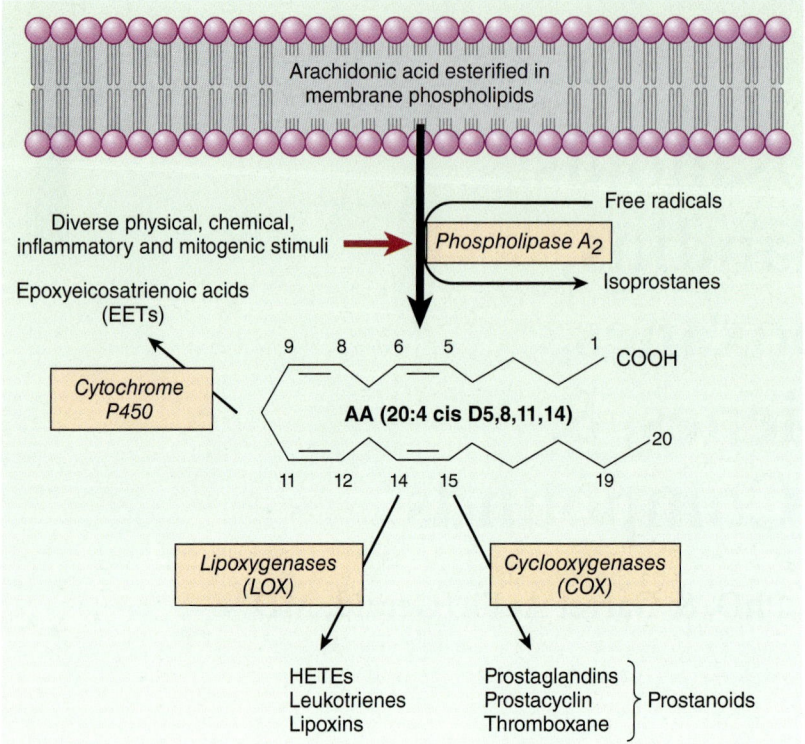

FIGURE 18–1 Pathways of arachidonic acid (AA) release and metabolism.

formed from precursors other than AA. For example, homo-γ-linoleic acid (C20:3–6) or eicosapentaenoic acid (C20:5–3, EPA) yields products that differ quantitatively and qualitatively from those derived from AA. This shift in product formation is the basis for using fatty acids obtained from cold-water fish or from plants as nutritional supplements in humans. For example, thromboxane (TXA$_2$), a powerful vasoconstrictor and platelet agonist, is synthesized from AA via the COX pathway. COX metabolism of EPA yields TXA$_3$, which is relatively inactive. 3-Series prostaglandins, such as prostaglandin E$_3$ (PGE$_3$), can also act as partial agonists or antagonists thereby reducing the activity of their AA-derived 2-series counterparts. The hypothesis that dietary eicosapentaenoate substitution for arachidonate could reduce the incidence of cardiovascular disease and cancer is a focus of current investigation.

SYNTHESIS OF EICOSANOIDS

Products of Prostaglandin Endoperoxide Synthases (Cyclooxygenases)

Two unique COX isozymes convert AA into prostaglandin endoperoxides. PGH synthase-1 (**COX-1**) is expressed constitutively in most cells. In contrast, PGH synthase-2 (**COX-2**) is inducible; its expression varies depending on the stimulus. COX-2 is an immediate early-response gene product that is markedly up-regulated by shear stress, growth factors, tumor promoters, and cytokines. COX-1 generates prostanoids for "housekeeping" such as gastric epithelial cytoprotection, whereas COX-2 is the major source of prostanoids in inflammation and cancer. This distinction is overly simplistic, however; there are both physiologic and pathophysiologic processes in which each enzyme is uniquely involved and others in which they function coordinately. For example, endothelial COX-2 is the primary source of vascular prostacyclin (PGI$_2$), whereas renal COX-2-derived prostanoids are important for normal renal development and maintenance of function. Nonsteroidal anti-inflammatory drugs (NSAIDs; see Chapter 36) exert their therapeutic effects through inhibition of the COXs. Indomethacin and sulindac are slightly selective for COX-1. Meclofenamate and ibuprofen are approximately equipotent on COX-1 and COX-2, whereas celecoxib = diclofenac < rofecoxib = lumiracoxib < etoricoxib in inhibition of COX-2 (listed in order of increasing average selectivity). Aspirin acetylates and inhibits both enzymes covalently. Low doses (< 100 mg/d) inhibit preferentially, but not exclusively, platelet COX-1, whereas higher doses inhibit both systemic COX-1 and COX-2.

Both COX-1 and COX-2 promote the uptake of two molecules of oxygen by cyclization of arachidonic acid to yield a C$_9$–C$_{11}$ endoperoxide C$_{15}$ hydroperoxide (Figure 18–2). This product is PGG$_2$, which is then rapidly modified by the peroxidase moiety of the COX enzyme to add a 15-hydroxyl group that is essential for biologic activity. This product is PGH$_2$. Both endoperoxides are highly unstable. Analogous families—PGH$_1$ and PGH$_3$ and all

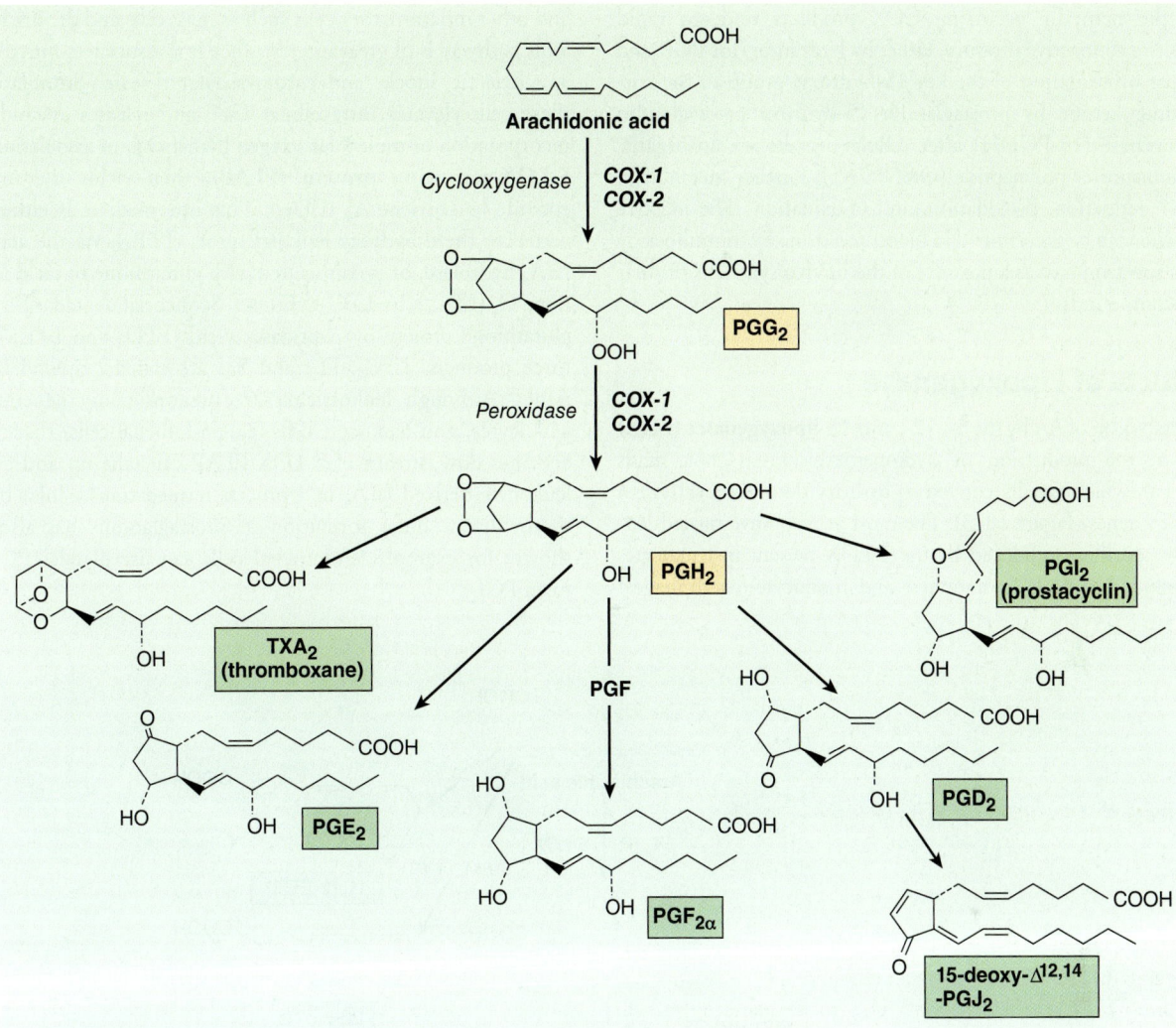

FIGURE 18–2 Prostanoid biosynthesis. Compound names are enclosed in boxes.

their subsequent products—are derived from homo-γ-linolenic acid and eicosapentaenoic acid, respectively.

The prostaglandins, thromboxane, and prostacyclin, collectively termed the prostanoids, are generated from PGH_2 through the action of downstream isomerases and synthases. These terminal enzymes are expressed in a relatively cell-specific fashion, such that most cells make one or two dominant prostanoids. The prostaglandins differ from each other in two ways: (1) in the substituents of the pentane ring (indicated by the last letter, eg, E and F in PGE and PGF) and (2) in the number of double bonds in the side chains (indicated by the subscript, eg, PGE_1, PGE_2). PGH_2 is metabolized by prostacyclin, thromboxane, and PGF synthases (PGIS, TXAS, and PGFS) to PGI_2, TXA_2, and $PGF_{2\alpha}$, respectively. Two additional enzymes, 9,11-endoperoxide reductase and 9-ketoreductase, provide for $PGF_{2\alpha}$ synthesis from PGH_2 and PGE_2, respectively. At least three PGE_2 synthases have been identified: microsomal (m) PGES-1, the more readily inducible mPGES-2, and cytosolic PGES. There are two distinct PGDS isoforms, the lipocalin-type PGDS and the hematopoietic PGDS.

Several products of the arachidonate series are of current clinical importance. **Alprostadil** (PGE_1) may be used for its smooth muscle relaxing effects to maintain the ductus arteriosus patent in some neonates awaiting cardiac surgery and in the treatment of impotence. **Misoprostol,** a PGE_1 derivative, is a cytoprotective prostaglandin used in preventing peptic ulcer and in combination with mifepristone (RU-486) for terminating early pregnancies. **PGE_2** and **PGF_2** are used in obstetrics to induce labor. **Latanoprost** and several similar compounds are topically active $PGF_{2\alpha}$ derivatives used in ophthalmology to treat open-angle glaucoma. **Prostacyclin** (PGI_2, epoprostenol) is synthesized mainly by the vascular endothelium and is a powerful vasodilator and inhibitor of platelet aggregation. It is used clinically to treat pulmonary hypertension and portopulmonary hypertension. In contrast, **thromboxane** (TXA_2) has undesirable properties (aggregation of platelets, vasoconstriction). Therefore TXA_2-receptor antagonists and synthesis inhibitors have been developed for cardiovascular indications, although these (except for aspirin) have yet to establish a place in clinical usage.

All the naturally occurring COX products undergo rapid metabolism to inactive products either by hydration (for PGI$_2$ and TXA$_2$) or by oxidation of the key 15-hydroxyl group to the corresponding ketone by prostaglandin 15-hydroxy prostaglandin dehydrogenase (15-PGDH) after cellular uptake via an organic anion transporter polypeptide (OATP 2A1). Further metabolism is by Δ^{13} reduction, β-oxidation, and ω-oxidation. The inactive metabolites can be determined in blood and urine by immunoassay or mass spectrometry as a measure of the in vivo synthesis of their parent compounds.

Products of Lipoxygenase

The metabolism of AA by the **5-, 12-, and 15-lipoxygenases (LOX)** results in the production of hydroperoxyeicosatetraenoic acids (HPETEs), which rapidly convert to hydroxy derivatives (HETEs) and leukotrienes (Figure 18–3). The most actively investigated leukotrienes are those produced by the 5-LOX present in leukocytes (neutrophils, basophils, eosinophils, and monocyte-macrophages)

and other inflammatory cells such as mast cells and dendritic cells. This pathway is of great interest since it is associated with asthma, anaphylactic shock, and cardiovascular disease. Stimulation of these cells elevates intracellular Ca^{2+} and releases arachidonate; incorporation of molecular oxygen by 5-LOX, in association with **5-LOX-activating protein (FLAP)**, then yields the unstable epoxide leukotriene A$_4$ (LTA$_4$). This intermediate is either converted to the dihydroxy leukotriene B$_4$ (LTB$_4$), via the action of LTA$_4$ hydrolase, or is conjugated with glutathione to yield leukotriene C$_4$ (LTC$_4$), by LTC$_4$ synthase. Sequential degradation of the glutathione moiety by peptidases yields LTD$_4$ and LTE$_4$. These three products, LTC$_4$, D$_4$, and E$_4$, are called cysteinyl leukotrienes. Although leukotrienes are predominantly generated in leukocytes, non-leukocyte cells (eg, endothelial cells) that express enzymes downstream of 5-LOX/FLAP can take up and convert leukocyte-derived LTA$_4$ in a process termed transcellular biosynthesis. Transcellular formation of prostaglandins has also been shown; for example, endothelial cells can use platelet PGH$_2$ to form PGI$_2$.

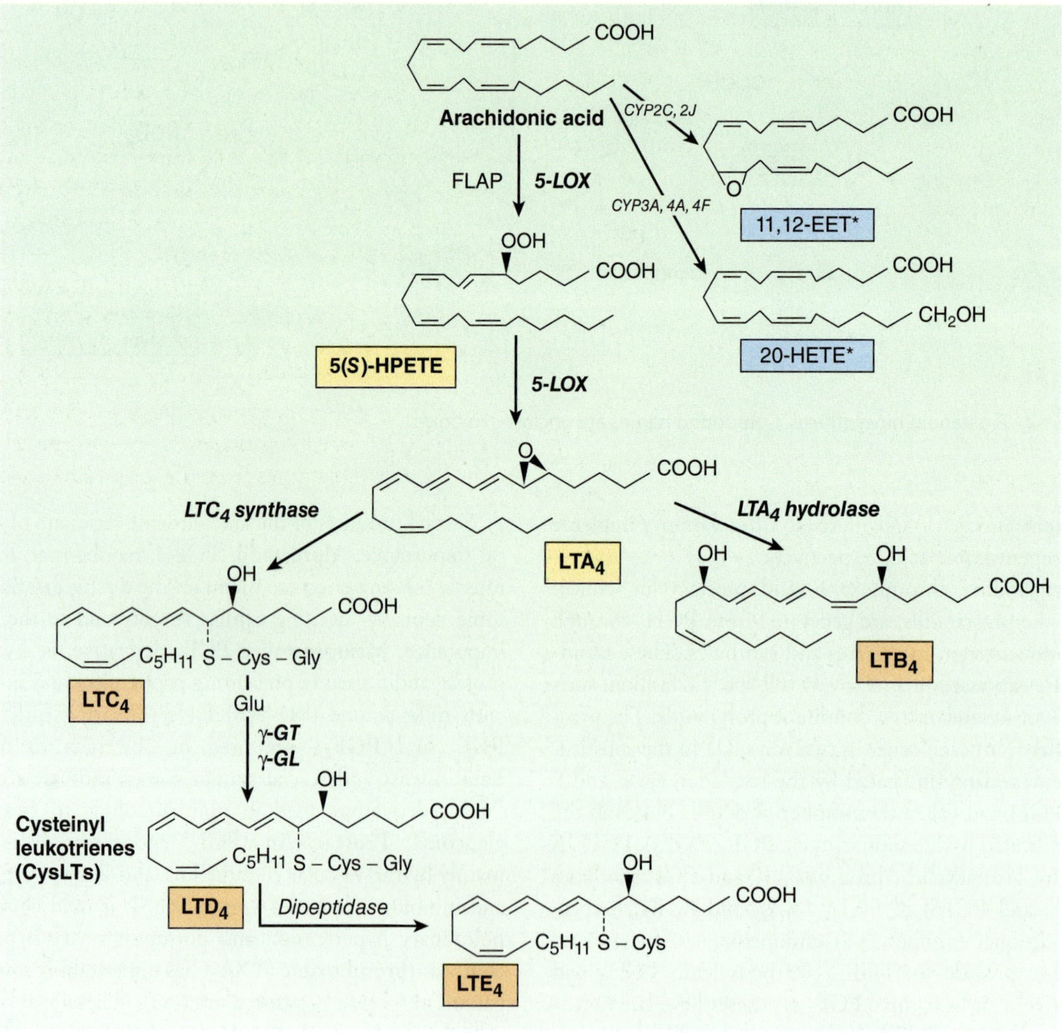

FIGURE 18–3 Leukotriene (LT) biosynthesis. LTC$_4$, LTD$_4$, and LTE$_4$ are known collectively as the cysteinyl (Cys) LTs. FLAP, 5-LOX-activating protein; GT, glutamyl transpeptidase; GL, glutamyl leukotrienase. *Additional products include 5,6-; 8,9-; and 14,15-EET; and 19-, 18-, 17-, and 16-HETE.

LTC$_4$ and **LTD$_4$** are potent bronchoconstrictors and are recognized as the primary components of the **slow-reacting substance of anaphylaxis (SRS-A)** that is secreted in asthma and anaphylaxis. There are four current approaches to antileukotriene drug development: 5-LOX enzyme inhibitors, leukotriene-receptor antagonists, inhibitors of FLAP, and phospholipase A$_2$ inhibitors.

LTA$_4$, the primary product of 5-LOX, can be converted with appropriate stimulation via 12-LOX in platelets to the **lipoxins** LXA$_4$ and LXB$_4$ in vitro. These mediators can also be generated through 5-LOX metabolism of 15-HETE, the product of 15-LOX-2 metabolism of arachidonic acid. 15-LOX-1 prefers linoleic acid as a substrate forming 15S-hydroxyoctadecadienoic acid. The stereochemical isomer, 15(R)-HETE, may be derived from the action of aspirin-acetylated COX-2 and further transformed in leukocytes by 5-LOX to 15-epi-LXA$_4$ or 15-epi-LXB$_4$, the so-called aspirin-triggered lipoxins. Synthetic lipoxins and epi-lipoxins exert anti-inflammatory actions when applied in vivo. Although these compounds can be formed from endogenous substrates in vitro and when synthesized may have potent biologic effects, the importance of the endogenous compounds in vivo in human biology remains ill defined. 12-HETE, a product of 12-LOX, can also undergo a catalyzed molecular rearrangement to epoxyhydroxyeicosatrienoic acids called **hepoxilins.** Proinflammatory effects of synthetic hepoxilins have been reported although their biologic relevance is unclear.

The LOXs located in epidermal cells are distinct from "conventional" enzymes—arachidonic acid and linoleic acid are apparently not the natural substrates for epidermal LOX. Epidermal accumulation of 12(R)-HETE is a feature of psoriasis and ichthyosis and inhibitors of 12(R)-LOX are under investigation for the treatment of these proliferative skin disorders.

Epoxygenase Products

Specific isozymes of microsomal cytochrome P450 monooxygenases convert AA to hydroxy- or epoxyeicosatrienoic acids (Figures 18–1 and 18–3). The products are 20-HETE, generated by the CYP hydroxylases (CYP3A, 4A, 4F) and the 5,6-, 8,9-, 11,12-, and 14,15-epoxyeicosatrienoic acids (EETs), which arise from the CYP epoxygenase (2J, 2C). Their biosynthesis can be altered by pharmacologic, nutritional, and genetic factors that affect P450 expression. The biologic actions of the EETs are reduced by their conversion to the corresponding, and biologically less active, dihydroxyeicosatrienoic acids (DHETs) through the action of soluble epoxide hydrolase (sEH). Unlike the prostaglandins, the EETs can be esterified into phospholipids, which then act as storage sites. Intracellular fatty acid-binding proteins promote EET uptake into cells, incorporation into phospholipids, and availability to sEH. EETs are synthesized in endothelial cells and cause vasodilation in a number of vascular beds by activating the smooth muscle large conductance Ca^{2+}-activated K$^+$ channels. This results in smooth muscle cell hyperpolarization and vasodilation, leading to reduced blood pressure. Substantial evidence indicates that EETs may function as **endothelium-derived hyperpolarizing factors,** particularly in the coronary circulation. Consequently there is interest in inhibitors of soluble sEH as potential antithrombotic and anti-

hypertensive drugs. An exception to the general response to EETs as vasodilators is the pulmonary vasculature where they cause vasoconstriction. It is unclear yet whether this activity of EETs may limit the potential clinical use of sEH inhibitors. Downregulation of pulmonary sEH may contribute to pulmonary hypertension. Anti-inflammatory, antiapoptotic, and proangiogenic actions of the EETs have also been reported.

Isoeicosanoids

The isoeicosanoids, a family of eicosanoid isomers, are formed nonenzymatically by direct free radical-based action on AA and related lipid substrates. Isoprostanes are prostaglandin stereoisomers. Because prostaglandins have many asymmetric centers, they have a large number of potential stereoisomers. COX is not needed for the formation of the isoprostanes, and its inhibition with aspirin or other NSAIDs should not affect the isoprostane pathway. The primary epimerization mechanism is peroxidation of arachidonate by free radicals. Peroxidation occurs while arachidonic acid is still esterified to the membrane phospholipids. Thus, unlike prostaglandins, these stereoisomers are "stored" as part of the membrane. They are then cleaved by phospholipases, circulate, and are excreted in urine. Isoprostanes are present in relatively large amounts (tenfold greater in blood and urine than the COX-derived prostaglandins). They have potent vasoconstrictor effects when infused into renal and other vascular beds and may activate prostanoid receptors. They also may modulate other aspects of vascular function, including leukocyte and platelet adhesive interactions and angiogenesis. It has been speculated that they may contribute to the pathophysiology of inflammatory responses in a manner insensitive to COX inhibitors. A particular difficulty in assessing the likely biologic functions of isoprostanes—several of which have been shown to serve as incidental ligands at prostaglandin receptors—is that while high concentrations of individual isoprostanes may be necessary to elicit a response, multiple compounds are formed coincidentally in vivo under conditions of oxidant stress. Analogous leukotriene and EET isomers have been described.

■ BASIC PHARMACOLOGY OF EICOSANOIDS

MECHANISMS & EFFECTS OF EICOSANOIDS

Receptor Mechanisms

As a result of their short half-lives, the eicosanoids act mainly in an autocrine and a paracrine fashion, ie, close to the site of their synthesis, and not as circulating hormones. These ligands bind to receptors on the cell surface, and pharmacologic specificity is determined by receptor density and type on different cells (Figure 18–4). A single gene product has been identified for the PGI$_2$ (IP), PGF$_{2\alpha}$ (FP), and TXA$_2$ (TP) receptors, while four distinct PGE$_2$ receptors (EPs 1–4) and two PGD$_2$ receptors (DP$_1$ and

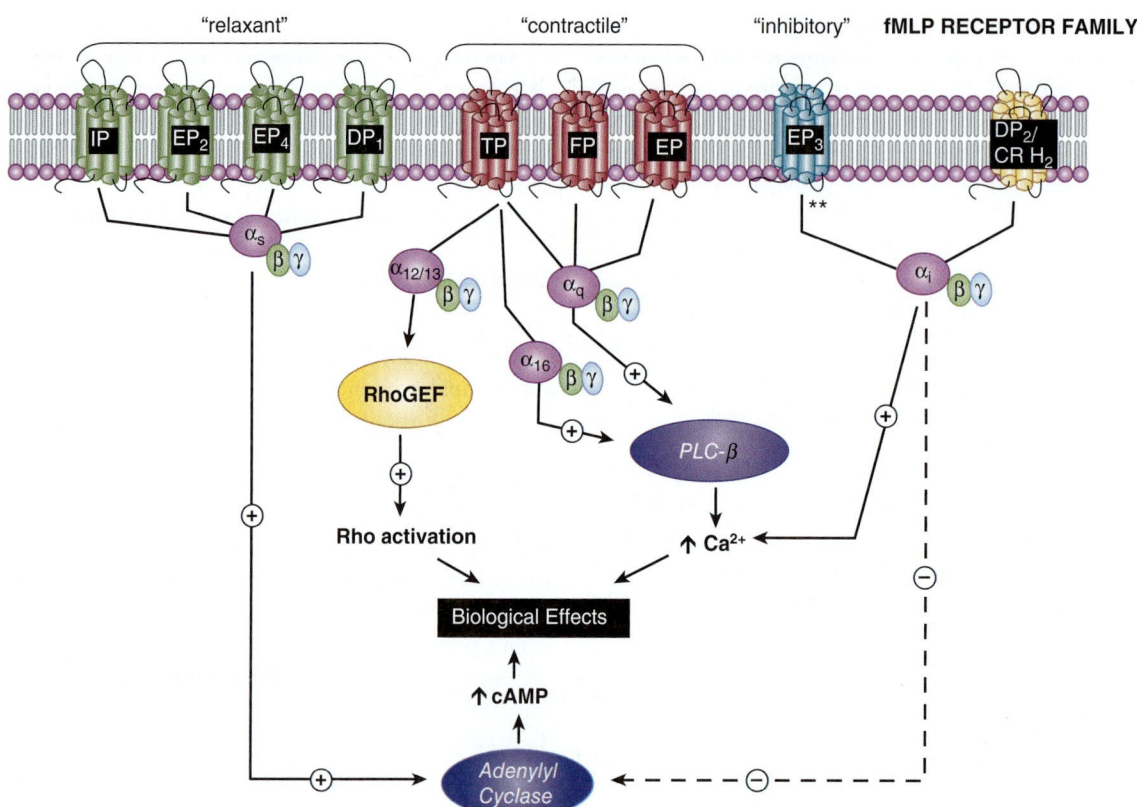

FIGURE 18–4 Prostanoid receptors and their signaling pathways. fMLP, formylated MetLeuPhe, a small peptide receptor; PLC-β, phospholipase C-β. All of the receptors shown are of the seven-transmembrane, G protein-coupled type. The terms "relaxant," "contractile," and "inhibitory" refer to the phylogenetic characterization of their primary effects. **All EP$_3$ isoforms couple through G$_i$ but some can also activate G$_s$ or G$_{12/13}$ pathways. RhoGEF, rho guanine nucleotide exchange factor. See text for additional details.

DP$_2$) have been cloned. Additional isoforms of the human TP (α and β), FP (A and B), and EP$_3$ (I, II, III, IV, V, VI, e, and f) receptors can arise through differential mRNA splicing. Two receptors exist for both LTB$_4$ (BLT$_1$ and BLT$_2$) and the cysteinyl leukotrienes (cysLT$_1$ and cysLT$_2$). The formyl peptide (fMLP)-1 receptor can be activated by lipoxin A4 and consequently has been termed the ALX receptor. All of these receptors are G protein-coupled; properties of the best-studied receptors are listed in Table 18–1.

EP$_2$, EP$_4$, IP, and DP$_1$ receptors activate adenylyl cyclase via G$_s$. This leads to increased intracellular cAMP levels, which in turn activate specific protein kinases (see Chapter 2). EP$_1$, FP, and TP activate phosphatidylinositol metabolism, leading to the formation of inositol trisphosphate, with subsequent mobilization of Ca^{2+} stores and an increase of free intracellular Ca^{2+}. TP also couples to multiple G proteins, including G$_{12/13}$ and G$_{16}$, to stimulate small G protein signaling pathways, and may activate or inhibit adenylyl cyclase via G$_s$ (TPα) or G$_i$ (TPβ), respectively. EP$_3$ isoforms can couple to both elevation of intracellular calcium and to increased or decreased cAMP. The DP$_2$ receptor (also known as the chemoattractant receptor-homologous molecule expressed on TH2 cells, or CRTH2), which is unrelated to the other prostanoid receptors, is a member of the fMLP (formylated MetLeuPhe) receptor superfamily. This receptor couples through

a G$_i$-type G protein and leads to inhibition of cAMP synthesis and increases in intracellular Ca^{2+} in a variety of cell types.

LTB$_4$ also causes inositol trisphosphate release via the BLT$_1$ receptor, causing activation, degranulation, and superoxide anion generation in leukocytes. The BLT$_2$ receptor, a low-affinity receptor for LTB$_4$, is also bound with reasonable affinity by 12(S)- and 12(R)-HETE, although the biologic relevance of this observation is not clear. CysLT$_1$ and cysLT$_2$ couple to G$_q$, leading to increased intracellular Ca^{2+}. Studies have also placed G$_i$ downstream of cysLT$_2$. An orphan receptor, GPR17, binds cysLTs and may negatively regulate the function of cysLT$_1$, but its physiologic role remains ill defined. As noted above, the EETs promote vasodilation via paracrine activation of calcium-activated potassium channels on smooth muscle cells leading to hyperpolarization and relaxation. This occurs in a manner consistent with activation of a G$_s$-coupled receptor, although a specific EET receptor has yet to be identified. EETs may also act in an autocrine manner directly activating endothelial transient receptor potential channels to cause endothelial hyperpolarization, which is then transferred to the smooth muscle cells by gap junctions or potassium ions. Specific receptors for isoprostanes have not been identified, and the biologic importance of their capacity to act as incidental ligands at prostaglandin receptors remains to be established.

TABLE 18–1 Eicosanoid receptors.[1]

Receptor (human)	Endogenous Ligand	Secondary Ligands	G Protein; Second Messenger	Major Phenotype(s) in Knockout Mice
DP_1	PGD_2		G_s; $\uparrow$cAMP	$\downarrow$Allergic asthma
DP_2, CRT_H2	PGD_2	15d-PGJ_2	G_i; $\uparrow Ca^{2+}_i$, $\downarrow$cAMP	$\uparrow$Allergic airway inflammation $\downarrow$Cutaneous inflammation
EP_1	PGE_2	PGI_2	G_q; $\uparrow Ca^{2+}_i$	$\downarrow$Colon carcinogenesis
EP_2	PGE_2		G_s; $\uparrow$cAMP	Impaired ovulation and fertilization
				Salt-sensitive hypertension
$EP_{3\ I, II, III, IV, V, VI, e, f}$	PGE_2		G_i; $\downarrow$cAMP, $\uparrow Ca^{2+}_i$	Resistance to pyrogens
			G_s; $\uparrow$cAMP	$\downarrow$Acute cutaneous inflammation
			G_q; $\uparrow$PLC, $\uparrow Ca^{2+}_i$	
EP_4	PGE_2		G_s; $\uparrow$cAMP	$\downarrow$Bone mass/density in aged mice
				$\uparrow$Bowel inflammatory/immune response
				$\downarrow$Colon carcinogenesis
				Patent ductus arteriosus
$FP_{A,B}$	$PGF_{2\alpha}$	isoPs	G_q; $\uparrow$PLC, $\uparrow Ca^{2+}_i$	Parturition failure
IP	PGI_2	PGE_2	G_s; $\uparrow$cAMP	$\uparrow$Thrombotic response
				$\uparrow$Response to vascular injury
				$\uparrow$Atherosclerosis
				$\uparrow$Cardiac fibrosis
				Salt-sensitive hypertension
				$\downarrow$Joint inflammation
$TP_{\alpha,\beta}$	TXA_2	isoPs	G_q, $G_{12/13}$, G_{16}; $\uparrow$PLC, $\uparrow Ca^{2+}_i$, Rho activation	$\uparrow$Bleeding time
				$\downarrow$Response to vascular injury
				$\downarrow$Atherosclerosis
				$\uparrow$Survival after cardiac allograft
BLT_1	LTB_4		G_{16}, G_i; $\uparrow Ca^{2+}_i$, $\downarrow$cAMP	Some suppression of inflammatory response
BLT_2	LTB_4	12(S)-HETE	G_q-like, G_i-like, G_{12}-like, $\uparrow Ca^{2+}_i$	Not known
		12(R)-HETE		
$CysLT_1$	LTD_4	LTC_4/LTE_4	G_q; $\uparrow$PLC, $\uparrow Ca^{2+}_i$	$\downarrow$Innate and adaptive immune vascular permeability response
				$\uparrow$Pulmonary inflammatory and fibrotic response
$CysLT_2$	LTC_4/LTD_4	LTE_4	G_q; $\uparrow$PLC, $\uparrow Ca^{2+}_i$	$\downarrow$Pulmonary inflammatory and fibrotic response

[1]Splice variants for the eicosanoid receptors are indicated where appropriate.

Ca^{2+}_i, intracellular calcium; cAMP, cyclic adenosine 3′,5′-monophosphate; PLC, phospholipase C; isoPs, isoprostanes; 15d-PGJ_2, 15-deoxy-$\Delta^{12,14}$-PGJ_2.

Although prostanoids can activate peroxisome proliferator-activated receptors (PPARs) if added in sufficient concentration in vitro, it remains questionable whether these compounds attain concentrations sufficient to function as endogenous nuclear-receptor ligands in vivo.

Effects of Prostaglandins & Thromboxanes

The prostaglandins and thromboxanes have major effects on smooth muscle in the vasculature, airways, and gastrointestinal and reproductive tracts. Contraction of smooth muscle is mediated by the release of calcium, while relaxing effects are mediated by the generation of cAMP. Many of the eicosanoids' contractile effects on smooth muscle can be inhibited by lowering extracellular calcium or by using calcium channel-blocking drugs. Other important targets include platelets and monocytes, kidneys, the central nervous system, autonomic presynaptic nerve terminals, sensory nerve endings, endocrine organs, adipose tissue, and the eye (the effects on the eye may involve smooth muscle).

A. Smooth Muscle

1. Vascular—TXA_2 is a potent vasoconstrictor. It is also a smooth muscle cell mitogen and is the only eicosanoid that has convincingly been shown to have this effect. The mitogenic effect is potentiated by exposure of smooth muscle cells to testosterone, which up-regulates smooth muscle cell TP expression. $PGF_{2\alpha}$ is also a vasoconstrictor but is not a smooth muscle mitogen. Another vasoconstrictor is the isoprostane 8-iso-$PGF_{2\alpha}$, also known as $iPF_{2\alpha}III$, which may act via the TP receptor.

Vasodilator prostaglandins, especially PGI_2 and PGE_2, promote vasodilation by increasing cAMP and decreasing smooth muscle intracellular calcium, primarily via the IP and EP_4 receptors. Vascular PGI_2 is synthesized by both smooth muscle and endothelial cells, with the COX-2 isoform in the latter cell type being the major contributor. In the microcirculation, PGE_2 is a vasodilator produced by endothelial cells. PGI_2 inhibits proliferation of smooth muscle cells, an action that may be particularly relevant in pulmonary hypertension. PGD_2 may also function as a vasodilator—in particular as a dominant mediator of flushing induced by the lipid-lowering drug niacin—although the role of this prostanoid in the cardiovascular system remains under investigation.

2. Gastrointestinal tract—Most of the prostaglandins and thromboxanes activate gastrointestinal smooth muscle. Longitudinal muscle is contracted by PGE_2 (via EP_3) and $PGF_{2\alpha}$ (via FP), whereas circular muscle is contracted strongly by $PGF_{2\alpha}$ and weakly by PGI_2, and is relaxed by PGE_2 (via EP_4). Administration of either PGE_2 or $PGF_{2\alpha}$ results in colicky cramps (see Clinical Pharmacology of Eicosanoids, below). The leukotrienes also have powerful contractile effects.

3. Airways—Respiratory smooth muscle is relaxed by PGE_2 and PGI_2 and contracted by PGD_2, TXA_2, and $PGF_{2\alpha}$. Studies of DP_1 and DP_2 receptor knockout mice suggest an important role of this prostanoid in asthma, although the DP_2 receptor appears more relevant to allergic airway diseases. The cysteinyl leukotrienes are also bronchoconstrictors. They act principally on smooth muscle in peripheral airways and are a thousand times more potent than histamine, both in vitro and in vivo. They also stimulate bronchial mucus secretion and cause mucosal edema. Bronchospasm occurs in about 10% of people taking NSAIDs, possibly because of a shift in arachidonate metabolism from COX metabolism to leukotriene formation.

4. Reproductive—The actions of prostaglandins on reproductive smooth muscle are discussed below under section D, Reproductive Organs.

B. Platelets

Platelet aggregation is markedly affected by eicosanoids. Low concentrations of PGE_2 enhance (via EP_3), whereas higher concentrations inhibit (via IP), platelet aggregation. Both PGD_2 and PGI_2 inhibit aggregation via, respectively, DP_1- and IP-dependent elevation in cAMP generation. Unlike their human counterparts, mouse platelets do not express DP_1. TXA_2 is the major product of COX-1, the only COX isoform expressed in mature platelets. Itself a platelet aggregator, TXA_2 amplifies the effects of other, more potent, platelet agonists such as thrombin. The TP-G_q signaling pathway elevates intracellular Ca^{2+} and activates protein kinase C, facilitating platelet aggregation and TXA_2 biosynthesis. Activation of G_{12}/G_{13} induces Rho/Rho-kinase–dependent regulation of myosin light chain phosphorylation leading to platelet shape change. Mutations in the human TP have been associated with mild bleeding disorders. The platelet actions of TXA_2 are restrained in vivo by PGI_2, which inhibits platelet aggregation by all recognized agonists. Platelet COX-1-derived TXA_2 biosynthesis is increased during platelet activation and aggregation and is irreversibly inhibited by chronic administration of aspirin at low doses. Urinary metabolites of TXA_2 increase in clinical syndromes of platelet activation such as myocardial infarction and stroke. Macrophage COX-2 appears to contribute roughly 10% of the increment in TXA_2 biosynthesis observed in smokers, while the rest is derived from platelet COX-1. A variable contribution, presumably from macrophage COX-2, may be insensitive to the effects of low-dose aspirin. In a single trial comparing low- and high-dose aspirin, no increase in benefit was associated with increased dose; in fact, this study, as well as indirect comparisons across placebo-controlled trials, suggests an inverse dose-response relationship, perhaps reflecting increasing inhibition of PGI_2 synthesis at higher doses of aspirin.

C. Kidney

Both the medulla and the cortex of the kidney synthesize prostaglandins, the medulla substantially more than the cortex. COX-1 is expressed mainly in cortical and medullary collecting ducts and mesangial cells, arteriolar endothelium, and epithelial cells of Bowman's capsule. COX-2 is restricted to the renal medullary interstitial cells, the macula densa, and the cortical thick ascending limb.

The major renal eicosanoid products are PGE_2 and PGI_2, followed by $PGF_{2\alpha}$ and TXA_2. The kidney also synthesizes several hydroxyeicosatetraenoic acids, leukotrienes, cytochrome P450 products, and epoxides. Prostaglandins play important roles in maintaining blood pressure and regulating renal function, particularly in marginally functioning kidneys and volume-contracted states. Under these circumstances, renal cortical COX-2-derived PGE_2 and PGI_2 maintain renal blood flow and glomerular filtration rate through their local vasodilating effects. These prostaglandins also modulate systemic blood pressure through regulation of water and sodium excretion. Expression of medullary COX-2 and mPGES-1 is increased under conditions of high salt intake. COX-2-derived prostanoids increase medullary blood flow and inhibit tubular sodium reabsorption, while COX-1-derived products promote salt excretion in the collecting ducts. Increased water clearance probably results from an attenuation of the action of antidiuretic hormone (ADH) on adenylyl cyclase. Loss of these effects may underlie the systemic or salt-sensitive hypertension often associated with COX inhibition. A common misperception—often articulated in discussion of the cardiovascular toxicity of drugs such as rofecoxib—is that hypertension secondary to NSAID administration is somehow independent of the inhibition of prostaglandins. Loop diuretics, eg, furosemide, produce some of their effect by stimulating COX activity. In the normal kidney, this increases the synthesis of the vasodilator prostaglandins. Therefore, patient response to a loop diuretic is diminished if a COX inhibitor is administered concurrently (see Chapter 15).

There is an additional layer of complexity associated with the effects of renal prostaglandins. In contrast to the medullary enzyme, cortical COX-2 expression is increased by low salt intake, leading to increased renin release. This elevates glomerular filtration rate and contributes to enhanced sodium reabsorption and a rise in blood pressure. PGE_2 is thought to stimulate renin release through activation of EP_4 or EP_2. PGI_2 can also stimulate renin release and this may be relevant to maintenance of blood pressure in volume-contracted conditions and to the pathogenesis of renovascular hypertension. Inhibition of COX-2 may reduce blood pressure in these settings.

TXA_2 causes intrarenal vasoconstriction (and perhaps an ADH-like effect), resulting in a decline in renal function. The normal kidney synthesizes only small amounts of TXA_2. However, in renal conditions involving inflammatory cell infiltration (such as glomerulonephritis and renal transplant rejection), the inflammatory cells (monocyte-macrophages) release substantial amounts of TXA_2. Theoretically, TXA_2 synthase inhibitors or receptor antagonists should improve renal function in these patients, but no such drug is clinically available. Hypertension is associated with increased TXA_2 and decreased PGE_2 and PGI_2 synthesis in some animal models, eg, the Goldblatt kidney model. It is not known whether these changes are primary contributing factors or secondary responses. Similarly, increased TXA_2 formation has been reported in cyclosporine-induced nephrotoxicity, but no causal relationship has been established. $PGF_{2\alpha}$ may elevate blood pressure by regulating renin release in the kidney. Although more research is necessary, FP antagonists have potential as novel antihypertensive drugs.

D. Reproductive Organs

1. Female reproductive organs—Animal studies demonstrate a role for PGE_2 and $PGF_{2\alpha}$ in early reproductive processes

such as ovulation, luteolysis, and fertilization. Uterine muscle is contracted by $PGF_{2\alpha}$, TXA_2, and low concentrations of PGE_2; PGI_2 and high concentrations of PGE_2 cause relaxation. $PGF_{2\alpha}$, together with oxytocin, is essential for the onset of parturition. The effects of prostaglandins on uterine function are discussed below (see Clinical Pharmacology of Eicosanoids).

2. Male reproductive organs—Despite the discovery of prostaglandins in seminal fluid, and their uterotropic effects, the role of prostaglandins in semen is still conjectural. The major source of these prostaglandins is the seminal vesicle; the prostate, despite the name "prostaglandin," and the testes synthesize only small amounts. The factors that regulate the concentration of prostaglandins in human seminal plasma are not known in detail, but testosterone does promote prostaglandin production. Thromboxane and leukotrienes have not been found in seminal plasma. Men with a low seminal fluid concentration of prostaglandins are relatively infertile.

Smooth muscle-relaxing prostaglandins such as PGE_1 enhance penile erection by relaxing the smooth muscle of the corpora cavernosa (see Clinical Pharmacology of Eicosanoids).

E. Central and Peripheral Nervous Systems

1. Fever—PGE_2 increases body temperature, predominantly via EP_3, although EP_1 also plays a role, especially when administered directly into the cerebral ventricles. Exogenous $PGF_{2\alpha}$ and PGI_2 induce fever, whereas PGD_2 and TXA_2 do not. Endogenous pyrogens release interleukin-1, which in turn promotes the synthesis and release of PGE_2. This synthesis is blocked by aspirin and other antipyretic compounds.

2. Sleep—When infused into the cerebral ventricles, PGD_2 induces natural sleep (as determined by electroencephalographic analysis) via activation of DP_1 receptors and secondary release of adenosine. PGE_2 infusion into the posterior hypothalamus causes wakefulness.

3. Neurotransmission—PGE compounds inhibit the release of norepinephrine from postganglionic sympathetic nerve endings. Moreover, NSAIDs increase norepinephrine release in vivo, suggesting that the prostaglandins play a physiologic role in this process. Thus, vasoconstriction observed during treatment with COX inhibitors may be due, in part, to increased release of norepinephrine as well as to inhibition of the endothelial synthesis of the vasodilators PGE_2 and PGI_2. PGE_2 and PGI_2 sensitize the peripheral nerve endings to painful stimuli by increasing their terminal membrane excitability. Prostaglandins also modulate pain centrally. Both COX-1 and COX-2 are expressed in the spinal cord and release prostaglandins in response to peripheral pain stimuli. PGE_2, and perhaps also PGD_2, PGI_2, and $PGF_{2\alpha}$, contribute to so-called central sensitization, an increase in excitability of spinal dorsal horn neurons, that augments pain intensity, widens the area of pain perception, and results in pain from normally innocuous stimuli.

F. Inflammation and Immunity

PGE_2 and PGI_2 are the predominant prostanoids associated with inflammation. Both markedly enhance edema formation and leukocyte infiltration by promoting blood flow in the inflamed region. PGE_2 and PGI_2, through activation of EP_2 and IP, respectively, increase vascular permeability and leukocyte infiltration. Through its action as a platelet agonist, TXA_2 can also increase platelet-leukocyte interactions. Although probably not made by lymphocytes, prostaglandins may contribute positively or negatively to lymphocyte function. PGE_2 and TXA_2 may play a role in T-lymphocyte development by regulating apoptosis of immature thymocytes. PGE_2 suppresses the immunologic response by inhibiting differentiation of B lymphocytes into antibody-secreting plasma cells, thus depressing the humoral antibody response. It also inhibits cytotoxic T-cell function, mitogen-stimulated proliferation of T lymphocytes, and the release of cytokines by sensitized TH1 lymphocytes. PGE_2 can modify myeloid cell differentiation promoting type 2 immune-suppressive macrophage and myeloid suppressor cell phenotypes. These effects likely contribute to immune escape in tumors where infiltrating myeloid-derived cells predominantly display type 2 phenotypes. PGD_2, a major product of mast cells, is a potent chemoattractant for eosinophils in which it also induces degranulation and leukotriene biosynthesis. PGD_2 also induces chemotaxis and migration of TH2 lymphocytes mainly via activation of DP_2, although a role for DP_1 has also been established. It remains unclear how these two receptors coordinate the actions of PGD_2 in inflammation and immunity. A degradation product of PGD_2, 15d-PGJ_2, at concentrations actually formed in vivo, may also activate eosinophils via the DP_2 (CRTH2) receptor.

G. Bone Metabolism

Prostaglandins are abundant in skeletal tissue and are produced by osteoblasts and adjacent hematopoietic cells. The major effect of prostaglandins (especially PGE_2, acting on EP_4) in vivo is to increase bone turnover, ie, stimulation of bone resorption and formation. EP_4 receptor deletion in mice results in an imbalance between bone resorption and formation, leading to a negative balance of bone mass and density in older animals. Prostaglandins may mediate the effects of mechanical forces on bones and changes in bone during inflammation. EP_4-receptor deletion and inhibition of prostaglandin biosynthesis have both been associated with impaired fracture healing in animal models. COX inhibitors can also slow skeletal muscle healing by interfering with prostaglandin effects on myocyte proliferation, differentiation, and fibrosis in response to injury. Prostaglandins may contribute to the bone loss that occurs at menopause; it has been speculated that NSAIDs may be of therapeutic value in osteoporosis and bone loss prevention in older women. However, controlled evaluation of such therapeutic interventions has not been carried out. NSAIDs, especially those specific for inhibition of COX-2, delay bone healing in experimental models of fracture.

H. Eye

PGE and PGF derivatives lower intraocular pressure. The mechanism of this action is unclear but probably involves increased outflow of aqueous humor from the anterior chamber via the uveoscleral pathway (see Clinical Pharmacology of Eicosanoids).

I. Cancer

There has been significant interest in the role of prostaglandins, and in particular the COX-2 pathway, in the development of malignancies. Pharmacologic inhibition or genetic deletion of COX-2 restrains tumor formation in models of colon, breast, lung, and other cancers. Large human epidemiologic studies have found that the incidental use of NSAIDs is associated with significant reductions in relative risk for developing these and other cancers. Chronic low-dose aspirin does not appear to have a substantial impact on cancer incidence; however, it is associated with reduced cancer death in a number of studies. In patients with familial polyposis coli, COX inhibitors significantly decrease polyp formation. Polymorphisms in COX-2 have been associated with increased risk of some cancers. Several studies have suggested that COX-2 expression is associated with markers of tumor progression in breast cancer. In mouse mammary tissue, COX-2 is oncogenic whereas NSAID use is associated with a reduced risk of breast cancer in women, especially for hormone receptor-positive tumors. Despite the support for COX-2 as the predominant source of oncogenic prostaglandins, randomized clinical trials have not been performed to determine whether superior anti-oncogenic effects occur with selective inhibition of COX-2, compared with nonselective NSAIDs. Indeed data from animal models and epidemiologic studies in humans are consistent with a role for COX-1 as well as COX-2 in the production of oncogenic prostanoids.

PGE_2, which is considered the principal oncogenic prostanoid, facilitates tumor initiation, progression, and metastasis through multiple biologic effects, increasing proliferation and angiogenesis, inhibiting apoptosis, augmenting cellular invasiveness, and modulating immunosuppression. Augmented expression of mPGES-1 is evident in tumors, and preclinical studies support the potential use of mPGES-1 inhibitors in chemoprevention or treatment. In tumors reduced levels of OATP2A1 and 15-PGDH, which mediate cellular uptake and metabolic inactivation of PGE_2, respectively, likely contribute to sustained PGE_2 activity. The pro- and anti-oncogenic roles of other prostanoids remain under investigation, with TXA_2 emerging as another likely procarcinogenic mediator, deriving either from macrophage COX-2 or platelet COX-1. Studies in mice lacking EP_1, EP_2, or EP_4 receptors confirm reduced disease in multiple carcinogenesis models. EP_3, in contrast, plays no role or may even play a protective role in some cancers. Transactivation of epidermal growth factor receptor (EGFR) has been linked with the oncogenic activity of PGE_2.

Effects of Lipoxygenase & Cytochrome P450-Derived Metabolites

The actions of lipoxygenases generate compounds that can regulate specific cellular responses important in inflammation and immunity. Cytochrome P450-derived metabolites affect nephron transport functions either directly or via metabolism to active compounds (see below). The biologic functions of the various forms of hydroxy- and hydroperoxyeicosaenoic acids are largely unknown, but their pharmacologic potency is impressive.

A. Blood Cells and Inflammation

LTB_4, acting at the BLT_1 receptor, is a potent chemoattractant for T lymphocytes, eosinophils, monocytes, and possibly mast cells; the cysteinyl leukotrienes are potent chemoattractants for eosinophils and T lymphocytes. Cysteinyl leukotrienes may also generate distinct sets of cytokines through activation of mast cell $cysLT_1$ and $cysLT_2$. At higher concentrations, these leukotrienes also promote eosinophil adherence, degranulation, cytokine or chemokine release, and oxygen radical formation. Cysteinyl leukotrienes also contribute to inflammation by increasing endothelial permeability, thus promoting migration of inflammatory cells to the site of inflammation. The leukotrienes have been strongly implicated in the pathogenesis of inflammation, especially in chronic diseases such as asthma and inflammatory bowel disease.

Lipoxins have diverse effects on leukocytes, including activation of monocytes and macrophages and inhibition of neutrophil, eosinophil, and lymphocyte activation. Both lipoxin A and lipoxin B inhibit natural killer cell cytotoxicity.

B. Heart and Smooth Muscle

1. Cardiovascular—12(*S*)-HETE promotes vascular smooth muscle cell proliferation and migration at low concentrations; it may play a role in myointimal proliferation that occurs after vascular injury such as that caused by angioplasty. Its stereoisomer, 12(*R*)-HETE, is not a chemoattractant, but is a potent inhibitor of the Na^+/K^+-ATPase in the cornea. LTC_4 and LTD_4 reduce myocardial contractility and coronary blood flow, leading to cardiac depression. Lipoxin A and lipoxin B exert coronary vasoconstrictor effects in vitro. In addition to their vasodilatory action, EETs may reduce cardiac hypertrophy as well as systemic and pulmonary vascular smooth muscle proliferation and migration.

2. Gastrointestinal—Human colonic epithelial cells synthesize LTB_4, a chemoattractant for neutrophils. The colonic mucosa of patients with inflammatory bowel disease contains substantially increased amounts of LTB_4.

3. Airways—The cysteinyl leukotrienes, particularly LTC_4 and LTD_4, are potent bronchoconstrictors and cause increased microvascular permeability, plasma exudation, and mucus secretion in the airways. Controversies exist over whether the pattern and specificity of the leukotriene receptors differ in animal models and humans. LTC_4-specific receptors have not been found in human lung tissue, whereas both high- and low-affinity LTD_4 receptors are present.

C. Renal System

There is substantial evidence for a role of the epoxygenase products in regulating renal function although their exact role in the human kidney remains unclear. Both 20-HETE and the EETs are generated in renal tissue. 20-HETE, which potently blocks the smooth muscle cell Ca^{2+}-activated K^+ channel and leads to vasoconstriction of the renal arteries, has been implicated in the pathogenesis of hypertension. In contrast, studies support an antihypertensive effect of the EETs because of their vasodilating and natriuretic actions. EETs increase renal blood flow and may protect against inflammatory renal damage by limiting glomerular macrophage infiltration. Inhibitors of soluble epoxide hydrolase, which prolong the biologic activities of the EETs, are being developed as potential new antihypertensive drugs. In vitro studies, and work in animal models, support targeting soluble epoxide hydrolase for blood pressure control, although the potential for pulmonary vasoconstriction and tumor promotion through antiapoptotic actions require careful investigation.

D. Miscellaneous

The effects of these products on the reproductive organs have not been elucidated. Similarly, actions on the nervous system have been suggested but not confirmed. 12-HETE stimulates the release of aldosterone from the adrenal cortex and mediates a portion of the aldosterone release stimulated by angiotensin II but not that by adrenocorticotropic hormone. Very low concentrations of LTC_4 increase and higher concentrations of arachidonate-derived epoxides augment luteinizing hormone (LH) and LH-releasing hormone release from isolated rat anterior pituitary cells.

INHIBITION OF EICOSANOID SYNTHESIS

Corticosteroids block all the known pathways of eicosanoid synthesis, perhaps in part by stimulating the synthesis of several inhibitory proteins collectively called annexins or lipocortins. They inhibit phospholipase A_2 activity, probably by interfering with phospholipid binding, thus preventing the release of arachidonic acid.

The NSAIDs (eg, **indomethacin, ibuprofen;** see Chapter 36) block both prostaglandin and thromboxane formation by reversibly inhibiting COX activity. The traditional NSAIDs are not selective for COX-1 or COX-2. Selective COX-2 inhibitors, which were developed more recently, vary—as do the older drugs—in their degree of selectivity. Indeed, there is considerable variability between (and within) individuals in the selectivity attained by the same dose of the same NSAID. Aspirin is an irreversible COX inhibitor. In platelets, which lack nuclei, COX-1 (the only isoform expressed in mature platelets) cannot be restored via protein biosynthesis, resulting in extended inhibition of TXA_2 biosynthesis.

EP-receptor agonists and antagonists are under evaluation in the treatment of bone fracture and osteoporosis, whereas TP-receptor antagonists are being investigated for usefulness in treatment of cardiovascular syndromes. Direct inhibition of PGE_2 biosynthesis through selective inhibition of the inducible mPGES-1 isoform is also under examination for potential therapeutic efficacy in pain and inflammation, cardiovascular disease, and chemoprevention of cancer.

Although they remain less effective than inhaled corticosteroids, a 5-LOX inhibitor (**zileuton**) and selective antagonists of the $CysLT_1$ receptor for leukotrienes (**zafirlukast, montelukast,** and **pranlukast;** see Chapter 20) are used clinically in mild to moderate asthma. Growing evidence for a role of the leukotrienes in cardiovascular disease has expanded the potential clinical applications of leukotriene modifiers. Conflicting data have been reported in animal studies depending on the disease model used and the molecular target (5-LOX versus FLAP). Human genetic studies initially demonstrated a link between cardiovascular disease and polymorphisms in the leukotriene biosynthetic enzymes, in particular FLAP, in some populations. However, these results have not been substantiated in more recent, larger studies.

NSAIDs usually do not inhibit lipoxygenase activity at concentrations that inhibit COX activity. In fact, by preventing arachidonic acid conversion via the COX pathway, NSAIDs may cause more substrate to be metabolized through the lipoxygenase pathways, leading to an increased formation of the inflammatory leukotrienes. Even among the COX-dependent pathways, inhibiting the synthesis of one derivative may increase the synthesis of an enzymatically related product. Therefore, drugs that inhibit both COX and lipoxygenase are being developed.

■ CLINICAL PHARMACOLOGY OF EICOSANOIDS

Several approaches have been used in the clinical application of eicosanoids. First, stable oral or parenteral long-acting analogs of the naturally occurring prostaglandins have been developed (Figure 18–5). Second, enzyme inhibitors and receptor antagonists have been developed to interfere with the synthesis or effects of the eicosanoids. The discovery of COX-2 as a major source of inflammatory prostanoids led to the development of selective COX-2 inhibitors in an effort to preserve the gastrointestinal and renal functions directed through COX-1, thereby reducing toxicity. However, it is apparent that the marked decrease in biosynthesis of PGI_2 that follows COX-2 inhibition occurring without a concurrent inhibition of platelet COX-1-derived TXA_2 removes a protective constraint on endogenous mediators of cardiovascular dysfunction and leads to an increase in cardiovascular events in patients taking selective COX-2 inhibitors. Third, efforts at dietary manipulation—to change the polyunsaturated fatty acid precursors in the cell membrane phospholipids and so change eicosanoid synthesis—is used extensively in over-the-counter products and in diets emphasizing increased consumption of cold-water fish.

Female Reproductive System

Studies with knockout mice have confirmed a role for prostaglandins in reproduction and parturition. COX-1-derived $PGF_{2\alpha}$ appears important for luteolysis, consistent with delayed parturition in COX-1-deficient mice. A complex interplay between $PGF_{2\alpha}$ and oxytocin is critical to the onset of labor. EP_2 receptor-deficient mice demonstrate a preimplantation defect, which underlies some of the breeding difficulties seen in COX-2 knockouts.

A. Abortion

PGE_2 and $PGF_{2\alpha}$ have potent oxytocic actions. The ability of the E and F prostaglandins and their analogs to terminate pregnancy at any stage by promoting uterine contractions has been adapted to common clinical use. Many studies worldwide have established that prostaglandin administration efficiently terminates pregnancy. The drugs are used for first- and second-trimester abortion and for priming or ripening the cervix before abortion. These prostaglandins appear to soften the cervix by increasing proteoglycan content and changing the biophysical properties of collagen.

Dinoprostone, a synthetic preparation of PGE_2, is administered vaginally for oxytocic use. In the USA, it is approved for inducing abortion in the second trimester of pregnancy, for missed abortion, for benign hydatidiform mole, and for ripening of the cervix for induction of labor in patients at or near term.

Dinoprostone stimulates the contraction of the uterus throughout pregnancy. As the pregnancy progresses, the uterus increases its contractile response, and the contractile effect of oxytocin is potentiated as well. Dinoprostone also directly affects the collagenase of the cervix, resulting in softening. The vaginal dose enters the maternal circulation, and a small amount is absorbed directly by the uterus via the cervix and the lymphatic system. Dinoprostone is metabolized in local tissues and on the first pass through the lungs (about 95%). The metabolites are mainly excreted in the urine. The plasma half-life is 2.5–5 minutes.

For the induction of labor, dinoprostone is used either as a gel (0.5 mg PGE_2) or as a controlled-release formulation (10 mg PGE_2) that releases PGE_2 in vivo at a rate of about 0.3 mg/h over 12 hours. An advantage of the controlled-release formulation is a lower incidence of gastrointestinal side effects (< 1%).

For abortifacient purposes, the recommended dosage is a 20-mg dinoprostone vaginal suppository repeated at 3- to 5-hour intervals depending on the response of the uterus. The mean time to abortion is 17 hours, but in more than 25% of cases, the abortion is incomplete and requires additional intervention.

For softening of the cervix at term, the preparations used are either a single vaginal insert containing 10 mg PGE_2 or a vaginal gel containing 0.5 mg PGE_2 administered every 6 hours. The softening of the cervix for induction of labor substantially shortens the time to onset of labor and the delivery time.

Antiprogestins (eg, **mifepristone**) have been combined with an oral oxytocic synthetic analog of PGE_1 (**misoprostol**) to produce early abortion. This regimen is available in the USA and Europe (see Chapter 40). The ease of use and the effectiveness of the combination have aroused considerable opposition in some quarters. The major toxicities are cramping pain and diarrhea. The oral and vaginal routes of administration are equally effective, but the vaginal route has been associated with an increased incidence of sepsis, so the oral route is now recommended.

An analog of $PGF_{2\alpha}$ is also used in obstetrics. This drug, **carboprost tromethamine** (15-methyl-$PGF_{2\alpha}$; the 15-methyl group prolongs the duration of action) is used to induce second-trimester abortions and to control postpartum hemorrhage that is not responding to conventional methods of management. The success rate is approximately 80%. It is administered as a single 250-mcg intramuscular injection, repeated if necessary. Vomiting and diarrhea occur commonly, probably because of gastrointestinal smooth muscle stimulation. In some patients transient bronchoconstriction can occur. Transient elevations in temperature are seen in approximately one eighth of patients.

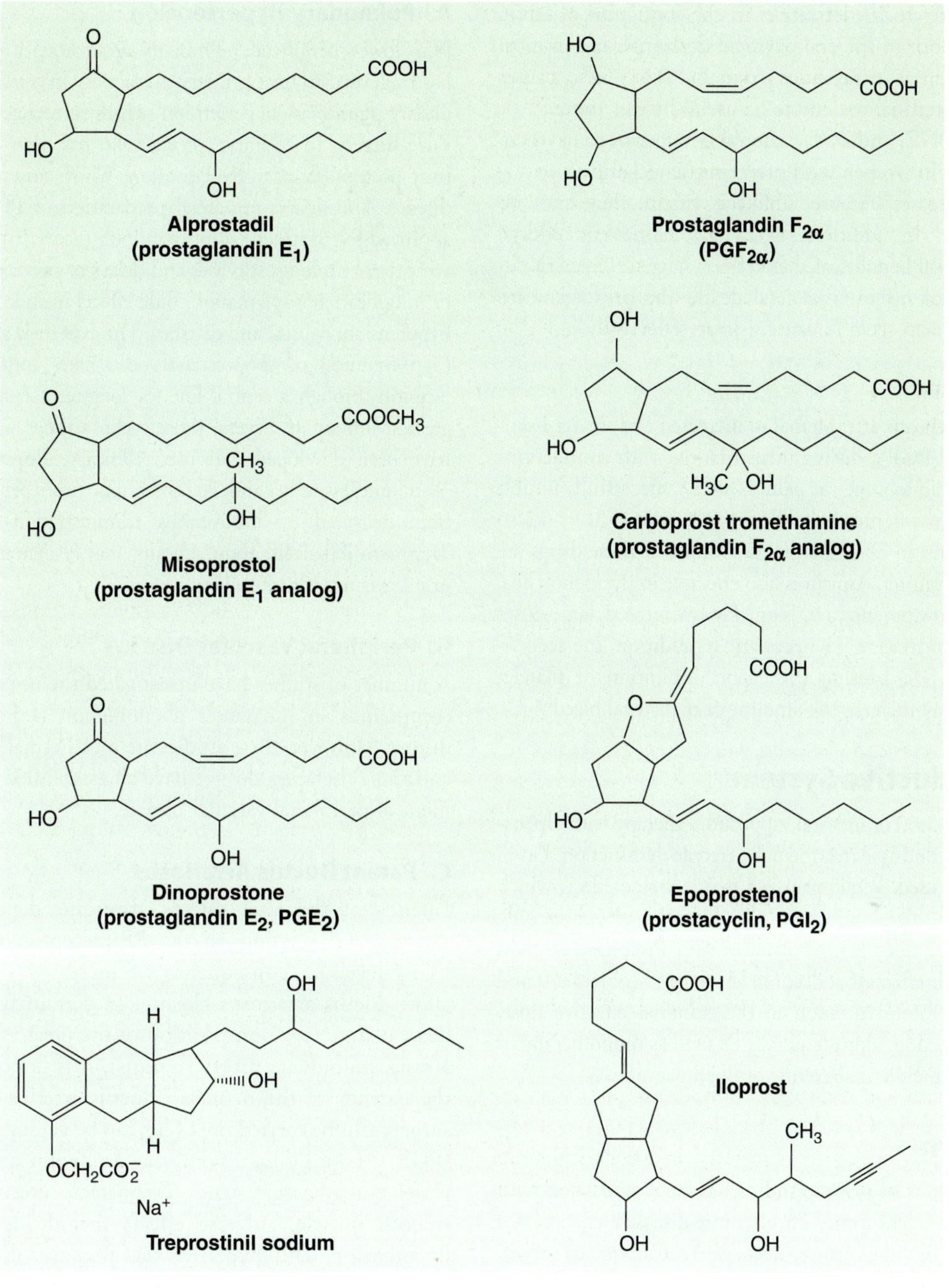

FIGURE 18–5 Chemical structures of some prostaglandins and prostaglandin analogs currently in clinical use.

B. Facilitation of Labor

Numerous studies have shown that PGE_2, $PGF_{2\alpha}$, and their analogs effectively initiate and stimulate labor, but $PGF_{2\alpha}$ is one tenth as potent as PGE_2. There appears to be no difference in the efficacy of PGE_2 and $PGF_{2\alpha}$ when they are administered intravenously; however, the most common usage is local application of PGE_2 analogs (dinoprostone) to promote labor through ripening of the cervix. These agents and oxytocin have similar success rates and comparable induction-to-delivery intervals. The adverse effects of the prostaglandins are moderate, with a slightly higher incidence of nausea, vomiting, and diarrhea than that produced by oxytocin.

$PGF_{2\alpha}$ has more gastrointestinal toxicity than PGE_2. Neither drug has significant maternal cardiovascular toxicity in the recommended doses. In fact, PGE_2 must be infused at a rate about 20 times faster than that used for induction of labor to decrease blood pressure and increase heart rate. $PGF_{2\alpha}$ is a bronchoconstrictor and should be used with caution in women with asthma; however, neither asthma attacks nor bronchoconstriction have been observed during the induction of labor. Although both PGE_2 and $PGF_{2\alpha}$ pass the fetoplacental barrier, fetal toxicity is uncommon.

The effects of oral PGE_2 administration (0.5–1.5 mg/h) have been compared with those of intravenous oxytocin and oral demoxytocin, an oxytocin derivative, in the induction of labor. Oral PGE_2 is superior to the oral oxytocin derivative and in most studies is as efficient as intravenous oxytocin. Oral $PGF_{2\alpha}$ causes too much gastrointestinal toxicity to be useful by this route.

Theoretically, PGE_2 and $PGF_{2\alpha}$ should be superior to oxytocin for inducing labor in women with preeclampsia-eclampsia or cardiac and renal diseases because, unlike oxytocin, they have no antidiuretic effect. In addition, PGE_2 has natriuretic effects. However, the clinical benefits of these effects have not been documented. In cases of intrauterine fetal death, the prostaglandins alone or with oxytocin seem to cause delivery effectively.

C. Dysmenorrhea

Primary dysmenorrhea is attributable to increased endometrial synthesis of PGE_2 and $PGF_{2\alpha}$ during menstruation, with contractions of the uterus that lead to ischemic pain. NSAIDs successfully inhibit the formation of these prostaglandins (see Chapter 36) and so relieve dysmenorrhea in 75–85% of cases. Some of these drugs are available over the counter. Aspirin is also effective in dysmenorrhea, but because it has low potency and is quickly hydrolyzed, large doses and frequent administration are necessary. In addition, the acetylation of platelet COX, causing irreversible inhibition of platelet TXA_2 synthesis, may increase the amount of menstrual bleeding.

Male Reproductive System

Intracavernosal injection or urethral suppository therapy with **alprostadil** (PGE_1) is a second-line treatment for erectile dysfunction. Doses of 2.5–25 mcg are used. Penile pain is a frequent side effect, which may be related to the algesic effects of PGE derivatives; however, only a few patients discontinue the use because of pain. Prolonged erection and priapism are side effects that occur in less than 4% of patients and are minimized by careful titration to the minimal effective dose. When given by injection, alprostadil may be used as monotherapy or in combination with either papaverine or phentolamine.

Renal System

Increased biosynthesis of prostaglandins has been associated with one form of Bartter's syndrome. This is a rare disease characterized by low-to-normal blood pressure, decreased sensitivity to angiotensin, hyperreninemia, hyperaldosteronism, and excessive loss of K^+. There also is an increased excretion of prostaglandins, especially PGE metabolites, in the urine. After long-term administration of COX inhibitors, sensitivity to angiotensin, plasma renin values, and the concentration of aldosterone in plasma return to normal. Although plasma K^+ rises, it remains low, and urinary wasting of K^+ persists. Whether an increase in prostaglandin biosynthesis is the cause of Bartter's syndrome or a reflection of a more basic physiologic defect is not yet known.

Cardiovascular System

The vasodilator effects of PGE compounds have been studied extensively in hypertensive patients. These compounds also promote sodium diuresis. Practical application will require derivatives with oral activity, longer half-lives, and fewer adverse effects.

A. Pulmonary Hypertension

PGI_2 lowers peripheral, pulmonary, and coronary vascular resistance. It has been used to treat primary pulmonary hypertension as well as secondary pulmonary hypertension, which sometimes occurs after mitral valve surgery. In addition, prostacyclin has been used successfully to treat portopulmonary hypertension, which arises secondary to liver disease. The first commercial preparation of PGI_2 (**epoprostenol**) approved for treatment of primary pulmonary hypertension improves symptoms, prolongs survival, and delays or prevents the need for lung or lung-heart transplantation. Side effects include flushing, headache, hypotension, nausea, and diarrhea. The extremely short plasma half-life (3–5 minutes) of epoprostenol necessitates continuous intravenous infusion through a central line for long-term treatment, which is its greatest limitation. Several prostacyclin analogs with longer half-lives have been developed and used clinically. **Iloprost** (half-life about 30 minutes) is usually inhaled six to nine times per day, although it has been delivered by intravenous administration outside the USA. **Treprostinil** (half-life about 4 hours) may be delivered by subcutaneous or intravenous infusion.

B. Peripheral Vascular Disease

A number of studies have investigated the use of PGE_1 and PGI_2 compounds in Raynaud's phenomenon and peripheral arterial disease. However, these studies are mostly small and uncontrolled, and these therapies do not have an established place in the treatment of peripheral vascular disease.

C. Patent Ductus Arteriosus

Patency of the fetal ductus arteriosus depends on COX-2-derived PGE_2 acting on the EP_4 receptor. At birth, reduced PGE_2 levels, a consequence of increased PGE_2 metabolism, allow ductus arteriosus closure. In certain types of congenital heart disease (eg, transposition of the great arteries, pulmonary atresia, pulmonary artery stenosis), it is important to maintain the patency of the neonate's ductus arteriosus until corrective surgery can be carried out. This can be achieved with alprostadil (PGE_1). Like PGE_2, PGE_1 is a vasodilator and an inhibitor of platelet aggregation, and it contracts uterine and intestinal smooth muscle. Adverse effects include apnea, bradycardia, hypotension, and hyperpyrexia. Because of rapid pulmonary clearance (the half-life is about 5–10 minutes in healthy adults and neonates), the drug must be continuously infused at an initial rate of 0.05–0.1 mcg/kg/min, which may be increased to 0.4 mcg/kg/min. Prolonged treatment has been associated with ductal fragility and rupture.

In delayed closure of the ductus arteriosus, COX inhibitors are often used to inhibit synthesis of PGE_2 and so close the ductus. Premature infants in whom respiratory distress develops due to failure of ductus closure can be treated with a high degree of success with indomethacin. This treatment often precludes the need for surgical closure of the ductus.

Blood

As noted above, eicosanoids are involved in thrombosis because TXA_2 promotes platelet aggregation while PGI_2, and perhaps also

PGE$_2$ and PGD$_2$, are platelet antagonists. Chronic administration of low-dose aspirin (81 mg/d) selectively and irreversibly inhibits platelet COX-1 without modifying the activity of systemic COX-1 or COX-2 (see Chapter 34). Because their effects are reversible within the typical dosing interval, nonselective NSAIDs (eg, ibuprofen) do not reproduce this effect, although naproxen, because of its variably prolonged half-life, may provide antiplatelet benefit in some individuals. TXA$_2$, in addition to activating platelets, amplifies the response to other platelet agonists; hence inhibition of its synthesis inhibits secondary aggregation of platelets induced by adenosine diphosphate, by low concentrations of thrombin and collagen, and by epinephrine. Not surprisingly, selective COX-2 inhibitors do not alter platelet TXA$_2$ biosynthesis and are not platelet inhibitors. However, COX-2-derived PGI$_2$ generation is substantially suppressed during selective COX-2 inhibition, removing a restraint on the cardiovascular action of TXA$_2$, and other platelet agonists. It is highly likely that selective depression of PGI$_2$ generation contributes to the increased thrombotic events in humans treated with selective COX-2 inhibitors.

Overview analyses have shown that low-dose aspirin reduces the secondary incidence of heart attack and stroke by about 25%. However, low-dose aspirin also elevates the low risk of serious gastrointestinal bleeding about twofold over placebo. Low-dose aspirin also reduces the incidence of first myocardial infarction. However, in this case, the benefit versus risk of gastrointestinal bleeding is less clear. The effects of aspirin on platelet function are discussed in greater detail in Chapter 34.

Respiratory System

PGE$_2$ is a powerful bronchodilator when given in aerosol form. Unfortunately, it also promotes coughing, and an analog that possesses only the bronchodilator properties has been difficult to obtain.

PGF$_{2\alpha}$ and TXA$_2$ are both strong bronchoconstrictors and were once thought to be primary mediators in asthma. Polymorphisms in the genes for PGD$_2$ synthase, both DP receptors, and the TP receptor have been linked with asthma in humans. DP antagonists, particularly those directed against DP$_2$, are being investigated as potential treatments for allergic diseases including asthma. However, the cysteinyl leukotrienes—LTC$_4$, LTD$_4$, and LTE$_4$—probably dominate during asthmatic constriction of the airways. As described in Chapter 20, leukotriene-receptor inhibitors (eg, **zafirlukast, montelukast**) are effective in asthma. A lipoxygenase inhibitor (**zileuton**) has also been used in asthma but is not as popular as the receptor inhibitors. It remains unclear whether leukotrienes are partially responsible for acute respiratory distress syndrome.

Corticosteroids and cromolyn are also useful in asthma. Corticosteroids inhibit eicosanoid synthesis and thus limit the amounts of eicosanoid mediator available for release. Cromolyn appears to inhibit the release of eicosanoids and other mediators such as histamine and platelet-activating factor from mast cells.

Gastrointestinal System

The word "cytoprotection" was coined to signify the remarkable protective effect of the E prostaglandins against peptic ulcers in animals at doses that do not reduce acid secretion. Since then, numerous experimental and clinical investigations have shown that the PGE compounds and their analogs protect against peptic ulcers produced by either steroids or NSAIDs. **Misoprostol** is an orally active synthetic analog of PGE$_1$. The FDA-approved indication is for prevention of NSAID-induced peptic ulcers. The drug is administered at a dosage of 200 mcg four times daily with food. This and other PGE analogs (eg, enprostil) are cytoprotective at low doses and inhibit gastric acid secretion at higher doses. Misoprostol use is low, probably because of its adverse effects including abdominal discomfort and occasional diarrhea. Dose-dependent bone pain and hyperostosis have been described in patients with liver disease who were given long-term PGE treatment.

Selective COX-2 inhibitors were developed in an effort to spare gastric COX-1 so that the natural cytoprotection by locally synthesized PGE$_2$ and PGI$_2$ is undisturbed (see Chapter 36). However, this benefit is seen only with highly selective inhibitors and may be offset by increased cardiovascular toxicity.

Immune System

Cells of the immune system contribute substantially to eicosanoid biosynthesis during an immune reaction. T and B lymphocytes are not primary synthetic sources; however, they may supply arachidonic acid to monocyte-macrophages for eicosanoid synthesis. In addition, there is evidence for eicosanoid-mediated cell-cell interaction by platelets, erythrocytes, leukocytes, and endothelial cells.

The eicosanoids modulate the effects of the immune system. PGE$_2$ and PGI$_2$ limit T-lymphocyte proliferation in vitro, as do corticosteroids. PGE$_2$ also inhibits B-lymphocyte differentiation and the antigen-presenting function of myeloid-derived cells, suppressing the immune response. T-cell clonal expansion is attenuated through inhibition of interleukin-1 and interleukin-2 and class II antigen expression by macrophages or other antigen-presenting cells. The leukotrienes, TXA$_2$, and platelet-activating factor stimulate T-cell clonal expansion. These compounds stimulate the formation of interleukin-1 and interleukin-2 as well as the expression of interleukin-2 receptors. The leukotrienes also promote interferon-γ release and can replace interleukin-2 as a stimulator of interferon-γ. PGD$_2$ induces chemotaxis and migration of T$_H$2 lymphocytes. These in vitro effects of the eicosanoids agree with in vivo findings in animals with acute organ transplant rejection, as described below.

A. Cell-Mediated Organ Transplant Rejection

Acute organ transplant rejection is a cell-mediated immune response (see Chapter 55). Administration of PGI$_2$ to renal transplant patients has reversed the rejection process in some cases. Experimental in vitro and in vivo data show that PGE$_2$ and PGI$_2$ can attenuate T-cell proliferation and rejection, which can also be seen with drugs that inhibit TXA$_2$ and leukotriene formation. In organ transplant patients, urinary excretion of metabolites of TXA$_2$ increases during acute rejection. Corticosteroids, the first-line drugs used for treatment of acute rejection because of their lymphotoxic effects, inhibit both phospholipase and COX-2 activity.

B. Inflammation

Aspirin has been used to treat arthritis of all types for approximately 100 years, but its mechanism of action—inhibition of COX activity—was not discovered until 1971. COX-2 appears to be the form of the enzyme most associated with cells involved in the inflammatory process, although, as outlined above, COX-1 also contributes significantly to prostaglandin biosynthesis during inflammation. Aspirin and other anti-inflammatory agents that inhibit COX are discussed in Chapter 36.

C. Rheumatoid Arthritis

In rheumatoid arthritis, immune complexes are deposited in the affected joints, causing an inflammatory response that is amplified by eicosanoids. Lymphocytes and macrophages accumulate in the synovium, whereas leukocytes localize mainly in the synovial fluid. The major eicosanoids produced by leukocytes are leukotrienes, which facilitate T-cell proliferation and act as chemoattractants. Human macrophages synthesize the COX products PGE_2 and TXA_2 and large amounts of leukotrienes.

D. Infection

The relationship of eicosanoids to infection is not well defined. The association between the use of the anti-inflammatory steroids and increased risk of infection is well established. However, NSAIDs do not seem to alter patient responses to infection.

Glaucoma

Latanoprost, a stable long-acting $PGF_{2\alpha}$ derivative, was the first prostanoid used for glaucoma. The success of latanoprost has stimulated development of similar prostanoids with ocular hypotensive effects, and **bimatoprost**, **travoprost**, and **unoprostone** are now available. These drugs act at the FP receptor and are administered as drops into the conjunctival sac once or twice daily. Adverse effects include irreversible brown pigmentation of the iris and eyelashes, drying of the eyes, and conjunctivitis.

DIETARY MANIPULATION OF ARACHIDONIC ACID METABOLISM

Because arachidonic acid is derived from dietary linoleic and α-linolenic acids, which are essential fatty acids, the effects of dietary manipulation on arachidonic acid metabolism have been extensively studied. Two approaches have been used. The first adds corn, safflower, and sunflower oils, which contain linoleic acid (C18:2), to the diet. The second approach adds oils containing eicosapentaenoic (C20:5) and docosahexaenoic acids (C22:6), so-called omega-3 fatty acids, from cold-water fish. Both types of diet change the phospholipid composition of cell membranes by replacing arachidonic acid with the dietary fatty acids. Diets high in fish oils have been shown to impact ex vivo indices of platelet and leukocyte function, blood pressure, and triglycerides with different dose-response relationships. There is an abundance of epidemiologic data relating diets high in fatty fish to a reduction in the incidence of myocardial infarction and sudden cardiac death although there is more ambiguity about stroke. Of course, epidemiologic data may confound such diets with a reduction in saturated fats and other elements of a "healthy" lifestyle. In addition, some data from prospective randomized trials suggest that such dietary interventions may reduce the incidence of sudden death. Experiments in vitro suggest that fish oils protect against experimentally induced arrhythmogenesis, platelet aggregation, vasomotor spasm, and dyslipidemias.

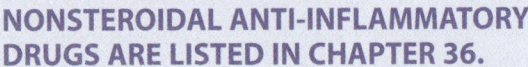

P R E P A R A T I O N S   A V A I L A B L E

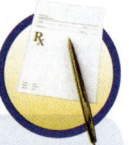

NONSTEROIDAL ANTI-INFLAMMATORY DRUGS ARE LISTED IN CHAPTER 36.

Alprostadil
   Penile injection (Caverject, Edex): 5, 10, 20, 40 mcg sterile powder for reconstitution
   Parenteral (Prostin VR Pediatric): 500 mcg/mL ampules

Bimatoprost (Lumigan)
   Ophthalmic drops: 0.03% solution

Carboprost tromethamine (Hemabate)
   Parenteral: 250 mcg carboprost and 83 mcg tromethamine per mL ampules

Dinoprostone [prostaglandin E₂](Prostin E2, Prepidil, Cervidil)
   Vaginal: 20 mg suppositories, 0.5 mg gel, 10 mg controlled-release system

Epoprostenol [prostacyclin] (Flolan)
   Intravenous: 0.5, 1.5 mg powder to reconstitute

Iloprost (Ventavis)
   Inhalation: 10 mcg/mL solution

Latanoprost (Xalatan)
   Topical: 0.005% ophthalmic solution

Misoprostol (generic, Cytotec)
   Oral: 100 and 200 mcg tablets

Montelukast (Singulair)
   Oral: 4, 5 mg chewable tablets, 10 mg tablets, 4 mg granules

Travoprost (Travatan)
   Ophthalmic solution: 0.004%

Treprostinil (Remodulin)
   Parenteral: 1, 2.5, 5, 10 mg/mL for intravenous infusion or subcutaneous

Zafirlukast (Accolate)
   Oral: 10, 20 mg tablets

Zileuton (Zyflo)
   Oral: 600 mg tablets

REFERENCES

Breyer RM et al: Prostanoid receptors: Subtypes and signaling. Annu Rev Pharmacol Toxicol 2001;41:661.

Brink C et al: International Union of Pharmacology XXXVII. Nomenclature for leukotriene and lipoxin receptors. Pharmacol Rev 2003;55:195.

Cheng HF, Harris RC: Cyclooxygenases, the kidney, and hypertension. Hypertension 2004;43:525.

Christin-Maitre S, Bouchard P, Spitz IM: Medical termination of pregnancy. N Engl J Med 2000;342:946.

Grosser T, Fries S, FitzGerald GA: Biological basis for the cardiovascular consequences of COX-2 inhibition: Therapeutic challenges and opportunities. J Clin Invest 2006;116:4.

Hao CM, Breyer MD: Physiological regulation of prostaglandins in the kidney. Annu Rev Physiol 2008;70:357.

Hata AN, Breyer RM: Pharmacology and signaling of prostaglandin receptors: Multiple roles in inflammation and immune modulation. Pharmacol Ther 2004;103:147.

Leonhardt A et al: Expression of prostanoid receptors in human ductus arteriosus. Br J Pharmacol 2003;138:655.

Martel-Pelletier J et al: Therapeutic role of dual inhibitors of 5-LOX and COX, selective and non-selective non-steroidal anti-inflammatory drugs. Ann Rheum Dis 2003;62:501.

Matsuoka T, Narumiya S: Prostaglandin receptor signaling in disease. Scientific World Journal 2007;7:1329.

Narumiya S, FitzGerald GA: Genetic and pharmacological analysis of prostanoid receptor function. J Clin Invest 2001;108:25.

Rokach J et al: Nomenclature of isoprostanes: A proposal. Prostaglandins 1997;54:853.

Smith WL, Dewitt DL, Garavito MR: Cyclooxygenases: Structural, cellular, and molecular biology. Annu Rev Biochem 2000;69:145.

Smyth EM, FitzGerald GA: Prostaglandin mediators. In: Bradshaw RD, Dennis EA (editors): *Handbook of Cell Signaling*. Elsevier, 2009.

Steiropoulos P, Trakada G, Bouros D: Current pharmacological treatment of pulmonary arterial hypertension. Curr Clin Pharmacol 2008;3:11.

Wang D, Dubois RN: Prostaglandins and cancer. Gut 2006;55:115.

Wang D, Mann JR, DuBois RN: The role of prostaglandins and other eicosanoids in the gastrointestinal tract. Gastroenterology 2005;128:1445.

Nitric Oxide

Samie R. Jaffrey, MD, PhD

Nitric oxide (NO) is a gaseous signaling molecule that readily diffuses across cell membranes and regulates a wide range of physiologic and pathophysiologic processes including cardiovascular, inflammatory, and neuronal functions. Nitric oxide should not be confused with nitrous oxide (N_2O), an anesthetic gas, nor with nitrogen dioxide (NO_2), a toxic pulmonary irritant gas.

■ DISCOVERY OF ENDOGENOUSLY GENERATED NITRIC OXIDE

Because NO is an environmental pollutant, the finding that NO is synthesized by cells and activates specific intracellular signaling pathways was unexpected. The first indication that NO is generated in cells came from studies of cultured macrophages, which showed that treatment with inflammatory mediators, such as bacterial endotoxin, resulted in the production of nitrate and nitrite, molecules that are byproducts of NO breakdown. Similarly, injection of endotoxin in animals elevated urinary nitrite and nitrate.

The second indication came from studies of vascular regulation. Several molecules, such as acetylcholine, were known to cause relaxation of blood vessels. This effect occurred only when the vessels were prepared so that the luminal endothelial cells covering the smooth muscle of the vessel wall were retained. Subsequent studies showed that endothelial cells respond to these vasorelaxants by releasing a soluble **endothelial-derived relaxing factor (EDRF)**. EDRF acts on vascular muscle to elicit relaxation. These findings prompted an intense search for the identity of EDRF.

At the same time, it was observed that exogenous application of NO or organic nitrates, which are metabolized to NO, elicit a variety of effects including inhibition of platelet aggregation and vasorelaxation. These effects were particularly intriguing, since they appeared to involve the activation of highly specific cellular responses, rather than more general cytotoxic responses. Comparison of the biochemical and pharmacological properties of EDRF and NO provided initial evidence that NO is the major bioactive component of EDRF. These findings also made it clear that exogenously applied NO and NO-releasing compounds (nitrates, nitrites, nitroprusside; see Chapters 11 and 12) elicited

their effects by recruiting physiologic signaling pathways that normally mediate the actions of endogenously generated NO.

■ NITRIC OXIDE SYNTHESIS, SIGNALING MECHANISMS, & INACTIVATION

Synthesis

NO, written as $NO^{\bullet}$ to indicate an unpaired electron in its chemical structure, or simply NO, is a highly reactive signaling molecule that is made by any of three closely related NO synthase (NOS, EC 1.14.13.49) isoenzymes, each of which is encoded by a separate gene and named for the initial cell type from which it was isolated (Table 19–1). These enzymes, neuronal NOS (nNOS or NOS-1), macrophage or inducible NOS (iNOS or NOS-2), and endothelial NOS (eNOS or NOS-3), despite their names, are each expressed in a wide variety of cell types, often with an overlapping distribution. These isoforms generate NO from the amino acid L-arginine in an O_2- and NADPH-dependent reaction (Figure 19–1). This enzymatic reaction involves enzyme-bound cofactors, including heme, tetrahydrobiopterin, and flavin adenine dinucleotide (FAD). In the case of nNOS and eNOS, NO synthesis is triggered by agents and processes that increase cytosolic calcium concentrations. Cytosolic calcium forms complexes with calmodulin, an abundant calcium-binding protein, which then binds and activates eNOS and nNOS. On the other hand, iNOS is not regulated by calcium, but is constitutively active. In macrophages and several other cell types, inflammatory mediators induce the transcriptional activation of the iNOS gene, resulting in accumulation of iNOS and increased synthesis of NO.

Signaling Mechanisms

NO mediates its effects by covalent modification of proteins. There are three major targets of NO (Figure 19–1):

1. Metalloproteins—NO interacts with metals, especially iron in heme. The major target of NO is soluble guanylyl cyclase (sGC),

TABLE 19–1 **Properties of the three isoforms of nitric oxide synthase (NOS).**

	Isoform Names		
Property	**NOS-1**	**NOS-2**	**NOS-3**
Other names	nNOS (neuronal NOS)	iNOS (inducible NOS)	eNOS (endothelial NOS)
Tissue	Neurons, skeletal muscle	Macrophages, smooth muscle cells	Endothelial cells, neurons
Expression	Constitutive	Transcriptional induction	Constitutive
Calcium regulation	Yes	No	Yes

a heme-containing enzyme that generates cyclic guanosine monophosphate (cGMP) from guanosine triphosphate (GTP). NO binds to the heme in sGC, resulting in enzyme activation and elevation in intracellular cGMP levels. cGMP activates protein kinase G (PKG), which phosphorylates specific proteins. In blood vessels, NO-dependent elevations in cGMP and PKG activity result in the phosphorylation of proteins that lead to reduced cytosolic calcium levels and subsequently reduced contraction of vascular smooth muscle. Interaction of NO with other metalloproteins mediates some of the cytotoxic effects of NO associated with NO overproduction, eg, by activated macrophages. For example, NO inhibits metalloproteins involved in cellular respiration, such as the citric acid cycle enzyme aconitase and the electron transport chain protein cytochrome oxidase. Inhibition of heme-containing cytochrome P450 enzymes by NO is a major pathogenic mechanism in inflammatory liver disease.

2. Thiols—NO reacts with thiols (compounds containing the –SH group) to form nitrosothiols. In proteins, the thiol moiety is found in the amino acid cysteine. This posttranslational modification, termed *S*-nitrosylation or *S*-nitrosation, requires either metals or O_2 to catalyze the formation of the nitrosothiol adduct. *S*-nitrosylation is highly specific, with only certain cysteine residues in proteins becoming *S*-nitrosylated. *S*-nitrosylation can alter the function, stability, or localization of target proteins. Although the physiologic roles of protein nitrosylation are not fully

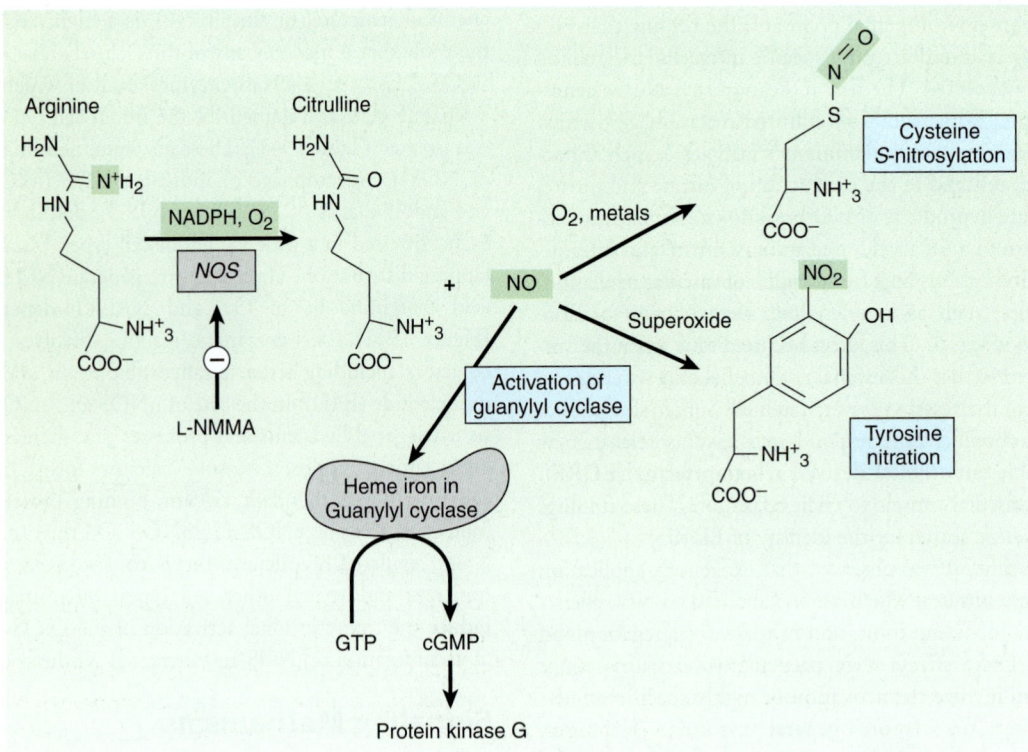

FIGURE 19–1 Synthesis and reactions of nitric oxide (NO). L-NMMA inhibits nitric oxide synthase. NO complexes with the iron in hemoproteins (eg, guanylyl cyclase), resulting in the activation of cyclic guanosine monophosphate (cGMP) synthesis and cGMP target proteins such as protein kinase G. Under conditions of oxidative stress, NO can react with superoxide to nitrate tyrosine. GTP, guanosine triphosphate.

TABLE 19–2 Oxides of nitrogen.

Name	Structure	Known Function
Nitric oxide (NO)	$N{=}O^{\bullet}$	Vasodilator, platelet inhibitor, immune regulator, neurotransmitter
Peroxynitrite (NO_3^{-})	$O{=}N{-}O{-}O^{-}$	Oxidant and nitrating agent
Nitroxyl anion (NO^{-})	$N^{-}{=}O$	Can form from nonspecific donation of an electron from metals to $NO^{\bullet}$
		Exhibits NO-like effects, possibly by first being oxidized to NO
Nitrous oxide (N_2O)	$N^{-}{=}N^{+}{=}O$	Anesthetic
Dinitrogen trioxide (N_2O_3)	$O{=}N{-}N^{+}{=}O$ $\underset{O^{-}}{\|}$	Auto-oxidation product of NO that can nitrosylate protein thiols
Nitrite (NO_2^{-})	$O{=}N{=}O^{-}$	Stable oxidation product of $NO^{\bullet}$
		Slowly metabolized to nitrosothiols, and decomposes to NO at acidic pH
Nitrate (NO_3^{-})	$O{=}N^{+}{-}O^{-}$ $\underset{O^{-}}{\|}$	Stable oxidation product of $NO^{\bullet}$

established, major targets of *S*-nitrosylation are H-ras, a regulator of cell proliferation that is activated by *S*-nitrosylation, and the metabolic enzyme glyceraldehyde-3-phosphate dehydrogenase, which is inhibited when it is *S*-nitrosylated. Denitrosylation of proteins is poorly understood but may involve enzymes, such as thioredoxin, or chemical reduction by intracellular reducing agents such as glutathione, an abundant intracellular sulfhydryl-containing compound. Glutathione can also be *S*-nitrosylated under physiologic conditions to generate *S*-nitrosoglutathione. *S*-nitrosoglutathione may serve as an endogenous stabilized form of NO or as a carrier of NO. Vascular glutathione is decreased in diabetes mellitus and atherosclerosis, and the resulting deficiency of *S*-nitrosoglutathione may account for the increased incidence of cardiovascular complications in these conditions.

3. Tyrosine nitration—NO undergoes both oxidative and reductive reactions, resulting in a variety of oxides of nitrogen that can nitrosylate thiols and nitrate tyrosines (described below) or are stable oxidation products (Table 19–2). NO reacts very efficiently with superoxide to form peroxynitrite ($ONOO^{-}$), a highly reactive oxidant that leads to DNA damage, nitration of tyrosine, and oxidation of cysteine to disulfides or to various sulfur oxides (SO_x). Several cellular enzymes synthesize superoxide, and the activity of these enzymes, as well as NO synthesis, is increased in numerous inflammatory and degenerative diseases, resulting in an increase in peroxynitrite levels. Numerous proteins are susceptible to peroxynitrite-catalyzed tyrosine nitration, and this irreversible modification can be associated with either activation or inhibition of protein function. Detection of tyrosine nitration in tissue is often used as a marker of oxidative stress and tissue damage, although a direct causal role of tyrosine nitration in the pathogenesis of any disease has not been definitively established. Peroxynitrite-mediated protein modification is mitigated by intracellular levels of glutathione, which can protect against tissue

damage by scavenging peroxynitrite. Factors that regulate the biosynthesis and decomposition of glutathione may have important consequences on the toxicity of NO.

Inactivation

NO is highly labile due to its rapid reaction with metals, O_2, and reactive oxygen species. NO can react with heme and hemoproteins, including oxyhemoglobin, which oxidizes NO to nitrate. The reaction of NO with hemoglobin may also lead to *S*-nitrosylation of hemoglobin, resulting in transport of NO throughout the vasculature. NO is also inactivated by reaction with O_2 to form nitrogen dioxide. NO reacts with superoxide, which results in the formation of the highly reactive oxidizing species, peroxynitrite. Scavengers of superoxide anion such as superoxide dismutase may protect NO, enhancing its potency and prolonging its duration of action.

■ PHARMACOLOGIC MANIPULATION OF NITRIC OXIDE

Inhibitors of Nitric Oxide Synthesis

The primary strategy to reduce NO generation in cells is to use NOS inhibitors. The majority of these inhibitors are arginine analogs that bind to the NOS arginine-binding site. Since each of the NOS isoforms has high structural similarity, most of these inhibitors do not exhibit selectivity for individual NOS isoforms. In inflammatory disorders and sepsis (see below), inhibition of the iNOS isoform is potentially beneficial, whereas nNOS-specific inhibitors may be useful for the treatment of neurodegenerative conditions. However, administration of nonselective NOS inhibitors leads to concurrent inhibition of eNOS, which impairs its homeostatic signaling and also results in vasoconstriction and potential ischemic damage. Thus, NOS isoform-selective inhibitors are being designed that exploit subtle differences in substrate binding sites between the isoforms, as well as newer isoform-selective inhibitors that prevent NOS dimerization, the conformation required for enzymatic activity. The efficacy of NOS isoform-selective inhibitors in medical conditions is under investigation.

Nitric Oxide Donors

NO donors, which release NO or related NO species, are used to elicit smooth muscle relaxation. Different classes of NO donors have differing biologic properties, depending on the nature of the NO species released and the mechanism that is responsible for its release.

1. Organic nitrates—Nitroglycerin, which dilates veins and coronary arteries, is metabolized to NO by mitochondrial aldehyde reductase, an enzyme enriched in venous smooth muscle, accounting for the potent venodilating activity of this molecule. Venous dilation decreases cardiac preload, which along with coronary artery dilation accounts for the antianginal effects of nitroglycerin. Other organic nitrates, such as isosorbide dinitrate, are metabolized to an NO-releasing species through a poorly understood enzymatic pathway. Unlike NO, organic nitrates have less significant effects on aggregation of platelets, which appear to lack the enzymatic pathways necessary for rapid metabolic activation. Organic nitrates exhibit rapid tolerance during continuous administration. This nitrate tolerance may derive from the generation of reactive oxygen species that inhibit mitochondrial aldehyde reductase, endogenous NO synthesis, and other pathways (see Chapter 12).

2. Organic nitrites—Organic nitrites, such as the antianginal inhalant amyl nitrite, also require metabolic activation to elicit vasorelaxation, although the responsible enzyme has not been identified. Nitrites are arterial vasodilators and do not exhibit the rapid tolerance seen with nitrates. Amyl nitrite is abused for euphoric effects and combining it with phosphodiesterase inhibitors, such as sildenafil, can cause lethal hypotension. Amyl nitrite has been largely replaced by nitrates, such as nitroglycerin, which are more easily administered.

3. Sodium nitroprusside—Sodium nitroprusside, which dilates arterioles and venules, is used for rapid pressure reduction in arterial hypertension. In response to light as well as chemical or enzymatic mechanisms in cell membranes, sodium nitroprusside breaks down to generate five cyanide molecules and a single NO. See Chapter 11 for additional details.

4. NO gas inhalation—NO itself can be used therapeutically. Inhalation of NO results in reduced pulmonary artery pressure and improved perfusion of ventilated areas of the lung. Inhaled NO is used for pulmonary hypertension, acute hypoxemia, and cardiopulmonary resuscitation, and there is evidence of short-term improvements in pulmonary function. Inhaled NO is stored as a compressed gas mixture with nitrogen, which does not readily react with NO, and further diluted to the desired concentration upon administration. NO can react with O_2 to form nitrogen dioxide, a pulmonary irritant that can cause deterioration of lung function (see Chapter 56). Additionally, NO can induce the formation of methemoglobin, a form of hemoglobin containing Fe^{3+} rather than Fe^{2+}, which does not bind O_2 (see also Chapter 12). Therefore, nitrogen dioxide and methemoglobin levels are monitored during inhaled NO treatment.

5. Alternate strategies—Another mechanism to potentiate the actions of NO is to inhibit the phosphodiesterase enzymes that degrade cGMP. Inhibitors of type 5 phosphodiesterase such as sildenafil result in prolongation of the duration of NO-induced cGMP elevations in a variety of tissues (see Chapter 12).

◼ NITRIC OXIDE IN DISEASE

VASCULAR EFFECTS

NO has a significant effect on vascular smooth muscle tone and blood pressure. Numerous endothelium-dependent vasodilators, such as acetylcholine and bradykinin, act by increasing intracellular calcium levels in endothelial cells, leading to the synthesis of NO. NO diffuses to vascular smooth muscle leading to vasorelaxation (Figure 19–2). Mice with a knockout mutation in the eNOS gene display increased vascular tone and elevated mean arterial pressure, indicating that eNOS is a fundamental regulator of blood pressure.

Apart from being a vasodilator and regulating blood pressure, NO also has antithrombotic effects. Both endothelial cells and platelets contain eNOS, which acts via an NO-cGMP pathway to inhibit platelet activation, an initiator of thrombus formation. Thus, in diseases associated with endothelial dysfunction, the associated decrease in NO generation leads to an increased propensity for abnormal platelet function and thrombosis. NO may have an additional inhibitory effect on blood coagulation by enhancing fibrinolysis via an effect on plasminogen.

NO also protects against atherogenesis. A major antiatherogenic mechanism of NO involves the inhibition of proliferation and migration of vascular smooth muscle cells. In animal models, myointimal proliferation following angioplasty can be blocked by NO donors, by NOS gene transfer, and by NO inhalation. NO reduces endothelial adhesion of monocytes and leukocytes, which are early steps in the development of atheromatous plaques. This effect is due to the inhibitory effect of NO on the expression of adhesion molecules on the endothelial surface. In addition, NO may act as an antioxidant, blocking the oxidation of low-density lipoproteins and thus preventing or reducing the formation of foam cells in the vascular wall. Plaque formation is also affected by NO-dependent reduction in endothelial cell permeability to lipoproteins. The importance of eNOS in cardiovascular disease is supported by experiments showing increased atherosclerosis in animals treated with eNOS inhibitors. Atherosclerosis risk factors,

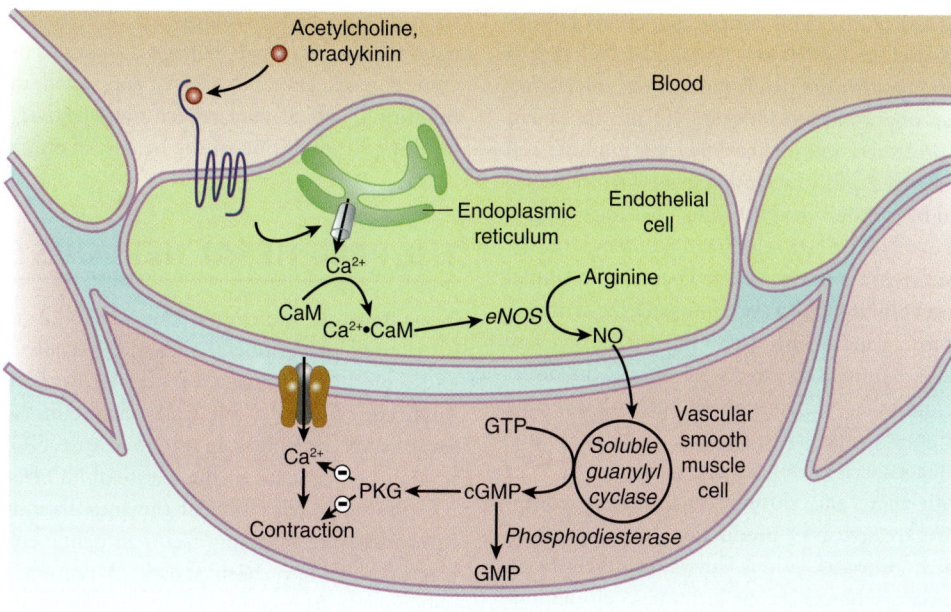

FIGURE 19–2 Regulation of vasorelaxation by endothelial-derived nitric oxide (NO). Endogenous vasodilators, eg, acetylcholine and bradykinin, activate NO synthesis in the luminal endothelial cells, leading to calcium (Ca^{2+}) efflux from the endoplasmic reticulum into the cytoplasm. Calcium binds to calmodulin (CaM), which activates endothelial NO synthase (eNOS), resulting in NO synthesis from L-arginine. NO diffuses into smooth muscle cells, where it activates soluble guanylyl cyclase and cyclic guanosine monophosphate (cGMP) synthesis from guanosine triphosphate (GTP). cGMP binds and activates protein kinase G (PKG), resulting in an overall reduction in calcium influx, and inhibition of calcium-dependent muscle contraction. PKG can also block other pathways that lead to muscle contraction. cGMP signaling is terminated by phosphodiesterases, which convert cGMP to GMP.

such as smoking, hyperlipidemia, diabetes, and hypertension, are associated with decreased endothelial NO production, and thus enhance atherogenesis.

SEPTIC SHOCK

Sepsis is a systemic inflammatory response caused by infection. Endotoxin components from the bacterial wall along with endogenously generated tumor necrosis factor-α and other cytokines induce synthesis of iNOS in macrophages, neutrophils, and T cells, as well as hepatocytes, smooth muscle cells, endothelial cells, and fibroblasts. This widespread generation of NO results in exaggerated hypotension, shock, and, in some cases, death. This hypotension is reduced or reversed by NOS inhibitors in humans as well as in animal models (Table 19–3). A similar reversal of hypotension is produced by compounds that prevent the action of NO, such as the sGC inhibitor methylene blue. Furthermore, knockout mice lacking a functional iNOS gene are more resistant to endotoxin than wild-type mice. However, despite the ability of NOS inhibitors to ameliorate hypotension in sepsis, there is no overall improvement in survival in patients with gram-negative sepsis treated with NOS inhibitors. The absence of benefit may reflect the inability of the NOS inhibitors used in these trials to differentiate between NOS isoforms, or may reflect concurrent inhibition of beneficial aspects of iNOS signaling.

INFECTION & INFLAMMATION

The generation of NO has both beneficial and detrimental roles in the host immune response and in inflammation. The host response to infection or injury involves the recruitment of leukocytes and the release of inflammatory mediators, such as tumor

TABLE 19–3 **Some inhibitors of nitric oxide synthesis or action.**

Inhibitor	Mechanism	Comment
N^{ω}-Monomethyl-L-arginine (L-NMMA)	Competitive inhibitor, binds arginine-binding site in NOS	Nonselective NOS inhibitor
N^{ω}-Nitro-L-arginine methyl ester (L-NAME)	Competitive inhibitor, binds arginine-binding site in NOS	Nonselective NOS inhibitor
7-Nitroindazole	Competitive inhibitor, binds both tetrahydrobiopterin and arginine-binding sites in NOS	Partially selective for NOS-1 in vivo
BBS-2	Inhibits iNOS dimerization	Also weakly inhibits nNOS and eNOS
Hemoglobin	NO scavenger	

NOS, nitric oxide SYNTHASE; BBS-2, a pyrimide imidazole.

necrosis factor and interleukin-1. This leads to induction of iNOS in leukocytes, fibroblasts, and other cell types. The NO that is produced, along with peroxynitrite that forms from its interaction with superoxide, is an important microbicide. NO also appears to play an important protective role in the body via immune cell function. When challenged with foreign antigens, TH1 cells (see Chapter 55) respond by synthesizing NO, which has roles in TH1 cells. The importance of NO in TH1 cell function is demonstrated by the impaired protective response to injected parasites in animal models after inhibition of iNOS. NO also stimulates the synthesis of inflammatory prostaglandins by activating cyclooxygenase isoenzyme 2 (COX-2). Through its effects on COX-2, its direct vasodilatory effects, and other mechanisms, NO generated during inflammation contributes to the erythema, vascular permeability, and subsequent edema associated with acute inflammation.

However, in both acute and chronic inflammatory conditions, prolonged or excessive NO production may exacerbate tissue injury. Indeed, psoriasis lesions, airway epithelium in asthma, and inflammatory bowel lesions in humans all demonstrate elevated levels of NO and iNOS, suggesting that persistent iNOS induction may contribute to disease pathogenesis. Moreover, these tissues also exhibit increased levels of nitrotyrosine, indicating excessive formation of peroxynitrite. In several animal models of arthritis, increasing NO production by dietary L-arginine supplementation exacerbates arthritis, whereas protection is seen with iNOS inhibitors. Thus, inhibition of the NO pathway may have a beneficial effect on a variety of acute and chronic inflammatory diseases.

THE CENTRAL NERVOUS SYSTEM

NO has an important role in the central nervous system as a neurotransmitter (see Chapter 21). Unlike classic transmitters such as glutamate or dopamine, which are stored in synaptic vesicles and released in the synaptic cleft upon vesicle fusion, NO is not stored, but rather is synthesized on demand and immediately diffuses to neighboring cells. NO synthesis is induced at postsynaptic sites in neurons, most commonly upon activation of the NMDA subtype of glutamate receptor, which results in calcium influx and activation of nNOS. In several neuronal subtypes, eNOS is also present and activated by neurotransmitter pathways that lead to calcium influx. NO synthesized postsynaptically may function as a retrograde messenger and diffuse to the presynaptic terminal to enhance the efficiency of neurotransmitter release, thereby regulating synaptic plasticity, the process of synapse strengthening that underlies learning and memory. Because aberrant NMDA receptor activation and excessive NO synthesis is linked to excitotoxic neuronal death in several neurologic diseases, including stroke, amyotrophic lateral

sclerosis, and Parkinson's disease, therapy with NOS inhibitors may reduce neuronal damage in these conditions. However, clinical trials have not clearly supported the benefit of NOS inhibition, which may reflect nonselectivity of the inhibitors, resulting in inhibition of the beneficial effects of eNOS.

THE PERIPHERAL NERVOUS SYSTEM

Nonadrenergic, noncholinergic (NANC) neurons are widely distributed in peripheral tissues, especially the gastrointestinal and reproductive tracts (see Chapter 6). Considerable evidence implicates NO as a mediator of certain NANC actions, and some NANC neurons appear to release NO. Penile erection is thought to be caused by the release of NO from NANC neurons; NO promotes relaxation of the smooth muscle in the corpora cavernosa—the initiating factor in penile erection—and inhibitors of NOS have been shown to prevent erection caused by pelvic nerve stimulation in the rat. An established approach in treating erectile dysfunction is to enhance the effect of NO signaling by inhibiting the breakdown of cGMP by the phosphodiesterase (PDE isoform 5) present in the smooth muscle of the corpora cavernosa with drugs such as sildenafil, tadalafil, and vardenafil (see Chapter 12).

RESPIRATORY DISORDERS

NO is administered by inhalation (see Preparations Available) to newborns with hypoxic respiratory failure associated with pulmonary hypertension. The current treatment for severely defective gas exchange in the newborn is with extracorporeal membrane oxygenation (ECMO), which does not directly affect pulmonary vascular pressures. NO inhalation dilates pulmonary vessels, resulting in decreased pulmonary vascular resistance and reduced pulmonary artery pressure. Inhaled NO also improves oxygenation by reducing mismatch of ventilation and perfusion in the lung. Inhalation of NO results in dilation of pulmonary vessels in areas of the lung with better ventilation, thereby redistributing pulmonary blood flow away from poorly ventilated areas. NO inhalation does not typically exert pronounced effects on the systemic circulation. Inhaled NO has also been shown to improve cardiopulmonary function in adult patients with pulmonary artery hypertension.

An additional approach for treating pulmonary hypertension is to potentiate the actions of NO in pulmonary vascular beds. Due to the enrichment of PDE-5 in pulmonary vascular beds, PDE-5 inhibitors such as sildenafil and tadalafil induce vasodilation and marked reductions in pulmonary hypertension (see also Chapter 12).

SUMMARY Nitric Oxide

Subclass	Mechanism of Action	Effects	Clinical Applications	Pharmacokinetics, Toxicity, Interactions
NITRIC OXIDE (NO)				
	NO activates soluble guanylyl cyclase to elevate cGMP levels in vascular smooth muscle	Vasodilator • relaxes other smooth muscle • inhalation of NO leads to increased blood flow to parts of the lung exposed to NO and decreased pulmonary vascular resistance	Hypoxic respiratory failure and pulmonary hypertension	Inhaled gas • *Toxicity:* Methemoglobinemia

PREPARATIONS AVAILABLE

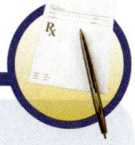

Nitric Oxide (INOmax)
 Inhalation: 100, 800 ppm gas

REFERENCES

Chen Z, Stamler JS: Bioactivation of nitroglycerin by the mitochondrial aldehyde dehydrogenase. Trends Cardiovasc Med 2006;16:259.

Griffiths MJ, Evans TW: Inhaled nitric oxide therapy in adults. N Engl J Med 2005;353:2683.

Guix FX et al: The physiology and pathophysiology of nitric oxide in the brain. Prog Neurobiol 2005;76:126.

McMillan K et al: Allosteric inhibitors of inducible nitric oxide synthase dimerization discovered via combinatorial chemistry. Proc Nat Acad Sci USA 2000;97:1506.

Moncada S, Higgs EA: The discovery of nitric oxide and its role in vascular biology. Br J Pharmacol 2006;147:S193.

Napoli C, Ignarro LJ: Nitric oxide-releasing drugs. Annu Rev Pharmacol Toxicol 2003;43:97.

Paige JS, Jaffrey, SR: Pharmacologic manipulation of nitric oxide signaling: Targeting NOS dimerization and protein-protein interactions. Curr Topics Med Chem 2007;7:97.

Ramani GV, Park MH: Update on the clinical utility of sildenafil in the treatment of pulmonary arterial hypertension. Drug Des Devel Ther 2010;4:61.

Wimalawansa SJ: Nitric oxide: New evidence for novel therapeutic indications. Expert Opin Pharmacother 2008;9:1935.

Drugs Used in Asthma

Homer A. Boushey, MD

C A S E   S T U D Y

A 10-year-old girl with a history of poorly controlled asthma presents to the emergency department with severe shortness of breath and audible inspiratory and expiratory wheezing. She is pale, refuses to lie down, and appears extremely frightened. Her pulse is 120 bpm and respirations 32/min. Her mother states that the girl has just recovered from a mild case of flu and had seemed comfortable until this afternoon. The girl uses an inhaler (albuterol) but "only when really needed" because her parents are afraid that she will become too dependent on medication. She administered two puffs from her inhaler just before coming to the hospital, but "the inhaler doesn't seem to have helped." What emergency measures are indicated? How should her long-term management be altered?

Asthma is characterized clinically by recurrent bouts of shortness of breath, chest tightness, and wheezing, often associated with coughing; physiologically by widespread, reversible narrowing of the bronchial airways and a marked increase in bronchial responsiveness to inhaled stimuli; and pathologically by lymphocytic, eosinophilic inflammation of the bronchial mucosa. It is also characterized pathologically by "remodeling" of the bronchial mucosa, with thickening of the lamina reticularis beneath the airway epithelium and hyperplasia of the cells of all structural elements of the airway wall—vessels, smooth muscle, and secretory glands and goblet cells.

In mild asthma, symptoms occur only occasionally, as on exposure to allergens or certain pollutants, on exercise, or after viral upper respiratory infection. More severe forms of asthma are associated with frequent attacks of wheezing dyspnea, especially at night, or with chronic airway narrowing, causing chronic respiratory impairment. These consequences of asthma are regarded as largely preventable, because effective treatments for relief of acute bronchoconstriction ("short-term relievers") and for reduction in symptoms and prevention of attacks ("long-term controllers") are available. The persistence of high medical costs for asthma care, driven largely by the costs of emergency department or hospital treatment of asthma exacerbations, are believed to reflect underutilization of the treatments available.

The causes of airway narrowing in acute asthmatic attacks, or "asthma exacerbations," include contraction of airway smooth muscle, inspissation of viscid mucus plugs in the airway lumen, and thickening of the bronchial mucosa from edema, cellular infiltration, and hyperplasia of secretory, vascular, and smooth muscle cells. Of these causes of airway obstruction, contraction of smooth muscle is most easily reversed by current therapy; reversal of the edema and cellular infiltration requires sustained treatment with anti-inflammatory agents.

Short-term relief is thus most effectively achieved by agents that relax airway smooth muscle, of which β-adrenoceptor stimulants (see Chapter 9) are the most effective and most widely used. Theophylline, a methylxanthine drug, and antimuscarinic agents (see Chapter 8) are sometimes also used for reversal of airway constriction.

Long-term control is most effectively achieved with an anti-inflammatory agent such as an inhaled corticosteroid. It can also be achieved, though less effectively, with a leukotriene pathway antagonist or an inhibitor of mast cell degranulation, such as cromolyn or nedocromil. Finally, clinical trials have established the efficacy of treatment for severe asthma with a humanized monoclonal antibody, omalizumab, which is specifically targeted against IgE, the antibody responsible for allergic sensitization.

The distinction between "short-term relievers" and "long-term controllers" is blurred. Inhaled corticosteroids, regarded as long-term controllers, produce modest immediate bronchodilation. Theophylline, regarded as a bronchodilator, inhibits some lymphocyte functions and modestly reduces airway mucosal inflammation. Theophylline may also enhance the anti-inflammatory action of inhaled corticosteroids. This is also true of long-acting β-adrenoceptor stimulants, like salmeterol and formoterol, which are effective in improving asthma control when added to inhaled corticosteroid treatment, though neither is anti-inflammatory when taken as a single agent.

This chapter presents the basic pharmacology of the methylxanthines, cromolyn, leukotriene pathway inhibitors, and monoclonal anti-IgE antibody—agents whose medical use is almost exclusively for pulmonary disease. The other classes of drugs listed above are discussed in relation to the therapy of asthma.

PATHOGENESIS OF ASTHMA

The classic immunologic model of asthma presents it as a disease mediated by reaginic immune globulin (IgE). Foreign materials that provoke IgE production are described as "allergens"; the most common are proteins from house dust mite, cockroach, animal danders, molds, and pollens. The tendency to produce IgE antibodies is genetically determined; asthma and other allergic diseases cluster in families. Once produced, IgE antibodies bind to mast cells in the airway mucosa (Figure 20–1). On reexposure to a specific allergen, antigen-antibody interaction on the surface of the mast cells triggers both the release of mediators stored in the cells' granules and the synthesis and release of other mediators. The histamine, tryptase, leukotrienes C_4 and D_4, and prostaglandin D_2 that are released diffuse through the airway mucosa, triggering the muscle contraction and vascular leakage responsible for the acute bronchoconstriction of the "early asthmatic response." This response is often followed in 3–6 hours by

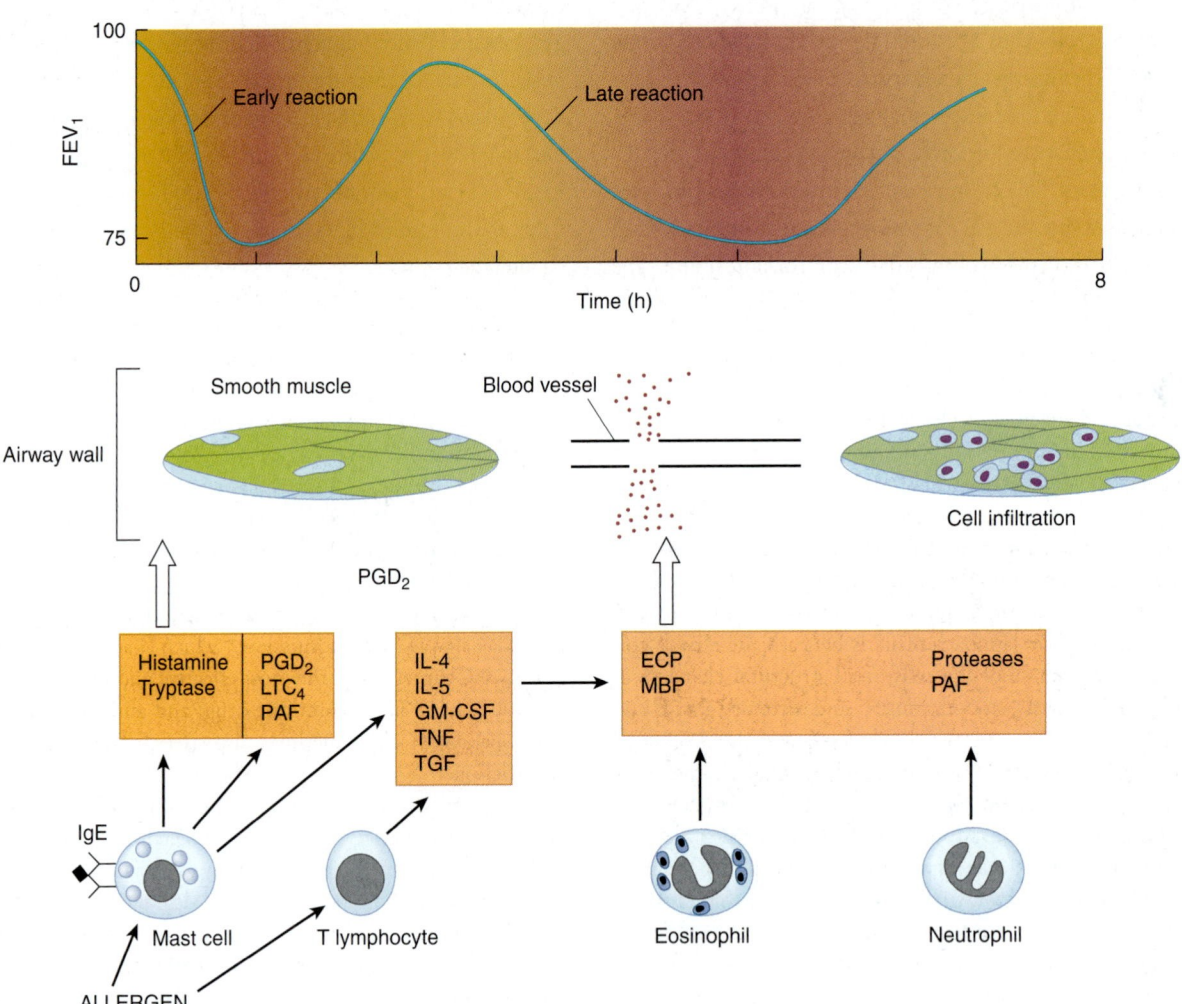

FIGURE 20–1 Conceptual model for the immunopathogenesis of asthma. Exposure to allergen causes synthesis of IgE, which binds to mast cells in the airway mucosa. On reexposure to allergen, antigen-antibody interaction on mast cell surfaces triggers release of mediators of anaphylaxis: histamine, tryptase, prostaglandin D_2 (PGD_2), leukotriene C_4, and platelet-activating factor (PAF). These agents provoke contraction of airway smooth muscle, causing the immediate fall in FEV_1. Reexposure to allergen also causes the synthesis and release of a variety of cytokines: interleukins 4 and 5, granulocyte-macrophage colony-stimulating factor (GM-CSF), tumor necrosis factor (TNF), and tissue growth factor (TGF) from T cells and mast cells. These cytokines in turn attract and activate eosinophils and neutrophils, whose products include eosinophil cationic protein (ECP), major basic protein (MBP), proteases, and platelet-activating factor. These mediators cause the edema, mucus hypersecretion, smooth muscle contraction, and increase in bronchial reactivity associated with the late asthmatic response, indicated by a second fall in FEV_1 3-6 hours after the exposure.

a second, more sustained phase of bronchoconstriction, the "late asthmatic response," which is associated with an influx of inflammatory cells into the bronchial mucosa and with an increase in bronchial reactivity that may last for several weeks after a single inhalation of allergen. The mediators responsible for this late response are thought to be cytokines characteristically produced by TH2 lymphocytes, especially interleukins 5, 9, and 13. These cytokines are thought to attract and activate eosinophils, stimulate IgE production by B lymphocytes, and stimulate mucus production by bronchial epithelial cells. It is not clear whether lymphocytes or mast cells in the airway mucosa are the primary source of the mediators responsible for the late inflammatory response, but the benefits of corticosteroid therapy are attributed to their inhibition of the production of pro-inflammatory cytokines in the airways.

The allergen challenge model does not reproduce all the features of asthma. Most asthma attacks are not triggered by inhalation of allergens. They are triggered by viral respiratory infection. Some adults with asthma have no evidence of allergic sensitivity to allergens, and even in people with allergic sensitivity, the severity of symptoms correlates poorly with levels of allergen in the atmosphere. Moreover, bronchospasm can be provoked by nonallergenic stimuli such as distilled water, exercise, cold air, sulfur dioxide, and rapid respiratory maneuvers.

This tendency to develop bronchospasm on encountering stimuli that do not affect healthy nonasthmatic airways is characteristic of asthma and is sometimes called "nonspecific bronchial hyperreactivity" to distinguish it from bronchial responsiveness to specific antigens. Bronchial reactivity is assessed by measuring the fall in forced expiratory volume in 1 second (FEV_1) provoked by inhaling serially increasing concentrations of aerosolized methacholine. The exaggerated reactivity of the airways appears to be fundamental to asthma's pathogenesis, because it is nearly ubiquitous in patients with asthma and its degree roughly correlates with the clinical severity of the disease.

The mechanisms underlying bronchial hyperreactivity are somehow related to inflammation of the airway mucosa. The agents that increase bronchial reactivity, such as ozone exposure, allergen inhalation, and infection with respiratory viruses, also cause airway inflammation. The increase in reactivity due to allergen inhalation is associated with an increase in both eosinophils and polymorphonuclear leukocytes in bronchial lavage fluid. The increase in reactivity that is associated with the late asthmatic response to allergen inhalation (Figure 20–1) is sustained and, because it is prevented by treatment with an inhaled corticosteroid, is thought to be caused by airway inflammation.

Whatever the mechanisms responsible for bronchial hyperreactivity, bronchoconstriction itself seems to result not simply from the direct effect of the released mediators but also from their activation of neural or humoral pathways. Evidence for the importance of neural pathways stems largely from studies of laboratory animals. The bronchospasm provoked in dogs by inhalation of histamine is reduced by pretreatment with an inhaled topical anesthetic agent, by transection of the vagus nerves, and by pretreatment with atropine. Studies of asthmatic humans, however, have shown that treatment with atropine causes only a reduction

in—not abolition of—the bronchospastic responses to antigens and to nonantigenic stimuli. It is possible that activity in another neural pathway, such as the nonadrenergic, noncholinergic system, contributes to bronchomotor responses to stimuli (Figure 20–2).

The hypothesis suggested by these studies—that asthmatic bronchospasm results from a combination of release of mediators and an exaggeration of responsiveness to their effects—predicts that asthma may be effectively treated by drugs with different modes of action. Asthmatic bronchospasm might be reversed or prevented, for example, by drugs that reduce the amount of IgE bound to mast cells (anti-IgE antibody), prevent mast cell degranulation (cromolyn or nedocromil, sympathomimetic agents, calcium channel blockers), block the action of the products released (antihistamines and leukotriene receptor antagonists), inhibit the effect of acetylcholine released from vagal motor nerves (muscarinic antagonists), or directly relax airway smooth muscle (sympathomimetic agents, theophylline).

The second approach to the treatment of asthma is aimed not only at preventing or reversing acute bronchospasm but at reducing the level of bronchial responsiveness. Because increased responsiveness appears to be linked to airway inflammation and because airway inflammation is a feature of late asthmatic responses, this strategy is implemented both by reducing exposure to the allergens that provoke inflammation and by prolonged therapy with anti-inflammatory agents, especially inhaled corticosteroids.

■ BASIC PHARMACOLOGY OF AGENTS USED IN THE TREATMENT OF ASTHMA

The drugs most used for management of asthma are adrenoceptor agonists, or sympathomimetic agents (used as "relievers" or bronchodilators) and inhaled corticosteroids (used as "controllers" or anti-inflammatory agents). Their basic pharmacology is presented elsewhere (see Chapters 9 and 39). In this chapter, we review their pharmacology relevant to asthma.

SYMPATHOMIMETIC AGENTS

The adrenoceptor agonists have several pharmacologic actions that are important in the treatment of asthma. They relax airway smooth muscle and inhibit release of bronchoconstricting mediators from mast cells. They may also inhibit microvascular leakage and increase mucociliary transport by increasing ciliary activity. As in other tissues, the β agonists stimulate adenylyl cyclase and increase the formation of intracellular cAMP (Figure 20–3).

The best-characterized action of the adrenoceptor agonists in the airways is relaxation of airway smooth muscle. Although there is no evidence for direct sympathetic innervation of human airway smooth muscle, ample evidence exists for the presence of adrenoceptors on airway smooth muscle. In general, stimulation of β_2

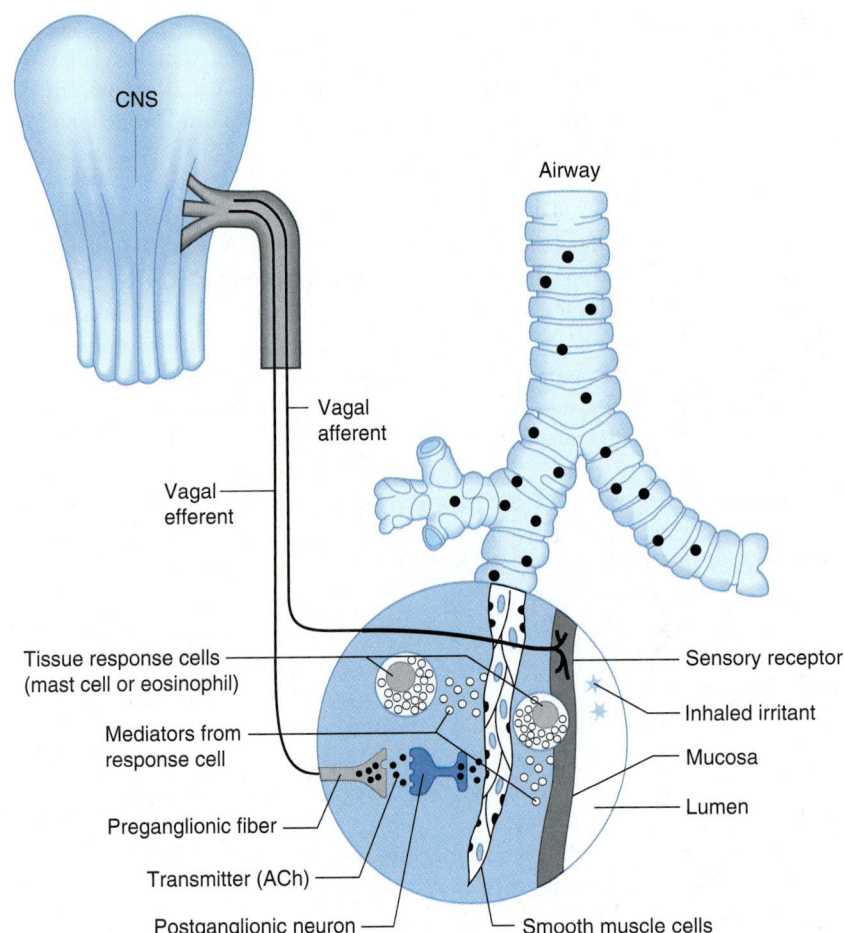

FIGURE 20–2 Mechanisms of response to inhaled irritants. The airway is represented microscopically by a cross-section of the wall with branching vagal sensory endings lying adjacent to the lumen. Afferent pathways in the vagus nerves travel to the central nervous system; efferent pathways from the central nervous system travel to efferent ganglia. Postganglionic fibers release acetylcholine (ACh), which binds to muscarinic receptors on airway smooth muscle. Inhaled materials may provoke bronchoconstriction by several possible mechanisms. First, they may trigger the release of chemical mediators from mast cells. Second, they may stimulate afferent receptors to initiate reflex bronchoconstriction or to release tachykinins (eg, substance P) that directly stimulate smooth muscle contraction.

receptors relaxes airway smooth muscle, inhibits mediator release, and causes tachycardia and skeletal muscle tremor as side effects.

The sympathomimetic agents that have been widely used in the treatment of asthma include epinephrine, ephedrine, isoproterenol, and albuterol and other β_2-selective agents (Figure 20–4). Because epinephrine and isoproterenol increase the rate and force of cardiac contraction (mediated mainly by β_1 receptors), they are reserved for special situations (see below).

In general, adrenoceptor agonists are best delivered by inhalation because this results in the greatest local effect on airway smooth muscle with the least systemic toxicity. Aerosol deposition depends on the particle size, the pattern of breathing, and the geometry of the airways. Even with particles in the optimal size range of 2–5 mm, 80–90% of the total dose of aerosol is deposited in the mouth or pharynx. Particles under 1–2 μm remain suspended and may be exhaled. Bronchial deposition of an aerosol is increased by slow inhalation of a nearly full breath and by more than 5 seconds of breath-holding at the end of inspiration.

Epinephrine is an effective, rapidly acting bronchodilator when injected subcutaneously (0.4 mL of 1:1000 solution) or inhaled as a microaerosol from a pressurized canister (320 mcg per puff). Maximal bronchodilation is achieved 15 minutes after inhalation and lasts 60–90 minutes. Because epinephrine stimulates α and β_1 as well as β_2 receptors, tachycardia, arrhythmias, and worsening of angina pectoris are troublesome adverse effects. The cardiovascular effects of epinephrine are of value for treating the acute vasodilation and shock as well as the bronchospasm of anaphylaxis, but its use in asthma has been displaced by other, more β_2-selective agents.

Ephedrine was used in China for more than 2000 years before its introduction into Western medicine in 1924. Compared with epinephrine, ephedrine has a longer duration, oral activity, more pronounced central effects, and much lower potency. Because of

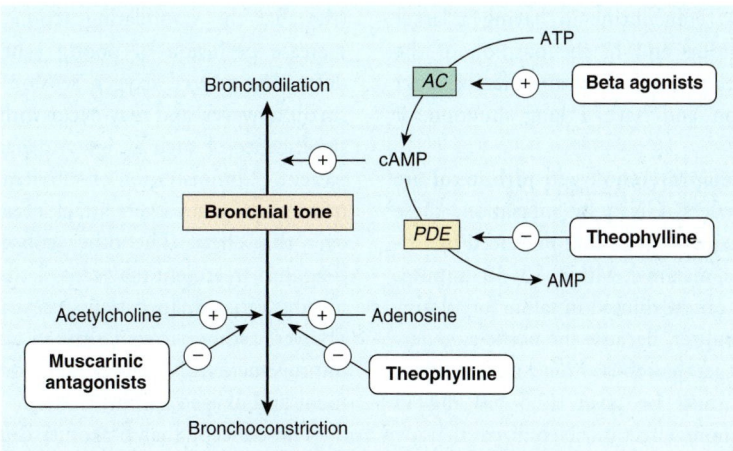

FIGURE 20–3 Bronchodilation is promoted by cAMP. Intracellular levels of cAMP can be increased by β-adrenoceptor agonists, which increase the rate of its synthesis by adenylyl cyclase (AC); or by phosphodiesterase (PDE) inhibitors such as theophylline, which slow the rate of its degradation. Bronchoconstriction can be inhibited by muscarinic antagonists and possibly by adenosine antagonists.

the development of more efficacious and β₂-selective agonists, ephedrine is now used infrequently in treating asthma.

Isoproterenol is a potent bronchodilator; when inhaled as a microaerosol from a pressurized canister, 80–120 mcg isoproterenol causes maximal bronchodilation within 5 minutes. Isoproterenol has a 60- to 90-minute duration of action. An increase in the asthma mortality rate that occurred in the United Kingdom in the mid-1960s was attributed to cardiac arrhythmias resulting

from the use of high doses of inhaled isoproterenol. It is now rarely used for asthma.

Beta₂-Selective Drugs

The β₂-selective adrenoceptor agonist drugs, particularly albuterol, are the most widely used sympathomimetics for the treatment of the bronchoconstriction of asthma at present (Figure 20–4). These

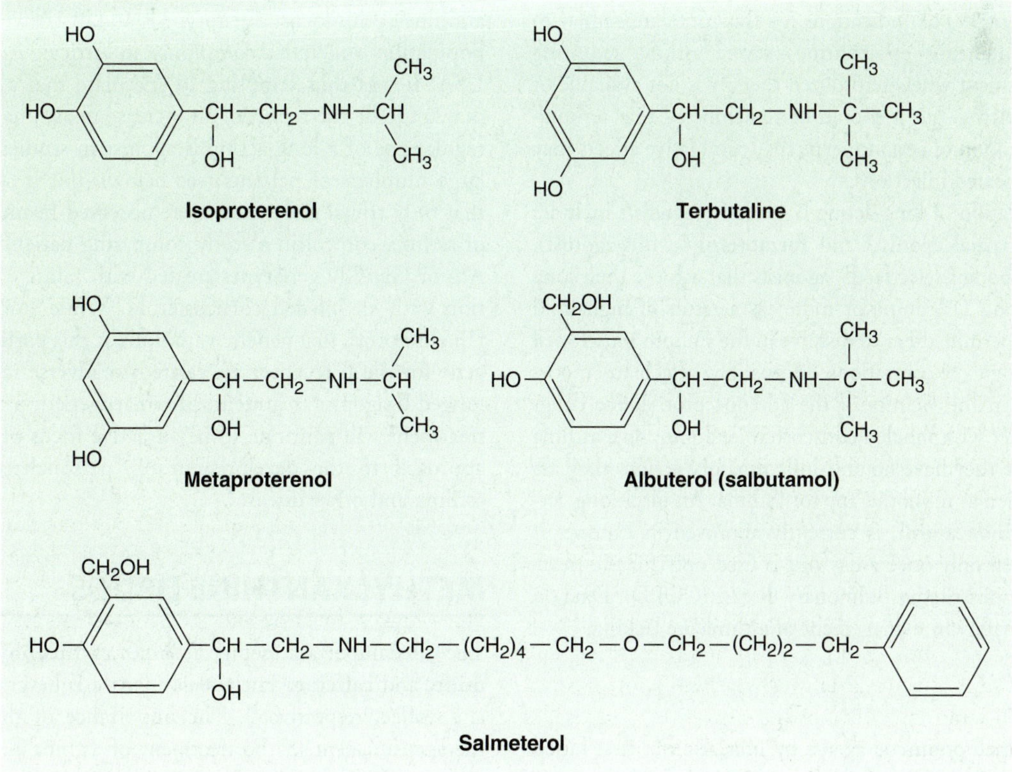

FIGURE 20–4 Structures of isoproterenol and several β₂-selective analogs.

agents differ structurally from epinephrine in having a larger substitution on the amino group and in the position of the hydroxyl groups on the aromatic ring. They are effective after inhaled or oral administration and have a long duration of action.

Albuterol, terbutaline, metaproterenol, and **pirbuterol** are available as metered-dose inhalers. Given by inhalation, these agents cause bronchodilation equivalent to that produced by isoproterenol. Bronchodilation is maximal within 15–30 minutes and persists for 3–4 hours. All can be diluted in saline for administration from a hand-held nebulizer. Because the particles generated by a nebulizer are much larger than those from a metered-dose inhaler, much higher doses must be given (2.5–5.0 mg vs 100–400 mcg) but are no more effective. Nebulized therapy should thus be reserved for patients unable to coordinate inhalation from a metered-dose inhaler.

Most preparations of β_2-selective drugs are a mixture of R and S isomers. Only the R isomer activates the β-agonist receptor. Reasoning that the S isomer may promote inflammation, a purified preparation of the R isomer of albuterol has been developed (levalbuterol). Whether this actually presents significant advantages in clinical use is unproven.

Albuterol and terbutaline are also available in tablet form. One tablet two or three times daily is the usual regimen; the principal adverse effects of skeletal muscle tremor, nervousness, and occasional weakness may be reduced by starting the patient on half-strength tablets for the first 2 weeks of therapy. This route of administration presents no advantage over inhaled treatment and is thus rarely prescribed.

Of these agents, only terbutaline is available for subcutaneous injection (0.25 mg). The indications for this route are similar to those for subcutaneous epinephrine—severe asthma requiring emergency treatment when aerosolized therapy is not available or has been ineffective—but it should be remembered that terbutaline's longer duration of action means that cumulative effects may be seen after repeated injections.

A new generation of long-acting β_2-selective agonists includes **salmeterol** (a partial agonist) and **formoterol** (a full agonist). Both drugs are potent selective β_2 agonists that achieve their long duration of action (12 hours or more) as a result of high lipid solubility. This permits them to dissolve in the smooth muscle cell membrane in high concentrations or, possibly, attach to "mooring" molecules in the vicinity of the adrenoceptor. These drugs appear to interact with inhaled corticosteroids to improve asthma control. Because they have no anti-inflammatory action, they are not recommended as monotherapy for asthma. An ultra-long acting β agonist, **indacaterol,** is currently approved in Europe. It needs to be taken only once a day but is used only for the treatment of chronic obstructive pulmonary disease (COPD). Data on its efficacy and safety in management of asthma are lacking.

Toxicities

The use of sympathomimetic agents by inhalation at first raised fears about possible cardiac arrhythmias and about hypoxemia acutely and tachyphylaxis or tolerance when given repeatedly. It is

true that the vasodilating action of β_2-agonist treatment may increase perfusion of poorly ventilated lung units, transiently decreasing arterial oxygen tension (PaO_2). This effect is usually small, however, and may occur with any bronchodilator drug; the significance of such an effect depends on the initial PaO_2 of the patient. Administration of supplemental oxygen, routine in treatment of an acute severe attack of asthma, eliminates any concern over this effect. The other concern, that customary doses of β-agonist treatment may cause lethal cardiac arrhythmias, appears unsubstantiated. In patients presenting for emergency treatment of severe asthma, irregularities in cardiac rhythm *improve* with the improvements in gas exchange effected by bronchodilator treatment and oxygen administration.

The concept that β-agonist drugs worsen clinical asthma by inducing tachyphylaxis to their own action has not been established. Most studies have shown only a small change in the bronchodilator response to β stimulation after prolonged treatment with β-agonist drugs, but some studies have shown a loss in the ability of β-agonist treatment to inhibit the response to subsequent challenge with exercise, methacholine, or antigen challenge (referred to as a loss of bronchoprotective action).

Although it is true that β_2-adrenoceptor agonists appear to be safe and effective bronchodilators when taken on an "as needed" basis for relief of symptoms, there is some evidence of risk of adverse effects from chronic treatment with long-acting β agonists. These risks were suspected to be greater for individuals carrying a genetic variant for the β receptor, specifically at the B-16 locus of the β receptor. Retrospective analyses of studies of regular treatment with an inhaled β agonist suggested that asthma control deteriorated among patients homozygous for arginine at this locus, a genotype found in 16% of the Caucasian population and more commonly in African Americans in the USA. It was thus tempting to speculate that a genetic variant may underlie the report of an increase in asthma mortality from regular use of a long-acting β agonist in studies involving very large numbers of patients (see below), but it should be noted that only trivial differences were observed in multiple measures of asthma control in a study comparing patients with the Arg/Arg or Gly/Gly genotypes treated with salmeterol in combination with an inhaled corticosteroid. While studies so far have failed to prove that genetic variations at this particular site in the gene for the β receptor are related to adverse responses to prolonged β-agonist treatment, pharmacogenetic studies of asthma treatment will continue to be an active focus of research, as an approach to the development of "personalized therapy" for asthma and other diseases.

METHYLXANTHINE DRUGS

The three important methylxanthines are **theophylline, theobromine,** and **caffeine.** Their major source is beverages (tea, cocoa, and coffee, respectively). The importance of theophylline as a therapeutic agent in the treatment of asthma has waned as the greater effectiveness of inhaled adrenoceptor agents for acute asthma and of inhaled anti-inflammatory agents for chronic asthma has been established, but theophylline's very low cost is an important advantage for economically disadvantaged patients in societies in which health care resources are limited.

Chemistry

As shown below, theophylline is 1,3-dimethylxanthine; theobromine is 3,7-dimethylxanthine; and caffeine is 1,3,7-trimethylxanthine. A theophylline preparation commonly used for therapeutic purposes is **aminophylline,** a theophylline-ethylenediamine complex. The pharmacokinetics of theophylline are discussed below (see Clinical Uses of Methylxanthines). The metabolic products, partially demethylated xanthines (not uric acid), are excreted in the urine.

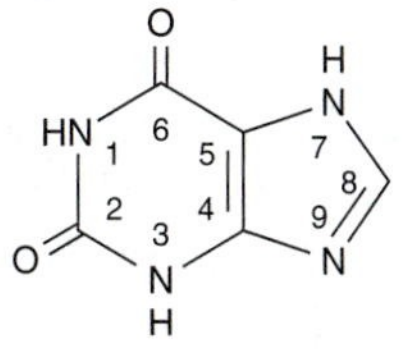

Xanthine

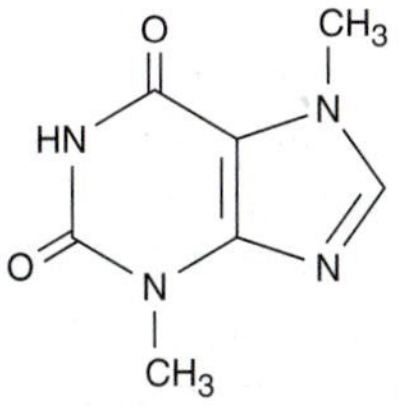

Theobromine

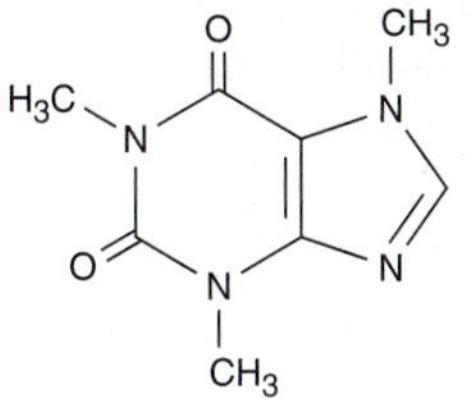

Caffeine

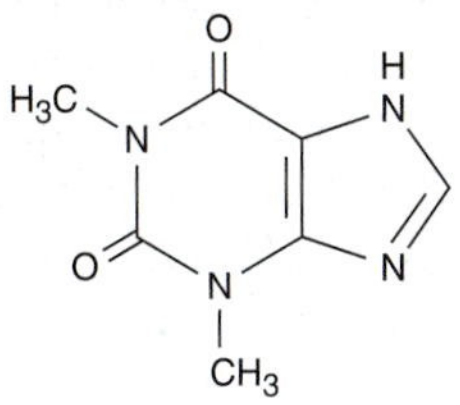

Theophylline

Mechanism of Action

Several mechanisms have been proposed for the actions of methylxanthines, but none has been firmly established. At high concentrations, they can be shown in vitro to inhibit several members of the phosphodiesterase (PDE) enzyme family (Figure 20–3). Because the phosphodiesterases hydrolyze cyclic nucleotides, this inhibition results in higher concentrations of intracellular cAMP and, in some tissues, cGMP. Cyclic AMP is responsible for a myriad of cellular functions including, but not limited to, stimulation of cardiac function, relaxation of smooth muscle, and reduction in the immune and inflammatory activity of specific cells.

Of the various isoforms of phosphodiesterase that have been identified, PDE4 appears to be the most directly involved in actions of methylxanthines on airway smooth muscle and on inflammatory cells. The inhibition of PDE4 in inflammatory cells reduces their release of cytokines and chemokines, which in turn results in a decrease in immune cell migration and activation.

In an effort to reduce toxicity while maintaining therapeutic efficacy, selective inhibitors of different isoforms of PDE4 were developed. Many were abandoned after clinical trials showed that their toxicities of nausea, headache, and diarrhea restricted dosing to subtherapeutic levels, but one, **roflumilast,** has recently been approved by the Food and Drug Administration (FDA) as a treatment for COPD, though not for asthma.

Another proposed mechanism is inhibition of cell surface receptors for adenosine. These receptors modulate adenylyl cyclase activity, and adenosine has been shown to provoke contraction of isolated airway smooth muscle and histamine release from airway mast cells. It has been shown, however, that xanthine derivatives devoid of adenosine antagonism (eg, enprofylline) may be potent in inhibiting bronchoconstriction in asthmatic subjects.

Some research suggests that the efficacy of theophyllines may be due to a third mechanism of action: enhancement of histone deacetylation. Acetylation of core histones is necessary for activation of inflammatory gene transcription. Corticosteroids act, at least in part, by recruiting histone deacetylactylases to the site of inflammatory gene transcription, an action enhanced by low-dose theophylline. This interaction should predict that low-dose theophylline treatment would enhance the effectiveness of corticosteroid treatment, and some clinical trials indeed support the idea that theophylline treatment is effective in restoring corticosteroid responsiveness in asthmatics who smoke and in patients with some forms of COPD.

Pharmacodynamics

The methylxanthines have effects on the central nervous system, kidney, and cardiac and skeletal muscle as well as smooth muscle. Of the three agents, theophylline is most selective in its smooth muscle effects, whereas caffeine has the most marked central nervous system effects.

A. Central Nervous System Effects

In low and moderate doses, the methylxanthines—especially caffeine—cause mild cortical arousal with increased alertness and deferral of fatigue. The caffeine contained in beverages—eg, 100 mg in a cup of coffee—is sufficient to cause nervousness and insomnia in sensitive individuals and slight bronchodilation in patients with asthma. The larger doses necessary for more effective bronchodilation commonly cause nervousness and tremor in some patients. Very high doses, from accidental or suicidal overdose, cause medullary stimulation and convulsions and may lead to death.

B. Cardiovascular Effects

The methylxanthines have positive chronotropic and inotropic effects. At low concentrations, these effects appear to result from inhibition of presynaptic adenosine receptors in sympathetic nerves increasing catecholamine release at nerve endings. The higher concentrations (> 10 μmol/L, 2 mg/L) associated with inhibition of phosphodiesterase and increases in cAMP may result in increased influx of calcium. At much higher concentrations (> 100 μmol/L), sequestration of calcium by the sarcoplasmic reticulum is impaired.

The clinical expression of these effects on cardiovascular function varies among individuals. Ordinary consumption of coffee and other methylxanthine-containing beverages usually produces slight tachycardia, an increase in cardiac output, and an increase in peripheral resistance, raising blood pressure slightly. In sensitive individuals, consumption of a few cups of coffee may result in arrhythmias.

In large doses, these agents also relax vascular smooth muscle except in cerebral blood vessels, where they cause contraction.

Methylxanthines decrease blood viscosity and may improve blood flow under certain conditions. The mechanism of this action is not well defined, but the effect is exploited in the treatment of intermittent claudication with **pentoxifylline,** a dimethylxanthine agent. However, no evidence suggests that this therapy is superior to other approaches.

C. Effects on Gastrointestinal Tract

The methylxanthines stimulate secretion of both gastric acid and digestive enzymes. However, even decaffeinated coffee has a potent stimulant effect on secretion, which means that the primary secretagogue in coffee is not caffeine.

D. Effects on Kidney

The methylxanthines—especially theophylline—are weak diuretics. This effect may involve both increased glomerular filtration and reduced tubular sodium reabsorption. The diuresis is not of sufficient magnitude to be therapeutically useful.

E. Effects on Smooth Muscle

The bronchodilation produced by the methylxanthines is the major therapeutic action in asthma. Tolerance does not develop, but adverse effects, especially in the central nervous system, may limit the dose (see below). In addition to their effect on airway smooth muscle, these agents—in sufficient concentration—inhibit antigen-induced release of histamine from lung tissue; their effect on mucociliary transport is unknown.

F. Effects on Skeletal Muscle

The respiratory actions of the methylxanthines may not be confined to the airways, for they also strengthen the contractions of isolated skeletal muscle in vitro and improve contractility and reverse fatigue of the diaphragm in patients with COPD. This effect on diaphragmatic performance—rather than an effect on the respiratory center—may account for theophylline's ability to improve the ventilatory response to hypoxia and to diminish dyspnea even in patients with irreversible airflow obstruction.

Clinical Uses

Of the xanthines, theophylline is the most effective bronchodilator, and it has been shown repeatedly both to relieve airflow obstruction in acute asthma and to reduce the severity of symptoms and time lost from work or school in patients with chronic asthma. Theophylline base is only slightly soluble in water, so it has been administered as several salts containing varying amounts of theophylline base. Most preparations are well absorbed from the gastrointestinal tract, but absorption of rectal suppositories is unreliable.

Improvements in theophylline preparations have come from alterations in the physical state of the drugs rather than from new chemical formulations. For example, the increased surface area of anhydrous theophylline in a microcrystalline form facilitates solubilization for complete and rapid absorption after oral administration. Numerous sustained-release preparations (see Preparations Available) are available and can produce therapeutic blood levels for 12 hours or more. These preparations offer the advantages of less frequent drug administration, less fluctuation of theophylline blood levels, and, in many cases, more effective treatment of nocturnal bronchospasm.

Theophylline should be used only where methods to measure theophylline blood levels are available because it has a narrow therapeutic window, and its therapeutic and toxic effects are related to its blood level. Improvement in pulmonary function is correlated with plasma concentration in the range of 5–20 mg/L. Anorexia, nausea, vomiting, abdominal discomfort, headache, and anxiety occur at concentrations of 15 mg/L in some patients and become common at concentrations greater than 20 mg/L. Higher levels (> 40 mg/L) may cause seizures or arrhythmias; these may not be preceded by gastrointestinal or neurologic warning symptoms.

The plasma clearance of theophylline varies widely. Theophylline is metabolized by the liver, so usual doses may lead to toxic concentrations of the drug in patients with liver disease. Conversely, clearance may be increased through the induction of hepatic enzymes by cigarette smoking or by changes in diet. In normal adults, the mean plasma clearance is 0.69 mL/kg/min. Children clear theophylline faster than adults (1–1.5 mL/kg/min). Neonates and young infants have the slowest clearance (see Chapter 60). Even when maintenance doses are altered to correct for the above factors, plasma concentrations vary widely.

Theophylline improves long-term control of asthma when taken as the sole maintenance treatment or when added to inhaled corticosteroids. It is inexpensive, and it can be taken orally. Its use, however, also requires occasional measurement of plasma levels; it often causes unpleasant minor side effects (especially insomnia); and accidental or intentional overdose can result in severe toxicity or death. For oral therapy with the prompt-release formulation, the usual dose is 3–4 mg/kg of theophylline every 6 hours. Changes in dosage result in a new steady-state concentration of theophylline in 1–2 days, so the dosage may be increased at intervals of 2–3 days until therapeutic plasma concentrations are achieved (10–20 mg/L) or until adverse effects develop.

ANTIMUSCARINIC AGENTS

Observation of the use of leaves from *Datura stramonium* for asthma treatment in India led to the discovery of atropine, a potent competitive inhibitor of acetylcholine at postganglionic muscarinic receptors, as a bronchodilator. Interest in the potential value of antimuscarinic agents increased with demonstration of the importance of the vagus nerves in bronchospastic responses of laboratory animals and with the development of a potent atropine analog that is poorly absorbed after aerosol administration and is therefore relatively free of systemic atropine-like effects.

Mechanism of Action

Muscarinic antagonists competitively inhibit the effect of acetylcholine at muscarinic receptors (see Chapter 8). In the airways, acetylcholine is released from efferent endings of the vagus nerves, and muscarinic antagonists block the contraction of airway smooth muscle and the increase in secretion of mucus that occurs in response to vagal activity (Figure 20–2). Very high concentrations—well above those achieved even with maximal therapy—are required to inhibit the response of airway smooth muscle to nonmuscarinic stimulation. This selectivity of muscarinic antagonists accounts for their usefulness as investigative tools in examining the role of parasympathetic pathways in bronchomotor responses but limits their usefulness in preventing bronchospasm. In the doses given, antimuscarinic agents inhibit only that portion of the response mediated by muscarinic receptors, which varies by stimulus, and which further appears to vary among individual responses to the same stimulus.

Clinical Uses

Antimuscarinic agents are effective bronchodilators. When given intravenously, atropine, the prototypical muscarinic antagonist, causes bronchodilation at a lower dose than that needed to cause an increase in heart rate. The selectivity of atropine's effect can be increased further by administering the drug by inhalation or by use of a more selective quaternary ammonium derivative of atropine, **ipratropium bromide.** Ipratropium can be delivered in high doses by this route because it is poorly absorbed into the circulation and does not readily enter the central nervous system. Studies with this agent have shown that the degree of involvement of parasympathetic pathways in bronchomotor responses varies among subjects. In some, bronchoconstriction is inhibited effectively; in others, only modestly. The failure of higher doses of the muscarinic antagonist to further inhibit the response in these individuals indicates that mechanisms other than parasympathetic reflex pathways must be involved.

Even in the subjects least protected by this antimuscarinic agent, however, the bronchodilation and partial inhibition of provoked bronchoconstriction are of potential clinical value, and antimuscarinic agents are valuable for patients intolerant of inhaled β-agonist agents. Although antimuscarinic drugs appear to be slightly less effective than β-agonist agents in reversing asthmatic bronchospasm, the addition of ipratropium enhances the bronchodilation produced by nebulized albuterol in acute severe asthma.

Ipratropium appears to be at least as effective in patients with COPD that includes a partially reversible component. A longer-acting, selective antimuscarinic agent, **tiotropium,** is approved as a treatment for COPD. It binds to M_1, M_2, and M_3 receptors with equal affinity, but dissociates most rapidly from M_2 receptors, expressed on the efferent nerve ending. This means that tiotropium does not inhibit the M_2-receptor–mediated auto–down-regulation of acetylcholine release, and thus confers a degree of receptor selectivity. Tiotropium is also taken by inhalation, and a single dose of 18 mcg has 24-hour duration of action. Daily inhalation of tiotropium has been shown not only to improve functional capacity of patients with COPD, but also to reduce the frequency of exacerbations of their condition, and tiotropium is approved by the FDA as a treatment for COPD. It has not been approved as a treatment for asthma, but the addition of tiotropium has recently been shown to be as effective as the addition of a long-acting β-agonist in asthmatic patients insufficiently controlled by inhaled corticosteroid therapy alone.

CORTICOSTEROIDS

Mechanism of Action

Corticosteroids have been used to treat asthma since 1950 and are presumed to act by their broad anti-inflammatory efficacy, mediated in part by inhibition of production of inflammatory cytokines (see Chapter 39). They do not relax airway smooth muscle directly but reduce bronchial reactivity and reduce the frequency of asthma exacerbations if taken regularly. Their effect on airway obstruction may be due in part to their contraction of engorged vessels in the bronchial mucosa and their potentiation of the effects of β-receptor agonists, but their most important action is inhibition of the infiltration of asthmatic airways by lymphocytes, eosinophils, and mast cells.

Clinical Uses

Clinical studies of corticosteroids consistently show them to be effective in improving all indices of asthma control—severity of symptoms, tests of airway caliber and bronchial reactivity, frequency of exacerbations, and quality of life. Because of severe adverse effects when given chronically, oral and parenteral corticosteroids are reserved for patients who require urgent treatment, ie, those who have not improved adequately with bronchodilators or who experience worsening symptoms despite maintenance therapy. Regular or "controller" therapy is maintained with aerosol corticosteroids.

Urgent treatment is often begun with an oral dose of 30–60 mg prednisone per day or an intravenous dose of 1 mg/kg methylprednisolone every 6–12 hours; the daily dose is decreased after airway obstruction has improved. In most patients, systemic corticosteroid therapy can be discontinued in 7–10 days, but in other patients symptoms may worsen as the dose is decreased to lower levels. Because adrenal suppression by corticosteroids is related to dose and because secretion of endogenous corticosteroids has a diurnal variation, it is customary to administer corticosteroids early in the morning after endogenous adrenocorticotropic hormone secretion has peaked. For prevention of nocturnal asthma, however, oral or inhaled corticosteroids are most effective when given in the late afternoon.

Aerosol treatment is the most effective way to avoid the systemic adverse effects of corticosteroid therapy. The introduction of corticosteroids such as **beclomethasone, budesonide, ciclesonide, flunisolide, fluticasone, mometasone,** and **triamcinolone** has made it possible to deliver corticosteroids to the airways with minimal systemic absorption. An average daily dose of four puffs twice daily of beclomethasone (400 mcg/d) is equivalent to about 10–15 mg/d of oral prednisone for the control of asthma, with far fewer systemic effects. Indeed, one of the cautions in switching patients from oral to inhaled corticosteroid therapy is to taper oral therapy slowly to avoid precipitation of adrenal insufficiency. In patients requiring continued prednisone treatment despite inhalation of standard doses of an aerosol corticosteroid, higher doses appear to be more effective; inhalation of high doses of both fluticasone and ciclesonide, for example, have been shown to be effective in weaning patients from chronic prednisone therapy. Although these high doses of inhaled steroids may cause adrenal suppression, the risks of systemic toxicity from chronic use appear negligible compared with those of the oral corticosteroid therapy they replace.

A special problem caused by inhaled topical corticosteroids is the occurrence of oropharyngeal candidiasis. The risk of this complication can be reduced by having patients gargle water and spit after each inhaled treatment. Hoarseness can also result from a direct local effect of inhaled corticosteroids on the vocal cords. These agents are remarkably free of other short-term complications in adults but may increase the risks of osteoporosis and cataracts over the long term. In children, inhaled corticosteroid therapy has been shown to slow the rate of growth by about 1 cm over the first year of treatment, but not the rate of growth thereafter, so that the effect on adult height is minimal.

A novel approach to minimizing the risk of toxicity from systemic absorption of an inhaled corticosteroid underlay the development of **ciclesonide.** This recently approved corticosteroid is inhaled as a prodrug activated by cleavage by esterases in bronchial epithelial cells. When absorbed into the circulation, the active product is tightly bound to serum proteins, and so has little access to glucocorticoid receptors in skin, eye, and bone, minimizing its risk of causing cutaneous thinning, cataracts, osteoporosis, or temporary slowing of growth. Ciclesonide has been shown to be effective in improving asthma control in clinical trials, but studies have not yet proven that its use is associated with the significant reduction in systemic toxicity predicted from its design as a prodrug with low corticosteroid activity, activated to a much more potent corticosteroid agonist by esterases at its site of deposition in the airways.

Chronic use of inhaled corticosteroids effectively reduces symptoms and improves pulmonary function in patients with mild asthma. Such use also reduces or eliminates the need for oral corticosteroids in patients with more severe disease. In contrast to β-stimulant agents and theophylline, chronic use of inhaled corticosteroids reduces bronchial reactivity. Because of the efficacy and safety of inhaled corticosteroids, national and international guidelines for asthma management recommend their prescription for patients who require more than occasional inhalations of a β agonist for relief of symptoms. This therapy is continued for 10–12 weeks and then withdrawn to determine whether more prolonged therapy is needed. Inhaled corticosteroids are not curative. In most patients, the manifestations of asthma return within a few weeks after stopping therapy even if they have been taken in high doses for 2 years or longer. A prospective, placebo-controlled study of the early, sustained use of an inhaled corticosteroids in young children with asthma showed significantly greater improvement in asthma symptoms,

pulmonary function, and frequency of asthma exacerbations over the 2 years of treatment, but no difference in overall asthma control 3 months after the end of the trial. Inhaled corticosteroids are thus properly labeled as "controllers." They are effective only so long as they are taken.

Another approach to reducing the risk of long-term, twice-daily use of inhaled corticosteroids is to administer them only intermittently, when symptoms of asthma flare. Taking a single inhalation of an inhaled corticosteroid with each inhalation of a short-acting β-agonist reliever (eg, an inhalation of beclomethasone for each inhalation of albuterol) or taking a 5–10 day course of twice-daily high-dose budesonide or beclomethasone when asthma symptoms worsen has been found to be as effective as regular daily therapy in adults and children with mild to moderate asthma, although these approaches to treatment are neither endorsed by guidelines for asthma management nor approved by the FDA.

CROMOLYN & NEDOCROMIL

Cromolyn sodium (disodium cromoglycate) and nedocromil sodium were once widely used for asthma management, especially in children, but have now been supplanted so completely by other therapies that they are mostly of historic interest. Both have low solubility, are poorly absorbed from the gastrointestinal tract, and must be inhaled as a microfine powder or microfine suspension. When taken by inhalation, they effectively inhibit both antigen- and exercise-induced asthma, and chronic use (four times daily) slightly reduces the overall level of bronchial reactivity. However, these drugs have no effect on airway smooth muscle tone and are ineffective in reversing asthmatic bronchospasm; they are only of value when taken prophylactically.

Cromolyn sodium

Nedocromil sodium

Mechanism of Action

Cromolyn and nedocromil are thought to alter the function of delayed chloride channels in the cell membranes, inhibiting cell activation. This action on airway nerves is thought to mediate nedocromil's inhibition of cough; on mast cells, the same mechanism is responsible for inhibition of the early response to antigen challenge and on eosinophils, for inhibition of the inflammatory response to inhalation of allergens. The inhibitory effect on mast cells appears to be specific for cell type, since cromolyn has little inhibitory effect on mediator release from human basophils. It may also be specific for different organs, since cromolyn inhibits mast cell degranulation in human and primate lung but not in skin. This in turn may reflect known differences in mast cells found in different sites, as in their neutral protease content.

At one time, the idea that cromolyn inhibits mast cell degranulation was so well accepted that the inhibition of a response by cromolyn was thought to indicate the involvement of mast cells in the response. This simplistic idea was overturned in part by the finding that cromolyn and nedocromil inhibit the function of cells other than mast cells and in part by the finding that nedocromil inhibits appearance of the late response even when given after the early response to antigen challenge, ie, after mast cell degranulation has occurred.

Clinical Uses

In short-term clinical trials, pretreatment with cromolyn or nedocromil blocks the bronchoconstriction caused by allergen inhalation, by exercise, by sulfur dioxide, and by a variety of causes of occupational asthma. This acute protective effect of a single treatment makes cromolyn useful for administration shortly before exercise or before unavoidable exposure to an allergen.

When taken regularly (two to four puffs two to four times daily) by patients with perennial (nonseasonal) asthma, both agents modestly but significantly reduce symptomatic severity and the need for bronchodilator medications, particularly in young patients with extrinsic asthma. These drugs are not as potent nor as predictably effective as inhaled corticosteroids, and the only way of determining whether a patient will respond is by a therapeutic trial of 4 weeks' duration.

Cromolyn and nedocromil solutions are also useful in reducing symptoms of **allergic rhinoconjunctivitis.** Applying the solution by nasal spray or eye drops several times a day is effective in about 75% of patients, even during the peak pollen season.

Because the drugs are so poorly absorbed, adverse effects of cromolyn and nedocromil are minor and are localized to the sites of deposition. These include such minor symptoms as throat irritation, cough, and mouth dryness, and, rarely, chest tightness, and wheezing. Some of these symptoms can be prevented by inhaling a β_2-adrenoceptor agonist before cromolyn or nedocromil treatment. Serious adverse effects are rare. Reversible dermatitis, myositis, or gastroenteritis occurs in less than 2% of patients, and a very few cases of pulmonary infiltration with eosinophilia and anaphylaxis have been reported. This lack of toxicity accounts for cromolyn's formerly widespread use in children, especially those at ages of rapid growth. Its place in treatment of childhood asthma has lately diminished, however, because of the significantly greater efficacy of even low-dose corticosteroid treatment and because of the availability of an alternate nonsteroidal controller class of medication, the leukotriene pathway inhibitors (see below).

LEUKOTRIENE PATHWAY INHIBITORS

Because of the evidence of leukotriene involvement in many inflammatory diseases (see Chapter 18) and in anaphylaxis, considerable effort has been expended on the development of drugs that block the synthesis of these arachidonic acid derivatives or their receptors. Leukotrienes result from the action of 5-lipoxygenase on arachidonic acid and are synthesized by a variety of inflammatory cells in the airways, including eosinophils, mast cells, macrophages, and basophils. Leukotriene B_4 (LTB_4) is a potent neutrophil chemoattractant, and LTC_4 and LTD_4 exert many effects known to occur in asthma, including bronchoconstriction, increased bronchial reactivity, mucosal edema, and mucus hypersecretion. Early studies established that antigen challenge of sensitized human lung tissue results in the generation of leukotrienes, whereas other studies of human subjects have shown that inhalation of leukotrienes causes not only bronchoconstriction but also an increase in bronchial reactivity to histamine that persists for several days.

Two approaches to interrupting the leukotriene pathway have been pursued: inhibition of 5-lipoxygenase, thereby preventing leukotriene synthesis; and inhibition of the binding of LTD_4 to its receptor on target tissues, thereby preventing its action. Efficacy in blocking airway responses to exercise and to antigen challenge has been shown for drugs in both categories: **zileuton**, a 5-lipoxygenase inhibitor, and **zafirlukast** and **montelukast**, LTD_4-receptor antagonists. All have been shown to improve asthma control and to reduce the frequency of asthma exacerbations in outpatient clinical trials. Their effects on symptoms, airway caliber, bronchial reactivity, and airway inflammation are less marked than the effects of inhaled corticosteroids, but they are more nearly equal in reducing the frequency of exacerbations. Their principal advantage is that they are taken orally; some patients—especially children—comply poorly with inhaled therapies. Montelukast is approved for children as young as 6 years of age.

Zafirlukast

Montelukast

Zileuton

Some patients appear to have particularly favorable responses, but no clinical features allow identification of "responders" before a trial of therapy. In the USA, zileuton is approved for use in an oral dosage of 1200 mg of the sustained-release form twice daily; zafirlukast, 20 mg twice daily; and montelukast, 10 mg (for adults) or 4 mg (for children) once daily.

Trials with leukotriene inhibitors have demonstrated an important role for leukotrienes in aspirin-induced asthma. It has long been known that 5–10% of asthmatics are exquisitely sensitive to aspirin, so that ingestion of even a very small dose causes profound bronchoconstriction and symptoms of systemic release of histamine, such as flushing and abdominal cramping. Because this reaction to aspirin is not associated with any evidence of allergic sensitization to aspirin or its metabolites and because it is produced by any of the nonsteroidal anti-inflammatory agents, it is thought to result from inhibition of prostaglandin synthetase (cyclooxygenase), shifting arachidonic acid metabolism from the prostaglandin to the leukotriene pathway. Support for this idea was provided by the demonstration that leukotriene pathway inhibitors impressively reduce the response to aspirin challenge and improve overall control of asthma on a day-to-day basis.

Of these agents, zileuton is the least prescribed because of reports of liver toxicity. The receptor antagonists appear to have little toxicity. Reports of Churg-Strauss syndrome (a systemic vasculitis accompanied by worsening asthma, pulmonary infiltrates, and eosinophilia) appear to have been coincidental, with the syndrome unmasked by the reduction in prednisone dosage made possible by the addition of zafirlukast or montelukast. Of these two, montelukast is the most prescribed, probably because it can be taken without regard to meals, and because of the convenience of once-daily treatment.

OTHER DRUGS IN THE TREATMENT OF ASTHMA

Anti-IgE Monoclonal Antibodies

An entirely new approach to the treatment of asthma exploits advances in molecular biology to target IgE antibody. From a collection of monoclonal antibodies raised in mice against IgE antibody itself, a monoclonal antibody was selected that is targeted against the portion of IgE that binds to its receptors (FCε-R1 and FCε-R2 receptors) on mast cells and other inflammatory cells. **Omalizumab** (an anti-IgE monoclonal antibody) inhibits the binding of IgE to mast cells but does not activate IgE already bound to these cells and thus does not provoke mast cell degranulation. The murine antibody has been genetically humanized by replacing all but a small fraction of its amino acids with those found in human proteins, and it does not appear to cause sensitization when given to human subjects.

Administration of omalizumab to asthmatic patients for 10 weeks lowers plasma IgE to undetectable levels and significantly reduces the magnitude of both early and late bronchospastic responses to antigen challenge. Repeated administration lessens asthma severity and reduces the corticosteroid requirement in patients with moderate to severe disease, especially those with a clear environmental antigen precipitating factor, and improves nasal and conjunctival symptoms in patients with perennial or seasonal allergic rhinitis. Omalizumab's most important effect is reduction of the frequency and severity of asthma exacerbations, even while enabling a reduction in corticosteroid requirements. Combined analysis of several clinical trials has shown that the patients most likely to respond are, fortunately, those with the greatest need: those with a history of repeated exacerbations, a high requirement for corticosteroid treatment, and poor pulmonary function. Similarly, the exacerbations most prevented are the ones most important to prevent: Omalizumab treatment reduced exacerbations requiring hospitalization by 88%. These benefits justify the high cost of this treatment in selected individuals with severe disease characterized by frequent exacerbations.

POSSIBLE FUTURE THERAPIES

The rapid advance in the scientific description of the immunopathogenesis of asthma has spurred the development of many new therapies targeting different sites in the immune cascade. These include monoclonal antibodies directed against cytokines (IL-4, IL-5, IL-13), antagonists of cell adhesion molecules, protease inhibitors, and immunomodulators aimed at shifting CD4 lymphocytes from the TH2 to the TH1 phenotype or at selective inhibition of the subset of TH2 lymphocytes directed against particular antigens. There is evidence that asthma may be aggravated—or even caused—by chronic airway infection with *Chlamydia pneumoniae* or *Mycoplasma pneumoniae*. This may explain the reports of benefit to some patients from treatment with macrolide antibiotics, but a recent trial of prolonged treatment with clarithromycin (500 mg twice daily for weeks) failed to improve asthma control in patients with moderately severe asthma.

■ CLINICAL PHARMACOLOGY OF DRUGS USED IN THE TREATMENT OF ASTHMA

Asthma is best thought of as a disease in two time domains. In the present domain, it is important for the distress it causes—cough, nocturnal awakenings, and shortness of breath that interferes with the ability to exercise or to pursue desired activities. For mild asthma, occasional inhalation of a bronchodilator may be all that is needed. For more severe asthma, treatment with a long-term controller, like an inhaled corticosteroid, is necessary to relieve symptoms and restore function. The second domain of asthma is the risk it presents of future events, such as exacerbations, or of progressive loss of pulmonary function. A patient's satisfaction with his or her ability to control symptoms and maintain function by frequent use of an inhaled β_2 agonist does not mean that the risk of future events is also controlled. In fact, use of two or more canisters of an inhaled β agonist per month is a marker of increased risk of asthma fatality.

The challenges of assessing severity and adjusting therapy for these two domains of asthma are different. For relief of distress in the present domain, the key information can be obtained by asking specific questions about the frequency and severity of symptoms, the frequency of use of an inhaled β_2 agonist for relief of symptoms, the frequency of nocturnal awakenings, and the ability to exercise. Estimating the risk for future exacerbations is more difficult. In general, patients with poorly controlled symptoms in the present have a heightened risk of exacerbations in the future, but some patients seem unaware of the severity of their underlying airflow obstruction (sometimes described as "poor perceivers") and can be identified only by measurement of pulmonary function, as by spirometry. Reductions in the FEV_1 correlate with heightened risk of attacks of asthma in the future. Other possible markers of heightened risk are unstable pulmonary function (large variations in FEV_1 from visit to visit, large change with bronchodilator treatment), extreme bronchial reactivity, or high numbers of eosinophils in sputum or of nitric oxide in exhaled air. Assessment of these features may identify patients who need increases in therapy for protection against exacerbations.

BRONCHODILATORS

Bronchodilators, such as inhaled albuterol, are rapidly effective, safe, and inexpensive. Patients with only occasional symptoms of asthma require no more than an inhaled β_2-receptor agonist taken on an as-needed basis. If symptoms require this "rescue" therapy more than twice a week, if nocturnal symptoms occur more than twice a month, or if the FEV_1 is less than 80% predicted, additional treatment is needed. The treatment first recommended is a low dose of an inhaled corticosteroid, although treatment with a leukotriene receptor antagonist or with cromolyn may be used. Theophylline is now largely reserved for patients in whom symptoms remain poorly controlled despite the combination of regular treatment with an inhaled anti-inflammatory agent and as-needed use of a β_2 agonist. If the addition of theophylline fails to improve symptoms or if adverse effects become bothersome, it is important to check the plasma level of theophylline to be sure it is in the therapeutic range (10–20 mg/L).

An important caveat for patients with mild asthma is that although the risk of a severe, life-threatening attack is lower than in patients with severe asthma, it is not zero. All patients with asthma should be instructed in a simple action plan for severe, frightening attacks: to take up to four puffs of albuterol every 20 minutes over 1 hour. If they do not note clear improvement after the first four puffs, they should take the additional treatments while on their way to an emergency department or some other higher level of care.

MUSCARINIC ANTAGONISTS

Inhaled muscarinic antagonists have so far earned a limited place in the treatment of asthma. The effects of short-acting agents (eg, ipratropium bromide) on baseline airway resistance is nearly as great as, but no greater than, those of the sympathomimetic

drugs, so they are used largely as alternative therapies for patients intolerant of β_2-adrenoceptor agonists. The airway effects of antimuscarinic and sympathomimetic drugs given in full doses have been shown to be additive only in patients with severe airflow obstruction who present for emergency care.

The long-acting antimuscarinic agent tiotropium has not yet earned a place in the treatment for asthma, although it has been shown to be as effective as a long-acting β_2-agonist when used in addition to an inhaled corticosteroid treatment for that condition. As a treatment for COPD, tiotropium both improves functional capacity, presumably through its action as a bronchodilator, and reduces the frequency of exacerbations, through mechanisms not yet defined.

Although it was predicted that muscarinic antagonists would dry airway secretions and interfere with mucociliary clearance, direct measurements of fluid volume secretion from single airway submucosal glands in animals show that atropine decreases baseline secretory rates only slightly. The drugs do, however, inhibit the increase in mucus secretion caused by vagal stimulation. No cases of inspissation of mucus have been reported following administration of these drugs.

CORTICOSTEROIDS

If asthmatic symptoms occur frequently or if significant airflow obstruction persists despite bronchodilator therapy, inhaled corticosteroids should be started. For patients with severe symptoms or severe airflow obstruction (eg, $FEV_1 < 50\%$ predicted), initial treatment with a combination of inhaled and oral corticosteroid (eg, 30 mg/d of prednisone for 3 weeks) is appropriate. Once clinical improvement is noted, usually after 7–10 days, the oral dose should be discontinued or reduced to the minimum necessary to control symptoms.

An issue for inhaled corticosteroid treatment is patient adherence. Analysis of prescription renewals shows that corticosteroids are taken regularly by a minority of patients. This may be a function of a general "steroid phobia" fostered by emphasis in the lay press on the hazards of long-term oral corticosteroid therapy and by ignorance of the difference between corticosteroids and anabolic steroids, taken to enhance muscle strength by now-infamous athletes. This fear of corticosteroid toxicity makes it hard to persuade patients whose symptoms have improved after starting treatment that they should continue it for protection against attacks. This context accounts for the interest in reports that instructing patients with mild but persistent asthma to take inhaled corticosteroid therapy only when their symptoms worsen is as effective in maintaining pulmonary function and preventing attacks as is taking the inhaled corticosteroid twice each day (see above).

In patients with more severe asthma whose symptoms are inadequately controlled by a standard dose of an inhaled corticosteroid, two options may be considered: to double the dose of inhaled corticosteroid or to combine it with another drug. The addition of theophylline or a leukotriene-receptor antagonist modestly increases asthma control, but the most impressive benefits are noted from addition of a *long-acting* inhaled β_2-receptor agonist (salmeterol or formoterol). Many studies have shown this combination therapy to be more effective than doubling the dose of the inhaled corticosteroid for reducing symptoms, reducing the "as-needed" use of albuterol, and preventing attacks of asthma. Combinations of an inhaled corticosteroid and a long-acting β agonist in a single inhaler are now commonly prescribed (eg, fluticasone and salmeterol [Advair]; budesonide and formoterol [Symbicort]). Offsetting the clear benefits is evidence of a statistically significant increase in the very low risk of fatal asthma attacks from use of a long-acting β agonist, perhaps even when taken in combination with an inhaled corticosteroid. This evidence prompted the FDA to issue a "black box" warning that the use of a long-acting β agonist is associated with a small but statistically significant increase in the risk of death or near-death from an asthma attack, especially in African Americans. The FDA did not withdraw approval of these drugs, for it recognizes that they are clinically effective. The major implications of the "black box" warning for the practitioner are: (1) that patients with mild to moderate asthma should be treated with a low-dose inhaled corticosteroid alone, and additional therapy considered only if their asthma is not well controlled; and, (2) that if their asthma is not well controlled, the possible increase in risk of a rare event, asthma fatality, should be discussed in presenting the options for treatment—an increase to a higher dose of the inhaled corticosteroid versus addition of a long-acting β agonist.

The FDA's warning has not so far had much effect on prescriptions for combinations of an inhaled corticosteroid with a long-acting β agonist, probably because their combination in a single inhaler offers several advantages. Combination inhalers are convenient; they ensure that the long-acting β agonist will not be taken as monotherapy (known not to protect against attacks); and they produce prompt, sustained improvements in clinical symptoms and pulmonary function and reduce the frequency of exacerbations requiring oral corticosteroid treatment. In patients prescribed such combination treatment, it is important to provide explicit instructions that a rapid-acting inhaled β$_2$ agonist, such as albuterol, should be used as needed for relief of acute symptoms.

An emerging approach to treatment takes advantage of the rapidity of onset of the bronchodilator action of the long-acting β agonist formoterol delivered in fixed-dose combination with the inhaled corticosteroid budesonide in Symbicort metered-dose inhalers. Several studies have confirmed that twice-daily and as-needed inhalation of this combination is as effective in preventing asthma exacerbations as a four-times-higher dose of budesonide twice daily with only albuterol for relief of symptoms. Use of this flexible dosing strategy is widespread in Europe, but is not approved in the USA.

LEUKOTRIENE ANTAGONISTS; CROMOLYN & NEDOCROMIL

A leukotriene receptor antagonist taken as an oral tablet may be considered as an alternative to inhaled corticosteroid treatment in patients with symptoms occurring more than twice a week or those who are awakened from sleep by asthma more than twice a month. This place in asthma therapy was once held by cromolyn and nedocromil, but neither is now available in the USA. Although these treatments are not as effective as even a low dose of an inhaled corticosteroid, both avoid the issue of "steroid phobia" described above and are commonly used in the treatment of children.

The leukotriene receptor antagonist montelukast (Singulair) is widely prescribed, especially by primary care providers. This drug, taken orally, is easy to administer and appears to be used more regularly than inhaled corticosteroids. Leukotriene receptor antagonists are rarely associated with troublesome side effects. Because of concerns over the possible long-term toxicity of systemic absorption of inhaled corticosteroids, this maintenance therapy is widely used for treating children in the USA.

ANTI-IGE MONOCLONAL ANTIBODY

Treatment with omalizumab, the monoclonal humanized anti-IgE antibody, is reserved for patients with chronic severe asthma inadequately controlled by high-dose inhaled corticosteroid plus long-acting β-agonist combination treatment (eg, fluticasone, 500 mcg, plus salmeterol, 50 mcg, inhaled twice daily). Omalizumab reduces lymphocytic, eosinophilic bronchial inflammation and effectively reduces the frequency and severity of exacerbations. It is reserved for patients with demonstrated IgE-mediated sensitivity (by positive skin test or radioallergosorbent test [RAST] to common allergens) and an IgE level within a range that can be reduced sufficiently by twice-weekly subcutaneous injection.

OTHER ANTI-INFLAMMATORY THERAPIES

Some reports suggest that agents commonly used to treat rheumatoid arthritis may also be used to treat patients with chronic steroid-dependent asthma. The development of an alternative treatment is important, because chronic treatment with oral corticosteroids may cause osteoporosis, cataracts, glucose intolerance, worsening of hypertension, and cushingoid changes in appearance. Initial studies suggested that oral methotrexate or gold salt injections were beneficial in prednisone-dependent asthmatic patients, but subsequent studies did not confirm this promise. In contrast, the benefit from treatment with cyclosporine seems real. However, this drug's great toxicity makes this finding only a source of hope that other immunomodulatory therapies will ultimately be developed for the small proportion of patients whose asthma can be managed only with high oral doses of prednisone. An immunomodulatory therapy recently reported to improve asthma is injection of etanercept, a TNF-α antagonist used in the treatment of ankylosing spondylitis and severe rheumatoid arthritis.

MANAGEMENT OF ACUTE ASTHMA

The treatment of acute attacks of asthma in patients reporting to the hospital requires close, continuous clinical assessment and repeated objective measurement of lung function. For patients with mild attacks, inhalation of a β$_2$-receptor agonist is as effective as subcutaneous injection of epinephrine. Both of these treatments are more effective than intravenous administration of aminophylline (a soluble salt of theophylline). Severe attacks require treatment with oxygen, frequent or continuous administration of aerosolized albuterol, and systemic treatment with prednisone or methylprednisolone (0.5 mg/kg every 6–12 hours). Even this aggressive treatment is not invariably effective, and patients must be watched closely for signs of deterioration. General anesthesia, intubation, and mechanical ventilation of asthmatic patients cannot be undertaken lightly but may be life-saving if respiratory failure supervenes.

PROSPECTS FOR PREVENTION

The high prevalence of asthma in the developed world and its rapid increases in the developing world call for a strategy for primary prevention. Strict antigen avoidance during infancy, once thought to be sensible, has now been shown to be ineffective. In fact, growing up from birth on a farm with domestic animals or in a household where cats or dogs are kept as pets appears to *protect* against developing asthma. The best hope seems to lie in understanding the mechanisms by which microbial exposures during infancy foster development of a balanced immune response and then mimicking the effects of natural environmental exposures through administration of harmless microbial commensals (probiotics) or of nutrients that foster their growth (prebiotics) in the intestinal tract during the critical period of immune development in early infancy.

TREATMENT OF CHRONIC OBSTRUCTIVE PULMONARY DISEASE (COPD)

COPD is characterized by airflow limitation that is not fully reversible with bronchodilator treatment. The airflow limitation is usually progressive and is believed to reflect an abnormal inflammatory response of the lung to noxious particles or gases. The condition is most often a consequence of prolonged habitual cigarette smoking, but approximately 15% of cases occur in nonsmokers. Although COPD is different from asthma, some of the same drugs are used in its treatment. This section discusses the drugs that are useful in both conditions.

Although asthma and COPD are both characterized by airway inflammation, reduction in maximum expiratory flow, and episodic exacerbations of airflow obstruction, most often triggered by viral respiratory infection, they differ in many important respects. Most important among them are differences in the populations affected, characteristics of airway inflammation, reversibility of airflow obstruction, responsiveness to corticosteroid treatment, and course and prognosis. Compared to asthma, COPD occurs in older patients, is associated with neutrophilic rather than eosinophilic inflammation, is poorly responsive even to high-dose inhaled corticosteroid therapy, and is associated with progressive, inexorable loss of pulmonary function over time, especially with continued cigarette smoking.

Despite these differences, the approaches to treatment are similar, although the benefits expected (and achieved) are less for COPD than for asthma. For relief of acute symptoms, inhalation of a short-acting β agonist (eg, albuterol), of an anticholinergic drug (eg, ipratropium bromide), or of the two in combination is usually effective. For patients with persistent symptoms of exertional dyspnea and limitation of activities, regular use of a long-acting bronchodilator, whether a long-acting β agonist (eg, salmeterol) or a long-acting anticholinergic (eg, tiotropium) is indicated. For patients with severe airflow obstruction or with a history of prior exacerbations, regular use of an inhaled corticosteroid reduces the frequency of future exacerbations. Theophylline may have a particular place in the treatment of COPD, as it may improve contractile function of the diaphragm, thus improving ventilatory capacity. The major difference in treatment of these conditions centers on management of exacerbations. The use of antibiotics in this context is routine in COPD, because such exacerbations involve bacterial infection of the lower airways far more often in COPD than in asthma.

SUMMARY Drugs Used in Asthma

Subclass	Mechanism of Action	Effects	Clinical Applications	Pharmacokinetics, Toxicities
BETA AGONISTS				
• Albuterol	Selective β_2 agonist	Prompt, efficacious bronchodilation	Asthma, chronic obstructive pulmonary disease (COPD) • drug of choice in acute asthmatic bronchospasm	Aerosol inhalation • duration several hours • also available for nebulizer and parenteral use • *Toxicity:* Tremor, tachycardia • overdose: arrhythmias
• Salmeterol	Selective β_2 agonist	Slow onset, primarily preventive action; potentiates corticosteroid effects	Asthma prophylaxis	Aerosol inhalation • duration 12–24 h • *Toxicity:* Tremor, tachycardia • overdose: arrhythmias
• *Metaproterenol, terbutaline: Similar to albuterol; terbutaline available as an oral drug*				
• *Formoterol: Similar to salmeterol*				
• Epinephrine	Nonselective α and β agonist	Bronchodilation plus all other sympathomimetic effects on cardiovascular and other organ systems (see Chapter 9)	Anaphylaxis, asthma, others (see Chapter 9) • rarely used for asthma (β_2-selective agents preferred)	Aerosol, nebulizer, or parenteral • see Chapter 9
• Isoproterenol	β_1 and β_2 agonist	Bronchodilation plus powerful cardiovascular effects	Asthma, but β_2-selective agents preferred	Aerosol, nebulizer, or parenteral • see Chapter 9
CORTICOSTEROIDS, INHALED				
• Fluticasone	Alters gene expression	Reduces mediators of inflammation • powerful prophylaxis of exacerbations	Asthma • adjunct in COPD • hay fever (nasal)	Aerosol • duration hours • *Toxicity:* Limited by aerosol application • candidal infection, vocal cord changes
• *Beclomethasone, budesonide, flunisolide, others: Similar to fluticasone*				
CORTICOSTEROIDS, SYSTEMIC				
• Prednisone	Like fluticasone	Like fluticasone	Asthma • adjunct in COPD	Oral • duration 12–24 hours • *Toxicity:* Multiple • see Chapter 39
• *Methylprednisolone: Parenteral agent like prednisone*				
STABILIZERS OF MAST AND OTHER CELLS				
• Cromolyn, nedocromil (no longer available in the USA)	Alter function of delayed chloride channels • inhibits inflammatory cell activation	Prevents acute bronchospasm	Asthma (other routes used for ocular, nasal, and gastrointestinal allergy)	Aerosol • duration 6–8 h • *Toxicity:* Cough • not absorbed so other toxicities are minimal
METHYLXANTHINES				
• Theophylline	Uncertain • phosphodiesterase inhibition • adenosine receptor antagonist	Bronchodilation, cardiac stimulation, increased skeletal muscle strength (diaphragm)	Asthma, COPD	Oral • duration 8–12 h but extended-release preparations often used • *Toxicity:* Multiple (see text)
LEUKOTRIENE ANTAGONISTS				
• Montelukast, zafirlukast	Block leukotriene D_4 receptors	Block airway response to exercise and antigen challenge	Prophylaxis of asthma, especially in children and in aspirin-induced asthma	Oral • duration hours • *Toxicity:* Minimal
• *Zileuton: Inhibits lipoxygenase, reduces synthesis of leukotrienes*				
IGE ANTIBODY				
• Omalizumab	Humanized IgE antibody reduces circulating IgE	Reduces frequency of asthma exacerbations	Severe asthma inadequately controlled by above agents	Parenteral • duration 2–4 d • *Toxicity:* Injection site reactions (anaphylaxis extremely rare)

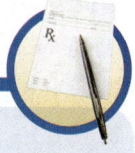

PREPARATIONS AVAILABLE

SYMPATHOMIMETICS USED IN ASTHMA

Albuterol (generic, Proventil, Ventolin)
Inhalant: 90 mcg/puff aerosol; 0.021, 0.042, 0.083, 0.5, 0.63% solution for nebulization
Oral: 2, 4 mg tablets; 2 mg/5 mL syrup
Oral sustained-release: 4, 8 mg tablets

Albuterol/Ipratropium (Combivent, DuoNeb)
Inhalant: 103 mcg albuterol + 18 mcg ipratropium/puff; 3 mg albuterol + 0.5 mg ipratropium/3 mL solution for nebulization

Arformoterol (Brovana)
Inhalant: 15 mcg/2 mL solution for nebulization

Bitolterol (Tornalate)
Inhalant: 0.2% solution for nebulization

Ephedrine (generic)
Oral: 25 mg capsules
Parenteral: 50 mg/mL for injection

Epinephrine (generic, Adrenalin)
Inhalant: 1, 10 mg/mL for nebulization; 0.22 mg/spray epinephrine base aerosol
Parenteral: 1:10,000 (0.1 mg/mL), 1:1000 (1 mg/mL)

Formoterol (Foradil)
Inhalant: 12 mcg/unit inhalant powder; 1% solution for nebulization

Formoterol/Budesonide (Symbicort)
Inhalant: 4.5 mcg/80 mcg, 4.5 mcg/160 mcg /puff

Isoetharine (generic)
Inhalant: 1% solution for nebulization

Isoproterenol (generic, Isuprel)
Inhalant: 0.5, 1% for nebulization; 80, 131 mcg/puff aerosols
Parenteral: 0.02, 0.2 mg/mL for injection

Levalbuterol (Xenopex)
Inhalant: 0.31, 0.63, 1.25 mg/3 mL solution

Metaproterenol (Alupent, generic)
Inhalant: 0.65 mg/puff aerosol in 7, 14 g containers; 0.4, 0.6, 5% for nebulization

Pirbuterol (Maxair)
Inhalant: 0.2 mg/puff aerosol in 80 and 300 dose containers

Salmeterol (Serevent)
Inhalant powder: 50 mcg/unit

Salmeterol/Fluticasone (Advair Diskus)
Inhalant: 100, 250, 500 mcg fluticasone + 50 mcg salmeterol/unit

Terbutaline (generic, Brethine)
Oral: 2.5, 5 mg tablets
Parenteral: 1 mg/mL for injection

AEROSOL CORTICOSTEROIDS (SEE ALSO CHAPTER 39)

Beclomethasone (QVAR)
Aerosol: 40, 80 mcg/puff in 100 dose containers

Budesonide (Pulmicort)
Aerosol powder (Turbuhaler): 160 mcg/activation
Inhalation suspension (Respules): 0.25, 0.5 mg/2 mL

Flunisolide (AeroBid, Aerospan)
Aerosol: 80, 250 mcg/puff in 80, 100, and 120 dose containers

Fluticasone (Flovent)
Aerosol: 44, 110, and 220 mcg/puff in 120 dose container; powder, 50, 100, 250 mcg/activation

Mometasone (Asmanex Twisthaler)
Inhalant: 110, 220 mcg/actuation in 14, 30, 60, 120 dose units

Triamcinolone (Azmacort)
Aerosol: 75 mcg/puff in 240 dose container

LEUKOTRIENE INHIBITORS

Montelukast (Singulair)
Oral: 10 mg tablets; 4, 5 mg chewable tablets; 4 mg/packet granules

Zafirlukast (Accolate)
Oral: 10, 20 mg tablets

Zileuton (Zyflo)
Oral: 600 mg tablets; 600 mg extended-release tablets

PHOSPHODIESTERASE INHIBITORS

Aminophylline (theophylline ethylenediamine, 79% theophylline) (generic)
Oral: 100, 200 mg tablets
Parenteral: 250 mg/10 mL for injection

Roflumilast (Daliresp)
Oral: 500 mcg tablets

Theophylline (generic, Elixophyllin, Slo-Phyllin, Uniphyl, Theo-Dur, Theo-24, others)
Oral: 50 mg/5 mL elixirs
Oral extended-release, 12 hours: 100, 200, 300, 450 mg tablets
Oral extended-release, 24 hours: 100, 200, 300 mg tablets and capsules; 400, 600 mg tablets
Parenteral: 0.08, 1.6, 2.0, 3.2, 4 mg/mL, theophylline and 5% dextrose for injection

OTHER METHYLXANTHINES

Dyphylline (Dylix, Lufyllin)
Oral: 200, 400 mg tablets; 100 mg/15 mL elixir

Pentoxifylline (generic, Trental)
Oral: 400 mg tablets and controlled-release tablets
Note: Pentoxifylline is labeled for use in intermittent claudication only.

ANTIMUSCARINIC DRUGS USED IN ASTHMA

Ipratropium (generic, Atrovent)
Aerosol: 17 (freon-free), 18 mcg/puff in 200 metered-dose inhaler; 0.02% (500 mcg/vial) for nebulization
Nasal spray: 21, 42 mcg/spray

Tiotropium (Spiriva)
Aerosol: 18 mcg/puff in 6 packs

ANTIBODY

Omalizumab (Xolair)
Powder for SC injection: 202.5 mg

REFERENCES

Pathophysiology of Airway Disease

Boushey H et al: Asthma. In Mason R et al (editors): *Textbook of Respiratory Medicine.* Elsevier Saunders, 2005:1168.

Locksley RM: Asthma and allergic inflammation. Cell 2010;140:777.

Asthma Treatment

Bateman ED et al: Overall asthma control: The relationship between current control and future risk. J Allergy Clin Immunol 2010;125:600.

Fanta CH: Drug therapy: Asthma. N Engl J Med 2009;360:1002.

Beta Agonists

Ducharme FM et al: Addition of long-acting beta2-agonists to inhaled corticosteroids versus same dose inhaled corticosteroids for chronic asthma in adults and children. Cochrane Database Syst Rev 2010;(5):CD005535.

Kelly HW, Harkins MS, Boushey H: The role of inhaled long-acting beta-2 agonists in the management of asthma. J Natl Med Assoc 2006;98:8.

Walters E, Walters J, Gibson P: Regular treatment with long acting beta agonists versus daily regular treatment with short acting beta agonists in adults and children with stable asthma. Cochrane Database Syst Rev 2002;(4):CD003901.

Methylxanthines & Roflumilast

Ito K et al: A molecular mechanism of action of theophylline: Induction of histone deacetylase activity to decrease inflammatory gene expression. Proc Natl Acad Sci USA 2002;99:8921.

Rabe KF: Roflumilast for the treatment of chronic obstructive pulmonary disease. Expert Rev Respir Med 2010;4:543.

Spina D: PDE4 inhibitors: Current status. Br J Pharmacol 2008;155:308.

Cromolyn & Nedocromil

Guevara J et al: Inhaled corticosteroids versus sodium cromoglycate in children and adults with asthma. Cochrane Database Syst Rev 2006;(2):CD003558.

Yoshihara S et al: Effects of early intervention with inhaled sodium cromoglycate in childhood asthma. Lung 2006;184:63.

Corticosteroids

Barnes P: How corticosteroids control inflammation: Quintiles Prize Lecture 2005. Br J Pharmacol 2006;148:245.

Boushey HA et al: Daily versus as-needed corticosteroids for mild persistent asthma. N Engl J Med 2005;352:1519.

O'Byrne PM et al: Budesonide/formoterol combination therapy as both maintenance and reliever medication in asthma. Am J Respir Crit Care Med 2005;171:129.

Suissa S et al: Low-dose inhaled corticosteroids and the prevention of death from asthma. N Engl J Med 2000;343:332.

Antimuscarinic Drugs

Gross N: Anticholinergic agents in asthma and COPD. Eur J Pharmacol 2006;8:533

Lee AM, Jacoby DB, Fryer AD: Selective muscarinic receptor antagonists for airway diseases. Curr Opin Pharmacol 2001;1:223.

Peters SP et al: Tiotropium bromide step-up therapy for adults with uncontrolled asthma. N Engl J Med 2010;363:1715.

Leukotriene Pathway Inhibitors

Calhoun WJ: Anti-leukotrienes for asthma. Curr Opin Pharmacol 2001;1:230.

Krawiec ME, Wenzel SE: Leukotriene inhibitors and non-steroidal therapies in the treatment of asthma. Exp Opin Invest Drugs 2001;2:47.

Wang L et al: Cost-effectiveness analysis of fluticasone versus montelukast in children with mild-to-moderate persistent asthma in the Pediatric Asthma Controller Trial. J Allergy Clin Immunol 2011;127:161.

Anti-IgE Therapy

Walker S et al: Anti-IgE for chronic asthma in adults and children. Cochrane Database Syst Rev 2006;(2):CD003559.

Clinical Management of Airway Disease

Barnes PJ: Drugs for asthma. Br J Pharmacol 2006;147(Suppl 1):S297.

Expert Panel Report 3 (EPR3): Guidelines for the diagnosis and management of asthma. National Institutes of Health, 2008; http://www.nhlbi.nih.gov/guidelines/asthma/asthgdln.htm.

Tattersfield AE et al: Asthma. Lancet 2002;360:1313.

Treatment of COPD

Buist S for the Executive Committee, Global Initiative for Chronic Obstructive Lung Disease: Global strategy for the diagnosis, management, and prevention of chronic obstructive pulmonary disease. Medical Communications Resources, 2007; http://www.goldcopd.com.

Matera MG, Page CP, Cazzola M: Novel bronchodilators for the treatment of chronic obstructive pulmonary disease. Trends Pharmacol Sci 2011;32:495.

Vogelmeier C et al: Tiotropium versus salmeterol for the prevention of exacerbations of COPD. N Engl J Med 2011;364;1093.

CASE STUDY ANSWER

This patient demonstrates the destabilizing effects of a respiratory infection on asthma, and the parents demonstrate the common (and dangerous) phobia about "overuse" of bronchodilator or steroid inhalers. The patient has signs of imminent respiratory failure, including her refusal to lie down, her fear, and her tachycardia—which cannot be attributed to her minimal treatment with albuterol. Critically important immediate steps are to administer high-flow oxygen and to start albuterol by nebulization. Adding ipratropium (Atrovent) to the nebulized solution is recommended. A corticosteroid (0.5–1.0 mg/kg of methylprednisolone) should be administered intravenously. It is also advisable to alert the intensive care unit, because a patient with severe bronchospasm who tires can slip into respiratory failure quickly, and intubation can be difficult.

Fortunately, most patients treated in hospital emergency departments do well. Asthma mortality is rare (fewer than 5000 deaths per year among a population of 20 million asthmatics in the USA), but when it occurs, it is often out of hospital. Presuming this patient recovers, she needs adjustments to her therapy before discharge. The strongest predictor of severe attacks of asthma is their occurrence in the past. Thus, this patient needs to be started on a long-term controller, especially an inhaled corticosteroid, and needs instruction in an action plan for managing severe symptoms. This can be as simple as advising her and her parents that if she has a severe attack that frightens her, she can take up to four puffs of albuterol every 15 minutes, but if the first treatment does not bring significant relief, she should take the next four puffs while on her way to an emergency department or urgent care clinic. She should also be given a prescription for prednisone, with instructions to take 40–60 mg orally for severe attacks, but not to wait for it to take effect if she remains severely short of breath even after albuterol inhalations. Asthma is a chronic disease, and good care requires close follow-up and creation of a provider-patient partnership for optimal management.

C H A P T E R

21

Introduction to the Pharmacology of CNS Drugs

Roger A. Nicoll, MD

Drugs acting in the central nervous system (CNS) were among the first to be discovered by primitive humans and are still the most widely used group of pharmacologic agents. In addition to their use in therapy, many drugs acting on the CNS are used without prescription to increase the sense of well-being.

The mechanisms by which various drugs act in the CNS have not always been clearly understood. In recent decades, however, dramatic advances have been made in the methodology of CNS pharmacology. It is now possible to study the action of a drug on individual cells and even single ion channels within synapses. The information obtained from such studies is the basis for several major developments in studies of the CNS.

First, it is clear that nearly all drugs with CNS effects act on specific receptors that modulate synaptic transmission. A very few agents such as general anesthetics and alcohol may have nonspecific actions on membranes (although these exceptions are not fully accepted), but even these non–receptor-mediated actions result in demonstrable alterations in synaptic transmission.

Second, drugs are among the most important tools for studying all aspects of CNS physiology, from the mechanism of convulsions to the laying down of long-term memory. As described below, agonists that mimic natural transmitters (and in many cases are more selective than the endogenous substances) and antagonists

are extremely useful in such studies. The Box, Natural Toxins: Tools for Characterizing Ion Channels, describes a few of these substances.

Third, unraveling the actions of drugs with known clinical efficacy has led to some of the most fruitful hypotheses regarding the mechanisms of disease. For example, information about the action of antipsychotic drugs on dopamine receptors has provided the basis for important hypotheses regarding the pathophysiology of schizophrenia. Studies of the effects of a variety of agonists and antagonists on γ-aminobutyric acid (GABA) receptors have resulted in new concepts pertaining to the pathophysiology of several diseases, including anxiety and epilepsy.

This chapter provides an introduction to the functional organization of the CNS and its synaptic transmitters as a basis for understanding the actions of the drugs described in the following chapters.

Methods for the Study of CNS Pharmacology

Like many areas of science, major progress in the study of CNS drugs has depended on the development of new experimental techniques. The first detailed description of synaptic transmission

Natural Toxins: Tools For Characterizing Ion Channels

Evolution is tireless in the development of natural toxins. A vast number of variations are possible with even a small number of amino acids in peptides, and peptides make up only one of a broad array of toxic compounds. For example, the predatory marine snail genus *Conus* is estimated to include at least 500 different species. Each species kills or paralyzes its prey with a venom that contains 50–200 different peptides or proteins. Furthermore, there is little duplication of peptides among *Conus* species. Other animals with useful toxins include snakes, frogs, spiders, bees, wasps, and scorpions. Plant species with toxic (or therapeutic) substances are too numerous to mention here; they are referred to in many chapters of this book.

Since many toxins act on ion channels, they provide a wealth of chemical tools for studying the function of these channels. In fact, much of our current understanding of the properties of ion channels comes from studies utilizing only a small percentage of the highly potent and selective toxins that are now available. The toxins typically target voltage-sensitive ion channels, but a number of very useful toxins block ionotropic neurotransmitter receptors. Table 21–1 lists some of the toxins most commonly used in research, their mode of action, and their source.

TABLE 21–1 Some toxins used to characterize ion channels.

Channel Types	Mode of Toxin Action	Source
Voltage-gated		
Sodium channels		
Tetrodotoxin (TTX)	Blocks channel from outside	Puffer fish
Batrachotoxin (BTX)	Slows inactivation, shifts activation	Colombian frog
Potassium channels		
Apamin	Blocks "small Ca-activated" K channel	Honeybee
Charybdotoxin	Blocks "big Ca-activated" K channel	Scorpion
Calcium channels		
Omega conotoxin (ω-CTX-GVIA)	Blocks N-type channel	Pacific cone snail
Agatoxin (ω-AGAIVA)	Blocks P-type channel	Funnel web spider
Ligand-gated		
Nicotinic ACh receptor		
α-Bungarotoxin	Irreversible antagonist	Marine snake
GABA$_A$ receptor		
Picrotoxin	Blocks channel	South Pacific plant
Glycine receptor		
Strychnine	Competitive antagonist	Indian plant
AMPA receptor		
Philanthotoxin	Blocks channel	Wasp

was made possible by the invention of glass microelectrodes, which permit intracellular recording. The development of the brain slice technique permitted an analysis of the physiology and pharmacology of synapses. Detailed electrophysiologic studies of the action of drugs on both voltage- and transmitter-operated channels were further facilitated by the introduction of the patch clamp technique, which permits the recording of current through single channels. Channels can be expressed in cultured cells and the currents evoked by their activation recorded (Figure 21–1). Histochemical, immunologic, and radioisotopic methods have made it possible to map the distribution of specific transmitters, their associated enzyme systems, and their receptors. Molecular cloning has had a major impact on our understanding of CNS receptors. These techniques make it possible to determine the precise molecular structure of the receptors and their associated channels. Finally, mice with mutated genes for specific receptors or enzymes (knockout mice) can provide important information regarding the physiologic and pharmacologic roles of these components.

ION CHANNELS & NEUROTRANSMITTER RECEPTORS

The membranes of nerve cells contain two types of channels defined on the basis of the mechanisms controlling their gating (opening and closing): **voltage-gated** and **ligand-gated** channels

(Figure 21–2A and B). Voltage-gated channels respond to changes in the membrane potential of the cell. The voltage-gated sodium channel described in Chapter 14 for the heart is an example of the first type of channel. In nerve cells, these channels are concentrated on the initial segment and the axon and are responsible for the fast action potential, which transmits the signal from cell body to nerve terminal. There are many types of voltage-sensitive calcium and potassium channels on the cell body, dendrites, and initial segment, which act on a much slower time scale and modulate the rate at which the neuron discharges. For example, some types of potassium channels opened by depolarization of the cell result in slowing of further depolarization and act as a brake to limit further action potential discharge.

Neurotransmitters exert their effects on neurons by binding to two distinct classes of receptor. The first class is referred to as **ligand-gated channels,** or **ionotropic receptors.** The receptor consists of subunits, and binding of ligand directly opens the channel, which is an integral parts of the receptor complex (see Figure 22–6). These channels are insensitive or only weakly sensitive to membrane potential. Activation of these channels typically

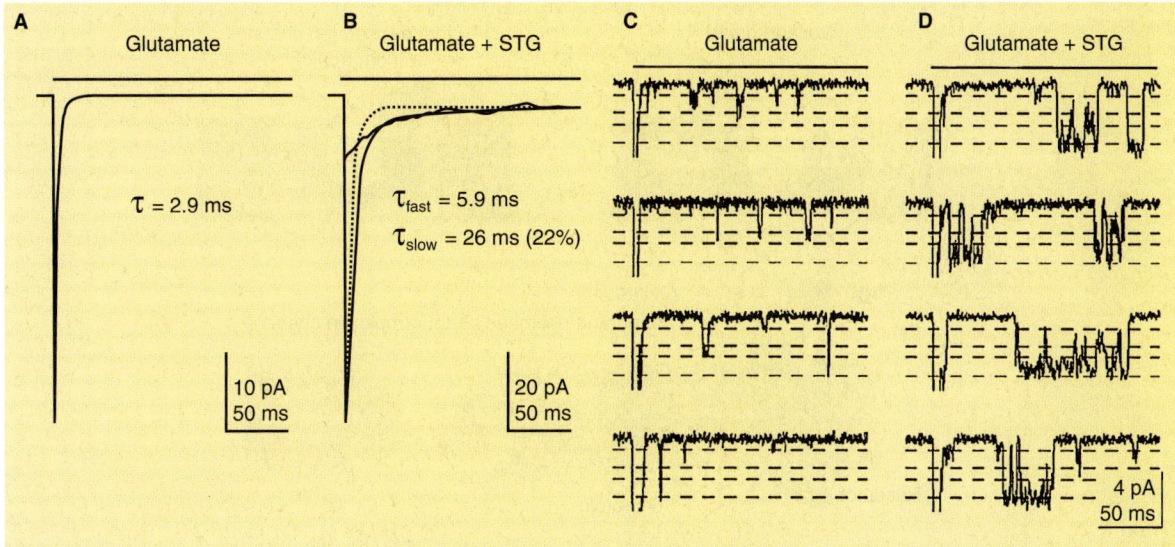

FIGURE 21–1 Whole-cell and single-channel currents. Modern techniques permit the recording of neuronal currents in response to the application of transmitters and modulators of transmission. **A:** Averaged and summed whole-cell currents evoked by the application of glutamate (inward currents are downward). **B:** Currents evoked by glutamate in the presence of a modulator (stargazin, STG). **C:** Single-channel currents evoked by glutamate alone. **D:** Single-channel currents evoked by glutamate plus stargazin. Note the prolonged channel openings in the presence of stargazin. (Reproduced, with permission, from Tomita et al: Stargazin modulates AMPA receptor gating and trafficking by distinct domains. Nature 2005;435:1052.)

results in a brief (a few milliseconds to tens of milliseconds) opening of the channel. Ligand-gated channels are responsible for fast synaptic transmission typical of hierarchical pathways in the CNS (see following text).

The second class of neurotransmitter receptor is referred to as **metabotropic receptors.** These are seven-transmembrane G protein-coupled receptors of the type described in Chapter 2. The binding of neurotransmitter to this type of receptor does not result in the direct gating of a channel. Rather, binding to the receptor engages a G protein, which results in the production of second messengers that modulate voltage-gated channels. These interactions can occur entirely with the plane of the membrane and are referred to as **membrane-delimited** pathways (Figure 21–2C). In this case, the G protein (often the βγ subunit) interacts directly with the voltage-gated ion channel. In general, two types of voltage-gated ion channels are the targets of this type of signaling: calcium channels and potassium channels. When G proteins interact with calcium channels, they inhibit channel function. This mechanism accounts for the presynaptic inhibition that occurs when presynaptic metabotropic receptors are activated. In contrast, when these receptors are postsynaptic, they activate (cause the opening of) potassium channels, resulting in a slow postsynaptic inhibition. Metabotropic receptors can also modulate voltage-gated channels less directly by the generation of **diffusible second messengers** (Figure 21–2D). A classic example of this type of action is provided by the β adrenoceptor, which generates cAMP via the activation of adenylyl cyclase (see Chapter 2). Whereas membrane-delimited actions occur within microdomains in the membrane, second messenger-mediated effects can occur over considerable distances. Finally, an important consequence of the involvement of G proteins in receptor signaling

is that, in contrast to the brief effect of ionotropic receptors, the effects of metabotropic receptor activation can last tens of seconds to minutes. Metabotropic receptors predominate in the diffuse neuronal systems in the CNS (see below).

THE SYNAPSE & SYNAPTIC POTENTIALS

The communication between neurons in the CNS occurs through chemical synapses in the majority of cases. (A few instances of electrical coupling between neurons have been documented, and such coupling may play a role in synchronizing neuronal discharge. However, it is unlikely that these electrical synapses are an important site of drug action.) The events involved in synaptic transmission can be summarized as follows.

An action potential in the presynaptic fiber propagates into the synaptic terminal and activates voltage-sensitive calcium channels in the membrane of the terminal (see Figure 6–3). The calcium channels responsible for the release of transmitter are generally resistant to the calcium channel-blocking agents discussed in Chapter 12 (verapamil, etc) but are sensitive to blockade by certain marine toxins and metal ions (see Tables 21–1 and 12–4). Calcium flows into the terminal, and the increase in intraterminal calcium concentration promotes the fusion of synaptic vesicles with the presynaptic membrane. The transmitter contained in the vesicles is released into the synaptic cleft and diffuses to the receptors on the postsynaptic membrane. Binding of the transmitter to its receptor causes a brief change in membrane conductance (permeability to ions) of the postsynaptic cell. The time delay from the arrival of the presynaptic action potential to the onset of the postsynaptic response is approximately

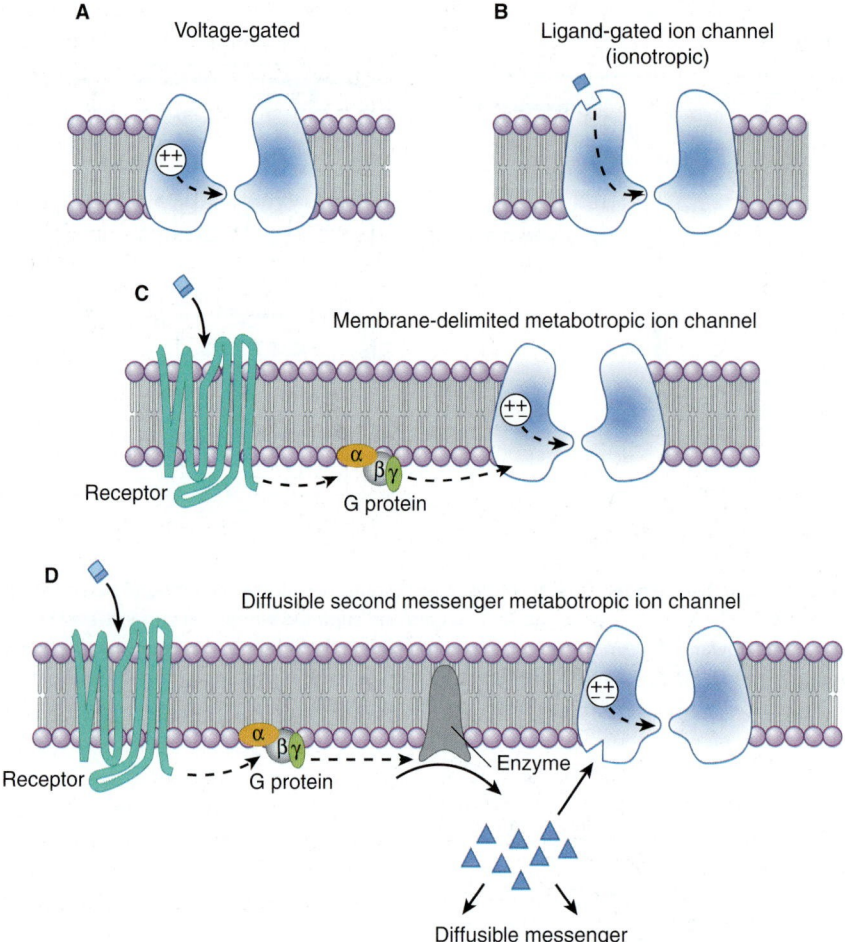

FIGURE 21–2 Types of ion channels and neurotransmitter receptors in the CNS. **A** shows a voltage-gated channel in which a voltage sensor component of the protein controls the gating (*broken arrow*) of the channel. **B** shows a ligand-gated channel in which the binding of the neurotransmitter to the ionotropic channel receptor controls the gating (*broken arrow*) of the channel. **C** shows a G protein-coupled (metabotropic) receptor, which, when bound, activates a G protein that then interacts directly to modulate an ion channel. **D** shows a G protein-coupled receptor, which, when bound, activates a G protein that then activates an enzyme. The activated enzyme generates a diffusible second messenger, eg, cAMP, which interacts to modulate an ion channel.

0.5 ms. Most of this delay is consumed by the release process, particularly the time required for calcium channels to open.

The first systematic analysis of synaptic potentials in the CNS was in the early 1950s by Eccles and associates, who recorded intracellularly from spinal motor neurons. When a microelectrode enters a cell, there is a sudden change in the potential recorded by the electrode, which is typically about –70 mV (Figure 21–3). This is the resting membrane potential of the neuron. Two types of pathways—excitatory and inhibitory—impinge on the motor neuron.

When an excitatory pathway is stimulated, a small depolarization or **excitatory postsynaptic potential (EPSP)** is recorded. This potential is due to the excitatory transmitter acting on an ionotropic receptor, causing an increase in cation permeability. Changing the stimulus intensity to the pathway, and therefore the number of presynaptic fibers activated, results in a graded change in the size of the depolarization. When a sufficient number of excitatory fibers are activated, the excitatory postsynaptic potential

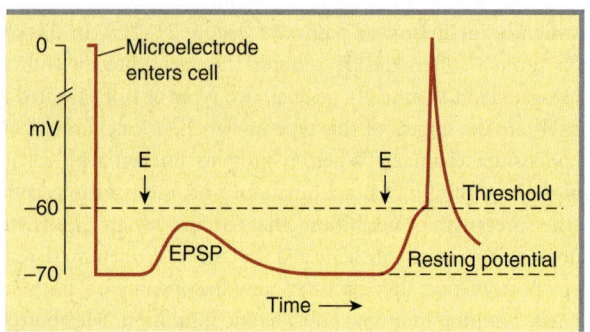

FIGURE 21–3 Excitatory postsynaptic potentials (EPSP) and spike generation. The figure shows entry of a microelectrode into a postsynaptic cell and subsequent recording of a resting membrane potential of –70 mV. Stimulation of an excitatory pathway (E) generates transient depolarization. Increasing the stimulus strength (second E) increases the size of the depolarization, so that the threshold for spike generation is reached.

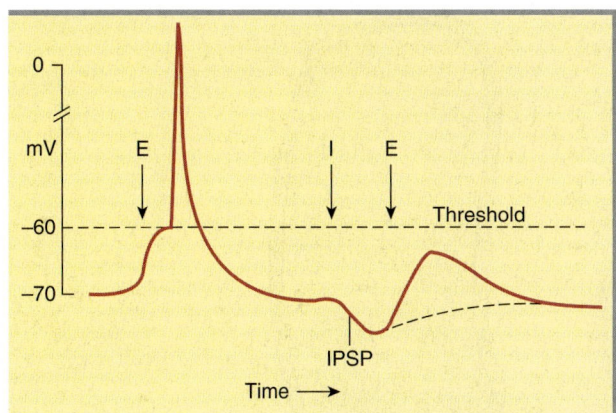

FIGURE 21–4 Interaction of excitatory and inhibitory synapses. On the left, a suprathreshold stimulus is given to an excitatory pathway (E) and an action potential is evoked. On the right, this same stimulus is given shortly after activating an inhibitory pathway (I), which results in an inhibitory postsynaptic potential (IPSP) that prevents the excitatory potential from reaching threshold.

depolarizes the postsynaptic cell to threshold, and an all-or-none action potential is generated.

When an inhibitory pathway is stimulated, the postsynaptic membrane is hyperpolarized owing to the selective opening of chloride channels, producing an **inhibitory postsynaptic potential (IPSP)** (Figure 21–4). However, because the equilibrium potential for chloride is only slightly more negative than the resting potential (~ –65 mV), the hyperpolarization is small and contributes only modestly to the inhibitory action. The opening of the chloride channel during the inhibitory postsynaptic potential makes the neuron "leaky" so that changes in membrane potential are more difficult to achieve. This shunting effect decreases the change in membrane potential during the excitatory postsynaptic potential. As a result, an excitatory postsynaptic potential that evoked an action potential under resting conditions fails to evoke an action potential during the inhibitory postsynaptic potential (Figure 21–4). A second type of inhibition is **presynaptic inhibition.** It was first described for sensory fibers entering the spinal cord, where excitatory synaptic terminals receive synapses called axoaxonic synapses (described later). When activated, axoaxonic synapses reduce the amount of transmitter released from the terminals of sensory fibers. It is interesting that presynaptic inhibitory receptors are present on almost all presynaptic terminals in the brain even though axoaxonic synapses appear to be restricted to the spinal cord. In the brain, transmitter spills over to neighboring synapses to activate the presynaptic receptors.

SITES OF DRUG ACTION

Virtually all the drugs that act in the CNS produce their effects by modifying some step in chemical synaptic transmission. Figure 21–5 illustrates some of the steps that can be altered. These transmitter-dependent actions can be divided into presynaptic and postsynaptic categories.

Drugs acting on the synthesis, storage, metabolism, and release of neurotransmitters fall into the presynaptic category. Synaptic transmission can be depressed by blockade of transmitter synthesis or storage. For example, reserpine depletes monoamine synapses of transmitters by interfering with intracellular storage. Blockade of transmitter catabolism inside the nerve terminal can increase transmitter concentrations and has been reported to increase the amount of transmitter released per impulse. Drugs can also alter the release of transmitters. The stimulant amphetamine induces the release of catecholamines from adrenergic synapses (see Chapters 6 and 32). Capsaicin causes the release of the peptide substance P from sensory neurons, and tetanus toxin blocks the release of transmitters. After a transmitter has been released into the synaptic cleft, its action is terminated either by uptake or by degradation. For most neurotransmitters, there are uptake mechanisms into the synaptic terminal and also into surrounding neuroglia. Cocaine, for example, blocks the uptake of catecholamines at adrenergic synapses and thus potentiates the action of these amines. However, acetylcholine is inactivated by enzymatic degradation, not reuptake. Anticholinesterases block the degradation of acetylcholine and thereby prolong its action. No uptake mechanism has been found for any of the numerous CNS peptides, and it has yet to be demonstrated whether specific enzymatic degradation terminates the action of peptide transmitters.

In the postsynaptic region, the transmitter receptor provides the primary site of drug action. Drugs can act either as neurotransmitter agonists, such as the opioids, which mimic the action of enkephalin, or they can block receptor function. Receptor antagonism is a common mechanism of action for CNS drugs. An example is strychnine's blockade of the receptor for the inhibitory transmitter glycine. This block, which underlies strychnine's convulsant action, illustrates how the blockade of inhibitory processes results in excitation. Drugs can also act directly on the ion channel of ionotropic receptors. For example, barbiturates can enter and block the channel of many excitatory ionotropic receptors. In the case of metabotropic receptors, drugs can act at any of the steps downstream of the receptor. Perhaps the best example is provided by the methylxanthines, which can modify neurotransmitter responses mediated through the second-messenger cAMP. At high concentrations, the methylxanthines elevate the level of cAMP by blocking its metabolism and thereby prolong its action.

The traditional view of the synapse is that it functions like a valve, transmitting information in one direction. However, it is now clear that the synapse can generate signals that feed back onto the presynaptic terminal to modify transmitter release. Endocannabinoids are the best documented example of such *retrograde* signaling. Postsynaptic activity leads to the synthesis and release of endocannabinoids, which then bind to receptors on the presynaptic terminal. Although the gas nitric oxide (NO) has long been proposed as a retrograde messenger, its physiologic role in the CNS is still not well understood.

The selectivity of CNS drug action is based almost entirely on the fact that different transmitters are used by different groups of

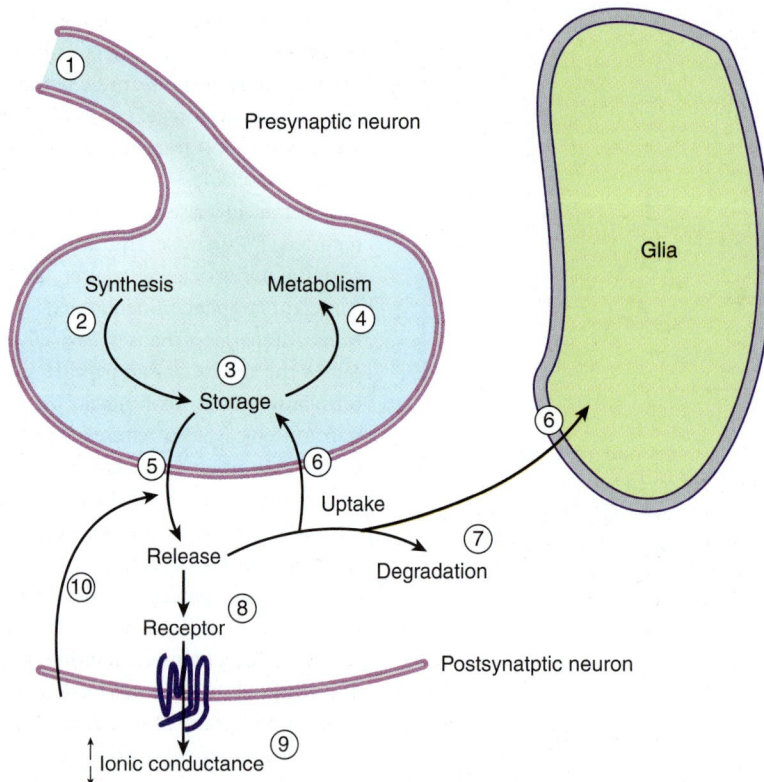

FIGURE 21–5 Sites of drug action. Schematic drawing of steps at which drugs can alter synaptic transmission. (1) Action potential in presynaptic fiber; (2) synthesis of transmitter; (3) storage; (4) metabolism; (5) release; (6) reuptake into the nerve ending or uptake into a glial cell; (7) degradation; (8) receptor for the transmitter; (9) receptor-induced increase or decrease in ionic conductance; (10) retrograde signaling.

neurons. Furthermore, these transmitters are often segregated into neuronal systems that subserve broadly different CNS functions. Without such segregation, it would be impossible to selectively modify CNS function, even if one had a drug that operated on a single neurotransmitter system. That such segregation does occur has provided neuroscientists with a powerful pharmacologic approach for analyzing CNS function and treating pathologic conditions.

IDENTIFICATION OF CENTRAL NEUROTRANSMITTERS

Because drug selectivity is based on the fact that different pathways use different transmitters, a primary goal of neuropharmacologists is to identify the transmitters in CNS pathways. Establishing that a chemical substance is a transmitter has been far more difficult for central synapses than for peripheral synapses. The following criteria have been established for transmitter identification.

Localization

Approaches that have been used to prove that a suspected transmitter resides in the presynaptic terminal of the pathway under study include biochemical analysis of regional concentrations of suspected transmitters and immunocytochemical techniques for enzymes and peptides.

Release

To determine whether the substance is released from a particular region, local collection (in vivo) of the extracellular fluid can sometimes be accomplished. In addition, slices of brain tissue can be electrically or chemically stimulated in vitro and the released substances measured. To determine whether the release is relevant to synaptic transmission, it is important to establish that the release is calcium-dependent.

Synaptic Mimicry

Finally, application of the suspected substance should produce a response that mimics the action of the transmitter released by nerve stimulation. Furthermore, application of a selective antagonist should block the response. Micro-iontophoresis, which permits highly localized drug administration, has been a valuable technique in assessing the action of suspected transmitters. Because of the complexity of the CNS, specific pharmacologic antagonism of a synaptic response provides a particularly powerful technique for transmitter identification.

CELLULAR ORGANIZATION OF THE BRAIN

Most of the neuronal systems in the CNS can be divided into two broad categories: **hierarchical** systems and **nonspecific** or **diffuse** neuronal systems.

Hierarchical Systems

Hierarchical systems include all the pathways directly involved in sensory perception and motor control. The pathways are generally clearly delineated, being composed of large myelinated fibers that can often conduct action potentials at a rate of more than 50 m/s. The information is typically phasic and occurs in bursts of action potentials. In sensory systems, the information is processed sequentially by successive integrations at each relay nucleus on its way to the cortex. A lesion at any link incapacitates the system. Within each nucleus and in the cortex, there are two types of cells: **relay** or **projection neurons** and **local circuit neurons** (Figure 21–6A). The projection neurons that form the interconnecting pathways transmit signals over long distances. The cell bodies are relatively large, and their axons emit collaterals that arborize extensively in the vicinity of the neuron. These neurons are excitatory, and their synaptic influences, which involve ionotropic receptors, are very short-lived.

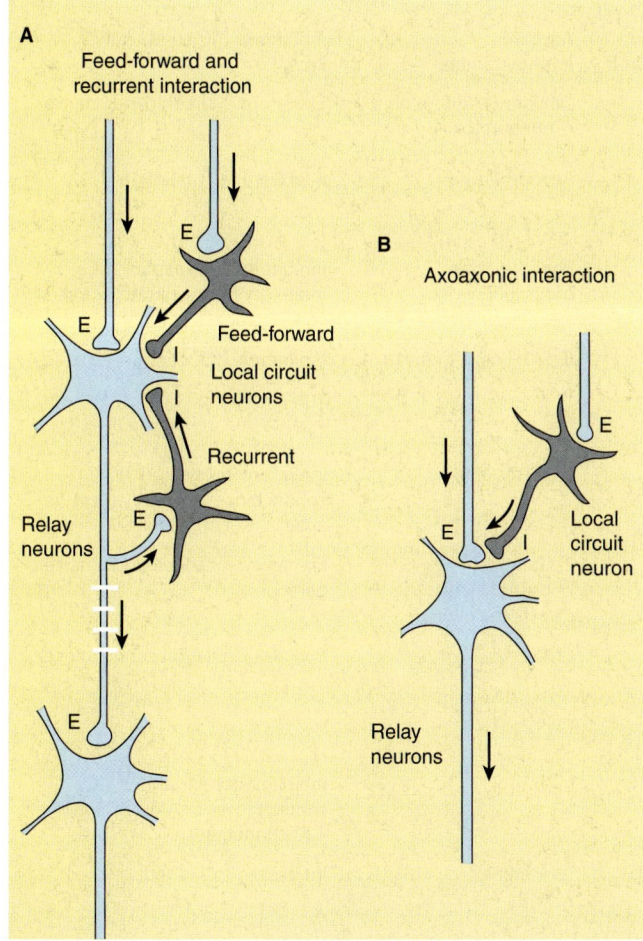

FIGURE 21–6 Pathways in the central nervous system. **A** shows parts of three relay neurons (blue) and two types of inhibitory pathways, recurrent and feed-forward. The inhibitory neurons are shown in gray. **B** shows the pathway responsible for presynaptic inhibition in which the axon of an inhibitory neuron (gray) synapses on the axon terminal of an excitatory fiber (blue).

The excitatory transmitter released from these cells is, in most instances, **glutamate.** Local circuit neurons are typically smaller than projection neurons, and their axons arborize in the immediate vicinity of the cell body. Most of these neurons are inhibitory, and they release either **GABA** or **glycine.** They synapse primarily on the cell body of the projection neurons but can also synapse on the dendrites of projection neurons as well as with each other. Two common types of pathways for these neurons (Figure 21–6A) include recurrent feedback pathways and feed-forward pathways. A special class of local circuit neurons in the spinal cord forms axoaxonic synapses on the terminals of sensory axons (Figure 21–6B). In some sensory pathways such as the retina and olfactory bulb, local circuit neurons may actually lack an axon and release neurotransmitter from dendritic synapses in a graded fashion in the absence of action potentials.

Although there is a great variety of synaptic connections in these hierarchical systems, the fact that a limited number of transmitters are used by these neurons indicates that any major pharmacologic manipulation of this system will have a profound effect on the overall excitability of the CNS. For instance, selectively blocking GABA$_A$ receptors with a drug such as picrotoxin results in generalized convulsions. Thus, although the mechanism of action of picrotoxin is specific in blocking the effects of GABA, the overall functional effect appears to be quite nonspecific, because GABA-mediated synaptic inhibition is so widely utilized in the brain.

Nonspecific or Diffuse Neuronal Systems

Neuronal systems that contain one of the monoamines—norepinephrine, dopamine, or 5-hydroxytryptamine (serotonin)—provide examples in this category. Certain other pathways emanating from the reticular formation and possibly some peptide-containing pathways also fall into this category. These systems differ in fundamental ways from the hierarchical systems, and the noradrenergic systems serve to illustrate the differences.

Noradrenergic cell bodies are found primarily in a compact cell group called the locus caeruleus located in the caudal pontine central gray matter. The number of neurons in this cell group is small, approximately 1500 on each side of the brain in the rat.

Because these axons are fine and unmyelinated, they conduct very slowly, at about 0.5 m/s. The axons branch repeatedly and are extraordinarily divergent. Branches from the same neuron can innervate several functionally different parts of the CNS. In the neocortex, these fibers have a tangential organization and therefore can monosynaptically influence large areas of cortex. The pattern of innervation by noradrenergic fibers in the cortex and nuclei of the hierarchical systems is diffuse, and these fibers form a very small percentage of the total number in the area. In addition, the axons are studded with periodic enlargements called varicosities, which contain large numbers of vesicles. In some instances, these varicosities do not form synaptic contacts, suggesting that norepinephrine may be released in a rather diffuse manner, as occurs with the noradrenergic autonomic innervation of smooth muscle. This indicates that the cellular targets of these systems are determined largely by the location of the receptors rather than by the location of the release sites. Finally, most neurotransmitters utilized by diffuse neuronal systems, including norepinephrine, act—perhaps exclusively—on metabotropic receptors and therefore initiate long-lasting synaptic effects. Based on these observations, it is clear that the monoamine systems cannot be conveying topographically specific types of information; rather, vast areas of the CNS must be affected simultaneously and in a rather uniform way. It is not surprising, then, that these systems have been implicated in such global functions as sleeping and waking, attention, appetite, and emotional states.

CENTRAL NEUROTRANSMITTERS

A vast number of small molecules have been isolated from the brain, and studies using a variety of approaches suggest that the agents listed in Table 21–2 are neurotransmitters. A brief summary of the evidence for some of these compounds follows.

Amino Acids

The amino acids of primary interest to the pharmacologist fall into two categories: the acidic amino acid glutamate and the neutral amino acids glycine and GABA. All these compounds are

TABLE 21–2 Summary of neurotransmitter pharmacology in the central nervous system.

Transmitter	Anatomy	Receptor Subtypes and Preferred Agonists	Receptor Antagonists	Mechanisms
Acetylcholine	Cell bodies at all levels; long and short connections	Muscarinic (M_1): muscarine	Pirenzepine, atropine	Excitatory: $\downarrow$ in K^+ conductance; $\uparrow IP_3$, DAG
		Muscarinic (M_2): muscarine, bethanechol	Atropine, methoctramine	Inhibitory: $\uparrow K^+$ conductance; $\downarrow$ cAMP
	Motoneuron-Renshaw cell synapse	Nicotinic: nicotine	Dihydro-β-erythroidine, α-bungarotoxin	Excitatory: $\uparrow$ cation conductance
Dopamine	Cell bodies at all levels; short, medium, and long connections	D_1	Phenothiazines	Inhibitory (?): $\uparrow$ cAMP
		D_2: bromocriptine	Phenothiazines, butyrophenones	Inhibitory (presynaptic): $\downarrow Ca^{2+}$; Inhibitory (postsynaptic): $\uparrow$ in K^+ conductance, $\downarrow$ cAMP
GABA	Supraspinal and spinal interneurons involved in pre- and postsynaptic inhibition	$GABA_A$: muscimol	Bicuculline, picrotoxin	Inhibitory: $\uparrow Cl^-$ conductance
		$GABA_B$: baclofen	2-OH saclofen	Inhibitory (presynaptic): $\downarrow Ca^{2+}$ conductance; Inhibitory (postsynaptic): $\uparrow K^+$ conductance
Glutamate	Relay neurons at all levels and some interneurons	N-Methyl-D-aspartate (NMDA): NMDA	2-Amino-5-phosphonovalerate, dizocilpine	Excitatory: $\uparrow$ cation conductance, particularly Ca^{2+}
		AMPA: AMPA	CNQX	Excitatory: $\uparrow$ cation conductance
		Kainate: kainic acid, domoic acid		
		Metabotropic: ACPD, quisqualate	MCPG	Inhibitory (presynaptic): $\downarrow Ca^{2+}$ conductance, $\downarrow$ cAMP; Excitatory: $\downarrow K^+$ conductance, $\uparrow IP_3$, DAG
Glycine	Spinal interneurons and some brainstem interneurons	Taurine, β-alanine	Strychnine	Inhibitory: $\uparrow Cl^-$ conductance
5-Hydroxytryptamine (serotonin)	Cell bodies in midbrain and pons project to all levels	$5-HT_{1A}$: LSD	Metergoline, spiperone	Inhibitory: $\uparrow K^+$ conductance, $\downarrow$ cAMP
		$5-HT_{2A}$: LSD	Ketanserin	Excitatory: $\downarrow K^+$ conductance, $\uparrow IP_3$, DAG

(continued)

TABLE 21–2 Summary of neurotransmitter pharmacology in the central nervous system. (Continued)

Transmitter	Anatomy	Receptor Subtypes and Preferred Agonists	Receptor Antagonists	Mechanisms
		5-HT$_3$: 2-methyl-5-HT	Ondansetron	Excitatory: ↑ cation conductance
		5-HT$_4$		Excitatory: ↓ K$^+$ conductance
Norepinephrine	Cell bodies in pons and brainstem project to all levels	α_1: phenylephrine	Prazosin	Excitatory: ↓ K$^+$ conductance, ↑ IP$_3$, DAG
		α_2: clonidine	Yohimbine	Inhibitory (presynaptic): ↓ Ca^{2+} conductance; Inhibitory: ↑ K$^+$ conductance, ↓ cAMP
		β_1: isoproterenol, dobutamine	Atenolol, practolol	Excitatory: ↓ K$^+$ conductance, ↑ cAMP
		β_2: albuterol	Butoxamine	Inhibitory: may involve ↑ in electrogenic sodium pump; ↑ cAMP
Histamine	Cells in ventral posterior hypothalamus	H$_1$: 2(m-fluorophenyl)-histamine	Mepyramine	Excitatory: ↓ K$^+$ conductance, ↑ IP$_3$, DAG
		H$_2$: dimaprit	Ranitidine	Excitatory: ↓ K$^+$ conductance, ↑ cAMP
		H$_3$: R-α-methyl-histamine	Thioperamide	Inhibitory autoreceptors
Opioid peptides	Cell bodies at all levels; long and short connections	Mu: bendorphin	Naloxone	Inhibitory (presynaptic): ↓ Ca^{2+} conductance, ↓ cAMP
		Delta: enkephalin	Naloxone	Inhibitory (postsynaptic): ↑ K$^+$ conductance, ↓ cAMP
		Kappa: dynorphin	Naloxone	
Tachykinins	Primary sensory neurons, cell bodies at all levels; long and short connections	NK1: substance P methylester, aprepitant	Aprepitant	Excitatory: ↓ K$^+$ conductance, ↑ IP$_3$, DAG
		NK2		
		NK3		
Endocannabinoids	Widely distributed	CB1: anandamide, 2-arachidonyglycerol	Rimonabant	Inhibitory (presynaptic): ↓ Ca^{2+} conductance, ↓ cAMP

Note: Many other central transmitters have been identified (see text).

ACPD, *trans*-1-amino-cyclopentyl-1,3-dicarboxylate; AMPA, DL-α-amino-3-hydroxy-5-methylisoxazole-4-propionate; cAMP, cyclic adenosine monophosphate; CQNX, 6-cyano-7-nitroquinoxaline-2,3-dione; DAG, diacylglycerol; IP$_3$, inositol trisphosphate; LSD, lysergic acid diethylamide; MCPG, α-methyl-4-carboxyphenylglycine.

present in high concentrations in the CNS and are extremely potent modifiers of neuronal excitability.

A. Glutamate

Excitatory synaptic transmission is mediated by glutamate, which is present in very high concentrations in excitatory synaptic vesicles (~100 mM). Glutamate is released into the synaptic cleft by Ca^{2+}-dependent exocytosis (Figure 21–7). The released glutamate acts on postsynaptic glutamate receptors and is cleared by glutamate transporters present on surrounding glia. In glia, glutamate is converted to glutamine by glutamine synthetase, released from the glia, taken up by the nerve terminal, and converted back to glutamate by the enzyme glutaminase. The high concentration of glutamate in synaptic vesicles is achieved by the **vesicular glutamate transporter (VGLUT)**.

Almost all neurons that have been tested are strongly excited by glutamate. This excitation is caused by the activation of both ionotropic and metabotropic receptors, which have been extensively characterized by molecular cloning. The ionotropic receptors can be further divided into three subtypes based on the action of selective agonists: α-amino-3-hydroxy-5-methylisoxazole-4-propionic acid **(AMPA)**, kainic acid **(KA)**, and *N*-methyl-D-aspartate

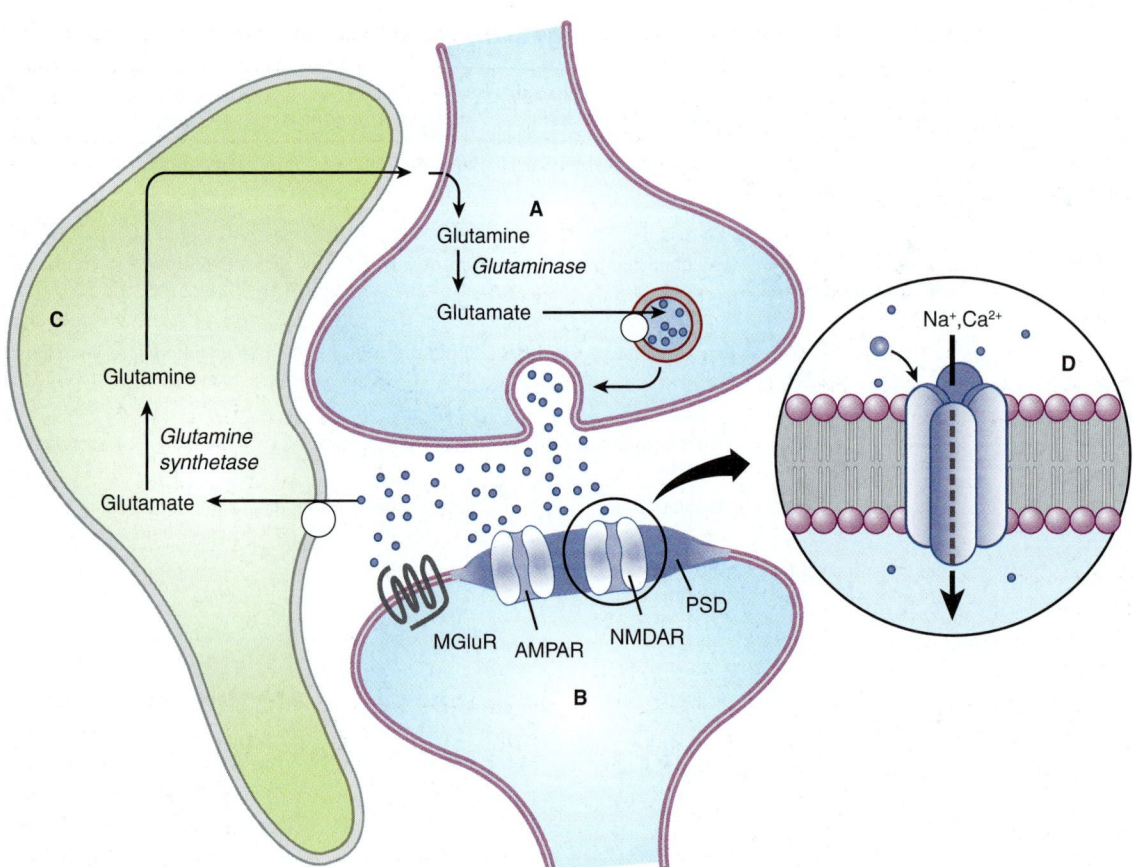

FIGURE 21–7 Schematic diagram of a glutamate synapse. Glutamine is imported into the glutamatergic neuron **(A)** and converted into glutamate by glutaminase. The glutamate is then concentrated in vesicles by the vesicular glutamate transporter. Upon release into the synapse, glutamate can interact with AMPA and NMDA ionotropic receptor channels (AMPAR, NMDAR) in the postsynaptic density (PSD) and with metabotropic receptors (MGluR) on the postsynaptic cell **(B)**. Synaptic transmission is terminated by active transport of the glutamate into a neighboring glial cell **(C)** by a glutamate transporter. It is synthesized into glutamine by glutamine synthetase and exported into the glutamatergic axon. **(D)** shows a model NMDA receptor channel complex consisting of a tetrameric protein that becomes permeable to Na^+ and Ca^{2+} when it binds a glutamate molecule.

(NMDA). All the ionotropic receptors are composed of four subunits. AMPA receptors, which are present on all neurons, are heterotetramers assembled from four subunits (GluA1–GluA4). The majority of AMPA receptors contain the GluA2 subunit and are permeable to Na^+ and K^+, but not to Ca^{2+}. Some AMPA receptors, typically present on inhibitory interneurons, lack the GluA2 subunit and are also permeable to Ca^{2+}.

Kainate receptors are not as uniformly distributed as AMPA receptors, being expressed at high levels in the hippocampus, cerebellum, and spinal cord. They are formed from a number of subunit combinations (GluK1–GluK5). Although GluK4 and GluK5 are unable to form channels on their own, their presence in the receptor changes the receptor's affinity and kinetics. Similar to AMPA receptors, kainate receptors are permeable to Na^+ and K^+ and in some subunit combinations can also be permeable to Ca^{2+}.

NMDA receptors are as ubiquitous as AMPA receptors, being present on essentially all neurons in the CNS. All NMDA receptors require the presence of the subunit GluN1. The channel also contains one or two NR2 subunits (GluN2A–GluN2D).

Unlike AMPA and kainate receptors, all NMDA receptors are highly permeable to Ca^{2+} as well as to Na^+ and K^+. NMDA receptor function is controlled in a number of intriguing ways. In addition to glutamate binding, the channel also requires the binding of glycine to a separate site. The physiologic role of glycine binding is unclear because the glycine site appears to be saturated at normal ambient levels of glycine. Another key difference between AMPA and kainate receptors on the one hand, and NMDA receptors on the other, is that AMPA and kainate receptor activation results in channel opening at resting membrane potential, whereas NMDA receptor activation does not. This is due to the voltage-dependent block of the NMDA pore by extracellular Mg^{2+}. When the neuron is strongly depolarized, as occurs with intense activation of the synapse or by activation of neighboring synapses, Mg^{2+} is expelled and the channel opens. Thus, there are two requirements for NMDA receptor channel opening: Glutamate must bind the receptor and the membrane must be depolarized. The rise in intracellular Ca^{2+} that accompanies channel opening results in a long-lasting enhancement in synaptic strength that is referred to as **long-term potentiation (LTP).** The change can last for many hours or even days and is generally accepted as an important cellular mechanism underlying learning and memory.

The metabotropic glutamate receptors are G protein-coupled receptors that act indirectly on ion channels via G proteins. Metabotropic receptors (mGluR1–mGluR8) have been divided into three groups (I, II, and III). A variety of agonists and antagonists have been developed that interact selectively with the different groups. Group I receptors are typically located postsynaptically and are thought to cause neuronal excitation by activating a nonselective cation channel. These receptors also activate phospholipase C, leading to inositol trisphosphate-mediated intracellular Ca^{2+} release. In contrast, group II and group III receptors are typically located on presynaptic nerve terminals and act as inhibitory autoreceptors. Activation of these receptors causes the inhibition of Ca^{2+} channels, resulting in inhibition of transmitter release. These receptors are activated only when the concentration of glutamate rises to high levels during repetitive stimulation of the synapse. Activation of these receptors causes the inhibition of adenylyl cyclase and decreases cAMP generation.

The postsynaptic membrane at excitatory synapses is thickened and referred to as the **postsynaptic density** (PSD; Figure 21–7). This is a highly complex structure containing glutamate receptors, signaling proteins, scaffolding proteins, and cytoskeletal proteins. A typical excitatory synapse contains AMPA receptors, which tend to be located toward the periphery, and NMDA receptors, which are concentrated in the center. Kainate receptors are present at a subset of excitatory synapses, but their exact location is unknown. Metabotropic glutamate receptors (group I), which are localized just outside the postsynaptic density, are also present at some excitatory synapses.

B. GABA and Glycine

Both GABA and glycine are inhibitory neurotransmitters, which are typically released from local interneurons. Interneurons that release glycine are restricted to the spinal cord and brainstem, whereas interneurons releasing GABA are present throughout the CNS, including the spinal cord. It is interesting that some interneurons in the spinal cord can release both GABA and glycine. Glycine receptors are pentameric structures that are selectively permeable to Cl^-. Strychnine, which is a potent spinal cord convulsant and has been used in some rat poisons, selectively blocks glycine receptors.

GABA receptors are divided into two main types: $GABA_A$ and $GABA_B$. Inhibitory postsynaptic potentials in many areas of the brain have a fast and slow component. The fast component is mediated by $GABA_A$ receptors and the slow component by $GABA_B$ receptors. The difference in kinetics stems from the differences in coupling of the receptors to ion channels. $GABA_A$ receptors are ionotropic receptors and, like glycine receptors, are pentameric structures that are selectively permeable to Cl^-. These receptors are selectively inhibited by picrotoxin and bicuculline, both of which cause generalized convulsions. A great many subunits for $GABA_A$ receptors have been cloned; this accounts for the large diversity in the pharmacology of $GABA_A$

receptors, making them key targets for clinically useful agents (see Chapter 22). $GABA_B$ receptors are metabotropic receptors that are selectively activated by the antispastic drug baclofen. These receptors are coupled to G proteins that, depending on their cellular location, either inhibit Ca^{2+} channels or activate K^+ channels. The $GABA_B$ component of the inhibitory postsynaptic potential is due to a selective increase in K^+ conductance. This inhibitory postsynaptic potential is long-lasting and slow because the coupling of receptor activation to K^+ channel opening is indirect and delayed. $GABA_B$ receptors are localized to the perisynaptic region and thus require the spillover of GABA from the synaptic cleft. $GABA_B$ receptors are also present on the axon terminals of many excitatory and inhibitory synapses. In this case, GABA spills over onto these presynaptic $GABA_B$ receptors, inhibiting transmitter release by inhibiting Ca^{2+} channels. In addition to their coupling to ion channels, $GABA_B$ receptors also inhibit adenylyl cyclase and decrease cAMP generation.

Acetylcholine

Acetylcholine was the first compound to be identified pharmacologically as a transmitter in the CNS. Eccles showed in the early 1950s that excitation of Renshaw cells by motor axon collaterals in the spinal cord was blocked by nicotinic antagonists. Furthermore, Renshaw cells were extremely sensitive to nicotinic agonists. These experiments were remarkable for two reasons. First, this early success at identifying a transmitter for a central synapse was followed by disappointment because it remained the sole central synapse for which the transmitter was known until the late 1960s, when comparable data became available for GABA and glycine. Second, the motor axon collateral synapse remains one of the best-documented examples of a cholinergic nicotinic synapse in the mammalian CNS, despite the rather widespread distribution of nicotinic receptors as defined by in situ hybridization studies. Most CNS responses to acetylcholine are mediated by a large family of G protein-coupled muscarinic receptors. At a few sites, acetylcholine causes slow inhibition of the neuron by activating the M_2 subtype of receptor, which opens potassium channels. A far more widespread muscarinic action in response to acetylcholine is a slow excitation that in some cases is mediated by M_1 receptors. These muscarinic effects are much slower than either nicotinic effects on Renshaw cells or the effect of amino acids. Furthermore, this M_1 muscarinic excitation is unusual in that acetylcholine produces it by *decreasing* the membrane permeability to potassium, ie, the opposite of conventional transmitter action.

A number of pathways contain acetylcholine, including neurons in the neostriatum, the medial septal nucleus, and the reticular formation. Cholinergic pathways appear to play an important role in cognitive functions, especially memory. Presenile dementia of the Alzheimer type is reportedly associated with a profound loss of cholinergic neurons. However, the specificity of this loss has been questioned because the levels of other putative transmitters, eg, somatostatin, are also decreased.

Monoamines

Monoamines include the catecholamines (dopamine and norepinephrine) and 5-hydroxytryptamine. Although these compounds are present in very small amounts in the CNS, they can be localized using extremely sensitive histochemical methods. These pathways are the site of action of many drugs; for example, the CNS stimulants cocaine and amphetamine appear to act primarily at catecholamine synapses. Cocaine blocks the reuptake of dopamine and norepinephrine, whereas amphetamines cause presynaptic terminals to release these transmitters.

A. Dopamine

The major pathways containing dopamine are the projection linking the substantia nigra to the neostriatum and the projection linking the ventral tegmental region to limbic structures, particularly the limbic cortex. The therapeutic action of the antiparkinsonism drug levodopa is associated with the former area (see Chapter 28), whereas the therapeutic action of the antipsychotic drugs is thought to be associated with the latter (see Chapter 29). Dopamine-containing neurons in the tuberobasal ventral hypothalamus play an important role in regulating hypothalamohypophysial function. Five dopamine receptors have been identified, and they fall into two categories: D_1-like (D_1 and D_5) and D_2-like (D_2, D_3, D_4). All dopamine receptors are metabotropic. Dopamine generally exerts a slow inhibitory action on CNS neurons. This action has been best characterized on dopamine-containing substantia nigra neurons, where D_2-receptor activation opens potassium channels via the G_i coupling protein.

B. Norepinephrine

Most noradrenergic neurons are located in the locus caeruleus or the lateral tegmental area of the reticular formation. Although the density of fibers innervating various sites differs considerably, most regions of the CNS receive diffuse noradrenergic input. All noradrenergic receptor subtypes are metabotropic. When applied to neurons, norepinephrine can hyperpolarize them by increasing potassium conductance. This effect is mediated by α_2 receptors and has been characterized most thoroughly on locus caeruleus neurons. In many regions of the CNS, norepinephrine actually enhances excitatory inputs by both indirect and direct mechanisms. The indirect mechanism involves disinhibition; that is, inhibitory local circuit neurons are inhibited. The direct mechanism involves blockade of potassium conductances that slow neuronal discharge. Depending on the type of neuron, this effect is mediated by either α_1 or β receptors. Facilitation of excitatory synaptic transmission is in accordance with many of the behavioral processes thought to involve noradrenergic pathways, eg, attention and arousal.

C. 5-Hydroxytryptamine

Most 5-hydroxytryptamine (5-HT, serotonin) pathways originate from neurons in the raphe or midline regions of the pons and upper brainstem. 5-HT is contained in unmyelinated fibers that diffusely innervate most regions of the CNS, but the density of the innervation varies. 5-HT acts on more than a dozen receptor subtypes. Except for the 5-HT_3 receptor, all of these receptors are metabotropic. The ionotropic 5-HT_3 receptor exerts a rapid excitatory action at a very limited number of sites in the CNS. In most areas of the CNS, 5-HT has a strong inhibitory action. This action is mediated by 5-HT_{1A} receptors and is associated with membrane hyperpolarization caused by an increase in potassium conductance. It has been found that 5-HT_{1A} receptors and $GABA_B$ receptors activate the same population of potassium channels. Some cell types are slowly excited by 5-HT owing to its blockade of potassium channels via 5-HT_2 or 5-HT_4 receptors. Both excitatory and inhibitory actions can occur on the same neuron. It has often been speculated that 5-HT pathways may be involved in the hallucinations induced by LSD (lysergic acid), since this compound can antagonize the peripheral actions of 5-HT. However, LSD does not appear to be a 5-HT antagonist in the CNS, and typical LSD-induced behavior is still seen in animals after raphe nuclei are destroyed. Other proposed regulatory functions of 5-HT-containing neurons include sleep, temperature, appetite, and neuroendocrine control.

Peptides

A great many CNS peptides have been discovered that produce dramatic effects both on animal behavior and on the activity of individual neurons. Many of the peptides have been mapped with immunohistochemical techniques and include opioid peptides (eg, enkephalins, endorphins), neurotensin, substance P, somatostatin, cholecystokinin, vasoactive intestinal polypeptide, neuropeptide Y, and thyrotropin-releasing hormone. As in the peripheral autonomic nervous system, peptides often coexist with a conventional nonpeptide transmitter in the same neuron. A good example of the approaches used to define the role of these peptides in the CNS comes from studies on substance P and its association with sensory fibers. Substance P is contained in and released from small unmyelinated primary sensory neurons in the spinal cord and brainstem and causes a slow excitatory postsynaptic potential in target neurons. These sensory fibers are known to transmit noxious stimuli, and it is therefore surprising that—although substance P receptor antagonists can modify responses to certain types of pain—they do not block the response. Glutamate, which is released with substance P from these synapses, presumably plays an important role in transmitting pain stimuli. Substance P is certainly involved in many other functions because it is found in many areas of the CNS that are unrelated to pain pathways.

Many of these peptides are also found in peripheral structures, including peripheral synapses. They are described in Chapters 6 and 17.

Nitric Oxide

The CNS contains a substantial amount of nitric oxide synthase (NOS) within certain classes of neurons. This neuronal

NOS is an enzyme activated by calcium-calmodulin, and activation of NMDA receptors, which increases intracellular calcium, results in the generation of nitric oxide. Although a physiologic role for nitric oxide has been clearly established for vascular smooth muscle, its role in synaptic transmission and synaptic plasticity remains controversial. Perhaps the strongest case for a role of nitric oxide in neuronal signaling in the CNS is for long-term depression of synaptic transmission in the cerebellum.

Endocannabinoids

The primary psychoactive ingredient in cannabis, Δ^9-tetrahydrocannabinol (Δ^9-THC), affects the brain mainly by activating a specific cannabinoid receptor, CB_1. CB_1 receptors are expressed at high levels in many brain regions, and they are primarily located on presynaptic terminals. Several endogenous brain lipids, including anandamide and 2-arachidonylglycerol (2-AG), have been identified as CB_1 ligands. These ligands are not stored, as are classic neurotransmitters, but instead are rapidly synthesized by neurons in response to depolarization and consequent calcium influx. Activation of metabotropic receptors (eg, by acetylcholine and glutamate) can also activate the formation of 2-AG. In further contradistinction to classic neurotransmitters, endogenous cannabinoids can function as retrograde synaptic messengers: They are released from postsynaptic neurons and travel backward across synapses, activating CB_1 receptors on presynaptic neurons and suppressing transmitter release. This suppression can be transient or long lasting, depending on the pattern of activity. Cannabinoids may affect memory, cognition, and pain perception by this mechanism.

REFERENCES

Aizenman CD et al: Use-dependent changes in synaptic strength at the Purkinje cell to deep nuclear synapse. Prog Brain Res 2000;124:257.

Bredt DS, Nicoll RA: AMPA receptor trafficking at excitatory synapses. Neuron 2003;40:361.

Catterall WA et al: Compendium of voltage-gated ion channels: Calcium channels. Pharmacol Rev 2003;55:579.

Catterall WA, Goldin AL, Waxman SG: Compendium of voltage-gated ion channels: Sodium channels. Pharmacol Rev 2003;55:575.

Clapham DE et al: Compendium of voltage-gated ion channels: Transient receptor potential channels. Pharmacol Rev 2003;55:591.

Fremeau RT, Jr et al: VGLUTs define subsets of excitatory neurons and suggest novel roles for glutamate. Trends Neurosci 2004;27:98.

Freund TF, Katona I, Piomelli D: Role of endogenous cannabinoids in synaptic signaling. Physiol Rev 2003;83:1017.

Gouaux E, MacKinnon R: Principles of selective ion transport in channels and pumps. Science 2005;310:1461.

Hall ZW: In: *An Introduction to Molecular Neurobiology.* Sinauer, 1992.

Hille B: *Ionic Channels of Excitable Membranes,* 3rd ed. Sinauer, 2001.

Julius D, Basbaum AI: Molecular mechanisms of nociception. Nature 2001;413:203.

Koles L, Furst S, Illes P: P2X and P2Y receptors as possible targets of therapeutic manipulations in CNS illnesses. Drug News Perspect 2005;18:85.

Malenka RC, Nicoll RA: Long-term potentiation—A decade of progress? Science 1999;285:1870.

Mody I, Pearce RA: Diversity of inhibitory neurotransmission through GABA(A) receptors. Trends Neurosci 2004;27:569.

Moran MM, Xu H, Clapham DE: TRP ion channels in the nervous system. Curr Opin Neurobiol 2004;14:362.

Nestler EJ, Hyman SE, Malenka RC: *Molecular Neuropharmacology,* 2nd ed. McGraw-Hill, 2009.

Rudolph U, Mohler H: Analysis of GABAA receptor function and dissection of the pharmacology of benzodiazepines and general anesthetics through mouse genetics. Annu Rev Pharmacol Toxicol 2004;44:475.

Sudhof TC: The synaptic vesicle cycle. Annu Rev Neurosci 2004;27:509.

Wilson RI, Nicoll RA: Endocannabinoid signaling in the brain. Science 2002;296:678.

Sedative-Hypnotic Drugs

Anthony J. Trevor, PhD, & Walter L. Way, MD

CASE STUDY

At her annual physical examination, a 53-year-old middle school teacher complains that she has been experiencing difficulty falling asleep and after falling asleep awakens several times during the night. These episodes occur almost nightly and are having a negative impact on her teaching functions. She has tried various over-the-counter sleep remedies, but they were of little help and she experienced "hangover" effects the next day. Her general health is good, she is not overweight, and she takes no prescription drugs. She drinks one cup of decaffeinated coffee in the morning; however, she drinks as many as six cans per day of diet cola. She drinks a glass of wine with her evening meal but does not like stronger spirits. What other aspects of this patient's history would you like to know? What therapeutic measures are appropriate for this patient? What drug, or drugs (if any), would you prescribe?

Assignment of a drug to the sedative-hypnotic class indicates that it is able to cause sedation (with concomitant relief of anxiety) or to encourage sleep. Because there is considerable chemical variation within the group, this drug classification is based on clinical uses rather than on similarities in chemical structure. Anxiety states and sleep disorders are common problems, and sedative-hypnotics are widely prescribed drugs worldwide.

■ BASIC PHARMACOLOGY OF SEDATIVE-HYPNOTICS

An effective **sedative** (anxiolytic) agent should reduce anxiety and exert a calming effect. The degree of central nervous system depression caused by a sedative should be the minimum consistent with therapeutic efficacy. A **hypnotic** drug should produce drowsiness and encourage the onset and maintenance of a state of sleep. Hypnotic effects involve more pronounced depression of the central nervous system than sedation, and this can be achieved with many drugs in this class simply by increasing the dose. Graded dose-dependent depression of central nervous system function is a characteristic of most sedative-hypnotics. However, individual drugs differ in the relationship between the dose and the degree of central nervous system depression. Two examples of such dose-response relationships are shown in Figure 22–1. The linear slope for drug A is typical of many of the older sedative-hypnotics, including the barbiturates and alcohols. With such drugs, an increase in dose higher than that needed for hypnosis may lead to a state of general anesthesia. At still higher doses, these sedative-hypnotics may depress respiratory and vasomotor centers in the medulla, leading to coma and death. Deviations from a linear dose-response relationship, as shown for drug B, require proportionately greater dosage increments to achieve central nervous system depression more profound than hypnosis. This appears to be the case for benzodiazepines and for certain newer hypnotics that have a similar mechanism of action.

Chemical Classification

The **benzodiazepines** are widely used sedative-hypnotics. All of the structures shown in Figure 22–2 are 1,4-benzodiazepines, and most contain a carboxamide group in the 7-membered heterocyclic ring structure. An electronegative substituent in the 7 position, such as a halogen or a nitro group, is required for sedative-hypnotic activity. The structures of triazolam and alprazolam include the addition of a triazole ring at the 1,2-position.

The chemical structures of some older and less commonly used sedative-hypnotics, including several **barbiturates**, are shown in Figure 22–3. Glutethimide and meprobamate are of distinctive chemical structure but are practically equivalent to barbiturates in their pharmacologic effects. They are rarely used. The sedative-

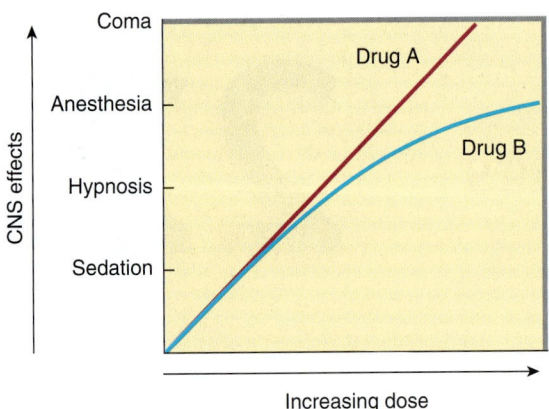

FIGURE 22–1 Dose-response curves for two hypothetical sedative-hypnotics.

hypnotic class also includes compounds of simpler chemical structure, including **ethanol** (see Chapter 23) and **chloral hydrate.**

Several drugs with novel chemical structures have been introduced more recently for use in sleep disorders. **Zolpidem**, an imidazopyridine, **zaleplon**, a pyrazolopyrimidine, and **eszopiclone**, a cyclopyrrolone (Figure 22–4), although structurally unrelated to benzodiazepines, share a similar mechanism of action, as described below. Eszopiclone is the *(S)*-enantiomer of zopiclone, a hypnotic drug that has been available outside the United States since 1989. **Ramelteon**, a melatonin receptor agonist, is a more recently introduced hypnotic drug (see Box: Ramelteon). **Buspirone** is a slow-onset anxiolytic agent whose actions are quite different from those of conventional sedative-hypnotics (see Box: Buspirone).

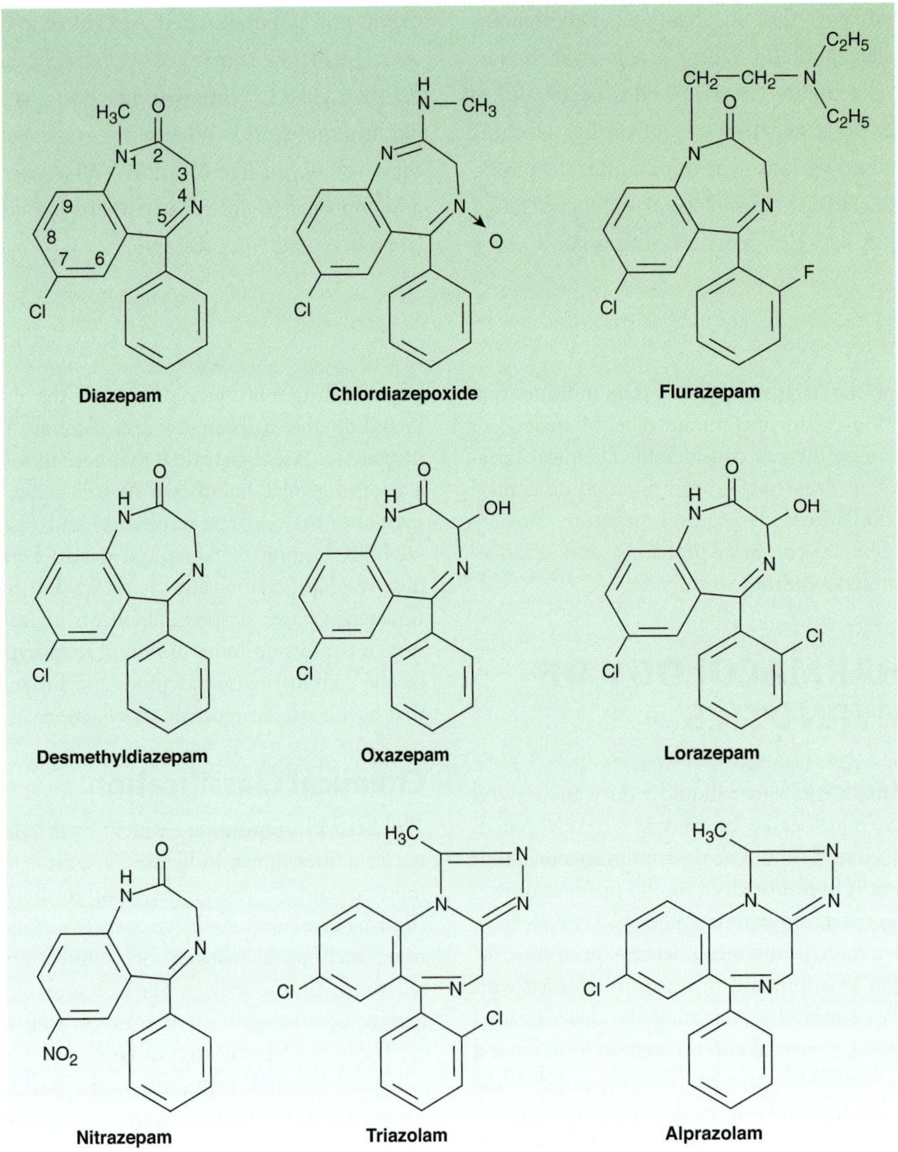

FIGURE 22–2 Chemical structures of some benzodiazepines.

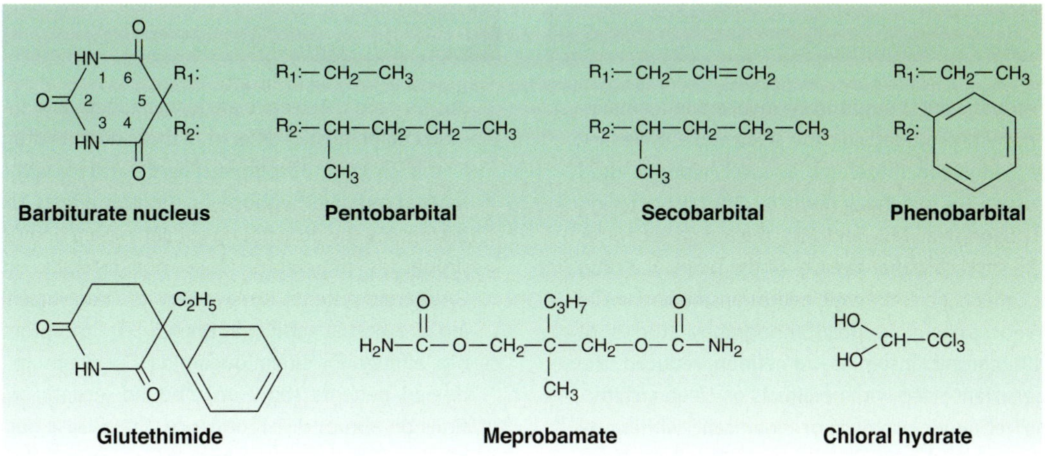

FIGURE 22–3 Chemical structures of some barbiturates and other sedative-hypnotics.

Other classes of drugs that exert sedative effects include anti-psychotics (see Chapter 29) and many antidepressant drugs (see Chapter 30). The latter are currently used widely in the management of chronic anxiety disorders. Certain antihistaminic agents including diphenhydramine, hydroxyzine, and promethazine (see Chapter 16) cause sedation but commonly also exert marked effects on the peripheral autonomic nervous system. Antihistaminic drugs with sedative effects are available as over-the-counter sleep aids.

Pharmacokinetics

A. Absorption and Distribution

The rates of oral absorption of sedative-hypnotics differ depending on a number of factors, including lipophilicity. For example, the absorption of triazolam is extremely rapid, and that of diazepam and the active metabolite of clorazepate is more rapid than other commonly used benzodiazepines. Clorazepate, a prodrug, is converted to its active form, desmethyldiazepam (nordiazepam), by acid hydrolysis in the stomach. Most of the barbiturates and other older sedative-hypnotics, as well as the newer hypnotics (eszopiclone, zaleplon, zolpidem), are absorbed rapidly into the blood following oral administration.

Lipid solubility plays a major role in determining the rate at which a particular sedative-hypnotic enters the central nervous system. This property is responsible for the rapid onset of central nervous system effects of triazolam, thiopental (see Chapter 25), and the newer hypnotics eszopiclone, zaleplon, and zolpidem.

All sedative-hypnotics cross the placental barrier during pregnancy. If sedative-hypnotics are given during the predelivery period, they may contribute to the depression of neonatal vital functions. Sedative-hypnotics are also detectable in breast milk and may exert depressant effects in the nursing infant.

B. Biotransformation

Metabolic transformation to more water-soluble metabolites is necessary for clearance of sedative-hypnotics from the body. The microsomal drug-metabolizing enzyme systems of the liver are

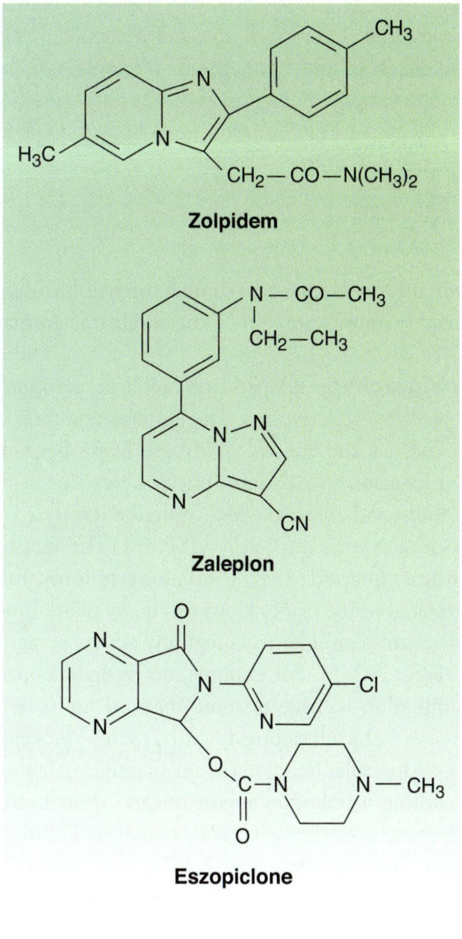

FIGURE 22–4 Chemical structures of newer hypnotics.

Ramelteon

Melatonin receptors are thought to be involved in maintaining circadian rhythms underlying the sleep-wake cycle (see Chapter 16). Ramelteon (Rozerem), a novel hypnotic drug specifically useful for patients who have difficulty in falling asleep, is an agonist at MT_1 and MT_2 melatonin receptors located in the suprachiasmatic nuclei of the brain. The drug has no direct effects on GABAergic neurotransmission in the central nervous system. In polysomnography studies of patients with chronic insomnia, ramelteon reduced the latency of persistent sleep with no effects on sleep architecture and no rebound insomnia or significant withdrawal symptoms. Ramelteon has minimal potential for abuse, is not a controlled substance, and regular use does not result in dependence. The drug is rapidly absorbed after oral administration and undergoes extensive first-pass metabolism, forming an active metabolite with longer half-life (2–5 hours) than the parent drug. The CYP1A2 isoform of cytochrome P450 is mainly responsible for the metabolism of ramelteon, but the CYP2C9 isoform is also involved. The drug should not be used in combination with inhibitors of CYP1A2 (eg, ciprofloxacin, fluvoxamine, tacrine, zileuton) or CYP2C9 (eg, fluconazole) and should be used with caution in patients with liver dysfunction. The CYP inducer rifampin markedly reduces the plasma levels of both ramelteon and its active metabolite. Adverse effects of ramelteon include dizziness, somnolence, fatigue, and endocrine changes as well as decreases in testosterone and increases in prolactin. Ramelteon is an FDA pregnancy category C drug.

Buspirone

Buspirone has selective anxiolytic effects, and its pharmacologic characteristics differ from those of other drugs described in this chapter. Buspirone relieves anxiety without causing marked sedative, hypnotic, or euphoric effects. Unlike benzodiazepines, the drug has no anticonvulsant or muscle relaxant properties. Buspirone does not interact directly with GABAergic systems. It may exert its anxiolytic effects by acting as a partial agonist at brain $5-HT_{1A}$ receptors, but it also has affinity for brain dopamine D_2 receptors. Buspirone-treated patients show no rebound anxiety or withdrawal signs on abrupt discontinuance. The drug is not effective in blocking the acute withdrawal syndrome resulting from abrupt cessation of use of benzodiazepines or other sedative-hypnotics. Buspirone has minimal abuse liability. In marked contrast to the benzodiazepines, the anxiolytic effects of buspirone may take more than a week to become established, making the drug unsuitable for management of acute anxiety states. The drug is used in generalized anxiety states but is less effective in panic disorders.

Buspirone is rapidly absorbed orally but undergoes extensive first-pass metabolism via hydroxylation and dealkylation reactions to form several active metabolites. The major metabolite is 1-(2-pyrimidyl)-piperazine (1-PP), which has α_2-adrenoceptor–blocking actions and which enters the central nervous system to reach higher levels than the parent drug. It is not known what role (if any) 1-PP plays in the central actions of buspirone. The elimination half-life of buspirone is 2–4 hours, and liver dysfunction may slow its clearance. Rifampin, an inducer of cytochrome P450, decreases the half-life of buspirone; inhibitors of CYP3A4 (eg, erythromycin, ketoconazole, grapefruit juice, nefazodone) can markedly increase its plasma levels.

Buspirone causes less psychomotor impairment than benzodiazepines and does not affect driving skills. The drug does not potentiate effects of conventional sedative-hypnotic drugs, ethanol, or tricyclic antidepressants, and elderly patients do not appear to be more sensitive to its actions. Nonspecific chest pain, tachycardia, palpitations, dizziness, nervousness, tinnitus, gastrointestinal distress, and paresthesias and a dose-dependent pupillary constriction may occur. Blood pressure may be significantly elevated in patients receiving MAO inhibitors. Buspirone is an FDA pregnancy category B drug.

most important in this regard, so elimination half-life of these drugs depends mainly on the rate of their metabolic transformation.

1. Benzodiazepines—Hepatic metabolism accounts for the clearance of all benzodiazepines. The patterns and rates of metabolism depend on the individual drugs. Most benzodiazepines undergo microsomal oxidation (phase I reactions), including *N*-dealkylation and aliphatic hydroxylation catalyzed by cytochrome P450 isozymes, especially CYP3A4. The metabolites are subsequently conjugated (phase II reactions) to form glucuronides that are excreted in the urine. However, many phase I metabolites of benzodiazepines are pharmacologically active, some with long half-lives (Figure 22–5). For example, desmethyldiazepam, which has an elimination half-life of more than 40 hours, is an active metabolite of chlordiazepoxide, diazepam, prazepam, and clorazepate. Alprazolam and triazolam undergo α-hydroxylation, and the resulting metabolites appear to exert short-lived pharmacologic effects because they are rapidly conjugated to form inactive glucuronides. The short elimination half-life of triazolam (2–3 hours) favors its use as a hypnotic rather than as a sedative drug.

The formation of active metabolites has complicated studies on the pharmacokinetics of the benzodiazepines in humans because the elimination half-life of the parent drug may have little relation to the time course of pharmacologic effects. Benzodiazepines for which the parent drug or active metabolites have long half-lives are predictably more likely to cause cumulative effects with multiple doses. Cumulative and residual effects such as excessive drowsiness appear to be less of a problem with such drugs as estazolam, oxazepam, and lorazepam, which have relatively short

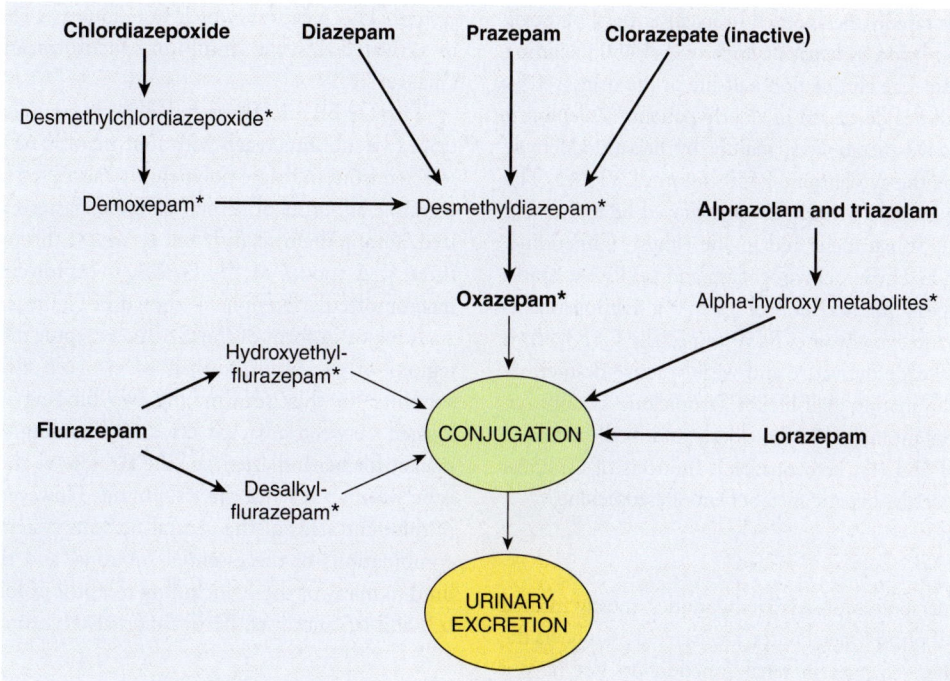

FIGURE 22–5 Biotransformation of benzodiazepines. (Boldface, drugs available for clinical use in various countries; *, active metabolite.)

half-lives and are metabolized directly to inactive glucuronides. Some pharmacokinetic properties of selected benzodiazepines are listed in Table 22–1. The metabolism of several commonly used benzodiazepines including diazepam, midazolam, and triazolam is affected by inhibitors and inducers of hepatic P450 isozymes (see Chapter 4).

2. Barbiturates—With the exception of phenobarbital, only insignificant quantities of the barbiturates are excreted unchanged. The major metabolic pathways involve oxidation by hepatic enzymes to form alcohols, acids, and ketones, which appear in the urine as glucuronide conjugates. The overall rate of hepatic metabolism in humans depends on the individual drug but (with the exception of the thiobarbiturates) is usually slow. The elimination half-lives of secobarbital and pentobarbital range from 18 to 48 hours in different individuals. The elimination half-life of phenobarbital in humans is 4–5 days. Multiple dosing with these agents can lead to cumulative effects.

3. Newer hypnotics—After oral administration of the standard formulation, zolpidem reaches peak plasma levels in 1.6 hours. A biphasic release formulation extends plasma levels by approximately

TABLE 22–1 Pharmacokinetic properties of some benzodiazepines and newer hypnotics in humans.

Drug	Peak Blood Level (hours)	Elimination Half-Life[1] (hours)	Comments
Alprazolam	1–2	12–15	Rapid oral absorption
Chlordiazepoxide	2–4	15–40	Active metabolites; erratic bioavailability from IM injection
Clorazepate	1–2 (nordiazepam)	50–100	Prodrug; hydrolyzed to active form in stomach
Diazepam	1–2	20–80	Active metabolites; erratic bioavailability from IM injection
Eszopiclone	1	6	Minor active metabolites
Flurazepam	1–2	40–100	Active metabolites with long half-lives
Lorazepam	1–6	10–20	No active metabolites
Oxazepam	2–4	10–20	No active metabolites
Temazepam	2–3	10–40	Slow oral absorption
Triazolam	1	2–3	Rapid onset; short duration of action
Zaleplon	< 1	1–2	Metabolized via aldehyde dehydrogenase
Zolpidem	1–3	1.5–3.5	No active metabolites

[1]Includes half-lives of major metabolites.

2 hours. Zolpidem is rapidly metabolized to inactive metabolites via oxidation and hydroxylation by hepatic cytochromes P450 including the CYP3A4 isozyme. The elimination half-life of the drug is 1.5–3.5 hours, with clearance decreased in elderly patients. Zaleplon is metabolized to inactive metabolites, mainly by hepatic aldehyde oxidase and partly by the cytochrome P450 isoform CYP3A4. The half-life of the drug is about 1 hour. Dosage should be reduced in patients with hepatic impairment and in the elderly. Cimetidine, which inhibits both aldehyde dehydrogenase and CYP3A4, markedly increases the peak plasma level of zaleplon. Eszopiclone is metabolized by hepatic cytochromes P450 (especially CYP3A4) to form the inactive *N*-oxide derivative and weakly active desmethyleszopiclone. The elimination half-life of eszopiclone is approximately 6 hours and is prolonged in the elderly and in the presence of inhibitors of CYP3A4 (eg, ketoconazole). Inducers of CYP3A4 (eg, rifampin) increase the hepatic metabolism of eszopiclone.

C. Excretion

The water-soluble metabolites of sedative-hypnotics, mostly formed via the conjugation of phase I metabolites, are excreted mainly via the kidney. In most cases, changes in renal function do not have a marked effect on the elimination of parent drugs. Phenobarbital is excreted unchanged in the urine to a certain extent (20–30% in humans), and its elimination rate can be increased significantly by alkalinization of the urine. This is partly due to increased ionization at alkaline pH, since phenobarbital is a weak acid with a pK_a of 7.4.

D. Factors Affecting Biodisposition

The biodisposition of sedative-hypnotics can be influenced by several factors, particularly alterations in hepatic function resulting from disease or drug-induced increases or decreases in microsomal enzyme activities (see Chapter 4).

In very old patients and in patients with severe liver disease, the elimination half-lives of these drugs are often increased significantly. In such cases, multiple normal doses of these sedative-hypnotics can result in excessive central nervous system effects.

The activity of hepatic microsomal drug-metabolizing enzymes may be increased in patients exposed to certain older sedative-hypnotics on a long-term basis (enzyme induction; see Chapter 4). Barbiturates (especially phenobarbital) and meprobamate are most likely to cause this effect, which may result in an increase in their own hepatic metabolism as well as that of other drugs. Increased biotransformation of other pharmacologic agents as a result of enzyme induction by barbiturates is a potential mechanism underlying drug interactions (see Chapter 66). In contrast, benzodiazepines and the newer hypnotics do not change hepatic drug-metabolizing enzyme activity with continuous use.

Pharmacodynamics of Benzodiazepines, Barbiturates, & Newer Hypnotics

A. Molecular Pharmacology of the GABA_A Receptor

The benzodiazepines, the barbiturates, zolpidem, zaleplon, eszopiclone, and many other drugs bind to molecular components of the GABA_A receptor in neuronal membranes in the central nervous system. This receptor, which functions as a chloride ion channel, is activated by the inhibitory neurotransmitter GABA (see Chapter 21).

The GABA_A receptor has a pentameric structure assembled from five subunits (each with four membrane-spanning domains) selected from multiple polypeptide classes (α, β, γ, δ, ε, π, ρ, etc). Multiple subunits of several of these classes have been characterized, among them six different α (eg, α1 through α6), four β, and three γ. A model of the GABA_A receptor-chloride ion channel macromolecular complex is shown in Figure 22–6.

A major isoform of the GABA_A receptor that is found in many regions of the brain consists of two α1, two β2, and one γ2 subunits. In this isoform, the two binding sites for GABA are located between adjacent α1 and β2 subunits, and the binding pocket for benzodiazepines (the **BZ site** of the GABA_A receptor) is between an α1 and the γ2 subunit. However, GABA_A receptors in different areas of the central nervous system consist of various combinations of the essential subunits, and the benzodiazepines bind to many of these, including receptor isoforms containing α2, α3, and α5 subunits. Barbiturates also bind to multiple isoforms

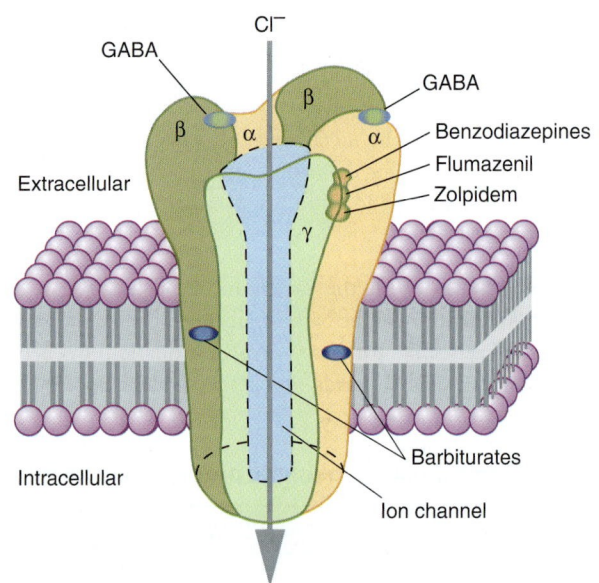

FIGURE 22–6 A model of the GABA_A receptor-chloride ion channel macromolecular complex. A hetero-oligomeric glycoprotein, the complex consists of five or more membrane-spanning subunits. Multiple forms of α, β, and γ subunits are arranged in different pentameric combinations so that GABA_A receptors exhibit molecular heterogeneity. GABA appears to interact at two sites between α and β subunits, triggering chloride channel opening with resulting membrane hyperpolarization. Binding of benzodiazepines and the newer hypnotic drugs such as zolpidem occurs at a single site between α and γ subunits, facilitating the process of chloride ion channel opening. The benzodiazepine antagonist flumazenil also binds at this site and can reverse the hypnotic effects of zolpidem. Note that these binding sites are distinct from those of the barbiturates. (See also text and Box: The Versatility of the Chloride Channel GABA Receptor Complex.)

of the $GABA_A$ receptor but at different sites from those with which benzodiazepines interact. In contrast to benzodiazepines, zolpidem, zaleplon, and eszopiclone bind more selectively because these drugs interact only with $GABA_A$-receptor isoforms that contain $\alpha 1$ subunits. The heterogeneity of $GABA_A$ receptors may constitute the molecular basis for the varied pharmacologic actions of benzodiazepines and related drugs (see Box: GABA Receptor Heterogeneity & Pharmacologic Selectivity).

In contrast to GABA itself, benzodiazepines and other sedative-hypnotics have a low affinity for $GABA_B$ receptors, which are activated by the spasmolytic drug baclofen (see Chapters 21 and 27).

B. Neuropharmacology

GABA (γ-aminobutyric acid) is a major inhibitory neurotransmitter in the central nervous system (see Chapter 21). Electrophysiologic studies have shown that benzodiazepines potentiate GABAergic inhibition at all levels of the neuraxis, including the spinal cord, hypothalamus, hippocampus, substantia nigra, cerebellar cortex, and cerebral cortex. Benzodiazepines appear to increase the efficiency of GABAergic synaptic inhibition. The benzodiazepines do not substitute for GABA but appear to enhance GABA's effects allosterically without directly activating $GABA_A$ receptors or opening the associated chloride channels. The enhancement in chloride ion conductance induced by the interaction of benzodiazepines with GABA takes the form of an increase in the *frequency* of channel-opening events.

Barbiturates also facilitate the actions of GABA at multiple sites in the central nervous system, but—in contrast to benzodiazepines—they appear to increase the *duration* of the GABA-gated chloride channel openings. At high concentrations, the barbiturates may also be GABA-mimetic, directly activating chloride channels. These effects involve a binding site or sites distinct from the benzodiazepine binding sites. Barbiturates are less selective in their actions than benzodiazepines, because they also depress the actions of the excitatory neurotransmitter glutamic acid via binding to the AMPA receptor. Barbiturates also exert nonsynaptic membrane effects in parallel with their effects on GABA and glutamate neurotransmission. This multiplicity of sites of action of barbiturates may be the basis for their ability to induce full surgical anesthesia (see Chapter 25) and for their more pronounced central depressant effects (which result in their low margin of safety) compared with benzodiazepines and the newer hypnotics.

C. Benzodiazepine Binding Site Ligands

The components of the $GABA_A$ receptor-chloride ion channel macromolecule that function as benzodiazepine binding sites exhibit heterogeneity (see Box: The Versatility of the Chloride Channel GABA Receptor Complex). Three types of ligand-benzodiazepine receptor interactions have been reported: (1) **Agonists** facilitate GABA actions, and this occurs at multiple BZ binding sites in the case of the benzodiazepines. As noted above, the nonbenzodiazepines zolpidem, zaleplon, and eszopiclone are selective agonists at the BZ sites that contain an $\alpha 1$ subunit. Endogenous agonist ligands for the BZ binding sites have been proposed, because benzodiazepine-like chemicals have been isolated from brain tissue of animals never exposed to these drugs. Nonbenzodiazepine molecules that have affinity for BZ sites on the $GABA_A$ receptor have also been detected in human brain. (2) **Antagonists** are typified by the synthetic benzodiazepine derivative **flumazenil,** which blocks the actions of benzodiazepines, eszopiclone, zaleplon, and zolpidem but does not antagonize the actions of barbiturates, meprobamate, or ethanol. Certain endogenous neuropeptides are also capable of blocking the interaction of benzodiazepines with BZ binding sites. (3) **Inverse agonists** act as negative allosteric modulators of GABA-receptor function (see Chapter 1). Their interaction with BZ sites on the $GABA_A$ receptor can *produce* anxiety and seizures, an action that has been demonstrated for several compounds, especially the β-carbolines, eg, *n*-butyl-β-carboline-3-carboxylate (β-CCB). In addition to their direct actions, these molecules can block the binding and the effects of benzodiazepines.

The physiologic significance of endogenous modulators of GABA functions in the central nervous system remains unclear. To date, it has not been established that the putative endogenous ligands of BZ binding sites play a role in the control of states of anxiety, sleep patterns, or any other characteristic behavioral expression of central nervous system function.

GABA Receptor Heterogeneity & Pharmacologic Selectivity

Studies involving strains of genetically engineered ("knockout") rodents have demonstrated that the specific pharmacologic actions elicited by benzodiazepines and other drugs that modulate GABA actions are influenced by the composition of the subunits assembled to form the $GABA_A$ receptor. Benzodiazepines interact primarily with brain $GABA_A$ receptors in which the α subunits (isoforms 1, 2, 3, and 5) have a conserved histidine residue in the N-terminal domain. Mice in which a point mutation has been inserted converting histidine to arginine in the $\alpha 1$ subunit show resistance to both the sedative and amnestic effects of benzodiazepines, but anxiolytic and muscle-relaxing effects are largely unchanged. These animals are also unresponsive to the hypnotic actions of zolpidem and zaleplon, drugs that bind selectively to $GABA_A$ receptors containing $\alpha 1$ subunits. In contrast, mice with selective histidine-arginine mutations in the $\alpha 2$ or $\alpha 3$ subunits of $GABA_A$ receptors show selective resistance to the antianxiety effects of benzodiazepines. Based on studies of this type, it has been suggested that $\alpha 1$ subunits in $GABA_A$ receptors mediate sedation, amnesia, and ataxic effects of benzodiazepines, whereas $\alpha 2$ and $\alpha 3$ subunits are involved in their anxiolytic and muscle-relaxing actions. Other mutation studies have led to suggestions that an $\alpha 5$ subtype is involved in at least some of the memory impairment caused by benzodiazepines. It should be emphasized that these studies involving genetic manipulations of the $GABA_A$ receptor utilize rodent models of the anxiolytic and amnestic actions of drugs.

The Versatility of the Chloride Channel GABA Receptor Complex

The GABA$_A$-chloride channel macromolecular complex is one of the most versatile drug-responsive machines in the body. In addition to the benzodiazepines, barbiturates, and the newer hypnotics (eg, zolpidem), many other drugs with central nervous system effects can modify the function of this important ionotropic receptor. These include alcohol and certain intravenous anesthetics (etomidate, propofol) in addition to thiopental. For example, etomidate and propofol (see Chapter 25) appear to act selectively at GABA$_A$ receptors that contain β2 and β3 subunits, the latter suggested to be the most important with respect to the hypnotic and muscle-relaxing actions of these anesthetic agents. The anesthetic steroid alphaxalone is thought to interact with GABA$_A$ receptors, and these receptors may also be targets for some of the actions of volatile anesthetics (eg, halothane). Most of these agents facilitate or mimic the action of GABA. However, it has not been shown that all these drugs act exclusively by this mechanism. Other drugs used in the management of seizure disorders indirectly influence the activity of the GABA$_A$-chloride channel macromolecular complex by inhibiting GABA metabolism (eg, vigabatrin) or reuptake of the transmitter (eg, tiagabine). Central nervous system excitatory agents that act on the chloride channel include picrotoxin and bicuculline. These convulsant drugs block the channel directly (picrotoxin) or interfere with GABA binding (bicuculline).

D. Organ Level Effects

1. Sedation—Benzodiazepines, barbiturates, and most older sedative-hypnotic drugs exert calming effects with concomitant reduction of anxiety at relatively low doses. In most cases, however, the anxiolytic actions of sedative-hypnotics are accompanied by some depressant effects on psychomotor and cognitive functions. In experimental animal models, benzodiazepines and older sedative-hypnotic drugs are able to disinhibit punishment-suppressed behavior. This disinhibition has been equated with antianxiety effects of sedative-hypnotics, and it is not a characteristic of all drugs that have sedative effects, eg, the tricyclic antidepressants and antihistamines. However, the disinhibition of previously suppressed behavior may be more related to behavioral disinhibitory effects of sedative-hypnotics, including euphoria, impaired judgment, and loss of self-control, which can occur at dosages in the range of those used for management of anxiety. The benzodiazepines also exert dose-dependent anterograde amnesic effects (inability to remember events occurring during the drug's duration of action).

2. Hypnosis—By definition, all of the sedative-hypnotics induce sleep if high enough doses are given. The effects of sedative-hypnotics on the stages of sleep depend on several factors, including the specific drug, the dose, and the frequency of its administration. The general effects of benzodiazepines and older sedative-hypnotics on patterns of normal sleep are as follows: (1) the latency of sleep onset is decreased (time to fall asleep); (2) the duration of stage 2 NREM (nonrapid eye movement) sleep is increased; (3) the duration of REM sleep is decreased; and (4) the duration of stage 4 NREM slow-wave sleep is decreased. The newer hypnotics all decrease the latency to persistent sleep. Zolpidem decreases REM sleep but has minimal effect on slow-wave sleep. Zaleplon decreases the latency of sleep onset with little effect on total sleep time, NREM, or REM sleep. Eszopiclone increases total sleep time, mainly via increases in stage 2 NREM sleep, and at low doses has little effect on sleep patterns. At the highest recommended dose, eszopiclone decreases REM sleep.

More rapid onset of sleep and prolongation of stage 2 are presumably clinically useful effects. However, the significance of sedative-hypnotic drug effects on REM and slow-wave sleep is not clear. Deliberate interruption of REM sleep causes anxiety and irritability followed by a rebound increase in REM sleep at the end of the experiment. A similar pattern of "REM rebound" can be detected following abrupt cessation of drug treatment with older sedative-hypnotics, especially when drugs with short durations of action (eg, triazolam) are used at high doses. With respect to zolpidem and the other newer hypnotics, there is little evidence of REM rebound when these drugs are discontinued after use of recommended doses. However, rebound insomnia occurs with both zolpidem and zaleplon if used at higher doses. Despite possible reductions in slow-wave sleep, there are no reports of disturbances in the secretion of pituitary or adrenal hormones when either barbiturates or benzodiazepines are used as hypnotics. The use of sedative-hypnotics for more than 1–2 weeks leads to some tolerance to their effects on sleep patterns.

3. Anesthesia—As shown in Figure 22–1, high doses of certain sedative-hypnotics depress the central nervous system to the point known as stage III of general anesthesia (see Chapter 25). However, the suitability of a particular agent as an adjunct in anesthesia depends mainly on the physicochemical properties that determine its rapidity of onset and duration of effect. Among the barbiturates, thiopental and methohexital are very lipid-soluble, penetrating brain tissue rapidly following intravenous administration, a characteristic favoring their use for the induction of anesthesia. Rapid tissue redistribution (not rapid elimination) accounts for the short duration of action of these drugs, a feature useful in recovery from anesthesia.

Benzodiazepines—including diazepam, lorazepam, and midazolam—are used intravenously in anesthesia (see Chapter 25), often in combination with other agents. Not surprisingly, benzodiazepines given in large doses as adjuncts to general anesthetics may contribute to a persistent postanesthetic respiratory depression. This is probably related to their relatively long half-lives and the formation of active metabolites. However, if necessary, such depressant actions of the benzodiazepines are usually reversible with flumazenil.

4. Anticonvulsant effects—Many sedative-hypnotics are capable of inhibiting the development and spread of epileptiform electrical activity in the central nervous system. Some selectivity exists in that some members of the group can exert anticonvulsant effects without marked central nervous system depression (although psychomotor function may be impaired). Several benzodiazepines—including clonazepam, nitrazepam, lorazepam, and diazepam—are sufficiently selective to be clinically useful in the management of seizures (see Chapter 24). Of the barbiturates, phenobarbital and metharbital (converted to phenobarbital in the body) are effective in the treatment of generalized tonic-clonic seizures, though not the drugs of first choice. Zolpidem, zaleplon, and eszopiclone lack anticonvulsant activity, presumably because of their more selective binding than that of benzodiazepines to GABA$_A$ receptor isoforms.

5. Muscle relaxation—Some sedative-hypnotics, particularly members of the carbamate (eg, meprobamate) and benzodiazepine groups, exert inhibitory effects on polysynaptic reflexes and internuncial transmission and at high doses may also depress transmission at the skeletal neuromuscular junction. Somewhat selective actions of this type that lead to muscle relaxation can be readily demonstrated in animals and have led to claims of usefulness for relaxing contracted voluntary muscle in muscle spasm (see Clinical Pharmacology). Muscle relaxation is not a characteristic action of zolpidem, zaleplon, and eszopiclone.

6. Effects on respiration and cardiovascular function—At hypnotic doses in healthy patients, the effects of sedative-hypnotics on respiration are comparable to changes during natural sleep. However, even at therapeutic doses, sedative-hypnotics can produce significant respiratory depression in patients with pulmonary disease. Effects on respiration are dose-related, and depression of the medullary respiratory center is the usual cause of death due to overdose of sedative-hypnotics.

At doses up to those causing hypnosis, no significant effects on the cardiovascular system are observed in healthy patients. However, in hypovolemic states, heart failure, and other diseases that impair cardiovascular function, normal doses of sedative-hypnotics may cause cardiovascular depression, probably as a result of actions on the medullary vasomotor centers. At toxic doses, myocardial contractility and vascular tone may both be depressed by central and peripheral effects, leading to circulatory collapse. Respiratory and cardiovascular effects are more marked when sedative-hypnotics are given intravenously.

Tolerance & Dependence

Tolerance—decreased responsiveness to a drug following repeated exposure—is a common feature of sedative-hypnotic use. It may result in the need for an increase in the dose required to maintain symptomatic improvement or to promote sleep. It is important to recognize that partial cross-tolerance occurs between the sedative-hypnotics described here and also with ethanol (see Chapter 23)—a feature of some clinical importance, as explained below. The mechanisms responsible for tolerance to sedative-hypnotics

are not well understood. An increase in the rate of drug metabolism (metabolic tolerance) may be partly responsible in the case of chronic administration of barbiturates, but changes in responsiveness of the central nervous system (pharmacodynamic tolerance) are of greater importance for most sedative-hypnotics. In the case of benzodiazepines, the development of tolerance in animals has been associated with down-regulation of brain benzodiazepine receptors. Tolerance has been reported to occur with the extended use of zolpidem. Minimal tolerance was observed with the use of zaleplon over a 5-week period and eszopiclone over a 6-month period.

The perceived desirable properties of relief of anxiety, euphoria, disinhibition, and promotion of sleep have led to the compulsive misuse of virtually all sedative-hypnotics. (See Chapter 32 for a detailed discussion.) For this reason, most sedative-hypnotic drugs are classified as Schedule III or Schedule IV drugs for prescribing purposes in the United States. The consequences of abuse of these agents can be defined in both psychological and physiologic terms. The psychological component may initially parallel simple neurotic behavior patterns difficult to differentiate from those of the inveterate coffee drinker or cigarette smoker. When the pattern of sedative-hypnotic use becomes compulsive (addiction, see Chapter 32), more serious complications develop, including dependence and tolerance.

Dependence can be described as an altered physiologic state that requires continuous drug administration to prevent an abstinence or withdrawal syndrome. In the case of sedative-hypnotics, this syndrome is characterized by states of increased anxiety, insomnia, and central nervous system excitability that may progress to convulsions. Most sedative-hypnotics—including benzodiazepines—are capable of causing dependence when used on a long-term basis. However, the severity of withdrawal symptoms differs among individual drugs and depends also on the magnitude of the dose used immediately before cessation of use. When higher doses of sedative-hypnotics are used, abrupt withdrawal leads to more serious withdrawal signs. Differences in the severity of withdrawal symptoms resulting from individual sedative-hypnotics relate in part to half-life, since drugs with long half-lives are eliminated slowly enough to accomplish gradual withdrawal with few physical symptoms. The use of drugs with very short half-lives for hypnotic effects may lead to signs of withdrawal even between doses. For example, triazolam, a benzodiazepine with a half-life of about 4 hours, has been reported to cause daytime anxiety when used to treat sleep disorders. The abrupt cessation of use of zolpidem, zaleplon, or eszopiclone may also result in withdrawal symptoms, though usually of less intensity than those seen with benzodiazepines.

BENZODIAZEPINE ANTAGONISTS: FLUMAZENIL

Flumazenil is one of several 1,4-benzodiazepine derivatives with a high affinity for the benzodiazepine binding site on the GABA$_A$ receptor that act as competitive antagonists. It blocks many of the actions of benzodiazepines, zolpidem, zaleplon, and eszopiclone, but does not antagonize the central nervous system effects of other sedative-hypnotics, ethanol, opioids, or general anesthetics. Flumazenil is approved for use in reversing the central nervous system depressant effects of benzodiazepine overdose and to hasten recovery following use of these drugs in anesthetic and diagnostic procedures. Although the drug reverses the sedative effects of benzodiazepines, antagonism of benzodiazepine-induced respiratory depression is less predictable. When given intravenously, flumazenil acts rapidly but has a short half-life (0.7–1.3 hours) due to rapid hepatic clearance. Because all benzodiazepines have a longer duration of action than flumazenil, sedation commonly recurs, requiring repeated administration of the antagonist.

Adverse effects of flumazenil include agitation, confusion, dizziness, and nausea. Flumazenil may cause a severe precipitated abstinence syndrome in patients who have developed marked benzodiazepine dependence. In patients who have ingested benzodiazepines with tricyclic antidepressants, seizures and cardiac arrhythmias may follow flumazenil administration.

■ CLINICAL PHARMACOLOGY OF SEDATIVE-HYPNOTICS

TREATMENT OF ANXIETY STATES

The psychological, behavioral, and physiological responses that characterize anxiety can take many forms. Typically, the psychic awareness of anxiety is accompanied by enhanced vigilance, motor tension, and autonomic hyperactivity. Anxiety is often secondary to organic disease states—acute myocardial infarction, angina pectoris, gastrointestinal ulcers, etc—which themselves require specific therapy. Another class of secondary anxiety states (situational anxiety) results from circumstances that may have to be dealt with only once or a few times, including anticipation of frightening medical or dental procedures and family illness or other stressful event. Even though situational anxiety tends to be self-limiting, the short-term use of sedative-hypnotics may be appropriate for the treatment of this and certain disease-associated anxiety states. Similarly, the use of a sedative-hypnotic as premedication prior to surgery or some unpleasant medical procedure is rational and proper (Table 22–2).

TABLE 22–2 Clinical uses of sedative-hypnotics.

For relief of anxiety
For insomnia
For sedation and amnesia before and during medical and surgical procedures
For treatment of epilepsy and seizure states
As a component of balanced anesthesia (intravenous administration)
For control of ethanol or other sedative-hypnotic withdrawal states
For muscle relaxation in specific neuromuscular disorders
As diagnostic aids or for treatment in psychiatry

Excessive or unreasonable anxiety about life circumstances (generalized anxiety disorder, GAD), panic disorders, and agoraphobia are also amenable to drug therapy, sometimes in conjunction with psychotherapy. The benzodiazepines continue to be used for the management of acute anxiety states and for rapid control of panic attacks. They are also used, though much less commonly than in the past, in the long-term management of GAD and panic disorders. Anxiety symptoms may be relieved by many benzodiazepines, but it is not always easy to demonstrate the superiority of one drug over another. Alprazolam has been used in the treatment of panic disorders and agoraphobia and appears to be more selective in these conditions than other benzodiazepines. The choice of benzodiazepines for the treatment of anxiety is based on several sound pharmacologic principles: (1) a rapid onset of action; (2) a relatively high therapeutic index (see drug B in Figure 22–1), plus availability of flumazenil for treatment of overdose; (3) a low risk of drug interactions based on liver enzyme induction; and (4) minimal effects on cardiovascular or autonomic functions.

Disadvantages of the benzodiazepines include the risk of dependence, depression of central nervous system functions, and amnestic effects. In addition, the benzodiazepines exert additive central nervous system depression when administered with other drugs, including ethanol. The patient should be warned of this possibility to avoid impairment of performance of any task requiring mental alertness and motor coordination. In the treatment of generalized anxiety disorders and certain phobias, newer antidepressants, including selective serotonin reuptake inhibitors (SSRIs) and serotonin-norepinephrine reuptake inhibitors (SNRIs), are now considered by many authorities to be drugs of first choice (see Chapter 30). However, these agents have a slow onset of action and thus, limited effectiveness in acute anxiety states.

Sedative-hypnotics should be used with appropriate caution so as to minimize adverse effects. A dose should be prescribed that does not impair mentation or motor functions during waking hours. Some patients may tolerate the drug better if most of the daily dose is given at bedtime, with smaller doses during the day. Prescriptions should be written for short periods, since there is little justification for long-term therapy (defined as use of therapeutic doses for 2 months or longer). The physician should make an effort to assess the efficacy of therapy from the patient's subjective responses. Combinations of antianxiety agents should be avoided, and people taking sedatives should be cautioned about the consumption of alcohol and the concurrent use of over-the-counter medications containing antihistaminic or anticholinergic drugs (see Chapter 63).

TREATMENT OF SLEEP PROBLEMS

Sleep disorders are common and often result from inadequate treatment of underlying medical conditions or psychiatric illness. True primary insomnia is rare. Nonpharmacologic therapies that are useful for sleep problems include proper diet and exercise, avoiding stimulants before retiring, ensuring a comfortable sleeping environment, and retiring at a regular time each night. In some cases, however, the patient will need and should be given a sedative-hypnotic for a limited period. It should be noted that the abrupt discontinuance of many drugs in this class can lead to rebound insomnia.

Benzodiazepines can cause a dose-dependent decrease in both REM and slow-wave sleep, though to a lesser extent than the barbiturates. The newer hypnotics zolpidem, zaleplon, and eszopiclone are less likely than the benzodiazepines to change sleep patterns. However, so little is known about the clinical impact of these effects that statements about the desirability of a particular drug based on its effects on sleep architecture have more theoretical than practical significance. Clinical criteria of efficacy in alleviating a particular sleeping problem are more useful. The drug selected should be one that provides sleep of fairly rapid onset (decreased sleep latency) and sufficient duration, with minimal "hangover" effects such as drowsiness, dysphoria, and mental or motor depression the following day. Older drugs such as chloral hydrate, secobarbital, and pentobarbital continue to be used occasionally, but zolpidem, zaleplon, eszopiclone, or benzodiazepines are generally preferred. Daytime sedation is more common with benzodiazepines that have slow elimination rates (eg, lorazepam) and those that are biotransformed to active metabolites (eg, flurazepam, quazepam). If benzodiazepines are used nightly, tolerance can occur, which may lead to dose increases by the patient to produce the desired effect. Anterograde amnesia occurs to some degree with all benzodiazepines used for hypnosis.

Eszopiclone, zaleplon, and zolpidem have efficacies similar to those of the hypnotic benzodiazepines in the management of sleep disorders. Favorable clinical features of zolpidem and the other newer hypnotics include rapid onset of activity and modest day-after psychomotor depression with few amnestic effects. Zolpidem, one of the most frequently prescribed hypnotic drugs in the United States, is available in a biphasic release formulation that provides sustained drug levels for sleep maintenance. Zaleplon acts rapidly, and because of its short half-life, the drug has value in the management of patients who awaken early in the sleep cycle. At recommended doses, zaleplon and eszopiclone (despite its relatively long half-life) appear to cause less amnesia or day-after somnolence than zolpidem or benzodiazepines. The drugs in this class commonly used for sedation and hypnosis are listed in Table 22–3 together with recommended doses.

Note: The failure of insomnia to remit after 7–10 days of treatment may indicate the presence of a primary psychiatric or medical illness that should be evaluated. Long-term use of hypnotics is an irrational and dangerous medical practice.

OTHER THERAPEUTIC USES

Table 22–2 summarizes several other important clinical uses of drugs in the sedative-hypnotic class. Drugs used in the management of seizure disorders and as intravenous agents in anesthesia are discussed in Chapters 24 and 25.

For sedative and possible amnestic effects during medical or surgical procedures such as endoscopy and bronchoscopy—as well as for premedication prior to anesthesia—oral formulations of shorter-acting drugs are preferred.

Long-acting drugs such as chlordiazepoxide and diazepam and, to a lesser extent, phenobarbital are administered in progressively decreasing doses to patients during withdrawal from physiologic dependence on ethanol or other sedative-hypnotics. Parenteral lorazepam is used to suppress the symptoms of delirium tremens.

Meprobamate and the benzodiazepines have frequently been used as central muscle relaxants, though evidence for general efficacy without accompanying sedation is lacking. A possible exception is diazepam, which has useful relaxant effects in skeletal muscle spasticity of central origin (see Chapter 27).

Psychiatric uses of benzodiazepines other than treatment of anxiety states include the initial management of mania and the control of drug-induced hyperexcitability states (eg, phencyclidine intoxication). Sedative-hypnotics are also used occasionally as diagnostic aids in neurology and psychiatry.

TABLE 22–3 Dosages of drugs used commonly for sedation and hypnosis.

Sedation		Hypnosis	
Drug	Dosage	Drug	Dosage (at Bedtime)
Alprazolam	0.25–0.5 mg 2–3 times daily	Chloral hydrate	500–1000 mg
Buspirone	5–10 mg 2–3 times daily	Estazolam	0.5–2 mg
Chlordiazepoxide	10–20 mg 2–3 times daily	Eszopiclone	1–3 mg
Clorazepate	5–7.5 mg twice daily	Lorazepam	2–4 mg
Diazepam	5 mg twice daily	Quazepam	7.5–15 mg
Halazepam	20–40 mg 3–4 times daily	Secobarbital	100–200 mg
Lorazepam	1–2 mg once or twice daily	Temazepam	7.5–30 mg
Oxazepam	15–30 mg 3–4 times daily	Triazolam	0.125–0.5 mg
Phenobarbital	15–30 mg 2–3 times daily	Zaleplon	5–20 mg
		Zolpidem	5–10 mg

CLINICAL TOXICOLOGY OF SEDATIVE-HYPNOTICS

Direct Toxic Actions

Many of the common adverse effects of sedative-hypnotics result from dose-related depression of the central nervous system. Relatively low doses may lead to drowsiness, impaired judgment, and diminished motor skills, sometimes with a significant impact on driving ability, job performance, and personal relationships. Sleep driving and other somnambulistic behavior with no memory of the event has occurred with the sedative-hypnotic drugs used in sleep disorders, prompting the Food and Drug Administration in 2007 to issue warnings of this potential hazard. Benzodiazepines may cause a significant dose-related anterograde amnesia; they can significantly impair ability to learn new information, particularly that involving effortful cognitive processes, while leaving the retrieval of previously learned information intact. This effect is utilized for uncomfortable clinical procedures, eg, endoscopy, because the patient is able to cooperate during the procedure but amnesic regarding it afterward. The criminal use of benzodiazepines in cases of "date rape" is based on their dose-dependent amnestic effects. Hangover effects are not uncommon following use of hypnotic drugs with long elimination half-lives. Because elderly patients are more sensitive to the effects of sedative-hypnotics, doses approximately half of those used in younger adults are safer and usually as effective. *The most common reversible cause of confusional states in the elderly is overuse of sedative-hypnotics.* At higher doses, toxicity may present as lethargy or a state of exhaustion or, alternatively, as gross symptoms equivalent to those of ethanol intoxication. The physician should be aware of variability among patients in terms of doses causing adverse effects. An increased sensitivity to sedative-hypnotics is more common in patients with cardiovascular disease, respiratory disease, or hepatic impairment and in older patients. Sedative-hypnotics can exacerbate breathing problems in patients with chronic pulmonary disease and in those with symptomatic sleep apnea.

Sedative-hypnotics are the drugs most frequently involved in deliberate overdoses, in part because of their general availability as very commonly prescribed pharmacologic agents. The benzodiazepines are considered to be safer drugs in this respect, since they have flatter dose-response curves. Epidemiologic studies on the incidence of drug-related deaths support this general assumption—eg, 0.3 deaths per million tablets of diazepam prescribed versus 11.6 deaths per million capsules of secobarbital in one study. Alprazolam is purportedly more toxic in overdose than other benzodiazepines. Of course, many factors other than the specific sedative-hypnotic could influence such data—particularly the presence of other central nervous system depressants, including ethanol. In fact, most serious cases of drug overdosage, intentional or accidental, do involve polypharmacy; and when combinations of agents are taken, the practical safety of benzodiazepines may be less than the foregoing would imply.

The lethal dose of any sedative-hypnotic varies with the patient and the circumstances (see Chapter 58). If discovery of the ingestion is made early and a conservative treatment regimen is started, the outcome is rarely fatal, even following very high doses. On the other hand, for most sedative-hypnotics—with the exception of benzodiazepines and possibly the newer hypnotic drugs that have a similar mechanism of action—a dose as low as ten times the hypnotic dose may be fatal if the patient is not discovered or does not seek help in time. With severe toxicity, the respiratory depression from central actions of the drug may be complicated by aspiration of gastric contents in the unattended patient—an even more likely occurrence if ethanol is present. Cardiovascular depression further complicates successful resuscitation. In such patients, treatment consists of ensuring a patent airway, with mechanical ventilation if needed, and maintenance of plasma volume, renal output, and cardiac function. Use of a positive inotropic drug such as dopamine, which preserves renal blood flow, is sometimes indicated. Hemodialysis or hemoperfusion may be used to hasten elimination of some of these drugs.

Flumazenil reverses the sedative actions of benzodiazepines, and those of eszopiclone, zaleplon, and zolpidem, although experience with its use in overdose of the newer hypnotics is limited. However, its duration of action is short, its antagonism of respiratory depression is unpredictable, and there is a risk of precipitation of withdrawal symptoms in long-term users of benzodiazepines (see below). Consequently, the use of flumazenil in benzodiazepine overdose *must* be accompanied by adequate monitoring and support of respiratory function. The extensive clinical use of triazolam has led to reports of serious central nervous system effects including behavioral disinhibition, delirium, aggression, and violence. Although behavioral disinhibition may occur with any sedative-hypnotic drug, it does not appear to be more prevalent with triazolam than with other benzodiazepines. Disinhibitory reactions during benzodiazepine treatment are more clearly associated with the use of very high doses and the pretreatment level of patient hostility.

Adverse effects of the sedative-hypnotics that are not referable to their central nervous system actions occur infrequently. Hypersensitivity reactions, including skin rashes, occur only occasionally with most drugs of this class. Reports of teratogenicity leading to fetal deformation following use of certain benzodiazepines have resulted in FDA assignment of individual benzodiazepines to either category D or X in terms of pregnancy risk. Most barbiturates are FDA pregnancy category D. Eszopiclone, ramelteon, zaleplon, and zolpidem are category C, while buspirone is a pregnancy category B drug. Because barbiturates enhance porphyrin synthesis, they are *absolutely contraindicated* in patients with a history of acute intermittent porphyria, variegate porphyria, hereditary coproporphyria, or symptomatic porphyria.

Alterations in Drug Response

Depending on the dosage and the duration of use, tolerance occurs in varying degrees to many of the pharmacologic effects of sedative-hypnotics. However, it should not be assumed that the degree of tolerance achieved is identical for all pharmacologic effects. There is evidence that the lethal dose range is not altered significantly by the long-term use of sedative-hypnotics. Cross-tolerance between the different sedative-hypnotics, including ethanol, can lead to an unsatisfactory therapeutic response when standard doses of a drug are used in a patient with a recent history of excessive use of these agents. However, there have been very few reports of tolerance development when eszopiclone, zolpidem, or zaleplon was used for less than 4 weeks.

With the long-term use of sedative-hypnotics, especially if doses are increased, a state of dependence can occur. This may develop to a degree unparalleled by any other drug group, *including the opioids*. Withdrawal from a sedative-hypnotic can have severe and life-threatening manifestations. Withdrawal symptoms range from restlessness, anxiety, weakness, and orthostatic hypotension to hyperactive reflexes and generalized seizures. Symptoms of withdrawal are usually more severe following discontinuance of sedative-hypnotics with shorter half-lives. However, eszopiclone, zolpidem, and zaleplon appear to be exceptions to this, because withdrawal symptoms are minimal following abrupt discontinuance of these newer short-acting agents. Symptoms are less pronounced with longer-acting drugs, which may partly accomplish their own tapered withdrawal by virtue of their slow elimination. Cross-dependence, defined as the ability of one drug to suppress abstinence symptoms from discontinuance of another drug, is quite marked among sedative-hypnotics. This provides the rationale for therapeutic regimens in the management of withdrawal states: Longer-acting drugs such as chlordiazepoxide, diazepam, and phenobarbital can be used to alleviate withdrawal symptoms of shorter-acting drugs, including ethanol.

Drug Interactions

The most common drug interactions involving sedative-hypnotics are interactions with other central nervous system depressant drugs, leading to additive effects. These interactions have some therapeutic usefulness when these drugs are used as adjuvants in anesthesia practice. However, if not anticipated, such interactions can lead to serious consequences, including enhanced depression with concomitant use of many other drugs. Additive effects can be predicted with concomitant use of alcoholic beverages, opioid analgesics, anticonvulsants, and phenothiazines. Less obvious but just as important is enhanced central nervous system depression with a variety of antihistamines, antihypertensive agents, and antidepressant drugs of the tricyclic class.

Interactions involving changes in the activity of hepatic drug-metabolizing enzyme systems have been discussed (see also Chapters 4 and 66).

SUMMARY Sedative-Hypnotics

Subclass and Examples	Mechanism of Action	Effects	Clinical Applications	Pharmacokinetics, Toxicities, Interactions
BENZODIAZEPINES • Alprazolam • Chlordiazepoxide • Clorazepate • Clonazepam • Diazepam • Estazolam • Flurazepam • Lorazepam • Midazolam • Oxazepam • Quazepam • Temazepam • Triazolam	Bind to specific GABA$_A$ receptor subunits at central nervous system (CNS) neuronal synapses facilitating frequency of GABA-mediated chloride ion channel opening—enhance membrane hyperpolarization	Dose-dependent depressant effects on the CNS including sedation and relief of anxiety • amnesia • hypnosis • anesthesia • coma and respiratory depression	Acute anxiety states • panic attacks • generalized anxiety disorder • insomnia and other sleep disorders • relaxation of skeletal muscle • anesthesia (adjunctive) • seizure disorders	Half-lives from 2–40 h • oral activity • Hepatic metabolism—some active metabolites • *Toxicity:* Extensions of CNS depressant effects • dependence liability • *Interactions:* Additive CNS depression with ethanol and many other drugs
BENZODIAZEPINE ANTAGONIST • Flumazenil	Antagonist at benzodiazepine binding sites on the GABA$_A$ receptor	Blocks actions of benzodiazepines and zolpidem but not other sedative-hypnotic drugs	Management of benzodiazepine overdose	IV • short half-life • *Toxicity:* Agitation • confusion • possible withdrawal symptoms in benzodiazepine dependence
BARBITURATES • Amobarbital • Butabarbital • Mephobarbital • Pentobarbital • Phenobarbital • Secobarbital	Bind to specific GABA$_A$ receptor subunits at CNS neuronal synapses increasing duration of GABA-mediated chloride ion channel opening • enhance membrane hyperpolarization	Dose-dependent depressant effects on the CNS including sedation and relief of anxiety • amnesia • hypnosis • anesthesia • coma and respiratory depression • steeper dose-response relationship than benzodiazepines	Anesthesia (thiopental) • insomnia (secobarbital) • seizure disorders (phenobarbital)	Half-lives from 4–60 h • oral activity • Hepatic metabolism—phenobarbital 20% renal elimination • *Toxicity:* Extensions of CNS depressant effects • dependence liability > benzodiazepines • *Interactions:* Additive CNS depression with ethanol and many other drugs • induction of hepatic drug-metabolizing enzymes
NEWER HYPNOTICS • Eszopiclone • Zaleplon • Zolpidem	Bind selectively to a sub-group of GABA$_A$ receptors, acting like benzodiazepines to enhance membrane hyperpolarization	Rapid onset of hypnosis with few amnestic effects or day-after psychomotor depression or somnolence	Sleep disorders, especially those categorized by difficulty in falling asleep	Oral activity • short half-lives • CYP substrates • *Toxicity:* Extensions of CNS depressant effects • dependence liability • *Interactions:* Additive CNS depression with ethanol and many other drugs
MELATONIN RECEPTOR AGONIST • Ramelteon	Activates MT$_1$ and MT$_2$ receptors in suprachiasmatic nuclei in the CNS	Rapid onset of sleep with minimal rebound insomnia or withdrawal symptoms	Sleep disorders, especially those categorized by difficulty in falling asleep • not a controlled substance	Oral activity • forms active metabolite via CYP1A2 • *Toxicity:* Dizziness • fatigue • endocrine changes • *Interactions:* Fluvoxamine inhibits metabolism
5-HT-RECEPTOR AGONIST • Buspirone	Mechanism uncertain: Partial agonist at 5-HT receptors but also affinity for D$_2$ receptors	Slow onset (1–2 weeks) of anxiolytic effects • minimal psychomotor impairment—no additive CNS depression with sedative-hypnotic drugs	Generalized anxiety states	Oral activity • forms active metabolite • short half-life • *Toxicity:* Tachycardia • paresthesias • gastrointestinal distress • *Interactions:* CYP3A4 inducers and inhibitors

PREPARATIONS AVAILABLE

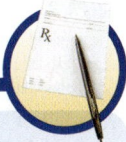

BENZODIAZEPINES

Alprazolam (generic, Xanax)
Oral: 0.25, 0.5, 1, 2 mg tablets, extended-release tablets, and orally disintegrating tablets; 1.0 mg/mL solution

Chlordiazepoxide (generic, Librium)
Oral: 5, 10, 25 mg capsules

Clorazepate (generic, Tranxene)
Oral: 3.75, 7.5, 15 mg tablets and capsules
Oral sustained-release: 11.25, 22.5 mg tablets

Clonazepam (generic, Klonopin)
Oral: 0.5, 1, 2 mg tablets; 0.125, 0.25, 0.5, 1, 2 mg orally disintegrating tablets

Diazepam (generic, Valium)
Oral: 2, 5, 10 mg tablets; 1, 5 mg/mL solutions
Parenteral: 5 mg/mL for injection

Estazolam (generic, ProSom)
Oral: 1, 2 mg tablets

Flurazepam (generic, Dalmane)
Oral: 15, 30 mg capsules

Lorazepam (generic, Ativan)
Oral: 0.5, 1, 2 mg tablets; 2 mg/mL solution
Parenteral: 2, 4 mg/mL for injection

Midazolam (Versed)
Oral: 2 mg/mL syrup
Parenteral: 1, 5 mg/mL in 1, 2, 5, 10 mL vials for injection

Oxazepam (generic)
Oral: 10, 15, 30 mg capsules

Quazepam (Doral)
Oral: 7.5, 15 mg tablets

Temazepam (generic, Restoril)
Oral: 7.5, 15, 22.5, 30 mg capsules

Triazolam (generic, Halcion)
Oral: 0.125, 0.25 mg tablets

BENZODIAZEPINE ANTAGONIST

Flumazenil (generic, Romazicon)
Parenteral: 0.1 mg/mL for IV injection

BARBITURATES

Amobarbital (Amytal)
Parenteral: powder in 250, 500 mg vials to reconstitute for injection

Mephobarbital (Mebaral)
Oral: 32, 50, 100 mg tablets

Pentobarbital (generic, Nembutal Sodium)
Oral: 50, 100 mg capsules; 4 mg/mL elixir
Rectal: 30, 60, 120, 200 mg suppositories
Parenteral: 50 mg/mL for injection

Phenobarbital (generic, Luminal Sodium)
Oral: 15, 16, 30, 60, 90, 100 mg tablets; 16 mg capsules; 15, 20 mg/5 mL elixirs
Parenteral: 30, 60, 65, 130 mg/mL for injection

Secobarbital (generic, Seconal)
Oral: 100 mg capsules

MISCELLANEOUS DRUGS

Buspirone (generic, BuSpar)
Oral: 5, 7.5, 10, 15, 30 mg tablets

Chloral hydrate (generic, Aquachloral Supprettes)
Oral: 500 mg capsules; 250, 500 mg/5 mL syrups
Rectal: 324, 648 mg suppositories

Eszopiclone (Lunesta)
Oral: 1, 2, 3 mg tablets

Hydroxyzine (generic, Atarax, Vistaril)
Oral: 10, 25, 50, 100 mg tablets; 25, 50, 100 mg capsules; 10 mg/5 mL syrup; 25 mg/5 mL suspension
Parenteral: 25, 50 mg/mL for injection

Meprobamate (generic, Equanil, Miltown)
Oral: 200, 400 mg tablets

Paraldehyde (generic)
Oral, rectal liquids: 1 g/mL

Ramelteon (Rozerem)
Oral: 8 mg tablets

Zaleplon (Sonata)
Oral: 5, 10 mg capsules

Zolpidem (generic, Ambien, Ambien-CR)
Oral: 5, 10 mg tablets; 6.25, 12.5 mg extended-release tablets

REFERENCES

Budur K et al: Advances in treating insomnia. Cleve Clin J Med 2007;74:251.

Chouinard G: Issues in the clinical use of benzodiazepines: Potency, withdrawal, and rebound. J Clin Psychiatry 2004;65(Suppl 5):7.

Clayton T et al: An updated unified pharmacophore model of the benzodiazepine binding site on gamma-aminobutyric acid(a) receptors: Correlation with comparative models. Curr Med Chem 2007;14:2755.

Cloos JM, Ferreira V: Current use of benzodiazepines in anxiety disorders. Curr Opin Psychiatry 2009;22:90.

Da Settimo F et al: GABA A/Bz receptor subtypes as targets for selective drugs. Curr Med Chem 2007;14:2680.

Drover DR: Comparative pharmacokinetics and pharmacodynamics of short-acting hypnosedatives: Zaleplon, zolpidem and zopiclone. Clin Pharmacokinet 2004;43:227.

Hanson SM, Czajkowski C: Structural mechanisms underlying benzodiazepine modulation of the GABA(A) receptor. J Neurosci 2008;28:3490.

Lader M et al: Withdrawing benzodiazepines in primary care. CNS Drugs 2009;23:19.

Miyamoto M: Pharmacology of ramelteon, a selective MT1/MT2 receptor agonist: A novel therapeutic drug for sleep disorders. CNS Neurosci Ther 2009;15:32.

Morin AK et al: Therapeutic options for sleep-maintenance and sleep-onset insomnia. Pharmacotherapy 2007;27:89.

Najib J: Eszopiclone, a nonbenzodiazepine sedative-hypnotic for the treatment of transient and chronic insomnia. Clin Ther 2006;28:491.

Neubauer DN: New directions in the pharmacologic treatment of insomnia. Primary Psychiatry 2006;13:51.

Ramakrishnan K et al: Treatment options for insomnia. Am Fam Physician 2007;76:526.

Rudolph U, Mohler H: GABA-based therapeutic approaches: GABA$_A$ receptor subtype functions. Curr Opin Pharmacol 2006;6:18.

Sanger DJ. The pharmacology and mechanism of action of new generation, non-benzodiazepine hypnotic agents. CNS Drugs 2004;18(Suppl 1):9.

Schutte-Rodin S et al: Clinical guideline for the evaluation and management of chronic insomnia in adults. J Clin Sleep Med 2008;4:487.

Simpson D, Curran MP: Ramelteon: A review of its use in insomnia. Drugs 2008:68:1901.

Siriwardena AN et al: Magic bullets for insomnia? Patient's use and experiences of newer (Z drugs) versus older (benzodiazepine) hypnotics for sleep problems in primary care. Br J Gen Pract 2008;58:417.

Verster JC et al: Residual effects of sleep medication on driving ability. Sleep Med Rev 2004;8:309.

CASE STUDY ANSWER

Common etiologies of insomnia include **situational** (eg, work or financial stress, interpersonal conflict), **medical** (eg, asthma, chronic pain), **psychiatric** (eg, mood, anxiety disorders), and **drug-induced** (eg, diuretics, steroids, stimulants). Such aspects of the patient's history would be of value in determining an appropriate course of action. For example, reducing this patient's consumption of diet cola (which commonly contains caffeine) might be of clinical value, as could nonpharmacologic approaches including stimulus control and sleep hygiene procedures. In terms of drug therapy (short term if possible), the pharmacokinetics of zolpidem and eszopiclone (but not zaleplon) are appropriate for a patient who has trouble both in falling asleep and staying asleep. Both drugs exhibit minimal next-day psychomotor performance or rebound insomnia on discontinuance.

The Alcohols

Susan B. Masters, PhD

CASE STUDY

An 18-year-old college freshman began drinking alcohol at 8:30 PM during a hazing event at his new fraternity. Between 8:30 and approximately midnight, he and several other pledges consumed beer and a bottle of whiskey, and then he consumed most of a bottle of rum at the urging of upperclassmen. The young man complained of feeling nauseated, lay down on a couch, and began to lose consciousness. Two upperclassmen carried him to his bedroom, placed him on his stomach, and positioned a trash can nearby. Approximately 10 minutes later, the freshman was found unconscious and covered with vomit. There was a delay in treatment because the upperclassmen called the college police instead of calling 911. After the call was transferred to 911, emergency medical technicians responded quickly and discovered that the young man was not breathing and that he had choked on his vomit. He was rushed to the hospital, where he remained in a coma for 2 days before ultimately being pronounced dead. The patient's blood alcohol concentration shortly after arriving at the hospital was 510 mg/dL. What was the cause of this patient's death? If he had received medical care sooner, what treatment might have prevented his death?

Alcohol, primarily in the form of ethyl alcohol (ethanol), has occupied an important place in the history of humankind for at least 8000 years. In Western society, beer and wine were a main staple of daily life until the 19th century. These relatively dilute alcoholic beverages were preferred over water, which was known to be associated with acute and chronic illness. They provided important calories and nutrients and served as a main source of daily liquid intake. As systems for improved sanitation and water purification were introduced in the 1800s, beer and wine became less important components of the human diet, and the consumption of alcoholic beverages, including distilled preparations with higher concentrations of alcohol, shifted toward their present-day role, in many societies, as a socially acceptable form of recreation.

Today, alcohol is widely consumed. Like other sedative-hypnotic drugs, alcohol in low to moderate amounts relieves anxiety and fosters a feeling of well-being or even euphoria. However, alcohol is also the most commonly abused drug in the world, and the cause of vast medical and societal costs. In the United States, approximately 75% of the adult population drinks alcohol regularly. The majority of this drinking population is able to enjoy the pleasurable effects of alcohol without allowing alcohol consumption to become a health risk. However, about 8% of the general population in the United States has an **alcohol-use disorder.** Individuals who use alcohol in dangerous situations (eg, drinking and driving or combining alcohol with other medications) or continue to drink alcohol in spite of adverse consequences related directly to their alcohol consumption suffer from **alcohol abuse.** Individuals with **alcohol dependence** have characteristics of alcohol abuse and additionally exhibit physical dependence on alcohol (tolerance to alcohol and signs and symptoms upon withdrawal). They also demonstrate an inability to control their drinking and devote much time to getting and using alcohol, or recovering from its effects. The alcohol-use disorders are complex, with genetic as well as environmental determinants.

The societal and medical costs of alcohol abuse are staggering. It is estimated that about 30% of all people admitted to hospitals have coexisting alcohol problems. Once in the hospital, people with chronic alcoholism generally have poorer outcomes. In addition, each year tens of thousands of children are born with morphologic and functional defects resulting from prenatal exposure to ethanol. Despite the investment of many resources and much basic research, alcoholism remains a common chronic disease that is difficult to treat.

Ethanol and many other alcohols with potentially toxic effects are used as fuels and in industry—some in enormous quantities. In addition to ethanol, methanol and ethylene glycol toxicity occurs with sufficient frequency to warrant discussion in this chapter.

■ BASIC PHARMACOLOGY OF ETHANOL

Pharmacokinetics

Ethanol is a small water-soluble molecule that is absorbed rapidly from the gastrointestinal tract. After ingestion of alcohol in the fasting state, peak blood alcohol concentrations are reached within 30 minutes. The presence of food in the stomach delays absorption by slowing gastric emptying. Distribution is rapid, with tissue levels approximating the concentration in blood. The volume of distribution for ethanol approximates total body water (0.5–0.7 L/kg). For an equivalent oral dose of alcohol, women have a higher peak concentration than men, in part because women have a lower total body water content and in part because of differences in first-pass metabolism. In the central nervous system (CNS), the concentration of ethanol rises quickly, since the brain receives a large proportion of total blood flow and ethanol readily crosses biologic membranes.

Over 90% of alcohol consumed is oxidized in the liver; much of the remainder is excreted through the lungs and in the urine. The excretion of a small but consistent proportion of alcohol by the lungs can be quantified with breath alcohol tests that serve as a basis for a legal definition of "driving under the influence" in many countries. At levels of ethanol usually achieved in blood, the rate of oxidation follows zero-order kinetics; that is, it is independent of time and concentration of the drug. The typical adult can metabolize 7–10 g (150–220 mmol) of alcohol per hour, the equivalent of approximately one "drink" [10 oz (300 mL) beer, 3.5 oz (105 mL) wine, or 1 oz (30 mL) distilled 80-proof spirits].

Two major pathways of alcohol metabolism to acetaldehyde have been identified (Figure 23–1). Acetaldehyde is then oxidized to acetate by a third metabolic process.

A. Alcohol Dehydrogenase Pathway

The primary pathway for alcohol metabolism involves alcohol dehydrogenase (ADH), a family of cytosolic enzymes that catalyze the conversion of alcohol to acetaldehyde (Figure 23–1, left). These enzymes are located mainly in the liver, but small amounts are found in other organs such as the brain and stomach. There is considerable genetic variation in ADH enzymes, affecting the rate of ethanol metabolism and also appearing to alter vulnerability to alcohol-abuse disorders. For example, one ADH allele (the *ADH1B*2* allele), which is associated with rapid conversion of ethanol to acetaldehyde, has been found to be protective against alcohol dependence in several ethnic populations and especially East Asians.

Some metabolism of ethanol by ADH occurs in the stomach in men, but a smaller amount occurs in women, who appear to have lower levels of the gastric enzyme. This difference in gastric

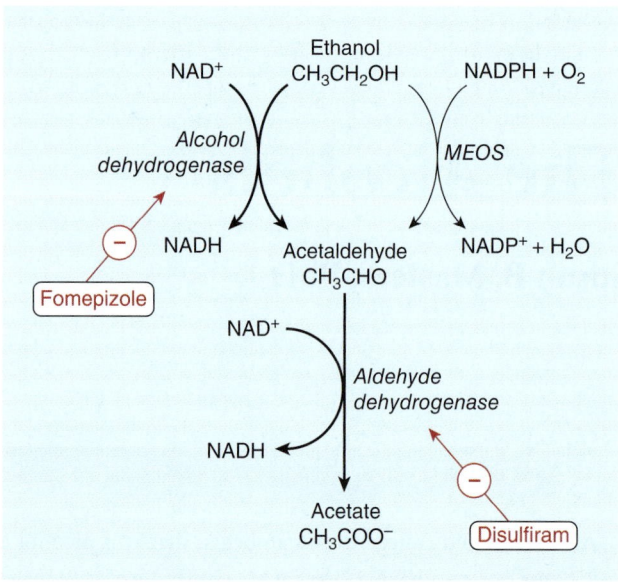

FIGURE 23–1 Metabolism of ethanol by alcohol dehydrogenase and the microsomal ethanol-oxidizing system (MEOS). Alcohol dehydrogenase and aldehyde dehydrogenase are inhibited by fomepizole and disulfiram, respectively. NAD^+, nicotinamide adenine dinucleotide; NADPH, nicotinamide adenine dinucleotide phosphate.

metabolism of alcohol in women probably contributes to the sex-related differences in blood alcohol concentrations noted above.

During conversion of ethanol by ADH to acetaldehyde, hydrogen ion is transferred from ethanol to the cofactor nicotinamide adenine dinucleotide (NAD^+) to form NADH. As a net result, alcohol oxidation generates an excess of reducing equivalents in the liver, chiefly as NADH. The excess NADH production appears to contribute to the metabolic disorders that accompany chronic alcoholism and to both the lactic acidosis and hypoglycemia that frequently accompany acute alcohol poisoning.

B. Microsomal Ethanol-Oxidizing System (MEOS)

This enzyme system, also known as the mixed function oxidase system, uses NADPH as a cofactor in the metabolism of ethanol (Figure 23–1, right) and consists primarily of cytochrome P450 2E1, 1A2, and 3A4 (see Chapter 4).

During chronic alcohol consumption, MEOS activity is induced. As a result, chronic alcohol consumption results in significant increases not only in ethanol metabolism but also in the clearance of other drugs eliminated by the cytochrome P450s that constitute the MEOS system, and in the generation of the toxic byproducts of cytochrome P450 reactions (toxins, free radicals, H_2O_2).

C. Acetaldehyde Metabolism

Much of the acetaldehyde formed from alcohol is oxidized in the liver in a reaction catalyzed by mitochondrial NAD-dependent aldehyde dehydrogenase (ALDH). The product of this reaction is acetate (Figure 23–1), which can be further metabolized to CO_2 and water, or used to form acetyl-CoA.

Oxidation of acetaldehyde is inhibited by **disulfiram,** a drug that has been used to deter drinking by patients with alcohol dependence. When ethanol is consumed in the presence of disulfiram, acetaldehyde accumulates and causes an unpleasant reaction of facial flushing, nausea, vomiting, dizziness, and headache. Several other drugs (eg, metronidazole, cefotetan, trimethoprim) inhibit ALDH and can cause a disulfiram-like reaction if combined with ethanol.

Some people, primarily of East Asian descent, have genetic deficiency in the activity of the mitochondrial form of ALDH, which is encoded by the *ALDH2* gene. When these individuals drink alcohol, they develop high blood acetaldehyde concentrations and experience a noxious reaction similar to that seen with the combination of disulfiram and ethanol. This form of ALDH, with reduced activity, is strongly protective against alcohol-use disorders.

Pharmacodynamics of Acute Ethanol Consumption

A. Central Nervous System

The CNS is markedly affected by acute alcohol consumption. Alcohol causes sedation, relief of anxiety and, at higher concentrations, slurred speech, ataxia, impaired judgment, and disinhibited behavior, a condition usually called intoxication or drunkenness (Table 23–1). These CNS effects are most marked as the blood level is rising, because acute tolerance to the effects of alcohol occurs after a few hours of drinking. For chronic drinkers who are tolerant to the effects of alcohol, higher concentrations are needed to elicit these CNS effects. For example, an individual with chronic alcoholism may appear sober or only slightly intoxicated with a blood alcohol concentration of 300–400 mg/dL, whereas this level is associated with marked intoxication or even coma in a nontolerant individual. The propensity of moderate doses of alcohol to inhibit the attention and information-processing skills as well as the motor skills required for operation of motor vehicles has profound effects. Approximately 30–40% of all traffic accidents resulting in a fatality in the United States involve at least one person with blood alcohol near or above the legal level of intoxication, and drunken driving is a leading cause of death in young adults.

TABLE 23–1 Blood alcohol concentration (BAC) and clinical effects in nontolerant individuals.

BAC (mg/dL)[1]	Clinical Effect
50–100	Sedation, subjective "high," slower reaction times
100–200	Impaired motor function, slurred speech, ataxia
200–300	Emesis, stupor
300–400	Coma
> 400	Respiratory depression, death

[1]In many parts of the United States, a blood level above 80–100 mg/dL for adults or 5–20 mg/dL for persons under 21 is sufficient for conviction of driving while "under the influence."

Like other sedative-hypnotic drugs, alcohol is a CNS depressant. At high blood concentrations, it induces coma, respiratory depression, and death.

Ethanol affects a large number of membrane proteins that participate in signaling pathways, including neurotransmitter receptors for amines, amino acids, opioids, and neuropeptides; enzymes such as Na^+/K^+-ATPase, adenylyl cyclase, phosphoinositide-specific phospholipase C; a nucleoside transporter; and ion channels. Much attention has focused on alcohol's effects on neurotransmission by glutamate and γ-aminobutyric acid (GABA), the main excitatory and inhibitory neurotransmitters in the CNS. Acute ethanol exposure enhances the action of GABA at $GABA_A$ receptors, which is consistent with the ability of GABA-mimetics to intensify many of the acute effects of alcohol and of $GABA_A$ antagonists to attenuate some of the actions of ethanol. Ethanol inhibits the ability of glutamate to open the cation channel associated with the *N*-methyl-D-aspartate (NMDA) subtype of glutamate receptors. The NMDA receptor is implicated in many aspects of cognitive function, including learning and memory. "Blackouts"—periods of memory loss that occur with high levels of alcohol—may result from inhibition of NMDA receptor activation. Experiments that use modern genetic approaches eventually will yield a more precise definition of ethanol's direct and indirect targets. In recent years, experiments with mutant strains of mice, worms, and flies have reinforced the importance of previously identified targets and helped identify new candidates, including a calcium-regulated and voltage-gated potassium channel that may be one of ethanol's direct targets (see Box: What Can Drunken Worms, Flies, and Mice Tell Us about Alcohol?).

B. Heart

Significant depression of myocardial contractility has been observed in individuals who acutely consume moderate amounts of alcohol, ie, at a blood concentration above 100 mg/dL.

C. Smooth Muscle

Ethanol is a vasodilator, probably as a result of both CNS effects (depression of the vasomotor center) and direct smooth muscle relaxation caused by its metabolite, acetaldehyde. In cases of severe overdose, hypothermia—caused by vasodilation—may be marked in cold environments. Ethanol also relaxes the uterus and—before the introduction of more effective and safer uterine relaxants (eg, calcium channel antagonists)—was used intravenously for the suppression of premature labor.

Consequences of Chronic Alcohol Consumption

Chronic alcohol consumption profoundly affects the function of several vital organs—particularly the liver—and the nervous, gastrointestinal, cardiovascular, and immune systems. Since ethanol has low potency, it requires concentrations thousands of times higher than other misused drugs (eg, cocaine, opiates, amphetamines) to produce its intoxicating effects. As a result, ethanol is consumed in quantities that are unusually large for a pharmacologically active

What Can Drunken Worms, Flies, and Mice Tell Us about Alcohol?

For a drug like ethanol, which exhibits low potency and specificity, and modifies complex behaviors, the precise roles of its many direct and indirect targets are difficult to define. Increasingly, ethanol researchers are employing genetic approaches to complement standard neurobiologic experimentation. Three experimental animal systems for which powerful genetic techniques exist—mice, flies, and worms—have yielded intriguing results.

Strains of mice with abnormal sensitivity to ethanol were identified many years ago by breeding and selection programs. Using sophisticated genetic mapping and sequencing techniques, researchers have made progress in identifying the genes that confer these traits. A more targeted approach is the use of transgenic mice to test hypotheses about specific genes. For example, after earlier experiments suggested a link between brain neuropeptide Y (NPY) and ethanol, researchers used two transgenic mouse models to further investigate the link. They found that a strain of mice that lacks the gene for NPY—NPY knockout mice—consume more ethanol than control mice and are less sensitive to ethanol's sedative effects. As would be expected if increased concentrations of NPY in the brain make mice more sensitive to ethanol, a strain of mice that overexpresses NPY drinks less alcohol than the controls even though their total consumption of food and liquid is normal. Work with other transgenic knockout mice supports the central role in ethanol responses of signaling molecules that have long been believed to be involved (eg, GABA$_A$, glutamate, dopamine, opioid, and serotonin receptors) and has helped build the case for newer candidates such as NPY and corticotropin-releasing hormone, cannabinoid receptors, ion channels, and protein kinase C.

It is easy to imagine mice having measurable behavioral responses to alcohol, but drunken worms and fruit flies are harder to imagine. Actually, both invertebrates respond to ethanol in ways that parallel mammalian responses. *Drosophila melanogaster* fruit flies exposed to ethanol vapor show increased locomotion at low concentrations but at higher concentrations, become poorly coordinated, sedated, and finally immobile. These behaviors can be monitored by sophisticated laser or video tracking methods or with an ingenious "chromatography" column that separates relatively insensitive flies from inebriated flies, which drop to the bottom of the column. The worm *Caenorhabditis elegans* similarly exhibits increased locomotion at low ethanol concentrations and, at higher concentrations, reduced locomotion, sedation, and—something that can be turned into an effective screen for mutant worms that are resistant to ethanol—impaired egg laying. The advantage of using flies and worms as genetic models for ethanol research is their relatively simple neuroanatomy, well-established techniques for genetic manipulation, an extensive library of well-characterized mutants, and completely or nearly completely solved genetic codes. Already, much information has accumulated about candidate proteins involved with the effects of ethanol in flies. In an elegant study on *C elegans,* researchers found evidence that a calcium-activated, voltage-gated BK potassium channel is a direct target of ethanol. This channel, which is activated by ethanol, has close homologs in flies and vertebrates, and evidence is accumulating that ethanol has similar effects in these homologs. Genetic experiments in these model systems should provide information that will help narrow and focus research into the complex and important effects of ethanol in humans.

drug. The tissue damage caused by chronic alcohol ingestion results from a combination of the direct effects of ethanol and acetaldehyde, and the metabolic consequences of processing a heavy load of a metabolically active substance. Specific mechanisms implicated in tissue damage include increased oxidative stress coupled with depletion of glutathione, damage to mitochondria, growth factor dysregulation, and potentiation of cytokine-induced injury.

Chronic consumption of large amounts of alcohol is associated with an increased risk of death. Deaths linked to alcohol consumption are caused by liver disease, cancer, accidents, and suicide.

A. Liver and Gastrointestinal Tract

Liver disease is the most common medical complication of alcohol abuse; an estimated 15–30% of chronic heavy drinkers eventually develop severe liver disease. Alcoholic fatty liver, a reversible condition, may progress to alcoholic hepatitis and finally to cirrhosis and liver failure. In the United States, chronic alcohol abuse is the leading cause of liver cirrhosis and of the need for liver transplantation. The risk of developing liver disease is related both to the average amount of daily consumption and to the duration

of alcohol abuse. Women appear to be more susceptible to alcohol hepatotoxicity than men. Concurrent infection with hepatitis B or C virus increases the risk of severe liver disease.

The pathogenesis of alcoholic liver disease is a multifactorial process involving metabolic repercussions of ethanol oxidation in the liver, dysregulation of fatty acid oxidation and synthesis, and activation of the innate immune system by a combination of direct effects of ethanol and its metabolites and by bacterial endotoxins that access the liver as a result of ethanol-induced changes in the intestinal tract. Tumor necrosis factor-α, a proinflammatory cytokine that is consistently elevated in animal models of alcoholic liver disease and in patients with alcoholic liver disease, appears to play a pivotal role in the progression of alcoholic liver disease and may be a fruitful therapeutic target.

Other portions of the gastrointestinal tract can also be injured. Chronic alcohol ingestion is by far the most common cause of chronic pancreatitis in the Western world. In addition to its direct toxic effect on pancreatic acinar cells, alcohol alters pancreatic epithelial permeability and promotes the formation of protein plugs and calcium carbonate-containing stones.

Individuals with chronic alcoholism are prone to gastritis and have increased susceptibility to blood and plasma protein loss during drinking, which may contribute to anemia and protein malnutrition. Alcohol also injures the small intestine, leading to diarrhea, weight loss, and multiple vitamin deficiencies.

Malnutrition from dietary deficiency and vitamin deficiencies due to malabsorption are common in alcoholism. Malabsorption of water-soluble vitamins is especially severe.

B. Nervous System

1. *Tolerance and dependence*—The consumption of alcohol in high doses over a long period results in tolerance and in physical and psychological dependence. Tolerance to the intoxicating effects of alcohol is a complex process involving poorly understood changes in the nervous system as well as the metabolic changes described earlier. As with other sedative-hypnotic drugs, there is a limit to tolerance, so that only a relatively small increase in the lethal dose occurs with increasing alcohol use.

Chronic alcohol drinkers, when forced to reduce or discontinue alcohol, experience a withdrawal syndrome, which indicates the existence of physical dependence. Alcohol withdrawal symptoms classically consist of hyperexcitability in mild cases and seizures, toxic psychosis, and **delirium tremens** in severe ones. The dose, rate, and duration of alcohol consumption determine the intensity of the withdrawal syndrome. When consumption has been very high, merely reducing the rate of consumption may lead to signs of withdrawal.

Psychological dependence on alcohol is characterized by a compulsive desire to experience the rewarding effects of alcohol and, for current drinkers, a desire to avoid the negative consequences of withdrawal. People who have recovered from alcoholism and become abstinent still experience periods of intense craving for alcohol that can be triggered by environmental cues associated in the past with drinking, such as familiar places, groups of people, or events.

The molecular basis of alcohol tolerance and dependence is not known with certainty, nor is it known whether the two phenomena reflect opposing effects on a shared molecular pathway. Tolerance may result from ethanol-induced up-regulation of a pathway in response to the continuous presence of ethanol. Dependence may result from overactivity of that same pathway after the ethanol effect dissipates and before the system has time to return to a normal ethanol-free state.

Chronic exposure of animals or cultured cells to alcohol elicits a multitude of adaptive responses involving neurotransmitters and their receptors, ion channels, and enzymes that participate in signal transduction pathways. Up-regulation of the NMDA subtype of glutamate receptors and voltage-sensitive Ca^{2+} channels may underlie the seizures that accompany the alcohol withdrawal syndrome. Based on the ability of sedative-hypnotic drugs that enhance GABAergic neurotransmission to substitute for alcohol during alcohol withdrawal and evidence of down-regulation of $GABA_A$-mediated responses with chronic alcohol exposure, changes in GABA neurotransmission are believed to play a central role in tolerance and withdrawal.

Like other drugs of abuse, ethanol modulates neural activity in the brain's mesolimbic dopamine reward circuit and increases dopamine release in the nucleus accumbens (see Chapter 32). Alcohol affects local concentrations of serotonin, opioids, and dopamine—neurotransmitters involved in the brain reward system—and has complex effects on the expression of receptors for these neurotransmitters and their signaling pathways. The discovery that naltrexone, a nonselective opioid receptor antagonist, helps patients who are recovering from alcoholism abstain from drinking supports the idea that a common neurochemical reward system is shared by very different drugs associated with physical and psychological dependence. There is also convincing evidence from animal models that ethanol intake and seeking behavior are reduced by antagonists of another important regulator of the brain reward system, the cannabinoid CB1 receptor, which is the molecular target of active ingredients in marijuana. Two other important neuroendocrine systems that appear to play key roles in modulating ethanol-seeking activity in experimental animals are the appetite-regulating system—which uses peptides such as leptin, ghrelin, and neuropeptide Y—and the stress response system, which is controlled by corticotropin-releasing factor.

2. *Neurotoxicity*—Consumption of large amounts of alcohol over extended periods (usually years) often leads to neurologic deficits. The most common neurologic abnormality in chronic alcoholism is generalized symmetric peripheral nerve injury, which begins with distal paresthesias of the hands and feet. Degenerative changes can also result in gait disturbances and ataxia. Other neurologic disturbances associated with alcoholism include dementia and, rarely, demyelinating disease.

Wernicke-Korsakoff syndrome is a relatively uncommon but important entity characterized by paralysis of the external eye muscles, ataxia, and a confused state that can progress to coma and death. It is associated with thiamine deficiency but is rarely seen in the absence of alcoholism. Because of the importance of thiamine in this pathologic condition and the absence of toxicity associated with thiamine administration, all patients suspected of having Wernicke-Korsakoff syndrome (including virtually all patients who present to the emergency department with altered consciousness, seizures, or both) should receive thiamine therapy. Often, the ocular signs, ataxia, and confusion improve promptly upon administration of thiamine. However, most patients are left with a chronic disabling memory disorder known as Korsakoff's psychosis.

Alcohol may also impair visual acuity, with painless blurring that occurs over several weeks of heavy alcohol consumption. Changes are usually bilateral and symmetric and may be followed by optic nerve degeneration. Ingestion of ethanol substitutes such as methanol (see Pharmacology of Other Alcohols) causes severe visual disturbances.

C. Cardiovascular System

1. *Cardiomyopathy and heart failure*—Alcohol has complex effects on the cardiovascular system. Heavy alcohol consumption of long duration is associated with a dilated cardiomyopathy with ventricular hypertrophy and fibrosis. In animals and humans, alcohol induces a number of changes in heart cells that may contribute to cardiomyopathy. They include membrane disruption, depressed function of mitochondria and sarcoplasmic reticulum, intracellular accumulation of phospholipids and fatty acids, and up-regulation of voltage-gated calcium channels. There is evidence that patients with alcohol-induced dilated cardiomyopathy do significantly worse than patients with idiopathic dilated cardiomyopathy, even though cessation of drinking is associated with a reduction in cardiac size and improved function. The poorer prognosis for patients who continue to drink appears to be due in part to interference by ethanol with the beneficial effects of β blockers and angiotensin-converting enzyme (ACE) inhibitors.

2. Arrhythmias—Heavy drinking—and especially "binge" drinking—are associated with both atrial and ventricular arrhythmias. Patients undergoing alcohol withdrawal syndrome can develop severe arrhythmias that may reflect abnormalities of potassium or magnesium metabolism as well as enhanced release of catecholamines. Seizures, syncope, and sudden death during alcohol withdrawal may be due to these arrhythmias.

3. Hypertension—A link between heavier alcohol consumption (more than three drinks per day) and hypertension has been firmly established in epidemiologic studies. Alcohol is estimated to be responsible for approximately 5% of cases of hypertension, making it one of the most common causes of reversible hypertension. This association is independent of obesity, salt intake, coffee drinking, and cigarette smoking. A reduction in alcohol intake appears to be effective in lowering blood pressure in hypertensives who are also heavy drinkers; the hypertension seen in this population is also responsive to standard blood pressure medications.

4. Coronary heart disease—Although the deleterious effects of excessive alcohol use on the cardiovascular system are well established, there is strong epidemiologic evidence that moderate alcohol consumption actually prevents coronary heart disease (CHD), ischemic stroke, and peripheral arterial disease. This type of relationship between mortality and the dose of a drug is called a "J-shaped" relationship. Results of these clinical studies are supported by ethanol's ability to raise serum levels of high-density lipoprotein (HDL) cholesterol (the form of cholesterol that appears to protect against atherosclerosis; see Chapter 35), by its ability to inhibit some of the inflammatory processes that underlie atherosclerosis while also increasing production of the endogenous anticoagulant tissue plasminogen activator (t-PA, see Chapter 34), and by the presence in alcoholic beverages (especially red wine) of antioxidants and other substances that may protect against atherosclerosis. These observational studies are intriguing, but randomized clinical trials examining the possible benefit of moderate alcohol consumption in prevention of CHD have not been carried out.

D. Blood

Alcohol indirectly affects hematopoiesis through metabolic and nutritional effects and may also directly inhibit the proliferation of all cellular elements in bone marrow. The most common hematologic disorder seen in chronic drinkers is mild anemia resulting from alcohol-related folic acid deficiency. Iron deficiency anemia may result from gastrointestinal bleeding. Alcohol has also been implicated as a cause of several hemolytic syndromes, some of which are associated with hyperlipidemia and severe liver disease.

E. Endocrine System and Electrolyte Balance

Chronic alcohol use has important effects on the endocrine system and on fluid and electrolyte balance. Clinical reports of gynecomastia and testicular atrophy in alcoholics with or without cirrhosis suggest a derangement in steroid hormone balance.

Individuals with chronic liver disease may have disorders of fluid and electrolyte balance, including ascites, edema, and effusions. Alterations of whole body potassium induced by vomiting and diarrhea, as well as severe secondary aldosteronism, may contribute to muscle weakness and can be worsened by diuretic therapy. The metabolic derangements caused by metabolism of large amounts of ethanol can result in hypoglycemia, as a result of impaired hepatic gluconeogenesis, and in ketosis, caused by excessive lipolytic factors, especially increased cortisol and growth hormone.

F. Fetal Alcohol Syndrome

Chronic maternal alcohol abuse during pregnancy is associated with teratogenic effects, and alcohol is a leading cause of mental retardation and congenital malformation. The abnormalities that have been characterized as fetal alcohol syndrome include (1) intrauterine growth retardation, (2) microcephaly, (3) poor coordination, (4) underdevelopment of midfacial region (appearing as a flattened face), and (5) minor joint anomalies. More severe cases may include congenital heart defects and mental retardation. Although the level of alcohol intake required to cause serious neurologic deficits appears quite high, the threshold for more subtle neurologic deficits is uncertain.

The mechanisms that underlie ethanol's teratogenic effects are unknown. Ethanol rapidly crosses the placenta and reaches concentrations in the fetus that are similar to those in maternal blood. The fetal liver has little or no alcohol dehydrogenase activity, so the fetus must rely on maternal and placental enzymes for elimination of alcohol.

The neuropathologic abnormalities seen in humans and in animal models of fetal alcohol syndrome indicate that ethanol triggers apoptotic neurodegeneration and also causes aberrant neuronal and glial migration in the developing nervous system. In tissue culture systems, ethanol causes a striking reduction in neurite outgrowth.

G. Immune System

The effects of alcohol on the immune system are complex; immune function in some tissues is inhibited (eg, the lung), whereas pathologic, hyperactive immune function in other tissues is triggered (eg, liver, pancreas). In addition, acute and chronic exposure to alcohol have widely different effects on immune function. The types of immunologic changes reported for the lung include suppression of the function of alveolar macrophages, inhibition of chemotaxis of granulocytes, and reduced number and function of T cells. In the liver, there is enhanced function of key cells of the innate immune system (eg, Kupffer cells, hepatic stellate cells) and increased cytokine production. In addition to the inflammatory damage that chronic heavy alcohol use precipitates in the liver and pancreas, it predisposes to infections, especially of the lung, and worsens the morbidity and increases the mortality risk of patients with pneumonia.

H. Increased Risk of Cancer

Chronic alcohol use increases the risk for cancer of the mouth, pharynx, larynx, esophagus, and liver. Evidence also points to a small increase in the risk of breast cancer in women. Much more information is required before a threshold level for alcohol consumption as it relates to cancer can be established. Alcohol itself does not appear to be a carcinogen in most test systems. However, its primary metabolite, acetaldehyde, can damage DNA, as can the reactive oxygen species produced by increased cytochrome P450 activity. Other factors implicated in the link between alcohol and cancer include changes in folate metabolism and the growth-promoting effects of chronic inflammation.

Alcohol-Drug Interactions

Interactions between ethanol and other drugs can have important clinical effects resulting from alterations in the pharmacokinetics or pharmacodynamics of the second drug.

The most common pharmacokinetic alcohol-drug interactions stem from alcohol-induced increases of drug-metabolizing enzymes, as described in Chapter 4. Thus, prolonged intake of alcohol without damage to the liver can enhance the metabolic biotransformation of other drugs. Ethanol-mediated induction of hepatic cytochrome P450 enzymes is particularly important with regard to acetaminophen. Chronic consumption of three or more drinks per day increases the risk of hepatotoxicity due to toxic or even high therapeutic levels of acetaminophen as a result of increased P450-mediated conversion of acetaminophen to reactive hepatotoxic metabolites (see Figure 4–4). In 1998, the Food and Drug Administration (FDA) announced that all over-the-counter products containing acetaminophen must carry a warning about the relation between chronic ethanol consumption and acetaminophen-induced hepatotoxicity.

In contrast, *acute* alcohol use can inhibit metabolism of other drugs because of decreased enzyme activity or decreased liver blood flow. Phenothiazines, tricyclic antidepressants, and sedative-hypnotic drugs are the most important drugs that interact with alcohol by this pharmacokinetic mechanism.

Pharmacodynamic interactions are also of great clinical significance. The additive CNS depression that occurs when alcohol is combined with other CNS depressants, particularly sedative-hypnotics, is most important. Alcohol also potentiates the pharmacologic effects of many nonsedative drugs, including vasodilators and oral hypoglycemic agents.

■ CLINICAL PHARMACOLOGY OF ETHANOL

Alcohol is the cause of more preventable morbidity and mortality than all other drugs combined with the exception of tobacco. The search for specific etiologic factors or the identification of significant predisposing variables for alcohol abuse has generally led to disappointing results. Personality type, severe life stresses, psychiatric disorders, and parental role models are not reliable predictors of alcohol abuse. Although environmental factors clearly play a role, evidence suggests that there is a large genetic contribution to the development of alcoholism. Not surprisingly, polymorphisms in alcohol dehydrogenase and aldehyde dehydrogenase that lead to increased aldehyde accumulation and its associated facial flushing, nausea, and hypotension appear to protect against alcoholism. Much attention in genetic mapping experiments has focused on membrane-signaling proteins known to be affected by ethanol and on protein constituents of reward pathways in the brain. Polymorphisms associated with a relative insensitivity to alcohol and presumably thereby a greater risk of alcohol abuse have been identified in genes encoding an α subunit of the $GABA_A$ receptor, an M_2 muscarinic receptor, a serotonin transporter, adenylyl cyclase, and a potassium channel. The link between a polymorphism in an opioid receptor gene and a blunted response to naltrexone raises the possibility of genotype-guided pharmacotherapy for alcohol dependence.

MANAGEMENT OF ACUTE ALCOHOL INTOXICATION

Nontolerant individuals who consume alcohol in large quantities develop typical effects of acute sedative-hypnotic drug overdose along with the cardiovascular effects previously described (vasodilation, tachycardia) and gastrointestinal irritation. Since tolerance is not absolute, even individuals with chronic alcohol dependence may become severely intoxicated if sufficient alcohol is consumed.

The most important goals in the treatment of acute alcohol intoxication are to prevent severe respiratory depression and aspiration of vomitus. Even with very high blood ethanol levels, survival is probable as long as the respiratory and cardiovascular systems can be supported. The average blood alcohol concentration in fatal cases is above 400 mg/dL; however, the lethal dose of alcohol varies because of varying degrees of tolerance.

Electrolyte imbalances often need to be corrected and metabolic alterations may require treatment of hypoglycemia and ketoacidosis by administration of **glucose. Thiamine** is given to protect against Wernicke-Korsakoff syndrome. Patients who are dehydrated and vomiting should also receive electrolyte solutions. If vomiting is severe, large amounts of potassium may be required as long as renal function is normal.

MANAGEMENT OF ALCOHOL WITHDRAWAL SYNDROME

Abrupt alcohol discontinuation in an individual with alcohol dependence leads to a characteristic syndrome of motor agitation, anxiety, insomnia, and reduction of seizure threshold. The severity of the syndrome is usually proportionate to the degree and duration of alcohol abuse. However, this can be greatly modified by the use of other sedatives as well as by associated factors (eg, diabetes,

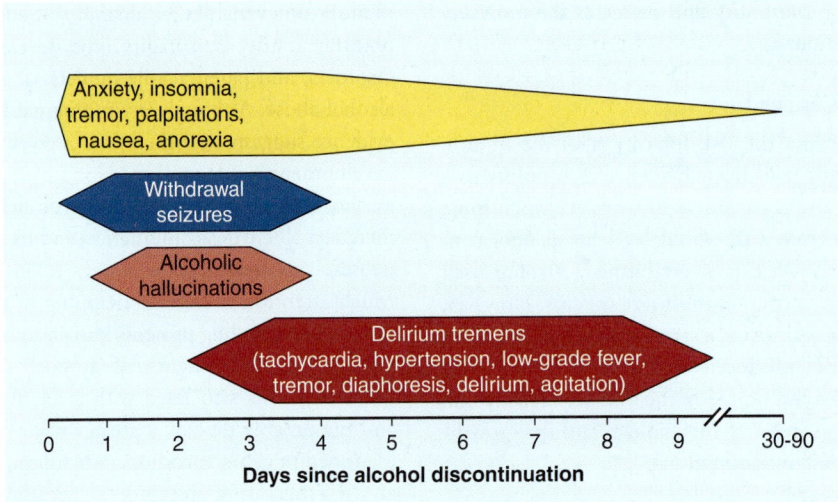

FIGURE 23–2 Time course of events during the alcohol withdrawal syndrome. The signs and symptoms that manifest earliest are anxiety, insomnia, tremor, palpitations, nausea, and anorexia as well as (in severe syndromes) hallucinations and seizures. Delirium tremens typically develops 48–72 hours after alcohol discontinuation. The earliest symptoms (anxiety, insomnia, etc) can persist, in a milder form, for several months after alcohol discontinuation.

injury). In its mildest form, the alcohol withdrawal syndrome of increased pulse and blood pressure, tremor, anxiety, and insomnia occurs 6–8 hours after alcohol consumption is stopped (Figure 23–2). These effects usually lessen in 1–2 days, although some such as anxiety and sleep disturbances can be seen at decreasing levels for several months. In some patients, more severe acute reactions occur, with patients at risk of withdrawal seizures or alcoholic hallucinations during the first 1–5 days of withdrawal. Alcohol withdrawal is one of the most common causes of seizures in adults. Several days later, individuals can develop the syndrome of delirium tremens, which is characterized by delirium, agitation, autonomic nervous system instability, low-grade fever, and diaphoresis.

The major objective of drug therapy in the alcohol withdrawal period is prevention of seizures, delirium, and arrhythmias. Potassium, magnesium, and phosphate balance should be restored as rapidly as is consistent with renal function. Thiamine therapy is initiated in all cases. Individuals in mild alcohol withdrawal do not need any other pharmacologic assistance.

Specific drug treatment for detoxification in more severe cases involves two basic principles: substituting a long-acting sedative-hypnotic drug for alcohol and then gradually reducing ("tapering") the dose of the long-acting drug. Because of their wide margin of safety, benzodiazepines are preferred. The choice of a specific agent in this class is generally based on pharmacokinetic or economic considerations. Long-acting benzodiazepines, including chlordiazepoxide and diazepam, have the advantage of requiring less frequent dosing. Since their pharmacologically active metabolites are eliminated slowly, the long-acting drugs provide a built-in tapering effect. A disadvantage of the long-acting drugs is that they and their active metabolites may accumulate, especially in patients with compromised liver function. Short-acting drugs such as lorazepam and oxazepam are rapidly converted to inactive water-soluble metabolites that will not accumulate, and for this

reason the short-acting drugs are especially useful in alcoholic patients with liver disease. Benzodiazepines can be administered orally in mild or moderate cases, or parenterally for patients with more severe withdrawal reactions.

After the alcohol withdrawal syndrome has been treated acutely, sedative-hypnotic medications must be tapered slowly over several weeks. Complete detoxification is not achieved with just a few days of alcohol abstinence. Several months may be required for restoration of normal nervous system function, especially sleep.

TREATMENT OF ALCOHOLISM

After detoxification, psychosocial therapy either in intensive inpatient or in outpatient rehabilitation programs serves as the primary treatment for alcohol dependence. Other psychiatric problems, most commonly depressive or anxiety disorders, often coexist with alcoholism and, if untreated, can contribute to the tendency of detoxified alcoholics to relapse. Treatment for these associated disorders with counseling and drugs can help decrease the rate of relapse for alcoholic patients.

Three drugs—disulfiram, naltrexone, and acamprosate—have FDA approval for adjunctive treatment of alcohol dependence.

Naltrexone

Naltrexone, a relatively long-acting opioid antagonist, blocks the effects at μ opioid receptors (see Chapter 31). Studies in experimental animals first suggested a link between alcohol consumption and opioids. Injection of small amounts of opioids was followed by an increase in alcohol drinking, whereas administration of opioid antagonists inhibited self-administration of alcohol.

Naltrexone, both alone and in combination with behavioral counseling, has been shown in a number of short-term (12- to 16-week) placebo-controlled trials to reduce the rate of relapse to either drinking or alcohol dependence and to reduce craving for alcohol, especially in patients with high rates of naltrexone adherence. Naltrexone was approved in 1994 by the FDA for treatment of alcohol dependence.

Naltrexone is generally taken once a day in an oral dose of 50 mg for treatment of alcoholism. An extended-release formulation administered as an IM injection once every 4 weeks is also effective. The drug can cause dose-dependent hepatotoxicity and should be used with caution in patients with evidence of mild abnormalities in serum aminotransferase activity. The combination of naltrexone plus disulfiram should be avoided, since both drugs are potential hepatotoxins. Administration of naltrexone to patients who are physically dependent on opioids precipitates an acute withdrawal syndrome, so patients must be opioid-free before initiating naltrexone therapy. Naltrexone also blocks the therapeutic analgesic effects of usual doses of opioids.

Acamprosate

Acamprosate has been used in Europe for a number of years to treat alcohol dependence and was approved for this use by the FDA in 2004. Like ethanol, acamprosate has many molecular effects including actions on GABA, glutamate, serotonergic, noradrenergic, and dopaminergic receptors. Probably its best-characterized actions are as a weak NMDA-receptor antagonist and a $GABA_A$-receptor activator. In European clinical trials, acamprosate reduced short-term and long-term (more than 6 months) relapse rates when combined with psychotherapy. In a large American trial that compared acamprosate with naltrexone and with combined acamprosate and naltrexone therapy (the COMBINE study), acamprosate did not show a statistically significant effect alone or in combination with naltrexone.

Acamprosate is administered as 1–2 enteric-coated 333 mg tablets three times daily. It is poorly absorbed, and food reduces its absorption even further. Acamprosate is widely distributed and is eliminated renally. It does not appear to participate in drug-drug interactions. The most common adverse effects are gastrointestinal (nausea, vomiting, diarrhea) and rash. It should not be used in patients with severe renal impairment.

Disulfiram

Disulfiram causes extreme discomfort in patients who drink alcoholic beverages. Disulfiram alone has little effect; however, flushing, throbbing headache, nausea, vomiting, sweating, hypotension, and confusion occur within a few minutes after an individual taking disulfiram drinks alcohol. The effects may last 30 minutes in mild cases or several hours in severe ones. Disulfiram acts by inhibiting aldehyde dehydrogenase. Thus, alcohol is metabolized as usual, but acetaldehyde accumulates.

Disulfiram is rapidly and completely absorbed from the gastrointestinal tract; however, a period of 12 hours is required for its full action. Its elimination rate is slow, so that its action may persist for several days after the last dose. The drug inhibits the metabolism of many other therapeutic agents, including phenytoin, oral anticoagulants, and isoniazid. It should not be administered with medications that contain alcohol, including nonprescription medications such as those listed in Table 63–3. Disulfiram can cause small increases in liver function tests. Its safety in pregnancy has not been demonstrated.

Because adherence to disulfiram therapy is low and because the evidence from clinical trials for its effectiveness is weak, disulfiram is no longer commonly used.

Other Drugs

Several other drugs have shown efficacy in maintaining abstinence and reducing craving in chronic alcoholism, although none has FDA approval yet for this use. Such drugs include ondansetron, a serotonin 5-HT_3-receptor antagonist (see Chapters 16, 62); topiramate, a drug used for partial and generalized tonic-clonic seizures (see Chapter 24); and baclofen, a $GABA_B$ receptor antagonist used as a spasmolytic (see Chapter 27). Based on evidence from model systems, efforts are underway to explore agents that modulate cannabinoid CB1 receptors, corticotropin-releasing factor receptors, and GABA receptor systems, as well as several other possible targets. Rimonabant, a CB1 receptor antagonist, has been shown to suppress alcohol-related behaviors in animal models and is being tested in clinical trials of alcoholism.

■ PHARMACOLOGY OF OTHER ALCOHOLS

Other alcohols related to ethanol have wide applications as industrial solvents and occasionally cause severe poisoning. Of these, **methanol** and **ethylene glycol** are two of the most common causes of intoxication.

METHANOL

Methanol (methyl alcohol, wood alcohol) is widely used in the industrial production of synthetic organic compounds and as a constituent of many commercial solvents. In the home, methanol is most frequently found in the form of "canned heat" or in windshield-washing products. Poisonings occur from accidental ingestion of methanol-containing products or when it is misguidedly ingested as an ethanol substitute.

Methanol can be absorbed through the skin or from the respiratory or gastrointestinal tract and is then distributed in body water. The primary mechanism of elimination of methanol in humans is by oxidation to formaldehyde, formic acid, and CO_2 (Figure 23–3).

Animal species show great variability in mean lethal doses of methanol. The special susceptibility of humans to methanol toxicity is due to metabolism to formate and formaldehyde, not to methanol itself. Since the conversion of methanol to its toxic metabolites is relatively slow, there is often a delay of 6–30 hours before the appearance of severe toxicity.

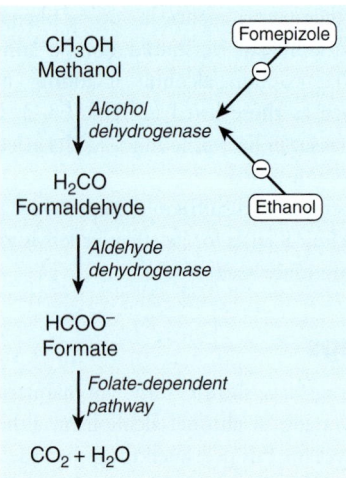

FIGURE 23–3 Methanol is converted to the toxic metabolites formaldehyde and formate by alcohol dehydrogenase and aldehyde dehydrogenase. By inhibiting alcohol dehydrogenase, fomepizole and ethanol reduce the formation of toxic metabolites.

Physical findings in early methanol poisoning are generally nonspecific, such as inebriation and gastritis, and possibly an elevated osmolar gap (see Chapter 58). In severe cases, the odor of formaldehyde may be present on the breath or in the urine. After a delay, the most characteristic symptom in methanol poisoning—visual disturbance—occurs along with anion gap metabolic acidosis. The visual disturbance is frequently described as "like being in a snowstorm" and can progress to blindness. Changes in the retina may sometimes be detected on examination, but these are usually late. The development of bradycardia, prolonged coma, seizures, and resistant acidosis all imply a poor prognosis. The cause of death in fatal cases is sudden cessation of respiration. A serum methanol concentration higher than 20 mg/dL warrants treatment, and a concentration higher than 50 mg/dL is considered serious enough to require hemodialysis. Serum formate levels are a better indication of clinical pathology but are not widely available.

The first treatment for methanol poisoning, as in all critical poisoning situations, is support of respiration. There are three specific modalities of treatment for severe methanol poisoning: suppression of metabolism by alcohol dehydrogenase to toxic products, hemodialysis to enhance removal of methanol and its toxic products, and alkalinization to counteract metabolic acidosis.

The enzyme chiefly responsible for methanol oxidation in the liver is alcohol dehydrogenase (Figure 23–3). **Fomepizole,** an alcohol dehydrogenase inhibitor, is approved for the treatment of methanol and ethylene glycol poisoning. It is administered intravenously in a loading dose of 15 mg/kg followed by 10 mg/kg every 12 hours for 48 hours and then 15 mg/kg every 12 hours thereafter until the serum methanol level falls below 20–30 mg/dL. The dosage increase after 48 hours is based on evidence that fomepizole rapidly induces its own metabolism by the cytochrome P450 system. Patients undergoing hemodialysis are given fomepizole more frequently (6 hours after the loading dose and every 4 hours thereafter). Fomepizole appears to be safe during the short time it is administered for treatment of methanol or ethylene glycol poisoning. The most common adverse effects are burning at the infusion site, headache, nausea, and dizziness. Intravenous ethanol is an alternative to fomepizole. It has a higher affinity than methanol for alcohol dehydrogenase; thus, saturation of the enzyme with ethanol reduces formate production. Ethanol is used intravenously as treatment for methanol and ethylene glycol poisoning. The dose-dependent characteristics of ethanol metabolism and the variability of ethanol metabolism require frequent monitoring of blood ethanol levels to ensure appropriate alcohol concentration.

In cases of severe poisoning, hemodialysis (discussed in Chapter 58) can be used to eliminate both methanol and formate from the blood. Two other measures are commonly taken. Because of profound metabolic acidosis in methanol poisoning, treatment with bicarbonate often is necessary. Since folate-dependent systems are responsible for the oxidation of formic acid to CO_2 in humans (Figure 23–3), folinic and folic acid are often administered to patients poisoned with methanol, although this has never been fully tested in clinical studies.

ETHYLENE GLYCOL

Polyhydric alcohols such as ethylene glycol (CH_2OHCH_2OH) are used as heat exchangers, in antifreeze formulations, and as industrial solvents. Young children and animals are sometimes attracted by the sweet taste of ethylene glycol and, rarely, it is ingested intentionally as an ethanol substitute or in attempted suicide. Although ethylene glycol itself is relatively harmless and eliminated by the kidney, it is metabolized to toxic aldehydes and oxalate.

Three stages of ethylene glycol overdose occur. Within the first few hours after ingestion, there is transient excitation followed by CNS depression. After a delay of 4–12 hours, severe metabolic acidosis develops from accumulation of acid metabolites and lactate. Finally, delayed renal insufficiency follows deposition of oxalate in renal tubules. The key to the diagnosis of ethylene glycol poisoning is recognition of anion gap acidosis, osmolar gap, and oxalate crystals in the urine in a patient without visual symptoms.

As with methanol poisoning, early fomepizole is the standard treatment for ethylene glycol poisoning. Intravenous treatment with fomepizole is initiated immediately, as described above for methanol poisoning, and continued until the patient's serum ethylene glycol concentration drops below a toxic threshold (20–30 mg/dL). Intravenous ethanol is an alternative to fomepizole in ethylene glycol poisoning. Hemodialysis effectively removes ethylene glycol and its toxic metabolites and is recommended for patients with a serum ethylene glycol concentration above 50 mg/dL, significant metabolic acidosis, and significant renal impairment. Fomepizole has reduced the need for hemodialysis, especially in patients with less severe acidosis and intact renal function.

SUMMARY The Alcohols and Associated Drugs

Subclass	Mechanism of Action	Clinical Applications	Pharmacokinetics, Toxicities, Interactions
ALCOHOLS			
• Ethanol	Multiple effects on neurotransmitter receptors, ion channels, and signaling pathways	Antidote in methanol and ethylene glycol poisoning	Zero-order metabolism • duration depends on dose • *Toxicity:* Acutely, central nervous system depression and respiratory failure • chronically, damage to many systems, including liver, pancreas, gastrointestinal tract, and central and peripheral nervous systems • *Interactions:* Induces CYP2E1 • increased conversion of acetaminophen to toxic metabolite

• *Methanol:* Poisonings result in toxic levels of formate, which causes characteristic visual disturbance plus coma, seizures, acidosis, and death due to respiratory failure

• *Ethylene glycol:* Poisoning creates toxic aldehydes and oxalate, which causes kidney damage and severe acidosis

Subclass	Mechanism of Action	Clinical Applications	Pharmacokinetics, Toxicities, Interactions
DRUGS USED IN ACUTE ETHANOL WITHDRAWAL			
• Benzodiazepines (eg, chlordiazepoxide, diazepam, lorazepam)	BDZ receptor agonists that facilitate GABA-mediated activation of GABA$_A$ receptors	Prevention and treatment of acute ethanol withdrawal syndrome	See Chapter 22
• Thiamine (vitamin B$_1$)	Essential vitamin required for synthesis of the coenzyme thiamine pyrophosphate	Administered to patients suspected of having alcoholism (those exhibiting acute alcohol intoxication or alcohol withdrawal syndrome) to prevent Wernicke-Korsakoff syndrome	Administered parenterally • *Toxicity:* None • *Interactions:* None

Subclass	Mechanism of Action	Clinical Applications	Pharmacokinetics, Toxicities, Interactions
DRUGS USED IN CHRONIC ALCOHOLISM			
• Naltrexone	Nonselective competitive antagonist of opioid receptors	Reduced risk of relapse in individuals with alcoholism	Available as an oral or long-acting parenteral formulation • *Toxicity:* GI effects and liver toxicity; will precipitate a withdrawal reaction in individuals physically dependent on opioids and will prevent the analgesic effect of opioids
• Acamprosate	Poorly understood NMDA receptor antagonist and GABA$_A$ agonist effects	Reduced risk of relapse in individuals with alcoholism	*Toxicity:* GI effects and rash
• Disulfiram	Inhibits aldehyde dehydrogenase, resulting in aldehyde accumulation during ethanol ingestion	Deterrent to drinking in individuals with alcohol dependence	*Toxicity:* Little effect alone but severe and potentially dangerous flushing, headache, nausea, vomiting, and hypotension when combined with ethanol

Subclass	Mechanism of Action	Clinical Applications	Pharmacokinetics, Toxicities, Interactions
DRUGS USED IN ACUTE METHANOL OR ETHYLENE GLYCOL TOXICITY			
• Fomepizole	Inhibits alcohol dehydrogenase, prevents conversion of methanol and ethylene glycol to toxic metabolites	Methanol and ethylene glycol poisoning	Orphan drug • *Toxicity:* Headache, nausea, dizziness, rare allergic reactions

• *Ethanol:* Higher affinity than methanol or ethylene glycol for alcohol dehydrogenase; used to reduce metabolism of methanol and ethylene glycol to toxic products

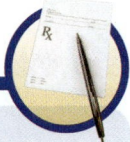

PREPARATIONS AVAILABLE

DRUGS FOR THE TREATMENT OF ACUTE ALCOHOL WITHDRAWAL SYNDROME (see also Chapter 22 for other benzodiazepines)

Chlordiazepoxide HCl (generic, Librium)
Oral: 5, 10, 25 mg tablets

Diazepam (generic, Valium)
Oral: 2, 5, 10 mg tablets; 1, 5 mg/mL solutions
Rectal: 2.5, 10, 20 mg gel
Parenteral: 5 mg/mL for injection

Lorazepam (generic, Ativan)
Oral: 0.5, 1, 2 mg tablets; 2 mg/mL solution
Parenteral: 2, 4 mg/mL for injection

Oxazepam (generic)
Oral: 10, 15, 30 mg capsules

Thiamine HCl (generic)
Oral: 50, 100, 250, 500 mg tablets or capsules
Parenteral: 100 mg/mL for injection

DRUGS FOR THE PREVENTION OF ALCOHOL ABUSE

Acamprosate Calcium (Campral)
Oral: 333 mg delayed-release tablets

Disulfiram (Antabuse)
Oral: 250, 500 mg tablets

Naltrexone HCl (generic, ReVia)
Oral: 50 mg tablets
Parenteral (Vivitrol): 380 mg for IM injection once per month

DRUGS FOR THE TREATMENT OF ACUTE METHANOL OR ETHYLENE GLYCOL POISONING

Ethanol (generic)
Parenteral: 5% or 10% ethanol and 5% dextrose in water for IV infusion

Fomepizole (generic, Antizol)
Parenteral: 1 g/mL concentrate for IV injection

REFERENCES

Anton RF: Naltrexone for the management of alcohol dependence. N Engl J Med 2008;359:715.

Anton RF et al: Combined pharmacotherapies and behavioral interventions for alcohol dependence: The COMBINE study: A randomized controlled trial. JAMA 2006;295:2003.

Brent J: Fomepizole for ethylene glycol and methanol poisoning. N Engl J Med 2009;360:2216.

Brodie MS et al: Ethanol interactions with calcium-dependent potassium channels. Alcohol Clin Exp Res 2007;31:1625.

CDC Fetal Alcohol Syndrome Website: http://www.cdc.gov/ncbddd/fas/

Chen YC et al: Polymorphism of ethanol-metabolism genes and alcoholism: Correlation of allelic variations with the pharmacokinetic and pharmacodynamic consequences. Chem Biol Interact 2009;178:2.

Colombo G et al: The cannabinoid CB1 receptor antagonist, rimonabant, as a promising pharmacotherapy for alcohol dependence: Preclinical evidence. Mol Neurobiol 2007;36:102.

Crabbe JC et al: Alcohol-related genes: Contributions from studies with genetically engineered mice. Addict Biol 2006;11:195.

Das SK, Vasudevan DM: Alcohol-induced oxidative stress. Life Sci 2007; 81:177.

Edenberg HJ: The genetics of alcohol metabolism: Role of alcohol dehydrogenase and aldehyde dehydrogenase variants. Alcohol Res Health 2007; 30:5.

Heilig M, Egli M: Pharmacologic treatment of alcohol dependence: Target symptoms and target mechanisms. Pharmacol Ther 2006;111:855.

Johnson BA: Update on neuropharmacological treatments for alcoholism: Scientific basis and clinical findings. Biochem Pharmacol 2008;75:34.

Lepik KJ et al: Adverse drug events associated with the antidotes for methanol and ethylene glycol poisoning: A comparison of ethanol and fomepizole. Ann Emerg Med 2009;53:439.

Lieber CS: Medical disorders of alcoholism. N Engl J Med 1995;333:1058.

Lobo IA, Harris RA: GABA(A) receptors and alcohol. Pharmacol Biochem Behav 2008;90:90.

Mayfield RD, Harris RA, Schuckit MA: Genetic factors influencing alcohol dependence. Br J Pharmacol 2008;154:275.

McIntire SL: Ethanol. WormBook 2010;29:1.

National Institute on Alcohol Abuse and Alcoholism Website: http://www.niaaa.nih.gov/

Olson KR et al (editors): *Poisoning and Drug Overdose,* 5th ed. McGraw-Hill, 2006.

Shuckit MA: Alcohol-use disorders. Lancet 2009;373:492.

Shuckit MA: *Drug and Alcohol Abuse: A Clinical Guide to Diagnosis and Treatment,* 6th ed. Springer, 2006.

Srisurapanont M, Jarusuraisin N: Opioid antagonists for alcohol dependence. Cochrane Database Syst Rev 2005;(1):CD001867.

Tetrault JM, O'Connor PG: Substance abuse and withdrawal in the critical care setting. Crit Care Clin 2008;24:767.

Wolf FW, Heberlein U: Invertebrate models of drug abuse. J Neurobiol 2003;54:161.

You M, Crabb DW: Recent advances in alcoholic liver disease II. Minireview: Molecular mechanisms of alcoholic fatty liver. Am J Physiol Gastrointest Liver Physiol 2004;287:G1.

CASE STUDY ANSWER

This young man exhibits classic signs and symptoms of acute alcohol poisoning, which is confirmed by the blood alcohol concentration. We do not know from the case whether the patient was tolerant to the effects of alcohol but note that his blood alcohol concentration was in the lethal range for a nontolerant individual. Death most likely resulted from respiratory and cardiovascular collapse prior to medical treatment, complicated by a chemical pneumonitis secondary to aspiration of vomitus. The treatment of acute alcohol poisoning includes standard supportive care of airway, breathing, and circulation (see Chapter 58). Intravenous access would be obtained and used to administer dextrose and thiamine, as well as other electrolytes and vitamins. If a young, previously healthy individual receives medical care in time, supportive care will most likely be highly effective. As the patient recovers, it is important to be vigilant for signs and symptoms of the alcohol withdrawal syndrome.

Antiseizure Drugs

Roger J. Porter, MD, &
Brian S. Meldrum, MB, PhD

CASE STUDY[*]

A 23-year-old woman presents to the office for consultation regarding her antiseizure medications. Seven years ago, this otherwise healthy young woman had a generalized tonic-clonic seizure (GTCS) at home. She was rushed to the emergency department, at which time she was alert but complained of headache. A consulting neurologist placed her on levetiracetam, 500 mg bid. Four days later, EEG showed rare right temporal sharp waves. MRI was normal. One year after this episode, a repeat EEG was unchanged, and levetiracetam was gradually increased to 1000 mg bid. The patient had no significant adverse effects from this dosage. At age 21, she had a second GTCS while in college; further discussion with her roommate at that time revealed a history of two recent episodes of 1–2 minutes of altered consciousness with lip smacking (complex partial seizures). A repeat EEG showed occasional right temporal spikes. Lamotrigine was gradually added to the regimen to a dosage of 200 mg bid. Since then, the patient has been seizure-free for almost 2 years but now comes to the office for a medication review. Gradual discontinuation of levetiracetam is planned if the patient continues to do well for another year, although risk of recurrent seizures is always present when medications are withdrawn.

Approximately 1% of the world's population has epilepsy, the second most common neurologic disorder after stroke. Although standard therapy permits control of seizures in 80% of these patients, millions (500,000 people in the USA alone) have uncontrolled epilepsy. Epilepsy is a heterogeneous symptom complex—a chronic disorder characterized by recurrent seizures. Seizures are finite episodes of brain dysfunction resulting from abnormal discharge of cerebral neurons. The causes of seizures are many and include the full range of neurologic diseases—from infection to neoplasm and head injury. In some subgroups, heredity has proved to be a predominant factor. Single gene defects, usually of an autosomal dominant nature involving genes coding voltage-gated ion channels or GABA$_A$ receptors, have been shown to account for a small number of familial generalized epilepsies. Commonly, one family shows multiple epilepsy syndromes including, for example, febrile seizures, absence attacks, and juvenile myoclonic epilepsy.

The antiseizure drugs described in this chapter are also used in patients with febrile seizures or with seizures occurring as part of an acute illness such as meningitis. The term "epilepsy" is not usually applied to such patients unless chronic seizures develop later. Seizures are occasionally caused by an acute underlying toxic or metabolic disorder, in which case appropriate therapy should be directed toward the specific abnormality, eg, hypocalcemia. In most cases of epilepsy, however, the choice of medication depends on the empiric seizure classification.

Drug Development for Epilepsy

For a long time it was assumed that a single **antiepileptic drug (AED)** could be developed for the treatment of all forms of epilepsy. However, the causes of epilepsy are extremely diverse, encompassing genetic and developmental defects and infective, traumatic, neoplastic, and degenerative disease processes. Drug therapy to date shows little evidence of etiologic specificity. There is some specificity according to seizure type (Table 24–1), which is most clearly seen with generalized seizures of the absence type. These are typically seen with 2–3 Hz spike-and-wave

---

[*]This case description includes the answers to implied questions regarding therapy.

TABLE 24–1 **Classification of seizure types.**

Partial seizures
Simple partial seizures
Complex partial seizures
Partial seizures secondarily generalized
Generalized seizures
Generalized tonic-clonic (grand mal) seizures
Absence (petit mal) seizures
Tonic seizures
Atonic seizures
Clonic and myoclonic seizures
Infantile spasms[1]

[1]An epileptic syndrome rather than a specific seizure type; drugs useful in infantile spasms will be reviewed separately.

discharges on the electroencephalogram, which respond to etho-suximide and valproate but can be exacerbated by phenytoin and carbamazepine. Drugs acting selectively on absence seizures can be identified by animal screens, using either threshold pentyle-netetrazol clonic seizures in mice or rats or mutant mice showing absence-like episodes (so-called lethargic, star-gazer, or tottering mutants). In contrast, the **maximal electroshock (MES)** test, with suppression of the tonic extensor phase, identifies drugs such as phenytoin, carbamazepine, and lamotrigine, which are active against generalized tonic-clonic seizures and complex par-tial seizures. The maximal electroshock test as the major initial screen for new drugs has led predominantly to the identification of drugs with a mechanism of action involving prolonged inac-tivation of the voltage-gated Na^+ channel. Limbic seizures induced in rats by the process of electrical kindling (involving repeated episodes of focal electrical stimulation) probably pro-vide a better screen for predicting efficacy in complex partial seizures.

Existing antiseizure drugs provide adequate seizure control in about two thirds of patients. So-called "drug resistance" may be observed from the onset of attempted therapy or may develop after a period of relatively successful therapy. Explanations are being sought in terms of impaired access of the drugs to target sites or insensitivity of target molecules to them. In children, some severe seizure syndromes associated with pro-gressive brain damage are very difficult to treat. In adults, some focal seizures are refractory to medications. Some, particularly in the temporal lobe, are amenable to surgical resection. Some of the drug-resistant population may respond to **vagus nerve stimulation (VNS)**, a nonpharmacologic treatment for epilepsy now widely approved for treatment of patients with partial sei-zures. VNS is indicated for refractory cases or for patients in whom antiseizure drugs are poorly tolerated. Stimulating elec-trodes are implanted on the left vagus nerve, and the pacemaker is implanted in the chest wall or axilla. Use of this device may permit seizure control with lower doses of drugs. Other devices,

using various paradigms of electrical stimulation, are in clinical development.

New antiseizure drugs are being sought not only by the screen-ing tests noted above but also by more focused approaches. Compounds are sought that act by one of three mechanisms: (1) enhancement of GABAergic (inhibitory) transmission, (2) diminution of excitatory (usually glutamatergic) transmission, or (3) modification of ionic conductances. Presynaptic effects on transmitter release appear particularly important, and some molecular targets are known, eg, SV_2A (see below).

Although it is widely recognized that current antiseizure drugs are palliative rather than curative, successful strategies for identify-ing drugs that are either disease modifying or that prevent epilep-togenesis have proved elusive. Neuronal targets for current and potential antiseizure drugs include both excitatory and inhibitory synapses. Figure 24–1 represents a glutamatergic (excitatory) synapse, and Figure 24–2 indicates targets in a GABAergic (inhibitory) synapse.

■ BASIC PHARMACOLOGY OF ANTISEIZURE DRUGS

Chemistry

Until 1990, approximately 16 antiseizure drugs were available, and 13 of them can be classified into five very similar chemical groups: barbiturates, hydantoins, oxazolidinediones, succinim-ides, and acetylureas. These groups have in common a similar heterocyclic ring structure with a variety of substituents (Figure 24–3). For drugs with this basic structure, the substitu-ents on the heterocyclic ring determine the pharmacologic class, either anti-MES or antipentylenetetrazol. Very small changes in structure can dramatically alter the mechanism of action and clinical properties of the compound. The remaining drugs in this older group—carbamazepine, valproic acid, and the benzo-diazepines—are structurally dissimilar, as are the newer com-pounds marketed since 1990, ie, eslicarbazepine, felbamate, gabapentin, lacosamide, lamotrigine, levetiracetam, oxcarba-zepine, pregabalin, retigabine, rufinamide, stiripentol, tiagabine, topiramate, vigabatrin, and zonisamide.

Pharmacokinetics

The antiseizure drugs exhibit many similar pharmacokinetic properties—even those whose structural and chemical properties are quite diverse—because most have been selected for oral activ-ity and all must enter the central nervous system. Although many of these compounds are only slightly soluble, absorption is usually good, with 80–100% of the dose reaching the circulation. Most antiseizure drugs (other than phenytoin, tiagabine, and valproic acid) are not highly bound to plasma proteins.

Antiseizure drugs are cleared chiefly by hepatic mechanisms, although they have low extraction ratios (see Chapter 3). Many are converted to active metabolites that are also cleared by the

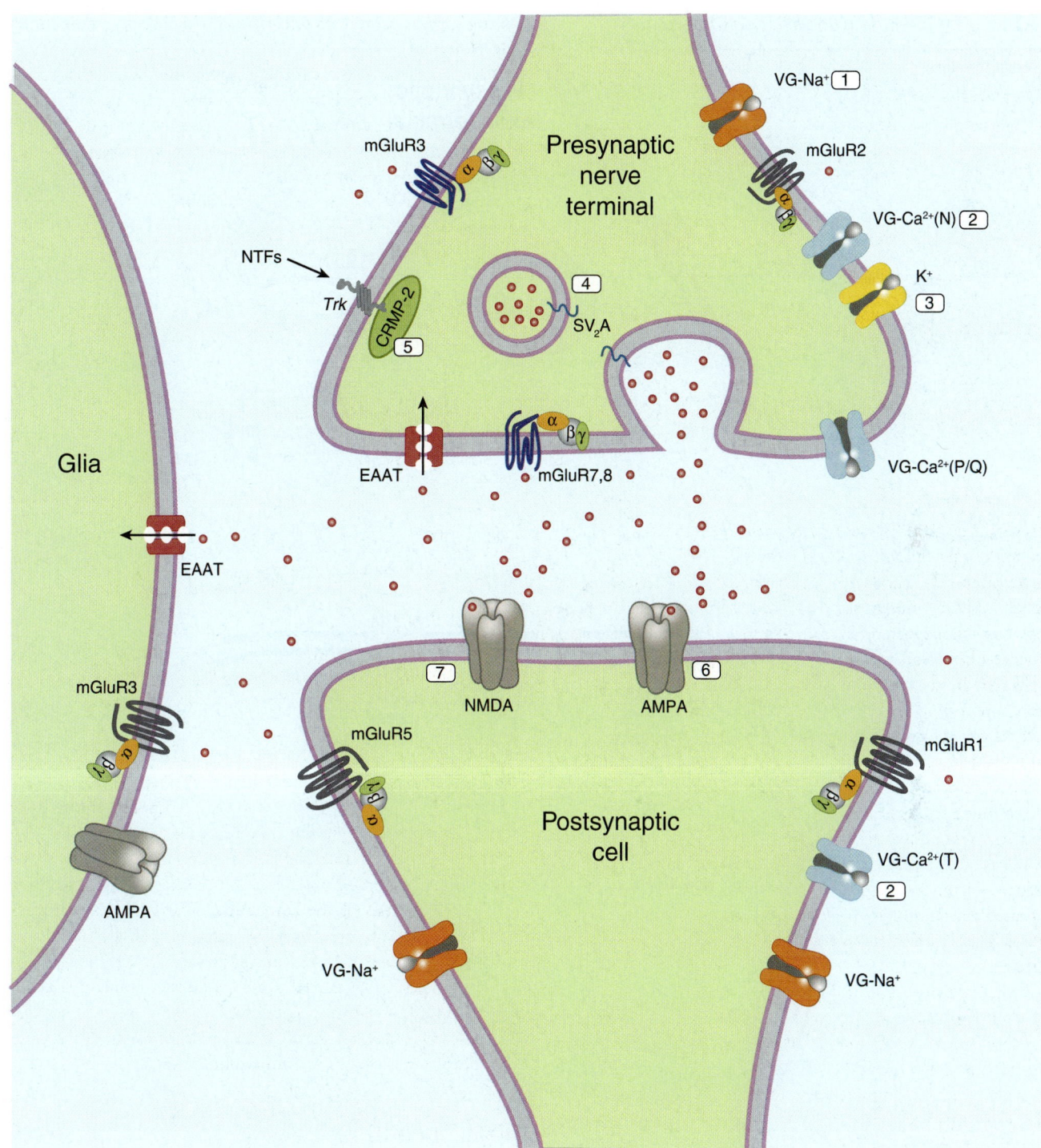

FIGURE 24–1 Molecular targets for antiseizure drugs at the excitatory, glutamatergic synapse. Presynaptic targets diminishing glutamate release include 1, voltage-gated (VG) Na$^+$ channels (phenytoin, carbamazepine, lamotrigine, and lacosamide); 2, VG-Ca^{2+} channels (ethosuximide, lamotrigine, gabapentin, and pregabalin); 3, K$^+$ channels (retigabine); synaptic vesicle proteins, 4, SV$_2$A (levetiracetam); and 5, CRMP-2, collapsin-response mediator protein-2 (lacosamide). Postsynaptic targets include 6, AMPA receptors (blocked by phenobarbital, topiramate, and lamotrigine) and 7, NMDA receptors (blocked by felbamate). EAAT, excitatory amino acid transporter. Red dots represent glutamate.

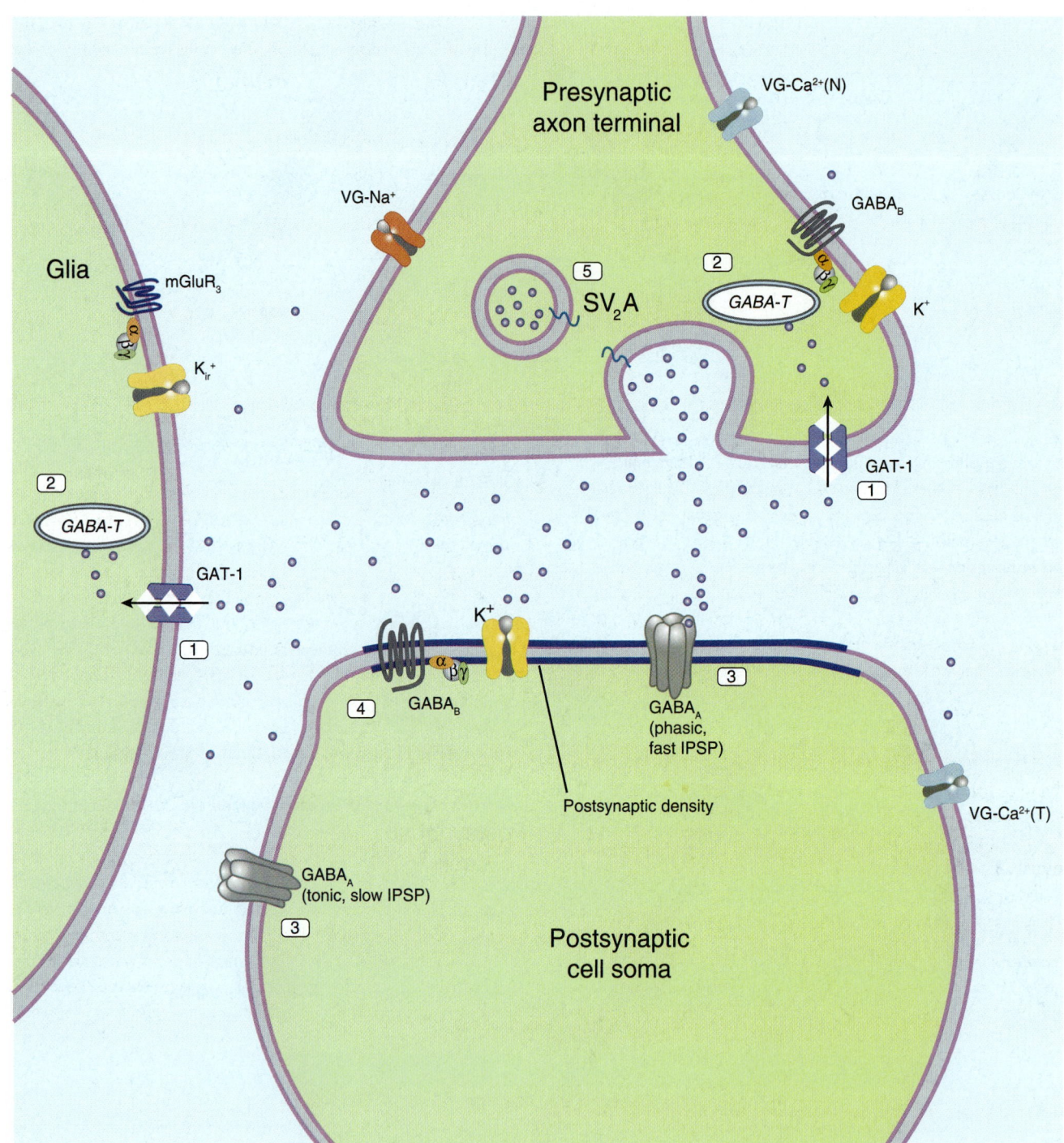

FIGURE 24–2 Molecular targets for antiseizure drugs at the inhibitory, GABAergic synapse. These include "specific" targets: 1, GABA transporters (especially GAT-1, tiagabine); 2, GABA-transaminase (GABA-T, vigabatrin); 3, GABA$_A$ receptors (benzodiazepines); potentially, 4, GABA$_B$ receptors; and 5, synaptic vesicular proteins (SVA$_2$). Effects may also be mediated by "nonspecific" targets such as by voltage-gated (VG) ion channels and synaptic proteins. IPSP, inhibitory postsynaptic potential. Blue dots represent GABA.

liver. These drugs are predominantly distributed into total body water. Plasma clearance is relatively slow; many antiseizure drugs are therefore considered to be medium to long acting. Some have half-lives longer than 12 hours. Many of the older

antiseizure drugs are potent inducers of hepatic microsomal enzyme activity. Compliance is better with less frequent administration; thus extended-release formulations permitting once- or twice-daily administration may offer an advantage.

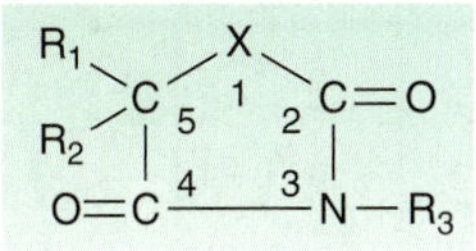

FIGURE 24–3 Antiseizure heterocyclic ring structure. The X varies as follows: hydantoin derivatives, –N–; barbiturates, –C–N–; oxazolidinediones, –O–; succinimides, –C–; acetylureas, –NH$_2$ (N connected to C$_2$). R$_1$, R$_2$, and R$_3$ vary within each subgroup.

DRUGS USED IN PARTIAL SEIZURES & GENERALIZED TONIC-CLONIC SEIZURES

The classic major drugs for partial and generalized tonic-clonic seizures are phenytoin (and congeners), carbamazepine, valproate, and the barbiturates. However, the availability of newer drugs—eslicarbazepine, lamotrigine, levetiracetam, gabapentin, oxcarbazepine, pregabalin, retigabine, topiramate, vigabatrin, lacosamide, and zonisamide—is altering clinical practice in countries where these compounds are available. The next section of the chapter is a description of major drugs from a historical and structural perspective. Factors involved in the clinical choice of drugs are described in the last section of the chapter.

PHENYTOIN

Phenytoin is the oldest nonsedative antiseizure drug, introduced in 1938 after a systematic evaluation of compounds such as phenobarbital that altered electrically induced seizures in laboratory animals. It was known for decades as **diphenylhydantoin.**

Chemistry

Phenytoin is a diphenyl-substituted hydantoin with the structure shown. It has much lower sedative properties than compounds with alkyl substituents at the 5 position. A more soluble prodrug

of phenytoin, **fosphenytoin,** is available for parenteral use; this phosphate ester compound is rapidly converted to phenytoin in the plasma.

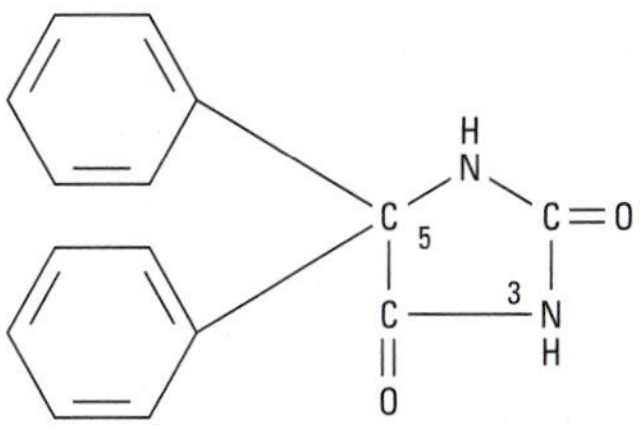

Phenytoin

Mechanism of Action

Phenytoin has major effects on several physiologic systems. It alters Na$^+$, K$^+$, and Ca^{2+} conductance, membrane potentials, and the concentrations of amino acids and the neurotransmitters norepinephrine, acetylcholine, and γ-aminobutyric acid (GABA). Studies with neurons in cell culture show that phenytoin blocks sustained high-frequency repetitive firing of action potentials (Figure 24–4). This effect is seen at therapeutically relevant concentrations. It is a use-dependent effect (see Chapter 14) on Na$^+$ conductance, arising from preferential binding to—and prolongation of—the inactivated state of the Na$^+$ channel. This effect is also seen with therapeutically relevant concentrations of carbamazepine, lamotrigine, and valproate and probably contributes to their antiseizure action in the electroshock model and in partial seizures. Phenytoin also blocks the persistent Na$^+$ current, as do several other AEDs including valproate, topiramate, and ethosuximide.

In addition, phenytoin paradoxically causes excitation in some cerebral neurons. A reduction of calcium permeability, with inhibition of calcium influx across the cell membrane, may explain the ability of phenytoin to inhibit a variety of calcium-induced secretory processes, including release of hormones and neurotransmitters. Recording of excitatory and inhibitory postsynaptic potentials show that phenytoin decreases the synaptic release of glutamate

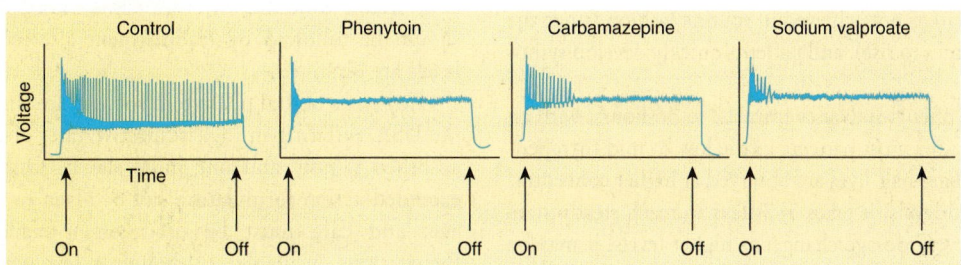

FIGURE 24–4 Effects of three antiseizure drugs on sustained high-frequency firing of action potentials by cultured neurons. Intracellular recordings were made from neurons while depolarizing current pulses, approximately 0.75 s in duration, were applied (on-off step changes indicated by arrows). In the absence of drug, a series of high-frequency repetitive action potentials filled the entire duration of the current pulse. Phenytoin, carbamazepine, and sodium valproate all markedly reduced the number of action potentials elicited by the current pulses.

(Modified and reproduced, with permission, from Macdonald RL, Meldrum BS: Principles of anti-epileptic drug action. In: Levy RH et al [editors]: *Antiepileptic Drugs*, 4th ed. Raven Press, 1995.)

and enhances the release of GABA. The mechanism of phenytoin's action probably involves a combination of actions at several levels. At therapeutic concentrations, the major action of phenytoin is to block Na^+ channels and inhibit the generation of rapidly repetitive action potentials. Presynaptic actions on glutamate and GABA release probably arise from actions other than those on voltage-gated Na^+ channels.

Clinical Uses

Phenytoin is effective against partial seizures and generalized tonic-clonic seizures. In the latter, it appears to be effective against attacks that are either primary or secondary to another seizure type.

Pharmacokinetics

Absorption of phenytoin is highly dependent on the formulation of the dosage form. Particle size and pharmaceutical additives affect both the rate and the extent of absorption. Absorption of phenytoin sodium from the gastrointestinal tract is nearly complete in most patients, although the time to peak may range from 3 to 12 hours. Absorption after intramuscular injection is unpredictable, and some drug precipitation in the muscle occurs; this route of administration is not recommended for phenytoin. In contrast, fosphenytoin, a more soluble phosphate prodrug of phenytoin, is well absorbed after intramuscular administration.

Phenytoin is highly bound to plasma proteins. The total plasma level decreases when the percentage that is bound decreases, as in uremia or hypoalbuminemia, but correlation of free levels with clinical states remains uncertain. Drug concentration in cerebrospinal fluid is proportionate to the free plasma level. Phenytoin accumulates in brain, liver, muscle, and fat.

Phenytoin is metabolized to inactive metabolites that are excreted in the urine. Only a very small proportion of the dose is excreted unchanged.

The elimination of phenytoin is dose-dependent. At very low blood levels, phenytoin metabolism follows first-order kinetics. However, as blood levels rise within the therapeutic range, the maximum capacity of the liver to metabolize phenytoin is approached. Further increases in dosage, though relatively small, may produce very large changes in phenytoin concentrations (Figure 24–5). In such cases, the half-life of the drug increases markedly, steady state is not achieved in routine fashion (since the plasma level continues to rise), and patients quickly develop symptoms of toxicity.

The half-life of phenytoin varies from 12 to 36 hours, with an average of 24 hours for most patients in the low to mid therapeutic range. Much longer half-lives are observed at higher concentrations. At low blood levels, it takes 5–7 days to reach steady-state blood levels after every dosage change; at higher levels, it may be 4–6 weeks before blood levels are stable.

Therapeutic Levels & Dosage

The therapeutic plasma level of phenytoin for most patients is between 10 and 20 mcg/mL. A loading dose can be given either orally or intravenously; the latter, using fosphenytoin, is the

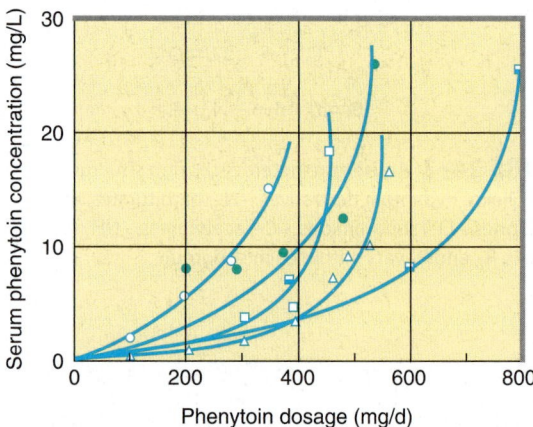

FIGURE 24–5 Nonlinear relationship of phenytoin dosage and plasma concentrations. Five patients (identified by different symbols) received increasing dosages of phenytoin by mouth, and the steady-state serum concentration was measured at each dosage. The curves are not linear, since, as the dosage increases, the metabolism is saturable. Note also the marked variation among patients in the serum levels achieved at any dosage. (Modified, with permission, from Jusko WJ: Bioavailability and disposition kinetics of phenytoin in man. In: Kellaway P, Peterson I [editors]: *Quantitative Analytic Studies in Epilepsy.* Raven Press, 1977.)

method of choice for convulsive status epilepticus (discussed later). When oral therapy is started, it is common to begin adults at a dosage of 300 mg/d, regardless of body weight. This may be acceptable in some patients, but it frequently yields steady-state blood levels below 10 mcg/mL, which is the minimum therapeutic level for most patients. If seizures continue, higher doses are usually necessary to achieve plasma levels in the upper therapeutic range. Because of its dose-dependent kinetics, some toxicity may occur with only small increments in dosage. The phenytoin dosage should be increased each time by only 25–30 mg in adults, and ample time should be allowed for the new steady state to be achieved before further increasing the dosage. A common clinical error is to increase the dosage directly from 300 mg/d to 400 mg/d; toxicity frequently occurs at a variable time thereafter. In children, a dosage of 5 mg/kg/d should be followed by readjustment after steady-state plasma levels are obtained.

Two types of oral phenytoin sodium are currently available in the USA, differing in their respective rates of dissolution; one is absorbed rapidly and one more slowly. Only the slow-release extended-action formulation can be given in a single daily dosage, and care must be used when changing brands (see Preparations Available). Although a few patients being given phenytoin on a long-term basis have been proved to have low blood levels from poor absorption or rapid metabolism, the most common cause of low levels is poor compliance. Fosphenytoin sodium is available for intravenous or intramuscular use and replaces intravenous phenytoin sodium, a much less soluble form of the drug.

Drug Interactions & Interference with Laboratory Tests

Drug interactions involving phenytoin are primarily related to protein binding or to metabolism. Since phenytoin is 90% bound to plasma proteins, other highly bound drugs, such as phenylbutazone and sulfonamides, can displace phenytoin from its binding site. In theory, such displacement may cause a transient increase in free drug. A decrease in protein binding—eg, from hypoalbuminemia—results in a decrease in the total plasma concentration of drug but not the free concentration. Intoxication may occur if efforts are made to maintain total drug levels in the therapeutic range by increasing the dose. The protein binding of phenytoin is decreased in the presence of renal disease. The drug has an affinity for thyroid-binding globulin, which confuses some tests of thyroid function; the most reliable screening test of thyroid function in patients taking phenytoin appears to be measurement of thyroid-stimulating hormone (TSH).

Phenytoin has been shown to induce microsomal enzymes responsible for the metabolism of a number of drugs. Autostimulation of its own metabolism, however, appears to be insignificant.

Toxicity

Dose-related adverse effects caused by phenytoin are often similar to those caused by other antiseizure drugs in this group, making differentiation difficult in patients receiving multiple drugs. Nystagmus occurs early, as does loss of smooth extraocular pursuit movements, but neither is an indication for decreasing the dose. Diplopia and ataxia are the most common dose-related adverse effects requiring dosage adjustment; sedation usually occurs only at considerably higher levels. Gingival hyperplasia and hirsutism occur to some degree in most patients; the latter can be especially unpleasant in women. Long-term use is associated in some patients with coarsening of facial features and with mild peripheral neuropathy, usually manifested by diminished deep tendon reflexes in the lower extremities. Long-term use may also result in abnormalities of vitamin D metabolism, leading to osteomalacia. Low folate levels and megaloblastic anemia have been reported, but the clinical importance of these observations is unknown.

Idiosyncratic reactions to phenytoin are relatively rare. A skin rash may indicate hypersensitivity of the patient to the drug. Fever may also occur, and in rare cases the skin lesions may be severe and exfoliative. Lymphadenopathy may be difficult to distinguish from malignant lymphoma, and although some studies suggest a causal relationship between phenytoin and Hodgkin's disease, the data are far from conclusive. Hematologic complications are exceedingly rare, although agranulocytosis has been reported in combination with fever and rash.

MEPHENYTOIN, ETHOTOIN, & PHENACEMIDE

Many congeners of phenytoin have been synthesized, but only three have been marketed in the USA, and one of these (phenacemide) has been withdrawn. The other two congeners,

mephenytoin and ethotoin, like phenytoin, appear to be most effective against generalized tonic-clonic seizures and partial seizures. No well-controlled clinical trials have documented their effectiveness. The incidence of severe reactions such as dermatitis, agranulocytosis, or hepatitis is higher for mephenytoin than for phenytoin.

Ethotoin may be recommended for patients who are hypersensitive to phenytoin, but larger doses are required. The adverse effects and toxicity are generally less severe than those associated with phenytoin, but the drug appears to be less effective.

Both ethotoin and mephenytoin share with phenytoin the property of saturable metabolism within the therapeutic dosage range. Careful monitoring of the patient during dosage alterations with either drug is essential. Mephenytoin is metabolized to 5,5-ethylphenylhydantoin via demethylation. This metabolite, **nirvanol,** contributes most of the antiseizure activity of mephenytoin. Both mephenytoin and nirvanol are hydroxylated and undergo subsequent conjugation and excretion. Therapeutic levels for mephenytoin range from 5 to 16 mcg/mL, and levels above 20 mcg/mL are considered toxic.

Therapeutic blood levels of nirvanol are between 25 and 40 mcg/mL. A therapeutic range for ethotoin has not been established.

CARBAMAZEPINE

Closely related to imipramine and other antidepressants, carbamazepine is a tricyclic compound effective in treatment of bipolar depression. It was initially marketed for the treatment of trigeminal neuralgia but has proved useful for epilepsy as well.

Chemistry

Although not obvious from a two-dimensional representation of its structure, carbamazepine has many similarities to phenytoin. The ureide moiety ($-N-CO-NH_2$) in the heterocyclic ring of most antiseizure drugs is also present in carbamazepine. Three-dimensional structural studies indicate that its spatial conformation is similar to that of phenytoin.

Carbamazepine

Mechanism of Action

The mechanism of action of carbamazepine appears to be similar to that of phenytoin. Like phenytoin, carbamazepine shows activity against maximal electroshock seizures. Carbamazepine, like phenytoin, blocks Na^+ channels at therapeutic concentrations and inhibits high-frequency repetitive firing in neurons in culture (Figure 24–4). It also acts presynaptically to decrease synaptic transmission. Potentiation of a voltage-gated K^+ current has also been described. These effects probably account for the anticonvulsant action of carbamazepine. Binding studies show that carbamazepine interacts with adenosine receptors, but the functional significance of this observation is not known.

Clinical Uses

Although carbamazepine has long been considered a drug of choice for both partial seizures and generalized tonic-clonic seizures, some of the newer antiseizure drugs are beginning to displace it from this role. Carbamazepine is not sedative in its usual therapeutic range. The drug is also very effective in some patients with trigeminal neuralgia, although older patients may tolerate higher doses poorly, with ataxia and unsteadiness. Carbamazepine is also useful for controlling mania in some patients with bipolar disorder.

Pharmacokinetics

The rate of absorption of carbamazepine varies widely among patients, although almost complete absorption apparently occurs in all. Peak levels are usually achieved 6–8 hours after administration. Slowing absorption by giving the drug after meals helps the patient tolerate larger total daily doses.

Distribution is slow, and the volume of distribution is roughly 1 L/kg. The drug is approximately 70% bound to plasma proteins; no displacement of other drugs from protein binding sites has been observed.

Carbamazepine has a very low systemic clearance of approximately 1 L/kg/d at the start of therapy. The drug has a notable ability to induce microsomal enzymes. Typically, the half-life of 36 hours observed in subjects after an initial single dose decreases to as little as 8–12 hours in subjects receiving continuous therapy. Considerable dosage adjustments are thus to be expected during the first weeks of therapy. Carbamazepine also alters the clearance of other drugs (see below).

Carbamazepine is completely metabolized in humans to several derivatives. One of these, carbamazepine-10,11-epoxide, has been shown to have anticonvulsant activity. The contribution of this and other metabolites to the clinical activity of carbamazepine is unknown.

Therapeutic Levels & Dosage

Carbamazepine is available only in oral form. The drug is effective in children, in whom a dosage of 15–25 mg/kg/d is appropriate. In adults, daily doses of 1 g or even 2 g are tolerated. Higher dosage is achieved by giving multiple divided doses daily. Extended-release preparations permit twice-daily dosing for most patients. In patients in whom the blood is drawn just before the morning dose (trough level), the therapeutic level is usually 4–8 mcg/mL. Although many patients complain of diplopia at drug levels above 7 mcg/mL, others can tolerate levels above 10 mcg/mL, especially with monotherapy. Extended-release formulations that overcome some of these issues are now available.

Drug Interactions

Drug interactions involving carbamazepine are almost exclusively related to the drug's enzyme-inducing properties. As noted previously, the increased metabolic capacity of the hepatic enzymes may cause a reduction in steady-state carbamazepine concentrations and an increased rate of metabolism of other drugs, eg, primidone, phenytoin, ethosuximide, valproic acid, and clonazepam. Other drugs such as valproic acid may inhibit carbamazepine clearance and increase steady-state carbamazepine blood levels. Other anticonvulsants, however, such as phenytoin and phenobarbital, may decrease steady-state concentrations of carbamazepine through enzyme induction. No clinically significant protein-binding interactions have been reported.

Toxicity

The most common dose-related adverse effects of carbamazepine are diplopia and ataxia. The diplopia often occurs first and may last less than an hour during a particular time of day. Rearrangement of the divided daily dose can often remedy this complaint. Other dose-related complaints include mild gastrointestinal upsets, unsteadiness, and, at much higher doses, drowsiness. Hyponatremia and water intoxication have occasionally occurred and may be dose related.

Considerable concern exists regarding the occurrence of idiosyncratic blood dyscrasias with carbamazepine, including fatal cases of aplastic anemia and agranulocytosis. Most of these have been in elderly patients with trigeminal neuralgia, and most have occurred within the first 4 months of treatment. The mild and persistent leukopenia seen in some patients is not necessarily an indication to stop treatment but requires careful monitoring. The most common idiosyncratic reaction is an erythematous skin rash; other responses such as hepatic dysfunction are unusual.

OXCARBAZEPINE

Oxcarbazepine is closely related to carbamazepine and is useful in the same seizure types, but it may have an improved toxicity profile. Oxcarbazepine has a half-life of only 1–2 hours. Its activity, therefore, resides almost exclusively in the 10-hydroxy metabolite (especially the $S(+)$ enantiomer, eslicarbazepine), to which it is rapidly converted and which has a half-life similar to that of carbamazepine, ie, 8–12 hours. The drug is mostly excreted as the glucuronide of the 10-hydroxy metabolite.

Oxcarbazepine

Oxcarbazepine is less potent than carbamazepine, both in animal models of epilepsy and in epileptic patients; clinical doses of oxcarbazepine may need to be 50% higher than those of carbamazepine to obtain equivalent seizure control. Some studies report fewer hypersensitivity reactions to oxcarbazepine, and cross-reactivity with carbamazepine does not always occur. Furthermore, the drug appears to induce hepatic enzymes to a lesser extent than carbamazepine, minimizing drug interactions. Although hyponatremia may occur more commonly with oxcarbazepine than with carbamazepine, most adverse effects that occur with oxcarbazepine are similar in character to reactions reported with carbamazepine.

ESLICARBAZINE

Eslicarbazepine acetate (ESL) is a prodrug that has been approved in Europe as adjunctive therapy in adults with partial-onset seizures, with or without secondary generalization. ESL is more rapidly converted to $S(+)$-licarbazine (eslicarbazine) than is oxcarbazepine; clearly both prodrugs have the same metabolite as active product. The mechanism of action of carbamazepine, oxcarbazepine, and ESL appears to be the same, ie, blocking of voltage-gated Na^+ channels. The $R(-)$ enantiomer has some activity, but much less than its counterpart.

Clinically, the drug is similar to carbamazepine and oxcarbazepine in its spectrum of action, but it is less well studied in other possible indications. The possible advantage of ESL is its once-daily dosing regimen. The measured half-life of the $S(+)$ enantiomer is 9–11 hours. The drug is administered at a dosage of 400–1200 mg/d; titration is typically required for the higher doses.

Minimal drug level effects are observed with coadministration of carbamazepine, levetiracetam, lamotrigine, topiramate, and valproate. Oral contraceptives may be less effective with concomitant ESL administration.

PHENOBARBITAL

Aside from the bromides, phenobarbital is the oldest of the currently available antiseizure drugs. Although it has long been considered one of the safest of the antiseizure agents, the use of other medications with lesser sedative effects has been urged. Many consider the barbiturates the drugs of choice for seizures only in infants.

Chemistry

The four derivatives of barbituric acid clinically useful as antiseizure drugs are phenobarbital, mephobarbital, metharbital, and primidone. The first three are so similar that they are considered together. Metharbital is methylated barbital, and mephobarbital is methylated phenobarbital; both are demethylated in vivo. The pK_as of these three weak acid compounds range from 7.3 to 7.9. Slight changes in the normal acid-base balance, therefore, can cause significant fluctuation in the ratio of the ionized to the nonionized species. This is particularly important for phenobarbital, the most commonly used barbiturate, whose pK_a is similar to the plasma pH of 7.4.

The three-dimensional conformations of the phenobarbital and N-methylphenobarbital molecules are similar to that of phenytoin. Both compounds possess a phenyl ring and are active against partial seizures.

Mechanism of Action

The exact mechanism of action of phenobarbital is unknown, but enhancement of inhibitory processes and diminution of excitatory transmission probably contribute significantly. Recent data indicate that phenobarbital may selectively suppress abnormal neurons, inhibiting the spread and suppressing firing from the foci. Like phenytoin, phenobarbital suppresses high-frequency repetitive firing in neurons in culture through an action on Na^+ conductance, but only at high concentrations. Also at high concentrations, barbiturates block some Ca^{2+} currents (L-type and N-type). Phenobarbital binds to an allosteric regulatory site on the $GABA_A$ receptor, and it enhances the GABA receptor-mediated current by prolonging the openings of the Cl^- channels (see Chapter 22). Phenobarbital can also decrease excitatory responses. An effect on glutamate release is probably more significant than blockade of AMPA responses (see Chapter 21). Both the enhancement of GABA-mediated inhibition and the reduction of glutamate-mediated excitation are seen with therapeutically relevant concentrations of phenobarbital.

Clinical Uses

Phenobarbital is useful in the treatment of partial seizures and generalized tonic-clonic seizures, although the drug is often tried for virtually every seizure type, especially when attacks are difficult to control. There is little evidence for its effectiveness in generalized seizures such as absence, atonic attacks, and infantile spasms; it may worsen certain patients with these seizure types.

Some physicians prefer either metharbital (no longer readily available) or mephobarbital (especially the latter) to phenobarbital because of supposed decreased adverse effects. Only anecdotal data are available to support such comparisons.

Pharmacokinetics, Therapeutic Levels, & Dosage

For pharmacokinetics, drug interactions, and toxicity of phenobarbital, see Chapter 22.

The therapeutic levels of phenobarbital in most patients range from 10 mcg/mL to 40 mcg/mL. Documentation of effectiveness is best in febrile seizures, and levels below 15 mcg/mL appear ineffective for prevention of febrile seizure recurrence. The upper end of the therapeutic range is more difficult to define because many patients appear to tolerate chronic levels above 40 mcg/mL.

PRIMIDONE

Primidone, or 2-desoxyphenobarbital (Figure 24–6), was first marketed in the early 1950s. It was later reported that primidone was metabolized to phenobarbital and phenylethylmalonamide (PEMA). All three compounds are active anticonvulsants.

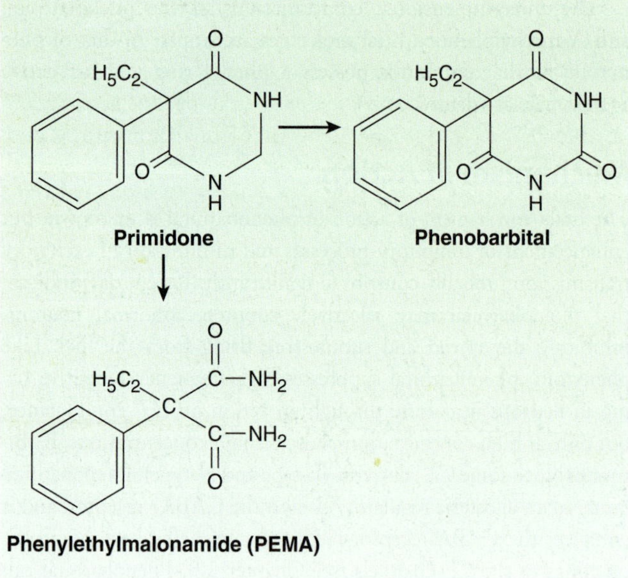

FIGURE 24–6 Primidone and its active metabolites.

Mechanism of Action

Although primidone is converted to phenobarbital, the mechanism of action of primidone itself may be more like that of phenytoin.

Clinical Uses

Primidone, like its metabolites, is effective against partial seizures and generalized tonic-clonic seizures and may be more effective than phenobarbital. It was previously considered to be the drug of choice for complex partial seizures, but later studies of partial seizures in adults strongly suggest that carbamazepine and phenytoin are superior to primidone. Attempts to determine the relative potencies of the parent drug and its two metabolites have been conducted in newborn infants, in whom drug-metabolizing enzyme systems are very immature and in whom primidone is only slowly metabolized. Primidone has been shown to be effective in controlling seizures in this group and in older patients beginning treatment with primidone; older patients show seizure control before phenobarbital concentrations reach the therapeutic range. Finally, studies of maximal electroshock seizures in animals suggest that primidone has an anticonvulsant action independent of its conversion to phenobarbital and PEMA (the latter is relatively weak).

Pharmacokinetics

Primidone is completely absorbed, usually reaching peak concentrations about 3 hours after oral administration, although considerable variation has been reported. Primidone is generally distributed in total body water, with a volume of distribution of 0.6 L/kg. It is not highly bound to plasma proteins; approximately 70% circulates as unbound drug.

Primidone is metabolized by oxidation to phenobarbital, which accumulates very slowly, and by scission of the heterocyclic ring to form PEMA (Figure 24–6). Both primidone and phenobarbital also undergo subsequent conjugation and excretion.

Primidone has a larger clearance than most other antiseizure drugs (2 L/kg/d), corresponding to a half-life of 6–8 hours. PEMA clearance is approximately half that of primidone, but phenobarbital has a very low clearance (see Table 3–1). The appearance of phenobarbital corresponds to the disappearance of primidone. Phenobarbital therefore accumulates very slowly but eventually reaches therapeutic concentrations in most patients when therapeutic doses of primidone are administered. During chronic therapy, phenobarbital levels derived from primidone are usually two to three times higher than primidone levels.

Therapeutic Levels & Dosage

Primidone is most efficacious when plasma levels are in the range of 8–12 mcg/mL. Concomitant levels of its metabolite, phenobarbital, at steady state usually vary from 15 to 30 mcg/mL. Dosages of 10–20 mg/kg/d are necessary to obtain these levels. It is very important, however, to start primidone at low doses and gradually increase over days to a few weeks to avoid prominent sedation and gastrointestinal complaints. When adjusting doses of the drug, it is important to remember that the parent drug reaches steady state rapidly (30–40 hours), but the active metabolites phenobarbital (20 days) and PEMA (3–4 days) reach steady state much more slowly.

Toxicity

The dose-related adverse effects of primidone are similar to those of its metabolite, phenobarbital, except that drowsiness occurs early in treatment and may be prominent if the initial dose is too large. Gradual increments are indicated when starting the drug in either children or adults.

FELBAMATE

Felbamate has been approved and marketed in the USA and in some European countries. Although it is effective in some patients with partial seizures, the drug causes aplastic anemia and severe hepatitis at unexpectedly high rates and has been relegated to the status of a third-line drug for refractory cases.

Felbamate appears to have multiple mechanisms of action. It produces a use-dependent block of the NMDA receptor, with selectivity for the NR1-2B subtype. It also produces a barbiturate-like potentiation of GABA$_A$ receptor responses. Felbamate has a half-life of 20 hours (somewhat shorter when administered with either phenytoin or carbamazepine) and is metabolized by hydroxylation and conjugation; a significant percentage of the drug is excreted unchanged in the urine. When added to treatment with other antiseizure drugs, felbamate increases plasma phenytoin and valproic acid levels but decreases levels of carbamazepine.

Felbamate

In spite of the seriousness of the adverse effects, thousands of patients worldwide utilize this medication. Usual dosages are 2000–4000 mg/d in adults, and effective plasma levels range from 30 mcg/mL to 100 mcg/mL. In addition to its usefulness in partial seizures, felbamate has proved effective against the seizures that occur in Lennox-Gastaut syndrome.

GABAPENTIN & PREGABALIN

Gabapentin is an amino acid, an analog of GABA, that is effective against partial seizures. Originally planned as a spasmolytic, it was found to be more effective as an antiseizure drug. Pregabalin is another GABA analog, closely related to gabapentin. This drug has been approved for both antiseizure activity and for its analgesic properties.

Gabapentin   **Pregabalin**

Mechanism of Action

In spite of their close structural resemblance to GABA, gabapentin and pregabalin do not act directly on GABA receptors. They may, however, modify the synaptic or nonsynaptic release of GABA. An increase in brain GABA concentration is observed in patients receiving gabapentin. Gabapentin is transported into the brain by the L-amino acid transporter. Gabapentin and pregabalin bind avidly to the $\alpha_2\delta$ subunit of voltage-gated Ca^{2+} channels. This appears to underlie the main mechanism of action, which is decreasing Ca^{2+} entry, with a predominant effect on presynaptic N-type channels. A decrease in the synaptic release of glutamate provides the antiepileptic effect.

Clinical Uses

Gabapentin is effective as an adjunct against partial seizures and generalized tonic-clonic seizures at dosages that range up to 2400 mg/d in controlled clinical trials. Open follow-up studies permitted dosages up to 4800 mg/d, but data are inconclusive on the effectiveness or tolerability of such doses. Monotherapy studies

also document some efficacy. Some clinicians have found that very high dosages are needed to achieve improvement in seizure control. Effectiveness in other seizure types has not been well demonstrated. Gabapentin has also been promoted for the treatment of neuropathic pain and is now indicated for postherpetic neuralgia in adults at doses of 1800 mg and above. The most common adverse effects are somnolence, dizziness, ataxia, headache, and tremor.

Pregabalin is approved for the adjunctive treatment of partial seizures, with or without secondary generalization; controlled clinical trials have documented its effectiveness. It is available only in oral form, and the dosage ranges from 150 to 600 mg/d, usually in two or three divided doses. Pregabalin is also approved for use in neuropathic pain, including painful diabetic peripheral neuropathy and postherpetic neuralgia. It is the first drug in the USA approved for fibromyalgia. In Europe it is approved for generalized anxiety disorder.

Pharmacokinetics

Gabapentin is not metabolized and does not induce hepatic enzymes. Absorption is nonlinear and dose-dependent at very high doses, but the elimination kinetics are linear. The drug is not bound to plasma proteins. Drug-drug interactions are negligible. Elimination is via renal mechanisms; the drug is excreted unchanged. The half-life is relatively short, ranging from 5 to 8 hours; the drug is typically administered two or three times per day.

Pregabalin, like gabapentin, is not metabolized and is almost entirely excreted unchanged in the urine. It is not bound to plasma proteins and has virtually no drug-drug interactions, again resembling the characteristics of gabapentin. Likewise, other drugs do not affect the pharmacokinetics of pregabalin. The half-life of pregabalin ranges from about 4.5 hours to 7.0 hours, thus requiring more than once-daily dosing in most patients.

LACOSAMIDE

Lacosamide is an amino acid-related compound that has been studied in both pain syndromes and partial seizures. The drug was approved in Europe and the USA in 2008 for the treatment of partial seizures.

Mechanism of Action

Activity resides in the R(–) enantiomer. Two effects relevant to the mechanism of action of lacosamide as an antiseizure drug have been described. Lacosamide enhances *slow* inactivation of voltage-gated Na^+ channels (in contrast to the prolongation of fast inactivation shown by other AEDs). It also binds to the collapsin-response mediator protein, CRMP-2, thereby blocking the effect of neurotrophic factors such as BDNF and NT3 on axonal and dendritic growth.

Clinical Uses

Lacosamide is approved as adjunctive therapy in the treatment of partial-onset seizures with or without secondary generalization in patients with epilepsy who are age 16–17 years and older. Clinical trials include three multicenter, randomized placebo-controlled studies with more than 1300 patients. Treatment was effective at both 200 and 400 mg/d. Adverse effects were dizziness, headache, nausea, and diplopia. In the open-label follow-up study, at dosages ranging from 100 to 800 mg/d, many patients continued lacosamide treatment for 24 to 30 months. The drug is typically administered twice daily, beginning with 50 mg doses and increasing by 100 mg increments weekly. An intravenous formulation provides short-term replacement for the oral drug.

Pharmacokinetics

Oral lacosamide is rapidly and completely absorbed in adults, with no food effect. Bioavailability is nearly 100%. The plasma concentrations are proportional to dosage up to 800 mg orally. Peak concentrations occur from 1 to 4 hours after oral dosing, with an elimination half-life of 13 hours. There are no active metabolites and protein binding is minimal. Lacosamide does not induce or inhibit cytochrome P450 isoenzymes, so drug interactions are negligible.

LAMOTRIGINE

Lamotrigine was developed when some investigators thought that the antifolate effects of certain antiseizure drugs (eg, phenytoin) might contribute to their effectiveness. Several phenyltriazines were developed, and though their antifolate properties were weak, some were active in seizure screening tests.

Lamotrigine

Mechanism of Action

Lamotrigine, like phenytoin, suppresses sustained rapid firing of neurons and produces a voltage- and use-dependent blockade of Na^+ channels. This action probably explains lamotrigine's efficacy in focal epilepsy. It appears likely that lamotrigine also inhibits voltage-gated Ca^{2+} channels, particularly the N- and P/Q-type channels, which would account for its efficacy in primary generalized seizures in childhood, including absence attacks. Lamotrigine also decreases the synaptic release of glutamate.

Clinical Uses

Although most controlled studies have evaluated lamotrigine as add-on therapy, it is generally agreed that the drug is effective as monotherapy for partial seizures, and lamotrigine is now widely prescribed for this indication. The drug is also active against absence

and myoclonic seizures in children and is approved for seizure control in the Lennox-Gastaut syndrome. Lamotrigine is also effective for bipolar disorder. Adverse effects include dizziness, headache, diplopia, nausea, somnolence, and skin rash. The rash is considered a typical hypersensitivity reaction. Although the risk of rash may be diminished by introducing the drug slowly, pediatric patients are at greatest risk, some studies suggest that a potentially life-threatening dermatitis will develop in 1–2% of pediatric patients.

Pharmacokinetics

Lamotrigine is almost completely absorbed and has a volume of distribution in the range of 1–1.4 L/kg. Protein binding is only about 55%. The drug has linear kinetics and is metabolized primarily by glucuronidation to the 2-N-glucuronide, which is excreted in the urine. Lamotrigine has a half-life of approximately 24 hours in normal volunteers; this decreases to 13–15 hours in patients taking enzyme-inducing drugs. Lamotrigine is effective against partial seizures in adults at dosages typically between 100 and 300 mg/d and with a therapeutic blood level near 3 mcg/mL. Valproate causes a twofold increase in the drug's half-life; in patients receiving valproate, the initial dosage of lamotrigine must be reduced to 25 mg every other day.

LEVETIRACETAM

Levetiracetam is a piracetam analog that is ineffective against seizures induced by maximum electroshock or pentylenetetrazol but has prominent activity in the kindling model. This is the first major drug with this unusual preclinical profile that is effective against partial seizures.

Levetiracetam

Mechanism of Action

Levetiracetam binds selectively to the synaptic vesicular protein SV_2A. The function of this protein is not understood but it is likely that levetiracetam modifies the synaptic release of glutamate and GABA through an action on vesicular function.

Clinical Uses

Levetiracetam is marketed for the adjunctive treatment of partial seizures in adults and children for primary generalized tonic-clonic seizures and for the myoclonic seizures of juvenile myoclonic epilepsy. Adult dosing can begin with 500 or 1000 mg/d. The dosage can be increased every 2–4 weeks by 1000 mg to a maximum dosage of 3000 mg/d. The drug is dosed twice daily. Adverse effects include somnolence, asthenia, ataxia, and dizziness. Less common but more serious are mood and behavioral changes; psychotic reactions are rare. Drug interactions are minimal; levetiracetam is not metabolized by cytochrome P450. Oral formulations include extended-release tablets; an intravenous preparation is also available.

Pharmacokinetics

Oral absorption of levetiracetam is nearly complete; it is rapid and unaffected by food, with peak plasma concentrations in 1.3 hours. Kinetics are linear. Protein binding is less than 10%. The plasma half-life is 6–8 hours, but may be longer in the elderly. Two thirds of the drug is excreted unchanged in the urine; the drug has no known active metabolites.

RETIGABINE (EZOGABINE)

Retigabine (ezogabine in the USA) was approved as an anti-seizure drug in Europe and the USA in 2010. It is a potassium-channel facilitator and unique in its mechanism of action. Absorption is not affected by food and kinetics are linear; drug interactions are minimal. Clinical trials demonstrated efficacy in partial seizures, and approval is for the adjunctive treatment of partial-onset seizures in adults. Doses range from 600 to 1200 mg/day, with 900 mg/day expected to be the median. The current dosage form requires three-times-per-day administration, and the dose must be titrated in most patients. Most adverse effects are dose-related and include dizziness, somnolence, blurred vision, confusion, and dysarthria. Bladder dysfunction, mostly mild and related to the drug's mechanism of action, was observed in 8-9% of patients in the clinical trials.

RUFINAMIDE

Rufinamide is a triazole derivative with little similarity to other antiseizure drugs.

Rufinamide

Mechanism of Action

Rufinamide is protective in the maximal electroshock and pentylenetetrazol tests in rats and mice. It decreases sustained high-frequency firing of neurons in vitro and is thought to prolong the inactive state of the Na^+ channel. Significant interactions with GABA systems or metabotropic glutamate receptors have not been seen.

Clinical Uses

Rufinamide is approved in the USA for adjunctive treatment of seizures associated with the Lennox-Gastaut syndrome in patients age 4 years and older. The drug is effective against all seizure types in this syndrome and specifically against tonic-atonic seizures. Recent data also suggest it may be effective against partial seizures. Treatment in children is typically started at 10 mg/kg/d in two equally divided doses and gradually increased to 45 mg/kg/d or 3200 mg/d, whichever is lower. Adults can begin with 400–800 mg/d in two equally divided doses up to a maximum of 3200 mg/d as tolerated. The drug should be given with food. The most common adverse events are somnolence, vomiting, pyrexia, and diarrhea.

Pharmacokinetics

Rufinamide is well absorbed, but plasma concentrations peak between 4 and 6 hours. The half-life is 6–10 hours, and minimal plasma protein binding is observed. Although cytochrome P450 enzymes are not involved, the drug is extensively metabolized to inactive products. Most of the drug is excreted in the urine; an acid metabolite accounts for about two thirds of the dose. In one study, rufinamide did not appear to significantly affect the plasma concentrations of other drugs used for the Lennox-Gastaut syndrome such as topiramate, lamotrigine, or valproic acid, but conflicting data suggest more robust interactions with other AEDs, including effects on rufinamide levels, especially in children.

STIRIPENTOL

Stiripentol, though not a new molecule, was approved in Europe in 2007 for a very specific type of epilepsy. The drug is used with clobazam and valproate in the adjunctive therapy of refractory generalized tonic-clonic seizures in patients with severe myoclonic epilepsy of infancy (SMEI, Dravet's syndrome) whose seizures are not adequately controlled with clobazam and valproate. The drug is legally imported into the USA on a compassionate use basis. The mechanism of action of stiripentol is not well understood but it has been shown to enhance GABAergic transmission in the brain, partly through a barbiturate-like effect, ie, prolonged opening of the Cl^- channels in $GABA_A$ receptors. It also increases GABA levels in the brain. It can increase the effect of other AEDs by slowing their inactivation by cytochrome P450.

Stiripentol is a potent inhibitor of CYP3A4, CYP1A2, and CYP2C19. Adverse effects of stiripentol itself are few, but the drug can dramatically increase the levels of valproate, clobazam, and the active metabolite of the latter, norclobazam. These drugs must be used cautiously together to avoid adverse effects. Dosing is complex, typically beginning with a reduction of the concomitant medication; stiripentol is then started at 10 mg/kg/d and increased gradually to tolerability or to much higher doses. The kinetics of stiripentol are nonlinear.

TIAGABINE

Tiagabine is a derivative of nipecotic acid and was "rationally designed" as an inhibitor of GABA uptake (as opposed to discovery through random screening).

Tiagabine

Mechanism of Action

Tiagabine is an inhibitor of GABA uptake in both neurons and glia. It preferentially inhibits the transporter isoform 1 (GAT-1) rather than GAT-2 or GAT-3 and increases extracellular GABA levels in the forebrain and hippocampus where GAT-1 is preferentially expressed. It prolongs the inhibitory action of synaptically released GABA, but its most significant effect may be potentiation of tonic inhibition. In rodents, it is potent against kindled seizures but weak against the maximal electroshock model, consistent with its predominant action in the forebrain and hippocampus.

Clinical Uses

Tiagabine is indicated for the adjunctive treatment of partial seizures and is effective in doses ranging from 16 to 56 mg/d. Divided doses as often as four times daily are sometimes required. Minor adverse events are dose related and include nervousness, dizziness, tremor, difficulty in concentrating, and depression. Excessive confusion, somnolence, or ataxia may require discontinuation. Psychosis occurs rarely. The drug can *cause* seizures in some patients, notably those taking the drug for other indications. Rash is an uncommon idiosyncratic adverse effect.

Pharmacokinetics

Tiagabine is 90–100% bioavailable, has linear kinetics, and is highly protein bound. The half-life is 5–8 hours and decreases in the presence of enzyme-inducing drugs. Food decreases the peak plasma concentration but not the area under the concentration curve (see Chapter 3). Hepatic impairment causes a slight decrease in clearance and may necessitate a lower dose. The drug is oxidized in the liver by CYP3A. Elimination is primarily in the feces (60–65%) and urine (25%).

TOPIRAMATE

Topiramate is a substituted monosaccharide that is structurally different from all other antiseizure drugs.

Topiramate

Mechanism of Action

Topiramate blocks repetitive firing of cultured spinal cord neurons, as do phenytoin and carbamazepine. Its mechanism of action, therefore, is likely to involve blocking of voltage-gated Na^+ channels. It also acts on high-voltage activated (L-type) Ca^{2+} channels. Topiramate potentiates the inhibitory effect of GABA, acting at a site different from the benzodiazepine or barbiturate sites. Topiramate also depresses the excitatory action of kainate on glutamate receptors. The multiple effects of topiramate may arise through a primary action on kinases altering the phosphorylation of voltage-gated and ligand-gated ion channels.

Clinical Uses

Clinical trials of topiramate as monotherapy demonstrated efficacy against partial and generalized tonic-clonic seizures. The drug is also approved for the Lennox-Gastaut syndrome, and may be effective in infantile spasms and even absence seizures. Topiramate is also approved for the treatment of migraine headaches. The use of the drug in psychiatric disorders is controversial; convincing controlled data are lacking. Dosages typically range from 200 to 600 mg/d, with a few patients tolerating dosages higher than 1000 mg/d. Most clinicians begin at a low dose (50 mg/d) and increase slowly to prevent adverse effects. Several studies have used topiramate in monotherapy with encouraging results. Although no idiosyncratic reactions have been noted, dose-related adverse effects occur most frequently in the first 4 weeks and include somnolence, fatigue, dizziness, cognitive slowing, paresthesias, nervousness, and confusion. Acute myopia and glaucoma may require prompt drug withdrawal. Urolithiasis has also been reported. The drug is teratogenic in animal models, and hypospadias has been reported in male infants exposed in utero to topiramate; no causal relationship, however, could be established.

Pharmacokinetics

Topiramate is rapidly absorbed (about 2 hours) and is 80% bioavailable. There is no food effect on absorption, minimal (15%) plasma protein binding, and only moderate (20–50%) metabolism; no active metabolites are formed. The drug is primarily excreted unchanged in the urine. The half-life is 20–30 hours. Although increased levels are seen with renal failure and hepatic impairment, there is no age or gender effect, no autoinduction, no inhibition of metabolism, and kinetics are linear. Drug interactions do occur and can be complex, but the major effect is on topiramate levels rather than on the levels of other antiseizure drugs. Birth control pills may be less effective in the presence of topiramate, and higher estrogen doses may be required.

VIGABATRIN

Current investigations that seek drugs to enhance the effects of GABA include efforts to find GABA agonists and prodrugs, GABA transaminase inhibitors, and GABA uptake inhibitors. Vigabatrin is one such drug.

Vigabatrin

Mechanism of Action

Vigabatrin is an irreversible inhibitor of GABA aminotransferase (GABA-T), the enzyme responsible for the degradation of GABA. It may also inhibit the vesicular GABA transporter. Vigabatrin produces a sustained increase in the extracellular concentration of GABA in the brain. This leads to some desensitization of synaptic GABA$_A$ receptors but prolonged activation of nonsynaptic GABA$_A$ receptors that provide tonic inhibition. A decrease in brain glutamine synthetase activity is probably secondary to the increased GABA concentrations. It is effective in a wide range of seizure models. Vigabatrin is marketed as a racemate; the S(+) enantiomer is active and the R(−) enantiomer appears to be inactive.

Clinical Uses

Vigabatrin is useful in the treatment of partial seizures and infantile spasms. The half-life is approximately 6–8 hours, but considerable evidence suggests that the pharmacodynamic activity of the drug is more prolonged and not well correlated with the plasma half-life. In infants, the dosage is 50–150 mg/d. In adults, vigabatrin should be started at an oral dosage of 500 mg twice daily; a total of 2–3 g (rarely more) daily may be required for full effectiveness.

Typical toxicities include drowsiness, dizziness, and weight gain. Less common but more troublesome adverse reactions are agitation, confusion, and psychosis; preexisting mental illness is a relative contraindication. The drug was delayed in its worldwide introduction by the appearance in rats and dogs of a reversible intramyelinic edema. This phenomenon has now been detected in infants taking the drug; the clinical significance is unknown. In addition, long-term therapy with vigabatrin has been associated with development of peripheral visual field defects in 30–50% of patients. The lesions are located in the retina, increase with drug exposure, and are usually not reversible. Newer techniques such as optical coherence tomography may better define the defect, which has proved difficult to quantify. Vigabatrin is usually reserved for use in patients with infantile spasms or with complex partial seizures refractory to other treatments.

ZONISAMIDE

Zonisamide is a sulfonamide derivative. Its primary site of action appears to be the Na$^+$ channel; it also acts on T-type voltage-gated Ca^{2+} channels. The drug is effective against partial and generalized tonic-clonic seizures and may also be useful against infantile spasms and certain myoclonias. It has good bioavailability, linear kinetics, low protein-binding, renal excretion, and a half-life of 1–3 days. Dosages range from 100 to 600 mg/d in adults and from 4 to 12 mg/d in children. Adverse effects include drowsiness, cognitive impairment, and potentially serious skin rashes. Zonisamide does not interact with other antiseizure drugs.

DRUGS USED IN GENERALIZED SEIZURES

ETHOSUXIMIDE

Ethosuximide was introduced in 1960 as the third of three marketed succinimides in the USA. Ethosuximide has very little activity against maximal electroshock but considerable efficacy against pentylenetetrazol seizures; it was introduced as a "pure petit mal" drug.

Chemistry

Ethosuximide is the last antiseizure drug to be marketed whose origin is in the cyclic ureide structure. The three antiseizure succinimides marketed in the USA are ethosuximide, phensuximide, and methsuximide. Methsuximide and phensuximide have phenyl substituents, whereas ethosuximide is 2-ethyl-2-methylsuccinimide.

Ethosuximide

Mechanism of Action

Ethosuximide has an important effect on Ca^{2+} currents, reducing the low-threshold (T-type) current. This effect is seen at therapeutically relevant concentrations in thalamic neurons. The T-type Ca^{2+} currents are thought to provide a pacemaker current in thalamic neurons responsible for generating the rhythmic cortical discharge of an absence attack. Inhibition of this current could therefore account for the specific therapeutic action of ethosuximide. A recently described effect on inwardly rectifying K$^+$ channels may also be significant.

Clinical Uses

As predicted from its activity in laboratory models, ethosuximide is particularly effective against absence seizures, but has a very narrow spectrum of clinical activity. Documentation of its effectiveness in human absence seizures was achieved with long-term electroencephalographic recording techniques. Data continue to show that ethosuximide and valproate are the drugs of choice for absence seizures and are more effective than lamotrigine.

Pharmacokinetics

Absorption is complete following administration of the oral dosage forms. Peak levels are observed 3–7 hours after oral administration of the capsules. Ethosuximide is not protein-bound. The drug is completely metabolized, principally by hydroxylation, to inactive metabolites. Ethosuximide has a very low total body clearance (0.25 L/kg/d). This corresponds to a half-life of approximately 40 hours, although values from 18 to 72 hours have been reported.

Therapeutic Levels & Dosage

Therapeutic levels of 60–100 mcg/mL can be achieved in adults with dosages of 750–1500 mg/d, although lower or higher dosages and blood levels (up to 125 mcg/mL) may be necessary and tolerated in some patients. Ethosuximide has a linear relationship between dose and steady-state plasma levels. The drug might be administered as a single daily dose were it not for its adverse gastrointestinal effects; twice-a-day dosage is common.

Drug Interactions & Toxicity

Administration of ethosuximide with valproic acid results in a decrease in ethosuximide clearance and higher steady-state concentrations owing to inhibition of metabolism. No other important drug interactions have been reported for the succinimides. The most common dose-related adverse effect of ethosuximide is gastric distress, including pain, nausea, and vomiting. When an adverse effect does occur, temporary dosage reductions may allow adaptation. Other dose-related adverse effects are transient lethargy or fatigue and, much less commonly, headache, dizziness, hiccup, and euphoria. Behavioral changes are usually in the direction of improvement. Non–dose-related or idiosyncratic adverse effects of ethosuximide are extremely uncommon.

PHENSUXIMIDE & METHSUXIMIDE

Phensuximide (no longer readily available) and methsuximide are phenylsuccinimides that were developed and marketed before ethosuximide. They are used primarily as anti-absence drugs. Methsuximide is generally considered more toxic, and phensuximide less effective, than ethosuximide. Unlike ethosuximide, these two compounds have some activity against maximal electroshock seizures, and methsuximide has been used for partial seizures by some investigators.

VALPROIC ACID & SODIUM VALPROATE

Sodium valproate, also used as the free acid, valproic acid, was found to have antiseizure properties when used as a solvent in the search for other drugs effective against seizures. It was marketed in France in 1969 but was not licensed in the USA until 1978. Valproic acid is fully ionized at body pH, and for that reason the active form of the drug may be assumed to be the valproate ion regardless of whether valproic acid or a salt of the acid is administered.

Chemistry

Valproic acid is one of a series of fatty carboxylic acids that have antiseizure activity; this activity appears to be greatest for carbon chain lengths of five to eight atoms. The amides and esters of valproic acid are also active antiseizure agents.

$$CH_3-CH_2-CH_2 \atop CH_3-CH_2-CH_2 \Big\rangle CH-COOH$$

Valproic acid

Mechanism of Action

The time course of valproate's anticonvulsant activity appears to be poorly correlated with blood or tissue levels of the parent drug, an observation giving rise to considerable speculation regarding both the active species and the mechanism of action of valproic acid. Valproate is active against both pentylenetetrazol and maximal electroshock seizures. Like phenytoin and carbamazepine, valproate blocks sustained high-frequency repetitive firing of neurons in culture at therapeutically relevant concentrations. Its action against partial seizures may be a consequence of this effect on Na^+ currents. Blockade of NMDA receptor-mediated excitation may also be important. Much attention has been paid to the effects of valproate on GABA. Several studies have shown increased levels of GABA in the brain after administration of valproate, although the mechanism for this increase remains unclear. An effect of valproate to facilitate glutamic acid decarboxylase (GAD), the enzyme responsible for GABA synthesis, has been described. An inhibitory effect on the GABA transporter GAT-1 may contribute. At very high concentrations, valproate inhibits GABA transaminase in the brain, thus blocking degradation of GABA. However, at the relatively low doses of valproate needed to abolish pentylenetetrazol seizures, brain GABA levels may remain unchanged. Valproate produces a reduction in the aspartate content of rodent brain, but the relevance of this effect to its anticonvulsant action is not known.

Valproic acid is a potent inhibitor of histone deacetylase and through this mechanism changes the transcription of many genes. A similar effect, but to a lesser degree, is shown by some other antiseizure drugs (topiramate, carbamazepine, and a metabolite of levetiracetam).

Clinical Uses

Valproate is very effective against absence seizures and is often preferred to ethosuximide when the patient has concomitant generalized tonic-clonic attacks. Valproate is unique in its ability to control certain types of myoclonic seizures; in some cases the effect is very dramatic. The drug is effective in tonic-clonic seizures, especially those that are primarily generalized. A few patients with atonic attacks may also respond, and some evidence suggests that the drug is effective in partial seizures. Its use in epilepsy is at least as broad as that of any other drug. Intravenous formulations are occasionally used to treat status epilepticus.

Other uses of valproate include management of bipolar disorder and migraine prophylaxis.

Pharmacokinetics

Valproate is well absorbed after an oral dose, with bioavailability greater than 80%. Peak blood levels are observed within 2 hours. Food may delay absorption, and decreased toxicity may result if the drug is given after meals.

Valproic acid is 90% bound to plasma proteins, although the fraction bound is somewhat reduced at blood levels greater than 150 mcg/mL. Since valproate is both highly ionized and highly protein-bound, its distribution is essentially confined to extracellular water, with a volume of distribution of approximately 0.15 L/kg. At higher doses, there is an increased free fraction of valproate, resulting in lower total drug levels than expected. It may be clinically useful, therefore, to measure both total and free drug levels. Clearance for valproate is low and dose dependent; its half-life varies from 9 to 18 hours. Approximately 20% of the drug is excreted as a direct conjugate of valproate.

The sodium salt of valproate is marketed in Europe as a tablet and is quite hygroscopic. In Central and South America, the magnesium salt is available, which is considerably less hygroscopic. The free acid of valproate was first marketed in the USA in a capsule containing corn oil; the sodium salt is also available in syrup, primarily for pediatric use. An enteric-coated tablet of divalproex sodium is also marketed in the USA. This improved product, a 1:1 coordination compound of valproic acid and sodium valproate, is as bioavailable as the capsule but is absorbed much more slowly and is preferred by many patients. Peak concentrations following administration of the enteric-coated tablets are seen in 3–4 hours. Various extended-release preparations are available; not all are bioequivalent and may require dosage adjustment.

Therapeutic Levels & Dosage

Dosages of 25–30 mg/kg/d may be adequate in some patients, but others may require 60 mg/kg/d or even more. Therapeutic levels of valproate range from 50 to 100 mcg/mL.

Drug Interactions

Valproate displaces phenytoin from plasma proteins. In addition to binding interactions, valproate inhibits the metabolism of several drugs, including phenobarbital, phenytoin, and carbamazepine, leading to higher steady-state concentrations of these agents. The inhibition of phenobarbital metabolism, for example, may cause levels of the barbiturate to rise steeply, causing stupor or coma. Valproate can dramatically decrease the clearance of lamotrigine.

Toxicity

The most common dose-related adverse effects of valproate are nausea, vomiting, and other gastrointestinal complaints such as abdominal pain and heartburn. The drug should be started gradually to avoid these symptoms. Sedation is uncommon with valproate alone but may be striking when valproate is added to phenobarbital. A fine tremor is frequently seen at higher levels. Other reversible adverse effects, seen in a small number of patients, include weight gain, increased appetite, and hair loss.

The idiosyncratic toxicity of valproate is largely limited to hepatotoxicity, but this may be severe; there seems little doubt that the hepatotoxicity of valproate has been responsible for more than 50 fatalities in the USA alone. The risk is greatest for patients under 2 years of age and for those taking multiple medications. Initial aspartate aminotransferase values may not be elevated in susceptible patients, although these levels do eventually become abnormal. Most fatalities have occurred within 4 months after

initiation of therapy. Some clinicians recommend treatment with oral or intravenous L-carnitine as soon as severe hepatotoxicity is suspected. Careful monitoring of liver function is recommended when starting the drug; the hepatotoxicity is reversible in some cases if the drug is withdrawn. The other observed idiosyncratic response with valproate is thrombocytopenia, although documented cases of abnormal bleeding are lacking. It should be noted that valproate is an effective and popular antiseizure drug and that only a very small number of patients have had severe toxic effects from its use.

Several epidemiologic studies of valproate have confirmed a substantial increase in the incidence of spina bifida in the offspring of women who took valproate during pregnancy. In addition, an increased incidence of cardiovascular, orofacial, and digital abnormalities has been reported. These observations must be strongly considered in the choice of drugs during pregnancy.

OXAZOLIDINEDIONES

Trimethadione, the first oxazolidinedione (Figure 24–3), was introduced as an antiseizure drug in 1945 and remained the drug of choice for absence seizures until the introduction of succinimides in the 1950s. Use of the oxazolidinediones—trimethadione, paramethadione, and dimethadione—is now very limited; the latter two are not readily available.

These compounds are active against pentylenetetrazol-induced seizures. Trimethadione raises the threshold for seizure discharges after repetitive thalamic stimulation. It—or, more notably, its active metabolite dimethadione—has the same effect on thalamic Ca^{2+} currents as ethosuximide (reducing the T-type Ca^{2+} current). Thus, suppression of absence seizures is likely to depend on inhibiting the pacemaker action of thalamic neurons.

Trimethadione is rapidly absorbed, with peak levels reached within 1 hour after drug administration. It is not bound to plasma proteins. Trimethadione is completely metabolized in the liver by demethylation to dimethadione, which may exert the major antiseizure activity. Dimethadione has an extremely long half-life (240 hours). The therapeutic plasma level range for trimethadione has never been established, although trimethadione blood levels higher than 20 mcg/mL and dimethadione levels higher than 700 mcg/mL have been suggested. A dosage of 30 mg/kg/d of trimethadione is necessary to achieve these levels in adults.

The most common and bothersome dose-related adverse effect of the oxazolidinediones is sedation. Trimethadione has been associated with many other toxic adverse effects, some of which are severe. These drugs should not be used during pregnancy.

OTHER DRUGS USED IN MANAGEMENT OF EPILEPSY

Some drugs not classifiable by application to seizure type are discussed in this section.

BENZODIAZEPINES

Six benzodiazepines play prominent roles in the therapy of epilepsy (see also Chapter 22). Although many benzodiazepines are similar chemically, subtle structural alterations result in differences in activity and pharmacokinetics. They have two mechanisms of antiseizure action, which are shown to different degrees by the six compounds. This is evident from the fact that diazepam is relatively more potent against electroshock and clonazepam against pentylenetetrazol (the latter effect correlating with an action at the GABA-benzodiazepine allosteric receptor sites). Possible mechanisms of action are discussed in Chapter 22.

Diazepam given intravenously or rectally is highly effective for stopping continuous seizure activity, especially generalized tonic-clonic status epilepticus (see below). The drug is occasionally given orally on a long-term basis, although it is not considered very effective in this application, probably because of the rapid development of tolerance. A rectal gel is available for refractory patients who need acute control of bouts of seizure activity. **Lorazepam** appears in some studies to be more effective and longer acting than diazepam in the treatment of status epilepticus and is preferred by some experts.

Clonazepam is a long-acting drug with documented efficacy against absence seizures; on a milligram basis, it is one of the most potent antiseizure agents known. It is also effective in some cases of myoclonic seizures and has been tried in infantile spasms. Sedation is prominent, especially on initiation of therapy; starting doses should be small. Maximal tolerated doses are usually in the range of 0.1–0.2 mg/kg, but many weeks of gradually increasing daily doses may be needed to achieve these dosages in some patients. **Nitrazepam** is not marketed in the USA but is used in many other countries, especially for infantile spasms and myoclonic seizures. It is less potent than clonazepam, and superiority to that drug has not been documented.

Clorazepate dipotassium is approved in the USA as an adjunct to treatment of complex partial seizures in adults. Drowsiness and lethargy are common adverse effects, but as long as the drug is increased gradually, dosages as high as 45 mg/d can be given.

Clobazam is not available in the USA but is marketed in most countries and is widely used in a variety of seizure types. It is a 1,5-benzodiazepine (other marketed benzodiazepines are 1,4-benzodiazepines) and reportedly has less sedative potential than benzodiazepines marketed in the USA. Whether the drug has significant clinical advantages is not clear. It has a half-life of 18 hours and is effective at dosages of 0.5–1 mg/kg/d. It does interact with some other antiseizure drugs and causes adverse effects typical of the benzodiazepines; efficacy, in some patients, is limited by the development of tolerance. It has an active metabolite, norclobazam.

Pharmacokinetics

See Chapter 22.

Limitations

Two prominent aspects of benzodiazepines limit their usefulness. The first is their pronounced sedative effect, which is unfortunate both in the treatment of status epilepticus and in chronic therapy. Children may manifest a paradoxical hyperactivity, as with barbiturates. The second problem is tolerance, in which seizures may respond initially but recur within a few months. The remarkable antiseizure potency of these compounds often cannot be realized because of these limiting factors.

ACETAZOLAMIDE

Acetazolamide is a diuretic whose main action is the inhibition of carbonic anhydrase (see Chapter 15). Mild acidosis in the brain may be the mechanism by which the drug exerts its antiseizure activity; alternatively, the depolarizing action of bicarbonate ions moving out of neurons via GABA receptor ion channels may be diminished by carbonic anhydrase inhibition. Acetazolamide has been used for all types of seizures but is severely limited by the rapid development of tolerance, with return of seizures usually within a few weeks. The drug may have a special role in epileptic women who experience seizure exacerbations at the time of menses; seizure control may be improved and tolerance may not develop because the drug is not administered continuously. The usual dosage is approximately 10 mg/kg/d to a maximum of 1000 mg/d.

Another carbonic anhydrase inhibitor, **sulthiame,** was not found to be effective as an anticonvulsant in clinical trials in the USA. It is marketed in a number of other countries.

■ CLINICAL PHARMACOLOGY OF ANTISEIZURE DRUGS

SEIZURE CLASSIFICATION

In general, the type of medication used for epilepsy depends on the empiric nature of the seizure. For this reason, considerable effort has been expended to classify seizures so that clinicians will be able to make a "seizure diagnosis" and on that basis prescribe appropriate therapy. Errors in seizure diagnosis cause use of the wrong drugs, and an unpleasant cycle ensues in which poor seizure control is followed by increasing drug doses and medication toxicity. As noted, seizures are divided into two groups: partial and generalized. Drugs used for partial seizures are more or less the same for all subtypes of partial seizures, but drugs used for generalized seizures are determined by the individual seizure subtype. A summary of the international classification of epileptic seizures is presented in Table 24–1.

Partial Seizures

Partial seizures are those in which a localized onset of the attack can be ascertained, either by clinical observation or by electroencephalographic recording; the attack begins in a specific locus in the brain. There are three types of partial seizures, determined to some extent by the degree of brain involvement by the abnormal discharge.

The least complicated partial seizure is the **simple partial seizure,** characterized by minimal spread of the abnormal discharge such that normal consciousness and awareness are preserved. For example, the patient may have a sudden onset of clonic jerking of an extremity lasting 60–90 seconds; residual weakness may last for 15–30 minutes after the attack. The patient is completely aware of the attack and can describe it in detail. The electroencephalogram may show an abnormal discharge highly localized to the involved portion of the brain.

The **complex partial seizure** also has a localized onset, but the discharge becomes more widespread (usually bilateral) and almost always involves the limbic system. Most complex partial seizures arise from one of the temporal lobes, possibly because of the susceptibility of this area of the brain to insults such as hypoxia or infection. Clinically, the patient may have a brief warning followed by an alteration of consciousness during which some patients stare and others stagger or even fall. Most, however, demonstrate fragments of integrated motor behavior called **automatisms** for which the patient has no memory. Typical automatisms are lip smacking, swallowing, fumbling, scratching, and even walking about. After 30–120 seconds, the patient makes a gradual recovery to normal consciousness but may feel tired or ill for several hours after the attack.

The last type of partial seizure is the **secondarily generalized attack,** in which a partial seizure immediately precedes a generalized tonic-clonic (grand mal) seizure. This seizure type is described in the text that follows.

Generalized Seizures

Generalized seizures are those in which there is no evidence of localized onset. The group is quite heterogeneous.

Generalized tonic-clonic (grand mal) seizures are the most dramatic of all epileptic seizures and are characterized by tonic rigidity of all extremities, followed in 15–30 seconds by a tremor that is actually an interruption of the tonus by relaxation. As the relaxation phases become longer, the attack enters the clonic phase, with massive jerking of the body. The clonic jerking slows over 60–120 seconds, and the patient is usually left in a stuporous state. The tongue or cheek may be bitten, and urinary incontinence is common. Primary generalized tonic-clonic seizures begin without evidence of localized onset, whereas secondary generalized tonic-clonic seizures are preceded by another seizure type, usually a partial seizure. The medical treatment of both primary and secondary generalized tonic-clonic seizures is the same and uses drugs appropriate for *partial* seizures.

The **absence (petit mal) seizure** is characterized by both sudden onset and abrupt cessation. Its duration is usually less than 10 seconds and rarely more than 45 seconds. Consciousness is altered; the attack may also be associated with mild clonic jerking of the eyelids or extremities, with postural tone changes, autonomic phenomena, and automatisms. The occurrence of automatisms can complicate the clinical differentiation from complex partial seizures in some patients. Absence attacks begin in childhood or adolescence and may occur up to hundreds of times a day. The electroencephalogram during the seizure shows a highly

characteristic 2.5–3.5 Hz spike-and-wave pattern. Atypical absence patients have seizures with postural changes that are more abrupt, and such patients are often mentally retarded; the electroencephalogram may show a slower spike-and-wave discharge, and the seizures may be more refractory to therapy.

Myoclonic jerking is seen, to a greater or lesser extent, in a wide variety of seizures, including generalized tonic-clonic seizures, partial seizures, absence seizures, and infantile spasms. Treatment of seizures that include myoclonic jerking should be directed at the primary seizure type rather than at the myoclonus. Some patients, however, have myoclonic jerking as the major seizure type, and some have frequent myoclonic jerking and occasional generalized tonic-clonic seizures without overt signs of neurologic deficit. Many kinds of myoclonus exist, and much effort has gone into attempts to classify this entity.

Atonic seizures are those in which the patient has sudden loss of postural tone. If standing, the patient falls suddenly to the floor and may be injured. If seated, the head and torso may suddenly drop forward. Although most often seen in children, this seizure type is not unusual in adults. Many patients with atonic seizures wear helmets to prevent head injury. Momentary *increased* tone may be observed in some patients, hence the use of the term "tonic-atonic seizure."

Infantile spasms are an epileptic syndrome and not a seizure type. The attacks, though sometimes fragmentary, are most often bilateral and are included for pragmatic purposes with the generalized seizures. These attacks are most often characterized clinically by brief, recurrent myoclonic jerks of the body with sudden flexion or extension of the body and limbs; the forms of infantile spasms are, however, quite heterogeneous. Ninety percent of affected patients have their first attack before the age of 1 year. Most patients are intellectually delayed, presumably from the same cause as the spasms. The cause is unknown in many patients, but such widely disparate disorders as infection, kernicterus, tuberous sclerosis, and hypoglycemia have been implicated. In some cases, the electroencephalogram is characteristic. Drugs used to treat infantile spasms are effective only in some patients; there is little evidence that the cognitive retardation is alleviated by therapy, even when the attacks disappear.

THERAPEUTIC STRATEGY

In designing a therapeutic strategy, the use of a single drug is preferred, especially in patients who are not severely affected and who can benefit from the advantage of fewer adverse effects using monotherapy. For patients with hard-to-control seizures, multiple drugs are usually utilized simultaneously.

For most of the older antiseizure drugs, relationships between blood levels and therapeutic effects have been characterized to a high degree. The same is true for the pharmacokinetics of these drugs. These relationships provide significant advantages in the development of therapeutic strategies for the treatment of epilepsy. The therapeutic index for most antiseizure drugs is low, and toxicity is not uncommon. Thus, effective treatment of seizures often requires an awareness of the therapeutic levels and pharmacokinetic

TABLE 24–2 Serum concentrations reference ranges for some antiseizure drugs.

Antiseizure Drug	Reference Range (μmol/L)[1]	Conversion Factor (F)[2]
OLDER DRUGS		
Carbamazepine	15–45	4.23
Clobazam	0.1–1.0	3.32
Clonazepam	60–220 nmol/L	3.17
Ethosuximide	300–600	7.08
Phenytoin	40–80	3.96
Phenobarbital	50–130	4.31
Valproate	300–600	7.08
NEWER DRUGS (Post-1990)		
Felbamate	125–250	4.20
Gabapentin	70–120	5.83
Lamotrigine	10–60	3.90
Levetiracetam	30–240	5.88
Oxcarbazepine[3]	50–140	3.96
Pregabalin[4]	1–50	6.33
Tiagabine	50–250 nmol/L	2.43
Topiramate	15–60	2.95
Zonisamide	45–180	4.71

[1] These data are provided only as a general guideline. Many patients will respond better at different levels and some patients may have drug-related adverse events within the listed average therapeutic ranges.
[2] To convert to mcg/mL or mg/L, divide μmol/L by the conversion factor F.
[3] Monohydroxy- metabolite.
[4] Not well established.

Modified and updated, with permission, from Johannessen SI, Landmark CJ: Value of therapeutic drug monitoring in epilepsy. Expert Rev Neurother 2008;8: 929.

properties as well as the characteristic toxicities of each agent. Measurements of antiseizure drug plasma levels can be very useful when combined with clinical observations and pharmacokinetic data (Table 24–2). The relationship between seizure control and plasma drug levels is variable and often less clear for the drugs marketed since 1990.

MANAGEMENT OF EPILEPSY

PARTIAL SEIZURES & GENERALIZED TONIC-CLONIC SEIZURES

For many years, the choice of drugs for partial and tonic-clonic seizures was usually limited to phenytoin, carbamazepine, or barbiturates. There was a strong tendency to limit the use of sedative antiseizure drugs such as barbiturates and benzodiazepines to patients who could not tolerate other medications; this trend led, in the 1980s, to increased use of carbamazepine. Although carbamazepine and phenytoin remain widely used, most newer drugs (marketed after 1990) are effective against these same seizure types. With the older drugs, efficacy and long-term adverse effects are well established; this creates a confidence level in spite of

questionable tolerability. Most newer drugs have a broader spectrum of activity, and many are well tolerated; therefore, the newer drugs are often preferred to the older ones. Although some data suggest that most of these newer drugs confer an increased risk of nontraumatic fractures, choosing a drug on this basis is not yet practical.

GENERALIZED SEIZURES

The issues (described above) related to choosing between old and new drugs apply to the generalized group of seizures as well.

The drugs used for generalized tonic-clonic seizures are the same as for partial seizures; in addition, valproate is clearly useful.

At least three drugs are effective against absence seizures. Two are nonsedating and therefore preferred: ethosuximide and valproate. Clonazepam is also highly effective but has disadvantages of dose-related adverse effects and development of tolerance. Lamotrigine and topiramate may also be useful.

Specific myoclonic syndromes are usually treated with valproate; an intravenous formulation can be used acutely if needed. It is nonsedating and can be dramatically effective. Other patients respond to clonazepam, nitrazepam, or other benzodiazepines, although high doses may be necessary, with accompanying drowsiness. Zonisamide and levetiracetam may be useful. Another specific myoclonic syndrome, juvenile myoclonic epilepsy, can be aggravated by phenytoin or carbamazepine; valproate is the drug of choice followed by lamotrigine and topiramate.

Atonic seizures are often refractory to all available medications, although some reports suggest that valproate may be beneficial, as may lamotrigine. Benzodiazepines have been reported to improve seizure control in some of these patients but may worsen the attacks in others. Felbamate has been demonstrated to be effective in some patients, although the drug's idiosyncratic toxicity limits its use. If the loss of tone appears to be part of another seizure type (eg, absence or complex partial seizures), every effort should be made to treat the other seizure type vigorously, hoping for simultaneous alleviation of the atonic component of the seizure. The ketogenic diet may also be useful.

DRUGS USED IN INFANTILE SPASMS

The treatment of infantile spasms is unfortunately limited to improvement of control of the seizures rather than other features of the disorder, such as retardation. Most patients receive a course of intramuscular corticotropin, although some clinicians note that prednisone may be equally effective and can be given orally. Clinical trials have been unable to settle the matter. In either case, therapy must often be discontinued because of adverse effects. If seizures recur, repeat courses of corticotropin or corticosteroids can be given, or other drugs may be tried. A repository corticotropin for injection is now approved in the USA for the treatment of infantile spasms, either of cryptogenic or symptomatic etiology. Other drugs widely used are the benzodiazepines such as clonazepam or nitrazepam; their efficacy in this heterogeneous syndrome may be nearly as good as that of corticosteroids. Vigabatrin is effective and is considered the drug of choice by many pediatric neurologists. The mechanism of action of corticosteroids or corticotropin in the treatment of infantile spasms is unknown but may involve reduction in inflammatory processes.

STATUS EPILEPTICUS

There are many forms of status epilepticus. The most common, generalized tonic-clonic status epilepticus, is a life-threatening emergency, requiring immediate cardiovascular, respiratory, and metabolic management as well as pharmacologic therapy. The latter virtually always requires intravenous administration of antiseizure medications. Diazepam is the most effective drug in most patients for stopping the attacks and is given directly by intravenous push to a maximum total dose of 20–30 mg in adults. Intravenous diazepam may depress respiration (less frequently, cardiovascular function), and facilities for resuscitation must be immediately at hand during its administration. The effect of diazepam is not lasting, but the 30- to 40-minute seizure-free interval allows more definitive therapy to be initiated. Some physicians prefer lorazepam, which is equivalent to diazepam in effect and perhaps somewhat longer acting. For patients who are not actually in the throes of a seizure, diazepam therapy can be omitted and the patient treated at once with a long-acting drug such as phenytoin.

Until the introduction of fosphenytoin, the mainstay of continuing therapy for status epilepticus was intravenous phenytoin, which is effective and nonsedating. It can be given as a loading dose of 13–18 mg/kg in adults; the usual error is to give too little. Administration should be at a maximum rate of 50 mg/min. It is safest to give the drug directly by intravenous push, but it can also be diluted in saline; it precipitates rapidly in the presence of glucose. Careful monitoring of cardiac rhythm and blood pressure is necessary, especially in elderly people. At least part of the cardiotoxicity is from the propylene glycol in which the phenytoin is dissolved. Fosphenytoin, which is freely soluble in intravenous solutions without the need for propylene glycol or other solubilizing agents, is a safer parenteral agent. Because of its greater molecular weight, this prodrug is two thirds to three quarters as potent as phenytoin on a milligram basis.

In previously treated epileptic patients, the administration of a large loading dose of phenytoin may cause some dose-related toxicity such as ataxia. This is usually a relatively minor problem during the acute status episode and is easily alleviated by later adjustment of plasma levels.

For patients who do not respond to phenytoin, phenobarbital can be given in large doses: 100–200 mg intravenously to a total of 400–800 mg. Respiratory depression is a common complication, especially if benzodiazepines have already been given, and there should be no hesitation in instituting intubation and ventilation.

Although other drugs such as lidocaine have been recommended for the treatment of generalized tonic-clonic status epilepticus, general anesthesia is usually necessary in highly resistant cases.

For patients in absence status, benzodiazepines are still drugs of first choice. Rarely, intravenous valproate may be required.

SPECIAL ASPECTS OF THE TOXICOLOGY OF ANTISEIZURE DRUGS

TERATOGENICITY

The potential teratogenicity of antiseizure drugs is controversial and important. It is important because teratogenicity resulting from long-term drug treatment of millions of people throughout the world may have a profound effect even if the effect occurs in only a small percentage of cases. It is controversial because both epilepsy and antiseizure drugs are heterogeneous, and few epileptic patients are available for study who are not receiving these drugs. Furthermore, patients with severe epilepsy, in whom genetic factors rather than drug factors may be of greater importance in the occurrence of fetal malformations, are often receiving multiple antiseizure drugs in high doses.

In spite of these limitations, it appears—from whatever cause—that children born to mothers taking antiseizure drugs have an increased risk, perhaps twofold, of congenital malformations. Phenytoin has been implicated in a specific syndrome called **fetal hydantoin syndrome,** although not all investigators are convinced of its existence and a similar syndrome has been attributed both to phenobarbital and to carbamazepine. Valproate, as noted above, has also been implicated in a specific malformation, spina bifida. It is estimated that a pregnant woman taking valproic acid or sodium valproate has a 1–2% risk of having a child with spina bifida. Topiramate has shown some teratogenicity in animal testing and, as noted earlier, in the human male fetus.

In dealing with the clinical problem of a pregnant woman with epilepsy, most epileptologists agree that although it is important to minimize exposure to antiseizure drugs, both in numbers and dosages, it is also important not to allow maternal seizures to go unchecked.

WITHDRAWAL

Withdrawal of antiseizure drugs, whether by accident or by design, can cause increased seizure frequency and severity. The two factors to consider are the effects of the withdrawal itself and the need for continued drug suppression of seizures in the individual patient. In many patients, both factors must be considered. It is important to note, however, that the abrupt discontinuance of antiseizure drugs ordinarily does not cause seizures in nonepileptic patients, provided that the drug levels are not above the usual therapeutic range when the drug is stopped.

Some drugs are more easily withdrawn than others. In general, withdrawal of anti-absence drugs is easier than withdrawal of drugs needed for partial or generalized tonic-clonic seizures. Barbiturates and benzodiazepines are the most difficult to discontinue; weeks or months may be required, with very gradual dosage decrements, to accomplish their complete outpatient removal.

Because of the heterogeneity of epilepsy, complete discontinuance of antiseizure drug administration is an especially difficult problem. If a patient is seizure-free for 3 or 4 years, a trial of gradual discontinuance is often warranted.

OVERDOSE

Antiseizure drugs are central nervous system depressants but are rarely lethal. Very high blood levels are usually necessary before overdoses can be considered life-threatening. The most dangerous effect of antiseizure drugs after large overdoses is respiratory depression, which may be potentiated by other agents, such as alcohol. Treatment of antiseizure drug overdose is supportive; stimulants should not be used. Efforts to hasten removal of antiseizure drugs, such as alkalinization of the urine (phenytoin is a weak acid), are usually ineffective.

SUICIDALITY

An FDA analysis of suicidal behavior during clinical trials of antiseizure drugs was carried out in 2008. The presence of either suicidal behavior or suicidal ideation was 0.37% in patients taking active drugs and 0.24% in patients taking placebo. This, according to one analyst, represents an additional 2 of 1000 patients with such thoughts or behaviors. It is noteworthy that, although the entire class may receive some changes in labeling, the odds ratios for carbamazepine and for valproate were less than 1, and no data were available for phenytoin. Whether this effect is real or inextricably associated with this serious, debilitating disorder—with its inherently high rate of suicidality—is unclear.

SUMMARY Antiseizure Drugs

Subclass	Mechanism of Action	Pharmacokinetics	Clinical Applications	Toxicities, Interactions
CYCLIC UREIDES				
• Phenytoin, fosphenytoin	Block high-frequency firing of neurons through action on voltage-gated (VG) Na$^+$ channels • decreases synaptic release of glutamate	Absorption is formulation dependent • highly bound to plasma proteins • no active metabolites • dose-dependent elimination, $t_{1/2}$ 12–36 h • fosphenytoin is for IV, IM routes	Generalized tonic-clonic seizures, partial seizures	*Toxicity:* Diplopia, ataxia, gingival hyperplasia, hirsutism, neuropathy • *Interactions:* Phenobarbital, carbamazepine, isoniazid, felbamate, oxcarbazepine, topiramate, fluoxetine, fluconazole, digoxin, quinidine, cyclosporine, steroids, oral contraceptives, others
• Primidone	Similar to phenytoin but converted to phenobarbital	Well absorbed orally • not highly bound to plasma proteins • peak concentrations in 2–6 h • $t_{1/2}$ 10–25 h • two active metabolites (phenobarbital and phenylethylmalonamide)	Generalized tonic-clonic seizures, partial seizures	*Toxicity:* Sedation, cognitive issues, ataxia, hyperactivity • *Interactions:* Similar to phenobarbital
• Phenobarbital	Enhances phasic GABA$_A$ receptor responses • reduces excitatory synaptic responses	Nearly complete absorption • not significantly bound to plasma proteins • peak concentrations in 0.5–4 h • no active metabolites • $t_{1/2}$ varies from 75 to 125 h	Generalized tonic-clonic seizures, partial seizures, myoclonic seizures, generalized seizures, neonatal seizures, status epilepticus	*Toxicity:* Sedation, cognitive issues, ataxia, hyperactivity • *Interactions:* Valproate, carbamazepine, felbamate, phenytoin, cyclosporine, felodipine, lamotrigine, nifedipine, nimodipine, steroids, theophylline, verapamil, others
• Ethosuximide	Reduces low-threshold Ca^{2+} currents (T-type)	Well absorbed orally, with peak levels in 3–7 h • not protein-bound • completely metabolized to inactive compounds • $t_{1/2}$ typically 40 h	Absence seizures	*Toxicity:* Nausea, headache, dizziness, hyperactivity • *Interactions:* Valproate, phenobarbital, phenytoin, carbamazepine, rifampicin
TRICYCLICS				
• Carbamazepine	Blocks high-frequency firing of neurons through action on VG Na$^+$ channels • decreases synaptic release of glutamate	Well absorbed orally, with peak levels in 6–8 h • no significant protein binding • metabolized in part to active 10-11-epoxide • $t_{1/2}$ of parent ranges from 8 to 12 h in treated patients to 36 h in normal subjects	Generalized tonic-clonic seizures, partial seizures	*Toxicity:* Nausea, diplopia, ataxia, hyponatremia, headache • *Interactions:* Phenytoin, carbamazepine, valproate, fluoxetine, verapamil, macrolide antibiotics, isoniazid, propoxyphene, danazol, phenobarbital, primidone, many others

• *Oxcarbazepine: Similar to carbamazepine; shorter half-life but active metabolite with longer duration and fewer interactions reported*
• *Eslicarbazepine acetate: Similar to oxcarbazepine but shown to be effective when given once daily and may be more rapidly converted to the active metabolite*

BENZODIAZEPINES				
• Diazepam	Potentiates GABA$_A$ responses	Well absorbed orally • rectal administration gives peak concentration in ~1 h with 90% bioavailability • IV for status epilepticus • highly protein-bound • extensively metabolized to several active metabolites • $t_{1/2}$ ~2 d	Status epilepticus, seizure clusters	*Toxicity:* Sedation • *Interactions:* Minimal
• Clonazepam	As for diazepam	>80% bioavailability • extensively metabolized but no active metabolites • $t_{1/2}$ 20–50 h	Absence seizures, myoclonic seizures, infantile spasms	*Toxicity:* Similar to diazepam • *Interactions:* Minimal

• *Lorazepam: Similar to diazepam*
• *Clobazam: Indications include absence seizures, myoclonic seizures, infantile spasms*

(continued)

Subclass	Mechanism of Action	Pharmacokinetics	Clinical Applications	Toxicities, Interactions
GABA DERIVATIVES				
• Gabapentin	Decreases excitatory transmission by acting on VG Ca^{2+} channels presynaptically ($\alpha_2\delta$ subunit)	Bioavailability 50%, decreasing with increasing doses • not bound to plasma proteins • not metabolized • $t_{1/2}$ 6–8 h	Generalized tonic-clonic seizures, partial seizures, generalized seizures	*Toxicity:* Somnolence, dizziness, ataxia • *Interactions:* Minimal
• Pregabalin	As for gabapentin	Well absorbed orally • not bound to plasma proteins • not metabolized • $t_{1/2}$ 6–7 h	Partial seizures	*Toxicity:* Somnolence, dizziness, ataxia • *Interactions:* Minimal
• Vigabatrin	Irreversibly inhibits GABA-transaminase	70% bioavailable • not bound to plasma proteins • not metabolized, $t_{1/2}$ 5–7 h (not relevant because of mechanism of action)	Partial seizures, infantile spasms	*Toxicity:* Drowsiness, dizziness, psychosis, visual field loss • *Interactions:* Minimal
OTHER				
• Valproate	Blocks high-frequency firing of neurons • modifies amino acid metabolism	Well absorbed from several formulations • highly bound to plasma proteins • extensively metabolized • $t_{1/2}$ 9–16 h	Generalized tonic-clonic seizures, partial seizures, generalized seizures, absence seizures, myoclonic seizures	*Toxicity:* Nausea, tremor, weight gain, hair loss, teratogenic, hepatotoxic • *Interactions:* Phenobarbital, phenytoin, carbamazepine, lamotrigine, felbamate, rifampin, ethosuximide, primidone
• Lamotrigine	Prolongs inactivation of VG Na^+ channels • acts presynaptically on VG Ca^{2+} channels, decreasing glutamate release	Well absorbed orally • no significant protein binding • extensively metabolized, but no active metabolites • $t_{1/2}$ 25–35 h	Generalized tonic-clonic seizures, generalized seizures, partial seizures, absence seizures	*Toxicity:* Dizziness, headache, diplopia, rash • *Interactions:* Valproate, carbamazepine, oxcarbazepine, phenytoin, phenobarbital, primidone, succinimides, sertraline, topiramate
• Levetiracetam	Action on synaptic protein SV_2A	Well absorbed orally • not bound to plasma proteins • metabolized to 3 inactive metabolites • $t_{1/2}$ 6–11 h	Generalized tonic-clonic seizures, partial seizures, generalized seizures	*Toxicity:* Nervousness, dizziness, depression, seizures • *Interactions:* Rare
• Retigabine	Enhances K^+ channel opening	Readily absorbed • requires 3-times daily dosing	Adjunctive treatment of partial seizures	*Toxicity:* Dizziness, somnolence, confusion, blurred vision • *Interactions:* minimal
• Rufinamide	Prolongs inactivation of VG Na^+ channels	Well absorbed orally • peak concentrations in 4–6 h • $t_{1/2}$ 6–10 h • minimal plasma protein binding • no active metabolites • mostly excreted in urine	Adjunctive treatment of the Lennox-Gastaut syndrome	*Toxicity:* Somnolence, vomiting, pyrexia, diarrhea • *Interactions:* Not metabolized via P450 enzymes, but antiseizure drug interactions may be present
• Tiagabine	Blocks GABA reuptake in forebrain by selective blockade of GAT-1	Well absorbed • highly bound to plasma proteins • extensively metabolized, but no active metabolites • $t_{1/2}$ 4–8 h	Partial seizures	*Toxicity:* Nervousness, dizziness, depression, seizures • *Interactions:* Phenobarbital, phenytoin, carbamazepine, primidone
• Topiramate	Multiple actions on synaptic function, probably via actions on phosphorylation	Well absorbed • not bound to plasma proteins • extensively metabolized, but 40% excreted unchanged in the urine • no active metabolites • $t_{1/2}$ 20 h, but decreases with concomitant drugs	Generalized tonic-clonic seizures, partial seizures, generalized seizures, absence seizures, migraine	*Toxicity:* Somnolence, cognitive slowing, confusion, paresthesias • *Interactions:* Phenytoin, carbamazepine, oral contraceptives, lamotrigine, lithium?
• Zonisamide	Blocks high-frequency firing via action on VG Na^+ channels	Approximately 70% bioavailable orally • minimally bound to plasma proteins • >50% metabolized • $t_{1/2}$ 50–70 h	Generalized tonic-clonic seizures, partial seizures, myoclonic seizures	*Toxicity:* Drowsiness, cognitive impairment, confusion, poor concentration • *Interactions:* Minimal
• Lacosamide	Enhances slow inactivation of Na^+ channels • blocks effect of neurotrophins (via CRMP-2)	Well absorbed • minimal protein binding • one major nonactive metabolite • $t_{1/2}$ 12–14 h	Generalized tonic-clonic seizures, partial seizures	*Toxicity:* Dizziness, headache, nausea • small increase in PR interval • *Interactions:* Minimal

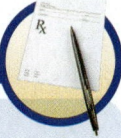

PREPARATIONS AVAILABLE

Carbamazepine (generic, Tegretol)
Oral: 200 mg tablets; 100 mg chewable tablets; 100 mg/5 mL suspension
Oral extended-release: 100, 200, 400 mg tablets; 200, 300 mg capsules

Clonazepam (generic, Klonopin)
Oral: 0.5, 1, 2 mg tablets

Clorazepate dipotassium (generic, Tranxene)
Oral: 3.75, 7.5, 15 mg tablets, capsules
Oral sustained-release (Tranxene-SD): 11.25, 22.5 mg tablets

Diazepam (generic, Valium, others)
Oral: 2, 5, 10 mg tablets; 5 mg/5 mL, 5 mg/mL solutions
Parenteral: 5 mg/mL for IV injection
Rectal: 2.5, 5, 10, 15, 20 mg viscous rectal solution

Eslicarbazepine (Stedesa)
Oral: 400 mg tablets

Ethosuximide (generic, Zarontin)
Oral: 250 mg capsules; 250 mg/5 mL syrup

Ethotoin (Peganone)
Oral: 250, 500 mg tablets

Felbamate (Felbatol)
Oral: 400, 600 mg tablets; 600 mg/5 mL suspension

Fosphenytoin (Cerebyx)
Parenteral: 75 mg/mL for IV or IM injection

Gabapentin (Neurontin)
Oral: 100, 300, 400 mg capsules; 600, 800 mg filmtabs; 50 mg/mL solution

Lacosamide (Vimpat)
Oral: 50, 100, 150, 200, 300 mg tablets, 15 mg/mL solution
Parenteral: 10 mg/mL for IV injection

Lamotrigine (generic, Lamictal)
Oral: 25, 100, 150, 200 mg tablets; 2, 5, 25 mg chewable tablets

Levetiracetam (generic, Keppra)
Oral: 250, 500, 750, 1000 mg tablets, 100 mg/mL solution
Parenteral: 100 mg/mL for injection

Lorazepam (generic, Ativan)
Oral: 0.5, 1, 2 mg tablets; 2 mg/mL solution
Parenteral: 2, 4 mg/mL for IV or IM injection

Mephenytoin (Mesantoin)
Oral: 100 mg tablets

Mephobarbital (Mebaral)
Oral: 32, 50, 100 mg tablets

Methsuximide (Celontin)
Oral: 150, 300 mg capsules

Oxcarbazepine (Trileptal)
Oral: 100, 300, 600 mg tablets; 60 mg/mL suspension

Pentobarbital sodium (generic, Nembutal)
Parenteral: 50 mg/mL for IV or IM injection

Phenobarbital (generic, Luminal Sodium, others)
Oral: 15, 16, 30, 60, 90, 100 mg tablets; 16 mg capsules; 15, 20 mg/5 mL elixirs
Parenteral: 30, 60, 65, 130 mg/mL for IV or IM injection

Phenytoin (generic, Dilantin, others)
Oral (prompt release): 100 mg capsules; 50 mg chewable tablets; 125 mg/5 mL suspension
Oral extended action: 30, 100 mg capsules
Oral slow release (Phenytek): 200, 300 mg capsules
Parenteral: 50 mg/mL for IV injection

Pregabalin (Lyrica)
Oral: 25, 50, 75, 100, 150, 200, 300 mg capsules

Primidone (generic, Mysoline)
Oral: 50, 250 mg tablets; 250 mg/5 mL suspension

Retigabine (Trobalt in Europe; ezogabine, Potiga in the USA)

Rufinamide (Banzel)
Oral: 200, 400 mg tablets

Stiripentol (Diacomit)
Oral: 250, 500 mg capsules

Tiagabine (Gabitril)
Oral: 2, 4, 12, 16, 20 mg tablets

Topiramate (Topamax)
Oral: 25, 50, 100, 200 mg tablets; 15, 25 mg sprinkle capsules

Trimethadione (Tridione)
Oral: 150 mg chewable tablets; 300 mg capsules; 40 mg/mL solution

Valproic acid (generic, Depakene)
Oral: 250 mg capsules; 250 mg/5 mL syrup (sodium valproate)
Oral sustained-release (Depakote): 125, 250, 500 mg tablets (as divalproex sodium)
Parenteral (Depacon): 100 mg/mL in 5 mL vial for IV injection

Vigabatrin (Sabril)
Oral: 500 mg tablets; 500 mg powder for solution

Zonisamide (generic, Zonegran)
Oral: 25, 50, 100 mg tablets

REFERENCES

Arroyo S: Rufinamide. Neurotherapeutics 2007;4:155.

Avorn J: Drug warnings that can cause fits—communicating risks in a data-poor environment. N Engl J Med 2008;359:991.

Bialer M: Progress report on new antiepileptic drugs: A summary of the tenth EILAT conference (EILAT X). Epilepsy Res 2010;92:89.

Brodie MJ et al: Rufinamide for the adjunctive treatment of partial seizures in adults and adolescents: A randomized placebo-controlled trial. Epilepsia 2009;50:1899.

Cross SA, Curran MP: Lacosamide in partial onset seizures. Drugs 2009;69:449.

Ettinger AB, Argoff CE: Use of antiepileptic drugs for non-epileptic conditions: Psychiatric disorders and chronic pain. Neurotherapeutics 2007;4:75.

Faught, E. Ezogabine: A new angle on potassium gates. Epilepsy Currents, 2011; 11:75.

French JA et al: Historical control monotherapy design in the treatment of epilepsy. Epilepsia 2010;51:1936.

Glauser TA et al: Ethosuximide, valproic acid, and lamotrigine in childhood absence epilepsy. N Engl J Med 2010;362:790.

Kaminski RM et al: SV2A is a broad-spectrum anticonvulsant target: Functional correlation between protein binding and seizure protection in models of both partial and generalized epilepsy. Neuropharmacol 2008;54:715.

Kobayashi T et al: Inhibitory effects of the antiepileptic drug ethosuximide on G-protein-activated inwardly rectifying K+ channels. Neuropharmacol 2009;56:499.

Meldrum BS, Rogawski MA: Molecular targets for antiepileptic drug development. Neurotherapeutics 2007;4:18.

Molgaard-Nielsen D, Hviid A: Newer-generation antiepileptic drugs and the risk of major birth defects. JAMA 2011;305:1996.

Porter RJ et al: Clinical development of drugs for epilepsy: A review of approaches in the United States and Europe. Epilepsy Research 2010;89:163.

General Anesthetics

Helge Eilers, MD, &
Spencer Yost, MD

CASE STUDY

An elderly man with type 2 diabetes mellitus and ischemic pain in the lower extremity is scheduled for femoral-to-popliteal bypass surgery. He has a history of hypertension and coronary artery disease with symptoms of stable angina and can walk only half a block before pain in his legs forces him to stop. He has a 50 pack-year smoking history but stopped 2 years ago. His medications include atenolol, atorvastatin, and hydrochlorothiazide. The nurse in the pre-operative holding area obtains the following vital signs: temperature 36.8°C (98.2°F), blood pressure 168/100 mm Hg, heart rate 78 bpm, oxygen saturation by pulse oximeter 96% while breathing room air, pain 5/10 in the right lower leg. What anesthetic agents will you choose and why? Does the choice of anesthetic make a difference?

For centuries, humankind has relied on natural medicines and physical methods to control surgical pain. Historical texts describe the sedative effects of cannabis, henbane, mandrake, and opium poppy. Physical methods such as cold, nerve compression, carotid artery occlusion, and cerebral concussion were also employed, with variable effect. Although surgery was performed under ether anesthesia as early as 1842, the first public demonstration of surgical general anesthesia in 1846 is usually considered to be the start of a new era of anesthesia. For the first time physicians had a reliable means to keep their patients from experiencing pain during surgical procedures.

The neurophysiologic state produced by general anesthetics is characterized by five primary effects: **unconsciousness, amnesia, analgesia, inhibition of autonomic reflexes**, and **skeletal muscle relaxation**. None of the currently available anesthetic agents when used alone can achieve all five of these desired effects. In addition, an ideal anesthetic drug should induce rapid, smooth loss of consciousness, be rapidly reversible upon discontinuation, and possess a wide margin of safety.

The modern practice of anesthesiology relies on the use of combinations of intravenous and inhaled drugs (**balanced anesthesia** techniques) to take advantage of the favorable properties of each agent while minimizing their adverse effects. The choice of anesthetic technique is determined by the type of diagnostic, therapeutic, or surgical intervention to be performed. For minor superficial surgery or for invasive diagnostic procedures, oral or parenteral sedatives can be used in combination with local anesthetics, so-called **monitored anesthesia care** techniques (see Box: Sedation & Monitored Anesthesia Care, and Chapter 26). These techniques provide profound analgesia, with retention of the patient's ability to maintain a patent airway and to respond to verbal commands. For more extensive surgical procedures, anesthesia may begin with preoperative benzodiazepines, be induced with an intravenous agent (eg, thiopental or propofol), and be maintained with a combination of inhaled (eg, volatile agents, nitrous oxide) or intravenous (eg, propofol, opioid analgesics) drugs, or both.

MECHANISM OF GENERAL ANESTHETIC ACTION

General anesthetics have been in clinical use for more than 160 years but their mechanism of action remains unknown. Initial research focused on identifying a single biologic site of action for these drugs. In recent years this "unitary theory" of anesthetic action has been supplanted by a more complex picture of molecular targets located at multiple levels of the central nervous system (CNS).

Anesthetics affect neurons at various cellular locations, but the primary focus has been on the synapse. A presynaptic action may alter the release of neurotransmitters, whereas a postsynaptic effect may change the frequency or amplitude of impulses exiting the synapse. At the organ level, the effect of anesthetics may result from

Sedation & Monitored Anesthesia Care

Many diagnostic and minor therapeutic surgical procedures can be performed without general anesthesia using sedation-based anesthetic techniques. In this setting, regional or local anesthesia supplemented with midazolam or propofol and opioid analgesics (or ketamine) may be a more appropriate and safer approach than general anesthesia for superficial surgical procedures. This anesthetic technique is known as monitored anesthesia care, often abbreviated as MAC, not to be confused with the minimal alveolar concentration for the comparison of potencies of inhaled anesthetics (see text and Box: What Does Anesthesia Represent & Where Does It Work?). The technique typically involves the use of intravenous midazolam for premedication (to provide anxiolysis, amnesia, and mild sedation) followed by a titrated, variable-rate propofol infusion (to provide moderate to deep levels of sedation). A potent opioid analgesic or ketamine may be added to minimize the discomfort associated with the injection of local anesthesia and the surgical manipulations.

Another approach, used primarily by nonanesthesiologists, is called **conscious sedation**. This technique refers to drug-induced alleviation of anxiety and pain in combination with an altered level of consciousness associated with the use of smaller doses of sedative medications. In this state the patient retains the ability to maintain a patent airway and is responsive to verbal commands. A wide variety of intravenous anesthetic drugs have proved to be useful drugs in conscious sedation techniques (eg, diazepam, midazolam, propofol). Use of benzodiazepines and opioid analgesics (eg, fentanyl) in conscious sedation protocols has the advantage of being reversible by the specific receptor antagonist drugs (flumazenil and naloxone, respectively).

A specialized form of sedation is occasionally required in the ICU, when patients are under severe stress and require mechanical ventilation for prolonged periods. In this situation, sedative-hypnotic drugs and low doses of intravenous anesthetics may be combined. Recently, dexmedetomidine has become a popular choice for this indication.

Deep sedation is similar to a light state of general (intravenous) anesthesia involving decreased consciousness from which the patient is not easily aroused. The transition from deep sedation to general anesthesia is fluid, and it is sometimes difficult to clearly determine where the transition is. Because deep sedation is often accompanied by a loss of protective reflexes, an inability to maintain a patent airway, and lack of verbal responsiveness to surgical stimuli, this state may be indistinguishable from intravenous anesthesia. Intravenous agents used in deep sedation protocols mainly include the sedative-hypnotics propofol and midazolam, sometimes in combination with potent opioid analgesics or ketamine, depending on the level of pain associated with the surgery or procedure.

---

strengthening inhibition or from diminishing excitation within the CNS. Studies on isolated spinal cord tissue have demonstrated that excitatory transmission is impaired more strongly by anesthetics than inhibitory effects are potentiated.

Chloride channels (γ-aminobutyric acid-A [GABA$_A$] and glycine receptors) and potassium channels (K$_{2P}$, possibly K$_v$, and K$_{ATP}$ channels) remain the primary *inhibitory* ion channels considered legitimate candidates of anesthetic action. *Excitatory* ion channel targets include those activated by acetylcholine (nicotinic and muscarinic receptors), by excitatory amino acids (amino-3-hydroxy-5-methyl-4-isoxazol-propionic acid [AMPA], kainate, and *N*-methyl-D-aspartate [NMDA] receptors), or by serotonin (5-HT$_2$ and 5-HT$_3$ receptors). Figure 25–1 depicts the relation of these inhibitory and excitatory targets of anesthetics within the context of the nerve terminal.

■ INHALED ANESTHETICS

A clear distinction should be made between volatile and gaseous anesthetics, both of which are administered by inhalation. Volatile anesthetics (halothane, enflurane, isoflurane, desflurane, sevoflurane) have low vapor pressures and thus high boiling points so that they are liquids at room temperature (20°C) and sea-level ambient pressure, whereas gaseous anesthetics (nitrous oxide, xenon) have high vapor pressures and low boiling points such that they are in gas form at room temperature. Figure 25–2 shows the chemical structures of important, clinically used, inhaled anesthetics.

PHARMACOKINETICS

Inhaled anesthetics, volatile as well as gaseous, are taken up through gas exchange in the alveoli. Uptake from the alveoli into the blood and distribution and partitioning into the effect compartments are important determinants of the kinetics of these agents. As previously mentioned, an ideal anesthetic should have a rapid onset (induction), and its effect should be rapidly terminated. To achieve this, the effect site concentration in the CNS (brain and spinal cord) will need to change rapidly. Several factors determine how quickly the CNS concentration changes.

Uptake & Distribution

A. Inspired Concentration and Ventilation

The driving force for uptake of an inhaled anesthetic is the alveolar concentration. Two parameters that can be controlled by the anesthesiologist determine how quickly the alveolar concentration changes: (1) *inspired concentration* or *partial pressure*, and (2) *alveolar ventilation*. The partial pressure of an inhaled anesthetic in the inspired gas mixture directly affects the maximum partial pressure that can be achieved in the alveoli and the rate of increase of

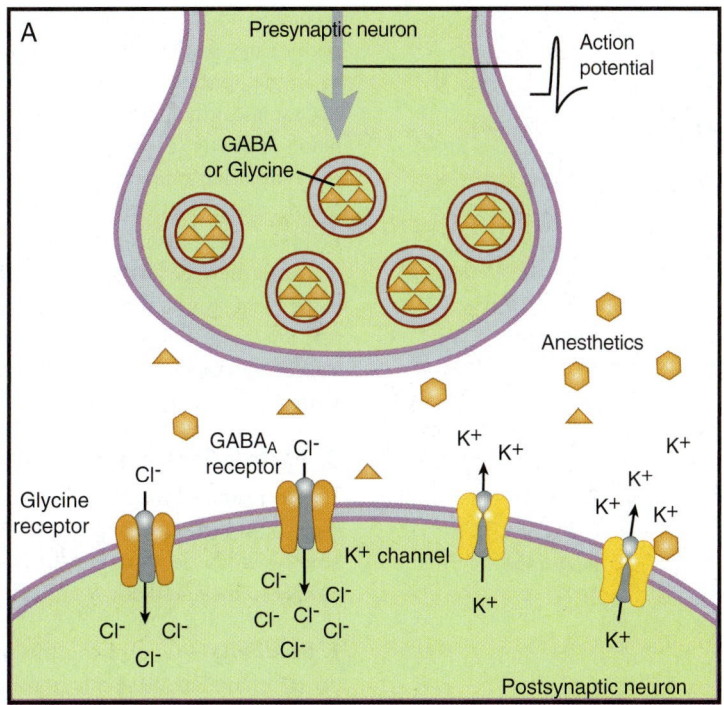

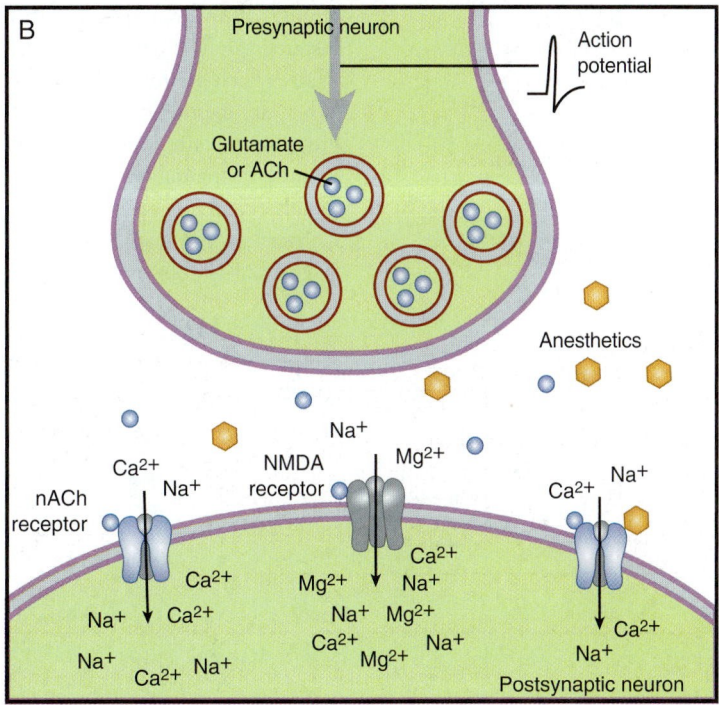

FIGURE 25–1 Putative targets of anesthetic action. Anesthetic drugs may increase inhibitory synaptic activity or diminish excitatory activity. ACh, acetylcholine; GABA$_A$, γ-aminobutyric acid-A.

the partial pressure in the alveoli and, ultimately, the blood. Increases in the inspired partial pressure increase the rate of rise in the alveoli and thus accelerate induction. The increase of partial pressure in the alveoli is usually expressed as a ratio of alveolar concentration (F_A) over inspired concentration (F_I); the faster F_A/F_I

approaches 1 (1 representing the equilibrium), the faster anesthesia will occur during an inhaled induction.

The other parameter that directly controls the rate by which F_A/F_I approaches 1 is alveolar ventilation. An increase in ventilation will increase the rate of rise. The magnitude of the effect varies

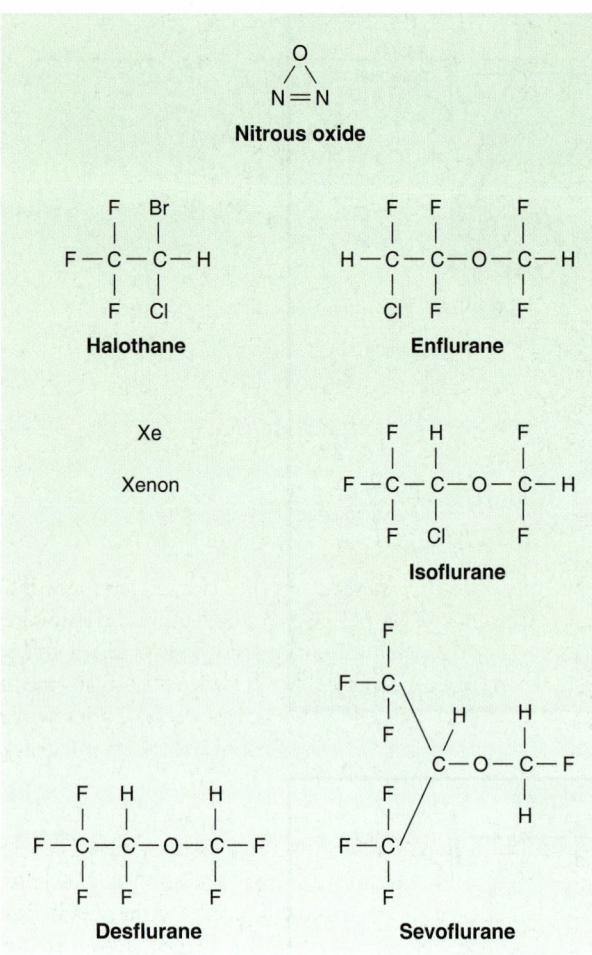

FIGURE 25–2 Chemical structures of inhaled anesthetics.

according to the blood:gas partition coefficient. An increase in pulmonary ventilation is accompanied by only a slight increase in arterial tension of an anesthetic with low blood solubility, but can significantly increase tension of agents with moderate to high blood solubility (Figure 25–3). For example, a fourfold increase in the ventilation rate almost doubles the F_A/F_I ratio for halothane during the first 10 minutes of administration but increases the F_A/F_I ratio for nitrous oxide by only 15%. Thus, hyperventilation increases the speed of induction of anesthesia with inhaled anesthetics that would normally have a slow onset. Depression of respiration by opioid analgesics slows the onset of anesthesia of inhaled anesthetics unless ventilation is manually or mechanically assisted.

B. Factors Controlling Uptake

The increase of F_A/F_I, which is an important determinant of the speed of induction, is opposed by the uptake of anesthetic into the blood, which is determined by pharmacokinetic parameters unique to the anesthetic agent as well as patient factors.

1. Solubility—One of the most important factors influencing the transfer of an anesthetic from the lungs to the arterial blood is its solubility characteristics (Table 25–1). The blood:gas partition coefficient is a useful index of solubility and defines the relative affinity of an anesthetic for the blood compared with that of inspired gas. The partition coefficients for desflurane and nitrous oxide, which are relatively insoluble in blood, are extremely low. When an anesthetic with low blood solubility diffuses from the lung into the arterial blood, relatively few molecules are required to raise its partial pressure; therefore, the arterial tension rises rapidly (Figure 25–4, top; nitrous oxide, desflurane, sevoflurane). Conversely, for anesthetics with moderate to high solubility (Figure 25–4, bottom; halothane, isoflurane), more molecules

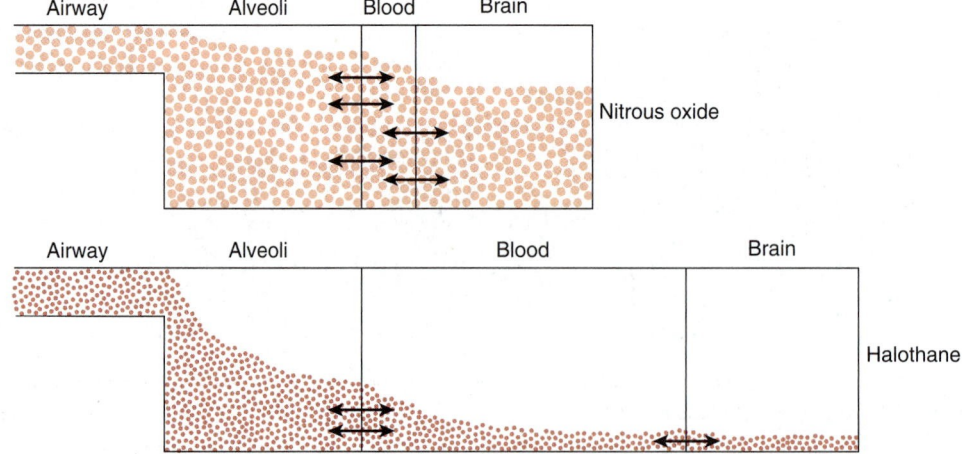

FIGURE 25–3 Why induction of anesthesia is slower with more soluble anesthetic gases. In this schematic diagram, solubility in blood is represented by the relative size of the blood compartment (the more soluble, the larger the compartment). Relative partial pressures of the agents in the compartments are indicated by the degree of filling of each compartment. For a given concentration or partial pressure of the two anesthetic gases in the inspired air, it will take much longer for the blood partial pressure of the more soluble gas (halothane) to rise to the same partial pressure as in the alveoli. Since the concentration of the anesthetic agent in the brain can rise no faster than the concentration in the blood, the onset of anesthesia will be slower with halothane than with nitrous oxide.

TABLE 25–1 Pharmacologic properties of inhaled anesthetics.

Anesthetic	Blood:Gas Partition Coefficient[1]	Brain:Blood Partition Coefficient[1]	Minimal Alveolar Concentration (MAC) (%)[2]	Metabolism	Comments
Nitrous oxide	0.47	1.1	> 100	None	Incomplete anesthetic; rapid onset and recovery
Desflurane	0.42	1.3	6–7	< 0.05%	Low volatility; poor induction agent (pungent); rapid recovery
Sevoflurane	0.69	1.7	2.0	2–5% (fluoride)	Rapid onset and recovery; unstable in soda-lime
Isoflurane	1.40	2.6	1.40	< 2%	Medium rate of onset and recovery
Enflurane	1.80	1.4	1.7	8%	Medium rate of onset and recovery
Halothane	2.30	2.9	0.75	> 40%	Medium rate of onset and recovery

[1] Partition coefficients (at 37°C) are from multiple literature sources.

[2] MAC is the anesthetic concentration that produces immobility in 50% of patients exposed to a noxious stimulus.

dissolve before partial pressure changes significantly, and arterial tension of the gas increases less rapidly. A blood:gas partition coefficient of 0.47 for nitrous oxide means that at equilibrium, the concentration in blood is 0.47 times the concentration in the alveolar space (gas). A larger blood:gas partition coefficient produces a greater uptake of anesthetic and therefore reduces the time required for F_A/F_I to approach 1 (equilibrium, Figure 25–4).

2. Cardiac output—Changes in pulmonary blood flow have obvious effects on the uptake of anesthetic gases from the alveolar space. An increase in pulmonary blood flow (ie, increased cardiac output) will increase the uptake of anesthetic, thereby decreasing the rate by which F_A/F_I rises, which will decrease the rate of induction of anesthesia. To better understand this mechanism, one should think about the effect of cardiac output in combination with the tissue distribution and uptake of anesthetic into other tissue compartments. An increase in cardiac output and pulmonary blood flow will increase uptake of anesthetic into the blood, but the anesthetic taken up will be distributed in all tissues, not just the CNS. Cerebral blood flow is well regulated and the increased cardiac output will therefore increase delivery of anesthetic to other tissues and not the brain.

3. Alveolar-venous partial pressure difference—The anesthetic partial pressure difference between alveolar and mixed venous blood is dependent mainly on uptake of the anesthetic by the tissues, including nonneural tissues. Depending on the rate and extent of tissue uptake, venous blood returning to the lungs may contain significantly less anesthetic than arterial blood. The greater this difference in anesthetic gas tensions, the more time it will take to achieve equilibrium with brain tissue. Anesthetic uptake into tissues is influenced by factors similar to those that determine transfer of the anesthetic from the lung to the intravascular space, including tissue:blood partition coefficients, rates of blood flow to the tissues, and concentration gradients.

During the induction phase of anesthesia (and the initial phase of the maintenance period), the tissues that exert greatest influence on the arteriovenous anesthetic concentration gradient are those that are highly perfused (eg, brain, heart, liver, kidneys, and splanchnic bed). Combined, these tissues receive over 75% of the resting cardiac output. In the case of volatile anesthetics with relatively high solubility in highly perfused tissues, venous blood concentration initially is very low, and equilibrium with the alveolar space is achieved slowly.

During maintenance of anesthesia with inhaled anesthetics, the drug continues to be transferred between various tissues at rates dependent on the solubility of the agent, the concentration gradient between the blood and the tissue, and the tissue blood flow. Although muscle and skin constitute 50% of the total body mass, anesthetics accumulate more slowly in these tissues than in highly perfused tissues (eg, brain) because they receive only one fifth of the resting cardiac output. Although most anesthetic agents are highly soluble in adipose (fatty) tissues, the relatively low blood

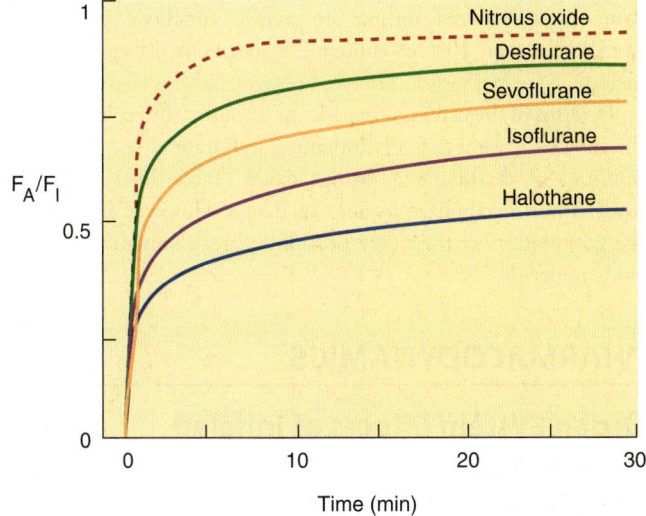

FIGURE 25–4 The alveolar anesthetic concentration (F_A) approaches the inspired anesthetic concentration (F_I) fastest for the least soluble agents.

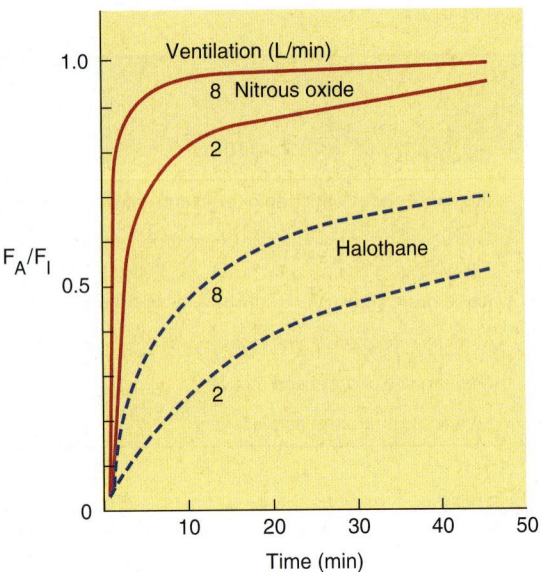

FIGURE 25–5 Effect of ventilation on F_A/F_I. Increased ventilation (8 versus 2 L/min) has a much greater effect on equilibration of halothane than nitrous oxide.

perfusion to these tissues delays accumulation, and equilibrium is unlikely to occur with most anesthetics during a typical 1- to 3-hour operation.

The combined effect of ventilation, solubility in the different tissues, cardiac output, and blood flow distribution determines the rate of rise of F_A/F_I characteristic of each drug (Figure 25–5). When inducing anesthesia by inhalation only, the rate by which F_A/F_I approaches 1 will determine the speed of induction.

Elimination

Recovery from inhalation anesthesia follows some of the same principles in reverse that are important during induction. The time to recovery from inhalation anesthesia depends on the rate of elimination of the anesthetic from the brain. One of the most important factors governing rate of recovery is the blood:gas partition coefficient of the anesthetic agent. Other factors controlling rate of recovery include pulmonary blood flow, magnitude of ventilation, and tissue solubility of the anesthetic. Two features differentiate the recovery phase from the induction phase. First, transfer of an anesthetic from the lungs to blood can be enhanced by increasing its concentration in inspired air, but the reverse transfer process cannot be enhanced because the concentration in the lungs cannot be reduced below zero. Second, at the beginning of the recovery phase, the anesthetic gas tension in different tissues may be quite variable, depending on the specific agent and the duration of anesthesia. In contrast, at the start of induction of anesthesia the initial anesthetic tension is zero in all tissues.

Inhaled anesthetics that are relatively insoluble in blood (ie, possess low blood:gas partition coefficients) and brain are eliminated at faster rates than the more soluble anesthetics. The washout

of nitrous oxide, desflurane, and sevoflurane occurs at a rapid rate, leading to a more rapid recovery from their anesthetic effects compared with halothane and isoflurane. Halothane is approximately twice as soluble in brain tissue and five times more soluble in blood than nitrous oxide and desflurane; its elimination therefore takes place more slowly, and recovery from halothane- and isoflurane-based anesthesia is predictably less rapid.

The duration of exposure to the anesthetic can also have a significant effect on the recovery time, especially in the case of the more soluble anesthetics (eg, halothane and isoflurane). Accumulation of anesthetics in muscle, skin, and fat increases with prolonged exposure (especially in obese patients), and blood tension may decline slowly during recovery as the anesthetic is slowly eliminated from these tissues. Although recovery may be rapid even with the more soluble agents following a short period of exposure, recovery is slow after prolonged administration of halothane or isoflurane.

A. Ventilation

Two parameters that can be manipulated by the anesthesiologist are useful in controlling the speed of induction of and recovery from inhaled anesthesia: (1) concentration of anesthetic in the inspired gas and (2) alveolar ventilation. Because the concentration of anesthetic in the inspired gas cannot be reduced below zero, ventilation is the only way to speed recovery.

B. Metabolism

Modern inhaled anesthetics are eliminated mainly by ventilation and are only metabolized to a very small extent; thus, metabolism of these drugs does not play a significant role in the termination of their effect. However, metabolism may have important implications for their toxicity (see Toxicity of Anesthetic Agents). Hepatic metabolism may also contribute to the elimination of and recovery from some older volatile anesthetics. For example, halothane is eliminated more rapidly during recovery than enflurane, which would not be predicted from their respective tissue solubility. This increased elimination occurs because over 40% of inspired halothane is metabolized during an average anesthetic procedure, whereas less than 10% of enflurane is metabolized over the same period.

In terms of the extent of hepatic metabolism, the rank order for the inhaled anesthetics is halothane > enflurane > sevoflurane > isoflurane > desflurane > nitrous oxide (Table 25–1). Nitrous oxide is not metabolized by human tissues. However, bacteria in the gastrointestinal tract may be able to break down the nitrous oxide molecule.

PHARMACODYNAMICS

Organ System Effects of Inhaled Anesthetics

A. Cerebral Effects

Anesthetic potency is currently described by the minimal alveolar concentration (MAC) required to prevent a response to a surgical

What Does Anesthesia Represent & Where Does It Work?

Anesthetic action has three principal components: immobility, amnesia, and unconsciousness.

Immobility

Immobility is the easiest anesthetic end point to measure. Edmond Eger and colleagues introduced the concept of minimal alveolar concentration (MAC) to quantify the potency of an inhalational anesthetic. They defined 1.0 MAC as the partial pressure of an inhalational anesthetic in the alveoli of the lungs at which 50% of a population of nonrelaxed patients remained immobile at the time of a skin incision. Anesthetic immobility is mediated primarily by neural inhibition within the spinal cord.

Amnesia

The ablation of memory arises from several locations in the CNS, including the hippocampus, amygdala, prefrontal cortex, and regions of the sensory and motor cortices. Memory researchers differentiate two types of memory: (1) explicit memory, ie, specific awareness or consciousness under anesthesia, and (2) implicit memory, the unconscious acquisition of information under adequate levels of anesthesia. Their studies have found that formation of both types of memory is reliably prevented at low MAC values (0.2–0.4 MAC). Prevention of explicit memory (awareness) has spurred the development of monitors such as the bispectral index, electroencephalogram, and entropy monitor of auditory evoked potentials to recognize inadequate planes of anesthesia.

Consciousness

The ability of anesthetic drugs to abolish consciousness requires action at anatomic locations responsible for the formation of human consciousness. Leading neuroscientists studying consciousness identify three regions in the brain involved in generating personal awareness: the cerebral cortex, the thalamus, and the reticular activating system. These regions seem to interact as a cortical system via identified pathways, producing a state in which humans are awake, aware, and perceiving.

Our current state of understanding supports the following framework: sensory stimuli conducted through the reticular formation of the brainstem into supratentorial signaling loops, connecting the thalamus with various regions of the cortex, are the foundation of consciousness. These neural pathways involved in the development of consciousness are disrupted by anesthetics.

---

incision (see Box: What Does Anesthesia Represent & Where Does It Work?).

Inhaled anesthetics (like intravenous anesthetics, discussed later) decrease the metabolic activity of the brain. Decreased cerebral metabolic rate (CMR) generally reduces blood flow within the brain. However, volatile anesthetics also cause cerebral vasodilation, which can increase cerebral blood flow. The net effect on cerebral blood flow (increase, decrease, or no change) depends on the concentration of anesthetic delivered. At 0.5 MAC, the reduction in CMR is greater than the vasodilation caused by the anesthetic, so cerebral blood flow is decreased. Conversely, at 1.5 MAC, vasodilation by the anesthetic is greater than the reduction in CMR, so cerebral blood flow is increased. In between, at 1.0 MAC, the effects are balanced and cerebral blood flow is unchanged. An increase in cerebral blood flow is clinically undesirable in patients who have increased intracranial pressure because of brain tumor, intracranial hemorrhage, or head injury. Therefore, administration of high concentrations of volatile anesthetics is undesirable in patients with increased intracranial pressure. Hyperventilation can be used to attenuate this response; decreasing the $PaCO_2$ (the partial pressure of carbon dioxide in arterial blood) through hyperventilation causes cerebral vasoconstriction. If the patient is hyperventilated before the volatile agent is started, the increase in intracranial pressure can be minimized.

Nitrous oxide can increase cerebral blood flow and cause increased intracranial pressure. This effect is most likely caused by activation of the sympathetic nervous system (as described above).

Therefore, nitrous oxide may be combined with other agents (intravenous anesthetics) or techniques (hyperventilation) that reduce cerebral blood flow in patients with increased intracranial pressure.

Potent inhaled anesthetics produce a basic pattern of change to brain electrical activity as recorded by standard electroencephalography (EEG). Isoflurane, desflurane, sevoflurane, halothane, and enflurane produce initial activation of the EEG at low doses and then slowing of electrical activity up to doses of 1.0–1.5 MAC. At higher concentrations, EEG suppression increases to the point of electrical silence with isoflurane at 2.0–2.5 MAC. Isolated epileptic-like patterns may also be seen between 1.0 and 2.0 MAC, especially with sevoflurane and enflurane, but frank clinical seizure activity has been observed only with enflurane. Nitrous oxide used alone causes fast electrical oscillations emanating from the frontal cortex at doses associated with analgesia and depressed consciousness.

Traditionally, anesthetic effects on the brain produce four stages or levels of increasing depth of CNS depression (Guedel's signs, derived from observations of the effects of inhaled diethyl ether): **Stage I—analgesia:** The patient initially experiences analgesia without amnesia. Later in stage I, both analgesia and amnesia are produced. **Stage II—excitement:** During this stage, the patient appears delirious, may vocalize but is completely amnesic. Respiration is rapid, and heart rate and blood pressure increase. Duration and severity of this light stage of anesthesia is shortened by rapidly increasing the concentration of the agent. **Stage III—surgical anesthesia:** This stage begins with slowing of respiration and heart rate and extends to complete cessation of spontaneous respiration (apnea). Four planes of stage III are described based on changes in ocular movements, eye reflexes, and pupil size, indicating increasing depth of anesthesia. **Stage IV—medullary depression:** This deep stage of anesthesia represents severe depression of the CNS, including the vasomotor center in the medulla and respiratory center in the brainstem. Without circulatory and respiratory support, death would rapidly ensue.

B. Cardiovascular Effects

Halothane, enflurane, isoflurane, desflurane, and sevoflurane all depress normal cardiac contractility (halothane and enflurane more so than isoflurane, desflurane, and sevoflurane). As a result, all volatile agents tend to decrease mean arterial pressure in direct proportion to their alveolar concentration. With halothane and enflurane, the reduced arterial pressure is caused primarily by myocardial depression (reduced cardiac output) and there is little change in systemic vascular resistance. In contrast, isoflurane, desflurane, and sevoflurane produce greater vasodilation with minimal effect on cardiac output. These differences may have important implications for patients with heart failure. Because isoflurane, desflurane, and sevoflurane better preserve cardiac output as well as reduce preload (ventricular filling) and afterload (systemic vascular resistance), these agents may be better choices for patients with impaired myocardial function.

Nitrous oxide also depresses myocardial function in a concentration-dependent manner. This depression may be significantly offset by a concomitant activation of the sympathetic nervous system resulting in preservation of cardiac output. Therefore, administration of nitrous oxide in combination with the more potent volatile anesthetics can minimize circulatory depressant effects by both anesthetic-sparing and sympathetic-activating actions.

Because all inhaled anesthetics produce a dose-dependent decrease in arterial blood pressure, activation of autonomic nervous system reflexes may trigger increased heart rate. However, halothane, enflurane, and sevoflurane have little effect on heart rate, probably because they attenuate baroreceptor input into the autonomic nervous system. Desflurane and isoflurane significantly increase heart rate because they cause less depression of the baroreceptor reflex. In addition, desflurane can trigger transient sympathetic activation—with elevated catecholamine levels—to cause marked increases in heart rate and blood pressure during administration of high desflurane concentrations or when desflurane concentrations are changed rapidly.

Inhaled anesthetics tend to reduce myocardial oxygen consumption, which reflects depression of normal cardiac contractility and decreased arterial blood pressure. In addition, inhaled anesthetics produce coronary vasodilation. The net effect of decreased oxygen demand and increased coronary flow (oxygen supply) is improved myocardial oxygenation. However, other factors such as surgical stimulation, intravascular volume status, blood oxygen levels, and withdrawal of perioperative β blockers, may tilt the oxygen supply-demand balance toward myocardial ischemia.

Halothane and, to a lesser extent, other volatile anesthetics sensitize the myocardium to epinephrine and circulating catecholamines. Ventricular arrhythmias may occur when patients under anesthesia with halothane are given sympathomimetic drugs or have high circulating levels of endogenous catecholamines (eg, anxious patients, administration of epinephrine-containing local anesthetics, inadequate intraoperative anesthesia or analgesia, patients with pheochromocytomas). This effect is less marked for isoflurane, sevoflurane, and desflurane.

C. Respiratory Effects

All volatile anesthetics possess varying degrees of bronchodilating properties, an effect of value in patients with active wheezing and in status asthmaticus. However, airway irritation, which may provoke coughing or breath-holding, is induced by the pungency of some volatile anesthetics. The pungency of isoflurane and desflurane makes these agents less suitable for induction of anesthesia in patients with active bronchospasm. These reactions rarely occur with halothane and sevoflurane, which are considered nonpungent. Therefore, the bronchodilating action of halothane and sevoflurane makes them the agents of choice in patients with underlying airway problems. Nitrous oxide is also nonpungent and can facilitate inhalational induction of anesthesia in a patient with bronchospasm.

The control of breathing is significantly affected by inhaled anesthetics. With the exception of nitrous oxide, all inhaled anesthetics in current use cause a dose-dependent decrease in tidal volume and an increase in respiratory rate (rapid shallow breathing pattern). However, the increase in respiratory rate varies among agents and does not fully compensate for the decrease in tidal volume, resulting in a decrease in alveolar ventilation. In addition, all volatile anesthetics are respiratory depressants, as defined by a reduced ventilatory response to increased levels of carbon dioxide in the blood. The degree of ventilatory depression varies among the volatile agents, with isoflurane and enflurane being the most depressant. By this hypoventilation mechanism, all volatile anesthetics increase the resting level of $PaCO_2$.

Volatile anesthetics also raise the apneic threshold ($PaCO_2$ level below which apnea occurs through lack of CO_2-driven respiratory stimulation) and decrease the ventilatory response to hypoxia. In practice, the respiratory depressant effects of anesthetics are overcome by assisting (controlling) ventilation mechanically. The ventilatory depression produced by inhaled anesthetics may be counteracted by surgical stimulation; however, low, subanesthetic concentrations of volatile anesthetic present after surgery in the early recovery period can continue to depress the compensatory increase in ventilation normally caused by hypoxia.

Inhaled anesthetics also depress mucociliary function in the airway. During prolonged exposure to inhaled anesthetics, mucus pooling and plugging may result in atelectasis and the development of postoperative respiratory complications, including hypoxemia and respiratory infections.

D. Renal Effects

Inhaled anesthetics tend to decrease glomerular filtration rate (GFR) and urine flow. Renal blood flow may also be decreased by some agents but filtration fraction is increased, implying that autoregulatory control of efferent arteriole tone helps compensate and limits the reduction in GFR. In general these anesthetic effects are minor compared with the stress of surgery itself and usually reversible after discontinuation of the anesthetic.

E. Hepatic Effects

Volatile anesthetics cause a concentration-dependent decrease in portal vein blood flow that parallels the decline in cardiac output produced by these agents. However, total hepatic blood flow may be relatively preserved as hepatic artery blood flow to the liver may increase or stay the same. Although transient changes in liver function tests may occur following exposure to volatile anesthetics, persistent elevation in liver enzymes is rare except following repeated exposures to halothane (see Toxicity of Anesthetic Agents).

F. Effects on Uterine Smooth Muscle

Nitrous oxide appears to have little effect on uterine musculature. However, the halogenated anesthetics are potent uterine muscle relaxants and produce this effect in a concentration-dependent fashion. This pharmacologic effect can be helpful when profound uterine relaxation is required for intrauterine fetal manipulation or manual extraction of a retained placenta during delivery. However, it can also lead to increased uterine bleeding.

Toxicity of Anesthetic Agents

A. Acute Toxicity

1. Nephrotoxicity—Metabolism of enflurane and sevoflurane may generate compounds that are potentially nephrotoxic. Although their metabolism can liberate nephrotoxic fluoride ions, significant renal injury has been reported only for enflurane with prolonged exposure. The insolubility and rapid elimination of sevoflurane may prevent toxicity. This drug may be degraded by carbon dioxide absorbents in anesthesia machines to form a nephrotoxic vinyl ether compound termed "compound A" which, in high concentrations, has caused proximal tubular necrosis in rats. Nevertheless, there have been no reports of renal injury in humans receiving sevoflurane anesthesia. Moreover, exposure to sevoflurane does not produce any change in standard markers of renal function.

2. Hematotoxicity—Prolonged exposure to nitrous oxide decreases methionine synthase activity, which theoretically could cause megaloblastic anemia. Megaloblastic bone marrow changes have been observed in patients after 12-hour exposure to 50% nitrous oxide. Chronic exposure of dental personnel to nitrous oxide in inadequately ventilated dental operating suites is a potential occupational hazard.

All inhaled anesthetics can produce some carbon monoxide (CO) from their interaction with strong bases in dry carbon dioxide absorbers. CO binds to hemoglobin with high affinity, reducing oxygen delivery to tissues. Desflurane produces the most CO, and intraoperative formation of CO has been reported. CO production can be avoided simply by using fresh carbon dioxide absorbent and by preventing its complete desiccation.

3. Malignant hyperthermia—Malignant hyperthermia is a heritable genetic disorder of skeletal muscle that occurs in susceptible individuals exposed to volatile anesthetics while undergoing general anesthesia (see Chapter 16 and Table 16–4). The depolarizing muscle relaxant succinylcholine may also trigger malignant hyperthermia. The malignant hyperthermia syndrome consists of muscle rigidity, hyperthermia, rapid onset of tachycardia and hypercapnia, hyperkalemia, and metabolic acidosis following exposure to one or more triggering agents. Malignant hyperthermia is a rare but important cause of anesthetic morbidity and mortality. The specific biochemical abnormality is an increase in free cytosolic calcium concentration in skeletal muscle cells. Treatment includes administration of **dantrolene** (to reduce calcium release from the sarcoplasmic reticulum) and appropriate measures to reduce body temperature and restore electrolyte and acid-base balance (see Chapter 27).

Malignant hyperthermia susceptibility is characterized by genetic heterogeneity, and several predisposing clinical myopathies have been identified. It has been associated with mutations in the gene coding for the skeletal muscle ryanodine receptor (RyR1), the calcium release channel on the sarcoplasmic reticulum, and mutant alleles of the gene encoding the α_1 subunit of the human skeletal muscle L-type voltage-dependent calcium channel. However, the genetic loci identified to date account for less than 50% of malignant hyperthermia-susceptible individuals, and genetic testing cannot definitively determine malignant hyperthermia susceptibility. Currently, the most reliable test to establish susceptibility is the in vitro caffeine-halothane contracture test using skeletal muscle biopsy samples.

4. Hepatotoxicity (halothane hepatitis)—Hepatic dysfunction following surgery and general anesthesia is most likely caused by hypovolemic shock, infection conferred by blood transfusion, or other surgical stresses rather than by volatile anesthetic toxicity. However, a small subset of individuals previously exposed to halothane has developed fulminant hepatic failure. The incidence of severe hepatotoxicity following exposure to halothane is estimated to be in the range of 1 in 20,000–35,000. The mechanisms underlying halothane hepatotoxicity remain unclear, but studies in animals implicate the formation of reactive metabolites that either cause direct hepatocellular damage (eg, free radicals) or initiate immune-mediated responses. Cases of hepatitis following exposure to other volatile anesthetics, including enflurane, isoflurane, and desflurane, have rarely been reported.

B. Chronic Toxicity

1. Mutagenicity, teratogenicity, and reproductive effects—Under normal conditions, inhaled anesthetics including nitrous oxide are neither mutagens nor carcinogens in patients. Nitrous oxide can be directly teratogenic in animals under conditions of extremely high exposure. Halothane, enflurane, isoflurane, desflurane, and sevoflurane may be teratogenic in rodents as a result of physiologic changes associated with the anesthesia rather than through a direct teratogenic effect.

The most consistent finding in surveys conducted to determine the reproductive success of female operating room personnel has been a questionably higher-than-expected incidence of miscarriages.

However, there are several problems in interpreting these studies. The association of obstetric problems with surgery and anesthesia in pregnant patients is also an important consideration. In the USA, at least 50,000 pregnant women each year undergo anesthesia and surgery for indications unrelated to pregnancy. The risk of abortion is clearly higher following this experience. It is not obvious, however, whether the underlying disease, surgery, anesthesia, or a combination of these factors is the cause of the increased risk

2. Carcinogenicity—Epidemiologic studies suggested an increase in the cancer rate in operating room personnel who were exposed to trace concentrations of anesthetic agents. However, no study has demonstrated the existence of a causal relationship between anesthetics and cancer. Many other factors might account for the questionably positive results seen after a careful review of epidemiologic data. Most operating rooms now use scavenging systems to remove trace concentrations of anesthetics released from anesthetic machines.

■ INTRAVENOUS ANESTHETICS

Intravenous nonopioid anesthetics play an important role in the practice of modern anesthesia. They are widely used to facilitate rapid induction of anesthesia and have replaced inhalation as the preferred method of anesthesia induction in most settings except for pediatric anesthesia. Intravenous agents are also commonly used to provide sedation during monitored anesthesia care and for patients in intensive care (ICU) settings. With the introduction of propofol, intravenous anesthesia also became an option for the maintenance of anesthesia. However, similar to the inhaled agents, the currently available intravenous anesthetics are not ideal anesthetic drugs in the sense of producing all and only the five desired effects (unconsciousness, amnesia, analgesia, inhibition of autonomic reflexes, and skeletal muscle relaxation). Therefore, **balanced anesthesia** with multiple drugs (inhaled anesthetics, sedative-hypnotics, opioids, neuromuscular blocking drugs) is generally used to minimize unwanted side effects.

The intravenous anesthetics used for induction of general anesthesia are lipophilic and preferentially partition into highly perfused lipophilic tissues (brain, spinal cord), which accounts for their rapid onset of action. Regardless of the extent and speed of their metabolism, termination of the effect of a single bolus is determined by redistribution of the drug into less perfused and inactive tissues such as skeletal muscle and fat. Thus, all drugs used for induction of anesthesia have a similar duration of action when administered as a single bolus dose despite significant differences in their metabolism. Figure 25–6 shows the chemical structures of common clinically used intravenous anesthetics. Table 25–2 lists pharmacokinetic properties of these and other intravenous agents.

PROPOFOL

In most countries, propofol is the most frequently administered drug for induction of anesthesia and has largely replaced barbiturates for this indication. Because its pharmacokinetic profile

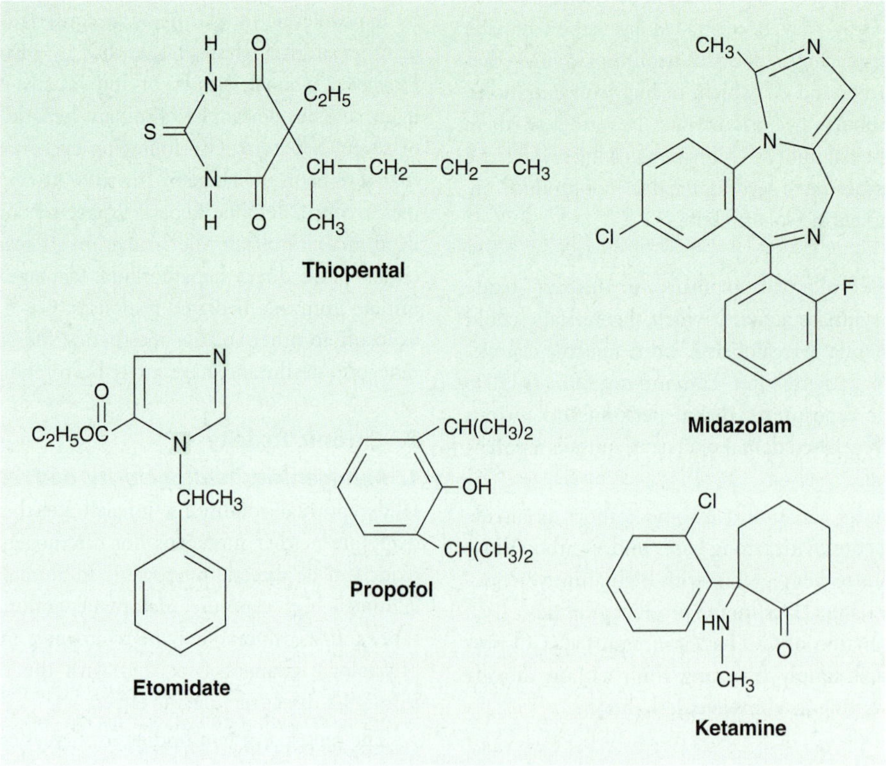

FIGURE 25–6 Chemical structures of some intravenous anesthetics.

TABLE 25–2 Pharmacokinetic properties of intravenous anesthetics.

Drug	Induction Dose (mg/kg IV)	Duration of Action (min)	V$_{dss}$ (L/kg)	$t_{1/2}$ Distribution (min)	Protein Binding (%)	CL (mL/kg/min)	$t_{1/2}$ Elimination (h)
Dexmedetomidine	NA	NA	2–3	6	94	10–30	2–3
Diazepam	0.3–0.6	15–30	0.7–1.7	10–5	98	0.2–0.5	20–50
Etomidate	0.2–0.3	3–8	2.5–4.5	2–4	77	18–25	2.9–5.3
Ketamine	1–2	5–10	3.1	11–16	12	12–17	2–4
Lorazepam	0.03–0.1	60–120	0.8–1.3	3–10	98	0.8–1.8	11–22
Methohexital	1–1.5	4–7	2.2	5–6	73	11	4
Midazolam	0.1–0.3	15–20	1.1–1.7	7–15	94	6.4–11	1.7–2.6
Propofol	1–2.5	3–8	2–10	2–4	97	20–30	4–23
Thiopental	3–5	5–10	2.5	2–4	83	3.4	11

Note: The duration of action reflects the duration after a typical single IV dose given for induction of anesthesia. Data are for average adult patients.

CL, clearance; NA, not applicable; V$_{dss}$, volume of distribution at steady state.

allows for continuous infusions, propofol is also used during maintenance of anesthesia and is a common choice for sedation in the setting of monitored anesthesia care. Increasingly, propofol is also used for sedation in the ICU as well as conscious sedation and short-duration general anesthesia in locations outside the operating room (eg, interventional radiology suites, emergency department; see Box: Sedation & Monitored Anesthesia Care, earlier).

Propofol (2,6-diisopropylphenol) is an alkyl phenol with hypnotic properties that is chemically distinct from other groups of intravenous anesthetics (Figure 25–6). Because of its poor solubility in water, it is formulated as an emulsion containing 10% soybean oil, 2.25% glycerol, and 1.2% lecithin, the major component of the egg yolk phosphatide fraction. Hence, susceptible patients may experience allergic reactions. The solution appears milky white and slightly viscous, has a pH of approximately 7, and a propofol concentration of 1% (10 mg/mL). In some countries, a 2% formulation is available. Although retardants of bacterial growth are added to the formulations, solutions should be used as soon as possible (no more than 8 hours after opening the vial) and proper sterile technique is essential. The addition of metabisulfite in one of the formulations has raised concern regarding its use in patients with reactive airway disease (eg, asthma) or sulfite allergies.

The presumed mechanism of action of propofol is through potentiation of the chloride current mediated through the GABA$_A$ receptor complex.

Pharmacokinetics

Propofol is rapidly metabolized in the liver; the resulting water-soluble compounds are presumed to be inactive and are excreted through the kidneys. Plasma clearance is high and exceeds hepatic blood flow, indicating the importance of extrahepatic metabolism, which is thought to occur to a significant extent in the lungs and may account for the elimination of up to 30% of a bolus dose of the drug (Table 25–2). The recovery from propofol is more complete,

with less "hangover" than that observed with thiopental, likely due to the high plasma clearance. However, as with other intravenous drugs, transfer of propofol from the plasma (central) compartment and the associated termination of drug effect after a single bolus dose are mainly the result of redistribution from highly perfused (brain) to less-well-perfused (skeletal muscle) compartments (Figure 25–7). As with other intravenous agents, awakening after an induction dose of propofol usually occurs within 8–10 minutes. The kinetics of propofol (and other intravenous anesthetics) after a single bolus dose or continuous infusion are best described by means of a three-compartment model. Such models have been used as the basis for developing systems of target-controlled infusions.

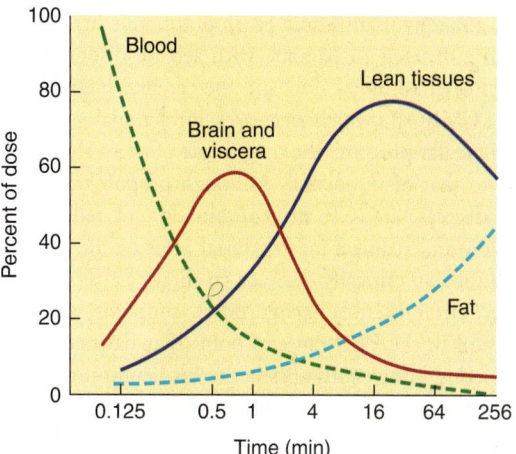

FIGURE 25–7 Redistribution of thiopental after an intravenous bolus administration. The redistribution curves for other intravenous anesthetics look similar after a bolus injection, explaining that the recovery times are similar despite remarkable differences in metabolism. Note that the time axis is not linear.

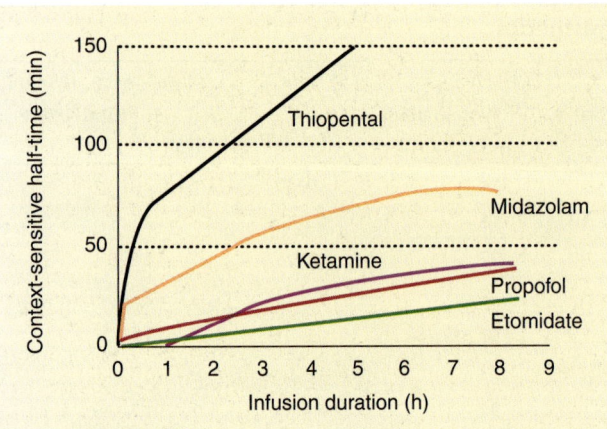

FIGURE 25–8 The context-sensitive half-time of common intravenous anesthetics. Even after a prolonged infusion, the half-time of propofol is relatively short, which makes propofol the preferred choice for intravenous anesthesia. Ketamine and etomidate have similar characteristics but their use is limited by other effects.

The **context-sensitive half-time** of a drug describes the elimination half-time after a continuous infusion as a function of the duration of the infusion and is an important factor in the suitability of a drug for use as maintenance anesthetic. The context-sensitive half-time of propofol is brief, even after a prolonged infusion, and recovery remains relatively prompt (Figure 25–8).

Organ System Effects

A. CNS Effects

Propofol acts as hypnotic but does not have analgesic properties. Although the drug leads to a general suppression of CNS activity, excitatory effects such as twitching or spontaneous movement are occasionally observed during induction of anesthesia. These effects may resemble seizure activity; however, most studies support an anticonvulsant effect of propofol, and the drug may be safely administered to patients with seizure disorders. Propofol decreases cerebral blood flow and the cerebral metabolic rate for oxygen (CMRO$_2$), which decreases intracranial pressure (ICP) and intraocular pressure; the magnitude of these changes is comparable to that of thiopental. Although propofol can produce a desired decrease in ICP, the combination of reduced cerebral blood flow and reduced mean arterial pressure due to peripheral vasodilation can critically decrease cerebral perfusion pressure.

When administered in large doses, propofol produces burst suppression in the EEG, an end point that has been used when administering intravenous anesthetics for neuroprotection during neurosurgical procedures. Evidence from animal studies suggests that propofol's neuroprotective effects during focal ischemia are similar to those of thiopental and isoflurane.

B. Cardiovascular Effects

Compared with other induction drugs, propofol produces the most pronounced decrease in systemic blood pressure; this is a result of profound vasodilation in both arterial and venous circulations

leading to reductions in preload and afterload. This effect on systemic blood pressure is more pronounced with increased age, in patients with reduced intravascular fluid volume, and with rapid injection. Because the hypotensive effects are further augmented by the inhibition of the normal baroreflex response, the vasodilation only leads to a small increase in heart rate. Profound bradycardia and asystole after the administration of propofol have been described in healthy adults despite prophylactic anticholinergic drugs.

C. Respiratory Effects

Propofol is a potent respiratory depressant and generally produces apnea after an induction dose. A maintenance infusion reduces minute ventilation through reductions in tidal volume and respiratory rate, with the effect on tidal volume being more pronounced. In addition, the ventilatory response to hypoxia and hypercapnia is reduced. Propofol causes a greater reduction in upper airway reflexes than thiopental does, which makes it well suited for instrumentation of the airway, such as placement of a laryngeal mask airway.

D. Other Effects

Although propofol, unlike volatile anesthetics, does not augment neuromuscular block, studies have found good intubating conditions after propofol induction without the use of neuromuscular blocking agents. Unexpected tachycardia occurring during propofol anesthesia should prompt laboratory evaluation for possible metabolic acidosis (propofol infusion syndrome). An interesting and desirable side effect of propofol is its antiemetic activity. Pain on injection is a common complaint and can be reduced by premedication with an opioid or coadministration with lidocaine. Dilution of propofol and the use of larger veins for injection can also reduce the incidence and severity of injection pain.

Clinical Uses & Dosage

The most common use of propofol is to facilitate induction of general anesthesia by bolus injection of 1–2.5 mg/kg IV. Increasing age, reduced cardiovascular reserve, or premedication with benzodiazepines or opioids reduces the required induction dose; children require higher doses (2.5–3.5 mg/kg IV). Generally, titration of the induction dose helps to prevent severe hemodynamic changes. Propofol is often used for maintenance of anesthesia either as part of a balanced anesthesia regimen in combination with volatile anesthetics, nitrous oxide, sedative-hypnotics, and opioids or as part of a total intravenous anesthetic technique, usually in combination with opioids. Therapeutic plasma concentrations for maintenance of anesthesia normally range between 3 and 8 mcg/mL (typically requiring a continuous infusion rate between 100 and 200 mcg/kg/min) when combined with nitrous oxide or opioids.

When used for sedation of mechanically ventilated patients in the ICU or for sedation during procedures, the required plasma concentration is 1–2 mcg/mL, which can be achieved with a continuous infusion at 25–75 mcg/kg/min. Because of its pronounced respiratory depressant effect and narrow therapeutic range, propofol should be administered only by individuals trained in airway management.

Subanesthetic doses of propofol can be used to treat postoperative nausea and vomiting (10–20 mg IV as bolus or 10 mcg/kg/min as an infusion).

FOSPROPOFOL

As previously noted, injection pain during administration of propofol is often perceived as severe, and the lipid emulsion has several disadvantages. Intense research has focused on finding alternative formulations or related drugs that would address some of these problems. Fospropofol is a water-soluble prodrug of propofol, chemically described as 2,6-diisopropylphenoxymethyl phosphate disodium salt, that was licensed by the Food and Drug Administration in 2008 as a sedating agent for use in adult patients during monitored anesthesia care. The prodrug is rapidly metabolized by alkaline phosphatase, producing propofol, phosphate, and formaldehyde. The formaldehyde is metabolized by aldehyde dehydrogenase in the liver and in erythrocytes. The available fospropofol formulation is a sterile, aqueous, colorless, and clear solution that is supplied in a single-dose vial at a concentration of 35 mg/mL under the trade name Lusedra.

Pharmacokinetics & Organ System Effects

Because the active compound is propofol and fospropofol is a prodrug that requires metabolism to form propofol, the pharmacokinetics are more complex than for propofol itself. Multicompartment models with two compartments for fospropofol and three for propofol have been used to describe the kinetics.

The effect profile is similar to that of propofol, but onset and recovery are prolonged compared with propofol because the prodrug must first be converted into an active form. Although patients receiving fospropofol do not appear to experience the injection pain typical of propofol, a common adverse effect is the experience of paresthesia, often in the perianal region, which occurs in up to 74% of patients. The mechanism for this effect is unknown.

Clinical Uses & Dosage

Fospropofol is approved for sedation during monitored anesthesia care. Supplemental oxygen must be administered to all patients receiving the drug. As with propofol, airway compromise is a major concern. Hence, it is recommended that fospropofol be administered only by personnel trained in airway management. The recommended standard dosage is an initial bolus dose of 6.5 mg/kg IV followed by supplemental doses of 1.6 mg/kg IV as needed. For patients weighing more than 90 kg or less than 60 kg, 90 or 60 kg should be used to calculate the dose, respectively. The dose should be reduced by 25% in patients older than 65 years and in those with an American Society of Anesthesiologists status of 3 or 4.

BARBITURATES

This section focuses on the use of thiopental and methohexital for induction of general anesthesia; however, these barbiturate hypnotics have been largely replaced as induction agents by propofol. Other

barbiturates as well as general barbiturate pharmacology are discussed in Chapter 22.

The anesthetic effect of barbiturates presumably involves a combination of enhancement of inhibitory and inhibition of excitatory neurotransmission. Although the effects on inhibitory transmission probably result from activation of the $GABA_A$ receptor complex, the effects on excitatory transmission are less well understood.

Pharmacokinetics

Thiopental and methohexital undergo hepatic metabolism, mostly by oxidation but also by N-dealkylation, desulfuration, and destruction of the barbituric acid ring structure. Barbiturates should not be administered to patients with acute intermittent porphyria because they increase the production of porphyrins through stimulation of aminolevulinic acid synthetase. Methohexital has a shorter elimination half-time than thiopental due to its larger plasma clearance (Table 25–2), leading to a faster and more complete recovery after bolus injection. Although thiopental is metabolized more slowly and has a long elimination half-time, recovery after a single bolus injection is comparable to that of methohexital and propofol because it depends on redistribution to inactive tissue sites rather than on metabolism (Figure 25–7). However, if administered through repeated bolus injections or continuous infusion, recovery will be markedly prolonged because elimination will depend on metabolism under these circumstances (see also context-sensitive half-time, Figure 25–8).

Organ System Effects

A. CNS Effects

Barbiturates produce dose-dependent CNS depression ranging from sedation to general anesthesia when administered as bolus injections. They do not produce analgesia; instead, some evidence suggests they may reduce the pain threshold causing hyperalgesia. Barbiturates are potent cerebral vasoconstrictors and produce predictable decreases in cerebral blood flow, cerebral blood volume, and ICP. As a result, they decrease $CMRO_2$ consumption in a dose-dependent manner up to a dose at which they suppress all EEG activity. The ability of barbiturates to decrease ICP and $CMRO_2$ makes these drugs useful in the management of patients with space-occupying intracranial lesions. They may provide neuroprotection from focal cerebral ischemia (stroke, surgical retraction, temporary clips during aneurysm surgery), but probably not from global cerebral ischemia (eg, from cardiac arrest). Except for methohexital, barbiturates decrease electrical activity on the EEG and can be used as anticonvulsants. In contrast, methohexital activates epileptic foci and may therefore be useful to facilitate electroconvulsive therapy or during the identification of epileptic foci during surgery.

B. Cardiovascular Effects

The decrease in systemic blood pressure associated with administration of barbiturates for induction of anesthesia is primarily due to peripheral vasodilation and is usually smaller than the blood pressure decrease associated with propofol. There are also direct negative inotropic effects on the heart. However, inhibition of the baroreceptor reflex is less pronounced than with propofol; thus, compensatory increases in heart rate limit the decrease in blood pressure and make it transient. The depressant effects on systemic blood pressure are increased in patients with hypovolemia, cardiac tamponade, cardiomyopathy, coronary artery disease, or cardiac valvular disease because such patients are less able to compensate for the effects of peripheral vasodilation. Hemodynamic effects are also more pronounced with larger doses and rapid injection.

C. Respiratory Effects

Barbiturates are respiratory depressants, and a usual induction dose of thiopental or methohexital typically produces transient apnea, which will be more pronounced if other respiratory depressants are also administered. Barbiturates lead to decreased minute ventilation through reduced tidal volumes and respiratory rate and also decrease the ventilatory responses to hypercapnia and hypoxia. Resumption of spontaneous breathing after an anesthetic induction dose of a barbiturate is characterized by a slow breathing rate and decreased tidal volume. Suppression of laryngeal reflexes and cough reflexes is probably not as profound as after an equianesthetic propofol administration, which makes barbiturates an inferior choice for airway instrumentation in the absence of neuromuscular blocking drugs. Furthermore, stimulation of the upper airway or trachea (eg, by secretions, laryngeal mask airway, direct laryngoscopy, tracheal intubation) during inadequate depression of airway reflexes may result in laryngospasm or bronchospasm. This phenomenon is not unique to barbiturates but is true whenever the drug dose is inadequate to suppress the airway reflexes.

D. Other Effects

Accidental intra-arterial injection of barbiturates results in excruciating pain and intense vasoconstriction, often leading to severe tissue injury involving gangrene. Approaches to treatment include blockade of the sympathetic nervous system (eg, stellate ganglion block) in the involved extremity. If extravasation occurs, some authorities recommend local injection of the area with 0.5% lidocaine (5–10 mL) in an attempt to dilute the barbiturate concentration. Life-threatening allergic reactions to barbiturates are rare, with an estimated occurrence of 1 in 30,000 patients. However, barbiturate-induced histamine release occasionally is seen.

Clinical Uses & Dosage

The principal clinical uses of thiopental (3–5 mg/kg IV) or methohexital (1–1.5 mg/kg IV) is for induction of anesthesia (unconsciousness), which usually occurs in less than 30 seconds. Patients may experience a garlic or onion taste after administration. Barbiturates such as methohexital (20–30 mg/kg) may be administered per rectum to facilitate induction of anesthesia in mentally challenged and uncooperative pediatric patients. When a barbiturate is administered with the goal of neuroprotection, an isoelectric EEG indicating maximal reduction of $CMRO_2$ has traditionally been used as the end point. More recent data demonstrating equal protection after smaller doses have challenged this practice. The use of smaller doses is less frequently associated with hypotension, thus

making it easier to maintain adequate cerebral perfusion pressure, especially in the setting of increased ICP.

BENZODIAZEPINES

Benzodiazepines commonly used in the perioperative period include midazolam, lorazepam, and less frequently, diazepam. Benzodiazepines are unique among the group of intravenous anesthetics in that their action can readily be terminated by administration of their selective antagonist, flumazenil. Their most desired effects are anxiolysis and anterograde amnesia, which are extremely useful for premedication.

The chemical structure and pharmacodynamics of the benzodiazepines are discussed in detail in Chapter 22.

Pharmacokinetics in the Anesthesia Setting

The highly lipid-soluble benzodiazepines rapidly enter the CNS, which accounts for their rapid onset of action, followed by redistribution to inactive tissue sites and subsequent termination of the drug effect. Additional information regarding the pharmacokinetics of the benzodiazepines may be found in Chapter 22.

Despite its prompt passage into the brain, midazolam is considered to have a slower effect-site equilibration time than propofol and thiopental. In this regard, intravenous doses of midazolam should be sufficiently spaced to permit the peak clinical effect to be recognized before a repeat dose is considered. Midazolam has the shortest context-sensitive half-time, which makes it the only one of the three benzodiazepine drugs suitable for continuous infusion (Figure 25–8).

Organ System Effects

A. CNS Effects

Similar to propofol and barbiturates, benzodiazepines decrease $CMRO_2$ and cerebral blood flow, but to a smaller extent. There appears to be a ceiling effect for benzodiazepine-induced decreases in $CMRO_2$ as evidenced by midazolam's inability to produce an isoelectric EEG. Patients with decreased intracranial compliance demonstrate little or no change in ICP after the administration of midazolam. Although neuroprotective properties have not been shown for benzodiazepines, these drugs are potent anticonvulsants used in the treatment of status epilepticus, alcohol withdrawal, and local anesthetic-induced seizures. The CNS effects of benzodiazepines can be promptly terminated by administration of the selective benzodiazepine antagonist flumazenil, which improves their safety profile.

B. Cardiovascular Effects

If used for the induction of anesthesia, midazolam produces a greater decrease in systemic blood pressure than comparable doses of diazepam. These changes are most likely due to peripheral vasodilation inasmuch as cardiac output is not changed. Similar to other intravenous induction agents, midazolam's effect on systemic blood pressure is exaggerated in hypovolemic patients.

C. Respiratory Effects

Benzodiazepines produce minimal depression of ventilation, although transient apnea may follow rapid intravenous administration of midazolam for induction of anesthesia, especially in the presence of opioid premedication. Benzodiazepines decrease the ventilatory response to carbon dioxide, but this effect is not usually significant if they are administered alone. More severe respiratory depression can occur when benzodiazepines are administered together with opioids. Another problem affecting ventilation is airway obstruction induced by the hypnotic effects of benzodiazepines.

D. Other Effects

Pain during intravenous and intramuscular injection and subsequent thrombophlebitis are most pronounced with diazepam and reflect the poor water solubility of this benzodiazepine, which requires an organic solvent in the formulation. Despite its better solubility (which eliminates the need for an organic solvent), midazolam may also produce pain on injection. Allergic reactions to benzodiazepines are rare to nonexistent.

Clinical Uses & Dosage

Benzodiazepines are most commonly used for preoperative medication, intravenous sedation, and suppression of seizure activity. Less frequently, midazolam and diazepam may also be used to induce general anesthesia. The slow onset and prolonged duration of action of lorazepam limit its usefulness for preoperative medication or induction of anesthesia, especially when rapid and sustained awakening at the end of surgery is desirable. Although flumazenil (8–15 mcg/kg IV) may be useful for treating patients experiencing delayed awakening, its duration of action is brief (about 20 minutes) and resedation may occur.

The amnestic, anxiolytic, and sedative effects of benzodiazepines make this class of drugs the most popular choice for preoperative medication. Midazolam (1–2 mg IV) is effective for premedication, sedation during regional anesthesia, and brief therapeutic procedures. Midazolam has a more rapid onset, with greater amnesia and less postoperative sedation, than diazepam. Midazolam is also the most commonly used oral premedication for children; 0.5 mg/kg administered orally 30 minutes before induction of anesthesia provides reliable sedation and anxiolysis in children without producing delayed awakening.

The synergistic effects between benzodiazepines and other drugs, especially opioids and propofol, can be used to achieve better sedation and analgesia but may also greatly enhance their combined respiratory depression and may lead to airway obstruction or apnea. Because benzodiazepine effects are more pronounced with increasing age, dose reduction and careful titration may be necessary in elderly patients.

General anesthesia can be induced by the administration of midazolam (0.1–0.3 mg/kg IV), but the onset of unconsciousness is slower than after the administration of thiopental, propofol, or etomidate. Delayed awakening is a potential disadvantage, limiting the usefulness of benzodiazepines for induction of general anesthesia despite their advantage of less pronounced circulatory effects.

ETOMIDATE

Etomidate (Figure 24–6) is an intravenous anesthetic with hypnotic but not analgesic effects and is often chosen for its minimal hemodynamic effects. Although its pharmacokinetics are favorable, endocrine side effects limit its use for continuous infusions. Etomidate is a carboxylated imidazole derivative that is poorly soluble in water and is therefore supplied as a 2 mg/mL solution in 35% propylene glycol. The solution has a pH of 6.9 and thus does not cause problems with precipitation as thiopental does. Etomidate appears to have GABA-like effects and seems to act primarily through potentiation of $GABA_A$-mediated chloride currents, like most other intravenous anesthetics.

Pharmacokinetics

An induction dose of etomidate produces rapid onset of anesthesia, and recovery depends on redistribution to inactive tissue sites, comparable to thiopental and propofol. Metabolism is primarily by ester hydrolysis to inactive metabolites, which are then excreted in urine (78%) and bile (22%). Less than 3% of an administered dose of etomidate is excreted as unchanged drug in urine. Clearance of etomidate is about five times that of thiopental, as reflected by a shorter elimination half-time (Table 25–2). The duration of action is linearly related to the dose, with each 0.1 mg/kg providing about 100 seconds of unconsciousness. Because of etomidate's minimal effects on hemodynamics and short context-sensitive half-time, larger doses, repeated boluses, or continuous infusions can safely be administered. Etomidate, like most other intravenous anesthetics, is highly protein bound (77%), primarily to albumin.

Organ System Effects

A. CNS Effects

Etomidate is a potent cerebral vasoconstrictor, as reflected by decreases in cerebral blood flow and ICP. These effects are similar to those produced by comparable doses of thiopental. Despite its reduction of $CMRO_2$, etomidate has failed to show neuroprotective properties in animal studies, and human studies are lacking. The frequency of excitatory spikes on the EEG after the administration of etomidate is greater than with thiopental. Similar to methohexital, etomidate may activate seizure foci, manifested as fast activity on the EEG. In addition, spontaneous movements characterized as myoclonus occur in more than 50% of patients receiving etomidate, and this myoclonic activity may be associated with seizure-like activity on the EEG.

B. Cardiovascular Effects

A characteristic and desired feature of induction of anesthesia with etomidate is cardiovascular stability after bolus injection. In this regard, decrease in systemic blood pressure is modest or absent and principally reflects a decrease in systemic vascular resistance. Therefore, the systemic blood pressure-lowering effects of etomidate are probably exaggerated in the presence of hypovolemia, and optimization of the patient's intravascular fluid volume status before induction of anesthesia should be achieved.

Etomidate produces minimal changes in heart rate and cardiac output. Its depressant effects on myocardial contractility are minimal at concentrations used for induction of anesthesia.

C. Respiratory Effects

The depressant effects of etomidate on ventilation are less pronounced than those of barbiturates, although apnea may occasionally follow rapid intravenous injection of the drug. Depression of ventilation may be exaggerated when etomidate is combined with inhaled anesthetics or opioids.

D. Endocrine Effects

Etomidate causes adrenocortical suppression by producing a dose-dependent inhibition of 11β-hydroxylase, an enzyme necessary for the conversion of cholesterol to cortisol. This suppression lasts 4–8 hours after an induction dose of the drug. Despite concerns regarding this finding, no outcome studies have demonstrated an adverse effect. However, because of its endocrine effects, etomidate is not used as continuous infusion.

Clinical Uses & Dosage

Etomidate is an alternative to propofol and barbiturates for the rapid intravenous induction of anesthesia, especially in patients with compromised myocardial contractility. After a standard induction dose (0.2–0.3 mg/kg IV), the onset of unconsciousness is comparable to that achieved by thiopental and propofol. Similar to propofol, during intravenous injection of etomidate there is a high incidence of pain, which may be followed by venous irritation. Involuntary myoclonic movements are also common but may be masked by the concomitant administration of neuromuscular blocking drugs. Awakening after a single intravenous dose of etomidate is rapid, with little evidence of any residual depressant effects. Etomidate does not produce analgesia, and postoperative nausea and vomiting may be more common than after the administration of thiopental or propofol.

KETAMINE

Ketamine (Figure 25–6) is a partially water-soluble and highly lipid-soluble phencyclidine derivative differing from most other intravenous anesthetics in that it produces significant analgesia. The characteristic state observed after an induction dose of ketamine is known as "dissociative anesthesia," wherein the patient's eyes remain open with a slow nystagmic gaze (cataleptic state). Of the two stereoisomers the $S(+)$ form is more potent than the $R(-)$ isomer, but only the racemic mixture of ketamine is available in the USA.

Ketamine's mechanism of action is complex, but the major effect is probably produced through inhibition of the NMDA receptor complex.

Pharmacokinetics

The high lipid solubility of ketamine ensures a rapid onset of its effect. As with other intravenous induction drugs, the effect of a single bolus injection is terminated by redistribution to inactive

tissue sites. Metabolism occurs primarily in the liver and involves *N*-demethylation by the cytochrome P450 system. Norketamine, the primary active metabolite, is less potent (one third to one fifth the potency of ketamine) and is subsequently hydroxylated and conjugated into water-soluble inactive metabolites that are excreted in urine. Ketamine is the only intravenous anesthetic that has low protein binding (12%) (Table 25–2).

Organ System Effects

If ketamine is administered as the sole anesthetic, amnesia is not as complete as with the benzodiazepines. Reflexes are often preserved, but it cannot be assumed that patients are able to protect the upper airway. The eyes remain open and the pupils are moderately dilated with a nystagmic gaze. Frequently, lacrimation and salivation are increased, and premedication with an anticholinergic drug may be indicated to limit this effect.

A. CNS Effects

In contrast to other intravenous anesthetics, ketamine is considered to be a cerebral vasodilator that *increases* cerebral blood flow, as well as $CMRO_2$. For these reasons, ketamine has traditionally not been recommended for use in patients with intracranial pathology, especially increased ICP. Nevertheless, these perceived undesirable effects on cerebral blood flow may be blunted by the maintenance of normocapnia. Despite the potential to produce myoclonic activity, ketamine is considered an anticonvulsant and may be recommended for treatment of status epilepticus when more conventional drugs are ineffective.

Unpleasant emergence reactions after administration are the main factor limiting ketamine's use. Such reactions may include vivid colorful dreams, hallucinations, out-of-body experiences, and increased and distorted visual, tactile, and auditory sensitivity. These reactions can be associated with fear and confusion, but a euphoric state may also be induced, which explains the potential for abuse of the drug. Children usually have a lower incidence of and less severe emergence reactions. Combination with a benzodiazepine may be indicated to limit the unpleasant emergence reactions and also increase amnesia.

B. Cardiovascular Effects

Ketamine can produce transient but significant *increases* in systemic blood pressure, heart rate, and cardiac output, presumably by centrally mediated sympathetic stimulation. These effects, which are associated with increased cardiac workload and myocardial oxygen consumption, are not always desirable and can be blunted by coadministration of benzodiazepines, opioids, or inhaled anesthetics. Though the effect is more controversial, ketamine is considered to be a direct myocardial depressant. This property is usually masked by its stimulation of the sympathetic nervous system but may become apparent in critically ill patients with limited ability to increase their sympathetic nervous system activity.

C. Respiratory Effects

Ketamine is not thought to produce significant respiratory depression. When it is used as a single drug, the respiratory response to hypercapnia is preserved and blood gases remain stable. Transient hypoventilation and, in rare cases, a short period of apnea can follow rapid administration of a large intravenous dose for induction of anesthesia. The ability to protect the upper airway in the presence of ketamine cannot be assumed despite the presence of active airway reflexes. Especially in children, the risk for laryngospasm because of increased salivation must be considered; this risk can be reduced by premedication with an anticholinergic drug. Ketamine relaxes bronchial smooth muscles and may be helpful in patients with reactive airways and in the management of patients experiencing bronchoconstriction.

Clinical Uses & Dosage

Its unique properties, including profound analgesia, stimulation of the sympathetic nervous system, bronchodilation, and minimal respiratory depression, make ketamine an important alternative to the other intravenous anesthetics and a desirable adjunct in many cases despite the unpleasant psychotomimetic effects. Moreover, ketamine can be administered by multiple routes (intravenous, intramuscular, oral, rectal, epidural), thus making it a useful option for premedication in mentally challenged and uncooperative pediatric patients.

Induction of anesthesia can be achieved with ketamine, 1–2 mg/kg intravenously or 4–6 mg/kg intramuscularly. Though the drug is not commonly used for maintenance of anesthesia, its short context-sensitive half-time makes ketamine a candidate for this purpose. For example, general anesthesia can be achieved with the infusion of ketamine, 15–45 mcg/kg/min, plus 50–70% nitrous oxide or by ketamine alone, 30–90 mcg/kg/min.

Small bolus doses of ketamine (0.2–0.8 mg/kg IV) may be useful during regional anesthesia when additional analgesia is needed (eg, cesarean delivery under neuraxial anesthesia with an insufficient regional block). Ketamine provides effective analgesia without compromise of the airway. An infusion of a subanalgesic dose of ketamine (3–5 mcg/kg/min) during general anesthesia and in the early postoperative period may be useful to produce analgesia or reduce opioid tolerance and opioid-induced hyperalgesia. The use of ketamine has always been limited by its unpleasant psychotomimetic side effects, but its unique features make it a very valuable alternative in certain settings, mostly because of the potent analgesia with minimal respiratory depression. Most recently it has become popular as an adjunct administered at subanalgesic doses to limit or reverse opioid tolerance.

DEXMEDETOMIDINE

Dexmedetomidine is a highly selective α_2-adrenergic agonist. Recognition of the usefulness of α_2 agonists is based on observations of decreased anesthetic requirements in patients receiving chronic clonidine therapy. The effects of dexmedetomidine can be antagonized with α_2-antagonist drugs. Dexmedetomidine is the active *S*-enantiomer of medetomidine, a highly selective α_2-adrenergic agonist imidazole derivative that is used in veterinary medicine. Dexmedetomidine is water soluble and available as a parenteral formulation.

Pharmacokinetics

Dexmedetomidine undergoes rapid hepatic metabolism involving conjugation, *N*-methylation, and hydroxylation, followed by conjugation. Metabolites are excreted in the urine and bile. Clearance is high, and the elimination half-time is short (Table 25–2). However, there is a significant increase in the context-sensitive half-time from 4 minutes after a 10-minute infusion to 250 minutes after an 8-hour infusion.

Organ System Effects

A. CNS Effects

Dexmedetomidine produces its selective α_2-agonist effects through activation of CNS α_2 receptors. Hypnosis presumably results from stimulation of α_2 receptors in the locus caeruleus, and the analgesic effect originates at the level of the spinal cord. The sedative effect produced by dexmedetomidine has a different quality than that produced by other intravenous anesthetics in that it more completely resembles a physiologic sleep state through activation of endogenous sleep pathways. Dexmedetomidine is likely to be associated with a decrease in cerebral blood flow without significant changes in ICP and $CMRO_2$. It has the potential to lead to the development of tolerance and dependence.

B. Cardiovascular Effects

Dexmedetomidine infusion results in moderate decreases in heart rate and systemic vascular resistance and, consequently, a decrease in systemic blood pressure. A bolus injection may produce a transient increase in systemic blood pressure and pronounced decrease in heart rate, an effect that is probably mediated through activation of peripheral α_2 adrenoceptors. Bradycardia associated with dexmedetomidine infusion may require treatment. Heart block, severe bradycardia, and asystole have been observed and may result from unopposed vagal stimulation. The response to anticholinergic drugs is unchanged.

C. Respiratory Effects

The effects of dexmedetomidine on the respiratory system are a small to moderate decrease in tidal volume and very little change in the respiratory rate. The ventilatory response to carbon dioxide is unchanged. Although the respiratory effects are mild, upper airway obstruction as a result of sedation is possible. In addition, dexmedetomidine has a synergistic sedative effect when combined with other sedative-hypnotics.

Clinical Uses & Dosage

Dexmedetomidine is principally used for the short-term sedation of intubated and ventilated patients in an ICU setting. In the operating room, dexmedetomidine may be used as an adjunct to general anesthesia or to provide sedation, eg, during awake fiberoptic tracheal intubation or regional anesthesia. When administered during general anesthesia, dexmedetomidine (0.5–1 mcg/kg loading dose over 10–15 minutes, followed by an infusion of 0.2–0.7 mcg/kg/h) decreases the dose requirements for inhaled and injected anesthetics. Awakening and the transition to the postoperative setting may benefit from dexmedetomidine-produced sedative and analgesic effects without respiratory depression.

OPIOID ANALGESICS

Opioids are analgesic agents and are distinct from general anesthetics and hypnotics. Even when high doses of opioid analgesics are administered, recall cannot be prevented reliably unless hypnotic agents such as benzodiazepines also are used. Opioid analgesics are routinely used to achieve postoperative analgesia and intraoperatively as part of a balanced anesthesia regimen as described earlier (see Intravenous Anesthetics). Their pharmacology and clinical use are described in greater detail in Chapter 31.

In addition to their use as part of a balanced anesthesia regimen, opioids in large doses have been used in combination with large doses of benzodiazepines to achieve a general anesthetic state, particularly in patients with limited circulatory reserve who undergo cardiac surgery. When administered in large doses, potent opioids such as fentanyl can induce chest wall (and laryngeal) rigidity, thereby acutely impairing mechanical ventilation. Furthermore, large doses of potent opioids may speed up the development of tolerance and complicate postoperative pain management.

CURRENT CLINICAL PRACTICE

The practice of clinical anesthesia requires integrating the pharmacology and the known adverse effects of these potent drugs with the pathophysiologic state of individual patients. The judgment and experience of the anesthesiologist is tested by every patient to produce the proper depth of anesthesia required to allow invasive surgery to proceed despite major medical problems present in the sickest patients.

P R E P A R A T I O N S   A V A I L A B L E *

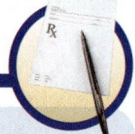

Desflurane (Suprane)
    Liquid: 240 mL for inhalation
Dexmedetomidine (Precedex)
    Parenteral: 100 mcg/mL for IV infusion
Diazepam (generic, Valium)
    Oral: 2, 5, 10 mg tablets; 1 mg/mL and 5 mg/mL solution
    Oral sustained-release: 15 mg capsules
    Rectal: 2.5, 10, 20 mg gel
    Parenteral: 5 mg/mL for injection
Droperidol (generic, Inapsine)
    Parenteral: 2.5 mg/mL for IV or IM injection
Enflurane (Enflurane, Ethrane)
    Liquid: 125, 250 mL for inhalation
Etomidate (Amidate)
    Parenteral: 2 mg/mL for injection
Fospropofol (Lusedra)
    Parenteral: 35 mg/mL in 30 mL vials
Halothane (generic, Fluothane)
    Liquid: 125, 250 mL for inhalation

Isoflurane (Isoflurane, Forane)
    Liquid: 100 mL for inhalation
Ketamine (generic, Ketalar)
    Parenteral: 10, 50, 100 mg/mL for injection
Lorazepam (generic, Ativan)
    Parenteral: 2, 4 mg/mL for injection
Methohexital (Brevital)
    Parenteral: 0.5, 2.5, 5 g powder to reconstitute for injection
Midazolam (generic, Versed)
    Parenteral: 1, 5 mg/mL for injection in 1, 2, 5, 10 mL vials
    Oral: 2 mg/mL syrup for children
Nitrous oxide (gas, supplied in blue cylinders)
Propofol (generic, Diprivan)
    Parenteral: 10 mg/mL for IV injection
Sevoflurane (generic, Ultane)
    Liquid: 250 mL for inhalation
Thiopental (generic, Pentothal)
    Parenteral: powder to reconstitute 20, 25 mg/mL for IV injection

*See Chapter 31 for formulations of opioid agents used in anesthesia.

REFERENCES

Eger EI II: The effect of inspired concentration on the rate of rise of alveolar concentration. Anesthesiology 1963;89:774.

Eger EI II: Uptake and distribution. In: Miller RD (editor): *Anesthesia,* 7th ed. Churchill Livingstone, 2010.

Eger EI II, Saidman LJ, Brandstater B: Minimum alveolar anesthetic concentration: A standard of anesthetic potency. Anesthesiology 1965;26:756.

Fragen RJ: *Drug Infusions in Anesthesiology.* Lippincott Williams & Wilkins, 2005.

Hemmings HC et al: Emerging molecular mechanisms of general anesthetic action. Trends Pharmacol Sci 2005;26:503.

Lugli AK, Yost CS, Kindler CH: Anesthetic mechanisms: Update on the challenge of unravelling the mystery of anaesthesia. Eur J Anaesth 2009;26:807.

Olkkola KT, Ahonen J: Midazolam and other benzodiazepines. Handb Exp Pharmacol 2008;182:335.

Reves JG et al: Intravenous anesthetics. In: Miller RD (editor): *Anesthesia,* 7th ed. Churchill Livingstone, 2010.

Rudolph U et al: Sedatives, anxiolytics, and amnestics. In: Evers AS, Maze M (editors): *Anesthetic Pharmacology: Physiologic Principles and Clinical Practice.* Churchill Livingstone, 2004.

Stoelting R, Hillier S: Barbiturates. In: Stoelting RK, Hillier SC (editors): *Pharmacology and Physiology in Anesthetic Practice.* Lippincott Williams & Wilkins, 2005.

Yasuda N et al: Kinetics of desflurane, isoflurane, and halothane in humans. Anesthesiology 1991;70:489.

CASE STUDY ANSWER

This patient has significant underlying cardiac risk involving major stressful surgery. Balanced anesthesia would begin with intravenous agents that cause minimal changes in blood pressure and heart rate such as propofol or etomidate, combined with potent analgesics such as fentanyl (see Chapter 31) to block undesirable stimulation of autonomic reflexes. Maintenance of anesthesia could incorporate inhaled anesthetics that ensure unconsciousness and amnesia, additional intravenous agents to provide intraoperative and postoperative analgesia, and, if needed, neuromuscular blocking drugs (see Chapter 27) to induce muscle relaxation. The choice of inhaled agent(s) would be made based on the desire to maintain sufficient myocardial contractility, systemic blood pressure, and cardiac output for adequate perfusion of critical organs throughout the operation. Rapid emergence from the combined effects of the chosen anesthetic drugs would facilitate the patient's return to a baseline state of heart function, breathing, and mentation.

26

Local Anesthetics

Kenneth Drasner, MD[*]

CASE STUDY

A 67-year-old woman is scheduled for elective total knee arthroplasty. What local anesthetic agents would be most appropriate if surgical anesthesia were to be administered using a spinal or an epidural technique, and what potential complications might arise from their use? What anesthetics would be most appropriate for providing postoperative analgesia via an indwelling epidural or peripheral nerve catheter?

Simply stated, local anesthesia refers to loss of sensation in a limited region of the body. This is accomplished by disruption of afferent neural traffic via inhibition of impulse generation or propagation. Such blockade may bring with it other physiologic changes such as muscle paralysis and suppression of somatic or visceral reflexes, and these effects might be desirable or undesirable depending on the particular circumstances. Nonetheless, in most cases, it is the loss of sensation, or at least the achievement of localized analgesia, that is the primary goal.

Although local anesthetics are often used as analgesics, it is their ability to provide complete loss of all sensory modalities that is their distinguishing characteristic. The contrast with general anesthesia should be obvious, but it is perhaps worthwhile to emphasize that with local anesthesia the drug is delivered directly to the target organ, and the systemic circulation serves only to diminish or terminate its effect. Local anesthesia can also be produced by various chemical or physical means. However, in routine clinical practice, it is achieved with a rather narrow spectrum of compounds, and recovery is normally spontaneous, predictable, and without residual effects. The development of these compounds has a rich history (see Box: Historical Development of Local Anesthesia), punctuated by serendipitous observations, delayed starts, and an evolution driven more by concerns for safety than improvements in efficacy.

■ BASIC PHARMACOLOGY OF LOCAL ANESTHETICS

Chemistry

Most local anesthetic agents consist of a lipophilic group (eg, an aromatic ring) connected by an intermediate chain via an ester or amide to an ionizable group (eg, a tertiary amine) (Table 26–1). In addition to the general physical properties of the molecules, specific stereochemical configurations are associated with differences in the potency of stereoisomers (eg, levobupivacaine, ropivacaine). Because ester links are more prone to hydrolysis than amide links, esters usually have a shorter duration of action.

Local anesthetics are weak bases and are usually made available clinically as salts to increase solubility and stability. In the body, they exist either as the uncharged base or as a cation (see Chapter 1, Ionization of Weak Acids and Weak Bases). The relative proportions of these two forms are governed by their pK_a and the pH of the body fluids according to the Henderson-Hasselbalch equation, which can be expressed as:

$$pK_a = pH - \log [base]/[conjugate\ acid]$$

If the concentration of base and conjugate acid are equal, the second portion of the right side of the equation drops out, as log 1 = 0, leaving:

$$pK_a = pH \text{ (where base = conjugate acid)}$$

[*]The author thanks Bertram G. Katzung, MD, PhD, and Paul F. White, PhD, MD, for contributions to this chapter in previous editions.

Historical Development of Local Anesthesia

Although the numbing properties of cocaine were recognized for centuries, one might consider September 15, 1884, to mark the "birth of local anesthesia." Based on work performed by Carl Koller, cocaine's numbing effect on the cornea was demonstrated before the Ophthalmological Congress in Heidelberg, ushering in the era of surgical anesthesia. Unfortunately, with widespread use came recognition of cocaine's significant CNS and cardiac toxicity, which along with its addiction potential, tempered enthusiasm for this application. As the early investigator Mattison commented, "the risk of untoward results have robbed this peerless drug of much favor in the minds of many surgeons, and so deprived them of a most valued ally." As cocaine was known to be a benzoic acid ester, the search for alternative local anesthetics focused on this class of compounds, resulting in the identification of benzocaine shortly before the turn of the last century. However, benzocaine proved to have limited utility due to its marked hydrophobicity, and was thus relegated to topical anesthesia, a use for which it still finds limited application in current clinical practice. The first useful injectable local anesthetic, procaine, was introduced shortly thereafter by Einhorn, and its structure has served as the template for the development of the most commonly used modern local anesthetics. The three basic structural elements of these compounds can be appreciated by review of Table 26–1: an aromatic ring, conferring lipophilicity, an ionizable tertiary amine, conferring hydrophilicity, and an intermediate chain connecting these via an ester or amide linkage.

One of procaine's limitations was its short duration of action, a drawback overcome with the introduction of tetracaine in 1928. Unfortunately, tetracaine demonstrated significant toxicity when employed for high-volume peripheral blocks, ultimately reducing its common usage to spinal anesthesia. Both procaine and tetracaine shared another drawback: their ester linkage conferred instability, and particularly in the case of procaine, the free aromatic acid released during ester hydrolysis of the parent compound was believed to be the source of relatively frequent allergic reactions.

Löfgren and Lundqvist circumvented the problem of instability with the introduction of lidocaine in 1948. Lidocaine was the first in a series of amino-amide local anesthetics that would come to dominate the second half of the 20th century. Lidocaine had a more favorable duration of action than procaine, and less systemic toxicity than tetracaine. To this day, it remains one of the most versatile and widely used anesthetics. Nonetheless, some applications required more prolonged block than that afforded by lidocaine, a pharmacologic void that was filled with the introduction of bupivacaine, a more lipophilic and more potent anesthetic. Unfortunately, bupivacaine was found to have greater propensity for significant effects on cardiac conduction and function, which at times proved lethal. Recognition of this potential for cardiac toxicity led to changes in anesthetic practice, and significant toxicity became sufficiently rare for it to remain a widely used anesthetic for nearly every regional technique in modern clinical practice. Nonetheless, this inherent cardiotoxicity would drive developmental work leading to the introduction of two recent additions to the anesthetic armamentarium, levobupivacaine and ropivacaine. The former is the $S(-)$ enantiomer of bupivacaine, which has less affinity for cardiac sodium channels than its $R(+)$ counterpart. Ropivacaine, another $S(-)$ enantiomer, shares this reduced affinity for cardiac sodium channels, while being slightly less potent than bupivacaine or levobupivacaine.

Thus, pK_a can be seen as an effective way to consider the tendency for compounds to exist in a charged or uncharged form, ie, the lower the pK_a, the greater the percentage of uncharged species at a given pH. Because the pK_a of most local anesthetics is in the range of 7.5–9.0, the charged, cationic form will constitute the larger percentage at physiologic pH. A glaring exception is benzocaine, which has a pK_a around 3.5, and thus exists solely as the nonionized base under normal physiologic conditions.

This issue of ionization is of critical importance because the cationic form is the most active at the receptor site. However, the story is a bit more complex, because the receptor site for local anesthetics is at the inner vestibule of the sodium channel, and the charged form of the anesthetic penetrates biologic membranes poorly. Thus, the uncharged form is important for cell penetration. After penetration into the cytoplasm, equilibration leads to formation and binding of the charged cation at the sodium channel, and hence the production of a clinical effect. Drug may also reach the receptor laterally through what has been termed the hydrophobic pathway (Figure 26–1). As a clinical consequence, local anesthetics are less effective when they are injected into infected tissues because the low extracellular pH favors the charged form, with less of the neutral base available for diffusion across the membrane. Conversely, adding bicarbonate to a local anesthetic—a strategy sometimes utilized in clinical practice—will raise the effective concentration of the nonionized form and thus shorten the onset time of a regional block.

Pharmacokinetics

When local anesthetics are used for local, peripheral, and central neuraxial anesthesia—their most common clinical applications—systemic absorption, distribution, and elimination serve only to diminish or terminate their effect. Thus, classic pharmacokinetics plays a lesser role than with systemic therapeutics, yet remains important to the anesthetic's duration and critical to the potential development of adverse reactions, specifically cardiac and central nervous system (CNS) toxicity.

Some pharmacokinetic properties of the commonly used amide local anesthetics are summarized in Table 26–2. The pharmacokinetics

TABLE 26–1 Structure and properties of some ester and amide local anesthetics.[1]

Structure	Potency (Procaine = 1)	Duration of Action
Esters		
Cocaine	2	Medium
Procaine (Novocain)	1	Short
Tetracaine (Pontocaine)	16	Long
Benzocaine	Surface use only	
Amides		
Lidocaine (Xylocaine)	4	Medium
Mepivacaine (Carbocaine, Isocaine)	2	Medium
Bupivacaine (Marcaine), Levobupivacaine (Chirocaine)	16	Long
Ropivacaine (Naropin)	16	Long
Articaine	nf[2]	Medium

[1]Other chemical types are available including ethers (pramoxine), ketones (dyclonine), and phenetidin derivatives (phenacaine).

[2]Data not found.

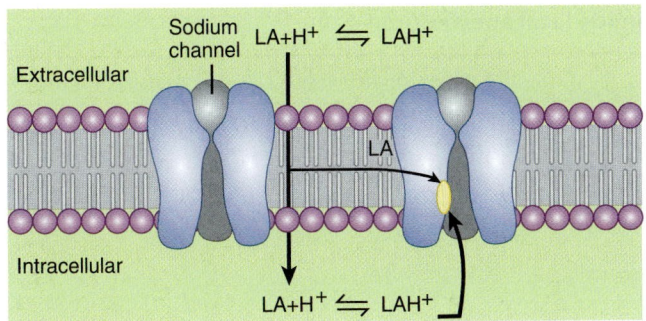

FIGURE 26–1 Schematic diagram depicting paths of local anesthetic (LA) to receptor sites. Extracellular anesthetic exists in equilibrium between charged and uncharged forms. The charged cation penetrates lipid membranes poorly; intracellular access is thus achieved by passage of the uncharged form. Intracellular re-equilibration results in formation of the more active charged species, which binds to the receptor at the inner vestibule of the sodium channel. Anesthetic may also gain access more directly by diffusing laterally within the membrane (hydrophobic pathway).

of the ester-based local anesthetics has not been extensively studied owing to their rapid breakdown in plasma (elimination half-life < 1 minute).

A. Absorption

Systemic absorption of injected local anesthetic from the site of administration is determined by several factors, including dosage, site of injection, drug-tissue binding, local tissue blood flow, use of a vasoconstrictor (eg, epinephrine), and the physicochemical properties of the drug itself. Anesthetics that are more lipid soluble are generally more potent, have a longer duration of action, and take longer to achieve their clinical effect. Extensive protein binding also serves to increase the duration of action.

Application of a local anesthetic to a highly vascular area such as the tracheal mucosa or the tissue surrounding intercostal nerves results in more rapid absorption and thus higher blood levels than if the local anesthetic is injected into a poorly perfused tissue such as subcutaneous fat. When used for major conduction blocks, the peak serum levels will vary as a function of the specific site of injection,

with intercostal blocks among the highest, and sciatic and femoral among the lowest (Figure 26–2). When vasoconstrictors are used with local anesthetics, the resultant reduction in blood flow serves to reduce the rate of systemic absorption and thus diminishes peak serum levels. This effect is generally most evident with the shorter-acting, less potent, and less lipid-soluble anesthetics.

B. Distribution

1. Localized—As local anesthetic is usually injected directly at the site of the target organ, distribution within this compartment plays an essential role with respect to achievement of clinical effect. For example, anesthetics delivered into the subarachnoid space will be diluted with cerebrospinal fluid (CSF) and the pattern of distribution will be dependent upon a host of factors, among the most critical being the specific gravity relative to that of CSF and the patient's position. Solutions are termed hyperbaric, isobaric, and hypobaric, and will respectively descend, remain relatively static, or ascend, within the subarachnoid space due to gravity when the patient sits upright. A review and analysis of relevant literature cited 25 factors that have been invoked as determinants of spread of local anesthetic in CSF, which can be broadly classified as characteristics of the anesthetic solution, CSF constituents, patient characteristics, and techniques of injection. Somewhat similar considerations apply to epidural and peripheral blocks.

2. Systemic—The peak blood levels achieved during major conduction anesthesia will be minimally affected by the concentration of anesthetic or the speed of injection. The disposition of these agents can be well approximated by a two-compartment model. The initial alpha phase reflects rapid distribution in blood and highly perfused organs (eg, brain, liver, heart, kidney), characterized by a steep exponential decline in concentration. This is followed by a slower declining beta phase reflecting distribution into less well perfused tissue (eg, muscle, gut), and may assume a nearly linear rate of decline. The potential toxicity of the local anesthetics is affected by the protective effect afforded by uptake by the lungs, which serve to attenuate the arterial concentration, though the time course and magnitude of this effect have not been adequately characterized.

C. Metabolism and Excretion

The amide local anesthetics are converted to more water-soluble metabolites in the liver (amide type) or in plasma (ester type),

TABLE 26–2 Pharmacokinetic properties of several amide local anesthetics.

Agent	$t_{1/2}$ Distribution (min)	$t_{1/2}$ Elimination (h)	V_{dss} (L)	CL (L/min)
Bupivacaine	28	3.5	72	0.47
Lidocaine	10	1.6	91	0.95
Mepivacaine	7	1.9	84	0.78
Prilocaine	5	1.5	261	2.84
Ropivacaine	23	4.2	47	0.44

CL, clearance; V_{dss}, volume of distribution at steady state.

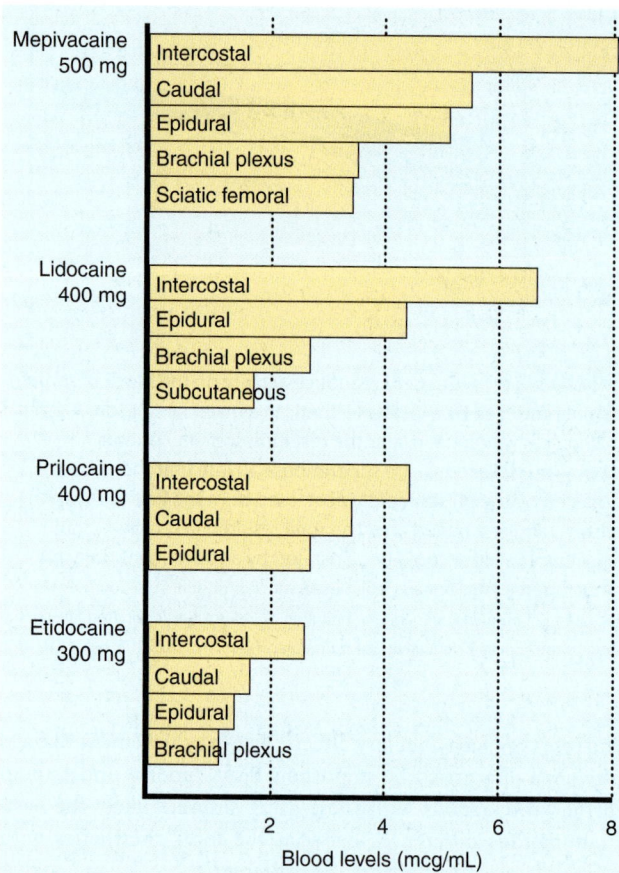

FIGURE 26–2 Comparative peak blood levels of several local anesthetic agents following administration into various anatomic sites. (Modified, with permission, from Covino BD, Vassals HG: *Local Anesthetics: Mechanism of Action in Clinical Use.* Grune & Stratton, 1976.)

which are excreted in the urine. Since local anesthetics in the uncharged form diffuse readily through lipid membranes, little or no urinary excretion of the neutral form occurs. Acidification of urine promotes ionization of the tertiary amine base to the more water-soluble charged form, leading to more rapid elimination. Ester-type local anesthetics are hydrolyzed very rapidly in the blood by circulating butyrylcholinesterase to inactive metabolites. For example, the half-lives of procaine and chloroprocaine in plasma are less than a minute. However, excessive concentrations may accumulate in patients with reduced or absent plasma hydrolysis secondary to atypical plasma cholinesterase.

The amide local anesthetics undergo complex biotransformation in the liver, which includes hydroxylation and *N*-dealkylation by liver microsomal cytochrome P450 isozymes. There is considerable variation in the rate of liver metabolism of individual amide compounds, with prilocaine (fastest) > lidocaine > mepivacaine > ropivacaine ≈ bupivacaine and levobupivacaine (slowest). As a result, toxicity from amide-type local anesthetics is more likely to occur in patients with hepatic disease. For example, the average elimination half-life of lidocaine may be increased from 1.6 hours in normal patients ($t_{1/2}$, Table 26–2) to more than 6 hours in patients with severe liver disease. Many other drugs used in anesthesia are metabolized by the same P450 isozymes, and concomitant

administration of these competing drugs may slow the hepatic metabolism of the local anesthetics. Decreased hepatic elimination of local anesthetics would also be anticipated in patients with reduced hepatic blood flow. For example, the hepatic elimination of lidocaine in patients anesthetized with volatile anesthetics (which reduce liver blood flow) is slower than in patients anesthetized with intravenous anesthetic techniques. Delayed metabolism due to impaired hepatic blood flow may likewise occur in patients with congestive heart failure.

Pharmacodynamics

A. Mechanism of Action

1. Membrane potential—The primary mechanism of action of local anesthetics is blockade of voltage-gated sodium channels (Figure 26–1). The excitable membrane of nerve axons, like the membrane of cardiac muscle (see Chapter 14) and neuronal cell bodies (see Chapter 21), maintains a resting transmembrane potential of –90 to –60 mV. During excitation, the sodium channels open, and a fast, inward sodium current quickly depolarizes the membrane toward the sodium equilibrium potential (+40 mV). As a result of this depolarization process, the sodium channels close (inactivate) and potassium channels open. The outward flow of potassium repolarizes the membrane toward the potassium equilibrium potential (about –95 mV); repolarization returns the sodium channels to the rested state with a characteristic recovery time that determines the refractory period. The transmembrane ionic gradients are maintained by the sodium pump. These ionic fluxes are similar to, but simpler than, those in heart muscle, and local anesthetics have similar effects in both tissues.

2. Sodium channel isoforms—Each sodium channel consists of a single alpha subunit containing a central ion-conducting pore associated with accessory beta subunits. The pore-forming alpha subunit is actually sufficient for functional expression, but the kinetics and voltage dependence of channel gating are modified by the beta subunit. A variety of different sodium channels have been characterized by electrophysiologic recording, and subsequently isolated and cloned, while mutational analysis has allowed for identification of the essential components of the local anesthetic binding site. Nine members of a mammalian family of sodium channels have been so characterized and classified as $Na_v1.1$–$Na_v1.9$, where the chemical symbol represents the primary ion, the subscript denotes the physiologic regulator (in this case voltage), the initial number denotes the gene, and the number following the period indicates the particular isoform.

3. Channel blockade—Biologic toxins such as batrachotoxin, aconitine, veratridine, and some scorpion venoms bind to receptors within the channel and prevent inactivation. This results in prolonged influx of sodium through the channel and depolarization of the resting potential. The marine toxins tetrodotoxin (TTX) and saxitoxin have clinical effects that largely resemble those of local anesthetics (ie, block of conduction without a change in the resting potential). However, in contrast to the

local anesthetics, their binding site is located near the extracellular surface. The sensitivity of these channels to TTX varies, and subclassification based on this pharmacologic sensitivity has important physiologic and therapeutic implications. Six of the aforementioned channels are sensitive to nanomolar concentration of this biotoxin (TTX-S), while three are resistant (TTX-R). Of the latter, $Na_v1.8$ and $Na_v1.9$ appear to be exclusively expressed in dorsal root ganglia nociceptors, which raises the developmental possibility of targeting these specific neuronal subpopulations. Such fine-tuned analgesic therapy has the theoretical potential of providing effective analgesia, while limiting the significant adverse effects produced by nonspecific sodium channel blockers.

When progressively increasing concentrations of a local anesthetic are applied to a nerve fiber, the threshold for excitation increases, impulse conduction slows, the rate of rise of the action potential declines, action potential amplitude decreases, and, finally, the ability to generate an action potential is completely abolished. These progressive effects result from binding of the local anesthetic to more and more sodium channels. If the sodium current is blocked over a critical length of the nerve, propagation across the blocked area is no longer possible. In myelinated nerves, the critical length appears to be two to three nodes of Ranvier. At the minimum dose required to block propagation, the resting potential is not significantly altered.

The blockade of sodium channels by most local anesthetics is both voltage and time dependent: Channels in the rested state, which predominate at more negative membrane potentials, have a much lower affinity for local anesthetics than activated (open state) and inactivated channels, which predominate at more positive membrane potentials (see Figure 14–10). Therefore, the effect of a given drug concentration is more marked in rapidly firing axons than in resting fibers (Figure 26–3). Between successive action potentials, a portion of the sodium channels will recover from the local anesthetic block (see Figure 14–10). The recovery from drug-induced block is 10–1000 times slower than the recovery of channels from normal inactivation (as shown for the cardiac membrane in Figure 14–4). As a result, the refractory period is lengthened and the nerve conducts fewer action potentials.

Elevated extracellular calcium partially antagonizes the action of local anesthetics owing to the calcium-induced increase in the surface potential on the membrane (which favors the low-affinity rested state). Conversely, increases in extracellular potassium depolarize the membrane potential and favor the inactivated state, enhancing the effect of local anesthetics.

4. Other effects—Currently used local anesthetics bind to the sodium channel with low affinity and poor specificity, and there are multiple other sites for which their affinity is nearly the same as that for sodium channel binding. Thus, at clinically relevant concentrations, local anesthetics are potentially active at countless other channels (eg, potassium and calcium), enzymes (eg, adenylate cyclase, carnitine-acylcarnitine translocase), and receptors (eg, *N*-methyl-D-aspartate [NMDA], G protein-coupled, 5-HT$_3$, neurokinin-1 [substance P receptor]).

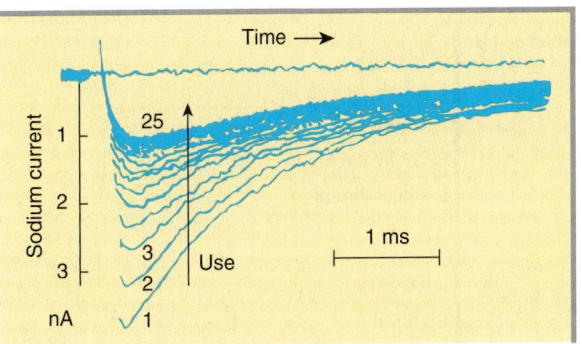

FIGURE 26–3 Effect of repetitive activity on the block of sodium current produced by a local anesthetic in a myelinated axon. A series of 25 pulses was applied, and the resulting sodium currents (downward deflections) are superimposed. Note that the current produced by the pulses rapidly decreased from the first to the 25th pulse. A long rest period after the train resulted in recovery from block, but the block could be reinstated by a subsequent train. nA, nanoamperes. (Modified and reproduced, with permission, from Courtney KR: Mechanism of frequency-dependent inhibition of sodium currents in frog myelinated nerve by the lidocaine derivative GEA. J Pharmacol Exp Ther 1975;195:225.)

The role that such ancillary effects play in achievement of local anesthesia appears to be important but is poorly understood. Further, interactions with these other sites are likely the basis for numerous differences between the local anesthetics with respect to anesthetic effects (eg, differential block) and toxicities that do not parallel anesthetic potency, and thus are not adequately accounted for solely by blockade of the voltage-gated sodium channel.

The actions of circulating local anesthetics at such diverse sites exert a multitude of effects, some of which go beyond pain control, including some that are also potentially beneficial. For example, there is evidence to suggest that the blunting of the stress response and improvements in perioperative outcome that may occur with epidural anesthesia derive in part from an action of the anesthetic beyond its sodium channel block. Circulating anesthetics also demonstrate antithrombotic effects having an impact on coagulation, platelet aggregation, and the microcirculation, as well as modulation of inflammation.

B. Structure-Activity Characteristics of Local Anesthetics

The smaller and more highly lipophilic local anesthetics have a faster rate of interaction with the sodium channel receptor. As previously noted, potency is also positively correlated with lipid solubility. Lidocaine, procaine, and mepivacaine are more water soluble than tetracaine, bupivacaine, and ropivacaine. The latter agents are more potent and have longer durations of local anesthetic action. These long-acting local anesthetics also bind more extensively to proteins and can be displaced from these binding sites by other protein-bound drugs. In the case of optically active agents (eg, bupivacaine), the *R*(+) isomer can usually be shown to be slightly more potent than the *S*(−) isomer (levobupivacaine).

C. Neuronal Factors Affecting Block

1. Differential block—Since local anesthetics are capable of blocking all nerves, their actions are not limited to the desired loss of sensation from sites of noxious (painful) stimuli. With central neuraxial techniques (spinal or epidural), motor paralysis may impair respiratory activity, and autonomic nerve blockade may promote hypotension. Further, while motor paralysis may be desirable during surgery, it may be disadvantageous in other settings. For example, motor weakness occurring as a consequence of epidural anesthesia during obstetrical labor may limit the ability of the patient to bear down (ie, "push") during delivery. Similarly, when used for postoperative analgesia, weakness may hamper ability to ambulate without assistance and pose a risk of falling, while residual autonomic blockade may interfere with bladder function, resulting in urinary retention and the need for bladder catheterization. These issues are particular problematic in the setting of ambulatory (same-day) surgery, which represents an ever-increasing percentage of surgical caseloads.

2. Intrinsic susceptibility of nerve fibers—Nerve fibers differ significantly in their susceptibility to local anesthetic blockade. It has been traditionally taught, and still often cited, that local anesthetics preferentially block smaller diameter fibers first because the distance over which such fibers can passively propagate an electrical impulse is shorter. However, a variable proportion of large fibers are blocked prior to the disappearance of the small fiber component of the compound action potential. Most notably, myelinated nerves tend to be blocked before unmyelinated nerves of the same diameter. For example, preganglionic B fibers are blocked before the smaller unmyelinated C fibers involved in pain transmission (Table 26–3).

Another important factor underlying differential block derives from the state- and use-dependent mechanism of action of local anesthetics. Blockade by these drugs is more marked at higher frequencies of depolarization. Sensory (pain) fibers have a high firing rate and relatively long action potential duration. Motor fibers fire at a slower rate and have a shorter action potential duration. As type A delta and C fibers participate in high-frequency pain transmission, this characteristic may favor blockade of these fibers earlier and with lower concentrations of local anesthetics. The potential impact of such effects mandates cautious interpretation of non-physiologic experiments evaluating intrinsic susceptibility of nerves to conduction block by local anesthetics.

3. Anatomic arrangement—In addition to the effect of intrinsic vulnerability to local anesthetic block, the anatomic organization of the peripheral nerve bundle may impact the onset and susceptibility of its components. As one would predict based on the necessity of having proximal sensory fibers join the nerve trunk last, the core will contain sensory fibers innervating the most distal sites. Anesthetic placed outside the nerve bundle will thus reach and anesthetize the proximal fibers located at the outer portion of the bundle first, and sensory block will occur in sequence from proximal to distal.

■ CLINICAL PHARMACOLOGY OF LOCAL ANESTHETICS

Local anesthetics can provide highly effective analgesia in well-defined regions of the body. The usual routes of administration include topical application (eg, nasal mucosa, wound [incision site] margins), injection in the vicinity of peripheral nerve endings (perineural infiltration) and major nerve trunks (blocks), and injection into the epidural or subarachnoid spaces surrounding the spinal cord (Figure 26–4).

Clinical Block Characteristics

In clinical practice, there is generally an orderly evolution of block components beginning with sympathetic transmission and

TABLE 26–3 Relative size and susceptibility of different types of nerve fibers to local anesthetics.

Fiber Type	Function	Diameter (µm)	Myelination	Conduction Velocity (m/s)	Sensitivity to Block
Type A					
Alpha	Proprioception, motor	12–20	Heavy	70–120	+
Beta	Touch, pressure	5–12	Heavy	30–70	++
Gamma	Muscle spindles	3–6	Heavy	15–30	++
Delta	Pain, temperature	2–5	Heavy	5–25	+++
Type B	Preganglionic autonomic	< 3	Light	3–15	++++
Type C					
Dorsal root	Pain	0.4–1.2	None	0.5–2.3	++++
Sympathetic	Postganglionic	0.3–1.3	None	0.7–2.3	++++

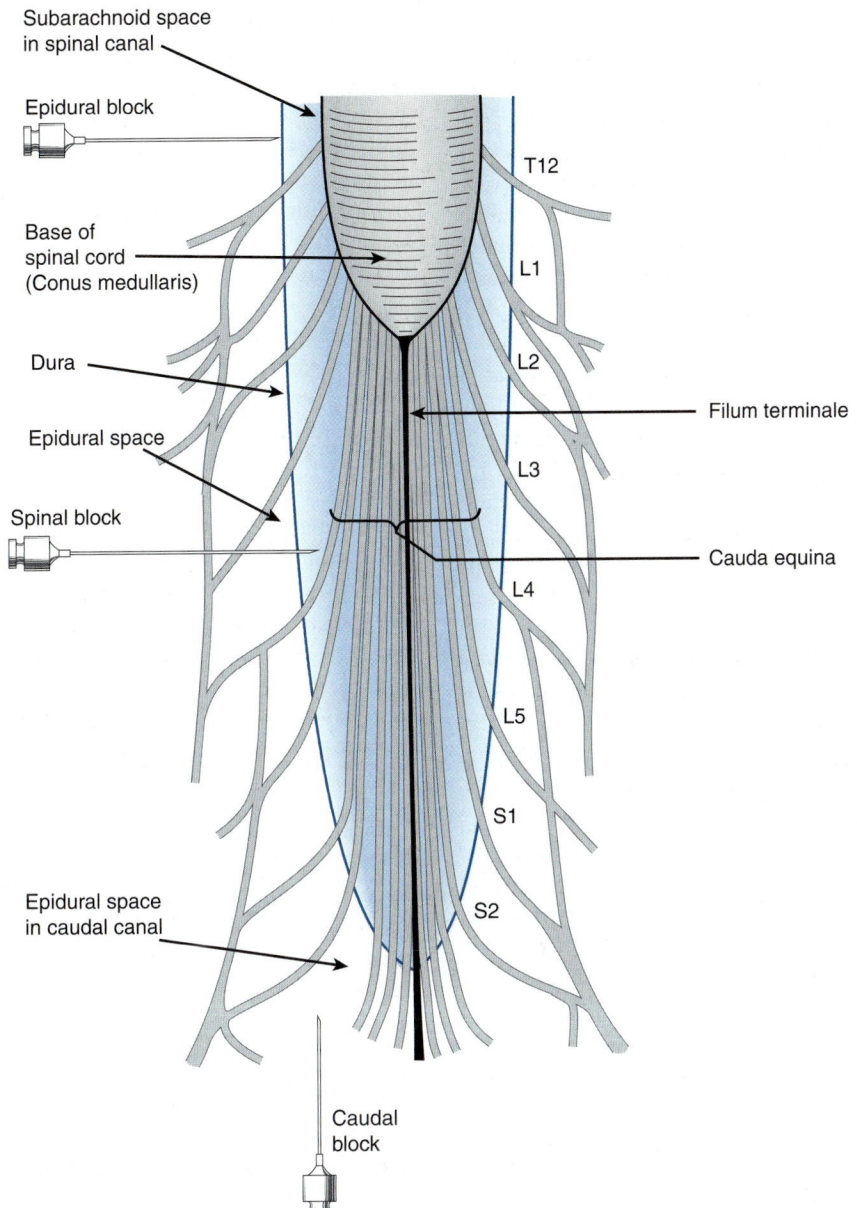

FIGURE 26–4 Schematic diagram of the typical sites of injection of local anesthetics in and around the spinal canal. When local anesthetics are injected extradurally, it is referred to as an epidural block. A caudal block is a specific type of epidural block in which a needle is inserted into the caudal canal via the sacral hiatus. Injections around peripheral nerves are known as perineural blocks (eg, paravertebral block). Finally, injection into cerebrospinal fluid in the subarachnoid (intrathecal) space is referred to as a spinal block.

progressing to temperature, pain, light touch, and finally motor block. This is most readily appreciated during onset of spinal anesthesia, where a spatial discrepancy can be detected in modalities, the most vulnerable components achieving greater dermatomal (cephalad) spread. Thus, loss of the sensation of cold (often assessed by a wet alcohol sponge) will be roughly two segments above the analgesic level for pinprick, which in turn will be roughly two segments rostral to loss of light touch recognition. However, because of the anatomic considerations noted earlier for peripheral nerve trunks, onset with peripheral blocks is more variable, and proximal motor weakness may precede onset of more distal sensory loss. Additionally, anesthetic solution is not generally deposited evenly around a nerve bundle, and longitudinal spread and radial penetration into the nerve trunk are far from uniform.

With respect to differential block, it is worth noting that "successful" surgical anesthesia may require loss of touch, not just ablation of pain, as some patients will find even the sensation of touch distressing during surgery, often fearing that the procedure may become painful. Further, while differences may exist in modalities, it is not possible with conventional techniques to produce surgical anesthesia without some loss of motor function.

A. Effect of Added Vasoconstrictors

Several benefits may be derived from addition of a vasoconstrictor to a local anesthetic. First, localized neuronal uptake is enhanced because of higher sustained local tissue concentrations that can translate clinically into a longer duration block. This may enable adequate anesthesia for more prolonged procedures, extended duration of postoperative pain control, and lower total anesthetic requirement. Second, peak blood levels will be lowered as absorption is more closely matched to metabolism and elimination, and the risk of systemic toxic effects is reduced. Moreover, when incorporated into a spinal anesthetic, epinephrine may not only contribute to prolongation of the local anesthetic effect via its vasoconstrictor properties, but also exert a direct analgesic effect mediated by postsynaptic α_2 adrenoceptors within the spinal cord. Recognition of this potential has led to the clinical use of the α_2 agonist clonidine as a local anesthetic adjuvant for spinal anesthesia.

Conversely, inclusion of epinephrine may have untoward effects. The addition of epinephrine to anesthetic solutions can potentiate the neurotoxicity of local anesthetics used for peripheral nerve blocks or spinal anesthesia. Further, the use of a vasoconstrictor agent in an area that lacks adequate collateral flow (eg, digital block) is generally avoided, though some have questioned the validity of this proscription.

B. Intentional Use of Systemic Local Anesthetics

Although the principal use of local anesthetics is to achieve anesthesia in a restricted area, these agents are sometimes deliberately administered systemically to take advantage of suppressive effects on pain processing. In addition to documented reductions in anesthetic requirement and postoperative pain, systemic administration of local anesthetics has been used with some success in the treatment of chronic pain, and this effect may outlast the duration of anesthetic exposure. The achievement of pain control by systemic administration of local anesthetics is thought to derive, at least in part, from the suppression of abnormal ectopic discharge, an effect observed at concentrations of local anesthetic an order of magnitude lower than those required for blockade of propagation of action potentials in normal nerves. Consequently, these effects can be achieved without the adverse effects that would derive from failure of normal nerve conduction. Escalating doses of anesthetic appear to exert the following systemic actions: (1) low concentrations may preferentially suppress ectopic impulse generation in chronically injured peripheral nerves; (2) moderate concentrations may suppress central sensitization, which would explain therapeutic benefit that may extend beyond the anesthetic exposure; and (3) higher concentrations will produce general analgesic effects and may culminate in serious toxicity.

Toxicity

Local anesthetic toxicity derives from two distinct processes: (1) systemic effects following inadvertent intravascular injection or absorption of the local anesthetic from the site of administration; and (2) neurotoxicity resulting from local effects produced by direct contact with neural elements.

A. Systemic Toxicity

The dose of local anesthetic used for epidural anesthesia or high-volume peripheral blocks is sufficient to produce major clinical toxicity, even death. To minimize risk, maximum recommended doses for each drug for each general application have been promulgated. The concept underlying this approach is that absorption from the site of injection should appropriately match metabolism, thereby preventing toxic serum levels. However, these recommendations do not consider patient characteristics or concomitant risk factors, nor do they take into account the specific peripheral nerve block performed, which has a significant impact on the rate of systemic uptake (Figure 26–2). Most importantly, they fail to afford protection from toxicity induced by inadvertent intravascular injection (occasionally into an artery, but more commonly a vein).

1. CNS toxicity—All local anesthetics have the ability to produce sedation, light-headedness, visual and auditory disturbances, and restlessness when high plasma concentrations result from rapid absorption or inadvertent intravascular administration. An early symptom of local anesthetic toxicity is circumoral and tongue numbness and a metallic taste. At higher concentrations, nystagmus and muscular twitching occur, followed by tonic-clonic convulsions. Local anesthetics apparently cause depression of cortical inhibitory pathways, thereby allowing unopposed activity of excitatory neuronal pathways. This transitional stage of unbalanced excitation (ie, seizure activity) is then followed by generalized CNS depression. However, this classic pattern of evolving toxicity has been largely characterized in human volunteer studies (which are ethically constrained to low doses), and by graded administration in animal models. Deviations from such classic progression are common in clinical toxicity and will be influenced by a host of factors, including patient vulnerability, the particular anesthetic administered, concurrent drugs, and rate of rise of serum drug levels. A recent literature review of reported clinical cases of local anesthetic cardiac toxicity found prodromal signs of CNS toxicity in only 18% of cases.

When large doses of a local anesthetic are required (eg, for major peripheral nerve block or local infiltration for major plastic surgery), premedication with a parenteral benzodiazepine (eg, diazepam or midazolam) will provide some prophylaxis against local anesthetic-induced CNS toxicity. However, such premedication will have little, if any, effect on cardiovascular toxicity, potentially delaying recognition of a life-threatening overdose. Of note, administration of a propofol infusion or general anesthesia accounted for 5 of the 10 cases presenting with isolated cardiovascular toxicity in the aforementioned literature review of reported clinical cases.

If seizures do occur, it is critical to prevent hypoxemia and acidosis, which potentiate anesthetic toxicity. Rapid tracheal intubation can facilitate adequate ventilation and oxygenation, and is essential to prevent pulmonary aspiration of gastric contents in patients at risk. The effect of hyperventilation is complex, and its role in resuscitation following anesthetic overdose is somewhat controversial, but it likely offers distinct benefit if used to counteract metabolic acidosis. Seizures induced by local anesthetics should be rapidly controlled to prevent patient harm and exacerbation of acidosis. A recent practice advisory from the American Society of Regional Anesthesia advocates benzodiazepines as first-line drugs (eg, midazolam, 0.03–0.06 mg/kg) because of their hemodynamic stability, but small doses of propofol (eg, 0.25–0.5 mg/kg) were considered acceptable alternatives, as they are often more immediately available in the setting of local anesthetic administration. The motor activity of the seizure can be effectively terminated by administration of a neuromuscular blocker, though this will not diminish the CNS manifestations, and efforts must include therapy directed at the underlying seizure activity.

2. Cardiotoxicity—The most feared complications associated with local anesthetic administration result from the profound effects these agents can have on cardiac conduction and function. In 1979, an editorial by Albright reviewed the circumstances of six deaths associated with the use of bupivacaine and etidocaine. This seminal piece suggested that these relatively new lipophilic and potent anesthetics had greater potential cardiotoxicity, and that cardiac arrest could occur concurrently or immediately following seizures and, most importantly, in the absence of hypoxia or acidosis. Although this suggestion was sharply criticized, subsequent clinical experience unfortunately reinforced Albright's concern—within 4 years the Food and Drug Administration (FDA) had received reports of 12 cases of cardiac arrest associated with the use of 0.75% bupivacaine for epidural anesthesia in obstetrics. Further support for enhanced cardiotoxicity of these anesthetics came from animal studies demonstrating that doses of bupivacaine and etidocaine as low as two thirds those producing convulsions could induce arrhythmias, while the margin between CNS and cardiac toxicity was less than half that for lidocaine. In response, the FDA banned the use of 0.75% bupivacaine in obstetrics. In addition, incorporation of a test dose became ingrained as a standard of anesthetic practice, along with the practice of fractionated administration of local anesthetic.

Although reduction in bupivacaine's anesthetic concentration and changes in anesthetic practice did much to reduce the risk of cardiotoxicity, the recognized differences in the toxicity of the stereoisomers comprising bupivacaine created an opportunity for the development of potentially safer anesthetics (see Chapter 1). Investigations demonstrated that the enantiomers of the racemic mixture bupivacaine were not equivalent with respect to cardiotoxicity, the S(–) enantiomer having better therapeutic advantage, leading to the subsequent marketing of levobupivacaine. This was followed shortly thereafter by ropivacaine, a slightly less potent anesthetic than bupivacaine. It should be noted, however, that the reduction in toxicity afforded by these compounds is only modest, and that risk of significant cardiotoxicity remains a very real concern when these anesthetics are administered for high-volume blocks.

3. Reversal of bupivacaine toxicity—Recently, a series of clinical events, serendipitous observations, systematic experimentation, and astute clinical decisions have identified a relatively simple, practical and apparently effective therapy for resistant bupivacaine cardiotoxicity using intravenous infusion of lipid. Furthermore, this therapy appears to have applications that extend

beyond bupivacaine cardiotoxicity to the cardiac or CNS toxicity induced by an overdose of any lipid-soluble drug (see Box: Lipid Resuscitation).

B. Localized Toxicity

1. Neural injury—From the early introduction of spinal anesthesia into clinical practice, sporadic reports of neurologic injury associated with this technique raised concern that local anesthetic agents were potentially neurotoxic. Following injuries associated with Durocaine—a spinal anesthetic formulation containing procaine—initial attention focused on the vehicle components. However, experimental studies found 10% procaine alone induced similar injuries in cats, whereas the vehicle did not. Concern for anesthetic neurotoxicity reemerged in the early 1980s with a series of reports of major neurologic injury occurring with the use of chloroprocaine for epidural anesthesia. In these cases, there was evidence that anesthetic intended for the epidural space was inadvertently administered intrathecally. As the dose required for spinal anesthesia is roughly an order of magnitude less than for epidural anesthesia, injury was apparently the result of excessive exposure of the more vulnerable subarachnoid neural elements.

With changes in vehicle formulation and in clinical practice, concern for toxicity again subsided, only to reemerge a decade later with reports of cauda equina syndrome associated with continuous spinal anesthesia (CSA). In contrast to the more common single-injection technique, CSA involves placing a catheter in the subarachnoid space to permit repetitive dosing to facilitate adequate anesthesia and maintenance of block for extended periods. In these cases the local anesthetic was evidently administered to a relatively restricted area of the subarachnoid space; in order to extend the block to achieve adequate surgical anesthesia, multiple repetitive doses of anesthetic were then administered. By the time the block was adequate, neurotoxic concentrations had accumulated in a restricted area of the caudal region of the subarachnoid space. Most notably, the anesthetic involved in the majority of these cases was lidocaine, a drug most clinicians considered to be the least toxic of agents. This was followed by reports of neurotoxic injury occurring with lidocaine intended for epidural administration that had inadvertently been administered intrathecally, similar to the cases involving chloroprocaine a decade earlier. The occurrence of neurotoxic injury with CSA and subarachnoid administration of epidural doses of lidocaine served to establish vulnerability whenever excessive anesthetic was administered intrathecally, regardless of the specific anesthetic used. Of even more concern, subsequent reports provided evidence for injury with spinal lidocaine administered at the high end of the recommended clinical dosage, prompting recommendations for a reduction in maximum dose. These clinical reports (as well as concurrent experimental studies) served to dispel the concept that modern local anesthetics administered at clinically relevant doses and concentrations were incapable of inducing neurotoxic injury.

The mechanism of local anesthetic neurotoxicity has been extensively investigated in cell culture, isolated axons, and in vivo models. These studies have demonstrated a myriad of deleterious effects including conduction failure, membrane damage, enzyme

Lipid Resuscitation

Based on a case of apparent cardiotoxicity from a very low dose of bupivacaine in a patient with carnitine deficiency, Weinberg postulated that this metabolic derangement led to enhanced toxicity due to the accumulation of fatty acids within the cardiac myocyte. He hypothesized that administration of lipid would similarly potentiate bupivacaine cardiotoxicity, but experiments performed to test this hypothesis demonstrated exactly the opposite effect. Accordingly, he began systematic laboratory investigations, which clearly demonstrated the potential efficacy of an intravenous lipid emulsion (ILE) for resuscitation from bupivacaine cardiotoxicity. Clinical confirmation came 8 years later with the report of the successful resuscitation of a patient who sustained an anesthetic-induced (bupivacaine plus mepivacaine) cardiac arrest refractory to standard advanced cardiac life support procedures (ACLS). Numerous similar reports of successful resuscitations soon followed, extending this clinical experience to other anesthetics including levobupivacaine and ropivacaine, anesthetic-induced CNS toxicity, as well as toxicity induced by other classes of compounds, eg, bupropion-induced cardiovascular collapse and multiform ventricular tachycardia provoked by

haloperidol. Laboratory investigations have likewise provided evidence of efficacy for treatment of diverse toxic challenges (eg, verapamil, clomipramine, and propranolol).

The mechanism by which lipid is effective is incompletely understood, but its predominant effect appears to stem from its ability to extract a lipophilic drug from aqueous plasma and tissue targets, a mechanism termed lipid sink. With respect to bupivacaine cardiotoxicity, there may be an additive effect of restoring energy to the myocardium by overcoming bupivacaine-induced inhibition of fatty acid transport. Although numerous questions remain, the evolving evidence is sufficient to warrant administration of lipid in cases of systemic anesthetic toxicity. Its use has been promulgated by a task force of the American Society of Regional Anesthesia, and administration of lipid has been incorporated into the most recent revision of ACLS guidelines for Cardiac Arrest in Special Situations. Importantly, propofol cannot be administered for this purpose, as the relatively enormous volume of this solution required for lipid therapy would deliver lethal quantities of propofol.

---

leakage, cytoskeletal disruption, accumulation of intracellular calcium, disruption of axonal transport, growth cone collapse, and apoptosis. It is not clear what role these factors or others play in clinical injury. It is clear, however, that injury does not result from blockade of the voltage-gated sodium channel per se, and thus clinical effect and toxicity are not tightly linked.

2. Transient neurologic symptoms (TNS)—In addition to the very rare but devastating neural complications that can occur with neuraxial (spinal and epidural) administration of local anesthetics, a syndrome of transient pain or dysesthesia, or both, has been recently linked to use of lidocaine for spinal anesthesia. Although these symptoms are not associated with sensory loss, motor weakness, or bowel and bladder dysfunction, the pain can be quite severe, often exceeding that induced by the surgical procedure. TNS occurs even at modest doses of anesthetic, and has been documented in as many as one third of patients receiving lidocaine, with increased risk associated with certain patient positions during surgery (eg, lithotomy), and with ambulatory anesthesia. Risk with other anesthetics varies considerably. For example, the incidence is only slightly reduced with procaine or mepivacaine but appears to be negligible with bupivacaine, prilocaine, and chloroprocaine. The etiology and significance of TNS remain to be established, but differences between factors affecting TNS and experimental animal toxicity argue strongly against a common mechanism mediating these symptoms and persistent or permanent neurologic deficits. Nonetheless, the high incidence of TNS has greatly contributed to dissatisfaction with lidocaine as a spinal anesthetic, leading to its near abandonment for this technique (although it remains a popular and appropriate anesthetic for all other applications, including epidural anesthesia). Chloroprocaine, once considered a

more toxic anesthetic, is now being explored for short-duration spinal anesthesia as an alternative to lidocaine, a compound that has been used for well over 50 million spinal anesthetic procedures.

■ COMMONLY USED LOCAL ANESTHETICS & THEIR APPLICATIONS

ARTICAINE

Approved for use in the USA as a dental anesthetic in April 2000, articaine is unique among the amino-amide anesthetics in having a thiophene, rather than a benzene ring, as well as an additional ester group that is subject to metabolism by plasma esterases (Table 26–1). The modification of the ring serves to enhance lipophilicity, and thus improve tissue penetration, while inclusion of the ester leads to a shorter plasma half-life (approximately 20 minutes) potentially imparting a better therapeutic index with respect to systemic toxicity. These characteristics have led to widespread popularity in dental anesthesia, where it is generally considered to be more effective, and possibly safer, than lidocaine, the prior standard. Balanced against these positive attributes are concerns that development of persistent paresthesias, while rare, may be three times more common with articaine. However, prilocaine has been associated with an even higher relative incidence (twice that of articaine). Importantly, these are the only two dental anesthetics that are formulated as 4% solutions; the others are all marketed at lower concentrations (eg, the maximum concentration of lidocaine used for dental anesthesia is 2%), and it is well established that anesthetic neurotoxicity is, to some extent, concentration-dependent. Thus, it is quite possible that enhanced risk derives from the formulation rather than from an intrinsic property of the anesthetic. In a recent survey of US and Canadian Dental Schools, over half of respondents indicated that 4% articaine is no longer used for mandibular nerve block.

BENZOCAINE

As previously noted, benzocaine's pronounced lipophilicity has relegated its application to topical anesthesia. However, despite over a century of use for this purpose, its popularity has recently diminished owing to increasing concerns regarding its potential to induce methemoglobinemia. Elevated levels can be due to inborn errors, or can occur with exposure to an oxidizing agent, and such is the case with significant exposure to benzocaine (or nitrites, see Chapter 12). Because methemoglobin does not transport oxygen, elevated levels pose serious risk, with severity obviously paralleling blood levels.

BUPIVACAINE

Based on concerns for cardiotoxicity, bupivacaine is often avoided for techniques that demand high volumes of concentrated anesthetic, such as epidural or peripheral nerve blocks performed for surgical anesthesia. In contrast, relatively low concentrations ($\leq 0.25\%$) are frequently used to achieve prolonged peripheral anesthesia and analgesia for postoperative pain control, and the drug enjoys similar popularity where anesthetic infiltration is used to control pain from a surgical incision. It is often the agent of choice for epidural infusions used for postoperative pain control and for labor analgesia. Finally, it has a comparatively unblemished record as a spinal anesthetic, with a relatively favorable therapeutic index with respect to neurotoxicity, and little, if any, risk of TNS. However, spinal bupivacaine is not well suited for outpatient or ambulatory surgery, because its relatively long duration of action can delay recovery, resulting in a longer stay prior to discharge to home.

CHLOROPROCAINE

The introduction of chloroprocaine into clinical practice in 1951 represented a reversion to the earlier amino-ester template. Chloroprocaine gained widespread use as an epidural agent in obstetric anesthesia, where its rapid hydrolysis served to minimize risk of systemic toxicity or fetal exposure. Subsequent reports of neurologic injury associated with apparent intrathecal misplacement of large doses intended for the epidural space led to its near abandonment. However, the frequent occurrence of TNS when lidocaine is administered as a spinal anesthetic has created an anesthetic void that chloroprocaine appears well suited to fill. Its onset and duration of action are even shorter than those of lidocaine, while presenting little, if any, risk of TNS. Although chloroprocaine was never exonerated with respect to the early neurologic injuries associated with epidural anesthesia, it is now well appreciated that high doses of any local anesthetic, which are not required to achieve spinal anesthesia, are capable of inducing neurotoxic injury. In addition to chloroprocaine's emerging use as a spinal anesthetic, the drug finds some current use as an epidural anesthetic, particularly in circumstances where there is an indwelling catheter and the need for quick attainment of surgical anesthesia, such as cesarean section in a laboring parturient with a compromised fetus.

COCAINE

Current clinical use of cocaine is largely restricted to topical anesthesia for ear, nose, and throat procedures, where its intense vasoconstriction can serve to reduce bleeding. Even here, use has diminished in favor of other anesthetics combined with vasoconstrictors because of concerns about systemic toxicity, as well as the inconvenience of dispensing and handling this controlled substance.

ETIDOCAINE

Introduced along with bupivacaine, etidocaine has had limited application due to its poor block characteristics. It has a tendency to produce an inverse differential block (ie, compared with other anesthetics such as bupivacaine, it produces excessive motor relative to sensory block), which is rarely a favorable attribute.

LEVOBUPIVACAINE

As previously discussed, this S(–) enantiomer of bupivacaine is somewhat less cardiotoxic than the racemic mixture. It is also less potent, and tends to have a longer duration of action, though the magnitude of these effects is too small to have any substantial clinical significance. Interestingly, recent work with lipid resuscitation suggests a potential advantage of levobupivacaine over ropivacaine, as the former is more effectively sequestered into a so-called lipid sink, implying greater ability to reverse toxic effects should they occur.

LIDOCAINE

Aside from the issue of a high incidence of TNS with spinal administration, lidocaine has had an excellent record as an intermediate duration anesthetic, and remains the reference standard against which most anesthetics are compared.

MEPIVACAINE

Although structurally similar to bupivacaine and ropivacaine (Table 26–1), mepivacaine displays clinical properties that are comparable to lidocaine. However, it differs from lidocaine with respect to vasoactivity, as it has a tendency toward vasoconstriction rather than vasodilation. This characteristic likely accounts for its slightly longer duration of action, which has made it a popular choice for major peripheral blocks. Lidocaine has retained its dominance over mepivacaine for epidural anesthesia, where the routine placement of a catheter negates the importance of a longer duration. More importantly, mepivacaine is slowly metabolized by the fetus, making it a poor choice for epidural anesthesia in the parturient. When used for spinal anesthesia, mepivacaine has a slightly lower incidence of TNS than lidocaine.

PRILOCAINE

Prilocaine has the highest clearance of the amino-amide anesthetics, imparting reduced risk of systemic toxicity. Unfortunately, this is somewhat offset by its propensity to induce methemoglobinemia, which results from accumulation of one its metabolites, ortho-toluidine, an oxidizing agent. As a spinal anesthetic, prilocaine's duration of action is slightly longer than that of lidocaine, and the limited data suggest it carries a low risk of TNS. It is gaining increasing use for spinal anesthesia in Europe, where it has been marketed specifically for this purpose. No approved formulation exists in the USA, nor is there any formulation that would be appropriate to use for spinal anesthesia as an off-label indication.

ROPIVACAINE

Ropivacaine is an S(–) enantiomer in a homologous series that includes bupivacaine and mepivacaine, distinguished by its chirality, and the propyl group off the piperidine ring (Table 26–1). Its perceived reduced cardiotoxicity has led to widespread use for high-volume peripheral blocks. It is also a popular choice for epidural infusions for control of labor and postoperative pain. Although there is some evidence to suggest that ropivacaine might produce a more favorable differential block than bupivacaine, the lack of equivalent clinical potency adds complexity to such comparisons.

EMLA

The term eutectic is applied to mixtures in which the combination of elements has a lower melting temperature than its component elements. Lidocaine and prilocaine can combine to form such a mixture, which is marketed as EMLA (**E**utectic **M**ixture of **L**ocal **A**nesthetics). This formulation, containing 2.5% of lidocaine and 2.5% prilocaine, permits anesthetic penetration of the keratinized layer of skin, producing localized numbness. It is commonly used in pediatrics to anesthetize the skin prior to venipuncture for intravenous catheter placement.

FUTURE DEVELOPMENTS

Sustained-Release Formulations

The provision of prolonged analgesia or anesthesia, as in the case of postoperative pain management, has traditionally been accomplished by placement of a catheter to permit continuous administration of anesthetic. More recently, efforts have focused on drug delivery systems that can slowly release anesthetic, thereby providing extended duration without the drawbacks of a catheter. Sustained-release delivery has the potential added advantage of reducing risk of systemic toxicity. Preliminary work encapsulating local anesthetic into microspheres, liposomes, and other microparticles has established proof of concept, although significant developmental problems, as well as questions regarding potential tissue toxicity, remain to be resolved.

Less Toxic Agents; More Selective Agents

It has been clearly demonstrated that anesthetic neurotoxicity does not result from blockade of the voltage-gated sodium channel. Thus, effect and tissue toxicity are not mediated by a common mechanism, establishing the possibility of developing compounds with considerably better therapeutic indexes.

As previously discussed, the identification and subclassification of families of neuronal sodium channels has spurred research aimed at development of more selective sodium channel blockers. The variable neuronal distribution of these isoforms and the unique role that some play in pain signaling suggests that selective blockade of these channels is feasible, and may greatly improve the therapeutic index of sodium channel modulators.

SUMMARY Drugs Used for Local Anesthesia

Subclass	Mechanism of Action	Effects	Clinical Applications	Pharmacokinetics, Toxicities
AMIDES				
• Lidocaine	Blockade of sodium channels	Slows, then blocks, action potential propagation	Short-duration procedures • topical (mucosal), intravenous, infiltration, spinal, epidural, minor and major peripheral blocks	Parenteral (eg, peripheral block, but varies significantly based on specific site) • duration 1–2 h • 2–4 h with epinephrine • *Toxicity:* Central nervous system (CNS) excitation (high-volume blocks) and local neurotoxicity
• Bupivacaine	Same as lidocaine	Same as lidocaine	Longer-duration procedures (but not used topically or intravenously)	Parenteral • duration 3–6 h • *Toxicity:* CNS excitation • cardiovascular collapse (high-volume blocks)
• *Prilocaine, mepivacaine: Like lidocaine (but also risk of methemoglobinemia with prilocaine)*				
• *Ropivacaine, levobupivacaine: Like bupivacaine*				
ESTERS				
• Chloroprocaine	Like lidocaine	Like lidocaine	Very short procedures (not generally used topically or intravenously)	Parenteral • duration 30–60 min • 60–90 min with epinephrine • *Toxicity:* Like lidocaine
• Cocaine	Same as above • also has sympathomimetic effects	Same as above	Procedures requiring high surface activity and vasoconstriction	Topical or parenteral • duration 1–2 h • *Toxicity:* CNS excitation, convulsions, cardiac arrhythmias, hypertension, stroke
• *Procaine: Like chloroprocaine (but not used epidurally)*				
• *Tetracaine: Used primarily for spinal anesthesia; duration 2–3 h*				

PREPARATIONS AVAILABLE

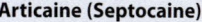

Articaine (Septocaine)
Parenteral: 4% with 1:100,000 epinephrine

Benzocaine (generic)
Topical: 5, 6% creams; 15, 20% gels; 5, 20% ointments; 0.8% lotion; 20% liquid; 20% spray

Bupivacaine (generic, Marcaine, Sensorcaine)
Parenteral: 0.25, 0.5, 0.75% for injection; 0.25, 0.5, 0.75% with 1:200,000 epinephrine

Chloroprocaine (generic, Nesacaine)
Parenteral: 1, 2, 3% for injection

Cocaine (generic)
Topical: 40, 100 mg/mL regular and viscous solutions; 5, 25 g powder

Dibucaine (generic, Nupercainal)
Topical: 1% ointment

Dyclonine (Dyclone)
Topical: 0.5, 1% solution

Levobupivacaine (Chirocaine)
Parenteral: 2.5, 5, 7.5 mg/mL

Lidocaine (generic, Xylocaine)
Parenteral: 0.5, 1, 1.5, 2, 4% for injection; 0.5, 1, 1.5, 2% with 1:200,000 epinephrine; 1, 2% with 1:100,000 epinephrine, 2% with 1:50,000 epinephrine
Topical: 2.5, 5% ointments; 0.5, 4% cream; 0.5, 2.5% gel; 2, 2.5, 4% solutions; 23, 46 mg/2 cm² patch

Lidocaine and hydrocortisone
Patch: 3% lidocaine plus 0.5% hydrocortisone

Lidocaine and bupivacaine mixture (Duocaine)
Parenteral: 10 mg/mL lidocaine plus 3.75 mg/mL bupivacaine for injection

Lidocaine and prilocaine eutectic mixture (EMLA cream)
Topical: lidocaine 2.5% plus prilocaine 2.5%

Mepivacaine (generic, Carbocaine)
Parenteral: 1, 1.5, 2, 3% for injection; 2% with 1:20,000 levonordefrin

Pramoxine (generic, Tronothane)
Topical: 1% cream, lotion, spray, and gel

Prilocaine (Citanest)
Parenteral: 4%; 4% with epinephrine

Procaine (generic, Novocain)
Parenteral: 1, 2, 10% for injection

Proparacaine (generic, Alcaine, others)
0.5% solution for ophthalmic use

Ropivacaine (Naropin)
Parenteral: 0.2, 0.5, 0.75, 1.0% solution for injection

Tetracaine (generic, Pontocaine)
Parenteral: 1% for injection; 0.2, 0.3% with 6% dextrose for spinal anesthesia
Topical: 1% ointment; 0.5% solution (ophthalmic); 1, 2% cream; 2% solution for nose and throat; 2% gel

REFERENCES

Adverse Reactions with Bupivacaine. FDA Drug Bulletin 1983;13:23

Albright GA: Cardiac arrest following regional anesthesia with etidocaine or bupivacaine. Anesthesiology 1979;51:285.

Andavan GS, Lemmens-Gruber R: Voltage-gated sodium channels: Mutations, channelopathies and targets. Curr Med Chem 2011;18:377.

Auroy Y et al: Serious complications related to regional anesthesia: Results of a prospective survey in France. Anesthesiology 1997;87:479.

Butterworth JF 4th, Strichartz GR: Molecular mechanisms of local anesthesia: A review. Anesthesiology 1990;72:711.

Catterall WA, Goldin AL, Waxman SG: International Union of Pharmacology. XLVII. Nomenclature and structure-function relationships of voltage-gated sodium channels. Pharmacol Rev 2005;57:397.

Cave G, Harvey M: Intravenous lipid emulsion as antidote beyond local anesthetic toxicity: A systematic review. Acad Emerg Med 2009;16:815.

de Jong RH, Ronfeld RA, DeRosa RA: Cardiovascular effects of convulsant and supraconvulsant doses of amide local anesthetics. Anesth Analg 1982;61:3.

Di Gregorio G et al: Clinical presentation of local anesthetic systemic toxicity: A review of published cases, 1979 to 2009. Reg Anesth Pain Med 2010;35:181.

Drasner K: Chloroprocaine spinal anesthesia: Back to the future? Anesth Analg 2005;100:549.

Drasner K: Lidocaine spinal anesthesia: A vanishing therapeutic index? Anesthesiology 1997;87:469.

Drasner K: Local anesthetic neurotoxicity: Clinical injury and strategies that may minimize risk. Reg Anesth Pain Med 2002;27:576.

Drasner K: Local anesthetic systemic toxicity: a historical perspective. Reg Anesth Pain Med 2010;35:162.

Drasner K et al: Cauda equina syndrome following intended epidural anesthesia. Anesthesiology 1992;77:582.

Drasner K et al: Persistent sacral sensory deficit induced by intrathecal local anesthetic infusion in the rat. Anesthesiology 1994;80:847.

Freedman JM et al: Transient neurologic symptoms after spinal anesthesia: An epidemiologic study of 1,863 patients. Anesthesiology 1998;89:633.

Gold MS et al: Lidocaine toxicity in primary afferent neurons from the rat. J Pharmacol Exp Ther 1998;285:413.

Groban L: Central nervous system and cardiac effects from long-acting amide local anesthetic toxicity in the intact animal model. Reg Anesth Pain Med 2003;28:3.

Hampl KF et al: Transient neurologic symptoms after spinal anesthesia. Anesth Analg 1995;81:1148.

Hashimoto K et al: Epinephrine increases the neurotoxic potential of intrathecally administered lidocaine in the rat. Anesthesiology 2001;94:876.

Heavner JE: Cardiac toxicity of local anesthetics in the intact isolated heart model: A review. Reg Anesth Pain Med 2002;27:545.

Hille B: Local anesthetics: Hydrophyilic and hydrophobic pathways for the drug-receptor interaction. J Gen Physiol 1977;69:497.

Holmdahl MH: Xylocain (lidocaine, lignocaine), its discovery and Gordh's contribution to its clinical use. Acta Anaesthesiol Scand Suppl 1998;113:8.

Kouri ME, Kopacz DJ: Spinal 2-chloroprocaine: A comparison with lidocaine in volunteers. Anesth Analg 2004;98(1):75-80.

Mattison JB: Cocaine poisoning. Med Surg Rep 1891;115:645.

Neal JM et al: ASRA practice advisory on local anesthetic systemic toxicity. Reg Anesth Pain Med 2010;35:152.

Pollock JE: Transient neurologic symptoms: Etiology, risk factors, and management. Reg Anesth Pain Med 2002;27:581.

Pollock JE et al: Prospective study of the incidence of transient radicular irritation in patients undergoing spinal anesthesia. Anesthesiology 1996;84:1361.

Pollock JE et al: Spinal nerve function in five volunteers experiencing transient neurologic symptoms after lidocaine subarachnoid anesthesia. Anesth Analg 2000;90:658.

Priest BT: Future potential and status of selective sodium channel blockers for the treatment of pain. Curr Opin Drug Discov Devel 2009;12:682.

Rigler ML et al: Cauda equina syndrome after continuous spinal anesthesia. Anesth Analg 1991;72:275.

Rose JS, Neal JM, Kopacz DJ: Extended-duration analgesia: Update on microspheres and liposomes. Reg Anesth Pain Med 2005;30:275.

Ruetsch YA, Boni T, Borgeat A: From cocaine to ropivacaine: The history of local anesthetic drugs. Curr Top Med Chem 2001;1:175.

Sakura S et al: Local anesthetic neurotoxicity does not result from blockade of voltage-gated sodium channels. Anesth Analg 1995;81:338.

Schneider M et al: Transient neurologic toxicity after hyperbaric subarachnoid anesthesia with 5% lidocaine. Anesth Analg 1993;76:1154.

Sirianni AJ et al: Use of lipid emulsion in the resuscitation of a patient with prolonged cardiovascular collapse after overdose of bupropion and lamotrigine. Ann Emerg Med 2008;51:412.

Taniguchi M, Bollen AW, Drasner K: Sodium bisulfite: Scapegoat for chloroprocaine neurotoxicity? Anesthesiology 2004;100:85.

Tremont-Lukats IW et al: Systemic administration of local anesthetics to relieve neuropathic pain: A systematic review and meta-analysis. Anesth Analg 2005;101:1738.

Weinberg GL et al: Pretreatment or resuscitation with a lipid infusion shifts the dose-response to bupivacaine-induced asystole in rats. Anesthesiology 1998;88:1071.

CASE STUDY ANSWER

If a spinal anesthetic technique were selected, bupivacaine would be an excellent choice. It has an adequately long duration of action and a relatively unblemished record with respect to neurotoxic injury and transient neurologic symptoms, which are the complications of most concern with spinal anesthetic technique. Although bupivacaine has greater potential for cardiotoxicity, this is not a concern when the drug is used for spinal anesthesia because of the extremely low doses required for intrathecal administration. If an epidural technique were chosen for the surgical procedure, the potential for systemic toxicity would need to be considered, making lidocaine or mepivacaine (generally with epinephrine) preferable to bupivacaine (or even ropivacaine or levobupivacaine) because of their better therapeutic indexes with respect to cardiotoxicity. However, this does not apply to epidural administration for postoperative pain control, which involves administration of more dilute anesthetic at a slower rate. The most common agents used for this indication are bupivacaine, ropivacaine, and levobupivacaine.

Skeletal Muscle Relaxants

27

Marieke Kruidering-Hall, PhD, &
Lundy Campbell, MD*

C A S E   S T U D Y

A 30-year-old woman is rushed to the emergency department at a major trauma center after a motor vehicle accident. Although in significant pain, she is awake, alert, and able to give a brief history. She states that she was the driver and was wearing a seatbelt. There were no passengers in the car. Her past medical history is significant only for asthma, for which she has been intubated once in the past. She has no allergies to medications. There are multiple lacerations on her face and extremities and a large open fracture of her right femur. An orthopedic surgeon has scheduled immediate operative repair of the femur fracture, and the plastic surgeon wants to suture the facial lacerations at the same time. You decide to intubate the patient for the procedure. What muscle relaxant would you choose? Would you choose the same agent if she had experienced a 30% total body burn in a fire at the time of the accident? What if the past medical history included right-sided hemiparesis of 10 years' duration?

Drugs that affect skeletal muscle function include two different therapeutic groups: those used during surgical procedures and in the intensive care unit (ICU) to produce muscle paralysis (ie, **neuromuscular blockers**), and those used to reduce spasticity in a variety of painful conditions (ie, **spasmolytics**). Neuromuscular blocking drugs interfere with transmission at the neuromuscular end plate and lack central nervous system activity. These compounds are used primarily as adjuncts during general anesthesia to facilitate endotracheal intubation and optimize surgical conditions while ensuring adequate ventilation. Drugs in the spasmolytic group have traditionally been called "centrally acting" muscle relaxants and are used primarily to treat chronic back pain and painful fibromyalgic conditions. Dantrolene, a spasmolytic agent that has no significant central effects and is used primarily to treat a rare anesthetic-related complication, malignant hyperthermia, is also discussed in this chapter.

NEUROMUSCULAR BLOCKING DRUGS

History

During the 16th century, European explorers found that natives in the Amazon Basin of South America were using curare, an arrow poison that produced skeletal muscle paralysis, to kill animals. The active compound, *d*-tubocurarine, and its modern synthetic derivatives have had a major influence on the practice of anesthesia and surgery and have proved useful in understanding the basic mechanisms involved in neuromuscular transmission.

Normal Neuromuscular Function

The mechanism of neuromuscular transmission at the motor end plate is similar to that described for preganglionic cholinergic nerves in Chapter 6. The arrival of an action potential at the motor nerve terminal causes an influx of calcium and release of the neurotransmitter acetylcholine. Acetylcholine then diffuses across the synaptic cleft to activate the nicotinic receptors located on the motor end plate. As noted in Chapter 7, the adult N_M receptor is composed of five peptides: two alpha peptides, one beta, one gamma, and one delta peptide (Figure 27–1). The binding of two acetylcholine

*The authors thank Paul F. White, PhD, MD, and Bertram G. Katzung, MD, PhD, for contributions to this chapter in previous editions.

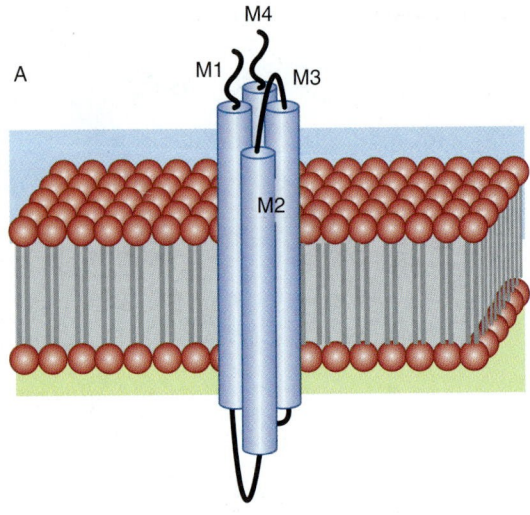

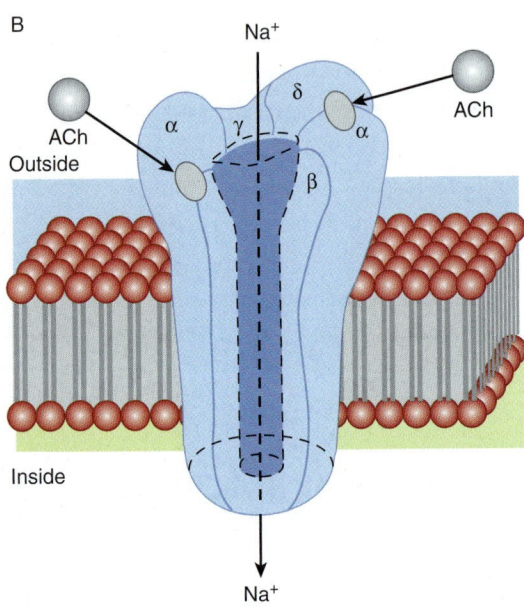

FIGURE 27–1 The adult nicotinic acetylcholine receptor (nAChR) is an intrinsic membrane protein with five distinct subunits ($\alpha_2\beta\delta\gamma$). **A:** Cartoon of the one of five subunits of the AChR in the end plate surface of adult mammalian muscle. Each subunit contains four helical domains labeled M1 to M4. The M2 domains line the channel pore. **B:** Cartoon of the full nAChR. The N termini of two subunits cooperate to form two distinct binding pockets for acetylcholine (ACh). These pockets occur at the α-β and the δ-α subunit interfaces.

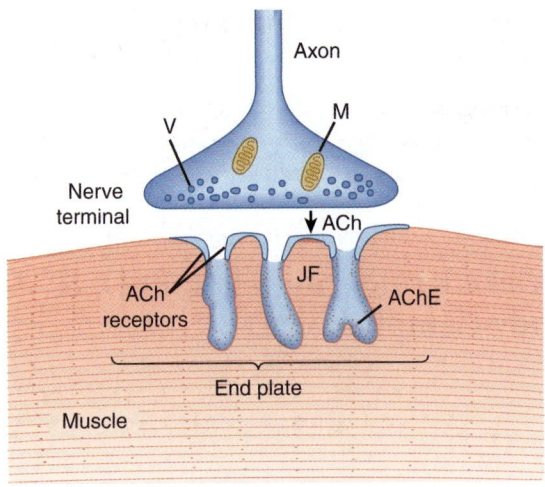

FIGURE 27–2 Schematic representation of the neuromuscular junction. ACh, acetylcholine; AChE, acetylcholinesterase; JF, junctional folds; M, mitochondrion; V, transmitter vesicle. (Reproduced, with permission, from Drachman DB: Myasthenia gravis. N Engl J Med 1978;298:135.)

However, if the end plate potential is large, the adjacent muscle membrane is depolarized, and an action potential will be propagated along the entire muscle fiber. Muscle contraction is then initiated by excitation-contraction coupling. The released acetylcholine is quickly removed from the end plate region by both diffusion and enzymatic destruction by the local acetylcholinesterase enzyme.

At least two additional types of acetylcholine receptors are found within the neuromuscular apparatus. One type is located on the presynaptic motor axon terminal, and activation of these receptors mobilizes additional transmitter for subsequent release by moving more acetylcholine vesicles toward the synaptic membrane. The second type of receptor is found on perijunctional cells and is not normally involved in neuromuscular transmission. However, under certain conditions (eg, prolonged immobilization, thermal burns), these receptors may proliferate sufficiently to affect subsequent neuromuscular transmission.

Skeletal muscle relaxation and paralysis can occur from interruption of function at several sites along the pathway from the central nervous system (CNS) to myelinated somatic nerves, unmyelinated motor nerve terminals, nicotinic acetylcholine receptors, the motor end plate, the muscle membrane, and the intracellular muscular contractile apparatus itself.

Blockade of end plate function can be accomplished by two basic mechanisms. Pharmacologic blockade of the physiologic agonist acetylcholine is characteristic of the antagonist neuromuscular blocking drugs (ie, nondepolarizing neuromuscular blocking drugs). These drugs prevent access of the transmitter to its receptor and thereby prevent depolarization. The prototype of this nondepolarizing subgroup is ***d*-tubocurarine.** The second type of blockade can be produced by an excess of a depolarizing agonist, such as acetylcholine. This seemingly paradoxical effect of acetylcholine also occurs at the ganglionic nicotinic acetylcholine receptor. The prototypical depolarizing blocking drug is **succinylcholine.** A similar depolarizing block can be produced by acetylcholine itself when high local concentrations are achieved in the synaptic

molecules to receptors on the α-β and δ-α subunits causes opening of the channel. The subsequent movement of sodium and potassium through the channel is associated with a graded depolarization of the end plate membrane (Figure 27–2). This change in voltage is termed the motor end plate potential. The magnitude of the end plate potential is directly related to the amount of acetylcholine released. If the potential is small, the permeability and the end plate potential return to normal without an impulse being propagated from the end plate region to the rest of the muscle membrane.

cleft (eg, by cholinesterase inhibitor intoxication) and by nicotine and other nicotinic agonists. However, the neuromuscular block produced by depolarizing drugs other than succinylcholine cannot be precisely controlled and is of no clinical value.

BASIC PHARMACOLOGY OF NEUROMUSCULAR BLOCKING DRUGS

Chemistry

All of the available neuromuscular blocking drugs bear a structural resemblance to acetylcholine. For example, succinylcholine is two acetylcholine molecules linked end-to-end (Figure 27–3). In contrast to the single linear structure of succinylcholine and other depolarizing drugs, the nondepolarizing agents (eg, pancuronium) conceal the "double-acetylcholine" structure in one of two types of bulky, semi-rigid ring systems (Figure 27–3). Examples of the two major families of nondepolarizing blocking drugs—the isoquinoline and steroid derivatives—are shown in Figures 27–4 and 27–5. Another feature common to all currently used neuromuscular blockers is the presence of one or two quaternary nitrogens, which makes them poorly lipid soluble and limits entry into the CNS.

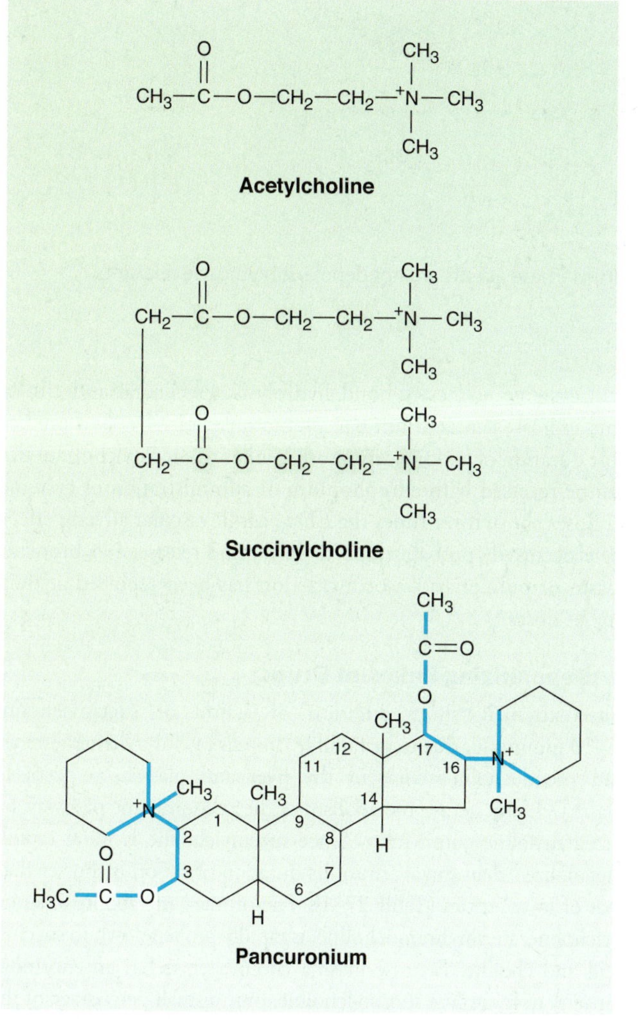

Pharmacokinetics of Neuromuscular Blocking Drugs

All of the neuromuscular blocking drugs are highly polar compounds and inactive orally; they must be administered parenterally.

A. Nondepolarizing Relaxant Drugs

The rate of disappearance of a nondepolarizing neuromuscular blocking drug from the blood is characterized by a rapid initial distribution phase followed by a slower elimination phase. Neuromuscular blocking drugs are highly ionized, do not readily cross cell membranes, and are not strongly bound in peripheral tissues. Therefore, their volume of distribution (80–140 mL/kg) is only slightly larger than the blood volume.

The duration of neuromuscular blockade produced by nondepolarizing relaxants is strongly correlated with the elimination half-life. Drugs that are excreted by the kidney typically have longer half-lives, leading to longer durations of action (> 35 minutes). Drugs eliminated by the liver tend to have shorter half-lives and durations of action (Table 27–1). All steroidal muscle relaxants are metabolized to their 3-hydroxy, 17-hydroxy, or 3,17-dihydroxy products in the liver. The 3-hydroxy metabolites are usually 40–80% as potent as the parent drug. Under normal circumstances, metabolites are not formed in sufficient quantities to produce a significant degree of neuromuscular blockade during or after anesthesia. However, if the parent compound is administered for several days in the ICU setting, the 3-hydroxy metabolite may accumulate and cause prolonged paralysis because it has a longer half-life than the parent compound. The remaining metabolites possess minimal neuromuscular blocking properties.

The intermediate-acting steroid muscle relaxants (eg, **vecuronium** and **rocuronium**) tend to be more dependent on biliary excretion or hepatic metabolism for their elimination. These muscle relaxants are more commonly used clinically than the long-acting steroid-based drugs (eg, pancuronium).

Atracurium (Figure 27–4) is an intermediate-acting isoquinoline nondepolarizing muscle relaxant. In addition to hepatic metabolism, atracurium is inactivated by a form of spontaneous breakdown known as Hofmann elimination. The main breakdown products are laudanosine and a related quaternary acid, neither of which possesses neuromuscular blocking properties. Laudanosine is slowly metabolized by the liver and has a longer elimination half-life (ie, 150 minutes). It readily crosses the blood-brain barrier, and high blood concentrations may cause seizures and an increase in the volatile anesthetic requirement. During surgical anesthesia, blood levels of laudanosine typically range from 0.2 to 1 mcg/mL;

FIGURE 27–3 Structural relationship of succinylcholine, a depolarizing agent, and pancuronium, a nondepolarizing agent, to acetylcholine, the neuromuscular transmitter. Succinylcholine, originally called diacetylcholine, is simply two molecules of acetylcholine linked through the acetate methyl groups. Pancuronium may be viewed as two acetylcholine-like fragments (outlined in color) oriented on a steroid nucleus.

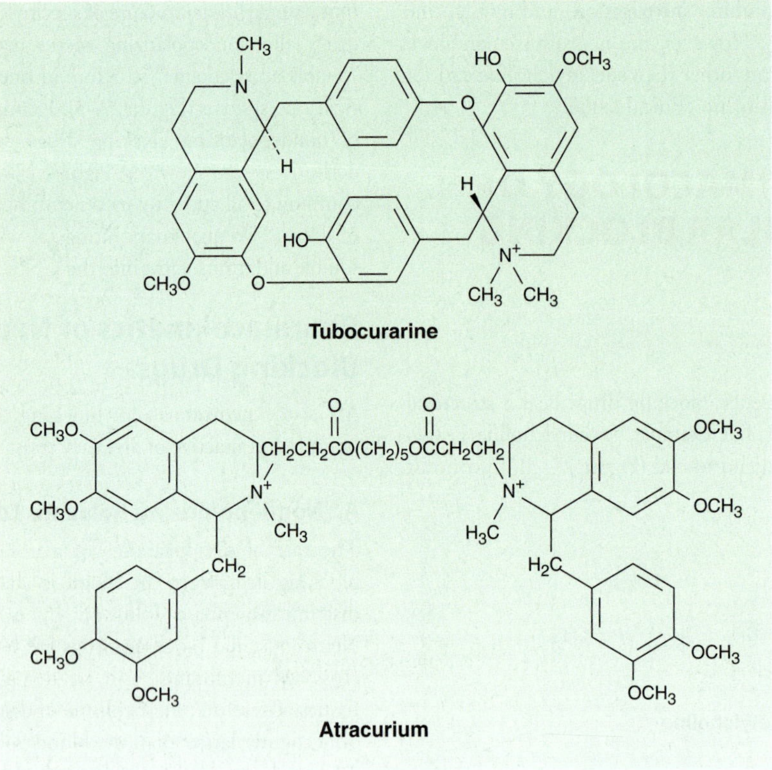

FIGURE 27–4 Structures of two isoquinoline neuromuscular blocking drugs. These agents are nondepolarizing muscle relaxants.

however, with prolonged infusions of atracurium in the ICU, laudanosine blood levels may exceed 5 mcg/mL.

Atracurium has several stereoisomers, and the potent isomer **cisatracurium** has become one of the most commonly used muscle relaxants in clinical practice. Although cisatracurium resembles atracurium, it has less dependence on hepatic inactivation, produces less laudanosine, and is less likely to release histamine. From the clinical perspective, cisatracurium has all the advantages of atracurium with fewer side effects. Therefore, cisatracurium has largely replaced atracurium in clinical practice.

Mivacurium, another isoquinoline compound, has the shortest duration of action of all nondepolarizing muscle relaxants (Table 27–1). However, its onset of action is significantly slower than that of succinylcholine. In addition, the use of a larger dose to speed the onset can be associated with profound histamine release leading to hypotension, flushing, and bronchospasm. Clearance of mivacurium by plasma cholinesterase is rapid and independent of the liver or kidney (Table 27–1). However, because patients with renal failure often have decreased levels of plasma cholinesterase, the short duration of action of mivacurium may be prolonged in patients with impaired renal function. Although mivacurium is no longer in widespread clinical use, an investigational ultra-short-acting isoquinoline nondepolarizing muscle relaxant, gantacurium, is currently in phase 3 clinical testing.

Gantacurium represents a new class of nondepolarizing neuromuscular blockers, called asymmetric mixed-onium chlorofumarates. It is degraded nonenzymatically by adduction of the amino acid cysteine and ester bond hydrolysis. Preclinical and clinical data indicate gantacurium has a rapid onset of effect and predictable duration of action (very short, similar to succinylcholine) that can be reversed with edrophonium or administration of cysteine. At doses above three times the ED_{95}, cardiovascular adverse effects have occurred, probably due to histamine release. No bronchospasm or pulmonary vasoconstriction has been reported at these higher doses.

B. Depolarizing Relaxant Drugs

The extremely short duration of action of succinylcholine (5–10 minutes) is due to its rapid hydrolysis by butyrylcholinesterase and pseudocholinesterase in the liver and plasma, respectively. Plasma cholinesterase metabolism is the predominant pathway for succinylcholine elimination. Since succinylcholine is more rapidly metabolized than mivacurium, its duration of action is shorter than that of mivacurium (Table 27–1). The primary metabolite of succinylcholine, succinylmonocholine, is rapidly broken down to succinic acid and choline. Because plasma cholinesterase has an enormous capacity to hydrolyze succinylcholine, only a small percentage of the original intravenous dose ever reaches the neuromuscular junction. In addition, because there is little if any plasma cholinesterase at the motor end plate, a succinylcholine-induced blockade is terminated by its diffusion away from the end plate into extracellular fluid. Therefore, the circulating levels of plasma cholinesterase influence the duration of action of succinylcholine by determining the amount of the drug that reaches the motor end plate.

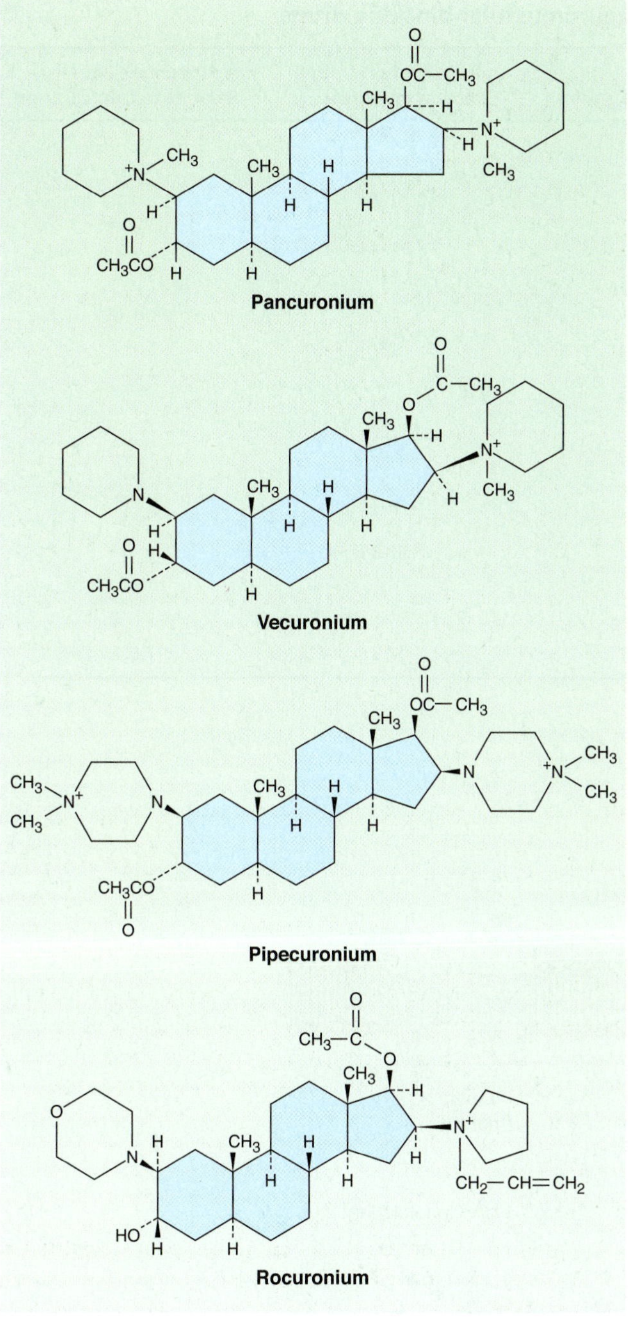

FIGURE 27–5 Structures of steroid neuromuscular blocking drugs (steroid nucleus in color). These agents are all nondepolarizing muscle relaxants.

Neuromuscular blockade produced by succinylcholine and mivacurium can be prolonged in patients with an abnormal genetic variant of plasma cholinesterase. The *dibucaine number* is a measure of the ability of a patient to metabolize succinylcholine and can be used to identify at-risk patients. Under standardized test conditions, dibucaine inhibits the normal enzyme by 80% and the abnormal enzyme by only 20%. Many genetic variants of plasma cholinesterase have been identified, although the dibucaine-related variants are the most important. Given the rarity of these genetic variants, plasma cholinesterase testing is not a routine clinical procedure.

Mechanism of Action

The interactions of drugs with the acetylcholine receptor-end plate channel have been described at the molecular level. Several modes of action of drugs on the receptor are illustrated in Figure 27–6.

A. Nondepolarizing Relaxant Drugs

All the neuromuscular blocking drugs in current use in the USA except succinylcholine are classified as nondepolarizing agents. Although it is no longer in widespread clinical use, *d*-tubocurarine is considered the prototype neuromuscular blocker. When small doses of nondepolarizing muscle relaxants are administered, they act predominantly at the nicotinic receptor site by competing with acetylcholine. The least potent nondepolarizing relaxants (eg, rocuronium) have the fastest onset and the shortest duration of action. In larger doses, nondepolarizing drugs can enter the pore of the ion channel (Figure 27–1) to produce a more intense motor blockade. This action further weakens neuromuscular transmission and diminishes the ability of the acetylcholinesterase inhibitors (eg, neostigmine, edrophonium, pyridostigmine) to antagonize the effect of nondepolarizing muscle relaxants.

Nondepolarizing relaxants can also block prejunctional sodium channels. As a result of this action, muscle relaxants interfere with the mobilization of acetylcholine at the nerve ending and cause fade (Figure 27–7). One consequence of the surmountable nature of the postsynaptic blockade produced by nondepolarizing muscle relaxants is the fact that tetanic stimulation, by releasing a large quantity of acetylcholine, is followed by transient posttetanic facilitation of the twitch strength (ie, relief of blockade). An important clinical consequence of this principle is the reversal of residual blockade by cholinesterase inhibitors. The characteristics of a nondepolarizing neuromuscular blockade are summarized in Table 27–2 and Figure 27–7.

B. Depolarizing Relaxant Drugs

1. Phase I block (depolarizing)—Succinylcholine is the only clinically useful depolarizing blocking drug. Its neuromuscular effects are like those of acetylcholine except that succinylcholine produces a longer effect at the myoneural junction. Succinylcholine reacts with the nicotinic receptor to open the channel and cause depolarization of the motor end plate, and this in turn spreads to the adjacent membranes, causing contractions of muscle motor units. Data from single-channel recordings indicate that depolarizing blockers can enter the channel to produce a prolonged "flickering" of the ion conductance (Figure 27–8). Because succinylcholine is not metabolized effectively at the synapse, the depolarized membranes remain depolarized and unresponsive to subsequent impulses (ie, a state of depolarizing blockade). Furthermore, because excitation-contraction coupling requires end plate repolarization ("repriming") and repetitive firing to maintain muscle tension, a flaccid paralysis results. In contrast to the nondepolarizing drugs, this so-called phase I (depolarizing) block is augmented, not reversed, by cholinesterase inhibitors.

The characteristics of a depolarizing neuromuscular blockade are summarized in Table 27–2 and Figure 27–7.

TABLE 27–1 Pharmacokinetic and dynamic properties of neuromuscular blocking drugs.

Drug	Elimination	Clearance (mL/kg/min)	Approximate Duration of Action (minutes)	Approximate Potency Relative to Tubocurarine
Isoquinoline derivatives				
Atracurium	Spontaneous[1]	6.6	20–35	1.5
Cisatracurium	Mostly spontaneous	5–6	25–44	1.5
Mivacurium	Plasma ChE[2]	70–95	10–20	4
Tubocurarine	Kidney (40%)	2.3–2.4	> 50	1
Steroid derivatives				
Pancuronium	Kidney (80%)	1.7–1.8	> 35	6
Rocuronium	Liver (75–90%) and kidney	2.9	20–35	0.8
Vecuronium	Liver (75–90%) and kidney	3–5.3	20–35	6
Depolarizing agent				
Succinylcholine	Plasma ChE[2] (100%)	> 100	< 8	0.4

[1]Nonenzymatic and enzymatic hydrolysis of ester bonds.

[2]Butyrylcholinesterase (pseudocholinesterase).

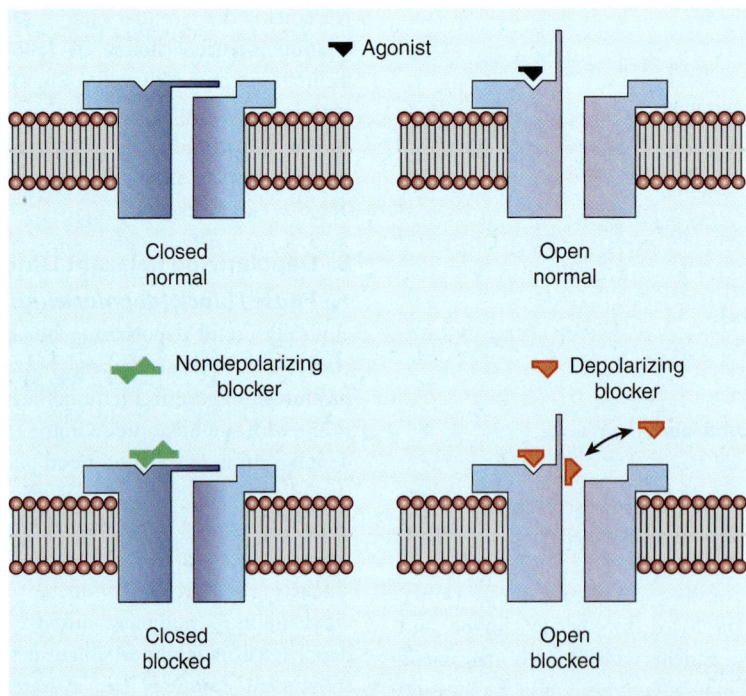

FIGURE 27–6 Schematic diagram of the interactions of drugs with the acetylcholine receptor on the end plate channel (structures are purely symbolic). **Top:** The action of the normal agonist, acetylcholine, in opening the channel. **Bottom, left:** A nondepolarizing blocker, eg, rocuronium, is shown as preventing the opening of the channel when it binds to the receptor. **Bottom, right:** A depolarizing blocker, eg, succinylcholine, both occupying the receptor and blocking the channel. Normal closure of the channel gate is prevented and the blocker may move rapidly in and out of the pore. Depolarizing blockers may desensitize the end plate by occupying the receptor and causing persistent depolarization. An additional effect of drugs on the end plate channel may occur through changes in the lipid environment surrounding the channel (not shown). General anesthetics and alcohols may impair neuromuscular transmission by this mechanism.

TABLE 27–2 Comparison of a typical nondepolarizing muscle relaxant (rocuronium) and a depolarizing muscle relaxant (succinylcholine).

	Rocuronium	Succinylcholine	
		Phase I	Phase II
Administration of tubocurarine	Additive	Antagonistic	Augmented[1]
Administration of succinylcholine	Antagonistic	Additive	Augmented[1]
Effect of neostigmine	Antagonistic	Augmented[1]	Antagonistic
Initial excitatory effect on skeletal muscle	None	Fasciculations	None
Response to a tetanic stimulus	Unsustained (fade)	Sustained[2] (no fade)	Unsustained (fade)
Posttetanic facilitation	Yes	No	Yes
Rate of recovery	30–60 min[3]	4–8 min	> 20 min[3]

[1]It is not known whether this interaction is additive or synergistic (superadditive).

[2]The amplitude is decreased, but the response is sustained.

[3]The rate depends on the dose and on the completeness of neuromuscular blockade.

2. Phase II block (desensitizing)—With prolonged exposure to succinylcholine, the initial end plate depolarization decreases and the membrane becomes repolarized. Despite this repolarization, the membrane cannot easily be depolarized again because it is *desensitized*. The mechanism for this desensitizing phase is unclear, but some evidence indicates that channel block may become more important than agonist action at the receptor in phase II of succinylcholine's neuromuscular blocking action. Regardless of the mechanism, the channels behave as if they are in a prolonged closed state (Figure 27–7). Later in phase II, the characteristics of the blockade are nearly identical to those of a nondepolarizing block (ie, a nonsustained twitch response to a tetanic stimulus) (Figure 27–7), with possible reversal by acetylcholinesterase inhibitors.

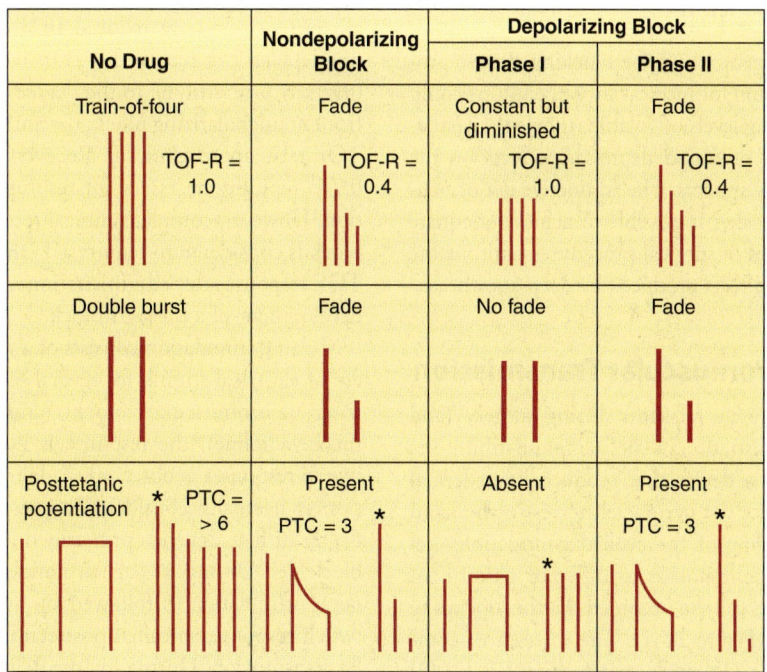

FIGURE 27–7 Muscle contraction responses to different patterns of nerve stimulation used in monitoring skeletal muscle relaxation. The alterations produced by a nondepolarizing blocker and depolarizing and desensitizing blockade by succinylcholine are shown. In the train-of-four (TOF) pattern, four stimuli are applied at 2 Hz. The TOF ratio (TOF-R) is calculated from the strength of the fourth contraction divided by that of the first. In the double-burst pattern, three stimuli are applied at 50 Hz, followed by a 700 ms rest period and then repeated. In the posttetanic potentiation pattern, several seconds of 50 Hz stimulation are applied, followed by several seconds of rest and then by single stimuli at a slow rate (eg, 0.5 Hz). The number of detectable posttetanic twitches is the posttetanic count (PTC). *, first posttetanic contraction.

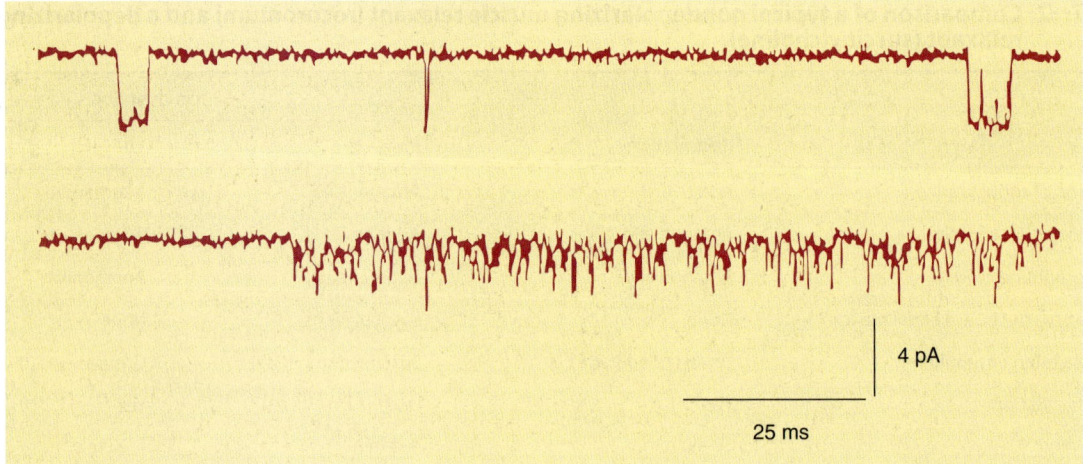

FIGURE 27–8 Action of succinylcholine on single-channel end plate receptor currents in frog muscle. Currents through a single AChR channel were recorded using the patch clamp technique. The upper trace was recorded in the presence of a low concentration of succinylcholine; the downward deflections represent openings of the channel and passage of inward (depolarizing) current. The lower trace was recorded in the presence of a much higher concentration of succinylcholine and shows prolonged "flickering" of the channel as it repetitively opens and closes or is "plugged" by the drug. (Reproduced, with permission, from Marshall CG, Ogden DC, Colquhoun D: The actions of suxamethonium (succinyldicholine) as an agonist and channel blocker at the nicotinic receptor of frog muscle. J Physiol [Lond] 1990;428:155.)

■ CLINICAL PHARMACOLOGY OF NEUROMUSCULAR BLOCKING DRUGS

Skeletal Muscle Paralysis

Before the introduction of neuromuscular blocking drugs, profound skeletal muscle relaxation for intracavitary operations could be achieved only by producing levels of volatile (inhaled) anesthesia deep enough to produce profound depressant effects on the cardiovascular and respiratory systems. The adjunctive use of neuromuscular blocking drugs makes it possible to achieve adequate muscle relaxation for all types of surgical procedures without the cardiorespiratory depressant effects produced by deep anesthesia.

Assessment of Neuromuscular Transmission

Monitoring the effect of muscle relaxants during surgery (and recovery following the administration of cholinesterase inhibitors) typically involves the use of a device that produces transdermal electrical stimulation of one of the peripheral nerves to the hand or facial muscles and recording of the evoked contractions (ie, twitch responses). The motor responses to different patterns of peripheral nerve stimulation can be recorded in the operating room during the procedure (Figure 27–7). The three most commonly used patterns include (1) single-twitch stimulation, (2) train-of-four (TOF) stimulation, and (3) tetanic stimulation. Two newer modalities are also available to monitor neuromuscular transmission: double-burst stimulation and posttetanic count.

With single-twitch stimulation, a single supramaximal electrical stimulus is applied to a peripheral nerve at frequencies from 0.1 Hz to 1.0 Hz. The higher frequency is often used during

induction and reversal to more accurately determine the peak (maximal) drug effect. TOF stimulation involves four successive supramaximal stimuli given at intervals of 0.5 second (2 Hz). Each stimulus in the TOF causes the muscle to contract, and the relative magnitude of the response of the fourth twitch compared with the first twitch is the TOF ratio. With a depolarizing block, all four twitches are reduced in a dose-related fashion. With a nondepolarizing block, the TOF ratio decreases ("fades") and is inversely proportional to the degree of blockade. During recovery from nondepolarizing block, the amount of fade decreases and the TOF ratio approaches 1.0. Recovery to a TOF ratio greater than 0.7 is typically necessary for resumption of spontaneous ventilation. However, complete clinical recovery from a nondepolarizing block is considered to require a TOF greater than 0.9. Fade in the TOF response after administration of succinylcholine signifies the development of a phase II block.

Tetanic stimulation consists of a very rapid (30–100 Hz) delivery of electrical stimuli for several seconds. During a nondepolarizing neuromuscular block (and a phase II block after succinylcholine), the response is not sustained and fade of the twitch responses is observed. Fade in response to tetanic stimulation is normally considered a presynaptic event. However, the degree of fade depends primarily on the degree of neuromuscular blockade. During a partial nondepolarizing blockade, tetanic nerve stimulation is followed by an increase in the posttetanic twitch response, so-called posttetanic facilitation of neuromuscular transmission. During intense neuromuscular blockade, there is no response to either tetanic or posttetanic stimulation. As the intensity of the block diminishes, the response to posttetanic twitch stimulation reappears. The time to reappearance of the first response to TOF stimulation is related to the posttetanic count and reflects the duration of profound (clinical) neuromuscular blockade. To determine the posttetanic count, 5 seconds of 50 Hz tetany is applied, followed by 3 seconds of rest, followed by 1 Hz pulses for about 10 seconds (10 pulses). The counted number of muscle twitches provides an estimation of the depth of blockade. For instance, a posttetanic count of 2 suggests no twitch response (by TOF) for about 20–30 minutes, and a posttetanic count of 5 correlates to a no-twitch response (by TOF) of about 10–15 minutes (Figure 27–7, bottom panel).

The double-burst stimulation pattern is a newer mode of electrical nerve stimulation developed with the goal of allowing for manual detection of residual neuromuscular blockade when it is not possible to record the responses to single-twitch, TOF, or tetanic stimulation. In this pattern, three nerve stimuli are delivered at 50 Hz followed by a 700 ms rest period and then by two or three additional stimuli at 50 Hz. It is easier to detect fade in the responses to double-burst stimulation than to TOF stimulation. The absence of fade in response to double-burst stimulation implies that clinically significant residual neuromuscular blockade does not exist.

The standard approach used for monitoring the clinical effects of muscle relaxants during surgery is to use a peripheral nerve stimulating device to elicit motor responses, which are visually observed by the anesthesiologist. A more quantitative approach to neuromuscular monitoring involves the use of acceleromyography or force-transduction for measuring the evoked response (ie, movement) of the thumb to TOF stimulation over the ulnar nerve at the wrist.

A. Nondepolarizing Relaxant Drugs

During anesthesia, administration of tubocurarine, 0.1–0.4 mg/kg IV, initially causes motor weakness, followed by the skeletal muscles becoming flaccid and inexcitable to electrical stimulation (Figure 27–9). In general, larger muscles (eg, abdominal, trunk, paraspinous, diaphragm) are more resistant to neuromuscular blockade and recover more rapidly than smaller muscles (eg, facial, foot, hand). The diaphragm is usually the last muscle to be paralyzed. Assuming that ventilation is adequately maintained, no adverse effects occur. When administration of muscle relaxants is discontinued, recovery of muscles usually occurs in reverse order, with the diaphragm regaining function first. The pharmacologic effect of tubocurarine, 0.3 mg/kg IV, usually lasts 45–60 minutes. However, subtle evidence of residual muscle paralysis detected using a neuromuscular monitor may last for another hour, increasing the likelihood of adverse outcomes, eg, aspiration and decreased hypoxic drive. Potency and duration of action of the other nondepolarizing drugs are shown in Table 27–1. In addition to the duration of action, the most important property distinguishing the nondepolarizing relaxants is the time to onset of the blocking effect, which determines how rapidly the patient's trachea can be intubated. Of the currently available nondepolarizing drugs, rocuronium has the most rapid onset time (60–120 seconds).

B. Depolarizing Relaxant Drugs

Following the administration of succinylcholine, 0.75–1.5 mg/kg IV, transient muscle fasciculations occur over the chest and abdomen within 30 seconds, although general anesthesia and the prior administration of a small dose of a nondepolarizing muscle relaxant tends to attenuate them. As paralysis develops rapidly (< 90 seconds), the arm, neck, and leg muscles are initially relaxed followed by the respiratory muscles. As a result of succinylcholine's rapid hydrolysis by cholinesterase in the plasma (and liver), the duration of neuromuscular block typically lasts less than 10 minutes (Table 27–1).

Cardiovascular Effects

Vecuronium, cisatracurium, and rocuronium have minimal, if any, cardiovascular effects. The other nondepolarizing muscle relaxants (ie, pancuronium, atracurium, mivacurium) produce cardiovascular effects that are mediated by either autonomic or

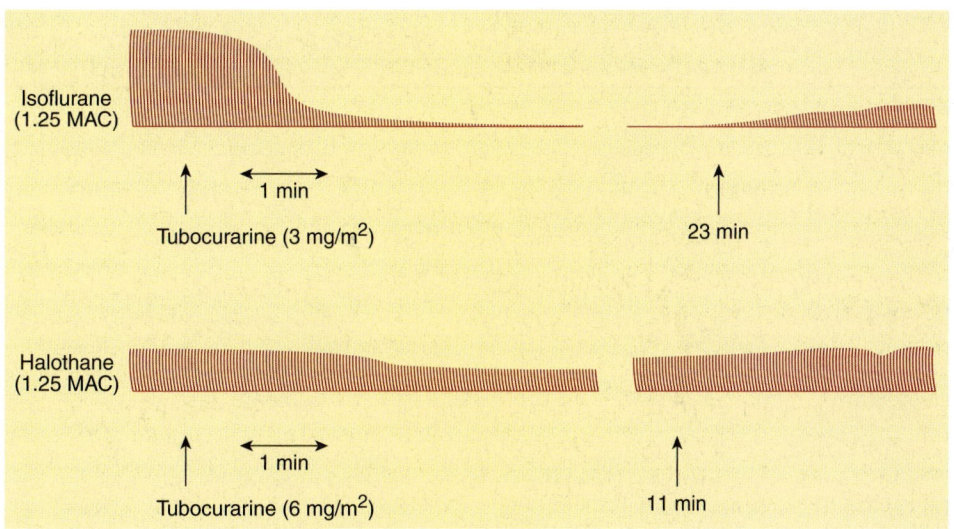

FIGURE 27–9 Neuromuscular blockade from tubocurarine during equivalent levels of isoflurane and halothane anesthesia in patients. Note that isoflurane augments the block far more than does halothane.

histamine receptors (Table 27–3). Tubocurarine and, to a lesser extent, metocurine, mivacurium, and atracurium can produce hypotension as a result of systemic histamine release, and with larger doses, ganglionic blockade may occur with tubocurarine and metocurine. Premedication with an antihistaminic compound attenuates tubocurarine- and mivacurium-induced hypotension. Pancuronium causes a moderate increase in heart rate and a smaller increase in cardiac output, with little or no change in systemic vascular resistance. Although pancuronium-induced tachycardia is primarily due to a vagolytic action, release of norepinephrine from adrenergic nerve endings and blockade of neuronal uptake of norepinephrine may be secondary mechanisms. Bronchospasm may be produced by neuromuscular blockers that release histamine (eg, mivacurium), but insertion of a endotracheal tube is the most common reason for bronchospasm after induction of general anesthesia.

Succinylcholine can cause cardiac arrhythmias when administered during halothane anesthesia. The drug stimulates autonomic cholinoceptors, including the nicotinic receptors at both sympathetic and parasympathetic ganglia and muscarinic receptors in the heart (eg, sinus node). The negative inotropic and chronotropic responses to succinylcholine can be attenuated by administration of an anticholinergic drug (eg, glycopyrrolate, atropine). With large doses of succinylcholine, positive inotropic and chronotropic effects may be observed. On the other hand, bradycardia has been repeatedly observed when a second dose of succinylcholine is given less than 5 minutes after the initial dose. This transient bradycardia can be prevented by thiopental, atropine, ganglionic-blocking drugs, and by pretreating with a small dose of a nondepolarizing muscle relaxant (eg, pancuronium). Direct myocardial effects, increased muscarinic stimulation, and ganglionic stimulation contribute to this bradycardic response.

Other Adverse Effects of Depolarizing Blockade

A. Hyperkalemia

Patients with burns, nerve damage or neuromuscular disease, closed head injury, and other trauma can respond to succinylcholine by releasing potassium into the blood, which, on rare occasions, results in cardiac arrest.

B. Increased Intraocular Pressure

Administration of succinylcholine may be associated with the rapid onset of an increase in intraocular pressure (< 60 seconds), peaking at 2–4 minutes, and declining after 5 minutes. The mechanism may involve tonic contraction of myofibrils or transient dilation of ocular choroidal blood vessels. Despite the increase in intraocular pressure, the use of succinylcholine for ophthalmologic operations is not contraindicated unless the anterior chamber is open ("open globe") due to trauma.

C. Increased Intragastric Pressure

In heavily muscled patients, the fasciculations associated with succinylcholine may cause an increase in intragastric pressure ranging from 5 to 40 cm H_2O, increasing the risk for regurgitation and aspiration of gastric contents. This complication is more likely to occur in patients with delayed gastric emptying (eg, those with diabetes), traumatic injury (eg, an emergency case), esophageal dysfunction, and morbid obesity.

D. Muscle Pain

Myalgias are a common postoperative complaint of heavily muscled patients and those who receive large doses (> 1.5 mg/kg) of succinylcholine. The true incidence of myalgias related to muscle fasciculations is difficult to establish because of confounding

TABLE 27–3 Effects of neuromuscular blocking drugs on other tissues.

Drug	Effect on Autonomic Ganglia	Effect on Cardiac Muscarinic Receptors	Tendency to Cause Histamine Release
Isoquinoline derivatives			
Atracurium	None	None	Slight
Cisatracurium	None	None	None
Mivacurium	None	None	Moderate
Tubocurarine	Weak block	None	Moderate
Steroid derivatives			
Pancuronium	None	Moderate block	None
Rocuronium[1]	None	Slight	None
Vecuronium	None	None	None
Other agents			
Gallamine	None	Strong block	None
Succinylcholine	Stimulation	Stimulation	Slight

[1]Allergic reactions have been reported.

factors, including the anesthetic technique, type of surgery, and positioning during the operation. However, the incidence of myalgias has been reported to vary from less than 1% to 20%. It occurs more frequently in ambulatory than in bedridden patients. The pain is thought to be secondary to the unsynchronized contractions of adjacent muscle fibers just before the onset of paralysis. However, there is controversy over whether the incidence of muscle pain following succinylcholine is actually higher than with nondepolarizing muscle relaxants when other potentially confounding factors are taken into consideration.

Interactions with Other Drugs

A. Anesthetics

Inhaled (volatile) anesthetics potentiate the neuromuscular blockade produced by nondepolarizing muscle relaxants in a dose-dependent fashion. Of the general anesthetics that have been studied, inhaled anesthetics augment the effects of muscle relaxants in the following order: isoflurane (most); sevoflurane, desflurane, enflurane, and halothane; and nitrous oxide (least) (Figure 27–9). The most important factors involved in this interaction are the following: (1) nervous system depression at sites proximal to the neuromuscular junction (ie, central nervous system); (2) increased muscle blood flow (ie, due to peripheral vasodilation produced by volatile anesthetics), which allows a larger fraction of the injected muscle relaxant to reach the neuromuscular junction; and (3) decreased sensitivity of the postjunctional membrane to depolarization.

A rare interaction of succinylcholine with volatile anesthetics results in **malignant hyperthermia**, a condition caused by abnormal release of calcium from stores in skeletal muscle. This condition is treated with dantrolene and is discussed below under Spasmolytic Drugs and in Chapter 16.

B. Antibiotics

Numerous reports have described enhancement of neuromuscular blockade by antibiotics (eg, aminoglycosides). Many of the antibiotics have been shown to cause a depression of evoked release of acetylcholine similar to that caused by administering magnesium. The mechanism of this prejunctional effect appears to be blockade of specific P-type calcium channels in the motor nerve terminal.

C. Local Anesthetics and Antiarrhythmic Drugs

In small doses, local anesthetics can depress posttetanic potentiation via a prejunctional neural effect. In large doses, local anesthetics can block neuromuscular transmission. With higher doses, local anesthetics block acetylcholine-induced muscle contractions as a result of blockade of the nicotinic receptor ion channels. Experimentally, similar effects can be demonstrated with sodium channel-blocking antiarrhythmic drugs such as quinidine. However, at the doses used for cardiac arrhythmias, this interaction is of little or no clinical significance. Higher concentrations of bupivacaine (0.75%) have been associated with cardiac arrhythmias independent of the muscle relaxant used.

D. Other Neuromuscular Blocking Drugs

The end plate-depolarizing effect of succinylcholine can be antagonized by administering a small dose of a nondepolarizing blocker. To prevent the fasciculations associated with succinylcholine administration, a small nonparalyzing dose of a nondepolarizing drug can be given before succinylcholine (eg, *d*-tubocurarine, 2 mg IV, or pancuronium, 0.5 mg IV). Although this dose usually reduces fasciculations and postoperative myalgias, it can increase the amount of succinylcholine required for relaxation by 50–90% and can produce a feeling of weakness in awake patients. Therefore, "pre-curarization" before succinylcholine is no longer widely practiced.

Effects of Diseases & Aging on the Neuromuscular Response

Several diseases can diminish or augment the neuromuscular blockade produced by nondepolarizing muscle relaxants. Myasthenia gravis enhances the neuromuscular blockade produced by these drugs. Advanced age is associated with a prolonged duration of action from nondepolarizing relaxants as a result of decreased clearance of the drugs by the liver and kidneys. As a result, the dosage of neuromuscular blocking drugs should be reduced in older patients (> 70 years).

Conversely, patients with severe burns and those with upper motor neuron disease are resistant to nondepolarizing muscle relaxants. This desensitization is probably caused by proliferation of extrajunctional receptors, which results in an increased dose requirement for the nondepolarizing relaxant to block a sufficient number of receptors.

Reversal of Nondepolarizing Neuromuscular Blockade

The cholinesterase inhibitors effectively antagonize the neuromuscular blockade caused by nondepolarizing drugs. Their general pharmacology is discussed in Chapter 7. **Neostigmine** and **pyridostigmine** antagonize nondepolarizing neuromuscular blockade by increasing the availability of acetylcholine at the motor end plate, mainly by inhibition of acetylcholinesterase. To a lesser extent, these cholinesterase inhibitors also increase the release of this transmitter from the motor nerve terminal. In contrast, **edrophonium** antagonizes neuromuscular blockade purely by inhibiting acetylcholinesterase activity. Edrophonium has a more rapid onset of action but may be less effective than neostigmine in reversing the effects of nondepolarizing blockers in the presence of a profound degree of neuromuscular blockade. These differences are important in determining recovery from *residual block*, the neuromuscular blockade remaining after completion of surgery and movement of the patient to the recovery room. Unsuspected residual block may result in hypoventilation, leading to hypoxia and even apnea, especially if patients have received central depressant medications in the early recovery period.

Since mivacurium is metabolized by plasma cholinesterase, its interaction with the anticholinesterase reversal drugs is less predictable. On the one hand, the neuromuscular blockade is antagonized because of increased acetylcholine concentrations in the synapse. On the other hand, mivacurium concentration may be higher because of decreased plasma cholinesterase breakdown of the muscle relaxant itself.

Sugammadex is a novel reversal agent approved in Europe but not yet approved for use in the USA. It is a modified γ-cyclodextran that binds tightly to rocuronium in a 1:1 ratio. By binding to plasma rocuronium, sugammadex decreases the free plasma rocuronium concentration and establishes a concentration gradient for rocuronium to diffuse away from the neuromuscular junction back into the circulation, where it is quickly bound by free sugammadex.

The optimum dose of sugammadex required to achieve adequate reversal of the neuromuscular blocking agent has yet to be definitively established. Clinical trials studying safety and efficacy have used doses ranging from 0.5 to 16 mg/kg. From 2 mg/kg upward, sugammadex dose-dependently reverses rocuronium with increasing speed and efficacy. These trials reported no difference in prevalence of untoward effects among sugammadex, placebo, and neostigmine. The data need to be confirmed in larger trials, especially the drug's potential to elicit allergic or hypersensitivity reactions.

The sugammadex-rocuronium complex is typically excreted unchanged in the urine within 24 hours in patients with normal renal function. In patients with renal insufficiency, complete urinary elimination may take much longer. However, due to the strong complex formation with rocuronium, no signs of recurrence of neuromuscular blockade have been noted up to 48 hours after use in such patients.

Further large-scale studies will be needed to evaluate the efficacy, safety, and clearance of sugammadex in patient populations with various levels of renal failure.

Uses of Neuromuscular Blocking Drugs

A. Surgical Relaxation

One of the most important applications of the neuromuscular blockers is in facilitating intracavitary surgery, especially in intra-abdominal and intrathoracic procedures.

B. Endotracheal Intubation

By relaxing the pharyngeal and laryngeal muscles, neuromuscular blocking drugs facilitate laryngoscopy and placement of the endotracheal tube. Placement of a endotracheal tube ensures an adequate airway and minimizes the risk of pulmonary aspiration during general anesthesia.

C. Control of Ventilation

In critically ill patients who have ventilatory failure from various causes (eg, severe bronchospasm, pneumonia, chronic obstructive airway disease), it may be necessary to control ventilation to provide adequate gas exchange and to prevent atelectasis. In the ICU, neuromuscular blocking drugs are frequently administered to reduce chest wall resistance (ie, improve thoracic compliance) and ineffective spontaneous ventilation in intubated patients.

D. Treatment of Convulsions

Neuromuscular blocking drugs (ie, succinylcholine) are occasionally used to attenuate the peripheral (motor) manifestations of convulsions associated with status epilepticus or local anesthetic toxicity. Although this approach is effective in eliminating the muscular manifestations of the seizures, it has no effect on the central processes because neuromuscular blocking drugs do not cross the blood-brain barrier.

■ SPASMOLYTIC DRUGS

Spasticity is characterized by an increase in tonic stretch reflexes and flexor muscle spasms (ie, increased basal muscle tone) together with muscle weakness. It is often associated with spinal injury, cerebral palsy, multiple sclerosis, and stroke. These conditions often involve abnormal function of the bowel and bladder as well as skeletal muscle. The mechanisms underlying clinical spasticity appear to involve not only the stretch reflex arc itself but also higher centers in the CNS (ie, upper motor neuron lesion), with damage to descending pathways in the spinal cord resulting in hyperexcitability of the alpha motoneurons in the cord. Pharmacologic therapy may ameliorate some of the symptoms of spasticity by modifying the stretch reflex arc or by interfering directly with skeletal muscle (ie, excitation-contraction coupling). The important components involved in these processes are shown in Figure 27–10.

Drugs that modify this reflex arc may modulate excitatory or inhibitory synapses (see Chapter 21). Thus, to reduce the hyperactive stretch reflex, it is desirable to reduce the activity of the Ia fibers that excite the primary motoneuron or to enhance the activity of the inhibitory internuncial neurons. These structures are shown in greater detail in Figure 27–11.

A variety of pharmacologic agents described as depressants of the spinal "polysynaptic" reflex arc (eg, barbiturates [phenobarbital] and glycerol ethers [mephenesin]) have been used to treat these conditions of excess skeletal muscle tone. However, as illustrated in Figure 27–11, nonspecific depression of synapses involved in the stretch reflex could reduce the desired GABAergic inhibitory activity, as well as the excitatory glutamatergic transmission. Currently available drugs can provide significant relief from painful muscle spasms, but they are less effective in improving meaningful function (eg, mobility and return to work).

DIAZEPAM

As described in Chapter 22, benzodiazepines facilitate the action of GABA in the central nervous system. Diazepam acts at $GABA_A$ synapses, and its action in reducing spasticity is at least partly mediated in the spinal cord because it is somewhat effective in patients with cord transection. Although diazepam can be used in patients with muscle spasm of almost any origin (including local muscle trauma), it also produces sedation at the doses required to reduce muscle tone. The initial dosage is 4 mg/d, and it is gradually increased to a maximum of 60 mg/d. Other benzodiazepines have been used as spasmolytics (eg, midazolam), but clinical experience with them is limited.

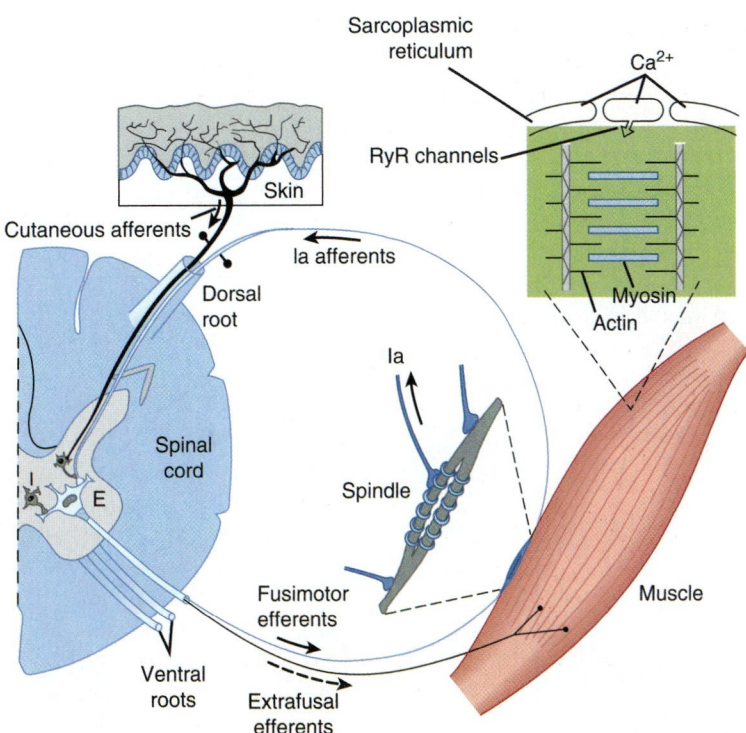

FIGURE 27–10 Diagram of the structures involved in the stretch reflex arc. *I* is an inhibitory interneuron; *E* indicates an excitatory presynaptic terminal; Ia is a primary intrafusal afferent fiber; Ca^{2+} denotes activator calcium stored in the sarcoplasmic reticulum of skeletal muscle; RyR channels indicates the Ca^{2+} release channels. (Reproduced, with permission, from Young RR, Delwaide PJ: Drug therapy: Spasticity. N Engl J Med 1981;304:28.)

BACLOFEN

Baclofen (*p*-chlorophenyl-GABA) was designed to be an orally active GABA-mimetic agent and is an agonist at $GABA_B$ receptors. Activation of these receptors by baclofen results in hyperpolarization, probably by increased K^+ conductance (see Figure 24–2). It has been suggested that hyperpolarization causes presynaptic inhibition by reducing calcium influx (Figure 27–11) and reduces the release of excitatory transmitters in both the brain and the spinal cord. Baclofen may also reduce pain in patients with spasticity, perhaps by inhibiting the release of substance P (neurokinin-1) in the spinal cord.

Baclofen is at least as effective as diazepam in reducing spasticity and causes less sedation. In addition, baclofen does not reduce overall muscle strength as much as dantrolene. It is rapidly and completely absorbed after oral administration and has a plasma half-life of 3–4 hours. Dosage is started at 15 mg twice daily, increasing as tolerated to 100 mg daily. Adverse effects of this drug include drowsiness; however, patients become tolerant to the sedative effect with chronic administration. Increased seizure activity has been reported in epileptic patients. Therefore, withdrawal from baclofen must be done very slowly.

Studies have confirmed that intrathecal administration of baclofen can control severe spasticity and muscle pain that is not responsive to medication by other routes of administration. Owing to the poor egress of baclofen from the spinal cord, peripheral symptoms are rare. Therefore, higher central concentrations of the drug may be tolerated. Partial tolerance to the effect of the drug may occur after several months of therapy, but can be overcome by upward dosage adjustments to maintain the beneficial effect. Excessive somnolence, respiratory depression, and even coma have been described. Although a major disadvantage of this therapeutic approach is the difficulty of maintaining the drug delivery catheter in the subarachnoid space, risking an acute withdrawal syndrome upon treatment interruption, long-term intrathecal baclofen therapy can improve the quality of life for patients with severe spastic disorders.

Oral baclofen has been studied in several other medical conditions, including patients with intractable low back pain. Preliminary studies suggest that it may also be effective in reducing craving in recovering alcoholics (see Chapter 32). Finally, it has been alleged to be effective in preventing migraine headaches in some patients.

TIZANIDINE

As noted in Chapter 11, α_2 agonists such as clonidine and other imidazoline compounds have a variety of effects on the CNS that are not fully understood. Among these effects is the ability to reduce muscle spasm. Tizanidine is a congener of clonidine that

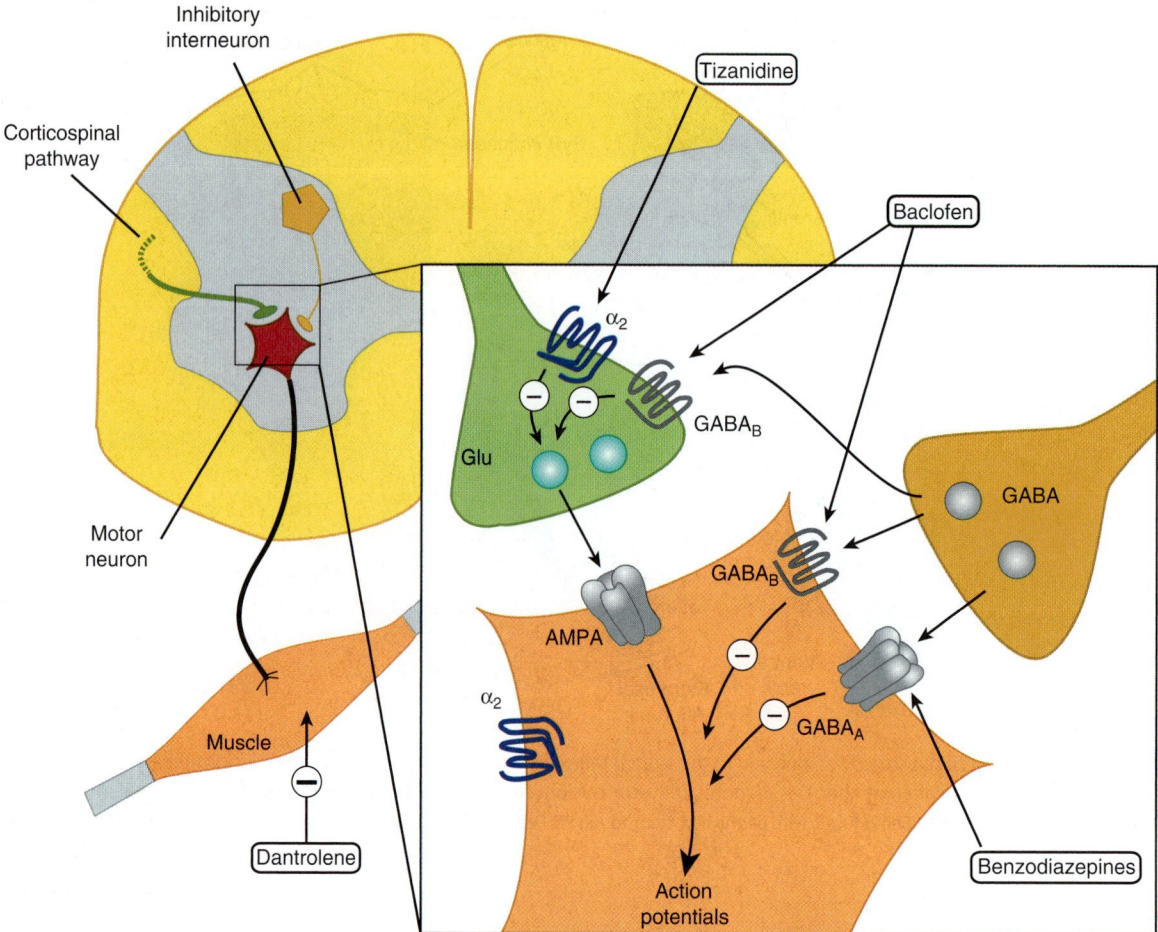

FIGURE 27–11 Postulated sites of spasmolytic action of tizanidine (α_2), benzodiazepines (GABA$_A$), and baclofen (GABA$_B$) in the spinal cord. Tizanidine may also have a postsynaptic inhibitory effect. Dantrolene acts on the sarcoplasmic reticulum in skeletal muscle. Glu, glutamatergic neuron.

has been studied for its spasmolytic actions. Tizanidine has significant α_2-adrenoceptor agonist effects, but it reduces spasticity in experimental models at doses that cause fewer cardiovascular effects than clonidine or dexmedetomidine. Tizanidine has approximately one tenth to one fifteenth of the blood pressure-lowering effects of clonidine. Neurophysiologic studies in animals and humans suggest that tizanidine reinforces both presynaptic and postsynaptic inhibition in the cord. It also inhibits nociceptive transmission in the spinal dorsal horn. Tizanidine's actions are believed to be mediated via restoration of inhibitory suppression of the group II spinal interneurons without inducing any changes in intrinsic muscle properties.

Clinical trials with oral tizanidine report comparable efficacy in relieving muscle spasm to diazepam, baclofen, and dantrolene. Tizanidine causes markedly less muscle weakness but produces a different spectrum of adverse effects, including drowsiness, hypotension, dizziness, dry mouth, asthenia, and hepatotoxicity. The drowsiness can be managed by taking the drug at night. Tizanidine displays linear pharmacokinetics, and dosage requirements vary considerably among patients. Dosage must be adjusted in patients with hepatic or renal impairment. In addition to its effectiveness in spastic conditions, tizanidine

also appears to be effective for management of chronic migraine.

OTHER CENTRALLY ACTING SPASMOLYTIC DRUGS

Gabapentin is an antiepileptic drug (see Chapter 24) that has shown considerable promise as a spasmolytic agent in several studies involving patients with multiple sclerosis. Pregabalin is a newer analog of gabapentin that may also prove useful in relieving painful disorders that involve a muscle spasm component. **Progabide** and **glycine** have also been found in preliminary studies to reduce spasticity. Progabide is a GABA$_A$ and GABA$_B$ agonist and has active metabolites, including GABA itself. Glycine is another inhibitory amino acid neurotransmitter (see Chapter 21) that appears to possess pharmacologic activity when given orally and readily passes the blood-brain barrier. **Idrocilamide** and **riluzole** are newer drugs for the treatment of amyotrophic lateral sclerosis (ALS) that appear to have spasm-reducing effects, possibly through inhibition of glutamatergic transmission in the central nervous system.

DANTROLENE

Dantrolene is a hydantoin derivative related to phenytoin that has a unique mechanism of spasmolytic activity. In contrast to the centrally acting drugs, dantrolene reduces skeletal muscle strength by interfering with excitation-contraction coupling in the muscle fibers. The normal contractile response involves release of calcium from its stores in the sarcoplasmic reticulum (see Figures 13–1 and 27–10). This activator calcium brings about the tension-generating interaction of actin with myosin. Calcium is released from the sarcoplasmic reticulum via a calcium channel, called the **ryanodine receptor** (**RyR**) **channel** because the plant alkaloid ryanodine combines with a receptor on the channel protein. In the case of the skeletal muscle RyR1 channel, ryanodine facilitates the open configuration.

Dantrolene

Dantrolene interferes with the release of activator calcium through this sarcoplasmic reticulum calcium channel by binding to the RyR1 and blocking the opening of the channel. Motor units that contract rapidly are more sensitive to the drug's effects than are slower-responding units. Cardiac muscle and smooth muscle are minimally depressed because the release of calcium from their sarcoplasmic reticulum involves a different RyR channel (RyR2).

Treatment with dantrolene is usually initiated with 25 mg daily as a single dose, increasing to a maximum of 100 mg four times daily as tolerated. Only about one third of an oral dose of dantrolene is absorbed, and the elimination half-life of the drug is approximately 8 hours. Major adverse effects are generalized muscle weakness, sedation, and occasionally hepatitis.

A special application of dantrolene is in the treatment of **malignant hyperthermia,** a rare heritable disorder that can be triggered by a variety of stimuli, including general anesthetics (eg, volatile anesthetics) and neuromuscular blocking drugs (eg, succinylcholine; see also Chapter 16). Patients at risk for this condition have a hereditary alteration in Ca^{2+}-induced Ca^{2+} release via the RyR1 channel or impairment in the ability of the sarcoplasmic reticulum to sequester calcium via the Ca^{2+} transporter (Figure 27–10). Several mutations associated with this risk have been identified. After administration of one of the triggering agents, there is a sudden and prolonged release of calcium, with massive muscle contraction, lactic acid production, and increased body temperature. Prompt treatment is essential to control acidosis and body temperature and to reduce calcium release. The latter is accomplished by administering intravenous dantrolene, starting with a dose of 1 mg/kg IV, and repeating as necessary to a maximum dose of 10 mg/kg.

BOTULINUM TOXIN

The therapeutic use of botulinum toxin for ophthalmic purposes and for local muscle spasm was mentioned in Chapter 6. Local facial injections of botulinum toxin are widely used for the short-term treatment (1–3 months per treatment) of wrinkles associated with aging around the eyes and mouth. Local injection of botulinum toxin has also become a useful treatment for generalized spastic disorders (eg, cerebral palsy). Most clinical studies to date have involved administration in one or two limbs, and the benefits appear to persist for weeks to several months after a single treatment. Most studies have used type A botulinum toxin, but type B is also available.

DRUGS USED TO TREAT ACUTE LOCAL MUSCLE SPASM

A large number of less well-studied, centrally active drugs (eg, **carisoprodol, chlorphenesin, chlorzoxazone, cyclobenzaprine, metaxalone, methocarbamol,** and **orphenadrine**) are promoted for the relief of acute muscle spasm caused by local tissue trauma or muscle strains. It has been suggested that these drugs act primarily at the level of the brainstem. Cyclobenzaprine may be regarded as the prototype of the group. Cyclobenzaprine is structurally related to the tricyclic antidepressants and produces antimuscarinic side effects. It is ineffective in treating muscle spasm due to cerebral palsy or spinal cord injury. As a result of its strong antimuscarinic actions, cyclobenzaprine may cause significant sedation, as well as confusion and transient visual hallucinations. The dosage of cyclobenzaprine for acute injury-related muscle spasm is 20–40 mg/d orally in divided doses.

SUMMARY Skeletal Muscle Relaxants

Subclass	Mechanism of Action	Effects	Clinical Applications	Pharmacokinetics, Toxicities, Interactions
DEPOLARIZING NEUROMUSCULAR BLOCKING AGENT				
• Succinylcholine	Agonist at nicotinic acetylcholine (ACh) receptors, especially at neuromuscular junctions • depolarizes • may stimulate ganglionic nicotinic ACh and cardiac muscarinic ACh receptors	Initial depolarization causes transient contractions, followed by prolonged flaccid paralysis • depolarization is then followed by repolarization that is also accompanied by paralysis	Placement of endotracheal tube at start of anesthetic procedure • rarely, control of muscle contractions in status epilepticus	Rapid metabolism by plasma cholinesterase • normal duration, ~5 min • *Toxicities:* Arrhythmias • hyperkalemia • transient increased intra-abdominal, intraocular pressure • postoperative muscle pain
NONDEPOLARIZING NEUROMUSCULAR BLOCKING AGENTS				
• *d*-Tubocurarine	Competitive antagonist at nACh receptors, especially at neuromuscular junctions	Prevents depolarization by ACh, causes flaccid paralysis • can cause histamine release with hypotension • weak block of cardiac muscarinic ACh receptors	Prolonged relaxation for surgical procedures • superseded by newer nondepolarizing agents	Renal excretion • duration, ~40–60 min • *Toxicities:* Histamine release • hypotension • prolonged apnea
• Cisatracurium	Similar to tubocurarine	Like tubocurarine but lacks histamine release and antimuscarinic effects	Prolonged relaxation for surgical procedures • relaxation of respiratory muscles to facilitate mechanical ventilation in intensive care unit	Not dependent on renal or hepatic function • duration, ~25–45 min • *Toxicities:* Prolonged apnea but less toxic than atracurium
• Rocuronium	Similar to cisatracurium	Like cisatracurium but slight antimuscarinic effect	Like cisatracurium • useful in patients with renal impairment	Hepatic metabolism • duration, ~20–35 min • *Toxicities:* Like cisatracurium
• *Mivacurium: Rapid onset, short duration (10–20 min); metabolized by plasma cholinesterase*				
• *Vecuronium: Intermediate duration; metabolized in liver*				
CENTRALLY ACTING SPASMOLYTIC DRUGS				
• Baclofen	GABA$_B$ agonist, facilitates spinal inhibition of motor neurons	Pre- and postsynaptic inhibition of motor output	Severe spasticity due to cerebral palsy, multiple sclerosis, stroke	Oral, intrathecal • *Toxicities:* Sedation, weakness
• Cyclobenzaprine	Poorly understood inhibition of muscle stretch reflex in spinal cord	Reduction in hyperactive muscle reflexes • antimuscarinic effects	Acute spasm due to muscle injury • inflammation	Hepatic metabolism • duration, ~4–6 h • *Toxicities:* Strong antimuscarinic effects
• *Chlorphenesin, methocarbamol, orphenadrine, others: Like cyclobenzaprine with varying degrees of antimuscarinic effect*				
• Diazepam	Facilitates GABAergic transmission in central nervous system (see Chapter 22)	Increases interneuron inhibition of primary motor afferents in spinal cord • central sedation	Chronic spasm due to cerebral palsy, stroke, spinal cord injury • acute spasm due to muscle injury	Hepatic metabolism • duration, ~12–24 h • *Toxicities:* See Chapter 22
• Tizanidine	α_2-Adrenoceptor agonist in the spinal cord	Presynaptic and postsynaptic inhibition of reflex motor output	Spasm due to multiple sclerosis, stroke, amyotrophic lateral sclerosis	Renal and hepatic elimination • duration, 3–6 h • *Toxicities:* Weakness, sedation • hypotension
DIRECT-ACTING MUSCLE RELAXANT				
• Dantrolene	Blocks RyR1 Ca^{2+}-release channels in the sarcoplasmic reticulum of skeletal muscle	Reduces actin-myosin interaction • weakens skeletal muscle contraction	IV: Malignant hyperthermia • Oral: Spasm due to cerebral palsy, spinal cord injury, multiple sclerosis	IV, oral • duration, 4–6 h • *Toxicities:* Muscle weakness

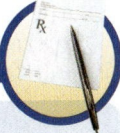

PREPARATIONS AVAILABLE

NEUROMUSCULAR BLOCKING DRUGS

Atracurium (generic)
Parenteral: 10 mg/mL for injection

Cisatracurium (Nimbex)
Parenteral: 2, 10 mg/mL for IV injection

Mivacurium (Mivacron)
Parenteral: 0.5, 2 mg/mL for injection

Pancuronium (generic)
Parenteral: 1, 2 mg/mL for injection

Rocuronium (generic, Zemuron)
Parenteral: 10 mg/mL for IV injection

Succinylcholine (generic, Anectine, Quelicin)
Parenteral: 20, 50, 100 mg/mL for injection; 500, 1000 mg per vial powder to reconstitute for injection

Tubocurarine (generic)
Parenteral: 3 mg (20 units)/mL for injection

Vecuronium (generic, Norcuron)
Parenteral: 10, 20 mg powder to reconstitute for injection

MUSCLE RELAXANTS (SPASMOLYTICS)

Baclofen (generic, Lioresal, Gablofen)
Oral: 10, 20 mg tablets
Intrathecal: 0.05, 0.5, 2 mg/mL

Botulinum toxin type A (Botox)
Parenteral: Powder for solution, 50, 100, 200 units/vial

Botulinum toxin type B (Myobloc)
Parenteral: 5000 units/mL for IM injection

Carisoprodol (generic, Soma)
Oral: 250, 350 mg tablets

Chlorzoxazone (generic)
Oral: 500 mg tablets, caplets

Cyclobenzaprine (generic, Amrix, Fexmid, Flexeril)
Oral: 5, 7.5, 10 mg tablets; 15, 30 mg capsules

Dantrolene (Dantrium, Revonto)
Oral: 25, 50, 100 mg capsules
Parenteral: 20 mg per vial powder to reconstitute for injection

Diazepam (generic, Diastat, Valium)
Oral: 2, 5, 10 mg tablets; 5 mg/5 mL, 5 mg/mL solutions
Parenteral: 5 mg/mL for injection
Rectal: 2.5, 5, 10 mg gel

Gabapentin (Neurontin)
Oral: 100, 300, 400 mg capsules; 600, 800 mg tablets; 50 mg/mL oral solution
Note: This drug is labeled for use only in epilepsy and postherpetic neuralgia.

Metaxalone (Skelaxin)
Oral: 800 mg tablets

Methocarbamol (generic, Robaxin)
Oral: 500, 750 mg tablets
Parenteral: 100 mg/mL for IM, IV injection

Orphenadrine (generic, Norflex)
Oral: 100 mg tablets; 100 mg sustained-release tablets
Parenteral: 30 mg/mL for IM, IV injection

Riluzole (Rilutek)
Oral: 50 mg tablets
Note: This drug is labeled only for use in amyotrophic lateral sclerosis.

Tizanidine (Zanaflex)
Oral: 2, 4 mg tablets, capsules; 6 mg capsules

REFERENCES

Neuromuscular Blockers

Brull SJ, Murphy GS: Residual neuromuscular block: Lessons unlearned. Part II: Methods to reduce the risk of residual weakness. Anesth Analg 2010;111:129.

De Boer HD et al: Reversal of rocuronium-induced (1.2 mg/kg) profound neuromuscular blockade by sugammadex. Anesthesiology 2007;107:239.

Gibb AJ, Marshall IG: Pre- and postjunctional effects of tubocurarine and other nicotinic antagonists during repetitive stimulation in the rat. J Physiol 1984;351:275.

Hemmerling TM, Russo G, Bracco D: Neuromuscular blockade in cardiac surgery: An update for clinicians. Ann Card Anaesth 2008;11:80.

Hirsch NP: Neuromuscular junction in health and disease. Br J Anaesth 2007;99:132.

Kampe S et al: Muscle relaxants. Best Prac Res Clin Anesthesiol 2003;17:137.

Lee C: Structure, conformation, and action of neuromuscular blocking drugs. Br J Anaesth 2001;87:755.

Lee C et al: Reversal of profound neuromuscular block by sugammadex administered three minutes after rocuronium. Anesthesiology 2009;110:1020.

Lien CA et al: Fumarates: Unique nondepolarizing neuromuscular blocking agents that are antagonized by cysteine. J Crit Care 2009;24:50.

Mace SE: Challenges and advances in intubation: rapid sequence intubation. Emerg Med Clin North Am 2008;26:1043.

Marshall CG, Ogden DC, Colquhoun D: The actions of suxamethonium (succinyldicholine) as an agonist and channel blocker at the nicotinic receptor of frog muscle. J Physiol (Lond) 1990;428:155.

Martyn JA: Neuromuscular physiology and pharmacology. In: Miller RD (editor): *Anesthesia*, 7th ed. Churchill Livingstone, 2010.

Meakin GH: Recent advances in myorelaxant therapy. Paed Anaesthesia 2001;11:523.

Murphy GS, Brull SJ: Residual neuromuscular block: Lessons unlearned. Part I: Definitions, incidence, and adverse physiologic effects of residual neuromuscular block. Anesth Analg 2010;111:120.

Naguib M: Sugammadex: Another milestone in clinical neuromuscular pharmacology. Anesth Analg 2007;104:575.

Naguib M, Brull SJ: Update on neuromuscular pharmacology. Curr Opin Anaesthesiol 2009;22:483.

Naguib M, Kopman AF, Ensor JE: Neuromuscular monitoring and postoperative residual curarisation: A meta-analysis. Br J Anaesth 2007;98:302.

Naguib M et al: Advances in neurobiology of the neuromuscular junction: Implications for the anesthesiologist. Anesthesiology 2002;96:202.

Nicholson WT, Sprung J, Jankowski CJ: Sugammadex: A novel agent for the reversal of neuromuscular blockade. Pharmacotherapy 2007;27:1181.

Pavlin JD, Kent CD: Recovery after ambulatory anesthesia. Curr Opin Anaesthesiol 2008;21:729.

Puhringer FK et al: Reversal of profound, high-dose rocuronium-induced neuromuscular blockade by sugammadex at two different time points. Anesthesiology 2008;109:188.

Sacan O, Klein K, White PF: Sugammadex reversal of rocuronium-induced neuromuscular blockade: A comparison with neostigmine-glycopyrrolate and edrophonium-atropine. Anesth Analg 2007;104:569.

Staals LM et al: Reduced clearance of rocuronium and sugammadex in patients with severe to end-stage renal failure: A pharmacokinetic study. Br J Anaesth 2010;104:31.

Sunaga H et al: Gantacurium and CW002 do not potentiate muscarinic receptor-mediated airway smooth muscle constriction in guinea pigs. Anesthesiology 2010;112:892.

Viby-Mogensen J: Neuromuscular monitoring. In: Miller RD (editor): *Anesthesia*, 5th ed. Churchill Livingstone, 2000.

Spasmolytics

Corcia P, Meininger V: Management of amyotrophic lateral sclerosis. Drugs 2008;68:1037.

Cutter NC et al: Gabapentin effect on spasticity in multiple sclerosis: A placebo-controlled, randomized trial. Arch Phys Med Rehabil 2000;81:164.

Gracies JM, Singer BJ, Dunne JW: The role of botulinum toxin injections in the management of muscle overactivity of the lower limb. Disabil Rehabil 2007;29:1789

Groves L, Shellenberger MK, Davis CS: Tizanidine treatment of spasticity: A meta-analysis of controlled, double-blind, comparative studies with baclofen and diazepam. Adv Ther 1998;15:241.

Krause T et al: Dantrolene—a review of its pharmacology, therapeutic use and new developments. Anaesthesia 2004;59:364.

Lopez JR et al: Effects of dantrolene on myoplasmic free $[Ca^{2+}]$ measured in vivo in patients susceptible to malignant hyperthermia. Anesthesiology 1992;76:711.

Lovell BV, Marmura MJ: New therapeutic developments in chronic migraine. Curr Opin Neurol 2010;23:254.

Malanga G, Reiter RD, Garay E: Update on tizanidine for muscle spasticity and emerging indications. Expert Opin Pharmacother 2008;9:2209

Mirbagheri MM, Chen D, Rymer WZ: Quantification of the effects of an alpha-2 adrenergic agonist on reflex properties in spinal cord injury using a system identification technique. J Neuroeng Rehabil 2010;7:29.

Nolan KW, Cole LL, Liptak GS: Use of botulinum toxin type A in children with cerebral palsy. Phys Ther 2006;86:573.

Ronan S, Gold JT: Nonoperative management of spasticity in children. Childs Nerv Syst 2007;23:943

Ross JC et al: Acute intrathecal baclofen withdrawal: A brief review of treatment options. Neurocrit Care 2011;14:103.

Vakhapova V, Auriel E, Karni A: Nightly sublingual tizanidine HCl in multiple sclerosis: Clinical efficacy and safety. Clin Neuropharmacol 2010;33:151.

Verrotti A et al: Pharmacotherapy of spasticity in children with cerebral palsy. Pediatr Neurol 2006;34:1.

Ward AB: Spasticity treatment with botulinum toxins. J Neural Transm 2008;115:607.

CASE STUDY ANSWER

Because of trauma and associated pain, it is assumed that gastric emptying will be significantly delayed. To avoid possible aspiration at the time of intubation, a very rapid-acting muscle relaxant should be used so the airway can be secured with an endotracheal tube. Therefore, succinylcholine is the agent of choice in this case. Despite its side effects, succinylcholine has the fastest mechanism of action of any currently available skeletal muscle relaxant. An alternative to succinylcholine is high-dose (up to 1.2 mg/kg) rocuronium, a nondepolarizing muscle relaxant. At this dose, rocuronium has a very rapid onset, which approaches but does not quite equal that of succinylcholine.

Both burns and neurologic injuries result in the expression of extrajunctional acetylcholine receptors. In patients with recent burns, succinylcholine use can lead to life-threatening hyperkalemia. Although the drug would not result in dangerous hyperkalemia if given immediately after a severe neurologic injury, in a patient with a chronic paralysis, its use may lead to hyperkalemia. Therefore, succinylcholine would also be contraindicated in a patient with long-standing hemiparesis.

28

Pharmacologic Management of Parkinsonism & Other Movement Disorders

Michael J. Aminoff, MD, DSc, FRCP

CASE STUDY

A 64-year-old architect complains of left-hand tremor at rest, which interferes with his writing and drawing. He also notes a stooped posture, a tendency to drag his left leg when walking, and slight unsteadiness on turning. He remains independent in all activities of daily living. Examination reveals hypomimia (flat facies), hypophonia, a rest tremor of the left arm and leg, mild rigidity in all limbs, and impaired rapid alternating movements in the left limbs. Neurologic and general examinations are otherwise normal. What is the likely diagnosis and prognosis, and how should his condition be managed?

Several types of abnormal movement are recognized. **Tremor** consists of a rhythmic oscillatory movement around a joint and is best characterized by its relation to activity. Tremor at rest is characteristic of parkinsonism, when it is often associated with rigidity and an impairment of voluntary activity. Tremor may occur during maintenance of sustained posture (postural tremor) or during movement (intention tremor). A conspicuous postural tremor is the cardinal feature of benign essential or familial tremor. Intention tremor occurs in patients with a lesion of the brainstem or cerebellum, especially when the superior cerebellar peduncle is involved; it may also occur as a manifestation of toxicity from alcohol or certain other drugs.

Chorea consists of irregular, unpredictable, involuntary muscle jerks that occur in different parts of the body and impair voluntary activity. In some instances, the proximal muscles of the limbs are most severely affected, and because the abnormal movements are then particularly violent, the term *ballismus* has been used to describe them. Chorea may be hereditary or may occur as a complication of a number of general medical disorders and of therapy with certain drugs.

Abnormal movements may be slow and writhing in character (**athetosis**) and in some instances are so sustained that they are more properly regarded as abnormal postures (**dystonia**). Athetosis or dystonia may occur with perinatal brain damage, with focal or generalized cerebral lesions, as an acute complication of certain drugs, as an accompaniment of diverse neurologic disorders, or as an isolated inherited phenomenon of uncertain cause known as idiopathic torsion dystonia or dystonia musculorum deformans. Various genetic loci have been reported (eg, 9q34, 8p21–q22, 18p, 1p36.32–p36.13, 14q22.1–q22.2, 19q13, Xq13) depending on the age of onset, mode of inheritance, and response to dopaminergic therapy. The physiologic basis is uncertain, and treatment is unsatisfactory.

Tics are sudden coordinated abnormal movements that tend to occur repetitively, particularly about the face and head, especially in children, and can be suppressed voluntarily for short periods of time. Common tics include repetitive sniffing or shoulder shrugging. Tics may be single or multiple and transient or chronic. Gilles de la Tourette's syndrome is characterized by chronic multiple tics; its pharmacologic management is discussed at the end of this chapter.

Many of the movement disorders have been attributed to disturbances of the basal ganglia. The basic circuitry of the basal ganglia involves three interacting neuronal loops that include the cortex and thalamus as well as the basal ganglia themselves (Figure 28–1). However, the precise function of these anatomic structures is not yet fully understood, and it is not possible to relate individual symptoms to involvement at specific sites.

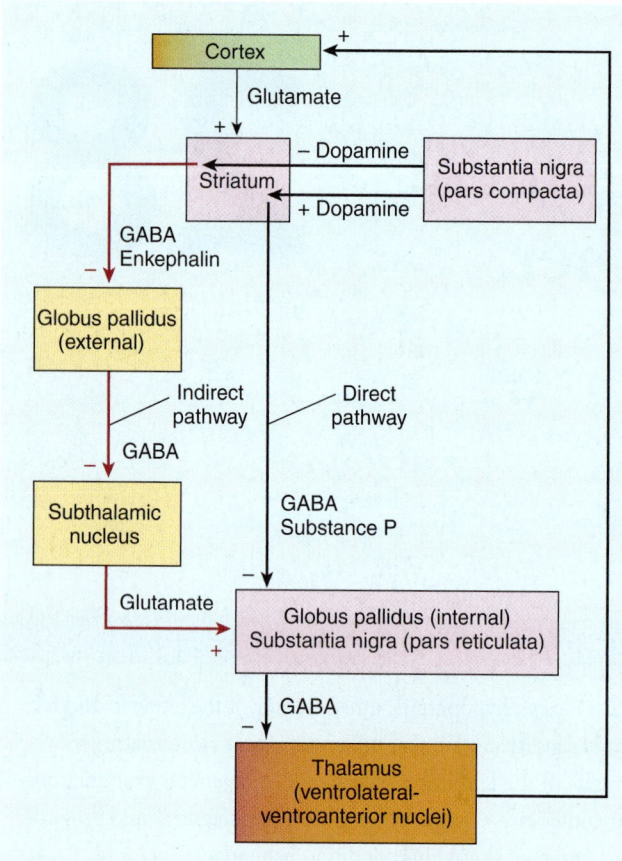

FIGURE 28–1 Functional circuitry between the cortex, basal ganglia, and thalamus. The major neurotransmitters are indicated. In Parkinson's disease, there is degeneration of the pars compacta of the substantia nigra, leading to overactivity in the indirect pathway (red) and increased glutamatergic activity by the subthalamic nucleus.

■ PARKINSONISM

Parkinsonism is characterized by a combination of rigidity, bradykinesia, tremor, and postural instability that can occur for a variety of reasons but is usually idiopathic (Parkinson's disease or paralysis agitans). Cognitive decline occurs in many patients as the disease advances. Other nonmotor symptoms—which are receiving increasing attention—are affective disorders (anxiety or depression), personality changes, abnormalities of autonomic function (sphincter or sexual functions; choking; sweating abnormalities; and disturbances of blood pressure regulation), sleep disorders, and sensory complaints or pain. The disease is generally progressive, leading to increasing disability unless effective treatment is provided.

Pathogenesis

The pathogenesis of parkinsonism seems to relate to a combination of impaired degradation of proteins, intracellular protein accumulation and aggregation, oxidative stress, mitochondrial damage, inflammatory cascades, and apoptosis. Studies in twins

suggest that genetic factors are important, especially when the disease occurs in patients under age 50. Recognized genetic abnormalities account for 10–15% of cases. Mutations of the α-synuclein gene at 4q21 or duplication and triplication of the normal synuclein gene are associated with Parkinson's disease, which is now widely recognized as a *synucleinopathy*. Mutations of the leucine-rich repeat kinase 2 (*LRRK2*) gene at 12cen, and the *UCHL1* gene may also cause autosomal dominant parkinsonism. Mutations in the *parkin* gene (6q25.2–q27) cause early-onset, autosomal recessive, familial parkinsonism, or sporadic juvenile-onset parkinsonism. Several other genes or chromosomal regions have been associated with familial forms of the disease. Environmental or endogenous toxins may also be important in the etiology of the disease. Epidemiologic studies reveal that cigarette smoking, coffee, anti-inflammatory drug use, and high serum uric acid levels are protective, whereas the incidence of the disease is increased in those working in teaching, health care, or farming, and in those with lead or manganese exposure or with vitamin D deficiency.

The finding of Lewy bodies (intracellular inclusion bodies containing α-synuclein) in fetal dopaminergic cells transplanted into the brain of parkinsonian patients some years previously has provided some support for suggestions that Parkinson's disease may represent a prion disease.

Staining for α-synuclein has revealed that pathology is more widespread than previously recognized, developing initially in the olfactory nucleus and lower brainstem (stage 1 of Braak), then the higher brainstem (stage 2), the substantia nigra (stage 3), the mesocortex and thalamus (stage 4), and finally the entire neocortex (stage 5). The motor features of Parkinson's disease develop at stage 3 on the Braak scale.

The normally high concentration of dopamine in the basal ganglia of the brain is reduced in parkinsonism, and pharmacologic attempts to restore dopaminergic activity with levodopa and dopamine agonists alleviate many of the motor features of the disorder. An alternative but complementary approach has been to restore the normal balance of cholinergic and dopaminergic influences on the basal ganglia with antimuscarinic drugs. The pathophysiologic basis for these therapies is that in idiopathic parkinsonism, dopaminergic neurons in the substantia nigra that normally inhibit the output of GABAergic cells in the corpus striatum are lost (Figure 28–2). Drugs that induce parkinsonian syndromes either are dopamine receptor antagonists (eg, antipsychotic agents; see Chapter 29) or lead to the destruction of the dopaminergic nigrostriatal neurons (eg, 1-methyl-4-phenyl-1-,2,3,6-tetrahydropyridine [MPTP]; see below). Various other neurotransmitters, such as norepinephrine, are also depleted in the brain in parkinsonism, but these deficiencies are of uncertain clinical relevance.

LEVODOPA

Dopamine does not cross the blood-brain barrier and if given into the peripheral circulation has no therapeutic effect in parkinsonism. However, (–)-3-(3,4-dihydroxyphenyl)-L-alanine (levodopa), the immediate metabolic precursor of dopamine, does enter the brain

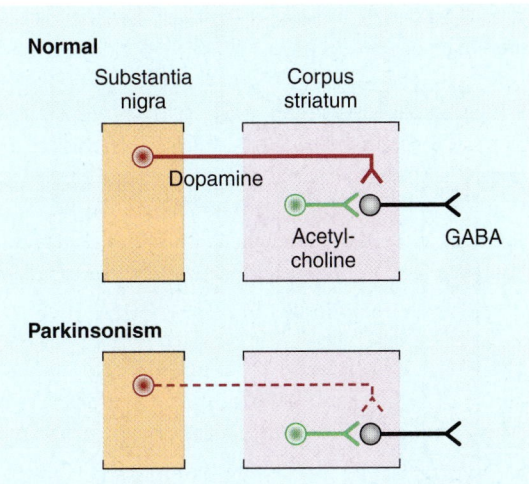

FIGURE 28–2 Schematic representation of the sequence of neurons involved in parkinsonism. **Top:** Dopaminergic neurons (red) originating in the substantia nigra normally inhibit the GABAergic output from the striatum, whereas cholinergic neurons (green) exert an excitatory effect. **Bottom:** In parkinsonism, there is a selective loss of dopaminergic neurons (dashed, red).

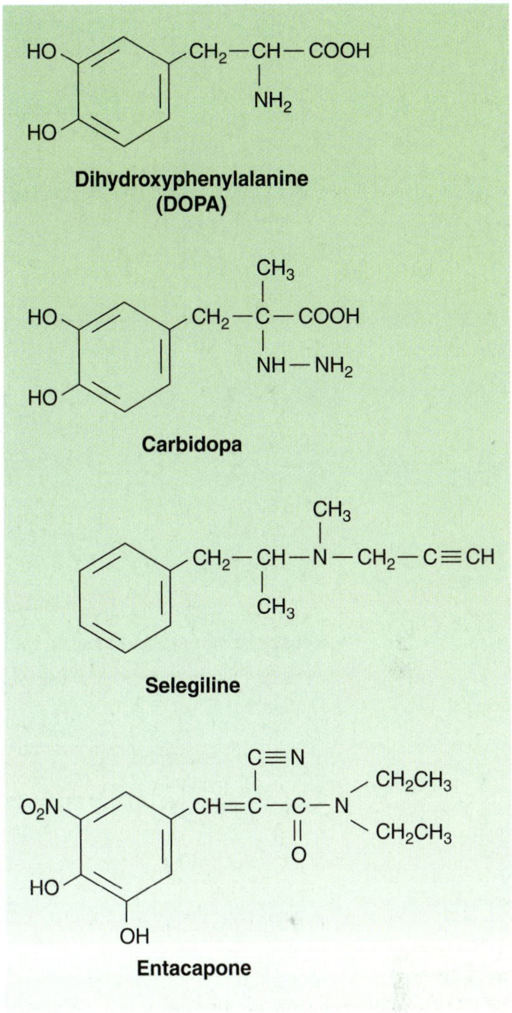

FIGURE 28–3 Some drugs used in the treatment of parkinsonism.

(via an L-amino acid transporter, LAT), where it is decarboxylated to dopamine (see Figure 6–5). Several noncatecholamine dopamine receptor agonists have also been developed and may lead to clinical benefit, as discussed in the text that follows.

Dopamine receptors are discussed in detail in Chapters 21 and 29. Dopamine receptors of the D_1 type are located in the pars compacta of the substantia nigra and presynaptically on striatal axons coming from cortical neurons and from dopaminergic cells in the substantia nigra. The D_2 receptors are located postsynaptically on striatal neurons and presynaptically on axons in the substantia nigra belonging to neurons in the basal ganglia. The benefits of dopaminergic antiparkinsonism drugs appear to depend mostly on stimulation of the D_2 receptors. However, D_1- receptor stimulation may also be required for maximal benefit and one of the newer drugs is D_3 selective. Dopamine agonist or partial agonist ergot derivatives such as lergotrile and bromocriptine that are powerful stimulators of the D_2 receptors have antiparkinsonism properties, whereas certain dopamine blockers that are selective D_2 antagonists can induce parkinsonism.

Chemistry

Dopa is the amino acid precursor of dopamine and norepinephrine (discussed in Chapter 6). Its structure is shown in Figure 28–3. Levodopa is the levorotatory stereoisomer of dopa.

Pharmacokinetics

Levodopa is rapidly absorbed from the small intestine, but its absorption depends on the rate of gastric emptying and the pH of the gastric contents. Ingestion of food delays the appearance of levodopa in the plasma. Moreover, certain amino acids from ingested food can compete with the drug for absorption from the gut and for transport from the blood to the brain. Plasma concentrations usually peak between 1 and 2 hours after an oral dose, and the plasma half-life is usually between 1 and 3 hours, although it varies considerably among individuals. About two thirds of the dose appears in the urine as metabolites within 8 hours of an oral dose, the main metabolic products being 3-methoxy-4-hydroxyphenyl acetic acid (homovanillic acid, HVA) and dihydroxyphenylacetic acid (DOPAC). Unfortunately, only about 1–3% of administered levodopa actually enters the brain unaltered; the remainder is metabolized extracerebrally, predominantly by decarboxylation to dopamine, which does not penetrate the blood-brain barrier. Accordingly, levodopa must be given in large amounts when used alone. However, when given in combination with a dopa decarboxylase inhibitor that does not penetrate the blood-brain barrier, the peripheral metabolism of levodopa is reduced, plasma levels of levodopa are higher, plasma half-life is longer, and more dopa is available for entry into the brain (Figure 28–4). Indeed, concomitant administration of a peripheral dopa decarboxylase inhibitor such as carbidopa may reduce the daily requirements of levodopa by approximately 75%.

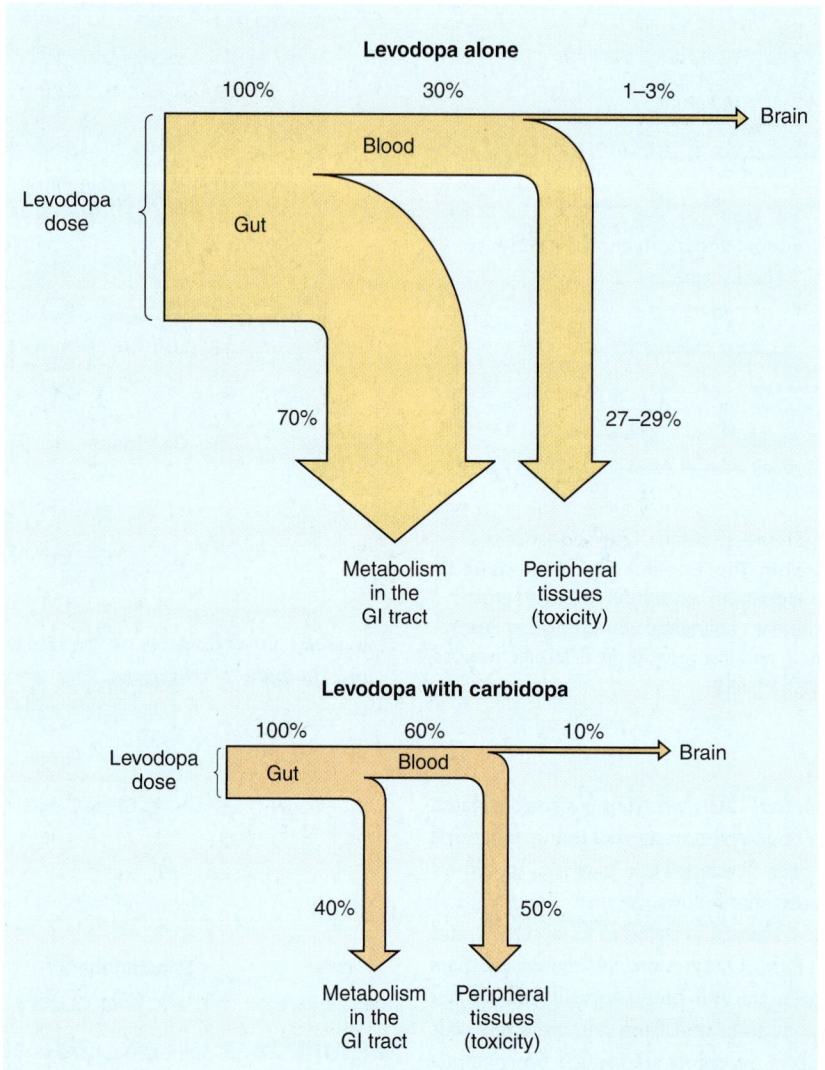

FIGURE 28–4 Fate of orally administered levodopa and the effect of carbidopa, estimated from animal data. The width of each pathway indicates the absolute amount of the drug at each site, whereas the percentages shown denote the relative proportion of the administered dose. The benefits of coadministration of carbidopa include reduction of the amount of levodopa required for benefit and of the absolute amount diverted to peripheral tissues and an increase in the fraction of the dose that reaches the brain. GI, gastrointestinal. (Data from Nutt JG, Fellman JH: Pharmacokinetics of levodopa. Clin Neuropharmacol 1984;7:35.)

Clinical Use

The best results of levodopa treatment are obtained in the first few years of treatment. This is sometimes because the daily dose of levodopa must be reduced over time to avoid adverse effects at doses that were well tolerated initially. Some patients become less responsive to levodopa, perhaps because of loss of dopaminergic nigrostriatal nerve terminals or some pathologic process directly involving striatal dopamine receptors. For such reasons, the benefits of levodopa treatment often begin to diminish after about 3 or 4 years of therapy, regardless of the initial therapeutic response. Although levodopa therapy does not stop the progression of parkinsonism, its early initiation lowers the mortality rate. However, long-term therapy may lead to a number of problems in management such as the on-off phenomenon discussed below. The most appropriate time to introduce levodopa therapy must therefore be determined individually.

When levodopa is used, it is generally given in combination with carbidopa (Figure 28–3), a peripheral dopa decarboxylase inhibitor, which reduces peripheral conversion to dopamine. Combination treatment is started with a small dose, eg, carbidopa 25 mg, levodopa 100 mg three times daily, and gradually increased. It should be taken 30–60 minutes before meals. Most patients ultimately require carbidopa 25 mg, levodopa 250 mg three or four times daily. It is generally preferable to keep treatment with this agent at a low level (eg, carbidopa-levodopa 25/100 three times daily) when possible, and to use a dopamine agonist instead, to reduce the risk of development of response fluctuations. A controlled-release formulation of carbidopa-levodopa is available and may be helpful in patients with established response fluctuations or as a means of reducing dosing frequency. A formulation of carbidopa-levodopa (10/100, 25/100, 25/250) that disintegrates in the mouth and is swallowed with the saliva (**Parcopa**) is now available commercially and is best taken about 1 hour before meals. The combination (**Stalevo**) of levodopa, carbidopa, and a catechol-*O*-methyltransferase (COMT) inhibitor (entacapone) is discussed in a later section. Finally, therapy by *intraduodenal infusion* of levodopa-carbidopa appears to be safe and is superior to a number of oral combination therapies in patients with response fluctuations. This approach has been used to a greater extent in Europe than the USA, but interest is growing.

Levodopa can ameliorate all the clinical features of parkinsonism, but it is particularly effective in relieving bradykinesia and any disabilities resulting from it. When it is first introduced, about one third of patients respond very well and one third less well. Most of the remainder either are unable to tolerate the medication or simply do not respond at all, especially if they do not have classic Parkinson's disease.

Adverse Effects

A. Gastrointestinal Effects

When levodopa is given without a peripheral decarboxylase inhibitor, anorexia and nausea and vomiting occur in about 80% of patients. These adverse effects can be minimized by taking the drug in divided doses, with or immediately after meals, and by increasing the total daily dose very slowly. Antacids taken 30–60 minutes before levodopa may also be beneficial. The vomiting has been attributed to stimulation of the chemoreceptor trigger zone located in the brainstem but outside the blood-brain barrier. Fortunately, tolerance to this emetic effect develops in many patients. Antiemetics such as phenothiazines should be avoided because they reduce the antiparkinsonism effects of levodopa and may exacerbate the disease.

When levodopa is given in combination with carbidopa, adverse gastrointestinal effects are much less frequent and troublesome, occurring in less than 20% of cases, so that patients can tolerate proportionately higher doses.

B. Cardiovascular Effects

A variety of cardiac arrhythmias have been described in patients receiving levodopa, including tachycardia, ventricular extrasystoles and, rarely, atrial fibrillation. This effect has been attributed to increased catecholamine formation peripherally. The incidence of such arrhythmias is low, even in the presence of established cardiac disease, and may be reduced still further if the levodopa is taken in combination with a peripheral decarboxylase inhibitor.

Postural hypotension is common, but often asymptomatic, and tends to diminish with continuing treatment. Hypertension may also occur, especially in the presence of nonselective monoamine oxidase inhibitors or sympathomimetics or when massive doses of levodopa are being taken.

C. Behavioral Effects

A wide variety of adverse mental effects have been reported, including depression, anxiety, agitation, insomnia, somnolence, confusion, delusions, hallucinations, nightmares, euphoria, and other changes in mood or personality. Such adverse effects are more common in patients taking levodopa in combination with a decarboxylase inhibitor rather than levodopa alone, presumably because higher levels are reached in the brain. They may be precipitated by intercurrent illness or operation. It may be necessary to reduce or withdraw the medication. Several atypical antipsychotic agents that have low affinity for dopamine D_2 receptors (clozapine, olanzapine, quetiapine, and risperidone; see Chapter 29) are now available and may be particularly helpful in counteracting such behavioral complications.

D. Dyskinesias and Response Fluctuations

Dyskinesias occur in up to 80% of patients receiving levodopa therapy for more than 10 years. The character of dopa dyskinesias varies between patients but tends to remain constant in individual patients. Choreoathetosis of the face and distal extremities is the most common presentation. The development of dyskinesias is dose related, but there is considerable individual variation in the dose required to produce them.

Certain fluctuations in clinical response to levodopa occur with increasing frequency as treatment continues. In some patients, these fluctuations relate to the timing of levodopa intake (**wearing-off** reactions or **end-of-dose akinesia**). In other instances, fluctuations in clinical state are unrelated to the timing of doses (**on-off phenomenon**). In the on-off phenomenon, off-periods of marked akinesia alternate over the course of a few hours with on-periods of improved mobility but often marked dyskinesia. For patients with severe off-periods who are unresponsive to other measures, subcutaneously injected apomorphine may provide temporary benefit. The phenomenon is most likely to occur in patients who responded well to treatment initially. The exact mechanism is unknown. The dyskinesias may relate to an unequal distribution of striatal dopamine. Dopaminergic denervation plus chronic pulsatile stimulation of dopamine receptors with levodopa has been associated with development of dyskinesias. A lower incidence of dyskinesias occurs when levodopa is administered continuously (eg, intraduodenally or intrajejunally), and with drug delivery systems that enable a more continuous delivery of dopaminergic medication.

E. Miscellaneous Adverse Effects

Mydriasis may occur and may precipitate an attack of acute glaucoma in some patients. Other reported but rare adverse effects include various blood dyscrasias; a positive Coombs' test with evidence of hemolysis; hot flushes; aggravation or precipitation of gout; abnormalities of smell or taste; brownish discoloration of saliva, urine, or vaginal secretions; priapism; and mild—usually transient—elevations of blood urea nitrogen and of serum transaminases, alkaline phosphatase, and bilirubin.

Drug Holidays

A drug holiday (discontinuance of the drug for 3–21 days) may temporarily improve responsiveness to levodopa and alleviate some of its adverse effects but is usually of little help in the management of the on-off phenomenon. Furthermore, a drug holiday carries the risks of aspiration pneumonia, venous thrombosis, pulmonary embolism, and depression resulting from the immobility accompanying severe parkinsonism. For these reasons and because of the temporary nature of any benefit, drug holidays are not recommended.

Drug Interactions

Pharmacologic doses of pyridoxine (vitamin B_6) enhance the extracerebral metabolism of levodopa and may therefore prevent its therapeutic effect unless a peripheral decarboxylase inhibitor is also taken. Levodopa should not be given to patients taking monoamine oxidase A inhibitors or within 2 weeks of their discontinuance because such a combination can lead to hypertensive crises.

Contraindications

Levodopa should not be given to psychotic patients because it may exacerbate the mental disturbance. It is also contraindicated in patients with angle-closure glaucoma, but those with chronic open-angle glaucoma may be given levodopa if intraocular pressure is well controlled and can be monitored. It is best given combined with carbidopa to patients with cardiac disease; even so, the risk of cardiac dysrhythmia is slight. Patients with active peptic ulcer must also be managed carefully, since gastrointestinal bleeding has occasionally occurred with levodopa. Because levodopa is a precursor of skin melanin and conceivably may activate malignant melanoma, it should be used with particular care in patients with a history of melanoma or with suspicious undiagnosed skin lesions; such patients should be monitored by a dermatologist regularly.

DOPAMINE RECEPTOR AGONISTS

Drugs acting directly on dopamine receptors may have a beneficial effect in addition to that of levodopa (Figure 28–5). Unlike levodopa, they do not require enzymatic conversion to an active metabolite, have no potentially toxic metabolites, and do not compete with other substances for active transport into the blood and across the blood-brain barrier. Moreover, drugs selectively affecting certain (but not all) dopamine receptors may have more limited adverse effects than levodopa. A number of dopamine agonists have antiparkinsonism activity. The older dopamine agonists (bromocriptine and pergolide) are ergot (ergoline) derivatives (see Chapter 16), and are rarely—if ever—used to treat parkinsonism. Their side effects are of more concern than those of the newer agents (pramipexole and ropinirole).

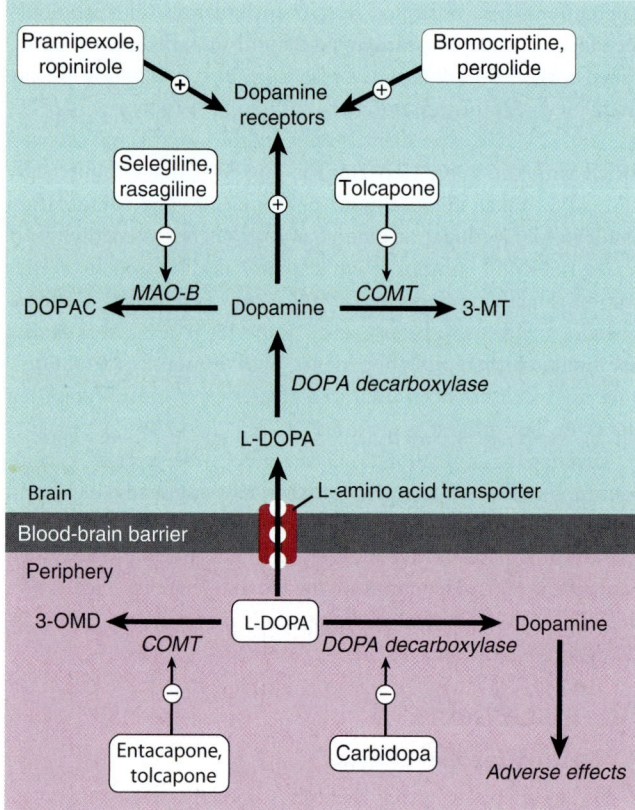

FIGURE 28–5 Pharmacologic strategies for dopaminergic therapy of Parkinson's disease. Drugs and their effects are indicated (see text). MAO, monoamine oxidase; COMT, catechol-*O*-methyltransferase; DOPAC, dihydroxyphenylacetic acid; L-DOPA, levodopa; 3-OMD, 3-*O*-methyldopa; 3-MT, 3-methoxytyramine.

There is no evidence that one agonist is superior to another; individual patients, however, may respond to one but not another of these agents. Apomorphine is a potent dopamine agonist but is discussed separately in a later section in this chapter because it is used primarily as a rescue drug for patients with disabling response fluctuations to levodopa.

Dopamine agonists have an important role as first-line therapy for Parkinson's disease, and their use is associated with a lower incidence of the response fluctuations and dyskinesias that occur with long-term levodopa therapy. In consequence, dopaminergic therapy may best be initiated with a dopamine agonist. Alternatively, a low dose of carbidopa plus levodopa (eg, Sinemet-25/100 three times daily) is introduced, and a dopamine agonist is then added. In either case, the dose of the dopamine agonist is built up gradually depending on response and tolerance. Dopamine agonists may also be given to patients with parkinsonism who are taking levodopa and who have end-of-dose akinesia or on-off phenomenon or are becoming resistant to treatment with levodopa. In such circumstances, it is generally necessary to lower the dose of levodopa to prevent intolerable adverse effects. The response to a dopamine agonist is generally disappointing in patients who have never responded to levodopa.

Bromocriptine

Bromocriptine is a D_2 agonist; its structure is shown in Table 16–6. This drug has been widely used to treat Parkinson's disease in the past but is now rarely used for this purpose, having been superseded by the newer dopamine agonists. The usual daily dose of bromocriptine for parkinsonism varies between 7.5 and 30 mg. To minimize adverse effects, the dose is built up slowly over 2 or 3 months depending on response or the development of adverse reactions.

Pergolide

Pergolide, another ergot derivative, directly stimulates both D_1 and D_2 receptors. It too has been widely used for parkinsonism but is no longer available in the United States because its use has been associated with the development of valvular heart disease.

Pramipexole

Pramipexole is not an ergot derivative, but it has preferential affinity for the D_3 family of receptors. It is effective as monotherapy for mild parkinsonism and is also helpful in patients with advanced disease, permitting the dose of levodopa to be reduced and smoothing out response fluctuations. Pramipexole may ameliorate affective symptoms. A possible neuroprotective effect has been suggested by its ability to scavenge hydrogen peroxide and enhance neurotrophic activity in mesencephalic dopaminergic cell cultures.

Pramipexole

Pramipexole is rapidly absorbed after oral administration, reaching peak plasma concentrations in approximately 2 hours, and is excreted largely unchanged in the urine. It is started at a dosage of 0.125 mg three times daily, doubled after 1 week, and again after another week. Further increments in the daily dose are by 0.75 mg at weekly intervals, depending on response and tolerance. Most patients require between 0.5 and 1.5 mg three times daily. Renal insufficiency may necessitate dosage adjustment. An extended-release preparation is now available and is taken once daily at a dose equivalent to the total daily dose of standard pramipexole. The extended-release preparation is generally more convenient for patients and avoids swings in blood levels of the drug over the day.

Ropinirole

Another nonergoline derivative, ropinirole (now available in a generic preparation) is a relatively pure D_2 receptor agonist that is effective as monotherapy in patients with mild disease and as a means of smoothing the response to levodopa in patients with more advanced disease and response fluctuations. It is introduced at 0.25 mg three times daily, and the total daily dose is then increased by 0.75 mg at weekly intervals until the fourth week and by 1.5 mg thereafter. In most instances, a dosage between 2 and 8 mg three times daily is necessary. Ropinirole is metabolized by CYP1A2; other drugs metabolized by this isoform may significantly reduce its clearance. A prolonged-release preparation taken once daily is now available.

Ropinirole

Rotigotine

The dopamine agonist rotigotine, delivered daily through a skin patch, was approved in 2007 by the Food and Drug Administration (FDA) for treatment of early Parkinson's disease. It supposedly provides more continuous dopaminergic stimulation than oral medication in early disease; its efficacy in more advanced disease is less clear. Benefits and side effects are similar to those of other dopamine agonists but reactions may also occur at the application site and are sometimes serious. The product was recalled in the United States in 2008 because of crystal formation on the patches, affecting the availability and efficacy of the agonist. It is still available in Europe.

Adverse Effects of Dopamine Agonists

A. Gastrointestinal Effects

Anorexia and nausea and vomiting may occur when a dopamine agonist is introduced and can be minimized by taking the medication with meals. Constipation, dyspepsia, and symptoms of reflux esophagitis may also occur. Bleeding from peptic ulceration has been reported.

B. Cardiovascular Effects

Postural hypotension may occur, particularly at the initiation of therapy. Painless digital vasospasm is a dose-related complication of long-term treatment with the ergot derivatives (bromocriptine or pergolide). When cardiac arrhythmias occur, they are an indication for discontinuing treatment. Peripheral edema is sometimes problematic. Cardiac valvulopathy may occur with pergolide.

C. Dyskinesias

Abnormal movements similar to those introduced by levodopa may occur and are reversed by reducing the total dose of dopaminergic drugs being taken.

D. Mental Disturbances

Confusion, hallucinations, delusions, and other psychiatric reactions are potential complications of dopaminergic treatment and are more common and severe with dopamine receptor agonists than with levodopa. Disorders of impulse control may lead to compulsive gambling, shopping, betting, sexual activity, and other behaviors (see Chapter 32). They clear on withdrawal of the offending medication.

E. Miscellaneous

Headache, nasal congestion, increased arousal, pulmonary infiltrates, pleural and retroperitoneal fibrosis, and erythromelalgia are other reported adverse effects of the ergot-derived dopamine agonists. Cardiac valvulopathies have occurred with pergolide. Erythromelalgia consists of red, tender, painful, swollen feet and, occasionally, hands, at times associated with arthralgia; symptoms and signs clear within a few days of withdrawal of the causal drug. In rare instances, an uncontrollable tendency to fall asleep at inappropriate times has occurred, particularly in patients receiving pramipexole or ropinirole; this requires discontinuation of the medication.

Contraindications

Dopamine agonists are contraindicated in patients with a history of psychotic illness or recent myocardial infarction, or with active peptic ulceration. The ergot-derived agonists are best avoided in patients with peripheral vascular disease.

MONOAMINE OXIDASE INHIBITORS

Two types of monoamine oxidase have been distinguished in the nervous system. Monoamine oxidase A metabolizes norepinephrine, serotonin, and dopamine; monoamine oxidase B metabolizes dopamine selectively. **Selegiline** (deprenyl) (Figure 28–3), a selective irreversible inhibitor of monoamine oxidase B at normal doses (at higher doses it inhibits monoamine oxidase A as well), retards the breakdown of dopamine (Figure 28–5); in consequence, it enhances and prolongs the antiparkinsonism effect of levodopa (thereby allowing the dose of levodopa to be reduced) and may reduce mild on-off or wearing-off phenomena. It is therefore used as adjunctive therapy for patients with a declining or fluctuating response to levodopa. The standard dose of selegiline is 5 mg with breakfast and 5 mg with lunch. Selegiline may cause insomnia when taken later during the day.

Selegiline has only a minor therapeutic effect on parkinsonism when given alone. Studies in animals suggest that it may reduce disease progression, but trials to test the effect of selegiline on the progression of parkinsonism in humans have yielded ambiguous results. The findings in a large multicenter study were taken to suggest a beneficial effect in slowing disease progression but may simply have reflected a symptomatic response.

Rasagiline, another monoamine oxidase B inhibitor, is more potent than selegiline in preventing MPTP-induced parkinsonism and is being used for early symptomatic treatment. The standard dosage is 1 mg/d. Rasagiline is also used as adjunctive therapy at a dosage of 0.5 or 1 mg/d to prolong the effects of levodopa-carbidopa in patients with advanced disease. A large double-blind,

placebo-controlled, delayed-start study (the ADAGIO trial) to evaluate whether it had neuroprotective benefit (ie, slowed the disease course) yielded unclear results: a daily dose of 1 mg met all the end points of the study and did seem to slow disease progression, but a 2-mg dose failed to do so. These findings are difficult to explain and the decision to use rasagiline for neuroprotective purposes therefore remains an individual one.

Neither selegiline nor rasagiline should be taken by patients receiving meperidine, tramadol, methadone, propoxyphene, cyclobenzaprine, or St. John's wort. The antitussive dextromethorphan should also be avoided by patients taking one of the monoamine oxidase B inhibitors; indeed, it is wise to advise patients to avoid all over-the-counter cold preparations. Rasagiline or selegiline should be used with care in patients receiving tricyclic antidepressants or serotonin reuptake inhibitors because of the theoretical risk of acute toxic interactions of the serotonin syndrome type (see Chapter 16), but this is rarely encountered in practice. The adverse effects of levodopa may be increased by these drugs.

The combined administration of levodopa and an inhibitor of both forms of monoamine oxidase (ie, a nonselective inhibitor) must be avoided, because it may lead to hypertensive crises, probably because of the peripheral accumulation of norepinephrine.

CATECHOL-O-METHYLTRANSFERASE INHIBITORS

Inhibition of dopa decarboxylase is associated with compensatory activation of other pathways of levodopa metabolism, especially catechol-O-methyltransferase (COMT), and this increases plasma levels of 3-O-methyldopa (3-OMD). Elevated levels of 3-OMD have been associated with a poor therapeutic response to levodopa, perhaps in part because 3-OMD competes with levodopa for an active carrier mechanism that governs its transport across the intestinal mucosa and the blood-brain barrier. Selective COMT inhibitors such as **tolcapone** and **entacapone** also prolong the action of levodopa by diminishing its peripheral metabolism (Figure 28–5). Levodopa clearance is decreased, and relative bioavailability of levodopa is thus increased. Neither the time to reach peak concentration nor the maximal concentration of levodopa is increased. These agents may be helpful in patients receiving levodopa who have developed response fluctuations—leading to a smoother response, more prolonged on-time, and the option of reducing total daily levodopa dose. Tolcapone and entacapone are both widely available, but entacapone is generally preferred because it has not been associated with hepatotoxicity.

The pharmacologic effects of tolcapone and entacapone are similar, and both are rapidly absorbed, bound to plasma proteins, and metabolized before excretion. However, tolcapone has both central and peripheral effects, whereas the effect of entacapone is peripheral. The half-life of both drugs is approximately 2 hours, but tolcapone is slightly more potent and has a longer duration of action. Tolcapone is taken in a standard dosage of 100 mg three times daily; some patients require a daily dose of twice that amount. By contrast, entacapone (200 mg) needs to be taken with each dose of levodopa, up to five times daily.

Adverse effects of the COMT inhibitors relate in part to increased levodopa exposure and include dyskinesias, nausea, and confusion. It is often necessary to lower the daily dose of levodopa by about 30% in the first 48 hours to avoid or reverse such complications. Other adverse effects include diarrhea, abdominal pain, orthostatic hypotension, sleep disturbances, and an orange discoloration of the urine. Tolcapone may cause an increase in liver enzyme levels and has been associated rarely with death from acute hepatic failure; accordingly, its use in the USA requires signed patient consent (as provided in the product labeling) plus monitoring of liver function tests every 2 weeks during the first year and less frequently thereafter. No such toxicity has been reported with entacapone.

A commercial preparation named Stalevo consists of a combination of levodopa with both carbidopa and entacapone. It is available in three strengths: Stalevo 50 (50 mg levodopa plus 12.5 mg carbidopa and 200 mg entacapone), Stalevo 100 (100 mg, 25 mg, and 200 mg, respectively), and Stalevo 150 (150 mg, 37.5 mg, and 200 mg). Use of this preparation simplifies the drug regimen and requires the consumption of a lesser number of tablets than otherwise. Stalevo is priced at or below the price of its individual components. The combination agent may provide greater symptomatic benefit than levodopa-carbidopa alone. However, despite the convenience of a single combination preparation, use of Stalevo rather than levodopa-carbidopa has been associated with earlier occurrence and increased frequency of dyskinesia. An investigation as to whether the use of Stalevo is associated with an increased risk for cardiovascular events (myocardial infarction, stroke, cardiovascular death) is ongoing.

APOMORPHINE

Subcutaneous injection of apomorphine hydrochloride (**Apokyn**), a potent dopamine agonist, is effective for the temporary relief ("rescue") of off-periods of akinesia in patients on optimized dopaminergic therapy. It is rapidly taken up in the blood and then the brain, leading to clinical benefit that begins within about 10 minutes of injection and persists for up to 2 hours. The optimal dose is identified by administering increasing test doses until adequate benefit is achieved or a maximum of 10 mg is reached. Most patients require a dose of 3–6 mg, and this should be given no more than about three times daily.

Nausea is often troublesome, especially at the initiation of apomorphine treatment; accordingly, pretreatment with the antiemetic trimethobenzamide (300 mg three times daily) for 3 days is recommended before apomorphine is introduced and is then continued for at least 1 month, if not indefinitely. Other adverse effects include dyskinesias, drowsiness, chest pain, sweating, hypotension, and bruising at the injection site. Apomorphine should be prescribed only by physicians familiar with its potential complications and interactions.

AMANTADINE

Amantadine, an antiviral agent, was by chance found to have antiparkinsonism properties. Its mode of action in parkinsonism is unclear, but it may potentiate dopaminergic function by influencing the synthesis, release, or reuptake of dopamine. It has been reported to antagonize the effects of adenosine at adenosine A_{2A} receptors, which are receptors that may inhibit D_2 receptor function. Release of catecholamines from peripheral stores has also been documented.

Pharmacokinetics

Peak plasma concentrations of amantadine are reached 1–4 hours after an oral dose. The plasma half-life is between 2 and 4 hours, most of the drug being excreted unchanged in the urine.

Clinical Use

Amantadine is less efficacious than levodopa, and its benefits may be short-lived, often disappearing after only a few weeks of treatment. Nevertheless, during that time it may favorably influence the bradykinesia, rigidity, and tremor of parkinsonism. The standard dosage is 100 mg orally two or three times daily. Amantadine may also help in reducing iatrogenic dyskinesias in patients with advanced disease.

Adverse Effects

Amantadine has a number of undesirable central nervous system effects, all of which can be reversed by stopping the drug. These include restlessness, depression, irritability, insomnia, agitation, excitement, hallucinations, and confusion. Overdosage may produce an acute toxic psychosis. With doses several times higher than recommended, convulsions have occurred.

Livedo reticularis sometimes occurs in patients taking amantadine and usually clears within 1 month after the drug is withdrawn. Other dermatologic reactions have also been described. Peripheral edema, another well-recognized complication, is not accompanied by signs of cardiac, hepatic, or renal disease and responds to diuretics. Other adverse reactions to amantadine include headache, heart failure, postural hypotension, urinary retention, and gastrointestinal disturbances (eg, anorexia, nausea, constipation, and dry mouth).

Amantadine should be used with caution in patients with a history of seizures or heart failure.

ACETYLCHOLINE-BLOCKING DRUGS

A number of centrally acting antimuscarinic preparations are available that differ in their potency and in their efficacy in different patients. Some of these drugs were discussed in Chapter 8. These agents may improve the tremor and rigidity of parkinsonism but have little effect on bradykinesia. Some of the more commonly used drugs are listed in Table 28–1.

TABLE 28–1 **Some drugs with antimuscarinic properties used in parkinsonism.**

Drug	Usual Daily Dose (mg)
Benztropine mesylate	1–6
Biperiden	2–12
Orphenadrine	150–400
Procyclidine	7.5–30
Trihexyphenidyl	6–20

Clinical Use

Treatment is started with a low dose of one of the drugs in this category, the dosage gradually being increased until benefit occurs or until adverse effects limit further increments. If patients do not respond to one drug, a trial with another member of the drug class is warranted and may be successful.

Adverse Effects

Antimuscarinic drugs have a number of undesirable central nervous system and peripheral effects (see Chapter 8) and are poorly tolerated by the elderly. Dyskinesias occur in rare cases. Acute suppurative parotitis sometimes occurs as a complication of dryness of the mouth.

If medication is to be withdrawn, this should be accomplished gradually rather than abruptly to prevent acute exacerbation of parkinsonism. For contraindications to the use of antimuscarinic drugs, see Chapter 8.

SURGICAL PROCEDURES

In patients with advanced disease that is poorly responsive to pharmacotherapy, worthwhile benefit may follow thalamotomy (for conspicuous tremor) or posteroventral pallidotomy. Ablative surgical procedures, however, have generally been replaced by functional, reversible lesions induced by high-frequency deep brain stimulation, which has a lower morbidity.

Stimulation of the subthalamic nucleus or globus pallidus by an implanted electrode and stimulator has yielded good results for the management of the clinical fluctuations occurring in advanced parkinsonism. The anatomic substrate for such therapy is indicated in Figure 28–1. Such procedures are contraindicated in patients with secondary or atypical parkinsonism, dementia, or failure to respond to dopaminergic medication.

In a controlled trial of the transplantation of dopaminergic tissue (fetal substantia nigra tissue), symptomatic benefit occurred in younger (less than 60 years old) but not older parkinsonian patients. In another trial, benefits were inconsequential. Furthermore, uncontrollable dyskinesias occurred in some patients in both studies, perhaps from a relative excess of dopamine from continued fiber outgrowth from the transplant. Additional basic studies are required before further trials of cellular therapies—in

particular, stem cell therapies—are undertaken, and such approaches therefore remain investigational.

NEUROPROTECTIVE THERAPY

Among the compounds under investigation as potential neuroprotective agents that may slow disease progression are antioxidants, antiapoptotic agents, glutamate antagonists, intraparenchymally administered glial-derived neurotrophic factor, coenzyme Q10, creatine, and anti-inflammatory drugs. The role of these agents remains to be established, however, and their use for therapeutic purposes is not indicated at this time. The possibility that rasagiline has a protective effect was discussed earlier.

GENE THERAPY

Three phase 1 (safety) trials of gene therapy for Parkinson's disease have now been completed in the USA. All trials involved infusion into the striatum of adeno-associated virus type 2 as the vector for the gene. The genes were for glutamic acid decarboxylase (GAD, to facilitate synthesis of GABA, an inhibitory neurotransmitter), infused into the subthalamic nucleus to cause inhibition; for aromatic acid decarboxylase (AADC), infused into the putamen to increase metabolism of levodopa to dopamine; and for neurturin (a growth factor that may enhance the survival of dopaminergic neurons), infused into the putamen. All agents were deemed safe and the data suggested efficacy. A phase 2 study of the GAD gene has been completed and the results are encouraging. A similar study of AADC is planned but has not yet started. A phase 2 study of neurturin failed to show significant benefit, but a new phase 2 study has been initiated in which neurturin is infused into the substantia nigra as well as the putamen.

THERAPY FOR NONMOTOR MANIFESTATIONS

Persons with cognitive decline may respond to rivastigmine (1.5–6 mg twice daily), memantine (5–10 mg daily), or donepezil (5–10 mg daily) (see Chapter 60); affective disorders to antidepressants or anxiolytic agents (see Chapter 30); excessive daytime sleepiness to modafinil (100–400 mg in the morning) (see Chapter 9); and bladder and bowel disorders to appropriate symptomatic therapy (see Chapter 8).

GENERAL COMMENTS ON DRUG MANAGEMENT OF PATIENTS WITH PARKINSONISM

Parkinson's disease generally follows a progressive course. Moreover, the benefits of levodopa therapy often diminish with time, and serious adverse effects may complicate long-term levodopa treatment. Nevertheless, dopaminergic therapy at a relatively early stage may be most effective in alleviating symptoms of parkinsonism and may also favorably affect the mortality rate due to the disease. Therefore, several strategies have evolved for optimizing dopaminergic therapy, as summarized in Figure 28–5. Symptomatic treatment of mild parkinsonism is probably best avoided until there is some degree of disability or until symptoms begin to have a significant impact on the patient's lifestyle. When symptomatic treatment becomes necessary, a trial of rasagiline, amantadine, or an antimuscarinic drug (in young patients) may be worthwhile. With disease progression, dopaminergic therapy becomes necessary. This can conveniently be initiated with a dopamine agonist, either alone or in combination with low-dose carbidopa-levodopa therapy. Alternatively, especially in older patients, a dopamine agonist can be omitted and the patient started immediately on carbidopa-levodopa. Physical therapy is helpful in improving mobility. In patients with severe parkinsonism and long-term complications of levodopa therapy such as the on-off phenomenon, a trial of treatment with a COMT inhibitor or rasagiline may be helpful. Regulation of dietary protein intake may also improve response fluctuations. Deep brain stimulation is often helpful in patients who fail to respond adequately to these measures. Treating patients who are young or have mild parkinsonism with rasagiline may delay disease progression and merits consideration.

DRUG-INDUCED PARKINSONISM

Reserpine and the related drug tetrabenazine deplete biogenic monoamines from their storage sites, whereas haloperidol, metoclopramide, and the phenothiazines block dopamine receptors. These drugs may therefore produce a parkinsonian syndrome, usually within 3 months after introduction. The disorder tends to be symmetric, with inconspicuous tremor, but this is not always the case. The syndrome is related to high dosage and clears over several weeks or months after withdrawal. If treatment is necessary, antimuscarinic agents are preferred. Levodopa is of no help if neuroleptic drugs are continued and may in fact aggravate the mental disorder for which antipsychotic drugs were prescribed originally.

In 1983, a drug-induced form of parkinsonism was discovered in individuals who attempted to synthesize and use a narcotic drug related to meperidine but actually synthesized and self-administered MPTP, as discussed in the Box: MPTP & Parkinsonism.

OTHER MOVEMENT DISORDERS

Tremor

Tremor consists of rhythmic oscillatory movements. Physiologic postural tremor, which is a normal phenomenon, is enhanced in amplitude by anxiety, fatigue, thyrotoxicosis, and intravenous epinephrine or isoproterenol. **Propranolol** reduces its amplitude and, if administered intra-arterially, prevents the response to isoproterenol in the perfused limb, presumably through some peripheral action. Certain drugs—especially the bronchodilators, valproate, tricyclic antidepressants, and lithium—may produce a dose-dependent exaggeration of the normal physiologic tremor that is reversed by discontinuing the drug. Although the tremor produced by sympathomimetics such as terbutaline (a bronchodilator) is blocked by propranolol, which antagonizes both β_1 and β_2 receptors, it is not blocked by metoprolol, a β_1-selective antagonist; this suggests that such tremor is mediated mainly by the β_2 receptors.

Essential tremor is a postural tremor, sometimes familial with autosomal dominant inheritance, which is clinically similar to physiologic tremor. At least three gene loci (*ETM1* on 3q13, *ETM2* on 2p24.1, and a locus on 6p23) have been described. Dysfunction of β_1 receptors has been implicated in some instances, since the tremor may respond dramatically to standard doses of metoprolol as well as to propranolol. The most useful approach is with propranolol, but whether the response depends on a central or

MPTP & Parkinsonism

Reports in the early 1980s of a rapidly progressive form of parkinsonism in young persons opened a new area of research in the etiology and treatment of parkinsonism. The initial report described apparently healthy young people who attempted to support their opioid habit with a meperidine analog synthesized by an amateur chemist. They unwittingly self-administered 1-methyl-4-phenyl-1,2,3,6-tetrahydropyridine (MPTP) and subsequently developed a very severe form of parkinsonism.

MPTP is a protoxin that is converted by monoamine oxidase B to *N*-methyl-4-phenylpyridinium (MPP+). MPP+ is selectively taken up by cells in the substantia nigra through an active mechanism normally responsible for dopamine reuptake. MPP+ inhibits mitochondrial complex I, thereby inhibiting oxidative phosphorylation. The interaction of MPP+ with complex I probably leads to cell death and thus to striatal dopamine depletion and parkinsonism.

Recognition of the effects of MPTP suggested that spontaneously occurring Parkinson's disease may result from exposure to an environmental toxin that is similarly selective in its target. However, no such toxin has yet been identified. It also suggested a successful means of producing an experimental model of Parkinson's disease in animals, especially nonhuman primates. This model is assisting in the development of new antiparkinsonism drugs. Pretreatment of exposed animals with a monoamine oxidase B inhibitor such as selegiline prevents the conversion of MPTP to MPP+ and thus protects against the occurrence of parkinsonism. This observation has provided one reason to believe that selegiline or rasagiline may retard the progression of Parkinson's disease in humans.

peripheral action is unclear. The pharmacokinetics, pharmacologic effects, and adverse reactions of propranolol are discussed in Chapter 10. Daily doses of propranolol on the order of 120 mg (range, 60–240 mg) are usually required, prescribed as 40–120 mg orally twice daily, and reported adverse effects have been few. Propranolol should be used with caution in patients with heart failure, heart block, asthma, and hypoglycemia. Patients can be instructed to take their own pulse and call the physician if significant bradycardia develops. Metoprolol is sometimes useful in treating tremor when patients have concomitant pulmonary disease that contraindicates use of propranolol. **Primidone** (an antiepileptic drug; see Chapter 24), in gradually increasing doses up to 250 mg three times daily, is also effective in providing symptomatic control in some cases. Patients with tremor are very sensitive to primidone and often cannot tolerate the doses used to treat seizures; they should be started on 50 mg once daily and the daily dose increased by 50 mg every 2 weeks depending on response.

Topiramate, another antiepileptic drug, may also be helpful in a dose of 400 mg daily, built up gradually. **Alprazolam** (in doses up to 3 mg daily) or **gabapentin** (100–2400 mg/d) is helpful in some patients. Others are helped by intramuscular injections of botulinum toxin. Thalamic stimulation by an implanted electrode and stimulator is often worthwhile in advanced cases refractory to pharmacotherapy. Diazepam, chlordiazepoxide, mephenesin, and antiparkinsonism agents have been advocated in the past but are generally worthless. Anecdotal reports of benefit from mirtazapine were not confirmed in a double-blind study, which found no effect on the tremor in most patients. Small quantities of alcohol may suppress essential tremor for a short time but should not be recommended as a treatment strategy because of possible behavioral and other complications of alcohol.

Intention tremor is present during movement but not at rest; sometimes it occurs as a toxic manifestation of alcohol or drugs such as phenytoin. Withdrawal or reduction in dosage provides dramatic relief. There is no satisfactory pharmacologic treatment for intention tremor due to other neurologic disorders.

Rest tremor is usually due to parkinsonism.

Huntington's Disease

Huntington's disease is an autosomal dominant inherited disorder caused by an abnormality (expansion of a CAG trinucleotide repeat that codes for a polyglutamine tract) of the *huntingtin* gene on chromosome 4. An autosomal recessive form may also occur. Huntington disease–like (HDL) disorders are not associated with an abnormal CAG trinucleotide repeat number of the *huntingtin* gene. Autosomal dominant (*HDL1*, 20pter-p12; *HDL2*, 16q24.3) and recessive forms (*HDL3*, 4p15.3) occur.

Huntington's disease is characterized by progressive chorea and dementia that usually begin in adulthood. The development of chorea seems to be related to an imbalance of dopamine, acetylcholine, GABA, and perhaps other neurotransmitters in the basal ganglia (Figure 28–6). Pharmacologic studies indicate that chorea results from functional overactivity in dopaminergic nigrostriatal pathways, perhaps because of increased responsiveness of postsynaptic dopamine receptors or deficiency of a neurotransmitter

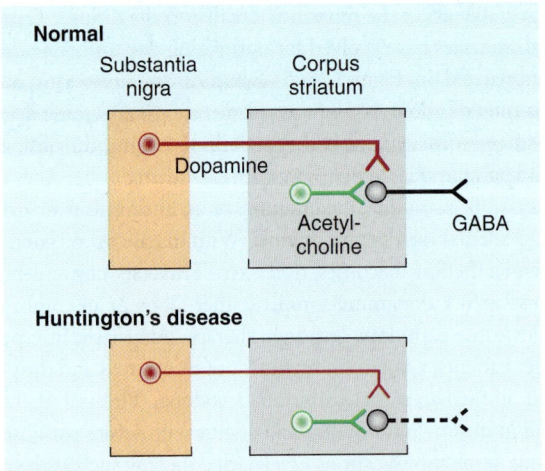

FIGURE 28–6 Schematic representation of the sequence of neurons involved in Huntington's chorea. **Top:** Dopaminergic neurons (red) originating in the substantia nigra normally inhibit the GABAergic output from the striatum, whereas cholinergic neurons (green) exert an excitatory effect. **Bottom:** In Huntington's chorea, some cholinergic neurons may be lost, but even more GABAergic neurons (black) degenerate.

that normally antagonizes dopamine. Drugs that impair dopaminergic neurotransmission, either by depleting central monoamines (eg, reserpine, tetrabenazine) or by blocking dopamine receptors (eg, phenothiazines, butyrophenones), often alleviate chorea, whereas dopamine-like drugs such as levodopa tend to exacerbate it.

Both GABA and the enzyme (glutamic acid decarboxylase) concerned with its synthesis are markedly reduced in the basal ganglia of patients with Huntington's disease, and GABA receptors are usually implicated in inhibitory pathways. There is also a significant decline in concentration of choline acetyltransferase, the enzyme responsible for synthesizing acetylcholine, in the basal ganglia of these patients. These findings may be of pathophysiologic significance and have led to attempts to alleviate chorea by enhancing central GABA or acetylcholine activity, but with disappointing results. As a consequence, the most commonly used drugs for controlling dyskinesia in patients with Huntington's disease are still those that interfere with dopamine activity. With all the latter drugs, however, reduction of abnormal movements may be associated with iatrogenic parkinsonism.

Reserpine depletes cerebral dopamine by preventing intraneuronal storage (see Chapter 6); it is introduced in low doses (eg, 0.25 mg daily), and the daily dose is then built up gradually (eg, by 0.25 mg every week) until benefit occurs or adverse effects become troublesome. A daily dose of 2–5 mg is often effective in suppressing abnormal movements, but adverse effects may include hypotension, depression, sedation, diarrhea, and nasal congestion. **Tetrabenazine** (12.5–50 mg orally three times daily) resembles reserpine in depleting cerebral dopamine and has less troublesome adverse effects. Treatment with postsynaptic dopamine receptor blockers such as phenothiazines and butyrophenones may also be helpful. **Haloperidol** is started in a small dose, eg, 1 mg twice daily, and increased every 4 days depending on the response. If haloperidol is not helpful, treatment with increasing doses of **perphenazine** up to a total of about 20 mg daily sometimes helps. Several recent reports suggest that **olanzapine** may also be useful; the dose varies with the patient, but 10 mg daily is often sufficient, although doses as high as 30 mg daily are sometimes required. The pharmacokinetics and clinical properties of these drugs are considered in greater detail elsewhere in this book. Selective serotonin reuptake inhibitors may reduce depression, aggression, and agitation.

Other Forms of Chorea

Benign hereditary chorea is inherited (usually autosomal dominant; possibly also autosomal recessive) or arises spontaneously. Chorea develops in early childhood and does not progress during adult life; dementia does not occur. In patients with *TITF-1* gene mutations, thyroid and pulmonary abnormalities may also be present (brain-thyroid-lung syndrome). Familial chorea may also occur as part of the chorea-acanthocytosis syndrome, together with orolingual tics, vocalizations, cognitive changes, seizures, peripheral neuropathy, and muscle atrophy; serum β-lipoproteins are normal. Mutations of the gene encoding chorein at 9q21 may be causal. Treatment of these hereditary disorders is symptomatic.

Treatment is directed at the underlying cause when chorea occurs as a complication of general medical disorders such as thyrotoxicosis, polycythemia vera rubra, systemic lupus erythematosus, hypocalcemia, and hepatic cirrhosis. Drug-induced chorea is managed by withdrawal of the offending substance, which may be levodopa, an antimuscarinic drug, amphetamine, lithium, phenytoin, or an oral contraceptive. Neuroleptic drugs may also produce an acute or tardive dyskinesia (discussed below). Sydenham's chorea is temporary and usually so mild that pharmacologic management of the dyskinesia is unnecessary, but dopamine-blocking drugs are effective in suppressing it.

Ballismus

The biochemical basis of ballismus is unknown, but the pharmacologic approach to management is the same as for chorea. Treatment with haloperidol, perphenazine, or other dopamine-blocking drugs may be helpful.

Athetosis & Dystonia

The pharmacologic basis of these disorders is unknown, and there is no satisfactory medical treatment for them. A subset of patients respond well to levodopa medication (dopa-responsive dystonia), which is therefore worthy of trial. Occasional patients with dystonia may respond to diazepam, amantadine, antimuscarinic drugs (in high dosage), carbamazepine, baclofen, haloperidol, or phenothiazines. A trial of these pharmacologic approaches is worthwhile, though often not successful. Patients with focal dystonias such as blepharospasm or torticollis often benefit from injection of botulinum toxin into the overactive muscles. Deep brain stimulation may be helpful in medically intractable cases.

Tics

The pathophysiologic basis of tics is unknown. Chronic multiple tics (**Gilles de la Tourette's syndrome**) may require symptomatic treatment if the disorder is severe or is having a significant impact on the patient's life. Education of patients, family, and teachers is important.

A common pharmacologic approach is with **haloperidol**. Patients are better able to tolerate this drug if treatment is started with a small dosage (eg, 0.25 or 0.5 mg daily) and then increased gradually (eg, by 0.25 mg every 4 or 5 days) over the following weeks depending on response and tolerance. Most patients ultimately require a total daily dose of 3–8 mg. Adverse effects include extrapyramidal movement disorders, sedation, dryness of the mouth, blurred vision, and gastrointestinal disturbances. **Pimozide**, another dopamine receptor antagonist, may be helpful in patients as a first-line treatment or in those who are either unresponsive to or intolerant of haloperidol. Treatment is started at 1 mg/d, and the dosage is increased by 1 mg every 5 days; most patients require 7–16 mg/d. It has similar side effects to haloperidol but may cause irregularities of cardiac rhythm.

Although not approved by the FDA for the treatment of tics or Tourette's syndrome, certain α-adrenergic agonists may be preferred as an initial treatment because they are less likely to cause extrapyramidal side effects than neuroleptics agents. **Clonidine** reduces motor or vocal tics in about 50% of children so treated. It may act by reducing activity in noradrenergic neurons in the locus caeruleus. It is introduced at a dose of 2–3 mcg/kg/d, increasing after 2 weeks to 4 mcg/kg/d and then, if required, to 5 mcg/kg/d. It may cause an initial transient fall in blood pressure. The most common adverse effect is sedation; other adverse effects include reduced or excessive salivation and diarrhea. **Guanfacine,** another α-adrenergic agonist, has also been used.

Phenothiazines such as fluphenazine sometimes help the tics, as do dopamine agonists. Atypical antipsychotics, such as risperidone and aripiprazole, have a more favorable side-effect profile and may be especially worthwhile in patients with significant behavioral problems. Clonazepam and carbamazepine have also been used. The pharmacologic properties of these drugs are discussed elsewhere in this book.

Injection of botulinum toxin A at the site of problematic tics is sometimes helpful. Treatment of any associated attention deficit disorder (eg, with clonidine patch, guanfacine, pemoline, methylphenidate, or dextroamphetamine) or obsessive-compulsive disorder (selective serotonin reuptake inhibitors or clomipramine) may be required. Deep brain stimulation is sometimes worthwhile in otherwise intractable cases but is best regarded as an investigational approach at this time.

Drug-Induced Dyskinesias

Levodopa or dopamine agonists produce diverse dyskinesias as a dose-related phenomenon in patients with Parkinson's disease; dose reduction reverses them. Chorea may also develop in patients receiving phenytoin, carbamazepine, amphetamines, lithium, and oral contraceptives, and it resolves with discontinuance of the offending medication. Dystonia has resulted from administration of dopaminergic agents, lithium, serotonin reuptake inhibitors, carbamazepine, and metoclopramide; and postural tremor from theophylline, caffeine, lithium, valproic acid, thyroid hormone, tricyclic antidepressants, and isoproterenol.

The pharmacologic basis of the acute dyskinesia or dystonia sometimes precipitated by the first few doses of a phenothiazine is not clear. In most instances, parenteral administration of an antimuscarinic drug such as benztropine (2 mg intravenously), diphenhydramine (50 mg intravenously), or biperiden (2–5 mg intravenously or intramuscularly) is helpful, whereas in other instances diazepam (10 mg intravenously) alleviates the abnormal movements.

Tardive dyskinesia, a disorder characterized by a variety of abnormal movements, is a common complication of long-term neuroleptic or metoclopramide drug treatment (see Chapter 29). Its precise pharmacologic basis is unclear. A reduction in dose of the offending medication, a dopamine receptor blocker, commonly worsens the dyskinesia, whereas an increase in dose may suppress it. The drugs most likely to provide immediate symptomatic benefit are those interfering with dopaminergic function, either by depletion (eg, reserpine, tetrabenazine) or receptor blockade (eg, phenothiazines, butyrophenones). Paradoxically, the receptor-blocking drugs are the very ones that also cause the dyskinesia.

Tardive dystonia is usually segmental or focal; generalized dystonia is less common and occurs in younger patients. Treatment is the same as for tardive dyskinesia, but anticholinergic drugs may also be helpful; focal dystonias may also respond to local injection of botulinum A toxin. **Tardive akathisia** is treated similarly to drug-induced parkinsonism. **Rabbit syndrome**, another neuroleptic-induced disorder, is manifested by rhythmic vertical movements about the mouth; it may respond to anticholinergic drugs.

Because the tardive syndromes that develop in adults are often irreversible and have no satisfactory treatment, care must be taken to reduce the likelihood of their occurrence. Antipsychotic medication should be prescribed only when necessary and should be withheld periodically to assess the need for continued treatment and to unmask incipient dyskinesia. Thioridazine, a phenothiazine with a piperidine side chain, is an effective antipsychotic agent that seems less likely than most to cause extrapyramidal reactions, perhaps because it has little effect on dopamine receptors in the striatal system. Finally, antimuscarinic drugs should not be prescribed routinely in patients receiving neuroleptics, because the combination may increase the likelihood of dyskinesia.

Neuroleptic malignant syndrome, a rare complication of treatment with neuroleptics, is characterized by rigidity, fever, changes in mental status, and autonomic dysfunction (see Table 16–4). Symptoms typically develop over 1–3 days (rather than minutes to hours as in malignant hyperthermia) and may occur at any time during treatment. Treatment includes withdrawal of antipsychotic drugs, lithium, and anticholinergics; reduction of body temperature; and rehydration. Dantrolene, dopamine agonists, levodopa, or amantadine may be helpful, but there is a high mortality rate (up to 20%) with neuroleptic malignant syndrome.

Restless Legs Syndrome

Restless legs syndrome is characterized by an unpleasant creeping discomfort that seems to arise deep within the legs and occasionally the arms. Symptoms occur particularly when patients are relaxed, especially when they are lying down or sitting, and they lead to an urge to move about. Such symptoms may delay the onset of sleep. A sleep disorder associated with periodic movements during sleep may also occur. The cause is unknown, but the disorder is especially common among pregnant women and also among uremic or diabetic patients with neuropathy. In most patients, no obvious predisposing cause is found, but several genetic loci have been associated with it (12q12-q21, 14q13-q31, 9p24-p22, 2q33, and 20p13).

Symptoms may resolve with correction of coexisting iron-deficiency anemia and often respond to dopamine agonists, levodopa, diazepam, clonazepam, gabapentin, or opiates. Dopaminergic therapy is the preferred treatment for restless legs syndrome and should be initiated with long-acting dopamine agonists (eg, **pramipexole** 0.125–0.75 mg or **ropinirole** 0.25–4.0 mg once daily) to avoid the augmentation that may be associated with levodopa-carbidopa (100/25 or 200/50 taken about 1 hour before bedtime). Augmentation refers to the earlier onset or enhancement of symptoms; earlier onset of symptoms at rest; and a briefer response to medication. When augmentation occurs with levodopa, the daily dose should be reduced or a dopamine agonist substituted. If it occurs in patients receiving an agonist, the daily dose should be lowered or divided, or opioids substituted. When opiates are required, those with long half-lives or low addictive potential should be used. Oxycodone is often effective; the dose is individualized. Gabapentin is an alternative to opioids and is taken once or twice daily (in the evening and before sleep); the starting dose is 300 mg daily, building up depending on response and tolerance (to approximately 1800 mg daily). A recent study suggests that pregabalin, a related drug, is also effective at a daily total dosage of 150–300 mg, taken in divided doses.

Wilson's Disease

A recessively inherited (13q14.3–q21.1) disorder of copper metabolism, Wilson's disease is characterized biochemically by reduced serum copper and ceruloplasmin concentrations, pathologically by markedly increased concentration of copper in the brain and viscera, and clinically by signs of hepatic and neurologic dysfunction. Neurologic signs include tremor, choreiform movements, rigidity, hypokinesia, and dysarthria and dysphagia. Siblings of affected patients should be screened for asymptomatic Wilson's disease.

Treatment involves the removal of excess copper, followed by maintenance of copper balance. Dietary copper should also be kept below 2 mg daily. **Penicillamine** (dimethylcysteine) has been used for many years as the primary agent to remove copper. It is a chelating agent that forms a ring complex with copper. It is readily absorbed from the gastrointestinal tract and rapidly excreted in the urine. A common starting dose in adults is 500 mg three or four times daily. After remission occurs, it may be possible to lower the maintenance dose, generally to not less than 1 g daily, which must thereafter be continued indefinitely. Adverse effects include nausea and vomiting, nephrotic syndrome, a lupus-like syndrome, pemphigus, myasthenia, arthropathy, optic neuropathy, and various blood dyscrasias. In about 10% of instances, neurologic worsening occurs with penicillamine. Treatment should be monitored by frequent urinalysis and complete blood counts.

Trientine hydrochloride, another chelating agent, is preferred by many over penicillamine because of the lesser likelihood of drug reactions or neurologic worsening. It may be used in a daily dose of 1–1.5 g. Trientine appears to have few adverse effects other than mild anemia due to iron deficiency in a few patients. **Tetrathiomolybdate** may be better than trientine for preserving neurologic function in

patients with neurologic involvement and is taken both with and between meals. It is not yet commercially available.

Zinc acetate administered orally increases the fecal excretion of copper and can be used in combination with these other agents. The dose is 50 mg three times a day. Zinc sulfate (200 mg/d orally) has also been used to decrease copper absorption. Zinc blocks copper absorption from the gastrointestinal tract by induction of intestinal cell metallothionein. Its main advantage is its low toxicity compared with that of other anticopper agents, although it may cause gastric irritation when introduced.

Liver transplantation is sometimes necessary. The role of hepatocyte transplantation and gene therapy is currently under investigation.

SUMMARY Drugs Used for Movement Disorders

Subclass	Mechanism of Action	Effects	Clinical Applications	Pharmacokinetics, Toxicities, Interactions
LEVODOPA AND COMBINATIONS				
• Levodopa	Transported into the central nervous system (CNS) and converted to dopamine (which does not enter the CNS); also converted to dopamine in the periphery	Ameliorates all symptoms of Parkinson's disease and causes significant peripheral dopaminergic effects (see text)	Parkinson's disease: Most efficacious therapy but not always used as the first drug due to development of disabling response fluctuations over time	Oral • ~ 6–8 h effect • *Toxicity:* Gastrointestinal upset, arrhythmias, dyskinesias, on-off and wearing-off phenomena, behavioral disturbances • *Interactions:* Use with carbidopa greatly diminishes required dosage • use with COMT or MAO-B inhibitors prolongs duration of effect
• Levodopa + carbidopa (Sinemet, others): Carbidopa inhibits peripheral metabolism of levodopa to dopamine and reduces required dosage and toxicity; carbidopa does not enter CNS				
• Levodopa + carbidopa + entacapone (Stalevo): Entacapone is a catechol-O-methyltransferase (COMT) inhibitor (see below)				
DOPAMINE AGONISTS				
• Pramipexole	Direct agonist at D_3 receptors, nonergot	Reduces symptoms of parkinsonism • smooths out fluctuations in levodopa response	Parkinson's disease: Can be used as initial therapy • also effective in on-off phenomenon	Oral • ~ 8 h effect • *Toxicity:* Nausea and vomiting, postural hypotension, dyskinesias, confusion, impulse control disorders, sleepiness
• Ropinirole: Similar to pramipexole; nonergot; relatively pure D_2 agonist				
• Bromocriptine: Ergot derivative; potent agonist at D_2 receptors; more toxic than pramipexole or ropinirole; now rarely used for antiparkinsonian effect				
• Apomorphine: Nonergot; subcutaneous route useful for rescue treatment in levodopa-induced dyskinesia; high incidence of nausea and vomiting				
MONOAMINE OXIDASE (MAO) INHIBITORS				
• Rasagiline	Inhibits MAO-B selectively; higher doses also inhibit MAO-A	Increases dopamine stores in neurons; may have neuroprotective effects	Parkinson's disease: Adjunctive to levodopa • smooths levodopa response	Oral • *Toxicity & interactions:* May cause serotonin syndrome with meperidine, and theoretically also with selective serotonin reuptake inhibitors, tricyclic antidepressants
• Selegiline: Like rasagiline, adjunctive use with levodopa; may be less potent than rasagiline				
COMT INHIBITORS				
• Entacapone	Inhibits COMT in periphery • does not enter CNS	Reduces metabolism of levodopa and prolongs its action	Parkinson's disease	Oral • *Toxicity:* Increased levodopa toxicity • nausea, dyskinesias, confusion
• Tolcapone: Like entacapone but enters CNS; some evidence of hepatotoxicity, elevation of liver enzymes				

(continued)

Subclass	Mechanism of Action	Effects	Clinical Applications	Pharmacokinetics, Toxicities, Interactions
ANTIMUSCARINIC AGENTS				
• Benztropine	Antagonist at M receptors in basal ganglia	Reduces tremor and rigidity • little effect on bradykinesia	Parkinson's disease	Oral • *Toxicity:* Typical antimuscarinic effects— sedation, mydriasis, urinary retention, constipation, confusion, dry mouth
• *Biperiden, orphenadrine, procyclidine, trihexyphenidyl: Similar antimuscarinic agents with CNS effects*				
DRUGS USED IN HUNTINGTON'S DISEASE				
• Tetrabenazine, reserpine	Deplete amine transmitters, especially dopamine, from nerve endings	Reduce chorea severity	Huntington's disease • other applications, see Chapter 11	Oral • *Toxicity:* Hypotension, sedation, depression, diarrhea • tetrabenazine somewhat less toxic
• *Haloperidol, other neuroleptics: Sometimes helpful*				
DRUGS USED IN TOURETTE'S SYNDROME				
• Haloperidol, pimozide	Block central D_2 receptors	Reduce vocal and motor tic frequency, severity	Tourette's syndrome • other applications, see Chapter 29	Oral • *Toxicity:* Parkinsonism, other dyskinesias • sedation • blurred vision • dry mouth • gastrointestinal disturbances • pimozide may cause cardiac rhythm disturbances
• *Clonidine: Effective in ~ 50% of patients; see Chapter 11 for basic pharmacology*				
• *Phenothiazines, benzodiazepines, carbamazepine: Sometimes of value*				

PREPARATIONS AVAILABLE

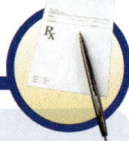

Amantadine (Symmetrel, others)
Oral: 100 mg capsules; 10 mg/mL syrup

Apomorphine (Apokyn)
Subcutaneous injection titration kit: 10 mg/mL

Benztropine (Cogentin, others)
Oral: 0.5, 1, 2 mg tablets
Parenteral: 1 mg/mL for injection

Biperiden (Akineton)
Oral: 2 mg tablets
Parenteral: 5 mg/mL for injection

Bromocriptine (Parlodel)
Oral: 2.5 mg tablets; 5 mg capsules

Carbidopa (Lodosyn)
Oral: 25 mg tablets

Carbidopa/levodopa (Sinemet, others)
Oral: 10 mg carbidopa and 100 mg levodopa, 25 mg carbidopa and 100 mg levodopa, 25 mg carbidopa and 250 mg levodopa tablets
Oral extended-release (Sinemet CR, others): 25 mg carbidopa and 100 mg levodopa; 50 mg carbidopa and 200 mg levodopa

Carbidopa/levodopa/entacapone (Stalevo)
Oral: 12.5 mg carbidopa, 50 mg levodopa, 200 mg entacapone; 18.75 mg carbidopa, 75 mg levodopa, 200 mg entacapone; 25 mg carbidopa, 100 mg levodopa, 200 mg entacapone; 31.25 mg carbidopa, 125 mg levodopa, 200 mg entacapone; 37.5 mg carbidopa, 150 mg levodopa, 200 mg entacapone; 50 mg carbidopa, 200 mg levodopa, 200 mg entacapone

Entacapone (Comtan)
Oral: 200 mg tablets

Levodopa (Dopar, others)
Oral: 100, 250, 500 mg tablets, capsules

Orphenadrine (various)
Oral: 100 mg tablets
Oral sustained-release: 100 mg tablets
Parenteral: 30 mg/mL for injection

Penicillamine (Cuprimine, Depen)
Oral: 125, 250 mg capsules; 250 mg tablets

Pergolide (Permax, other)[1]
Oral: 0.05, 0.25, 1 mg tablets

Pramipexole (Mirapex)
Oral: 0.125, 0.25, 0.75, 1, 1.5 mg tablets; 0.375, 0.75, 1.5, 3.0, 4.5 mg extended-release tablets

Procyclidine (Kemadrin)
Oral: 5 mg tablets

Rasagiline (Azilect)
Oral: 0.5, 1 mg tablets

Ropinirole (Requip, Requip XL)
Oral: 0.25, 0.5, 1, 2, 3, 4, 5 mg tablets; 2, 4, 6, 8, 12 mg extended-release tablets

Selegiline (deprenyl) (generic, Eldepryl)
Oral: 5 mg tablets, capsules; 6, 9, 12 mg transdermal patch

Tetrabenazine (Xenazine)
Oral: 12.5, 25 mg tablets

Tolcapone (Tasmar)
Oral: 100, 200 mg tablets

Trientine (Syprine)
Oral: 250 mg capsules

Trihexyphenidyl (Artane, others)
Oral: 2, 5 mg tablets; 2 mg/5 mL elixir
Oral sustained-release (Artane Sequels): 5 mg capsules

[1] Not available in the USA.

REFERENCES

Allain H et al: Disease-modifying drugs and Parkinson's disease. Prog Neurobiol 2008;84:25.

Aminoff MJ: Treatment should not be initiated too soon in Parkinson's disease. Ann Neurol 2006;59:562.

Angot E et al: Are synucleinopathies prion-like disorders? Lancet Neurol 2010;9:1128.

Antonini A et al: Role of pramipexole in the management of Parkinson's disease. CNS Drugs 2010;24:829.

Baldwin CM, Keating GM: Rotigotine transdermal patch: A review of its use in the management of Parkinson's disease. CNS Drugs 2007;21:1039.

Bestha DP et al: Management of tics and Tourette's disorder: An update. Expert Opin Pharmacother 2010;11:1813.

Bhidayasiri R, Tarsy D: Treatment of dystonia. Expert Rev Neurother 2006;6:863.

Brewer GJ: The use of copper-lowering therapy with tetrathiomolybdate in medicine. Expert Opin Investig Drugs 2009;18:89.

Bronstein JM et al: Deep brain stimulation for Parkinson disease: An expert consensus and review of key issues. Arch Neurol 2010;68:165.

Christine CW et al: Safety and tolerability of putaminal AADC gene therapy for Parkinson disease. Neurology 2009;73:1662.

Cummings J, Winblad B: A rivastigmine patch for the treatment of Alzheimer's disease and Parkinson's disease dementia. Expert Rev Neurother 2007;7:1457.

Deng H et al: Genetics of essential tremor. Brain 2007;130:1456.

Earley CJ et al: Restless legs syndrome and periodic leg movements in sleep. Handb Clin Neurol 2011;99:913.

Follett KA et al: Pallidal versus subthalamic deep-brain stimulation for Parkinson's disease. N Engl J Med 2010;362:2077.

Frank S: Tetrabenazine as anti-chorea therapy in Huntington disease: An open-label continuation study. Huntington Study Group/TETRA-HD Investigators. BMC Neurol 2009;9:62.

Frank S, Jankovic J: Advances in the pharmacological management of Huntington's disease. Drugs 2010;70:561.

Garcia-Borreguero D et al: Augmentation as a treatment complication of restless legs syndrome: Concept and management. Mov Disord 2007;22 (Suppl 18):S476.

Garcia-Borreguero D et al: Treatment of restless legs syndrome with pregabalin: A double-blind, placebo-controlled study. Neurology 2010;74:1897.

Gasser T: Update on the genetics of Parkinson's disease. Mov Disord 2007;22 (Suppl 17):S343.

Haq IU et al: Apomorphine therapy in Parkinson's disease: A review. Expert Opin Pharmacother 2007;8:2799.

Hauser RA et al: Double-blind trial of levodopa/carbidopa/entacapone versus levodopa/carbidopa in early Parkinson's disease. Mov Disord 2009;24:541.

Huster D: Wilson disease. Best Pract Res Clin Gastroenterol 2010;24:531.

Jankovic J: Treatment of dystonia. Lancet Neurol 2006;5:864.

Jankovic J, Stacy M: Medical management of levodopa-associated motor complications in patients with Parkinson's disease. CNS Drugs 2007;21:677.

Kenney C et al: Long-term tolerability of tetrabenazine in the treatment of hyperkinetic movement disorders. Mov Disord 2007;22:193.

Kimber TE: An update on Tourette syndrome. Curr Neurol Neurosci Rep 2010;10:286.

Kordower JH et al: Transplanted dopaminergic neurons develop PD pathologic changes: A second case report. Mov Disord 2008;23:2303.

Lavenstein BL: Treatment approaches for children with Tourette's syndrome. Curr Neurol Neurosci Rep 2003;3:143.

LeWitt PA et al: AAV2-GAD gene therapy for advanced Parkinson's disease: a double-blind, sham-surgery controlled, randomised trial. Lancet Neurol 2011;10:309.

Lorenz D, Deuschl G: Update on pathogenesis and treatment of essential tremor. Curr Opin Neurol 2007;20:447.

Lorincz MT: Neurologic Wilson's disease. Ann N Y Acad Sci 2010;1184:173.

Maciunas RJ et al: Prospective randomized double-blind trial of bilateral thalamic deep brain stimulation in adults with Tourette syndrome. J Neurosurg 2007;107:1004.

Mak CM, Lam CW: Diagnosis of Wilson's disease: A comprehensive review. Crit Rev Clin Lab Sci 2008;45:263.

Marks WJ Jr et al: Gene delivery of AAV2-neurturin for Parkinson's disease: A double-blind, randomised, controlled trial. Lancet Neurol 2010;9:1164.

Mink JW et al: Patient selection and assessment recommendations for deep brain stimulation in Tourette syndrome. Mov Disord 2006;21:1831.

Nakamura K, Aminoff MJ. Huntington's disease: Clinical characteristics, pathogenesis and therapies. Drugs Today (Barc) 2007;43:97.

Oertel WH et al: State of the art in restless legs syndrome therapy: Practice recommendations for treating restless legs syndrome. Mov Disord 2007;22(Suppl 18):S466.

Olanow CW et al: A double-blind, delayed-start trial of rasagiline in Parkinson's disease. N Engl J Med 2009;361:1268.

Olanow CW et al: A randomized, double-blind, placebo-controlled, delayed start study to assess rasagiline as a disease modifying therapy in Parkinson's disease (the ADAGIO study): Rationale, design, and baseline characteristics. Mov Disord 2008;23:2194.

Pahwa R et al: Ropinirole 24-hour prolonged release: Randomized, controlled study in advanced Parkinson disease. Neurology 2007;68:1108.

Perlmutter JS, Mink JW: Deep brain stimulation. Annu Rev Neurosci 2006;29:229.

Potenza MN et al: Drug insight: Impulse control disorders and dopamine therapies in Parkinson's disease. Nat Clin Pract Neurol 2007;3:664.

Sadeghi R, Ondo WG: Pharmacological management of essential tremor. Drugs 2010;70:2215.

Schapira AH: Treatment options in the modern management of Parkinson disease. Arch Neurol 2007;64:1083.

Schilsky ML: Wilson disease: Current status and the future. Biochimie 2009;91:1278.

Schwartz M, Hocherman S: Antipsychotic-induced rabbit syndrome: Epidemiology, management and pathophysiology. CNS Drugs 2004;18:213.

Seeberger LC, Hauser RA: Levodopa/carbidopa/entacapone in Parkinson's disease. Expert Rev Neurother 2009;9:929.

Servello D et al: Deep brain stimulation in 18 patients with severe Gilles de la Tourette syndrome refractory to treatment: The surgery and stimulation. J Neurol Neurosurg Psychiatry 2008;79:136.

Singer HS: Treatment of tics and Tourette syndrome. Curr Treat Options Neurol 2010;12:539.

Soares-Weiser KV, Joy C: Miscellaneous treatments for neuroleptic-induced tardive dyskinesia. Cochrane Database Syst Rev 2003;(2):CD000208.

Stocchi F et al: Initiating levodopa/carbidopa therapy with and without entacapone in early Parkinson disease: The STRIDE-PD study. Ann Neurol 2010;68:18.

Suchowersky O et al. Practice parameter: Neuroprotective strategies and alternative therapies for Parkinson disease (an evidence-based review). Report of the Quality Standards Subcommittee of the American Academy of Neurology. Neurology 2006;66:976.

Taylor RM et al: Triethylene tetramine dihydrochloride (trientine) in children with Wilson disease: Experience at King's College Hospital and review of the literature. Eur J Pediatr 2009;168:1061.

Trenkwalder C, Paulus W: Restless legs syndrome: Pathophysiology, clinical presentation and management. Nat Rev Neurol 2010;6:337.

Weaver FM et al: Bilateral deep brain stimulation vs best medical therapy for patients with advanced Parkinson disease: A randomized controlled trial. JAMA 2009;301:63.

Weintraub D et al: Impulse control disorders in Parkinson disease: A cross-sectional study of 3090 patients. Arch Neurol 2010;67:589.

Welter ML et al: Internal pallidal and thalamic stimulation in patients with Tourette syndrome. Arch Neurol 2008; 65:952.

Wiggelinkhuizen M et al: Systematic review: Clinical efficacy of chelator agents and zinc in the initial treatment of Wilson disease. Aliment Pharmacol Ther 2009;29:947.

Zesiewicz TA et al: Practice parameter: Therapies for essential tremor: Report of the Quality Standards Subcommittee of the American Academy of Neurology. Neurology 2005;64:2008.

CASE STUDY ANSWER

The relation of the tremor to activity (rest tremor) in this case is characteristic of parkinsonism. Examination reveals the classic findings of Parkinson's disease—rest tremor, rigidity, bradykinesia, and a gait disturbance; an asymmetry of the abnormalities is common in Parkinson's disease. The prognosis is that symptoms will become more generalized with time. Pharmacologic treatment would involve a dopamine agonist (pramipexole or ropinirole) but may not need to be started now unless the patient is disturbed by his symptoms. Although the evidence is incomplete, rasagiline may slow disease progression and could also be introduced.

Antipsychotic Agents & Lithium

Herbert Meltzer, MD, PhD[*]

A 17-year-old male high school student is referred to the psychiatry clinic for evaluation of suspected schizophrenia. After a diagnosis is made, haloperidol is prescribed at a gradually increasing dose on an outpatient basis. The drug improves the patient's positive symptoms but ultimately causes intolerable side effects. Although more costly, risperidone is then prescribed, which, over the course of several weeks of treatment, improves his symptoms and is tolerated by the patient. What signs and symptoms would support an initial diagnosis of schizophrenia? In the treatment of schizophrenia, what benefits do the atypical antipsychotic drugs offer over the traditional agents such as haloperidol? In addition to the management of schizophrenia, what other clinical indications warrant consideration of the use of drugs nominally classified as antipsychotics?

◼ ANTIPSYCHOTIC AGENTS

Antipsychotic drugs are able to reduce psychotic symptoms in a wide variety of conditions, including schizophrenia, bipolar disorder, psychotic depression, senile psychoses, various organic psychoses, and drug-induced psychoses. They are also able to improve mood and reduce anxiety and sleep disturbances, but they are not the treatment of choice when these symptoms are the primary disturbance in nonpsychotic patients. A **neuroleptic** is a subtype of antipsychotic drug that produces a high incidence of extrapyramidal side effects (EPS) at clinically effective doses, or catalepsy in laboratory animals. The **"atypical" antipsychotic drugs,** are now the most widely used type of antipsychotic drug.

History

Reserpine and chlorpromazine were the first drugs found to be useful to reduce psychotic symptoms in schizophrenia. Reserpine was used only briefly for this purpose and is no longer of interest as an antipsychotic agent. Chlorpromazine is a neuroleptic agent; that is, it produces catalepsy in rodents and EPS in humans. The discovery that its antipsychotic action was related to dopamine (D or DA)-receptor blockade led to the identification of other compounds as antipsychotics between the 1950s and 1970s. The discovery of clozapine in 1959 led to the realization that antipsychotic drugs need not cause EPS in humans at clinically effective doses. Clozapine was called an atypical antipsychotic drug because of this dissociation; it produces fewer EPS at equivalent antipsychotic doses in man and laboratory animals. As a result, there has been a major shift in clinical practice away from typical antipsychotic drugs towards the use of an ever increasing number of atypical drugs, which have other advantages as well. The introduction of antipsychotic drugs led to massive changes in disease management, including brief instead of life-long hospitalizations. These drugs have also proved to be of great value in studying the pathophysiology of schizophrenia and other psychoses. It should be noted that schizophrenia and bipolar disorder are no longer believed by many to be separate disorders but rather to be part of a continuum of brain disorders with psychotic features.

---

[*]The author acknowledges the contributions of the previous author of this chapter, William Z. Potter, MD, PhD.

Nature of Psychosis & Schizophrenia

The term "psychosis" denotes a variety of mental disorders: the presence of delusions (false beliefs), various types of hallucinations, usually auditory or visual, but sometimes tactile or olfactory, and grossly disorganized thinking in a clear sensorium. Schizophrenia is a particular kind of psychosis characterized mainly by a clear sensorium but a marked thinking disturbance. Psychosis is not unique to schizophrenia and is not present in all patients with schizophrenia at all times.

Schizophrenia is considered to be a neurodevelopmental disorder. This implies that structural and functional changes in the brain are present even in utero in some patients, or that they develop during childhood and adolescence, or both. Twin, adoption, and family studies have established that schizophrenia is a genetic disorder with high heritability. No single gene is involved. Current theories involve multiple genes with common and rare mutations, including large deletions and insertions (copy number variations), combining to produce a very variegated clinical presentation and course.

THE SEROTONIN HYPOTHESIS OF SCHIZOPHRENIA

The discovery that indole hallucinogens such as LSD (lysergic acid diethylamide) and mescaline are serotonin (5-HT) agonists led to the search for endogenous hallucinogens in the urine, blood, and brains of patients with schizophrenia. This proved fruitless, but the identification of many 5-HT-receptor subtypes led to the pivotal discovery that 5-HT$_{2A}$-receptor and possibly 5-HT$_{2C}$ stimulation was the basis for the hallucinatory effects of these agents.

It has been found that 5-HT$_{2A}$-receptor blockade is a key factor in the mechanism of action of the main class of atypical antipsychotic drugs, of which clozapine is the prototype, and includes, in order of their introduction around the world, melperone, risperidone, zotepine, blonanseine olanzapine, quetiapine, ziprasidone, aripiprazole, sertindole, paliperidone, iloperidone, asenapine, and lurasidone. These drugs are *inverse agonists* of the 5-HT$_{2A}$ receptor; that is, they block the constitutive activity of these receptors. These receptors modulate the release of dopamine, norepinephrine, glutamate, GABA and acetylcholine, among other neurotransmiters in the cortex, limbic region, and striatum. Stimulation of 5-HT$_{2A}$ receptors leads to depolarization of glutamate neurons, but also stabilization of N-methyl-D-aspartate (NMDA) receptors on postsynaptic neurons. Recently, it has been found that hallucinogens can modulate the stability of a complex consisting of 5-HT$_{2A}$ and NMDA receptors.

5-HT$_{2C}$-receptor stimulation provides a further means of modulating cortical and limbic dopaminergic activity. Stimulation of 5-HT$_{2C}$ receptors leads to inhibition of cortical and limbic dopamine release. Many atypical antipsychotic drugs, eg, clozapine, asenapine, olanzapine are 5-HT$_{2C}$ inverse agonists. 5-HT$_{2C}$ agonists are currently being studied as antipsychotic agents.

THE DOPAMINE HYPOTHESIS OF SCHIZOPHRENIA

The dopamine hypothesis for schizophrenia was the second neurotransmitter-based concept to be developed but is no longer considered adequate to explain all aspects of schizophrenia, especially the cognitive impairment. Nevertheless, it is still highly relevant to understanding the major dimensions of schizophrenia, such as positive and negative symptoms (emotional blunting, social withdrawal, lack of motivation), cognitive impairment, and possibly depression. It is also essential to understanding the mechanisms of action of most and probably all antipsychotic drugs.

Several lines of evidence suggest that excessive limbic dopaminergic activity plays a role in psychosis. (1) Many antipsychotic drugs strongly block postsynaptic D$_2$ receptors in the central nervous system, especially in the mesolimbic and striatal-frontal system; this includes partial dopamine agonists, such as aripiprazole and bifeprunox. (2) Drugs that increase dopaminergic activity, such as levodopa, amphetamines, and bromocriptine and apomorphine, either aggravate schizophrenia psychosis or produce psychosis de novo in some patients. (3) Dopamine-receptor density has been found postmortem to be increased in the brains of schizophrenics who have not been treated with antipsychotic drugs. (4) Some but not all postmortem studies of schizophrenic subjects have reported increased dopamine levels and D$_2$-receptor density in the nucleus accumbens, caudate, and putamen. (5) Imaging studies have shown increased amphetamine-induced striatal dopamine release, increased baseline occupancy of striatal D$_2$ receptors by extracellular dopamine, and other measures consistent with increased striatal dopamine synthesis and release.

However, the dopamine hypothesis is far from a complete explanation of all aspects of schizophrenia. *Diminished* cortical or hippocampal dopaminergic activity has been suggested to underlie the cognitive impairment and negative symptoms of schizophrenia. Postmortem and in vivo imaging studies of cortical, limbic, nigral, and striatal dopaminergic neurotransmission in schizophrenic subjects have reported findings consistent with diminished dopaminergic activity in these regions. Decreased dopaminergic innervation in medial temporal cortex, dorsolateral prefrontal cortex, and hippocampus, and decreased levels of DOPAC, a metabolite of dopamine, in the anterior cingulate have been reported in postmortem studies. Imaging studies have found increased prefrontal D$_1$-receptor levels that correlated with working memory impairments.

The fact that several of the atypical antipsychotic drugs have much less effect on D$_2$ receptors and yet are effective in schizophrenia has redirected attention to the role of other dopamine receptors and to nondopamine receptors. Serotonin receptors—particularly the 5-HT$_{2A}$-receptor subtype—may mediate synergistic effects or protect against the extrapyramidal consequences of D$_2$ antagonism. As a result of these considerations, the direction of research has changed to a greater focus on compounds that may act on several transmitter-receptor systems, eg, serotonin and glutamate. The atypical antipsychotic drugs share the property of weak D_2-receptor antagonism and more potent 5-HT_{2A}-receptor blockade.

THE GLUTAMATE HYPOTHESIS OF SCHIZOPHRENIA

Glutamate is the major excitatory neurotransmitter in the brain (see Chapter 21). Phencyclidine and ketamine are noncompetitive inhibitors of the NMDA receptor that exacerbate both cognitive impairment and psychosis in patients with schizophrenia. PCP and a related drug, MK-801, increase locomotor activity and, acutely or chronically, a variety of cognitive impairments in rodents and primates. These effects are widely employed as a means to develop novel antipsychotic and cognitive-enhancing drugs. Selective 5-HT_{2A} antagonists, as well as atypical antipsychotic drugs, are much more potent than D_2 antagonists in blocking these effects of PCP and MK-801. This was the starting point for the hypothesis that hypofunction of NMDA receptors, located on GABAergic interneurons, leading to diminished inhibitory influences on neuronal function, contributed to schizophrenia. The diminished GABAergic activity can induce disinhibition of downstream glutamatergic activity, which can lead to hyperstimulation of cortical neurons through non-NMDA receptors. Preliminary evidence suggests that LY2140023, a drug that acts as an agonist of the metabotropic 2/3 glutamate receptor (mGLuR2/3), may be effective in schizophrenia.

The NMDA receptor, an ion channel, requires glycine for full activation. It has been suggested that in patients with schizophrenia, the glycine site of the NMDA receptor is not fully saturated. There have been several trials of high doses of glycine to promote glutamatergic activity, but the results are far from convincing. Currently, glycine transport inhibitors are in development as possible antipsychotic agents.

Ampakines are drugs that potentiate currents mediated by AMPA-type glutamate receptors. In behavioral tests, ampakines are effective in correcting behaviors in various animal models of schizophrenia and depression. They protect neurons against neurotoxic insults, in part by mobilizing growth factors such as brain-derived neurotrophic factor (BDNF, see also Chapter 30).

BASIC PHARMACOLOGY OF ANTIPSYCHOTIC AGENTS

Chemical Types

A number of chemical structures have been associated with antipsychotic properties. The drugs can be classified into several groups as shown in Figures 29–1 and 29–2.

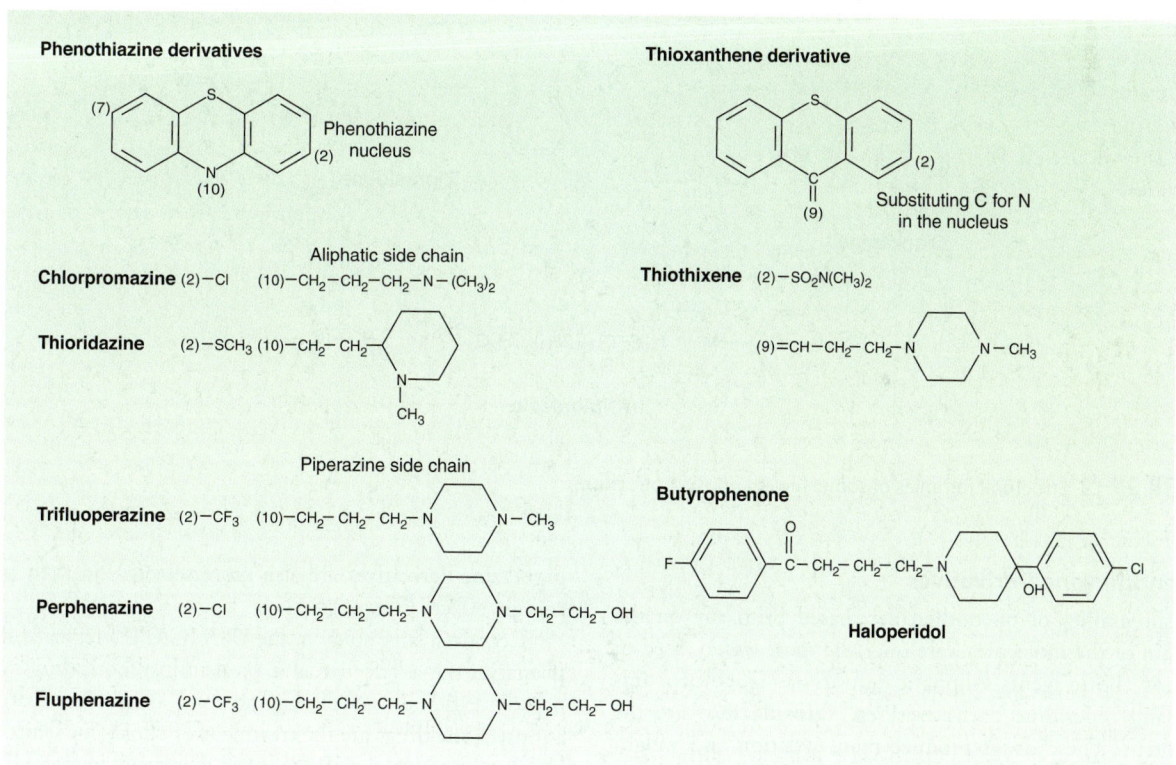

FIGURE 29–1 Structural formulas of some older antipsychotic drugs: phenothiazines, thioxanthenes, and butyrophenones. Only representative members of each type are shown.

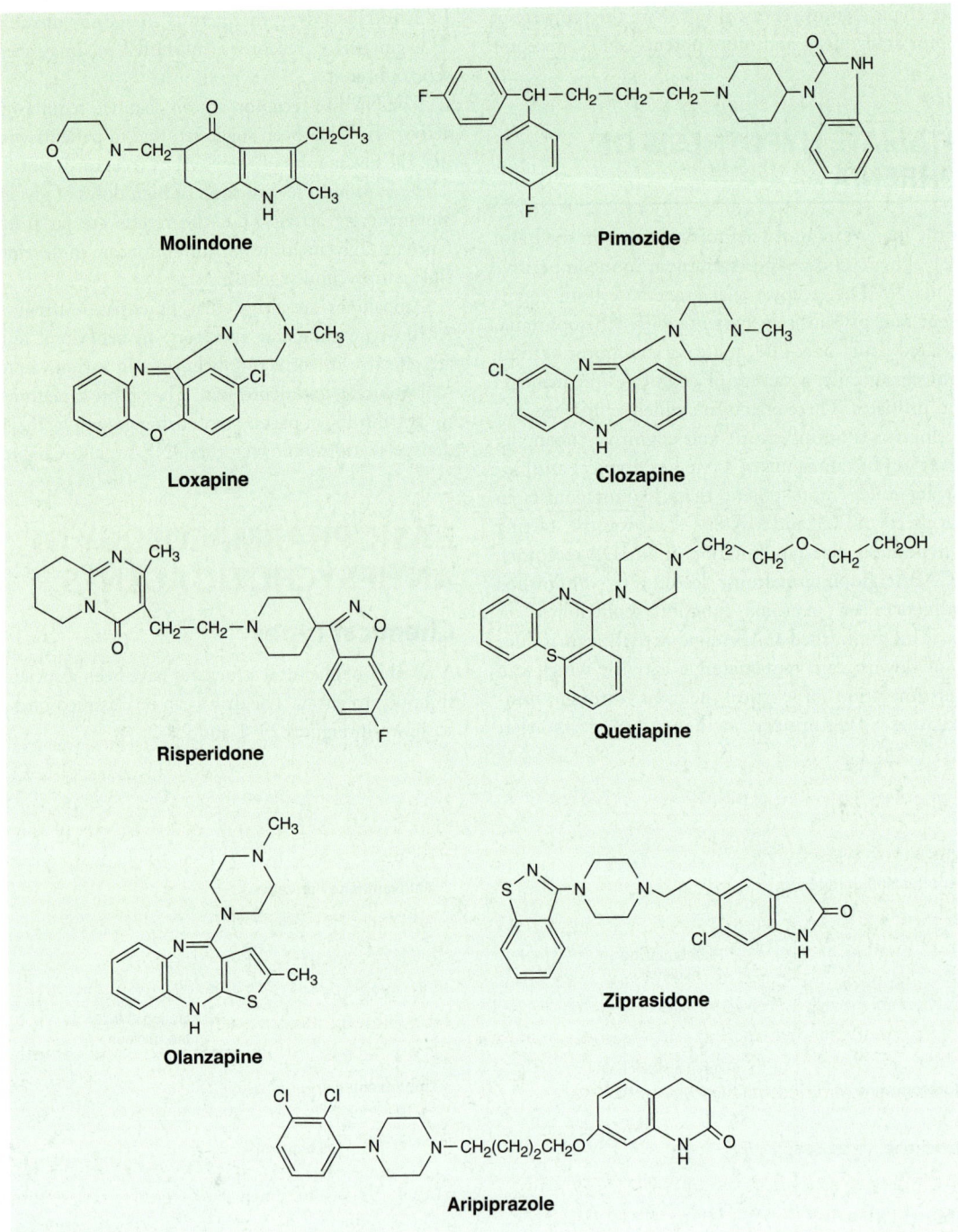

FIGURE 29–2 Structural formulas of some newer antipsychotic drugs.

A. Phenothiazine Derivatives

Three subfamilies of phenothiazines, based primarily on the side chain of the molecule, were once the most widely used of the antipsychotic agents. Aliphatic derivatives (eg, **chlorpromazine**) and piperidine derivatives (eg, **thioridazine**) are the least potent. These drugs produce more sedation and weight gain. Piperazine derivatives are more potent (effective in lower doses) but not necessarily more efficacious. Perphenazine, a piperazine derivative, was the typical antipsychotic drug used in the CATIE study described in the following text. The

piperazine derivatives are also more selective in their pharmacologic effects (Table 29–1).

Recently, a large study in the USA (CATIE) reported that perphenazine was as effective as atypical antipsychotic drugs, with the modest exception of olanzapine, and concluded that typical antipsychotic drugs are the treatment of choice for schizophrenia based on their lower cost. However, there were numerous flaws in the design, execution and analysis of this study, leading to it having only modest impact on clinical practice. In particular, it failed to consider issues such as dosage of olanzapine, inclusion of treatment

TABLE 29–1 Antipsychotic drugs: Relation of chemical structure to potency and toxicities.

Chemical Class	Drug	$D_2/5$-HT_{2A} Ratio[1]	Clinical Potency	Extrapyramidal Toxicity	Sedative Action	Hypotensive Actions
Phenothiazines						
Aliphatic	Chlorpromazine	High	Low	Medium	High	High
Piperazine	Fluphenazine	High	High	High	Low	Very low
Thioxanthene	Thiothixene	Very high	High	Medium	Medium	Medium
Butyrophenone	Haloperidol	Medium	High	Very high	Low	Very low
Dibenzodiazepine	Clozapine	Very low	Medium	Very low	Low	Medium
Benzisoxazole	Risperidone	Very low	High	Low[2]	Low	Low
Thienobenzodiazepine	Olanzapine	Low	High	Very low	Medium	Low
Dibenzothiazepine	Quetiapine	Low	Low	Very low	Medium	Low to medium
Dihydroindolone	Ziprasidone	Low	Medium	Very low	Low	Very low
Dihydrocarbostyril	Aripiprazole	Medium	High	Very low	Very low	Low

[1]Ratio of affinity for D_2 receptors to affinity for 5-HT_{2A} receptors.

[2]At dosages below 8 mg/d.

resistant patients, encouragement of patients to switch medications inherent in the design, risk for tardive dyskinesia following long term use of even low dose typical antipsychotics, and the necessity of large sample sizes in equivalency studies.

B. Thioxanthene Derivatives

This group of drugs is exemplified primarily by thiothixene.

C. Butyrophenone Derivatives

This group, of which **haloperidol** is the most widely used, has a very different structure from those of the two preceding groups. Haloperidol, a butyrophenone, is the most widely used typical antipsychotic drug, despite its high level of EPS relative to typical antipsychotic drugs. Diphenylbutylpiperidines are closely related compounds. The butyrophenones and congeners tend to be more potent and to have fewer autonomic effects but greater extrapyramidal effects than phenothiazines (Table 29–1).

D. Miscellaneous Structures

Pimozide and molindone are typical antipsychotic drugs. There is no significant difference in efficacy between these newer typical and the older typical antipsychotic drugs.

E. Atypical Antipsychotic Drugs

Clozapine, asenapine, olanzapine, quetiapine, paliperidone, risperidone, sertindole, ziprasidone, zotepine, and **aripiprazole** are atypical antipsychotic drugs (Figure 29–2). Clozapine is the prototype. Paliperidone is 9-hydroxyrisperidone, the active metabolite of risperidone. Risperidone is rapidly converted to 9-hydroxyrisperidone in vivo in most patients, except for about 10% of patients who are poor metabolizers. Sertindole is approved in some European countries but not in the USA.

These drugs have complex pharmacology but they share a greater ability to alter 5-HT_{2A}-receptor activity than to interfere with D_2-receptor action. In most cases, they act as partial agonists

at the 5-HT_{1A} receptor, which produces synergistic effects with 5-HT_{2A} receptor antagonism. Most are either 5-HT_6 or 5-HT_7 receptor antagonists.

Sulpride and sulpiride constitute another class of atypical agents. They have equivalent potency for D_2 and D_3 receptors, but they are also 5-HT_7 antagonists. They dissociate EPS and antipsychotic efficacy. However, they also produce marked increases in serum prolactin levels and are not as free of the risk of tardive dyskinesia as are drugs such as clozapine and quetiapine.

Pharmacokinetics

A. Absorption and Distribution

Most antipsychotic drugs are readily but incompletely absorbed. Furthermore, many undergo significant first-pass metabolism. Thus, oral doses of chlorpromazine and thioridazine have systemic availability of 25–35%, whereas haloperidol, which has less first-pass metabolism, has an average systemic availability of about 65%.

Most antipsychotic drugs are highly lipid soluble and protein bound (92–99%). They tend to have large volumes of distribution (usually more than 7 L/kg). They generally have a much longer clinical duration of action than would be estimated from their plasma half-lives. This is paralleled by prolonged occupancy of D_2 dopamine receptors in the brain by the typical antipsychotic drugs.

Metabolites of chlorpromazine may be excreted in the urine weeks after the last dose of chronically administered drug. Long-acting injectable formulations may cause some blockade of D_2 receptors 3–6 months after the last injection. Time to recurrence of psychotic symptoms is highly variable after discontinuation of antipsychotic drugs. The average time for relapse in stable patients with schizophrenia who discontinue their medication is 6 months. Clozapine is an exception in that relapse after discontinuation is usually rapid and severe. Thus, clozapine should never be discontinued abruptly unless clinically needed because of adverse effects such as myocarditis or agranulocytosis, which are true medical emergencies.

B. Metabolism

Most antipsychotic drugs are almost completely metabolized by oxidation or demethylation, catalyzed by liver microsomal cytochrome P450 enzymes. CYP2D6, CYP1A2, and CYP3A4 are the major isoforms involved (see Chapter 4). Drug-drug interactions should be considered when combining antipsychotic drugs with various other psychotropic drugs or drugs—such as ketoconazole—that inhibit various cytochrome P450 enzymes. At the typical clinical doses, antipsychotic drugs do not usually interfere with the metabolism of other drugs.

Pharmacodynamics

The first phenothiazine antipsychotic drugs, with chlorpromazine as the prototype, proved to have a wide variety of central nervous system, autonomic, and endocrine effects. Although efficacy of these drugs is primarily driven by D_2-receptor blockade, their adverse actions were traced to blocking effects at a wide range of receptors including α adrenoceptors and muscarinic, H_1 histaminic, and 5-HT_2 receptors.

A. Dopaminergic Systems

Five dopaminergic systems or pathways are important for understanding schizophrenia and the mechanism of action of antipsychotic drugs. The first pathway—the one most closely related to behavior and psychosis—is the **mesolimbic-mesocortical** pathway, which projects from cell bodies in the ventral tegmentum in separate bundles of axons to the limbic system and neocortex. The second system—the **nigrostriatal** pathway—consists of neurons that project from the substantia nigra to the dorsal striatum, which includes the caudate and putamen; it is involved in the coordination of voluntary movement. Blockade of the D_2 receptors in the nigrostriatal pathway is responsible for EPS. The third pathway—the **tuberoinfundibular** system—arises in the arcuate nuclei and periventricular neurons and releases dopamine into the pituitary portal circulation. Dopamine released by these neurons physiologically inhibits prolactin secretion from the anterior pituitary. The fourth dopaminergic system— the **medullary-periventricular** pathway—consists of neurons in the motor nucleus of the vagus whose projections are not well defined. This system may be involved in eating behavior. The fifth pathway—the **incertohypothalamic** pathway—forms connections from the medial zona incerta to the hypothalamus and the amygdala. It appears to regulate the anticipatory motivational phase of copulatory behavior in rats.

After dopamine was identified as a neurotransmitter in 1959, it was shown that its effects on electrical activity in central synapses and on production of the second messenger cAMP synthesized by adenylyl cyclase could be blocked by antipsychotic drugs such as chlorpromazine, haloperidol, and thiothixene. This evidence led to the conclusion in the early 1960s that these drugs should be considered **dopamine-receptor antagonists** and was a key factor in the development of dopamine hypothesis of schizophrenia described earlier in this chapter. The antipsychotic action is now

thought to be produced (at least in part) by their ability to block the effect of dopamine to inhibit the activity of adenylyl cyclase in the mesolimbic system.

B. Dopamine Receptors and Their Effects

At present, five dopamine receptors have been described, consisting of two separate families, the D_1-like and D_2-like receptor groups. The D_1 receptor is coded by a gene on chromosome 5, increases cAMP by G_s-coupled activation of adenylyl cyclase, and is located mainly in the putamen, nucleus accumbens, and olfactory tubercle and cortex. The other member of this family, D_5, is coded by a gene on chromosome 4, also increases cAMP, and is found in the hippocampus and hypothalamus. The therapeutic potency of antipsychotic drugs does not correlate with their affinity for binding to the D_1 receptor (Figure 29–3, top)

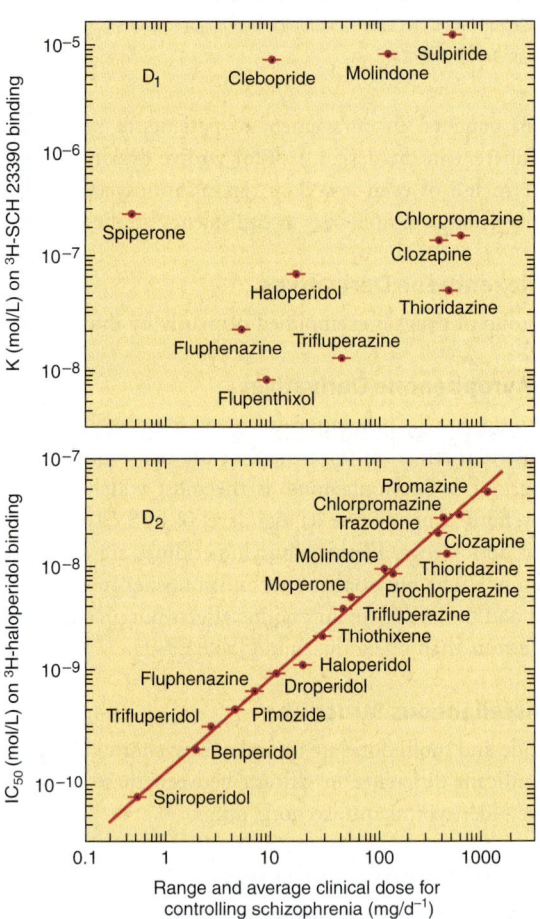

FIGURE 29–3 Correlations between the therapeutic potency of antipsychotic drugs and their affinity for binding to dopamine D_1 (*top*) or D_2 receptors (*bottom*). Potency is indicated on the horizontal axes; it decreases to the right. Binding affinity for D_1 receptors was measured by displacing the selective D_1 ligand SCH 23390; affinity for D_2 receptors was similarly measured by displacing the selective D_2 ligand haloperidol. Binding affinity decreases upward. (Modified and reproduced, with permission, from Seeman P: Dopamine receptors and the dopamine hypothesis of schizophrenia. Synapse 1987;1:133.)

nor did a selective D_1 antagonist prove to be an effective antipsychotic in patients with schizophrenia. The D_2 receptor is coded on chromosome 11, decreases cAMP (by G_i-coupled inhibition of adenylyl cyclase), and inhibits calcium channels but opens potassium channels. It is found both pre- and postsynaptically on neurons in the caudate-putamen, nucleus accumbens, and olfactory tubercle. A second member of this family, the D_3 receptor, also coded by a gene on chromosome 11, is thought to also decrease cAMP and is located in the frontal cortex, medulla, and midbrain. D_4 receptors also decrease cAMP and are concentrated in the cortex.

The typical antipsychotic agents block D_2 receptors stereoselectively for the most part, and their binding affinity is very strongly correlated with clinical antipsychotic and extrapyramidal potency (Figure 29–3, bottom). In vivo imaging studies of D_2-receptor occupancy indicate that for antipsychotic efficacy, the typical antipsychotic drugs must be given in sufficient doses to achieve at least 60% occupancy of striatal D_2 receptors. This is not required for the atypical antipsychotic drugs such as clozapine and olanzapine, which are effective at lower occupancy levels of 30–50%, most likely because of their concurrent high occupancy of $5\text{-}HT_{2A}$ receptors. The typical antipsychotic drugs produce EPS when the occupancy of striatal D_2 receptors reaches 80% or higher.

Positron emission tomography (PET) studies with aripiprazole show very high occupancy of D_2 receptors, but this drug does not cause EPS because it is a partial D_2-receptor agonist. Aripiprazole also gains therapeutic efficacy through its $5\text{-}HT_{2A}$ antagonism and possibly $5\text{-}HT_{1A}$ partial agonism.

These findings have been incorporated into the dopamine hypothesis of schizophrenia. However, additional factors complicate interpretation of dopamine receptor data. For example, dopamine receptors exist in both high- and low-affinity forms, and it is not known whether schizophrenia or the antipsychotic drugs alter the proportions of receptors in these two forms.

It has not been convincingly demonstrated that antagonism of any dopamine receptor other than the D_2 receptor plays a role in the action of antipsychotic drugs. Selective and relatively specific D_1, D_3-, and D_4-receptor antagonists have been tested repeatedly with no evidence of antipsychotic action. Most of the newer atypical antipsychotic agents and some of the traditional ones have a higher affinity for the $5\text{-}HT_{2A}$ receptor than for the D_2 receptor (Table 29–1), suggesting an important role for the serotonin 5-HT system in the etiology of schizophrenia and the action of these drugs.

C. Differences among Antipsychotic Drugs

Although all effective antipsychotic drugs block D_2 receptors, the degree of this blockade in relation to other actions on receptors varies considerably among drugs. Vast numbers of ligand-receptor binding experiments have been performed in an effort to discover a single receptor action that would best predict antipsychotic efficacy. A summary of the relative receptor-binding affinities of several key agents in such comparisons illustrates the difficulty in drawing simple conclusions from such experiments:

Chlorpromazine: $\alpha_1 = 5\text{-}HT_{2A} > D_2 > D_1$
Haloperidol: $D_2 > \alpha_1 > D_4 > 5\text{-}HT_{2A} > D_1 > H_1$
Clozapine: $D_4 = \alpha_1 > 5\text{-}HT_{2A} > D_2 = D_1$
Olanzapine: $5\text{-}HT_{2A} > H_1 > D_4 > D_2 > \alpha_1 > D_1$
Aripiprazole: $D_2 = 5\text{-}HT_{2A} > D_4 > \alpha_1 = H_1 >> D_1$
Quetiapine: $H_1 > \alpha_1 > M_{1,3} > D_2 > 5\text{-}HT_{2A}$

Thus, most of the atypical and some typical antipsychotic agents are at least as potent in inhibiting $5\text{-}HT_2$ receptors as they are in inhibiting D_2 receptors. The newest, aripiprazole, appears to be a partial agonist of D_2 receptors. Varying degrees of antagonism of α_2 adrenoceptors are also seen with risperidone, clozapine, olanzapine, quetiapine, and aripiprazole.

Current research is directed toward discovering atypical antipsychotic compounds that are either more selective for the mesolimbic system (to reduce their effects on the extrapyramidal system) or have effects on central neurotransmitter receptors—such as those for acetylcholine and excitatory amino acids—that have been proposed as new targets for antipsychotic action.

In contrast to the difficult search for receptors responsible for antipsychotic *efficacy*, the differences in receptor effects of various antipsychotics do explain many of their *toxicities* (Tables 29–1 and 29–2). In particular, extrapyramidal toxicity appears to be consistently associated with high D_2 potency.

D. Psychological Effects

Most antipsychotic drugs cause unpleasant subjective effects in nonpsychotic individuals. The mild to severe EPS, including akathisia, sleepiness, restlessness, and autonomic effects are unlike any associated with more familiar sedatives or hypnotics.

TABLE 29–2 Adverse pharmacologic effects of antipsychotic drugs.

Type	Manifestations	Mechanism
Autonomic nervous system	Loss of accommodation, dry mouth, difficulty urinating, constipation	Muscarinic cholinoceptor blockade
	Orthostatic hypotension, impotence, failure to ejaculate	α-Adrenoceptor blockade
Central nervous system	Parkinson's syndrome, akathisia, dystonias	Dopamine-receptor blockade
	Tardive dyskinesia	Supersensitivity of dopamine receptors
	Toxic-confusional state	Muscarinic blockade
Endocrine system	Amenorrhea-galactorrhea, infertility, impotence	Dopamine-receptor blockade resulting in hyperprolactinemia
Other	Weight gain	Possibly combined H_1 and $5\text{-}HT_2$ blockade

Nevertheless, low doses of some of these drugs, particularly quetiapine, are used to promote sleep onset and maintenance, although there is no approved indication for such usage.

People without psychiatric illness given antipsychotic drugs, even at low doses, experience impaired performance as judged by a number of psychomotor and psychometric tests. Psychotic individuals, however, may actually show improvement in their performance as the psychosis is alleviated. The ability of the atypical antipsychotic drugs to improve some domains of cognition in patients with schizophrenia and bipolar disorder is controversial. Some individuals experience marked improvement, and for that reason, cognition should be assessed in all patients with schizophrenia and a trial of an atypical agent considered, even if positive symptoms are well controlled by typical agents.

E. Electroencephalographic Effects

Antipsychotic drugs produce shifts in the pattern of electroencephalographic (EEG) frequencies, usually slowing them and increasing their synchronization. The slowing (hypersynchrony) is sometimes focal or unilateral, which may lead to erroneous diagnostic interpretations. Both the frequency and the amplitude changes induced by psychotropic drugs are readily apparent and can be quantitated by sophisticated electrophysiologic techniques. Some of the neuroleptic agents lower the seizure threshold and induce EEG patterns typical of seizure disorders; however, with careful dosage titration, most can be used safely in epileptic patients.

F. Endocrine Effects

Older typical antipsychotic drugs, as well as risperidone and paliperidone, produce elevations of prolactin, see Adverse Effects, below. Newer antipsychotics such as olanzapine, quetiapine, and aripiprazole cause no or minimal increases of prolactin and reduced risks of extrapyramidal system dysfunction and tardive dyskinesia, reflecting their *diminished* D_2 antagonism.

G. Cardiovascular Effects

The low-potency phenothiazines frequently cause orthostatic hypotension and tachycardia. Mean arterial pressure, peripheral resistance, and stroke volume are decreased. These effects are predictable from the autonomic actions of these agents (Table 29–2). Abnormal electrocardiograms have been recorded, especially with thioridazine. Changes include prolongation of QT interval and abnormal configurations of the ST segment and T waves. These changes are readily reversed by withdrawing the drug. Thioridazine, however, is *not* associated with increased risk of torsades more than other typical antipsychotics, whereas haloperidol, which does not increase QT_c, is.

Among the newest atypical antipsychotics, prolongation of the QT or QT_c interval has received much attention. Because this was believed to indicate an increased risk of dangerous arrhythmias, approval of sertindole has been delayed and ziprasidone and quetiapine are accompanied by warnings. There is, however, no evidence that this has actually translated into increased incidence of arrhythmias.

H. Animal Screening Tests

Inhibition of conditioned (but not unconditioned) avoidance behavior is one of the most predictive tests of antipsychotic action. Another is the inhibition of amphetamine- or apomorphine-induced stereotyped behavior. Other tests that may predict antipsychotic action are reduction of exploratory behavior without undue sedation, induction of a cataleptic state, inhibition of intracranial self-stimulation of reward areas, and prevention of apomorphine-induced vomiting. Most of these tests are difficult to relate to any model of clinical psychosis.

The psychosis produced by phencyclidine (PCP) has been used as a model for schizophrenia. Because this drug is an antagonist of the NMDA glutamate receptor, attempts have been made to develop antipsychotic drugs that work as NMDA agonists. Sigma receptor and cholecystokinin type b (CCK_b) antagonism have also been suggested as potential targets. Thus far, NMDA receptor-based models have pointed to agents that modulate glutamate release as potential antipsychotics. $5-HT_{2A}$ inverse agonists such as pimavanserin, ritanserin, and M100907 are potent inhibitors of PCP-induced locomotor activity, whereas D_2 antagonists are relatively weak in comparison. Thus, atypical antipsychotic drugs that act as $5-HT_{2A}$ antagonists appear much more potent than typical antipsychotic drugs in PCP models.

CLINICAL PHARMACOLOGY OF ANTIPSYCHOTIC AGENTS

Indications

A. Psychiatric Indications

Schizophrenia is the primary indication for antipsychotic agents. Antipsychotic drugs are also used very extensively in patients with psychotic bipolar disorder (BP1), psychotic depression, and treatment-resistant depression.

Catatonic forms of schizophrenia are best managed by intravenous benzodiazepines. Antipsychotic drugs may be needed to treat psychotic components of that form of the illness after catatonia has ended, and they remain the mainstay of treatment for this condition. Unfortunately, many patients show little response, and virtually none show a complete response.

Antipsychotic drugs are also indicated for **schizoaffective disorders,** which share characteristics of both schizophrenia and affective disorders. No fundamental difference between these two diagnoses has been reliably demonstrated. It is most likely that they are part of a continuum with bipolar psychotic disorder. The psychotic aspects of the illness require treatment with antipsychotic drugs, which may be used with other drugs such as antidepressants, lithium, or valproic acid. The manic phase in **bipolar affective disorder** often requires treatment with antipsychotic agents, although lithium or valproic acid supplemented with high-potency benzodiazepines (eg, lorazepam or clonazepam) may suffice in milder cases. Recent controlled trials support the efficacy of monotherapy with atypical antipsychotics in the acute phase (up to 4 weeks) of mania. Aripiprazole, olanzapine, quetiapine, risperidone and ziprasidone have been approved for treatment of various phases of bipolar disorder. They are most effective for the manic phase and for maintenance treatment.

As mania subsides, the antipsychotic drug may be withdrawn, although maintenance treatment with atypical antipsychotic agents has become more common. Nonmanic excited states may also be managed by antipsychotics, often in combination with benzodiazepines.

Other indications for the use of antipsychotics include **Tourette's syndrome,** disturbed behavior in patients with **Alzheimer's disease,** and, with antidepressants, **psychotic depression.** Antipsychotics are not indicated for the treatment of various withdrawal syndromes, eg, opioid withdrawal. In small doses, antipsychotic drugs have been promoted (wrongly) for the relief of anxiety associated with minor emotional disorders. The antianxiety sedatives (see Chapter 22) are preferred in terms of both safety and acceptability to patients.

B. Nonpsychiatric Indications

Most older typical antipsychotic drugs, with the exception of thioridazine, have a strong **antiemetic** effect. This action is due to dopamine-receptor blockade, both centrally (in the chemoreceptor trigger zone of the medulla) and peripherally (on receptors in the stomach). Some drugs, such as prochlorperazine and benzquinamide, are promoted solely as antiemetics.

Phenothiazines with shorter side chains have considerable H_1-**receptor-blocking** action and have been used for relief of pruritus or, in the case of promethazine, as preoperative sedatives. The butyrophenone droperidol is used in combination with an opioid, fentanyl, in **neuroleptanesthesia.** The use of these drugs in anesthesia practice is described in Chapter 25.

Drug Choice

Choice among antipsychotic drugs is based mainly on differences in adverse effects and possible differences in efficacy. Since use of the older drugs is still widespread, especially for patients treated in the public sector, knowledge of such agents as chlorpromazine and haloperidol remains relevant. Thus, one should be familiar with one member of each of the three subfamilies of phenothiazines, a member of the thioxanthene and butyrophenone group, and all of the newer compounds—clozapine, risperidone, olanzapine, quetiapine, ziprasidone, and aripiprazole. Each may have special benefits for selected patients. A representative group of antipsychotic drugs is presented in Table 29–3.

TABLE 29–3 Some representative antipsychotic drugs.

Drug Class	Drug	Advantages	Disadvantages
Phenothiazines			
Aliphatic	Chlorpromazine[1]	Generic, inexpensive	Many adverse effects, especially autonomic
Piperidine	Thioridazine[2]	Slight extrapyramidal syndrome; generic	800 mg/d limit; no parenteral form; cardiotoxicity
Piperazine	Fluphenazine[3]	Depot form also available (enanthate, decanoate)	(?) Increased tardive dyskinesia
Thioxanthene	Thiothixene	Parenteral form also available; (?) decreased tardive dyskinesia	Uncertain
Butyrophenone	Haloperidol	Parenteral form also available; generic	Severe extrapyramidal syndrome
Dibenzoxazepine	Loxapine	(?) No weight gain	Uncertain
Dibenzodiazepine	Clozapine	May benefit treatment-resistant patients; little extrapyramidal toxicity	May cause agranulocytosis in up to 2% of patients; dose-related lowering of seizure threshold
Benzisoxazole	Risperidone	Broad efficacy; little or no extrapyramidal system dysfunction at low doses	Extrapyramidal system dysfunction and hypotension with higher doses
Thienobenzodiazepine	Olanzapine	Effective against negative as well as positive symptoms; little or no extrapyramidal system dysfunction	Weight gain; dose-related lowering of seizure threshold
Dibenzothiazepine	Quetiapine	Similar to olanzapine; perhaps less weight gain	May require high doses if there is associated hypotension; short $t_{1/2}$ and twice-daily dosing
Dihydroindolone	Ziprasidone	Perhaps less weight gain than clozapine, parenteral form available	QT_c prolongation
Dihydrocarbostyril	Aripiprazole	Lower weight gain liability, long half-life, novel mechanism potential	Uncertain, novel toxicities possible

[1]Other aliphatic phenothiazines: promazine, triflupromazine.

[2]Other piperidine phenothiazines: piperacetazine, mesoridazine.

[3]Other piperazine phenothiazines: acetophenazine, perphenazine, carphenazine, prochlorperazine, trifluoperazine.

For approximately 70% of patients with schizophrenia, and probably for a similar proportion of patients with bipolar disorder with psychotic features, typical and atypical antipsychotic drugs are of equal efficacy for treating positive symptoms. However, the evidence favors atypical drugs for benefit for negative symptoms and cognition, for diminished risk of tardive dyskinesia and other forms of EPS, and for lesser increases in prolactin levels.

Some of the atypical antipsychotic drugs produce more weight gain and increases in lipids than some typical antipsychotic drugs. A small percentage of patients develop diabetes mellitus, most often seen with clozapine and olanzapine. Ziprasidone is the atypical drug causing the least weight gain. Risperidone, paliperidone, and aripiprazole usually produce small increases in weight and lipids. Asenapine and quetiapine have an intermediate effect. Clozapine and olanzapine frequently result in large increases in weight and lipids. Thus, these drugs should be considered as second-line drugs unless there is a specific indication. That is the case with clozapine, which at high doses (300–900 mg/d) is effective in the majority of patients with schizophrenia refractory to other drugs, provided that treatment is continued for up to 6 months. Case reports and several clinical trials suggest that high-dose olanzapine, ie, doses of 30–45 mg/d, may also be efficacious in refractory schizophrenia when given over a 6-month period. Clozapine is the only atypical antipsychotic drug indicated to reduce the risk of suicide. All patients with schizophrenia who have made life-threatening suicide attempts should be seriously evaluated for switching to clozapine.

New antipsychotic drugs have been shown in some trials to be more effective than older ones for treating negative symptoms. The floridly psychotic form of the illness accompanied by uncontrollable behavior probably responds equally well to all potent antipsychotics but is still frequently treated with older drugs that offer intramuscular formulations for acute and chronic treatment. Moreover, the low cost of the older drugs contributes to their widespread use despite their risk of adverse EPS effects. Several of the newer antipsychotics, including clozapine, risperidone, and olanzapine, show superiority over haloperidol in terms of overall response in some controlled trials. More comparative studies with aripiprazole are needed to evaluate its relative efficacy. Moreover, the superior adverse-effect profile of the newer agents and low to absent risk of tardive dyskinesia suggest that these should provide the first line of treatment.

The best guide for selecting a drug for an individual patient is the patient's past responses to drugs. At present, clozapine is limited to those patients who have failed to respond to substantial doses of conventional antipsychotic drugs. The agranulocytosis and seizures associated with this drug prevent more widespread use. Risperidone's superior side-effect profile (compared with that of haloperidol) at dosages of 6 mg/d or less and the lower risk of tardive dyskinesia have contributed to its widespread use. Olanzapine and quetiapine may have even lower risk and have also achieved widespread use.

Dosage

The range of effective dosages among various antipsychotic agents is broad. Therapeutic margins are substantial. At appropriate

TABLE 29–4 Dose relationships of antipsychotics.

	Minimum Effective Therapeutic Dose (mg)	Usual Range of Daily Doses (mg)
Chlorpromazine	100	100–1000
Thioridazine	100	100–800
Trifluoperazine	5	5–60
Perphenazine	10	8–64
Fluphenazine	2	2–60
Thiothixene	2	2–120
Haloperidol	2	2–60
Loxapine	10	20–160
Molindone	10	20–200
Clozapine	50	300–600
Olanzapine	5	10–30
Quetiapine	150	150–800
Risperidone	4	4–16
Ziprasidone	40	80–160
Aripiprazole	10	10–30

dosages, antipsychotics—with the exception of clozapine and perhaps olanzapine—are of equal efficacy in broadly selected groups of patients. However, some patients who fail to respond to one drug may respond to another; for this reason, several drugs may have to be tried to find the one most effective for an individual patient. Patients who have become refractory to two or three antipsychotic agents given in substantial doses become candidates for treatment with clozapine or high-dose olanzapine. Thirty to fifty percent of patients previously refractory to standard doses of other antipsychotic drugs respond to these drugs. In such cases, the increased risk of clozapine can well be justified.

Some dosage relationships between various antipsychotic drugs, as well as possible therapeutic ranges, are shown in Table 29–4.

Parenteral Preparations

Well-tolerated parenteral forms of the high-potency older drugs haloperidol and fluphenazine are available for rapid initiation of treatment as well as for maintenance treatment in noncompliant patients. Since the parenterally administered drugs may have much greater bioavailability than the oral forms, doses should be only a fraction of what might be given orally, and the manufacturer's literature should be consulted. Fluphenazine decanoate and haloperidol decanoate are suitable for long-term parenteral maintenance therapy in patients who cannot or will not take oral medication.

Dosage Schedules

Antipsychotic drugs are often given in divided daily doses, titrating to an effective dosage. The low end of the dosage range in Table 29–4 should be tried for at least several weeks. After an effective daily dosage has been defined for an individual patient, doses can be given less frequently. Once-daily doses, usually given at night, are feasible for many patients during chronic maintenance treatment. Simplification of dosage schedules leads to better compliance.

Maintenance Treatment

A very small minority of schizophrenic patients may recover from an acute episode and require no further drug therapy for prolonged periods. In most cases, the choice is between "as needed" increased doses or the addition of other drugs for exacerbations versus continual maintenance treatment with full therapeutic dosage. The choice depends on social factors such as the availability of family or friends familiar with the symptoms of early relapse and ready access to care.

Drug Combinations

Combining antipsychotic drugs confounds evaluation of the efficacy of the drugs being used. Use of combinations, however, is widespread, with more emerging experimental data supporting such practices. Tricyclic antidepressants or, more often, selective serotonin reuptake inhibitors (SSRIs) are often used with antipsychotic agents for symptoms of depression complicating schizophrenia. The evidence for the usefulness of this polypharmacy is minimal. Electroconvulsive therapy (ECT) is a useful adjunct for antipsychotic drugs, not only for treating mood symptoms, but for positive symptom control as well. Electroconvulsive therapy can augment clozapine when maximum doses of clozapine are ineffective. In contrast, adding risperidone to clozapine is not beneficial. Lithium or valproic acid is sometimes added to antipsychotic agents with benefit to patients who do not respond to the latter drugs alone. There is some evidence that lamotrigine is more effective than any of the other mood stabilizers for this indication (see below). It is uncertain whether instances of successful combination therapy represent misdiagnosed cases of mania or schizoaffective disorder. Benzodiazepines may be useful for patients with anxiety symptoms or insomnia not controlled by antipsychotics.

Adverse Reactions

Most of the unwanted effects of antipsychotic drugs are extensions of their known pharmacologic actions (Tables 29–1 and 29–2), but a few effects are allergic in nature and some are idiosyncratic.

A. Behavioral Effects

The older typical antipsychotic drugs are unpleasant to take. Many patients stop taking these drugs because of the adverse effects, which may be mitigated by giving small doses during the day and the major portion at bedtime. A "pseudodepression" that may be due to drug-induced akinesia usually responds to treatment with antiparkinsonism drugs. Other pseudodepressions may be due to higher doses than needed in a partially remitted patient,

in which case decreasing the dose may relieve the symptoms. Toxic-confusional states may occur with very high doses of drugs that have prominent antimuscarinic actions.

B. Neurologic Effects

Extrapyramidal reactions occurring early during treatment with older agents include typical **Parkinson's syndrome, akathisia** (uncontrollable restlessness), and **acute dystonic reactions** (spastic retrocollis or torticollis). Parkinsonism can be treated, when necessary, with conventional antiparkinsonism drugs of the antimuscarinic type or, in rare cases, with amantadine. (Levodopa should never be used in these patients.) Parkinsonism may be self-limiting, so that an attempt to withdraw antiparkinsonism drugs should be made every 3–4 months. Akathisia and dystonic reactions also respond to such treatment, but many clinicians prefer to use a sedative antihistamine with anticholinergic properties, eg, diphenhydramine, which can be given either parenterally or orally.

Tardive dyskinesia, as the name implies, is a late-occurring syndrome of abnormal choreoathetoid movements. It is the most important unwanted effect of antipsychotic drugs. It has been proposed that it is caused by a relative cholinergic deficiency secondary to supersensitivity of dopamine receptors in the caudate-putamen. The prevalence varies enormously, but tardive dyskinesia is estimated to have occurred in 20–40% of chronically treated patients before the introduction of the newer atypical antipsychotics. Early recognition is important, since advanced cases may be difficult to reverse. Any patient with tardive dyskinesia treated with a typical antipsychotic drug or possibly risperidone or paliperidone should be switched to quetiapine or clozapine, the atypical agents with the least likelihood of causing tardive dyskinesia. Many treatments have been proposed, but their evaluation is confounded by the fact that the course of the disorder is variable and sometimes self-limited. Reduction in dosage may also be considered. Most authorities agree that the first step should be to discontinue or reduce the dose of the current antipsychotic agent or switch to one of the newer atypical agents. A logical second step would be to eliminate all drugs with central anticholinergic action, particularly antiparkinsonism drugs and tricyclic antidepressants. These two steps are often enough to bring about improvement. If they fail, the addition of diazepam in doses as high as 30–40 mg/d may add to the improvement by enhancing GABAergic activity.

Seizures, though recognized as a complication of chlorpromazine treatment, were so rare with the high-potency older drugs as to merit little consideration. However, de novo seizures may occur in 2–5% of patients treated with clozapine. Use of an anticonvulsant is able to control seizures in most cases.

C. Autonomic Nervous System Effects

Most patients are able to tolerate the antimuscarinic adverse effects of antipsychotic drugs. Those who are made too uncomfortable or who develop urinary retention or other severe symptoms can be switched to an agent without significant antimuscarinic action. Orthostatic hypotension or impaired ejaculation—common complications of therapy with chlorpromazine or mesoridazine—should be managed by switching to drugs with less marked adrenoceptor-blocking actions.

D. Metabolic and Endocrine Effects

Weight gain is very common, especially with clozapine and olanzapine, and requires monitoring of food intake, especially carbohydrates. Hyperglycemia may develop, but whether secondary to weight gain-associated insulin resistance or to other potential mechanisms remains to be clarified. Hyperlipidemia may occur. The management of weight gain, insulin resistance, and increased lipids should include monitoring of weight at each visit and measurement of fasting blood sugar and lipids at 3–6 month intervals. Measurement of hemoglobin A_{1C} may be useful when it is impossible to be sure of obtaining a fasting blood sugar. Diabetic ketoacidosis has been reported in a few cases. The triglyceride:HDL ratio should be less than 3.5 in fasting samples. Levels higher than that indicate increased risk of atherosclerotic cardiovascular disease.

Hyperprolactinemia in women results in the amenorrhea-galactorrhea syndrome and infertility; in men, loss of libido, impotence, and infertility may result. Hyperprolactinemia may cause osteoporosis, particularly in women. If dose reduction is not indicated, or ineffective in controlling this pattern, switching to one of the atypical agents that do not raise prolactin levels, eg, aripiprazole, may be indicated.

E. Toxic or Allergic Reactions

Agranulocytosis, cholestatic jaundice, and skin eruptions occur rarely with the high-potency antipsychotic drugs currently used.

In contrast to other antipsychotic agents, clozapine causes agranulocytosis in a small but significant number of patients—approximately 1–2% of those treated. This serious, potentially fatal effect can develop rapidly, usually between the 6th and 18th weeks of therapy. It is not known whether it represents an immune reaction, but it appears to be reversible upon discontinuance of the drug. *Because of the risk of agranulocytosis, patients receiving clozapine must have weekly blood counts for the first 6 months of treatment and every 3 weeks thereafter.*

F. Ocular Complications

Deposits in the anterior portions of the eye (cornea and lens) are a common complication of chlorpromazine therapy. They may accentuate the normal processes of aging of the lens. Thioridazine is the only antipsychotic drug that causes retinal deposits, which in advanced cases may resemble retinitis pigmentosa. The deposits are usually associated with "browning" of vision. The maximum daily dose of thioridazine has been limited to 800 mg/d to reduce the possibility of this complication.

G. Cardiac Toxicity

Thioridazine in doses exceeding 300 mg daily is almost always associated with minor abnormalities of T waves that are easily reversible. Overdoses of thioridazine are associated with major ventricular arrhythmias, eg, torsades de pointes, cardiac conduction block, and sudden death; it is not certain whether thioridazine

can cause these same disorders when used in therapeutic doses. In view of possible additive antimuscarinic and quinidine-like actions with various tricyclic antidepressants, thioridazine should be combined with the latter drugs only with great care. Among the atypical agents, ziprasidone carries the greatest risk of QT prolongation and therefore should not be combined with other drugs that prolong the QT interval, including thioridazine, pimozide, and group 1A or 3 antiarrhythmic drugs. Clozapine is sometimes associated with myocarditis and must be discontinued if myocarditis manifests. Sudden death due to arrhythmias is common in schizophrenia. It is not always drug-related, and there are no studies that definitively show increased risk with particular drugs. Monitoring of QT_c prolongation has proved to be of little use unless the values increase to more than 500 ms and this is manifested in multiple rhythm strips or a Holter monitor study. A 20,000 patient study of ziprasidone versus olanzapine showed minimal or no increased risk of torsades de pointes or sudden death in patients who were randomized to ziprasidone.

H. Use in Pregnancy; Dysmorphogenesis

Although antipsychotic drugs appear to be relatively safe in pregnancy, a small increase in teratogenic risk could be missed. Questions about whether to use these drugs during pregnancy and whether to abort a pregnancy in which the fetus has already been exposed must be decided individually. If a pregnant woman could manage to be free of antipsychotic drugs during pregnancy, this would be desirable because of their effects on the neurotransmitters involved in neurodevelopment.

I. Neuroleptic Malignant Syndrome

This life-threatening disorder occurs in patients who are extremely sensitive to the extrapyramidal effects of antipsychotic agents (see also Chapter 16). The initial symptom is marked muscle rigidity. If sweating is impaired, as it often is during treatment with anticholinergic drugs, fever may ensue, often reaching dangerous levels. The stress leukocytosis and high fever associated with this syndrome may erroneously suggest an infectious process. Autonomic instability, with altered blood pressure and pulse rate, is often present.

Muscle-type creatine kinase levels are usually elevated, reflecting muscle damage. This syndrome is believed to result from an excessively rapid blockade of postsynaptic dopamine receptors. A severe form of extrapyramidal syndrome follows. Early in the course, vigorous treatment of the extrapyramidal syndrome with antiparkinsonism drugs is worthwhile. Muscle relaxants, particularly diazepam, are often useful. Other muscle relaxants, such as dantrolene, or dopamine agonists, such as bromocriptine, have been reported to be helpful. If fever is present, cooling by physical measures should be tried. Various minor forms of this syndrome are now recognized. Switching to an atypical drug after recovery is indicated.

Drug Interactions

Antipsychotics produce more important pharmacodynamic than pharmacokinetic interactions because of their multiple effects.

Additive effects may occur when these drugs are combined with others that have sedative effects, α-adrenoceptor–blocking action, anticholinergic effects, and—for thioridazine and ziprasidone—quinidine-like action.

A variety of pharmacokinetic interactions have been reported, but none are of major clinical significance.

Overdoses

Poisonings with antipsychotic agents (unlike tricyclic antidepressants) are rarely fatal, with the exception of those due to mesoridazine and thioridazine. In general, drowsiness proceeds to coma, with an intervening period of agitation. Neuromuscular excitability may be increased and proceed to convulsions. Pupils are miotic, and deep tendon reflexes are decreased. Hypotension and hypothermia are the rule, although fever may be present later in the course. The lethal effects of mesoridazine and thioridazine are related to induction of ventricular tachyarrhythmias. Patients should be given the usual "ABCD" treatment for poisonings (see Chapter 58) and treated supportively. Management of overdoses of thioridazine and mesoridazine, which are complicated by cardiac arrhythmias, is similar to that for tricyclic antidepressants (see Chapter 30).

Psychosocial Treatment & Cognitive Remediation

Patients with schizophrenia need psychosocial support based around activities of daily living, including housing, social activities, returning to school, obtaining the optimal level of work they may be capable of, and restoring social interactions. Unfortunately, funding for this crucial component of treatment has been minimized in recent years. Case management and therapy services are a vital part of the treatment program that should be provided to patients with schizophrenia. First-episode patients are particularly needful of this support because they often deny their illness and are noncompliant with medication.

Benefits & Limitations of Drug Treatment

As noted at the beginning of this chapter, antipsychotic drugs have had a major impact on psychiatric treatment. First, they have shifted the vast majority of patients from long-term hospitalization to the community. For many patients, this shift has provided a better life under more humane circumstances and in many cases has made possible life without frequent use of physical restraints. For others, the tragedy of an aimless existence is now being played out in the streets of our communities rather than in mental institutions.

Second, these antipsychotic drugs have markedly shifted psychiatric thinking to a more biologic orientation. Partly because of research stimulated by the effects of these drugs on schizophrenia, we now know much more about central nervous system physiology and pharmacology than was known before the introduction of these agents. However, despite much research, schizophrenia remains a scientific mystery and a personal disaster for the patient. Although most schizophrenic patients obtain some degree of benefit from these drugs—in some cases substantial benefit—none are made well by them.

■ LITHIUM, MOOD-STABILIZING DRUGS, & OTHER TREATMENT FOR BIPOLAR DISORDER

Bipolar disorder, once known as manic-depressive illness, was conceived of as a psychotic disorder distinct from schizophrenia at the end of the 19th century. Before that both of these disorders were considered part of a continuum. It is ironic that the weight of the evidence today is that there is profound overlap in these disorders. This is not to say that there are no pathophysiologically important differences or that some drug treatments are differentially effective in these disorders. According to *DSM-IV*, they are separate disease entities while research continues to define the dimensions of these illnesses and their genetic and other biologic markers.

Lithium was the first agent shown to be useful in the treatment of the manic phase of bipolar disorder that was not also an antipsychotic drug. Lithium has no known use in schizophrenia. Lithium continues to be used for acute-phase illness as well as for prevention of recurrent manic and depressive episodes.

A group of mood-stabilizing drugs that are also anticonvulsant agents has become more widely used than lithium. It includes **carbamazepine** and **valproic acid** for the treatment of acute mania and for prevention of its recurrence. **Lamotrigine** is approved for prevention of recurrence. **Gabapentin, oxcarbazepine,** and **topiramate** are sometimes used to treat bipolar disorder but are not approved by the Food and Drug Administration for this indication. **Aripiprazole, chlorpromazine, olanzapine, quetiapine, risperidone,** and **ziprasidone** are approved by the FDA for treatment of the manic phase of bipolar disorder. Olanzapine plus fluoxetine in combination and quetiapine are approved for treatment of bipolar depression.

Nature of Bipolar Affective Disorder

Bipolar affective (manic-depressive) disorder occurs in 1–3% of the adult population. It may begin in childhood, but most cases are first diagnosed in the third and fourth decades of life. The key symptoms of bipolar disorder in the manic phase are excitement, hyperactivity, impulsivity, disinhibition, aggression, diminished need for sleep, psychotic symptoms in some (but not all) patients, and cognitive impairment. Depression in bipolar patients is phenomenologically similar to that of major depression, with the key features being depressed mood, diurnal variation, sleep disturbance, anxiety, and sometimes, psychotic symptoms. Mixed manic and depressive symptoms are also seen. Patients with bipolar disorder are at high risk for suicide.

The sequence, number, and intensity of manic and depressive episodes are highly variable. The cause of the mood swings characteristic of bipolar affective disorder is unknown, although a preponderance of catecholamine-related activity may be present. Drugs that increase this activity tend to exacerbate mania, whereas those that reduce activity of dopamine or norepinephrine relieve mania. Acetylcholine or glutamate may also be involved. The nature of the abrupt switch from mania to depression experienced by some patients is uncertain. Bipolar disorder has a strong familial component, and there is abundant evidence that bipolar disorder is genetically determined.

Many of the genes that increase vulnerability to bipolar disorder are common to schizophrenia but some genes appear to be unique to each disorder. Genome-wide association studies of psychotic bipolar disorder have shown replicated linkage to chromosomes 8p and 13q. Several candidate genes have shown association with bipolar disorder with psychotic features and with schizophrenia. These include genes for dysbindin, *DAOA/G30*, disrupted-inschizophrenia-1 (*DISC-1*), and neuregulin 1.

BASIC PHARMACOLOGY OF LITHIUM

Lithium was first used therapeutically in the mid-19th century in patients with gout. It was briefly used as a substitute for sodium chloride in hypertensive patients in the 1940s but was banned after it proved too toxic for use without monitoring. In 1949, Cade discovered that lithium was an effective treatment for bipolar disorder, engendering a series of controlled trials that confirmed its efficacy as monotherapy for the manic phase of bipolar disorder.

Pharmacokinetics

Lithium is a small monovalent cation. Its pharmacokinetics are summarized in Table 29–5.

Pharmacodynamics

Despite considerable investigation, the biochemical basis for mood stabilizer therapies including lithium and anticonvulsant mood stabilizers is not clearly understood. Lithium directly inhibits two signal transduction pathways. It both suppresses inositol signaling through depletion of intracellular inositol and inhibits glycogen synthase kinase-3 (GSK-3), a multifunctional protein kinase. GSK-3 is a component of diverse intracellular signaling pathways. These include signaling via insulin/insulin-like growth factor, brain-derived neurotrophic factor (BDNF), and the Wnt pathway. All of these lead to inhibition of GSK-3. GSK-3 phosphorylates β-catenin, resulting in interaction with transcription factors. The pathways that are facilitated in this manner modulate energy metabolism, provide neuroprotection, and increase neuroplasticity.

Studies on the enzyme prolyl oligopeptidase and the sodium myoinositol transporter support an inositol depletion mechanism for mood-stabilizer action. Valproic acid may indirectly reduce GSK-3 activity and can up-regulate gene expression through inhibition of histone deacetylase. Valproic acid also inhibits inositol signaling through an inositol depletion mechanism. There is no evidence of GSK-3 inhibition by carbamazepine, a second antiepileptic mood stabilizer. In contrast, this drug alters neuronal morphology through an inositol depletion mechanism, as seen with lithium and valproic acid. The mood stabilizers may also have indirect effects on neurotransmitters and their release.

A. Effects on Electrolytes and Ion Transport

Lithium is closely related to sodium in its properties. It can substitute for sodium in generating action potentials and in Na^+-Na^+ exchange across the membrane. It inhibits the latter process; that is, Li^+-Na^+ exchange is gradually slowed after lithium is introduced into the body. At therapeutic concentrations (around 1 mmol/L), it does not significantly affect the Na^+-Ca^{2+} exchanger or the Na^+/K^+-ATPase pump.

B. Effects on Second Messengers

Some of the enzymes affected by lithium are listed in Table 29–6. One of the best-defined effects of lithium is its action on inositol

TABLE 29–5 Pharmacokinetics of lithium.

Absorption	Virtually complete within 6–8 hours; peak plasma levels in 30 minutes to 2 hours
Distribution	In total body water; slow entry into intracellular compartment. Initial volume of distribution is 0.5 L/kg, rising to 0.7–0.9 L/kg; some sequestration in bone. No protein binding.
Metabolism	None
Excretion	Virtually entirely in urine. Lithium clearance about 20% of creatinine. Plasma half-life about 20 hours.
Target plasma concentration	0.6–1.4 mEq/L
Dosage	0.5 mEq/kg/d in divided doses

TABLE 29–6 Enzymes affected by lithium at therapeutic concentrations.

Enzyme	Enzyme Function; Action of Lithium
Inositol monophosphatase	The rate-limiting enzyme in inositol recycling; inhibited by lithium, resulting in depletion of substrate for IP_3 production (Figure 29–4)
Inositol polyphosphate 1-phosphatase	Another enzyme in inositol recycling; inhibited by lithium, resulting in depletion of substrate for IP_3 production (Figure 29–4)
Bisphosphate nucleotidase	Involved in AMP production; inhibited by lithium; may be target that results in lithium-induced nephrogenic diabetes insipidus
Fructose 1,6-biphosphatase	Involved in gluconeogenesis; inhibition by lithium of unknown relevance
Phosphoglucomutase	Involved in glycogenolysis; inhibition by lithium of unknown relevance
Glycogen synthase kinase-3	Constitutively active enzyme that appears to limit neurotrophic and neuroprotective processes; lithium inhibits

AMP, adenosine monophosphate; IP_3, inositol 1,4,5-trisphosphate.

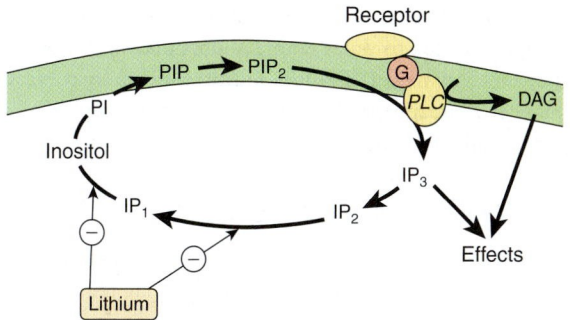

FIGURE 29–4 Effect of lithium on the IP_3 (inositol trisphosphate) and DAG (diacylglycerol) second-messenger system. The schematic diagram shows the synaptic membrane of a neuron. (PIP_2, phosphatidylinositol-4,5-bisphosphate; PLC, phospholipase C; G, coupling protein; Effects, activation of protein kinase C, mobilization of intracellular Ca^{2+}, etc.) Lithium, by inhibiting the recycling of inositol substrates, may cause depletion of the second-messenger source PIP_2 and therefore reduce the release of IP_3 and DAG. Lithium may also act by other mechanisms.

phosphates. Early studies of lithium demonstrated changes in brain inositol phosphate levels, but the significance of these changes was not appreciated until the second-messenger roles of inositol-1,4,5-trisphosphate (IP_3) and diacylglycerol (DAG) were discovered. As described in Chapter 2, inositol trisphosphate and diacylglycerol are important second messengers for both α-adrenergic and muscarinic transmission. Lithium inhibits inositol monophosphatase (IMPase) and other important enzymes in the normal recycling of membrane phosphoinositides, including conversion of IP_2 (inositol diphosphate) to IP_1 (inositol monophosphate) and the conversion of IP_1 to inositol (Figure 29–4). This block leads to a depletion of free inositol and ultimately of phosphatidylinositol-4,5-bisphosphate (PIP_2), the membrane precursor of IP_3 and DAG. Over time, the effects of transmitters on the cell diminish in proportion to the amount of activity in the PIP_2-dependent pathways. The activity of these pathways is postulated to be markedly increased during a manic episode. Treatment with lithium would be expected to diminish the activity in these circuits.

Studies of noradrenergic effects in isolated brain tissue indicate that lithium can inhibit norepinephrine-sensitive adenylyl cyclase. Such an effect could relate to both its antidepressant and its antimanic effects. The relationship of these effects to lithium's actions on IP_3 mechanisms is currently unknown.

Because lithium affects second-messenger systems involving both activation of adenylyl cyclase and phosphoinositol turnover, it is not surprising that G proteins are also found to be affected. Several studies suggest that lithium may uncouple receptors from their G proteins; indeed, two of lithium's most common side effects, polyuria and subclinical hypothyroidism, may be due to uncoupling of the vasopressin and thyroid-stimulating hormone (TSH) receptors from their G proteins.

The major current working hypothesis for lithium's therapeutic mechanism of action supposes that its effects on phosphoinositol

turnover, leading to an early relative reduction of myoinositol in human brain, are part of an initiating cascade of intracellular changes. Effects on specific isoforms of protein kinase C may be most relevant. Alterations of protein kinase C-mediated signaling alter gene expression and the production of proteins implicated in long-term neuroplastic events that could underlie long-term mood stabilization.

CLINICAL PHARMACOLOGY OF LITHIUM

Bipolar Affective Disorder

Until recently, lithium carbonate was the universally preferred treatment for bipolar disorder, especially in the manic phase. With the approval of valproate, aripiprazole, olanzapine, quetiapine, risperidone, and ziprasidone for this indication, a smaller percentage of bipolar patients now receive lithium. This trend is reinforced by the slow onset of action of lithium, which has often been supplemented with concurrent use of antipsychotic drugs or potent benzodiazepines in severely manic patients. The overall success rate for achieving remission from the manic phase of bipolar disorder can be as high as 80% but lower among patients who require hospitalization. A similar situation applies to maintenance treatment, which is about 60% effective overall but less in severely ill patients. These considerations have led to increased use of combined treatment in severe cases. After mania is controlled, the antipsychotic drug may be stopped and benzodiazepines and lithium continued as maintenance therapy.

The depressive phase of manic-depressive disorder often requires concurrent use of an antidepressant drug (see Chapter 30). Tricyclic antidepressant agents have been linked to precipitation of mania, with more rapid cycling of mood swings, although most patients do not show this effect. Selective serotonin reuptake inhibitors are less likely to induce mania but may have limited efficacy. Bupropion has shown some promise but—like tricyclic antidepressants—may induce mania at higher doses. As shown in recent controlled trials, the anticonvulsant lamotrigine is effective for many patients with bipolar depression. For some patients, however, one of the older monoamine oxidase inhibitors may be the antidepressant of choice. Quetiapine and the combination of olanzapine and fluoxetine has been approved for use in bipolar depression.

Unlike antipsychotic or antidepressant drugs, which exert several actions on the central or autonomic nervous system, lithium ion at therapeutic concentrations is devoid of autonomic blocking effects and of activating or sedating effects, although it can produce nausea and tremor. Most important is that the prophylactic use of lithium can prevent both mania and depression. Many experts believe that the aggressive marketing of newer drugs has inappropriately produced a shift to drugs that are less effective than lithium for substantial numbers of patients.

Other Applications

Recurrent endogenous depression with a cyclic pattern is controlled by either lithium or imipramine, both of which are superior to placebo.

Schizoaffective disorder, another condition with an affective component characterized by a mixture of schizophrenic symptoms and depression or excitement, is treated with antipsychotic drugs alone or combined with lithium. Various antidepressants are added if depression is present.

Lithium alone is rarely successful in treating **schizophrenia,** but adding it to an antipsychotic may salvage an otherwise treatment-resistant patient. Carbamazepine may work equally well when added to an antipsychotic drug.

An interesting application of lithium that is relatively well supported by controlled studies is as an adjunct to tricyclic antidepressants and SSRIs in patients with **unipolar depression** who do not respond fully to monotherapy with the antidepressant. For this application, concentrations of lithium at the lower end of the recommended range for manic-depressive illness appear to be adequate.

Monitoring Treatment

Clinicians rely on measurements of serum lithium concentrations for assessing both the dosage required for treatment of acute mania and for prophylactic maintenance. These measurements are customarily taken 10–12 hours after the last dose, so all data in the literature pertaining to these concentrations reflect this interval.

An initial determination of serum lithium concentration should be obtained about 5 days after the start of treatment, at which time steady-state conditions should have been attained. If the clinical response suggests a change in dosage, simple arithmetic (new dose equals present dose times desired blood level divided by present blood level) should produce the desired level. The serum concentration attained with the adjusted dosage can be checked after another 5 days. Once the desired concentration has been achieved, levels can be measured at increasing intervals unless the schedule is influenced by intercurrent illness or the introduction of a new drug into the treatment program.

Maintenance Treatment

The decision to use lithium as *prophylactic* treatment depends on many factors: the frequency and severity of previous episodes, a crescendo pattern of appearance, and the degree to which the patient is willing to follow a program of indefinite maintenance therapy. If the present attack was the patient's first or if the patient is unreliable, one might prefer to terminate treatment after the episode has subsided. Patients who have one or more episodes of illness per year are candidates for maintenance treatment. Although some patients can be maintained with serum levels as low as 0.6 mEq/L, the best results have been obtained with higher levels, such as 0.9 mEq/L.

Drug Interactions

Renal clearance of lithium is reduced about 25% by diuretics (eg, thiazides), and doses may need to be reduced by a similar amount. A similar reduction in lithium clearance has been noted with several of the newer nonsteroidal anti-inflammatory drugs that block synthesis of prostaglandins. This interaction

has not been reported for either aspirin or acetaminophen. All neuroleptics tested to date, with the possible exception of clozapine and the newer atypical antipsychotics, may produce more severe extrapyramidal syndromes when combined with lithium.

Adverse Effects & Complications

Many adverse effects associated with lithium treatment occur at varying times after treatment is started. Some are harmless, but it is important to be alert to adverse effects that may signify impending serious toxic reactions.

A. Neurologic and Psychiatric Adverse Effects

Tremor is one of the most common adverse effects of lithium treatment, and it occurs with therapeutic doses. Propranolol and atenolol, which have been reported to be effective in essential tremor, also alleviate lithium-induced tremor. Other reported neurologic abnormalities include choreoathetosis, motor hyperactivity, ataxia, dysarthria, and aphasia. Psychiatric disturbances at toxic concentrations are generally marked by mental confusion and withdrawal. Appearance of any new neurologic or psychiatric symptoms or signs is a clear indication for temporarily stopping treatment with lithium and for close monitoring of serum levels.

B. Decreased Thyroid Function

Lithium probably decreases thyroid function in most patients exposed to the drug, but the effect is reversible or nonprogressive. Few patients develop frank thyroid enlargement, and fewer still show symptoms of hypothyroidism. Although initial thyroid testing followed by regular monitoring of thyroid function has been proposed, such procedures are not cost-effective. Obtaining a serum TSH concentration every 6–12 months, however, is prudent.

C. Nephrogenic Diabetes Insipidus and Other Renal Adverse Effects

Polydipsia and polyuria are common but reversible concomitants of lithium treatment, occurring at therapeutic serum concentrations. The principal physiologic lesion involved is loss of responsiveness to antidiuretic hormone (nephrogenic diabetes insipidus). Lithium-induced diabetes insipidus is resistant to vasopressin but responds to amiloride.

Extensive literature has accumulated concerning other forms of renal dysfunction during long-term lithium therapy, including chronic interstitial nephritis and minimal-change glomerulopathy with nephrotic syndrome. Some instances of decreased glomerular filtration rate have been encountered but no instances of marked azotemia or renal failure.

Patients receiving lithium should avoid dehydration and the associated increased concentration of lithium in urine. Periodic tests of renal concentrating ability should be performed to detect changes.

D. Edema

Edema is a common adverse effect of lithium treatment and may be related to some effect of lithium on sodium retention. Although weight gain may be expected in patients who become edematous, water retention does not account for the weight gain observed in up to 30% of patients taking lithium.

E. Cardiac Adverse Effects

The bradycardia-tachycardia ("sick sinus") syndrome is a definite contraindication to the use of lithium because the ion further depresses the sinus node. T-wave flattening is often observed on the electrocardiogram but is of questionable significance.

F. Use During Pregnancy

Renal clearance of lithium increases during pregnancy and reverts to lower levels immediately after delivery. A patient whose serum lithium concentration is in a good therapeutic range during pregnancy may develop toxic levels after delivery. Special care in monitoring lithium levels is needed at these times. Lithium is transferred to nursing infants through breast milk, in which it has a concentration about one third to one half that of serum. Lithium toxicity in newborns is manifested by lethargy, cyanosis, poor suck and Moro reflexes, and perhaps hepatomegaly.

The issue of lithium-induced dysmorphogenesis is not settled. An earlier report suggested an increase in cardiac anomalies—especially Ebstein's anomaly—in lithium babies, and it is listed as such in Table 59–1 in this book. However, more recent data suggest that lithium carries a relatively low risk of teratogenic effects. Further research is needed in this important area.

G. Miscellaneous Adverse Effects

Transient acneiform eruptions have been noted early in lithium treatment. Some of them subside with temporary discontinuance of treatment and do not recur with its resumption. Folliculitis is less dramatic and probably occurs more frequently. Leukocytosis is always present during lithium treatment, probably reflecting a direct effect on leukopoiesis rather than mobilization from the marginal pool. This adverse effect has now become a therapeutic effect in patients with low leukocyte counts.

Overdoses

Therapeutic overdoses of lithium are more common than those due to deliberate or accidental ingestion of the drug. Therapeutic overdoses are usually due to accumulation of lithium resulting from some change in the patient's status, such as diminished serum sodium, use of diuretics, or fluctuating renal function. Since the tissues will have already equilibrated with the blood, the plasma concentrations of lithium may not be excessively high in proportion to the degree of toxicity; any value over 2 mEq/L must be considered as indicating likely toxicity. Because lithium is a small ion, it is dialyzed readily. Both peritoneal dialysis and hemodialysis are effective, although the latter is preferred.

VALPROIC ACID

Valproic acid (valproate), discussed in detail in Chapter 24 as an antiepileptic, has been demonstrated to have antimanic effects and

is now being widely used for this indication in the USA. (Gabapentin is not effective, leaving the mechanism of action of valproate unclear.) Overall, valproic acid shows efficacy equivalent to that of lithium during the early weeks of treatment. It is significant that valproic acid has been effective in some patients who have failed to respond to lithium. Moreover, its side-effect profile is such that one can rapidly increase the dosage over a few days to produce blood levels in the apparent therapeutic range, with nausea being the only limiting factor in some patients. The starting dosage is 750 mg/d, increasing rapidly to the 1500–2000 mg range with a recommended maximum dosage of 60 mg/kg/d.

Combinations of valproic acid with other psychotropic medications likely to be used in the management of either phase of bipolar illness are generally well tolerated. Valproic acid is an appropriate first-line treatment for mania, although it is not clear that it will be as effective as lithium as a maintenance treatment in all subsets of patients. Many clinicians advocate combining valproic acid and lithium in patients who do not fully respond to either agent alone.

CARBAMAZEPINE

Carbamazepine has been considered to be a reasonable alternative to lithium when the latter is less than optimally efficacious. The mode of action of carbamazepine is unclear, and oxcarbazepine is not effective. Carbamazepine may be used to treat acute mania and also for prophylactic therapy. Adverse effects (discussed in Chapter 24) are generally no greater and sometimes less than those associated with lithium. Carbamazepine may be used alone or, in refractory patients, in combination with lithium or, rarely, valproate.

The use of carbamazepine as a mood stabilizer is similar to its use as an anticonvulsant (see Chapter 24). Dosage usually begins with 200 mg twice daily, with increases as needed. Maintenance dosage is similar to that used for treating epilepsy, ie, 800–1200 mg/d. Plasma concentrations between 3 and 14 mg/L are considered desirable, although no therapeutic range has been established. Blood dyscrasias have figured prominently in the adverse effects of carbamazepine when it is used as an anticonvulsant, but they have not been a major problem with its use as a mood stabilizer. Overdoses of carbamazepine are a major emergency and should generally be managed like overdoses of tricyclic antidepressants (see Chapter 58).

OTHER DRUGS

Lamotrigine has been reported to be useful in preventing the depression that often follows the manic phase of bipolar disorder. A number of novel agents are under investigation for bipolar depression, including riluzole, a neuroprotective agent that is approved for use in amyotrophic lateral sclerosis; ketamine, a noncompetitive NMDA antagonist previously discussed as a drug believed to model schizophrenia but thought to act by producing relative enhancement of AMPA receptor activity; and AMPA receptor potentiators.

SUMMARY   Antipsychotic Drugs & Lithium

Subclass	Mechanism of Action	Effects	Clinical Applications	Pharmacokinetics, Toxicities, Interactions
PHENOTHIAZINES • Chlorpromazine • Fluphenazine • Thioridazine **THIOXANTHENE** • Thiothixene	Blockade of D_2 receptors >> 5-HT_{2A} receptors	α-Receptor blockade (fluphenazine least) • muscarinic (M)-receptor blockade (especially chlorpromazine and thioridazine) • H_1-receptor blockade (chlorpromazine, thiothixene) • central nervous system (CNS) depression (sedation) • decreased seizure threshold • QT prolongation (thioridazine)	Psychiatric: schizophrenia (alleviate positive symptoms), bipolar disorder (manic phase) • nonpsychiatric: antiemesis, preoperative sedation (promethazine) • pruritus	Oral and parenteral forms, long half-lives with metabolism-dependent elimination • *Toxicity*: Extensions of effects on α- and M-receptors • blockade of dopamine receptors may result in akathisia, dystonia, parkinsonian symptoms, tardive dyskinesia, and hyperprolactinemia
BUTYROPHENONE • Haloperidol	Blockade of D_2 receptors >> 5-HT_{2A} receptors	Some α blockade, but minimal M-receptor blockade and much less sedation than the phenothiazines	Schizophrenia (alleviates positive symptoms), bipolar disorder (manic phase), Huntington's chorea, Tourette's syndrome	Oral and parenteral forms with metabolism-dependent elimination • *Toxicity*: Extrapyramidal dysfunction is major adverse effect
ATYPICAL ANTIPSYCHOTICS • Aripiprazole • Clozapine • Olanzapine • Quetiapine • Risperidone • Ziprasidone	Blockade of 5-HT_{2A} receptors > blockade of D_2 receptors	Some α blockade (clozapine, risperidone, ziprasidone) and M-receptor blockade (clozapine, olanzapine) • variable H_1-receptor blockade (all)	Schizophrenia—improve both positive and negative symptoms • bipolar disorder (olanzapine or risperidone adjunctive with lithium) • agitation in Alzheimer's and Parkinson's patients (low doses) • major depression (aripiprazole)	*Toxicity*: Agranulocytosis (clozapine), diabetes (clozapine, olanzapine), hypercholesterolemia (clozapine, olanzapine), hyperprolactinemia (risperidone), QT prolongation (ziprasidone), weight gain (clozapine, olanzapine)
LITHIUM	Mechanism of action uncertain • suppresses inositol signaling and inhibits glycogen synthase kinase-3 (GSK-3), a multifunctional protein kinase	No significant antagonistic actions on autonomic nervous system receptors or specific CNS receptors • no sedative effects	Bipolar affective disorder—prophylactic use can prevent mood swings between mania and depression	Oral absorption, renal elimination • half-life 20 h • narrow therapeutic window (monitor blood levels) • *Toxicity*: Tremor, edema, hypothyroidism, renal dysfunction, dysrhythmias • pregnancy category D • *Interactions*: Clearance decreased by thiazides and some NSAIDs
NEWER AGENTS FOR BIPOLAR DISORDER • Carbamazepine • Lamotrigine • Valproic acid	Mechanism of action in bipolar disorder unclear (see Chapter 24 for putative actions in seizure disorders)	Carbamazepine causes dose-related diplopia and ataxia • lamotrigine causes nausea, dizziness, and headache • valproic acid causes gastrointestinal distress, possible weight gain, alopecia	Valproic acid is increasingly used as first choice in acute mania • carbamazepine and lamotrigine are also used both in acute mania and for prophylaxis in depressive phase	Oral absorption • once-daily dosing • carbamazepine forms active metabolite • lamotrigine and valproic acid form conjugates • *Toxicity*: Hematotoxicity and induction of P450 drug metabolism (carbamazepine), rash (lamotrigine), tremor, liver dysfunction, weight gain, inhibition of drug metabolism (valproic acid)

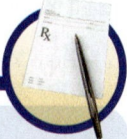

PREPARATIONS AVAILABLE

ANTIPSYCHOTIC AGENTS

Aripiprazole (Abilify)
Oral: 2, 5, 10, 15, 20, 30 mg tablets; 1 mg/mL solution
Parenteral: 7.5 mg/mL for IM injection

Asenapine (Saphris)
Oral: 5, 10 mg sublingual tablets

Chlorpromazine (generic, Thorazine)
Oral: 10, 25, 50, 100, 200 mg tablets; 100 mg/mL concentrate
Rectal: 100 mg suppositories
Parenteral: 25 mg/mL for IM injection

Clozapine (generic, Clozaril)
Oral: 12.5, 25, 50, 100, 200 mg tablets; 25, 100 mg orally disinte-grating tablets

Fluphenazine (generic, Prolixin)
Oral: 1, 2.5, 5, 10 mg tablets; 2.5 mg/5 mL elixir
Parenteral: (fluphenazine HCl): 2.5 mg/mL for IM injection

Fluphenazine decanoate (generic, Prolixin)
Parenteral: 25 mg/mL for IM or SC injection

Haloperidol (generic, Haldol)
Oral: 0.5, 1, 2, 5, 10, 20 mg tablets; 2 mg/mL concentrate
Parenteral: 5 mg/mL for IM injection

Haloperidol ester (Haldol Decanoate)
Parenteral: 50, 100 mg/mL for IM injection

Loxapine (generic, Loxitane)
Oral: 5, 10, 25, 50 mg capsules

Molindone (Moban)
Oral: 5, 10, 25, 50 mg tablets

Olanzapine (Zyprexa)
Oral: 2.5, 5, 7.5, 10, 15, 20 mg tablets; 5, 10, 15, 20 mg orally disin-tegrating tablets
Parenteral: 10 mg powder for injection

Paliperidone (Invega)
Oral: 3, 6, 9 mg extended-release tablets

Perphenazine (generic)
Oral: 2, 4, 8, 16 mg tablets; 16 mg/5 mL concentrate

Pimozide (Orap)
Oral: 1, 2 mg tablets
Prochlorperazine (generic, Compazine)
Oral: 5, 10 mg tablets; 5 mg/5 mL syrup

Oral sustained-release: 10, 15 mg capsules
Rectal: 2.5, 5, 25 mg suppositories
Parenteral: 5 mg/mL for IM injection

Quetiapine (Seroquel)
Oral: 25, 50, 100, 200, 300, 400 mg tablets; 200, 300, 400 mg extend-ed-release tablets

Risperidone (Risperdal)
Oral: 0.25, 0.5, 1, 2, 3, 4 mg tablets; 0.5, 1, 2, 3, 4 mg orally disinte-grating tablets; 1 mg/mL oral solution
Parenteral: 12.5, 25, 37.5, 50 mg powder for injection; long-acting injectable 25, 37.5, 50 mg

Thioridazine (generic, Mellaril)
Oral: 10, 15, 25, 50, 100, 150, 200 mg tablets; 30 mg/mL concentrate

Thiothixene (generic, Navane)
Oral: 1, 2, 5, 10, 20 mg capsules

Trifluoperazine (generic)
Oral: 1, 2, 5, 10 mg tablets

Ziprasidone (Geodon)
Oral: 20, 40, 60, 80 mg capsules
Parenteral: 20 mg powder for IM injection

MOOD STABILIZERS

Carbamazepine (generic, Tegretol)
Oral: 200 mg tablets, 100 mg chewable tablets; 100 mg/5 mL oral suspension
Oral extended-release: 100, 200, 400 mg tablets; 100, 200, 300 mg capsules

Divalproex (Depakote)
Oral: 125, 250, 500 mg delayed-release tablets

Lamotrigine (Lamictal)
Oral: 2, 5, 25, 100, 150, 200 mg tablets

Lithium carbonate (generic, Eskalith) (*Note:* 300 mg lithium carbonate = 8.12 mEq Li$^+$.)
Oral: 150, 300, 600 mg capsules; 300 mg tablets; 8 mEq/5 mL syrup
Oral sustained-release: 300, 450 mg tablets

Topiramate (Topamax)
Oral: 25, 50, 100, 200 mg tablets

Valproic acid (generic, Depakene)
Oral: 250 mg capsules; 250 mg/5 mL syrup

REFERENCES

Antipsychotic Drugs

Bhattacharjee J, El-Sayeh HG: Aripiprazole versus typical antipsychotic drugs for schizophrenia. Cochrane Database Syst Rev 2008;16;(3):CD006617.

Breier A, Berg PH: The psychosis of schizophrenia: Prevalence, response to atypical antipsychotics, and prediction of outcome. Biol Psychiatry 1999;46:361.

Carlsson A, Waters N, Carlsson ML: Neurotransmitter interactions in schizophrenia—therapeutic implications. Biol Psychiatry 1999;46:1388.

Coyle JT: Glutamate and schizophrenia: Beyond the dopamine hypothesis. Cell Mol Neurobiol 2006;26:365.

Ertugrul A, Meltzer HY: Antipsychotic drugs in bipolar disorder. Int J Neuropsychopharmacol 2003;6:277.

Escamilla MA, Zavala JM: Genetics of bipolar disorder. Dialogues Clin Neurosci 2008;10:141.

Farde L et al: Central D$_2$-dopamine receptor occupancy in schizophrenic patients treated with antipsychotic drugs. Arch Gen Psychiatry 1987;45:71.

Freudenreich O, Goff DC: Antipsychotic combination therapy in schizophrenia. A review of efficacy and risks of current combinations. Acta Psychiatr Scand 2002;106:323.

Fountoulakis KN, Vieta E: Treatment of bipolar disorder: a systematic review of available data and clinical perspectives. Int J Neuropsychopharmacol. 2008 11(7):999-1029.

Glassman AH: Schizophrenia, antipsychotic drugs, and cardiovascular disease. J Clin Psychiatry 2005;66(Suppl 6):5.

Grunder G, Nippius H, Carlsson A: The 'atypicality' of antipsychotics: A concept re-examined and re-defined. Nat Rev Drug Discov 2009;8:197.

Haddad PM, Anderson IM: Antipsychotic-related QT_c prolongation, torsade de pointes and sudden death. Drugs 2002;62:1649.

Harrison PJ, Weinberger DR: Schizophrenia genes, gene expression, and neuropathology: On the matter of their convergence. Mol Psychiatry 2005; 10:40.

Karam CS et al: Signaling pathways in schizophrenia: Emerging targets and therapeutic strategies. Trend Pharmacol Sci 2010;31:381.

Large CH, Webster EL, Goff DC: The potential role of lamotrigine in schizophrenia. Psychopharmacology (Berl) 2005;181:415.

Lieberman JA et al: Effectiveness of antipsychotic drugs in patients with chronic schizophrenia. N Engl J Med 2005;353:1209.

Lieberman JA et al: Antipsychotic drugs: Comparison in animal models of efficacy, neurotransmitter regulation, and neuroprotection. Pharmacol Rev 2008;60:358.

McGavin JK, Goa KL: Aripiprazole. CNS Drugs 2002;16:779.

McKeage K, Plosker GL: Amisulpride: A review of its use in the management of schizophrenia. CNS Drugs 2004;18:933.

Meltzer HY: Treatment of schizophrenia and spectrum disorders: Pharmacotherapy, psychosocial treatments, and neurotransmitter interactions. Biol Psychiatry 1999;46:1321.

Meltzer HY, Massey BW: The role of serotonin receptors in the action of atypical antipsychotic drugs. Curr Opin Pharmacol 2011;11:59.

Meltzer HY et al: Serotonin receptors: Their key role in drugs to treat schizophrenia. Prog Neuropsychopharmacol Biol Psychiatry 2003;27:1159.

Meltzer HY et al: A randomized, double-blind comparison of clozapine and high-dose olanzapine in treatment-resistant patients with schizophrenia. *Journal of Clinical Psychiatry* 2008;69:274.

Newcomer JW, Haupt DW: The metabolic effects of antipsychotic medications. Can J Psychiatry 2006;51:480.

Patil ST et al: Activation of mGlu2/3 receptors as a new approach to treat schizophrenia: A randomized Phase 2 clinical trial. Nat Med 2007;13:1102.

Schwarz C et al: Valproate for schizophrenia. Cochrane Database Syst Rev 2008;(3):CD004028.

Urichuk L et al: Metabolism of atypical antipsychotics: Involvement of cytochrome p450 enzymes and relevance for drug-drug interactions. Curr Drug Metab 2008;9:410.

Walsh T et al: Rare structural variants disrupt multiple genes in neurodevelopmental pathways in schizophrenia. Science 2008;320:539.

Woodward ND et al: A meta-analysis of neuropsychological change to clozapine, olanzapine, quetiapine, and risperidone in schizophrenia. Int J Neuropsychopharmacol 2005;8:457.

Zhang A, Neumeyer JL, Baldessarini RJ: Recent progress in development of dopamine receptor subtype-selective agents: Potential therapeutics for neurological and psychiatric disorders. Chem Rev 2007;107:274.

Mood Stabilizers

Baraban JM, Worley PF, Snyder SH: Second messenger systems and psychoactive drug action: Focus on the phosphoinositide system and lithium. Am J Psychiatry 1989;146:1251.

Bauer MS, Mitchner L: What is a "mood stabilizer"? An evidence-based response. Am J Psychiatry 2004;161:3.

Bowden CL, Singh V: Valproate in bipolar disorder: 2000 onwards. Acta Psychiatr Scand Suppl 2005;(426):13.

Catapano LA, Manji HK: Kinases as drug targets in the treatment of bipolar disorder. Drug Discov Today 2008;13:295.

Fountoulakis KN, Vieta E: Treatment of bipolar disorder: A systematic review of available data and clinical perspectives. Int J Neuropsychopharmacol 2008;11:999.

Goes FS, Sanders LL, Potash JB: The genetics of psychotic bipolar disorder. Curr Psychiatry Rep 2008;10:178.

Gould TD, Manji HK: Glycogen synthase kinase-3: A putative molecular target for lithium mimetic drugs. Neuropsychopharmacology 2005;30:1223.

Jope RS: Anti-bipolar therapy: Mechanism of action of lithium. Mol Psychiatry 1999;4:117.

Mathew SJ, Manji HK, Charney DS: Novel drugs and therapeutic targets for severe mood disorders. Neuropsychopharmacology 2008;33:2080.

Quiroz JA et al: Emerging experimental therapeutics for bipolar disorder: Clues from the molecular pathophysiology. Mol Psychiatry 2004;9:756.

Schou M: Lithium treatment at 52. J Affect Disord 2001;67:21.

Vieta E, Sanchez-Moreno J: Acute and long-term treatment of mania. Dialogues Clin Neurosci 2008;10:165.

Yatham LN et al: Third generation anticonvulsants in bipolar disorder: a review of efficacy and summary of clinical recommendations. J Clin Psychiatry 2002;63:275.

CASE STUDY ANSWER*

Schizophrenia is characterized by a disintegration of thought processes and emotional responsiveness. Symptoms commonly include auditory hallucinations, paranoid or bizarre delusions, disorganized thinking and speech, and social and occupational dysfunction. For many patients, typical (eg, haloperidol) and atypical agents (eg, risperidone) are of equal efficacy for treating positive symptoms. Atypical agents are often more effective for treating negative symptoms and cognitive dysfunction and have lower risk of tardive dyskinesia and hyperprolactinemia. Other indications for the use of selected antipsychotics include bipolar disorder, psychotic depression, Tourette's syndrome, disturbed behavior in patients with Alzheimer's disease and in the case of older drugs (eg, chlorpromazine), treatment of emesis and pruritus.

*Case Study Answer contributed by A.J. Trevor

Antidepressant Agents

Charles DeBattista, MD

CASE STUDY

A 47-year-old woman presents to her primary care physician with a chief complaint of fatigue. She indicates that she was promoted to senior manager in her company approximately 11 months earlier. Although her promotion was welcome and came with a sizable raise in pay, it resulted in her having to move away from an office and group of colleagues she very much enjoyed. In addition, her level of responsibility increased dramatically. The patient reports that for the last 7 weeks, she has been waking up at 3 AM every night and been unable to go back to sleep. She dreads the day and the stresses of the workplace. As a consequence, she is not eating as well as she might and has dropped 7% of her body weight in the last 3 months. She also reports being so stressed that she breaks down crying in the office occasionally and has been calling in sick frequently. When she comes home, she finds she is less motivated to attend to chores around the house and has no motivation, interest, or energy to pursue recreational activities that she once enjoyed such as hiking. She describes herself as "chronically miserable and worried all the time." Her medical history is notable for chronic neck pain from a motor vehicle accident for which she is being treated with tramadol and meperidine. In addition, she is on hydrochlorothiazide and propranolol for hypertension. The patient has a history of one depressive episode after a divorce that was treated successfully with fluoxetine. Medical workup including complete blood cell count, thyroid function tests, and a chemistry panel reveals no abnormalities. She is started on fluoxetine for a presumed major depressive episode and referred for cognitive behavioral psychotherapy. What CYP450 and pharmacodynamic interactions might be associated with fluoxetine use in this patient? Which class of antidepressants would be contraindicated in this patient?

The diagnosis of depression still rests primarily on the clinical interview. Major depressive disorder (MDD) is characterized by depressed mood most of the time for at least 2 weeks and/or loss of interest or pleasure in most activities. In addition, depression is characterized by disturbances in sleep and appetite as well as deficits in cognition and energy. Thoughts of guilt, worthlessness, and suicide are common. Coronary artery disease, diabetes, and stroke appear to be more common in depressed patients, and depression may considerably worsen the prognosis for patients with a variety of comorbid medical conditions.

According to a 2007 report by the Centers for Disease Control and Prevention, antidepressant drugs were the most commonly prescribed medications in the USA at the time of the survey. The wisdom of such widespread use of antidepressants is debated. However, it is clear that American physicians have been increasingly inclined to use antidepressants to treat a host of conditions and that patients have been increasingly receptive to their use.

The primary indication for antidepressant agents is the treatment of MDD. Major depression, with a lifetime prevalence of around 17% in the USA and a point prevalence of 5%, is associated with substantial morbidity and mortality. MDD represents one of the most common causes of disability in the developed world. In addition, major depression is commonly associated with a variety of medical conditions—from chronic pain to coronary artery disease. When depression coexists with other medical conditions, the patient's disease burden increases, and the quality of life—and often the prognosis for effective treatment—decreases significantly.

Some of the growth in antidepressant use may be related to the broad application of these agents for conditions other than major depression. For example, antidepressants have received Food and Drug Administration (FDA) approvals for the treatment of panic disorder, generalized anxiety disorder (GAD), posttraumatic stress disorder (PTSD), and obsessive-compulsive disorder (OCD). In addition, antidepressants are commonly used to treat pain disorders such as neuropathic pain and the pain associated with fibromyalgia. Some antidepressants are used for treating premenstrual dysphoric disorder (PMDD), mitigating the vasomotor symptoms of menopause, and treating stress urinary incontinence. Thus, antidepressants have a broad spectrum of use in medical practice. However, their primary use remains the treatment for MDD.

Pathophysiology of Major Depression

There has been a marked shift in the last decade in our understanding of the pathophysiology of major depression. In addition to the older idea that a deficit in function or amount of monoamines (the **monoamine hypothesis**) is central to the biology of depression, there is evidence that neurotrophic and endocrine factors play a major role (the **neurotrophic hypothesis**). Histologic studies, structural and functional brain imaging research, genetic

findings, and steroid research all suggest a complex pathophysiology for MDD with important implications for drug treatment.

Neurotrophic Hypothesis

There is substantial evidence that nerve growth factors such as **brain-derived neurotrophic factor (BDNF)** are critical in the regulation of neural plasticity, resilience, and neurogenesis. The evidence suggests that depression is associated with the loss of neurotrophic support and that effective antidepressant therapies increase neurogenesis and synaptic connectivity in cortical areas such as the hippocampus. BDNF is thought to exert its influence on neuronal survival and growth effects by activating the tyrosine kinase receptor B in both neurons and glia (Figure 30–1).

Several lines of evidence support the neurotrophic hypothesis. Animal and human studies indicate that stress and pain are associated with a drop in BDNF levels and that this loss of neurotrophic support contributes to atrophic structural changes in the hippocampus and perhaps other areas such as the medial frontal cortex and anterior cingulate. The hippocampus is known to be

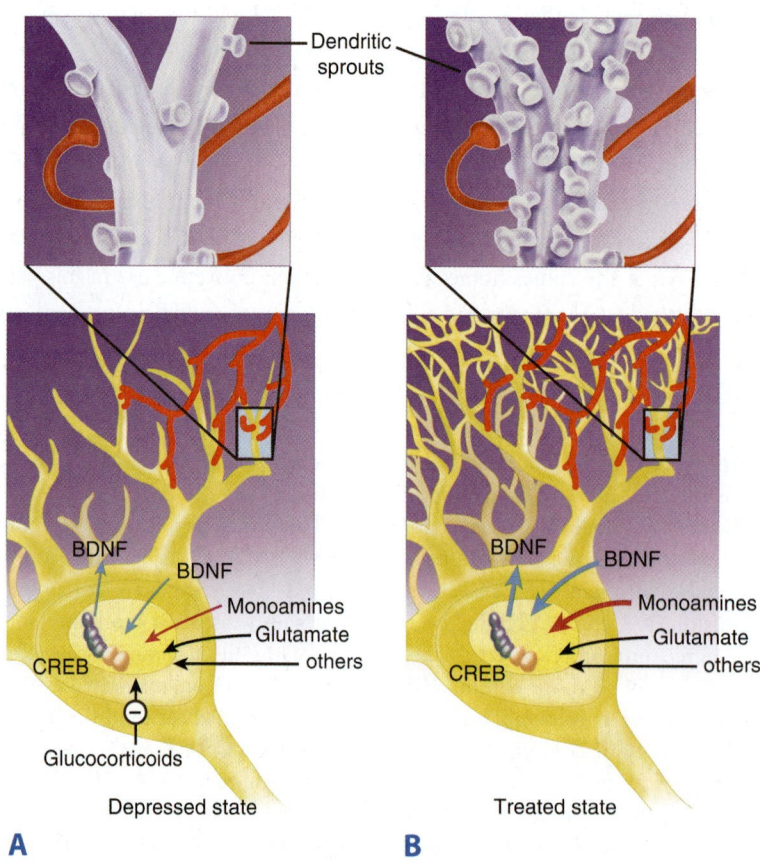

FIGURE 30–1 The neurotrophic hypothesis of major depression. Changes in trophic factors (especially brain-derived neurotrophic factor, BDNF) and hormones appear to play a major role in the development of major depression (**A**). Successful treatment results in changes in these factors (**B**). CREB, cAMP response element-binding (protein). BDNF, brain-derived neurotrophic factor. (Redrawn, with permission, from Nestler EJ: Neurobiology of depression. Neuron 2002;34[1]:13–25.)

important both in contextual memory and regulation of the hypothalamic-pituitary-adrenal (HPA) axis. Likewise, the anterior cingulate plays a role in the integration of emotional stimuli and attention functions, whereas the medial orbital frontal cortex is also thought to play a role in memory, learning, and emotion.

Over 30 structural imaging studies suggest that major depression is associated with a 5–10% loss of volume in the hippocampus, although some studies have not replicated this finding. Depression and chronic stress states have also been associated with a substantial loss of volume in the anterior cingulate and medial orbital frontal cortex. Loss of volume in structures such as the hippocampus also appears to increase as a function of the duration of illness and the amount of time that the depression remains untreated.

Another source of evidence supporting the neurotrophic hypothesis of depression comes from studies of the direct effects of BDNF on emotional regulation. Direct infusion of BDNF into the midbrain, hippocampus, and lateral ventricles of rodents has an antidepressant-like effect in animal models. Moreover, all known classes of antidepressants are associated with an increase in BDNF levels in animal models with chronic (but not acute) administration. This increase in BDNF levels is consistently associated with increased neurogenesis in the hippocampus in these animal models. Other interventions thought to be effective in the treatment of major depression, including electroconvulsive therapy, also appear to robustly stimulate BDNF levels and hippocampus neurogenesis in animal models.

Human studies seem to support the animal data on the role of neurotrophic factors in stress states. Depression appears to be associated with a drop in BDNF levels in the cerebrospinal fluid and serum as well as with a decrease in tyrosine kinase receptor B activity. Conversely, administration of antidepressants increases BDNF levels in clinical trials and may be associated with an increase in hippocampus volume in some patients.

Much evidence supports the neurotrophic hypothesis of depression, but not all evidence is consistent with this concept. Animal studies in BDNF knockout mice have not always suggested an increase in depressive or anxious behaviors that would be expected with a deficiency of BDNF. In addition, some animal studies have found an increase in BDNF levels after some types of social stress and an increase rather than a decrease in depressive behaviors with lateral ventricle injections of BDNF.

A proposed explanation for the discrepant findings on the role of neurotrophic factors in depression is that there are polymorphisms for BDNF that may yield very different effects. Mutations in the *BDNF* gene have been found to be associated with altered anxiety and depressive behavior in both animal and human studies.

Thus, the neurotrophic hypothesis continues to be intensely investigated and has yielded new insights and potential targets in the treatment of MDD.

Monoamines and Other Neurotransmitters

The monoamine hypothesis of depression (Figure 30–2) suggests that depression is related to a deficiency in the amount or function of cortical and limbic serotonin (5-HT), norepinephrine (NE), and dopamine (DA).

Evidence to support the monoamine hypothesis comes from several sources. It has been known for many years that reserpine treatment, which is known to deplete monoamines, is associated with depression in a subset of patients. Similarly, depressed patients who respond to serotonergic antidepressants such as fluoxetine often rapidly suffer relapse when given diets free of tryptophan, a precursor of serotonin synthesis. Patients who respond to noradrenergic antidepressants such as desipramine are less likely to relapse on a tryptophan-free diet. Moreover, depleting catecholamines in depressed patients who have previously responded to noradrenergic agents likewise tends to be associated with relapse. Administration of an inhibitor of norepinephrine synthesis is also associated with a rapid return of depressive symptoms in patients who respond to noradrenergic but not necessarily in patients who had responded to serotonergic antidepressants.

Another line of evidence supporting the monoamine hypothesis comes from genetic studies. A functional polymorphism exists for the promoter region of the serotonin transporter gene, which regulates how much of the transporter protein is available. Subjects who are homozygous for the s (short) allele may be more vulnerable to developing major depression and suicidal behavior in response to stress. In addition, homozygotes for the s allele may also be less likely to respond to and tolerate serotonergic antidepressants. Conversely, subjects with the l (long) allele tend to be more resistant to stress and may be more likely to respond to serotonergic antidepressants.

Studies of depressed patients have sometimes shown an alteration in monoamine function. For example, some studies have found evidence of alteration in serotonin receptor numbers ($5-HT_{1A}$ and $5-HT_{2C}$) or norepinephrine (α_2) receptors in depressed and suicidal patients, but these findings have not been consistent. A reduction in the primary serotonin metabolite 5-hydroxyindoleacetic acid in the cerebrospinal fluid is associated with violent and impulsive behavior, including violent suicide attempts. However, this finding is not specific to major depression and is associated more generally with violent and impulsive behavior.

Finally, perhaps the most convincing line of evidence supporting the monoamine hypothesis is the fact that (at the time of this writing) all available antidepressants appear to have significant effects on the monoamine system. All classes of antidepressants appear to enhance the synaptic availability of 5-HT, norepinephrine, or dopamine. Attempts to develop antidepressants that work on other neurotransmitter systems have not been effective to date.

The monoamine hypothesis, like the neurotrophic hypothesis, is at best incomplete. Many studies have not found an alteration in function or levels of monoamines in depressed patients. In addition, some candidate antidepressant agents under study do not act directly on the monoamine system. These include glutamate antagonists, melatonin agonists, and glucocorticoid-specific agents. Thus, monoamine function appears to be an important but not exclusive factor in the pathophysiology of depression.

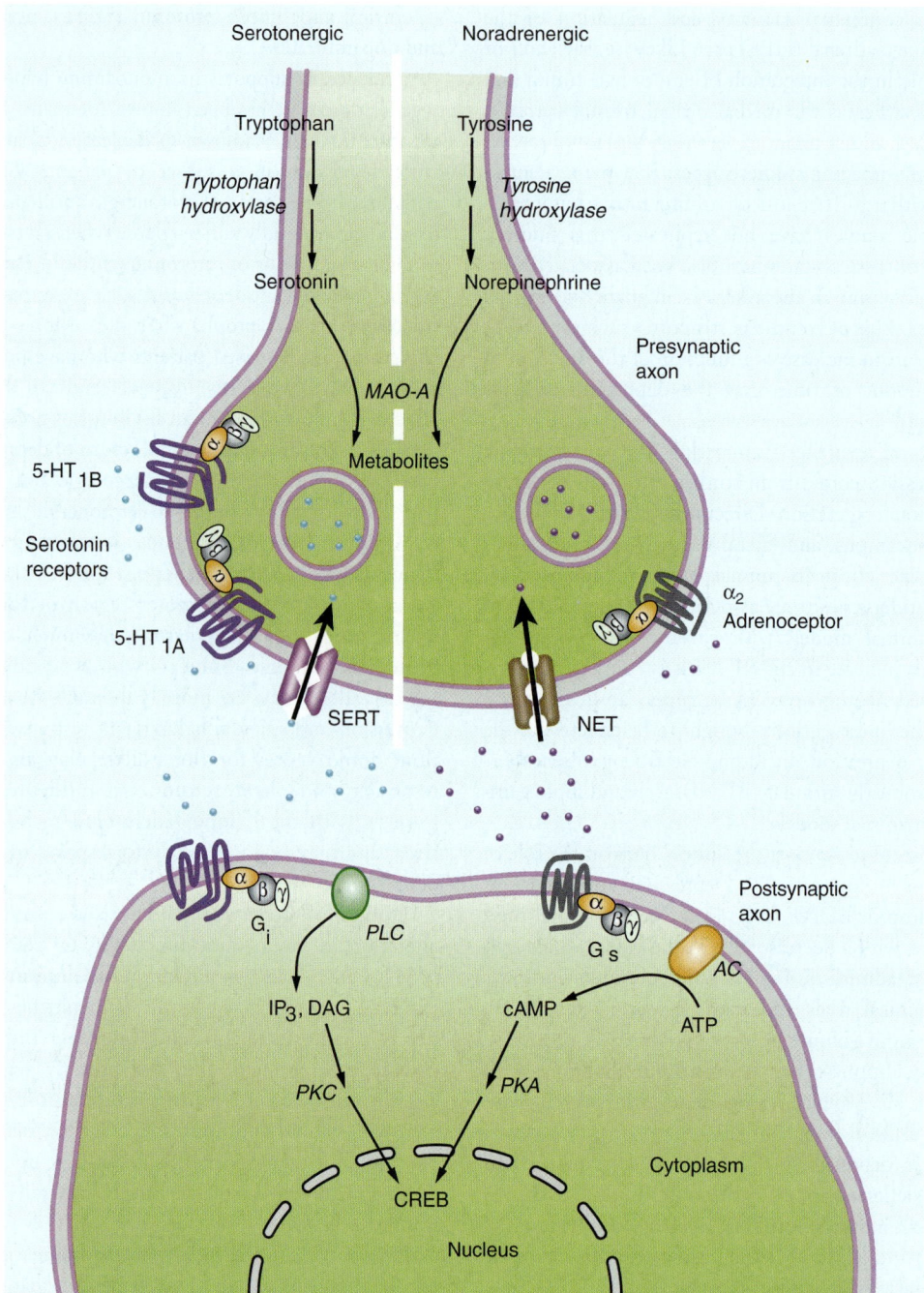

FIGURE 30–2 The amine hypothesis of major depression. Depression appears to be associated with changes in serotonin or norepinephrine signaling in the brain (or both) with significant downstream effects. Most antidepressants cause changes in amine signaling. AC, adenylyl cyclase; 5-HT, serotonin; CREB, cAMP response element-binding (protein); DAG, diacyl glycerol; IP_3, inositol trisphosphate; MAO, monoamine oxidase; NET, norepinephrine transporter; PKC, protein kinase C; PLC, phospholipase C; SERT, serotonin transporter. (Redrawn, with permission, from Belmaker R, Agam G: Major depressive disorder. N Engl J Med 2008;358:59.)

Neuroendocrine Factors in the Pathophysiology of Depression

Depression is known to be associated with a number of hormonal abnormalities. Among the most replicated of these findings are abnormalities in the HPA axis in patients with MDD. Moreover, MDD is associated with elevated cortisol levels (Figure 30–1),

nonsuppression of adrenocorticotropic hormone (ACTH) release in the dexamethasone suppression test, and chronically elevated levels of corticotropin-releasing hormone. The significance of these HPA abnormalities is unclear, but they are thought to indicate a dysregulation of the stress hormone axis. More severe types of depression, such as psychotic depression, tend to be associated with HPA abnormalities more commonly than milder forms of major depression. It is well known that both exogenous glucocorticoids and endogenous elevation of cortisol are associated with mood symptoms and cognitive deficits similar to those seen in MDD.

Thyroid dysregulation has also been reported in depressed patients. Up to 25% of depressed patients are reported to have abnormal thyroid function. These include a blunting of response of thyrotropin to thyrotropin-releasing hormone, and elevations in circulating thyroxine during depressed states. Clinical hypothyroidism often presents with depressive symptoms, which resolve with thyroid hormone supplementation. Thyroid hormones are also commonly used in conjunction with standard antidepressants to augment therapeutic effects of the latter.

Finally, sex steroids are also implicated in the pathophysiology of depression. Estrogen deficiency states, which occur in the postpartum and postmenopausal periods, are thought to play a role in the etiology of depression in some women. Likewise, severe testosterone deficiency in men is sometimes associated with depressive symptoms. Hormone replacement therapy in hypogonadal men and women may be associated with an improvement in mood and depressive symptoms.

Integration of Hypotheses Regarding the Pathophysiology of Depression

The several pathophysiologic hypotheses just described are not mutually exclusive. It is evident that the monoamine, neuroendocrine, and neurotrophic systems are interrelated in important ways. For example, HPA and steroid abnormalities may contribute to suppression of transcription of the *BDNF* gene. Glucocorticoid receptors are found in high density in the hippocampus. Binding of these hippocampal glucocorticoid receptors by cortisol during chronic stress states such as major depression may decrease BDNF synthesis and may result in volume loss in stress-sensitive regions such as the hippocampus. The chronic activation of monoamine receptors by antidepressants appears to have the opposite effect of stress and results in an increase in BDNF transcription. In addition, activation of monoamine receptors appears to down-regulate the HPA axis and may normalize HPA function.

One of the weaknesses of the monoamine hypothesis is the fact that amine levels increase immediately with antidepressant use, but maximum beneficial effects of antidepressants are not seen for many weeks. The time required to synthesize neurotrophic factors has been proposed as an explanation for this delay of antidepressant effects. Appreciable protein synthesis of products such as BDNF typically takes 2 weeks or longer and coincides with the clinical course of antidepressant treatment.

■ BASIC PHARMACOLOGY OF ANTIDEPRESSANTS

Chemistry & Subgroups

The currently available antidepressants make up a remarkable variety of chemical types. These differences and the differences in

their molecular targets provide the basis for distinguishing several subgroups.

A. Selective Serotonin Reuptake Inhibitors

The selective serotonin reuptake inhibitors (SSRIs) represent a chemically diverse class of agents that have as their primary action the inhibition of the serotonin transporter (SERT) (Figure 30–3). Fluoxetine was introduced in the United States in 1988 and quickly became one of the most commonly prescribed medications in medical practice. The development of fluoxetine emerged out of the search for chemicals that had high affinity for monoamine receptors but lacked the affinity for histamine, acetylcholine, and α adrenoceptors that is seen with the tricyclic antidepressants (TCAs). There are currently six available SSRIs, and they are the most common antidepressants in clinical use. In addition to their use in major depression, SSRIs have indications in GAD, PTSD, OCD, panic disorder, PMDD, and bulimia. **Fluoxetine, sertraline,** and **citalopram** exist as isomers and are formulated in the racemic forms, whereas **paroxetine** and **fluvoxamine** are not optically active. **Escitalopram** is the *S* enantiomer of citalopram. As with all antidepressants, SSRIs are highly lipophilic. The popularity of SSRIs stems largely from their ease of use, safety in overdose, relative tolerability, cost (all except escitalopram are generically available), and broad spectrum of uses.

B. Serotonin-Norepinephrine Reuptake Inhibitors

Two classes of antidepressants act as combined serotonin and norepinephrine reuptake inhibitors: selective **serotonin-norepinephrine reuptake inhibitors (SNRIs)** and **TCAs.**

1. Selective serotonin-norepinephrine reuptake inhibitors—The SNRIs include **venlafaxine,** its metabolite **desvenlafaxine,** and **duloxetine.** Another SNRI, **milnacipran,** has been approved for the treatment of fibromyalgia in the USA but has been studied extensively as an antidepressant. It has been available in Europe for several years. In addition to their use in major depression, other applications of the SNRIs include the treatment of pain disorders including neuropathies and fibromyalgia. SNRIs are also used in the treatment of generalized anxiety, stress urinary incontinence, and vasomotor symptoms of menopause.

R = CH₃ : **Venlafaxine**
R = H : **Desvenlafaxine**

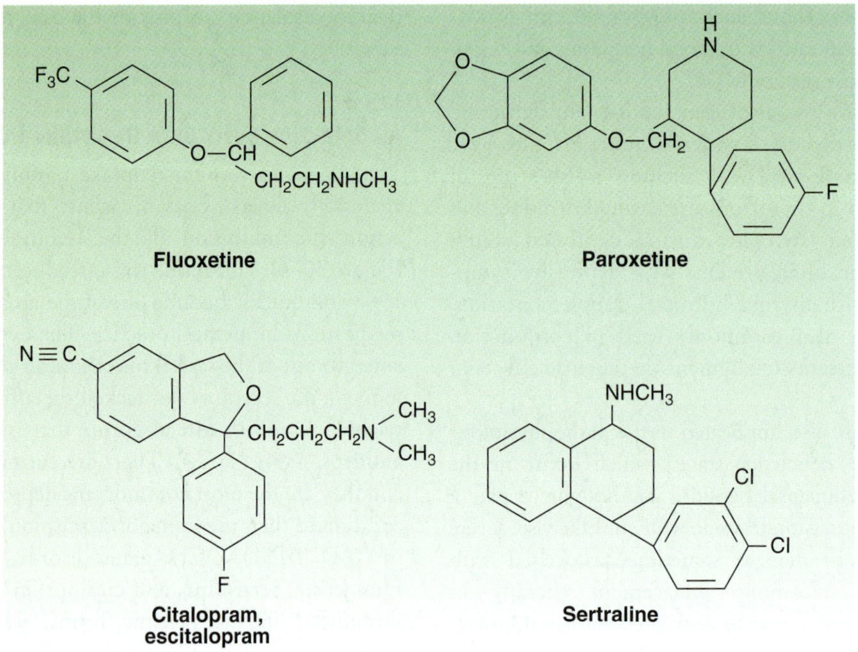

FIGURE 30–3 Structures of several selective serotonin reuptake inhibitors.

SNRIs are chemically unrelated to each other. Venlafaxine was discovered in the process of evaluating chemicals that inhibit binding of imipramine. Venlafaxine's in vivo effects are similar to those of imipramine but with a more favorable adverse-effect profile. All SNRIs bind the serotonin (SERT) and norepinephrine (NET) transporters, as do the TCAs. However, unlike the TCAs, the SNRIs do not have much affinity for other receptors. Venlafaxine and desvenlafaxine are bicyclic compounds, whereas duloxetine is a three-ring structure unrelated to the TCAs. Milnacipran contains a cyclopropane ring and is provided as a racemic mixture.

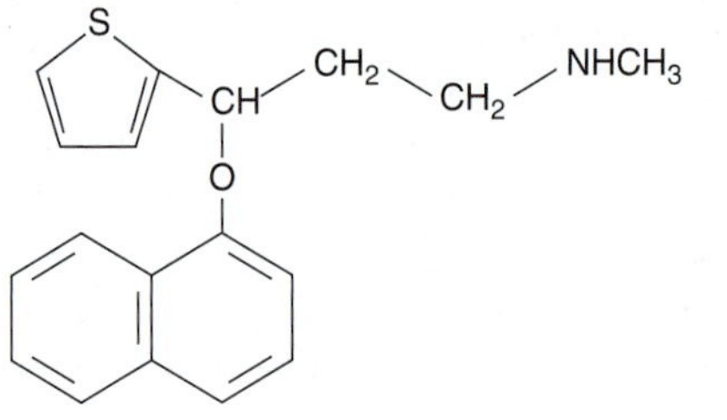

Duloxetine

2. Tricyclic antidepressants—The TCAs were the dominant class of antidepressants until the introduction of SSRIs in the 1980s and 1990s. Nine TCAs are available in the USA, and they all have an iminodibenzyl (tricyclic) core (Figure 30–4). The chemical differences between the TCAs are relatively subtle. For example, the prototype TCA **imipramine** and its metabolite, **desipramine,** differ by only a methyl group in the propylamine side chain. However, this minor difference results in a substantial change in their pharmacologic profiles. Imipramine is highly

anticholinergic and is a relatively strong serotonin as well as norepinephrine reuptake inhibitor. In contrast, desipramine is much less anticholinergic and is a more potent and somewhat more selective norepinephrine reuptake inhibitor than is imipramine.

At the present time, the TCAs are used primarily in depression that is unresponsive to more commonly used antidepressants such as the SSRIs or SNRIs. Their loss of popularity stems in large part from relatively poorer tolerability compared with newer agents, to difficulty of use, and to lethality in overdose. Other uses for TCAs include the treatment of pain conditions, enuresis, and insomnia.

C. 5-HT₂ Antagonists

Two antidepressants are thought to act primarily as antagonists at the 5-HT$_2$ receptor: **trazodone** and **nefazodone**. Trazodone's structure includes a triazolo moiety that is thought to impart antidepressant effects. Its primary metabolite, m-chlorophenylpiperazine (m-cpp), is a potent 5-HT$_2$ antagonist. Trazodone was among the most commonly prescribed antidepressants until it was supplanted by the SSRIs in the late 1980s. The most common use of trazodone in current practice is as an unlabeled hypnotic, since it is highly sedating and not associated with tolerance or dependence.

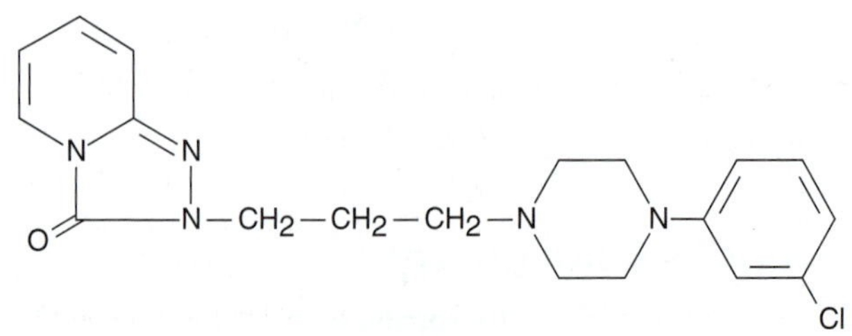

Trazodone

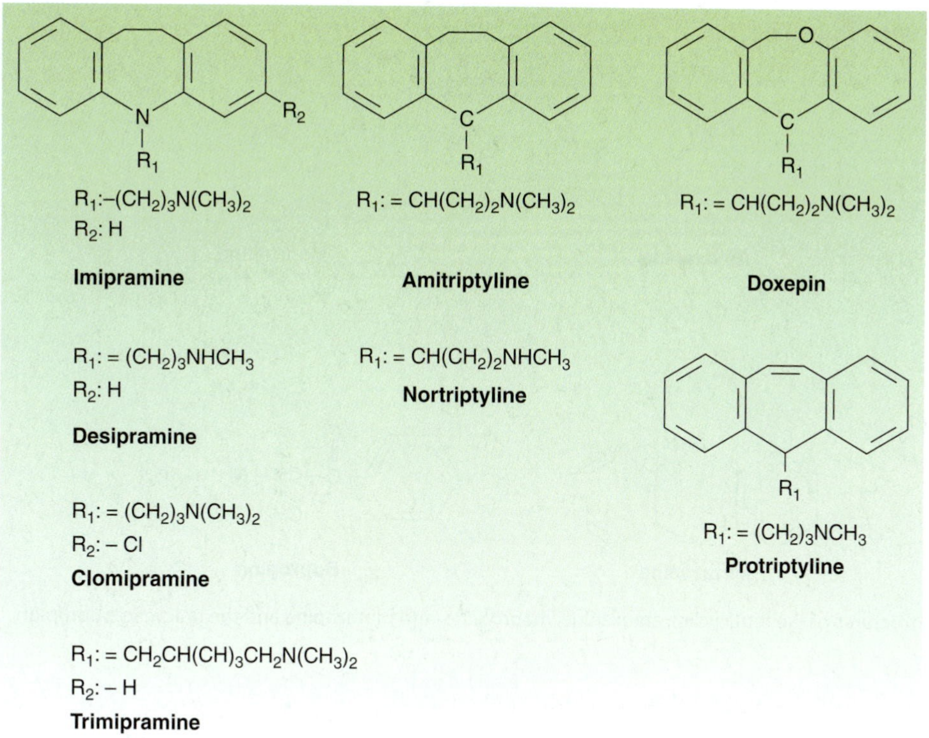

FIGURE 30–4 Structures of the tricyclic antidepressants (TCAs).

Nefazodone is chemically related to trazodone. Its primary metabolites, hydroxynefazodone and m-cpp are both inhibitors of the 5-HT$_2$ receptor. Nefazodone received an FDA black box warning in 2001 implicating it in hepatotoxicity, including lethal cases of hepatic failure. Though still available generically, nefazodone is no longer commonly prescribed. The primary indications for both nefazodone and trazodone are major depression, although both have also been used in the treatment of anxiety disorders.

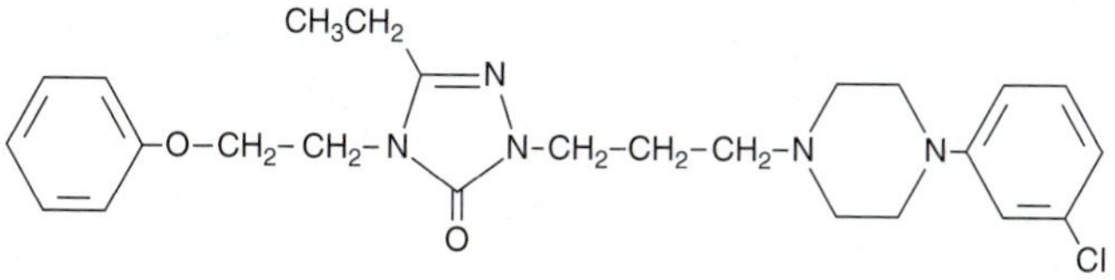

Nefazodone

D. Tetracyclic and Unicyclic Antidepressants

A number of antidepressants do not fit neatly into the other classes. Among these are **bupropion, mirtazapine, amoxapine,** and **maprotiline** (Figure 30–5). Bupropion has a unicyclic aminoketone structure. Its unique structure results in a different side-effect profile than most antidepressants (described below). Bupropion somewhat resembles amphetamine in chemical structure and, like the stimulant, has central nervous system (CNS) activating properties.

Mirtazapine was introduced in 1994 and, like bupropion, is one of the few antidepressants not commonly associated with sexual side effects. It has a tetracyclic chemical structure and belongs to the piperazino-azepine group of compounds.

Mirtazapine, amoxapine, and maprotiline have tetracyclic structures. Amoxapine is the N-methylated metabolite of loxapine, an older antipsychotic drug. Amoxapine and maprotiline share structural similarities and side effects comparable to the TCAs. As a result, these tetracyclics are not commonly prescribed in current practice. Their primary use is in MDD that is unresponsive to other agents.

E. Monoamine Oxidase Inhibitors

Arguably the first modern class of antidepressants, monoamine oxidase inhibitors (MAOIs) were introduced in the 1950s but are now rarely used in clinical practice because of toxicity and potentially lethal food and drug interactions. Their primary use now is in the treatment of depression unresponsive to other antidepressants. However, MAOIs have also been used historically to treat anxiety states, including social anxiety and panic disorder. In addition, selegiline is used for the treatment of Parkinson's disease (see Chapter 28).

Current MAOIs include the hydrazine derivatives **phenelzine** and **isocarboxazid** and the non-hydrazines **tranylcypromine, selegiline,** and **moclobemide** (the latter is not available in the USA). The hydrazines and tranylcypromine bind irreversibly and nonselectively with MAO-A and -B, whereas other MAOIs may have more selective or reversible properties. Some of the MAOIs

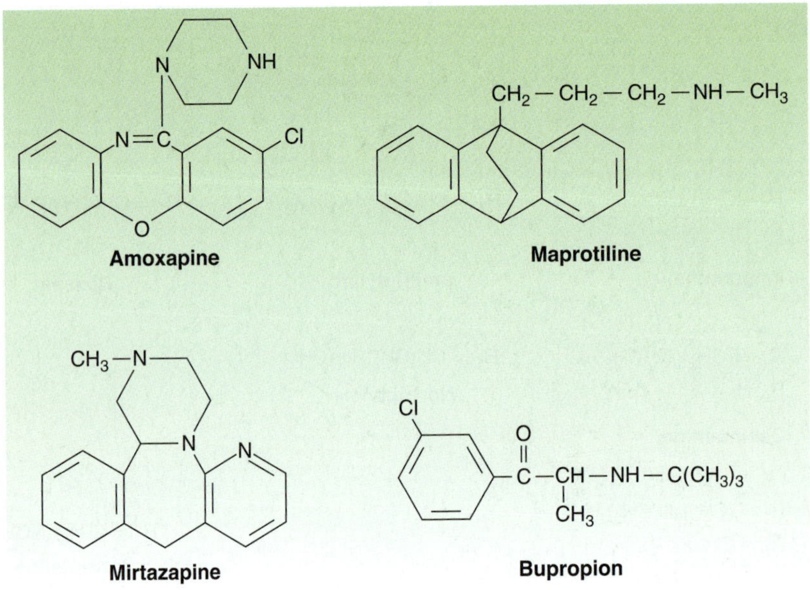

FIGURE 30–5 Structures of the tetracyclics, amoxapine, maprotiline, and mirtazapine and the unicyclic, bupropion.

such as tranylcypromine resemble amphetamine in chemical structure, whereas other MAOIs such as selegiline have amphetamine-like metabolites. As a result, these MAOIs tend to have substantial CNS-stimulating effects.

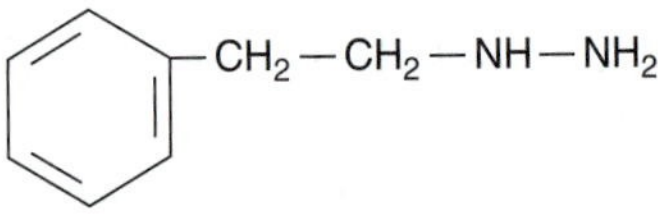

Phenelzine

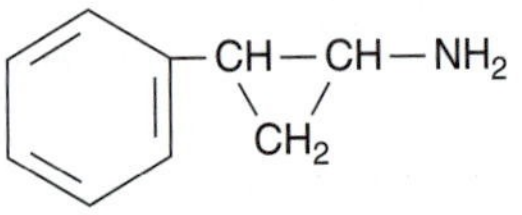

Tranylcypromine

Pharmacokinetics

The antidepressants share several pharmacokinetic features (Table 30–1). Most have fairly rapid oral absorption, achieve peak plasma levels within 2–3 hours, are tightly bound to plasma proteins, undergo hepatic metabolism, and are renally cleared. However, even within classes, the pharmacokinetics of individual antidepressants varies considerably.

A. Selective Serotonin Reuptake Inhibitors

The prototype SSRI, fluoxetine, differs from other SSRIs in some important respects (Table 30–1). Fluoxetine is metabolized to an active product, norfluoxetine, which may have plasma concentrations greater than those of fluoxetine. The elimination half-life of norfluoxetine is about three times longer than fluoxetine and contributes to the longest half-life of all the SSRIs. As a result,

fluoxetine has to be discontinued 4 weeks or longer before an MAOI can be administered to mitigate the risk of serotonin syndrome.

Fluoxetine and paroxetine are potent inhibitors of the CYP2D6 isoenzyme, and this contributes to potential drug interactions (see Drug Interactions). In contrast, fluvoxamine is an inhibitor of CYP3A4, whereas citalopram, escitalopram, and sertraline have more modest CYP interactions.

B. Serotonin-Norepinephrine Reuptake Inhibitors

1. Selective serotonin-norepinephrine reuptake inhibitors—Venlafaxine is extensively metabolized in the liver via the CYP2D6 isoenzyme to *O*-desmethylvenlafaxine (desvenlafaxine). Both have similar half-lives of about 11 hours. Despite the relatively short half-lives, both drugs are available in formulations that allow once-daily dosing. Venlafaxine and desvenlafaxine have the lowest protein binding of all antidepressants (27–30%). Unlike most antidepressants, desvenlafaxine is conjugated and does not undergo extensive oxidative metabolism. At least 45% of desvenlafaxine is excreted unchanged in the urine compared with 4–8% of venlafaxine.

Duloxetine is well absorbed and has a half-life of about 12 hours but is dosed once daily. It is tightly bound to protein (97%) and undergoes extensive oxidative metabolism via CYP2D6 and CYP1A2. Hepatic impairment significantly alters duloxetine levels unlike desvenlafaxine.

2. Tricyclic antidepressants—The TCAs tend to be well absorbed and have long half-lives (Table 30–1). As a result, most are dosed once daily at night because of their sedating effects. TCAs undergo extensive metabolism via demethylation, aromatic hydroxylation, and glucuronide conjugation. Only about 5% of TCAs are excreted unchanged in the urine. The TCAs are

TABLE 30–1 Pharmacokinetic profiles of selected antidepressants.

Class, Drug	Bioavailability (%)	Plasma $t_{1/2}$ (hours)	Active Metabolite $t_{1/2}$ (hours)	Volume of Distribution (L/kg)	Protein Binding (%)
SSRIs					
Citalopram	80	33–38	ND	15	80
Escitalopram	80	27–32	ND	12–15	80
Fluoxetine	70	48–72	180	12–97	95
Fluvoxamine	90	14–18	14–16	25	80
Paroxetine	50	20–23	ND	28–31	94
Sertraline	45	22–27	62–104	20	98
SNRIs					
Duloxetine	50	12–15	ND	10–14	90
Milnacipran	85–90	6–8	ND	5–6	13
Venlafaxine[1]	45	8–11	9–13	4–10	27
Tricyclics					
Amitriptyline	45	31–46	20–92	5–10	90
Clomipramine	50	19–37	54–77	7–20	97
Imipramine	40	9–24	14–62	15–30	84
5-HT$_2$ antagonists					
Nefazodone	20	2–4	ND	0.5–1	99
Trazodone	95	3–6	ND	1–3	96
Tetracyclics and unicyclic					
Amoxapine	ND	7–12	5–30	0.9–1.2	90
Bupropion	70	11–14	15–25	20–30	84
Maprotiline	70	43–45	ND	23–27	88
Mirtazapine	50	20–40	20–40	3–7	85
MAOIs					
Phenelzine	ND	11	ND	ND	ND
Selegiline	4	8–10	9–11	8–10	99

[1]Desvenlafaxine has similar properties but is less completely metabolized.

MAOIs, monoamine oxidase inhibitors; ND, no data found; SNRIs, serotonin-norepinephrine reuptake inhibitors; SSRIs, selective serotonin reuptake inhibitors.

substrates of the CYP2D6 system, and the serum levels of these agents tend to be substantially influenced by concurrent administration of drugs such as fluoxetine. In addition, genetic polymorphism for CYP2D6 may result in low or extensive metabolism of the TCAs.

The secondary amine TCAs, including desipramine and nortriptyline, lack active metabolites and have fairly linear kinetics. These TCAs have a wide therapeutic window, and serum levels are reliable in predicting response and toxicity.

C. 5-HT$_2$ Antagonists

Trazodone and nefazodone are rapidly absorbed and undergo extensive hepatic metabolism. Both drugs are extensively bound to protein and have limited bioavailability because of extensive metabolism. Their short half-lives generally require split dosing when used as antidepressants. However, trazodone is often prescribed as a single dose at night as a hypnotic in lower doses than are used in the treatment of depression. Both trazodone and nefazodone have active metabolites that also exhibit 5-HT$_2$ antagonism. Nefazodone is a potent inhibitor of the CYP3A4 system and may interact with drugs metabolized by this enzyme (see Drug Interactions).

D. Tetracyclic and Unicyclic Agents

Bupropion is rapidly absorbed and has a mean protein binding of 85%. It undergoes extensive hepatic metabolism and has a substantial first-pass effect. It has three active metabolites including hydroxybupropion; the latter is being developed as an antidepressant. Bupropion has a biphasic elimination with the first phase lasting about 1 hour and the second phase lasting 14 hours.

Amoxapine is also rapidly absorbed with protein binding of about 85%. The half-life is variable, and the drug is often given in divided doses. Amoxapine undergoes extensive hepatic metabolism. One of the active metabolites, 7-hydroxyamoxapine, is a potent D_2 blocker and is associated with antipsychotic effects. Maprotiline is similarly well absorbed orally and 88% bound to protein. It undergoes extensive hepatic metabolism.

Mirtazapine is demethylated followed by hydroxylation and glucuronide conjugation. Several CYP isozymes are involved in the metabolism of mirtazapine, including 2D6, 3A4, and 1A2. The half-life of mirtazapine is 20–40 hours, and it is usually dosed once in the evening because of its sedating effects.

E. Monoamine Oxidase Inhibitors

The different MAOIs are metabolized via different pathways but tend to have extensive first-pass effects that may substantially decrease bioavailability. Tranylcypromine is ring hydroxylated and N-acetylated, whereas acetylation appears to be a minor pathway for phenelzine. Selegiline is N-demethylated and then hydroxylated. The MAOIs are well absorbed from the gastrointestinal tract.

Because of the prominent first-pass effects and their tendency to inhibit MAO in the gut (resulting in tyramine pressor effects), alternative routes of administration are being developed. For example, selegiline is available in both transdermal and sublingual forms that bypass both gut and liver. These routes decrease the risk of food interactions and provide substantially increased bioavailability.

Pharmacodynamics

As previously noted, all currently available antidepressants enhance monoamine neurotransmission by one of several mechanisms. The most common mechanism is inhibition of the activity of SERT, NET, or both monoamine transporters (Table 30–2). Antidepressants that inhibit SERT, NET, or both include the SSRIs and SNRIs (by definition), and the TCAs. Another mechanism for increasing the availability of monoamines is inhibition of their enzymatic degradation (the MAOIs). Additional strategies for enhancing monoamine tone include binding presynaptic autoreceptors (mirtazapine) or specific postsynaptic receptors (5-HT$_2$ antagonists and mirtazapine). Ultimately, the increased availability of monoamines for binding in the synaptic cleft results in a cascade of events that enhance the transcription of some proteins and the inhibition of others. It is the net production of these proteins, including BDNF, glucocorticoid receptors, β adrenoceptors, and other proteins, that appears to determine the benefits as well as the toxicity of a given agent.

TABLE 30–2 Antidepressant effects on several receptors and transporters.

Antidepressant	ACh M	α₁	H₁	5-HT₂	NET	SERT
Amitriptyline	+++	+++	++	0/+	+	++
Amoxapine	+	++	+	+++	++	+
Bupropion	0	0	0	0	0/+	0
Citalopram, escitalopram	0	0	0		0	+++
Clomipramine	+	++	+	+	+	+++
Desipramine	+	+	+	0/+	+++	+
Doxepin	++	+++	+++	0/+	+	+
Fluoxetine	0	0	0	0/+	0	+++
Fluvoxamine	0	0	0	0	0	+++
Imipramine	++	+	+	0/+	+	++
Maprotiline	+	+	++	0/+	++	0
Mirtazapine	0	0	+++	+	+	0
Nefazodone	0	+	0	++	0/+	+
Nortriptyline	+	+	+	+	++	+
Paroxetine	+	0	0	0	+	+++
Protriptyline	+++	+	+	+	+++	+
Sertraline	0	0	0	0	0	+++
Trazodone	0	++	0/+	++	0	+
Trimipramine	++	++	+++	0/+	0	0
Venlafaxine	0	0	0	0	+	++

ACh M, acetylcholine muscarinic receptor; α₁, alpha₁-adrenoceptor; H₁, histamine₁ receptor; 5-HT₂, serotonin 5-HT₂ receptor; NET, norepinephrine transporter; SERT, serotonin transporter.

0/+, minimal affinity; +, mild affinity; ++, moderate affinity; +++, high affinity.

A. Selective Serotonin Reuptake Inhibitors

The serotonin transporter (SERT) is a glycoprotein with 12 transmembrane regions embedded in the axon terminal and cell body membranes of serotonergic neurons. When extracellular serotonin binds to receptors on the transporter, conformational changes occur in the transporter and serotonin, Na^+, and Cl^- are moved into the cell. Binding of intracellular K^+ then results in return of the transporter to its original conformation and the release of serotonin inside the cell. SSRIs allosterically inhibit the transporter by binding the receptor at a site other than active binding site for serotonin. At therapeutic doses, about 80% of the activity of the transporter is inhibited. Functional polymorphisms exist for SERT that determine the activity of the transporter.

SSRIs have modest effects on other neurotransmitters. Unlike TCAs and SNRIs, there is little evidence that SSRIs have prominent effects on β adrenoceptors or the norepinephrine transporter, NET. Binding to the serotonin transporter is associated with tonic inhibition of the dopamine system, although there is substantial interindividual variability in this effect. The SSRIs do not bind aggressively to histamine, muscarinic, or other receptors.

B. Drugs That Block Both Serotonin and Norepinephrine Transporters

A large number of antidepressants have mixed inhibitory effects on both serotonin and norepinephrine transporters. The newer agents in this class (venlafaxine and duloxetine) are denoted by the acronym SNRIs, whereas the agents in the older group are termed TCAs.

1. Serotonin-norepinephrine reuptake inhibitors—SNRIs
bind both the serotonin and the norepinephrine transporters. The NET is structurally very similar to the 5-HT transporter. Like the serotonin transporter, it is a 12-transmembrane domain complex that allosterically binds norepinephrine. The NET also has a moderate affinity for dopamine.

Venlafaxine is a weak inhibitor of NET, whereas desvenlafaxine, duloxetine, and milnacipran are more balanced inhibitors of both SERT and NET. Nonetheless, the affinity of most SNRIs tends to be much greater for SERT than for NET. The SNRIs differ from the TCAs in that they lack the potent antihistamine, α-adrenergic blocking, and anticholinergic effects of the TCAs. As a result, the SNRIs tend to be favored over the TCAs in the treatment of MDD and pain syndromes because of their better tolerability.

2. Tricyclic antidepressants—The TCAs resemble the SNRIs
in function, and their antidepressant activity is thought to relate primarily to their inhibition of 5-HT and norepinephrine reuptake. Within the TCAs, there is considerable variability in affinity for SERT versus NET. For example, clomipramine has relatively very little affinity for NET but potently binds SERT. This selectivity for the serotonin transporter contributes to clomipramine's known benefits in the treatment of OCD. On the other hand, the secondary amine TCAs, desipramine and nortriptyline, are relatively more selective for NET. Although the tertiary amine TCA imipramine has more serotonin effects initially, its metabolite, desipramine, then balances this effect with more NET inhibition.

Common adverse effects of the TCAs, including dry mouth and constipation, are attributable to the potent antimuscarinic effects of many of these drugs. The TCAs also tend to be potent antagonists of the histamine H_1 receptor. TCAs such as doxepin are sometimes prescribed as hypnotics and used in treatments for pruritus because of their antihistamine properties. The blockade of α adrenoceptors can result in substantial orthostatic hypotension, particularly in older patients.

C. 5-HT$_2$ Antagonists

The principle action of both nefazodone and trazodone appears to be blockade of the $5\text{-}HT_{2A}$ receptor. Inhibition of this receptor in both animal and human studies is associated with substantial antianxiety, antipsychotic, and antidepressant effects. Conversely, agonists of the $5\text{-}HT_{2A}$ receptor, eg, lysergic acid (LSD) and mescaline, are often hallucinogenic and anxiogenic. The $5\text{-}HT_{2A}$ receptor is a G protein-coupled receptor and is distributed throughout the neocortex.

Nefazodone is a weak inhibitor of both SERT and NET but is a potent antagonist of the postsynaptic $5\text{-}HT_{2A}$ receptor, as are its metabolites. Trazodone is also a weak but selective inhibitor of SERT with little effect on NET. Its primary metabolite, m-cpp, is a potent $5\text{-}HT_2$ antagonist, and much of trazodone's benefits as an antidepressant might be attributed to this effect. Trazodone also has weak-to-moderate presynaptic α-adrenergic–blocking properties and is a modest antagonist of the H_1 receptor.

D. Tetracyclic and Unicyclic Antidepressants

The actions of bupropion remain poorly understood. Bupropion and its major metabolite hydroxybupropion are modest-to-moderate inhibitors of norepinephrine and dopamine reuptake in animal studies. However, these effects seem less than are typically associated with antidepressant benefit. A more significant effect of bupropion is presynaptic release of catecholamines. In animal studies, bupropion appears to substantially increase the presynaptic availability of norepinephrine, and dopamine to a lesser extent. Bupropion has virtually no direct effects on the serotonin system.

Mirtazapine has a complex pharmacology. It is an antagonist of the presynaptic α_2 autoreceptor and enhances the release of both norepinephrine and 5-HT. In addition, mirtazapine is an antagonist of $5\text{-}HT_2$ and $5\text{-}HT_3$ receptors. Finally, mirtazapine is a potent H_1 antagonist, which is associated with the drug's sedative effects.

The actions of amoxapine and maprotiline resemble those of TCAs such as desipramine. Both are potent NET inhibitors and less potent SERT inhibitors. In addition, both possess anticholinergic properties. Unlike the TCAs or other antidepressants, amoxapine is a moderate inhibitor of the postsynaptic D_2 receptor. As such, amoxapine possesses some antipsychotic properties.

E. Monoamine Oxidase Inhibitors

MAOIs act by mitigating the actions of monoamine oxidase in the neuron and increasing monoamine content. There are two forms of monoamine oxidase. MAO-A is present in both dopamine and norepinephrine neurons and is found primarily in the brain, gut, placenta, and liver; its primary substrates are norepinephrine,

epinephrine, and serotonin. MAO-B is found primarily in serotonergic and histaminergic neurons and is distributed in the brain, liver, and platelets. MAO-B acts primarily on tyramine, phenylethylamine, and benzylamine. Both MAO-A and -B metabolize tryptamine and dopamine.

MAOIs are classified by their specificity for MAO-A or -B and whether their effects are reversible or irreversible. Phenelzine and tranylcypromine are examples of irreversible, nonselective MAOIs. Moclobemide is a reversible and selective inhibitor of MAO-A but is not available in the USA. Moclobemide can be displaced from MAO-A by tyramine, and this mitigates the risk of food interactions. In contrast, selegiline is an irreversible MAO-B–specific agent at low doses. Selegiline is useful in the treatment of Parkinson's disease at these low doses, but at higher doses it becomes a nonselective MAOI similar to other agents.

■ CLINICAL PHARMACOLOGY OF ANTIDEPRESSANTS

Clinical Indications

A. Depression

The FDA indication for the use of the antidepressants in the treatment of major depression is fairly broad. Most antidepressants are approved for both acute and long-term treatment of major depression. Acute episodes of MDD tend to last about 6–14 months untreated, but at least 20% of episodes last 2 years or longer.

The goal of acute treatment of MDD is remission of all symptoms. Since antidepressants may not achieve their maximum benefit for 1–2 months or longer, it is not unusual for a trial of therapy to last 8–12 weeks at therapeutic doses. The antidepressants are successful in achieving remission in about 30–40% of patients within a single trial of 8–12 weeks. If an inadequate response is obtained, therapy is often switched to another agent or augmented by addition of another drug. For example, bupropion, an atypical antipsychotic, or mirtazapine might be added to an SSRI or SNRI to augment antidepressant benefit if monotherapy is unsuccessful. Seventy to eighty percent of patients are able to achieve remission with sequenced augmentation or switching strategies. Once an adequate response is achieved, continuation therapy is recommended for a minimum of 6–12 months to reduce the substantial risk of relapse.

Approximately 85% of patients who have a single episode of MDD will have at least one recurrence in a lifetime. Many patients have multiple recurrences, and these recurrences may progress to more serious, chronic, and treatment-resistant episodes. Thus, it is not unusual for patients to require maintenance treatment to prevent recurrences. Although maintenance treatment studies of more than 5 years are uncommon, long-term studies with TCAs, SNRIs, and SSRIs suggest a significant protective benefit when given chronically. Thus, it is commonly recommended that patients be considered for long-term maintenance treatment if they have had two or more serious MDD episodes in the previous 5 years or three or more serious episodes in a lifetime.

It is not clear whether antidepressants are useful for all subtypes of depression. For example, patients with bipolar depression may not benefit much from antidepressants even when added to mood stabilizers. In fact, the antidepressants are sometimes associated with switches into mania or more rapid cycling. There has also been some debate about the overall efficacy of antidepressants in unipolar depression, with some meta-analyses showing large effects and others showing more modest effects. Although this debate is not likely to be settled immediately, there is little debate that antidepressants have important benefits for most patients.

Psychotherapeutic interventions such as cognitive behavior therapy appear to be as effective as antidepressant treatment for mild to moderate forms of depression. However, cognitive behavior therapy tends to take longer to be effective and is generally more expensive than antidepressant treatment. Psychotherapy is often combined with antidepressant treatment, and the combination appears more effective than either strategy alone.

B. Anxiety Disorders

After major depression, anxiety disorders represent the most common application of antidepressants. A number of SSRIs and SNRIs have been approved for all the major anxiety disorders, including PTSD, OCD, social anxiety disorder, GAD, and panic disorder. Panic disorder is characterized by recurrent episodes of brief overwhelming anxiety, which often occur without precipitant. Patients may begin to fear having an attack, or they avoid situations in which they might have an attack. In contrast, GAD is characterized by a chronic, free-floating anxiety and undue worry that tends to be chronic in nature. Although older antidepressants and drugs of the sedative-hypnotic class are still occasionally used for the treatment of anxiety disorders, SSRIs and SNRIs have largely replaced them.

The benzodiazepines (see Chapter 22) provide much more rapid relief of both generalized anxiety and panic than do any of the antidepressants. However, the antidepressants appear to be at least as effective and perhaps more effective than benzodiazepines in the long-term treatment of these anxiety disorders. Furthermore, antidepressants do not carry the risks of dependence and tolerance that may occur with the benzodiazepines.

OCD is known to respond to serotonergic antidepressants. It is characterized by repetitive anxiety-provoking thoughts (obsessions) or repetitive behaviors aimed at reducing anxiety (compulsions). Clomipramine and several of the SSRIs are approved for the treatment of OCD, and they are moderately effective. Behavior therapy is usually combined with the antidepressant for additional benefits.

Social anxiety disorder is an uncommonly diagnosed but a fairly common condition in which the patient experiences severe anxiety in social interactions. This anxiety may limit their ability to function adequately in their jobs or interpersonal relationships. Several SSRIs and venlafaxine are approved for the treatment of social anxiety. The efficacy of the SSRIs in the treatment of social anxiety is greater in some studies than their efficacy in the treatment of MDD.

PTSD is manifested when a traumatic or life-threatening event results in intrusive anxiety-provoking thoughts or imagery, hypervigilance, nightmares, and avoidance of situations that remind the patient of the trauma. SSRIs are considered first-line treatment for PTSD and can benefit a number of symptoms including anxious thoughts and hypervigilance. Other treatments, including psychotherapeutic interventions, are usually required in addition to antidepressants.

C. Pain Disorders

It has been known for over 40 years that antidepressants possess analgesic properties independent of their mood effects. TCAs have been used in the treatment of neuropathic and other pain conditions since the 1960s. Medications that possess both norepinephrine and 5-HT reuptake blocking properties are often useful in treating pain disorders. Ascending corticospinal monoamine pathways appear to be important in the endogenous analgesic system. In addition, chronic pain conditions are commonly associated with major depression. TCAs continue to be commonly used for some of these conditions, and SNRIs are increasingly used. In 2010, duloxetine was approved for the treatment of chronic joint and muscle pain. As mentioned earlier, milnacipran has been approved for the treatment of fibromyalgia. Other SNRIs, eg, desvenlafaxine, are being investigated for a variety of pain conditions from postherpetic neuralgia to chronic back pain.

D. Premenstrual Dysphoric Disorder

Approximately 5% of women in the child-bearing years will have prominent mood and physical symptoms during the late luteal phase of almost every cycle; these may include anxiety, depressed mood, irritability, insomnia, fatigue, and a variety of other physical symptoms. These symptoms are more severe than those typically seen in premenstrual syndrome (PMS) and can be quite disruptive to vocational and interpersonal activities. The SSRIs are known to be beneficial to many women with PMDD, and fluoxetine and sertraline have been approved for this indication. Treating for 2 weeks out of the month in the luteal phase may be as effective as continuous treatment. The rapid effects of SSRIs in PMDD may be associated with rapid increases in pregnenolone levels.

E. Smoking Cessation

Bupropion was approved in 1997 as a treatment for smoking cessation. Approximately twice as many people treated with bupropion as with placebo have a reduced urge to smoke. In addition, patients taking bupropion appear to experience fewer mood symptoms and possibly less weight gain while withdrawing from nicotine dependence. Bupropion appears to be about as effective as nicotine patches in smoking cessation. The mechanism by which bupropion is helpful in this application is unknown, but the drug may mimic nicotine's effects on dopamine and norepinephrine and may antagonize nicotinic receptors. Nicotine is also known to have antidepressant effects in some people, and bupropion may substitute for this effect.

Other antidepressants may also have a role in the treatment of smoking cessation. Nortriptyline has been shown to be helpful in smoking cessation, but the effects have not been as consistent as those seen with bupropion.

F. Eating Disorders

Bulimia nervosa and anorexia nervosa are potentially devastating disorders. Bulimia is characterized by episodic intake of large amounts of food (binges) followed by ritualistic purging through emesis, the use of laxatives, or other methods. Medical complications of the purging, such as hypokalemia, are common and dangerous. Anorexia is a disorder in which reduced food intake results in a loss of weight of 15% or more of ideal body weight, and the person has a morbid fear of gaining weight and a highly distorted body image. Anorexia is often chronic and may be fatal in 10% or more of cases.

Antidepressants appear to be helpful in the treatment of bulimia but not anorexia. Fluoxetine was approved for the treatment of bulimia in 1996, and other antidepressants have shown benefit in reducing the binge-purge cycle. The primary treatment for anorexia at this time is refeeding, family therapy, and cognitive behavioral therapy.

Bupropion may have some benefits in treating obesity. Nondepressed, obese patients treated with bupropion were able to lose somewhat more weight and maintain the loss relative to a similar population treated with placebo. However, the weight loss was not robust, and there appear to be more effective options for weight loss.

G. Other Uses for Antidepressants

Antidepressants are used for many other on- and off-label applications. Enuresis in children is an older labeled use for some TCAs, but they are less commonly used now because of their side effects. The SNRI duloxetine is approved in Europe for the treatment of urinary stress incontinence. Many of the serotonergic antidepressants appear to be helpful for treating vasomotor symptoms in perimenopause. Desvenlafaxine is under consideration for FDA approval for the treatment of these vasomotor symptoms, and studies have suggested that SSRIs, venlafaxine, and nefazodone may also provide benefit. Although serotonergic antidepressants are commonly associated with inducing sexual adverse effects, some of these effects might prove useful for some sexual disorders. For example, SSRIs are known to delay orgasm in some patients. For this reason, SSRIs are sometimes used to treat premature ejaculation. In addition, bupropion has been used to treat sexual adverse effects associated with SSRI use, although its efficacy for this use has not been consistently demonstrated in controlled trials.

Choosing an Antidepressant

The choice of an antidepressant depends first on the indication. Not all conditions are equally responsive to all antidepressants. However, in the treatment of MDD, it is difficult to demonstrate that one antidepressant is consistently more effective than another.

Thus, the choice of an antidepressant for the treatment of depression rests primarily on practical considerations such as cost, availability, adverse effects, potential drug interactions, the patient's history of response or lack thereof, and patient preference. Other factors such as the patient's age, gender, and medical status may also guide antidepressant selection. For example, older patients are particularly sensitive to the anticholinergic effects of the TCAs. On the other hand, the CYP3A4-inhibiting effects of the SSRI fluvoxamine may make this a problematic choice in some older patients because fluvoxamine may interact with many other medications that an older patient may require. There is some suggestion that female patients may respond to and tolerate serotonergic better than noradrenergic or TCA antidepressants, but the data supporting this gender difference have not been consistent. Patients with narrow-angle glaucoma may have an exacerbation with noradrenergic antidepressants, whereas bupropion and other antidepressants are known to lower the seizure threshold in epilepsy patients.

At present, SSRIs are the most commonly prescribed first-line agents in the treatment of both MDD and anxiety disorders. Their popularity comes from their ease of use, tolerability, and safety in overdose. The starting dose of the SSRIs is usually the same as the therapeutic dose for most patients, and so titration may not be required. In addition, most SSRIs are now generically available and inexpensive. Other agents, including the SNRIs, bupropion, and mirtazapine, are also reasonable first-line agents for the treatment of MDD. Bupropion, mirtazapine, and nefazodone are the antidepressants with the least association with sexual side effects and are often prescribed for this reason. However, bupropion is not thought to be effective in the treatment of the anxiety disorders and may be poorly tolerated in anxious patients. The primary indication for bupropion is in the treatment of major depression, including seasonal (winter) depression. Off-label uses of bupropion include the treatment of attention deficit hyperkinetic disorder (ADHD), and bupropion is commonly combined with other antidepressants to augment therapeutic response. The primary indication for mirtazapine is in the treatment of major depression. However, its strong antihistamine properties have contributed to its occasional use as a hypnotic and as an adjunctive treatment to more activating antidepressants.

The TCAs and MAOIs are now relegated to second- or third-line treatments for MDD. Both the TCAs and the MAOIs are potentially lethal in overdose, require titration to achieve a therapeutic dose, have serious drug interactions, and have many troublesome adverse effects. As a consequence, their use in the treatment of MDD or anxiety is now reserved for patients who have been unresponsive to other agents. Clearly, there are patients whose depression responds only to MAOIs or TCAs. Thus, TCAs and MAOIs are probably underused in treatment-resistant depressed patients.

The use of antidepressants outside the treatment of MDD tends to require specific agents. For example, the TCAs and SNRIs appear to be useful in the treatment of pain conditions, but other antidepressant classes appear to be far less effective. SSRIs and the highly serotonergic TCA, clomipramine, are effective in the treatment of OCD, but noradrenergic antidepressants have not proved to be as helpful for this condition. Bupropion and nortriptyline have usefulness in the treatment of smoking cessation, but SSRIs have not been proven useful. Thus, outside the treatment of depression, the choice of antidepressant is primarily dependent on the known benefit of a particular antidepressant or class for a particular indication.

Dosing

The optimal dose of an antidepressant depends on the indication and on the patient. For SSRIs, SNRIs, and a number of newer agents, the starting dose for the treatment of depression is usually a therapeutic dose (Table 30–3). Patients who show little or no benefit after at least 4 weeks of treatment may benefit from a higher dose even though it has been difficult to show a clear advantage for higher doses with SSRIs, SNRIs, and other newer antidepressants. The dose is generally titrated to the maximum dosage recommended or to the highest dosage tolerated if the patient is not responsive to lower doses. Some patients may benefit from doses lower than the usual minimum recommended therapeutic dose. TCAs and MAOIs typically require titration to a therapeutic dosage over several weeks. Dosing of the TCAs may be guided by monitoring TCA serum levels.

Some anxiety disorders may require higher doses of antidepressants than are used in the treatment of major depression. For example, patients treated for OCD often require maximum or somewhat higher than maximum recommended MDD doses to achieve optimal benefits. Likewise, the minimum dose of paroxetine for the effective treatment of panic disorder is higher than the minimum dose required for the effective treatment of depression.

In the treatment of pain disorders, modest doses of TCAs are often sufficient. For example, 25–50 mg/d of imipramine might be beneficial in the treatment of pain associated with a neuropathy, but this would be a subtherapeutic dose in the treatment of MDD. In contrast, SNRIs are usually prescribed in pain disorders at the same doses used in the treatment of depression.

Adverse Effects

Although some potential adverse effects are common to all antidepressants, most of their adverse effects are specific to a subclass of agents and to their pharmacodynamic effects. An FDA warning applied to all antidepressants is the risk of increased suicidality in patients under the age 25. The warning suggests that use of antidepressants is associated with suicidal ideation and gestures, but not completed suicides, in up to 4% of patients under 25 years who were prescribed antidepressant in clinical trials. This rate is about twice the rate seen with placebo treatment. For those over 25, there is either no increased risk or a reduced risk of suicidal thoughts and gestures on antidepressants, particularly after age 65. Although a small minority of patients may experience a treatment-emergent increase in suicidal ideation with antidepressants, the absence of treatment of a major depressive episode in all age groups is a particularly important risk factor in completed suicides.

TABLE 30–3 Antidepressant dose ranges.

Drug	Usual Therapeutic Dosage (mg/d)
SSRIs	
Citalopram	20–60
Escitalopram	10–30
Fluoxetine	20–60
Fluvoxamine	100–300
Paroxetine	20–60
Sertraline	50–200
SNRIs	
Venlafaxine	75–375
Desvenlafaxine	50–200
Duloxetine	40–120
Milnacipran	100–200
Tricyclics	
Amitriptyline	150–300
Clomipramine	100–250
Desipramine	150–300
Doxepin	150–300
Imipramine	150–300
Nortriptyline	50–150
Protriptyline	15–60
Trimipramine maleate	150–300
5-HT$_2$ antagonists	
Nefazodone	300–500
Trazodone	150–300
Tetracyclics and unicyclics	
Amoxapine	150–400
Bupropion	200–450
Maprotiline	150–225
Mirtazapine	15–45
MAOIs	
Isocarboxazid	30–60
Phenelzine	45–90
Selegiline	20–50
Tranylcypromine	30–60

MAOIs, monoamine oxidase inhibitors; SNRIs, serotonin-norepinephrine reuptake inhibitors; SSRIs, selective serotonin reuptake inhibitors.

A. Selective Serotonin Reuptake Inhibitors

The adverse effects of the most commonly prescribed antidepressants—the SSRIs—can be predicted from their potent inhibition of SERT. SSRIs enhance serotonergic tone, not just in the brain but throughout the body. Increased serotonergic activity in the gut is commonly associated with nausea, gastrointestinal upset, diarrhea, and other gastrointestinal symptoms. Gastrointestinal adverse effects usually emerge early in the course of treatment and tend to improve after the first week. Increasing serotonergic tone at the level of the spinal cord and above is associated with diminished sexual function and interest. As a result, at least 30–40% of patients treated with SSRIs report loss of libido, delayed orgasm, or diminished arousal. The sexual effects often persist as long as the patient remains on the antidepressant but may diminish with time.

Other adverse effects related to the serotonergic effects of SSRIs include an increase in headaches and insomnia or hypersomnia. Some patients gain weight while taking SSRIs, particularly paroxetine. Sudden discontinuation of short half-life SSRIs such as paroxetine and sertraline is associated with a *discontinuation syndrome* in some patients characterized by dizziness, paresthesias, and other symptoms beginning 1 or 2 days after stopping the drug and persisting for 1 week or longer.

Most antidepressants are category C agents by the FDA teratogen classification system. There is an association of paroxetine with cardiac septal defects in first trimester exposures. Thus, paroxetine is a category D agent. Other possible associations of SSRIs with post-birth complications, including pulmonary hypertension, have not been clearly established.

B. Serotonin-Norepinephrine Reuptake Inhibitors and Tricyclic Antidepressants

SNRIs have many of the serotonergic adverse effects associated with SSRIs. In addition, SNRIs may also have noradrenergic effects, including increased blood pressure and heart rate, and CNS activation, such as insomnia, anxiety, and agitation. The hemodynamic effects of SNRIs tend not to be problematic in most patients. A dose-related increase in blood pressure has been seen more commonly with the immediate-release form of venlafaxine than with other SNRIs. Likewise, there are more reports of cardiac toxicity with venlafaxine overdose than with either the other SNRIs or SSRIs. Duloxetine is rarely associated with hepatic toxicity in patients with a history of liver damage. All the SNRIs have been associated with a discontinuation syndrome resembling that seen with SSRI discontinuation.

The primary adverse effects of TCAs have been described in the previous text. Anticholinergic effects are perhaps the most common. These effects result in dry mouth, constipation, urinary retention, blurred vision, and confusion. They are more common with tertiary amine TCAs such as amitriptyline and imipramine than with the secondary amine TCAs desipramine and nortriptyline. The potent α-blocking property of TCAs often results in orthostatic hypotension. H$_1$ antagonism by the TCAs is associated with weight gain and sedation. The TCAs are class 1A antiarrhythmic agents (see Chapter 14) and are arrhythmogenic at higher doses. Sexual effects are common, particularly with highly serotonergic TCAs such as clomipramine. The TCAs have a prominent discontinuation syndrome characterized by cholinergic rebound and flulike symptoms.

C. 5-HT₂ Antagonists

The most common adverse effects associated with the 5-HT$_2$ antagonists are sedation and gastrointestinal disturbances. Sedative effects, particularly with trazodone, can be quite pronounced. Thus, it is not surprising that the treatment of insomnia is currently the primary application of trazodone. The gastrointestinal effects appear to be dose-related and are less pronounced than those seen with SNRIs or SSRIs. Sexual effects are uncommon with nefazodone or trazodone treatment as a result of the relatively selective serotonergic effects of these drugs on the 5-HT$_2$ receptor rather than on SERT. However, trazodone has rarely been associated with inducing priapism. Both nefazodone and trazodone are α-blocking agents and may result in a dose-related orthostatic hypotension in some patients. Nefazodone has been associated with hepatotoxicity, including rare fatalities and cases of fulminant hepatic failure requiring transplantation. The rate of serious hepatotoxicity with nefazodone has been estimated at 1 in 250,000 to 1 in 300,000 patient-years of nefazodone treatment.

D. Tetracyclics and Unicyclics

Amoxapine is sometimes associated with a parkinsonian syndrome due to its D$_2$-blocking action. Mirtazapine has significant sedative effect. Maprotiline has a moderately high affinity for NET and may cause TCA-like adverse effects and, rarely, seizures. Bupropion is occasionally associated with agitation, insomnia, and anorexia.

E. Monoamine Oxidase Inhibitors

The most common adverse effects of the MAOIs leading to discontinuation of these drugs are orthostatic hypotension and weight gain. In addition, the irreversible nonselective MAOIs are associated with the highest rates of sexual effects of all the antidepressants. Anorgasmia is fairly common with therapeutic doses of some MAOIs. The amphetamine-like properties of some MAOIs contributes to activation, insomnia, and restlessness in some patients. Phenelzine tends to be more sedating than either selegiline or tranylcypromine. Confusion is also sometimes associated with higher doses of MAOIs. Because they block metabolism of tyramine and similar ingested amines, MAOIs may cause dangerous interactions with certain foods and with serotonergic drugs (see Interactions). Finally, MAOIs have been associated with a sudden discontinuation syndrome manifested in a delirium-like presentation with psychosis, excitement, and confusion.

Overdose

Suicide attempts are a common and unfortunate consequence of major depression. The lifetime risk of completing suicide in patients previously hospitalized with MDD may be as high as 15%. Overdose is the most common method used in suicide attempts, and antidepressants, especially the TCAs, are frequently involved. Overdose can induce lethal arrhythmias, including ventricular tachycardia and fibrillation. In addition, blood pressure changes and anticholinergic effects including altered mental status and seizures are sometimes seen in TCA overdoses. A 1500 mg dose of imipramine or amitriptyline (less than 7 days' supply at antidepressant doses) is enough to be lethal in many patients.

Toddlers taking 100 mg will likely show evidence of toxicity. Treatment typically involves cardiac monitoring, airway support, and gastric lavage. Sodium bicarbonate is often administered to uncouple the TCA from cardiac sodium channels.

An overdose with an MAOI can produce a variety of effects including autonomic instability, hyperadrenergic symptoms, psychotic symptoms, confusion, delirium, fever, and seizures. Management of MAOI overdoses usually involves cardiac monitoring, vital signs support, and lavage.

Compared with TCAs and MAOIs, the other antidepressants are generally much safer in overdose. Fatalities with SSRI overdose alone are extremely uncommon. Similarly, SNRIs tend to be much safer in overdose than the TCAs. However, venlafaxine has been associated with some cardiac toxicity in overdose and appears to be less safe than SSRIs. Bupropion is associated with seizures in overdose, and mirtazapine may be associated with sedation, disorientation, and tachycardia. With the newer agents, fatal overdoses often involve the combination of the antidepressant with other drugs, including alcohol. Management of overdose with the newer antidepressants usually involves emptying of gastric contents and vital sign support as the initial intervention.

Drug Interactions

Antidepressants are commonly prescribed with other psychotropic and nonpsychotropic agents. There is potential for drug interactions with all antidepressants, but the most serious of these involve the MAOIs and to a lesser extent the TCAs.

A. Selective Serotonin Reuptake Inhibitors

The most common interactions with SSRIs are pharmacokinetic interactions. For example, paroxetine and fluoxetine are potent CYP2D6 inhibitors (Table 30–4). Thus, administration with 2D6 substrates such as TCAs can lead to dramatic and sometimes unpredictable elevations in the tricyclic drug concentration. The result may be toxicity from the TCA. Similarly, fluvoxamine, a CYP3A4 inhibitor, may elevate the levels of concurrently administered substrates for this enzyme such as diltiazem and induce bradycardia or hypotension. Other SSRIs, such as citalopram and escitalopram, are relatively free of pharmacokinetic interactions. The most serious interaction with the SSRIs are pharmacodynamic interactions with MAOIs that produce a serotonin syndrome (see below).

B. Selective Serotonin-Norepinephrine Reuptake Inhibitors and Tricyclic Antidepressants

The SNRIs have relatively fewer CYP450 interactions than the SSRIs. Venlafaxine is a substrate but not an inhibitor of CYP2D6 or other isoenzymes, whereas desvenlafaxine is a minor substrate for CYP3A4. Duloxetine is a moderate inhibitor of CYP2D6 and so may elevate TCA and levels of other CYP2D6 substrates. Like all serotonergic antidepressants, SNRIs are contraindicated in combination with MAOIs.

Elevations of TCA levels may occur when combined with CYP2D6 inhibitors or from constitutional factors. About 7% of the Caucasian population in the USA has a CYP2D6

TABLE 30–4 Some antidepressant–CYP450 drug interactions.

Enzyme	Substrates	Inhibitors	Inducers
1A2	Tertiary amine tricyclic antidepressants (TCAs), duloxetine, theophylline, phenacetin, TCAs (demethylation), clozapine, diazepam, caffeine	Fluvoxamine, fluoxetine, moclobemide, ramelteon	Tobacco, omeprazole
2C19	TCAs, citalopram (partly), warfarin, tolbutamide, phenytoin, diazepam	Fluoxetine, fluvoxamine, sertraline, imipramine, ketoconazole, omeprazole	Rifampin
2D6	TCAs, benztropine, perphenazine, clozapine, haloperidol, codeine/oxycodone, risperidone, class Ic antiarrhythmics, β blockers, trazodone, paroxetine, maprotiline, amoxapine, duloxetine, mirtazapine (partly), venlafaxine, bupropion	Fluoxetine, paroxetine, duloxetine, hydroxybupropion, methadone, cimetidine, haloperidol, quinidine, ritonavir	Phenobarbital, rifampin
3A4	Citalopram, escitalopram, TCAs, glucocorticoids, androgens/estrogens, carbamazepine, erythromycin, Ca^{2+} channel blockers, protease inhibitors, sildenafil, alprazolam, triazolam, vincristine/vinblastine, tamoxifen, zolpidem	Fluvoxamine, nefazodone, sertraline, fluoxetine, cimetidine, fluconazole, erythromycin, protease inhibitors, ketoconazole, verapamil	Barbiturates, glucocorticoids, rifampin, modafinil, carbamazepine

polymorphism that is associated with slow metabolism of TCAs and other 2D6 substrates. Combination of a known CYP2D6 inhibitor and a TCA in a patient who is a slow metabolizer may result in additive effects. Such an interaction has been implicated, though rarely, in cases of TCA toxicity. There may also be additive TCA effects such as anticholinergic or antihistamine effects when combined with other agents that share these properties such as benztropine or diphenhydramine. Similarly, antihypertensive drugs may exacerbate the orthostatic hypotension induced by TCAs.

C. 5-HT₂ Antagonists

Nefazodone is an inhibitor of the CYP3A4 isoenzyme, so it can raise the level and thus exacerbate adverse effects of many 3A4-dependent drugs. For example, triazolam levels are increased by concurrent administration of nefazodone such that a reduction in triazolam dosage by 75% is recommended. Likewise, administration of nefazodone with simvastatin has been associated with 20-fold increase in plasma levels of simvastatin.

Trazodone is a substrate but not a potent inhibitor of CYP3A4. As a result, combining trazodone with potent inhibitors of CYP3A4, such as ritonavir or ketoconazole, may lead to substantial increases in trazodone levels.

D. Tetracyclic and Unicyclic Antidepressants

Bupropion is metabolized primarily by CYP2B6, and its metabolism may be altered by drugs such as cyclophosphamide, which is a substrate of 2B6. The major metabolite of bupropion, hydroxybupropion, is a moderate inhibitor of CYP2D6 and so can raise desipramine levels. Bupropion should be avoided in patients taking MAOIs.

Mirtazapine is a substrate for several CYP450 enzymes including 2D6, 3A4, and 1A2. Consequently, drugs that inhibit these isozymes may raise mirtazapine levels. However, mirtazapine is not an inhibitor of these enzymes. The sedating effects of mirtazapine may be additive with those of CNS depressants such as alcohol and benzodiazepines.

Amoxapine and maprotiline share most drug interactions common to the TCA group. Both are CYP2D6 substrates and should

be used with caution in combination with inhibitors such as fluoxetine. Amoxapine and maprotiline also both have anticholinergic and antihistaminic properties that may be additive with drugs that share a similar profile.

E. Monoamine Oxidase Inhibitors

MAOIs are associated with two classes of serious drug interactions. The first of these is the pharmacodynamic interaction of MAOIs with serotonergic agents including SSRIs, SNRIs, and most TCAs along with some analgesic agents such as meperidine. These combinations of an MAOI with a serotonergic agent may result in a life-threatening **serotonin syndrome** (see Chapter 16). The serotonin syndrome is thought to be caused by overstimulation of 5-HT receptors in the central gray nuclei and the medulla. Symptoms range from mild to lethal and include a triad of cognitive (delirium, coma), autonomic (hypertension, tachycardia, diaphoreses), and somatic (myoclonus, hyperreflexia, tremor) effects. Most serotonergic antidepressants should be discontinued at least 2 weeks before starting an MAOI. Fluoxetine, because of its long half-life, should be discontinued for 4–5 weeks before an MAOI is initiated. Conversely, an MAOI must be discontinued for at least 2 weeks before starting a serotonergic agent.

The second serious interaction with MAOIs occurs when an MAOI is combined with tyramine in the diet or with sympathomimetic substrates of MAO. An MAOI prevents the breakdown of tyramine in the gut, and this results in high serum levels that enhance peripheral noradrenergic effects, including raising blood pressure dramatically. Patients on an MAOI who ingest large amounts of dietary tyramine may experience malignant hypertension and subsequently a stroke or myocardial infarction. Thus, patients taking MAOIs require a low-tyramine diet and should avoid foods such as aged cheeses, tap beer, soy products, and dried sausages, which contain high amounts of tyramine (see Chapter 9). Similar sympathomimetics also may cause significant hypertension when combined with MAOIs. Thus, over-the-counter cold preparations that contain pseudoephedrine and phenylpropanolamine are contraindicated in patients taking MAOIs.

SUMMARY Antidepressants

Subclass	Mechanism of Action	Effects	Clinical Applications	Pharmacokinetics, Toxicities, Interactions
SELECTIVE SEROTONIN REUPTAKE INHIBITORS (SSRIs)				
• Fluoxetine • Citalopram • Escitalopram • Paroxetine • Sertraline	Highly selective blockade of serotonin transporter (SERT) • little effect on norepinephrine transporter (NET)	Acute increase of serotonergic synaptic activity • slower changes in several signaling pathways and neurotrophic activity	Major depression, anxiety disorders • panic disorder • obsessive-compulsive disorder • post-traumatic stress disorder • perimenopausal vasomotor symptoms • eating disorder (bulimia)	Half-lives from 15–75 h • oral activity • *Toxicity:* Well tolerated but cause sexual dysfunction • risk of serotonin syndrome with MAOIs • *Interactions:* Some CYP inhibition (fluoxetine 2D6, 3A4; fluvoxamine 1A2; paroxetine 2D6)
• *Fluvoxamine:* Similar to above but approved only for obsessive-compulsive behavior				
SEROTONIN-NOREPINEPHRINE REUPTAKE INHIBITORS (SNRIs)				
• Duloxetine • Venlafaxine	Moderately selective blockade of NET and SERT	Acute increase in serotonergic and adrenergic synaptic activity • otherwise like SSRIs	Major depression, chronic pain disorders • fibromyalgia, perimenopausal symptoms	*Toxicity:* Anticholinergic, sedation, hypertension (venlafaxine) • *Interactions:* Some CYP2D6 inhibition (duloxetine, desvenlafaxine)
• *Desvenlafaxine:* Desmethyl metabolite of venlafaxine, metabolism is by phase II rather than CYP phase I • *Milnacipran:* Significantly more selective for NET than SERT; little effect on DAT				
TRICYCLIC ANTIDEPRESSANTS (TCAs)				
• Imipramine • Many others	Mixed and variable blockade of NET and SERT	Like SNRIs plus significant blockade of autonomic nervous system and histamine receptors	Major depression not responsive to other drugs • chronic pain disorders • incontinence • obsessive-compulsive disorder (clomipramine)	Long half-lives • CYP substrates • active metabolites • *Toxicity:* Anticholinergic, α-blocking effects, sedation, weight gain, arrhythmias, and seizures in overdose • *Interactions:* CYP inducers and inhibitors
5-HT$_2$ ANTAGONISTS				
• Nefazodone • Trazodone	Inhibition of 5-HT$_{2A}$ receptor • nefazodone also blocks SERT weakly	Trazodone forms a metabolite (m-cpp) that blocks 5-HT$_{2A,2C}$ receptors	Major depression • sedation and hypnosis (trazodone)	Relatively short half-lives • active metabolites • *Toxicity:* Modest α- and H$_1$-receptor blockade (trazodone) • *Interactions:* Nefazodone inhibits CYP3A4
TETRACYCLICS, UNICYCLIC				
• Bupropion • Amoxapine • Maprotiline • Mirtazapine	Increased norepinephrine and dopamine activity (bupropion) • NET > SERT inhibition (amoxapine, maprotiline) • increased release of norepinephrine, 5-HT (mirtazapine)	Presynaptic release of catecholamines but no effect on 5-HT (bupropion) • amoxapine and maprotiline resemble TCAs	Major depression • smoking cessation (bupropion) • sedation (mirtazapine) • amoxapine and maprotiline rarely used	Extensive metabolism in liver • *Toxicity:* Lowers seizure threshold (amoxapine, bupropion); sedation and weight gain (mirtazepine) • *Interactions:* CYP2D6 inhibitor (bupropion)
MONOAMINE OXIDASE INHIBITORS (MAOIs)				
• Phenelzine • Tranylcypromine • Selegiline	Blockade of MAO-A and MAO-B (phenelzine, nonselective) • MAO-B irreversible selective MAO-B inhibition (low-dose selegiline)	Transdermal absorption of selegiline achieves levels that inhibit MAO-A	Major depression unresponsive to other drugs	Very slow elimination • *Toxicity:* Hypotension, insomnia • *Interactions:* Hypertensive crisis with tyramine, other indirect sympathomimetics • serotonin syndrome with serotonergic agents, meperidine

PREPARATIONS AVAILABLE

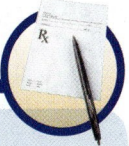

SELECTIVE SEROTONIN REUPTAKE INHIBITORS

Citalopram (generic, Celexa)
Oral: 10, 20, 40 mg tablets; 10 mg/5 mL solution

Escitalopram (Lexapro)
Oral: 5, 10, 20 mg tablets; 5 mg/5 mL solution

Fluoxetine (generic, Prozac)
Oral: 10, 20, 40 mg capsules; 10, 20 mg tablets; 20 mg/5 mL liquid
Oral delayed-release (Prozac Weekly): 90 mg capsules

Fluvoxamine (generic, labeled only for obsessive-compulsive disorder)
Oral: 25, 50, 100 mg tablets

Paroxetine (generic, Paxil)
Oral: 10, 20, 30, 40 mg tablets; 10 mg/5 mL suspension; 12.5, 25, 37.5 mg controlled-release tablets

Sertraline (generic, Zoloft)
Oral: 25, 50, 100 mg tablets; 20 mg/mL oral concentrate

Vilazodone (Viibryd)
Oral: 10, 20, 40 mg tablets

SELECTIVE NOREPINEPHRINE REUPTAKE INHIBITORS

Desvenlafaxine (Pristiq)
Oral: 50, 100 mg capsules

Duloxetine (Cymbalta)
Oral: 20, 30, 50 mg capsules

Milnacipran (Savella; labeled only for fibromyalgia)
Oral: 12.5, 25, 50, 100 mg tablets

Venlafaxine (Effexor)
Oral: 25, 37.5, 50, 75, 100 mg tablets; 37.5, 75, 150 mg extended-release capsules

5-HT$_2$ ANTAGONISTS

Nefazodone (generic)
Oral: 50, 100, 150, 200, 250 mg tablets

Trazodone (generic, Desyrel)
Oral: 50, 100, 150, 300 mg tablets

TRICYCLICS

Amitriptyline (generic, Elavil)
Oral: 10, 25, 50, 75, 100, 150 mg tablets
Parenteral: 10 mg/mL for IM injection

Amoxapine (generic)
Oral: 25, 50, 100, 150 mg tablets

Clomipramine (generic, Anafranil; labeled only for obsessive-compulsive disorder)
Oral: 25, 50, 75 mg capsules

Desipramine (generic, Norpramin)
Oral: 10, 25, 50, 75, 100, 150 mg tablets

Doxepin (generic, Sinequan)
Oral: 10, 25, 50, 75, 100, 150 mg capsules; 10 mg/mL concentrate

Imipramine (generic, Tofranil)
Oral: 10, 25, 50 mg tablets (as hydrochloride); 75, 100, 125, 150 mg capsules (as pamoate)

Nortriptyline (generic, Pamelor)
Oral: 10, 25, 50, 75 mg capsules; 2 mg/mL solution

Protriptyline (generic, Vivactil)
Oral: 5, 10 mg tablets

Trimipramine (Surmontil)
Oral: 25, 50, 100 mg capsules

TETRACYCLIC AND UNICYCLIC AGENTS

Amoxipine (generic)
Oral: 25, 50, 100, 150 mg tablets

Bupropion (generic, Wellbutrin)
Oral: 75, 100 mg tablets; 100, 150, 200 mg 12-hour sustained-release tablets; 150, 300 mg 24-hour sustained-release tablets
Oral: 25, 50, 75 mg tablets

Maprotiline (generic)
Oral: 7.5, 15, 30, 45 mg tablets; 15, 30, 45 mg oral disintegrating tablets

Mirtazapine (generic, Remeron)
Oral: 7.5, 15, 30, 45 mg tablets; 15, 30, 45 mg disintegrating tablets

MONOAMINE OXIDASE INHIBITORS

Isocarboxazid (generic, Marplan)
Oral: 10 mg tablets

Phenelzine (generic, Nardil)
Oral: 15 mg tablets

Selegiline
Oral (generic, Eldepryl): 5 mg tablets, capsules; 1.25 oral disintegrating tablets

Tranylcypromine (generic, Parnate)
Oral: 10 mg tablets

REFERENCES

Alessandro S, Kato M: The serotonin transporter gene and effectiveness of SSRIs. Expert Rev Neurother 2008;8(1):111.

Bab I, Yirmiya R: Depression, selective serotonin reuptake inhibitors, and osteoporosis. Curr Osteoporos Rep 2010;8:185.

Barrera AZ, Torres LD, Munoz RF: Prevention of depression: The state of the science at the beginning of the 21st century. Int Rev Psychiatry 2007;19(6):655.

Bellingham GA, Peng PW: Duloxetine: A review of its pharmacology and use in chronic pain management. Reg Anesth Pain Med 2010;35:294.

Belmaker R, Agam G: Major depressive disorder. N Engl J Med 2008;358:55.

Bockting CL et al: Continuation and maintenance use of antidepressants in recurrent depression. Psychother Psychosom 2008;77(1):17.

Bonisch H, Bruss M: The norepinephrine transporter in physiology and disease. Handb Exp Pharmacol 2006;175:485.

Castren E, Voikar V, Rantamaki T: Role of neurotrophic factors in depression. Curr Opin Pharmacol 2007;7(1):18.

Chappell AS et al: A double-blind, randomized, placebo-controlled study of the efficacy and safety of duloxetine for the treatment of chronic pain due to osteoarthritis of the knee. Pain Pract 2011;11:33.

Cipriani A et al: Fluoxetine versus other types of pharmacotherapy for depression. Cochrane Database Syst Rev 2005;(4):CD004185.

Cipriani A et al: Metareview on short-term effectiveness and safety of antidepressants for depression: An evidence-based approach to inform clinical practice. Can J Psychiatry 2007;52(9):553.

de Beaurepaire R: Questions raised by the cytokine hypothesis of depression. Brain Behav Immun 2002;16(5):610.

Delgado PL: How antidepressants help depression: Mechanisms of action and clinical response. J Clin Psychiatry 2004;65(Suppl 4):25.

Dhillon S, Scott LJ, Plosker GL: Escitalopram: A review of its use in the management of anxiety disorders. CNS Drugs 2006;20(9):763.

Dhillon S, Yang LP, Curran MP: Bupropion: A review of its use in the management of major depressive disorder. Drugs 2008;68(5):653.

Duman RS: Role of neurotrophic factors in the etiology and treatment of mood disorders. Neuromolecular Med 2004;5(1):11.

Duman RS, Monteggia LM: A neurotrophic model for stress-related mood disorders. Biol Psychiatry 2006;59(12):1116.

Dvir Y, Smallwood P: Serotonin syndrome: A complex but easily avoidable condition. Gen Hosp Psychiatry 2008;30(3):284.

Fontenelle LF et al: An update on the pharmacological treatment of obsessive-compulsive disorder. Expert Opin Pharmacother 2007;8(5):563.

Geisser ME et al: A pooled analysis of two randomized, double-blind, placebo-controlled trials of milnacipran monotherapy in thetreatment of fibromyalgia. Pain Pract 2011;11:120.

Gether U et al: Neurotransmitter transporters: Molecular function of important drug targets. Trends Pharmacol Sci 2006;27(7):375.

Gillespie CF, Nemeroff CB: Hypercortisolemia and depression. Psychosom Med 2005;67(Suppl 1):S26.

Gillman PK: A review of serotonin toxicity data: Implications for the mechanisms of antidepressant drug action. Biol Psychiatry 2006;59(11):1046.

Gillman PK: Tricyclic antidepressant pharmacology and therapeutic drug interactions updated. Br J Pharmacol 2007;151(6):737.

Giner L et al: Selective serotonin reuptake inhibitors and the risk for suicidality in adolescents: An update. Int J Adolesc Med Health 2005;17(3):211.

Gutman DA, Owens MJ: Serotonin and norepinephrine transporter binding profile of SSRIs. Essent Psychopharmacol 2006;7(1):35.

Heninger GR, Delgado PL, Charney DS: The revised monoamine theory of depression: A modulatory role for monoamines, based on new findings from monoamine depletion experiments in humans. Pharmacopsychiatry 1996;29(1):2.

Hirschfeld RM: Antidepressants in long-term therapy: A review of tricyclic antidepressants and selective serotonin reuptake inhibitors. Acta Psychiatr Scand Suppl 2000;403:35.

Hirschfeld RM: History and evolution of the monoamine hypothesis of depression. J Clin Psychiatry 2000;61(Suppl 6):4.

Holma KM et al: Long-term outcome of major depressive disorder in psychiatric patients is variable. J Clin Psychiatry 2008;69(2):196.

Jann MW, Slade JH: Antidepressant agents for the treatment of chronic pain and depression. Pharmacotherapy 2007;27(11):1571.

Kalia M: Neurobiological basis of depression: An update. Metabolism 2005;54(5 Suppl 1):24.

Katz LY et al: Effect of regulatory warnings on antidepressant prescription rates, use of health services and outcomes among children, adolescents and young adults. CMAJ 2008;178(8):1005.

Kozisek ME, Middlemas D, Bylund DB: Brain-derived neurotrophic factor and its receptor tropomyosin-related kinase B in the mechanism of action of antidepressant therapies. Pharmacol Ther 2008;117(1):30.

Lee AL, Ogle WO, Sapolsky RM: Stress and depression: Possible links to neuron death in the hippocampus. Bipolar Disord 2002;4(2):117.

Lesch KP, Gutknecht L: Pharmacogenetics of the serotonin transporter. Prog Neuropsychopharmacol Biol Psychiatry 2005;29(6):1062.

Maletic V et al: Neurobiology of depression: An integrated view of key findings. Int J Clin Pract 2007;61(12):2030.

Manji HK, Drevets WC, Charney DS: The cellular neurobiology of depression. Nat Med 2001;7(5):541.

McCleane G: Antidepressants as analgesics. CNS Drugs 2008;22(2):139.

McEwen BS: Glucocorticoids, depression, and mood disorders: Structural remodeling in the brain. Metabolism 2005;54(5 Suppl 1):20.

Mendelson WB: A review of the evidence for the efficacy and safety of trazodone in insomnia. J Clin Psychiatry 2005;66(4):469.

Moller HJ: Evidence for beneficial effects of antidepressants on suicidality in depressive patients: A systematic review. Eur Arch Psychiatry Clin Neurosci 2006;256(6):329.

Nestler EJ et al: Neurobiology of depression. Neuron 2002;34(1):13.

Pace TW, Hu F, Miller AH: Cytokine-effects on glucocorticoid receptor function: Relevance to glucocorticoid resistance and the pathophysiology and treatment of major depression. Brain Behav Immun 2007;21(1):9.

Perugi G, Frare F, Toni C: Diagnosis and treatment of agoraphobia with panic disorder. CNS Drugs 2007;21(9):741.

Sakinofsky I: Treating suicidality in depressive illness. Part 2: Does treatment cure or cause suicidality? Can J Psychiatry 2007;52(6 Suppl 1):85S.

Schatzberg AF, Cole JO, DeBattista C: *Manual of Clinical Psychopharmacology*, 6th ed. American Psychiatric Publishing, Inc., 2007.

Shapiro JR et al: Bulimia nervosa treatment: A systematic review of randomized controlled trials. Int J Eat Disord 20207;40(4):321.

Soomro GM et al: Selective serotonin reuptake inhibitors (SSRIs) versus placebo for obsessive compulsive disorder (OCD). Cochrane Database Syst Rev 2008;(1):CD001765.

Stein DJ, Kupfer DJ, Schatzberg AF: *American Psychiatric Publishing Textbook of Mood Disorders*. American Psychiatric Publishing, Inc., 2006.

Stein MB, Stein DJ: Social anxiety disorder. Lancet 2008;371(9618):1115.

Stone EA, Lin Y, Quartermain D: A final common pathway for depression? Progress toward a general conceptual framework. Neurosci Biobehav Rev 2008;32(3):508.

Szegedi A, Schwertfeger N: Mirtazapine: A review of its clinical efficacy and tolerability. Expert Opin Pharmacother 2005;6(4):631.

Tang SW, Helmeste D: Paroxetine. Expert Opin Pharmacother 2008;9(5):787.

Tuccori M et al: Use of selective serotonin reuptake inhibitors during pregnancy and risk of major and cardiovascular malformations: An update. Postgrad Med 2010;122:49.

Warden D et al: The STAR*D Project results: A comprehensive review of findings. Curr Psychiatry Rep 2007;9(6):449.

Wheeler BW et al: The population impact on incidence of suicide and non-fatal self harm of regulatory action against the use of selective serotonin reuptake inhibitors in under 18s in the United Kingdom: Ecological study. Br Med J 2008;336(7643):542.

Wilson KL et al: Persistent pulmonary hypertension of the newborn is associated with mode of delivery and not with maternal use of selective serotonin reuptake inhibitors. Am J Perinatol 2010 Jul 6. [Epub ahead of print]

Yu S, Holsboer F, Almeida OF: Neuronal actions of glucocorticoids: Focus on depression. J Steroid Biochem Mol Biol 2008;108(3-5):300.

CASE STUDY ANSWER

Fluoxetine, the prototype SSRI, has a number of pharmacokinetic and pharmacodynamic interactions. Fluoxetine is a CYP450 2D6 inhibitor and thus can inhibit the metabolism of 2D6 substrates such as propranolol and other β blockers, tricyclic antidepressants, tramadol, opioids such as methadone, codeine, and oxycodone, antipsychotics such as haloperidol and thioridazine, and many other drugs. This inhibition of metabolism can result in significantly higher plasma levels of the concurrent drug, and this may lead to an increase in adverse reactions associated with that drug.

As a potent inhibitor of the serotonin transporter, fluoxetine is associated with a number of pharmacodynamic interactions involving serotonergic neurotransmission. The combination of tramadol with fluoxetine has occasionally been associated with a serotonin syndrome, characterized by diaphoreses, autonomic instability, myoclonus, seizures, and coma. The combination of fluoxetine with an MAOI is contraindicated because of the risk of a fatal serotonin syndrome. In addition, meperidine is specifically contraindicated in combination with an MAOI.

Opioid Analgesics & Antagonists

Mark A. Schumacher, PhD, MD, Allan I. Basbaum, PhD, & Walter L. Way, MD[*]

CASE STUDY

A 60-year-old man with a history of moderate chronic obstructive pulmonary disease presents in the emergency department with a broken hip suffered in an automobile accident. He complains of severe pain. What is the most appropriate immediate treatment for his pain? Are any special precautions needed?

Morphine, the prototypical opioid agonist, has long been known to relieve severe pain with remarkable efficacy. The opium poppy is the source of crude opium from which Sertürner in 1803 isolated morphine, the pure alkaloid, naming it after Morpheus, the Greek god of dreams. It remains the standard against which all drugs that have strong analgesic action are compared. These drugs are collectively known as opioid analgesics and include not only the natural and semisynthetic alkaloid derivatives from opium but also synthetic surrogates, other opioid-like drugs whose actions are blocked by the nonselective antagonist naloxone, plus several endogenous peptides that interact with the different subtypes of opioid receptors.

■ BASIC PHARMACOLOGY OF THE OPIOID ANALGESICS

Source

Opium, the source of morphine, is obtained from the poppy, *Papaver somniferum* and *P album*. After incision, the poppy seed pod exudes a white substance that turns into a brown gum that is crude opium. Opium contains many alkaloids, the principal one being morphine, which is present in a concentration of about 10%. Codeine is synthesized commercially from morphine.

Classification & Chemistry

Opioid drugs include full agonists, partial agonists, and antagonists. Morphine is a full agonist at the **μ (mu)-opioid receptor,** the major analgesic opioid receptor (Table 31–1). In contrast, codeine functions as a partial (or "weak") μ-receptor agonist. Other opioid receptor subtypes include **δ (delta)** and **κ (kappa)** receptors. Simple substitution of an allyl group on the nitrogen of the full *agonist* morphine plus addition of a single hydroxyl group results in naloxone, a strong μ-receptor *antagonist*. The structures of some of these compounds are shown later in this chapter. Some opioids, eg, nalbuphine, are capable of producing an agonist (or partial agonist) effect at one opioid receptor subtype and an antagonist effect at another. The receptor activating properties and affinities of opioid analgesics can be manipulated by pharmaceutical chemistry; in addition, certain opioid analgesics are modified in the liver, resulting in compounds with greater analgesic action. Chemically, the opioids derived from opium are phenanthrene derivatives and include four or more fused rings, while most of the synthetic opioids are simpler molecules.

Endogenous Opioid Peptides

Opioid alkaloids (eg, morphine) produce analgesia through actions at receptors in the central nervous system (CNS) that respond to certain endogenous peptides with opioid-like pharmacologic properties. The general term currently used for these endogenous substances is **endogenous opioid peptides.**

---

[*]Deceased

TABLE 31–1 Opioid receptor subtypes, their functions, and their endogenous peptide affinities.

Receptor Subtype	Functions	Endogenous Opioid Peptide Affinity
μ (mu)	Supraspinal and spinal analgesia; sedation; inhibition of respiration; slowed gastrointestinal transit; modulation of hormone and neurotransmitter release	Endorphins > enkephalins > dynorphins
δ (delta)	Supraspinal and spinal analgesia; modulation of hormone and neurotransmitter release	Enkephalins > endorphins and dynorphins
κ (kappa)	Supraspinal and spinal analgesia; psychotomimetic effects; slowed gastrointestinal transit	Dynorphins > > endorphins and enkephalins

Three families of endogenous opioid peptides have been described in detail: the **endorphins,** the pentapeptide **enkephalins** methionine-enkephalin (**met-enkephalin**) and leucine-enkephalin (**leu-enkephalin**), and the **dynorphins.** The three families of opioid receptors have overlapping affinities for these endogenous peptides (Table 31–1).

The endogenous opioid peptides are derived from three precursor proteins: prepro-opiomelanocortin (POMC), preproenkephalin (proenkephalin A), and preprodynorphin (proenkephalin B). POMC contains the met-enkephalin sequence, β-endorphin, and several nonopioid peptides, including adrenocorticotropic hormone (ACTH), β-lipotropin, and melanocyte-stimulating hormone. Preproenkephalin contains six copies of met-enkephalin and one copy of leu-enkephalin. Leu- and met-enkephalin have slightly higher affinity for the δ (delta) than for the μ-opioid receptor (Table 31–1). Preprodynorphin yields several active opioid peptides that contain the leu-enkephalin sequence. These are **dynorphin A, dynorphin B,** and α and β **neoendorphins.** The endogenous peptides **endomorphin-1** and **endomorphin-2** also possess many of the properties of opioid peptides, notably analgesia and high-affinity binding to the μ receptor. Endomorphin-1 and -2 selectively activate central and peripheral μ-opioid receptors but much about them remains unknown, including the identity of their preproendomorphin gene. Both the endogenous opioid precursor molecules and the endomorphins are present at CNS sites that have been implicated in pain modulation. Evidence suggests that they can be released during stressful conditions such as pain or the anticipation of pain and diminish the sensation of noxious stimuli. Whether acupuncture releases endogenous opioid peptides is under investigation.

In contrast to the analgesic role of leu- and met-enkephalin, an analgesic action of dynorphin A—through its binding to κ (kappa)-opioid receptors—remains controversial. Dynorphin A is also found in the dorsal horn of the spinal cord, where it may play a critical role in the *sensitization* of nociceptive neurotransmission. Increased levels of dynorphin can be found in the dorsal horn after tissue injury and inflammation. This elevated dynorphin level is proposed to increase pain and induce a state of long-lasting hyperalgesia. The pronociceptive action of dynorphin in the spinal cord appears to be independent of the opioid receptor system but dependent on the activation of the bradykinin receptor. Moreover, dynorphin A can bind and activate the *N*-methyl-D-aspartate (NMDA)-receptor complex, a site of action that is the focus of intense therapeutic development.

Recently, a novel receptor-ligand system homologous to the opioid peptides has been found. The principal receptor for this system is the G protein-coupled **orphanin opioid-receptor-like subtype 1 (ORL1).** Its endogenous ligand has been termed *nociceptin* by one group of investigators and **orphanin FQ** by another group. This ligand-receptor system is currently known as the *N/OFQ* system. Nociceptin is structurally similar to dynorphin except for the absence of an N-terminal tyrosine; it acts only at the ORL1 receptor, now known as **NOP.** The N/OFQ system is widely expressed in the CNS and periphery, reflecting its equally diverse biology and pharmacology. As a result of experiments using highly selective NOP receptor ligands, the N/OFQ system has been implicated in both pro- and anti-nociceptive activity as well as in the modulation of drug reward, learning, mood, anxiety, and cough processes, and of parkinsonism.

Pharmacokinetics

Some properties of clinically important opioids are summarized in Table 31–2.

A. Absorption

Most opioid analgesics are well absorbed when given by subcutaneous, intramuscular, and oral routes. However, because of the first-pass effect, the oral dose of the opioid (eg, morphine) may need to be much higher than the parenteral dose to elicit a therapeutic effect. Considerable interpatient variability exists in first-pass opioid metabolism, making prediction of an effective oral dose difficult. Certain analgesics such as codeine and oxycodone are effective orally because they have reduced first-pass metabolism. Nasal insufflation of certain opioids can result in rapid therapeutic blood levels by avoiding first-pass metabolism. Other routes of opioid administration include oral mucosa via lozenges, and transdermal via transdermal patches. The latter can provide delivery of potent analgesics over days. Recently an iontophoretic transdermal system has been introduced, allowing needle-free delivery of fentanyl for patient-controlled analgesia.

B. Distribution

The uptake of opioids by various organs and tissues is a function of both physiologic and chemical factors. Although all opioids bind to plasma proteins with varying affinity, the drugs rapidly leave the blood compartment and localize in highest concentrations in tissues that are highly perfused such as the brain, lungs, liver, kidneys, and spleen. Drug concentrations in skeletal muscle may be much lower, but this tissue serves as the main reservoir because of its greater bulk. Even though blood flow to fatty tissue is much lower than to the highly perfused tissues, accumulation

TABLE 31–2 Common opioid analgesics.

Generic Name	Receptor Effects[1] μ	δ	κ	Approximately Equivalent Dose (mg)	Oral:Parenteral Potency Ratio	Duration of Analgesia (hours)	Maximum Efficacy
Morphine[2]	+++		+	10	Low	4–5	High
Hydromorphone	+++			1.5	Low	4–5	High
Oxymorphone	+++			1.5	Low	3–4	High
Methadone	+++			10	High	4–6	High
Meperidine	+++			60–100	Medium	2–4	High
Fentanyl	+++			0.1	Low	1–1.5	High
Sufentanil	+++	+	+	0.02	Parenteral only	1–1.5	High
Alfentanil	+++			Titrated	Parenteral only	0.25–0.75	High
Remifentanil	+++			Titrated[3]	Parenteral only	0.05[4]	High
Levorphanol	+++			2–3	High	4–5	High
Codeine	±			30–60	High	3–4	Low
Hydrocodone[5]	±			5–10	Medium	4–6	Moderate
Oxycodone[2,6]	++			4.5	Medium	3–4	Mod-High
Pentazocine	±		+	30–50	Medium	3–4	Moderate
Nalbuphine	––		++	10	Parenteral only	3–6	High
Buprenorphine	±	––	––	0.3	Low	4–8	High
Butorphanol	±		+++	2	Parenteral only	3–4	High

[1]+++, ++, +, strong agonist; ±, partial agonist; ––, antagonist.

[2]Available in sustained-release forms, morphine (MS Contin); oxycodone (Oxy Contin).

[3]Administered as an infusion at 0.025–0.2 mcg/kg/min.

[4]Duration is dependent on a context-sensitive half-time of 3–4 minutes.

[5]Available in tablets containing acetaminophen (Norco, Vicodin, Lortab, others).

[6]Available in tablets containing acetaminophen (Percocet); aspirin (Percodan).

can be very important, particularly after frequent high-dose administration or continuous infusion of highly lipophilic opioids that are slowly metabolized, eg, fentanyl.

C. Metabolism

The opioids are converted in large part to polar metabolites (mostly glucuronides), which are then readily excreted by the kidneys. For example, morphine, which contains free hydroxyl groups, is primarily conjugated to morphine-3-glucuronide (M3G), a compound with neuroexcitatory properties. The neuroexcitatory effects of M3G do not appear to be mediated by μ receptors but rather by the GABA/glycinergic system. In contrast, approximately 10% of morphine is metabolized to morphine-6-glucuronide (M6G), an active metabolite with analgesic potency four to six times that of its parent compound. However, these relatively polar metabolites have limited ability to cross the blood-brain barrier and probably do not contribute significantly to the usual CNS effects of morphine given acutely. Nevertheless, accumulation of these metabolites may produce unexpected adverse effects in patients with renal failure or when exceptionally large doses of morphine are administered or high doses are administered over long periods. This can result in M3G-induced CNS excitation (seizures) or enhanced and prolonged opioid action produced

by M6G. CNS uptake of M3G and, to a lesser extent, M6G can be enhanced by co-administration with probenecid or with drugs that inhibit the P-glycoprotein drug transporter. Like morphine, hydromorphone is metabolized by conjugation, yielding hydromorphone-3-glucuronide (H3G), which has CNS excitatory properties. However, hydromorphone has not been shown to form significant amounts of a 6-glucuronide metabolite.

The effects of these active metabolites should be considered in patients with renal impairment before the administration of morphine or hydromorphone, especially when given at high doses.

Esters (eg, heroin, remifentanil) are rapidly hydrolyzed by common tissue esterases. Heroin (diacetylmorphine) is hydrolyzed to monoacetylmorphine and finally to morphine, which is then conjugated with glucuronic acid.

Hepatic oxidative metabolism is the primary route of degradation of the phenylpiperidine opioids (meperidine, fentanyl, alfentanil, sufentanil) and eventually leaves only small quantities of the parent compound unchanged for excretion. However, accumulation of a demethylated metabolite of meperidine, normeperidine, may occur in patients with decreased renal function and in those receiving multiple high doses of the drug. In high concentrations, normeperidine may cause seizures. In contrast, no active metabolites of fentanyl have been reported. The P450 isozyme CYP3A4 metabolizes fentanyl by *N*-dealkylation in the liver. CYP3A4 is also present in the mucosa of the small intestine and contributes to the first-pass metabolism of fentanyl when it is taken orally. Codeine, oxycodone, and hydrocodone undergo metabolism in the liver by P450 isozyme CYP2D6, resulting in the production of metabolites of greater potency. For example, codeine is demethylated to morphine. Genetic polymorphism of CYP2D6 has been documented and linked to the variation in analgesic response seen among patients. Nevertheless, the metabolites of oxycodone and hydrocodone may be of minor consequence; the parent compounds are currently believed to be directly responsible for the majority of their analgesic actions. However, oxycodone and its metabolites can accumulate under conditions of renal failure and have been associated with prolonged action and sedation. In the case of codeine, conversion to morphine may be of greater importance because codeine itself has relatively low affinity for opioid receptors. As a result, patients may experience either no significant analgesic effect or an exaggerated response based on differences in metabolic conversion. For this reason, routine use of codeine, especially in pediatric age groups, is being reconsidered.

D. Excretion

Polar metabolites, including glucuronide conjugates of opioid analgesics, are excreted mainly in the urine. Small amounts of unchanged drug may also be found in the urine. In addition, glucuronide conjugates are found in the bile, but enterohepatic circulation represents only a small portion of the excretory process.

Pharmacodynamics

A. Mechanism of Action

Opioid agonists produce analgesia by binding to specific G protein-coupled receptors that are located in brain and spinal cord regions involved in the transmission and modulation of pain (Figure 31–1). Some effects may be mediated by opioid receptors on peripheral sensory nerve endings.

1. Receptor types—As noted previously, three major classes of opioid receptors (μ, δ, and κ) have been identified in various nervous system sites and in other tissues (Table 31–1). Each of the three major receptors has now been cloned. All are members of the G protein-coupled family of receptors and show significant amino acid sequence homologies. Multiple receptor subtypes have been proposed based on pharmacologic criteria, including μ_1, μ_2; δ_1, δ_2; and κ_1, κ_2, and κ_3. However, genes encoding only one subtype from each of the μ, δ, and κ receptor families have been isolated and characterized thus far. One plausible explanation is that μ-receptor subtypes arise from alternate splice variants of a common gene. This idea has been supported by the identification of receptor splice variants in mice and humans. Since an opioid may function with different potencies as an agonist, partial agonist, or antagonist at more than one receptor class or subtype, it is not surprising that these agents are capable of diverse pharmacologic effects.

2. Cellular actions—At the molecular level, opioid receptors form a family of proteins that physically couple to G proteins and

through this interaction affect ion channel gating, modulate intracellular Ca^{2+} disposition, and alter protein phosphorylation (see Chapter 2). The opioids have two well-established direct G protein-coupled actions on neurons: (1) they close voltage-gated Ca^{2+} channels on presynaptic nerve terminals and thereby reduce transmitter release, and (2) they hyperpolarize and thus inhibit postsynaptic neurons by opening K^+ channels. Figure 31–1 schematically illustrates these effects. The presynaptic action—depressed transmitter release—has been demonstrated for release of a large number of neurotransmitters including glutamate, the principal excitatory amino acid released from nociceptive nerve terminals, as well as acetylcholine, norepinephrine, serotonin, and substance P.

3. Relation of physiologic effects to receptor type—The majority of currently available opioid analgesics act primarily at the μ-opioid receptor (Table 31–2). Analgesia and the euphoriant, respiratory depressant, and physical dependence properties of morphine result principally from actions at μ receptors. In fact, the μ receptor was originally defined using the relative potencies for clinical analgesia of a series of opioid alkaloids. However, opioid analgesic effects are complex and include interaction with δ and κ receptors. This is supported by the study of genetic knockouts of the μ, δ, and κ genes in mice. Delta-receptor agonists retain analgesic properties in δ receptor knockout mice. The development of μ-receptor–selective agonists could be clinically useful if their side-effect profiles (respiratory depression, risk of dependence) were more favorable than those found with current μ-receptor agonists, such as morphine. Although morphine does act at κ and δ receptor sites, it is unclear to what extent this contributes to its analgesic action. The endogenous opioid peptides differ from most of the alkaloids in their affinity for the δ and κ receptors (Table 31–1).

In an effort to develop opioid analgesics with a reduced incidence of respiratory depression or propensity for addiction and dependence, compounds that show preference for κ opioid receptors have been developed. Butorphanol and nalbuphine have shown some clinical success as analgesics, but they can cause dysphoric reactions and have limited potency. It is interesting that butorphanol has also been shown to cause significantly greater analgesia in women than in men. In fact, gender-based differences in analgesia mediated by μ- and δ-receptor activation have been widely reported.

4. Receptor distribution and neural mechanisms of analgesia—Opioid receptor binding sites have been localized autoradiographically with high-affinity radioligands and with antibodies to unique peptide sequences in each receptor subtype. All three major receptors are present in high concentrations in the dorsal horn of the spinal cord. Receptors are present both on spinal cord pain transmission neurons and on the primary afferents that relay the pain message to them (Figure 31–2, sites A and B). Although opioid agonists directly inhibit the dorsal horn pain transmission neurons, they also inhibit the release of excitatory transmitters from the primary afferents. Within the presynaptic terminals, there is evidence that heterodimerization of the μ-opioid

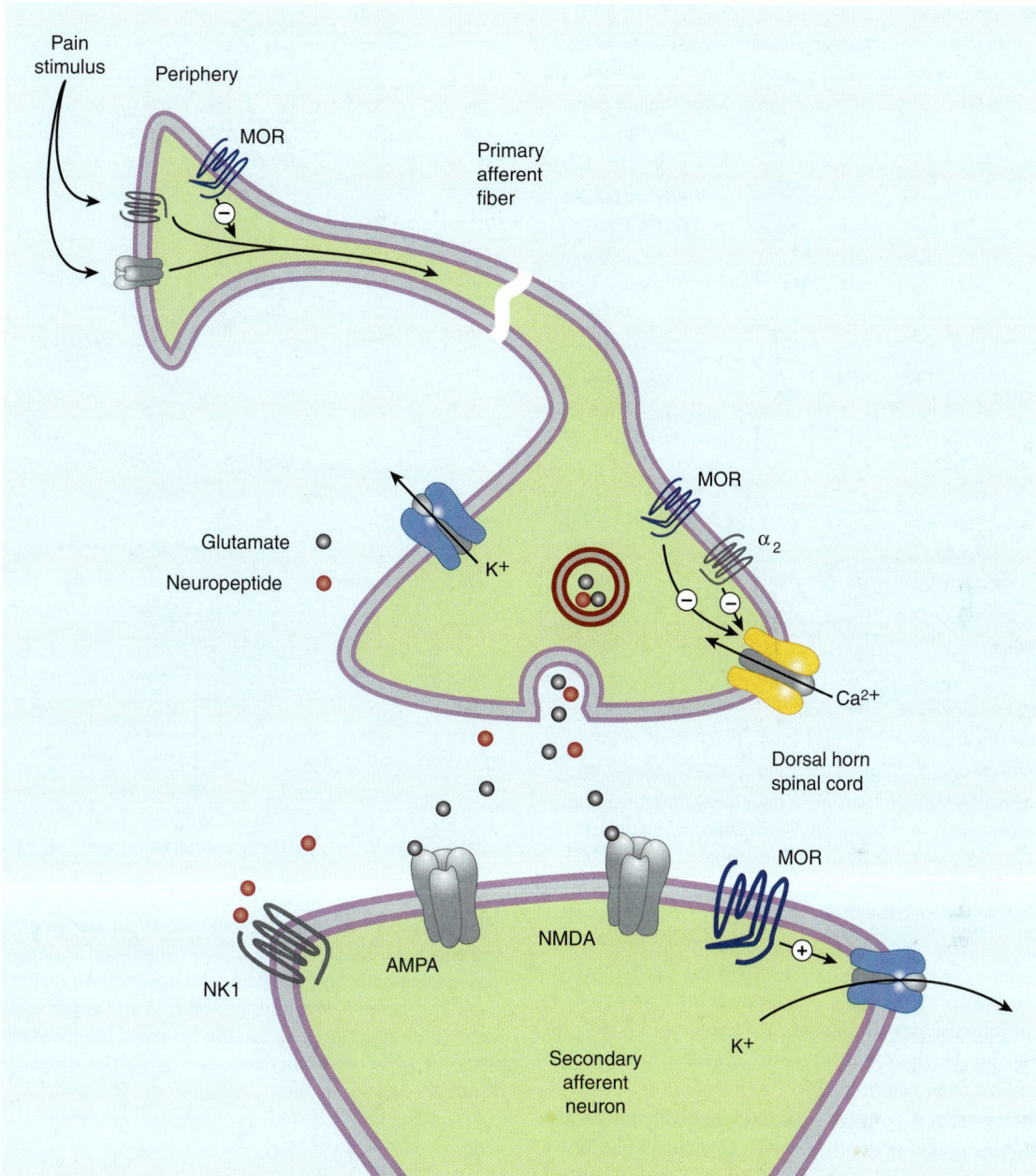

FIGURE 31–1 Potential receptor mechanisms of analgesic drugs. The primary afferent neuron (cell body not shown) originates in the periphery and carries pain signals to the dorsal horn of the spinal cord, where it synapses via glutamate and neuropeptide transmitters with the secondary neuron. Pain stimuli can be attenuated in the periphery (under inflammatory conditions) by opioids acting at μ-opioid receptors (MOR) or blocked in the afferent axon by local anesthetics (not shown). Action potentials reaching the dorsal horn can be attenuated at the presynaptic ending by opioids and by calcium blockers (ziconotide), α_2 agonists, and possibly, by drugs that increase synaptic concentrations of norepinephrine by blocking reuptake (tapentadol). Opioids also inhibit the postsynaptic neuron, as do certain neuropeptide antagonists acting at tachykinin (NK1) and other neuropeptide receptors.

and δ-opioid receptors contribute to μ-agonist efficacy (eg, inhibition of presynaptic voltage-gated calcium channel activity). On the other hand, a recent study using a transgenic mouse that expresses a δ–receptor-enhanced green fluorescent protein (eGFP) fusion protein shows little overlap of μ receptor and δ receptor in the dorsal root ganglion neurons. Importantly, the μ receptor is associated with TRPV1 and peptide (substance P)-expressing nociceptors, whereas δ-receptor expression predominates in the non-peptidergic population of nociceptors, including many primary afferents with myelinated axons. This is consistent with the action of intrathecal μ-receptor– and δ-receptor–selective ligands that are found to block heat versus mechanical pain processing, respectively. To what

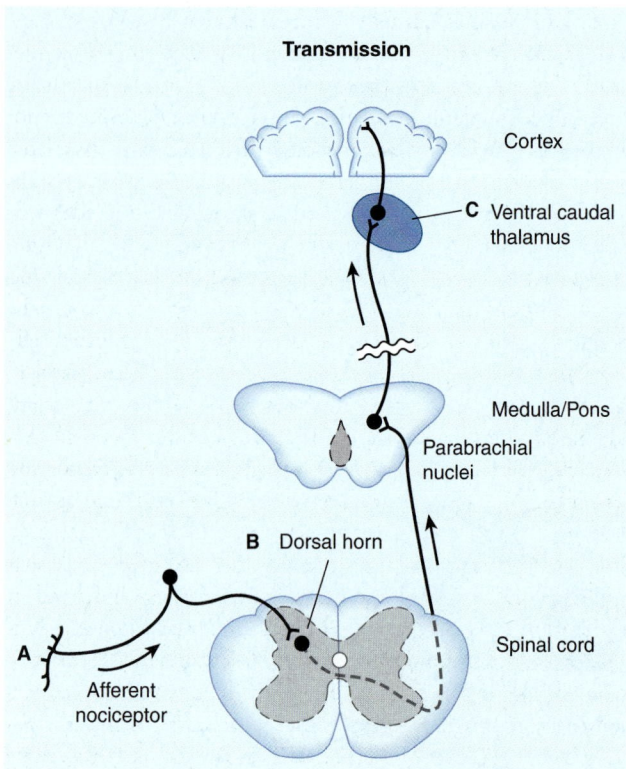

FIGURE 31–2 Putative sites of action of opioid analgesics. Sites of action on the afferent pain transmission pathway from the periphery to the higher centers are shown. **A:** Direct action of opioids on inflamed or damaged peripheral tissues (see Figure 31–1 for detail). **B:** Inhibition also occurs in the spinal cord (see Figure 31–1). **C:** Possible sites of action in the thalamus.

extent the differential expression of the μ receptor and δ receptor in the dorsal root ganglia is characteristic of neurons throughout the CNS remains to be determined.

Thus, opioids exert a powerful analgesic effect directly on the spinal cord. This *spinal action* has been exploited clinically by direct application of opioid agonists to the spinal cord, which provides a regional analgesic effect while reducing the unwanted respiratory depression, nausea and vomiting, and sedation that may occur from the *supraspinal actions* of systemically administered opioids.

Under most circumstances, opioids are given systemically and so act simultaneously at multiple sites. These include not only the ascending pathways of pain transmission beginning with specialized peripheral sensory terminals that transduce painful stimuli (Figure 31–2) but also descending (modulatory) pathways (Figure 31–3). At these sites as at others, opioids directly inhibit neurons; yet this action results in the *activation* of descending inhibitory neurons that send processes to the spinal cord and inhibit pain transmission neurons. This activation has been shown to result from the inhibition of inhibitory neurons in several locations (Figure 31–4). Taken together, interactions at these sites increase the overall analgesic effect of opioid agonists.

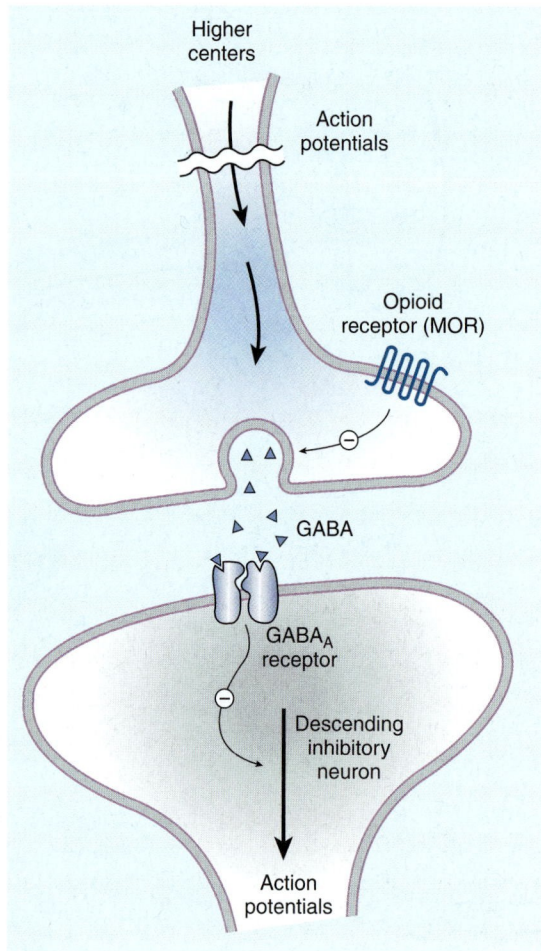

FIGURE 31–3 Brainstem local circuitry underlying the modulating effect of μ-opioid receptor (MOR)–mediated analgesia on descending pathways. The pain-inhibitory neuron is indirectly activated by opioids (exogenous or endogenous), which inhibit an inhibitory (GABAergic) interneuron. This results in *enhanced* inhibition of nociceptive processing in the dorsal horn of the spinal cord (see Figure 31–4).

When pain-relieving opioid drugs are given systemically, they presumably act upon neuronal circuits normally regulated by endogenous opioid peptides. Part of the pain-relieving action of exogenous opioids involves the release of endogenous opioid peptides. An exogenous opioid agonist (eg, morphine) may act primarily and directly at the μ receptor, but this action may evoke the release of endogenous opioids that additionally act at δ and κ receptors. Thus, even a receptor-selective ligand can initiate a complex sequence of events involving multiple synapses, transmitters, and receptor types.

Animal and human clinical studies demonstrate that both endogenous and exogenous opioids can also produce opioid-mediated analgesia at sites *outside* the CNS. Pain associated with inflammation seems especially sensitive to these peripheral opioid actions. The presence of functional μ receptors on the peripheral terminals of sensory neurons supports this hypothesis.

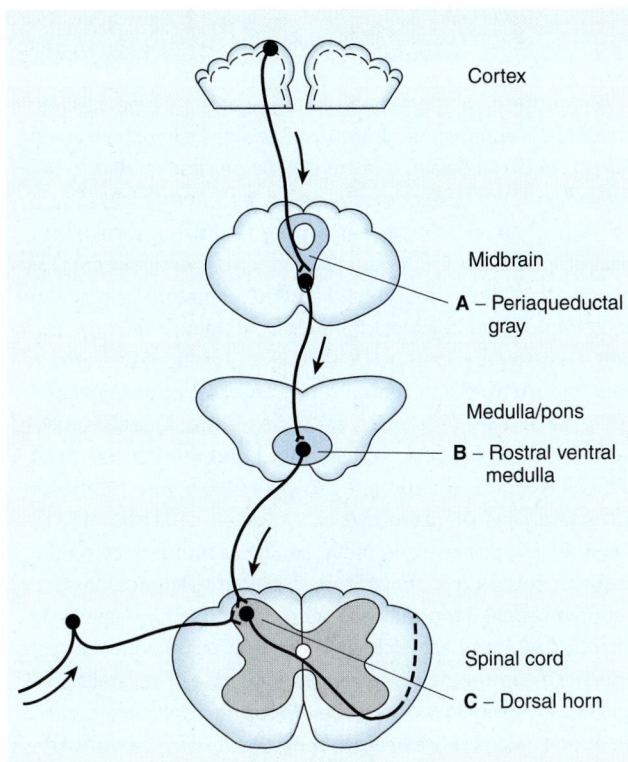

FIGURE 31–4 Opioid analgesic action on the descending inhibitory pathway. Sites of action of opioids on pain-modulating neurons in the midbrain and medulla including the midbrain periaqueductal gray area **(A)**, rostral ventral medulla **(B)**, and the locus caeruleus indirectly control pain transmission pathways by enhancing descending inhibition to the dorsal horn **(C)**.

Cortex

Midbrain

A – Periaqueductal gray

Medulla/pons

B – Rostral ventral medulla

Spinal cord

C – Dorsal horn

Furthermore, activation of peripheral μ receptors results in a decrease in sensory neuron activity and transmitter release. The endogenous release of β-endorphin produced by immune cells within injured or inflamed tissue represents one source of physiologic peripheral μ-receptor activation. Peripheral administration of opioids, eg, into the knees of patients following arthroscopic knee surgery, has shown clinical benefit up to 24 hours after administration. If they can be developed, opioids selective for a peripheral site would be useful adjuncts in the treatment of inflammatory pain (see Box: Ion Channels & Novel Analgesic Targets). Such compounds could have the additional benefit of reducing unwanted effects such as constipation.

5. Tolerance and dependence—With frequently repeated therapeutic doses of morphine or its surrogates, there is a gradual loss in effectiveness; this loss of effectiveness is denoted tolerance. To reproduce the original response, a larger dose must be administered. Along with tolerance, physical dependence develops. Physical dependence is defined as a characteristic **withdrawal** or **abstinence syndrome** when a drug is stopped or an antagonist is administered (see also Chapter 32).

The mechanism of development of tolerance and physical dependence is poorly understood, but persistent activation of

μ receptors such as occurs with the treatment of severe chronic pain appears to play a primary role in its induction and maintenance. Current concepts have shifted away from tolerance being driven by a simple up-regulation of the cyclic adenosine monophosphate (cAMP) system. Although this process is associated with tolerance, it is not sufficient to explain it. A second hypothesis for the development of opioid tolerance and dependence is based on the concept of **receptor recycling.** Normally, activation of μ receptors by endogenous ligands results in endocytosis followed by resensitization and recycling of the receptor to the plasma membrane (see Chapter 2). However, using genetically modified mice, research now shows that the *failure* of morphine to induce endocytosis of the μ-opioid receptor is an important component of tolerance and dependence. In contrast, methadone, a μ-receptor agonist used for the *treatment* of opioid tolerance and dependence, does induce receptor endocytosis. This suggests that maintenance of normal sensitivity of μ receptors requires reactivation by endocytosis and recycling. Another area of research suggests that the δ opioid receptor functions as an independent component in the maintenance of tolerance. In addition, the concept of **receptor uncoupling** has gained prominence. Under this hypothesis, tolerance is due to a dysfunction of structural interactions between the μ receptor and G proteins, second-messenger systems, and their target ion channels. Uncoupling and recoupling of μ receptor function is likely linked to receptor recycling. Moreover, the NMDA-receptor ion channel complex has been shown to play a critical role in tolerance development and maintenance because NMDA-receptor antagonists such as ketamine can block tolerance development. Although a role in endocytosis is not yet clearly defined, the development of novel NMDA-receptor antagonists or other strategies to recouple μ receptors to their target ion channels provides hope for achieving a clinically effective means to prevent or reverse opioid analgesic tolerance.

In addition to the development of tolerance, persistent administration of opioid analgesics has been observed to *increase* the sensation of pain leading to a state of hyperalgesia. This phenomenon has been observed with several opioid analgesics, including morphine, fentanyl, and remifentanil. Spinal dynorphin and activation of the bradykinin receptor have emerged as important candidates for the mediation of opioid-induced hyperalgesia.

B. Organ System Effects of Morphine and Its Surrogates

The actions described below for morphine, the prototypic opioid agonist, can also be observed with other opioid agonists, partial agonists, and those with mixed receptor effects. Characteristics of specific members of these groups are discussed below.

1. Central nervous system effects—The principal effects of opioid analgesics with affinity for μ receptors are on the CNS; the more important ones include analgesia, euphoria, sedation, and respiratory depression. With repeated use, a high degree of tolerance occurs to all of these effects (Table 31–3).

a. Analgesia—Pain consists of both sensory and affective (emotional) components. Opioid analgesics are unique in that they can reduce both aspects of the pain experience, especially the affective

Ion Channels & Novel Analgesic Targets

Even the most severe *acute* pain (lasting hours to days) can usually be well controlled—with significant but tolerable adverse effects—using currently available analgesics, especially the opioids. *Chronic* pain (lasting weeks to months), however, is not very satisfactorily managed with opioids. It is now known that in chronic pain, receptors on sensory nerve terminals in the periphery contribute to increased excitability of sensory nerve endings (peripheral sensitization). The hyperexcitable sensory neuron bombards the spinal cord, leading to increased excitability and synaptic alterations in the dorsal horn (central sensitization). Such changes appear to be important in chronic inflammatory and neuropathic pain states.

In the effort to discover better analgesic drugs for chronic pain, renewed attention is being paid to synaptic transmission in nociception and peripheral sensory transduction. Potentially important ion channels associated with these processes in the periphery include members of the transient receptor potential family such as the **capsaicin receptor, TRPV1** (which is activated by multiple noxious stimuli such as heat, protons, and products of inflammation) as well as TRPA1, activated by inflammatory mediators; and P2X receptors (which are responsive to purines released from tissue damage). Special types of tetrodotoxin-resistant voltage-gated sodium channels **(Nav 1.7, 1.8, 1.9)** are uniquely associated with nociceptive neurons in dorsal root ganglia. **Lidocaine** and **mexiletine,** which are useful in some chronic pain states, may act by blocking this class of channels. Genetic polymorphisms of Nav 1.7 are associated with either absence or predisposition to pain. Because of the importance of their peripheral sites of action, therapeutic strategies that deliver agents that block peripheral pain transduction or transmission have been introduced in the form of transdermal patches and balms. Such products that specifically target peripheral capsaicin receptors and sodium channel function are becoming available.

Ziconotide, a blocker of voltage-gated N-type calcium channels, is approved for intrathecal analgesia in patients with refractory chronic pain. It is a synthetic peptide related to the marine snail toxin ω-conotoxin, which selectively blocks these calcium channels. **Gabapentin/pregabalin,** anticonvulsant analogs of GABA (see Chapter 24), are effective treatments for neuropathic (nerve injury) pain and inflammatory pain acting at voltage-gated calcium channels containing the $\alpha_2\delta_1$ subunit. *N*-methyl-D-aspartate (NMDA) receptors appear to play a very important role in central sensitization at both spinal and supraspinal levels. Although certain NMDA antagonists have demonstrated analgesic activity (eg, **ketamine**), it has been difficult to find agents with an acceptably low profile of adverse effects or neurotoxicity. However, ketamine at very small doses appears to improve analgesia and reduce opioid requirements under conditions of opioid tolerance. In fact, ketamine applied topically has been claimed to have analgesic effects. GABA and acetylcholine (through nicotinic receptors) appear to control the central synaptic release of several transmitters involved in nociception. **Nicotine** itself and certain nicotine analogs cause analgesia, and their use for postoperative analgesia is under investigation. Finally, work on cannabinoids and vanilloids and their receptors suggest that **Δ9- tetrahydrocannabinol,** which acts primarily on CB_1 cannabinoid receptors, can synergize with μ-receptor analgesics and interact with the TRPV1 capsaicin receptor to produce analgesia under certain circumstances.

As our understanding of peripheral and central pain transduction improves, additional therapeutic targets and strategies will become available. Combined with our present knowledge of opioid analgesics, a "multimodal" approach to pain therapy is emerging, which allows the use of complementary compounds resulting in improved analgesia with fewer adverse effects.

---

aspect. In contrast, nonsteroidal anti-inflammatory analgesic drugs have no significant effect on the emotional aspects of pain.

b. Euphoria—Typically, patients or intravenous drug users who receive intravenous morphine experience a pleasant floating sensation with lessened anxiety and distress. However, dysphoria, an unpleasant state characterized by restlessness and malaise, may sometimes occur.

c. Sedation—Drowsiness and clouding of mentation are common effects of opioids. There is little or no amnesia. Sleep is induced by opioids more frequently in the elderly than in young, healthy individuals. Ordinarily, the patient can be easily aroused from this sleep. However, the combination of morphine with other central depressant drugs such as the sedative-hypnotics may result in very deep sleep. Marked sedation occurs more frequently with compounds closely related to the phenanthrene derivatives and less frequently with the synthetic agents such as meperidine and fentanyl. In standard analgesic doses, morphine (a phenanthrene) disrupts normal rapid eye movement (REM) and non-REM sleep patterns. This disrupting effect is probably characteristic of all opioids. In contrast to humans, a number of

TABLE 31–3 Degrees of tolerance that may develop to some of the effects of the opioids.

High	Moderate	Minimal or None
Analgesia	Bradycardia	Miosis
Euphoria, dysphoria		Constipation
Mental clouding		Convulsions
Sedation		
Respiratory depression		
Antidiuresis		
Nausea and vomiting		
Cough suppression		

species (cats, horses, cows, pigs) may manifest excitation rather than sedation when given opioids. These paradoxic effects are at least partially dose-dependent.

d. Respiratory depression—All of the opioid analgesics can produce significant respiratory depression by inhibiting brainstem respiratory mechanisms. Alveolar P_{CO_2} may increase, but the most reliable indicator of this depression is a depressed response to a carbon dioxide challenge. The respiratory depression is dose-related and is influenced significantly by the degree of sensory input occurring at the time. For example, it is possible to partially overcome opioid-induced respiratory depression by stimulation of various sorts. When strongly painful stimuli that have prevented the depressant action of a large dose of an opioid are relieved, respiratory depression may suddenly become marked. A small to moderate decrease in respiratory function, as measured by $PaCO_2$ elevation, may be well tolerated in the patient without prior respiratory impairment. However, in individuals with increased intracranial pressure, asthma, chronic obstructive pulmonary disease, or cor pulmonale, this decrease in respiratory function may not be tolerated. Opioid-induced respiratory depression remains one of the most difficult clinical challenges in the treatment of severe pain. Research is ongoing to understand and develop analgesic agents and adjuncts that avoid this effect. Research to overcome this problem is focused on μ-receptor pharmacology and serotonin signaling pathways in the brainstem respiratory control centers.

e. Cough suppression—Suppression of the cough reflex is a well-recognized action of opioids. Codeine in particular has been used to advantage in persons suffering from pathologic cough and in patients in whom it is necessary to maintain ventilation via an endotracheal tube. However, cough suppression by opioids may allow accumulation of secretions and thus lead to airway obstruction and atelectasis.

f. Miosis—Constriction of the pupils is seen with virtually all opioid agonists. Miosis is a pharmacologic action to which little or no tolerance develops (Table 31–3); thus, it is valuable in the diagnosis of opioid overdose. Even in highly tolerant addicts, miosis is seen. This action, which can be blocked by opioid antagonists, is mediated by parasympathetic pathways, which, in turn, can be blocked by atropine.

g. Truncal rigidity—An intensification of tone in the large trunk muscles has been noted with a number of opioids. It was originally believed that truncal rigidity involved a spinal cord action of these drugs, but there is now evidence that it results from an action at supraspinal levels. Truncal rigidity reduces thoracic compliance and thus interferes with ventilation. The effect is most apparent when high doses of the highly lipid-soluble opioids (eg, fentanyl, sufentanil, alfentanil, remifentanil) are rapidly administered intravenously. Truncal rigidity may be overcome by administration of an opioid antagonist, which of course will also antagonize the analgesic action of the opioid. Preventing truncal rigidity while preserving analgesia requires the concomitant use of neuromuscular blocking agents.

h. Nausea and vomiting—The opioid analgesics can activate the brainstem chemoreceptor trigger zone to produce nausea and vomiting. There may also be a vestibular component in this effect because ambulation seems to increase the incidence of nausea and vomiting.

i. Temperature—Homeostatic regulation of body temperature is mediated in part by the action of endogenous opioid peptides in the brain. This has been supported by experiments demonstrating that administration of μ-opioid receptor agonists such as morphine administered to the anterior hypothalamus produces hyperthermia, whereas administration of κ agonists induces hypothermia.

2. Peripheral effects

a. Cardiovascular system—Most opioids have no significant direct effects on the heart and, other than bradycardia, no major effects on cardiac rhythm. Meperidine is an exception to this generalization because its antimuscarinic action can result in tachycardia. Blood pressure is usually well maintained in subjects receiving opioids unless the cardiovascular system is stressed, in which case hypotension may occur. This hypotensive effect is probably due to peripheral arterial and venous dilation, which has been attributed to a number of mechanisms including central depression of vasomotor-stabilizing mechanisms and release of histamine. No consistent effect on cardiac output is seen, and the electrocardiogram is not significantly affected. However, caution should be exercised in patients with decreased blood volume, because the above mechanisms make these patients susceptible to hypotension. Opioid analgesics affect cerebral circulation minimally except when P_{CO_2} rises as a consequence of respiratory depression. Increased P_{CO_2} leads to cerebral vasodilation associated with a decrease in cerebral vascular resistance, an increase in cerebral blood flow, and an increase in intracranial pressure.

b. Gastrointestinal tract—Constipation has long been recognized as an effect of opioids, an effect that does not diminish with continued use. That is, tolerance does not develop to opioid-induced constipation (Table 31–3). Opioid receptors exist in high density in the gastrointestinal tract, and the constipating effects of the opioids are mediated through an action on the enteric nervous system (see Chapter 6) as well as the CNS. In the stomach, motility (rhythmic contraction and relaxation) may decrease but tone (persistent contraction) may increase—particularly in the central portion; gastric secretion of hydrochloric acid is decreased. Small intestine resting tone is increased, with periodic spasms, but the amplitude of nonpropulsive contractions is markedly decreased. In the large intestine, propulsive peristaltic waves are diminished and tone is increased; this delays passage of the fecal mass and allows increased absorption of water, which leads to constipation. The large bowel actions are the basis for the use of opioids in the management of diarrhea, and constipation is a major problem in the use of opioids for control of severe cancer pain.

c. Biliary tract—The opioids contract biliary smooth muscle, which can result in biliary colic. The sphincter of Oddi may constrict, resulting in reflux of biliary and pancreatic secretions and elevated plasma amylase and lipase levels.

d. Renal—Renal function is depressed by opioids. It is believed that in humans this is chiefly due to decreased renal plasma flow. In addition, μ opioids have been found to have an antidiuretic effect in humans. Mechanisms may involve both the CNS and peripheral sites. Opioids also enhance renal tubular sodium reabsorption. The role of opioid-induced changes in antidiuretic hormone (ADH) release is controversial. Ureteral and bladder tone are increased by therapeutic doses of the opioid analgesics. Increased sphincter tone may precipitate urinary retention, especially in postoperative patients. Occasionally, ureteral colic caused by a renal calculus is made worse by opioid-induced increase in ureteral tone.

e. Uterus—The opioid analgesics may prolong labor. The mechanism for this action is unclear, but both peripheral and central actions of the opioids can reduce uterine tone.

f. Neuroendocrine—Opioid analgesics stimulate the release of ADH, prolactin, and somatotropin but inhibit the release of luteinizing hormone. These effects suggest that endogenous opioid peptides, through effects in the hypothalamus, regulate these systems (Table 31–1).

g. Pruritus—Therapeutic doses of the opioid analgesics produce flushing and warming of the skin accompanied sometimes by sweating and itching; CNS effects and peripheral histamine release may be responsible for these reactions. Opioid-induced pruritus and occasionally urticaria appear more frequently when opioid analgesics are administered parenterally. In addition, when opioids such as morphine are administered to the neuraxis by the spinal or epidural route, their usefulness may be limited by intense pruritus over the lips and torso.

h. Miscellaneous—The opioids modulate the immune system by effects on lymphocyte proliferation, antibody production, and chemotaxis. In addition, leucocytes migrate to the site of tissue injury and release opioid peptides, which in turn help counter inflammatory pain. However, natural killer cell cytolytic activity and lymphocyte proliferative responses to mitogens are usually inhibited by opioids. Although the mechanisms involved are complex, activation of central opioid receptors could mediate a significant component of the changes observed in peripheral immune function. In general, these effects are mediated by the sympathetic nervous system in the case of acute administration and by the hypothalamic-pituitary-adrenal system in the case of prolonged administration of opioids.

C. Effects of Opioids with Both Agonist and Antagonist Actions

Buprenorphine is an opioid agonist that displays high binding affinity but low intrinsic activity at the μ receptor. Its slow rate of dissociation from the μ receptor has also made it an attractive alternative to methadone for the management of opioid withdrawal. It functions as an *antagonist* at the δ and κ receptors and for this reason is referred to as a "mixed agonist-antagonist." Although buprenorphine is used as an analgesic, it can antagonize the action of more potent μ agonists such as morphine. Buprenorphine also binds to ORL1, the orphanin receptor. Whether this property also participates in opposing μ receptor function is under study. Pentazocine and nalbuphine are other examples of opioid analgesics with mixed agonist-antagonist properties. Psychotomimetic effects, with hallucinations, nightmares, and anxiety, have been reported after use of drugs with mixed agonist-antagonist actions.

A combined buprenorphine HCl/naloxone HCl dihydrate preparation is now available as sublingual tablets and a sublingual film for use in a maintenance treatment plan that includes counseling, psychosocial support, and direction by physicians qualified under the Drug Addiction Treatment Act. Both formulations can be abused in a manner similar to other opioids, legal or illicit. The combination formulations can cause serious respiratory depression and death, particularly when extracted and injected intravenously in combination with benzodiazepines or other CNS depressants (ie, sedatives, tranquilizers, or alcohol). It is extremely dangerous to self-administer benzodiazepines or other CNS depressants while taking the buprenorphine-naloxone combination.

■ CLINICAL PHARMACOLOGY OF THE OPIOID ANALGESICS

Successful treatment of pain is a challenging task that begins with careful attempts to assess the source and magnitude of the pain. The amount of pain experienced by the patient is often measured by means of a pain Numeric Rating Scale (NRS) or less frequently by marking a line on a Visual Analog Scale (VAS) with word descriptors ranging from no pain (0) to excruciating pain (10). In either case, values indicate the magnitude of pain as: mild (1–3), moderate (4–6), or severe (7–10). A similar scale can be used with children and with patients who cannot speak; this scale depicts five faces ranging from smiling (no pain) to crying (maximum pain).

For a patient in severe pain, the administration of an opioid analgesic is usually considered a primary part of the overall management plan. Determining the route of administration (oral, parenteral, neuraxial), duration of drug action, ceiling effect (maximal intrinsic activity), duration of therapy, potential for adverse effects, and the patient's past experience with opioids all should be addressed. One of the principal errors made by physicians in this setting is failure to adequately assess a patient's pain and to match its severity with an appropriate level of therapy. Just as important is the principle that following delivery of the therapeutic plan, its effectiveness must be reevaluated and the plan modified, if necessary, if the response was excessive or inadequate.

Use of opioid drugs in acute situations may be contrasted with their use in chronic pain management, in which a multitude of other factors must be considered, including the development of tolerance to and physical dependence on opioid analgesics.

Clinical Use of Opioid Analgesics

A. Analgesia

Severe, *constant* pain is usually relieved with opioid analgesics with high intrinsic activity (see Table 31–2), whereas sharp, intermittent pain does not appear to be as effectively controlled.

The pain associated with cancer and other terminal illnesses must be treated aggressively and often requires a multidisciplinary approach for effective management. Such conditions may require continuous use of potent opioid analgesics and are associated with some degree of tolerance and dependence. *However, this should not be used as a barrier to providing patients with the best possible care and quality of life.* Research in the hospice movement has demonstrated that fixed-interval administration of opioid medication (ie, a regular dose at a scheduled time) is more effective in achieving pain relief than dosing on demand. New dosage forms of opioids that allow slower release of the drug are now available, eg, sustained-release forms of morphine (MS Contin) and oxycodone (OxyContin). Their purported advantage is a longer and more stable level of analgesia.

If disturbances of gastrointestinal function prevent the use of oral sustained-release morphine, the fentanyl transdermal system (fentanyl patch) can be used over long periods. Furthermore, buccal transmucosal fentanyl can be used for short episodes of breakthrough pain (see Alternative Routes of Administration). Administration of strong opioids by nasal insufflation has been shown to be efficacious, and nasal preparations are now available in some countries. Approval of such formulations in the USA is growing. In addition, stimulant drugs such as the amphetamines have been shown to enhance the analgesic actions of the opioids and thus may be very useful adjuncts in the patient with chronic pain.

Opioid analgesics are often used during obstetric labor. Because opioids cross the placental barrier and reach the fetus, care must be taken to minimize neonatal depression. If it occurs, immediate injection of the antagonist naloxone will reverse the depression. The phenylpiperidine drugs (eg, meperidine) appear to produce less depression, particularly respiratory depression, in newborn infants than does morphine; this may justify their use in obstetric practice.

The acute, severe pain of renal and biliary colic often requires a strong agonist opioid for adequate relief. However, the drug-induced increase in smooth muscle tone may cause a paradoxical *increase* in pain secondary to increased spasm. An increase in the dose of opioid is usually successful in providing adequate analgesia.

B. Acute Pulmonary Edema

The relief produced by intravenous morphine in dyspnea from pulmonary edema associated with left ventricular heart failure is remarkable. Proposed mechanisms include reduced anxiety (*perception* of shortness of breath) and reduced cardiac preload (reduced venous tone) and afterload (decreased peripheral resistance). However, if respiratory depression is a problem, furosemide may be preferred for the treatment of pulmonary edema. On the other hand, morphine can be particularly useful when treating painful myocardial ischemia with pulmonary edema.

C. Cough

Suppression of cough can be obtained at doses lower than those needed for analgesia. However, in recent years the use of opioid analgesics to allay cough has diminished largely because a number of effective synthetic compounds have been developed that are neither analgesic nor addictive. These agents are discussed below.

D. Diarrhea

Diarrhea from almost any cause can be controlled with the opioid analgesics, but if diarrhea is associated with infection such use must not substitute for appropriate chemotherapy. Crude opium preparations (eg, paregoric) were used in the past to control diarrhea, but now synthetic surrogates with more selective gastrointestinal effects and few or no CNS effects, eg, diphenoxylate or loperamide, are used. Several preparations are available specifically for this purpose (see Chapter 62).

E. Shivering

Although all opioid agonists have some propensity to reduce shivering, meperidine is reported to have the most pronounced anti-shivering properties. Meperidine apparently blocks shivering mainly through an action on subtypes of the α_2 adrenoceptor.

F. Applications in Anesthesia

The opioids are frequently used as premedicant drugs before anesthesia and surgery because of their sedative, anxiolytic, and analgesic properties. They are also used intraoperatively both as adjuncts to other anesthetic agents and, in high doses (eg, 0.02–0.075 mg/kg of fentanyl), as a primary component of the anesthetic regimen (see Chapter 25). Opioids are most commonly used in cardiovascular surgery and other types of high-risk surgery in which a primary goal is to minimize cardiovascular depression. In such situations, mechanical respiratory assistance must be provided.

Because of their direct action on the superficial neurons of the spinal cord dorsal horn, opioids can also be used as regional analgesics by administration into the epidural or subarachnoid spaces of the spinal column. A number of studies have demonstrated that long-lasting analgesia with minimal adverse effects can be achieved by epidural administration of 3–5 mg of morphine, followed by slow infusion through a catheter placed in the epidural space. It was initially assumed that the epidural application of opioids might selectively produce analgesia without impairment of motor, autonomic, or sensory functions other than pain. However, respiratory depression can occur after the drug is injected into the epidural space and may require reversal with naloxone. Effects such as pruritus and nausea and vomiting are common after epidural and subarachnoid administration of opioids and may also be reversed with naloxone if necessary. Currently, the epidural route is favored over subarachnoid administration because adverse effects are less common and robust outcome studies have shown a significant reduction in perioperative mortality and morbidity with the use of thoracic epidural analgesia. The use of low doses of local anesthetics in combination with fentanyl infused through a thoracic epidural catheter has become an accepted method of pain control in patients recovering from thoracic and major upper abdominal surgery. In rare cases, chronic pain management specialists may elect to surgically implant a programmable infusion pump connected to a spinal catheter for continuous infusion of opioids or other analgesic compounds.

G. Alternative Routes of Administration

Rectal suppositories of morphine and hydromorphone have been used when oral and parenteral routes are undesirable. The **transdermal patch** provides stable blood levels of drug and better pain control while avoiding the need for repeated parenteral injections. Fentanyl has been the most successful opioid in transdermal application and is indicated for the management of persistent unremitting pain. Because of the complication of fentanyl-induced respiratory depression, the Food and Drug Administration (FDA) recommends that introduction of a transdermal fentanyl patch (25 mcg/h) be reserved for patients with an established oral morphine requirement of at least 60 mg/d for 1 week or more. Extreme caution must be exercised in any patient initiating therapy or undergoing a dose increase because the peak effects may not be realized until 24–48 hours after patch application. The **intranasal** route avoids repeated parenteral drug injections and the first-pass metabolism of orally administered drugs. Butorphanol is the only opioid currently available in the USA in a nasal formulation, but more are expected. Another alternative to parenteral administration is the **buccal transmucosal** route, which uses a fentanyl citrate lozenge or a "lollipop" mounted on a stick.

Another type of pain control called **patient-controlled analgesia (PCA)** is now in widespread use for the management of breakthrough pain. With PCA, the patient controls a parenteral (usually intravenous) infusion device by pressing a button to deliver a preprogrammed dose of the desired opioid analgesic. Claims of better pain control using less opioid are supported by well-designed clinical trials, making this approach very useful in postoperative pain control. However, health care personnel must be very familiar with the use of PCAs to avoid overdosage secondary to misuse or improper programming. There is a proven risk of PCA-associated respiratory depression and hypoxia that requires careful monitoring of vital signs and sedation level, and provision of supplemental oxygen. This risk is increased if patients are concurrently prescribed medications with sedative properties such as benzodiazepines.

Toxicity & Undesired Effects

Direct toxic effects of the opioid analgesics that are extensions of their acute pharmacologic actions include respiratory depression, nausea, vomiting, and constipation (Table 31–4). In addition, tolerance and dependence, diagnosis and treatment of overdosage, and contraindications must be considered.

A. Tolerance and Dependence

Drug dependence of the opioid type is marked by a relatively specific withdrawal or abstinence syndrome. Just as there are pharmacologic differences between the various opioids, there are also differences in psychological dependence and the severity of withdrawal effects. For example, withdrawal from dependence on a strong agonist is associated with more severe withdrawal signs and symptoms than withdrawal from a mild or moderate agonist. Administration of an opioid *antagonist* to an opioid-dependent person is followed by brief but severe withdrawal symptoms (see antagonist-precipitated withdrawal, below). The potential for physical and psychological dependence of the partial agonist-antagonist opioids appears to be less than that of the strong agonist drugs.

1. Tolerance—Although development of tolerance begins with the first dose of an opioid, tolerance generally does not become clinically manifest until after 2–3 weeks of frequent exposure to ordinary therapeutic doses. Nevertheless, perioperative and critical care use of ultrapotent opioid analgesics such as remifentanil have been shown to induce opioid tolerance within hours. Tolerance develops most readily when large doses are given at short intervals and is minimized by giving small amounts of drug with longer intervals between doses.

Depending on the compound and the effect measured, the degree of tolerance may be as great as 35-fold. Marked tolerance may develop to the analgesic, sedating, and respiratory depressant effects. It is possible to produce respiratory arrest in a non-tolerant

TABLE 31–4 Adverse effects of the opioid analgesics.

Behavioral restlessness, tremulousness, hyperactivity (in dysphoric reactions)
Respiratory depression
Nausea and vomiting
Increased intracranial pressure
Postural hypotension accentuated by hypovolemia
Constipation
Urinary retention
Itching around nose, urticaria (more frequent with parenteral and spinal administration)

person with a dose of 60 mg of morphine, whereas in addicts maximally tolerant to opioids as much as 2000 mg of morphine taken over a 2- or 3-hour period may not produce significant respiratory depression. Tolerance also develops to the antidiuretic, emetic, and hypotensive effects but not to the miotic, convulsant, and constipating actions (Table 31–3).

Tolerance to the sedating and respiratory effects of the opioids dissipates within a few days after the drugs are discontinued. Tolerance to the emetic effects may persist for several months after withdrawal of the drug. The rates at which tolerance appears and disappears, as well as the degree of tolerance, may also differ considerably among the different opioid analgesics and among individuals using the same drug. For instance, tolerance to methadone develops more slowly and to a lesser degree than to morphine.

Tolerance also develops to analgesics with mixed receptor effects but to a lesser extent than to the agonists. Such effects as hallucinations, sedation, hypothermia, and respiratory depression are reduced after repeated administration of the mixed receptor drugs. However, tolerance to the latter agents does not generally include cross-tolerance to the agonist opioids. It is also important to note that tolerance does not develop to the antagonist actions of the mixed agents or to those of the pure antagonists.

Cross-tolerance is an extremely important characteristic of the opioids, ie, patients tolerant to morphine often show a reduction in analgesic response to other agonist opioids. This is particularly true of those agents with primarily μ-receptor agonist activity. Morphine and its congeners exhibit cross-tolerance not only with respect to their analgesic actions but also to their euphoriant, sedative, and respiratory effects. However, the cross-tolerance existing among the μ-receptor agonists can often be partial or incomplete. This clinical observation has led to the concept of "opioid rotation," which has been used in the treatment of cancer pain for many years. A patient who is experiencing decreasing effectiveness of one opioid analgesic regimen is "rotated" to a different opioid analgesic (eg, morphine to hydromorphone; hydromorphone to methadone) and typically experiences significantly improved analgesia at a reduced overall equivalent dosage. Another approach is to "recouple" opioid receptor function through the use of adjunctive nonopioid agents. NMDA-receptor antagonists (eg, ketamine) have shown promise in preventing or reversing opioid-induced tolerance in animals and humans. Use of ketamine is increasing because well-controlled studies have shown clinical efficacy in reducing postoperative pain and opioid requirements in opioid-tolerant patients. Agents that independently enhance μ-receptor recycling may also hold promise to improve analgesia in the opioid-tolerant patient.

The novel use of δ-receptor antagonists with μ-receptor agonists is also emerging as a strategy to avoid the development of tolerance. This idea has developed around the observation that mice lacking the δ-opioid receptor fail to develop tolerance to morphine.

2. Dependence

The development of physical dependence is an invariable accompaniment of tolerance to repeated administration of an opioid of the μ type. Failure to continue administering the drug results in a characteristic withdrawal or abstinence syndrome that reflects an exaggerated rebound from the acute pharmacologic effects of the opioid.

The signs and symptoms of withdrawal include rhinorrhea, lacrimation, yawning, chills, gooseflesh (piloerection), hyperventilation, hyperthermia, mydriasis, muscular aches, vomiting, diarrhea, anxiety, and hostility. The number and intensity of the signs and symptoms are largely dependent on the degree of physical dependence that has developed. Administration of an opioid at this time suppresses abstinence signs and symptoms almost immediately.

The time of onset, intensity, and duration of abstinence syndrome depend on the drug previously used and may be related to its biologic half-life. With morphine or heroin, withdrawal signs usually start within 6–10 hours after the last dose. Peak effects are seen at 36–48 hours, after which most of the signs and symptoms gradually subside. By 5 days, most of the effects have disappeared, but some may persist for months. In the case of meperidine, the withdrawal syndrome largely subsides within 24 hours, whereas with methadone several days are required to reach the peak of the abstinence syndrome, and it may last as long as 2 weeks. The slower subsidence of methadone effects is associated with a less intense immediate syndrome, and this is the basis for its use in the detoxification of heroin addicts. However, despite the loss of physical dependence on the opioid, craving for it may persist. In addition to methadone, buprenorphine and clonidine (an α_2-noradrenergic receptor agonist) are FDA-approved treatments for opioid analgesic detoxification (see Chapter 32).

A transient, explosive abstinence syndrome—**antagonist-precipitated withdrawal**—can be induced in a subject physically dependent on opioids by administering naloxone or another antagonist. Within 3 minutes after injection of the antagonist, signs and symptoms similar to those seen after abrupt discontinuance appear, peaking in 10–20 minutes and largely subsiding after 1 hour. Even in the case of methadone, withdrawal of which results in a relatively mild abstinence syndrome, the antagonist-precipitated abstinence syndrome may be very severe.

In the case of agents with mixed effects, withdrawal signs and symptoms can be induced after repeated administration followed by abrupt discontinuance of pentazocine, cyclazocine, or nalorphine, but the syndrome appears to be somewhat different from that produced by morphine and other agonists. Anxiety, loss of appetite and body weight, tachycardia, chills, increase in body temperature, and abdominal cramps have been noted.

3. Addiction

The euphoria, indifference to stimuli, and sedation usually caused by the opioid analgesics, especially when injected intravenously, tend to promote their compulsive use. In addition, the addict experiences abdominal effects that have been likened to an intense sexual orgasm. These factors constitute the primary reasons for opioid abuse liability and are strongly reinforced by the development of physical dependence. This disorder has been linked to dysregulation of brain regions mediating reward and stress (see Chapter 32).

Obviously, the risk of causing dependence is an important consideration in the therapeutic use of these drugs. *Despite that risk, under no circumstances should adequate pain relief ever be withheld simply because an opioid exhibits potential for abuse or because legislative controls complicate the process of prescribing narcotics.* Furthermore, certain principles can be observed by the clinician to minimize problems presented by tolerance and dependence when using opioid analgesics:

- Establish therapeutic goals before starting opioid therapy. This tends to limit the potential for physical dependence. The patient and his or her family should be included in this process.
- Once an effective dose is established, attempt to limit dosage to this level. This goal is facilitated by use of a written treatment contract that specifically prohibits early refills and having multiple prescribing physicians.
- Instead of opioid analgesics—especially in chronic management—consider using other types of analgesics or compounds exhibiting less pronounced withdrawal symptoms on discontinuance.
- Frequently evaluate continuing analgesic therapy and the patient's need for opioids.

B. Diagnosis and Treatment of Opioid Overdosage

Intravenous injection of naloxone dramatically reverses coma due to opioid overdose but not that due to other CNS depressants. Use of the antagonist should not, of course, delay the institution of other therapeutic measures, especially respiratory support.

See also the Antagonists section below and Chapter 58.

C. Contraindications and Cautions in Therapy

1. Use of pure agonists with weak partial agonists—When a weak partial agonist such as pentazocine is given to a patient also receiving a full agonist (eg, morphine), there is a risk of diminishing analgesia or even inducing a state of withdrawal; combining full agonist with partial agonist opioids should be avoided.

2. Use in patients with head injuries—Carbon dioxide retention caused by respiratory depression results in cerebral vasodilation. In patients with elevated intracranial pressure, this may lead to lethal alterations in brain function.

3. Use during pregnancy—In pregnant women who are chronically using opioids, the fetus may become physically dependent in utero and manifest withdrawal symptoms in the early postpartum period. A daily dose as small as 6 mg of heroin (or equivalent) taken by the mother can result in a mild withdrawal syndrome in the infant, and twice that much may result in severe signs and symptoms, including irritability, shrill crying, diarrhea, or even seizures. Recognition of the problem is aided by a careful history and physical examination. When withdrawal symptoms are judged to be relatively mild, treatment is aimed at control of these symptoms using such drugs as diazepam; with more severe withdrawal, camphorated tincture of opium (paregoric; 0.4 mg of morphine/mL) in an oral dose of 0.12–0.24 mL/kg is used. Oral doses of methadone (0.1–0.5 mg/kg) have also been used.

4. Use in patients with impaired pulmonary function—In patients with borderline respiratory reserve, the depressant properties of the opioid analgesics may lead to acute respiratory failure.

5. Use in patients with impaired hepatic or renal function—Because morphine and its congeners are metabolized primarily in the liver, their use in patients in prehepatic coma may be questioned. Half-life is prolonged in patients with impaired renal function, and morphine and its active glucuronide metabolite may accumulate; dosage can often be reduced in such patients.

6. Use in patients with endocrine disease—Patients with adrenal insufficiency (Addison's disease) and those with hypothyroidism (myxedema) may have prolonged and exaggerated responses to opioids.

Drug Interactions

Because seriously ill or hospitalized patients may require a large number of drugs, there is always a possibility of drug interactions when the opioid analgesics are administered. Table 31–5 lists some of these drug interactions and the reasons for not combining the named drugs with opioids.

SPECIFIC AGENTS

The following section describes the most important and widely used opioid analgesics, along with features peculiar to specific agents. Data about doses approximately equivalent to 10 mg of intramuscular morphine, oral versus parenteral efficacy, duration of analgesia, and intrinsic activity (maximum efficacy) are presented in Table 31–2.

STRONG AGONISTS

Phenanthrenes

Morphine, hydromorphone, and **oxymorphone** are strong agonists useful in treating severe pain. These prototypic agents have been described in detail above.

TABLE 31–5 Opioid drug interactions.

Drug Group	Interaction with Opioids
Sedative-hypnotics	Increased central nervous system depression, particularly respiratory depression.
Antipsychotic tranquilizers	Increased sedation. Variable effects on respiratory depression. Accentuation of cardiovascular effects (antimuscarinic and α-blocking actions).
Monoamine oxidase inhibitors	Relative contraindication to all opioid analgesics because of the high incidence of hyperpyrexic coma; hypertension has also been reported.

Morphine

Heroin (diamorphine, diacetylmorphine) is potent and fast-acting, but its use is prohibited in the USA and Canada. In recent years, there has been considerable agitation to revive its use. However, double-blind studies have not supported the claim that heroin is more effective than morphine in relieving severe chronic pain, at least when given by the intramuscular route.

Phenylheptylamines

Methadone has undergone a dramatic revival as a potent and clinically useful analgesic. It can be administered by the oral, intravenous, subcutaneous, spinal, and rectal routes. It is well absorbed from the gastrointestinal tract and its bioavailability far exceeds that of oral morphine.

Methadone

Methadone is not only a potent μ-receptor agonist but its racemic mixture of D- and L-methadone isomers can also block both NMDA receptors and monoaminergic reuptake transporters. These nonopioid receptor properties may help explain its ability to relieve difficult-to-treat pain (neuropathic, cancer pain), especially when a previous trial of morphine has failed. In this regard, when analgesic tolerance or intolerable side effects have developed with the use of increasing doses of morphine or hydromorphone, "opioid rotation" to methadone has provided superior analgesia at 10–20% of the morphine-equivalent daily dose. In contrast to its use in suppressing symptoms of opioid withdrawal, use of methadone as an analgesic typically requires administration at intervals of no more than 8 hours. However, given methadone's highly variable pharmacokinetics and long half-life (25–52 hours), initial administration should be closely monitored to avoid potentially harmful adverse effects, especially respiratory depression. Because methadone is metabolized by CYP3A4 and CYP2B6 isoforms in the liver, inhibition of its metabolic pathway or hepatic dysfunction has also been associated with overdose effects, including respiratory depression or, more rarely, prolonged QT-based cardiac arrhythmias.

Methadone is widely used in the treatment of opioid abuse. Tolerance and physical dependence develop more slowly with methadone than with morphine. The withdrawal signs and symptoms occurring after abrupt discontinuance of methadone are milder, although more prolonged, than those of morphine. These properties make methadone a useful drug for detoxification and for maintenance of the chronic relapsing heroin addict.

For detoxification of a heroin-dependent addict, low doses of methadone (5–10 mg orally) are given two or three times daily for 2 or 3 days. Upon discontinuing methadone, the addict experiences a mild but endurable withdrawal syndrome.

For maintenance therapy of the opioid recidivist, tolerance to 50–100 mg/d of oral methadone may be deliberately produced; in this state, the addict experiences cross-tolerance to heroin, which prevents most of the addiction-reinforcing effects of heroin. One rationale of maintenance programs is that blocking the reinforcement obtained from abuse of illicit opioids removes the drive to obtain them, thereby reducing criminal activity and making the addict more amenable to psychiatric and rehabilitative therapy. The pharmacologic basis for the use of methadone in maintenance programs is sound and the sociologic basis is rational, but some methadone programs fail because nonpharmacologic management is inadequate.

The concurrent administration of methadone to heroin addicts known to be recidivists has been questioned because of the increased risk of overdose death secondary to respiratory arrest. Not only has the number of patients prescribed methadone for persistent pain increased, but the incidence of accidental overdose and complications related to respiratory depression have also increased. Buprenorphine, a partial μ-receptor agonist with long-acting properties, has been found to be effective in opioid detoxification and maintenance programs and is presumably associated with a lower risk of such overdose fatalities.

Phenylpiperidines

Fentanyl is one of the most widely used agents in the family of synthetic opioids. The fentanyl subgroup now includes **sufentanil, alfentanil,** and **remifentanil** in addition to the parent compound, fentanyl.

Fentanyl

These opioids differ mainly in their potency and biodisposition. Sufentanil is five to seven times more potent than fentanyl. Alfentanil is considerably less potent than fentanyl, but acts more rapidly and has a markedly shorter duration of action. Remifentanil is metabolized very rapidly by blood and nonspecific tissue esterases, making its pharmacokinetic and pharmacodynamic half-lives extremely short. Such properties are useful when these compounds are used in anesthesia practice. Although fentanyl is now the predominant analgesic in the phenylpiperidine class, **meperidine** continues to be used. This older opioid has significant antimuscarinic effects, which may be a contraindication if tachycardia would be a problem. Meperidine is also reported to have a negative inotropic action on the heart. In addition, it has the potential for producing seizures secondary to accumulation of its metabolite, normeperidine, in patients receiving high doses or with concurrent renal failure. Given this undesirable profile, use of meperidine as a first-line analgesic is becoming increasingly rare.

Morphinans

Levorphanol is a synthetic opioid analgesic closely resembling morphine in its action.

MILD TO MODERATE AGONISTS

Phenanthrenes

Codeine, dihydrocodeine, and **hydrocodone** are all somewhat less efficacious than morphine and often have adverse effects that limit the maximum tolerated dose when one attempts to achieve analgesia comparable to that of morphine. **Oxycodone is more potent and is prescribed alone in higher doses as immediate-release or controlled-release forms for the treatment of moderate to severe pain.** Combinations of hydrocodone or oxycodone with acetaminophen are the predominant formulations of orally administered analgesics for the treatment of mild to moderate pain. However, there has been a large increase in the use of controlled-release oxycodone at the highest dose range.

Since each controlled-release tablet of oxycodone contains a large quantity of oxycodone to allow for prolonged action, those intent on abusing the old formulation have modified the tablets, achieving high levels instantly, resulting in abuse and possible fatal overdose. The FDA recently approved a new formulation of the controlled-release form of oxycodone that reportedly prevents the tablets from being cut, broken, chewed, crushed, or dissolved to release more oxycodone. This new formulation will hopefully lead to less abuse by snorting or injection. Approximately half a million people used a controlled-release form of oxycodone for the first time in 2008, which prompted the FDA to require the manufacturer to collect data on abuse or misuse of the drug. The FDA is also requiring a Risk Evaluation and Mitigation Strategy (REMS) that will include the issuance of a medication guide to patients and a requirement for prescriber education regarding the appropriate use of opioid analgesics in the treatment of pain. (See Box: Educating Opioid Prescribers.)

Codeine

Phenylheptylamines

Propoxyphene is chemically related to methadone but has extremely low analgesic activity. Its low efficacy makes it unsuitable, even in combination with aspirin, for severe pain. The increasing incidence of deaths associated with its use and misuse caused it to be withdrawn in the United States.

Phenylpiperidines

Diphenoxylate and its metabolite, **difenoxin,** are not used for analgesia but for the treatment of diarrhea. They are scheduled for minimal control (difenoxin is Schedule IV, diphenoxylate Schedule V; see inside front cover) because the likelihood of their abuse is remote. The poor solubility of the compounds limits their use for parenteral injection. As antidiarrheal drugs, they are used in combination with atropine. The atropine is added in a concentration

too low to have a significant antidiarrheal effect but is presumed to further reduce the likelihood of abuse.

Loperamide is a phenylpiperidine derivative used to control diarrhea. However, due to action on peripheral μ-opioid receptors and lack of effect on CNS receptors, there is renewed interest in its potential for the treatment of neuropathic pain. Its potential for abuse is considered very low because of its limited access to the brain. It is therefore available without a prescription.

The usual dose with all of these antidiarrheal agents is two tablets to start and then one tablet after each diarrheal stool.

OPIOIDS WITH MIXED RECEPTOR ACTIONS

Care should be taken not to administer any partial agonist or drug with mixed opioid receptor actions to patients receiving pure agonist drugs because of the unpredictability of both drugs' effects; reduction of analgesia or precipitation of an explosive abstinence syndrome may result.

Phenanthrenes

Nalbuphine is a strong κ-receptor *agonist* and a μ-receptor *antagonist;* it is given parenterally. At higher doses there seems to be a definite ceiling—not noted with morphine—to the respiratory depressant effect. Unfortunately, when respiratory depression does occur, it may be relatively resistant to naloxone reversal.

Buprenorphine is a potent and long-acting phenanthrene derivative that is a partial μ-receptor agonist and a κ–receptor antagonist. Administration by the sublingual route is preferred to avoid significant first-pass effect. Its long duration of action is due to its slow dissociation from μ receptors. This property renders its effects resistant to naloxone reversal. Its clinical applications are much like those of nalbuphine. In addition, studies continue to suggest that buprenorphine is as effective as methadone in the detoxification and maintenance of heroin abusers. Buprenorphine was approved by the FDA in 2002 for the management of opioid dependence. In contrast to methadone, high-dose administration of buprenorphine results in a μ-opioid *antagonist* action, limiting its properties of analgesia and respiratory depression. Moreover, buprenorphine is also available combined with a pure μ-opioid antagonist (Suboxone) to help prevent its diversion for illicit intravenous abuse. A slow-release transdermal patch preparation that releases drug over a 1-week period is also available.

Morphinans

Butorphanol produces analgesia equivalent to nalbuphine and buprenorphine but appears to produce more sedation at equianalgesic doses. Butorphanol is considered to be predominantly a κ agonist. However, it may also act as a partial agonist or antagonist at the μ receptor.

Benzomorphans

Pentazocine is a κ agonist with weak μ-antagonist or partial agonist properties. It is the oldest mixed agent available. It may be used orally or parenterally. However, because of its irritant properties, the injection of pentazocine subcutaneously is not recommended.

MISCELLANEOUS

Tramadol is a centrally acting analgesic whose mechanism of action is predominantly based on blockade of serotonin reuptake. Tramadol has also been found to inhibit norepinephrine transporter function. Because it is only partially antagonized by naloxone, it is believed to be only a weak μ-receptor agonist. The recommended dosage is 50–100 mg orally four times daily. Toxicity includes association with seizures; the drug is relatively contraindicated in patients with a history of epilepsy and for use with other drugs that lower the seizure threshold. Another serious risk is the development of serotonin syndrome, especially if selective serotonin reuptake inhibitor (SSRI) antidepressants are being administered (see Chapter 16). Other side effects include nausea and dizziness, but these symptoms typically abate after several days of therapy. It is surprising that no clinically significant effects on respiration or the cardiovascular system have thus far been reported. Given the fact that the analgesic action of tramadol is largely independent of μ-receptor action, tramadol may serve as an adjunct with pure opioid agonists in the treatment of chronic neuropathic pain.

Tapentadol is a newer analgesic with modest μ-opioid receptor affinity and significant norepinephrine reuptake-inhibiting action. In animal models, its analgesic effects were only moderately reduced by naloxone but strongly reduced by an α_2-adrenoceptor antagonist. Furthermore, its binding to the norepinephrine transporter (NET, see Chapter 6) was stronger than that of tramadol, whereas its binding to the serotonin transporter (SERT) was less than that of tramadol. Tapentadol was approved in 2008 and has been shown to be as effective as oxycodone in the treatment of moderate to severe pain but with a reduced profile of gastrointestinal complaints such as nausea. Tapentadol carries risk for seizures in patients with seizure disorders and for the development of serotonin syndrome. It is unknown how tapentadol compares in clinical utility to tramadol or other analgesics whose mechanism of action is not based primarily on opioid receptor pharmacology.

ANTITUSSIVES

The opioid analgesics are among the most effective drugs available for the suppression of cough. This effect is often achieved at doses below those necessary to produce analgesia. The receptors involved in the antitussive effect appear to differ from those associated with the other actions of opioids. For example, the antitussive effect is also produced by stereoisomers of opioid molecules that are devoid of analgesic effects and addiction liability (see below).

The physiologic mechanism of cough is complex, and little is known about the specific mechanism of action of the opioid antitussive drugs. It appears likely that both central and peripheral effects play a role.

The opioid derivatives most commonly used as antitussives are **dextromethorphan, codeine, levopropoxyphene,** and **noscapine** (levopropoxyphene and noscapine are not available in the USA). They should be used with caution in patients taking monoamine oxidase inhibitors (see Table 31–5). Antitussive preparations usually also contain expectorants to thin and liquefy respiratory secretions. Importantly, due to increasing reports of death in young children taking dextromethorphan in formulations of over-the-counter "cold/cough" medications, its use in children less than 6 years of age has been banned by the FDA. Moreover, because of variations in the metabolism of codeine, its use for any purpose in young children is being reconsidered.

Dextromethorphan is the dextrorotatory stereoisomer of a methylated derivative of levorphanol. It is purported to be free of addictive properties and produces less constipation than codeine. The usual antitussive dose is 15–30 mg three or four times daily. It is available in many over-the-counter products. Dextromethorphan has also been found to enhance the analgesic action of morphine and presumably other μ-receptor agonists. However, abuse of its purified (powdered) form has been reported to lead to serious adverse events including death.

Codeine, as noted, has a useful antitussive action at doses lower than those required for analgesia. Thus, 15 mg is usually sufficient to relieve cough.

Levopropoxyphene is the stereoisomer of the weak opioid agonist dextropropoxyphene. It is devoid of opioid effects, although sedation has been described as a side effect. The usual antitussive dose is 50–100 mg every 4 hours.

THE OPIOID ANTAGONISTS

The pure opioid antagonist drugs **naloxone, naltrexone,** and **nalmefene** are morphine derivatives with bulkier substituents at the N_17 position. These agents have a relatively high affinity for μ-opioid binding sites. They have lower affinity for the other receptors but can also reverse agonists at δ and κ sites.

Naloxone

Pharmacokinetics

Naloxone is usually given by injection and has a short duration of action (1–2 hours) when given by this route. Metabolic disposition is chiefly by glucuronide conjugation like that of the agonist opioids with free hydroxyl groups. Naltrexone is well absorbed after oral administration but may undergo rapid first-pass metabolism. It has a half-life of 10 hours, and a single oral dose of 100 mg blocks the effects of injected heroin for up to 48 hours. Nalmefene, the newest of these agents, is a derivative of naltrexone but is available only for intravenous administration. Like naloxone, nalmefene is used for opioid overdose but has a longer half-life (8–10 hours).

Pharmacodynamics

When given in the absence of an agonist drug, these antagonists are almost inert at doses that produce marked antagonism of agonist opioid effects.

When given intravenously to a morphine-treated subject, the antagonist completely and dramatically reverses the opioid effects within 1–3 minutes. In individuals who are acutely depressed by an overdose of an opioid, the antagonist effectively normalizes respiration, level of consciousness, pupil size, bowel activity, and awareness of pain. In dependent subjects who appear normal while taking opioids, naloxone or naltrexone almost instantaneously precipitates an abstinence syndrome.

There is no tolerance to the antagonistic action of these agents, nor does withdrawal after chronic administration precipitate an abstinence syndrome.

Clinical Use

Naloxone is a pure antagonist and is preferred over older weak agonist-antagonist agents that had been used primarily as antagonists, eg, nalorphine and levallorphan.

The major application of naloxone is in the treatment of acute opioid overdose (see also Chapter 58). *It is very important that the*

relatively short duration of action of naloxone be borne in mind, because a severely depressed patient may recover after a single dose of naloxone and appear normal, only to relapse into coma after 1–2 hours.

The usual initial dose of naloxone is 0.1–0.4 mg intravenously for life-threatening respiratory and CNS depression. Maintenance is with the same drug, 0.4–0.8 mg given intravenously, and repeated whenever necessary. In using naloxone in the severely opioid-depressed newborn, it is important to start with doses of 5–10 mcg/kg and to consider a second dose of up to a total of 25 mcg/kg if no response is noted.

Low-dose naloxone (0.04 mg) has an increasing role in the treatment of adverse effects that are commonly associated with intravenous or epidural opioids. Careful titration of the naloxone dosage can often eliminate the itching, nausea, and vomiting while sparing the analgesia. For this purpose, oral naloxone, and more recently modified analogs of naloxone and naltrexone, have been approved by the FDA. These include **methylnaltrexone bromide** (Relistor) for the treatment of constipation in patients with late-stage advanced illness and **alvimopan** (Entereg) for the treatment of postoperative ileus following bowel resection surgery. The principal mechanism for this selective therapeutic effect is believed to be inhibition of peripheral μ receptors in the gut with minimal CNS penetration.

Because of its long duration of action, naltrexone has been proposed as a maintenance drug for addicts in treatment programs. A single dose given on alternate days blocks virtually all of the effects of a dose of heroin. It might be predicted that this approach to rehabilitation would not be popular with a large percentage of drug users unless they are motivated to become drug-free. A related use is in combination with morphine sulfate in a controlled-release formulation (Embeda) in which 20–100 mg of morphine is slowly released over 8–12 hours or longer for the control of prolonged postoperative pain. Naltrexone, 0.4–4 mg, is sequestered in the center of the formulation pellets and is present to prevent the abuse of the morphine (by grinding and extraction of the morphine from the capsules).

There is evidence that naltrexone decreases the craving for alcohol in chronic alcoholics by increasing baseline β-endorphin release, and it has been approved by the FDA for this purpose (see Chapter 23). Naltrexone also facilitates abstinence from nicotine (cigarette smoking) with reduced weight gain. In fact, a combination of naltrexone plus bupropion (Chapter 30) may also offer an effective and synergistic strategy for weight loss. If current trials demonstrate cardiovascular safety during prolonged use, this and other weight-loss medications compounded with naltrexone may eventually win FDA approval.

SUMMARY Opioids, Opioid Substitutes, and Opioid Antagonists

Subclass	Mechanism of Action	Effects	Clinical Applications	Pharmacokinetics, Toxicities
STRONG OPIOID AGONISTS				
• Morphine • Methadone • Fentanyl	Strong μ-receptor agonists • variable affinity for δ and κ receptors	Analgesia • relief of anxiety • sedation • slowed gastro-intestinal transit	Severe pain • adjunct in anesthesia (fentanyl, morphine) • pulmonary edema (morphine only) • maintenance in rehabilitation programs (methadone only)	First-pass effect • duration 1–4 h except methadone, 4–6 h • *Toxicity:* Respiratory depression • severe constipation • addiction liability • convulsions
• *Hydromorphone, oxymorphone: Like morphine in efficacy, but higher potency*				
• *Meperidine: Strong agonist with anticholinergic effects*				
• *Oxycodone: Dose-dependent analgesia*				
• *Sufentanil, alfentanil, remifentanil: Like fentanyl but shorter durations of action*				
PARTIAL AGONISTS				
• Codeine • Hydrocodone	Less efficacious than morphine • can antagonize strong agonists	Like strong agonists • weaker effects	Mild-moderate pain • cough (codeine)	Like strong agonists, toxicity dependent on genetic variation of metabolism
MIXED OPIOID AGONIST-ANTAGONISTS				
• Buprenorphine	Partial μ agonist • κ antagonist	Like strong agonists but can antagonize their effects • also reduces craving for alcohol	Moderate pain • some maintenance rehabilitation programs	Long duration of action 4–8 h • may precipitate abstinence syndrome
• Nalbuphine	κ Agonist • μ antagonist	Similar to buprenorphine	Moderate pain	Like buprenorphine
ANTITUSSIVES				
• Dextromethorphan	Poorly understood but strong and partial μ agonists are also effective antitussives	Reduces cough reflex	Acute debilitating cough	30–60 min duration • *Toxicity:* Minimal when taken as directed
• *Codeine, levopropoxyphene: Similar to dextromethorphan*				
OPIOID ANTAGONISTS				
• Naloxone	Antagonist at μ, δ, and κ receptors	Rapidly antagonizes all opioid effects	Opioid overdose	Duration 1–2 h (may have to be repeated when treating overdose) • *Toxicity:* Precipitates abstinence syndrome in dependent users
• *Naltrexone, nalmefene: Like naloxone but longer durations of action (10+ h); naltrexone is used in maintenance programs and can block heroin effects for up to 48 h; naltrexone is also used for alcohol and nicotine dependence; when combined with bupropion, may be effective in weight loss programs*				
• *Alvimopan, methylnaltrexone bromide: Potent μ antagonists with poor entry into the central nervous system; can be used to treat severe opioid-induced constipation without precipitating an abstinence syndrome*				
OTHER ANALGESICS USED IN MODERATE PAIN				
• Tapentadol	Moderate μ agonist, strong NET inhibitor	Analgesia	Moderate pain	Duration 4–6 h • *Toxicity:* Headache; nausea and vomiting; possible dependence
• Tramadol	Mixed effects: weak μ agonist, moderate SERT inhibitor, weak NET inhibitor	Analgesia	Moderate pain • adjunct to opioids in chronic pain syndromes	Duration 4–6 h • *Toxicity:* Seizures • risk of serotonin syndrome

NET, norepinephrine reuptake transporter; SERT, serotonin reuptake transporter.

PREPARATIONS AVAILABLE[1]

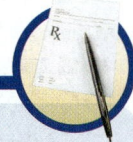

ANALGESIC OPIOIDS

Alfentanil (generic, Alfenta)
Parenteral: 0.5 mg/mL for injection

Buprenorphine (Buprenex, others)
Oral: 2, 8 mg sublingual tablets
Transdermal (Butrans): 5, 10, 20 mcg/h release rate for 1 week/patch
Parenteral: 0.3 mg/mL for injection

Butorphanol (generic, Stadol)
Parenteral: 1, 2 mg/mL for injection
Nasal (generic, Stadol NS): 10 mg/mL nasal spray

Codeine (sulfate or phosphate) (generic)
Oral: 15, 30, 60 mg tablets; 15 mg/5 mL solution
Parenteral: 15, 30 mg/mL for injection

Fentanyl (generic, other)
Parenteral (generic, Sublimaze): 50 mcg/mL for injection
Fentanyl Transdermal System (Duragesic): 12.5, 25, 50, 75, 100 mcg/h delivery
Fentanyl Buccal: 100, 200, 400, 600, 800 mcg oral lozenge
Fentanyl Actiq: 200, 400, 600, 800, 1200, 1600 mcg lozenge on a stick
Patient Controlled Transdermal Iontophoretic Fentanyl System: 40 mcg per dose for delivery

Hydromorphone (generic, Dilaudid)
Oral: 2, 8 mg tablets; 1 mg/mL liquid
Parenteral: 1, 2, 4, 10 mg/mL for injection

Levomethadyl acetate (Orlaam)
Oral: 10 mg/mL solution. Note: Orphan drug approved only for the treatment of narcotic addiction.

Levorphanol (generic, Levo-Dromoran)
Oral: 2 mg tablets
Parenteral: 2 mg/mL for injection

Meperidine (generic, Demerol)
Oral: 50, 100 mg tablets; 50 mg/5 mL syrup
Parenteral: 10, 25, 50, 75, 100 mg per dose for injection

Methadone (generic, Dolophine)
Oral: 5, 10 mg tablets; 40 mg dispersible tablets; 1, 2, 10 mg/mL solutions
Parenteral: 10 mg/mL for injection

Morphine sulfate (generic, others)
Oral: 15, 30 mg tablets; 15, 30 mg capsules; 10, 20, 100 mg/5 mL solution
Oral sustained-release tablets (MS Contin, others): 15, 30, 60, 100, 200 mg tablets
Oral sustained-release capsules (Avinza, Kadian): 20, 30, 50, 60, 90, 100, 120 mg capsules
Oral extended-release capsules (Embeda) (morphine sulfate/naltrexone HCl): 20/0.8, 30/1.2, 50/2, 60/2.4, 80/3.2, 100/4 mg
Parenteral: 0.5, 1, 2, 4, 5, 8, 10, 15, 25, 50 mg/mL for injection
Rectal: 5, 10, 20, 30 mg suppositories

Nalbuphine (generic, Nubain)
Parenteral: 10, 20 mg/mL for injection

Oxycodone (generic)
Oral: 5, 10, 15, 20, 30 mg tablets, capsules; 1, 20 mg/mL solutions
Oral sustained-release (generic, Oxy Contin): 10, 20, 40, 80 mg tablets

Oxymorphone (Numorphan)
Parenteral: 1, 1.5 mg/mL for injection
Rectal: 5 mg suppositories

Pentazocine (Talwin)
Oral: See combinations
Parenteral: 30 mg/mL for injection

Remifentanil (Ultiva)
Parenteral: 1, 2, 5 mg powder for reconstitution for injection

Sufentanil (generic, Sufenta)
Parenteral: 50 mcg/mL for injection

OTHER ANALGESICS

Tapentadol (Nucynta)
Oral: 50, 75, 100 mg tablets

Tramadol (generic, Ultram)
Oral: 50 mg tablets; 100, 200, 300 mg extended-release tablets

Ziconotide (Prialt)
Intrathecal: 25, 100 mcg/mL for programmable pump

ANALGESIC COMBINATIONS[2]

Codeine/acetaminophen (generic, Tylenol with Codeine, others)
Oral: 15, 30, 60 mg codeine plus 300 or 325 mg acetaminophen tablets or capsules; 12 mg codeine plus 120 mg acetaminophen tablets

Codeine/aspirin (generic, Empirin Compound, others)
Oral: 30, 60 mg codeine plus 325 mg aspirin tablets

Hydrocodone/acetaminophen (generic, Norco, Vicodin, Lortab, others)
Oral: 2.5, 5, 7.5, 10 mg hydrocodone plus 500 or 650 mg acetaminophen tablets

Hydrocodone/ibuprofen (Vicoprofen)
Oral: 7.5 mg hydrocodone plus 200 mg ibuprofen

Oxycodone/acetaminophen (generic, Percocet, Tylox, others)
Oral: 5 mg oxycodone plus 325 or 500 mg acetaminophen tablets
Note: High-dose acetaminophen has potential for hepatic toxicity with repeated use.

Oxycodone/aspirin (generic, Percodan)
Oral: 4.9 mg oxycodone plus 325 mg aspirin

OPIOID ANTAGONISTS

Alvimopan (Entereg)
Oral: 12 mg capsules

Methylnaltrexone (Relistor)
Parenteral: 12 mg/0.6 mL for injection

Nalmefene (Revex)
Parenteral: 0.1, 1 mg/mL for injection

Naloxone (generic, Narcan)
Parenteral: 0.4, 1 mg/mL; 0.02 mg/mL (for neonatal use) for injection

Naltrexone (generic, ReVia, Depade)
Oral: 50 mg tablets
Parenteral: 380 mg suspension for injection

ANTITUSSIVES

Codeine (generic)

Oral: 15, 30, 60 mg tablets; constituent of many proprietary syrups[2]

Dextromethorphan (generic, Benylin DM, Delsym, others)

Oral: 5, 7.5 mg lozenges; 7.5, 10, 15, 30 mg/5 mL syrup; 30 mg sustained-action liquid; constituent of many proprietary syrups[2]

[1]Antidiarrheal opioid preparations are listed in Chapter 62.

[2]Dozens of combination products are available; only a few of the most commonly prescribed are listed here. Codeine combination products available in several strengths are usually denoted No. 2 (15 mg codeine), No. 3 (30 mg codeine), and No. 4 (60 mg codeine). Prescribers should be aware of the possible danger of renal and hepatic injury with acetaminophen, aspirin, and nonsteroidal anti-inflammatory drugs contained in these analgesic combinations.

REFERENCES

Angst MS, Clark JD: Opioid-induced hyperalgesia. Anesthesiology 2006; 104:570.

Anton RF: Naltrexone for the management of alcohol dependence. N Eng J Med 2008;359:715.

Basbaum AI et al: Cellular and molecular mechanisms of pain. Cell 2009;139:267.

Basbaum AI, Jessel T: The perception of pain. In: Kandel ER et al (editors): *Principles of Neural Science,* 4th ed. McGraw-Hill, 2000.

Benedetti C, Premuda L: The history of opium and its derivatives. In: Benedetti C et al (editors): *Advances in Pain Research and Therapy,* vol 14. Raven Press, 1990.

Bolan EA, Tallarida RJ, Pasternak GW: Synergy between mu opioid ligands: Evidence for functional interactions among mu opioid receptor subtypes. J Pharmacol Exp Ther 2002;303:557.

Chu LF, Angst MS, Clark D: Opioid-induced hyperalgesia in humans: Molecular mechanisms and clinical considerations. Clin J Pain 2008;24:479.

Curran MP et al: Alvimopan. Drugs 2008;68:2011.

Dahan A et al: Sex-specific responses to opiates: Animal and human studies. Anesth Analg 2008;107:83.

Davis MP, Walsh D: Methadone for relief of cancer pain: A review of pharmacokinetics, pharmacodynamics, drug interactions and protocols of administration. Support Care Cancer 2001;9:73.

Ferner RE, Daniels AM: Office-based treatment of opioid-dependent patients. N Engl J Med 2003;348:81.

Ferrante FM: Principles of opioid pharmacotherapy: Practical implications of basic mechanisms. J Pain Symptom Manage 1996;11:265.

Fields HL, Basbaum AI: Central nervous system mechanisms of pain modulation. In: Wall PD, Melzack R (editors): *Textbook of Pain.* Churchill Livingstone, 1999.

Fillingim RB, Gear RW: Sex differences in opioid analgesia: Clinical and experimental findings. Eur J Pain 2004;8:413.

Fischer BD, Carrigan KA, Dykstra LA: Effects of N-methyl-D-aspartate receptor antagonists on acute morphine-induced and L-methadone-induced antinociception in mice. J Pain 2005;6:425.

Goldman D, Barr CS: Restoring the addicted brain. N Engl J Med 2002;347:843.

Joly V et al: Remifentanil-induced postoperative hyperalgesia and its prevention with small-dose ketamine. Anesthesiology 2005;103:147.

Julius D, Basbaum AI: Molecular mechanisms of nociception. Nature 2001;413:203.

Kalso E et al: No pain, no gain: Clinical excellence and scientific rigour—lessons learned from IA morphine. Pain 2002;98:269.

Kiefer BL: Opioids: First lessons from knockout mice. Trends Pharmacol Sci 1999;20:19.

Kim JA et al: Morphine-induced receptor endocytosis in a novel knockin mouse reduces tolerance and dependence. Curr Biol 2008;18:129.

King T et al: Role of NK-1 neurotransmission in opioid-induced hyperalgesia. Pain 2005;116:276.

Lai J et al: Pronociceptive actions of dynorphin via bradykinin receptors. Neurosci Lett 2008;437:175.

Lambert DG: The nociceptin/orphanin FQ receptor: A target with broad therapeutic potential. Nat Rev Drug Discov 2008;7:694.

Laughlin TM, Larson AA, Wilcox GL: Mechanisms of induction of persistent nociception by dynorphin. J Pharmacol Exp Ther 2001;299:6.

Liaw WI et al: Distinct expression of synaptic NR2A and NR2B in the central nervous system and impaired morphine tolerance and physical dependence in mice deficient in postsynaptic density-93 protein. Mol Pain 2008;4:45.

McGaraughty S, Heinricher MM: Microinjection of morphine into various amygdaloid nuclei differentially affects nociceptive responsiveness and RVM neuronal activity. Pain 2002;96:153.

Mercadante S, Arcuri E: Opioids and renal function. J Pain 2004;5:2.

Meunier J, Mouledous L, Topham CM: The nociceptin (ORL1) receptor: Molecular cloning and functional architecture. Peptides 2000;21:893.

Mitchell JM, Basbaum AI, Fields HL: A locus and mechanism of action for associative morphine tolerance. Nat Neurosci 2000;3:47.

Okie S: A flood of opioids, a rising tide of deaths. N Engl J Med 2010;363:1981.

Pan YX: Diversity and complexity of the mu opioid receptor gene: Alternate pre-mRNA splicing and promoters. DNA Cell Biol 2005;24:736.

Reimann F et al: Pain perception is altered by a nucleotide polymorphism in SCN9A. Proc Natl Acad Sci USA 2010;107:5148.

Reynolds SM et al: The pharmacology of cough. Trends Pharmacol Sci 2004;25:569.

Rittner HL, Brack A, Stein C: Pain and the immune system. Br J Anaesth 2008;101:40.

Skarke C, Geisslinger G, Lotsch J: Is morphine-3-glucuronide of therapeutic relevance? Pain 2005;116:177.

Smith MT: Neuroexcitatory effects of morphine and hydromorphone: Evidence implicating the 3-glucuronide metabolites. Clin Exp Pharmacol Physiol 2000;27:524.

Smith MT: Differences between and combinations of opioids revisited. Curr Opin Anaesthesiol 2008;21:596.

Stein C, Schafer M, Machelska H: Attacking pain at its source: New perspectives on opioids. Nat Med 2003;9:1003.

Vanderah TW et al: Mechanisms of opioid-induced pain and antinociceptive tolerance: Descending facilitation and spinal dynorphin. Pain 2001;92:5.

Waldhoer M et al: A heterodimer-selective agonist shows in vivo relevance of G protein-coupled receptor dimers. Proc Natl Acad Sci USA 2005;102:9050.

Wang Z et al: Pronociceptive actions of dynorphin maintain chronic neuropathic pain. J Neurosci 2001;21:1779.

Wild JE et al: Long-term safety and tolerability of tapentadol extended release for the management of chronic low back pain or osteoarthritis pain. Pain Pract 2010;10:416.

Williams JT, Christie MJ, Manzoni O: Cellular and synaptic adaptations mediating opioid dependence. Physiol Rev 2001;81:299.

Woolf CJ, Salter MW: Neuronal plasticity: Increasing the gain in pain. Science 2000;288:1765.

Zhao GM et al: Profound spinal tolerance after repeated exposure to a highly selective mu-opioid peptide agonist: Role of delta-opioid receptors. J Pharmacol Exp Ther 2002;302:188.

Zubieta JK et al: Regional mu opioid receptor regulation of sensory and affective dimensions of pain. Science 2001;293:311.

CASE STUDY ANSWER

In this case, the treatment of severe pain should be managed with the administration of a potent intravenous opioid analgesic such as morphine, hydromorphone, or fentanyl. It is expected that he will require frequent reevaluation of both the severity of his pain and the presence of potential side effects before an additional dose of an opioid analgesic is administered. Given his history of pulmonary disease, he is also at increased risk of developing respiratory depression. Frequent reevaluation of his level of consciousness, respiratory rate, fractional oxygen saturation, and other vital parameters can help achieve the goal of pain relief and minimize respiratory depression. Concurrent use of sedative agents such as benzodiazepines should be avoided if possible and used only with great caution.

Drugs of Abuse

Christian Lüscher, MD

A retired accountant developed a tremor and slowing of movements and was diagnosed with Parkinson's disease at age 67. At that time, his neurologist prescribed levodopa to restore dopamine levels. Two years later, motor symptoms start to fluctuate and the dopamine receptor agonist ropinirole is added to his treatment.[*] A few months later, he developed a strong interest in gambling, first buying lottery tickets and then visiting a casino almost every day. He concealed his gambling activity until he had lost more than $100,000. When he came for a consultation 5 weeks ago, ropinirole was replaced with monoamine oxidase inhibitor therapy. He now reports that his interest in gambling has disappeared. Is there a link between the dopamine agonist treatment and gambling addiction?

Drugs are abused (used in ways that are not medically approved) because they cause strong feelings of euphoria or alter perception. However, repetitive exposure induces widespread adaptive changes in the brain. As a consequence, drug use may become compulsive—the hallmark of addiction.

■ BASIC NEUROBIOLOGY OF DRUG ABUSE

DEPENDENCE VERSUS ADDICTION

Recent neurobiologic research has led to the conceptual and mechanistic separation of "dependence" and "addiction." The older term "physical dependence" is now denoted as **dependence,** whereas "psychological dependence" is more simply called **addiction.**

Every addictive drug causes its own characteristic spectrum of acute effects, but all have in common that they induce strong feelings of euphoria and reward. With repetitive exposure, addictive drugs induce adaptive changes such as tolerance (ie, escalation of dose to maintain effect). Once the abused drug is no longer available, signs of withdrawal become apparent. A combination of such signs, referred to as the **withdrawal syndrome,** defines *dependence.* Dependence is not always a correlate of drug abuse—it can also occur with many classes of nonpsychoactive drugs, eg, sympathomimetic vasoconstrictors and bronchodilators, and organic nitrate vasodilators. *Addiction,* on the other hand, consists of compulsive, relapsing drug use despite negative consequences, at times triggered by cravings that occur in response to contextual cues (see Box: Animal Models in Addiction Research). Although dependence invariably occurs with chronic exposure, only a small percentage of subjects develop a habit, lose control, and become addicted. For example, very few patients who receive opioids as analgesics desire the drug after withdrawal. And only one person out of six becomes addicted within 10 years of first use of cocaine. Conversely, relapse is very common in addicts after a successful withdrawal when, by definition, they are no longer dependent.

ADDICTIVE DRUGS INCREASE THE LEVEL OF DOPAMINE: REINFORCEMENT

To understand the long-term changes induced by drugs of abuse, their initial molecular and cellular targets must be identified. A combination of approaches in animals and humans, including functional imaging, has revealed the mesolimbic dopamine system as the prime target of addictive drugs. This system originates in the **ventral tegmental area (VTA),** a tiny structure at the tip of the brainstem, which projects to the **nucleus accumbens,** the amygdala, the hippocampus,

---

[*]The treatment of Parkinson's disease is discussed in Chapter 28.

Animal Models in Addiction Research

Many of the recent advances in addiction research have been made possible by the use of animal models. Since drugs of abuse are not only rewarding but also reinforcing, an animal will learn a behavior (eg, press a lever) when paired with drug administration. In such a self-administration paradigm, the number of times an animal is willing to press the lever in order to obtain a single dose reflects the strength of reinforcement and is therefore a measure of the rewarding properties of a drug. Observing withdrawal signs specific for rodents (eg, escape jumps or "wet-dog" shakes after abrupt termination of chronic morphine administration) allows the quantification of dependence. Behavioral tests for addiction in the rodent have proven difficult to develop, and so far no test fully captures the complexity of the disease. However it is possible to model core components of addiction, for example by monitoring behavioral sensitization and conditioned place preference. In the first test, an increase in locomotor activity is observed with intermittent drug exposure. The latter tests for the preference of a particular environment associated with drug exposure by measuring the time an animal spends in the compartment where a drug was received compared with the compartment where only saline was injected (conditioned place preference). Both tests have in common that they are sensitive to cue-conditioned effects of addictive drugs. Subsequent exposures to the environment without the drug lead to extinction of the place preference, which can be reinstated with a low dose of the drug or the presentation of a conditioned stimulus. These persistent changes serve as a model of relapse and have been linked to synaptic plasticity of excitatory transmission in the ventral tegmental area, nucleus accumbens and prefrontal cortex (see also Box: The Dopamine Hypothesis of Addiction). Recent findings suggest that prolonged self-administration of cocaine leads to behaviors in rats that closely resemble human addiction. Such "addicted rats" are very strongly motivated to seek cocaine, continue looking for the drug even when no longer available, and self-administer cocaine in spite of negative consequences, such as an electric foot shock. These findings suggest that addiction is a disease that does not respect species boundaries.

and the prefrontal cortex (Figure 32–1). Most projection neurons of the VTA are dopamine-producing neurons. When the dopamine neurons of the VTA begin to fire in bursts, large quantities of dopamine are released in the nucleus accumbens and the prefrontal cortex. Early animal studies pairing electrical stimulation of the VTA with operant responses (eg, lever pressing) that result in strong reinforcement established the central role of the mesolimbic dopamine system in reward processing. Direct application of drugs into

the VTA also acts as a strong reinforcer, and systemic administration of drugs of abuse causes release of dopamine. Even selective activation of dopamine neurons is sufficient to elicit behavioral changes typically observed with addictive drugs. These very selective interventions use optogenetic methods. Blue light is delivered in a freely moving mouse through light guides to activate channelrhodopsin, a light-gated cation channel that is artificially expressed in dopamine neurons.

As a general rule, all addictive drugs activate the mesolimbic dopamine system. The behavioral significance of this increase of dopamine is still debated. An appealing hypothesis is that mesolimbic dopamine codes for the difference between expected and actual reward and thus constitutes a strong learning signal (see Box: The Dopamine Hypothesis of Addiction).

Since each addictive drug has a specific molecular target that engages distinct cellular mechanisms to activate the mesolimbic system, three classes can be distinguished: A first group binds to **G$_{io}$ protein-coupled receptors,** a second group interacts with **ionotropic receptors or ion channels,** and a third group targets the **dopamine transporter** (Table 32–1 and Figure 32–2). G protein-coupled receptors (GPCRs) of the G$_{io}$ family inhibit neurons through postsynaptic hyperpolarization and presynaptic regulation of transmitter release. In the VTA, the action of these drugs is preferentially on the γ-aminobutyric acid (GABA) neurons that act as local inhibitory interneurons. Addictive drugs that bind to ionotropic receptors and ion channels can have combined effects on dopamine neurons and GABA neurons, eventually leading to enhanced release of dopamine. Finally, addictive drugs that interfere with monoamine transporters block reuptake or stimulate nonvesicular release of dopamine, causing an accumulation of extracellular dopamine in target structures. Since neurons of the VTA also express somatodendritic transporters, which normally clear dopamine released by the dendrites, class III drugs also increase dopamine level in the VTA. Although drugs of this class also affect transporters of other monoamines (norepinephrine, serotonin), action on the dopamine transporter remains central for addiction. This is consistent with the observations that antidepressants that block serotonin and norepinephrine uptake, but not dopamine uptake, do not cause addiction even after prolonged use.

DEPENDENCE: TOLERANCE & WITHDRAWAL

With chronic exposure to addictive drugs, the brain shows signs of adaptation. For example, if morphine is used at short intervals, the dose has to be progressively increased over the course of several days to maintain rewarding or analgesic effects. This phenomenon is called tolerance. It may become a serious problem because of increasing side effects—eg, respiratory depression—that do not show much tolerance and may lead to fatalities associated with overdose.

Tolerance to opioids may be due to a reduction of the concentration of a drug or a shorter duration of action in a target system

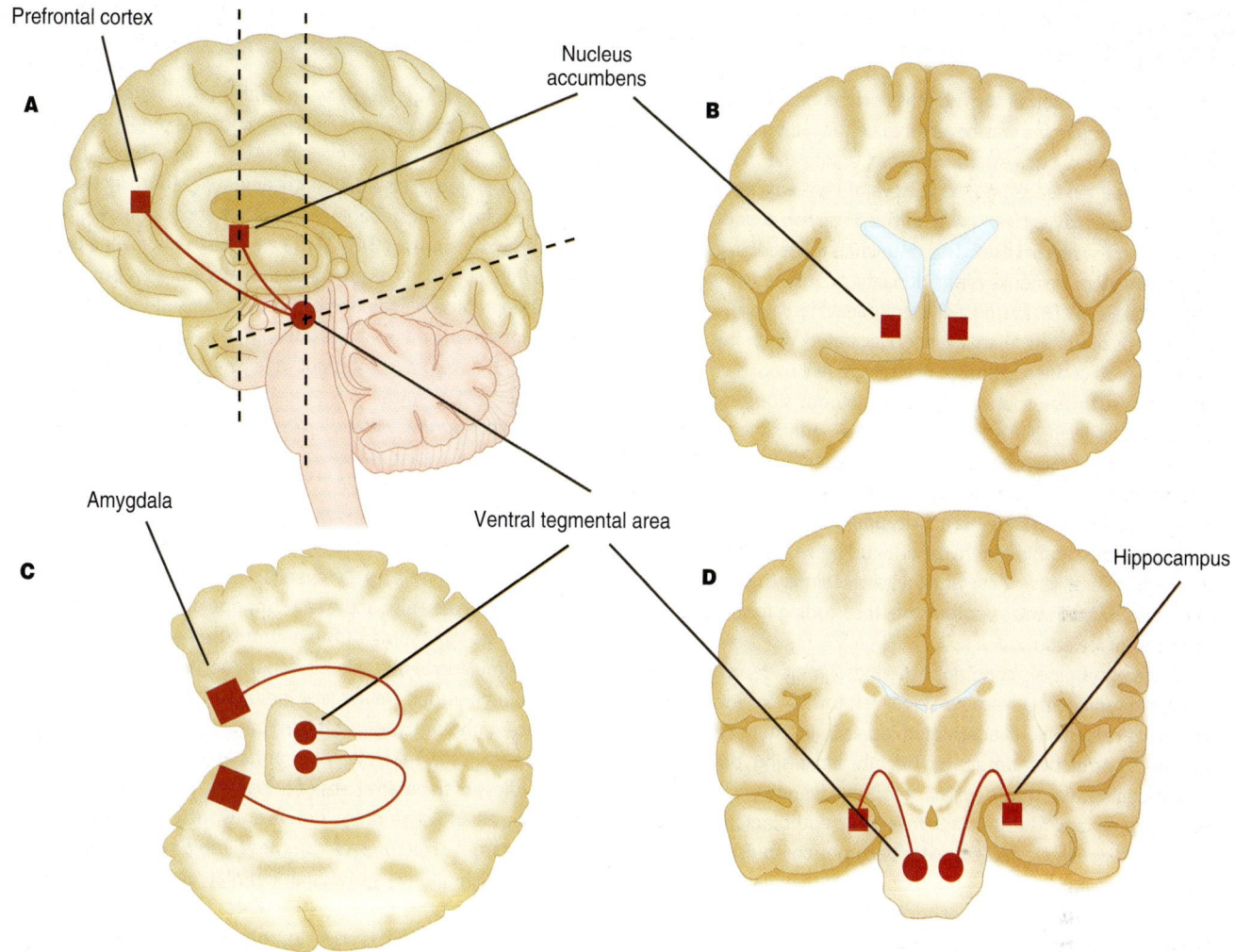

FIGURE 32–1 Major connections of the mesolimbic dopamine system in the brain. Schematic diagram of brain sections illustrating that the dopamine projections originate in the ventral tegmental area and target the nucleus accumbens, prefrontal cortex, amygdala, and hippocampus. The dashed lines on the sagittal section indicate where the horizontal and coronal sections were made.

(pharmacokinetic tolerance). Alternatively, it may involve changes of μ-opioid receptor function (pharmacodynamic tolerance). In fact, many μ-opioid receptor agonists promote strong receptor phosphorylation that triggers the recruitment of the adaptor protein β-arrestin, causing G proteins to uncouple from the receptor and to internalize within minutes (see Chapter 2). Since this decreases signaling, it is tempting to explain tolerance by such a mechanism. However, morphine, which strongly induces tolerance, does not recruit β-arrestins and fails to promote receptor internalization. Conversely, other agonists that drive receptor internalization very efficiently induce only modest tolerance. Based on these observations, it has been hypothesized that desensitization and receptor internalization actually protect the cell from overstimulation. In this model, morphine, by failing to trigger receptor endocytosis, disproportionally stimulates adaptive processes, which

eventually cause tolerance. Although the molecular identity of these processes is still under investigation, they may be similar to the ones involved in withdrawal (see below).

Adaptive changes become fully apparent once drug exposure is terminated. This state is called **withdrawal** and is observed to varying degrees after chronic exposure to most drugs of abuse. Withdrawal from opioids in humans is particularly strong (described below). Studies in rodents have added significantly to our understanding of the neural and molecular mechanisms that underlie dependence. For example, signs of dependence, as well as analgesia and reward, are abolished in knockout mice lacking the μ-opioid receptor, but not in mice lacking other opioid receptors (δ, κ). Although activation of the μ-opioid receptor initially strongly inhibits adenylyl cyclase, this inhibition becomes weaker after several days of repeated exposure. The reduction of the

The Dopamine Hypothesis of Addiction

In the earliest version of the hypothesis described in this chapter, mesolimbic dopamine was believed to be the neurochemical correlate of pleasure and reward. However, during the past decade, experimental evidence has led to several revisions. Phasic dopamine release may actually code for the *prediction error* of reward rather than the reward itself. This distinction is based on pioneering observations in monkeys that dopamine neurons in the ventral tegmental area (VTA) are most efficiently activated by a reward (eg, a few drops of fruit juice) that is not anticipated. When the animal learns to predict the occurrence of a reward (eg, by pairing it with a stimulus such as a sound), dopamine neurons stop responding to the reward itself (juice), but increase their firing rate when the conditioned stimulus (sound) occurs. Finally, if reward is predicted but not delivered (sound but no juice), dopamine neurons are inhibited below their baseline activity and become silent. In other words, the mesolimbic system continuously scans the reward situation. It increases its activity when reward is larger than expected, and shuts down in the opposite case, thus coding for the prediction error of reward.

Under physiologic conditions the mesolimbic dopamine signal could represent a learning signal responsible for reinforcing constructive behavioral adaptation (eg, learning to press a lever for food). Addictive drugs, by directly increasing dopamine, would generate a strong but inappropriate learning signal, thus hijacking the reward system and leading to pathologic reinforcement. As a consequence, behavior becomes compulsive; that is decisions are no longer planned and under control, but automatic, which is the hallmark of addiction.

This appealing hypothesis has been challenged based on the observation that some reward and drug-related learning is still possible in the absence of dopamine. Another intriguing observation is that mice genetically modified to lack the primary molecular target of cocaine, the dopamine transporter DAT, still self-administer the drug. Only when transporters of other biogenic amines are also knocked out does cocaine completely lose its rewarding properties. However, in $DAT^{-/-}$ mice, in which basal synaptic dopamine levels are high, cocaine still leads to increased dopamine release, presumably because other cocaine-sensitive monoamine transporters (NET, SERT) are able to clear some dopamine. When cocaine is given, these transporters are also inhibited and dopamine is again increased. As a consequence of this substitution among monoamine transporters, fluoxetine (a selective serotonin reuptake inhibitor, see Chapter 30) becomes addictive in $DAT^{-/-}$ mice. This concept is supported by newer evidence showing that deletion of the cocaine binding site on DAT leaves basal dopamine levels unchanged but abolishes the rewarding effect of cocaine.

The dopamine hypothesis of addiction has also been challenged by the observation that salient stimuli that are not rewarding (they may actually even be aversive and therefore negative reinforcers) also activate a subpopulation of dopamine neurons in the VTA. Some of the neurons that are activated by aversive stimuli do in fact release dopamine, while the majority of dopamine neurons are actually inhibited by aversive stimuli. These recent findings suggest that in parallel to the reward system, a system for aversion-learning originates in the VTA.

Regardless of the many roles of dopamine under physiologic conditions, all addictive drugs significantly increase its concentration in target structures of the mesolimbic projection. This suggests that high levels of dopamine may actually be at the origin of the adaptive changes that underlie dependence and addiction, a concept that is now supported by novel techniques that allow controlling the activity of dopamine neurons in vivo. In fact manipulations that drive sustained activity of VTA dopamine neurons cause the same cellular adaptations and behavioral changes typically observed with addictive drug exposure.

inhibition of adenylyl cyclase is due to a counter-adaptation of the enzyme system during exposure to the drug, which results in over-production of cAMP during subsequent withdrawal. Several mechanisms exist for this adenylyl cyclase compensatory response, including up-regulation of transcription of the enzyme. Increased cAMP concentrations in turn strongly activate the transcription factor cyclic AMP response element binding protein (CREB), leading to the regulation of downstream genes. Of the few such genes identified to date, one of the most interesting is the gene for the endogenous κ-opioid ligand dynorphin. During withdrawal, neurons of the nucleus accumbens produce high levels of dynorphin, which is then co-released with GABA onto the projection neurons of the VTA (Figure 32–3). These cells express κ-opioid receptors on their synaptic terminals and on the dendrites. As a consequence, they are inhibited and dopamine release is reduced. This mechanism exemplifies the adaptive processes engaged during dependence and may underlie the intense dysphoria typically observed during withdrawal.

ADDICTION: A DISEASE OF MALADAPTIVE LEARNING

Addiction is characterized by a high motivation to obtain and use a drug despite negative consequences. With time, drug use becomes compulsive ("wanting without liking"). Addiction is a recalcitrant, chronic, and stubbornly relapsing disease that is very difficult to treat.

TABLE 32–1 The mechanistic classification of drugs of abuse.[1]

Name	Main Molecular Target	Pharmacology	Effect on Dopamine (DA) Neurons	RR[2]
Drugs That Activate G Protein-Coupled Receptors				
Opioids	μ-OR (G_{io})	Agonist	Disinhibition	4
Cannabinoids	CB_1R (G_{io})	Agonist	Disinhibition	2
γ-Hydroxybutyric acid (GHB)	$GABA_BR$ (G_{io})	Weak agonist	Disinhibition	?
LSD, mescaline, psilocybin	$5\text{-}HT_{2A}R$ (G_q)	Partial agonist	...	1
Drugs That Bind to Ionotropic Receptors and Ion Channels				
Nicotine	nAChR ($\alpha_2\beta_2$)	Agonist	Excitation	4
Alcohol	$GABA_AR$, $5\text{-}HT_3R$, nAChR, NMDAR, Kir3 channels		Excitation, disinhibition (?)	3
Benzodiazepines	$GABA_AR$	Positive modulator	Disinhibition	3
Phencyclidine, ketamine	NMDAR	Antagonist	...	1
Drugs That Bind to Transporters of Biogenic Amines				
Cocaine	DAT, SERT, NET	Inhibitor	Blocks DA uptake	5
Amphetamine	DAT, NET, SERT, VMAT	Reverses transport	Blocks DA uptake , synaptic depletion	5
Ecstasy	SERT > DAT, NET	Reverses transport	Blocks DA uptake, synaptic depletion	?

$5\text{-}HT_xR$, serotonin receptor; CB_1R, cannabinoid-1; DAT, dopamine transporter; GABA, γ-aminobutyric acid; Kir3 channels, G protein-coupled inwardly rectifying potassium channels; LSD, lysergic acid diethylamide; μ-OR, μ-opioid receptor; nAChR, nicotinic acetylcholine receptor; NET, norepinephrine transporter; NMDAR, N-methyl-D-aspartate receptor; SERT, serotonin transporter; VMAT, vesicular monoamine transporter; ? indicates data not available.

[1]Drugs fall into one of three categories, targeting either G protein-coupled receptors, ionotropic receptors or ion channels, or biogenic amine transporters.

[2]RR, relative risk of addiction; 1 = nonaddictive; 5 = highly addictive.

The central problem is that even after successful withdrawal and prolonged drug-free periods, addicted individuals have a high risk of relapsing. Relapse is typically triggered by one of the following three conditions: reexposure to the addictive drug, stress, or a context that recalls prior drug use. It appears that when paired with drug use, a neutral stimulus may undergo a switch and motivate ("trigger") addiction-related behavior. This phenomenon may involve synaptic plasticity in the target nuclei of the mesolimbic projection (eg, nucleus accumbens). Several recent studies suggest that the recruitment of the dorsal striatum is responsible for the

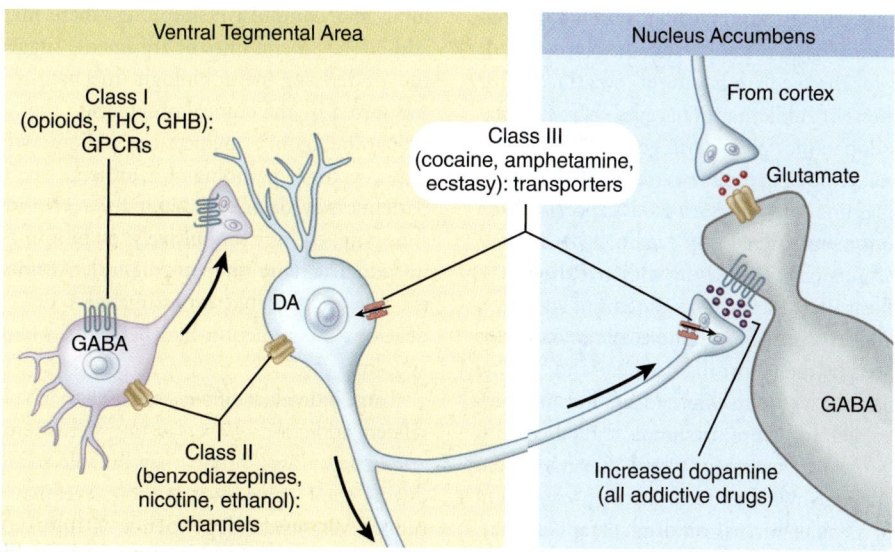

FIGURE 32–2 Neuropharmacologic classification of addictive drugs by primary target (see text and Table 32–1). DA, dopamine; GABA, γ-aminobutyric acid; GHB, γ-hydroxybutyric acid; GPCRs, G protein-coupled receptors; THC, Δ^9-tetrahydrocannabinol.

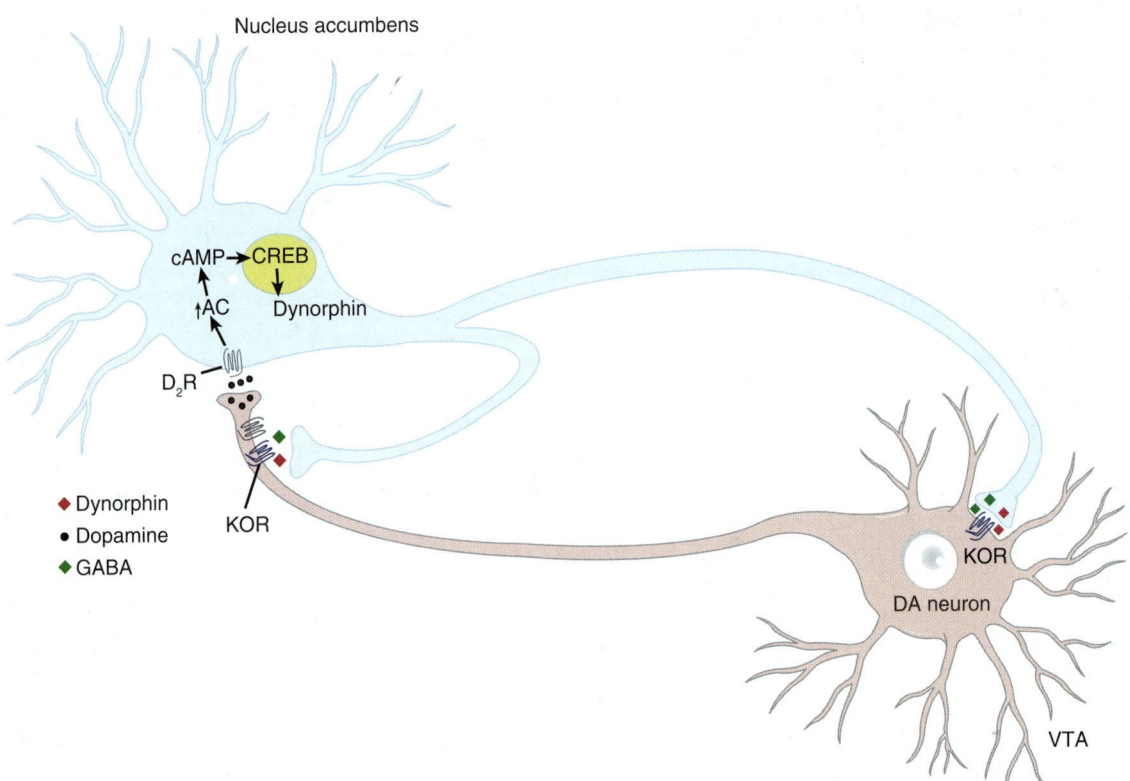

FIGURE 32–3 CREB-mediated up-regulation of dynorphin during withdrawal from dependence. Supersensitization of adenylyl cyclase (AC) leads to an increase of cAMP concentration in medium spiny neurons of the accumbens. This activates the transcription factor CREB, which turns on several genes, including that for dynorphin. Dynorphin is then co-released with γ-aminobutyric acid (GABA), activating the κ-opioid receptor (KOR) located on dopamine neurons of the ventral tegmental area (VTA), thereby leading to pre- and postsynaptic inhibition. D_2R, dopamine D_2 receptor.

compulsion. This switch may depend on synaptic plasticity in the nucleus accumbens of the ventral striatum, where mesolimbic dopamine afferents and cortical glutamatergic afferents converge. If dopamine release codes for the prediction error of reward (see Box: The Dopamine Hypothesis of Addiction), pharmacologic stimulation of the mesolimbic dopamine systems will generate an unusually strong learning signal. Unlike natural rewards, addictive drugs continue to increase dopamine even when reward is expected. Such overriding of the prediction error signal may eventually be responsible for the usurping of memory processes by addictive drugs.

The involvement of learning and memory systems in addiction is also suggested by clinical studies. For example, the role of context in relapse is supported by the report that soldiers who became addicted to heroin during the Vietnam War had significantly better outcomes when treated after their return home, compared with addicts who remained in the environment where they had taken the drug. In other words, cravings may recur at the presentation of contextual cues (eg, people, places, or drug paraphernalia). Current research therefore focuses on the effects of drugs on associative forms of synaptic plasticity, such as long-term potentiation (LTP), which underlie learning and memory (see Box: Synaptic Plasticity & Addiction).

Non-substance-dependent disorders, such as pathologic gambling and compulsive shopping, share many clinical features of addiction. Several lines of arguments suggest that they also share the underlying neurobiologic mechanisms. This conclusion is supported by the clinical observation that, as an adverse effect of dopamine agonist medication, patients with Parkinson's disease may become pathologic gamblers (see Case Study). Other patients may develop a habit for recreational activities, such as shopping, eating compulsively, or becoming excessively involved in sexual activity (hypersexuality). Although large-scale studies are not yet available, an estimated 1 of 7 parkinsonian patients develops an addiction-like behavior when receiving dopamine agonists.

Large individual differences exist also in vulnerability to substance-related addiction. Whereas one person may become "hooked" after a few doses, others may be able to use a drug occasionally during their entire lives without ever having difficulty in stopping. Even when dependence is induced with chronic exposure, only a small percentage of dependent users progress to addiction. Recent studies in rats suggest that impulsivity or excessive anxiety may be crucial traits that represent a risk for addiction. The transition to addiction is determined by a combination

Synaptic Plasticity & Addiction

Long-term potentiation (LTP) is a form of experience-dependent synaptic plasticity that is induced by activating glutamate receptors of the N-methyl-D-aspartate (NMDA) type. Since NMDA receptors are blocked by magnesium at negative potentials, their activation requires the concomitant release of glutamate (presynaptic activity) onto a receiving neuron that is depolarized (postsynaptic activity). Correlated pre- and postsynaptic activity durably enhances synaptic efficacy and triggers the formation of new connections. Because associativity is a critical component, LTP has become a leading candidate mechanism underlying learning and memory. LTP can be elicited at glutamatergic synapses of the mesolimbic reward system and is modulated by dopamine. Drugs of abuse could therefore interfere with LTP at sites of convergence of dopamine and glutamate projections (eg, ventral tegmental area [VTA], nucleus accumbens, or prefrontal cortex). Interestingly, exposure to an addictive drug triggers a specific form of synaptic plasticity at excitatory afferents (drug-evoked synaptic plasticity) and reduces GABA$_A$ receptor-mediated inhibition of the VTA. As a consequence, the excitability of dopamine neurons is increased, the synaptic calcium sources altered, and the rules for subsequent LTP inverted. Genetic manipulations in mice that prevent drug-evoked plasticity at this synapse also have effects on persistent changes of drug-associated behavioral paradigms such as reinstatement of conditioned place preference, further supporting the idea that synaptic plasticity is involved in context-dependent components of relapse.

of environmental and genetic factors. Heritability of addiction, as determined by comparing monozygotic with dizygotic twins, is relatively modest for cannabinoids but very high for cocaine. It is of interest that the relative risk for addiction (addiction liability) of a drug (Table 32–1) correlates with its heritability, suggesting that the neurobiologic basis of addiction common to all drugs is what is being inherited. Further genomic analysis indicates that only a few alleles (or perhaps even a single recessive allele) need to function in combination to produce the phenotype. However, identification of the genes involved remains elusive. Although some substance-specific candidate genes have been identified (eg, alcohol dehydrogenase), future research will also focus on genes implicated in the neurobiologic mechanisms common to all addictive drugs.

NONADDICTIVE DRUGS OF ABUSE

Some drugs of abuse do not lead to addiction. This is the case for substances that alter perception without causing sensations of reward and euphoria, such as the hallucinogens and the dissociative anesthetics (Table 32–1). Unlike addictive drugs, which primarily target the mesolimbic dopamine system, these agents primarily target cortical and thalamic circuits. Lysergic acid diethylamide (LSD), for example, activates the serotonin 5-HT$_{2A}$ receptor in the prefrontal cortex, enhancing glutamatergic transmission onto pyramidal neurons. These excitatory afferents mainly come from the thalamus and carry sensory information of varied modalities, which may constitute a link to enhanced perception. Phencyclidine (PCP) and ketamine produce a feeling of separation of mind and body (which is why they are called dissociative anesthetics) and, at higher doses, stupor and coma. The principal mechanism of action is a use-dependent inhibition of glutamate receptors of the N-methyl-D-aspartate (NMDA) type.

The classification of NMDA antagonists as nonaddictive drugs was based on early assessments, which, in the case of PCP, have recently been questioned. In fact, animal research shows that PCP can increase mesolimbic dopamine concentrations and has some reinforcing properties in rodents. Concurrent effects on both thalamocortical and mesolimbic systems also exist for other addictive drugs. Psychosis-like symptoms can be observed with cannabinoids, amphetamines, and cocaine, which may reflect their effects on thalamocortical structures. For example, cannabinoids, in addition to their documented effects on the mesolimbic dopamine system, also enhance excitation in cortical circuits through presynaptic inhibition of GABA release.

Hallucinogens and NMDA antagonists, even if they do not produce dependence or addiction, can still have long-term effects. Flashbacks of altered perception can occur years after LSD use. Moreover, chronic use of PCP may lead to an irreversible schizophrenia-like psychosis.

■ BASIC PHARMACOLOGY OF DRUGS OF ABUSE

Since all addictive drugs increase dopamine concentrations in target structures of the mesolimbic projections, we classify them on the basis of their molecular targets and the underlying mechanisms (Table 32–1 and Figure 32–2). The first group contains the **opioids, cannabinoids, γ-hydroxybutyric acid (GHB),** and the **hallucinogens,** which all exert their action through G$_{io}$ protein-coupled receptors. The second group includes **nicotine, alcohol, the benzodiazepines, dissociative anesthetics,** and some **inhalants,** which interact with ionotropic receptors or ion channels. The last group comprises **cocaine, amphetamines,** and **ecstasy,** which all bind to monoamine transporters. The nonaddictive drugs are classified using the same criteria.

DRUGS THAT ACTIVATE G$_{IO}$-COUPLED RECEPTORS

OPIOIDS

Opioids may have been the first drugs to be abused (preceding stimulants), and are still among the most commonly used for nonmedical purposes.

Pharmacology & Clinical Aspects

As described in Chapter 31, opioids comprise a large family of endogenous and exogenous agonists at three G protein-coupled receptors: the μ-, κ-, and δ-opioid receptors. Although all three receptors couple to inhibitory G proteins (ie, they all inhibit adenylyl cyclase), they have distinct, sometimes even opposing effects, mainly because of the cell type-specific expression throughout the brain. In the VTA, for example, μ-opioid receptors are selectively expressed on GABA neurons (which they inhibit), whereas κ-opioid receptors are expressed on and inhibit dopamine neurons. This may explain why μ-opioid agonists cause euphoria, whereas κ agonists induce dysphoria.

In line with the latter observations, the rewarding effects of morphine are absent in knockout mice lacking μ receptors but persist when either of the other opioid receptors are ablated. In the VTA, μ opioids cause an inhibition of GABAergic inhibitory interneurons, which leads eventually to a disinhibition of dopamine neurons.

The most commonly abused μ opioids include **morphine, heroin** (diacetylmorphine, which is rapidly metabolized to morphine), **codeine,** and **oxycodone. Meperidine** abuse is common among health professionals. All of these drugs induce strong tolerance and dependence. The withdrawal syndrome may be very severe (except for codeine) and includes intense dysphoria, nausea or vomiting, muscle aches, lacrimation, rhinorrhea, mydriasis, piloerection, sweating, diarrhea, yawning, and fever. Beyond the withdrawal syndrome, which usually lasts no longer than a few days, individuals who have received opioids as analgesics only rarely develop addiction. In contrast, when taken for recreational purposes, opioids are highly addictive. The relative risk of addiction is 4 out of 5 on a scale of 1 = nonaddictive, 5 = highly addictive.

Treatment

The opioid antagonist **naloxone** reverses the effects of a dose of morphine or heroin within minutes. This may be life-saving in the case of a massive overdose (see Chapters 31 and 58). Naloxone administration also provokes an acute withdrawal (precipitated abstinence) syndrome in a dependent person who has recently taken an opioid.

In the treatment of opioid addiction, a long-acting opioid (eg, **methadone, buprenorphine)** is often substituted for the shorter-acting, more rewarding, opioid (eg, heroin). For substitution therapy, methadone is given orally once daily, facilitating supervised intake. Using a partial agonist (buprenorphine) and the much longer half-life (methadone and buprenorphine) may also

have some beneficial effects (eg, weaker drug sensitization, which typically requires intermittent exposures), but it is important to realize that abrupt termination of methadone administration invariably precipitates a withdrawal syndrome; that is, the subject on substitution therapy remains dependent. Some countries (eg, Switzerland, Netherlands) even allow substitution of heroin by heroin. A follow-up of a cohort of addicts who receive heroin injections in a controlled setting and have access to counseling indicates that addicts under heroin substitution have an improved health status and are better integrated in society.

CANNABINOIDS

Endogenous cannabinoids that act as neurotransmitters include 2-arachidonyl glycerol (2-AG) and anandamide, both of which bind to CB$_1$ receptors. These very lipid-soluble compounds are released at the postsynaptic somatodendritic membrane, and diffuse through the extracellular space to bind at presynaptic CB$_1$ receptors, where they inhibit the release of either glutamate or GABA. Because of such backward signaling, endocannabinoids are called retrograde messengers. In the hippocampus, release of endocannabinoids from pyramidal neurons selectively affects inhibitory transmission and may contribute to the induction of synaptic plasticity during learning and memory formation.

Exogenous cannabinoids, eg in **marijuana,** include several pharmacologically active substances including Δ^9-**tetrahydrocannabinol (THC),** a powerful psychoactive substance. Like opioids, THC causes disinhibition of dopamine neurons, mainly by presynaptic inhibition of GABA neurons in the VTA. The half-life of THC is about 4 hours. The onset of effects of THC after smoking marijuana occurs within minutes and reaches a maximum after 1–2 hours. The most prominent effects are euphoria and relaxation. Users also report feelings of well-being, grandiosity, and altered perception of passage of time. Dose-dependent perceptual changes (eg, visual distortions), drowsiness, diminished coordination, and memory impairment may occur. Cannabinoids can also create a dysphoric state and, in rare cases following the use of very high doses, eg, in **hashish,** result in visual hallucinations, depersonalization, and frank psychotic episodes. Additional effects of THC, eg, increased appetite, attenuation of nausea, decreased intraocular pressure, and relief of chronic pain, have led to the use of cannabinoids in medical therapeutics. The justification of medicinal use of marijuana was comprehensively examined by the Institute of Medicine (IOM) of the National Academy of Sciences in its 1999 report, *Marijuana & Medicine.* This continues to be a controversial issue, mainly because of the fear that cannabinoids may serve as a gateway to the consumption of "hard" drugs or cause schizophrenia in individuals with a predisposition.

Chronic exposure to marijuana leads to dependence, which is revealed by a distinctive, but mild and short-lived, withdrawal syndrome that includes restlessness, irritability, mild agitation, insomnia, nausea, and cramping. The relative risk for addiction is 2.

The synthetic Δ^9-THC analog **dronabinol** is a Food and Drug Administration (FDA)-approved cannabinoid agonist currently marketed in the USA and some European countries. **Nabilone,** an older commercial Δ^9-THC analog, was recently reintroduced in the USA for adjunctive therapy in chronic pain management. The cannabinoid system is likely to emerge as an important drug target in the future because of its apparent involvement in several therapeutically desirable effects.

GAMMA-HYDROXYBUTYRIC ACID

Gamma-hydroxybutyric acid (GHB) is produced during the metabolism of GABA, but the function of this endogenous agent is unknown at present. The pharmacology of GHB is complex because there are two distinct binding sites. The protein that contains a high-affinity binding site (1 μM) for GHB has been cloned, but its involvement in the cellular effects of GHB at pharmacologic concentrations remains unclear. The low-affinity binding site (1 mM) has been identified as the GABA_B receptor. In mice that lack GABA_B receptors, even very high doses of GHB have no effect; this suggests that GABA_B receptors are the sole mediators of GHB's pharmacologic action.

GHB was first synthesized in 1960 and introduced as a general anesthetic. Because of its narrow safety margin and its addictive potential, it is not available in the USA for this purpose at present. It can however be prescribed (under restricted access rules) to treat narcolepsy, because GHB decreases daytime sleepiness and episodes of cataplexy through a mechanism unrelated to the reward system. Before causing sedation and coma, GHB causes euphoria, enhanced sensory perceptions, a feeling of social closeness, and amnesia. These properties have made it a popular "club drug" that goes by colorful street names such as "liquid ecstasy," "grievous bodily harm," or "date rape drug." As the latter name suggests, GHB has been used in date rapes because it is odorless and can be readily dissolved in beverages. It is rapidly absorbed after ingestion and reaches a maximal plasma concentration 20–30 minutes after ingestion of a 10–20 mg/kg dose. The elimination half-life is about 30 minutes.

Although GABA_B receptors are expressed on all neurons of the VTA, GABA neurons are much more sensitive to GHB than are dopamine neurons (Figure 32–4). This is reflected by the EC_{50}s, which differ by about one order of magnitude, and indicates the difference in coupling efficiency of the GABA_B receptor and the potassium channels responsible for the hyperpolarization. Because GHB is a weak agonist, only GABA neurons are inhibited at the concentrations typically obtained with recreational use. This feature may underlie the reinforcing effects of GHB and the basis for addiction to the drug. At higher doses, however, GHB also hyperpolarizes dopamine neurons, eventually completely inhibiting dopamine release. Such an inhibition of the VTA may in turn preclude its activation by other addictive drugs and may explain why GHB might have some usefulness as an "anticraving" compound.

LSD, MESCALINE, & PSILOCYBIN

LSD, mescaline, and psilocybin are commonly called hallucinogens because of their ability to alter consciousness such that the individual senses things that are not present. They induce, often in an unpredictable way, perceptual symptoms, including shape and color distortion. Psychosis-like manifestations (depersonalization, hallucinations, distorted time perception) have led some to classify these drugs as psychotomimetics. They also produce somatic symptoms (dizziness, nausea, paresthesias, and blurred vision). Some users have reported intense reexperiencing of perceptual effects (flashbacks) up to several years after the last drug exposure.

Hallucinogens differ from most other drugs described in this chapter in that they induce neither dependence nor addiction. However, repetitive exposure still leads to rapid tolerance (also called tachyphylaxis). Animals do not self-administer hallucinogens, suggesting that they are not rewarding to them. Additional studies show that these drugs also fail to stimulate dopamine release, further supporting the idea that only drugs that activate the mesolimbic dopamine system are addictive. Instead, hallucinogens increase glutamate release in the cortex, presumably by enhancing excitatory afferent input via presynaptic serotonin receptors (eg, $5HT_{2A}$) from the thalamus.

LSD is an ergot alkaloid. After synthesis, blotter paper or sugar cubes are sprinkled with the liquid and allowed to dry. When LSD is swallowed, psychoactive effects typically appear after 30 minutes and last 6–12 hours. During this time, subjects have impaired ability to make rational judgments and understand common dangers, which puts them at risk for accidents and personal injury.

In an adult, a typical dose is 20–30 mcg. LSD is considered neurotoxic and like most ergot alkaloids, may lead to strong contractions of the uterus that can induce abortion (see Chapter 16).

The main molecular target of LSD and other hallucinogens is the $5-HT_{2A}$ receptor. This receptor couples to G proteins of the G_q type and generates inositol trisphosphate (IP_3), leading to a release of intracellular calcium. Although hallucinogens, and LSD in particular, have been proposed for several therapeutic indications, efficacy has never been demonstrated.

DRUGS THAT MEDIATE THEIR EFFECTS VIA IONOTROPIC RECEPTORS

NICOTINE

In terms of numbers affected, addiction to nicotine exceeds all other forms of addiction, touching more than 50% of all adults in some countries. Nicotine exposure occurs primarily through smoking of tobacco, which causes associated diseases that are responsible for many preventable deaths. The chronic use of chewing tobacco and snuff tobacco is also addictive.

Nicotine is a selective agonist of the nicotinic acetylcholine receptor (nAChR) that is normally activated by acetylcholine (see Chapters 6 and 7). Based on nicotine's enhancement of cognitive performance and the association of Alzheimer's dementia with a loss of ACh-releasing neurons from the nucleus basalis of Meynert, nAChRs are believed to play an important role in many cognitive processes. The rewarding effect of nicotine requires involvement of

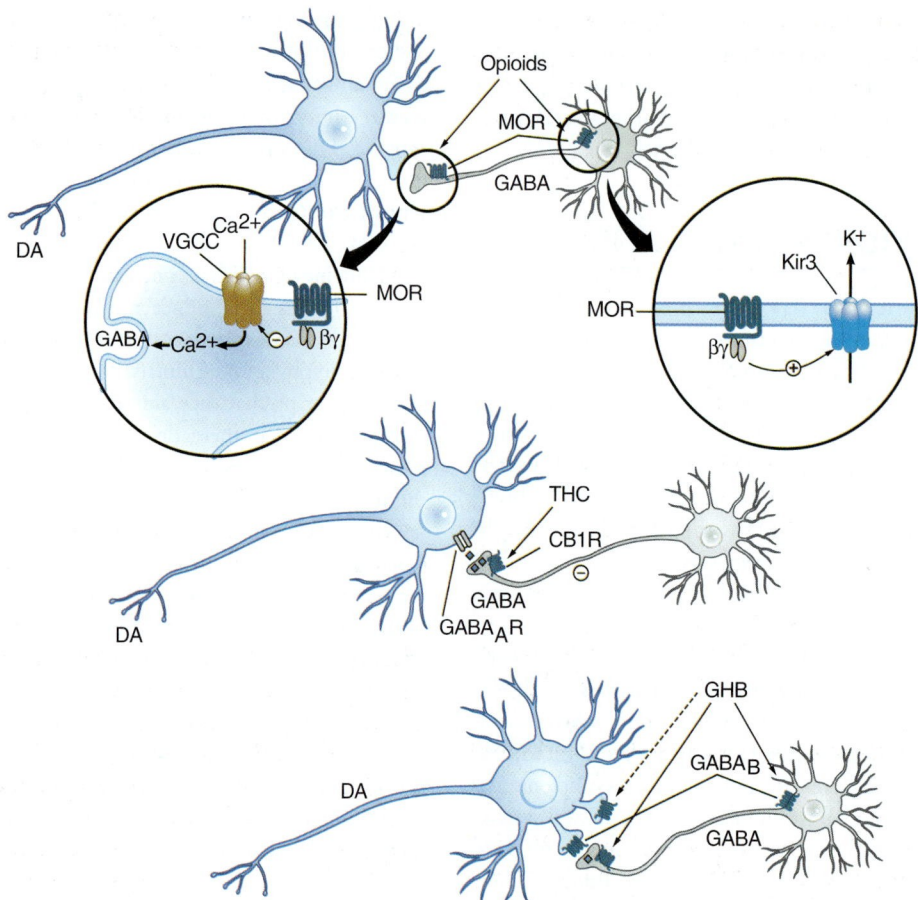

FIGURE 32–4 Disinhibition of dopamine (DA) neurons in the ventral tegmental area (VTA) through drugs that act via G_{io}-coupled receptors. **Top:** Opioids target μ-opioid receptors (MORs) that in the VTA are located exclusively on γ-aminobutyric acid (GABA) neurons. MORs are expressed on the presynaptic terminal of these cells and the somatodendritic compartment of the postsynaptic cells. Each compartment has distinct effectors (*insets*). G protein-βγ-mediated inhibition of voltage-gated calcium channels (VGCC) is the major mechanism in the presynaptic terminal. Conversely, in dendrites MORs activate K channels. **Middle:** Δ^9-tetrahydrocannabinol (THC) and other cannabinoids mainly act through presynaptic inhibition. **Bottom:** Gama-hydroxybutyric acid (GHB) targets $GABA_B$ receptors, which are located on both cell types. However, GABA neurons are more sensitive to GHB than are DA neurons, leading to disinhibition at concentrations typically obtained with recreational use. CB_1R, cannabinoid receptors.

the VTA, in which nAChRs are expressed on dopamine neurons. When nicotine excites projection neurons, dopamine is released in the nucleus accumbens and the prefrontal cortex, thus fulfilling the dopamine requirement of addictive drugs. Recent work has identified α4β2-containing channels in the VTA as the nAChRs that are required for the rewarding effects of nicotine. This statement is based on the observation that knockout mice deficient for the β2 subunit lose interest in self-administering nicotine, and that in these mice, this behavior can be restored through an in vivo transfection of the β2 subunit in neurons of the VTA. Electrophysiologic evidence suggests that homomeric nAChRs made exclusively of α7 subunits also contribute to the reinforcing effects of nicotine. These receptors are mainly expressed on synaptic terminals of excitatory afferents projecting onto the dopamine neurons. They also contribute to nicotine-evoked dopamine release and the long-term changes induced by the drugs related to addiction (eg, long-term synaptic potentiation of excitatory inputs).

Nicotine withdrawal is mild compared with opioid withdrawal and involves irritability and sleep problems. However, nicotine is among the most addictive drugs (relative risk 4), and relapse after attempted cessation is very common.

Treatment

Treatments for nicotine addiction include nicotine itself in forms that are slowly absorbed and several other drugs. Nicotine that is chewed, inhaled, or transdermally delivered can be substituted for the nicotine in cigarettes, thus slowing the pharmacokinetics and eliminating the many complications associated with the toxic substances found in tobacco smoke. Recently, two partial agonists of α4β2-containing nAChRs have been characterized; the plant-extract **cytisine** and its synthetic derivative **varenicline.** Both work by occupying nAChRs on dopamine neurons of the VTA, thus preventing nicotine from exerting its action. Varenicline may impair the capacity to drive and has been associated with suicidal ideation. The antidepressant **bupropion** is approved for nicotine cessation therapy. It is most effective when combined with behavioral therapies.

Many countries have banned smoking in public places to create smoke-free environments. This important step not only reduces passive smoking and the hazards of secondhand smoke, but also the risk that ex-smokers will be exposed to smoke, which as a contextual cue, may trigger relapse.

BENZODIAZEPINES

Benzodiazepines are commonly prescribed as anxiolytics and sleep medications. They represent a moderate risk for abuse, which has to be weighed against their beneficial effects. Benzodiazepines are abused by some persons for their euphoriant effects, but most often abuse occurs concomitant with other drugs, eg, to attenuate anxiety during withdrawal from opioids.

Barbiturates, which preceded benzodiazepines as the most commonly abused sedative hypnotics (after ethanol), are now rarely prescribed to outpatients and therefore constitute a less common prescription drug problem than they did in the past. Street sales of barbiturates, however, continue. Management of barbiturate withdrawal and addiction is similar to that of benzodiazepines.

Benzodiazepine dependence is very common, and diagnosis of addiction probably often missed. Withdrawal from benzodiazepines occurs within days of stopping the medication and varies as a function of the half-life of elimination. Symptoms include irritability, insomnia, phonophobia and photophobia, depression, muscle cramps, and even seizures. Typically, these symptoms taper off within 1–2 weeks.

Benzodiazepines are positive modulators of the GABA$_A$ receptor, increasing both single-channel conductance and open-channel probability. GABA$_A$ receptors are pentameric structures consisting of α, β, and γ subunits (see Chapter 22). GABA receptors on dopamine neurons of the VTA lack α1, a subunit isoform that is present in GABA neurons nearby (ie, interneurons). Because of this difference, unitary synaptic currents in interneurons are larger than those in dopamine neurons, and when this difference is amplified by benzodiazepines, interneurons fall silent. GABA is no longer released, and benzodiazepines lose their effect on dopamine neurons, ultimately leading to disinhibition of the dopamine neurons. The rewarding effects of benzodiazepines are, therefore, mediated by α1-containing GABA$_A$ receptors expressed on VTA neurons. Receptors containing α5 subunits seem to be required for tolerance to the sedative effects of benzodiazepines, and studies in humans link α2β3-containing receptors to alcohol dependence (the GABA$_A$ receptor is also a target of alcohol, see following text). Taken together, a picture is emerging linking GABA$_A$ receptors that contain the α1 subunit isoform to their addiction liability. By extension, α1-sparing compounds, which at present remain experimental and are not approved for human use, may eventually be preferred to treat anxiety disorders because of their reduced risk to induced addiction.

ALCOHOL

Alcohol (ethanol, see Chapter 23) is regularly used by a majority of the population in many Western countries. Although only a minority becomes dependent and addicted, abuse is a very serious public health problem because of the many diseases associated with alcoholism.

Pharmacology

The pharmacology of alcohol is complex, and no single receptor mediates all of its effects. On the contrary, alcohol alters the function of several receptors and cellular functions, including GABA$_A$ receptors, Kir3/GIRK channels, adenosine reuptake (through the equilibrative nucleoside transporter, ENT1), glycine receptor, NMDA receptor, and 5-HT$_3$ receptor. They are all, with the exception of ENT1, either ionotropic receptors or ion channels. It is not clear which of these targets is responsible for the increase of dopamine release from the mesolimbic reward system. The inhibition of ENT1 is probably not responsible for the rewarding effects (ENT1 knockout mice drink more than controls) but seems to be involved in alcohol dependence through an accumulation of adenosine, stimulation of adenosine A$_2$ receptors, and ensuing enhanced CREB signaling.

Dependence becomes apparent 6–12 hours after cessation of heavy drinking as a withdrawal syndrome that may include tremor (mainly of the hands), nausea and vomiting, excessive sweating, agitation, and anxiety. In some individuals, this is followed by visual, tactile, and auditory hallucinations 12–24 hours after cessation. Generalized seizures may manifest after 24–48 hours. Finally, 48–72 hours after cessation, an alcohol withdrawal delirium (delirium tremens) may become apparent in which the person hallucinates, is disoriented, and shows evidence of autonomic instability. Delirium tremens is associated with 5–15% mortality.

Treatment

Treatment of ethanol withdrawal is supportive and relies on **benzodiazepines,** taking care to use compounds such as oxazepam and lorazepam, which are not as dependent on hepatic metabolism as most other benzodiazepines. In patients in whom monitoring is not reliable and liver function is adequate, a longer-acting benzodiazepine such as chlordiazepoxide is preferred.

As in the treatment of all chronic drug abuse problems, heavy reliance is placed on psychosocial approaches to alcohol addiction. This is perhaps even more important for the alcoholic patient because of the ubiquitous presence of alcohol in many social contexts.

The pharmacologic treatment of alcohol addiction is limited, although several compounds, with different goals, have been used. Therapy is discussed in Chapter 23.

KETAMINE & PHENCYCLIDINE (PCP)

Ketamine and PCP were developed as general anesthetics (see Chapter 25), but only ketamine is still used for this application. Both drugs, along with others, are now classified as "club drugs" and sold under names such as "angel dust," "Hog," and "Special K." They owe their effects to their use-dependent, noncompetitive antagonism of the NMDA receptor. The effects of these substances became apparent when patients undergoing surgery reported unpleasant vivid dreams and hallucinations after anesthesia. Ketamine and PCP are white crystalline powders in their pure forms, but on the street they are also sold as liquids, capsules, or pills, which can be snorted, ingested, injected, or smoked. Psychedelic effects last for about 1 hour and also include increased blood pressure, impaired memory function, and visual alterations. At high doses, unpleasant out-of-body and near-death experiences have been reported. Although ketamine and phencyclidine do not cause dependence and addiction (relative risk = 1), chronic exposure, particularly to PCP, may lead to long-lasting psychosis closely resembling schizophrenia, which may persist beyond drug exposure.

INHALANTS

Inhalant abuse is defined as recreational exposure to chemical vapors, such as **nitrates, ketones,** and aliphatic and aromatic **hydrocarbons.** These substances are present in a variety of household and industrial products that are inhaled by "sniffing," "huffing," or "bagging." Sniffing refers to inhalation from an open container, huffing to the soaking of a cloth in the volatile substance before inhalation, and bagging to breathing in and out of a paper or plastic bag filled with fumes. It is common for novices to start with sniffing and progress to huffing and bagging as addiction develops. Inhalant abuse is particularly prevalent in children and young adults.

The exact mechanism of action of most volatile substances remains unknown. Altered function of ionotropic receptors and ion channels throughout the central nervous system has been demonstrated for a few. Nitrous oxide, for example, binds to NMDA receptors and fuel additives enhance $GABA_A$ receptor function. Most inhalants produce euphoria; increased excitability of the VTA has been documented for toluene and may underlie its addiction risk. Other substances, such as amyl nitrite ("poppers"), primarily produce smooth muscle relaxation and enhance erection, but are not addictive. With chronic exposure to the aromatic hydrocarbons (eg, benzene, toluene), toxic effects can be observed in many organs, including white matter lesions in the central nervous system. Management of overdose remains supportive.

DRUGS THAT BIND TO TRANSPORTERS OF BIOGENIC AMINES

Cocaine

The prevalence of cocaine abuse has increased greatly over the last decade and now represents a major public health problem worldwide. Cocaine is highly addictive (relative risk = 5), and its use is associated with a number of complications.

Cocaine is an alkaloid found in the leaves of *Erythroxylon coca*, a shrub indigenous to the Andes. For more than 100 years, it has been extracted and used in clinical medicine, mainly as a local anesthetic and to dilate pupils in ophthalmology. Sigmund Freud famously proposed its use to treat depression and alcohol dependence, but addiction quickly brought an end to this idea.

Cocaine hydrochloride is a water-soluble salt that can be injected or absorbed by any mucosal membrane (eg, nasal snorting). When heated in an alkaline solution, it is transformed into the free base, "crack cocaine," which can then be smoked. Inhaled crack cocaine is rapidly absorbed in the lungs and penetrates swiftly into the brain, producing an almost instantaneous "rush."

In the peripheral nervous system, cocaine inhibits voltage-gated sodium channels, thus blocking initiation and conduction of action potentials (see Chapter 26). This effect, however, seems responsible for neither the acute rewarding nor the addictive effects. In the central nervous system, cocaine blocks the uptake of dopamine, noradrenaline, and serotonin through their respective transporters. The block of the **dopamine transporter (DAT),** by increasing dopamine concentrations in the nucleus accumbens, has been implicated in the rewarding effects of cocaine (Figure 32–5). In fact, the rewarding effects of cocaine are abolished in mice with a cocaine-insensitive DAT. The activation of the sympathetic nervous system results mainly from blockage of the norepinephrine transporter (NET) and leads to an acute increase in arterial pressure, tachycardia, and often, ventricular arrhythmias. Users typically lose their appetite, are hyperactive, and sleep little. Cocaine exposure increases the risk for intracranial hemorrhage, ischemic stroke, myocardial infarction, and seizures. Cocaine overdose may lead to hyperthermia, coma, and death.

Susceptible individuals may become dependent and addicted after only a few exposures to cocaine. Although a withdrawal syndrome is reported, it is not as strong as that observed with opioids. Tolerance may develop, but in some users a reverse tolerance is observed; that is, they become sensitized to small doses of cocaine. This behavioral sensitization is in part context-dependent. Cravings are very strong and underline the very high addiction liability of cocaine. To date, no specific antagonist is available, and the management of intoxication remains supportive. Developing a pharmacologic treatment for cocaine addiction is a top priority.

AMPHETAMINES

Amphetamines are a group of synthetic, indirect-acting sympathomimetic drugs that cause the release of endogenous biogenic amines, such as dopamine and noradrenaline (see Chapters 6 and 9). Amphetamine, methamphetamine, and their many derivatives exert their effects by reversing the action of biogenic amine transporters at the plasma membrane. Amphetamines are substrates of these transporters and are taken up into the cell (Figure 32–5). Once in the cell, amphetamines interfere with the vesicular monoamine transporter (VMAT; see Figure 6–4), depleting synaptic vesicles of their neurotransmitter content. As a consequence, levels of dopamine (or other transmitter amine) in the cytoplasm increase and quickly become sufficient to cause release into the

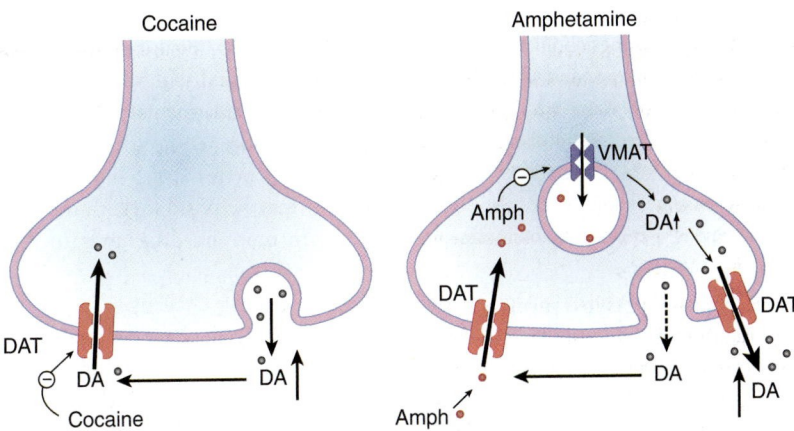

FIGURE 32–5 Mechanism of action of cocaine and amphetamine on synaptic terminal of dopamine (DA) neurons. **Left:** Cocaine inhibits the dopamine transporter (DAT), decreasing DA clearance from the synaptic cleft and causing an increase in extracellular DA concentration. **Right:** Since amphetamine (Amph) is a substrate of the DAT, it competitively inhibits DA transport. In addition, once in the cell, amphetamine interferes with the vesicular monoamine transporter (VMAT) and impedes the filling of synaptic vesicles. As a consequence, vesicles are depleted and cytoplasmic DA increases. This leads to a reversal of DAT direction, strongly increasing nonvesicular release of DA, and further increasing extracellular DA concentrations.

synapse by reversal of the plasma membrane DAT. Normal vesicular release of dopamine consequently decreases (because synaptic vesicles contain less transmitter), whereas nonvesicular release increases. Similar mechanisms apply for other biogenic amines (serotonin and norepinephrine).

Together with GHB and ecstasy, amphetamines are often referred to as "club drugs," because they are increasingly popular in the club scene. They are often produced in small clandestine laboratories, which makes their precise chemical identification difficult. They differ from ecstasy chiefly in the context of use: intravenous administration and "hard core" addiction is far more common with amphetamines, especially methamphetamine. In general, amphetamines lead to elevated catecholamine levels that increase arousal and reduce sleep, whereas the effects on the dopamine system mediate euphoria but may also cause abnormal movements and precipitate psychotic episodes. Effects on serotonin transmission may play a role in the hallucinogenic and anorexigenic functions as well as in the hyperthermia often caused by amphetamines.

Unlike many other abused drugs, amphetamines are neurotoxic. The exact mechanism is not known, but neurotoxicity depends on the NMDA receptor and affects mainly serotonin and dopamine neurons.

Amphetamines are typically taken initially in pill form by abusers, but can also be smoked or injected. Heavy users often progress rapidly to intravenous administration. Within hours after oral ingestion, amphetamines increase alertness and cause euphoria, agitation, and confusion. Bruxism (tooth grinding) and skin flushing may occur. Effects on heart rate may be minimal with some compounds (eg, methamphetamine), but with increasing dosage these agents often lead to tachycardia and dysrhythmias. Hypertensive crisis and vasoconstriction may lead to stroke. Spread of HIV and hepatitis infection in inner cities has been closely associated with needle sharing by intravenous users of methamphetamine.

With chronic use, amphetamine tolerance may develop, leading to dose escalation. Withdrawal consists of dysphoria, drowsiness (in some cases, insomnia), and general irritability.

ECSTASY (MDMA)

Ecstasy is the name of a class of drugs that includes a large variety of derivatives of the amphetamine-related compound methylenedioxymethamphetamine (MDMA). MDMA was originally used in some forms of psychotherapy, but no medically useful effects were documented. This is perhaps not surprising, because the main effect of ecstasy appears to be to foster feelings of intimacy and empathy without impairing intellectual capacities. Today, MDMA and its many derivatives are often produced in small quantities in ad hoc laboratories and distributed at parties or "raves," where it is taken orally. Ecstasy therefore is the prototypical designer drug and, as such, is increasingly popular.

Similar to the amphetamines, MDMA causes release of biogenic amines by reversing the action of their respective transporters. It has a preferential affinity for the **serotonin transporter (SERT)** and therefore most strongly increases the extracellular concentration of serotonin. This release is so profound that there is a marked intracellular depletion for 24 hours after a single dose. With repetitive administration, serotonin depletion may become permanent, which has triggered a debate on its neurotoxicity. Although direct proof from animal models for neurotoxicity remains weak, several studies report long-term cognitive impairment in heavy users of MDMA.

In contrast, there is a wide consensus that MDMA has several acute toxic effects, in particular hyperthermia, which along with dehydration (eg, caused by an all-night dance party) may be fatal. Other complications include serotonin syndrome (mental status change, autonomic hyperactivity, and neuromuscular abnormalities, see Chapter 16) and seizures. Following warnings about the dangers of MDMA, some users have attempted to compensate for hyperthermia by drinking excessive amounts of water, causing water intoxication involving severe hyponatremia, seizures, and even death.

Withdrawal is marked by a mood "offset" characterized by depression lasting up to several weeks. There have also been reports of increased aggression during periods of abstinence in chronic MDMA users.

Taken together, the evidence for irreversible damage to the brain, although not completely convincing, implies that even occasional recreational use of MDMA cannot be considered safe.

■ CLINICAL PHARMACOLOGY OF DEPENDENCE & ADDICTION

To date no single pharmacologic treatment (even in combination with behavioral interventions) efficiently eliminates addiction. This is not to say that addiction is irreversible. Pharmacologic interventions may in fact be useful at all stages of the disease. This is particularly true in the case of a massive overdose, in which reversal of drug action may be a life-saving measure. However, in this regard, FDA-approved antagonists are available only for opioids and benzodiazepines.

Pharmacologic interventions may also aim to alleviate the withdrawal syndrome, particularly after opioid exposure. On the assumption that withdrawal reflects at least in part a hyperactivity of central adrenergic systems, the α_2-adrenoceptor agonist clonidine (also used as a centrally active antihypertensive drug, see Chapter 11) has been used with some success to attenuate withdrawal. Today, most clinicians prefer to manage opioid withdrawal by very slowly tapering the administration of long-acting opioids.

Another widely accepted treatment is substitution of a legally available agonist that acts at the same receptor as the abused drug. This approach has been approved for opioids and nicotine. For example, heroin addicts may receive methadone to replace heroin; smoking addicts may receive nicotine continuously via a transdermal patch system to replace smoking. In general, a rapid-acting substance is replaced with one that acts or is absorbed more slowly. Substitution treatments are largely justified by the benefits of reducing associated health risks, the reduction of drug-associated crime, and better social integration. Although dependence persists, it may be possible, with the support of behavioral interventions, to motivate drug users to gradually reduce the dose and become abstinent.

The biggest challenge is the treatment of addiction itself. Several approaches have been proposed, but all remain experimental. One approach is to pharmacologically reduce cravings. The μ-opioid receptor antagonist and partial agonist **naltrexone** is FDA-approved for this indication in opioid and alcohol addiction. Its effect is modest and may involve a modulation of endogenous opioid systems.

Clinical trials are currently being conducted with a number of drugs, including the high-affinity $GABA_B$-receptor agonist **baclofen,** and initial results have shown a significant reduction of craving. This effect may be mediated by the inhibition of the dopamine neurons of the VTA, which is possible at baclofen concentrations obtained by oral administration because of its very high affinity for the $GABA_B$ receptor.

Rimonabant is an inverse agonist of the CB_1 receptor that behaves like an antagonist of cannabinoids. It was developed for smoking cessation and to facilitate weight loss. Because of frequent adverse effects—most notably severe depression carrying a substantial risk of suicide—this drug is no longer used clinically. It was initially used in conjunction with diet and exercise for patients with a body mass index above 30 kg/m^2 (27 kg/m^2 if associated risk factors, such as type 2 diabetes or dyslipidemia are present). Although a recent large-scale study confirmed that rimonabant is effective for smoking cessation and the prevention of weight gain in smokers who quit, this indication has never been approved. Although the cellular mechanism of rimonabant remains to be elucidated, data in rodents convincingly demonstrate that this compound can reduce self-administration in naive as well as drug-experienced animals.

SUMMARY Drugs Used to Treat Dependence and Addiction

Subclass	Mechanism of Action	Effects	Clinical Application	Pharmacokinetics, Toxicities, Interactions
OPIOID RECEPTOR ANTAGONIST				
• Naloxone	Nonselective antagonist of opioid receptors	Reverses the acute effects of opioids; can precipitate severe abstinence syndrome	Opioid overdose	Effect much shorter than morphine (1–2 h); therefore several injections required
• Naltrexone	Antagonist of opioid receptors	Blocks effects of illicit opioids	Treatment of alcoholism	Half-life ~ 4 h
SYNTHETIC OPIOID				
• Methadone	Slow-acting agonist of μ-opioid receptor	Acute effects similar to morphine (see text)	Substitution therapy for opioid addicts	High oral bioavailability • half-life highly variable among individuals (range 4–130 h) • *Toxicity:* Respiratory depression, constipation, miosis, tolerance, dependence, and withdrawal symptoms
PARTIAL μ-OPIOID RECEPTOR AGONIST				
• Buprenorphine	Partial agonist at μ-opioid receptors	Attenuates acute effects of morphine	Oral substitution therapy for opioid addicts	Long half-life (40 h) • formulated together with naloxone to avoid illicit IV injections
NICOTINIC RECEPTOR PARTIAL AGONIST				
• Varenicline	Partial agonist of nicotinic acetylcholine receptor of the α4β2-type	Occludes "rewarding" effects of smoking • heightened awareness of colors	Smoking cessation	*Toxicity:* Nausea and vomiting, convulsions, psychiatric changes
• *Cytisine: Natural analog (extracted from laburnum flowers) of varenicline*				
BENZODIAZEPINES				
• Oxazepam, others	Positive modulators of the GABA$_A$ receptors, increase frequency of channel opening	Enhances GABAergic synaptic transmission; attenuates withdrawal symptoms (tremor, hallucinations, anxiety) in alcoholics • prevents withdrawal seizures	Delirium tremens	Half-life 4–15 h • pharmacokinetics not affected by decreased liver function
• *Lorazepam: Alternate to oxazepam with similar properties*				
N-METHYL-D-ASPARTATE (NMDA)				
• Acamprosate	Antagonist of NMDA glutamate receptors	May interfere with forms of synaptic plasticity that depend on NMDA receptors	Treatment of alcoholism • effective only in combination with counseling	Allergic reactions, arrhythmia, and low or high blood pressure, headaches, insomnia, and impotence • hallucinations, particularly in elderly patients
CANNABINOID RECEPTOR AGONIST				
• Rimonabant	CB$_1$ receptor inverse agonist	Decreases neurotransmitter release at GABAergic and glutamatergic synapses	Approved in Europe from 2006 to 2008 to treat obesity, then withdrawn because of major side effects • Smoking cessation has never been approved, but remains an off-label indication	Major depression, including increased risk of suicide

REFERENCES

General

Goldman D, Oroszi G, Ducci F: The genetics of addictions: Uncovering the genes. Nat Rev Genet 2005;6:521.

Hyman SE: Addiction: A disease of learning and memory. Am J Psychiatry 2005;162:1414.

Lüscher C, Malenka RC: Synaptic plasticity in addiction: From molecular changes to circuit remodeling. Neuron 2011;69:650.

Lüscher C, Ungless MA: The mechanistic classification of addictive drugs. PLoS Med 2006;3:e437.

Redish AD, Jensen S, Johnson A: A unified framework for addiction: Vulnerabilities in the decision process. Behav Brain Sci 2008;31:461.

Pharmacology of Drugs of Abuse

Benowitz NL: Nicotine addiction. N Engl J Med 2010;362:2295.

Mansvelder HD, Keath JR, McGehee DS: Synaptic mechanisms underlie nicotine-induced excitability of brain reward areas. Neuron 2002;33:905.

Maskos U et al: Nicotine reinforcement and cognition restored by targeted expression of nicotinic receptors. Nature 2005;436:103.

Morton J: Ecstasy: Pharmacology and neurotoxicity. Curr Opin Pharmacol 2005;5:79.

Nichols DE: Hallucinogens. Pharmacol Ther 2004;101:131.

Snead OC, Gibson KM: Gamma-hydroxybutyric acid. N Engl J Med 2005;352:2721.

Sulzer D: How addictive drugs disrupt presynaptic dopamine transmission. Neuron 2011; 69:628.

Sulzer D et al: Mechanisms of neurotransmitter release by amphetamines: A review. Prog Neurobiol 2005;75:406.

Tan KR et al: Neural basis for addictive properties of benzodiazepines. Nature 2010;463:769.

CASE STUDY ANSWER

The patient was diagnosed with pathologic gambling secondary to the dopamine agonist prescription. Compulsive behavior including gambling, binge eating, or hypersexuality is observed in about 15% of patients who receive dopamine agonist treatment. The condition is not related to Parkinson's disease, as compulsive behaviors also occur in patients with restless legs syndrome who are treated with the same medication. The incidence with levodopa is lower, and compulsive behavior is sometimes preceded by dose escalation.

SECTION VI DRUGS USED TO TREAT DISEASES OF THE BLOOD, INFLAMMATION, & GOUT

CHAPTER 33

Agents Used in Anemias; Hematopoietic Growth Factors

Susan B. Masters, PhD

CASE STUDY

A 65-year-old woman with a long-standing history of poorly controlled type 2 diabetes mellitus presents with increasing numbness and paresthesias in her extremities, generalized weakness, a sore tongue, and gastrointestinal discomfort. Physical examination reveals a frail-looking, pale woman with diminished vibration sensation, diminished spinal reflexes, and a positive Babinski sign. Examination of her oral cavity reveals Hunter's glossitis, in which the tongue appears deep red in color and abnormally smooth and shiny due to atrophy of the lingual papillae. Laboratory testing reveals a macrocytic anemia based on a hematocrit of 30% (normal for women, 37–48%), a hemoglobin concentration of 9.4 g/dL (normal for elderly women, 11.7–13.8 g/dL), an erythrocyte mean cell volume (MCV) of 123 fL (normal, 84–99 fL), an erythrocyte mean cell hemoglobin concentration (MCHC) of 34% (normal, 31–36%), and a low reticulocyte count. Further laboratory testing reveals a normal serum folate concentration and a serum vitamin B_{12} (cobalamin) concentration of 98 pg/mL (normal, 250–1100 pg/mL). Results of a Schilling test indicate a diagnosis of pernicious anemia. Once megaloblastic anemia was identified, why was it important to measure serum concentrations of both folic acid and cobalamin? Should this patient be treated with oral or parenteral vitamin B_{12}?

Hematopoiesis, the production from undifferentiated stem cells of circulating erythrocytes, platelets, and leukocytes, is a remarkable process that produces over 200 billion new blood cells per day in the normal person and even greater numbers of cells in people with conditions that cause loss or destruction of blood cells. The hematopoietic machinery resides primarily in the bone marrow in adults and requires a constant supply of three essential nutrients—**iron, vitamin B_{12},** and **folic acid**—as well as the presence of **hematopoietic growth factors,** proteins that regulate the proliferation and differentiation of hematopoietic cells. Inadequate supplies of either the essential nutrients or the growth factors result in deficiency of functional blood cells. **Anemia,** a deficiency in

Sickle Cell Disease and Hydroxyurea

Sickle cell disease is an important genetic cause of hemolytic anemia, a form of anemia due to increased erythrocyte destruction, instead of the reduced mature erythrocyte production seen with iron, folic acid, and vitamin B_{12} deficiency. Patients with sickle cell disease are homozygous for the aberrant β-hemoglobin S (HbS) allele or heterozygous for HbS and a second mutated β-hemoglobin gene such as hemoglobin C (*HbC*) or β-thalassemia. Sickle cell disease has an increased prevalence in individuals of African descent because the heterozygous trait confers resistance to malaria.

In the majority of patients with sickle cell disease, anemia is not the major problem; the anemia is generally well compensated even though such individuals have a chronically low hematocrit (20–30%), a low serum hemoglobin level (7–10 g/dL), and an elevated reticulocyte count. Instead, the primary problem is that deoxygenated HbS chains form polymeric structures that dramatically change erythrocyte shape, reduce deformability, and elicit membrane permeability changes that further promote hemoglobin polymerization. Abnormal erythrocytes aggregate in the microvasculature—where oxygen tension is low and hemoglobin is deoxygenated—and cause veno-occlusive damage. The clinical manifestations of sickle cell disease reflect organ damage by veno-occlusive events. In the musculoskeletal system, this results in characteristic, extremely painful bone and joint pain. In the cerebral vascular system, it causes ischemic stroke. Damage to the spleen increases the risk of infection, particularly by encapsulated bacteria such as *Streptococcus pneumoniae*. In the pulmonary system, there is an increased risk of infection and, in adults, an increase in embolism and pulmonary hypertension. Supportive treatment includes analgesics, antibiotics, pneumococcal vaccination, and blood transfusions. In addition, the cancer chemotherapeutic drug **hydroxyurea** (hydroxycarbamide) reduces veno-occlusive events. It is approved in the United States for treatment of adults with recurrent sickle cell crises and approved in Europe in adults and children with recurrent vaso-occlusive events. As an anticancer drug used in the treatment of chronic and acute myelogenous leukemia, hydroxyurea inhibits ribonucleotide reductase and thereby depletes deoxynucleoside triphosphate and arrests cells in the S phase of the cell cycle (see Chapter 54). In the treatment of sickle cell disease, hydroxyurea acts through poorly defined pathways to increase the production of fetal hemoglobin γ (HbF), which interferes with the polymerization of HbS. Clinical trials have shown that hydroxyurea decreases painful crises in adults and children with severe sickle cell disease. Its adverse effects include hematopoietic depression, gastrointestinal effects, and teratogenicity in pregnant women.

---

oxygen-carrying erythrocytes, is the most common and several forms are easily treated. Sickle cell anemia, a condition resulting from a genetic alteration in the hemoglobin molecule, is common but is not easily treated. It is discussed in the Box: Sickle Cell Disease and Hydroxyurea. **Thrombocytopenia** and **neutropenia** are not rare, and some forms are amenable to drug therapy. In this chapter, we first consider treatment of anemia due to deficiency of iron, vitamin B_{12}, or folic acid and then turn to the medical use of hematopoietic growth factors to combat anemia, thrombocytopenia, and neutropenia, and to support stem cell transplantation.

■ AGENTS USED IN ANEMIAS

IRON

Basic Pharmacology

Iron deficiency is the most common cause of chronic anemia. Like other forms of chronic anemia, iron deficiency anemia leads to pallor, fatigue, dizziness, exertional dyspnea, and other generalized symptoms of tissue hypoxia. The cardiovascular adaptations to chronic anemia—tachycardia, increased cardiac output, vasodilation—can worsen the condition of patients with underlying cardiovascular disease.

Iron forms the nucleus of the iron-porphyrin heme ring, which together with globin chains forms hemoglobin. Hemoglobin reversibly binds oxygen and provides the critical mechanism for oxygen delivery from the lungs to other tissues. In the absence of adequate iron, small erythrocytes with insufficient hemoglobin are formed, giving rise to **microcytic hypochromic anemia.** Iron-containing heme is also an essential component of myoglobin, cytochromes, and other proteins with diverse biologic functions.

Pharmacokinetics

Free inorganic iron is extremely toxic, but iron is required for essential proteins such as hemoglobin; therefore, evolution has provided an elaborate system for regulating iron absorption, transport, and storage (Figure 33–1). The system uses specialized transport, storage, ferrireductase, and ferroxidase proteins whose concentrations are controlled by the body's demand for hemoglobin synthesis and adequate iron stores (Table 33–1). A peptide called hepcidin, produced primarily by liver cells, serves as a key central regulator of the system. Nearly all of the iron used to support hematopoiesis is reclaimed from catalysis of the hemoglobin in senescent or damaged erythrocytes. Normally, only a small amount of iron is lost from the body each day, so dietary

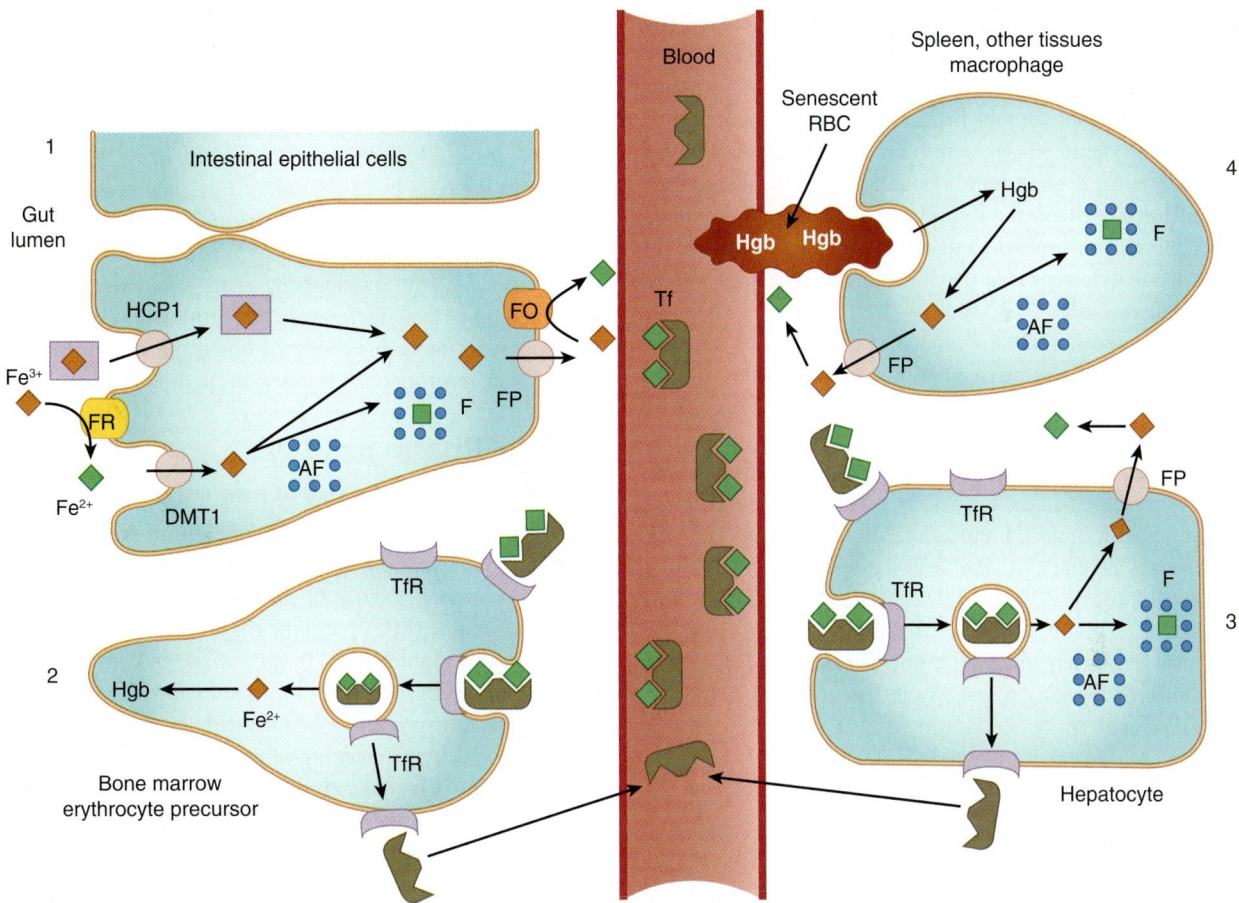

FIGURE 33–1 Absorption, transport, and storage of iron. Intestinal epithelial cells actively absorb inorganic iron via the divalent metal transporter 1 (DMT1) and heme iron via the heme carrier protein 1 (HCP1). Iron that is absorbed or released from absorbed heme iron in the intestine (**1**) is actively transported into the blood by ferroportin (FP) or complexed with apoferritin (AF) and stored as ferritin (F). In the blood, iron is transported by transferrin (Tf) to erythroid precursors in the bone marrow for synthesis of hemoglobin (Hgb) (**2**) or to hepatocytes for storage as ferritin (**3**). The transferrin-iron complex binds to transferrin receptors (TfR) in erythroid precursors and hepatocytes and is internalized. After release of iron, the TfR-Tf complex is recycled to the plasma membrane and Tf is released. Macrophages that phagocytize senescent erythrocytes (RBC) reclaim the iron from the RBC hemoglobin and either export it or store it as ferritin (**4**). Hepatocytes use several mechanisms to take up iron and store the iron as ferritin. FO, ferroxidase. (Modified and reproduced, with permission, from Trevor A et al: *Pharmacology Examination & Board Review*, 9th ed. McGraw-Hill, 2010.)

TABLE 33–1 Iron distribution in normal adults.[1]

	Iron Content (mg)	
	Men	*Women*
Hemoglobin	3050	1700
Myoglobin	430	300
Enzymes	10	8
Transport (transferrin)	8	6
Storage (ferritin and other forms)	750	300
Total	4248	2314

[1]Values are based on data from various sources and assume that normal men weigh 80 kg and have a hemoglobin level of 16 g/dL and that normal women weigh 55 kg and have a hemoglobin level of 14 g/dL.

Adapted, with permission, from Brown EB: Iron deficiency anemia. In: Wyngaarden JB, Smith LH (editors). *Cecil Textbook of Medicine*, 16th ed. Saunders, 1982.

requirements are small and easily fulfilled by the iron available in a wide variety of foods. However, in special populations with either increased iron requirements (eg, growing children, pregnant women) or increased losses of iron (eg, menstruating women), iron requirements can exceed normal dietary supplies and iron deficiency can develop.

A. Absorption

The average American diet contains 10–15 mg of elemental iron daily. A normal individual absorbs 5–10% of this iron, or about 0.5–1 mg daily. Iron is absorbed in the duodenum and proximal jejunum, although the more distal small intestine can absorb iron if necessary. Iron absorption increases in response to low iron stores or increased iron requirements. Total iron absorption increases to 1–2 mg/d in menstruating women and may be as high as 3–4 mg/d in pregnant women.

Iron is available in a wide variety of foods but is especially abundant in meat. The iron in meat protein can be efficiently absorbed, because heme iron in meat hemoglobin and myoglobin can be absorbed intact without first having to be dissociated into elemental iron (Figure 33–1). Iron in other foods, especially vegetables and grains, is often tightly bound to organic compounds and is much less available for absorption. Nonheme iron in foods and iron in inorganic iron salts and complexes must be reduced by a ferrireductase to ferrous iron (Fe^{2+}) before it can be absorbed by intestinal mucosal cells.

Iron crosses the luminal membrane of the intestinal mucosal cell by two mechanisms: active transport of ferrous iron by the divalent metal transporter DMT1, and absorption of iron complexed with heme (Figure 33–1). Together with iron split from absorbed heme, the newly absorbed iron can be actively transported into the blood across the basolateral membrane by a transporter known as ferroportin and oxidized to ferric iron (Fe^{3+}) by the ferroxidase hephaestin. The liver-derived hepcidin inhibits intestinal cell iron release by binding to ferroportin and triggering its internalization and destruction. Excess iron is stored in intestinal epithelial cells as ferritin, a water-soluble complex consisting of a core of ferric hydroxide covered by a shell of a specialized storage protein called apoferritin.

B. Transport

Iron is transported in the plasma bound to **transferrin,** a β-globulin that can bind two molecules of ferric iron (Figure 33–1). The transferrin-iron complex enters maturing erythroid cells by a specific receptor mechanism. Transferrin receptors—integral membrane glycoproteins present in large numbers on proliferating erythroid cells—bind and internalize the transferrin-iron complex through the process of receptor-mediated endocytosis. In endosomes, the ferric iron is released, reduced to ferrous iron, and transported by DMT1 into the cytoplasm, where it is funneled into hemoglobin synthesis or stored as ferritin. The transferrin-transferrin receptor complex is recycled to the cell membrane, where the transferrin dissociates and returns to the plasma. This process provides an efficient mechanism for supplying the iron required by developing red blood cells.

Increased erythropoiesis is associated with an increase in the number of transferrin receptors on developing erythroid cells and a reduction in hepatic hepcidin release. Iron store depletion and iron deficiency anemia are associated with an increased concentration of serum transferrin.

C. Storage

In addition to the storage of iron in intestinal mucosal cells, iron is also stored, primarily as ferritin, in macrophages in the liver, spleen, and bone, and in parenchymal liver cells (Figure 33–1). The mobilization of iron from macrophages and hepatocytes is primarily controlled by hepcidin regulation of ferroportin activity. Low hepcidin concentrations result in iron release from these storage sites; high hepcidin concentrations inhibit iron release. Ferritin is detectable in serum. Since the ferritin present in serum is in equilibrium with storage ferritin in reticuloendothelial tissues, the serum ferritin level can be used to estimate total body iron stores.

D. Elimination

There is no mechanism for excretion of iron. Small amounts are lost in the feces by exfoliation of intestinal mucosal cells, and trace amounts are excreted in bile, urine, and sweat. These losses account for no more than 1 mg of iron per day. Because the body's ability to excrete iron is so limited, regulation of iron balance must be achieved by changing intestinal absorption and storage of iron, in response to the body's needs. As noted below, impaired regulation of iron absorption leads to serious pathology.

Clinical Pharmacology

A. Indications for the Use of Iron

The only clinical indication for the use of iron preparations is the treatment or prevention of iron deficiency anemia. This manifests as a hypochromic, microcytic anemia in which the erythrocyte mean cell volume (MCV) and the mean cell hemoglobin concentration are low (Table 33–2). Iron deficiency is commonly seen in populations with increased iron requirements. These include infants, especially premature infants; children during rapid growth periods; pregnant and lactating women; and patients with chronic kidney disease who lose erythrocytes at a relatively high rate during hemodialysis and also form them at a high rate as a result of treatment with the erythrocyte growth factor erythropoietin (see below). Inadequate iron absorption can also cause iron deficiency. This is seen after gastrectomy and in patients with severe small bowel disease that results in generalized malabsorption.

The most common cause of iron deficiency in adults is blood loss. Menstruating women lose about 30 mg of iron with each

TABLE 33–2 Distinguishing features of the nutritional anemias.

Nutritional Deficiency	Type of Anemia	Laboratory Abnormalities
Iron	Microcytic, hypochromic with MCV <80 fL and MCHC <30%	Low SI <30 mcg/dL with increased TIBC, resulting in a % transferrin saturation (SI/TIBC) of <10%; low serum ferritin level (<20 mcg/L)
Folic acid Vitamin B$_{12}$	Macrocytic, normochromic with MCV >100 fL and normal or elevated MCHC	Low serum folic acid (<4 ng/mL) Low serum cobalamin (<150 pmol/L) accompanied by increased serum homocysteine (>13 μmol/L), and increased serum (>0.4 μmol/L) and urine (>3.6 μmol/mol creatinine) methylmalonic acid

MCV, mean cell volume; MCHC, mean cell hemoglobin concentration; SI, serum iron; TIBC, transferrin iron-binding capacity.

menstrual period; women with heavy menstrual bleeding may lose much more. Thus, many premenopausal women have low iron stores or even iron deficiency. In men and postmenopausal women, the most common site of blood loss is the gastrointestinal tract. Patients with unexplained iron deficiency anemia should be evaluated for occult gastrointestinal bleeding.

B. Treatment

Iron deficiency anemia is treated with oral or parenteral iron preparations. Oral iron corrects the anemia just as rapidly and completely as parenteral iron in most cases if iron absorption from the gastrointestinal tract is normal. An exception is the high requirement for iron of patients with advanced chronic kidney disease who are undergoing hemodialysis and treatment with erythropoietin; for these patients, parenteral iron administration is preferred.

1. Oral iron therapy—A wide variety of oral iron preparations is available. Because ferrous iron is most efficiently absorbed, ferrous salts should be used. Ferrous sulfate, ferrous gluconate, and ferrous fumarate are all effective and inexpensive and are recommended for the treatment of most patients.

Different iron salts provide different amounts of elemental iron, as shown in Table 33–3. In an iron-deficient individual, about 50–100 mg of iron can be incorporated into hemoglobin daily, and about 25% of oral iron given as ferrous salt can be absorbed. Therefore, 200–400 mg of elemental iron should be given daily to correct iron deficiency most rapidly. Patients unable to tolerate such large doses of iron can be given lower daily doses of iron, which results in slower but still complete correction of iron deficiency. Treatment with oral iron should be continued for 3–6 months after correction of the cause of the iron loss. This corrects the anemia and replenishes iron stores.

Common adverse effects of oral iron therapy include nausea, epigastric discomfort, abdominal cramps, constipation, and diarrhea. These effects are usually dose-related and can often be overcome by lowering the daily dose of iron or by taking the tablets immediately after or with meals. Some patients have less severe gastrointestinal adverse effects with one iron salt than another and

benefit from changing preparations. Patients taking oral iron develop black stools; this has no clinical significance in itself but may obscure the diagnosis of continued gastrointestinal blood loss.

2. Parenteral iron therapy—Parenteral therapy should be reserved for patients with documented iron deficiency who are unable to tolerate or absorb oral iron and for patients with extensive chronic anemia who cannot be maintained with oral iron alone. This includes patients with advanced chronic renal disease requiring hemodialysis and treatment with erythropoietin, various postgastrectomy conditions and previous small bowel resection, inflammatory bowel disease involving the proximal small bowel, and malabsorption syndromes.

The challenge with parenteral iron therapy is that parenteral administration of inorganic free ferric iron produces serious dose-dependent toxicity, which severely limits the dose that can be administered. However, when the ferric iron is formulated as a colloid containing particles with a core of iron oxyhydroxide surrounded by a core of carbohydrate, bioactive iron is released slowly from the stable colloid particles. In the United States, the three available forms of parenteral iron are **iron dextran, sodium ferric gluconate complex,** and **iron sucrose.**

Iron dextran is a stable complex of ferric oxyhydroxide and dextran polymers containing 50 mg of elemental iron per milliliter of solution. It can be given by deep intramuscular injection or by intravenous infusion, although the intravenous route is used most commonly. Intravenous administration eliminates the local pain and tissue staining that often occur with the intramuscular route and allows delivery of the entire dose of iron necessary to correct the iron deficiency at one time. Adverse effects of intravenous iron dextran therapy include headache, light-headedness, fever, arthralgias, nausea and vomiting, back pain, flushing, urticaria, bronchospasm, and, rarely, anaphylaxis and death. Owing to the risk of a hypersensitivity reaction, a small test dose of iron dextran should always be given before full intramuscular or intravenous doses are given. Patients with a strong history of allergy and patients who have previously received parenteral iron dextran are more likely to have hypersensitivity reactions after treatment with parenteral iron dextran. The iron dextran formulations used clinically are distinguishable as high-molecular-weight and low-molecular-weight forms. In the United States, the InFeD preparation is a low-molecular-weight form while DexFerrum is a high-molecular-weight form. Clinical data—primarily from observational studies—indicate that the risk of anaphylaxis is largely associated with high-molecular-weight formulations.

Sodium ferric gluconate complex and **iron-sucrose complex** are alternative parenteral iron preparations. These agents can be given only by the intravenous route. They appear to be less likely than high-molecular-weight iron dextran to cause hypersensitivity reactions.

For patients treated chronically with parenteral iron, it is important to monitor iron storage levels to avoid the serious toxicity associated with iron overload. Unlike oral iron therapy, which is subject to the regulatory mechanism provided by the intestinal uptake system, parenteral administration—which bypasses this

TABLE 33–3 Some commonly used oral iron preparations.

Preparation	Tablet Size	Elemental Iron per Tablet	Usual Adult Dosage for Treatment of Iron Deficiency (Tablets per Day)
Ferrous sulfate, hydrated	325 mg	65 mg	2–4
Ferrous sulfate, desiccated	200 mg	65 mg	2–4
Ferrous gluconate	325 mg	36 mg	3–4
Ferrous fumarate	325 mg	106 mg	2–3

regulatory system—can deliver more iron than can be safely stored. Iron stores can be estimated on the basis of serum concentrations of ferritin and the transferrin saturation, which is the ratio of the total serum iron concentration to the total iron-binding capacity (TIBC).

Clinical Toxicity

A. Acute Iron Toxicity

Acute iron toxicity is seen almost exclusively in young children who accidentally ingest iron tablets. As few as 10 tablets of any of the commonly available oral iron preparations can be lethal in young children. Adult patients taking oral iron preparations should be instructed to store tablets in child-proof containers out of the reach of children. Children who are poisoned with oral iron experience necrotizing gastroenteritis, with vomiting, abdominal pain, and bloody diarrhea followed by shock, lethargy, and dyspnea. Subsequently, improvement is often noted, but this may be followed by severe metabolic acidosis, coma, and death. Urgent treatment is necessary. **Whole bowel irrigation** (see Chapter 58) should be performed to flush out unabsorbed pills. **Deferoxamine,** a potent iron-chelating compound, can be given intravenously to bind iron that has already been absorbed and to promote its excretion in urine and feces. Activated charcoal, a highly effective adsorbent for most toxins, does **not** bind iron and thus is ineffective. Appropriate supportive therapy for gastrointestinal bleeding, metabolic acidosis, and shock must also be provided.

B. Chronic Iron Toxicity

Chronic iron toxicity (iron overload), also known as **hemochromatosis,** results when excess iron is deposited in the heart, liver, pancreas, and other organs. It can lead to organ failure and death. It most commonly occurs in patients with inherited hemochromatosis, a disorder characterized by excessive iron absorption, and in patients who receive many red cell transfusions over a long period of time (eg, individuals with β-thalassemia).

Chronic iron overload in the absence of anemia is most efficiently treated by intermittent phlebotomy. One unit of blood can be removed every week or so until all of the excess iron is removed. Iron chelation therapy using parenteral **deferoxamine** or the oral iron chelator **deferasirox** (see Chapter 57) is less efficient as well as more complicated, expensive, and hazardous, but it may be the only option for iron overload that cannot be managed by phlebotomy, as is the case for many individuals with inherited and acquired causes of refractory anemia such as thalassemia major, sickle cell anemia, aplastic anemia, etc.

VITAMIN B$_{12}$

Vitamin B$_{12}$ (cobalamin) serves as a cofactor for several essential biochemical reactions in humans. Deficiency of vitamin B$_{12}$ leads to megaloblastic anemia (Table 33–2), gastrointestinal symptoms, and neurologic abnormalities. Although deficiency of vitamin B$_{12}$ due to an inadequate supply in the diet is unusual, deficiency of B$_{12}$ in adults—especially older adults—due to inadequate absorption

of dietary vitamin B$_{12}$ is a relatively common and easily treated disorder.

Chemistry

Vitamin B$_{12}$ consists of a porphyrin-like ring with a central cobalt atom attached to a nucleotide. Various organic groups may be covalently bound to the cobalt atom, forming different cobalamins. Deoxyadenosylcobalamin and methylcobalamin are the active forms of the vitamin in humans. **Cyanocobalamin** and **hydroxocobalamin** (both available for therapeutic use) and other cobalamins found in food sources are converted to the active forms. The ultimate source of vitamin B$_{12}$ is from microbial synthesis; the vitamin is not synthesized by animals or plants. The chief dietary source of vitamin B$_{12}$ is microbially derived vitamin B$_{12}$ in meat (especially liver), eggs, and dairy products. Vitamin B$_{12}$ is sometimes called **extrinsic factor** to differentiate it from **intrinsic factor,** a protein secreted by the stomach that is required for gastrointestinal uptake of dietary vitamin B$_{12}$.

Pharmacokinetics

The average American diet contains 5–30 mcg of vitamin B$_{12}$ daily, 1–5 mcg of which is usually absorbed. The vitamin is avidly stored, primarily in the liver, with an average adult having a total vitamin B$_{12}$ storage pool of 3000–5000 mcg. Only trace amounts of vitamin B$_{12}$ are normally lost in urine and stool. Because the normal daily requirements of vitamin B$_{12}$ are only about 2 mcg, it would take about 5 years for all of the stored vitamin B$_{12}$ to be exhausted and for megaloblastic anemia to develop if B$_{12}$ absorption were stopped. Vitamin B$_{12}$ is absorbed after it complexes with intrinsic factor, a glycoprotein secreted by the parietal cells of the gastric mucosa. Intrinsic factor combines with the vitamin B$_{12}$ that is liberated from dietary sources in the stomach and duodenum, and the intrinsic factor-vitamin B$_{12}$ complex is subsequently absorbed in the distal ileum by a highly selective receptor-mediated transport system. Vitamin B$_{12}$ deficiency in humans most often results from malabsorption of vitamin B$_{12}$ due either to lack of intrinsic factor or to loss or malfunction of the absorptive mechanism in the distal ileum. Nutritional deficiency is rare but may be seen in strict vegetarians after many years without meat, eggs, or dairy products.

Once absorbed, vitamin B$_{12}$ is transported to the various cells of the body bound to a family of specialized glycoproteins, transcobalamin I, II, and III. Excess vitamin B$_{12}$ is stored in the liver.

Pharmacodynamics

Two essential enzymatic reactions in humans require vitamin B$_{12}$ (Figure 33–2). In one, methylcobalamin serves as an intermediate in the transfer of a methyl group from N^5-methyltetrahydrofolate to homocysteine, forming methionine (Figure 33–2A; Figure 33–3, section 1). Without vitamin B$_{12}$, conversion of the major dietary and storage folate—N^5-methyltetrahydrofolate—to tetrahydrofolate, the precursor of folate cofactors, cannot occur. As a result, vitamin B$_{12}$ deficiency leads to deficiency of folate cofactors necessary for several biochemical reactions involving the transfer of one-carbon

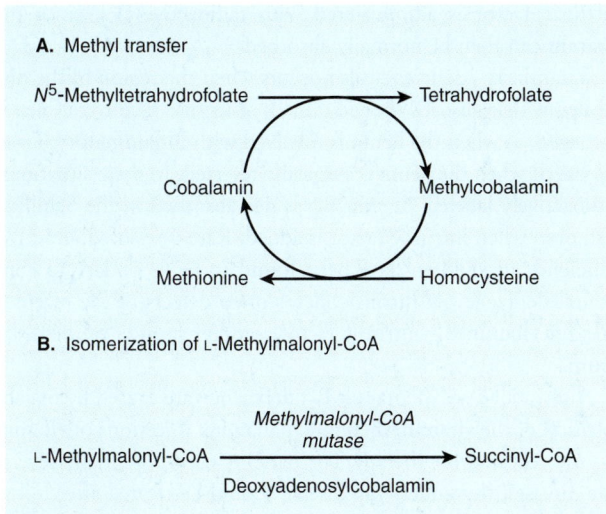

FIGURE 33–2 Enzymatic reactions that use vitamin B_{12}. See text for details.

groups. In particular, the depletion of tetrahydrofolate prevents synthesis of adequate supplies of the deoxythymidylate (dTMP) and purines required for DNA synthesis in rapidly dividing cells, as shown in Figure 33–3, section 2. The accumulation of folate as N^5-methyltetrahydrofolate and the associated depletion of tetrahydrofolate cofactors in vitamin B_{12} deficiency have been referred to as the "methylfolate trap." This is the biochemical step whereby vitamin B_{12} and folic acid metabolism are linked, and it explains why the megaloblastic anemia of vitamin B_{12} deficiency can be partially corrected by ingestion of large amounts of folic acid. Folic acid can be reduced to dihydrofolate by the enzyme dihydrofolate reductase (Figure 33–3, section 3) and thereby serve as a source of the tetrahydrofolate required for synthesis of the purines and dTMP required for DNA synthesis.

Vitamin B_{12} deficiency causes the accumulation of homocysteine due to reduced formation of methylcobalamin, which is required for the conversion of homocysteine to methionine (Figure 33–3, section 1). The increase in serum homocysteine can be used to help establish a diagnosis of vitamin B_{12} deficiency (Table 33–2). There is evidence from observational studies that

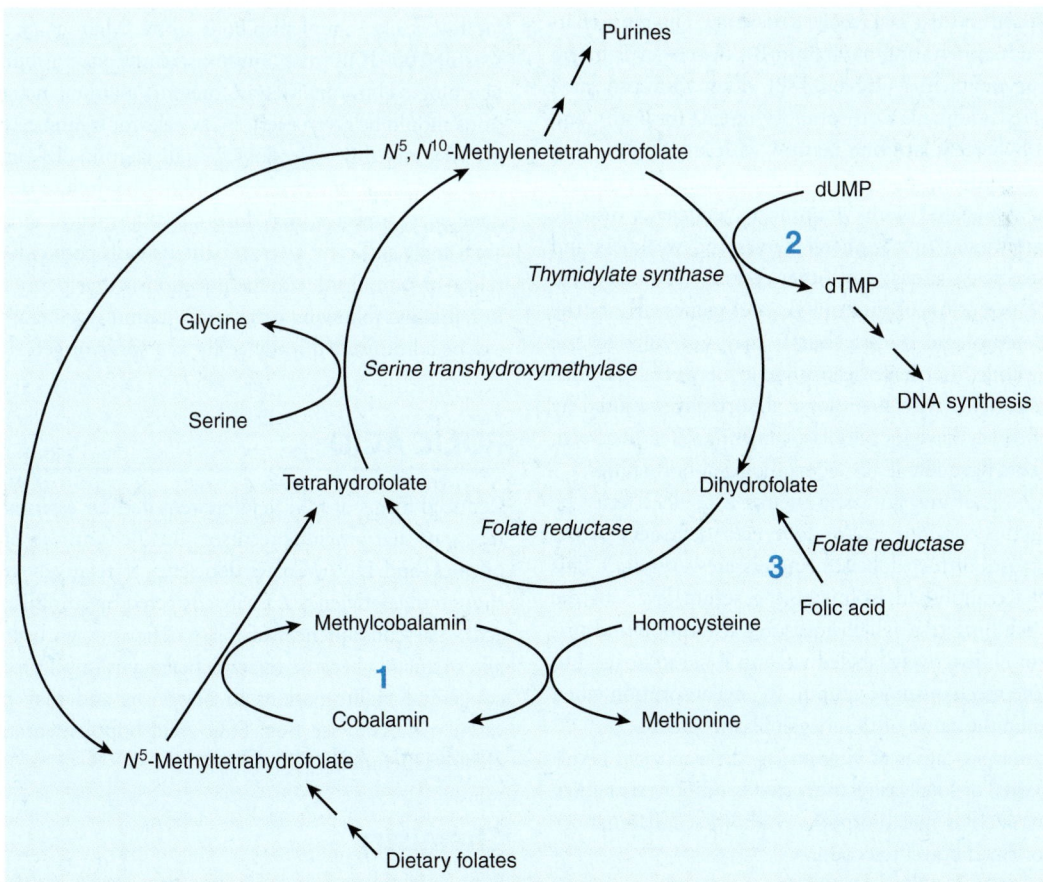

FIGURE 33–3 Enzymatic reactions that use folates. **Section 1** shows the vitamin B_{12}-dependent reaction that allows most dietary folates to enter the tetrahydrofolate cofactor pool and becomes the "folate trap" in vitamin B_{12} deficiency. **Section 2** shows the dTMP cycle. **Section 3** shows the pathway by which folic acid enters the tetrahydrofolate cofactor pool. Double arrows indicate pathways with more than one intermediate step.

elevated serum homocysteine increases the risk of atherosclerotic cardiovascular disease. However, randomized clinical trials have not shown a definitive reduction in cardiovascular events (myocardial infarction, stroke) in patients receiving vitamin supplementation that lowers serum homocysteine.

The other reaction that requires vitamin B_{12} is isomerization of methylmalonyl-CoA to succinyl-CoA by the enzyme methylmalonyl-CoA mutase (Figure 33–2B). In vitamin B_{12} deficiency, this conversion cannot take place and the substrate, methylmalonyl-CoA, as well as methylmalonic acid accumulate. The increase in serum and urine concentrations of methylmalonic acid can be used to support a diagnosis of vitamin B_{12} deficiency (Table 33–2). In the past, it was thought that abnormal accumulation of methylmalonyl-CoA causes the neurologic manifestations of vitamin B_{12} deficiency. However, newer evidence instead implicates the disruption of the methionine synthesis pathway as the cause of neurologic problems. Whatever the biochemical explanation for neurologic damage, the important point is that administration of folic acid in the setting of vitamin B_{12} deficiency will not prevent neurologic manifestations even though it will largely correct the anemia caused by the vitamin B_{12} deficiency.

Clinical Pharmacology

Vitamin B_{12} is used to treat or prevent deficiency. The most characteristic clinical manifestation of vitamin B_{12} deficiency is megaloblastic, macrocytic anemia (Table 33–2), often with associated mild or moderate leukopenia or thrombocytopenia (or both), and a characteristic hypercellular bone marrow with an accumulation of megaloblastic erythroid and other precursor cells. The neurologic syndrome associated with vitamin B_{12} deficiency usually begins with paresthesias in peripheral nerves and weakness and progresses to spasticity, ataxia, and other central nervous system dysfunctions. Correction of vitamin B_{12} deficiency arrests the progression of neurologic disease, but it may not fully reverse neurologic symptoms that have been present for several months. Although most patients with neurologic abnormalities caused by vitamin B_{12} deficiency have megaloblastic anemia when first seen, occasional patients have few if any hematologic abnormalities.

Once a diagnosis of megaloblastic anemia is made, it must be determined whether vitamin B_{12} or folic acid deficiency is the cause. (Other causes of megaloblastic anemia are very rare.) This can usually be accomplished by measuring serum levels of the vitamins. The Schilling test, which measures absorption and urinary excretion of radioactively labeled vitamin B_{12}, can be used to further define the mechanism of vitamin B_{12} malabsorption when this is found to be the cause of the megaloblastic anemia.

The most common causes of vitamin B_{12} deficiency are pernicious anemia, partial or total gastrectomy, and conditions that affect the distal ileum, such as malabsorption syndromes, inflammatory bowel disease, or small bowel resection.

Pernicious anemia results from defective secretion of intrinsic factor by the gastric mucosal cells. Patients with pernicious anemia have gastric atrophy and fail to secrete intrinsic factor (as well as hydrochloric acid). The Schilling test shows diminished absorption of radioactively labeled vitamin B_{12}, which is corrected when intrinsic factor is administered with radioactive B_{12}, since the vitamin can then be normally absorbed.

Vitamin B_{12} deficiency also occurs when the region of the distal ileum that absorbs the vitamin B_{12}-intrinsic factor complex is damaged, as when the ileum is involved with inflammatory bowel disease or when the ileum is surgically resected. In these situations, radioactively labeled vitamin B_{12} is not absorbed in the Schilling test, even when intrinsic factor is added. Rare cases of vitamin B_{12} deficiency in children have been found to be secondary to congenital deficiency of intrinsic factor or to defects of the receptor sites for vitamin B_{12}-intrinsic factor complex located in the distal ileum.

Almost all cases of vitamin B_{12} deficiency are caused by malabsorption of the vitamin; therefore, parenteral injections of vitamin B_{12} are required for therapy. For patients with potentially reversible diseases, the underlying disease should be treated after initial treatment with parenteral vitamin B_{12}. Most patients, however, do not have curable deficiency syndromes and require lifelong treatment with vitamin B_{12}.

Vitamin B_{12} for parenteral injection is available as cyanocobalamin or hydroxocobalamin. Hydroxocobalamin is preferred because it is more highly protein-bound and therefore remains longer in the circulation. Initial therapy should consist of 100–1000 mcg of vitamin B_{12} intramuscularly daily or every other day for 1–2 weeks to replenish body stores. Maintenance therapy consists of 100–1000 mcg intramuscularly once a month for life. If neurologic abnormalities are present, maintenance therapy injections should be given every 1–2 weeks for 6 months before switching to monthly injections. Oral vitamin B_{12}-intrinsic factor mixtures and liver extracts should not be used to treat vitamin B_{12} deficiency; however, oral doses of 1000 mcg of vitamin B_{12} daily are usually sufficient to treat patients with pernicious anemia who refuse or cannot tolerate the injections. After pernicious anemia is in remission following parenteral vitamin B_{12} therapy, the vitamin can be administered intranasally as a spray or gel.

FOLIC ACID

Reduced forms of folic acid are required for essential biochemical reactions that provide precursors for the synthesis of amino acids, purines, and DNA. Folate deficiency is relatively common, even though the deficiency is easily corrected by administration of folic acid. The consequences of folate deficiency go beyond the problem of anemia because folate deficiency is implicated as a cause of congenital malformations in newborns and may play a role in vascular disease (see Box: Folic Acid Supplementation: A Public Health Dilemma).

Chemistry

Folic acid (pteroylglutamic acid) is composed of a heterocycle (pteridine), *p*-aminobenzoic acid, and glutamic acid (Figure 33–4). Various numbers of glutamic acid moieties are attached to the pteroyl portion of the molecule, resulting in monoglutamates, triglutamates, or polyglutamates. Folic acid undergoes reduction,

Folic Acid Supplementation: A Public Health Dilemma

Starting in January 1998, all products made from enriched grains in the United States and Canada were required to be supplemented with folic acid. These rulings were issued to reduce the incidence of congenital neural tube defects (NTDs). Epidemiologic studies show a strong correlation between maternal folic acid deficiency and the incidence of NTDs such as spina bifida and anencephaly. The requirement for folic acid supplementation is a public health measure aimed at the significant number of women who do not receive prenatal care and are not aware of the importance of adequate folic acid ingestion for preventing birth defects in their infants. Observational studies from countries that supplement grains with folic acid have found that supplementation is associated with a significant (20–25%) reduction in NTD rates. Observational studies also suggest that rates of other types of congenital anomalies (heart and orofacial) have fallen since supplementation began.

There may be an added benefit for adults. N^5-Methyltetrahydrofolate is required for the conversion of homocysteine to methionine (Figure 33–2; Figure 33–3, reaction 1). Impaired synthesis of N^5-methyltetrahydrofolate results in elevated serum concentrations of homocysteine. Data from several sources suggest a positive correlation between elevated serum homocysteine and occlusive vascular diseases such as ischemic heart disease and stroke. Clinical data suggest that the folate supplementation program has improved the folate status and reduced the prevalence of hyperhomocysteinemia in a population of middle-aged and older adults who did not use vitamin supplements. There is also evidence that adequate folic acid protects against several cancers, including colorectal, breast, and cervical cancer.

Although the potential benefits of supplemental folic acid during pregnancy are compelling, the decision to require folic acid in grains was controversial. As described in the text, ingestion of folic acid can partially or totally correct the anemia caused by vitamin B_{12} deficiency. However, folic acid supplementation does not prevent the potentially irreversible neurologic damage caused by vitamin B_{12} deficiency. People with pernicious anemia and other forms of vitamin B_{12} deficiency are usually identified because of signs and symptoms of anemia, which typically occur before neurologic symptoms. Some opponents of folic acid supplementation were concerned that increased folic acid intake in the general population would mask vitamin B_{12} deficiency and increase the prevalence of neurologic disease in the elderly population. To put this in perspective, approximately 4000 pregnancies, including 2500 live births, in the United States each year are affected by NTDs. In contrast, it is estimated that over 10% of the elderly population in the United States, or several million people, are at risk for the neuropsychiatric complications of vitamin B_{12} deficiency. In acknowledgment of this controversy, the FDA kept its requirements for folic acid supplementation at a somewhat low level. There is also concern based on observational and prospective clinical trials that high folic acid levels can increase the risk of some diseases, such as colorectal cancer, for which folic acid may exhibit a bell-shaped curve. Further research is needed to more accurately define the optimal level of folic acid fortification in food and recommendations for folic acid supplementation in different populations and age groups.

catalyzed by the enzyme dihydrofolate reductase ("folate reductase"), to give dihydrofolic acid (Figure 33–3, section 3). Tetrahydrofolate is subsequently transformed to folate cofactors possessing one-carbon units attached to the 5-nitrogen, to the 10-nitrogen, or to both positions (Figure 33–3). Folate cofactors are interconvertible by various enzymatic reactions and serve the important biochemical function of donating one-carbon units at various levels of oxidation. In most of these, tetrahydrofolate is regenerated and becomes available for reutilization.

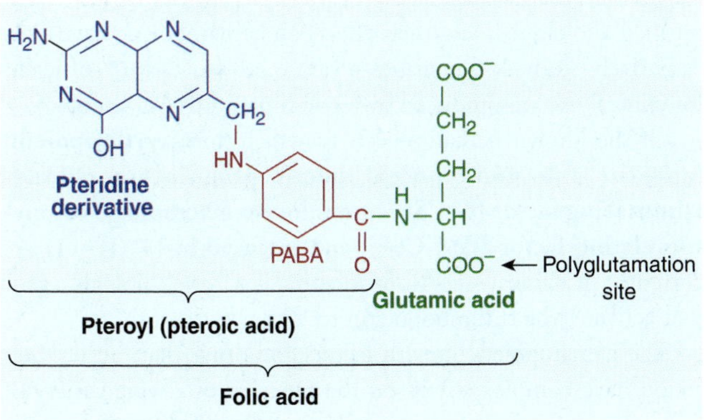

Pharmacokinetics

The average American diet contains 500–700 mcg of folates daily, 50–200 mcg of which is usually absorbed, depending on metabolic requirements. Pregnant women may absorb as much as 300–400 mcg of folic acid daily. Various forms of folic acid are present in a wide variety of plant and animal tissues; the richest sources are yeast, liver, kidney, and green vegetables. Normally, 5–20 mg of folates is stored in the liver and other tissues. Folates are excreted in the urine and stool and are also destroyed by catabolism, so serum levels fall within a few days when intake is diminished. Because body stores of folates are relatively low and daily requirements high, folic acid deficiency and megaloblastic anemia can develop within 1–6 months after the intake of folic acid stops, depending on the patient's nutritional status and the rate of folate utilization.

Unaltered folic acid is readily and completely absorbed in the proximal jejunum. Dietary folates, however, consist primarily of

FIGURE 33–4 The structure of folic acid. (Reproduced, with permission, from Murray RK et al: *Harper's Biochemistry*, 24th ed. McGraw-Hill, 1996.)

polyglutamate forms of N^5-methyltetrahydrofolate. Before absorption, all but one of the glutamyl residues of the polyglutamates must be hydrolyzed by the enzyme α-1-glutamyl transferase ("conjugase") within the brush border of the intestinal mucosa. The monoglutamate N^5-methyltetrahydrofolate is subsequently transported into the bloodstream by both active and passive transport and is then widely distributed throughout the body. Inside cells, N^5-methyltetrahydrofolate is converted to tetrahydrofolate by the demethylation reaction that requires vitamin B_{12} (Figure 33–3, section 1).

Pharmacodynamics

Tetrahydrofolate cofactors participate in one-carbon transfer reactions. As described earlier in the discussion of vitamin B_{12}, one of these essential reactions produces the dTMP needed for DNA synthesis. In this reaction, the enzyme thymidylate synthase catalyzes the transfer of the one-carbon unit of N^5, N^{10}-methylenetetrahydrofolate to deoxyuridine monophosphate (dUMP) to form dTMP (Figure 33–3, section 2). Unlike all the other enzymatic reactions that use folate cofactors, in this reaction the cofactor is oxidized to dihydrofolate, and for each mole of dTMP produced, 1 mole of tetrahydrofolate is consumed. In rapidly proliferating tissues, considerable amounts of tetrahydrofolate are consumed in this reaction, and continued DNA synthesis requires continued regeneration of tetrahydrofolate by reduction of dihydrofolate, catalyzed by the enzyme dihydrofolate reductase. The tetrahydrofolate thus produced can then reform the cofactor N^5, N^{10}-methylenetetrahydrofolate by the action of serine transhydroxymethylase and thus allow for the continued synthesis of dTMP. The combined catalytic activities of dTMP synthase, dihydrofolate reductase, and serine transhydroxymethylase are referred to as the *dTMP synthesis cycle*. Enzymes in the dTMP cycle are the targets of two anticancer drugs; methotrexate inhibits dihydrofolate reductase, and a metabolite of 5-fluorouracil inhibits thymidylate synthase (see Chapter 54).

Cofactors of tetrahydrofolate participate in several other essential reactions. N^5-Methylenetetrahydrofolate is required for the vitamin B_{12}-dependent reaction that generates methionine from homocysteine (Figure 33–2A; Figure 33–3, section 1). In addition, tetrahydrofolate cofactors donate one-carbon units during the de novo synthesis of essential purines. In these reactions, tetrahydrofolate is regenerated and can reenter the tetrahydrofolate cofactor pool.

Clinical Pharmacology

Folate deficiency results in a megaloblastic anemia that is microscopically indistinguishable from the anemia caused by vitamin B_{12} deficiency (see above). However, folate deficiency does not cause the characteristic neurologic syndrome seen in vitamin B_{12} deficiency. In patients with megaloblastic anemia, folate status is assessed with assays for serum folate or for red blood cell folate. Red blood cell folate levels are often of greater diagnostic value than serum levels, because serum folate levels tend to be labile and do not necessarily reflect tissue levels.

Folic acid deficiency is often caused by inadequate dietary intake of folates. Patients with alcohol dependence and patients with liver disease can develop folic acid deficiency because of poor diet and diminished hepatic storage of folates. Pregnant women and patients with hemolytic anemia have increased folate requirements and may become folic acid-deficient, especially if their diets are marginal. Evidence implicates maternal folic acid deficiency in the occurrence of fetal neural tube defects. (See Box: Folic Acid Supplementation: A Public Health Dilemma.) Patients with malabsorption syndromes also frequently develop folic acid deficiency. Patients who require renal dialysis are at risk of folic acid deficiency because folates are removed from the plasma during the dialysis procedure.

Folic acid deficiency can be caused by drugs. Methotrexate and, to a lesser extent, trimethoprim and pyrimethamine, inhibit dihydrofolate reductase and may result in a deficiency of folate cofactors and ultimately in megaloblastic anemia. Long-term therapy with phenytoin can also cause folate deficiency, but only rarely causes megaloblastic anemia.

Parenteral administration of folic acid is rarely necessary, since oral folic acid is well absorbed even in patients with malabsorption syndromes. A dose of 1 mg folic acid orally daily is sufficient to reverse megaloblastic anemia, restore normal serum folate levels, and replenish body stores of folates in almost all patients. Therapy should be continued until the underlying cause of the deficiency is removed or corrected. Therapy may be required indefinitely for patients with malabsorption or dietary inadequacy. Folic acid supplementation to prevent folic acid deficiency should be considered in high-risk patients, including pregnant women, patients with alcohol dependence, hemolytic anemia, liver disease, or certain skin diseases, and patients on renal dialysis.

■ HEMATOPOIETIC GROWTH FACTORS

The hematopoietic growth factors are glycoprotein hormones that regulate the proliferation and differentiation of hematopoietic progenitor cells in the bone marrow. The first growth factors to be identified were called colony-stimulating factors because they could stimulate the growth of colonies of various bone marrow progenitor cells in vitro. Many of these growth factors have been purified and cloned, and their effects on hematopoiesis have been extensively studied. Quantities of these growth factors sufficient for clinical use are produced by recombinant DNA technology.

Of the known hematopoietic growth factors, **erythropoietin (epoetin alfa and epoetin beta), granulocyte colony-stimulating factor (G-CSF), granulocyte-macrophage colony-stimulating factor (GM-CSF),** and **interleukin-11 (IL-11)** are currently in clinical use. **Romiplostim** is a novel biologic agent that activates the thrombopoietin receptor.

The hematopoietic growth factors and drugs that mimic their action have complex effects on the function of a wide variety of cell types, including nonhematologic cells. Their usefulness in other areas of medicine, particularly as potential anticancer and anti-inflammatory drugs, is being investigated.

ERYTHROPOIETIN

Chemistry & Pharmacokinetics

Erythropoietin, a 34–39 kDa glycoprotein, was the first human hematopoietic growth factor to be isolated. It was originally purified from the urine of patients with severe anemia. Recombinant human erythropoietin (rHuEPO, epoetin alfa) is produced in a mammalian cell expression system. After intravenous administration, erythropoietin has a serum half-life of 4–13 hours in patients with chronic renal failure. It is not cleared by dialysis. It is measured in international units (IU). Darbepoetin alfa is a modified form of erythropoietin that is more heavily glycosylated as a result of changes in amino acids. Darbepoetin alfa has a twofold to threefold longer half-life than epoetin alfa. Methoxy polyethylene glycol-epoetin beta is an isoform of erythropoietin covalently attached to a long polyethylene glycol polymer. This long-lived recombinant product is administered as a single intravenous or subcutaneous dose at 2-week or monthly intervals, whereas epoetin alfa is generally administered three times a week and darbepoetin is administered weekly.

Pharmacodynamics

Erythropoietin stimulates erythroid proliferation and differentiation by interacting with erythropoietin receptors on red cell progenitors. The erythropoietin receptor is a member of the JAK/STAT superfamily of cytokine receptors that use protein phosphorylation and transcription factor activation to regulate cellular function (see Chapter 2). Erythropoietin also induces release of reticulocytes from the bone marrow. Endogenous erythropoietin is primarily produced in the kidney. In response to tissue hypoxia, more erythropoietin is produced through an increased rate of transcription of the erythropoietin gene. This results in correction of the anemia, provided that the bone marrow response is not impaired by red cell nutritional deficiency (especially iron deficiency), primary bone marrow disorders (see below), or bone marrow suppression from drugs or chronic diseases.

Normally, an inverse relationship exists between the hematocrit or hemoglobin level and the serum erythropoietin level. Nonanemic individuals have serum erythropoietin levels of less than 20 IU/L. As the hematocrit and hemoglobin levels fall and anemia becomes more severe, the serum erythropoietin level rises exponentially. Patients with moderately severe anemia usually have erythropoietin levels in the 100–500 IU/L range, and patients with severe anemia may have levels of thousands of IU/L. The most important exception to this inverse relationship is in the anemia of chronic renal failure. In patients with renal disease, erythropoietin levels are usually low because the kidneys cannot produce the growth factor. These are the patients most likely to respond to treatment with exogenous erythropoietin. In most primary bone marrow disorders (aplastic anemia, leukemias, myeloproliferative and myelodysplastic disorders, etc) and most nutritional and secondary anemias, endogenous erythropoietin levels are high, so there is less likelihood of a response to exogenous erythropoietin (but see below).

Clinical Pharmacology

The availability of erythropoiesis-stimulating agents (ESAs) has had a significant positive impact for patients with several types of anemia (Table 33–4). The ESAs consistently improve the

TABLE 33–4 Clinical uses of hematopoietic growth factors and agents that mimic their actions.

Hematopoietic Growth Factor	Clinical Condition Being Treated or Prevented	Recipients
Erythropoietin, darbepoetin alfa	Anemia	Patients with chronic renal failure
		HIV-infected patients treated with zidovudine
		Cancer patients treated with myelosuppressive cancer chemotherapy
		Patients scheduled to undergo elective, noncardiac, nonvascular surgery
Granulocyte colony-stimulating factor (G-CSF; filgrastim) and granulocyte-macrophage colony-stimulating factor (GM-CSF; sargramostim)	Neutropenia	Cancer patients treated with myelosuppressive cancer chemotherapy
		Patients with severe chronic neutropenia
		Patients recovering from bone marrow transplantation
	Stem cell or bone marrow transplantation	Patients with nonmyeloid malignancies or other conditions being treated with stem cell or bone marrow transplantation
	Mobilization of peripheral blood progenitor cells (PBPCs)	Donors of stem cells for allogeneic or autologous transplantation
Interleukin-11 (IL-11, oprelvekin)	Thrombocytopenia	Patients with nonmyeloid malignancies who receive myelosuppressive cancer chemotherapy
Romiplostim	Thrombocytopenia	Patients with idiopathic thrombocytopenic purpura

hematocrit and hemoglobin level, often eliminate the need for transfusions, and reliably improve quality of life indices. The ESAs are used routinely in patients with anemia secondary to chronic kidney disease. In patients treated with an ESA, an increase in reticulocyte count is usually observed in about 10 days and an increase in hematocrit and hemoglobin levels in 2–6 weeks. Dosages of ESAs are adjusted to maintain a target hemoglobin up to, but not exceeding, 10–12 g/dL. To support the increased erythropoiesis, nearly all patients with chronic kidney disease require oral or parenteral iron supplementation. Folate supplementation may also be necessary in some patients.

In selected patients, erythropoietin is also used to reduce the need for red blood cell transfusion in patients undergoing myelosuppressive cancer chemotherapy who have a hemoglobin level <10 mg/dL, and for selected patients with low-risk myelodysplastic syndromes and anemia requiring red blood cell transfusion. Patients who have disproportionately low serum erythropoietin levels for their degree of anemia are most likely to respond to treatment. Patients with endogenous erythropoietin levels of less than 100 IU/L have the best chance of response, although patients with erythropoietin levels between 100 and 500 IU/L respond occasionally. Methoxy polyethylene glycol-epoetin beta should not be used for treatment of anemia caused by cancer chemotherapy because a clinical trial found significantly more deaths among patients receiving this form of erythropoietin.

Erythropoietin has been used successfully to offset the anemia produced by zidovudine treatment in patients with HIV infection and in the treatment of the anemia of prematurity. It can also be used to reduce the need for transfusion in high-risk patients undergoing elective, non-cardiac, nonvascular surgery.

Erythropoietin is one of the drugs banned by the International Olympic Committee. The use of erythropoietin by athletes is based on their hope that increased red blood cell concentration will increase oxygen delivery to muscles and improve performance.

Toxicity

The most common adverse effects of erythropoietin are hypertension and thrombotic complications. In March 2007, the FDA issued a warning that patients with chronic renal failure or cancer whose serum hemoglobin is raised to more than 12 g/dL with an ESA face a greater risk of a thrombotic event or, in patients with advanced head and neck cancers, faster tumor growth. The warning was primarily based on clinical trial data from patients with chronic kidney disease indicating an increased rate of mortality and cardiovascular events (stroke, myocardial infarction, worsening congestive heart failure, and hypertension) in patients dosed with an ESA to a target hemoglobin level of 12–16 g/dL or dosed to maintain a normal hematocrit (42%) versus a lower target hematocrit of 30%. In addition, a meta-analysis of 51 placebo-controlled trials of ESAs in cancer patients reported an increased rate of all-cause mortality and venous thrombosis in those receiving an ESA. Based on the accumulated evidence, it is recommended that the hemoglobin level not exceed 12 g/dL in patients with chronic kidney disease receiving an ESA, and that ESAs be used conservatively in cancer patients (eg, when

hemoglobin levels are <10 g/dL) and with the lowest dose needed to avoid transfusion.

Allergic reactions to ESAs have been infrequent. There have been a small number of cases of pure red cell aplasia (PRCA) accompanied by neutralizing antibodies to erythropoietin. PRCA was most commonly seen in dialysis patients treated subcutaneously for a long period with a particular form of epoetin alfa (Eprex with a polysorbate 80 stabilizer rather than human serum albumin) that is not available in the United States. After regulatory agencies required that Eprex be administered intravenously rather than subcutaneously, the rate of ESA-associated PRCA diminished. However, rare cases have still been seen with all ESAs administered subcutaneously for long periods to patients with chronic kidney disease.

MYELOID GROWTH FACTORS

Chemistry & Pharmacokinetics

G-CSF and **GM-CSF,** the two myeloid growth factors currently available for clinical use, were originally purified from cultured human cell lines (Table 33–4). Recombinant human G-CSF (**rHuG-CSF; filgrastim**) is produced in a bacterial expression system. It is a nonglycosylated peptide of 175 amino acids, with a molecular weight of 18 kDa. Recombinant human GM-CSF (**rHuGM-CSF; sargramostim**) is produced in a yeast expression system. It is a partially glycosylated peptide of 127 amino acids, with three molecular species with molecular weights of 15,500; 15,800; and 19,500. These preparations have serum half-lives of 2–7 hours after intravenous or subcutaneous administration. **Pegfilgrastim,** a covalent conjugation product of filgrastim and a form of polyethylene glycol, has a much longer serum half-life than recombinant G-CSF, and it can be injected once per myelosuppressive chemotherapy cycle instead of daily for several days. **Lenograstim,** used widely in Europe, is a glycosylated form of recombinant G-CSF.

Pharmacodynamics

The myeloid growth factors stimulate proliferation and differentiation by interacting with specific receptors found on myeloid progenitor cells. Like the erythropoietin receptor, these receptors are members of the JAK/STAT superfamily (see Chapter 2). G-CSF stimulates proliferation and differentiation of progenitors already committed to the neutrophil lineage. It also activates the phagocytic activity of mature neutrophils and prolongs their survival in the circulation. G-CSF also has a remarkable ability to mobilize hematopoietic stem cells, ie, to increase their concentration in peripheral blood. This biologic effect underlies a major advance in transplantation—the use of **peripheral blood stem cells (PBSCs)** rather than bone marrow stem cells for autologous and allogeneic hematopoietic stem cell transplantation (see below).

GM-CSF has broader biologic actions than G-CSF. It is a multipotential hematopoietic growth factor that stimulates proliferation and differentiation of early and late granulocytic progenitor cells as well as erythroid and megakaryocyte progenitors.

Like G-CSF, GM-CSF also stimulates the function of mature neutrophils. GM-CSF acts together with interleukin-2 to stimulate T-cell proliferation and appears to be a locally active factor at the site of inflammation. GM-CSF mobilizes peripheral blood stem cells, but it is significantly less efficacious and more toxic than G-CSF in this regard.

Clinical Pharmacology

A. Cancer Chemotherapy-Induced Neutropenia

Neutropenia is a common adverse effect of the cytotoxic drugs used to treat cancer and increases the risk of serious infection in patients receiving chemotherapy. Unlike the treatment of anemia and thrombocytopenia, transfusion of neutropenic patients with granulocytes collected from donors is performed rarely and with limited success. The introduction of G-CSF in 1991 represented a milestone in the treatment of chemotherapy-induced neutropenia. This growth factor dramatically accelerates the rate of neutrophil recovery after dose-intensive myelosuppressive chemotherapy (Figure 33–5). It reduces the duration of neutropenia and usually raises the nadir count, the lowest neutrophil count seen following a cycle of chemotherapy.

The ability of G-CSF to increase neutrophil counts after myelosuppressive chemotherapy is nearly universal, but its impact on clinical outcomes is more variable. Many, but not all, clinical trials and meta-analyses have shown that G-CSF reduces episodes of febrile neutropenia, requirements for broad-spectrum antibiotics, infections, and days of hospitalization. Clinical trials have not shown improved survival in cancer patients treated with G-CSF. Clinical guidelines for the use of G-CSF after cytotoxic chemotherapy recommend reserving G-CSF for patients at high risk for febrile neutropenia based on age, medical history, and disease characteristics; patients receiving dose-intensive chemotherapy regimens that carry a greater than 40% risk of causing febrile neutropenia; patients with a prior episode of febrile neutropenia after cytotoxic chemotherapy; patients at high risk for febrile neutropenia; and patients who are unlikely to survive an episode of febrile neutropenia. Pegfilgrastim is an alternative to G-CSF for prevention of chemotherapy-induced febrile neutropenia. Pegfilgrastim can be administered once per chemotherapy cycle, and it may shorten the period of severe neutropenia slightly more than G-CSF.

Like G-CSF and pegfilgrastim, GM-CSF also reduces the duration of neutropenia after cytotoxic chemotherapy. It has been more difficult to show that GM-CSF reduces the incidence of febrile neutropenia, probably because GM-CSF itself can induce fever. In the treatment of chemotherapy-induced neutropenia, G-CSF, 5 mcg/kg/d, or GM-CSF, 250 mcg/m²/d, is usually started within 24–72 hours after completing chemotherapy and is continued until the absolute neutrophil count is greater than 10,000 cells/μL. Pegfilgrastim is given as a single dose of 6 mg.

The utility and safety of the myeloid growth factors in the postchemotherapy supportive care of patients with acute myeloid leukemia (AML) have been the subject of a number of clinical trials. Because leukemic cells arise from progenitors whose proliferation and differentiation are normally regulated by hematopoietic growth factors, including GM-CSF and G-CSF, there was concern that myeloid growth factors could stimulate leukemic cell growth and increase the rate of relapse. The results of randomized clinical trials suggest that both G-CSF and GM-CSF are safe following induction and consolidation treatment of myeloid and lymphoblastic leukemia. There has been no evidence that these growth factors reduce the rate of remission or increase relapse rate. On the contrary, the growth factors accelerate neutrophil recovery and reduce infection rates and days of hospitalization. Both G-CSF and GM-CSF have FDA approval for treatment of patients with AML.

B. Other Applications

G-CSF and GM-CSF have also proved to be effective in treating the neutropenia associated with **congenital neutropenia, cyclic neutropenia, myelodysplasia,** and **aplastic anemia.** Many patients with these disorders respond with a prompt and sometimes dramatic increase in neutrophil count. In some cases, this results in a decrease in the frequency of infections. Because neither G-CSF nor GM-CSF stimulates the formation of erythrocytes and platelets, they are sometimes combined with other growth factors for treatment of pancytopenia.

The myeloid growth factors play an important role in **autologous stem cell transplantation** for patients undergoing high-dose chemotherapy. High-dose chemotherapy with autologous stem cell support is increasingly used to treat patients with tumors that are resistant to standard doses of chemotherapeutic drugs. The high-dose regimens produce extreme myelosuppression; the myelosuppression is then counteracted by reinfusion of the patient's own hematopoietic stem cells (which are collected prior to chemotherapy). The administration of G-CSF or GM-CSF early after autologous stem cell transplantation reduces the time to engraftment and to recovery from neutropenia in patients receiving stem cells obtained either from bone marrow or from

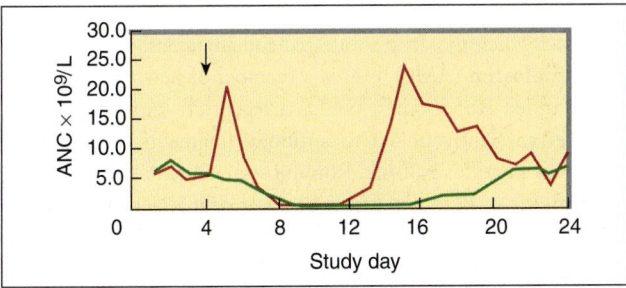

FIGURE 33–5 Effects of granulocyte colony-stimulating factor (G-CSF; *red line*) or placebo (*green line*) on absolute neutrophil count (ANC) after cytotoxic chemotherapy for lung cancer. Doses of chemotherapeutic drugs were administered on days 1 and 3. G-CSF or placebo injections were started on day 4 and continued daily through day 12 or 16. The first peak in ANC reflects the recruitment of mature cells by G-CSF. The second peak reflects a marked increase in new neutrophil production by the bone marrow under stimulation by G-CSF. (Normal ANC is 2.2–8.6 × 10⁹/L.) (Modified and reproduced, with permission, from Crawford J et al: Reduction by granulocyte colony-stimulating factor of fever and neutropenia induced by chemotherapy in patients with small-cell lung cancer. N Engl J Med 1991;325:164.)

peripheral blood. These effects are seen in patients being treated for lymphoma or for solid tumors. G-CSF and GM-CSF are also used to support patients who have received allogeneic bone marrow transplantation for treatment of hematologic malignancies or bone marrow failure states. In this setting, the growth factors speed the recovery from neutropenia without increasing the incidence of acute graft-versus-host disease.

Perhaps the most important role of the myeloid growth factors in transplantation is for mobilization of PBSCs. Stem cells collected from peripheral blood have nearly replaced bone marrow as the hematopoietic preparation used for autologous and allogeneic transplantation. The cells can be collected in an outpatient setting with a procedure that avoids much of the risk and discomfort of bone marrow collection, including the need for general anesthesia. In addition, there is evidence that PBSC transplantation results in more rapid engraftment of all hematopoietic cell lineages and in reduced rates of graft failure or delayed platelet recovery.

G-CSF is the cytokine most commonly used for PBSC mobilization because of its increased efficacy and reduced toxicity compared with GM-CSF. To mobilize stem cells for autologous transplantation, donors are given 5–10 mcg/kg/d subcutaneously for 4 days. On the fifth day, they undergo leukapheresis. The success of PBSC transplantation depends on transfusion of adequate numbers of stem cells. CD34, an antigen present on early progenitor cells and absent from later, committed, cells, is used as a marker for the requisite stem cells. The goal is to infuse at least 5×10^6 CD34 cells/kg; this number of CD34 cells usually results in prompt and durable engraftment of all cell lineages. It may take several separate leukaphereses to collect enough CD34 cells, especially from older patients and patients who have been exposed to radiation therapy or chemotherapy.

For patients with multiple myeloma or non-Hodgkin's lymphoma who respond suboptimally to G-CSF alone, the novel hematopoietic stem cell mobilizer **plerixafor** can be added to G-CSF. Plerixafor is a bicyclam molecule originally developed as an anti-HIV drug because of its ability to inhibit the CXC chemokine receptor 4 (CXCR4), a co-receptor for HIV entry into CD4+ T lymphocytes (see Chapter 49). Early clinical trials of plerixafor revealed a remarkable ability to increase CD34 cells in peripheral blood. Plerixafor mobilizes CD34 cells by preventing chemokine stromal cell-derived factor-1α (SDF-1α) from binding to CXCR4 and directing the CD34 cells to "home" to the bone marrow. Plerixafor is administered by subcutaneous injection after four days of G-CSF treatment and 11 hours prior to leukapheresis; it can be used with G-CSF for up to four continuous days. Plerixafor is eliminated primarily by the renal route and must be dose-adjusted for patients with renal impairment. The drug is well-tolerated; the most common adverse effects associated with its use are injection site reactions, GI disturbances, dizziness, fatigue, and headache.

Toxicity

Although the three growth factors have similar effects on neutrophil counts, G-CSF and pegfilgrastim are used more frequently than GM-CSF because they are better tolerated. G-CSF and pegfilgrastim can cause bone pain, which clears when the drugs are discontinued. GM-CSF can cause more severe side effects, particularly at higher doses. These include fever, malaise, arthralgias, myalgias, and a capillary leak syndrome characterized by peripheral edema and pleural or pericardial effusions. Allergic reactions may occur but are infrequent. Splenic rupture is a rare but serious complication of the use of G-CSF for PBSC.

MEGAKARYOCYTE GROWTH FACTORS

Patients with thrombocytopenia have a high risk of hemorrhage. Although platelet transfusion is commonly used to treat thrombocytopenia, this procedure can cause adverse reactions in the recipient; furthermore, a significant number of patients fail to exhibit the expected increase in platelet count. **Thrombopoietin** and **IL-11** both appear to be key endogenous regulators of platelet production. A recombinant form of IL-11 was the first agent to gain FDA approval for treatment of thrombocytopenia. Recombinant human thrombopoietin and a pegylated form of a shortened human thrombopoietin protein underwent extensive clinical investigation in the 1990s. However, further development was abandoned after autoantibodies to the native thrombopoietin formed in healthy human subjects and caused thrombocytopenia. Efforts shifted to investigation of novel, nonimmunogenic peptide agonists of the thrombopoietin receptor, which is known as Mpl. The first of these—**romiplostim**—was approved by the FDA for idiopathic thrombocytopenic purpura in 2008.

Chemistry & Pharmacokinetics

Interleukin-11 is a 65–85 kDa protein produced by fibroblasts and stromal cells in the bone marrow. **Oprelvekin,** the recombinant form of IL-11 approved for clinical use (Table 33–4), is produced by expression in *Escherichia coli*. The half-life of IL-11 is 7–8 hours when the drug is injected subcutaneously.

Romiplostim (AMG 531) is a member of new class of therapeutics called "peptibodies," which are peptides with key biologic activities covalently linked to antibody fragments that serve to extend the peptide's half-life. Romiplostim contains two disulfide-bonded human F_c fragments, each covalently attached through a polyglycine sequence to a peptide chain containing two Mpl-binding peptides that are linked to one another by a second polyglycine sequence. The Mpl-binding peptide was selected from a peptide library based on its ability in cell assays to activate the thrombopoietin receptor. The Mpl-binding peptide has no sequence homology with human thrombopoietin and there is no evidence in animal or human studies that the Mpl-binding peptide or romiplostim induces antibodies to thrombopoietin. After subcutaneous administration, romiplostim is eliminated by the reticuloendothelial system with an average half-life of 3–4 days. Its half-life is inversely related to the serum platelet count; it has a longer half-life in patients with thrombocytopenia and a shorter half-life in patients whose platelet counts have recovered to normal levels.

Eltrombopag, an orally active small molecule agonist at the thrombopoietin receptor, was licensed in 2008 for use in patients with severe idiopathic thrombocytopenia who have failed to respond adequately to first-line treatments. Because of concerns about hepatotoxicity and hemorrhage, eltrombopag is restricted to use by registered physicians and patients and its use requires close monitoring of liver enzymes.

Pharmacodynamics

Interleukin-11 acts through a specific cell surface cytokine receptor to stimulate the growth of multiple lymphoid and myeloid cells. It acts synergistically with other growth factors to stimulate the growth of primitive megakaryocytic progenitors and, most importantly, increases the number of peripheral platelets and neutrophils.

Romiplostim has high affinity for the human Mpl receptor. It causes a dose-dependent increase in platelet count that begins on day 5 after subcutaneous administration and peaks at days 12–15.

Clinical Pharmacology

Interleukin-11 is approved for the secondary prevention of thrombocytopenia in patients receiving cytotoxic chemotherapy for treatment of nonmyeloid cancers. Clinical trials show that it reduces the number of platelet transfusions required by patients who experience severe thrombocytopenia after a previous cycle of chemotherapy. Although IL-11 has broad stimulatory effects on hematopoietic cell lineages in vitro, it does not appear to have significant effects on the leukopenia caused by myelosuppressive chemotherapy. Interleukin-11 is given by subcutaneous injection at a dose of 50 mcg/kg/d. It is started 6–24 hours after completion of chemotherapy and continued for 14–21 days or until the platelet count passes the nadir and rises to more than 50,000 cells/μL.

In patients with chronic idiopathic thrombocytopenia (ITP) who failed to respond adequately to previous treatment with steroids, immunoglobulins, or splenectomy, romiplostim significantly increased platelet count in most patients. In a 6-week placebo-controlled study in which patients were treated weekly with 1 or 3 mcg/kg, 12 of 16 patients reached the targeted platelet range of 50,000–450,000 platelets/μL. Romiplostim does not appear to decrease the rate of platelet destruction in ITP as platelet counts returned to pretreatment levels after the drug's discontinuation. An open label trial found that many patients maintained a platelet count of 100,000 platelets/μL or higher over a 48-week period and that over half of the patients were able to discontinue other therapies. Romiplostim is initiated as a weekly subcutaneous dose of 1 mcg/kg and then continued at the lowest dose required to maintain a platelet count of at least 50,000 platelets/μL.

Toxicity

The most common adverse effects of IL-11 are fatigue, headache, dizziness, and cardiovascular effects. The cardiovascular effects include anemia (due to hemodilution), dyspnea (due to fluid accumulation in the lungs), and transient atrial arrhythmias. Hypokalemia has also been seen in some patients. All of these adverse effects appear to be reversible.

Romiplostim appears to be well tolerated except for a mild headache on the day of administration. A potential long-term concern is that two patients treated with romiplostim had an increase in bone marrow reticulin, a possible marker of myelodysplastic or myeloproliferative processes. However, neither patient had evidence of increased collagen fibrosis or of abnormal bone marrow cytogenetics.

by causing the release of lipoprotein lipase from tissues, and long-term use is associated with mineralocorticoid deficiency.

B. Heparin-Induced Thrombocytopenia

Heparin-induced thrombocytopenia (HIT) is a systemic hypercoagulable state that occurs in 1–4% of individuals treated with UFH for a minimum of 7 days. Surgical patients are at greatest risk. The reported incidence of HIT is lower in pediatric populations outside the critical care setting and is relatively rare in pregnant women. The risk of HIT may be higher in individuals treated with UFH of bovine origin compared with porcine heparin and is lower in those treated exclusively with LMWH.

Morbidity and mortality in HIT are related to thrombotic events. Venous thrombosis occurs most commonly, but occlusion of peripheral or central arteries is not infrequent. If an indwelling catheter is present, the risk of thrombosis is increased in that extremity. Skin necrosis has been described, particularly in individuals treated with warfarin in the absence of a direct thrombin inhibitor, presumably due to acute depletion of the vitamin K-dependent anticoagulant protein C occurring in the presence of high levels of procoagulant proteins and an active hypercoagulable state.

The following points should be considered in all patients receiving heparin: Platelet counts should be performed frequently; thrombocytopenia appearing in a time frame consistent with an immune response to heparin should be considered suspicious for HIT; and any new thrombus occurring in a patient receiving heparin therapy should raise suspicion of HIT. Patients who develop HIT are treated by discontinuance of heparin and administration of a direct thrombin inhibitor.

Contraindications

Heparin is contraindicated in patients with HIT, hypersensitivity to the drug, active bleeding, hemophilia, significant thrombocytopenia, purpura, severe hypertension, intracranial hemorrhage, infective endocarditis, active tuberculosis, ulcerative lesions of the gastrointestinal tract, threatened abortion, visceral carcinoma, or advanced hepatic or renal disease. Heparin should be avoided in patients who have recently had surgery of the brain, spinal cord, or eye, and in patients who are undergoing lumbar puncture or regional anesthetic block. Despite the apparent lack of placental transfer, heparin should be used in pregnant women only when clearly indicated.

Administration & Dosage

The indications for the use of heparin are described in the section on clinical pharmacology. A plasma concentration of heparin of 0.2–0.4 unit/mL (by protamine titration) or 0.3–0.7 unit/mL (anti-Xa units) usually prevents pulmonary emboli in patients with established venous thrombosis. This concentration generally corresponds to a PTT of 2–3 times baseline. However, the use of the PTT for heparin monitoring is problematic. There is no standardization scheme for the PTT as there is for the prothrombin time (PT) and its international normalized ratio (INR). Currently

more than 300 reagent-instrument combinations are in use, and the actual ratios required to obtain an anti-Xa activity of 0.3–0.7 units/mL are variable, ranging from 1.6 to 6 times control PTT. Thus, if the PTT is used for monitoring, the laboratory should determine the clotting time that corresponds to the therapeutic range by protamine titration or anti-Xa activity, as listed above.

In addition, some patients have a prolonged baseline PTT due to factor deficiency or inhibitors (which could increase bleeding risk) or lupus anticoagulant (which is not associated with bleeding risk but may be associated with thrombosis risk). Using the PTT to assess heparin effect in such patients is very difficult. An alternative is to use anti-Xa activity to assess heparin concentration, a test now widely available on automated coagulation instruments. This approach more accurately measures the heparin concentration; however, it does not provide the global assessment of intrinsic pathway integrity of the PTT.

The following strategy is recommended: prior to initiating anticoagulant therapy of any type, the integrity of the patient's hemostatic system should be assessed by a careful history of prior bleeding events, and baseline PT and PTT. If there is a prolonged clotting time, the cause of this (deficiency or inhibitor) should be determined prior to initiating therapy, and treatment goals stratified to a risk-benefit assessment. In high-risk patients measuring both the PTT and anti-Xa activity may be useful. When *intermittent* heparin administration is used, the aPTT or anti-Xa activity should be measured 6 hours after the administered dose to maintain prolongation of the aPTT to 2–2.5 times that of the control value. However, LMW heparin therapy is the preferred option in this case, as no monitoring is required in most patients.

Continuous intravenous administration of heparin is accomplished via an infusion pump. After an initial bolus injection of 80–100 units/kg, a continuous infusion of about 15–22 units/kg/h is required to maintain the anti-Xa activity in the range of 0.3–0.7 units/mL. Low-dose prophylaxis is achieved with subcutaneous administration of heparin, 5000 units every 8–12 hours. Because of the danger of hematoma formation at the injection site, heparin must never be administered intramuscularly.

Prophylactic enoxaparin is given subcutaneously in a dosage of 30 mg twice daily or 40 mg once daily. Full-dose enoxaparin therapy is 1 mg/kg subcutaneously every 12 hours. This corresponds to a therapeutic anti-factor Xa level of 0.5–1 unit/mL. Selected patients may be treated with enoxaparin 1.5 mg/kg once a day, with a target anti-Xa level of 1.5 units/mL. The prophylactic dose of dalteparin is 5000 units subcutaneously once a day; therapeutic dosing is 200 units/kg once a day for venous disease or 120 units/kg every 12 hours for acute coronary syndrome. LMWH should be used with caution in patients with renal insufficiency or body weight greater than 150 kg. Measurement of the anti-Xa level is useful to guide dosing in these individuals.

The synthetic pentasaccharide molecule **fondaparinux** (Figure 34–4) avidly binds antithrombin with high specific activity, resulting in efficient inactivation of factor Xa. Fondaparinux has a long half-life of 15 hours, allowing for once-daily dosing by subcutaneous administration. Fondaparinux is effective in the

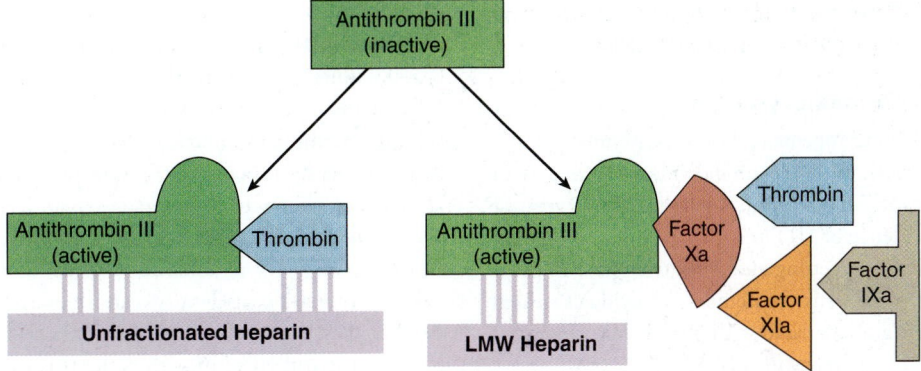

FIGURE 34–4 Cartoon illustrating differences between fondaparinux, low-molecular-weight heparins (LMWH), and high-molecular-weight heparin (HMWH, unfractionated heparin). Activated antithrombin III (AT III) degrades thrombin, factor X, and several other factors. Binding of these drugs to AT III can increase the catalytic action of AT III 1000-fold. The combination of AT III with unfractionated heparin increases degradation of both factor Xa and thrombin. Combination with fondaparinux or LMWH more selectively increases degradation of Xa.

accelerated 1000-fold. Only about a third of the molecules in commercial heparin preparations have an accelerating effect because the remainder lack the unique pentasaccharide sequence needed for high-affinity binding to antithrombin. The active heparin molecules bind tightly to antithrombin and cause a conformational change in this inhibitor. The conformational change of antithrombin exposes its active site for more rapid interaction with the proteases (the activated clotting factors). Heparin functions as a cofactor for the antithrombin-protease reaction without being consumed. Once the antithrombin-protease complex is formed, heparin is released intact for renewed binding to more antithrombin.

The antithrombin binding region of commercial unfractionated heparin consists of repeating sulfated disaccharide units composed of D-glucosamine-L-iduronic acid and D-glucosamine-D-glucuronic acid. High-molecular-weight (HMW), also known as UFH, fractions of heparin with high affinity for antithrombin markedly inhibit blood coagulation by inhibiting all three factors, especially thrombin and factor Xa. Unfractionated heparin has a molecular weight range of 5000–30,000. In contrast, the shorter-chain low-molecular-weight (LMW) fractions of heparin inhibit activated factor X but have less effect on thrombin than the HMW species. Nevertheless, numerous studies have demonstrated that LMW heparins such as **enoxaparin, dalteparin,** and **tinzaparin** are effective in several thromboembolic conditions. In fact, these LMW heparins—in comparison with UFH—have equal efficacy, increased bioavailability from the subcutaneous site of injection, and less frequent dosing requirements (once or twice daily is sufficient).

Because commercial heparin consists of a family of molecules of different molecular weights extracted from porcine intestinal mucosa and bovine lung, the correlation between the concentration of a given heparin preparation and its effect on coagulation often is poor. Therefore, UFH is standardized by bioassay. Heparin was reformulated in 2009 in response to heparin contamination events in 2007 and 2008. The contaminant was identified as over-sulfated chondroitin sulfate and linked to more than150 adverse events in patients, most commonly hypotension, nausea, and dyspnea within 30 minutes of infusion. In response

to this event, heparin sodium was reformulated with stricter quality control measures and bioassays to make detection of contaminants easier. This reformulation led to a decrease in potency of approximately 10% from the previous formulation. USP heparin is now harmonized to the World Health Organization International Standard (IS) unit dose. Enoxaparin is obtained from the same sources as regular unfractionated heparin, but doses are specified in milligrams. Dalteparin, tinzaparin, and danaparoid (an LMW heparanoid containing heparan sulfate, dermatan sulfate, and chondroitin sulfate), on the other hand, are specified in anti-factor Xa units.

Monitoring of Heparin Effect

Close monitoring of the **activated partial thromboplastin time (aPTT or PTT)** is necessary in patients receiving UFH. Levels of UFH may also be determined by protamine titration (therapeutic levels 0.2–0.4 unit/mL) or anti-Xa units (therapeutic levels 0.3–0.7 unit/mL). Weight-based dosing of the LMW heparins results in predictable pharmacokinetics and plasma levels in patients with normal renal function. Therefore, LMW heparin levels are not generally measured except in the setting of renal insufficiency, obesity, and pregnancy. LMW heparin levels can be determined by anti-Xa units. Peak therapeutic levels should be 0.5–1 unit/mL for twice-daily dosing, determined 4 hours after administration, and approximately 1.5 units/mL for once-daily dosing.

Toxicity

A. Bleeding and Miscellaneous Effects

The major adverse effect of heparin is bleeding. This risk can be decreased by scrupulous patient selection, careful control of dosage, and close monitoring. Elderly women and patients with renal failure are more prone to hemorrhage. Heparin is of animal origin and should be used cautiously in patients with allergy. Increased loss of hair and reversible alopecia have been reported. Long-term heparin therapy is associated with osteoporosis and spontaneous fractures. Heparin accelerates the clearing of postprandial lipemia by causing the release of lipoprotein lipase from tissues, and long-term use is associated with mineralocorticoid deficiency.

B. Heparin-Induced Thrombocytopenia

Heparin-induced thrombocytopenia (HIT) is a systemic hypercoagulable state that occurs in 1–4% of individuals treated with UFH for a minimum of 7 days. Surgical patients are at greatest risk. The reported incidence of HIT is lower in pediatric populations outside the critical care setting and is relatively rare in pregnant women. The risk of HIT may be higher in individuals treated with UFH of bovine origin compared with porcine heparin and is lower in those treated exclusively with LMWH.

Morbidity and mortality in HIT are related to thrombotic events. Venous thrombosis occurs most commonly, but occlusion of peripheral or central arteries is not infrequent. If an indwelling catheter is present, the risk of thrombosis is increased in that extremity. Skin necrosis has been described, particularly in individuals treated with warfarin in the absence of a direct thrombin inhibitor, presumably due to acute depletion of the vitamin K-dependent anticoagulant protein C occurring in the presence of high levels of procoagulant proteins and an active hypercoagulable state.

The following points should be considered in all patients receiving heparin: Platelet counts should be performed frequently; thrombocytopenia appearing in a time frame consistent with an immune response to heparin should be considered suspicious for HIT; and any new thrombus occurring in a patient receiving heparin therapy should raise suspicion of HIT. Patients who develop HIT are treated by discontinuance of heparin and administration of a direct thrombin inhibitor.

Contraindications

Heparin is contraindicated in patients with HIT, hypersensitivity to the drug, active bleeding, hemophilia, significant thrombocytopenia, purpura, severe hypertension, intracranial hemorrhage, infective endocarditis, active tuberculosis, ulcerative lesions of the gastrointestinal tract, threatened abortion, visceral carcinoma, or advanced hepatic or renal disease. Heparin should be avoided in patients who have recently had surgery of the brain, spinal cord, or eye, and in patients who are undergoing lumbar puncture or regional anesthetic block. Despite the apparent lack of placental transfer, heparin should be used in pregnant women only when clearly indicated.

Administration & Dosage

The indications for the use of heparin are described in the section on clinical pharmacology. A plasma concentration of heparin of 0.2–0.4 unit/mL (by protamine titration) or 0.3–0.7 unit/mL (anti-Xa units) usually prevents pulmonary emboli in patients with established venous thrombosis. This concentration generally corresponds to a PTT of 2–3 times baseline. However, the use of the PTT for heparin monitoring is problematic. There is no standardization scheme for the PTT as there is for the prothrombin time (PT) and its international normalized ratio (INR). Currently

more than 300 reagent-instrument combinations are in use, and the actual ratios required to obtain an anti-Xa activity of 0.3–0.7 units/mL are variable, ranging from 1.6 to 6 times control PTT. Thus, if the PTT is used for monitoring, the laboratory should determine the clotting time that corresponds to the therapeutic range by protamine titration or anti-Xa activity, as listed above.

In addition, some patients have a prolonged baseline PTT due to factor deficiency or inhibitors (which could increase bleeding risk) or lupus anticoagulant (which is not associated with bleeding risk but may be associated with thrombosis risk). Using the PTT to assess heparin effect in such patients is very difficult. An alternative is to use anti-Xa activity to assess heparin concentration, a test now widely available on automated coagulation instruments. This approach more accurately measures the heparin concentration; however, it does not provide the global assessment of intrinsic pathway integrity of the PTT.

The following strategy is recommended: prior to initiating anticoagulant therapy of any type, the integrity of the patient's hemostatic system should be assessed by a careful history of prior bleeding events, and baseline PT and PTT. If there is a prolonged clotting time, the cause of this (deficiency or inhibitor) should be determined prior to initiating therapy, and treatment goals stratified to a risk-benefit assessment. In high-risk patients measuring both the PTT and anti-Xa activity may be useful. When *intermittent* heparin administration is used, the aPTT or anti-Xa activity should be measured 6 hours after the administered dose to maintain prolongation of the aPTT to 2–2.5 times that of the control value. However, LMW heparin therapy is the preferred option in this case, as no monitoring is required in most patients.

Continuous intravenous administration of heparin is accomplished via an infusion pump. After an initial bolus injection of 80–100 units/kg, a continuous infusion of about 15–22 units/kg/h is required to maintain the anti-Xa activity in the range of 0.3–0.7 units/mL. Low-dose prophylaxis is achieved with subcutaneous administration of heparin, 5000 units every 8–12 hours. Because of the danger of hematoma formation at the injection site, heparin must never be administered intramuscularly.

Prophylactic enoxaparin is given subcutaneously in a dosage of 30 mg twice daily or 40 mg once daily. Full-dose enoxaparin therapy is 1 mg/kg subcutaneously every 12 hours. This corresponds to a therapeutic anti-factor Xa level of 0.5–1 unit/mL. Selected patients may be treated with enoxaparin 1.5 mg/kg once a day, with a target anti-Xa level of 1.5 units/mL. The prophylactic dose of dalteparin is 5000 units subcutaneously once a day; therapeutic dosing is 200 units/kg once a day for venous disease or 120 units/kg every 12 hours for acute coronary syndrome. LMWH should be used with caution in patients with renal insufficiency or body weight greater than 150 kg. Measurement of the anti-Xa level is useful to guide dosing in these individuals.

The synthetic pentasaccharide molecule **fondaparinux** (Figure 34–4) avidly binds antithrombin with high specific activity, resulting in efficient inactivation of factor Xa. Fondaparinux has a long half-life of 15 hours, allowing for once-daily dosing by subcutaneous administration. Fondaparinux is effective in the increased risk of venous thrombosis. The most common defect in the natural anticoagulant system is a mutation in factor V (factor V Leiden), which results in resistance to inactivation by the protein C, protein S mechanism.

Fibrinolysis

Fibrinolysis refers to the process of fibrin digestion by the fibrin-specific protease, plasmin. The fibrinolytic system is similar to the coagulation system in that the precursor form of the serine protease plasmin circulates in an inactive form as plasminogen. In response to injury, endothelial cells synthesize and release tissue plasminogen activator (t-PA), which converts plasminogen to plasmin (Figure 34–3). Plasmin remodels the thrombus and limits its extension by proteolytic digestion of fibrin.

Both plasminogen and plasmin have specialized protein domains (kringles) that bind to exposed lysines on the fibrin clot and impart clot specificity to the fibrinolytic process. It should be noted that this clot specificity is only observed at *physiologic* levels of t-PA. At the *pharmacologic* levels of t-PA used in thrombolytic therapy, clot specificity is lost and a systemic lytic state is created, with attendant increase in bleeding risk. As in the coagulation cascade, there are negative regulators of fibrinolysis: endothelial cells synthesize and release plasminogen activator inhibitor (PAI), which inhibits t-PA; in addition α_2 antiplasmin circulates in the blood at high concentrations and under physiologic conditions

will rapidly inactivate any plasmin that is not clot-bound. However, this regulatory system is overwhelmed by therapeutic doses of plasminogen activators.

If the coagulation and fibrinolytic systems are pathologically activated, the hemostatic system may careen out of control, leading to generalized intravascular clotting and bleeding. This process is called **disseminated intravascular coagulation (DIC)** and may follow massive tissue injury, advanced cancers, obstetric emergencies such as abruptio placentae or retained products of conception, or bacterial sepsis. The treatment of DIC is to control the underlying disease process; if this is not possible, DIC is often fatal.

Regulation of the fibrinolytic system is useful in therapeutics. Increased fibrinolysis is effective therapy for thrombotic disease. **Tissue plasminogen activator, urokinase,** and **streptokinase** all activate the fibrinolytic system (Figure 34–3). Conversely, decreased fibrinolysis protects clots from lysis and reduces the bleeding of hemostatic failure. **Aminocaproic acid** is a clinically useful inhibitor of fibrinolysis. Heparin and the oral anticoagulant drugs do not affect the fibrinolytic mechanism.

■ BASIC PHARMACOLOGY OF THE ANTICOAGULANT DRUGS

The ideal anticoagulant drug would prevent pathologic thrombosis and limit reperfusion injury, yet allow a normal response to vascular injury and limit bleeding. Theoretically this could be accomplished by preservation of the TF-VIIa initiation phase of the clotting mechanism with attenuation of the secondary intrinsic pathway propagation phase of clot development. At this time such a drug does not exist; all anticoagulants and fibrinolytic drugs have an increased bleeding risk as their principle toxicity.

INDIRECT THROMBIN INHIBITORS

The indirect thrombin inhibitors are so-named because their antithrombotic effect is exerted by their interaction with a separate protein, antithrombin. **Unfractionated heparin (UFH), low-molecular-weight heparin (LMWH),** and the synthetic penta-saccharide **fondaparinux** bind to antithrombin and enhance its inactivation of factor Xa (Figure 34–4). Unfractionated heparin and to a lesser extent LMWH also enhance antithrombin's inactivation of thrombin.

HEPARIN

Chemistry & Mechanism of Action

Heparin is a heterogeneous mixture of sulfated mucopolysaccharides. It binds to endothelial cell surfaces and a variety of plasma proteins. Its biologic activity is dependent upon the endogenous anticoagulant **antithrombin**. Antithrombin inhibits clotting factor proteases, especially thrombin (IIa), IXa, and Xa, by forming equimolar stable complexes with them. In the absence of heparin, these reactions are slow; in the presence of heparin, they are

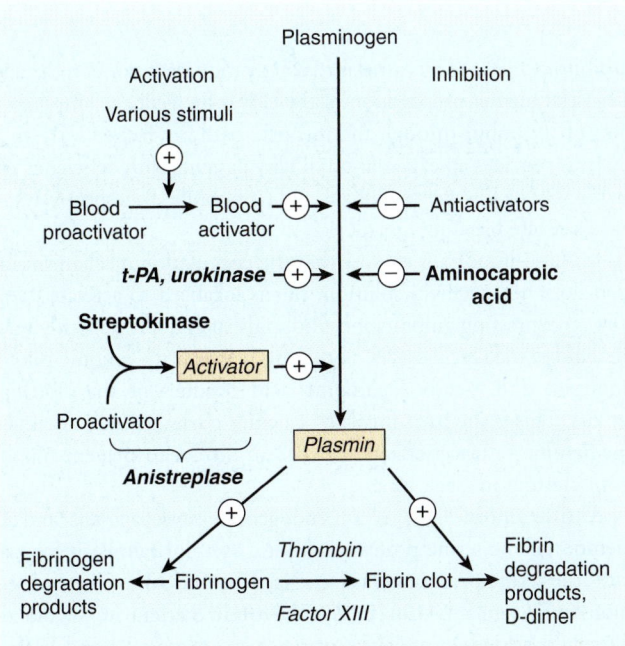

FIGURE 34–3 Schematic representation of the fibrinolytic system. Plasmin is the active fibrinolytic enzyme. Several clinically useful activators are shown on the left in bold. Anistreplase is a combination of streptokinase and the proactivator plasminogen. Aminocaproic acid (right) inhibits the activation of plasminogen to plasmin and is useful in some bleeding disorders. t-PA, tissue plasminogen activator.

Clotting in the Lab

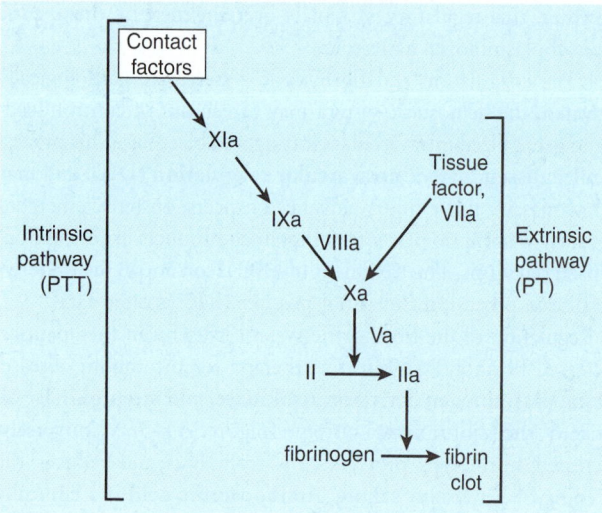

Clotting in Vivo

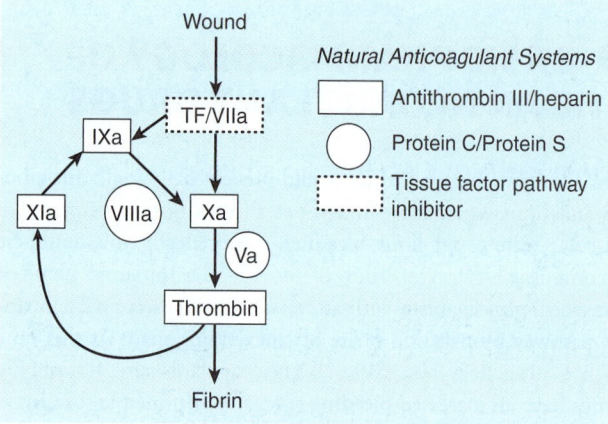

FIGURE 34–2 A model of blood coagulation. With tissue factor (TF), factor VII forms an activated complex (VIIa-TF) that catalyzes the activation of factor IX to factor IXa. Activated factor XIa also catalyzes this reaction. Tissue factor pathway inhibitor (TFPI) inhibits the catalytic action of the VIIa-TF complex. The cascade proceeds as shown, resulting ultimately in the conversion of fibrinogen to fibrin, an essential component of a functional clot. The two major anticoagulant drugs, heparin and warfarin, have very different actions. Heparin, acting in the blood, directly activates anticlotting factors, specifically antithrombin, which inactivates the factors enclosed in rectangles. Warfarin, acting in the liver, inhibits the synthesis of the factors enclosed in circles. Proteins C and S exert anticlotting effects by inactivating activated factors Va and VIIIa.

The exposure of TF on damaged endothelium or to blood that has extravasated into tissue binds TF to factor VIIa. This complex, in turn, activates factors X and IX. Factor Xa along with factor Va forms the prothrombinase complex on activated cell surfaces, which catalyzes the conversion of prothrombin (factor II) to thrombin (factor IIa). Thrombin, in turn, activates upstream clotting factors, primarily factors V, VIII, and XI, resulting in amplification of thrombin generation. The TF-factor VIIa-catalyzed activation of factor Xa is regulated by tissue factor pathway

TABLE 34–1 Blood clotting factors and drugs that affect them.[1]

Component or Factor	Common Synonym	Target for the Action of:
I	Fibrinogen	
II	Prothrombin	Heparin (IIa); warfarin (synthesis)
III	Tissue thromboplastin	
IV	Calcium	
V	Proaccelerin	
VII	Proconvertin	Warfarin (synthesis)
VIII	Antihemophilic factor (AHF)	
IX	Christmas factor, plasma thromboplastin component (PTC)	Warfarin (synthesis)
X	Stuart-Prower factor	Heparin (Xa); warfarin (synthesis)
XI	Plasma thromboplastin antecedent (PTA)	
XII	Hageman factor	
XIII	Fibrin-stabilizing factor	
Proteins C and S		Warfarin (synthesis)
Plasminogen		Thrombolytic enzymes, aminocaproic acid

[1]See Figure 34–2 and text for additional details.

inhibitor (TFPI). Thus after initial activation of factor X to Xa by TF-VIIa, further propagation of the clot is by feedback amplification of thrombin through the intrinsic pathway factors VIII and IX (this provides an explanation of why patients with deficiency of factor VIII or IX—hemophilia A and hemophilia B, respectively—have a severe bleeding disorder).

It is also important to note that the coagulation mechanism in vivo does not occur in solution, but is localized to activated *cell surfaces* expressing anionic phospholipids such as phosphatidylserine, and is mediated by Ca^{2+} bridging between the anionic phospholipids and γ-carboxyglutamic acid residues of the clotting factors. This is the basis for using calcium chelators such as ethylenediamine tetraacetic acid (EDTA) or citrate to prevent blood from clotting in a test tube.

Antithrombin (AT) is an endogenous anticoagulant and a member of the serine protease inhibitor (serpin) family; it inactivates the serine proteases IIa, IXa, Xa, XIa, and XIIa. The endogenous anticoagulants **protein C** and **protein S** attenuate the blood clotting cascade by proteolysis of the two cofactors Va and VIIIa. From an evolutionary standpoint, it is of interest that factors V and VIII have an identical overall domain structure and considerable homology, consistent with a common ancestor gene; likewise the serine proteases are descendants of a trypsin-like common ancestor. Thus, the TF–VIIa initiating complex, serine proteases, and cofactors each have their own lineage-specific attenuation mechanism (Figure 34–2). Defects in natural anticoagulants result in an

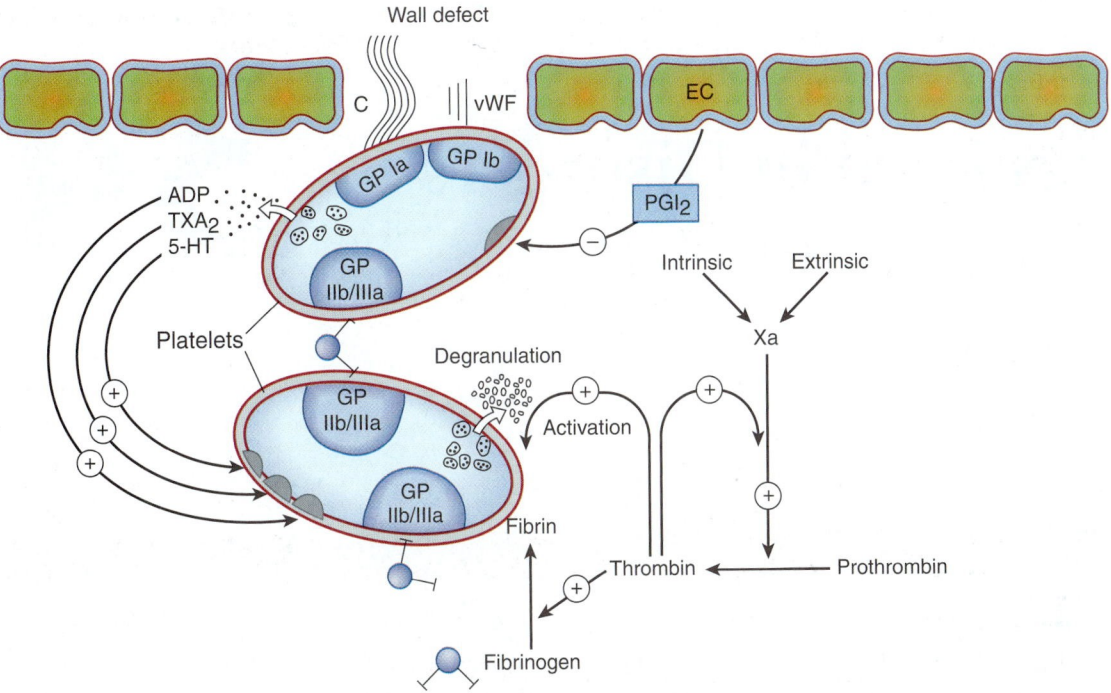

FIGURE 34–1 Thrombus formation at the site of the damaged vascular wall (EC, endothelial cell) and the role of platelets and clotting factors. Platelet membrane receptors include the glycoprotein (GP) Ia receptor, binding to collagen (C); GP Ib receptor, binding von Willebrand factor (vWF); and GP IIb/IIIa, which binds fibrinogen and other macromolecules. Antiplatelet prostacyclin (PGI$_2$) is released from the endothelium. Aggregating substances released from the degranulating platelet include adenosine diphosphate (ADP), thromboxane A$_2$ (TXA$_2$), and serotonin (5-HT). Production of factor Xa is detailed in Figure 34–2. (Redrawn and reproduced, with permission, from Simoons ML, Decker JW: New directions in anticoagulant and antiplatelet treatment. [Editorial.] Br Heart J 1995;74:337.)

amputation or organ failure. Venous clots tend to be more fibrin-rich, contain large numbers of trapped red blood cells, and are recognized pathologically as **red thrombi.** Venous thrombi can cause severe swelling and pain of the affected extremity, but the most feared consequence is pulmonary embolism. This occurs when part or all of the clot breaks off from its location in the deep venous system and travels as an embolus through the right side of the heart and into the pulmonary arterial circulation. Sudden occlusion of a large pulmonary artery can cause acute right heart failure and sudden death. In addition lung ischemia or infarction will occur distal to the occluded pulmonary arterial segment. Such emboli usually arise from the deep venous system of the proximal lower extremities or pelvis. Although all thrombi are mixed, the platelet nidus dominates the arterial thrombus and the fibrin tail dominates the venous thrombus.

BLOOD COAGULATION CASCADE

Blood coagulates due to the transformation of soluble fibrinogen into insoluble fibrin by the enzyme thrombin. Several circulating proteins interact in a cascading series of limited proteolytic reactions (Figure 34–2). At each step, a clotting factor zymogen undergoes limited proteolysis and becomes an active protease (eg, factor VII is converted to factor VIIa). Each protease factor activates the next clotting factor in the sequence, culminating in

the formation of thrombin (factor IIa). Several of these factors are targets for drug therapy (Table 34–1).

Thrombin has a central role in hemostasis and has many functions. In clotting, thrombin proteolytically cleaves small peptides from fibrinogen, allowing fibrinogen to polymerize and form a fibrin clot. Thrombin also activates many upstream clotting factors, leading to more thrombin generation, and activates factor XIII, a transaminase that cross-links the fibrin polymer and stabilizes the clot. Thrombin is a potent platelet activator and mitogen. Thrombin also exerts *anti*coagulant effects by activating the protein C pathway, which attenuates the clotting response (Figure 34–2). It should therefore be apparent that the response to vascular injury is a complex and precisely modulated process that ensures that under normal circumstances, repair of vascular injury occurs without thrombosis and downstream ischemia; that is, the response is proportionate and reversible. Eventually vascular remodeling and repair occur with reversion to the quiescent resting anticoagulant endothelial cell phenotype.

Initiation of Clotting: The Tissue Factor-VIIa Complex

The main initiator of blood coagulation in vivo is the tissue factor (TF)-factor VIIa pathway (Figure 34–2). Tissue factor is a transmembrane protein ubiquitously expressed outside the vasculature, but not normally expressed in an active form within vessels.

Drugs Used in Disorders of Coagulation

34

James L. Zehnder, MD

CASE STUDY

A 25-year-old woman presents to the emergency department complaining of acute onset of shortness of breath and pleuritic pain. She had been in her usual state of health until 2 days prior when she noted that her left leg was swollen and red. Her only medication was oral contraceptives. Family history was significant for a history of "blood clots" in multiple members of the maternal side of her family. Physical examination demonstrates an anxious woman with stable vital signs. The left lower extremity demonstrates erythema and edema and is tender to touch. Ultrasound reveals a deep vein thrombosis in the left lower extremity; chest computed tomography scan confirms the presence of pulmonary emboli. Laboratory blood tests indicate elevated D-dimer levels. What therapy is indicated acutely? What are the long-term therapy options? How long should she be treated? Should this individual use oral contraceptives?

Hemostasis refers to the finely regulated dynamic process of maintaining fluidity of the blood, repairing vascular injury, and limiting blood loss while avoiding vessel occlusion (thrombosis) and inadequate perfusion of vital organs. Either extreme—excessive bleeding or thrombosis—represents a breakdown of the hemostatic mechanism. Common causes of dysregulated hemostasis include hereditary or acquired defects in the clotting mechanism and secondary effects of infection or cancer. The drugs used to inhibit thrombosis and to limit abnormal bleeding are the subjects of this chapter.

MECHANISMS OF BLOOD COAGULATION

The vascular endothelial cell layer lining blood vessels has an anticoagulant phenotype, and circulating blood platelets and clotting factors do not normally adhere to it to an appreciable extent. In the setting of vascular injury, the endothelial cell layer rapidly undergoes a series of changes resulting in a more procoagulant phenotype. Injury exposes reactive subendothelial matrix proteins such as collagen and von Willebrand factor, which results in platelet adherence and activation, and secretion and synthesis of vasoconstrictors and platelet-recruiting and activating molecules. Thus, **thromboxane A_2 (TXA$_2$)** is synthesized from arachidonic acid within platelets and is a platelet activator and potent vasoconstrictor. Products secreted from platelet granules include **adenosine diphosphate (ADP)**, a powerful inducer of platelet aggregation, and **serotonin (5-HT),** which stimulates aggregation and vasoconstriction. Activation of platelets results in a conformational change in the $\alpha_{IIb}\beta_{III}$ integrin (IIb/IIIa) receptor, enabling it to bind fibrinogen, which cross-links adjacent platelets, resulting in aggregation and formation of a platelet plug (Figure 34–1). Simultaneously, the coagulation system cascade is activated, resulting in thrombin generation and a fibrin clot, which stabilizes the platelet plug (see below). Knowledge of the hemostatic mechanism is important for diagnosis of bleeding disorders. Patients with defects in the formation of the primary platelet plug (defects in primary hemostasis, eg, platelet function defects, von Willebrand disease) typically bleed from surface sites (gingiva, skin, heavy menses) with injury. In contrast, patients with defects in the clotting mechanism (secondary hemostasis, eg, hemophilia A) tend to bleed into deep tissues (joints, muscle, retroperitoneum), often with no apparent inciting event, and bleeding may recur unpredictably.

The platelet is central to normal hemostasis and thromboembolic disease, and is the target of many therapies discussed in this chapter. Platelet-rich thrombi (**white thrombi**) form in the high flow rate and high shear force environment of arteries. Occlusive arterial thrombi cause serious disease by producing downstream ischemia of extremities or vital organs, and can result in limb

CASE STUDY ANSWER

This patient's megaloblastic anemia appears to be due to vitamin B_{12} (cobalamin) deficiency secondary to impaired production of intrinsic factor resulting in insufficient absorption of vitamin B_{12} from the GI tract. It is important to measure serum concentrations of both folic acid and cobalamin because megaloblastic anemia can result from deficiency of either nutrient. It is especially important to diagnose vitamin B_{12} deficiency because this deficiency, if untreated, can lead to irreversible neurologic damage. Folate supplementation, which can compensate for vitamin B_{12}-derived anemia, does not prevent B_{12}-deficiency neurologic damage. To correct this patient's vitamin B_{12} deficiency, she would probably be treated parenterally with cobalamin because of her impaired oral absorption of vitamin B_{12}. Several weeks of daily administration would be followed with weekly doses until her hematocrit returned to normal. Monthly doses would then be given to maintain her body stores of vitamin B_{12}.

PREPARATIONS AVAILABLE

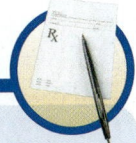

Darbepoetin alfa (Aranesp)
Parenteral: 25, 40, 60, 100, 200, 300, 500 mcg/mL solution for IV or SC injection

Deferasirox (Exjade)
Oral: 125, 250, 500 mg tablets

Deferoxamine (generic, Desferal)
Parenteral: 500, 2000 mg powder for reconstitution for IM, SC, or IV injection

Eltrombopag (Promacta)
Oral: 25, 50, 75 mg tablet

Epoetin alfa (erythropoietin, EPO) (Epogen, Procrit)
Parenteral: 2000, 3000, 4000, 10,000, 20,000, 40,000 IU/mL solution for IV or SC injection

Epoetin beta (Methoxy polyethylene glycol-epoetin beta) (Mircera)
Parenteral: 50, 100, 200, 300, 400, 600, 1000 mcg/mL solution in vials and prefilled syringes for IV or SC injection

Filgrastim (G-CSF) (Neupogen)
Parenteral: 300 mcg/mL, 600 mcg/mL solution in vials and prefilled syringes for IV or SC injection

Folic acid (folacin, pteroylglutamic acid) (generic)
Oral: 0.4, 0.8, 1 mg tablets
Parenteral: 5 mg/mL solution for injection

Iron (generic)
Oral: See Table 33–3.

Parenteral (Iron dextran) (InFeD, DexFerrum): 50 mg elemental iron/mL solution for IM or IV injection
Parenteral (Sodium ferric gluconate complex) (Ferrlecit): 12.5 mg elemental iron/mL solution for IV injection
Parenteral (Iron sucrose) (Venofer): 20 mg elemental iron/mL solution for IV injection

Oprelvekin (IL-11) (Neumega)
Parenteral: 5 mg powder for reconstitution for SC injection

Pegfilgrastim (Neulasta)
Parenteral: 6 mg/0.6 mL solution in single-dose syringe

Plerixafor (Mozobil)
Parenteral: 20 mg/mL solution for SC injection

Romiplostim (Nplate)
Parenteral: 250, 500 mcg powder for reconstitution for SC injection

Sargramostim (GM-CSF) (Leukine)
Parenteral: 250 mcg powder for reconstitution; 500 mcg/mL solution

Vitamin B$_{12}$ (generic cyanocobalamin or hydroxocobalamin)
Oral (cyanocobalamin): 50, 100, 250, 500, 1000 mcg regular tablets or lozenges; 500, 1000, 2500, 5000, 6000 mg sublingual tablets or lozenges; 1000, 1500 mg controlled-release tablets
Nasal (Nascobal, CaloMist): 500 mcg/spray
Parenteral (cyanocobalamin): 1000, 5000 mcg/mL for IM or SC injection
Parenteral (hydroxocobalamin): 1000 mcg/mL solution for IM injection; 2.5 g powder for reconstitution (antidote for cyanide poisoning) for IV injection

REFERENCES

Auerbach M, Al Talib K: Low-molecular weight iron dextran and iron sucrose have similar comparative safety profiles in chronic kidney disease. Kidney Int 2008;73:528.

Barzi A, Sekeres MA: Myelodysplastic syndromes: a practical approach to diagnosis and treatment. Cleve Clin J Med 2010;77:37.

Bhana N: Granulocyte colony-stimulating factors in the management of chemotherapy-induced neutropenia: Evidence based review. Curr Opin Oncol 2007;19:328.

Brittenham GM: Iron-chelating therapy for transfusional iron overload. N Engl J Med 2011;364:146.

Clark SF: Iron deficiency anemia: diagnosis and management. Curr Opin Gastroenterol 2009;25:122.

Crawford J et al: Reduction by granulocyte colony-stimulating factor of fever and neutropenia induced by chemotherapy in patients with small-cell lung cancer. N Engl J Med 1991;325:164.

Darshan D, Fraer DM, Anderson GJ: Molecular basis of iron-loading disorders. Expert Rev Mol Med 2010;12:e36.

Gertz MA: Current status of stem cell mobilization. Br J Haematol 2010;150:647.

Kessans MR, Gatesman ML, Kockler DR: Plerixafor: A peripheral blood stem cell mobilizer. Pharmacotherapy 2010;30:485.

McKoy JM et al: Epoetin-associated pure red cell aplasia: Past, present, and future considerations. Transfusion 2008;48:1754.

Rees DC, Williams TN, Gladwin MT: Sickle-cell disease. Lancet 2010;376:2018.

Rizzo JD et al: American Society of Clinical Oncology/American Society of Hematology clinical practice guideline update on the use of epoetin and darbepoetin in adult patients with cancer. J Clin Oncol 2010;28:4996.

Sauer J, Mason JB, Choi SW: Too much folate: a risk factor for cancer and cardiovascular disease? Curr Opin Clin Nutr Metab Care 2009;12:30.

Solomon LR: Disorders of cobalamin (vitamin B12) metabolism: Emerging concepts in pathophysiology, diagnosis and treatment. Blood Rev 2007;21:113.

Stasi R et al: Thrombopoietic agents. Blood Rev 2010;24:179.

Winkelmayer WC: Confusion about the appropriate use of erythropoiesis-stimulating agents in patients undergoing maintenance dialysis. Semin Dial 2010;23:486.

Wolff T et al: Folic acid supplementation for the prevention of neural tube defects: An update of the evidence for the U.S. Preventive Services Task Force. Ann Intern Med 2009;150:632.

Subclass	Mechanism of Action	Effects	Clinical Applications	Pharmacokinetics, Toxicities, Interactions
ERYTHROCYTE-STIMULATING AGENTS				
• Epoetin alfa	Agonist of erythropoietin receptors expressed by red cell progenitors	Stimulates erythroid proliferation and differentiation, and induces the release of reticulocytes from the bone marrow	Anemia, especially anemia associated with chronic renal failure, HIV infection, cancer, and prematurity • prevention of the need for transfusion in patients undergoing certain types of elective surgery	IV or SC administration 1–3 times per week • *Toxicity:* Hypertension, thrombotic complications, and, very rarely, pure red cell aplasia • to reduce the risk of serious CV events, hemoglobin levels should be maintained <12 g/dL
• *Darbepoetin alfa: Long-acting glycosylated form administered weekly*				
• *Methoxy polyethylene glycol-epoetin beta: Long-acting form administered 1–2 times per month*				
MYELOID GROWTH FACTORS				
• Granulocyte-macrophage colony-stimulating factor (GM-CSF; filgrastim)	Stimulates G-CSF receptors expressed on mature neutrophils and their progenitors	Stimulates neutrophil progenitor proliferation and differentiation • activates phagocytic activity of mature neutrophils and extends their survival • mobilizes hematopoietic stem cells	Neutropenia associated with congenital neutropenia, cyclic neutropenia, myelodysplasia, and aplastic anemia • secondary prevention of neutropenia in patients undergoing cytotoxic chemotherapy • mobilization of peripheral blood cells in preparation for autologous and allogeneic stem cell transplantation	Daily SC administration • *Toxicity:* Bone pain • rarely, splenic rupture
• *Pegfilgrastim: Long-acting form of filgrastim that is covalently linked to a type of polyethylene glycol*				
• *GM-CSF (sargramostim): Myeloid growth factor that acts through a distinct GM-CSF receptor to stimulate proliferation and differentiation of early and late granulocytic progenitor cells, and erythroid and megakaryocyte progenitors; clinical uses are similar to those of G-CSF, but it is more likely than GM-CSF to cause fever, arthralgia, myalgia, and capillary leak syndrome*				
• *Plerixafor: Antagonist of CXCR4 used in combination with G-CSF for mobilization of peripheral blood cells prior to autologous transplantation in patients with multiple myeloma or non-Hodgkin's lymphoma who responded suboptimally to G-CSF alone*				
MEGAKARYOCYTE GROWTH FACTORS				
• Oprelvekin (interleukin-11; IL-11)	Recombinant form of an endogenous cytokine • activates IL-11 receptors	Stimulates growth of multiple lymphoid and myeloid cells, including megakaryocyte progenitors • increases the number of circulating platelets and neutrophils	Secondary prevention of thrombocytopenia in patients undergoing cytotoxic chemotherapy for nonmyeloid cancers	Daily SC injection • *Toxicity:* Fatigue, headache, dizziness, anemia, fluid accumulation in the lungs, and transient atrial arrhythmias
• *Romiplostim: Genetically engineered protein in which F_c components of a human antibody are fused to multiple copies of a peptide that stimulates the thrombopoietin receptors; approved for treatment of idiopathic thrombocytopenic purpura*				
• *Eltrombopag: Orally active, restricted use*				

Eltrombopag, an orally active small molecule agonist at the thrombopoietin receptor, was licensed in 2008 for use in patients with severe idiopathic thrombocytopenia who have failed to respond adequately to first-line treatments. Because of concerns about hepatotoxicity and hemorrhage, eltrombopag is restricted to use by registered physicians and patients and its use requires close monitoring of liver enzymes.

Pharmacodynamics

Interleukin-11 acts through a specific cell surface cytokine receptor to stimulate the growth of multiple lymphoid and myeloid cells. It acts synergistically with other growth factors to stimulate the growth of primitive megakaryocytic progenitors and, most importantly, increases the number of peripheral platelets and neutrophils.

Romiplostim has high affinity for the human Mpl receptor. It causes a dose-dependent increase in platelet count that begins on day 5 after subcutaneous administration and peaks at days 12–15.

Clinical Pharmacology

Interleukin-11 is approved for the secondary prevention of thrombocytopenia in patients receiving cytotoxic chemotherapy for treatment of nonmyeloid cancers. Clinical trials show that it reduces the number of platelet transfusions required by patients who experience severe thrombocytopenia after a previous cycle of chemotherapy. Although IL-11 has broad stimulatory effects on hematopoietic cell lineages in vitro, it does not appear to have significant effects on the leukopenia caused by myelosuppressive chemotherapy. Interleukin-11 is given by subcutaneous injection at a dose of 50 mcg/kg/d. It is started 6–24 hours after completion

of chemotherapy and continued for 14–21 days or until the platelet count passes the nadir and rises to more than 50,000 cells/μL.

In patients with chronic idiopathic thrombocytopenia (ITP) who failed to respond adequately to previous treatment with steroids, immunoglobulins, or splenectomy, romiplostim significantly increased platelet count in most patients. In a 6-week placebo-controlled study in which patients were treated weekly with 1 or 3 mcg/kg, 12 of 16 patients reached the targeted platelet range of 50,000–450,000 platelets/μL. Romiplostim does not appear to decrease the rate of platelet destruction in ITP as platelet counts returned to pretreatment levels after the drug's discontinuation. An open label trial found that many patients maintained a platelet count of 100,000 platelets/μL or higher over a 48-week period and that over half of the patients were able to discontinue other therapies. Romiplostim is initiated as a weekly subcutaneous dose of 1 mcg/kg and then continued at the lowest dose required to maintain a platelet count of at least 50,000 platelets/μL.

Toxicity

The most common adverse effects of IL-11 are fatigue, headache, dizziness, and cardiovascular effects. The cardiovascular effects include anemia (due to hemodilution), dyspnea (due to fluid accumulation in the lungs), and transient atrial arrhythmias. Hypokalemia has also been seen in some patients. All of these adverse effects appear to be reversible.

Romiplostim appears to be well tolerated except for a mild headache on the day of administration. A potential long-term concern is that two patients treated with romiplostim had an increase in bone marrow reticulin, a possible marker of myelodysplastic or myeloproliferative processes. However, neither patient had evidence of increased collagen fibrosis or of abnormal bone marrow cytogenetics.

SUMMARY Agents Used in Anemias and Hematopoietic Growth Factors

Subclass	Mechanism of Action	Effects	Clinical Applications	Pharmacokinetics, Toxicities, Interactions
IRON				
• Ferrous sulfate	Required for biosynthesis of heme and heme-containing proteins, including hemoglobin and myoglobin	Adequate supplies required for normal heme synthesis • deficiency results in inadequate heme production	Iron deficiency, which manifests as microcytic anemia • oral preparation	Complicated endogenous system for absorbing, storing, and transporting iron • *Toxicity:* Acute overdose results in necrotizing gastroenteritis, abdominal pain, bloody diarrhea, shock, lethargy, and dyspnea • chronic iron overload results in hemochromatosis, with damage to the heart, liver, pancreas, and other organs • organ failure and death can ensue

• *Ferrous gluconate and ferrous fumarate: Oral iron preparations*
• *Iron dextran, iron sucrose complex, and sodium ferric gluconate complex: Parenteral preparations; can cause pain, hypersensitivity reactions*

Subclass	Mechanism of Action	Effects	Clinical Applications	Pharmacokinetics, Toxicities, Interactions
IRON CHELATORS				
• Deferoxamine (see also Chapters 57 and 58)	Chelates excess iron	Reduces toxicity associated with acute or chronic iron overload	Acute iron poisoning; inherited or acquired hemochromatosis	Preferred route of administration is IM or SC • *Toxicity:* Rapid IV administration may cause hypotension • neurotoxicity and increased susceptibility to certain infections have occurred with long-term use

• *Deferasirox: Orally administered iron chelator for treatment of hemochromatosis*

Subclass	Mechanism of Action	Effects	Clinical Applications	Pharmacokinetics, Toxicities, Interactions
VITAMIN B$_{12}$				
• Cyanocobalamin • Hydroxocobalamin	Cofactor required for essential enzymatic reactions that form tetrahydrofolate, convert homocysteine to methionine, and metabolize L-methylmalonyl-CoA	Adequate supplies required for amino acid and fatty acid metabolism, and DNA synthesis	Vitamin B$_{12}$ deficiency, which manifests as megaloblastic anemia and is the basis of pernicious anemia	Parenteral vitamin B$_{12}$ is required for pernicious anemia and other malabsorption syndromes • *Toxicity:* No toxicity associated with excess vitamin B$_{12}$
FOLIC ACID				
• Folacin (pteroylglutamic acid)	Precursor of an essential donor of methyl groups used for synthesis of amino acids, purines, and deoxynucleotide	Adequate supplies required for essential biochemical reactions involving amino acid metabolism, and purine and DNA synthesis	Folic acid deficiency, which manifests as megaloblastic anemia, and prevention of congenital neural tube defects	Oral; well-absorbed; need for parenteral administration is rare • *Toxicity:* Folic acid is not toxic in overdose, but large amounts can partially compensate for vitamin B$_{12}$ deficiency and put people with unrecognized B$_{12}$ deficiency at risk of neurologic consequences of vitamin B$_{12}$ deficiency, which are not compensated by folic acid

prevention and treatment of venous thromboembolism, and appears to not cross-react with pathologic HIT antibodies in most individuals. The use of fondaparinux as an alternative anticoagulant in HIT is currently being tested in clinical trials.

A major focus of drug development has been to develop orally active anticoagulants that do not require monitoring. **Rivaroxaban** is the first oral factor Xa inhibitor to reach phase III clinical trials. The safety and efficacy of rivaroxaban appears to be at least equivalent, and possibly superior, to LMW heparins (see below).

Reversal of Heparin Action

Excessive anticoagulant action of heparin is treated by discontinuance of the drug. If bleeding occurs, administration of a specific antagonist such as **protamine sulfate** is indicated. Protamine is a highly basic, positively charged peptide that combines with negatively charged heparin as an ion pair to form a stable complex devoid of anticoagulant activity. For every 100 units of heparin remaining in the patient, 1 mg of protamine sulfate is given intravenously; the rate of infusion should not exceed 50 mg in any 10-minute period. Excess protamine must be avoided; it also has an anticoagulant effect. Neutralization of LMW heparin by protamine is incomplete. Limited experience suggests that 1 mg of protamine sulfate may be used to partially neutralize 1 mg of enoxaparin. Protamine will not reverse the activity of fondaparinux. Excess danaparoid can be removed by plasmapheresis.

ORAL DIRECT FACTOR XA INHIBITORS

Oral Xa inhibitors, including rivaroxaban and apixaban, are approved or in advanced stages of development and along with oral thrombin inhibitors (discussed below) are likely to have a major impact on antithrombotic pharmacotherapy. These drugs inhibit factor Xa, in the final common pathway of clotting (see Figure 34–2). These drugs are given as fixed doses and do not require monitoring. They have a rapid onset of action and shorter half-lives than warfarin (approximately 10 hours but half-life may be prolonged in elderly patients or those with renal impairment).

Rivaroxaban is approved for prevention of venous thromboembolism following hip or knee surgery. The prophylactic dose is 10 mg orally per day. A recent large randomized clinical trial of DVT treatment compared a higher dose of rivaroxaban (15 mg bid for 3 weeks, followed by 20 mg daily) to a standard treatment regimen of enoxaparin followed by warfarin. This trial demonstrated non-inferiority of rivaroxaban in preventing recurrent venous thromboembolism and showed no difference in bleeding risk. Another trial reported non-inferiority of rivaroxaban to warfarin for prevention of stroke in patients with atrial fibrillation.

Apixaban is currently in clinical development. A recent study of patients undergoing total hip replacement compared apixaban 2.5 mg orally once per day with enoxaparin 40 mg subcutaneously once per day. This trial demonstrated the apixaban arm had lower rates of venous thromboembolism and similar bleeding

rates. Another multicenter study randomized patients with recent myocardial infarction to apixaban 5 mg or placebo. This trial was stopped early because of an increase in bleeding risk without a significant decrease in ischemic events. Another trial comparing apixaban to aspirin for stroke prevention in atrial fibrillation was stopped early because of evidence of increased efficacy in the apixaban arm.

Thus, it appears that the primary target populations for development of both rivaroxaban and apixaban will be prevention and treatment of patients with venous thromboembolism and stroke prevention in patients with atrial fibrillation. Both of these drugs are excreted in part by the kidneys; therefore, the dosage may need to be reduced in patients with renal impairment. In such patients, use of a hepatically metabolized drug such as warfarin may be a better alternative. No antidotes exist for direct Xa inhibitors.

DIRECT THROMBIN INHIBITORS

The direct thrombin inhibitors (DTIs) exert their anticoagulant effect by directly binding to the active site of thrombin, thereby inhibiting thrombin's downstream effects. This is in contrast to indirect thrombin inhibitors such as heparin and LMWH (see above), which act through antithrombin. **Hirudin** and **bivalirudin** are bivalent DTIs in that they bind at both the catalytic or active site of thrombin as well as at a substrate recognition site. **Argatroban** and **melagatran** are small molecules that bind only at the thrombin active site.

PARENTERAL DIRECT THROMBIN INHIBITORS

Leeches have been used for bloodletting since the age of Hippocrates. More recently, surgeons have used medicinal leeches (*Hirudo medicinalis*) to prevent thrombosis in the fine vessels of reattached digits. **Hirudin** is a specific, irreversible thrombin inhibitor from leech saliva that is now available in recombinant form as **lepirudin.** Its action is independent of antithrombin, which means it can reach and inactivate fibrin-bound thrombin in thrombi. Lepirudin has little effect on platelets or the bleeding time. Like heparin, it must be administered parenterally and is monitored by the aPTT. Lepirudin is approved by the FDA for use in patients with thrombosis related to heparin-induced thrombocytopenia. Lepirudin is excreted by the kidney and should be used with great caution in patients with renal insufficiency as no antidote exists. Up to 40% of patients who receive long-term infusions develop an antibody directed against the thrombin-lepirudin complex. These antigen-antibody complexes are not cleared by the kidney and may result in an enhanced anticoagulant effect. Some patients re-exposed to the drug have developed life-threatening anaphylactic reactions.

Bivalirudin, another bivalent inhibitor of thrombin, is administered intravenously, with a rapid onset and offset of action. The drug has a short half-life with clearance that is 20% renal and the remainder metabolic. Bivalirudin also inhibits platelet activation and has been FDA-approved for use in percutaneous coronary angioplasty.

Argatroban is a small molecule thrombin inhibitor that is FDA-approved for use in patients with HIT with or without thrombosis and coronary angioplasty in patients with HIT. It, too, has a short half-life, is given by continuous intravenous infusion, and is monitored by aPTT. Its clearance is not affected by renal disease but is dependent on liver function; dose reduction is required in patients with liver disease. Patients on argatroban will demonstrate elevated INRs, rendering the transition to warfarin difficult (ie, the INR will reflect contributions from both warfarin and argatroban). (INR is discussed in detail in the discussion of warfarin administration.) A nomogram is supplied by the manufacturer to assist in this transition. No properly designed head-to-head trials have been performed to determine whether argatroban or lepirudin is superior in the treatment of HIT. However, in practice, the choice of which DTI to use in a patient with HIT is usually dictated by the condition of the clearing organ. If the patient has severe renal insufficiency, then argatroban would be preferred. If there is severe hepatic insufficiency, then lepirudin would be a better choice.

ORAL DIRECT THROMBIN INHIBITORS

Advantages of oral direct thrombin inhibitors include predictable pharmacokinetics and bioavailability, which allow for fixed dosing and predictable anticoagulant response, and make routine coagulation monitoring unnecessary. In addition, these agents do not interact with P450-interacting drugs, and their rapid onset and offset of action allow for immediate anticoagulation, thus avoiding the need for overlap with additional anticoagulant drugs.

Dabigatran etexilate mesylate is the first oral direct thrombin inhibitor approved by the FDA. Dabigatran was approved in 2010 to reduce risk of stroke and systemic embolism with nonvalvular atrial fibrillation. In the EU, dabigatran is approved for prevention of venous thromboembolism in patients who have undergone hip or knee replacement surgery. The pivotal trial leading to FDA approval was a study of > 18,000 patients with nonvalvular atrial fibrillation and at least one other defined risk factor. Dabigatran at a dose of 150 mg bid was shown to be superior to warfarin with an INR target of 2–3 in preventing stroke and systemic embolization.

Pharmacology

Dabigatran and its metabolites are direct thrombin inhibitors. Following oral administration, dabigatran etexilate mesylate is converted to dabigatran. The oral bioavailability is 3–7% in normal volunteers. The drug is a substrate for the P-glycoprotein efflux pump; however, P-glycoprotein inhibitors or inducers do not have a significant effect on drug clearance. Concomitant use of ketoconazole, amiodarone, quinidine, and clopidogrel increases the effect of dabigatran. The half-life of the drug in normal volunteers is 12–17 hours. Renal impairment results in prolonged drug

clearance and may require dose adjustment; the drug should be avoided in patients with severe renal impairment.

Administration & Dosage

For prevention of stroke and systemic embolism in nonvalvular atrial fibrillation, 150 mg should be given bid to patients with creatinine clearance > 30 mL/min. For decreased creatinine clearance of 15–30 mL/min, the dose is 75 mg bid. No monitoring is required. Dabigatran will prolong the PTT and thrombin time, which can be used to estimate drug effect if necessary.

Toxicity

As with any anticoagulant drug, the primary toxicity of dabigatran is bleeding. In the RE-LY study, there was an increase in gastrointestinal adverse reactions and gastrointestinal bleeding compared to warfarin. There was also a trend toward increased bleeding with dabigatran in patients older than 75 years. There is no antidote for dabigatran. In a drug overdose situation, it is important to maintain renal function or dialyze if necessary. Use of recombinant factor VIIa or prothrombin complex concentrates may be considered as an unproven, off-label use in cases of life-threatening bleeding associated with dabigatran use.

Oral direct thrombin inhibitors and oral direct Xa inhibitors offer significant advantages over warfarin (discussed next), which has a narrow therapeutic window, is affected by diet and many drugs, and requires monitoring for dosage adjustment. It appears that the oral anti-Xa drugs and oral direct thrombin inhibitors are poised to challenge warfarin's dominance in the prevention and therapy of thrombotic disease.

WARFARIN & OTHER COUMARIN ANTICOAGULANTS

Chemistry & Pharmacokinetics

The clinical use of the coumarin anticoagulants began with the discovery of an anticoagulant substance formed in spoiled sweet clover silage which caused hemorrhagic disease in cattle. At the behest of local farmers, a chemist at the University of Wisconsin identified the toxic agent as bishydroxycoumarin. A synthesized derivative, dicumarol and its congeners, most notably warfarin (**W**isconsin **A**lumni **R**esearch **F**oundation, with "arin" from coumarin added; Figure 34–5), were initially used as rodenticides. In the 1950s warfarin (under the brand name Coumadin) was introduced as an antithrombotic agent in humans. Warfarin is one of the most commonly prescribed drugs, used by approximately 1.5 million individuals, and several studies have indicated that the drug is significantly underused in clinical situations where it has proven benefit.

Warfarin is generally administered as the sodium salt and has 100% bioavailability. Over 99% of racemic warfarin is bound to plasma albumin, which may contribute to its small volume of distribution (the albumin space), its long half-life in plasma (36 hours), and the lack of urinary excretion of unchanged drug. Warfarin used

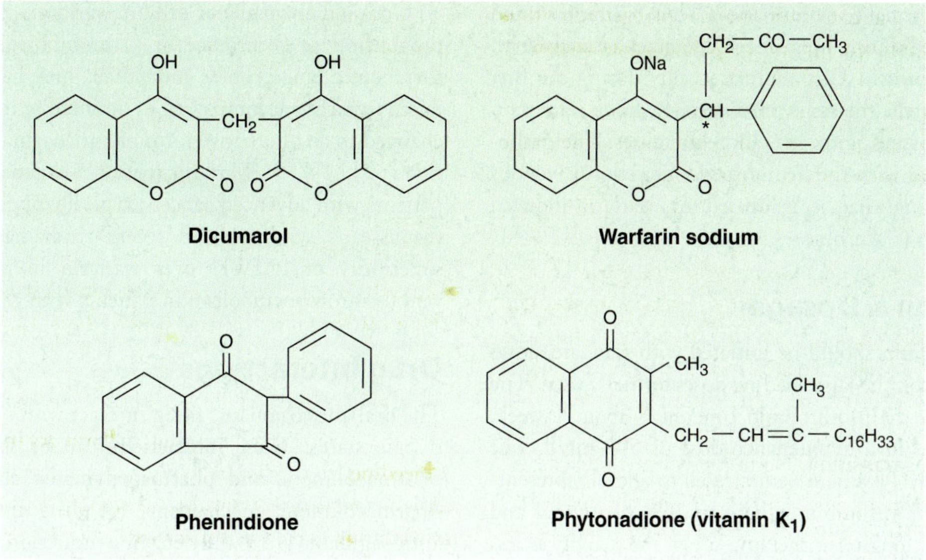

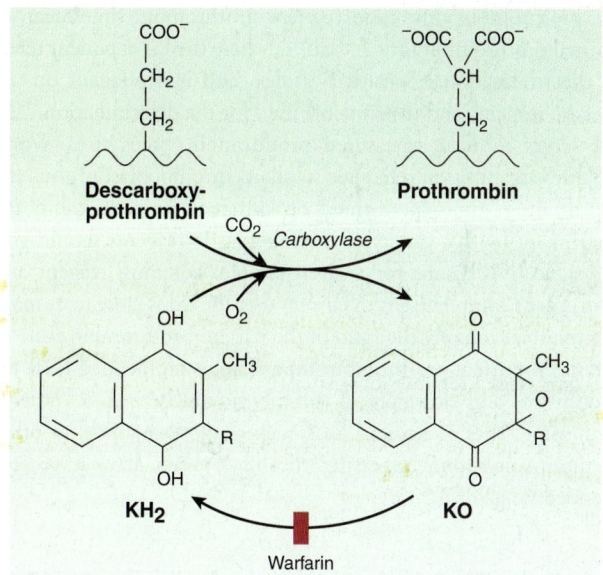

FIGURE 34–5 Structural formulas of several oral anticoagulant drugs and of vitamin K. The carbon atom of warfarin shown at the asterisk is an asymmetric center.

clinically is a racemic mixture composed of equal amounts of two enantiomorphs. The levorotatory *S*-warfarin is four times more potent than the dextrorotatory *R*-warfarin. This observation is useful in understanding the stereoselective nature of several drug interactions involving warfarin.

Mechanism of Action

Coumarin anticoagulants block the γ-carboxylation of several glutamate residues in prothrombin and factors VII, IX, and X as well as the endogenous anticoagulant proteins C and S (Figure 34–2, Table 34–1). The blockade results in incomplete coagulation factor molecules that are biologically inactive. The protein carboxylation reaction is coupled to the oxidation of vitamin K. The vitamin must then be reduced to reactivate it. Warfarin prevents reductive metabolism of the inactive vitamin K epoxide back to its active hydroquinone form (Figure 34–6). Mutational change of the responsible enzyme, vitamin K epoxide reductase, can give rise to genetic resistance to warfarin in humans and especially in rats.

There is an 8- to 12-hour delay in the action of warfarin. Its anticoagulant effect results from a balance between partially inhibited synthesis and unaltered degradation of the four vitamin K-dependent clotting factors. The resulting inhibition of coagulation is dependent on their degradation half-lives in the circulation. These half-lives are 6, 24, 40, and 60 hours for factors VII, IX, X, and II, respectively. Larger initial doses of warfarin—up to about 0.75 mg/kg—hasten the onset of the anticoagulant effect. Beyond this dosage, the speed of onset is independent of the dose size. The only effect of a larger loading dose is to prolong the time that the plasma concentration of drug remains above that required for suppression of clotting factor synthesis. The only difference among oral anticoagulants in producing and maintaining hypoprothrombinemia is the half-life of each drug.

FIGURE 34–6 Vitamin K cycle—metabolic interconversions of vitamin K associated with the synthesis of vitamin K–dependent clotting factors. Vitamin K_1 or K_2 is activated by reduction to the hydroquinone form (KH_2). Stepwise oxidation to vitamin K epoxide (KO) is coupled to prothrombin carboxylation by the enzyme carboxylase. The reactivation of vitamin K epoxide is the warfarin-sensitive step (warfarin). The R on the vitamin K molecule represents a 20-carbon phytyl side chain in vitamin K_1 and a 30- to 65-carbon polyprenyl side chain in vitamin K_2.

Toxicity

Warfarin crosses the placenta readily and can cause a hemorrhagic disorder in the fetus. Furthermore, fetal proteins with γ-carboxyglutamate residues found in bone and blood may be affected by warfarin; the drug can cause a serious birth defect characterized by abnormal bone formation. Thus, warfarin should never be administered during pregnancy. Cutaneous necrosis with reduced activity of protein C sometimes occurs during the first weeks of therapy. Rarely, the same process causes frank infarction of the breast, fatty tissues, intestine, and extremities. The pathologic lesion associated with the hemorrhagic infarction is venous thrombosis, suggesting that it is caused by warfarin-induced depression of protein C synthesis.

Administration & Dosage

Treatment with warfarin should be initiated with standard doses of 5–10 mg rather than the large loading doses formerly used. The initial adjustment of the prothrombin time takes about 1 week, which usually results in a maintenance dose of 5–7 mg/d. The **prothrombin time (PT)** should be increased to a level representing a reduction of prothrombin activity to 25% of normal and maintained there for long-term therapy. When the activity is less than 20%, the warfarin dosage should be reduced or omitted until the activity rises above 20%.

The therapeutic range for oral anticoagulant therapy is defined in terms of an international normalized ratio (INR). The INR is the prothrombin time ratio (patient prothrombin time/mean of normal prothrombin time for lab)^{ISI}, where the ISI exponent refers to the International Sensitivity Index, and is dependent on the specific reagents and instruments used for the determination. The ISI serves to relate measured prothrombin times to a World Health Organization reference standard thromboplastin; thus the prothrombin times performed on different properly calibrated instruments with a variety of thromboplastin reagents should give the same INR results for a given sample. For most reagent and instrument combinations in current use, the ISI is close to 1, making the INR roughly the ratio of the patient prothrombin time to the mean normal prothrombin time. The recommended INR for prophylaxis and treatment of thrombotic disease is 2–3. Patients with some types of artificial heart valves (eg, tilting disk) or other medical conditions increasing thrombotic risk have a recommended range of 2.5–3.5.

Occasionally patients exhibit warfarin resistance, defined as progression or recurrence of a thrombotic event while in the therapeutic range. These individuals may have their INR target raised (which is accompanied by an increase in bleeding risk) or be changed to an alternative form of anticoagulation (eg, daily injections of LMWH). Warfarin resistance is most commonly seen in patients with advanced cancers, typically of gastrointestinal origin (Trousseau's syndrome). A recent study has demonstrated the superiority of LMWH over warfarin in preventing recurrent venous thromboembolism in patients with cancer.

Drug Interactions

The oral anticoagulants often interact with other drugs and with disease states. These interactions can be broadly divided into pharmacokinetic and pharmacodynamic effects (Table 34–2). Pharmacokinetic mechanisms for drug interaction with oral anticoagulants are mainly enzyme induction, enzyme inhibition, and reduced plasma protein binding. Pharmacodynamic mechanisms for interactions with warfarin are synergism (impaired hemostasis, reduced clotting factor synthesis, as in hepatic disease), competitive antagonism (vitamin K), and an altered physiologic control loop for vitamin K (hereditary resistance to oral anticoagulants).

The most serious interactions with warfarin are those that increase the anticoagulant effect and the risk of bleeding. The most dangerous of these interactions are the pharmacokinetic interactions with the mostly obsolete pyrazolones phenylbutazone and sulfinpyrazone. These drugs not only augment the hypoprothrombinemia but also inhibit platelet function and may induce peptic ulcer disease (see Chapter 36). The mechanisms for their hypoprothrombinemic interaction are a stereoselective inhibition of oxidative metabolic transformation of S-warfarin (the more potent isomer) and displacement of albumin-bound warfarin, increasing the free fraction. For this and other reasons, neither phenylbutazone nor sulfinpyrazone is in common use in the USA. Metronidazole, fluconazole, and trimethoprim-sulfamethoxazole also stereoselectively inhibit the

TABLE 34–2 Pharmacokinetic and pharmacodynamic drug and body interactions with oral anticoagulants.

Increased Prothrombin Time		Decreased Prothrombin Time	
Pharmacokinetic	*Pharmacodynamic*	*Pharmacokinetic*	*Pharmacodynamic*
Amiodarone	**Drugs**	Barbiturates	**Drugs**
Cimetidine	Aspirin (high doses)	Cholestyramine	Diuretics
Disulfiram	Cephalosporins, third-generation	Rifampin	Vitamin K
Metronidazole[1]	Heparin		**Body factors**
Fluconazole[1]	**Body factors**		Hereditary resistance
Phenylbutazone[1]	Hepatic disease		Hypothyroidism
Sulfinpyrazone[1]	Hyperthyroidism		
Trimethoprim-sulfamethoxazole			

[1]Stereoselectively inhibits the oxidative metabolism of the *S*-warfarin enantiomorph of racemic warfarin.

metabolic transformation of *S*-warfarin, whereas amiodarone, disulfiram, and cimetidine inhibit metabolism of both enantiomorphs of warfarin. Aspirin, hepatic disease, and hyperthyroidism augment warfarin's effects—aspirin by its effect on platelet function and the latter two by increasing the turnover rate of clotting factors. The third-generation cephalosporins eliminate the bacteria in the intestinal tract that produce vitamin K and, like warfarin, also directly inhibit vitamin K epoxide reductase.

Barbiturates and rifampin cause a marked *decrease* of the anticoagulant effect by induction of the hepatic enzymes that transform racemic warfarin. Cholestyramine binds warfarin in the intestine and reduces its absorption and bioavailability.

Pharmacodynamic reductions of anticoagulant effect occur with vitamin K (increased synthesis of clotting factors), the diuretics chlorthalidone and spironolactone (clotting factor concentration), hereditary resistance (mutation of vitamin K reactivation cycle molecules), and hypothyroidism (decreased turnover rate of clotting factors).

Drugs with *no* significant effect on anticoagulant therapy include ethanol, phenothiazines, benzodiazepines, acetaminophen, opioids, indomethacin, and most antibiotics.

Reversal of Warfarin Action

Excessive anticoagulant effect and bleeding from warfarin can be reversed by stopping the drug and administering oral or parenteral vitamin K_1 (phytonadione), fresh-frozen plasma, prothrombin complex concentrates such as Bebulin and Proplex T, and recombinant factor VIIa (rFVIIa). The disappearance of excessive effect is not correlated with plasma warfarin concentrations but rather with re-establishment of normal activity of the clotting factors. A modest excess of anticoagulant effect without bleeding may require no more than cessation of the drug. The warfarin effect can be rapidly reversed in the setting of severe bleeding with the administration of prothrombin complex or rFVIIa coupled with intravenous vitamin K. It is important to note that due to the long half-life of warfarin, a single dose of vitamin K or rFVIIa may not be sufficient.

■ BASIC PHARMACOLOGY OF THE FIBRINOLYTIC DRUGS

Fibrinolytic drugs rapidly lyse thrombi by catalyzing the formation of the serine protease **plasmin** from its precursor zymogen, plasminogen (Figure 34–3). These drugs create a generalized lytic state when administered intravenously. Thus, both protective hemostatic thrombi and target thromboemboli are broken down. The Box: Thrombolytic Drugs for Acute Myocardial Infarction describes the use of these drugs in one major application.

Pharmacology

Streptokinase is a protein (but not an enzyme in itself) synthesized by streptococci that combines with the proactivator plasminogen. This enzymatic complex catalyzes the conversion of inactive plasminogen to active plasmin. **Urokinase** is a human enzyme synthesized by the kidney that directly converts plasminogen to active plasmin. Plasmin itself cannot be used because naturally occurring inhibitors in plasma prevent its effects. However, the absence of inhibitors for urokinase and the streptokinase-proactivator complex permits their use clinically. Plasmin formed inside a thrombus by these activators is protected from plasma antiplasmins, which allows it to lyse the thrombus from within.

Thrombolytic Drugs for Acute Myocardial Infarction

The paradigm shift in 1980 on the causation of acute myocardial infarction to acute coronary occlusion by a thrombus created the rationale for thrombolytic therapy of this common lethal disease. At that time—and for the first time—intravenous thrombolytic therapy for acute myocardial infarction in the European Cooperative Study Group trial was found to reduce mortality significantly. Later studies, with thousands of patients in each trial, provided enough statistical power for the 20% reduction in mortality to be considered statistically significant. Although the standard of care in areas with adequate facilities and experience in percutaneous coronary intervention (PCI) now favors catheterization and placement of a stent, thrombolytic therapy is still very important where PCI is not readily available.

The proper selection of patients for thrombolytic therapy is critical. The diagnosis of acute myocardial infarction is made clinically and is confirmed by electrocardiography. Patients with ST-segment elevation and bundle branch block on electrocardiography have the best outcomes. All trials to date show the greatest benefit for thrombolytic therapy when it is given early, within 6 hours after symptomatic onset of acute myocardial infarction.

Thrombolytic drugs reduce the mortality of acute myocardial infarction. The early and appropriate use of any thrombolytic drug probably transcends possible advantages of a particular drug. Adjunctive drugs such as aspirin, heparin, β blockers, and angiotensin-converting enzyme (ACE) inhibitors reduce mortality even further. The principles of management are outlined in Antman, et al, 2008 (see References).

Anistreplase (anisoylated plasminogen streptokinase activator complex; APSAC) consists of a complex of purified human plasminogen and bacterial streptokinase that has been acylated to protect the enzyme's active site. When administered, the acyl group spontaneously hydrolyzes, freeing the activated streptokinase-proactivator complex. This product (now discontinued in the USA) allows for rapid intravenous injection, greater clot selectivity (ie, more activity on plasminogen associated with clots than on free plasminogen in the blood), and more thrombolytic activity.

Plasminogen can also be activated endogenously by **tissue plasminogen activators (t-PAs).** These activators preferentially activate plasminogen that is bound to fibrin, which (in theory) confines fibrinolysis to the formed thrombus and avoids systemic activation. Human t-PA is manufactured as **alteplase** by means of recombinant DNA technology. **Reteplase** is another recombinant human t-PA from which several amino acid sequences have been deleted. Reteplase is less expensive to produce than t-PA. Because it lacks the major fibrin-binding domain, reteplase is less fibrin-specific than t-PA. **Tenecteplase** is a mutant form of t-PA that has a longer half-life, and it can be given as an intravenous bolus. Tenecteplase is slightly more fibrin-specific than t-PA.

Indications & Dosage

Administration of fibrinolytic drugs by the intravenous route is indicated in cases of **pulmonary embolism with hemodynamic instability,** severe **deep venous thrombosis** such as the superior vena caval syndrome, and **ascending thrombophlebitis** of the iliofemoral vein with severe lower extremity edema. These drugs are also given intra-arterially, especially for peripheral vascular disease.

Thrombolytic therapy in the management of **acute myocardial infarction** requires careful patient selection, the use of a specific thrombolytic agent, and the benefit of adjuvant therapy. Streptokinase is administered by intravenous infusion of a loading dose of 250,000 units, followed by 100,000 units/h for 24–72 hours. Patients with antistreptococcal antibodies can develop fever, allergic reactions, and therapeutic resistance. Urokinase requires a loading dose of 300,000 units given over 10 minutes and a maintenance dose of 300,000 units/h for 12 hours. Alteplase (t-PA) is given by intravenous infusion of 60 mg over the first hour and then 40 mg at a rate of 20 mg/h. Reteplase is given as two intravenous bolus injections of 10 units each, separated by 30 minutes. Tenecteplase is given as a single intravenous bolus of 0.5 mg/kg. Anistreplase (where available) is given as a single intravenous injection of 30 units over 3–5 minutes. A single course of fibrinolytic drugs is expensive: hundreds of dollars for streptokinase and thousands for urokinase and t-PA.

Recombinant t-PA has also been approved for use in acute ischemic stroke within 3 hours of symptom onset. In patients without hemorrhagic infarct or other contraindications, this therapy has been demonstrated to provide better outcomes in several randomized clinical trials. The recommended dose is 0.9 mg/kg, not to exceed 90 mg, with 10% given as a bolus and the remainder during a 1 hour infusion. Streptokinase has been associated with increased bleeding risk in acute ischemic stroke when given at a dose of 1.5 million units, and its use is not recommended in this setting.

■ BASIC PHARMACOLOGY OF ANTIPLATELET AGENTS

Platelet function is regulated by three categories of substances. The first group consists of agents generated outside the platelet that interact with platelet membrane receptors, eg, catecholamines, collagen, thrombin, and prostacyclin. The second category contains agents generated within the platelet that interact with membrane receptors, eg, ADP, prostaglandin D_2, prostaglandin E_2, and serotonin. The third group comprises agents generated within the platelet that act within the platelet, eg, prostaglandin endoperoxides and thromboxane A_2, the cyclic nucleotides cAMP and cGMP, and calcium ion. From this list of agents, several targets for platelet inhibitory drugs have been identified (Figure 34–1): inhibition of prostaglandin synthesis (aspirin), inhibition of ADP-induced platelet aggregation (clopidogrel, prasugrel, ticlopidine), and blockade of glycoprotein IIb/IIIa receptors on platelets (abciximab, tirofiban, and eptifibatide). Dipyridamole and cilostazol are additional antiplatelet drugs.

ASPIRIN

The prostaglandin **thromboxane A_2** is an arachidonate product that causes platelets to change shape, release their granules, and aggregate (see Chapter 18). Drugs that antagonize this pathway interfere with platelet aggregation in vitro and prolong the bleeding time in vivo. Aspirin is the prototype of this class of drugs.

As described in Chapter 18, aspirin inhibits the synthesis of thromboxane A_2 by irreversible acetylation of the enzyme cyclooxygenase. Other salicylates and nonsteroidal anti-inflammatory drugs also inhibit cyclooxygenase but have a shorter duration of inhibitory action because they cannot acetylate cyclooxygenase; that is, their action is reversible.

The FDA has approved the use of 325 mg/d aspirin for *primary* prophylaxis of myocardial infarction but urges caution in this use of aspirin by the general population except when prescribed as an adjunct to risk factor management by smoking cessation and lowering of blood cholesterol and blood pressure. Meta-analysis of many published trials of aspirin and other antiplatelet agents confirms the value of this intervention in the *secondary* prevention of vascular events among patients with a history of vascular events.

TICLOPIDINE, CLOPIDOGREL, & PRASUGREL

Ticlopidine, clopidogrel, and prasugrel reduce platelet aggregation by inhibiting the ADP pathway of platelets. These drugs irreversibly block the ADP receptor on platelets. Unlike aspirin, these drugs have no effect on prostaglandin metabolism. Use of ticlopidine, clopidogrel, or prasugrel to prevent thrombosis is now considered standard practice in patients undergoing placement of a coronary stent. As the indications and adverse effects of these drugs are different, they will be considered individually.

Ticlopidine is approved for prevention of stroke in patients with a history of a transient ischemic attack (TIA) or thrombotic stroke, and in combination with aspirin for prevention of coronary stent thrombosis. Adverse effects of ticlopidine include nausea, dyspepsia, and diarrhea in up to 20% of patients, hemorrhage in 5%, and, most seriously, leukopenia in 1%. The leukopenia is detected by regular monitoring of the white blood cell count during the first 3 months of treatment. Development of thrombotic thrombocytopenic purpura has also been associated with the ingestion of ticlopidine. The dosage of ticlopidine is 250 mg twice daily. Because of the significant side effect profile, the use of ticlopidine for stroke prevention should be restricted to those who are intolerant of or have failed aspirin therapy. Doses of ticlopidine less than 500 mg/d may be efficacious with fewer adverse effects.

Clopidogrel is approved for patients with unstable angina or non-ST-elevation acute myocardial infarction (NSTEMI) in combination with aspirin; for patients with ST-elevation myocardial infarction (STEMI); or recent myocardial infarction, stroke, or established peripheral arterial disease. For NSTEMI, the dosage is a 300 mg loading dose followed by 75 mg daily of clopidogrel, with a daily aspirin dose of 75–325 mg. For patients with STEMI, the dose is 75 mg daily of clopidogrel, in association with aspirin as above; and for recent myocardial infarction, stroke, or peripheral vascular disease, the dose is 75 mg/d.

Clopidogrel has fewer adverse effects than ticlopidine and is rarely associated with neutropenia. Thrombotic thrombocytopenic purpura has been reported. Because of its superior side effect profile and dosing requirements, clopidogrel is frequently preferred over ticlopidine. The antithrombotic effects of clopidogrel are dose-dependent; within 5 hours after an oral loading dose of 300 mg, 80% of platelet activity will be inhibited. The maintenance dose of clopidogrel is 75 mg/d, which achieves maximum platelet inhibition. The duration of the antiplatelet effect is 7–10 days. Clopidogrel is a prodrug that requires activation via the cytochrome P450 enzyme isoform CYP2C19. Depending on the single nucleotide polymorphism inheritance pattern in CYP2C19, individuals may be poor metabolizers of clopidogrel, and these patients may be at increased risk of cardiovascular events due to inadequate drug effect. The FDA has recommended CYP2C19 genotyping to identify such patients and advises prescribers to consider alternative therapies in poor metabolizers. However, more recent studies have questioned the impact of CYP2C19 metabolizer status on outcomes. Drugs that impair CYP2C19 function, such as omeprazole, should be used with caution pending clarification of the importance of CYP2C19 status.

Prasugrel, similar to clopidogrel, is approved for patients with acute coronary syndromes. The drug is given as a 60-mg loading dose and then 10 mg/d in combination with aspirin as outlined for clopidogrel. The Trial to assess Improvement in Therapeutic Outcomes by Optimizing Platelet Inhibition with Prasugrel (TRITON-TIMI38) compared prasugrel with clopidogrel in a randomized, double-blind trial with aspirin and other standard therapies managed with percutaneous coronary interventions. This trial showed a reduction in the primary composite cardiovascular endpoint (cardiovascular death, nonfatal stroke or nonfatal myocardial infarction) for prasugrel in comparison with clopidogrel. However, the major and minor bleeding risk was increased with prasugrel. Prasugrel is contraindicated in patients with history of TIA or stroke because of increased bleeding risk. Although cytochrome P450 genotype status is an issue with clopidogrel, it does not have an impact on the use of prasugrel.

Aspirin & Clopidogrel Resistance

The reported incidence of resistance to these drugs varies greatly, from less than 5% to 75%. In part this tremendous variation in incidence reflects the definition of resistance (recurrent thrombosis while on antiplatelet therapy vs in vitro testing), methods by which drug response is measured, and patient compliance. Several methods for testing aspirin and clopidogrel resistance in vitro are now FDA-approved. However, the incidence of drug resistance varies considerably by testing method. These tests may be useful in selected patients to assess compliance or the cause of a recurrent thrombotic event, but their utility in routine clinical decision making outside of clinical trials remains controversial.

BLOCKADE OF PLATELET GLYCOPROTEIN IIB/IIIA RECEPTORS

The glycoprotein IIb/IIIa inhibitors are used in patients with acute coronary syndromes. These drugs target the platelet IIb/IIIa receptor complex (Figure 34–1). The IIb/IIIa complex functions as a receptor mainly for fibrinogen and vitronectin but also for fibronectin and von Willebrand factor. Activation of this receptor complex is the "final common pathway" for platelet aggregation. There are approximately 50,000 copies of this complex on the surface of each platelet. Persons lacking this receptor have a bleeding disorder called Glanzmann's thrombasthenia.

Abciximab, a chimeric monoclonal antibody directed against the IIb/IIIa complex including the vitronectin receptor, was the first agent approved in this class of drugs. It has been approved for use in percutaneous coronary intervention and in acute coronary syndromes. Eptifibatide is an analog of the sequence at the extreme carboxyl terminal of the delta chain of fibrinogen, which mediates the binding of fibrinogen to the receptor. Tirofiban is a smaller molecule with similar properties. Eptifibatide and tirofiban inhibit ligand binding to the IIb/IIIa receptor by their occupancy of the receptor but do not block the vitronectin receptor.

The three agents described above are administered parenterally. Oral formulations of IIb/IIIa antagonists are in various stages of development.

ADDITIONAL ANTIPLATELET-DIRECTED DRUGS

Dipyridamole is a vasodilator that also inhibits platelet function by inhibiting adenosine uptake and cGMP phosphodiesterase activity. Dipyridamole by itself has little or no beneficial effect. Therefore, therapeutic use of this agent is primarily in combination with aspirin to prevent cerebrovascular ischemia. It may also be used in combination with warfarin for primary prophylaxis of thromboemboli in patients with prosthetic heart valves. A combination of dipyridamole complexed with 25 mg of aspirin is now available for secondary prophylaxis of cerebrovascular disease.

Cilostazol is a newer phosphodiesterase inhibitor that promotes vasodilation and inhibition of platelet aggregation. Cilostazol is used primarily to treat intermittent claudication.

■ CLINICAL PHARMACOLOGY OF DRUGS USED TO PREVENT CLOTTING

VENOUS THROMBOSIS

Risk Factors

A. Inherited Disorders

The inherited disorders characterized by a tendency to form thrombi (thrombophilia) derive from either quantitative or qualitative abnormalities of the natural anticoagulant system. Deficiencies (loss of function mutations) in the natural anticoagulants antithrombin, protein C, and protein S account for approximately 15% of selected patients with juvenile or recurrent thrombosis and 5–10% of unselected cases of acute venous thrombosis. Additional causes of thrombophilia include gain of function mutations such as the factor V Leiden mutation and the prothrombin 20210 mutation, elevated clotting factor and cofactor levels, and hyperhomocysteinemia that together account for the greater number of hypercoagulable patients. Although the loss of function mutations is less common, they are associated with the greatest thrombosis risk. Some patients have multiple inherited risk factors or combinations of inherited and acquired risk factors as discussed below. These individuals are at higher risk for recurrent thrombotic events and are often considered candidates for lifelong therapy.

B. Acquired Disease

The increased risk of thromboembolism associated with atrial fibrillation and with the placement of mechanical heart valves has long been recognized. Similarly, prolonged bed rest, high-risk surgical procedures, and the presence of cancer are clearly associated with an increased incidence of deep venous thrombosis and embolism. Antiphospholipid antibody syndrome is another important acquired risk factor. Drugs may function as synergistic risk factors in concert with inherited risk factors. For example, women who have the factor V Leiden mutation and take oral contraceptives have a synergistic increase in risk.

Antithrombotic Management

A. Prevention

Primary prevention of venous thrombosis reduces the incidence of and mortality rate from pulmonary emboli. Heparin and warfarin may be used to prevent venous thrombosis. Subcutaneous administration of low-dose unfractionated heparin, LMWH, or fondaparinux provides effective prophylaxis. Warfarin is also effective but requires laboratory monitoring of the prothrombin time.

B. Treatment of Established Disease

Treatment for established venous thrombosis is initiated with unfractionated or LMWH for the first 5–7 days, with an overlap with warfarin. Once therapeutic effects of warfarin have been established, therapy with warfarin is continued for a minimum of 3–6 months. Patients with recurrent disease or identifiable, non-reversible risk factors may be treated indefinitely. Small thrombi confined to the calf veins may be managed without anticoagulants if there is documentation over time that the thrombus is not extending.

Warfarin readily crosses the placenta. It can cause hemorrhage at any time during pregnancy as well as developmental defects when administered during the first trimester. Therefore, venous thromboembolic disease in pregnant women is generally treated with heparin, best administered by subcutaneous injection.

ARTERIAL THROMBOSIS

Activation of platelets is considered an essential process for arterial thrombosis. Thus, treatment with platelet-inhibiting drugs such as aspirin and clopidogrel or ticlopidine is indicated in patients with TIAs and strokes or unstable angina and acute myocardial infarction. Prasugrel is an alternative to clopidogrel for patients with acute coronary syndromes managed with percutaneous coronary interventions. In angina and infarction, these drugs are often used in conjunction with β blockers, calcium channel blockers, and fibrinolytic drugs.

■ DRUGS USED IN BLEEDING DISORDERS

VITAMIN K

Vitamin K confers biologic activity upon prothrombin and factors VII, IX, and X by participating in their postribosomal modification. Vitamin K is a fat-soluble substance found primarily in leafy green vegetables. The dietary requirement is low, because the vitamin is additionally synthesized by bacteria that colonize the human intestine. Two natural forms exist: vitamins K_1 and K_2. Vitamin K_1 (phytonadione; Figure 34–5) is found in food. Vitamin K_2 (menaquinone) is found in human tissues and is synthesized by intestinal bacteria.

Vitamins K_1 and K_2 require bile salts for absorption from the intestinal tract. Vitamin K_1 is available clinically in oral and parenteral forms. Onset of effect is delayed for 6 hours but the effect is complete by 24 hours when treating depression of prothrombin activity by excess warfarin or vitamin K deficiency. Intravenous administration of vitamin K_1 should be slow, because rapid infusion can produce dyspnea, chest and back pain, and even death. Vitamin K repletion is best achieved with intravenous or oral administration, because its bioavailability after subcutaneous administration is erratic. Vitamin K_1 is currently administered to all newborns to prevent the hemorrhagic disease of vitamin K deficiency, which is especially common in premature infants.

The water-soluble salt of vitamin K₃ (menadione) should never be used in therapeutics. It is particularly ineffective in the treatment of warfarin overdosage. Vitamin K deficiency frequently occurs in hospitalized patients in intensive care units because of poor diet, parenteral nutrition, recent surgery, multiple antibiotic therapy, and uremia. Severe hepatic failure results in diminished protein synthesis and a hemorrhagic diathesis that is unresponsive to vitamin K.

PLASMA FRACTIONS

Sources & Preparations

Deficiencies in plasma coagulation factors can cause bleeding (Table 34–3). Spontaneous bleeding occurs when factor activity is less than 5–10% of normal. Factor VIII deficiency (**classic hemophilia,** or **hemophilia A**) and factor IX deficiency (**Christmas disease,** or **hemophilia B**) account for most of the heritable coagulation defects. Concentrated plasma fractions are available for the treatment of these deficiencies. Administration of plasma-derived, heat- or detergent-treated factor concentrates and recombinant factor concentrates are the standard treatments for bleeding associated with hemophilia. Lyophilized factor VIII concentrates are prepared from large pools of plasma. Transmission of viral diseases such as hepatitis B and C and HIV is reduced or eliminated by pasteurization and by extraction of plasma with solvents and detergents. However, this treatment does not remove other potential causes of transmissible diseases such as prions. For this reason, recombinant clotting factor preparations are recommended whenever possible for factor replacement. The best use of these therapeutic materials requires diagnostic specificity of the deficient factor and quantitation of its activity in plasma. Intermediate purity factor VIII concentrates (as opposed to recombinant or high purity concentrates) contain significant amounts of von Willebrand factor. Humate-P is a factor VIII concentrate that is approved by the FDA for the treatment of bleeding associated with von Willebrand disease.

Clinical Uses

An uncomplicated hemorrhage into a joint should be treated with sufficient factor VIII or factor IX replacement to maintain a level of at least 30–50% of the normal concentration for 24 hours. Soft tissue hematomas require a minimum of 100% activity for 7 days. Hematuria requires at least 10% activity for 3 days. Surgery and

TABLE 34–3 Therapeutic products for the treatment of coagulation disorders.

Factor	Deficiency State	Hemostatic Levels	Half-Life of Infused Factor	Replacement Source
I	Hypofibrinogenemia	1 g/dL	4 days	Cryoprecipitate FFP
II	Prothrombin deficiency	30–40%	3 days	Prothrombin complex concentrates (intermediate purity factor IX concentrates)
V	Factor V deficiency	20%	1 day	FFP
VII	Factor VII deficiency	30%	4–6 hours	FFP Prothrombin complex concentrates (intermediate purity factor IX concentrates) Recombinant factor VIIa
VIII	Hemophilia A	30–50% 100% for major bleeding or trauma	12 hours	Recombinant factor VIII products Plasma-derived high purity concentrates Cryoprecipitate[1] Some patients with mild deficiency will respond to DDAVP
IX	Hemophilia B Christmas disease	30–50% 100% for major bleeding or trauma	24 hours	Recombinant factor IX products Plasma-derived high purity concentrates
X	Stuart-Prower defect	25%	36 hours	FFP Prothrombin complex concentrates
XI	Hemophilia C	30–50%	3 days	FFP
XII	Hageman defect	Not required		Treatment not necessary
von Willebrand	von Willebrand disease	30%	Approximately 10 hours	Intermediate purity factor VIII concentrates that contain von Willebrand factor Some patients respond to DDAVP Cryoprecipitate[1]
XIII	Factor XIII deficiency	5%	6 days	FFP Cryoprecipitate

FFP, fresh frozen plasma; DDAVP, 1-deamino-8-D-arginine vasopressin.

Antithrombin and activated protein C concentrates are available for the appropriate indications that include thrombosis in the setting of antithrombin deficiency and sepsis respectively.

[1]Cryoprecipitate should be used to treat bleeding in the setting of factor VIII deficiency and von Willebrand disease only in an emergency in which pathogen-inactivated products are not available.

major trauma require a minimum of 100% activity for 10 days. The initial loading dose for factor VIII is 50 units/kg of body weight to achieve 100% activity of factor VIII from a baseline of 1% or less, assuming a normal hemoglobin. Each unit of factor VIII per kilogram of body weight raises its activity in plasma 2%. Replacement should be administered every 12 hours. Factor IX therapy requires twice the dose of factor VIII, but with an administration of about every 24 hours because of its longer half-life. Recombinant factor IX has only 80% recovery compared with plasma-derived factor IX products. Therefore, dosing with recombinant factor IX requires 120% of the dose used with the plasma-derived product.

Desmopressin acetate increases the factor VIII activity of patients with mild hemophilia A or von Willebrand disease. It can be used in preparation for minor surgery such as tooth extraction without any requirement for infusion of clotting factors if the patient has a documented adequate response. High-dose intranasal desmopressin (see Chapter 17) is available and has been shown to be efficacious and well tolerated by patients.

Freeze-dried concentrates of plasma containing prothrombin, factors IX and X, and varied amounts of factor VII (Proplex, etc) are commercially available for treating deficiencies of these factors (Table 34–3). Each unit of factor IX per kilogram of body weight raises its activity in plasma 1.5%. Heparin is often added to inhibit coagulation factors activated by the manufacturing process. However, addition of heparin does not eliminate all thromboembolic risk.

Some preparations of factor IX concentrate contain *activated* clotting factors, which has led to their use in treating patients with inhibitors or antibodies to factor VIII or factor IX. Two products are available expressly for this purpose: **Autoplex** (with factor VIII correctional activity) and **FEIBA** (**F**actor **E**ight **I**nhibitor **B**ypassing **A**ctivity). These products are not uniformly successful in arresting hemorrhage, and the factor IX inhibitor titers often rise after treatment with them. Acquired inhibitors of coagulation factors may also be treated with porcine factor VIII (for factor VIII inhibitors) and recombinant activated factor VII. Recombinant activated factor VII (**NovoSeven**) is being increasingly used to treat coagulopathy associated with liver disease and major blood loss in trauma and surgery. These recombinant and plasma-derived factor concentrates are very expensive, and the indications for them are very precise. Therefore, close consultation with a hematologist knowledgeable in this area is essential.

Cryoprecipitate is a plasma protein fraction obtainable from whole blood. It is used to treat deficiencies or qualitative abnormalities of fibrinogen, such as that which occurs with disseminated intravascular coagulation and liver disease. A single unit of cryoprecipitate contains 300 mg of fibrinogen.

Cryoprecipitate may also be used for patients with factor VIII deficiency and von Willebrand disease if desmopressin is not indicated and a pathogen-inactivated, recombinant, or plasma-derived product is not available. The concentration of factor VIII and von Willebrand factor in cryoprecipitate is not as great as that found in the concentrated plasma fractions. Moreover, cryoprecipitate is not treated in any manner to decrease the risk of viral exposure. For infusion, the frozen cryoprecipitate unit is thawed and dissolved in a small volume of sterile citrate-saline solution and pooled with other units. Rh-negative women with potential for childbearing should receive only Rh-negative cryoprecipitate because of possible contamination of the product with Rh-positive blood cells.

RECOMBINANT FACTOR VIIA

Recombinant factor VIIa is approved for treatment of inherited or acquired hemophilia A or B with inhibitors, treatment of bleeding associated with invasive procedures in congenital or acquired hemophilia, or factor VII deficiency. In the EU, the drug is also approved for treatment of Glanzmann's thrombasthenia.

Factor VIIa initiates activation of the clotting pathway by activating factor IX and factor X in association with tissue factor (see Figure 34–2). The drug is given by bolus injection. For hemophilia A or B with inhibitors and bleeding, the dose is 90 mg/kg every 2 hours until hemostasis is achieved, and then continued at 3–6 hour intervals until stable. For congenital factor VII deficiency, the recommended dosage is 15–30 mg/kg every 4–6 hours until hemostasis is achieved.

Factor VIIa has been widely used for off-label indications, including bleeding with trauma, surgery, intracerebral hemorrhage, and warfarin toxicity. A major concern of off-label use has been the possibility that thrombotic events may be increased. A recent study examined rates of thromboembolic events in 35 placebo-controlled trials where factor VIIa was administered for nonapproved indications. This study found an increase in arterial, but not venous, thrombotic events, particularly among elderly individuals.

FIBRINOLYTIC INHIBITORS: AMINOCAPROIC ACID

Aminocaproic acid (EACA), which is chemically similar to the amino acid lysine, is a synthetic inhibitor of fibrinolysis. It competitively inhibits plasminogen activation (Figure 34–3). It is rapidly absorbed orally and is cleared from the body by the kidney. The usual oral dosage of EACA is 6 g four times a day. When the drug is administered intravenously, a 5 g loading dose should be infused over 30 minutes to avoid hypotension. **Tranexamic acid** is an analog of aminocaproic acid and has the same properties. It is administered orally with a 15 mg/kg loading dose followed by 30 mg/kg every 6 hours.

Clinical uses of EACA are as adjunctive therapy in hemophilia, as therapy for bleeding from fibrinolytic therapy, and as prophylaxis for rebleeding from intracranial aneurysms. Treatment success has also been reported in patients with postsurgical gastrointestinal bleeding and postprostatectomy bleeding and bladder hemorrhage secondary to radiation- and drug-induced cystitis. Adverse effects of the drug include intravascular thrombosis from inhibition of plasminogen activator, hypotension, myopathy, abdominal discomfort, diarrhea, and nasal stuffiness. The drug should not be used in patients with disseminated intravascular coagulation or genitourinary bleeding of the upper tract, eg, kidney and ureters, because of the potential for excessive clotting.

SERINE PROTEASE INHIBITORS: APROTININ

Aprotinin is a serine protease inhibitor (serpin) that inhibits fibrinolysis by free plasmin and may have other antihemorrhagic effects as well. It also inhibits the plasmin-streptokinase complex in patients who have received that thrombolytic agent. Aprotinin was shown to reduce bleeding—by as much as 50%—from many types of surgery, especially that involving extracorporeal circulation for open heart procedures and liver transplantation. However, clinical trials and internal data from the manufacturer suggested that use of the drug was associated with an increased risk of renal failure, heart attack, and stroke. A prospective trial was initiated in Canada but halted early because of concerns that use of the drug was associated with increased mortality. The drug was removed from the market in 2007.

PREPARATIONS AVAILABLE

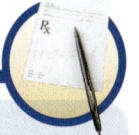

Abciximab (ReoPro)
Parenteral: 2 mg/mL for IV injection

Alteplase recombinant [t-PA] (Activase*)
Parenteral: 50, 100 mg lyophilized powder to reconstitute for IV injection; 2 mg for catheter clots

Aminocaproic acid (generic, Amicar)
Oral: 500 mg tablets; 250 mg/mL syrup
Parenteral: 250 mg/mL for IV injection

Anisindione (Miradon)
Oral: 50 mg tablets

Antihemophilic factor [factor VIII, AHF] (Alphanate, Bioclate,* Helixate,* Hemofil M, Koate-HP, Kogenate,* Monoclate, Recombinate,* others)
Parenteral: in vials

Anti-inhibitor coagulant complex (Autoplex T, Feiba VH Immuno)
Parenteral: in vials

Antithrombin III (Thrombate III)
Parenteral: 500, 1000 IU powder to reconstitute for IV injection

Argatroban
Parenteral: 100 mg/mL in 2.5 mL vials

Bivalirudin (Angiomax)
Parenteral: 250 mg per vial

Cilostazol (generic, Pletal)
Oral: 50, 100 mg tablets

Clopidogrel (generic, Plavix)
Oral: 75, 300 mg tablets

Coagulation factor VIIa recombinant (Novo-Seven*)
Parenteral: 1.2, 4.8 mg powder/vial for IV injection

Dabigatran (Pradaxa)
Oral: 75, 150 mg capsules

Dalteparin (Fragmin)
Parenteral: 2500, 5000, 10,000, 15,000, 18,000 anti-factor Xa units/0.2 mL for SC injection only

Danaparoid (Orgaran)
Parenteral: 750 anti-Xa units/vial

Desirudin (Iprivask)
Parenteral: 15 mg for injection

Dipyridamole (generic, Persantine)
Oral: 25, 50, 75 mg tablets
Oral combination product (Aggrenox): 200 mg extended-release dipyridamole plus 25 mg extended-release dipyridamole plus 25 mg aspirin

Enoxaparin (low-molecular-weight heparin, Lovenox)
Parenteral: pre-filled, multiple-dose syringes for SC injection only

Eptifibatide (Integrilin)
Parenteral: 0.75, 2 mg/mL for IV infusion

Factor VIIa: see Coagulation factor VIIa recombinant

Factor VIII: see Antihemophilic factor

Factor IX complex, human (AlphaNine SD, Bebulin VH, BeneFix*, Konyne 80, Mononine, Profilnine SD, Proplex T, Proplex SX-T)
Parenteral: in vials

Fondaparinux (Arixtra)
Parenteral: 2.5, 5, 7.5, 10 mg in single-dose pre-filled syringes

Heparin sodium (generic, Liquaemin)
Parenteral: 1000, 2000, 2500, 5000, 10,000, 20,000, 40,000 units/mL for injection

Lepirudin (Refludan*)
Parenteral: 50 mg powder for IV injection

Prasugrel (Effient)
Oral: 5, 10 mg tablets

Protamine (generic)
Parenteral: 10 mg/mL for injection

Reteplase (Retavase*)
Parenteral: 10.4 IU powder for injection

Rivaroxaban (Xarelto)
Oral: 10 mg tablets

Streptokinase (Streptase)
Parenteral: 250,000, 750,000, 1,500,000 IU per vial powders to reconstitute for injection

Tenecteplase (TNKase*)
Parenteral: 50 mg powder for injection

Ticlopidine (Ticlid)
Oral: 250 mg tablets

Tinzaparin (Innohep)
Parenteral: 20,000 anti-Xa units/mL for subcutaneous injection only

Tirofiban (Aggrastat)
Parenteral: 50, 250 mcg/mL for IV infusion

Tranexamic acid (Cyklokapron, Lysteda)
Oral: 500 mg tablets
Parenteral: 100 mg/mL for IV infusion

Urokinase (Abbokinase)
Parenteral: 250,000 IU per vial for systemic use

Vitamin K (generic, various)
Oral: 5 mg tablets
Parenteral: 2, 10 mg/mL solution for injection

Warfarin (generic, Coumadin)
Oral: 1, 2, 2.5, 3, 4, 5, 6, 7.5, 10 mg tablets

*Recombinant product.

REFERENCES

Blood Coagulation & Bleeding Disorders

Dahlback B: Advances in understanding pathogenic mechanisms of thrombophilic disorders. Blood 2008;112:19.

Greaves M, Watson HG: Approach to the diagnosis and management of mild bleeding disorders. J Thromb Haemost 2007;5(Suppl 1):167.

Mannucci PM, Levi M: Prevention and treatment of major blood loss. N Engl J Med 2007;356:2301.

Drugs Used in Thrombotic Disorders

Antman E et al: 2007 Focused update of the ACC/AHA guidelines for the management of patients with ST-elevation myocardial infarction. Circulation 2008;117:296.

Crowther MA, Warkentin TE: Bleeding risk and the management of bleeding complications in patients undergoing anticoagulant therapy: Focus on new anticoagulant agents. Blood 2008;111:4871.

Hirsh J et al (editors): Antithrombotic and Thrombolytic Therapy: American College of Chest Physicians Evidence-Based Clinical Practice Guidelines (8th Edition). Chest 2008;133(Suppl):110S.

Hyek EM: Therapeutic potential of oral factor Xa inhibitors. N Engl J Med 2010;363:2559.

Kishimoto TK et al: Contaminated heparin associated with adverse clinical events and activation of the contact system. N Engl J Med 2008;358:2457.

Lohrmann J, Becker RC: New anticoagulants—the path from discovery to clinical practice. N Engl J Med 2008;358:2827.

van Ryn J et al: Dabigatran etexilate—a novel, reversible, oral direct thrombin inhibitor: interpretation of coagulation assays and reversal of anticoagulant activity. Thromb Haemost 2010;103:1116.

CASE STUDY ANSWER

This patient has pulmonary embolism secondary to a deep venous thrombosis (DVT). Immediate therapy with intravenous heparin is indicated. If hemodynamic instability or pulmonary function deteriorates, suggesting further embolization to the lung, percutaneous placement of an inferior vena cava filter may be considered. Long-term therapy with warfarin is traditional standard of care, using a target of 2–3 international normalized ratio. This patient should be advised to use other methods of contraception.

Agents Used in Dyslipidemia

Mary J. Malloy, MD, & John P. Kane, MD, PhD

CASE STUDY

RL, a 42-year-old man with moderately severe coronary artery disease, has a body mass index (BMI) of 29, increased abdominal girth, and hypertension that is well controlled. In addition to medicine for hypertension, he is taking 40 mg atorvastatin. Current lipid panel (mg/dL): cholesterol 184, triglycerides 200, low-density lipoprotein cholesterol (LDL-C) 110, HDL-C 34, non–HDL-C 150. Lipoprotein(a) (Lp[a]) is twice normal. Fasting glucose is 102 mg/dL, and fasting insulin is 38 μU/mL.

Liver enzymes are normal. Creatine kinase level is mildly elevated. The patient is referred for help with management of his dyslipidemia. You advise dietary measures, exercise, and weight loss. Which additional drugs would help him achieve his lipoprotein treatment goals: LDL-C 60–70 mg/dL; triglycerides < 120 mg/dL; HDL-C > 45 mg/dL; and reduced level of Lp(a)? Would this patient also benefit from a drug to manage insulin resistance? If so, which drug?

Plasma lipids are transported in complexes called **lipoproteins.** Metabolic disorders that involve elevations in any lipoprotein species are termed **hyperlipoproteinemias** or **hyperlipidemias.** **Hyperlipemia** denotes increased levels of triglycerides.

The two major clinical sequelae of hyperlipidemias are acute pancreatitis and atherosclerosis. The former occurs in patients with marked hyperlipemia. Control of triglycerides can prevent recurrent attacks of this life-threatening disease.

Atherosclerosis is the leading cause of death for both genders in the USA and other Western countries. Lipoproteins that contain **apolipoprotein (apo) B-100** convey lipids into the artery wall. These are **low-density (LDL), intermediate-density (IDL), very-low-density (VLDL),** and **lipoprotein(a) (Lp[a]).** Remnant lipoproteins formed during the catabolism of chylomicrons that contain the B-48 protein (apo B-48) can also enter the artery wall, contributing to atherosclerosis.

Cellular components in atherosclerotic plaques include foam cells, which are transformed macrophages, and smooth muscle cells filled with **cholesteryl esters.** These cellular alterations result from endocytosis of modified lipoproteins via at least four species of **scavenger receptors.** Chemical modification of lipoproteins by free radicals creates ligands for these receptors. The atheroma

grows with the accumulation of foam cells, collagen, fibrin, and frequently calcium. Whereas such lesions can slowly occlude coronary vessels, clinical symptoms are more frequently precipitated by rupture of unstable atheromatous plaques, leading to activation of platelets and formation of occlusive thrombi.

Although treatment of hyperlipidemia can cause slow physical regression of plaques, the well-documented reduction in acute coronary events that follows vigorous lipid-lowering treatment is attributable chiefly to mitigation of the inflammatory activity of macrophages and is evident within 2–3 months after starting therapy.

High-density lipoproteins (HDL) exert several *anti*atherogenic effects. They participate in retrieval of cholesterol from the artery wall and inhibit the oxidation of atherogenic lipoproteins. Low levels of HDL (hypoalphalipoproteinemia) are an independent risk factor for atherosclerotic disease and thus are a target for intervention.

Cigarette smoking is a major risk factor for coronary disease. It is associated with reduced levels of HDL, impairment of cholesterol retrieval, cytotoxic effects on the endothelium, increased oxidation of lipoproteins, and stimulation of thrombogenesis. Diabetes, also a major risk factor, is another source of oxidative stress.

Normal coronary arteries can dilate in response to ischemia, increasing delivery of oxygen to the myocardium. This process is mediated by nitric oxide, acting on smooth muscle cells of the arterial media. This function is impaired by atherogenic lipoproteins, thus aggravating ischemia. Reducing levels of atherogenic lipoproteins and inhibiting their oxidation restores endothelial function.

Because atherogenesis is multifactorial, therapy should be directed toward all modifiable risk factors. Atherogenesis is a dynamic process. Quantitative angiographic trials have demonstrated net regression of plaques during aggressive lipid-lowering therapy. Primary and secondary prevention trials have shown significant reduction in mortality from new coronary events and in all-cause mortality.

■ PATHOPHYSIOLOGY OF HYPERLIPOPROTEINEMIA

NORMAL LIPOPROTEIN METABOLISM

Structure

Lipoproteins have hydrophobic core regions containing cholesteryl esters and triglycerides surrounded by unesterified cholesterol, phospholipids, and apoproteins. Certain lipoproteins contain very high-molecular-weight B proteins that exist in two forms: **B-48,** formed in the intestine and found in chylomicrons and their remnants; and **B-100,** synthesized in liver and found in **VLDL, VLDL remnants (IDL), LDL** (formed from VLDL), and **Lp(a) lipoproteins.** HDL consist of at least 20 discrete molecular species. All species contain apolipoprotein A-I (apo A-I). Fifty-three other proteins are known to be distributed variously among the HDL species.

Synthesis & Catabolism

A. Chylomicrons

Chylomicrons are formed in the intestine and carry **triglycerides** of dietary origin, **unesterified cholesterol,** and **cholesteryl esters.** They transit the thoracic duct to the bloodstream.

ACRONYMS

Apo	Apolipoprotein
CETP	Cholesteryl ester transfer protein
CK	Creatine kinase
HDL	High-density lipoproteins
HMG-CoA	3-Hydroxy-3-methylglutaryl-coenzyme A
IDL	Intermediate-density lipoproteins
LCAT	Lecithin:cholesterol acyltransferase
LDL	Low-density lipoproteins
Lp(a)	Lipoprotein(a)
LPL	Lipoprotein lipase
PPAR	Peroxisome proliferator-activated receptor
VLDL	Very-low-density lipoproteins

Triglycerides are removed in extrahepatic tissues through a pathway shared with VLDL that involves hydrolysis by the **lipoprotein lipase (LPL)** system. Decrease in particle diameter occurs as triglycerides are depleted. Surface lipids and small apoproteins are transferred to HDL. The resultant chylomicron remnants are taken up by receptor-mediated endocytosis into hepatocytes.

B. Very-Low-Density Lipoproteins

VLDL are secreted by liver and export triglycerides to peripheral tissues (Figure 35–1). VLDL triglycerides are hydrolyzed by LPL, yielding free fatty acids for storage in adipose tissue and for oxidation in tissues such as cardiac and skeletal muscle. Depletion of triglycerides produces remnants (IDL), some of which undergo endocytosis directly by liver. The remainder is converted to LDL by further removal of triglycerides mediated by hepatic lipase. This process explains the "beta shift" phenomenon, the increase of LDL (beta-lipoprotein) in serum as hypertriglyceridemia subsides. Increased levels of LDL can also result from increased secretion of VLDL and from decreased LDL catabolism.

C. Low-Density Lipoproteins

LDL is catabolized chiefly in hepatocytes and other cells by receptor-mediated endocytosis. Cholesteryl esters from LDL are hydrolyzed, yielding free cholesterol for the synthesis of cell membranes. Cells also obtain cholesterol by synthesis via a pathway involving the formation of mevalonic acid by HMG-CoA reductase. Production of this enzyme and of LDL receptors is transcriptionally regulated by the content of cholesterol in the cell. Normally, about 70% of LDL is removed from plasma by hepatocytes. Even more cholesterol is delivered to the liver via IDL and chylomicrons. Unlike other cells, hepatocytes can eliminate cholesterol by secretion in bile and by conversion to bile acids.

D. Lp(a) Lipoprotein

Lp(a) lipoprotein is formed from LDL and the (a) protein, linked by a disulfide bridge. The (a) protein is highly homologous with plasminogen but is not activated by tissue plasminogen activator. It occurs in a number of isoforms of different molecular weights. Levels of Lp(a) vary from nil to over 500 mg/dL and are determined chiefly by genetic factors. Lp(a) can be found in atherosclerotic plaques and may also contribute to coronary disease by inhibiting thrombolysis. Levels are elevated in certain inflammatory states. The risk of coronary disease is strongly related to the level of Lp(a). A common variant (I4399M) in the coding region is associated with elevated levels.

E. High-Density Lipoproteins

The apoproteins of HDL are secreted by the liver and intestine. Much of the lipid comes from the surface monolayers of chylomicrons and VLDL during lipolysis. HDL also acquires cholesterol from peripheral tissues, protecting the cholesterol homeostasis of cells. Free cholesterol is transported from the cell membrane by a

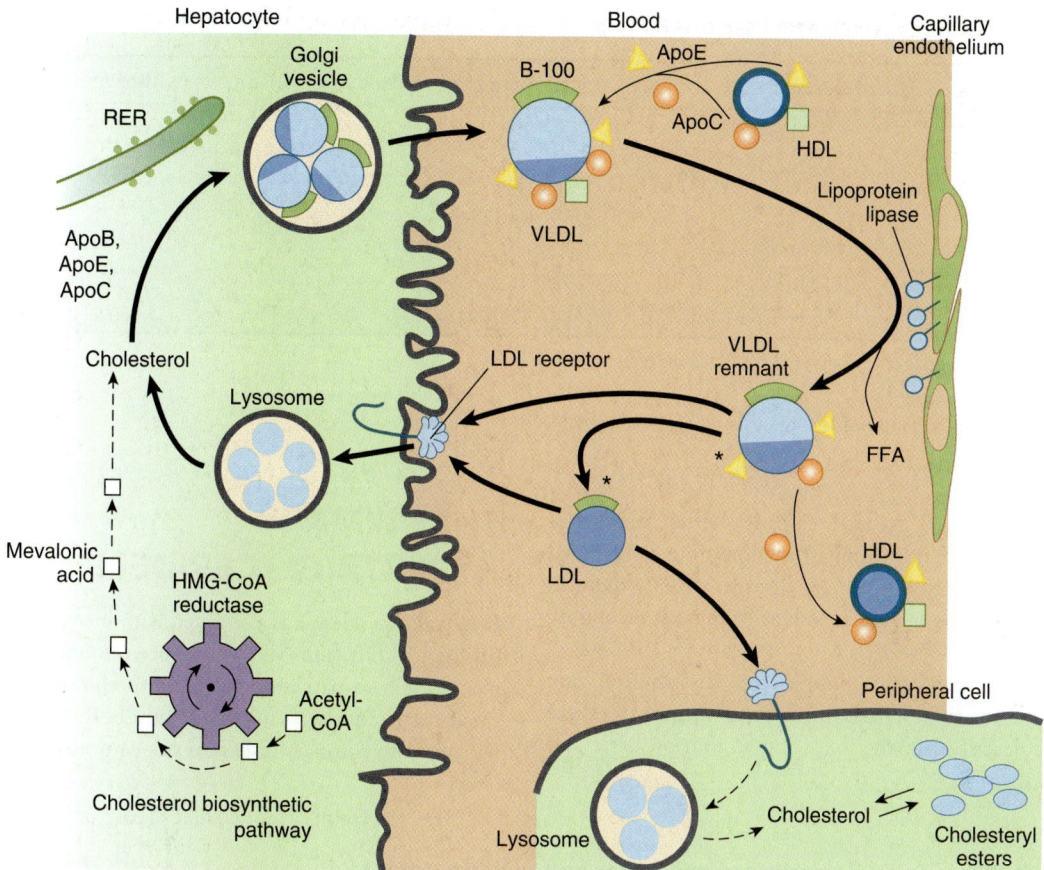

FIGURE 35–1 Metabolism of lipoproteins of hepatic origin. The heavy arrows show the primary pathways. Nascent VLDL are secreted via the Golgi apparatus. They acquire additional apo C lipoproteins and apo E from HDL. Very-low-density lipoproteins (VLDL) are converted to VLDL remnants (IDL) by lipolysis via lipoprotein lipase in the vessels of peripheral tissues. In the process, C apolipoproteins and a portion of the apo E are given back to high-density lipoproteins (HDL). Some of the VLDL remnants are converted to LDL by further loss of triglycerides and loss of apo E. A major pathway for LDL degradation involves the endocytosis of LDL by LDL receptors in the liver and the peripheral tissues, for which apo B-100 is the ligand. Dark color denotes cholesteryl esters; light color denotes triglycerides; the asterisk denotes a functional ligand for LDL receptors; triangles indicate apo E; circles and squares represent C apolipoproteins. FFA, free fatty acid; RER, rough endoplasmic reticulum. (Modified and redrawn, with permission, from Kane J, Malloy M: Disorders of lipoproteins. In: Rosenberg RN et al [editors]: *The Molecular and Genetic Basis of Neurological Disease.* Butterworth-Heinemann, 1993.)

transporter, ABCA1, acquired by a small particle termed prebeta-1 HDL, and then esterified by lecithin:cholesterol acyltransferase (LCAT), leading to the formation of larger HDL species. Cholesterol is also exported from macrophages by the ABCG1 transporter to large HDL particles. The cholesteryl esters are transferred to VLDL, IDL, LDL, and chylomicron remnants with the aid of cholesteryl ester transfer protein (CETP). Much of the cholesteryl ester thus transferred is ultimately delivered to the liver by endocytosis of the acceptor lipoproteins. HDL can also deliver cholesteryl esters directly to the liver via a docking receptor (scavenger receptor, SR-BI) that does not cause endocytosis of the lipoproteins. HDL-C levels relate inversely to risk at the population level. Among individuals, the capacity to accept exported cholesterol can vary widely at identical levels of HDL-C. The ability of peripheral tissues to export cholesterol via the transporter

mechanism and the acceptor capacity of HDL are emerging as major determinants of coronary atherosclerosis.

LIPOPROTEIN DISORDERS

Lipoprotein disorders are detected by measuring lipids in serum after a 10-hour fast. Risk of heart disease increases with concentrations of the atherogenic lipoproteins, is inversely related to levels of HDL, and is modified by other risk factors (Table 35–1). Evidence from clinical trials suggests that LDL cholesterol levels of 60 mg/dL may be optimal for patients with coronary disease. Ideally, triglycerides should be below 120 mg/dL. Although LDL-C is still the primary target of treatment, reducing the levels of VLDL and IDL is also important. Calculation of non-HDL cholesterol provides a means of assessing levels of all the

TABLE 35–1 National Cholesterol Education Program: Adult Treatment Guidelines (2001).

	Desirable	Borderline to High[1]	High
Total cholesterol	< 200 (5.2)[2]	200–239 (5.2–6.2)[2]	> 240 (6.2)[2]
LDL cholesterol	< 130 (3.4)[3]	130–159 (3.4–4.1)	> 160 (4.1)
HDL cholesterol			> 60 (1.55)
Men	> 40 (1.04)		
Women	> 50 (1.30)		
Triglycerides	< 120 (1.4)	120–199 (1.4–2.3)	> 200 (2.3)

[1]Consider as high if coronary disease or more than two risk factors are present.

[2]mg/dL (mmol/L).

[3]Optimal level is < 100 (2.6); if known atherosclerotic disease, goal is 60–70 mg/dL.

lipoproteins in the VLDL to LDL cascade. Differentiation of the disorders requires identification of the lipoproteins involved (Table 35–2). Diagnosis of a primary disorder usually requires further clinical and genetic data as well as ruling out secondary hyperlipidemias (Table 35–3).

Phenotypes of abnormal lipoprotein distribution are described in this section. Drugs mentioned for use in these conditions are described in the following section on basic and clinical pharmacology.

THE PRIMARY HYPERTRIGLYCERIDEMIAS

Hypertriglyceridemia is associated with increased risk of coronary disease. VLDL and IDL have been found in atherosclerotic plaques. These patients tend to have cholesterol-rich VLDL of small-particle diameter and small, dense LDL. Hypertriglyceridemic patients with coronary disease or risk equivalents should be treated

TABLE 35–2 The primary hyperlipoproteinemias and their treatment.

Disorder	Manifestations	Diet + Single Drug[1]	Drug Combination
Primary chylomicronemia (familial lipoprotein lipase or cofactor deficiency; others)	Chylomicrons, VLDL increased	Dietary management (omega-3 fatty acids, niacin, or fibrate)	Niacin plus fibrate
Familial hypertriglyceridemia-Severe	VLDL, chylomicrons increased	Omega-3 fatty acids, niacin, or fibrate	Niacin plus fibrate
Moderate	VLDL increased; chylomicrons may be increased	Omega-3 fatty acids, niacin, or fibrate	Niacin plus fibrate
Familial combined hyperlipoproteinemia	VLDL predominantly increased	Omega-3 fatty acids, niacin, fibrate, or reductase inhibitor	Two or three of the individual drugs
	LDL predominantly increased	Niacin, reductase inhibitor, or ezetimibe	Two or three of the individual drugs
	VLDL, LDL increased	Omega-3 fatty acids, niacin, or reductase inhibitor	Niacin or fibrate plus reductase inhibitor[2]
Familial dysbetalipoproteinemia	VLDL remnants, chylomicron remnants increased	Omega-3 fatty acids, fibrate, or niacin	Fibrate plus niacin, or either plus reductase inhibitor
Familial hypercholesterolemia			
Heterozygous	LDL increased	Reductase inhibitor, resin, niacin, or ezetimibe	Two or three of the individual drugs
Homozygous	LDL increased	Niacin, atorvastatin, rosuvastatin, or ezetimibe	Niacin plus reductase inhibitor plus ezetimibe
Familial ligand-defective apo B	LDL increased	Niacin, reductase inhibitor, or ezetimibe	Niacin plus reductase inhibitor or ezetimibe
Lp(a) hyperlipoproteinemia	Lp(a) increased	Niacin	

[1]Single-drug therapy with marine omega-3 dietary supplement should be evaluated before drug combinations are used.

[2]Select pharmacologically compatible reductase inhibitor (see text).

TABLE 35–3 Secondary causes of hyperlipoproteinemia.

Hypertriglyceridemia	Hypercholesterolemia
Diabetes mellitus	Hypothyroidism
Alcohol ingestion	Early nephrosis
Severe nephrosis	Resolving lipemia
Estrogens	Immunoglobulin-lipoprotein complex disorders
Uremia	Anorexia nervosa
Corticosteroid excess	Cholestasis
Myxedema	Hypopituitarism
Glycogen storage disease	Corticosteroid excess
Hypopituitarism	
Acromegaly	
Immunoglobulin-lipoprotein complex disorders	
Lipodystrophy	
Protease inhibitors	

aggressively. Patients with triglycerides above 700 mg/dL should be treated to prevent acute pancreatitis because the LPL clearance mechanism is saturated at about this level.

Hypertriglyceridemia is an essential component of the metabolic syndrome, which also includes low levels of HDL-C, insulin resistance, hypertension, and abdominal obesity. Hyperuricemia is also frequently present. Insulin resistance appears to be central to this process. Management of these patients frequently requires, in addition to a fibrate or niacin, the use of metformin or a peroxisome proliferator-activated receptor-gamma (PPAR-γ) agonist or both (see Chapter 41). In the latter case, pioglitazone is the drug of choice because it reduces triglycerides and does not increase levels of LDL. The severity of hypertriglyceridemia of any cause is increased in the presence of the metabolic syndrome or type 2 diabetes.

Primary Chylomicronemia

Chylomicrons are not present in the serum of normal individuals who have fasted 10 hours. The recessive traits of deficiency of LPL or its cofactor, apo C-II, are usually associated with severe lipemia (2000–3000 mg/dL of triglycerides when the patient is consuming a typical American diet). These disorders might not be diagnosed until an attack of acute pancreatitis occurs. Patients may have eruptive xanthomas, hepatosplenomegaly, hypersplenism, and lipid-laden foam cells in bone marrow, liver, and spleen. The lipemia is aggravated by estrogens because they stimulate VLDL production, and pregnancy may cause marked increases in triglycerides despite strict dietary control. Although these patients have a predominant chylomicronemia, they may also have moderately elevated VLDL, presenting with a pattern called mixed lipemia (fasting chylomicronemia and elevated VLDL). LPL deficiency is

diagnosed by assay of lipolytic activity after intravenous injection of heparin. A presumptive diagnosis is made by demonstrating a pronounced decrease in triglycerides a few days after reduction of daily fat intake below 15 g. Marked restriction of total dietary fat is the basis of effective long-term treatment. Niacin, a fibrate, or marine omega-3 fatty acids may be of some benefit if VLDL levels are increased. Genetic variants at other loci that participate in intravascular lipolysis, including LMF1, apo A-V, GPI-HDL BP1, and apo C-III, can have profound effects on triglyceride levels.

Familial Hypertriglyceridemia

A. Severe (Usually Mixed Lipemia)

Mixed lipemia usually results from impaired removal of triglyceride-rich lipoproteins. Factors that increase VLDL production aggravate the lipemia because VLDL and chylomicrons are competing substrates for LPL. The primary mixed lipemias probably reflect a variety of genetic determinants. Most patients have centripetal obesity with insulin resistance. Other factors that increase secretion of VLDL also worsen the lipemia. Eruptive xanthomas, lipemia retinalis, epigastric pain, and pancreatitis are variably present depending on the severity of the lipemia. Treatment is primarily dietary, with restriction of total fat, avoidance of alcohol and exogenous estrogens, weight reduction, exercise, and supplementation with marine omega-3 fatty acids. Most patients also require treatment with a fibrate or niacin.

B. Moderate

Primary increases of VLDL also reflect a genetic predisposition and are worsened by factors that increase the rate of VLDL secretion from liver, ie, obesity, alcohol, diabetes, and estrogens. Treatment includes addressing these issues and the use of fibrates or niacin as needed. Marine omega-3 fatty acids are a valuable adjuvant.

Familial Combined Hyperlipoproteinemia

In this common disorder associated with an increased incidence of coronary disease, individuals may have elevated levels of VLDL, LDL, or both, and the pattern may change with time. Familial combined hyperlipoproteinemia involves an approximate doubling in VLDL secretion and appears to be transmitted as a semidominant trait. Triglycerides can be increased by the factors noted above. Elevations of cholesterol and triglycerides are generally moderate, and xanthomas are usually absent. Diet alone does not normalize lipid levels. A reductase inhibitor alone, or in combination with niacin or fenofibrate, is usually required to treat these patients. When fenofibrate is combined with a reductase inhibitor, either pravastatin or rosuvastatin is recommended because neither is metabolized via CYP3A4.

Familial Dysbetalipoproteinemia

In this disorder, remnants of chylomicrons and VLDL accumulate and levels of LDL are decreased. Because remnants are rich in cholesteryl esters, the level of cholesterol may be as high as that of triglycerides. Diagnosis is confirmed by the absence of the ε3 and ε4 alleles of apo E, the ε2/ε2 genotype. Patients often develop tuberous or tuberoeruptive xanthomas, or characteristic planar xanthomas of the palmar creases. They tend to be obese, and some have impaired glucose tolerance. These factors, as well as hypothyroidism, can aggravate the lipemia. Coronary and peripheral atherosclerosis occurs with increased frequency. Weight loss, together with decreased fat, cholesterol, and alcohol consumption, may be sufficient, but a fibrate or niacin is usually needed to control the condition. These agents can be given together in more resistant cases, or a reductase inhibitor may be added.

Apo E is also secreted by glia in the central nervous system and plays a role in sterol transport. The ε4 allele is associated in a dose-dependent manner with early-onset Alzheimer's disease (see Chapter 60).

THE PRIMARY HYPERCHOLESTEROLEMIAS

Familial Hypercholesterolemia

Familial hypercholesterolemia is an autosomal dominant trait. Although levels of LDL tend to increase throughout childhood, the diagnosis can often be made on the basis of elevated umbilical cord blood cholesterol. In most heterozygotes, cholesterol levels range from 260 to 500 mg/dL. Triglycerides are usually normal, tendon xanthomas are often present, and arcus corneae and xanthelasma may appear in the third decade. Coronary disease tends to occur prematurely. In homozygous familial hypercholesterolemia, which can lead to coronary disease in childhood, levels of cholesterol often exceed 1000 mg/dL and early tuberous and tendinous xanthomas occur. These patients may also develop elevated plaque-like xanthomas of the aortic valve, digital webs, buttocks, and extremities.

Defects of LDL receptors underlie familial hypercholesterolemia. Some individuals have combined heterozygosity for alleles producing nonfunctional and kinetically impaired receptors. In heterozygous patients, LDL can be normalized with combined drug regimens (Figure 35–2). Homozygotes and those with combined heterozygosity whose receptors retain even minimal function may partially respond to niacin, ezetimibe, or reductase inhibitors.

Familial Ligand-Defective Apolipoprotein B-100

Defects in the domain of apo B-100 that binds to the LDL receptor impair the endocytosis of LDL, leading to hypercholesterolemia of moderate severity. Tendon xanthomas may occur. These disorders are as prevalent as familial hypercholesterolemia. Response to reductase inhibitors is variable. Up-regulation of LDL receptors in liver increases endocytosis of LDL precursors but does not increase uptake of ligand-defective LDL particles. Niacin often has beneficial effects by reducing VLDL production.

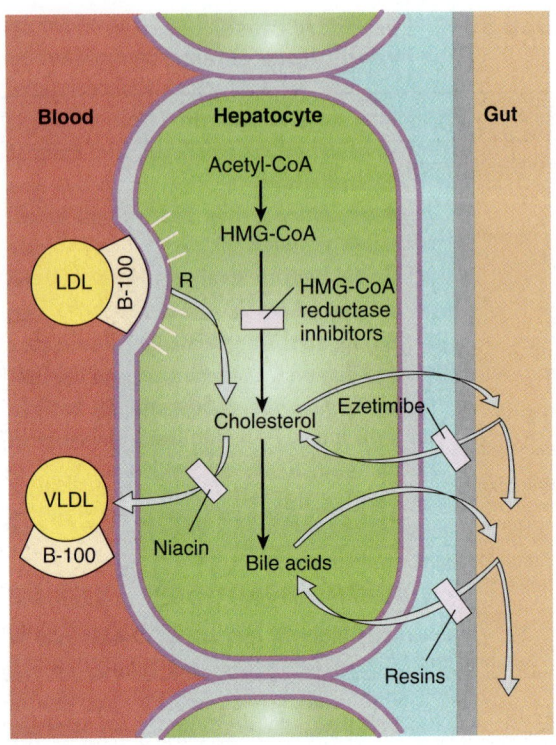

FIGURE 35–2 Sites of action of HMG-CoA reductase inhibitors, niacin, ezetimibe, and resins used in treating hyperlipidemias. Low-density lipoprotein (LDL) receptors are increased by treatment with resins and HMG-CoA reductase inhibitors. VLDL, very-low-density lipoproteins; R, LDL receptor.

Familial Combined Hyperlipoproteinemia

As described, some persons with familial combined hyperlipoproteinemia have only an elevation in LDL. Serum cholesterol is usually less than 350 mg/dL. Dietary and drug treatment, usually with a reductase inhibitor, is indicated. It may be necessary to add niacin or ezetimibe to normalize LDL.

Lp(a) Hyperlipoproteinemia

This familial disorder, which is associated with increased atherogenesis, is determined chiefly by alleles that dictate increased production of the (a) protein moiety. Lp(a) can be secondarily elevated in patients with severe nephrosis and certain other inflammatory states. Niacin reduces levels of Lp(a) in many patients.

Other Disorders

Deficiency of cholesterol 7α-hydroxylase can increase LDL in the heterozygous state. Homozygotes can also have elevated triglycerides, resistance to reductase inhibitors, and increased risk of gallstones and coronary disease. Autosomal recessive hypercholesterolemia is due to mutations in a protein that normally assists in endocytosis of LDL. Some mutations in the *PCSK9* gene also cause isolated elevations of LDL. Niacin, ezetimibe, and reductase inhibitors may be useful, variably, in these disorders.

HDL Deficiency

Rare genetic disorders, including Tangier disease and LCAT (lecithin:cholesterol acyltransferase) deficiency, are associated with extremely low levels of HDL. Familial hypoalphalipoproteinemia is a more common disorder with levels of HDL cholesterol usually below 35 mg/dL in men and 45 mg/dL in women. These patients tend to have premature atherosclerosis, and the low HDL may be the only identified risk factor. Management should include special attention to avoidance or treatment of other risk factors. Niacin increases HDL in many of these patients. Reductase inhibitors and fibric acid derivatives exert lesser effects.

In the presence of hypertriglyceridemia, HDL cholesterol is low because of exchange of cholesteryl esters from HDL into triglyceride-rich lipoproteins. Treatment of the hypertriglyceridemia may increase or normalize the HDL level.

SECONDARY HYPERLIPOPROTEINEMIA

Before primary disorders can be diagnosed, secondary causes of the phenotype must be considered. The more common conditions are summarized in Table 35–3. The lipoprotein abnormality usually resolves if the underlying disorder can be treated successfully.

■ DIETARY MANAGEMENT OF HYPERLIPOPROTEINEMIA

Dietary measures are initiated first—unless the patient has evident coronary or peripheral vascular disease—and may obviate the need for drugs. Patients with familial hypercholesterolemia or familial combined hyperlipidemia always require drug therapy. Cholesterol and saturated and *trans*-fats are the principal factors that increase LDL, whereas total fat, alcohol, and excess calories increase triglycerides.

Sucrose and fructose raise VLDL. Alcohol can cause significant hypertriglyceridemia by increasing hepatic secretion of VLDL. Synthesis and secretion of VLDL are increased by excess calories. During weight loss, LDL and VLDL levels may be much lower than can be maintained during neutral caloric balance. The conclusion that diet suffices for management can be made only after weight has stabilized for at least 1 month.

General recommendations include limiting total calories from fat to 20–25% of daily intake, saturated fats to less than 8%, and cholesterol to less than 200 mg/d. Reductions in serum cholesterol range from 10% to 20% on this regimen. Use of complex carbohydrates and fiber is recommended, and *cis*-monounsaturated fats should predominate. Weight reduction, caloric restriction, and avoidance of alcohol are especially important for patients with elevated VLDL and IDL.

The effect of dietary fats on hypertriglyceridemia is dependent on the disposition of double bonds in the fatty acids. Omega-3 fatty acids found in fish oils, but not those from plant sources, activate peroxisome proliferator-activated receptor-alpha (PPAR-α)

and can induce profound reduction of triglycerides in some patients. They also have anti-inflammatory and antiarrhythmic activities. Omega-3 fatty acids are available over the counter as triglycerides from marine sources or as a prescription medication (Lovaza) containing ethyl esters of omega-3 fatty acids. The recommended dose of Lovaza is 4 g/d. It is necessary to determine the content of docosahexaenoic acid and eicosapentaenoic acid in over-the-counter preparations. Appropriate amounts should be taken to provide up to 3–4 g of these fatty acids daily. It is important to select preparations free of mercury and other contaminants. The omega-6 fatty acids present in vegetable oils may cause triglycerides to increase.

Patients with primary chylomicronemia and some with mixed lipemia must consume a diet severely restricted in total fat (10–20 g/d, of which 5 g should be vegetable oils rich in essential fatty acids), and fat-soluble vitamins should be given.

Homocysteine, which initiates proatherogenic changes in endothelium, can be reduced in many patients by restriction of total protein intake to the amount required for amino acid replacement. Supplementation with folic acid plus other B vitamins is indicated in severe homocysteinemia.

■ BASIC & CLINICAL PHARMACOLOGY OF DRUGS USED IN HYPERLIPIDEMIA

The decision to use drug therapy for hyperlipidemia is based on the specific metabolic defect and its potential for causing atherosclerosis or pancreatitis. Suggested regimens for the principal lipoprotein disorders are presented in Table 35–2. Diet should be continued to achieve the full potential of the drug regimen. These drugs should be avoided in pregnant and lactating women and those likely to become pregnant. All drugs that alter plasma lipoprotein concentrations may require adjustment of doses of warfarin and indandione anticoagulants. Children with heterozygous familial hypercholesterolemia may be treated with a resin or reductase inhibitor, usually after 7 or 8 years of age, when myelination of the central nervous system is essentially complete. The decision to treat a child should be based on the level of LDL, other risk factors, the family history, and the child's age. Drugs are rarely indicated before age 16 in the absence of multiple risk factors or compound genetic dyslipidemias.

COMPETITIVE INHIBITORS OF HMG-COA REDUCTASE (REDUCTASE INHIBITORS; "STATINS")

These compounds are structural analogs of HMG-CoA (3-hydroxy-3-methylglutaryl-coenzyme A, Figure 35–3). **Lovastatin, atorvastatin, fluvastatin, pravastatin, simvastatin, rosuvastatin,** and **pitavastatin** belong to this class. They are most effective in reducing LDL. Other effects include decreased oxidative stress and vascular inflammation with increased stability of atherosclerotic

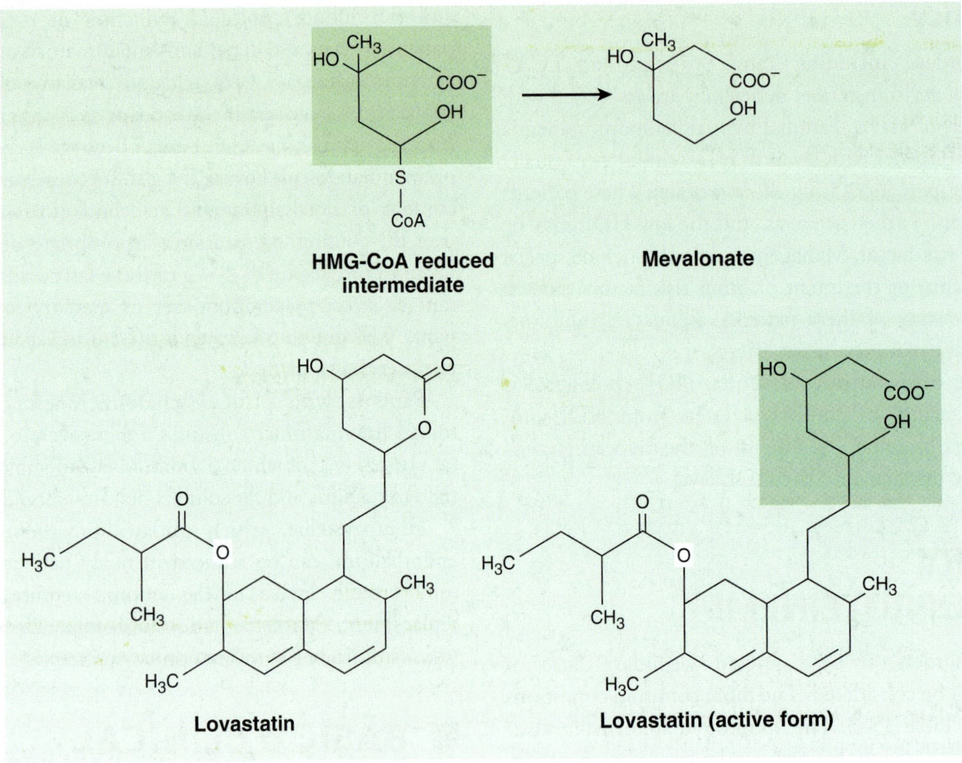

FIGURE 35–3 Inhibition of HMG-CoA reductase. **Top:** The HMG-CoA intermediate that is the immediate precursor of mevalonate, a critical compound in the synthesis of cholesterol. **Bottom:** The structure of lovastatin and its active form, showing the similarity to the normal HMG-CoA intermediate (shaded areas).

lesions. It has become standard practice to initiate reductase inhibitor therapy immediately after acute coronary syndromes, regardless of lipid levels.

Chemistry & Pharmacokinetics

Lovastatin and simvastatin are inactive lactone prodrugs that are hydrolyzed in the gastrointestinal tract to the active β-hydroxyl derivatives, whereas pravastatin has an open, active lactone ring. Atorvastatin, fluvastatin, and rosuvastatin are fluorine-containing congeners that are active as given. Absorption of the ingested doses of the reductase inhibitors varies from 40% to 75% with the exception of fluvastatin, which is almost completely absorbed. All have high first-pass extraction by the liver. Most of the absorbed dose is excreted in the bile; 5–20% is excreted in the urine. Plasma half-lives of these drugs range from 1 to 3 hours except for atorvastatin (14 hours), pitavastatin (12 hours), and rosuvastatin (19 hours).

Mechanism of Action

HMG-CoA reductase mediates the first committed step in sterol biosynthesis. The active forms of the reductase inhibitors are structural analogs of the HMG-CoA intermediate (Figure 35–3) that is formed by HMG-CoA reductase in the synthesis of mevalonate. These analogs cause partial inhibition of the enzyme and thus may impair the synthesis of isoprenoids such as ubiquinone and dolichol and the prenylation of proteins. It is not known whether

this has biologic significance. However, the reductase inhibitors clearly induce an increase in high-affinity LDL receptors. This effect increases both the fractional catabolic rate of LDL and the liver's extraction of LDL precursors (VLDL remnants) from the blood, thus reducing LDL (Figure 35–2). Because of marked first-pass hepatic extraction, the major effect is on the liver. Preferential activity in liver of some congeners appears to be attributable to tissue-specific differences in uptake. Modest decreases in plasma triglycerides and small increases in HDL also occur.

Clinical trials involving many of the statins have demonstrated significant reduction of new coronary events and atherothrombotic stroke. Mechanisms other than reduction of lipoprotein levels appear to be involved. The availability of isoprenyl groups from the HMG-CoA pathway for prenylation of proteins is reduced by statins, resulting in reduced prenylation of Rho and Rab proteins. Prenylated Rho activates Rho kinase, which mediates a number of mechanisms in vascular biology. The observation that reduction in new coronary events occurs more rapidly than changes in morphology of arterial plaques suggests that these pleiotropic effects may be important. Likewise, decreased prenylation of Rab reduces the accumulation of Aβ protein in neurons, possibly mitigating the manifestations of Alzheimer's disease.

Therapeutic Uses & Dosage

Reductase inhibitors are useful alone or with resins, niacin, or ezetimibe in reducing levels of LDL. Women with hyperlipidemia who are pregnant, lactating, or likely to become pregnant should not be given these agents. Use in children is restricted to selected patients with familial hypercholesterolemia or familial combined hyperlipidemia.

Because cholesterol synthesis occurs predominantly at night, reductase inhibitors—except atorvastatin and rosuvastatin—should be given in the evening if a single daily dose is used. Absorption generally (with the exception of pravastatin) is enhanced by food. Daily doses of lovastatin vary from 10 to 80 mg. Pravastatin is nearly as potent on a mass basis as lovastatin with a maximum recommended daily dose of 80 mg. Simvastatin is twice as potent and is given in doses of 5–80 mg daily. Because of increased risk of myopathy with the 80 mg/day dose, the FDA issued labelling for scaled dosing of simvastatin and Vytorin in June 2011. Fluvastatin appears to be about half as potent as lovastatin on a mass basis and is given in doses of 10–80 mg daily. Atorvastatin is given in doses of 10–80 mg/d, and rosuvastatin, the most efficacious agent for severe hypercholesterolemia, at 5–40 mg/d. The dose-response curves of pravastatin and especially of fluvastatin tend to level off in the upper part of the dosage range in patients with moderate to severe hypercholesterolemia. Those of other statins are somewhat more linear.

Toxicity

Elevations of serum aminotransferase activity (up to three times normal) occur in some patients. This is often intermittent and usually not associated with other evidence of hepatic toxicity. Therapy may be continued in such patients in the absence of symptoms if aminotransferase levels are monitored and stable. In some patients, who may have underlying liver disease or a history of alcohol abuse, levels may exceed three times normal. This finding portends more severe hepatic toxicity. These patients may present with malaise, anorexia, and precipitous decreases in LDL. Medication should be discontinued immediately in these patients and in asymptomatic patients whose aminotransferase activity is persistently elevated to more than three times the upper limit of normal. These agents should be used with caution and in reduced dosage in patients with hepatic parenchymal disease, Asians, and the elderly. Severe hepatic disease may preclude their use. In general, aminotransferase activity should be measured at baseline, at 1–2 months, and then every 6–12 months (if stable). Monitoring of liver enzymes should be more frequent if the patient is taking other drugs that have potential interactions with the statin. Fasting plasma glucose levels tend to increase 5–7 mg/dL with statin treatment.

Minor increases in creatine kinase (CK) activity in plasma are observed in some patients receiving reductase inhibitors, frequently associated with heavy physical activity. Rarely, patients may have marked elevations in CK activity, often accompanied by generalized discomfort or weakness in skeletal muscles. If the drug is not discontinued, myoglobinuria can occur, leading to renal injury. Myopathy may occur with monotherapy, but there is an increased incidence in patients also receiving certain other drugs. Genetic variation in an anion transporter (OATP1B1) is associated with severe myopathy and rhabdomyolysis induced by statins.

The catabolism of lovastatin, simvastatin, and atorvastatin proceeds chiefly through CYP3A4, whereas that of fluvastatin and rosuvastatin, and to a lesser extent pitavastatin, is mediated by CYP2C9. Pravastatin is catabolized through other pathways, including sulfation. The 3A4-dependent reductase inhibitors tend to accumulate in plasma in the presence of drugs that inhibit or compete for the 3A4 cytochrome. These include the macrolide antibiotics, cyclosporine, ketoconazole and its congeners, some HIV protease inhibitors, tacrolimus, nefazodone, fibrates, paroxetine, venlafaxine, and others (see Chapter 4). Concomitant use of reductase inhibitors with amiodarone or verapamil also causes an increased risk of myopathy.

Conversely, drugs such as phenytoin, griseofulvin, barbiturates, rifampin, and thiazolidinediones increase expression of CYP3A4 and can reduce the plasma concentrations of the 3A4-dependent reductase inhibitors. Inhibitors of CYP2C9 such as ketoconazole and its congeners, metronidazole, sulfinpyrazone, amiodarone, and cimetidine may increase plasma levels of fluvastatin and rosuvastatin. Pravastatin and rosuvastatin appear to be the statins of choice for use with verapamil, the ketoconazole group of antifungal agents, macrolides, and cyclosporine. Doses should be kept low and the patient monitored frequently. Plasma levels of lovastatin, simvastatin, and atorvastatin may be elevated in patients ingesting more than 1 liter of grapefruit juice daily. All statins undergo glycosylation, thus creating an interaction with gemfibrozil.

Creatine kinase activity should be measured in patients receiving potentially interacting drug combinations. In all patients, CK should be measured at baseline. If muscle pain, tenderness, or weakness appears, CK should be measured immediately and the drug discontinued if activity is elevated significantly over baseline. The myopathy usually reverses promptly upon cessation of therapy. If the association is unclear, the patient can be rechallenged under close surveillance. Myopathy in the absence of elevated CK can occur. Rarely, hypersensitivity syndromes have been reported that include a lupus-like disorder and peripheral neuropathy.

Reductase inhibitors should be temporarily discontinued in the event of serious illness, trauma, or major surgery.

NIACIN (NICOTINIC ACID)

Niacin (but not niacinamide) decreases VLDL and LDL levels, and Lp(a) in most patients. It often increases HDL levels significantly.

Chemistry & Pharmacokinetics

Niacin (vitamin B_3) is converted in the body to the amide, which is incorporated into niacinamide adenine dinucleotide (NAD). It is excreted in the urine unmodified and as several metabolites.

Mechanism of Action

Niacin inhibits VLDL secretion, in turn decreasing production of LDL (Figure 35–2). Increased clearance of VLDL via the LPL pathway contributes to reduction of triglycerides. Niacin has no effect on bile acid production. Excretion of neutral sterols in the stool is increased acutely as cholesterol is mobilized from tissue pools and a new steady state is reached. The catabolic rate for HDL is decreased. Fibrinogen levels are reduced, and levels of tissue plasminogen activator appear to increase. Niacin inhibits the intracellular lipase of adipose tissue via receptor-mediated signaling, possibly reducing VLDL production by decreasing the flux of free fatty acids to the liver. Sustained inhibition of lipolysis has not been established, however.

Therapeutic Uses & Dosage

In combination with a resin or reductase inhibitor, niacin normalizes LDL in most patients with heterozygous familial hypercholesterolemia and other forms of hypercholesterolemia. These combinations are also indicated in some cases of nephrosis. In severe mixed lipemia that is incompletely responsive to diet, niacin often produces marked reduction of triglycerides, an effect enhanced by marine omega-3 fatty acids. It is useful in patients with combined hyperlipidemia and in those with dysbetalipoproteinemia. It is clearly the most effective agent for increasing HDL and the only agent that may reduce Lp(a).

For treatment of heterozygous familial hypercholesterolemia, most patients require 2–6 g of niacin daily; more than this should not be given. For other types of hypercholesterolemia and for hypertriglyceridemia, 1.5–3.5 g daily is often sufficient. Crystalline niacin should be given in divided doses with meals, starting with 100 mg two or three times daily and increasing gradually.

Toxicity

Most persons experience a harmless cutaneous vasodilation and sensation of warmth after each dose when niacin is started or the dose increased. Taking 81–325 mg of aspirin one half hour beforehand blunts this prostaglandin-mediated effect. Ibuprofen, once daily, also mitigates the flush. Tachyphylaxis to flushing usually occurs within a few days at doses above 1.5–3 g daily. Patients should be warned to expect the flush and understand that it is a harmless side effect. Pruritus, rashes, dry skin or mucous membranes, and acanthosis nigricans have been reported. The latter contraindicates use of niacin because of its association with insulin resistance. Some patients experience nausea and abdominal discomfort. Many can continue the drug at reduced dosage, with inhibitors of gastric acid secretion or with antacids not containing aluminum. Niacin should be avoided in most patients with severe peptic disease.

Reversible elevations in aminotransferases up to twice normal may occur, usually not associated with liver toxicity. However, liver function should be monitored at baseline and at appropriate intervals. Rarely, true hepatotoxicity may occur, and in these cases the drug should be discontinued. The association of severe hepatic dysfunction, including acute necrosis, with the use of over-the-counter sustained-release preparations of niacin has been reported. This effect has not been noted to date with an extended-release preparation, Niaspan, given at bedtime in doses of 2 g or less. Carbohydrate tolerance may be moderately impaired, especially in obese patients, but this is usually reversible except in some patients with latent diabetes. Niacin may be given to diabetics who are receiving insulin and to some receiving oral agents. Niacin may increase insulin resistance in some patients. This can often be addressed by increasing the dose of insulin or the oral agents. Hyperuricemia occurs in some patients and occasionally precipitates gout. Allopurinol can be given with niacin if needed. Red cell macrocytosis is frequently observed with higher doses of niacin and is not an indication for discontinuing treatment. Significant platelet deficiency can occur rarely and is reversible on cessation of treatment. Rarely, niacin is associated with arrhythmias, mostly atrial, and with macular edema. Patients should be instructed to report blurring of distance vision. Niacin may potentiate the action of antihypertensive agents, requiring adjustment of their dosages. Birth defects have been reported in animals given very high doses.

FIBRIC ACID DERIVATIVES (FIBRATES)

Gemfibrozil and fenofibrate decrease levels of VLDL and, in some patients, LDL as well. Another fibrate, bezafibrate, is not yet available in the USA.

Chemistry & Pharmacokinetics

Gemfibrozil is absorbed quantitatively from the intestine and is tightly bound to plasma proteins. It undergoes enterohepatic circulation and readily passes the placenta. The plasma half-life is 1.5 hours. Seventy percent is eliminated through the kidneys, mostly unmodified. The liver modifies some of the drug to hydroxymethyl, carboxyl, or quinol derivatives. Fenofibrate is an isopropyl ester that is hydrolyzed completely in the intestine. Its plasma half-life is 20 hours. Sixty percent is excreted in the urine as the glucuronide, and about 25% in feces.

Gemfibrozil

Fenofibrate

Mechanism of Action

Fibrates function primarily as ligands for the nuclear transcription receptor, PPAR-α. They transcriptionally up-regulate LPL, apo A-I and apo A-II, and down-regulate apo C-III, an inhibitor of lipolysis. A major effect is an increase in oxidation of fatty acids in liver and striated muscle (Figure 35–4). They increase lipolysis of lipoprotein triglyceride via LPL. Intracellular lipolysis in adipose

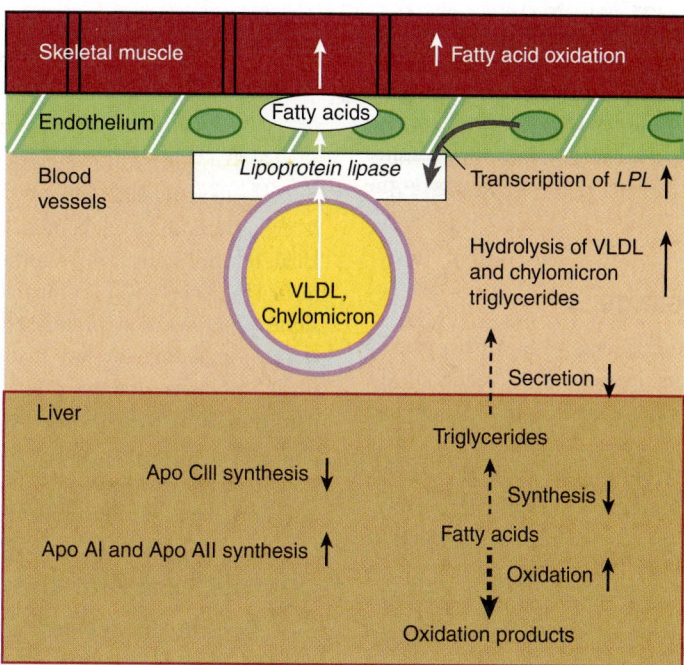

FIGURE 35–4 Hepatic and peripheral effects of fibrates. These effects are mediated by activation of peroxisome proliferator-activated receptor-α, which modulates the expression of several proteins. LPL, lipoprotein lipase; VLDL, very-low-density lipoproteins.

tissue is decreased. Levels of VLDL decrease, in part as a result of decreased secretion by the liver. Only modest reductions of LDL occur in most patients. In others, especially those with combined hyperlipidemia, LDL often increases as triglycerides are reduced. HDL cholesterol increases moderately. Part of this apparent increase is a consequence of decreasing triglycerides in plasma, with reduction in exchange of triglycerides into HDL in place of cholesteryl esters.

Therapeutic Uses & Dosage

Fibrates are useful drugs in hypertriglyceridemias in which VLDL predominate and in dysbetalipoproteinemia. They also may be of benefit in treating the hypertriglyceridemia that results from treatment with viral protease inhibitors. The usual dose of gemfibrozil is 600 mg orally once or twice daily. The dosage of fenofibrate (as Tricor) is one to three 48 mg tablets (or a single 145 mg tablet) daily. Absorption of gemfibrozil is improved when the drug is taken with food.

Toxicity

Rare adverse effects of fibrates include rashes, gastrointestinal symptoms, myopathy, arrhythmias, hypokalemia, and high blood levels of aminotransferases or alkaline phosphatase. A few patients show decreases in white blood count or hematocrit. Both agents potentiate the action of coumarin and indanedione anticoagulants, and doses of these agents should be adjusted. Rhabdomyolysis has occurred rarely. Risk of myopathy increases when fibrates are given with reductase inhibitors. Fenofibrate is the fibrate of choice for use in combination with a statin. Fibrates should be avoided in patients

with hepatic or renal dysfunction. There appears to be a modest increase in the risk of cholesterol gallstones, reflecting an increase in the cholesterol content of bile. Therefore, fibrates should be used with caution in patients with biliary tract disease or in those at high risk such as women, obese patients, and Native Americans.

BILE ACID-BINDING RESINS

Colestipol, cholestyramine, and colesevelam are useful only for isolated increases in LDL. In patients who also have hypertriglyceridemia, VLDL levels may be further increased during treatment with resins.

Chemistry & Pharmacokinetics

The bile acid-binding agents are large polymeric cationic exchange resins that are insoluble in water. They bind bile acids in the intestinal lumen and prevent their reabsorption. The resin itself is not absorbed.

Mechanism of Action

The bile acids, metabolites of cholesterol, are normally efficiently reabsorbed in the jejunum and ileum (Figure 35–2). Excretion is increased up to tenfold when resins are given, resulting in enhanced conversion of cholesterol to bile acids in liver via 7α-hydroxylation, which is normally controlled by negative feedback by bile acids. Decreased activation of the FXR receptor by bile acids may result in a modest increase in plasma triglycerides but can also improve glucose metabolism in patients with diabetes. The latter effect is due to increased secretion of the incretin glucagon-like peptide-1 from the intestine, thus increasing insulin secretion. Increased uptake of LDL and IDL from plasma results from up-regulation of LDL receptors, particularly in liver. Therefore, the resins are without effect in patients with homozygous familial hypercholesterolemia who have no functioning receptors but may be useful in patients with receptor-defective combined heterozygous states.

Therapeutic Uses & Dosage

The resins are used in treatment of patients with primary hypercholesterolemia, producing approximately 20% reduction in LDL cholesterol in maximal dosage. If resins are used to treat LDL elevations in persons with combined hyperlipidemia, they may cause an increase in VLDL, requiring the addition of a second agent such as niacin. Resins are also used in combination with other drugs to achieve further hypocholesterolemic effect (see below). They may be helpful in relieving pruritus in patients who have cholestasis and bile salt accumulation. Because the resins bind digitalis glycosides, they may be useful in digitalis toxicity.

Colestipol and cholestyramine are available as granular preparations. A gradual increase of dosage of granules from 4 or 5 g/d to 20 g/d is recommended. Total dosages of 30–32 g/d may be needed for maximum effect. The usual dosage for a child is 10–20 g/d. Granular resins are mixed with juice or water and allowed to hydrate for 1 minute. Colestipol is also available in 1 g tablets that must be swallowed whole, with a maximum dose of 16 g daily. Colesevelam is available in 625 mg tablets and as a suspension (1875-mg or 3750-mg packets). The maximum dose is six tablets or 3750 mg as suspension, daily. Resins should be taken in two or three doses with meals. They lack effect when taken between meals.

Toxicity

Common complaints are constipation and bloating, usually relieved by increasing dietary fiber or mixing psyllium seed with the resin. Resins should be avoided in patients with diverticulitis. Heartburn and diarrhea are occasionally reported. In patients who have preexisting bowel disease or cholestasis, steatorrhea may occur. Malabsorption of vitamin K occurs rarely, leading to hypoprothrombinemia. Prothrombin time should be measured frequently in patients who are taking resins and anticoagulants. Malabsorption of folic acid has been reported rarely. Increased formation of gallstones, particularly in obese persons, was an anticipated adverse effect but has rarely occurred in practice.

Absorption of certain drugs, including those with neutral or cationic charge as well as anions, may be impaired by the resins. These include digitalis glycosides, thiazides, warfarin, tetracycline, thyroxine, iron salts, pravastatin, fluvastatin, ezetimibe, folic acid, phenylbutazone, aspirin, and ascorbic acid, among others. In general, additional medication (except niacin) should be given 1 hour before or at least 2 hours after the resin to ensure adequate absorption. Colesevelam does not bind digoxin, warfarin, or reductase inhibitors.

INHIBITORS OF INTESTINAL STEROL ABSORPTION

Ezetimibe is the first member of a group of drugs that inhibit intestinal absorption of phytosterols and cholesterol. Its primary clinical effect is reduction of LDL levels. In one trial, patients receiving ezetimibe in combination with simvastatin had marginal, but not statistically significant, increases in carotid intimal-medial thickness (IMT) compared with those receiving simvastatin alone. Interpretation of this observation is difficult for several reasons, including the fact that baseline IMT was unexpectedly small, probably due to prior lipid-lowering therapy. Because reducing LDL levels by virtually every modality has been associated with reduced risk of coronary events, it is reasonable to assume that reduction of LDL by ezetimibe will have a similar impact. Further studies are pending.

Chemistry & Pharmacokinetics

Ezetimibe is readily absorbed and conjugated in the intestine to an active glucuronide, reaching peak blood levels in 12–14 hours. It undergoes enterohepatic circulation, and its half-life is 22 hours. Approximately 80% of the drug is excreted in feces. Plasma concentrations are substantially increased when it is administered with fibrates and reduced when it is given with cholestyramine. Other resins may also decrease its absorption. There are no significant interactions with warfarin or digoxin.

Ezetimibe

Mechanism of Action

Ezetimibe is a selective inhibitor of intestinal absorption of cholesterol and phytosterols. A transport protein, NPC1L1, appears to be the target of the drug. It is effective even in the absence of dietary cholesterol because it inhibits reabsorption of cholesterol excreted in the bile.

Therapeutic Uses & Dosage

The effect of ezetimibe on cholesterol absorption is constant over the dosage range of 5–20 mg/d. Therefore, a single daily dose of 10 mg is used. Average reduction in LDL cholesterol with ezetimibe alone in patients with primary hypercholesterolemia is about 18%, with minimal increases in HDL cholesterol. It is also effective in patients with phytosterolemia. Ezetimibe is synergistic with reductase inhibitors, producing decrements as great as 25% in LDL cholesterol beyond that achieved with the reductase inhibitor alone.

Toxicity

Ezetimibe does not appear to be a substrate for cytochrome P450 enzymes. Experience to date reveals a low incidence of reversible impaired hepatic function with a small increase in incidence when given with a reductase inhibitor. Myositis has been reported rarely.

CETP INHIBITORS

Cholesteryl ester transfer protein (CETP) inhibitors are under active investigation. The first drug in this class, **torcetrapib**, aroused great interest because it markedly increased HDL and reduced LDL. However, it was withdrawn from clinical trials because it increased cardiovascular events and deaths in the treatment group. **Anacetrapib** and **dalcetrapib** are analogs currently in clinical trials.

TREATMENT WITH DRUG COMBINATIONS

Combined drug therapy is useful (1) when VLDL levels are significantly increased during treatment of hypercholesterolemia with a resin; (2) when LDL and VLDL levels are both elevated initially; (3) when LDL or VLDL levels are not normalized with a single agent, or (4) when an elevated level of Lp(a) or an HDL deficiency coexists with other hyperlipidemias. The lowest effective doses should be used in combination therapy and the patient should be monitored more closely for evidence of toxicity.

FIBRIC ACID DERIVATIVES & BILE ACID-BINDING RESINS

This combination is sometimes useful in treating patients with familial combined hyperlipidemia who are intolerant of niacin or statins. However, it may increase the risk of cholelithiasis.

HMG-COA REDUCTASE INHIBITORS & BILE ACID-BINDING RESINS

This synergistic combination is useful in the treatment of familial hypercholesterolemia but may not control levels of VLDL in some patients with familial combined hyperlipoproteinemia. Statins should be given 1 hour before or at least 2 hours after the resin to ensure their absorption.

NIACIN & BILE ACID-BINDING RESINS

This combination effectively controls VLDL levels during resin therapy of familial combined hyperlipoproteinemia or other disorders involving both increased VLDL and LDL levels. When VLDL and LDL levels are both initially increased, doses of niacin as low as 1–3 g/d may be sufficient in combination with a resin. The niacin-resin combination is effective for treating heterozygous familial hypercholesterolemia.

The drugs may be taken together, because niacin does not bind to the resins. LDL levels in patients with heterozygous familial hypercholesterolemia require daily doses of up to 6 g of niacin with 24–30 g of resin.

NIACIN & REDUCTASE INHIBITORS

This regimen is more effective than either agent alone in treating hypercholesterolemia. Experience indicates that it is an efficacious and practical combination for treatment of familial combined hyperlipoproteinemia.

REDUCTASE INHIBITORS & EZETIMIBE

This combination is highly synergistic in treating primary hypercholesterolemia and has some use in the treatment of patients with homozygous familial hypercholesterolemia who have some receptor function.

REDUCTASE INHIBITORS & FENOFIBRATE

Fenofibrate appears to be complementary with most statins in the treatment of familial combined hyperlipoproteinemia and other conditions involving elevations of both LDL and VLDL. The combination of fenofibrate with rosuvastatin appears to be well tolerated. Some other statins may interact unfavorably owing to effects on cytochrome P450 metabolism. In any case, particular vigilance for liver and muscle toxicity is indicated.

COMBINATIONS OF RESINS, EZETIMIBE, NIACIN, & REDUCTASE INHIBITORS

These agents act in a complementary fashion to normalize cholesterol in patients with severe disorders involving elevated LDL. The effects are sustained, and little compound toxicity has been observed. Effective doses of the individual drugs may be lower than when each is used alone; for example, as little as 1–2 g of niacin may substantially increase the effects of the other agents.

PREPARATIONS AVAILABLE

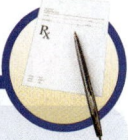

Atorvastatin (Lipitor)
Oral: 10, 20, 40, 80 mg tablets

Cholestyramine (generic, Questran, Questran Light)
Oral: 4 g packets anhydrous granules cholestyramine resin

Colesevelam (WelChol)
Oral: 625 mg tablets; 1.875 g and 3.75 g packets powder

Colestipol (Colestid)
Oral: 5 g packets granules; 1 g tablets

Ezetimibe (Zetia)
Oral: 10 mg tablets

Fenofibrate (generic, Tricor, Antara, Lofibra)
Oral: 48, 50, 54, 107, 145, 160 mg tablets; 45, 50, 67, 100, 130, 134, 135 150, 200 mg capsules

Fluvastatin (Lescol)
Oral: 20, 40 mg capsules; extended-release (Lescol XL): 80 mg capsules

Gemfibrozil (generic, Lopid)
Oral: 600 mg tablets

Lovastatin (generic, Mevacor)
Oral: 10, 20, 40 mg tablets; extended-release (Altoprev): 20, 40, 60 mg

Niacin, nicotinic acid, vitamin B₃ (generic, others)
Oral: 100, 250, 500, 1000 mg tablets; extended-release (Niaspan): 500, 750, 1000 mg

Omega-3 fatty acids-marine (generic, Lovaza)
Oral: 1 g (300 mg PUFA, generic) or 1 g (900 mg PUFA, Lovaza) capsules

Pitavastatin (Livalo)
Oral: 1, 2, 4 mg tablets

Pravastatin (generic, Pravachol)
Oral: 10, 20, 40, 80 mg tablets

Rosuvastatin (Crestor)
Oral: 5, 10, 20, 40 mg tablets

Simvastatin (generic, Zocor)
Oral: 5, 10, 20, 40, 80 mg tablets

COMBINATION TABLETS

Advicor (extended-release niacin/lovastatin)
Oral: 500/20, 750/20, 1000/20, 1000/40 mg tablets

Simcor (extended-release niacin/simvastatin)
Oral: 500/20, 750/20, 1000/20 mg tablets

Vytorin (ezetimibe/simvastatin)
Oral: 10/10, 10/20, 10/40, 10/80 mg tablets

PUFA, polyunsaturated fatty acid.

REFERENCES

Ballantyne CM et al; Asteroid Investigators. Effect of rosuvastatin therapy on coronary artery stenoses assessed by quantitative coronary angiography: A study to evaluate the effect of rosuvastatin on intravascular ultrasound-derived coronary atheroma burden. Circulation 2008;117:2458.

Bruckert E, Labreuche J, Amarenco P: Meta-analysis of the effect of nicotinic acid alone or in combination on cardiovascular events and atherosclerosis. Atherosclerosis 2010;210:353.

Brunzell JD et al: Lipoprotein management in patients with cardiometabolic risk: Consensus conference report from the ADA and the American College of Cardiology Foundation. J Am Coll Cardiol 2008;51(15):1512.

Elam M, Lovato E, Ginsberg H: The role of fibrates in cardiovascular disease prevention, The ACCORD–lipid perspective. Curr Opin Lipidol 2011;22:55.

Forrester JS: Redefining normal low-density lipoprotein cholesterol: A strategy to unseat coronary disease as the nation's leading killer. J Am Coll Cardiol 2010;56:630.

Grundy SM et al, for the Coordinating Committee of the National Cholesterol Education Program: Implications of recent clinical trials for the National Cholesterol Education Adult Treatment Panel III guidelines. Circulation 2004;110:227.

Harper CR, Jacobson TA: Evidence-based management of statin myopathy. Curr Atheroscler Rep 2010;12:322.

Polonsky TS, Davidson MH: Reducing the residual risk of 3-hydroxy-3-methylglutaryl coenzyme A reductase inhibitor therapy with combination therapy. Am J Cardiol 2008;101(Suppl):27B.

Steinberg D et al: Evidence mandating earlier and more aggressive treatment of hypercholesterolemia. Circulation 2008;118:672.

CASE STUDY ANSWER

This patient has combined hyperlipidemia. The statin should be continued. A drug that reduces VLDL production would be beneficial (niacin or fenofibrate). Niacin is the preferred agent to increase HDL-C and to reduce triglycerides and Lp(a). However, increased insulin resistance may occur, necessitating frequent monitoring and, if necessary, the addition of metformin. If the LDL-C goal is not reached with the addition of niacin (or fenofibrate), the statin dose should be increased. Creatine kinase should be monitored. Marine omega-3 fatty acids will help to reduce triglycerides.

Toxicity

Ezetimibe does not appear to be a substrate for cytochrome P450 enzymes. Experience to date reveals a low incidence of reversible impaired hepatic function with a small increase in incidence when given with a reductase inhibitor. Myositis has been reported rarely.

CETP INHIBITORS

Cholesteryl ester transfer protein (CETP) inhibitors are under active investigation. The first drug in this class, **torcetrapib,** aroused great interest because it markedly increased HDL and reduced LDL. However, it was withdrawn from clinical trials because it increased cardiovascular events and deaths in the treatment group. **Anacetrapib** and **dalcetrapib** are analogs currently in clinical trials.

TREATMENT WITH DRUG COMBINATIONS

Combined drug therapy is useful (1) when VLDL levels are significantly increased during treatment of hypercholesterolemia with a resin; (2) when LDL and VLDL levels are both elevated initially; (3) when LDL or VLDL levels are not normalized with a single agent, or (4) when an elevated level of Lp(a) or an HDL deficiency coexists with other hyperlipidemias. The lowest effective doses should be used in combination therapy and the patient should be monitored more closely for evidence of toxicity.

FIBRIC ACID DERIVATIVES & BILE ACID-BINDING RESINS

This combination is sometimes useful in treating patients with familial combined hyperlipidemia who are intolerant of niacin or statins. However, it may increase the risk of cholelithiasis.

HMG-COA REDUCTASE INHIBITORS & BILE ACID-BINDING RESINS

This synergistic combination is useful in the treatment of familial hypercholesterolemia but may not control levels of VLDL in some patients with familial combined hyperlipoproteinemia. Statins should be given 1 hour before or at least 2 hours after the resin to ensure their absorption.

NIACIN & BILE ACID-BINDING RESINS

This combination effectively controls VLDL levels during resin therapy of familial combined hyperlipoproteinemia or other disorders involving both increased VLDL and LDL levels. When VLDL and LDL levels are both initially increased, doses of niacin as low as 1–3 g/d may be sufficient in combination with a resin. The niacin-resin combination is effective for treating heterozygous familial hypercholesterolemia.

The drugs may be taken together, because niacin does not bind to the resins. LDL levels in patients with heterozygous familial hypercholesterolemia require daily doses of up to 6 g of niacin with 24–30 g of resin.

NIACIN & REDUCTASE INHIBITORS

This regimen is more effective than either agent alone in treating hypercholesterolemia. Experience indicates that it is an efficacious and practical combination for treatment of familial combined hyperlipoproteinemia.

REDUCTASE INHIBITORS & EZETIMIBE

This combination is highly synergistic in treating primary hypercholesterolemia and has some use in the treatment of patients with homozygous familial hypercholesterolemia who have some receptor function.

REDUCTASE INHIBITORS & FENOFIBRATE

Fenofibrate appears to be complementary with most statins in the treatment of familial combined hyperlipoproteinemia and other conditions involving elevations of both LDL and VLDL. The combination of fenofibrate with rosuvastatin appears to be well tolerated. Some other statins may interact unfavorably owing to effects on cytochrome P450 metabolism. In any case, particular vigilance for liver and muscle toxicity is indicated.

COMBINATIONS OF RESINS, EZETIMIBE, NIACIN, & REDUCTASE INHIBITORS

These agents act in a complementary fashion to normalize cholesterol in patients with severe disorders involving elevated LDL. The effects are sustained, and little compound toxicity has been observed. Effective doses of the individual drugs may be lower than when each is used alone; for example, as little as 1–2 g of niacin may substantially increase the effects of the other agents.

SUMMARY Drugs Used in Dyslipidemia

Subclass	Mechanism of Action	Effects	Clinical Applications	Pharmacokinetics, Toxicities, Interactions
STATINS				
• Atorvastatin, simvastatin, rosuvastatin, pitavastatin	Inhibit HMG-CoA reductase	Reduce cholesterol synthesis and up-regulate low-density lipoprotein (LDL) receptors on hepatocytes • modest reduction in triglycerides	Atherosclerotic vascular disease (primary and secondary prevention) • acute coronary syndromes	Oral • duration 12–24 h • *Toxicity:* Myopathy, hepatic dysfunction • *Interactions:* CYP-dependent metabolism (3A4, 2C9) interacts with CYP inhibitors
• *Fluvastatin, pravastatin, lovastatin: Similar but somewhat less efficacious*				
FIBRATES				
• Fenofibrate, gemfibrozil	Peroxisome proliferator-activated receptor-alpha (PPAR-α) agonists	Decrease secretion of very-low-density lipoproteins (VLDL) • increase lipoprotein lipase activity • increase high-density lipoproteins (HDL)	Hypertriglyceridemia, low HDL	Oral • duration 3–24 h • *Toxicity:* Myopathy, hepatic dysfunction
BILE ACID SEQUESTRANTS				
• Colestipol	Binds bile acids in gut • prevents reabsorption • increases cholesterol catabolism • up-regulates LDL receptors	Decreases LDL	Elevated LDL, digitalis toxicity, pruritus	Oral • taken with meals • not absorbed • *Toxicity:* Constipation, bloating • interferes with absorption of some drugs and vitamins
• *Cholestyramine, colesevelam: Similar to colestipol*				
STEROL ABSORPTION INHIBITOR				
• Ezetimibe	Blocks sterol transporter NPC1L1 in intestine brush border	Inhibits reabsorption of cholesterol excreted in bile • decreases LDL and phytosterols	Elevated LDL, phytosterolemia	Oral • duration 24 h • *Toxicity:* Low incidence of hepatic dysfunction, myositis
NIACIN				
	Decreases catabolism of apo AI • reduces VLDL secretion from liver	Increases HDL • decreases lipoprotein(a) [Lp(a)], LDL, and triglycerides	Low HDL • elevated VLDL, LDL, Lp(a)	Oral • large doses • *Toxicity:* Gastric irritation, flushing, low incidence of hepatic toxicity • may reduce glucose tolerance
• *Extended-release niacin: Similar to regular niacin*				
• *Sustained-release niacin (not the same as extended-release product): Should be avoided*				

Nonsteroidal Anti-Inflammatory Drugs, Disease-Modifying Antirheumatic Drugs, Nonopioid Analgesics, & Drugs Used in Gout

Daniel E. Furst, MD, Robert W. Ulrich, PharmD, & Shraddha Prakash, MD

CASE STUDY

A 48-year-old man presents with complaints of bilateral morning stiffness in his wrists and knees and pain in these joints on exercise. On physical examination, the joints are slightly swollen. The rest of the examination is unremarkable. His laboratory findings are also negative except for slight anemia, elevated erythrocyte sedimentation rate, and positive rheumatoid factor. With the diagnosis of rheumatoid arthritis, he is started on a regimen of naproxen, 220 mg twice daily. After 1 week, the dosage is increased to 440 mg twice daily. His symptoms are reduced at this dosage, but he complains of significant heartburn that is not controlled by antacids. He is then switched to celecoxib, 200 mg twice daily, and on this regimen his joint symptoms and heartburn resolve. Two years later, he returns with increased joint symptoms. His hands, wrists, elbows, feet, and knees are all now involved and appear swollen, warm, and tender. What therapeutic options should be considered at this time? What are the possible complications?

THE IMMUNE RESPONSE

The immune response occurs when immunologically competent cells are activated in response to foreign organisms or antigenic substances liberated during the acute or chronic inflammatory response. The outcome of the immune response for the host may be deleterious if it leads to chronic inflammation without resolution of the underlying injurious process (see Chapter 55). Chronic inflammation involves the release of a number of mediators that are not prominent in the acute response. One of the most important conditions involving these mediators is rheumatoid arthritis, in which chronic inflammation results in pain and destruction of bone and cartilage that can lead to severe disability and in which systemic changes occur that can result in shortening of life.

The cell damage associated with inflammation acts on cell membranes to release leukocyte lysosomal enzymes; arachidonic acid is then liberated from precursor compounds, and various eicosanoids are synthesized. As discussed in Chapter 18, the cyclooxygenase (COX) pathway of arachidonate metabolism produces prostaglandins, which have a variety of effects on blood vessels, on nerve endings, and on cells involved in inflammation. The lipoxygenase pathway of arachidonate metabolism yields leukotrienes, which have a powerful chemotactic effect on eosinophils, neutrophils, and macrophages and promote bronchoconstriction and alterations in vascular permeability.

The discovery of two cyclooxygenase isoforms (COX-1 and COX-2) led to the concept that the constitutive COX-1 isoform tends to be homeostatic, while COX-2 is induced during inflammation and facilitates the inflammatory response. On this basis, highly selective COX-2 inhibitors have been developed and marketed on the assumption that such selective inhibitors would be safer than nonselective COX-1 inhibitors but without loss of efficacy.

Kinins, neuropeptides, and histamine are also released at the site of tissue injury, as are complement components, cytokines, and other products of leukocytes and platelets. Stimulation of the neutrophil membranes produces oxygen-derived free radicals and other reactive molecules such as hydrogen peroxide and hydroxyl radicals. The interaction of these substances with arachidonic acid results in the generation of chemotactic substances, thus perpetuating the inflammatory process.

THERAPEUTIC STRATEGIES

The treatment of patients with inflammation involves two primary goals: first, the relief of symptoms and the maintenance of function, which are usually the major continuing complaints of the patient; and second, the slowing or arrest of the tissue-damaging process. In rheumatoid arthritis, response to therapy can be quantitated using several measures such as the Disease Activity Scale (DAS), the Clinical Disease Activity Index (CDAI), and the American College of Rheumatology Response index (ACR Response). The first two are continuous variables denoting both state and change, while the latter is solely a change measure. In the latter, the scoring values of ACR20, ACR50, and ACR70 denote the percentage of patients showing an improvement of 20%, 50%, or 70%, respectively, in a global assessment of signs and symptoms.

Reduction of inflammation with **nonsteroidal anti-inflammatory drugs (NSAIDs)** often results in relief of pain for significant periods. Furthermore, most of the nonopioid analgesics (aspirin, etc) have anti-inflammatory effects, so they are appropriate for the treatment of both acute and chronic inflammatory conditions.

The **glucocorticoids** also have powerful anti-inflammatory effects and when first introduced were considered to be the ultimate answer to the treatment of inflammatory arthritis. Although there are data that low-dose corticosteroids have disease-modifying properties, their toxicity makes them less favored than other medications, when it is possible to use the others. However, the glucocorticoids continue to have a significant role in the long-term treatment of arthritis.

Another important group of agents is characterized as **disease-modifying antirheumatic drugs (DMARDs)** and **biologics** (a subset of the DMARDs). They decrease inflammation, improve symptoms, and slow the bone damage associated with rheumatoid arthritis. They affect more basic inflammatory mechanisms than do glucocorticoids or the NSAIDs. They may also be more toxic than those alternative medications.

■ NONSTEROIDAL ANTI-INFLAMMATORY DRUGS

Salicylates and other similar agents used to treat rheumatic disease share the capacity to suppress the signs and symptoms of inflammation. These drugs also exert antipyretic and analgesic effects, but it is their anti-inflammatory properties that make them most useful in the management of disorders in which pain is related to the intensity of the inflammatory process.

Since aspirin, the original NSAID, has a number of adverse effects, many other NSAIDs have been developed in attempts to improve upon aspirin's efficacy and decrease its toxicity.

Chemistry & Pharmacokinetics

The NSAIDs are grouped in several chemical classes, as shown in Figure 36–1. This chemical diversity yields a broad range of pharmacokinetic characteristics (Table 36–1). Although there are many differences in the kinetics of NSAIDs, they have some general properties in common. All but one of the NSAIDs are weak organic acids as given; the exception, nabumetone, is a ketone prodrug that is metabolized to the acidic active drug.

Most of these drugs are well absorbed, and food does not substantially change their bioavailability. Most of the NSAIDs are highly metabolized, some by phase I followed by phase II mechanisms and others by direct glucuronidation (phase II) alone. NSAID metabolism proceeds, in large part, by way of the CYP3A or CYP2C families of P450 enzymes in the liver. While renal excretion is the most important route for final elimination, nearly all undergo varying degrees of biliary excretion and reabsorption (enterohepatic circulation). In fact, the degree of lower gastrointestinal (GI) tract irritation correlates with the amount of enterohepatic circulation. Most of the NSAIDs are highly protein-bound (~ 98%), usually to albumin. Most of the NSAIDs (eg, ibuprofen, ketoprofen) are racemic mixtures, while one, naproxen, is provided as a single enantiomer and a few have no chiral center (eg, diclofenac).

All NSAIDs can be found in synovial fluid after repeated dosing. Drugs with short half-lives remain in the joints longer than would be predicted from their half-lives, while drugs with longer half-lives disappear from the synovial fluid at a rate proportionate to their half-lives.

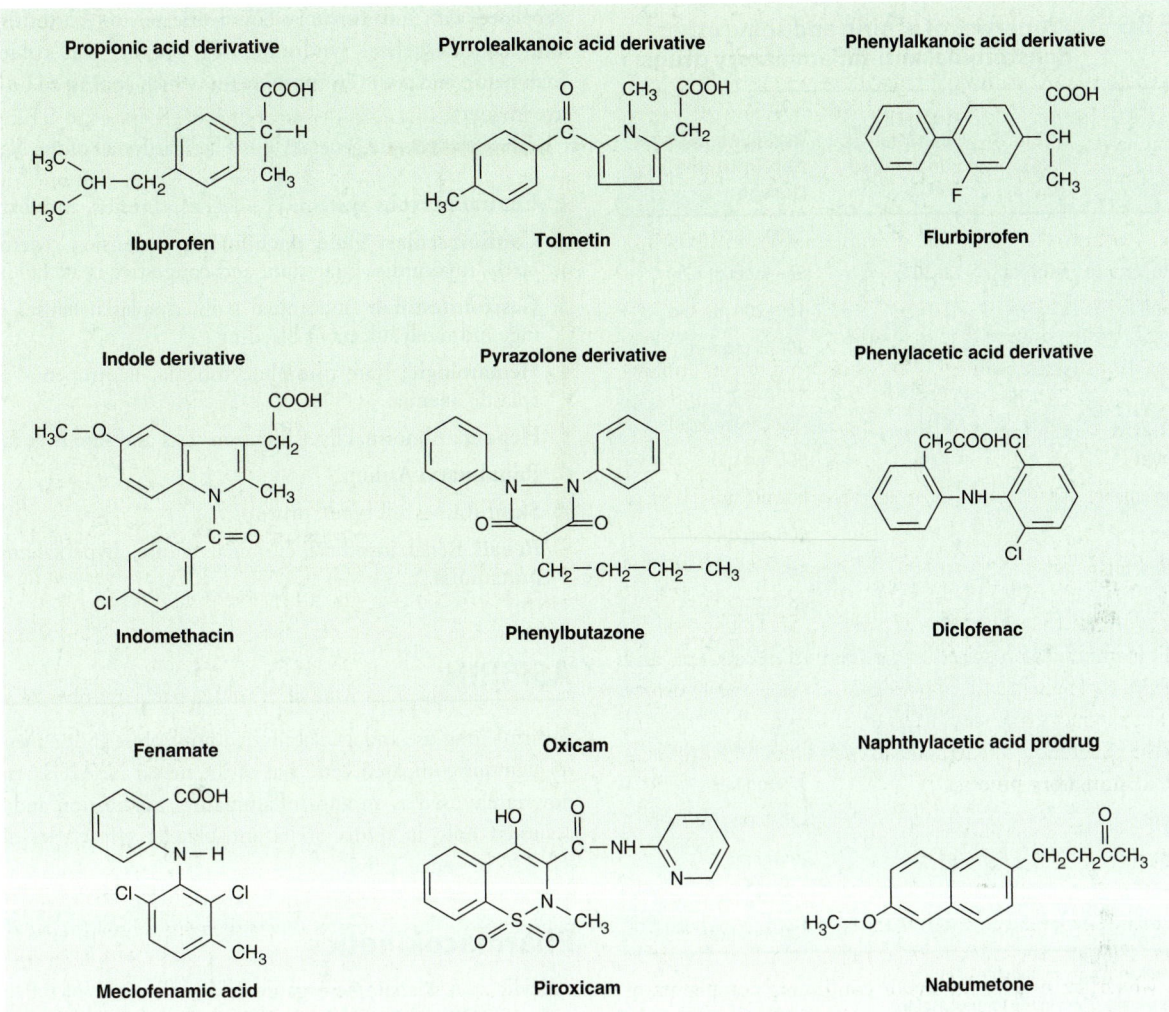

FIGURE 36–1 Chemical structures of some NSAIDs.

Pharmacodynamics

NSAID anti-inflammatory activity is mediated chiefly through inhibition of prostaglandin biosynthesis (Figure 36–2). Various NSAIDs have additional possible mechanisms of action, including inhibition of chemotaxis, down-regulation of interleukin-1 production, decreased production of free radicals and superoxide, and interference with calcium-mediated intracellular events. Aspirin irreversibly acetylates and blocks platelet cyclooxygenase, while the non-COX-selective NSAIDs are reversible inhibitors.

Selectivity for COX-1 versus COX-2 is variable and incomplete for the older NSAIDs, but selective COX-2 inhibitors have been synthesized. The selective COX-2 inhibitors do not affect platelet function at their usual doses. In testing using human whole blood, aspirin, ibuprofen, indomethacin, piroxicam, and sulindac are somewhat more effective in inhibiting COX-1. The efficacy of COX-2-selective drugs equals that of the older NSAIDs, while GI safety may be improved. On the other hand, selective COX-2 inhibitors may increase the incidence of edema and hypertension. As of August 2011, celecoxib and the less selective meloxicam were the only COX-2 inhibitors marketed in the USA. Rofecoxib and valdecoxib, two previously marketed, selective COX-2 inhibitors, were withdrawn from the market because of their association with increased cardiovascular thrombotic events. Celecoxib has a Food and Drug Administration initiated "black box" warning concerning cardiovascular risks. It has been recommended that all NSAID product labels be revised to mention cardiovascular risks.

The NSAIDs decrease the sensitivity of vessels to bradykinin and histamine, affect lymphokine production from T lymphocytes, and reverse the vasodilation of inflammation. To varying degrees, all newer NSAIDs are analgesic, anti-inflammatory, and antipyretic, and all (except the COX-2-selective agents and the nonacetylated salicylates) inhibit platelet aggregation. NSAIDs are all gastric irritants and can be associated with GI ulcers and bleeds as well, although as a group the newer agents tend to cause less GI irritation than aspirin. Nephrotoxicity has been observed for all of

TABLE 36–1 Properties of aspirin and some other nonsteroidal anti-inflammatory drugs.

Drug	Half-Life (hours)	Urinary Excretion of Unchanged Drug	Recommended Anti-inflammatory Dosage
Aspirin	0.25	<2%	1200–1500 mg tid
Salicylate[1]	2–19	2–30%	See footnote 2
Celecoxib	11	27%[3]	100–200 mg bid
Diclofenac	1.1	<1%	50–75 mg qid
Diflunisal	13	3–9%	500 mg bid
Etodolac	6.5	<1%	200–300 mg qid
Fenoprofen	2.5	30%	600 mg qid
Flurbiprofen	3.8	<1%	300 mg tid
Ibuprofen	2	<1%	600 mg qid
Indomethacin	4–5	16%	50–70 mg tid
Ketoprofen	1.8	<1%	70 mg tid
Ketorolac	4–10	58%	10 mg qid[4]
Meloxicam	20	Data not found	7.5–15 mg qd
Nabumetone[5]	26	1%	1000–2000 mg qd[6]
Naproxen	14	<1%	375 mg bid
Oxaprozin	58	1–4%	1200–1800 mg qd[6]
Piroxicam	57	4–10%	20 mg qd[6]
Sulindac	8	7%	200 mg bid
Tolmetin	1	7%	400 mg qid

[1]Major anti-inflammatory metabolite of aspirin.

[2]Salicylate is usually given in the form of aspirin.

[3]Total urinary excretion including metabolites.

[4]Recommended for treatment of acute (eg, surgical) pain only.

[5]Nabumetone is a prodrug; the half-life and urinary excretion are for its active metabolite.

[6]A single daily dose is sufficient because of the long half-life.

the drugs for which extensive experience has been reported. Nephrotoxicity is due, in part, to interference with the autoregulation of renal blood flow, which is modulated by prostaglandins. Hepatotoxicity can also occur with any NSAID.

Although these drugs effectively inhibit inflammation, there is no evidence that—in contrast to drugs such as methotrexate and other DMARDs—they alter the course of any arthritic disorder.

Several NSAIDs (including aspirin) reduce the incidence of colon cancer when taken chronically. Several large epidemiologic studies have shown a 50% reduction in relative risk when the drugs are taken for 5 years or longer. The mechanism for this protective effect is unclear.

The NSAIDs have a number of commonalities. Although not all NSAIDs are approved by the FDA for the whole range of rheumatic diseases, most are probably effective in rheumatoid arthritis, seronegative spondyloarthropathies (eg, psoriatic arthritis and arthritis associated with inflammatory bowel disease), osteoarthritis, localized musculoskeletal syndromes (eg, sprains and strains, low back pain), and gout (except tolmetin, which appears to be ineffective in gout).

Adverse effects are generally quite similar for all of the NSAIDs:

1. **Central nervous system:** Headaches, tinnitus, and dizziness.
2. **Cardiovascular:** Fluid retention, hypertension, edema, and rarely, myocardial infarction, and congestive heart failure.
3. **Gastrointestinal:** Abdominal pain, dysplasia, nausea, vomiting, and rarely, ulcers or bleeding.
4. **Hematologic:** Rare thrombocytopenia, neutropenia, or even aplastic anemia.
5. **Hepatic:** Abnormal liver function tests and rare liver failure.
6. **Pulmonary:** Asthma.
7. **Skin:** Rashes, all types, pruritus.
8. **Renal:** Renal insufficiency, renal failure, hyperkalemia, and proteinuria.

ASPIRIN

Aspirin's long use and availability without prescription diminishes its glamour compared with that of the newer NSAIDs. Aspirin is now rarely used as an anti-inflammatory medication and will be reviewed only in terms of its anti-platelet effects (ie, doses of 81–325 mg once daily).

Pharmacokinetics

Salicylic acid is a simple organic acid with a pK_a of 3.0. Aspirin (acetylsalicylic acid; ASA) has a pK_a of 3.5 (see Table 1–3). The salicylates are rapidly absorbed from the stomach and upper small intestine yielding a peak plasma salicylate level within 1–2 hours. Aspirin is absorbed as such and is rapidly hydrolyzed (serum half-life 15 minutes) to acetic acid and salicylate by esterases in tissue and blood (Figure 36–3). Salicylate is nonlinearly bound to albumin. Alkalinization of the urine increases the rate of excretion of free salicylate and its water-soluble conjugates.

Mechanisms of Action

Aspirin irreversibly inhibits platelet COX so that aspirin's anti-platelet effect lasts 8–10 days (the life of the platelet). In other tissues, synthesis of new COX replaces the inactivated enzyme so that ordinary doses have a duration of action of 6–12 hours.

Clinical Uses

Aspirin decreases the incidence of transient ischemic attacks, unstable angina, coronary artery thrombosis with myocardial infarction, and thrombosis after coronary artery bypass grafting (see Chapter 34).

Epidemiologic studies suggest that long-term use of aspirin at low dosage is associated with a lower incidence of colon cancer, possibly related to its COX-inhibiting effects.

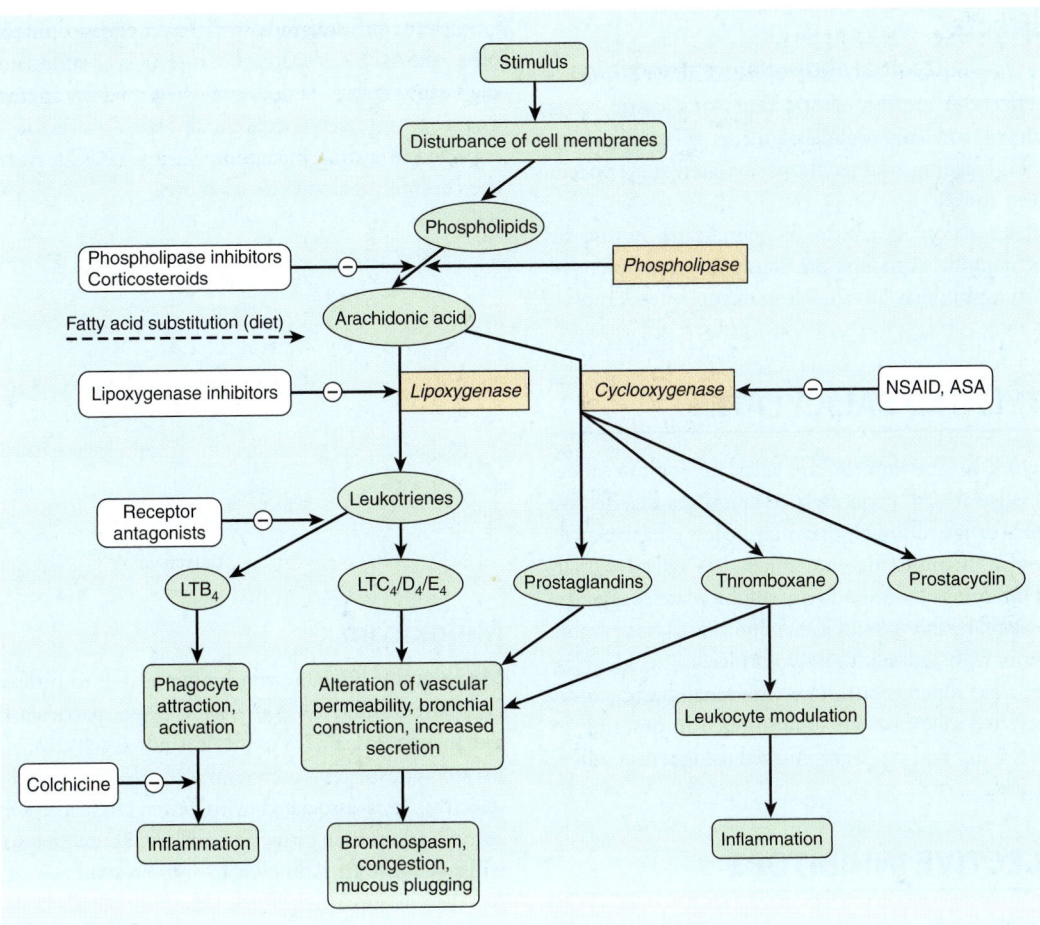

FIGURE 36–2 Prostanoid mediators derived from arachidonic acid and sites of drug action. ASA, acetylsalicylic acid (aspirin); LT, leukotriene; NSAID, nonsteroidal anti-inflammatory drug.

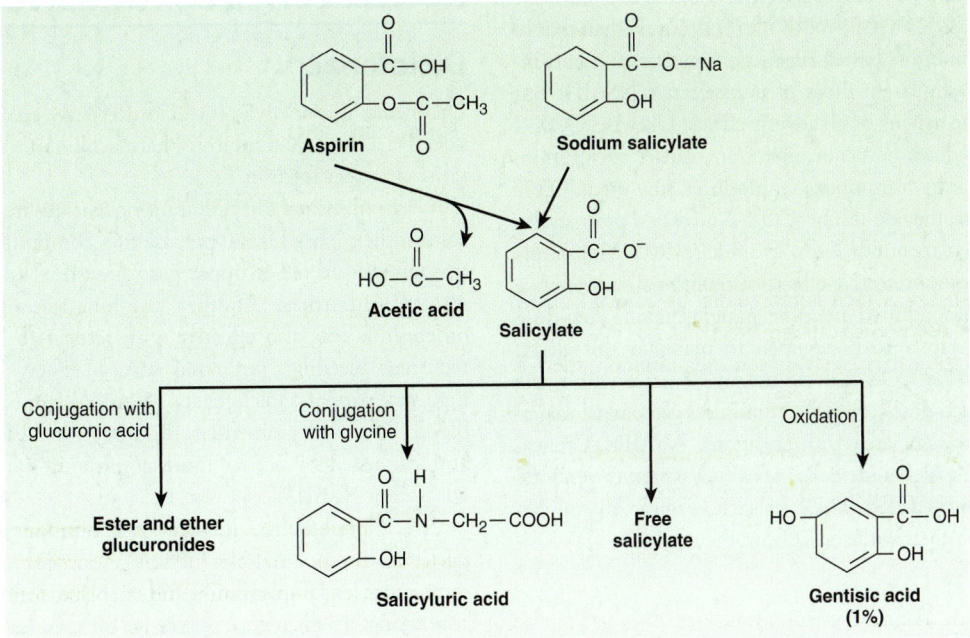

FIGURE 36–3 Structure and metabolism of the salicylates. (Modified and reproduced, with permission, from Meyers FH, Jawetz E, Goldfien A: *Review of Medical Pharmacology*, 7th ed. McGraw-Hill, 1980.)

Adverse Effects

In addition to the common side effects listed above, aspirin's main adverse effects at antithrombotic doses are gastric upset (intolerance) and gastric and duodenal ulcers. Hepatotoxicity, asthma, rashes, GI bleeding, and renal toxicity rarely if ever occur at antithrombotic doses.

The antiplatelet action of aspirin contraindicates its use by patients with hemophilia. Although previously not recommended during pregnancy, aspirin may be valuable in treating preeclampsia-eclampsia.

NONACETYLATED SALICYLATES

These drugs include magnesium choline salicylate, sodium salicylate, and salicyl salicylate. All nonacetylated salicylates are effective anti-inflammatory drugs, although they may be less effective analgesics than aspirin. Because they are much less effective than aspirin as COX inhibitors and they do not inhibit platelet aggregation, they may be preferable when COX inhibition is undesirable such as in patients with asthma, those with bleeding tendencies, and even (under close supervision) those with renal dysfunction.

The nonacetylated salicylates are administered in doses up to 3–4 g of salicylate a day and can be monitored using serum salicylate measurements.

COX-2 SELECTIVE INHIBITORS

COX-2 selective inhibitors, or coxibs, were developed in an attempt to inhibit prostaglandin synthesis by the COX-2 isozyme induced at sites of inflammation without affecting the action of the constitutively active "housekeeping" COX-1 isozyme found in the GI tract, kidneys, and platelets. Coxibs selectively bind to and block the active site of the COX-2 enzyme much more effectively than that of COX-1. COX-2 inhibitors have analgesic, antipyretic, and anti-inflammatory effects similar to those of non-selective NSAIDs but with an approximate halving of GI adverse effects. Likewise, COX-2 inhibitors at usual doses have no impact on platelet aggregation, which is mediated by thromboxane produced by the COX-1 isozyme. In contrast, they do inhibit COX-2-mediated prostacyclin synthesis in the vascular endothelium. As a result, COX-2 inhibitors do not offer the cardioprotective effects of traditional nonselective NSAIDs, which has resulted in some patients taking low-dose aspirin in addition to a coxib regimen to maintain this effect. Unfortunately, because COX-2 is constitutively active within the kidney, recommended doses of COX-2 inhibitors cause renal toxicities similar to those associated with traditional NSAIDs. Clinical data have suggested a higher incidence of cardiovascular thrombotic events associated with COX-2 inhibitors such as rofecoxib and valdecoxib, resulting in their withdrawal from the market.

Celecoxib

Celecoxib is a selective COX-2 inhibitor—about 10–20 times more selective for COX-2 than for COX-1. Pharmacokinetic and dosage considerations are given in Table 36–1.

Celecoxib is associated with fewer endoscopic ulcers than most other NSAIDs. Probably because it is a sulfonamide, celecoxib may cause rashes. It does not affect platelet aggregation at usual doses. It interacts occasionally with warfarin—as would be expected of a drug metabolized via CYP2C9. Adverse effects are the common toxicities listed above.

Celecoxib

Meloxicam

Meloxicam is an enolcarboxamide related to piroxicam that preferentially inhibits COX-2 over COX-1, particularly at its lowest therapeutic dose of 7.5 mg/d. It is not as selective as celecoxib and may be considered "preferentially" selective rather than "highly" selective. It is associated with fewer clinical GI symptoms and complications than piroxicam, diclofenac, and naproxen. Similarly, while meloxicam is known to inhibit synthesis of thromboxane A_2, even at supratherapeutic doses, its blockade of thromboxane A_2 does not reach levels that result in decreased in vivo platelet function (see common adverse effects above).

NONSELECTIVE COX INHIBITORS

Diclofenac

Diclofenac is a phenylacetic acid derivative that is relatively nonselective as a COX inhibitor. Pharmacokinetic and dosage characteristics are set forth in Table 36–1.

Gastrointestinal ulceration may occur less frequently than with some other NSAIDs. A preparation combining diclofenac and misoprostol decreases upper gastrointestinal ulceration but may result in diarrhea. Another combination of diclofenac and omeprazole was also effective with respect to the prevention of recurrent bleeding, but renal adverse effects were common in high-risk patients. Diclofenac, 150 mg/d, appears to impair renal blood flow and glomerular filtration rate. Elevation of serum aminotransferases occurs more commonly with this drug than with other NSAIDs.

A 0.1% ophthalmic preparation is promoted for prevention of postoperative ophthalmic inflammation and can be used after intraocular lens implantation and strabismus surgery. A topical gel containing 3% diclofenac is effective for solar keratoses. Diclofenac in rectal suppository form can be considered for preemptive analgesia and postoperative nausea. In Europe, diclofenac is also available as an oral mouthwash and for intramuscular administration.

Diflunisal

Although diflunisal is derived from salicylic acid, it is not metabolized to salicylic acid or salicylate. It undergoes an enterohepatic cycle with reabsorption of its glucuronide metabolite followed by cleavage of the glucuronide to again release the active moiety. Diflunisal is subject to capacity-limited metabolism, with serum half-lives at various dosages approximating that of salicylates (Table 36–1). In rheumatoid arthritis the recommended dose is 500–1000 mg daily in two divided doses. It is claimed to be particularly effective for cancer pain with bone metastases and for pain control in dental (third molar) surgery. A 2% diflunisal oral ointment is a clinically useful analgesic for painful oral lesions.

Because its clearance depends on renal function as well as hepatic metabolism, diflunisal's dosage should be limited in patients with significant renal impairment.

Etodolac

Etodolac is a racemic acetic acid derivative with an intermediate half-life (Table 36–1). Etodolac does not undergo chiral inversion in the body. The dosage of etodolac is 200–400 mg three to four times daily.

Flurbiprofen

Flurbiprofen is a propionic acid derivative with a possibly more complex mechanism of action than other NSAIDs. Its (S)(–) enantiomer inhibits COX nonselectively, but it has been shown in rat tissue to also affect tumor necrosis factor-α (TNF-α) and nitric oxide synthesis. Hepatic metabolism is extensive; its (R)(+) and (S) (–) enantiomers are metabolized differently, and it does not undergo chiral conversion. It does demonstrate enterohepatic circulation.

Flurbiprofen is also available in a topical ophthalmic formulation for inhibition of intraoperative miosis. Flurbiprofen intravenously is effective for perioperative analgesia in minor ear, neck, and nose surgery and in lozenge form for sore throat.

Although its adverse effect profile is similar to that of other NSAIDs in most ways, flurbiprofen is also rarely associated with cogwheel rigidity, ataxia, tremor, and myoclonus.

Ibuprofen

Ibuprofen is a simple derivative of phenylpropionic acid (Figure 36–1). In doses of about 2400 mg daily, ibuprofen is equivalent to 4 g of aspirin in anti-inflammatory effect. Pharmacokinetic characteristics are given in Table 36–1.

Oral ibuprofen is often prescribed in lower doses (<2400 mg/d), at which it has analgesic but not anti-inflammatory efficacy. It is available over the counter in low-dose forms under several trade names.

Ibuprofen is effective in closing patent ductus arteriosus in preterm infants, with much the same efficacy and safety as indomethacin. The oral and intravenous routes are equally effective for this indication. A topical cream preparation appears to be absorbed

into fascia and muscle; an (S)(–) formulation has been tested. Ibuprofen cream was more effective than placebo cream in the treatment of primary knee osteoarthritis. A liquid gel preparation of ibuprofen, 400 mg, provides prompt relief and good overall efficacy in postsurgical dental pain.

In comparison with indomethacin, ibuprofen decreases urine output less and also causes less fluid retention. The drug is relatively contraindicated in individuals with nasal polyps, angioedema, and bronchospastic reactivity to aspirin. Aseptic meningitis (particularly in patients with systemic lupus erythematosus), and fluid retention have been reported. Interaction with anticoagulants is uncommon. The concomitant administration of ibuprofen and aspirin antagonizes the irreversible platelet inhibition induced by aspirin. Thus, treatment with ibuprofen in patients with increased cardiovascular risk may limit the cardioprotective effects of aspirin. Furthermore, the use of ibuprofen concomitantly with aspirin may *decrease* the total anti-inflammatory effect. Common adverse effects are listed on page 638; rare hematologic effects include agranulocytosis and aplastic anemia.

Indomethacin

Indomethacin, introduced in 1963, is an indole derivative (Figure 36–1). It is a potent nonselective COX inhibitor and may also inhibit phospholipase A and C, reduce neutrophil migration, and decrease T-cell and B-cell proliferation.

It differs somewhat from other NSAIDs in its indications and toxicities.

It has been used to accelerate closure of patent ductus arteriosus. Indomethacin has been tried in numerous small or uncontrolled trials for many other conditions, including Sweet's syndrome, juvenile rheumatoid arthritis, pleurisy, nephrotic syndrome, diabetes insipidus, urticarial vasculitis, postepisiotomy pain, and prophylaxis of heterotopic ossification in arthroplasty.

An ophthalmic preparation is efficacious for conjunctival inflammation and to reduce pain after traumatic corneal abrasion. Gingival inflammation is reduced after administration of indomethacin oral rinse. Epidural injections produce a degree of pain relief similar to that achieved with methylprednisolone in postlaminectomy syndrome.

At usual doses, indomethacin has the common side effects listed above. The GI effects may include pancreatitis. Headache is experienced by 15–25% of patients and may be associated with dizziness, confusion, and depression. Rarely, psychosis with hallucinations has been reported. Renal papillary necrosis has also been observed. A number of interactions with other drugs have been reported (see Chapter 66). Probenecid prolongs indomethacin's half-life by inhibiting both renal and biliary clearance.

Ketoprofen

Ketoprofen is a propionic acid derivative that inhibits both COX (nonselectively) and lipoxygenase. Its pharmacokinetic characteristics are given in Table 36–1. Concurrent administration of probenecid elevates ketoprofen levels and prolongs its plasma half-life.

The effectiveness of ketoprofen at dosages of 100–300 mg/d is equivalent to that of other NSAIDs. In spite of its dual effect on prostaglandins and leukotrienes, ketoprofen is not superior to other NSAIDs in clinical efficacy. Its major adverse effects are on the GI tract and the central nervous system (see common adverse effects above).

Ketorolac

Ketorolac is an NSAID promoted for systemic use mainly as an analgesic, not as an anti-inflammatory drug (although it has typical NSAID properties). Pharmacokinetics are presented in Table 36–1. The drug is an effective analgesic and has been used successfully to replace morphine in some situations involving mild to moderate postsurgical pain. It is most often given intramuscularly or intravenously, but an oral dose formulation is available. When used with an opioid, it may decrease the opioid requirement by 25–50%. An ophthalmic preparation is available for ocular inflammatory conditions. Toxicities are similar to those of other NSAIDs (see page 638), although renal toxicity may be more common with chronic use.

Nabumetone

Nabumetone is the only nonacid NSAID in current use; it is converted to the active acetic acid derivative in the body. It is given as a ketone prodrug that resembles naproxen in structure (Figure 36–1). Its half-life of more than 24 hours (Table 36–1) permits once-daily dosing, and the drug does not appear to undergo enterohepatic circulation. Renal impairment results in a doubling of its half-life and a 30% increase in the area under the curve.

Its properties are very similar to those of other NSAIDs, though it may be less damaging to the stomach than some other NSAIDs when given at a dosage of 1000 mg/d. Unfortunately, higher dosages (eg, 1500–2000 mg/d) are often needed, and this is a very expensive NSAID. Like naproxen, nabumetone has been associated with pseudoporphyria and photosensitivity in some patients. Other adverse effects mirror those of other NSAIDs.

Naproxen

Naproxen is a naphthylpropionic acid derivative. It is the only NSAID presently marketed as a single enantiomer. Naproxen's free fraction is significantly higher in women than in men, but half-life is similar in both sexes (Table 36–1). Naproxen is effective for the usual rheumatologic indications and is available in a slow-release formulation, as an oral suspension, and over the counter. A topical preparation and an ophthalmic solution are also available.

The incidence of upper GI bleeding in over-the-counter use is low but still double that of over-the-counter ibuprofen (perhaps due to a dose effect). Rare cases of allergic pneumonitis, leukocytoclastic vasculitis, and pseudoporphyria as well as the common NSAID-associated adverse effects have been noted.

Oxaprozin

Oxaprozin is another propionic acid derivative NSAID. As noted in Table 36–1, its major difference from the other members of this

subgroup is a very long half-life (50–60 hours), although oxaprozin does not undergo enterohepatic circulation. It is mildly uricosuric, making it potentially more useful in gout than some other NSAIDs. Otherwise, the drug has the same benefits and risks that are associated with other NSAIDs.

Piroxicam

Piroxicam, an oxicam (Figure 36–1), is a nonselective COX inhibitor that at high concentrations also inhibits polymorphonuclear leukocyte migration, decreases oxygen radical production, and inhibits lymphocyte function. Its long half-life (Table 36–1) permits once-daily dosing.

Piroxicam can be used for the usual rheumatic indications. When piroxicam is used in dosages higher than 20 mg/d, an increased incidence of peptic ulcer and bleeding is encountered. Epidemiologic studies suggest that this risk is as much as 9.5 times higher with piroxicam than with other NSAIDs (see common adverse effects above).

Sulindac

Sulindac is a sulfoxide prodrug. It is reversibly metabolized to the active sulfide metabolite, which is excreted in bile and then reabsorbed from the intestine. The enterohepatic cycling prolongs the duration of action to 12–16 hours.

In addition to its rheumatic disease indications, sulindac suppresses familial intestinal polyposis and it may inhibit the development of colon, breast, and prostate cancer in humans. It appears to inhibit the occurrence of GI cancer in rats. The latter effect may be caused by the sulfone rather than the sulfide.

Among the more severe adverse reactions, Stevens-Johnson epidermal necrolysis syndrome, thrombocytopenia, agranulocytosis, and nephrotic syndrome have all been observed. Like diclofenac, sulindac may have some propensity to cause elevation of serum aminotransferases; it is also sometimes associated with cholestatic liver damage, which disappears when the drug is stopped.

Tolmetin

Tolmetin is a nonselective COX inhibitor with a short half-life (1–2 hours) and is not often used. Its efficacy and toxicity profiles are similar to those of other NSAIDs with the following exceptions: it is ineffective (for unknown reasons) in the treatment of gout, and it may cause (rarely) thrombocytopenic purpura.

Other NSAIDs

Azapropazone, carprofen, meclofenamate, and **tenoxicam** are rarely used and are not reviewed here.

CHOICE OF NSAID

All NSAIDs, including aspirin, are about equally efficacious with a few exceptions—tolmetin seems not to be effective for gout, and aspirin is less effective than other NSAIDs (eg, indomethacin) for ankylosing spondylitis.

Thus, NSAIDs tend to be differentiated on the basis of toxicity and cost-effectiveness. For example, the GI and renal side effects of ketorolac limit its use. Some surveys suggest that indomethacin and tolmetin are the NSAIDs associated with the greatest toxicity, while salsalate, aspirin, and ibuprofen are least toxic. The selective COX-2 inhibitors were not included in these analyses.

For patients with renal insufficiency, nonacetylated salicylates may be best. Diclofenac and sulindac are associated with more liver function test abnormalities than other NSAIDs. The relatively expensive, selective COX-2 inhibitor celecoxib is probably safest for patients at high risk for GI bleeding but may have a higher risk of cardiovascular toxicity. Celecoxib or a nonselective NSAID plus omeprazole or misoprostol may be appropriate in patients at highest risk for GI bleeding; in this subpopulation of patients, they are cost-effective despite their high acquisition costs.

The choice of an NSAID thus requires a balance of efficacy, cost-effectiveness, safety, and numerous personal factors (eg, other drugs also being used, concurrent illness, compliance, medical insurance coverage), so that there is no best NSAID for all patients. There may, however, be one or two best NSAIDs for a specific person.

■ DISEASE-MODIFYING ANTIRHEUMATIC DRUGS

Rheumatoid arthritis is an immunologic disease that causes significant systemic effects, shortens life, and reduces mobility and quality of life. Interest has centered on finding treatments that might arrest—or at least slow—this progression by modifying the disease itself. The effects of disease-modifying therapies may take 6 weeks to 6 months to become clinically evident, although some biologics are effective within 2 weeks or less.

These therapies include nonbiologic disease-modifying antirheumatic drugs (usually designated "DMARDs") such as methotrexate, azathioprine, chloroquine and hydroxychloroquine, cyclophosphamide, cyclosporine, leflunomide, mycophenolate mofetil, and sulfasalazine. Gold salts, which were once extensively used, are no longer recommended because of their significant toxicities and questionable efficacy.

There are also several biologic DMARDs (designated "biologics") marketed for rheumatoid arthritis: a T-cell-modulating biologic (abatacept), a B-cell cytotoxic agent (rituximab), an anti-IL-6 receptor antibody (tocilizumab), and the TNF-α-blocking agents (five drugs).

These DMARDs and biologics are discussed alphabetically, independent of origin.

ABATACEPT

Mechanism of Action

Abatacept is a co-stimulation modulator biologic that inhibits the activation of T cells (see also Chapter 55). After a T cell has engaged an antigen-presenting cell (APC), a second signal is produced by CD28 on the T cell that interacts with CD80 or CD86 on the APC, leading to T-cell activation. Abatacept (which contains the endogenous ligand CTLA-4) binds to CD80 and 86, thereby inhibiting the binding to CD28 and preventing the activation of T cells.

Pharmacokinetics

Abatacept is given as three intravenous infusion "induction" doses (day 0, week 2, and week 4), followed by monthly infusions. The dose is based on body weight; patients weighing less than 60 kg receiving 500 mg, those 60–100 kg receiving 750 mg, and those more than 100 kg receiving 1000 mg. Dosing regimens in any adult group can be increased if needed. The terminal serum half-life is 13–16 days. Co-administration with methotrexate, NSAIDs, and corticosteroids does not influence abatacept clearance.

Indications

Abatacept can be used as monotherapy or in combination with other DMARDs in patients with moderate to severe rheumatoid arthritis who have had an inadequate response to other DMARDs. It reduces the clinical signs and symptoms of rheumatoid arthritis, including slowing of radiographic progression. It is also being tested in early rheumatoid arthritis.

Adverse Effects

There is a slightly increased risk of infection (as with other biologic DMARDs), predominantly of the upper respiratory tract. Concomitant use with TNF-α antagonists is not recommended due to the increased incidence of serious infection. Infusion-related reactions and hypersensitivity reactions, including anaphylaxis, have been reported but are rare. Anti-abatacept antibody formation is infrequent (<5%) and has no effect on clinical outcomes. There is a possible increase in lymphomas but not in other malignancies when using abatacept.

AZATHIOPRINE

Mechanism of Action

Azathioprine is a synthetic DMARD that acts through its major metabolite, 6-thioguanine. 6-Thioguanine suppresses inosinic acid synthesis, B-cell and T-cell function, immunoglobulin production, and interleukin-2 secretion (see Chapter 55).

Pharmacokinetics

The metabolism of azathioprine is bimodal in humans, with rapid metabolizers clearing the drug four times faster than slow metabolizers. Production of 6-thioguanine is dependent on thiopurine methyltransferase (TPMT), and patients with low or absent TPMT activity (0.3% of the population) are at particularly high risk of myelosuppression by excess concentrations of the parent drug, if dosage is not adjusted.

Indications

Azathioprine is approved for use in rheumatoid arthritis and is used at a dosage of 2 mg/kg/d. Controlled trials show efficacy in psoriatic arthritis, reactive arthritis, polymyositis, systemic lupus erythematosus, and Behçet's disease.

Adverse Effects

Azathioprine's toxicity includes bone marrow suppression, GI disturbances, and some increase in infection risk. As noted in Chapter 55, lymphomas may be increased with azathioprine use. Rarely, fever, rash, and hepatotoxicity signal acute allergic reactions.

CHLOROQUINE & HYDROXYCHLOROQUINE

Mechanism of Action

Chloroquine and hydroxychloroquine are nonbiologic drugs mainly used for malaria (see Chapter 52) and in the rheumatic diseases. The mechanism of the anti-inflammatory action of these drugs in rheumatic diseases is unclear. The following mechanisms have been proposed: suppression of T-lymphocyte responses to mitogens, decreased leukocyte chemotaxis, stabilization of lysosomal enzymes, inhibition of DNA and RNA synthesis, and the trapping of free radicals.

Pharmacokinetics

Antimalarials are rapidly absorbed and 50% protein-bound in the plasma. They are very extensively tissue-bound, particularly in melanin-containing tissues such as the eyes. The drugs are deaminated in the liver and have blood elimination half-lives of up to 45 days.

Indications

Antimalarials are approved for rheumatoid arthritis, but they are not considered very effective DMARDs. Dose-response and serum concentration-response relationships have been documented for hydroxychloroquine and dose-loading may increase rate of response. Although antimalarials improve symptoms, there is no evidence that these compounds alter bony damage in rheumatoid arthritis at their usual dosages (up to 6.4 mg/kg/d for hydroxychloroquine or 200 mg/d for chloroquine). It usually takes 3–6 months to obtain a response. Antimalarials are often used in the treatment of the skin manifestations, serositis, and joint pains of systemic lupus erythematosus, and they have been used in Sjögren's syndrome.

Adverse Effects

Although ocular toxicity (see Chapter 52) may occur at dosages greater than 250 mg/d for chloroquine and greater than 6.4 mg/kg/d for hydroxychloroquine, it rarely occurs at lower doses. Nevertheless, ophthalmologic monitoring every 12 months is advised. Other toxicities include dyspepsia, nausea, vomiting, abdominal pain, rashes, and nightmares. These drugs appear to be relatively safe in pregnancy.

CYCLOPHOSPHAMIDE

Mechanism of Action

Cyclophosphamide is a synthetic DMARD. Its major active metabolite is phosphoramide mustard, which cross-links DNA to prevent cell replication. It suppresses T-cell and B-cell function by 30–40%; T-cell suppression correlates with clinical response in the rheumatic diseases. Its pharmacokinetics and toxicities are discussed in Chapter 54.

Indications

Cyclophosphamide is active against rheumatoid arthritis when given orally at dosages of 2 mg/kg/d but not intravenously. It is used regularly to treat systemic lupus erythematosus, vasculitis, Wegener's granulomatosis, and other severe rheumatic diseases.

CYCLOSPORINE

Mechanism of Action

Cyclosporine is a peptide antibiotic but is considered a nonbiologic DMARD. Through regulation of gene transcription, it inhibits interleukin-1 and interleukin-2 production and secondarily inhibits macrophage–T-cell interaction and T-cell responsiveness (see Chapter 55). T-cell-dependent B-cell function is also affected.

Pharmacokinetics

Cyclosporine absorption is incomplete and somewhat erratic, although a microemulsion formulation improves its consistency and provides 20–30% bioavailability. Grapefruit juice increases cyclosporine bioavailability by as much as 62%. Cyclosporine is metabolized by CYP3A and consequently is subject to a large number of drug interactions (see Chapters 55 and 66).

Indications

Cyclosporine is approved for use in rheumatoid arthritis and retards the appearance of new bony erosions. Its usual dosage is 3–5 mg/kg/d divided into two doses. Anecdotal reports suggest that it may be useful in systemic lupus erythematosus, polymyositis and dermatomyositis, Wegener's granulomatosis, and juvenile chronic arthritis.

Adverse Effects

Leukopenia, thrombocytopenia, and to a lesser extent, anemia, are predictable. High doses can be cardiotoxic and sterilty may occur after chronic dosing at anti-rheumatic doses, especially in women. Bladder cancer is very rare but must be looked for, even 5 years after cessation of use.

LEFLUNOMIDE

Mechanism of Action

Leflunomide, another nonbiologic DMARD, undergoes rapid conversion, both in the intestine and in the plasma, to its active metabolite, A77-1726. This metabolite inhibits dihydroorotate dehydrogenase, leading to a decrease in ribonucleotide synthesis and the arrest of stimulated cells in the G_1 phase of cell growth. Consequently, leflunomide inhibits T-cell proliferation and production of autoantibodies by B cells. Secondary effects include increases of interleukin-10 receptor mRNA, decreased interleukin-8 receptor type A mRNA, and decreased TNF-α-dependent nuclear factor kappa B (NF-κB) activation.

Pharmacokinetics

Leflunomide is completely absorbed and has a mean plasma half-life of 19 days. Its active metabolite, A77-1726, is thought to have approximately the same half-life and is subject to enterohepatic recirculation. Cholestyramine can enhance leflunomide excretion and increases total clearance by approximately 50%.

Indications

Leflunomide is as effective as methotrexate in rheumatoid arthritis, including inhibition of bony damage. In one study, combined treatment with methotrexate and leflunomide resulted in a 46.2% ACR20 response compared with 19.5% in patients receiving methotrexate alone.

Adverse Effects

Diarrhea occurs in approximately 25% of patients given leflunomide, although only about 3–5% discontinue the drug because of this side effect. Elevation in liver enzymes can occur. Both effects can be reduced by decreasing the dose of leflunomide. Other adverse effects associated with leflunomide are mild alopecia, weight gain, and increased blood pressure. Leukopenia and thrombocytopenia occur rarely. This drug is contraindicated in pregnancy.

METHOTREXATE

Methotrexate, a synthetic antimetabolite, is now considered the first-line DMARD for treatment of rheumatoid arthritis and is used in 50–70% of patients. It is active in this condition at much lower doses than those needed in cancer chemotherapy (see Chapter 54).

Mechanism of Action

Methotrexate's principal mechanism of action at the low doses used in the rheumatic diseases probably relates to inhibition of aminoimidazolecarboxamide ribonucleotide (AICAR) transformylase and thymidylate synthetase. AICAR, which accumulates intracellularly, competitively inhibits AMP deaminase, leading to an accumulation of AMP. The AMP is released and converted extracellularly to adenosine, which is a potent inhibitor of inflammation. As a result,

the inflammatory functions of neutrophils, macrophages, dendritic cells, and lymphocytes are suppressed. Methotrexate has secondary effects on polymorphonuclear chemotaxis. There is some effect on dihydrofolate reductase and this affects lymphocyte and macrophage function, but this is not its principal mechanism of action. Methotrexate has direct inhibitory effects on proliferation and stimulates apoptosis in immune-inflammatory cells. Additionally, it has also been shown to have inhibition of proinflammatory cytokines linked to rheumatoid synovitis.

Pharmacokinetics

The drug is approximately 70% absorbed after oral administration (see Chapter 54). It is metabolized to a less active hydroxylated metabolite. Both the parent compound and the metabolite are polyglutamated within cells where they stay for prolonged periods. Methotrexate's serum half-life is usually only 6–9 hours, although it may be as long as 24 hours in some individuals. Methotrexate's concentration is increased in the presence of hydroxychloroquine, which can reduce the clearance or increase the tubular reabsorption of methotrexate. This drug is excreted principally in the urine, but up to 30% may be excreted in bile.

Indications

Although the most common methotrexate dosing regimen for the treatment of rheumatoid arthritis is 15–25 mg weekly, there is an increased effect up to 30–35 mg weekly. The drug decreases the rate of appearance of new erosions. Evidence supports its use in juvenile chronic arthritis, and it has been used in psoriasis, psoriatic arthritis, ankylosing spondylitis, polymyositis, dermatomyositis, Wegener's granulomatosis, giant cell arteritis, systemic lupus erythematosus, and vasculitis.

Adverse Effects

Nausea and mucosal ulcers are the most common toxicities. Additionally, many other side effects such as leukopenia, anemia, stomatitis, GI ulcerations, and alopecia are probably the result of inhibiting cellular proliferation. Progressive dose-related hepatotoxicity in the form of enzyme elevation occurs frequently, but cirrhosis is rare (<1%). Liver toxicity is not related to serum methotrexate concentrations. Rare hypersensitivity-like lung reaction with acute shortness of breath has been documented, as have pseudo-lymphomatous reactions. The incidence of GI and liver function test abnormalities can be reduced by the use of leucovorin 24 hours after each weekly dose or by the use of daily folic acid, although this may decrease the efficacy of the methotrexate by about 10%. This drug is contraindicated in pregnancy.

MYCOPHENOLATE MOFETIL

Mechanism of Action

Mycophenolate mofetil (MMF), a semisynthetic DMARD, is converted to mycophenolic acid, the active form of the drug. The active product inhibits inosine monophosphate dehydrogenase, leading to suppression of T- and B-lymphocyte proliferation. Downstream, it interferes with leukocyte adhesion to endothelial cells through inhibition of E-selectin, P-selectin, and intercellular adhesion molecule 1. MMF's pharmacokinetics and toxicities are discussed in Chapter 55.

Indications

MMF is effective for the treatment of renal disease due to systemic lupus erythematosus and may be useful in vasculitis and Wegener's granulomatosis. Although MMF is occasionally used at a dosage of 2 g/d to treat rheumatoid arthritis, there are no well-controlled data regarding its efficacy in this disease.

Adverse Effects

MMF is associated with nausea, dyspepsia and abdominal pain. Like azathioprine, it can cause hepatotoxicity although it is not associated with the acute febrile hepatotoxicity of that drug. MMF can cause leukopenia, thrombocytopenia, and anemia. MMF is associated with an increased incidence of infections. It is only rarely associated with malignancy.

RITUXIMAB

Mechanism of Action

Rituximab is a chimeric monoclonal antibody biologic agent that targets CD20 B lymphocytes (see Chapter 55). This depletion takes place through cell-mediated and complement-dependent cytotoxicity and stimulation of cell apoptosis. Depletion of B lymphocytes reduces inflammation by decreasing the presentation of antigens to T lymphocytes and inhibiting the secretion of proinflammatory cytokines. Rituximab rapidly depletes peripheral B cells, although this depletion correlates neither with efficacy nor with toxicity.

Pharmacokinetics

Rituximab is given as two intravenous infusions of 1000 mg, separated by 2 weeks. It may be repeated every 6–9 months, as needed. Repeated courses remain effective. Pretreatment with intravenous glucocorticoids given 30 minutes prior to infusion (usually 100 mg of methylprednisolone) decreases the incidence and severity of infusion reactions.

Indications

Rituximab is indicated for the treatment of moderately to severely active rheumatoid arthritis in combination with methotrexate in patients with an inadequate response to one or more TNF-α antagonists.

Adverse Effects

About 30% of patients develop rash with the first 1000 mg treatment; this incidence decreases to about 10% with the second infusion and progressively decreases with each course of therapy

thereafter. These rashes do not usually require discontinuation of therapy but of course an urticarial or anaphylactoid reaction precludes further therapy. Immunoglobulins (particularly IgG and IgM) may decrease with repeated courses of therapy and infections can occur, although they do not seem directly associated with the decreases in immunoglobulins. Rituximab has not been associated with either activation of tuberculosis or the occurrence of lymphomas or other tumors (see Chapter 55). Other adverse effects, like cardiovascular events, are rare.

SULFASALAZINE

Mechanism of Action

Sulfasalazine, a synthetic DMARD, is metabolized to sulfapyridine and 5-aminosalicylic acid. The sulfapyridine is probably the active moiety when treating rheumatoid arthritis (unlike inflammatory bowel disease, see Chapter 62). Some authorities believe that the parent compound, sulfasalazine, also has an effect. In treated arthritis patients, IgA and IgM rheumatoid factor production are decreased. Suppression of T-cell responses to concanavalin and inhibition of in vitro B-cell proliferation have also been documented. In vitro, sulfasalazine or its metabolites inhibit the release of inflammatory cytokines, including those produced by monocytes or macrophages, eg, interleukins-1, -6, and -12, and TNF-α. These findings suggest a possible mechanism for the clinical efficacy of sulfasalazine in rheumatoid arthritis.

Pharmacokinetics

Only 10–20% of orally administered sulfasalazine is absorbed, although a fraction undergoes enterohepatic recirculation into the bowel where it is reduced by intestinal bacteria to liberate sulfapyridine and 5-aminosalicylic acid (see Figure 62–8). Sulfapyridine is well absorbed while 5-aminosalicylic acid remains unabsorbed. Some sulfasalazine is excreted unchanged in the urine whereas sulfapyridine is excreted after hepatic acetylation and hydroxylation. Sulfasalazine's half-life is 6–17 hours.

Indications

Sulfasalazine is effective in rheumatoid arthritis and reduces radiologic disease progression. It has also been used in juvenile chronic arthritis and in ankylosing spondylitis and its associated uveitis. The usual regimen is 2–3 g/d.

Adverse Effects

Approximately 30% of patients using sulfasalazine discontinue the drug because of toxicity. Common adverse effects include nausea, vomiting, headache, and rash. Hemolytic anemia and methemoglobinemia also occur, but rarely. Neutropenia occurs in 1–5% of patients, while thrombocytopenia is very rare. Pulmonary toxicity and positive double-stranded DNA (dsDNA) are occasionally seen, but drug-induced lupus is rare. Reversible infertility occurs in men, but sulfasalazine does not affect fertility in women. The drug does not appear to be teratogenic.

TOCILIZUMAB

Mechanism of Action

Tocilizumab, a newer biologic humanized antibody, binds to soluble and membrane-bound IL-6 receptors, and inhibit the IL-6-mediated signaling via these receptors. IL-6 is a proinflammatory cytokine produced by different cell types including T cells, B cells, monocytes, fibroblasts, and synovial and endothelial cells. IL-6 is involved in a variety of physiologic processes such as T-cell activation, hepatic acute-phase protein synthesis, and stimulation of the inflammatory processes involved in diseases such as rheumatoid arthritis.

Pharmacokinetics

The half-life of tocilizumab is dose-dependent, approximately 11 days for the 4 mg/kg dose and 13 days for the 8 mg/kg dose. IL-6 can suppress several CYP450 isoenzymes; thus, inhibiting IL-6 may restore CYP450 activities to higher levels. This may be clinically relevant for drugs that are CYP450 substrates and have a narrow therapeutic window (eg, cyclosporine or warfarin), and dosage adjustment of these medications may be needed.

Tocilizumab can be used in combination with nonbiologic DMARDs or as monotherapy. The recommended starting dose is 4 mg/kg intravenously every 4 weeks followed by an increase to 8 mg/kg dependent on clinical response. Additionally, dosage modifications are recommended on the basis of certain laboratory changes, elevated liver enzymes, neutropenia, and thrombocytopenia.

Indications

Tocilizumab is indicated for adult patients with moderately to severely active rheumatoid arthritis who have had an inadequate response to one or more TNF antagonists.

Adverse Effects

Serious infections including tuberculosis, fungal, viral, and other opportunistic infections have occurred. Screening for tuberculosis should be done prior to beginning tocilizumab. The most common adverse reactions were upper respiratory tract infections, headache, hypertension, and elevated liver enzymes.

Neutropenia and reduction in platelet counts occur occasionally, and lipids (eg, cholesterol, triglycerides, LDL, and HDL) should be monitored. GI perforation has been reported when using tocilizumab in patients with diverticulitis or who are using corticosteroids.

TNF-α-BLOCKING AGENTS

Cytokines play a central role in the immune response (see Chapter 55) and in rheumatoid arthritis. Although a wide range of cytokines are expressed in the joints of rheumatoid arthritis patients, TNF-α appears to be particularly important in the inflammatory process.

TNF-α affects cellular function via activation of specific membrane-bound TNF receptors (TNFR$_1$, TNFR$_2$). Five biologic DMARDs interfering with TNF-α have been approved for the treatment of rheumatoid arthritis and other rheumatic diseases (Figure 36–4).

Adalimumab

A. Mechanism of Action

Adalimumab is a fully human IgG$_1$ anti-TNF monoclonal antibody. This compound complexes with soluble TNF-α and prevents its interaction with p55 and p75 cell surface receptors. This results in down-regulation of macrophage and T-cell function.

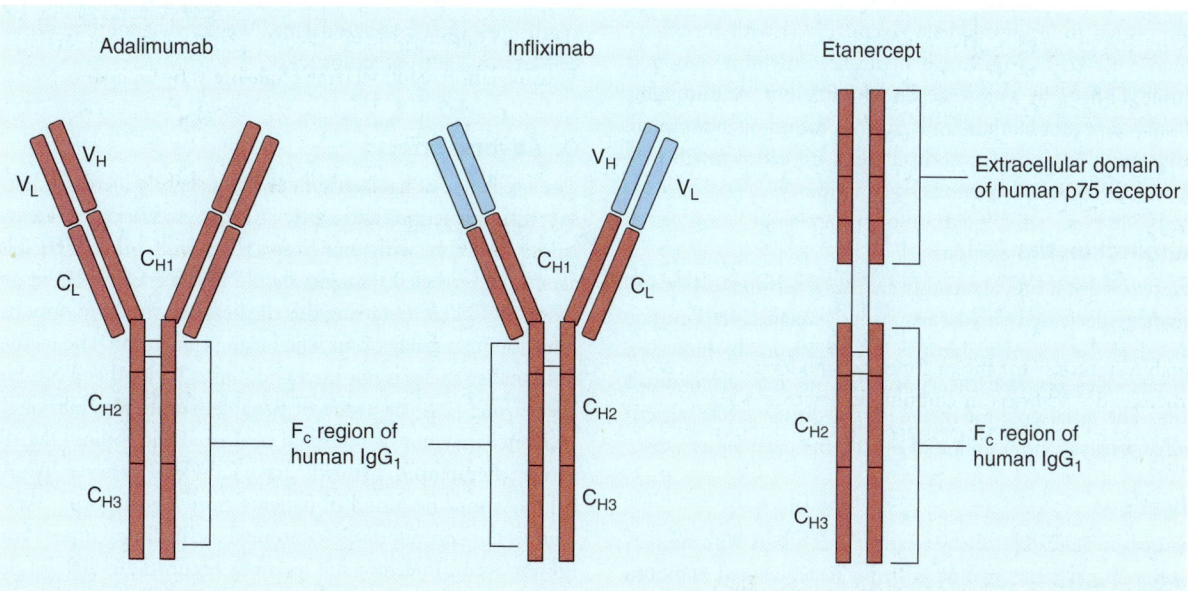

FIGURE 36–4 Structures of TNF-α antagonists used in rheumatoid arthritis. C$_H$, constant heavy chain; C$_L$, constant light chain; F$_c$, complex immunoglobulin region; V$_H$, variable heavy chain; V$_L$, variable light chain. Red regions, human derived; blue regions, mouse derived.

B. Pharmacokinetics

Adalimumab is given subcutaneously and has a half-life of 10–20 days. Its clearance is decreased by more than 40% in the presence of methotrexate, and the formation of human anti-monoclonal antibody is decreased when methotrexate is given at the same time. The usual dose in rheumatoid arthritis is 40 mg every other week; increased responses may be evident with the higher weekly dosing regimen. In psoriasis, 80 mg is given at week 0, 40 mg at week 1, and then 40 mg every other week thereafter.

C. Indications

The compound is approved for rheumatoid arthritis, ankylosing spondylitis, psoriatic arthritis, juvenile idiopathic arthritis, plaque psoriasis, and Crohn's disease. It decreases the rate of formation of new erosions. It is effective both as monotherapy and in combination with methotrexate and other DMARDs.

D. Adverse Effects

In common with the other TNF-α-blocking agents, the risk of bacterial infections and macrophage-dependent infection (including tuberculosis and other opportunistic infections) is increased, although it remains very low. Patients should be screened for latent or active tuberculosis before starting adalimumab or other TNF-α-blocking agents. There is no evidence of an increased incidence of solid malignancies. It is not clear if the incidence of lymphomas is increased by adalimumab. A low incidence of newly formed dsDNA antibodies and antinuclear antibodies (ANAs) has been documented when using adalimumab, but clinical lupus is extremely rare. Rare cases of leukopenia and vasculitis associated with adalimumab have been documented.

Certolizumab

A. Mechanism of Action

Certolizumab is a recombinant, humanized antibody Fab fragment conjugated to a polyethylene glycol (PEG) with specificity for human TNF-α. Certolizumab neutralizes membrane-bound and soluble TNF-α in a dose-dependent manner. Additionally, certolizumab does not contain an F_c region, found on a complete antibody, and does not fix complement or cause antibody-dependent cell-mediated cytotoxicity in vitro.

B. Pharmacokinetics

Certolizumab is given subcutaneously and has a half-life of 14 days. The clearance is decreased with decreasing body weight. Methotrexate does not alter the pharmacokinetics of certolizumab. However, methotrexate does decrease the appearance of anti-certolizumab antibodies. The usual dose for rheumatoid arthritis is 400 mg initially and at weeks 2 and 4, followed by 200 mg every other week.

C. Indications

Certolizumab is indicated for the treatment of adults with moderately to severely active rheumatoid arthritis. It can be used as monotherapy or in combination with nonbiologic DMARDs. Additionally, certolizumab is approved to reduce signs and symptoms and maintain clinical response in adult patients with Crohn's disease.

D. Adverse Effects

Consistent with other TNF-α blockers, the risk of serious infections, including tuberculosis, fungal, and other opportunistic pathogens, is increased and patients should be monitored closely. Prior to initiation of treatment, testing for latent tuberculosis should be performed. The association of lymphoma and other tumors with TNF-α blockers as a class, of which certolizumab is a member, is not fully understood.

Etanercept

A. Mechanism of Action

Etanercept is a recombinant fusion protein consisting of two soluble TNF p75 receptor moieties linked to the F_c portion of human IgG$_1$ (Figure 36–4); it binds TNF-α molecules and also inhibits lymphotoxin-α.

B. Pharmacokinetics

Etanercept is given subcutaneously in a dosage of 25 mg twice weekly or 50 mg weekly. In psoriasis, 50 mg is given twice weekly for 12 weeks followed by 50 mg weekly. The drug is slowly absorbed, with peak concentration 72 hours after drug administration. Etanercept has a mean serum elimination half-life of 4.5 days. Fifty milligrams given once weekly gives the same area under the curve and minimum serum concentrations as 25 mg twice weekly.

C. Indications

Etanercept is approved for the treatment of rheumatoid arthritis, juvenile chronic arthritis, psoriasis, psoriatic arthritis, and ankylosing spondylitis. It can be used as monotherapy, although over 70% of patients taking etanercept are also using methotrexate. Etanercept decreases the rate of formation of new erosions relative to methotrexate alone. It is also being used in other rheumatic syndromes such as scleroderma, Wegener's granulomatosis, giant cell arteritis, and sarcoidosis.

D. Adverse Effects

The incidence of bacterial infections is slightly increased, especially soft tissue infections and septic arthritis. Activation of latent tuberculosis is lower with etanercept than with other TNF-blocking agents. Nevertheless, patients should be screened for latent or active tuberculosis before starting this medication. Similarly, opportunistic infections can rarely occur when using etanercept. The incidence of solid malignancies is not increased, but as with other TNF-blocking agents, one must be aware of possible lymphomas (although their incidence may not be increased compared with other DMARDs or active rheumatoid arthritis itself). While positive ANAs and dsDNAs may be found in patients receiving this drug, these findings do not contraindicate continued use if clinical lupus symptoms do not occur. Injection site reactions occur in 20–40% of patients, although they rarely result in discontinuation of therapy. Anti-etanercept antibodies are present in up to 16% of treated patients, but they do not interfere with efficacy or predict toxicity.

Golimumab

A. Mechanism of Action

Golimumab is a human monoclonal antibody with a high affinity for soluble and membrane-bound TNF-α. Golimumab effectively neutralizes the inflammatory effects produced by TNF-α seen in diseases such as rheumatoid arthritis.

B. Pharmacokinetics

Golimumab is administered subcutaneously and has a half-life of approximately 14 days. Concomitant use with methotrexate showed increased serum levels of golimumab as well as a decrease in anti-golimumab antibodies. The recommended dose is 50 mg given every 4 weeks.

C. Indications

Golimumab, given with methotrexate, is indicated for the treatment of moderately to severely active rheumatoid arthritis in adult patients. It is also indicated for the treatment of psoriatic arthritis and ankylosing spondylitis.

D. Adverse Events

TNF-α blockers, including golimumab, increase the risk of serious infections, including tuberculosis, fungal, and other opportunistic pathogens. Prior to initiation of treatment, testing for latent tuberculosis should be performed. As with other TNF-α-blocking agents, there is a potential association with lymphoma; there is no association with other solid tumors (except possibly non-melanotic skin cancers).

Infliximab

A. Mechanism of Action

Infliximab (Figure 36–4) is a chimeric (25% mouse, 75% human) IgG$_1$ monoclonal antibody that binds with high affinity to soluble and possibly membrane-bound TNF-α. Its mechanism of action probably is the same as that of adalimumab.

B. Pharmacokinetics

Infliximab is given as an intravenous infusion with "induction" at 0, 2, and 6 weeks and maintenance every 8 weeks thereafter. Dosing is 3–10 mg/kg, although the usual dose is 3–5 mg/kg every 8 weeks. There is a relationship between serum concentration and effect, although individual clearances vary markedly. The terminal half-life is 9–12 days without accumulation after repeated dosing at the recommended interval of 8 weeks. After intermittent therapy, infliximab elicits human antichimeric antibodies in up to 62% of patients. Concurrent therapy with methotrexate markedly decreases the prevalence of human antichimeric antibodies.

C. Indications

Infliximab is approved for use in rheumatoid arthritis, ankylosing spondylitis, psoriatic arthritis, and Crohn's disease. It is being used in other diseases, including psoriasis, ulcerative colitis, juvenile chronic arthritis, Wegener's granulomatosis, giant cell arteritis, and sarcoidosis. In rheumatoid arthritis, a regimen of infliximab plus methotrexate decreases the rate of formation of new erosions more than methotrexate alone over 12–24 months. Although it is recommended that methotrexate be used in conjunction with infliximab, a number of other DMARDs, including antimalarials, azathioprine, leflunomide, and cyclosporine, can be used as background therapy for this drug. Infliximab is also used as monotherapy, although this is neither approved by regulatory agencies nor advisable.

D. Adverse Effects

Like other TNF-α-blocking agents, infliximab is associated with an increased incidence of bacterial infections, including upper respiratory tract infections. As a potent macrophage inhibitor, infliximab can be associated with activation of latent tuberculosis, and patients should be screened for latent or active tuberculosis before starting therapy. Other infections have been documented, though rarely. There is no evidence of an increased incidence of solid malignancies and it is not clear whether the incidence of lymphoma is increased with infliximab. Because rare demyelinating syndromes have been reported, patients with multiple sclerosis or neuro-uveitis should not use infliximab. Rare cases of leukopenia, hepatitis, activation of hepatitis B, and vasculitis have been documented. The incidence of positive ANA and dsDNA antibodies is increased, although clinical lupus erythematosus remains an extremely rare occurrence and the presence of ANA and dsDNA does not contraindicate the use of infliximab. Infusion site reactions correlate with anti-infliximab antibodies. These reactions occur in approximately 3–11% of patients, and the combined use of antihistamines and H$_2$-blocking agents apparently prevents some of these reactions.

COMBINATION THERAPY WITH DMARDS

In a 1998 study, approximately half of North American rheumatologists treated moderately aggressive rheumatoid arthritis with combination therapy, and the use of drug combinations is probably much higher now. Combinations of DMARDs can be designed rationally on the basis of complementary mechanisms of action, non-overlapping pharmacokinetics, and non-overlapping toxicities.

When added to methotrexate background therapy, cyclosporine, chloroquine, hydroxychloroquine, leflunomide, infliximab, adalimumab, rituximab, and etanercept have all shown improved efficacy. In contrast, azathioprine, auranofin, or sulfasalazine plus methotrexate results in no additional therapeutic benefit. Other combinations have occasionally been used, including the combination of intramuscular gold with hydroxychloroquine.

While it might be anticipated that combination therapy could result in more toxicity, this is often not the case. Combination therapy for patients not responding adequately to monotherapy is becoming the rule in the treatment of rheumatoid arthritis.

GLUCOCORTICOID DRUGS

The general pharmacology of corticosteroids, including mechanism of action, pharmacokinetics, and other applications, is discussed in Chapter 39.

Indications

Corticosteroids have been used in 60–70% of rheumatoid arthritis patients. Their effects are prompt and dramatic, and they are capable of slowing the appearance of new bone erosions. Corticosteroids may be administered for certain serious extra-articular manifestations of rheumatoid arthritis such as pericarditis or eye involvement or during periods of exacerbation. When prednisone is required for long-term therapy, the dosage should not exceed 7.5 mg daily, and gradual reduction of the dose should be encouraged. Alternate-day corticosteroid therapy is usually unsuccessful in rheumatoid arthritis.

Other rheumatic diseases in which the corticosteroids' potent anti-inflammatory effects may be useful include vasculitis, systemic lupus erythematosus, Wegener's granulomatosis, psoriatic arthritis, giant cell arteritis, sarcoidosis, and gout.

Intra-articular corticosteroids are often helpful to alleviate painful symptoms and, when successful, are preferable to increasing the dosage of systemic medication.

Adverse Effects

Prolonged use of these drugs leads to serious and disabling toxic effects as described in Chapter 39. There is controversy over whether many of these side effects occur at doses below 7.5 mg prednisone equivalent daily, although many experts believe that even 3–5 mg/d can cause these effects in susceptible individuals when this class of drugs is used over prolonged periods.

■ OTHER ANALGESICS

Acetaminophen is one of the most important drugs used in the treatment of mild to moderate pain when an anti-inflammatory effect is not necessary. Phenacetin, a prodrug that is metabolized to acetaminophen, is more toxic than its active metabolite and has no rational indications.

ACETAMINOPHEN

Acetaminophen is the active metabolite of phenacetin and is responsible for its analgesic effect. It is a weak COX-1 and COX-2 inhibitor in peripheral tissues and possesses no significant anti-inflammatory effects.

N-Acetyl-*p*-aminophenol
(acetaminophen)

Pharmacokinetics

Acetaminophen is administered orally. Absorption is related to the rate of gastric emptying, and peak blood concentrations are usually reached in 30–60 minutes. Acetaminophen is slightly bound to plasma proteins and is partially metabolized by hepatic microsomal enzymes and converted to acetaminophen sulfate and glucuronide, which are pharmacologically inactive (see Figure 4–5). Less than 5% is excreted unchanged. A minor but highly reactive metabolite (*N*-acetyl-*p*-benzoquinone) is important in large doses because it is toxic to both liver and kidney (see Chapter 4). The half-life of acetaminophen is 2–3 hours and is relatively unaffected by renal function. With toxic doses or liver disease, the half-life may be increased twofold or more.

Indications

Although said to be equivalent to aspirin as an analgesic and antipyretic agent, acetaminophen differs in that it lacks anti-inflammatory properties. It does not affect uric acid levels and lacks platelet-inhibiting effects. The drug is useful in mild to moderate pain such as headache, myalgia, postpartum pain, and other circumstances in which aspirin is an effective analgesic. Acetaminophen alone is inadequate therapy for inflammatory conditions such as rheumatoid arthritis, although it may be used as an analgesic adjunct to anti-inflammatory therapy. For mild analgesia, acetaminophen is the preferred drug in patients allergic to aspirin or when salicylates are poorly tolerated. It is preferable to aspirin in patients with hemophilia or a history of peptic ulcer and in those in whom bronchospasm is precipitated by aspirin. Unlike aspirin, acetaminophen does not antagonize the effects of uricosuric agents; it may be used concomitantly with probenecid in the treatment of gout. It is preferred to aspirin in children with viral infections.

Adverse Effects

In therapeutic doses, a mild increase in hepatic enzymes may occasionally occur in the absence of jaundice; this is reversible when the drug is withdrawn. With larger doses, dizziness, excitement, and disorientation may occur. Ingestion of 15 g of acetaminophen may be fatal, death being caused by severe hepatotoxicity with centrilobular necrosis, sometimes associated with acute renal tubular necrosis (see Chapters 4 and 58). Present data indicate that 4–6 g acetaminophen is associated with increased liver function test abnormalities. Doses greater than 4 g/d are not usually recommended and a history of alcoholism contraindicates even this dose. Early symptoms of hepatic damage include nausea, vomiting, diarrhea, and abdominal pain. Cases of renal damage without hepatic damage have occurred, even after usual doses of acetaminophen. Therapy is much less satisfactory than for aspirin overdose. In addition to supportive therapy, the measure that has proved most useful is the provision of sulfhydryl groups in the form of acetylcysteine to neutralize the toxic metabolites (see Chapter 58).

Hemolytic anemia and methemoglobinemia are very rare adverse events. Interstitial nephritis and papillary necrosis—serious complications of phenacetin—have not occurred nor has GI bleeding. Caution is necessary in patients with any type of liver disease.

Dosage

Acute pain and fever may be effectively treated with 325–500 mg four times daily and proportionately less for children. Dosing in adults is now recommended not to exceed 4 g/d, in most cases.

DRUGS USED IN GOUT

Gout is a metabolic disease characterized by recurrent episodes of acute arthritis due to deposits of monosodium urate in joints and cartilage. Uric acid renal calculi, tophi, and interstitial nephritis may also occur. Gout is usually associated with a high serum uric acid level (hyperuricemia), a poorly soluble substance that is the major end product of purine metabolism. In most mammals, uricase converts uric acid to the more soluble allantoin; this enzyme is absent in humans. While clinical gouty episodes are associated with hyperuricemia, most individuals with hyperuricemia may never develop a clinical event from urate crystal deposition.

The treatment of gout aims to relieve acute gouty attacks and prevent recurrent gouty episodes and urate lithiasis. Therapies for acute gout are based on our current understanding of the pathophysiologic events that occur in this disease (Figure 36–5). Urate crystals are initially phagocytosed by synoviocytes, which then release prostaglandins, lysosomal enzymes, and interleukin-1. Attracted by these chemotactic mediators, polymorphonuclear leukocytes migrate into the joint space and amplify the ongoing inflammatory process. In the later phases of the attack, increased numbers of mononuclear phagocytes (macrophages) appear, ingest the urate crystals, and release more inflammatory mediators. This sequence of events suggests that the most effective agents for the management of acute urate crystal-induced inflammation are those that suppress different phases of leukocyte activation.

Before starting chronic urate-lowering therapy for gout, patients in whom hyperuricemia is associated with gout and urate lithiasis must be clearly distinguished from individuals with only hyperuricemia. The efficacy of long-term drug treatment in an asymptomatic hyperuricemic person is unproved. In some individuals, uric acid levels may be elevated up to 2 standard deviations above the mean for a lifetime without adverse consequences. Many different agents have been used for the treatment of acute and chronic gout. However, non-adherence to these drugs is exceedingly common; adherence has been documented to be as low as 26–18%, especially in younger patients. Providers should be aware of compliance as an important issue.

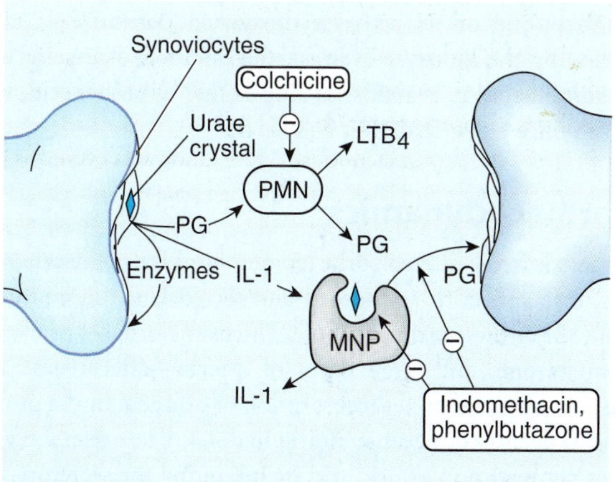

COLCHICINE

Although NSAIDs are now the first-line drugs for acute gout, colchicine was the primary treatment for many years. Colchicine is an alkaloid isolated from the autumn crocus, *Colchicum autumnale*. Its structure is shown in Figure 36–6.

Pharmacokinetics

Colchicine is absorbed readily after oral administration, reaches peak plasma levels within 2 hours, and is eliminated with a serum half-life of 9 hours. Metabolites are excreted in the intestinal tract and urine.

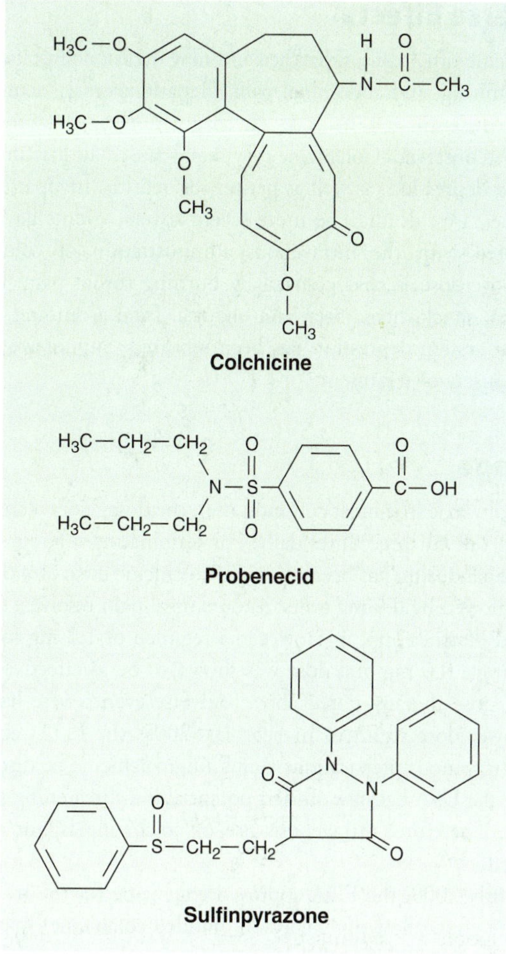

FIGURE 36–5 Pathophysiologic events in a gouty joint. Synoviocytes phagocytose urate crystals and then secrete inflammatory mediators, which attract and activate polymorphonuclear leukocytes (PMN) and mononuclear phagocytes (MNP) (macrophages). Drugs active in gout inhibit crystal phagocytosis and polymorphonuclear leukocyte and macrophage release of inflammatory mediators. PG, prostaglandin; IL-1, interleukin-1; LTB_4, leukotriene B_4.

FIGURE 36–6 Colchicine and uricosuric drugs.

Pharmacodynamics

Colchicine relieves the pain and inflammation of gouty arthritis in 12–24 hours without altering the metabolism or excretion of urates and without other analgesic effects. Colchicine produces its anti-inflammatory effects by binding to the intracellular protein tubulin, thereby preventing its polymerization into microtubules and leading to the inhibition of leukocyte migration and phagocytosis. It also inhibits the formation of leukotriene B_4. Several of colchicine's adverse effects are produced by its inhibition of tubulin polymerization and cell mitosis.

Indications

Although colchicine is more specific in gout than the NSAIDs, NSAIDs (eg, indomethacin and other NSAIDs [except aspirin]) are sometimes used in its stead because of the troublesome diarrhea associated with colchicine therapy. Colchicine is now used between attacks (the "intercritical period") for prolonged prophylaxis (at low doses). It is effective in preventing attacks of acute Mediterranean fever and may have a mild beneficial effect in sarcoid arthritis and in hepatic cirrhosis. (Although it has been given intravenously, this route is no longer approved by the FDA [2009].)

Adverse Effects

Colchicine often causes diarrhea and may occasionally cause nausea, vomiting, and abdominal pain. Hepatic necrosis, acute renal failure, disseminated intravascular coagulation, and seizures have also been observed. Colchicine may rarely cause hair loss and bone marrow depression, as well as peripheral neuritis, myopathy, and, in some cases, death. The more severe adverse events have been associated with the intravenous administration of colchicine. Acute overdose is characterized by burning throat pain, bloody diarrhea, shock, hematuria, and oliguria. Fatal ascending central nervous system depression has been reported. Supportive care is the mainstay of treatment.

Dosage

In prophylaxis (the most common use), the dosage of colchicine is 0.6 mg one to three times daily. For terminating a gouty attack, traditional dosing has been an initial colchicine dose of 0.6 or 1.2 mg, followed by 0.6 mg every 2 hours until pain resolves, or nausea and diarrhea appear. However, a regimen of 1.2 mg followed by a single 0.6 mg oral dose was shown to be as effective as the higher dose therapy noted above. Adverse events were less with this lower dose regimen. In February 2008, the FDA requested that intravenous preparations containing colchicine be discontinued in the USA because of their potential life-threatening adverse effects. Therefore, intravenous use of colchicine is not recommended.

In July 2009, the FDA approved colchicine for the treatment of acute gout, allowing Colcrys (a branded colchicine) marketing exclusivity in the USA. Colchicine, per se, rather than Colcrys, is available throughout the rest of the world in a generic form.

NSAIDS IN GOUT

In addition to inhibiting prostaglandin synthase, indomethacin and other NSAIDs also inhibit urate crystal phagocytosis. Aspirin is not used because it causes renal retention of uric acid at low doses (≤ 2.6 g/d). It is uricosuric at doses greater than 3.6 g/d. Indomethacin is commonly used in the initial treatment of gout as a replacement for colchicine. For acute gout, 50 mg is given three times daily; when a response occurs, the dosage is reduced to 25 mg three times daily for 5–7 days.

All other NSAIDs except aspirin, salicylates, and tolmetin have been successfully used to treat acute gouty episodes. Oxaprozin, which lowers serum uric acid, is theoretically a good choice, although it should not be given to patients with uric acid stones because it increases uric acid excretion in the urine. These agents appear to be as effective and safe as the older drugs.

URICOSURIC AGENTS

Probenecid and sulfinpyrazone are uricosuric drugs employed to decrease the body pool of urate in patients with tophaceous gout or in those with increasingly frequent gouty attacks. In a patient who excretes large amounts of uric acid, the uricosuric agents should not be used.

Chemistry

Uricosuric drugs are organic acids (Figure 36–6) and, as such, act at the anionic transport sites of the renal tubule (see Chapter 15). Sulfinpyrazone is a metabolite of an analog of phenylbutazone.

Pharmacokinetics

Probenecid is completely reabsorbed by the renal tubules and is metabolized slowly with a terminal serum half-life of 5–8 hours. Sulfinpyrazone or its active hydroxylated derivative is rapidly excreted by the kidneys. Even so, the duration of its effect after oral administration is almost as long as that of probenecid, which is given once or twice daily.

Pharmacodynamics

Uric acid is freely filtered at the glomerulus. Like many other weak acids, it is also both reabsorbed and secreted in the middle segment (S2) of the proximal tubule. Uricosuric drugs—probenecid, sulfinpyrazone, and large doses of aspirin—affect these active transport sites so that net reabsorption of uric acid in the proximal tubule is decreased. Because aspirin in doses of less than 2.6 g daily causes net retention of uric acid by inhibiting the secretory transporter, it should not be used for analgesia in patients with gout. The secretion of other weak acids (eg, penicillin) is also reduced by uricosuric agents. Probenecid was originally developed to prolong penicillin blood levels.

As the urinary excretion of uric acid increases, the size of the urate pool decreases, although the plasma concentration may not be greatly reduced. In patients who respond favorably, tophaceous deposits of urate are reabsorbed, with relief of arthritis and remineralization of bone. With the ensuing increase in uric acid excretion, a predisposition to the formation of renal stones is augmented rather than decreased; therefore, the urine volume should be maintained at a high level, and at least early in treatment, the urine pH should be kept above 6.0 by the administration of alkali.

Indications

Uricosuric therapy should be initiated in gouty patients with underexcretion of uric acid when allopurinol or febuxostat is contraindicated or when tophi are present. Therapy should not be started until 2–3 weeks after an acute attack.

Adverse Effects

Adverse effects do not provide a basis for preferring one or the other of the uricosuric agents. Both of these organic acids cause GI irritation, but sulfinpyrazone is more active in this regard. A rash may appear after the use of either compound. Nephrotic syndrome has occurred after the use of probenecid. Both sulfinpyrazone and probenecid may rarely cause aplastic anemia.

Contraindications & Cautions

It is essential to maintain a large urine volume to minimize the possibility of stone formation.

Dosage

Probenecid is usually started at a dosage of 0.5 g orally daily in divided doses, progressing to 1 g daily after 1 week. Sulfinpyrazone is started at a dosage of 200 mg orally daily, progressing to 400–800 mg daily. It should be given in divided doses with food to reduce adverse GI effects.

ALLOPURINOL

The preferred and standard-of-care therapy for gout during the period between acute episodes is allopurinol, which reduces total uric acid body burden by inhibiting xanthine oxidase.

Chemistry

The structure of allopurinol, an isomer of hypoxanthine, is shown in Figure 36–7.

Pharmacokinetics

Allopurinol is approximately 80% absorbed after oral administration and has a terminal serum half-life of 1–2 hours. Like uric acid, allopurinol is metabolized by xanthine oxidase, but the resulting compound, alloxanthine, retains the capacity to inhibit xanthine oxidase and has a long enough duration of action so that allopurinol is given only once a day.

Pharmacodynamics

Dietary purines are not an important source of uric acid. Quantitatively important amounts of purine are formed from amino acids, formate, and carbon dioxide in the body. Those purine ribonucleotides not incorporated into nucleic acids and derived from nucleic acid degradation are converted to xanthine or hypoxanthine and oxidized to uric acid (Figure 36–7). Allopurinol inhibits this last step, resulting in a fall in the plasma urate level and a decrease in the overall urate burden. The more soluble xanthine and hypoxanthine are increased.

Indications

Allopurinol is often the first-line agent for the treatment of chronic gout in the period between attacks and it aims to prolong

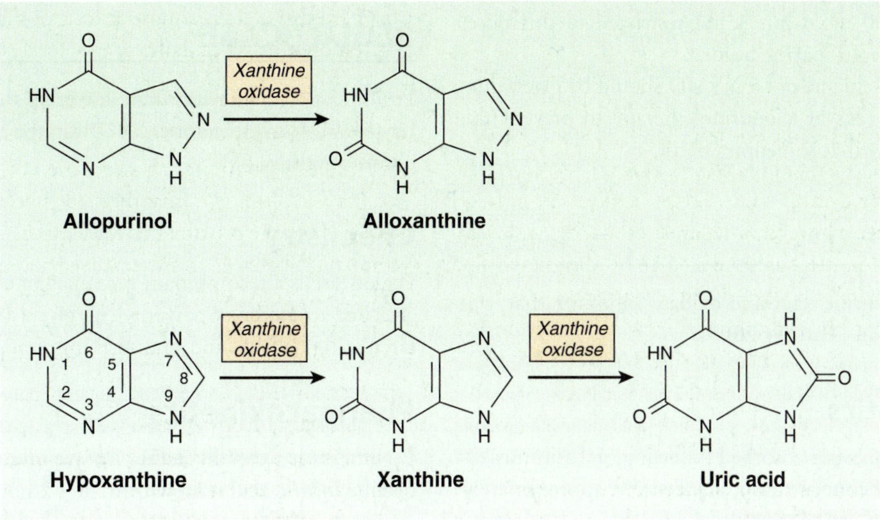

FIGURE 36–7 Inhibition of uric acid synthesis by allopurinol. (Modified and reproduced, with permission, from Meyers FH, Jawetz E, Goldfien A: *Review of Medical Pharmacology*, 7th ed. McGraw-Hill, 1980.)

the intercritical period. As with uricosuric agents, the therapy is begun with the expectation that it will be continued for years if not for life. When initiating allopurinol, colchicine or NSAID should be used until steady-state serum uric acid is normalized or decreased to less than 6 mg/dL and they should be continued for 3-6 months or even longer if required. Thereafter, colchicine or the NSAID can be cautiously stopped while continuing allopurinol therapy. In addition to gout, allopurinol is also used as an antiprotozoal agent (see Chapter 52) and is indicated to prevent the massive uricosuria following therapy of blood dyscrasias that could otherwise lead to renal calculi.

Adverse Effects

See above for prophylaxis against an acute attack during the initiation of allopurinol, which can occur as a result of acute changes in the serum uric acid level. Among the side effects, GI intolerance including nausea, vomiting, and diarrhea, peripheral neuritis and necrotizing vasculitis, bone marrow suppression, and rarely aplastic anemia may also occur. Hepatic toxicity and interstitial nephritis have been reported. An allergic skin reaction characterized by pruritic maculopapular lesions occurs in 3% of patients. Isolated cases of exfoliative dermatitis have been reported. In very rare cases, allopurinol has become bound to the lens, resulting in cataracts.

Interactions & Cautions

When chemotherapeutic purines (eg, azathioprine) are given concomitantly with allopurinol, their dosage must be reduced by about 75%. Allopurinol may also increase the effect of cyclophosphamide. Allopurinol inhibits the metabolism of probenecid and oral anticoagulants and may increase hepatic iron concentration. Safety in children and during pregnancy has not been established.

Dosage

The initial dosage of allopurinol is 100 mg/d. It should be titrated upward until serum uric acid is below 6 mg/dL; this level is commonly achieved at 300 mg/d but is not restricted to this dose; doses as high as 800 mg/d may be needed.

As noted above, colchicine or an NSAID should be given during the first several weeks of allopurinol therapy to prevent the gouty arthritis episodes that sometimes occur.

FEBUXOSTAT

Febuxostat is a non-purine xanthine oxidase inhibitor that was approved by the FDA in February 2009.

Pharmacokinetics

Febuxostat is more than 80% absorbed following oral administration. With maximum concentration achieved in approximately 1 hour and a half-life of 4–18 hours, once-daily dosing is effective. Febuxostat is extensively metabolized in the liver. All of the drug and its inactive metabolites appear in the urine, although less than 5% appears as unchanged drug.

Pharmacodynamics

Febuxostat is a potent and selective inhibitor of xanthine oxidase, thereby reducing the formation of xanthine and uric acid without affecting other enzymes in the purine or pyrimidine metabolic pathway. In clinical trials, febuxostat at daily dosing of 80 mg or 120 mg was more effective in lowering serum urate levels than allopurinol at a standard 300 mg daily dose. The urate-lowering effect was comparable regardless of the pathogenic cause of hyperuricemia—overproduction or underexcretion.

Indications

Febuxostat is approved at doses of 40, 80, or 120 mg the treatment of chronic hyperuricemia in gout patients. Although it appeared to be more effective then allopurinol as urate-lowering therapy, the allopurinol dosing was limited to 300 mg/d, thus not reflecting the actual dosing regimens used in clinical practice. At this time, the dose equivalence of allopurinol and febuxostat is unknown.

Adverse Effects

As with allopurinol, prophylactic treatment with colchicine or NSAIDs should be started at the beginning of therapy to avoid gout flares. The most frequent treatment-related adverse events are liver function abnormalities, diarrhea, headache, and nausea. Febuxostat appears to be well tolerated in patients with a history of allopurinol intolerance. There does not appear to be an increased risk of cardiovascular events.

Dosage

The recommended starting dose of febuxostat is 40 mg daily. Because of the concern for cardiovascular events in the original phase 3 trials, the FDA approved only 40 mg and 80 mg dosing. No dose adjustment is necessary for patients with renal impairment since it is highly metabolized into an inactive metabolite by the liver.

PEGLOTICASE

Pegloticase is the newest urate-lowering therapy; it was approved by the FDA in September 2010 for the treatment of refractory chronic gout.

Chemistry

Pegloticase is a recombinant mammalian uricase that is covalently attached to methoxy polyethylene glycol (mPEG) to prolong the circulating half-life and diminish immunogenic response.

Pharmacokinetics

Pegloticase is a rapidly acting intravenous drug, achieving a peak decline in uric acid level within 24–72 hours. The serum half-life ranges from 6.4 to 13.8 days. Several studies have shown earlier clearance of PEG-uricase (mean of 11 days) due to antibody response when compared to PEG-uricase antibody-negative subjects (mean of 16.1 days).

Pharmacodynamics

Urate oxidase enzyme, absent in humans and some higher primates, converts uric acid to allantoin. This product is highly soluble and can be easily eliminated by kidney. Pegloticase has been shown to maintain low urate levels for up to 21 days at doses of 4–12 mg, allowing for IV dosing every 2 weeks.

Adverse Effects

The most common adverse events include infusion reactions and gout flare (especially during the first 3 months of treatment). Nephrolithiasis, arthralgia, muscle spasm, headache, anemia, and nausea may occur. Other less frequent side effects noted include upper respiratory tract infection, peripheral edema, urinary tract infection, and diarrhea. There is some concern for hemolytic anemia in patients with glucose-6-phosphate dehydrogenase because of the formation of hydrogen peroxide by uricase; therefore, pegloticase should be avoided in these patients. Large numbers of patients show immune responses to pegloticase. The presence of antibody is associated with shortened circulating half-life, loss of response leading to a rise in plasma urate levels, and a higher rate of infusion reactions. Monitoring of plasma uric acid level, with rising level as an indicator of antibody production, allows for safer administration and monitoring of efficacy.

Dosage

The recommended dose for pegloticase is 8 mg IV every 2 weeks. As noted for other urate-lowering therapy, patients should be started on prophylaxis for acute gout flares (using colchicine) while initiating pegloticase.

GLUCOCORTICOIDS

Corticosteroids are sometimes used in the treatment of severe symptomatic gout, by intra-articular, systemic, or subcutaneous routes, depending on the degree of pain and inflammation.

The most commonly used oral corticosteroid is prednisone. The recommended dose is 30–50 mg/d for 1–2 days, tapered over 7–10 days. Intra-articular injection of 10 mg (small joints), 30 mg (wrist, ankle, elbow), and 40 mg (knee) of triamcinolone acetonide can be given if the patient is unable to take oral medications.

INTERLEUKIN-1 INHIBITORS

Drugs targeting the interleukin-1 pathway, such as anakinra, canakinumab, and rilonacept, are being investigated for the treatment of gout. Although the data are limited, these agents may provide a promising treatment option for acute gout in patients with contraindications to, or who are refractory to, traditional therapies like NSAIDs and/or colchicine. A recent study suggests that canakinumab, a fully human anti-IL-1β monoclonal antibody, can provide rapid and sustained pain relief at a dose of 150 mg subcutaneously. These medications are also being evaluated as therapies for prevention of gout flares while initiating urate-lowering therapy.

P R E P A R A T I O N S   A V A I L A B L E

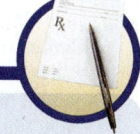

NONSTEROIDAL ANTI-INFLAMMATORY DRUGS

Aspirin, acetylsalicylic acid (generic, Easprin, others)
Oral (regular, enteric-coated, buffered): 81, 165, 325, 500, 650, 800 mg tablets; 81, 650, 800 mg timed- or extended-release tablets
Rectal: 120, 200, 300, 600 mg suppositories

Bromfenac (Xibrom)
Ophthalmic: 0.09% solution

Celecoxib (Celebrex)
Oral: 50, 100, 200, 400 mg capsules

Choline salicylate (various)
Oral: 870 mg/5 mL liquid

Diclofenac (generic, Cataflam, Voltaren)
Oral: 50 mg tablets; 25, 50, 75 mg delayed-release tablets; 100 mg extended-release tablets
Ophthalmic: 0.1% solution

Diflunisal (generic, Dolobid)
Oral: 500 mg tablets

Etodolac (generic, Lodine)
Oral: 200, 300 mg capsules; 400, 500 mg tablets; 400, 500, 600 mg extended-release tablets

Fenoprofen (generic, Nalfon)
Oral: 200, 300 mg capsules; 600 mg tablets

Flurbiprofen (generic, Ansaid)
Oral: 50, 100 mg tablets
Ophthalmic (generic, Ocufen): 0.03% solution

Ibuprofen (generic, Motrin, Rufen, Advil [OTC], Nuprin [OTC], others)
Oral: 100, 200, 400, 600, 800 mg tablets; 50, 100 mg chewable tablets; 200 mg capsules; 100 mg/2.5 mL suspension, 100 mg/5 mL suspension; 40 mg/mL drops

Indomethacin (generic, Indocin)
Oral: 25, 50 mg capsules; 75 mg sustained-release capsules; 25 mg/5 mL suspension
Rectal: 50 mg suppositories

Ketoprofen (generic, Orudis)
Oral: 12.5 mg tablets; 25, 50, 75 mg capsules; 100, 150, 200 mg extended-release capsules

Ketorolac tromethamine (generic, Toradol)
Oral: 10 mg tablets
Parenteral: 15, 30 mg/mL for IM injection
Ophthalmic: 0.4, 0.5% solution

Magnesium salicylate (Doan's Pills, Magan, Mobidin)
Oral: 545, 600 mg tablets; 467, 500, 580 mg caplets

Meclofenamate sodium (generic)
Oral: 50, 100 mg capsules

Mefenamic acid (Ponstel)
Oral: 250 mg capsules

Meloxicam (Mobic)
Oral: 7.5, 15 mg tablets; 7.5 mg/5 mL suspension

Nabumetone (generic)
Oral: 500, 750 mg tablets

Naproxen (generic, Naprosyn, Anaprox, Aleve [OTC])
Oral: 200, 220, 250, 375, 500 mg tablets; 375, 550 mg controlled-release tablets; 375, 500 mg delayed-release tablets; 125 mg/5 mL suspension

Oxaprozin (generic, Daypro)
Oral: 600 mg tablets, capsules

Piroxicam (generic, Feldene)
Oral: 10, 20 mg capsules

Salsalate, salicylsalicylic acid (generic, Disalcid)
Oral: 500, 750 mg tablets; 500 mg capsules

Sodium salicylate (generic)
Oral: 325, 650 mg enteric-coated tablets

Sodium thiosalicylate (generic, Rexolate)
Parenteral: 50 mg/mL for IM injection

Sulindac (generic, Clinoril)
Oral: 150, 200 mg tablets

Suprofen (Profenal)
Topical: 1% ophthalmic solution

Tolmetin (generic, Tolectin)
Oral: 200, 600 mg tablets; 400 mg capsules

DISEASE-MODIFYING ANTIRHEUMATIC DRUGS

Abatacept (Orencia)
Parenteral: 250 mg/vial lyophilized, for reconstitution for IV injection

Adalimumab (Humira)
Parenteral: 40 mg/0.8 mL for SC injection

Auranofin (Ridaura)
Oral: 3 mg capsules

Aurothioglucose (Solganal)
Parenteral: 50 mg/mL suspension for injection

Certolizumab (Cimzia)
Parenteral: 200 mg powder for solution for subcutaneous injection

Cyclophosphamide: see Chapter 54

Cyclosporine: see Chapter 55

Etanercept (Enbrel)
Parenteral: 50 mg/mL, 25 mg powder for SC injection

Gold sodium thiomalate (generic, Aurolate)
Parenteral: 50 mg/mL for injection

Golimumab (Simponi)
Parenteral: 50 mg per 0.5 mL solution for SC injection

Infliximab (Remicade)
Parenteral: 100 mg powder for IV infusion

Leflunomide (Arava)
Oral: 10, 20, 100 mg tablets

Methotrexate (generic, Rheumatrex)
Oral: 2.5 mg tablet dose packs; 5, 7.5, 10, 15 mg tablets

Mycophenolate mofetil: see Chapter 55

Penicillamine (Cuprimine, Depen)
Oral: 125, 250 mg capsules; 250 mg tablets

Rituximab (Rituxan)
Parenteral: 10 mg/mL for IV infusion

Sulfasalazine (generic, Azulfidine)
Oral: 500 mg tablets; 500 mg delayed-release tablets

Tocilizumab (Actemra)
Parenteral: 20 mg/mL concentrate for IV administration

ACETAMINOPHEN

Acetaminophen (generic, Tylenol, Tempra, Panadol, Acephen, others)
Oral: 160, 325, 500, 650 mg tablets; 80 mg chewable tablets; 160, 500, 650 mg caplets; 325, 500 mg capsules; 80, 120, 160 mg/5 mL elixir; 500 mg/15 mL elixir; 80 mg/1.66 mL, 100 mg/mL solution
Rectal: 80, 120, 125, 300, 325, 650 mg suppositories

DRUGS USED IN GOUT

Allopurinol (generic, Zyloprim)
Oral: 100, 300 mg tablets

Colchicine (generic, Colchrys)
Oral: 0.6 mg tablets

Febuxostat (Uloric)
Oral: 40, 80 mg tablets

Pegloticase (Krystexxa)
Parenteral: 8 mg/mL solution for IV infusion

Probenecid (generic)
Oral: 500 mg tablets

Sulfinpyrazone (generic, Anturane)
Oral: 100 mg tablets; 200 mg capsules

REFERENCES

General

Hellman DB, Imboden JB Jr: Arthritis and musculoskeletal disorders. In: McPhee ST, Papadakis MA (editors). *Current Medical Diagnosis & Treatment*, 2011. McGraw-Hill, 2011.

NSAIDs

Bombardier C et al: Comparison of upper gastrointestinal toxicity of rofecoxib and naproxen in patients with rheumatoid arthritis. VIGOR Study Group. N Engl J Med 2000;343:1520.

Chan FK et al: Celecoxib versus diclofenac and omeprazole in reducing the risk of recurrent ulcer bleeding in patients with arthritis. N Engl J Med 2002;347:2104.

Clevers H: Colon cancer—Understanding how NSAIDs work. N Engl J Med 2006;354:761.

Deeks JJ, Smith LA, Bradley MD: Efficacy, tolerability, and upper gastrointestinal safety of celecoxib for treatment of osteoarthritis and rheumatoid arthritis: Systematic review of randomised controlled trials. BMJ 2002;325:619.

FitzGerald GA: COX-2 in play at the AHA and FDA. Trends Pharmacol Sci 2007;28:303.

Furst DE et al: Dose response and safety study of meloxicam up to 22.5 mg daily in rheumatoid arthritis: A 12 week multi-center, double blind, dose response study versus placebo and diclofenac. J Rheumatol 2002;29:436.

Knijff-Dutmer EA et al: Platelet function is inhibited by non-selective non-steroidal anti-inflammatory drugs but not by cyclooxygenase-2-selective inhibitors in patients with rheumatoid arthritis. Rheumatology (Oxford) 2002;41:458.

Lago P et al: Safety and efficacy of ibuprofen versus indomethacin in preterm infants treated for patent ductus arteriosus: A randomized controlled trial. Eur J Pediatr 2002;161:202.

Laine L et al: Serious lower gastrointestinal clinical events with non-selective NSAID or coxib use. Gastroenterology 2003;124:288.

Moran EM: Epidemiological and clinical aspects of nonsteroidal anti-inflammatory drugs and cancer risks. J Environ Pathol Toxicol Oncol 2002;21:193.

Niccoli L, Bellino S, Cantini F: Renal tolerability of three commonly employed non-steroidal anti-inflammatory drugs in elderly patients with osteoarthritis. Clin Exp Rheumatol 2002;20:201.

Ray WA et al: COX-2 selective non-steroidal anti-inflammatory drugs and risk of serious coronary heart disease. Lancet 2002;360:1071.

Rovensky J et al: Treatment of knee osteoarthritis with a topical nonsteroidal anti-inflammatory drug. Results of a randomized, double-blind, placebo-controlled study on the efficacy and safety of a 5% ibuprofen cream. Drugs Exp Clin Res 2001;27:209.

Vane J, Botting R: Inflammation and the mechanism of action of anti-inflammatory drugs. FASEB J 1987;1:89.

http://www.rheumatology.org/publications/hotline/0305NSAIDs.asp

Disease-Modifying Antirheumatic Drugs & Glucocorticoids

Bongartz T et al: Anti-TNF antibody therapy in rheumatoid arthritis and the risk of serious infections and malignancies. JAMA 2006;295:2275.

Cronstein B: How does methotrexate suppress inflammation? Clin Exp Rheumatol 2010:28(Suppl 61):S21.

Emery P et al: Golimumab, a human anti-tumor necrosis factor α monoclonal antibody, injected subcutaneously every four weeks in methotrexate-naïve patients with active rheumatoid arthritis. Arthritis Rheum 2009;60(8):2272.

Emery P et al: IL-6 receptor inhibition with tocilizumab improves treatment outcomes in patients with rheumatoid arthritis refractory to anti-tumour necrosis factor biologicals: results from a 24-week multicentre randomized placebo-controlled trial. Ann Rheum Dis 2008;67:1516.

Furst DE: Rational use of disease-modifying antirheumatic drugs. Drugs 1990;39:19.

Genovese MC et al: Abatacept for rheumatoid arthritis refractory to tumor necrosis factor α inhibition. N Engl J Med 2005;353:1114.

Keystone E et al: Improvement in patient-reported outcomes in a rituximab trial in patients with severe rheumatoid arthritis refractory to anti-tumor necrosis factor therapy. Arthritis Rheum 2008;59:785.

Kremer J: Toward a better understanding of methotrexate. Arthritis Rheum 2004;50:1370.

Plosker G, Croom K: Sulfasalazine: A review of its use in the management of rheumatoid arthritis. Drugs 2006;65:1825.

Scott DL, Kingsley GH: Tumor necrosis factor inhibitors for rheumatoid arthritis. N Engl J Med 2006;355:704.

Smolen J et al: Efficacy and safety of certolizumab pegol plus methotrexate in active rheumatoid arthritis: the RAPID 2 study. A randomized controlled trial. Ann Rheum Dis 2009;68:797.

Teng GG, Turkiewicz AM, Moreland LW: Abatacept: A costimulatory inhibitor for treatment of rheumatoid arthritis. Expert Opin Biol Ther 2005;5:1245.

Weinblatt M et al: Adalimumab, a fully human anti-tumor necrosis factor α monoclonal antibody, for the treatment of rheumatoid arthritis in patients taking concomitant methotrexate. Arthritis Rheum 2003;48(1):35.

Other Analgesics

Chandrasekharan NV et al: COX-3, a cyclooxygenase-1 variant inhibited by acetaminophen and other analgesic/antipyretic drugs: Cloning, structure, and expression. Proc Natl Acad Sci USA 2002;99:13926.

Styrt B, Sugarman B: Antipyresis and fever. Arch Intern Med 1990;150:1589.

Drugs Used in Gout

Becker MA et al: Febuxostat compared with allopurinol in patients with hyperuricemia and gout. N Engl J Med 2005;353:2450.

Getting SJ et al: Activation of melanocortin type 3 receptor as a molecular mechanism for adrenocorticotropic hormone efficacy in gouty arthritis. Arthritis Rheum 2002;46:2765.

Pacher P, Nivorozhkin A, Szabo C: Therapeutic effects of xanthine oxidase inhibitors: Renaissance half a century after the discovery of allopurinol. Pharmacol Rev 2006;58:87.

Schumacher HR: Febuxostat: A non-purine, selective inhibitor of xanthine oxidase for the management of hyperuricaemia in patients with gout. Expert Opin Investig Drugs 2005;14:893.

So A et al: A pilot study of IL-1 inhibition by anakinra in acute gout. Arthritis Res Ther 2007;9:R28.

Wallace SL, Singer JZ: Systemic toxicity associated with intravenous administration of colchicine—Guidelines for use. J Rheumatol 1988;15:495.

http://www.fda.gov/cder/drugs/unapproved_drugs/colchicine_qa.htm (Restriction on drugs containing colchicine)

CASE STUDY ANSWER

This patient had good control of his symptoms for 1 year but now has a prolonged flare, probably denoting worsening disease (not just a temporary flare). In addition to physical findings and measurement of acute-phase reactants such as sedimentation rate or C-reactive protein, it would be wise to get hand and feet radiographs to document whether he has developed joint damage. Assuming such damage is found, the appropriate approach would be either a combination of nonbiologic DMARDs (eg, adding sulfasalazine and hydroxychloroquine) or adding a biologic medication, usually a tumor necrosis factor inhibitor. Follow-up should be every 1–3 months to gauge response and toxicity. Adverse events requiring caution are an increased risk of infection, possible appearance of lymphoma and rare liver function test or hematologic abnormalities. Importantly, close follow-up should ensue, including changing medications every 3–6 months until full disease control is achieved.

C H A P T E R

37

Hypothalamic & Pituitary Hormones

Susan B. Masters, PhD, & Stephen M. Rosenthal, MD

CASE STUDY

A 3-year-old boy [height 85 cm, –3 standard deviations (SD); weight 13 kg, approximately 10th percentile) presents with short stature. Review of the past history and growth chart demonstrates normal birth weight and birth length, but a progressive fall off in height velocity relative to age-matched normal ranges starting at 6 months of age. Physical examination demonstrates short stature and mild generalized obesity. Genital examination reveals descended but small testes and a phallic length of –2 SD. Laboratory evaluation demonstrates growth hormone (GH) deficiency and a delayed bone age of 18 months. The patient is started on replacement with recombinant human GH at a dose of 40 mcg/kg/d subcutaneously. After 1 year of treatment, his height velocity has increased from 5 cm/yr to 11 cm/yr. How does GH stimulate growth in children? What other hormone deficiencies are suggested by the patient's physical examination? What other hormone supplementation is this patient likely to require?

The control of metabolism, growth, and reproduction is mediated by a combination of neural and endocrine systems located in the hypothalamus and pituitary gland. The pituitary weighs about 0.6 g and rests at the base of the brain in the bony sella turcica near the optic chiasm and the cavernous sinuses. The pituitary consists of an anterior lobe (adenohypophysis) and a posterior lobe (neurohypophysis) (Figure 37–1). It is connected to the overlying hypothalamus by a stalk of neurosecretory fibers and blood vessels, including a portal venous system that drains the hypothalamus and perfuses the anterior pituitary. The portal venous system carries small regulatory hormones (Figure 37–1, Table 37–1) from the hypothalamus to the anterior pituitary.

The posterior lobe hormones are synthesized in the hypothalamus and transported via the neurosecretory fibers in the stalk of the pituitary to the posterior lobe, from which they are released into the circulation.

Drugs that mimic or block the effects of hypothalamic and pituitary hormones have pharmacologic applications in three primary areas: (1) as replacement therapy for hormone deficiency states; (2) as antagonists for diseases caused by excess production of pituitary hormones; and (3) as diagnostic tools for identifying several endocrine abnormalities.

■ ANTERIOR PITUITARY HORMONES & THEIR HYPOTHALAMIC REGULATORS

All the hormones produced by the anterior pituitary except prolactin (PRL) are key participants in hormonal systems in which they regulate the production of hormones and autocrine-paracrine factors by endocrine glands and other peripheral tissues. In these systems, the secretion of the pituitary hormone is under the control of one or more hypothalamic hormones. Each hypothalamic-pituitary-endocrine gland system or axis provides multiple opportunities for complex neuroendocrine regulation of growth and development, metabolism, and reproductive function.

ANTERIOR PITUITARY & HYPOTHALAMIC HORMONE RECEPTORS

The anterior pituitary hormones can be classified according to hormone structure and the types of receptors that they activate. **Growth hormone (GH)** and **prolactin**, single-chain protein hormones with significant homology, form one group. Both hormones activate receptors of the JAK/STAT superfamily (see

ACRONYMS

ACTH	Adrenocorticotropic hormone (corticotropin)
CRH	Corticotropin-releasing hormone
FSH	Follicle-stimulating hormone
GH	Growth hormone
GHRH	Growth hormone-releasing hormone
GnRH	Gonadotropin-releasing hormone
hCG	Human chorionic gonadotropin
hMG	Human menopausal gonadotropin
IGF	Insulin-like growth factor
LH	Luteinizing hormone
PRL	Prolactin
rhGH	Recombinant human growth hormone
SST	Somatostatin
TRH	Thyrotropin-releasing hormone
TSH	Thyroid-stimulating hormone (thyrotropin)

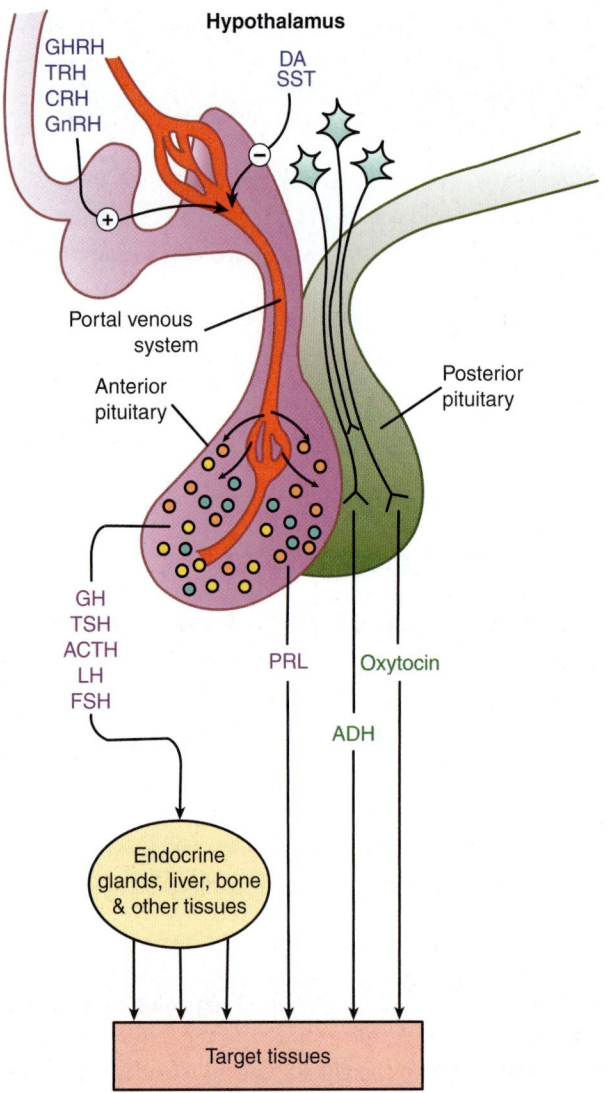

FIGURE 37–1 The hypothalamic-pituitary endocrine system. Except for prolactin, hormones released from the anterior pituitary stimulate the production of hormones by a peripheral endocrine gland, the liver, or other tissues. Prolactin and the hormones released from the posterior pituitary (vasopressin and oxytocin) act directly on target tissues. Hypothalamic factors regulate the release of anterior pituitary hormones. ACTH, adrenocorticotropin; ADH, antidiuretic hormone [vasopressin]; CRH, corticotropin-releasing hormone; DA, dopamine; FSH, follicle-stimulating hormone; GH, growth hormone; GHRH, growth hormone-releasing hormone; GnRH, gonadotropin-releasing hormone; LH, luteinizing hormone; PRL, prolactin; SST, somatostatin; TRH, thyrotropin-releasing hormone; TSH, thyroid-stimulating hormone.

Chapter 2). Three pituitary hormones—**thyroid-stimulating hormone (TSH, thyrotropin)**, **follicle-stimulating hormone (FSH)**, and **luteinizing hormone (LH)**—are dimeric proteins that activate G protein-coupled receptors (see Chapter 2). TSH, FSH, and LH share a common α chain. Their β chains, though somewhat similar to each other, differ enough to confer receptor

TABLE 37–1 Links between hypothalamic, anterior pituitary, and target organ hormone or mediator.[1]

Anterior Pituitary Hormone	Hypothalamic Hormone	Target Organ	Primary Target Organ Hormone or Mediator
Growth hormone (GH, somatotropin)	Growth hormone-releasing hormone (GHRH) (+) Somatostatin (−)	Liver, bone, muscle, kidney, and others	Insulin-like growth factor-I (IGF-I)
Thyroid-stimulating hormone (TSH)	Thyrotropin-releasing hormone (TRH) (+)	Thyroid	Thyroxine, triiodothyronine
Adrenocorticotropin (ACTH)	Corticotropin-releasing hormone (CRH) (+)	Adrenal cortex	Cortisol
Follicle-stimulating hormone (FSH) Luteinizing hormone (LH)	Gonadotropin-releasing hormone (GnRH) (+)[2]	Gonads	Estrogen, progesterone, testosterone
Prolactin (PRL)	Dopamine (−)	Breast	—

[1]All of these hormones act through G protein-coupled receptors except growth hormone and prolactin, which act through JAK/STAT receptors.

[2]Endogenous GnRH, which is released in pulses, stimulates LH and FSH release. When administered continuously as a drug, GnRH and its analogs inhibit LH and FSH release through down-regulation of GnRH receptors.

(+), stimulant; (−), inhibitor.

specificity. Finally, **adrenocorticotropic hormone (ACTH)**, a single peptide cleaved from a larger precursor that also contains the peptide β-endorphin (see Chapter 31), represents a third category. Like TSH, LH, and FSH, ACTH acts through a G protein-coupled receptor. A unique feature of the ACTH receptor (also known as the melanocortin 2 receptor) is that a transmembrane protein, melanocortin 2 receptor accessory protein, is essential for normal ACTH receptor trafficking and signaling.

TSH, FSH, LH, and ACTH share similarities in the regulation of their release from the pituitary. Each is under the control of a distinctive hypothalamic peptide that stimulates their production by acting on G protein-coupled receptors (Table 37–1). TSH release is regulated by **thyrotropin-releasing hormone (TRH)**, whereas the release of LH and FSH (known collectively as gonadotropins) is stimulated by pulses of **gonadotropin-releasing hormone (GnRH).** ACTH release is stimulated by **corticotropin-releasing hormone (CRH).** An important regulatory feature shared by these four structurally related hormones is that they and their hypothalamic releasing factors are subject to feedback inhibitory regulation by the hormones whose production they control. TSH and TRH production are inhibited by the two key thyroid hormones, thyroxine and triiodothyronine (see Chapter 38). Gonadotropin and GnRH production is inhibited in women by estrogen and progesterone, and in men by testosterone and other androgens. ACTH and CRH production are inhibited by cortisol. Feedback regulation is critical to the physiologic control of thyroid, adrenal cortical, and gonadal function and is also important in pharmacologic treatments that affect these systems.

The hypothalamic hormonal control of GH and prolactin differs from the regulatory systems for TSH, FSH, LH, and ACTH. The hypothalamus secretes two hormones that regulate GH; **growth hormone-releasing hormone (GHRH)** stimulates GH production, whereas the peptide **somatostatin (SST)** inhibits GH production. GH and its primary peripheral mediator, **insulin-like growth factor-I (IGF-I)**, also provide feedback to inhibit GH release. Prolactin production is inhibited by the catecholamine **dopamine** acting through the D_2 subtype of dopamine receptors. The hypothalamus does not produce a hormone that specifically stimulates prolactin secretion, although TRH can stimulate

prolactin release, particularly when TRH concentrations are high in the setting of primary hypothyroidism.

Whereas all the pituitary and hypothalamic hormones described previously are available for use in humans, only a few are of major clinical importance. Because of the greater ease of administration of target endocrine gland hormones or their synthetic analogs, the related hypothalamic and pituitary hormones (TRH, TSH, CRH, ACTH, GHRH) are used infrequently as treatments. Some, such as ACTH, are used for specialized diagnostic testing. These agents are described in Tables 37–2 and 37–3 and are not discussed further in this chapter. In contrast, GH, SST, LH, FSH, GnRH, and dopamine or analogs of these hormones are commonly used and are described in the following text.

TABLE 37–2 Clinical uses of hypothalamic hormones and their analogs.

Hypothalamic Hormone	Clinical Uses
Growth hormone-releasing hormone (GHRH)	Used rarely as a diagnostic test for GH and GHRH sufficiency
Thyrotropin-releasing hormone (TRH, protirelin)	May be used to diagnose TRH or TSH deficiencies
Corticotropin-releasing hormone (CRH)	Used rarely to distinguish Cushing's disease from ectopic ACTH secretion
Gonadotropin-releasing hormone (GnRH)	May be used in pulses to treat infertility caused by GnRH deficiency
	Analogs used in long-acting formulations to inhibit gonadal function in children with precocious puberty, in some transgender/gender variant early pubertal adolescents (to block endogenous puberty), in men with prostate cancer and women undergoing assisted reproductive technology (ART) or women who require ovarian suppression for a gynecologic disorder
Dopamine	Dopamine agonists (eg, bromocriptine, cabergoline) used for treatment of hyperprolactinemia

TABLE 37–3 Diagnostic uses of thyroid-stimulating hormone and adrenocorticotropin.

Hormone	Diagnostic Use
Thyroid-stimulating hormone (TSH; thyrotropin)	In patients who have been treated surgically for thyroid carcinoma, to test for recurrence by assessing TSH-stimulated whole-body ^{131}I scans and serum thyroglobulin determinations
Adrenocorticotropin (ACTH)	In patients suspected of adrenal insufficiency, either central (CRH/ACTH deficiency) or peripheral (cortisol deficiency), in particular in suspected cases of congenital adrenal hyperplasia. (See Figure 39–1 and Chapter 39.)

GROWTH HORMONE (SOMATOTROPIN)

Growth hormone, an anterior pituitary hormone, is required during childhood and adolescence for attainment of normal adult size and has important effects throughout postnatal life on lipid and carbohydrate metabolism, and on lean body mass and bone density. Its growth-promoting effects are primarily mediated via **IGF-I** (also known as **somatomedin C**). Individuals with congenital or acquired deficiency of GH during childhood or adolescence fail to reach their predicted adult height and have disproportionately increased body fat and decreased muscle mass. Adults with GH deficiency also have disproportionately low lean body mass.

Chemistry & Pharmacokinetics

A. Structure

Growth hormone is a 191-amino-acid peptide with two sulfhydryl bridges. Its structure closely resembles that of prolactin. In the past, medicinal GH was isolated from the pituitaries of human cadavers. However, this form of GH was found to be contaminated with prions that could cause Creutzfeldt-Jakob disease. For this reason, it is no longer used. **Somatropin**, the recombinant form of GH, has a 191-amino-acid sequence that is identical with the predominant native form of human GH.

B. Absorption, Metabolism, and Excretion

Circulating endogenous GH has a half-life of 20–25 minutes and is predominantly cleared by the liver. Recombinant human GH (rhGH) is administered subcutaneously 6–7 times per week. Peak levels occur in 2–4 hours and active blood levels persist for approximately 36 hours.

Pharmacodynamics

Growth hormone mediates its effects via cell surface receptors of the JAK/STAT cytokine receptor superfamily. Growth hormone has two distinct GH receptor binding sites. Dimerization of two GH receptors is stimulated by a single GH molecule and activates signaling cascades mediated by receptor-associated JAK tyrosine kinases and STATs (see Chapter 2). GH has complex effects on growth, body composition, and carbohydrate, protein, and lipid metabolism. The growth-promoting effects are mediated principally through an increase in the production of IGF-I. Much of the circulating IGF-I is produced in the liver. GH also stimulates production of IGF-I in bone, cartilage, muscle, kidney, and other tissues, where it plays autocrine or paracrine roles. GH stimulates longitudinal bone growth until the epiphyses close—near the end of puberty. In both children and adults, GH has anabolic effects in muscle and catabolic effects in lipid cells that shift the balance of body mass to an increase in muscle mass and a reduction in adiposity. The direct and indirect effects of GH on carbohydrate metabolism are mixed, in part because GH and IGF-I have opposite effects on insulin sensitivity. GH reduces insulin sensitivity, which results in mild hyperinsulinemia, whereas IGF-I has insulin-like effects on glucose transport. In patients who are unable to respond to GH because of severe GH resistance (caused by GH receptor mutations, post-GH receptor signaling mutations, or GH antibodies), the administration of recombinant human IGF-I may cause hypoglycemia because of its insulin-like effects.

Clinical Pharmacology

A. Growth Hormone Deficiency

GH deficiency can have a genetic basis, may be associated with midline developmental defect syndromes (eg, septo-optic dysplasia), or can be acquired as a result of damage to the pituitary or hypothalamus by a trauma (including breech or traumatic delivery), intracranial tumors, infection, infiltrative or hemorrhagic processes, or irradiation. Neonates with isolated GH deficiency are typically of normal size at birth because prenatal growth is not GH-dependent. In contrast, IGF-I is essential for normal prenatal and postnatal growth. Through poorly understood mechanisms, IGF-I expression and postnatal growth become GH-dependent during the first year of life. In childhood, GH deficiency typically presents as short stature, often with mild adiposity. Another early sign of GH deficiency is hypoglycemia due to unopposed action of insulin, to which young children are especially sensitive. Criteria for diagnosis of GH deficiency usually include (1) a subnormal height velocity for age and (2) a subnormal serum GH response following stimulation with at least two GH secretagogues. The prevalence of GH deficiency is approximately 1:5000. Therapy with rhGH permits many children with short stature due to GH deficiency to achieve normal adult height.

In the past, it was believed that adults with GH deficiency do not exhibit a significant syndrome. However, more detailed studies suggest that adults with GH deficiency often have generalized obesity, reduced muscle mass, asthenia, and reduced cardiac output. GH-deficient adults who have been treated with GH have been shown to experience a reversal of many of these manifestations.

B. Growth Hormone Treatment of Pediatric Patients with Short Stature

Although the greatest improvement in growth occurs in patients with GH deficiency, exogenous GH has some effect on height in

TABLE 37–4 Clinical uses of recombinant human growth hormone.

Primary Therapeutic Objective	Clinical Condition
Growth	Growth failure in pediatric patients associated with:
	Growth hormone deficiency
	Chronic renal insufficiency pre-transplant
	Noonan syndrome
	Prader-Willi syndrome
	Short stature homeobox-containing gene (SHOX) deficiency
	Turner syndrome
	Small for gestational age with failure to catch up by age 2 years
	Idiopathic short stature
Improved metabolic state, increased lean body mass, sense of well-being	Growth hormone deficiency in adults
Increased lean body mass, weight, and physical endurance	Wasting in patients with HIV infection
Improved gastrointestinal function	Short bowel syndrome in patients who are also receiving specialized nutritional support

children with short stature caused by factors other than GH deficiency. GH has been approved for several conditions (Table 37–4) and has been used experimentally or off-label in many others. **Prader-Willi syndrome** is an autosomal dominant genetic disease associated with growth failure, obesity, and carbohydrate intolerance. In children with Prader-Willi syndrome and growth failure, GH treatment decreases body fat and increases lean body mass, linear growth, and energy expenditure.

GH treatment has also been shown to have a strong beneficial effect on final height of girls with **Turner syndrome** (45 X karyotype and variants). In clinical trials, GH treatment has been shown to increase final height in girls with Turner syndrome by 10–15 cm (4–6 inches). Because girls with Turner syndrome also have either absent or rudimentary ovaries, GH must be judiciously combined with gonadal steroids to achieve maximal height. Other conditions of pediatric growth failure for which GH treatment is FDA-approved include chronic renal insufficiency pre-transplant and small-for-gestational-age at birth in which the child's height remains more than 2 standard deviations below the norm at 2 years of age.

A controversial but approved use of GH is for children with **idiopathic short stature** (ISS). This is a heterogeneous population that has in common no identifiable cause of the short stature. Some have arbitrarily defined ISS clinically as having a height at least 2.25 standard deviations below the norm for children of the same age and an unlikelihood of achieving an adult height that will be less than 2.25 standard deviations below the norm. In this

group of children, many years of GH therapy result in an average increase in adult height of 4–7 cm (1.57–2.76 inches) at a cost of $5000–$40,000 per year. The complex issues involved in the cost-risk-benefit relationship of this use of GH are important because an estimated 400,000 children in the United States fit the diagnostic criteria for ISS.

Treatment of children with short stature should be carried out by specialists experienced in GH administration. GH dose requirements vary with the condition being treated, with GH-deficient children typically being most responsive. Children must be observed closely for slowing of growth velocity, which could indicate a need to increase the dosage or the possibility of epiphyseal fusion or intercurrent problems such as hypothyroidism or malnutrition.

Other Uses of Growth Hormone

Growth hormone affects many organ systems and also has a net anabolic effect. It has been tested in a number of conditions that are associated with a severe catabolic state and is approved for the treatment of wasting in patients with AIDS. In 2004, GH was approved for treatment of patients with short bowel syndrome who are dependent on total parenteral nutrition (TPN). After intestinal resection or bypass, the remaining functional intestine in many patients undergoes extensive adaptation that allows it to adequately absorb nutrients. However, other patients fail to adequately adapt and develop a malabsorption syndrome. GH has been shown to increase intestinal growth and improve its function in experimental animals. Benefits of GH treatment for patients with short bowel syndrome and dependence on total parenteral nutrition have mostly been short-lived in the clinical studies that have been published to date. Growth hormone is administered with glutamine, which also has trophic effects on the intestinal mucosa.

GH is a popular component of "anti-aging" programs. Serum levels of GH normally decline with aging; anti-aging programs claim that injection of GH or administration of drugs purported to increase GH release are effective anti-aging remedies. These claims are largely unsubstantiated. In contrast studies in mice and the nematode *C elegans* have clearly demonstrated that analogs of human GH and IGF-I consistently *shorten* life span and that loss-of-function mutations in the signaling pathways for the GH and IGF-I analogs lengthen life span. Another use of GH is by athletes for a purported increase in muscle mass and athletic performance. GH is one of the drugs banned by the Olympic Committee.

Although GH has important effects on lipid and carbohydrate metabolism and on lean body mass, it does not seem likely to be a fruitful direct target for efforts to develop new drugs to treat obesity. However, some of the hormonal and neuroendocrine systems that regulate GH secretion are being investigated as possible targets for antiobesity drugs (see Box: Treatment of Obesity).

In 1993, the FDA approved the use of recombinant bovine growth hormone (rbGH) in dairy cattle to increase milk production. Although milk and meat from rbGH-treated cows appear to be safe, these cows have a higher incidence of mastitis, which could increase antibiotic use and result in greater antibiotic residues in milk and meat.

TREATMENT OF OBESITY[1]

It is said that the developed world is experiencing an "epidemic of obesity." This statement is based on statistics showing that in the USA, for example, 30–40% of the population is above optimal weight and that the excess weight (especially abdominal fat) is often associated with the **metabolic syndrome** and increased risks of cardiovascular disease and diabetes. Since eating behavior is an expression of endocrine, neurophysiologic, and psychological processes, prevention and treatment of obesity are complex. It is not surprising that there is considerable scientific and financial interest in developing pharmacologic therapy for the condition.

Although obesity can be defined as excess adipose tissue, it is currently quantitated by means of the body mass index (BMI), calculated from BMI = weight (in kilograms)/height^2 (in meters). Using this measure, a normal BMI is defined as 18.5–24.9; overweight, 25–29.9; obese, 30–39.9; and morbidly obese (ie, at very high risk), ≥ 40. Some extremely muscular individuals may have a BMI higher than 25 and no excess fat; however, the BMI scale generally correlates with the degree of obesity and with risk.

Although the cause of obesity can be simply stated as energy intake (dietary calories) exceeding energy output (resting metabolism plus exercise), the actual physiology of weight control is extremely complex, and the pathophysiology of obesity is still poorly understood. Many hormones and neuronal mechanisms regulate intake (appetite, satiety), processing (absorption, conversion to fat, glycogen, etc), and output (thermogenesis, muscle work). The fact that a large number of hormones reduce appetite (Table 37–4.1, see online version of this book) might appear to offer many targets for weight-reducing drug therapy, but despite intensive research, no available pharmacologic therapy has succeeded in maintaining a weight loss of over 10% for 1 year. Furthermore, the social and psychological aspects of eating are powerful influences that are independent of or only partially dependent on the physiologic control mechanisms. In contrast, bariatric (weight-reducing) surgery readily achieves a sustained weight loss of 10–40%. Furthermore, surgery that bypasses the stomach and upper small intestine (but not simple restrictive banding) rapidly reverses some aspects of the metabolic syndrome even before significant weight is lost. However, even a 5–10% loss of weight is associated with a reduction in blood pressure and improved glycemic control.

Until approximately 15 years ago, the most popular and successful appetite suppressants were the nonselective 5-HT$_2$ agonists: fenfluramine and dexfenfluramine. Combined with phentermine as Fen-Phen and Dex-Phen, they were moderately effective. However, these drugs were found to cause pulmonary hypertension and cardiac valve defects and were withdrawn.

Older drugs still available in the United States and some other countries include phenylpropanolamine, benzphetamine, amphetamine, methamphetamine, phentermine, diethylpropion, mazindol, and phendimetrazine. These drugs are all amphetamine mimics and are central nervous system appetite suppressants; they are generally helpful only during the first few weeks of therapy. Their toxicity is significant and includes hypertension (with a risk of cerebral hemorrhage) and addiction liability.

Orlistat is the only non-amphetamine drug currently approved in the United States for the treatment of obesity. Two other drugs that have been intensely studied are listed in Table 37–5. Clinical trials and phase 4 reports suggest that orlistat is modestly effective for the duration of therapy (up to 1 year) and is probably safer than the amphetamine mimics. However, it does not produce more than a 5–10% loss of weight. Sibutramine was marketed for several years but was withdrawn because of increasing evidence of cardiovascular toxicity. Lorcaserin received intense study through 2010 and was submitted for approval to the FDA, but this was denied on the basis of considerations of inadequate safety and effectiveness.

Because of the low efficacy of the drugs listed in Table 37–5, intensive research continues. (Some drugs approved for other indications that reduce appetite and possible future weight loss drugs are set forth in Table 37–5.1, see online version of this book). Because of the redundancy of the physiologic mechanisms for control of body weight, it seems likely that polypharmacy targeting multiple pathways will be needed to achieve success.

[1]Contributed by B.G. Katzung.

Toxicity & Contraindications

Children generally tolerate GH treatment well. Adverse events are relatively rare and include pseudotumor cerebri; slipped capital femoral epiphysis; progression of scoliosis; edema; hyperglycemia; and increased risk of asphyxiation in severely obese patients with Prader-Willi syndrome and upper airway obstruction or sleep apnea. Patients with Turner syndrome have an increased risk of otitis media while taking GH. In children with GH deficiency, periodic evaluation of the other anterior pituitary hormones may reveal concurrent deficiencies, which also require treatment (eg, with hydrocortisone, levothyroxine, or gonadal hormones). Pancreatitis, gynecomastia, and nevus growth have occurred in patients receiving GH. Adults tend to have more adverse effects from GH therapy. Peripheral edema, myalgias, and arthralgias (especially in the hands and wrists) occur commonly but remit with dosage reduction. Carpal tunnel syndrome can occur. GH treatment increases the activity of cytochrome P450 isoforms, which may reduce the serum levels of drugs

TABLE 37–5 Newer anti-obesity drugs and their effects.

	Orlistat	Sibutramine	Lorcaserin
Target organ	Gut	CNS	CNS (peripheral ?)
Target molecule	GI lipase inhibitor	SERT and NET inhibitor	Selective 5-HT$_{2C}$ receptor agonist
Mechanism of action	Reduces absorption of fats since triglycerides not split	Reduces appetite	Reduces appetite
Toxicity	GI: Flatulence, steatorrhea, fecal incontinence	Tachycardia, hypertension, infarction	Headache; tumorigenesis in rats
Dosage	130 mg tid	10–15 mg qd	10–20 mg qd
Availability	Over the counter	Prescription; withdrawn in 2010	NDA approval denied by FDA

CNS, central nervous system; GI, gastrointestinal; SERT, serotonin reuptake transporter; NET, norepinephrine reuptake transporter; tid, three times daily; qd, daily.

metabolized by that enzyme system (see Chapter 4). There has been no increased incidence of malignancy among patients receiving GH therapy, but GH treatment is contraindicated in a patient with a known active malignancy. Proliferative retinopathy may rarely occur. GH treatment of critically ill patients appears to *increase* mortality.

MECASERMIN

A small number of children with growth failure have severe IGF-I deficiency that is not responsive to exogenous GH. Causes include mutations in the GH receptor and in the GH receptor signaling pathway, neutralizing antibodies to GH, and IGF-I gene defects. In 2005, the FDA approved two forms of recombinant human IGF-I (rhIGF-I) for treatment of severe IGF-I deficiency that is not responsive to GH: mecasermin and mecasermin rinfabate. Mecasermin is rhIGF-I alone, while mecasermin rinfabate is a complex of recombinant human IGF-I (rhIGF-I) and recombinant human insulin-like growth factor-binding protein-3 (rhIGFBP-3). This binding protein significantly increases the circulating half-life of rhIGF-I. Normally, the great majority of the circulating IGF-I is bound to IGFBP-3, which is produced principally by the liver under the control of GH. Mecasermin rinfabate is not currently available in the United States. Mecasermin is administered subcutaneously twice daily at a recommended starting dosage of 0.04–0.08 mg/kg and increased weekly up to a maximum twice-daily dosage of 0.12 mg/kg.

The most important adverse effect observed with mecasermin is hypoglycemia. To avoid hypoglycemia, the prescribing instructions require consumption of a carbohydrate-containing meal or snack 20 minutes before or after mecasermin administration. Several patients have experienced intracranial hypertension and asymptomatic elevation of liver enzymes.

GROWTH HORMONE ANTAGONISTS

The need for antagonists of GH stems from the tendency of GH-producing cells (somatotrophs) in the anterior pituitary to form GH-secreting tumors. Pituitary adenomas occur most commonly in adults. In adults, GH-secreting adenomas cause **acromegaly**, which is characterized by abnormal growth of cartilage and bone tissue, and

many organs including skin, muscle, heart, liver, and the gastrointestinal tract. Acromegaly adversely affects the skeletal, muscular, cardiovascular, respiratory, and metabolic systems. When a GH-secreting adenoma occurs before the long bone epiphyses close, it leads to the rare condition, **gigantism**. Small GH-secreting adenomas can be treated with GH antagonists. These include somatostatin analogs and dopamine receptor agonists, which reduce the production of GH, and the novel GH receptor antagonist **pegvisomant**, which prevents GH from activating GH signaling pathways. Larger pituitary adenomas produce greater amounts of GH and also can impair visual and central nervous system function by encroaching on nearby brain structures. These are treated with transsphenoidal surgery or radiation.

Somatostatin Analogs

Somatostatin, a 14-amino-acid peptide (Figure 37–2), is found in the hypothalamus, other parts of the central nervous system, the pancreas, and other sites in the gastrointestinal tract. It inhibits the release of GH, TSH, glucagon, insulin, and gastrin.

Exogenous somatostatin is rapidly cleared from the circulation, with an initial half-life of 1–3 minutes. The kidney appears to play an important role in its metabolism and excretion.

Somatostatin has limited therapeutic usefulness because of its short duration of action and multiple effects in many secretory

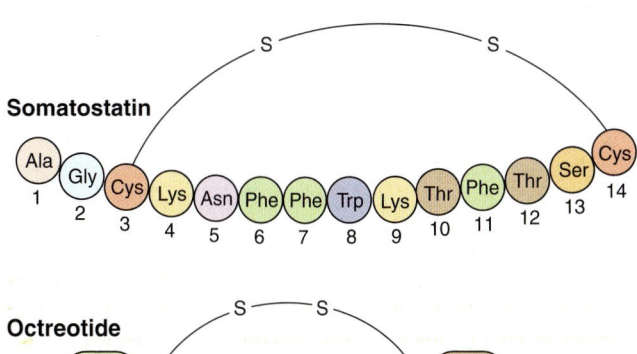

FIGURE 37–2 **Above:** Amino acid sequence of somatostatin. **Below:** Sequence of the synthetic analog, octreotide.

systems. A series of longer-acting somatostatin analogs that retain biologic activity have been developed. **Octreotide**, the most widely used somatostatin analog (Figure 37–2), is 45 times more potent than somatostatin in inhibiting GH release but only twice as potent in reducing insulin secretion. Because of this relatively reduced effect on pancreatic beta cells, hyperglycemia rarely occurs during treatment. The plasma elimination half-life of octreotide is about 80 minutes, 30 times longer than that of somatostatin.

Octreotide, 50–200 mcg given subcutaneously every 8 hours, reduces symptoms caused by a variety of hormone-secreting tumors: acromegaly; the carcinoid syndrome; gastrinoma; glucagonoma; nesidioblastosis; the watery diarrhea, hypokalemia, and achlorhydria (WDHA) syndrome; and diabetic diarrhea. Somatostatin receptor scintigraphy, using radiolabeled octreotide, is useful in localizing neuroendocrine tumors having somatostatin receptors and helps predict the response to octreotide therapy. Octreotide is also useful for the acute control of bleeding from esophageal varices.

Octreotide acetate injectable long-acting suspension is a slow-release microsphere formulation. It is instituted only after a brief course of shorter-acting octreotide has been demonstrated to be effective and tolerated. Injections into alternate gluteal muscles are repeated at 4-week intervals in doses of 20–40 mg.

Adverse effects of octreotide therapy include nausea, vomiting, abdominal cramps, flatulence, and steatorrhea with bulky bowel movements. Biliary sludge and gallstones may occur after 6 months of use in 20–30% of patients. However, the yearly incidence of symptomatic gallstones is about 1%. Cardiac effects include sinus bradycardia (25%) and conduction disturbances (10%). Pain at the site of injection is common, especially with the long-acting octreotide suspension. Vitamin B_{12} deficiency may occur with long-term use of octreotide.

A long-acting formulation of **lanreotide**, another octapeptide somatostatin analog, was approved by the FDA in 2007 for treatment of acromegaly. Lanreotide appears to have effects comparable to those of octreotide on reducing GH levels and normalizing IGF-I concentrations.

Pegvisomant

Pegvisomant is a GH receptor antagonist used to treat acromegaly. It is the polyethylene glycol (PEG) derivative of a mutant GH, B2036. Like native GH, pegvisomant has two GH receptor binding sites. However, one of the pegvisomant GH receptor binding sites has increased affinity for the GH receptor, whereas its second GH receptor binding site has reduced affinity. This differential receptor affinity allows the initial step (GH receptor dimerization) but blocks the conformational changes required for signal transduction. Pegvisomant is a less potent GH receptor antagonist than is B2036, but pegylation reduces its clearance and improves its overall clinical effectiveness. When pegvisomant was administered subcutaneously to 160 patients with acromegaly daily for 12 months or more, serum levels of IGF-I fell into the normal range in 97%; two patients experienced growth of their GH-secreting pituitary tumors and two patients developed increases in liver enzymes.

THE GONADOTROPINS (FOLLICLE-STIMULATING HORMONE & LUTEINIZING HORMONE) & HUMAN CHORIONIC GONADOTROPIN

The gonadotropins are produced by a single type of pituitary cell, the gonadotroph. These hormones serve complementary functions in the reproductive process. In women, the principal function of FSH is to direct ovarian follicle development. Both FSH and LH are needed for ovarian steroidogenesis. In the ovary, LH stimulates androgen production by theca cells in the follicular stage of the menstrual cycle, whereas FSH stimulates the conversion by granulosa cells of androgens to estrogens. In the luteal phase of the menstrual cycle, estrogen and progesterone production is primarily under the control first of LH and then, if pregnancy occurs, under the control of human chorionic gonadotropin (hCG). Human chorionic gonadotropin is a placental protein nearly identical with LH; its actions are mediated through LH receptors.

In men, FSH is the primary regulator of spermatogenesis, whereas LH is the main stimulus for testosterone synthesis in Leydig cells. FSH helps maintain high local androgen concentrations in the vicinity of developing sperm by stimulating the production of androgen-binding protein in Sertoli cells. FSH also stimulates the conversion by Sertoli cells of testosterone to estrogen.

FSH, LH, and hCG are available in several pharmaceutical forms. They are used in states of infertility to stimulate spermatogenesis in men and to induce ovulation in women. Their most common clinical use is for the controlled ovulation hyperstimulation that is the cornerstone of assisted reproductive technologies such as in vitro fertilization (IVF, see below).

Chemistry & Pharmacokinetics

All three hormones—FSH, LH, and hCG—are heterodimers that share an identical α chain in addition to a distinct β chain that confers receptor specificity. The β chains of hCG and LH are nearly identical, and these two hormones are used interchangeably. All the gonadotropin preparations are administered by subcutaneous or intramuscular injection, usually on a daily basis. Half-lives vary by preparation and route of injection from 10 to 40 hours.

A. Menotropins

The first commercial gonadotropin product was extracted from the urine of postmenopausal women, which contains a substance with FSH-like properties (but with 4% of the potency of FSH) and an LH-like substance. This purified extract of FSH and LH is known as **menotropins**, or human menopausal gonadotropins (**hMG**).

B. Follicle-Stimulating Hormone

Three forms of purified FSH are available. **Urofollitropin**, also known as uFSH, is a purified preparation of human FSH extracted from the urine of postmenopausal women. Virtually all the LH activity has been removed through a form of immuno-affinity chromatography that uses anti-hCG antibodies. Two recombinant forms of FSH (**rFSH**) are also available: **follitropin alfa** and **follitropin beta.** The amino acid sequences of these two products are identical to that of human FSH. They differ from each other and urofollitropin in the composition of carbohydrate side chains. The rFSH preparations have a shorter half-life than preparations derived from human urine but stimulate estrogen secretion at least as efficiently and, in some studies, more efficiently. The rFSH preparations are considerably more expensive.

C. Luteinizing Hormone

Lutropin alfa, the recombinant form of human LH, was introduced in the United States in 2004. When given by subcutaneous injection, it has a half-life of about 10 hours. Lutropin has only been approved for use in combination with follitropin alfa for stimulation of follicular development in infertile women with profound LH deficiency. It has not been approved for use with the other preparations of FSH nor for simulating the endogenous LH surge that is needed to complete follicular development and precipitate ovulation.

D. Human Chorionic Gonadotropin

hCG is produced by the human placenta and excreted into the urine, whence it can be extracted and purified. It is a glycoprotein consisting of a 92-amino-acid α chain virtually identical to that of FSH, LH, and TSH, and a β chain of 145 amino acids that resembles that of LH except for the presence of a carboxyl terminal sequence of 30 amino acids not present in LH. **Choriogonadotropin alfa** (rhCG) is a recombinant form of hCG. Because of its greater consistency in biologic activity, rhCG is packaged and dosed on the basis of weight rather than units of activity. All of the other gonadotropins, including rFSH, are packaged and dosed on the basis of units of activity. The preparation of hCG that is purified from human urine is administered by intramuscular injection, whereas rhCG is administered by subcutaneous injection.

Pharmacodynamics

The gonadotropins and hCG exert their effects through G protein-coupled receptors. LH and FSH have complex effects on reproductive tissues in both sexes. In women, these effects change over the time course of a menstrual cycle as a result of a complex interplay between concentration-dependent effects of the gonadotropins, cross-talk between LH, FSH, and gonadal steroids, and the influence of other ovarian hormones. A coordinated pattern of FSH and LH secretion during the menstrual cycle (see Figure 40–1) is required for normal follicle development, ovulation, and pregnancy.

During the first 8 weeks of pregnancy, the progesterone and estrogen required to maintain pregnancy are produced by the ovarian corpus luteum. For the first few days after ovulation, the corpus luteum is maintained by maternal LH. However, as maternal LH concentrations fall owing to increasing concentrations of progesterone and estrogen, the corpus luteum will continue to

function only if the role of maternal LH is taken over by hCG produced by the embryo and its new placenta.

Clinical Pharmacology

A. Ovulation Induction

The gonadotropins are used to induce ovulation in women with anovulation that is secondary to hypogonadotropic hypogonadism, polycystic ovary syndrome, obesity, and other causes. Because of the high cost of gonadotropins and the need for close monitoring during their administration, they are generally reserved for anovulatory women who fail to respond to other less complicated forms of treatment (eg, clomiphene; see Chapter 40). Gonadotropins are also used for **controlled ovarian hyperstimulation** in assisted reproductive technology procedures. A number of protocols make use of gonadotropins in ovulation induction and controlled ovulation hyperstimulation, and new protocols are continually being developed to improve the rates of success and to decrease the two primary risks of ovulation induction: multiple pregnancies and the **ovarian hyperstimulation syndrome** (OHSS; see below).

Although the details differ, all of these protocols are based on the complex physiology that underlies a normal menstrual cycle. Like a menstrual cycle, ovulation induction is discussed in relation to a cycle that begins on the first day of a menstrual bleed (Figure 37–3). Shortly after the first day (usually on day 3), daily injections with one of the FSH preparations (hMG, urofollitropin) are begun and are continued for approximately 7–12 days. In women with hypogonadotropic hypogonadism, follicle development requires treatment with a combination of FSH and LH because these women do not produce the basal level of LH that is required for adequate ovarian estrogen production and normal follicle development. The dose and duration of FSH treatment are based on the response as measured by the serum estradiol concentration and by ultrasound evaluation of ovarian follicle development and endometrial thickness. When exogenous gonadotropins are used to stimulate follicle development, there is risk of a premature endogenous surge in LH owing to the rapidly changing hormonal milieu. To prevent this, gonadotropins are almost always administered in conjunction with a drug that blocks the effects of endogenous GnRH—either continuous administration of a GnRH agonist, which down-regulates GnRH receptors or a GnRH receptor antagonist (see below and Figure 37–3).

When appropriate follicular maturation has occurred, the FSH and the GnRH agonist or GnRH antagonist injections are discontinued; the following day, hCG (5000–10,000 IU) is administered intramuscularly to induce final follicular maturation and, in ovulation induction protocols, ovulation. The hCG administration is followed by insemination in ovulation induction and by oocyte retrieval in assisted reproductive technology procedures. Because use of GnRH agonists or antagonists during the follicular phase of ovulation induction suppresses endogenous LH production, it is important to provide exogenous hormonal support of the luteal phase. In clinical trials, exogenous progesterone, hCG, or a combination of the two have been effective at providing adequate luteal support. However, progesterone is preferred for luteal

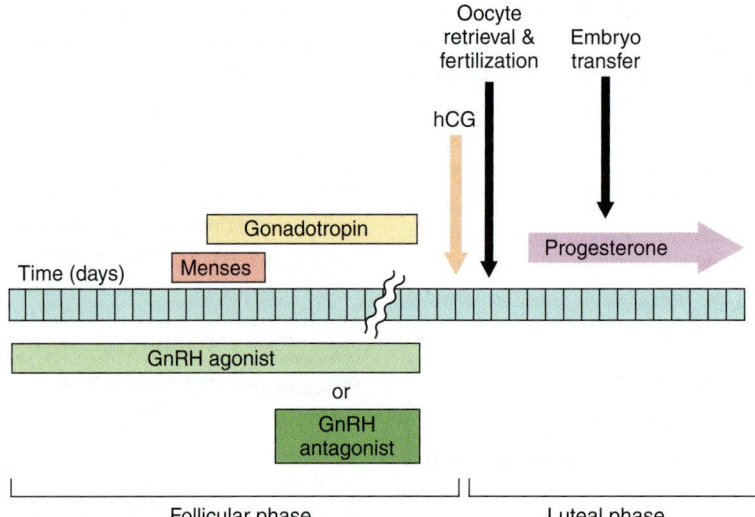

FIGURE 37–3 Controlled ovarian hyperstimulation in preparation for an assisted reproductive technology such as in vitro fertilization. Follicular phase: Follicle development is stimulated with gonadotropin injections that begin about 3 days after menses begin. When the follicles are ready, as assessed by measurement of serum estrogen concentration and ultrasound measurement of follicle size, final oocyte maturation is induced by an injection of hCG. Luteal phase: Shortly thereafter oocytes are retrieved and fertilized in vitro. The recipient's luteal phase is supported with injections of progesterone. To prevent a premature luteinizing-hormone surge, endogenous gonadotropin secretion is inhibited during the follicular phase with either a GnRH agonist or a GnRH antagonist. In most protocols, the GnRH agonist is started midway through the preceding luteal cycle.

support because hCG carries a higher risk of the ovarian hyperstimulation syndrome (see below).

B. Male Infertility

Most of the signs and symptoms of hypogonadism in males (eg, delayed puberty, retention of prepubertal secondary sex characteristics after puberty) can be adequately treated with exogenous androgen; however, treatment of infertility in hypogonadal men requires the activity of both LH and FSH. For many years, conventional therapy has consisted of initial treatment for 8–12 weeks with injections of 1000–2500 IU hCG several times per week. After the initial phase, hMG is injected at a dose of 75–150 units three times per week. In men with hypogonadal hypogonadism, it takes an average of 4–6 months of such treatment for sperm to appear in the ejaculate. With the more recent availability of urofollitropin, rFSH, and rLH, a number of alternative protocols have been developed. An advance that has indirectly benefited gonadotropin treatment of male infertility is intracytoplasmic sperm injection (ICSI), in which a single sperm is injected directly into a mature oocyte that has been retrieved after controlled ovarian hyperstimulation of a female partner. With the advent of ICSI, the minimum threshold of spermatogenesis required for pregnancy is greatly lowered.

C. Outdated Uses

Chorionic gonadotropin is approved for the treatment of prepubertal cryptorchidism. Prepubertal boys generally between 4 and 9 years of age were treated with IM injections of hCG for 2–6 weeks.

However, this clinical use is no longer supported because the long-term efficacy of hormonal treatment of cryptorchidism (~ 20%) is much lower than the long-term efficacy of surgical treatment (> 95%), and because of concerns that early childhood treatment with hCG treatment has a negative impact on germ cells in addition to increasing the risk of precocious puberty.

In the United States, chorionic gonadotropin has a black-box warning against its use for weight loss. The use of hCG plus severe calorie restriction for weight loss was popularized by a publication in the 1950s claiming that the hCG selectively mobilizes body fat stores. This practice continues today, despite a preponderance of subsequent scientific evidence from placebo-controlled trials that hCG does not provide any weight loss benefit beyond the weight loss associated with severe calorie restriction alone.

Toxicity & Contraindications

In women treated with gonadotropins and hCG, the two most serious complications are the **ovarian hyperstimulation syndrome** and **multiple pregnancies.** Overstimulation of the ovary during ovulation induction often leads to uncomplicated ovarian enlargement that usually resolves spontaneously. The ovarian hyperstimulation syndrome is a more serious complication that occurs in 0.5–4% of patients. It is characterized by ovarian enlargement, ascites, hydrothorax, and hypovolemia, sometimes resulting in shock. Hemoperitoneum (from a ruptured ovarian cyst), fever, and arterial thromboembolism can occur.

The probability of multiple pregnancies is greatly increased when ovulation induction and assisted reproductive technologies are used. In ovulation induction, the risk of a multiple pregnancy is estimated to be 15–20%, whereas the percentage of multiple pregnancies in the general population is closer to 1%. Multiple pregnancies carry an increased risk of complications, such as gestational diabetes, preeclampsia, and preterm labor. For in vitro fertilization procedures, the risk of a multiple pregnancy is primarily determined by the number of embryos transferred to the recipient. A strong trend in recent years has been to transfer fewer embryos.

Other reported adverse effects of gonadotropin treatment are headache, depression, edema, precocious puberty, and (rarely) production of antibodies to hCG. In men treated with gonadotropins, the risk of gynecomastia is directly correlated with the level of testosterone produced in response to treatment. An association between ovarian cancer, infertility, and fertility drugs has been reported. However, it is not known which, if any, fertility drugs are causally related to cancer.

GONADOTROPIN-RELEASING HORMONE & ITS ANALOGS

Gonadotropin-releasing hormone is secreted by neurons in the hypothalamus. It travels through the hypothalamic-pituitary venous portal plexus to the anterior pituitary, where it binds to G protein-coupled receptors on the plasma membranes of gonadotroph cells. *Pulsatile* GnRH secretion is required to stimulate the gonadotroph cell to produce and release LH and FSH.

Sustained *nonpulsatile* administration of GnRH or GnRH analogs *inhibits* the release of FSH and LH by the pituitary in both women and men, resulting in hypogonadism. GnRH agonists are used to produce gonadal suppression in men with prostate cancer. They are also used in women who are undergoing assisted reproductive technology procedures or who have a gynecologic problem that is benefited by ovarian suppression.

Chemistry & Pharmacokinetics

A. Structure

GnRH is a decapeptide found in all mammals. **Gonadorelin** is an acetate salt of synthetic human GnRH. Synthetic analogs of GnRH include **goserelin, histrelin, leuprolide, nafarelin,** and **triptorelin.** These analogs all have D-amino acids at position 6, and all but nafarelin have ethylamide substituted for glycine at position 10. Both modifications make them more potent and longer-lasting than native GnRH and gonadorelin.

B. Pharmacokinetics

Gonadorelin can be administered intravenously or subcutaneously. GnRH analogs can be administered subcutaneously, intramuscularly, via nasal spray (nafarelin), or as a subcutaneous implant. The half-life of intravenous gonadorelin is 4 minutes, and the half-lives of subcutaneous and intranasal GnRH analogs are approximately 3 hours. The duration of clinical uses of GnRH agonists varies from a few days for ovulation induction to a number of years for treatment of metastatic prostate cancer. Therefore,

preparations have been developed with a range of durations of action from several hours (for daily administration) to 1, 4, 6, or 12 months (depot forms).

Pharmacodynamics

The physiologic actions of GnRH exhibit complex dose-response relationships that change dramatically from the fetal period through the end of puberty. This is not surprising in view of the complex role that GnRH plays in normal reproduction, particularly in female reproduction. Pulsatile GnRH release occurs and is responsible for stimulating LH and FSH production during the fetal and neonatal period. Subsequently, from the age of 2 years until the onset of puberty, GnRH secretion falls off and the pituitary simultaneously exhibits very low sensitivity to GnRH. Just before puberty, an increase in the frequency and amplitude of GnRH release occurs and then, in early puberty, pituitary sensitivity to GnRH increases, which is due in part to the effect of increasing concentrations of gonadal steroids. In females, it usually takes several months to a year after the onset of puberty for the hypothalamic-pituitary system to produce an LH surge and ovulation. By the end of puberty, the system is well established so that menstrual cycles proceed at relatively constant intervals. The amplitude and frequency of GnRH pulses vary in a regular pattern through the menstrual cycle with the highest amplitudes occurring during the luteal phase and the highest frequency occurring late in the follicular phase. Lower pulse frequencies favor FSH secretion, whereas higher pulse frequencies favor LH secretion. Gonadal steroids as well as the peptide hormones activin and inhibin have complex modulatory effects on the gonadotropin response to GnRH.

In the pharmacologic use of GnRH and its analogs, pulsatile intravenous administration of gonadorelin every 1–4 hours stimulates FSH and LH secretion. Continuous administration of gonadorelin or its longer-acting analogs produces a biphasic response. During the first 7–10 days, an agonist effect results in increased concentrations of gonadal hormones in males and females; this initial phase is referred to as a *flare*. After this period, the continued presence of GnRH results in an inhibitory action that manifests as a drop in the concentration of gonadotropins and gonadal steroids. The inhibitory action is due to a combination of receptor down-regulation and changes in the signaling pathways activated by GnRH.

Clinical Pharmacology

The GnRH agonists are occasionally used for stimulation of gonadotropin production. They are used far more commonly for suppression of gonadotropin release.

A. Stimulation

1. Female infertility—In the current era of widespread availability of gonadotropins and assisted reproductive technology, the use of pulsatile GnRH administration to treat infertility is uncommon. Although pulsatile GnRH is less likely than gonadotropins to cause multiple pregnancies and the ovarian hyperstimulation syndrome, the inconvenience and cost associated with continuous use of an intravenous pump and difficulties obtaining native GnRH (gonadorelin) are barriers to pulsatile GnRH. When this approach is used, a portable battery-powered programmable pump and intravenous tubing deliver pulses of gonadorelin every 90 minutes.

Gonadorelin or a GnRH agonist analog can be used to initiate an LH surge and ovulation in women with infertility who are undergoing ovulation induction with gonadotropins. Traditionally, hCG has been used to initiate ovulation in this situation. However, there is some evidence that gonadorelin or a GnRH agonist is less likely than hCG to cause multiple ova to be released and less likely to cause the ovarian hyperstimulation syndrome.

2. Male infertility

It is possible to use pulsatile gonadorelin for infertility in men with hypothalamic hypogonadotropic hypogonadism. A portable pump infuses gonadorelin intravenously every 90 minutes. Serum testosterone levels and semen analyses must be done regularly. At least 3–6 months of pulsatile infusions are required before significant numbers of sperm are seen. As described above, treatment of hypogonadotropic hypogonadism is more commonly done with hCG and hMG or their recombinant equivalents.

3. Diagnosis of LH responsiveness

GnRH can be useful in determining whether delayed puberty in a hypogonadotropic adolescent is due to constitutional delay or to hypogonadotropic hypogonadism. The LH response (but not the FSH response) to a single dose of GnRH can distinguish between these two conditions. Serum LH levels are measured before and at various times after an intravenous or subcutaneous bolus of GnRH. An increase in serum LH with a peak that exceeds 15.6 mIU/mL is normal and suggests impending puberty. An impaired LH response suggests hypogonadotropic hypogonadism due to either pituitary or hypothalamic disease, but does not rule out constitutional delay of adolescence.

B. Suppression of Gonadotropin Production

1. Controlled ovarian hyperstimulation

In the controlled ovarian hyperstimulation that provides multiple mature oocytes for assisted reproductive technologies such as in vitro fertilization, it is critical to suppress an endogenous LH surge that could prematurely trigger ovulation. This suppression is most commonly achieved by daily subcutaneous injections of leuprolide or daily nasal applications of nafarelin. For leuprolide, treatment is commonly initiated with 1.0 mg daily for about 10 days or until menstrual bleeding occurs. At that point, the dose is reduced to 0.5 mg daily until hCG is administered (Figure 37–3). For nafarelin, the beginning dosage is generally 400 mcg twice a day, which is decreased to 200 mcg when menstrual bleeding occurs. In women who respond poorly to the standard protocol, alternative protocols that use shorter courses and lower doses of GnRH agonists may improve the follicular response to gonadotropins.

2. Endometriosis

Endometriosis is a syndrome of cyclical abdominal pain in premenopausal women that is due to the presence of estrogen-sensitive endometrium-like tissue outside the uterus. The pain of endometriosis is often reduced by abolishing exposure to the cyclical changes in the concentrations of estrogen and progesterone that are a normal part of the menstrual cycle. The ovarian suppression induced by continuous treatment with a GnRH agonist greatly reduces estrogen and progesterone concentrations and prevents cyclical changes. The preferred duration of treatment with a GnRH agonist is limited to 6 months because ovarian suppression beyond this period can result in decreased bone density. Leuprolide, goserelin, and nafarelin are approved for this indication. Leuprolide and goserelin are administered as depot preparations that provide 1 or 3 months of continuous GnRH agonist activity. Nafarelin is administered twice daily as a nasal spray at a dose of 0.2 mg per spray.

3. Uterine leiomyomata (uterine fibroids)

Uterine leiomyomata are benign, estrogen-sensitive, fibrous growths in the uterus that can cause menorrhagia, with associated anemia and pelvic pain. Treatment for 3–6 months with a GnRH agonist reduces fibroid size and, when combined with supplemental iron, improves anemia. Leuprolide, goserelin, and nafarelin are approved for this indication. The doses and routes of administration are similar to those described for treatment of endometriosis.

4. Prostate cancer

Antiandrogen therapy is the primary medical therapy for prostate cancer. Combined antiandrogen therapy with continuous GnRH agonist and an androgen receptor antagonist such as flutamide (see Chapter 40) is as effective as surgical castration in reducing serum testosterone concentrations and effects. Leuprolide, goserelin, histrelin, and triptorelin are approved for this indication. The preferred formulation is one of the long-acting depot forms that provide 1, 3, 4, 6, or 12 months of active drug therapy. During the first 7–10 days of GnRH analog therapy, serum testosterone levels increase because of the agonist action of the drug; this can precipitate pain in patients with bone metastases, and tumor growth and neurologic symptoms in patients with vertebral metastases. It can also temporarily worsen symptoms of urinary obstruction. Such tumor flares can usually be avoided with the concomitant administration of bicalutamide or one of the other androgen receptor antagonists (see Chapter 40). Within about 2 weeks, serum testosterone levels fall to the hypogonadal range.

5. Central precocious puberty

Continuous administration of a GnRH agonist is indicated for treatment of central precocious puberty (onset of secondary sex characteristics before 7–8 years in girls or 9 years in boys). Before embarking on treatment with a GnRH agonist, one must confirm central precocious puberty by demonstrating a pubertal gonadotropin response to GnRH or a "test dose" of a GnRH analog. Treatment is typically indicated in a child whose final height would be otherwise significantly compromised (as evidenced by a significantly advanced bone age) or in whom the development of pubertal secondary sexual characteristics

or menses causes significant emotional distress. While central precocious puberty is most often idiopathic, it is important to rule out central nervous system pathology with MRI imaging of the hypothalamic-pituitary area.

Treatment is most commonly carried out with either a monthly intramuscular depot injection of leuprolide acetate or with a once-yearly implant of histrelin acetate. Daily subcutaneous regimens and multiple daily nasal spray regimens of GnRH agonists are also available. Treatment with a GnRH agonist is generally continued to age 11 in females and age 12 in males.

6. Other—Other clinical uses for the gonadal suppression provided by continuous GnRH agonist treatment include advanced breast and ovarian cancer; thinning of the endometrial lining in preparation for an endometrial ablation procedure in women with dysfunctional uterine bleeding; and treatment of amenorrhea and infertility in women with polycystic ovary disease. Recently published clinical practice guidelines recommend the use of continuous GnRH agonist administration in early pubertal transgender adolescents to block endogenous puberty prior to subsequent treatment with cross-gender gonadal hormones.

Toxicity

Gonadorelin can cause headache, light-headedness, nausea, and flushing. Local swelling often occurs at subcutaneous injection sites. Generalized hypersensitivity dermatitis has occurred after long-term subcutaneous administration. Rare acute hypersensitivity reactions include bronchospasm and anaphylaxis. Sudden pituitary apoplexy and blindness have been reported following administration of GnRH to a patient with a gonadotropin-secreting pituitary tumor.

Continuous treatment of women with a GnRH analog (leuprolide, nafarelin, goserelin) causes the typical symptoms of menopause, which include hot flushes, sweats, and headaches. Depression, diminished libido, generalized pain, vaginal dryness, and breast atrophy may also occur. Ovarian cysts may develop within the first 2 months of therapy and generally resolve after an additional 6 weeks; however, the cysts may persist and require discontinuation of therapy. Reduced bone density and osteoporosis may occur with prolonged use, so patients should be monitored with bone densitometry before repeated treatment courses. Depending on the condition being treated with the GnRH agonist, it may be possible to ameliorate the signs and symptoms of the hypoestrogenic state without losing clinical efficacy by adding back a small dose of a progestin alone or in combination with a low dose of an estrogen. Contraindications to the use of GnRH agonists in women include pregnancy and breast-feeding.

In men treated with continuous GnRH agonist administration, adverse effects include hot flushes and sweats, edema, gynecomastia, decreased libido, decreased hematocrit, reduced bone density, asthenia, and injection site reactions. GnRH analog treatment of children is generally well tolerated. However, temporary exacerbation of precocious puberty may occur during the first few weeks of therapy. Nafarelin nasal spray may cause or aggravate sinusitis.

GNRH RECEPTOR ANTAGONISTS

Three synthetic decapeptides that function as competitive antagonists of GnRH receptors are available for clinical use. **Ganirelix, cetrorelix,** and **degarelix** inhibit the secretion of FSH and LH in a dose-dependent manner. Ganirelix and cetrorelix are approved for use in controlled ovarian hyperstimulation procedures, whereas degarelix is approved for men with advanced prostate cancer.

Pharmacokinetics

Ganirelix and cetrorelix are absorbed rapidly after subcutaneous injection. Administration of 0.25 mg daily maintains GnRH antagonism. Alternatively, a single 3.0-mg dose of cetrorelix suppresses LH secretion for 96 hours. Degarelix therapy is initiated with 240 mg administered as two subcutaneous injections. Maintenance dosing is with an 80-mg subcutaneous injection every 28 days.

Clinical Pharmacology

A. Suppression of Gonadotropin Production

GnRH antagonists are approved for preventing the LH surge during controlled ovarian hyperstimulation. They offer several advantages over continuous treatment with a GnRH agonist. Because GnRH antagonists produce an immediate antagonist effect, their use can be delayed until day 6–8 of the in vitro fertilization cycle (Figure 37–3), and thus the duration of administration is shorter. They also appear to have a less negative impact on the ovarian response to gonadotropin stimulation, which permits a decrease in the total duration and dose of gonadotropin. Finally, GnRH antagonists are associated with a lower risk of ovarian hyperstimulation syndrome, which can lead to cycle cancellation. On the other hand, because their antagonist effects reverse more quickly after their discontinuation, adherence to the treatment regimen is critical. The antagonists produce a more complete suppression of gonadotropin secretion than agonists. There is concern that the suppression of LH may inhibit ovarian steroidogenesis to an extent that impairs follicular development when recombinant or the purified form of FSH is used during the follicular phase of an in vitro fertilization cycle. Clinical trials have shown a slightly lower rate of pregnancy in in vitro fertilization cycles that used GnRH antagonist treatment compared with cycles that used GnRH agonist treatment.

B. Advanced Prostate Cancer

Degarelix is approved for the treatment of symptomatic advanced prostate cancer. This GnRH antagonist reduces concentrations of gonadotropins and androgens more rapidly than GnRH agonists and avoids the testosterone surge seen with GnRH agonist therapy.

Toxicity

When used for controlled ovarian hyperstimulation, ganirelix and cetrorelix are well tolerated. The most common adverse effects are

nausea and headache. During the treatment of men with prostate cancer, degarelix caused injection-site reactions and increases in liver enzymes. Like continuous treatment with a GnRH agonist, degarelix leads to signs and symptoms of androgen deprivation, including hot flushes and weight gain.

PROLACTIN

Prolactin is a 198-amino-acid peptide hormone produced in the anterior pituitary. Its structure resembles that of GH. Prolactin is the principal hormone responsible for lactation. Milk production is stimulated by prolactin when appropriate circulating levels of estrogens, progestins, corticosteroids, and insulin are present. A deficiency of prolactin—which can occur in rare states of pituitary deficiency—is manifested by failure to lactate or by a luteal phase defect. In rare cases of hypothalamic destruction, prolactin levels may be elevated as a result of impaired transport of dopamine (prolactin-inhibiting hormone) to the pituitary. Much more commonly, however, prolactin is elevated as a result of prolactin-secreting adenomas. Hyperprolactinemia produces a syndrome of amenorrhea and galactorrhea in women, and loss of libido and infertility in men. In the case of large tumors (macroadenomas), it can be associated with symptoms of a pituitary mass, including visual changes due to compression of the optic nerves. The hypogonadism and infertility associated with hyperprolactinemia result from inhibition of GnRH release.

No preparation of prolactin is available for use in prolactin-deficient patients. For patients with symptomatic hyperprolactinemia, inhibition of prolactin secretion can be achieved with dopamine agonists, which act in the pituitary to inhibit prolactin release.

DOPAMINE AGONISTS

Adenomas that secrete excess prolactin usually retain the sensitivity to inhibition by dopamine exhibited by the normal pituitary. **Bromocriptine** and **cabergoline** are ergot derivatives (see Chapters 16 and 28) with a high affinity for dopamine D_2 receptors. **Quinagolide,** a drug approved in Europe, is a nonergot agent with similarly high D_2 receptor affinity. The chemical structure and pharmacokinetic features of ergot alkaloids are presented in Chapter 16.

Dopamine agonists suppress prolactin release very effectively in patients with hyperprolactinemia. GH release is reduced in patients with acromegaly, although not as effectively. Bromocriptine has also been used in Parkinson's disease to improve motor function and reduce levodopa requirements (see Chapter 28). Newer, nonergot D_2 agonists used in Parkinson's disease (pramipexole and ropinirole; see Chapter 28) have been reported to interfere with lactation, but they are not approved for use in hyperprolactinemia.

Pharmacokinetics

All available dopamine agonists are active as oral preparations, and all are eliminated by metabolism. They can also be absorbed systemically after vaginal insertion of tablets. Cabergoline, with a half-life of approximately 65 hours, has the longest duration of action. Quinagolide has a half-life of about 20 hours, whereas the half-life of bromocriptine is about 7 hours. After vaginal administration, serum levels peak more slowly.

Clinical Pharmacology

A. Hyperprolactinemia

A dopamine agonist is the standard medical treatment for hyperprolactinemia. These drugs shrink pituitary prolactin-secreting tumors, lower circulating prolactin levels, and restore ovulation in approximately 70% of women with microadenomas and 30% of women with macroadenomas (Figure 37–4). Cabergoline is initiated at 0.25 mg twice weekly orally or vaginally. It can be increased gradually, according to serum prolactin determinations, up to a maximum of 1 mg twice weekly. Bromocriptine is generally taken daily after the evening meal at the initial dose of 1.25 mg; the dose

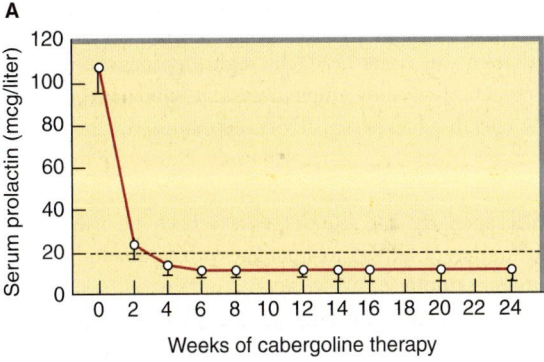

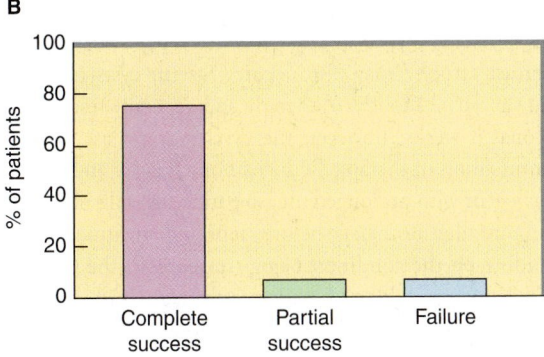

FIGURE 37–4 Results from a clinical trial of cabergoline in women with hyperprolactinemia and anovulation. **A:** The dotted line indicates the upper limit of normal serum prolactin concentrations. **B:** Complete success was defined as pregnancy or at least two consecutive menses with evidence of ovulation at least once. Partial success was two menstrual cycles without evidence of ovulation or just one ovulatory cycle. The most common reasons for withdrawal from the trial were nausea, headache, dizziness, abdominal pain, and fatigue. (Modified and reproduced, with permission, from Webster J et al: A comparison of cabergoline and bromocriptine in the treatment of hyperprolactinemic amenorrhea. N Engl J Med 1994;331:904.)

is then increased as tolerated. Most patients require 2.5–7.5 mg daily. Long-acting oral bromocriptine formulations (Parlodel SRO) and intramuscular formulations (Parlodel L.A.R.) are available outside the United States.

B. Physiologic Lactation

Dopamine agonists were used in the past to prevent breast engorgement when breast-feeding was not desired. Their use for this purpose has been discouraged because of toxicity (see Toxicity & Contraindications).

C. Acromegaly

A dopamine agonist alone or in combination with pituitary surgery, radiation therapy, or octreotide administration can be used to treat acromegaly. The doses required are higher than those used to treat hyperprolactinemia. For example, patients with acromegaly require 20–30 mg/d of bromocriptine and seldom respond adequately to bromocriptine alone unless the pituitary tumor secretes prolactin as well as GH.

Toxicity & Contraindications

Dopamine agonists can cause nausea, headache, light-headedness, orthostatic hypotension, and fatigue. Psychiatric manifestations occasionally occur, even at lower doses, and may take months to resolve. Erythromelalgia occurs rarely. High dosages of ergot-derived preparations can cause cold-induced peripheral digital vasospasm. Pulmonary infiltrates have occurred with chronic high-dosage therapy. Cabergoline appears to cause nausea less often than bromocriptine. Vaginal administration can reduce nausea, but may cause local irritation.

Dopamine agonist therapy during the early weeks of pregnancy has not been associated with an increased risk of spontaneous abortion or congenital malformations. Although there has been a longer experience with the safety of bromocriptine during early pregnancy, there is growing evidence that cabergoline is also safe in women with macroadenomas who must continue a dopamine agonist during pregnancy. In patients with small pituitary adenomas, dopamine agonist therapy is discontinued upon conception because growth of microadenomas during pregnancy is rare. Patients with very large adenomas require vigilance for tumor progression and often require a dopamine agonist throughout pregnancy. There have been rare reports of stroke or coronary thrombosis in postpartum women taking bromocriptine to suppress postpartum lactation.

■ POSTERIOR PITUITARY HORMONES

The two posterior pituitary hormones—vasopressin and oxytocin—are synthesized in neuronal cell bodies in the hypothalamus and transported via their axons to the posterior pituitary, where they are stored and then released into the circulation. Each has limited but important clinical uses.

OXYTOCIN

Oxytocin is a peptide hormone secreted by the posterior pituitary that participates in labor and delivery and elicits milk ejection in lactating women. During the second half of pregnancy, uterine smooth muscle shows an increase in the expression of oxytocin receptors and becomes increasingly sensitive to the stimulant action of endogenous oxytocin. Pharmacologic concentrations of oxytocin powerfully stimulate uterine contraction.

Chemistry & Pharmacokinetics

A. Structure

Oxytocin is a 9-amino-acid peptide with an intrapeptide disulfide cross-link (Figure 37–5). Its amino acid sequence differs from that of vasopressin at positions 3 and 8.

B. Absorption, Metabolism, and Excretion

Oxytocin is administered intravenously for initiation and augmentation of labor. It also can be administered intramuscularly for control of postpartum bleeding. Oxytocin is not bound to plasma proteins and is eliminated by the kidneys and liver, with a circulating half-life of 5 minutes.

Pharmacodynamics

Oxytocin acts through G protein-coupled receptors and the phosphoinositide-calcium second-messenger system to contract uterine smooth muscle. Oxytocin also stimulates the release of prostaglandins and leukotrienes that augment uterine contraction. Oxytocin in small doses increases both the frequency and the force of uterine contractions. At higher doses, it produces sustained contraction.

Oxytocin also causes contraction of myoepithelial cells surrounding mammary alveoli, which leads to milk ejection. Without

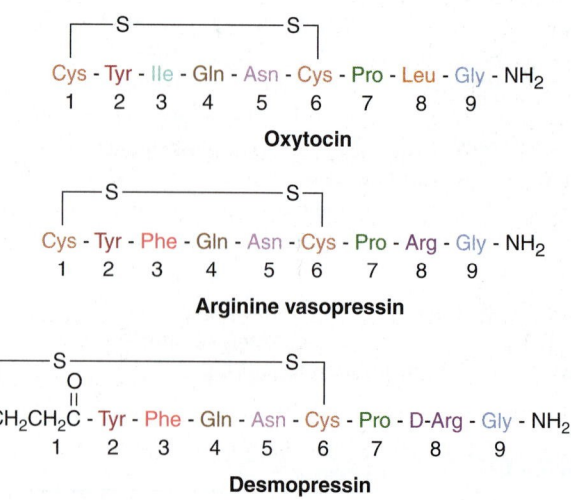

FIGURE 37–5 Posterior pituitary hormones and desmopressin. (Modified and reproduced, with permission, from Ganong WF: *Review of Medical Physiology*, 21st ed. McGraw-Hill, 2003.)

oxytocin-induced contraction, normal lactation cannot occur. At high concentrations, oxytocin has weak antidiuretic and pressor activity due to activation of vasopressin receptors.

Clinical Pharmacology

Oxytocin is used to induce labor for conditions requiring early vaginal delivery such as Rh problems, maternal diabetes, pre-eclampsia, or ruptured membranes. It is also used to augment abnormal labor that is protracted or displays an arrest disorder. Oxytocin has several uses in the immediate postpartum period, including the control of uterine hemorrhage after vaginal or cesarean delivery. It is sometimes used during second-trimester abortions.

Before delivery, oxytocin is usually administered intravenously via an infusion pump with appropriate fetal and maternal monitoring. For induction of labor, an initial infusion rate of 0.5–2 mU/min is increased every 30–60 minutes until a physiologic contraction pattern is established. The maximum infusion rate is 20 mU/min. For postpartum uterine bleeding, 10–40 units are added to 1 L of 5% dextrose, and the infusion rate is titrated to control uterine atony. Alternatively, 10 units of oxytocin can be administered by intramuscular injection after delivery of the placenta.

During the antepartum period, oxytocin induces uterine contractions that transiently reduce placental blood flow to the fetus. The oxytocin challenge test measures the fetal heart rate response to a standardized oxytocin infusion and provides information about placental circulatory reserve. An abnormal response, seen as late decelerations in the fetal heart rate, indicates fetal hypoxia and may warrant immediate cesarean delivery.

Toxicity & Contraindications

When oxytocin is used judiciously, serious toxicity is rare. The toxicity that does occur is due either to excessive stimulation of uterine contractions or to inadvertent activation of vasopressin receptors. Excessive stimulation of uterine contractions before delivery can cause fetal distress, placental abruption, or uterine rupture. These complications can be detected early by means of standard fetal monitoring equipment. High concentrations of oxytocin with activation of vasopressin receptors can cause excessive fluid retention, or water intoxication, leading to hyponatremia, heart failure, seizures, and death. Bolus injections of oxytocin can cause hypotension. To avoid hypotension, oxytocin is administered intravenously as dilute solutions at a controlled rate.

Contraindications to oxytocin include fetal distress, prematurity, abnormal fetal presentation, cephalopelvic disproportion, and other predispositions for uterine rupture.

OXYTOCIN ANTAGONIST

Atosiban is an antagonist of the oxytocin receptor that has been approved outside the United States as a treatment for preterm labor (tocolysis). Atosiban is a modified form of oxytocin that is administered by IV infusion for 2–48 hours. In a small number of published clinical trials, atosiban appears to be as effective as β-adrenoceptor-agonist tocolytics and to produce fewer adverse effects. In 1998, however, the FDA decided not to approve atosiban based on concerns about efficacy and safety.

VASOPRESSIN (ANTIDIURETIC HORMONE, ADH)

Vasopressin is a peptide hormone released by the posterior pituitary in response to rising plasma tonicity or falling blood pressure. Vasopressin possesses antidiuretic and vasopressor properties. A deficiency of this hormone results in diabetes insipidus (see Chapters 15 and 17).

Chemistry & Pharmacokinetics

A. Structure

Vasopressin is a nonapeptide with a 6-amino-acid ring and a 3-amino-acid side chain. The residue at position 8 is arginine in humans and in most other mammals except pigs and related species, whose vasopressin contains lysine at position 8 (Figure 37–5). Desmopressin acetate (DDAVP, 1-desamino-8-D-arginine vasopressin) is a long-acting synthetic analog of vasopressin with minimal pressor activity and an antidiuretic-to-pressor ratio 4000 times that of vasopressin. **Desmopressin** is modified at position 1 and contains a D-amino acid at position 8. Like vasopressin and oxytocin, desmopressin has a disulfide linkage between positions 1 and 6.

B. Absorption, Metabolism, and Excretion

Vasopressin is administered by intravenous or intramuscular injection. The half-life of circulating vasopressin is approximately 15 minutes, with renal and hepatic metabolism via reduction of the disulfide bond and peptide cleavage.

Desmopressin can be administered intravenously, subcutaneously, intranasally, or orally. The half-life of circulating desmopressin is 1.5–2.5 hours. Nasal desmopressin is available as a unit dose spray that delivers 0.1 mL per spray; it is also available with a calibrated nasal tube that can be used to deliver a more precise dose. Nasal bioavailability of desmopressin is 3–4%, whereas oral bioavailability is less than 1%.

Pharmacodynamics

Vasopressin activates two subtypes of G protein-coupled receptors (see Chapter 17). V_1 receptors are found on vascular smooth muscle cells and mediate vasoconstriction via the coupling protein G_q. V_2 receptors are found on renal tubule cells and reduce diuresis through increased water permeability and water resorption in the collecting tubules via G_s. Extrarenal V_2-like receptors regulate the release of coagulation factor VIII and von Willebrand factor.

Clinical Pharmacology

Vasopressin and desmopressin are treatments of choice for pituitary diabetes insipidus. The dosage of desmopressin is 10–40 mcg

(0.1–0.4 mL) in two to three divided doses as a nasal spray or, as an oral tablet, 0.1–0.2 mg two to three times daily. The dosage by injection is 1–4 mcg (0.25–1 mL) every 12–24 hours as needed for polyuria, polydipsia, or hypernatremia. Bedtime desmopressin therapy, by intranasal or oral administration, ameliorates nocturnal enuresis by decreasing nocturnal urine production. Vasopressin infusion is effective in some cases of esophageal variceal bleeding and colonic diverticular bleeding.

Desmopressin is also used for the treatment of coagulopathy in hemophilia A and von Willebrand's disease (see Chapter 34).

Toxicity & Contraindications

Headache, nausea, abdominal cramps, agitation, and allergic reactions occur rarely. Overdosage can result in hyponatremia and seizures.

Vasopressin (but not desmopressin) can cause vasoconstriction and should be used cautiously in patients with coronary artery disease. Nasal insufflation of desmopressin may be less effective when nasal congestion is present.

VASOPRESSIN ANTAGONISTS

A group of nonpeptide antagonists of vasopressin receptors is being investigated for use in patients with hyponatremia or acute heart failure, which is often associated with elevated concentrations of vasopressin. **Conivaptan** has high affinity for both V_{1a} and V_2 receptors. **Tolvaptan** has a 30-fold higher affinity for V_2 than for V_1 receptors. In several clinical trials, both agents relieved symptoms and reduced objective signs of hyponatremia and heart failure. Conivaptan and tolvaptan are approved by the FDA for intravenous administration in hyponatremia. Several other nonselective nonpeptide vasopressin receptor antagonists are being investigated for these conditions (see Chapter 15).

SUMMARY Hypothalamic & Pituitary Hormones[1]

Subclass	Mechanism of Action	Effects	Clinical Applications	Pharmacokinetics, Toxicities, Interactions
GROWTH HORMONE (GH)				
• Somatropin	Recombinant form of human GH • acts through GH receptors to increase production of IGF-I	Restores normal growth and metabolic GH effects in GH-deficient individuals • increases final adult height in some children with short stature not due to GH deficiency	Replacement in GH deficiency • increased final adult height in children with certain conditions associated with short stature (see Table 37–4) • wasting in HIV infection • short bowel syndrome	SC injection • Toxicity: Pseudotumor cerebri, slipped capital femoral epiphysis, edema, hyperglycemia, progression of scoliosis, risk of asphyxia in severely obese patients with Prader-Willi syndrome and upper airway obstruction or sleep apnea
IGF-I AGONIST				
• Mecasermin	Recombinant form of IGF-I that stimulates IGF-I receptors	Improves growth and metabolic IGF-I effects in individuals with IGF-I deficiency due to severe GH resistance	Replacement in IGF-I deficiency that is not responsive to exogenous GH	SC injection • Toxicity: Hypoglycemia, intracranial hypertension, increased liver enzymes
SOMATOSTATIN ANALOGS				
• Octreotide	Agonist at somatostatin receptors	Inhibits production of GH and, to a lesser extent, of TSH, glucagon, insulin, and gastrin	Acromegaly and several other hormone-secreting tumors • acute control of bleeding from esophageal varices	SC or IV injection • long-acting formulation injected IM monthly • Toxicity: Gastrointestinal disturbances, gallstones, bradycardia, cardiac conduction problems
• Lanreotide: Similar to octreotide; available as a long-acting formulation for acromegaly				
GH RECEPTOR ANTAGONIST				
• Pegvisomant	Blocks GH receptors	Ameliorates effects of excess GH production	Acromegaly	SC injection • Toxicity: Increased liver enzymes

(continued)

Subclass	Mechanism of Action	Effects	Clinical Applications	Pharmacokinetics, Toxicities, Interactions
GONADOTROPINS: FOLLICLE-STIMULATING HORMONE (FSH) ANALOGS				
• Follitropin alfa	Activates FSH receptors	Mimics effects of endogenous FSH	Controlled ovulation hyperstimulation in women • infertility due to hypogonadotropic hypogonadism in men	SC injection • *Toxicity:* Ovarian hyperstimulation syndrome and multiple pregnancies in women • gynecomastia in men • headache, depression, edema in both sexes
• *Follitropin beta: A recombinant product with the same peptide sequence as follitropin alfa but differs in its carbohydrate side chains*				
• *Urofollitropin: Human FSH purified from the urine of postmenopausal women*				
• *Menotropins (hMG): Extract of the urine of postmenopausal women; contains both FSH and LH activity*				
GONADOTROPINS: LUTEINIZING HORMONE (LH) ANALOGS				
• Human chorionic gonadotropin (hCG)	Agonist at LH receptors	Mimics effects of endogenous LH	Initiation of ovulation during controlled ovulation hyperstimulation • ovarian follicle development in women with hypogonadotropic hypogonadism • male hypogonadotropic hypogonadism	IM injection • *Toxicity:* Ovarian hyperstimulation syndrome and multiple pregnancies in women • gynecomastia in men • headache, depression, edema in both sexes
• *Choriogonadotropin alfa: Recombinant form of hCG*				
• *Lutropin: Recombinant form of human LH*				
• *Menotropins (hMG): Extract of the urine of postmenopausal women that contains both FSH and LH activity*				
GONADOTROPIN-RELEASING HORMONE (GNRH) ANALOGS				
• Leuprolide	Agonist of GnRH receptors	Increased LH and FSH secretion with intermittent administration • reduced LH and FSH secretion with prolonged continuous administration	Ovarian suppression • controlled ovarian hyperstimulation • central precocious puberty • block of endogenous puberty in some transgender/gender variant early pubertal adolescents • advanced prostate cancer	Administered IV, SC, IM, or intranasally • depot formulations are available • *Toxicity:* Headache, light-headedness, nausea, injection site reactions • symptoms of hypogonadism with continuous treatment
• *Gonadorelin: Synthetic human GnRH*				
• *Other GnRH analogs: Goserelin, histrelin, nafarelin, and triptorelin*				
GONADOTROPIN-RELEASING HORMONE (GNRH) RECEPTOR ANTAGONISTS				
• Ganirelix	Blocks GnRH receptors	Reduces endogenous production of LH and FSH	Prevention of premature LH surges during controlled ovulation hyperstimulation	SC injection • *Toxicity:* Nausea, headache
• *Cetrorelix: Similar to ganirelix, approved for controlled ovarian hyperstimulation*				
• *Degarelix: Approved for advanced prostate cancer*				
DOPAMINE AGONISTS				
• Bromocriptine	Activates dopamine D_2 receptors	Suppresses pituitary secretion of prolactin and, less effectively, GH • dopaminergic effects on CNS motor control and behavior	Treatment of hyperprolactinemia • acromegaly • Parkinson's disease (see Chapter 28)	Administered orally or, for hyperprolactinemia, vaginally • *Toxicity:* Gastrointestinal disturbances, orthostatic hypotension, headache, psychiatric disturbances, vasospasm and pulmonary infiltrates in high doses
• *Cabergoline: Another ergot derivative with similar effects*				
OXYTOCIN	Activates oxytocin receptors	Increased uterine contractions	Induction and augmentation of labor • control of uterine hemorrhage after delivery	IV infusion or IM injection • *Toxicity:* Fetal distress, placental abruption, uterine rupture, fluid retention, hypotension
OXYTOCIN RECEPTOR ANTAGONIST				
• Atosiban	Blocks oxytocin receptors	Decreased uterine contractions	Tocolysis for preterm labor	IV infusion • *Toxicity:* Concern about increased rates of infant death; not FDA approved

(continued)

Subclass	Mechanism of Action	Effects	Clinical Applications	Pharmacokinetics, Toxicities, Interactions
VASOPRESSIN RECEPTOR AGONISTS				
• Desmopressin	Relatively selective vasopressin V_2 receptor agonist	Acts in the kidney collecting duct cells to decrease the excretion of water • acts on extrarenal V_2 receptors to increase factor VIII and von Willebrand factor	Pituitary diabetes insipidus • pediatric primary nocturnal enuresis • hemophilia A and von Willebrand disease	Oral, IV, SC, or intranasal • *Toxicity:* Gastrointestinal disturbances, headache, hyponatremia, allergic reactions
• *Vasopressin: Available for treatment of diabetes insipidus and sometimes used to control bleeding from esophageal varices*				
VASOPRESSIN RECEPTOR ANTAGONIST				
• Conivaptan	Antagonist of vasopressin V_{1a} and V_2 receptors	Reduced renal excretion of water in conditions associated with increased vasopressin	Hyponatremia in hospitalized patients	IV infusion • *Toxicity:* Infusion site reactions
• *Tolvaptan: Similar but more selective for vasopressin V_2 receptors; oral administration*				

[1]See Tables 37-2 and 37-3 for summaries of the clinical uses of the rarely used hypothalamic and pituitary hormones not described in this table.

P R E P A R A T I O N S   A V A I L A B L E

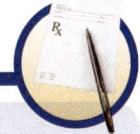

GROWTH FACTOR AGONISTS & ANTAGONISTS

Lanreotide acetate (Somatuline Depot)
Parenteral: 60, 90, 120 mg in single-use prefilled syringe for SC injection

Mecasermin (Increlex)
Parenteral: 10 mg/mL solution for SC injection

Octreotide acetate (generic, Sandostatin)
Parenteral: 0.05, 0.1, 0.2, 0.5, 1.0 mg/mL solution for SC or IV injection
Parenteral depot injection (Sandostatin LAR Depot): 10, 20, 30 mg powder in single-use vials to reconstitute for IM injection

Pegvisomant (Somavert)
Parenteral: 10, 15, 20 mg powder in single-use vials to reconstitute for SC injection

Somatropin (various)
Parenteral: many dose strengths between 0.2 to 24 mg available to reconstitute for SC or IM injection

GONADOTROPIN AGONISTS & ANTAGONISTS

Cetrorelix acetate (Cetrotide)
Parenteral: 0.25, 3.0 mg in single-use vials for SC injection

Choriogonadotropin alfa [rhCG] (Ovidrel)
Parenteral: 250 mcg in single-dose prefilled syringes for SC injection

Chorionic gonadotropin [hCG] (generic, Profasi, Pregnyl)
Parenteral: 10,000 unit powder to reconstitute for IM injection

Degarelix (Firmagon)
Parenteral: 80, 120 mg powder to reconstitute for SC injection

Follitropin alfa [rFSH] (Gonal-f)
Parenteral: 75, 450, 1050 unit powder in vials to reconstitute or 300, 450, 900 units in prefilled pens with needles for SC injection

Follitropin beta [rFSH] (Follistim)
Parenteral: 37.5, 150 units/mL solution in single-use vials for 175, 350, 650, 975 units in cartridges for SC injection

Ganirelix acetate (Antagon)
Parenteral: 500 mcg/mL solution in prefilled syringes for SC injection

Gonadorelin hydrochloride [GnRH] (Factrel)
Parenteral: 100, 500 mcg powder to reconstitute for SC or intravenous injection

Goserelin acetate (Zoladex)
Parenteral: 3.6, 10.8 mg in prefilled syringes for SC implantation

Histrelin acetate (Supprelin LA, Vantas)
Parenteral: 50 mg SC implant

Leuprolide acetate (generic, Eligard, Lupron)
Parenteral: 5 mg/mL solution in multiple-dose vials for SC injection
Parenteral depot polymeric delivery system: 7.5, 22.5, 30, 45 mg in a single-dose kit for SC injection
Parenteral depot microsphere suspension: 3.75, 7.5, 11.25, 15, 22.5, 30 mg in a single-dose kit for IM injection

Lutropin alfa [rLH] (Luveris)
Parenteral: 75 unit powder to reconstitute for SC injection

Menotropins [hMG] (Menopur, Repronex)
Parenteral: 75 IU FSH and 75 IU LH powder to reconstitute for SC or IM injection

Nafarelin acetate (Synarel)
Nasal: 2 mg/mL solution

Triptorelin pamoate (Trelstar)
Parenteral: 3.75, 11.25, 22.5 mg powder to reconstitute for IM injection

Urofollitropin (Bravelle)
Parenteral: 75 IU FSH powder to reconstitute for SC injection

PROLACTIN ANTAGONISTS (DOPAMINE AGONISTS)

Bromocriptine mesylate (generic, Parlodel)
Oral: 2.5 mg tablets, 5 mg capsules

Cabergoline (generic, Dostinex)
Oral: 0.5 mg tablets

OXYTOCIN

Oxytocin (generic, Pitocin)
Parenteral: 10 units/mL solution for intravenous or IM injection

VASOPRESSIN AGONISTS AND ANTAGONISTS

Conivaptan HCl (Vaprisol)
Parenteral: 0.2 mg/mL solution for IV injection

Desmopressin acetate (DDAVP, generic, Minirin, Stimate)
Nasal: 0.1, 1.5 mg/mL solution
Parenteral: 4 mcg/mL solution for IV or SC injection
Oral: 0.1, 0.2 mg tablets

Tolvaptan (Samsca)
Oral: 15, 30 mg tablets

Vasopressin (generic, Pitressin)
Parenteral: 20 IU/mL solution for IM, SC or nasal administration

OTHER

Corticorelin ovine triflutate (Acthrel)
Parenteral: 100 mcg powder to reconstitute for IV injection

Corticotropin (H.P. Acthar Gel)
Parenteral: 80 units/mL gelatin for IM or SC administration

Cosyntropin (generic, Cortrosyn)
Parenteral: 0.25 mg powder to reconstitute or 0.25 mg/mL solution for IV or IM injection

Thyrotropin alfa (Thyrogen)
Parenteral: 1.1 mg powder to reconstitute for IM injection

REFERENCES

Barlier A, Jaquet P: Quinagolide—a valuable treatment option for hyperprolactinaemia. Eur J Endocrinol 2006;154:187.

Carel JC et al: Consensus statement on the use of gonadotropin-releasing hormone analogs in children. Pediatrics 2009;123:752.

Carter-Su C, Schwartz J, Smit LS: Molecular mechanism of growth hormone action. Annu Rev Physiol 1996;58:187.

Chandraharan E, Arulkumaran S: Acute tocolysis. Curr Opin Obstet Gynecol 2005;17:151.

Colaro A: The prolactinoma. Best Pract Res Clin Endocrinol Metab 2009;23:575.

Collett-Solberg PF et al: The role of recombinant human insulin-like growth factor-I in treating children with short stature. J Clin Endocrinol Metab 2008;93(1):10.

de Heus R et al: Acute tocolysis for uterine activity reduction in term labor: a review. Obstet Gynecol Surv 2008;63(6):383.

Devroey P et al: Reproductive biology and IVF: Ovarian stimulation and endometrial receptivity. Trends Endocrinol Metab 2004;15:84.

Dong Q, Rosenthal SM: Endocrine disorders of the hypothalamus and pituitary. In: Swaiman KF, Ashwal S, Ferriero DM (editors): *Pediatric Neurology*, 5th ed. Mosby, Inc. (Elsevier, Inc.) 2011, in press.

Ebling FJ: The neuroendocrine timing of puberty. Neuroendocrine 2005;129:675.

Gabe SG, Neibyl JR, Simpson JL: *Obstetrics: Normal and Problem Pregnancies*, 5th ed. Churchill Livingstone, 2007.

Han TS, Bouloux PM: What is the optimal therapy for young males with hypogonadatropic hypogonadism? Clin Endocrinol 2010;72:731.

Hapgood JP et al: Regulation of expression of mammalian gonadotropin-releasing hormone receptor genes. J Neuroendocrinol 2005;17:619.

Huirne JA, Homburg R, Lambalk CB: Are GnRH antagonists comparable to agonists for use in IVF? Hum Reprod 2007;22 (11):2805.

Larson PR et al: *Williams Textbook of Endocrinology*, 11th ed. Saunders, 2007.

Macklon NS et al: The science behind 25 years of ovulation stimulation for in vitro fertilization. Endocr Rev 2006;27:170.

Mammen AA, Ferrer FA: Nocturnal enuresis: Medical management. Urol Clin North Am 2004;31:491.

Manjila S et al: Pharmacological management of acromegaly: A current perspective. Neurosurg Focus 2010;29:E14.

Maughan KL, Heim SW, Galazka SS: Preventing postpartum hemorrhage: Managing the third stage of labor. Am Fam Physician 2006;73:1025.

Papatsonis D et al: Oxytocin receptor antagonists for inhibiting pre-term labour. Cochrane Database Syst Rev 2005;20:CD004452.

Richmond E, Rogol AD: Current indications for growth hormone therapy for children and adolescents. Endocr Dev 2010;18:92.

Ritzén EM: Undescended testes: A consensus on management. Eur J Endocrinol 2008;159 (Suppl 1):S87.

Rosenfeld RG, Hwa V: The growth hormone cascade and its role in mammalian growth. Horm Res 2009;71(Suppl 2):36.

Speroff L, Fritz MA: *Clinical Gynecologic Endocrinology and Infertility*, 7th ed. Lippincott Williams & Wilkins, 2005.

Steinberg M: Degarelix: A gonadotropin-releasing hormone antagonist for the management of prostate cancer. Clin Ther 2009;31(Pt 2):2312.

Takala J et al: Increased mortality associated with growth hormone treatment in critically ill adults. N Engl J Med 1999;341:785.

Wales PW et al: Human growth hormone and glutamine for patients with short bowel syndrome. Cochrane Database Syst Rev 2010;16:CD006321.

Webster J et al: A comparison of cabergoline and bromocriptine in the treatment of hyperprolactinemic amenorrhea. N Engl J Med 1994;331:904.

Wit JM et al: Idiopathic short stature: Definition, epidemiology, and diagnostic evaluation. Growth Horm IGF Res 2008;18:89.

Obesity

Adan RAH et al: Anti-obesity drugs and neural circuits of feeding. Trends Pharmacol Sci 2008;29:208.

Bloom SR et al: The obesity epidemic: Pharmacological challenges. Molec Interventions 2008;8:82.

Hofbauer KG, Nicholson JR, Boss O: The obesity epidemic: current and future pharmacological treatments. Annu Rev Pharmacol Toxicol 2007;47:565.

CASE STUDY ANSWER

While GH may have some direct growth-promoting effects, GH is thought to mediate skeletal growth principally through epiphyseal production of insulin-like growth factor-I (IGF-I), which acts principally in an autocrine/paracrine manner. IGF-I may also promote statural growth through endocrine mechanisms. The findings of small testes and a microphallus in this patient suggest a diagnosis of hypogonadism, likely as a consequence of gonadotropin deficiency. This patient is at risk for multiple hypothalamic/pituitary deficiencies. This patient may already have or may subsequently develop ACTH/cortisol and TSH/thyroid hormone deficiencies and thus may require supplementation with hydrocortisone and levothyroxine, in addition to supplementation with GH and testosterone. The patient should also be evaluated for the presence of central diabetes insipidus and, if present, treated with desmopressin, a V_2 vasopressin receptor-selective analog.

Thyroid & Antithyroid Drugs

Betty J. Dong, PharmD, FASHP, FCCP, &
Francis S. Greenspan, MD, FACP

CASE STUDY

A 33-year-old woman presents with complaints of fatigue, sluggishness, weight gain, cold intolerance, dry skin, and muscle weakness for the last 2 months. She is so tired that she has to take several naps during the day to complete her tasks. These complaints are new for her since she used to feel warm all the time, had boundless energy causing her some insomnia, and states she felt like her heart was going to jump out of her chest. She also states that she would like to become pregnant in the near future. Her past medical history is significant for radioactive iodine therapy (RAI) about 1 year ago after a short trial of methimazole and propranolol therapy.

She underwent RAI due to her poor medication adherence and did not attend routine scheduled appointments afterward. On physical examination, her blood pressure is 130/89 mm Hg with a pulse of 50 bpm. Her weight is 136 lb (61.8 kg), an increase of 10 lb (4.5 kg) in the last year. Her thyroid gland is not palpable and her reflexes are delayed. Laboratory findings include a thyroid-stimulating hormone (TSH) level of 24.9 μIU/mL and a free thyroxine level of 8 pmol/L. Evaluate the management of her past history of hyperthyroidism. Identify the available treatment options for control of her current thyroid status.

THYROID PHYSIOLOGY

The normal thyroid gland secretes sufficient amounts of the thyroid hormones—**triiodothyronine (T_3)** and **tetraiodothyronine (T_4, thyroxine)**—to normalize growth and development, body temperature, and energy levels. These hormones contain 59% and 65% (respectively) of iodine as an essential part of the molecule. Calcitonin, the second type of thyroid hormone, is important in the regulation of calcium metabolism and is discussed in Chapter 42.

Iodide Metabolism

The recommended daily adult iodide (I^-)* intake is 150 mcg (200 mcg during pregnancy).

Iodide, ingested from food, water, or medication, is rapidly absorbed and enters an extracellular fluid pool. The thyroid gland removes about 75 mcg a day from this pool for hormone synthesis, and the balance is excreted in the urine. If iodide intake is increased, the fractional iodine uptake by the thyroid is diminished.

Biosynthesis of Thyroid Hormones

Once taken up by the thyroid gland, iodide undergoes a series of enzymatic reactions that incorporate it into active thyroid hormone (Figure 38–1). The first step is the transport of iodide into the thyroid gland by an intrinsic follicle cell basement membrane protein called the sodium/iodide symporter (NIS). This can be inhibited by such anions as thiocyanate (SCN^-), pertechnetate (TcO_4^-), and perchlorate (ClO_4^-). At the apical cell membrane a second I^- transport enzyme called pendrin controls the flow of iodide across the membrane. Pendrin is also found in the cochlea of the inner ear. If pendrin is deficient or absent, a hereditary syndrome of goiter and

---

*In this chapter, the term "iodine" denotes all forms of the element; the term "iodide" denotes only the ionic form, I^-.

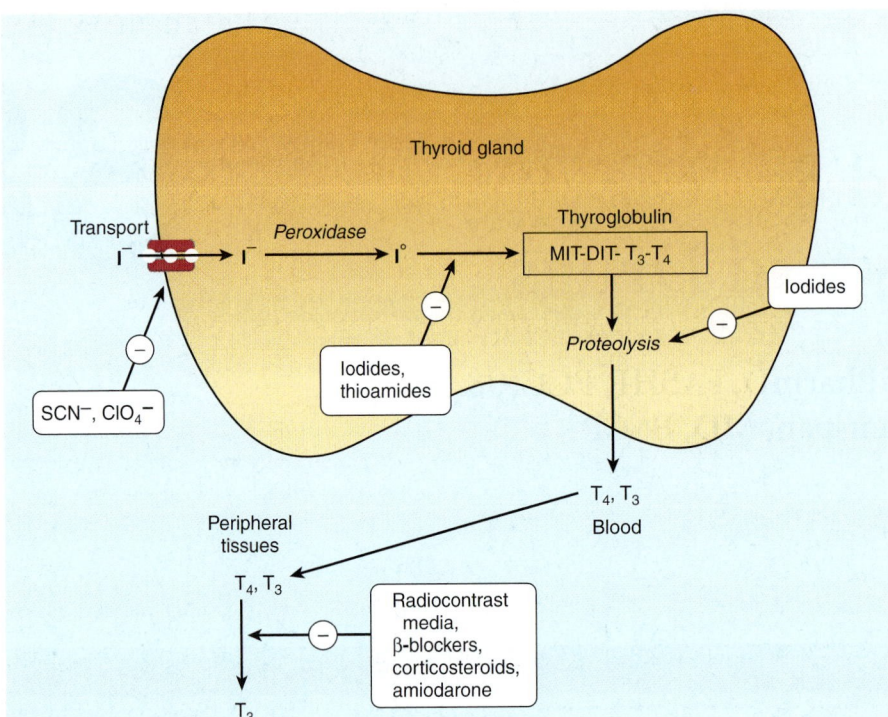

FIGURE 38-1 Biosynthesis of thyroid hormones. The sites of action of various drugs that interfere with thyroid hormone biosynthesis are shown.

deafness, called Pendred's syndrome, ensues. At the apical cell membrane, iodide is oxidized by thyroidal peroxidase to iodine, in which form it rapidly iodinates tyrosine residues within the thyroglobulin molecule to form **monoiodotyrosine (MIT)** and **diiodotyrosine (DIT).** This process is called **iodide organification.** Thyroidal peroxidase is transiently blocked by high levels of intrathyroidal iodide and blocked more persistently by thioamide drugs.

Two molecules of DIT combine within the thyroglobulin molecule to form L-thyroxine (T_4). One molecule of MIT and one molecule of DIT combine to form T_3. In addition to thyroglobulin, other proteins within the gland may be iodinated, but these iodoproteins do not have hormonal activity. Thyroxine, T_3, MIT, and DIT are released from thyroglobulin by exocytosis and proteolysis of thyroglobulin at the apical colloid border. The MIT and DIT are then deiodinated within the gland, and the iodine is reutilized. This process of proteolysis is also blocked by high levels of intrathyroidal iodide. The ratio of T_4 to T_3 within thyroglobulin is approximately 5:1, so that most of the hormone released is thyroxine. Most of the T_3 circulating in the blood is derived from peripheral metabolism of thyroxine (see below, Figure 38-2).

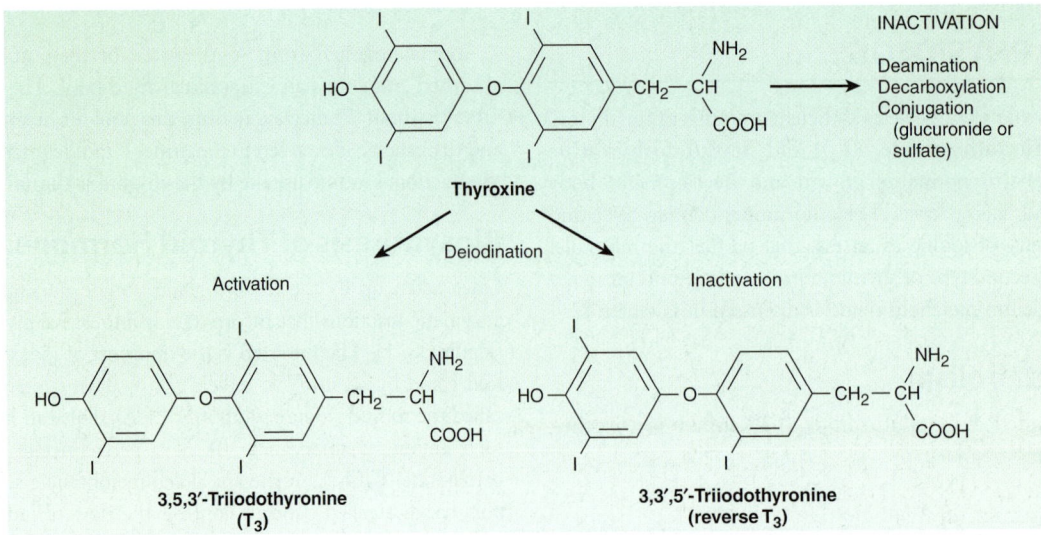

FIGURE 38-2 Peripheral metabolism of thyroxine. (Modified and reproduced, with permission, from Gardner DG, Shoback D [editors]: *Greenspan's Basic & Clinical Endocrinology*, 8th ed. McGraw-Hill, 2007.)

TABLE 38–1 Summary of thyroid hormone kinetics.

Variable	T_4	T_3
Volume of distribution	10 L	40 L
Extrathyroidal pool	800 mcg	54 mcg
Daily production	75 mcg	25 mcg
Fractional turnover per day	10%	60%
Metabolic clearance per day	1.1 L	24 L
Half-life (biologic)	7 days	1 day
Serum levels		
Total	4.8–10.4 mcg/dL	60–181 ng/dL
	(62–134 nmol/L)	(0.92–2.79 nmol/L)
Free	0.8–2.7 ng/dL	230–420 pg/dL
	(10.3–34.7 pmol/L)	(3.5–6.47 pmol/L)
Amount bound	99.96%	99.6%
Biologic potency	1	4
Oral absorption	80%	95%

Transport of Thyroid Hormones

T_4 and T_3 in plasma are reversibly bound to protein, primarily thyroxine-binding globulin (TBG). Only about 0.04% of total T_4 and 0.4% of T_3 exist in the free form. Many physiologic and pathologic states and drugs affect T_4, T_3, and thyroid transport. However, the actual levels of free hormone generally remain normal, reflecting feedback control.

Peripheral Metabolism of Thyroid Hormones

The primary pathway for the peripheral metabolism of thyroxine is deiodination. Deiodination of T_4 may occur by monodeiodination of the outer ring, producing 3,5,3'-triiodothyronine (T_3), which is three to four times more potent than T_4. Alternatively, deiodination may occur in the inner ring, producing 3,3',5'-triiodothyronine (reverse T_3, or rT_3), which is metabolically inactive (Figure 38–2). Drugs such as amiodarone, iodinated contrast media, β blockers, and corticosteroids, and severe illness or starvation inhibit the 5'-deiodinase necessary for the conversion of T_4 to T_3, resulting in low T_3 and high rT_3 levels in the serum. The pharmacokinetics of thyroid hormones are listed in Table 38–1. The low serum levels of T_3 and rT_3 in normal individuals are due to the high metabolic clearances of these two compounds.

Evaluation of Thyroid Function

The tests used to evaluate thyroid function are listed in Table 38–2.

A. Thyroid-Pituitary Relationships

Control of thyroid function via thyroid-pituitary feedback is also discussed in Chapter 37. Briefly, hypothalamic cells secrete thyrotropin-releasing hormone (TRH) (Figure 38–3). TRH is secreted into capillaries of the pituitary portal venous system, and in the pituitary gland, TRH stimulates the synthesis and release of thyrotropin (thyroid-stimulating hormone, TSH). TSH in turn stimulates an adenylyl cyclase–mediated mechanism in the thyroid cell to increase the synthesis and release of T_4 and T_3. These thyroid hormones act in a negative feedback fashion in the

TABLE 38–2 Typical values for thyroid function tests.

Name of Test	Normal Value[1]	Results in Hypothyroidism	Results in Hyperthyroidism
Total thyroxine (T_4)	4.8–10.4 mcg/dL (62–134 nmol/L)	Low	High
Total triiodothyronine (T_3)	60–181 ng/dL (0.92–2.79 nmol/L)	Normal or low	High
Free T_4 (FT_4)	0.8–2.7 ng/dL (10.3–34.7 pmol/L)	Low	High
Free T_3 (FT_3)	230–420 pg/dL (3.5–6.47 pmol/L)	Low	High
Thyrotropic hormone (TSH)	0.4–4 μIU/mL (0.4–4 mIU/L)	High[2]	Low
^{123}I uptake at 24 hours	5–35%	Low	High
Thyroglobulin autoantibodies (Tg-ab)	< 20 IU/mL	Often present	Usually present
Thyroid peroxidase antibodies (TPA)	< 0.8 IU/mL	Often present	Usually present
Isotope scan with ^{123}I or $^{99m}TcO_4$	Normal pattern	Test not indicated	Diffusely enlarged gland
Fine-needle aspiration biopsy (FNA)	Normal pattern	Test not indicated	Test not indicated
Serum thyroglobulin	< 56 ng/mL	Test not indicated	Test not indicated
Serum calcitonin	Men: < 8 ng/L (< 2.3 pmol/L); women: < 4 ng/L (< 1.17 pmol/L)	Test not indicated	Test not indicated
TSH receptor-stimulating antibody or thyroid-stimulating immunoglobulin (TSI)	< 125%	Test not indicated	Elevated in Graves' disease

[1]Results may vary with different laboratories.

[2]Exception is central hypothyroidism.

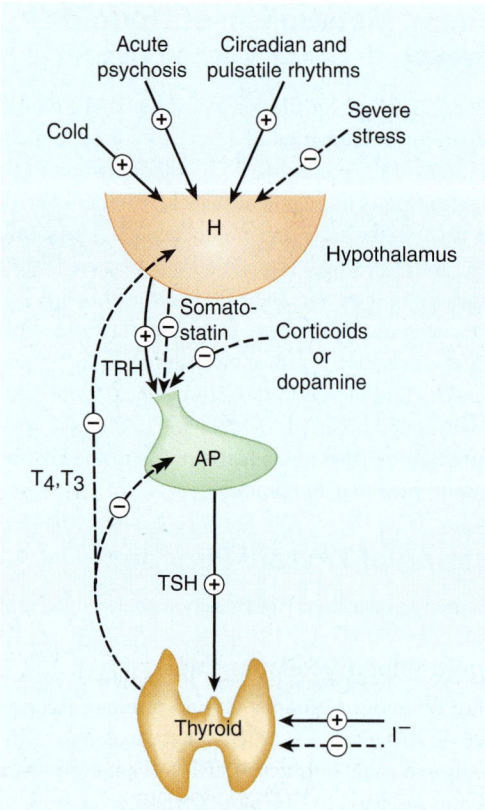

FIGURE 38–3 The hypothalamic-pituitary-thyroid axis. Acute psychosis or prolonged exposure to cold may activate the axis. Hypothalamic thyroid-releasing hormone (TRH) stimulates pituitary thyroid-stimulating hormone (TSH) release, while somatostatin and dopamine inhibit it. TSH stimulates T_4 and T_3 synthesis and release from the thyroid, and they in turn inhibit both TRH and TSH synthesis and release. Small amounts of iodide are necessary for hormone production, but large amounts inhibit T_3 and T_4 production and release. Solid arrows, stimulatory influence; dashed arrows, inhibitory influence. H, hypothalamus; AP, anterior pituitary.

pituitary to block the action of TRH and in the hypothalamus to inhibit the synthesis and secretion of TRH. Other hormones or drugs may also affect the release of TRH or TSH.

B. Autoregulation of the Thyroid Gland

The thyroid gland also regulates its uptake of iodide and thyroid hormone synthesis by intrathyroidal mechanisms that are independent of TSH. These mechanisms are primarily related to the level of iodine in the blood. Large doses of iodine inhibit iodide organification (Wolff-Chaikoff block, see Figure 38–1). In certain disease states (eg, Hashimoto's thyroiditis), this can inhibit thyroid hormone synthesis and result in hypothyroidism. Hyperthyroidism can result from the loss of the Wolff-Chaikoff block in susceptible individuals (eg, multinodular goiter).

C. Abnormal Thyroid Stimulators

In Graves' disease (see below), lymphocytes secrete a TSH receptor-stimulating antibody (TSH-R Ab [stim]), also known as

thyroid-stimulating immunoglobulin (TSI). This immunoglobulin binds to the TSH receptor and stimulates the gland in the same fashion as TSH itself. The duration of its effect, however, is much longer than that of TSH. TSH receptors are also found in orbital fibrocytes, which may be stimulated by high levels of TSH-R Ab [stim] and can cause ophthalmopathy.

■ BASIC PHARMACOLOGY OF THYROID & ANTITHYROID DRUGS

THYROID HORMONES

Chemistry

The structural formulas of thyroxine and triiodothyronine as well as reverse triiodothyronine (rT_3) are shown in Figure 38–2. All of these naturally occurring molecules are levo (L) isomers. The synthetic dextro (D) isomer of thyroxine, dextrothyroxine, has approximately 4% of the biologic activity of the L-isomer as evidenced by its lesser ability to suppress TSH secretion and correct hypothyroidism.

Pharmacokinetics

Thyroxine is absorbed best in the duodenum and ileum; absorption is modified by intraluminal factors such as food, drugs, gastric acidity, and intestinal flora. Oral bioavailability of current preparations of L-thyroxine averages 80% (Table 38–1). In contrast, T_3 is almost completely absorbed (95%). T_4 and T_3 absorption appears not to be affected by mild hypothyroidism but may be impaired in severe myxedema with ileus. These factors are important in switching from oral to parenteral therapy. For parenteral use, the intravenous route is preferred for both hormones.

In patients with hyperthyroidism, the metabolic clearances of T_4 and T_3 are increased and the half-lives decreased; the opposite is true in patients with hypothyroidism. Drugs that induce hepatic microsomal enzymes (eg, rifampin, phenobarbital, carbamazepine, phenytoin, tyrosine kinase inhibitors, HIV protease inhibitors) increase the metabolism of both T_4 and T_3 (Table 38–3). Despite this change in clearance, the normal hormone concentration is maintained in the majority of euthyroid patients as a result of compensatory hyperfunction of the thyroid. However, patients dependent on T_4 replacement medication may require increased dosages to maintain clinical effectiveness. A similar compensation occurs if binding sites are altered. If TBG sites are increased by pregnancy, estrogens, or oral contraceptives, there is an initial shift of hormone from the free to the bound state and a decrease in its rate of elimination until the normal free hormone concentration is restored. Thus, the concentration of total and bound hormone will increase, but the concentration of free hormone and the steady-state elimination will remain normal. The reverse occurs when thyroid binding sites are decreased.

Mechanism of Action

A model of thyroid hormone action is depicted in Figure 38–4, which shows the free forms of thyroid hormones, T_4 and T_3,

TABLE 38–3 Drug effects and thyroid function.

Drug Effect	Drugs
Change in thyroid hormone synthesis	
Inhibition of TRH or TSH secretion without induction of hypothyroidism or hyperthyroidism	Dopamine, bromocriptine, levodopa, corticosteroids, somatostatin, metformin
Inhibition of thyroid hormone synthesis or release with the induction of hypothyroidism (or occasionally hyperthyroidism)	Iodides (including amiodarone), lithium, aminoglutethimide, thioamides, ethionamide, tyrosine kinase inhibitors (eg, sunitinib, sorafenib, imatinib), HIV protease inhibitors
Alteration of thyroid hormone transport and serum total T_3 and T_4 levels, but usually no modification of FT_4 or TSH	
Increased TBG	Estrogens, tamoxifen, heroin, methadone, mitotane, fluorouracil
Decreased TBG	Androgens, glucocorticoids
Displacement of T_3 and T_4 from TBG with transient hyperthyroxinemia	Salicylates, fenclofenac, mefenamic acid, furosemide
Alteration of T_4 and T_3 metabolism with modified serum T_3 and T_4 levels but not TSH levels (unless receiving thyroxine replacement therapy)	
Increased hepatic metabolism, enhanced degradation of thyroid hormone	Nicardipine, bexarotene, phenytoin, carbamazepine, phenobarbital, rifampin, rifabutin, tyrosine kinase inhibitors (eg, sunitinib, sorafenib, imatinib)
Inhibition of 5'-deiodinase with decreased T_3, increased rT_3	Iopanoic acid, ipodate, amiodarone, β blockers, corticosteroids, propylthiouracil, flavonoids
Other interactions	
Interference with T_4 absorption	Cholestyramine, chromium picolinate, colestipol, ciprofloxacin, proton pump inhibitors, sucralfate, sodium polystyrene sulfonate, raloxifene, sevelamer hydrochloride, aluminum hydroxide, ferrous sulfate, calcium carbonate, bran, soy, coffee
Induction of autoimmune thyroid disease with hypothyroidism or hyperthyroidism	Interferon-α, interleukin-2, interferon-β, lithium, amiodarone, tyrosine kinase inhibitors (eg, sunitinib, sorafenib, imatinib)
Effect of thyroid function on drug effects	
Anticoagulation	Lower doses of warfarin required in hyperthyroidism, higher doses in hypothyroidism
Glucose control	Increased hepatic glucose production and glucose intolerance in hyperthyroidism; impaired insulin action and glucose disposal in hypothyroidism
Cardiac drugs	Higher doses of digoxin required in hyperthyroidism; lower doses in hypothyroidism
Sedatives; analgesics	Increased sedative and respiratory depressant effects from sedatives and opioids in hypothyroidism; converse in hyperthyroidism

dissociated from thyroid-binding proteins, entering the cell by active transport. Within the cell, T_4 is converted to T_3 by 5'-deiodinase, and the T_3 enters the nucleus, where T_3 binds to a specific T_3 receptor protein, a member of the c-*erb* oncogene family. (This family also includes the steroid hormone receptors and receptors for vitamins A and D.) The T_3 receptor exists in two forms, α and β. Differing concentrations of receptor forms in different tissues may account for variations in T_3 effect on different tissues.

Most of the effects of thyroid on metabolic processes appear to be mediated by activation of nuclear receptors that lead to increased formation of RNA and subsequent protein synthesis, eg, increased formation of Na^+/K^+-ATPase. This is consistent with the observation that the action of thyroid is manifested in vivo with a time lag of hours or days after its administration.

Large numbers of thyroid hormone receptors are found in the most hormone-responsive tissues (pituitary, liver, kidney, heart, skeletal muscle, lung, and intestine), while few receptor sites occur in hormone-unresponsive tissues (spleen, testes). The brain, which lacks an anabolic response to T_3, contains an intermediate number of receptors. In congruence with their biologic potencies, the affinity of the receptor site for T_4 is about ten times lower than that for T_3. Under some conditions, the number of nuclear receptors may be altered to preserve body homeostasis. For example, starvation lowers both circulating T_3 hormone and cellular T_3 receptors.

Effects of Thyroid Hormones

The thyroid hormones are responsible for optimal growth, development, function, and maintenance of all body tissues. Excess or inadequate amounts result in the signs and symptoms of hyperthyroidism or hypothyroidism, respectively (Table 38–4). Since T_3 and T_4 are qualitatively similar, they may be considered as one hormone in the discussion that follows.

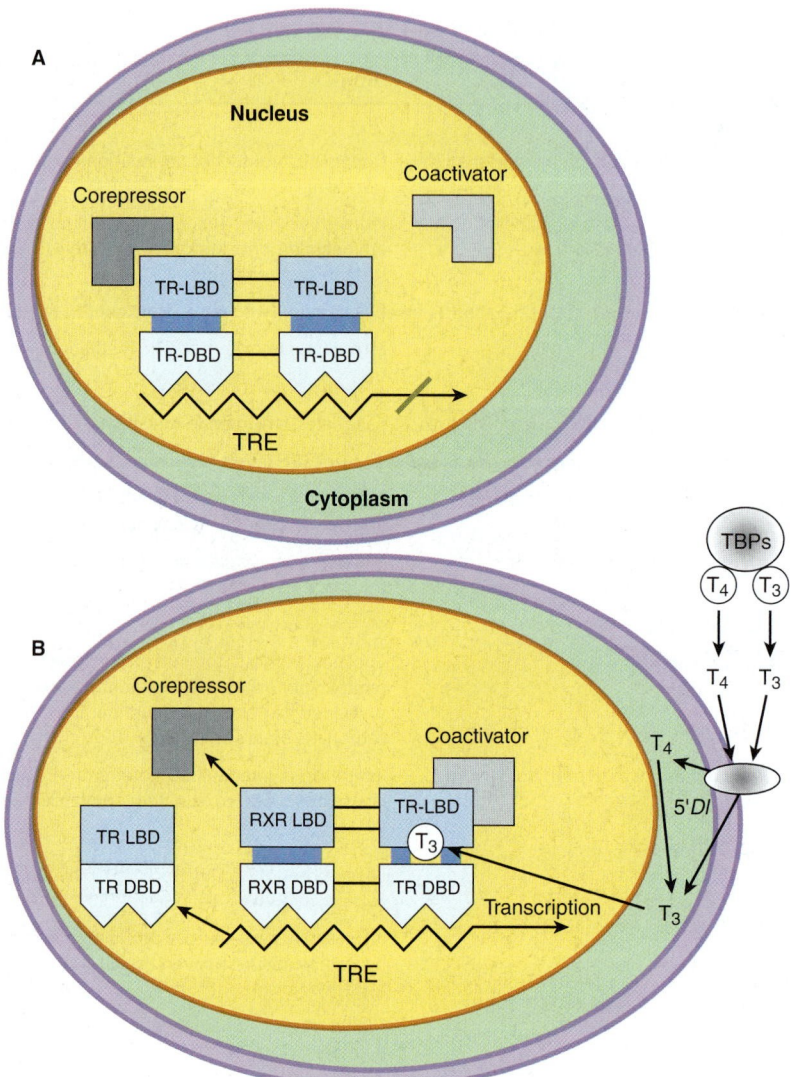

FIGURE 38–4 Model of the interaction of T_3 with the T_3 receptor. **A:** *Inactive phase*—the unliganded T_3 receptor dimer bound to the thyroid hormone response element (TRE) along with corepressors acts as a suppressor of gene transcription. **B:** *Active phase*—T_3 and T_4 circulate bound to thyroid-binding proteins (TBPs). The free hormones are transported into the cell by a specific transport system. Within the cytoplasm, T_4 is converted to T_3 by 5′-deiodinase (5′DI); T_3 then moves into the nucleus. There it binds to the ligand-binding domain of the thyroid receptor (TR) monomer. This promotes disruption of the TR homodimer and heterodimerization with retinoid X receptor (RXR) on the TRE, displacement of corepressors, and binding of coactivators. The TR-coactivator complex activates gene transcription, which leads to alteration in protein synthesis and cellular phenotype. TR-LBD, T_3 receptor ligand-binding domain; TR-DBD, T_3 receptor DNA-binding domain; RXR-LBD, retinoid X receptor ligand-binding domain; RXR-DBD, retinoid X receptor DNA-binding domain; T_3, triiodothyronine; T_4, tetraiodothyronine, L-thyroxine. (Modified and reproduced, with permission, from Gardner DG, Shoback D [editors]: *Greenspan's Basic & Clinical Endocrinology*, 8th ed. McGraw-Hill, 2007.)

Thyroid hormone is critical for the development and functioning of nervous, skeletal, and reproductive tissues. Its effects depend on protein synthesis as well as potentiation of the secretion and action of growth hormone. Thyroid deprivation in early life results in irreversible mental retardation and dwarfism—typical of congenital cretinism.

Effects on growth and calorigenesis are accompanied by a pervasive influence on metabolism of drugs as well as carbohydrates, fats, proteins, and vitamins. Many of these changes are dependent upon or modified by activity of other hormones. Conversely, the secretion and degradation rates of virtually all other hormones, including catecholamines, cortisol, estrogens, testosterone, and insulin, are affected by thyroid status.

Many of the manifestations of thyroid hyperactivity resemble sympathetic nervous system overactivity (especially in the cardiovascular system), although catecholamine levels are not increased. Changes in catecholamine-stimulated adenylyl cyclase activity as measured by cAMP are found with changes in thyroid activity.

TABLE 38–4 Manifestations of thyrotoxicosis and hypothyroidism.

System	Thyrotoxicosis	Hypothyroidism
Skin and appendages	Warm, moist skin; sweating; heat intolerance; fine, thin hair; Plummer's nails; pretibial dermopathy (Graves' disease)	Pale, cool, puffy skin; dry and brittle hair; brittle nails
Eyes, face	Retraction of upper lid with wide stare; periorbital edema; exophthalmos; diplopia (Graves' disease)	Drooping of eyelids; periorbital edema; loss of temporal aspects of eyebrows; puffy, nonpitting facies; large tongue
Cardiovascular system	Decreased peripheral vascular resistance; increased heart rate, stroke volume, cardiac output, pulse pressure; high-output heart failure; increased inotropic and chronotropic effects; arrhythmias; angina	Increased peripheral vascular resistance; decreased heart rate, stroke volume, cardiac output, pulse pressure; low-output heart failure; ECG: bradycardia, prolonged PR interval, flat T wave, low voltage; pericardial effusion
Respiratory system	Dyspnea; decreased vital capacity	Pleural effusions; hypoventilation and CO_2 retention
Gastrointestinal system	Increased appetite; increased frequency of bowel movements; hypoproteinemia	Decreased appetite; decreased frequency of bowel movements; ascites
Central nervous system	Nervousness; hyperkinesia; emotional lability	Lethargy; general slowing of mental processes; neuropathies
Musculoskeletal system	Weakness and muscle fatigue; increased deep tendon reflexes; hypercalcemia; osteoporosis	Stiffness and muscle fatigue; decreased deep tendon reflexes; increased alkaline phosphatase, LDH, AST
Renal system	Mild polyuria; increased renal blood flow; increased glomerular filtration rate	Impaired water excretion; decreased renal blood flow; decreased glomerular filtration rate
Hematopoietic system	Increased erythropoiesis; anemia[1]	Decreased erythropoiesis; anemia[1]
Reproductive system	Menstrual irregularities; decreased fertility; increased gonadal steroid metabolism	Hypermenorrhea; infertility; decreased libido; impotence; oligospermia; decreased gonadal steroid metabolism
Metabolic system	Increased basal metabolic rate; negative nitrogen balance; hyperglycemia; increased free fatty acids; decreased cholesterol and triglycerides; increased hormone degradation; increased requirements for fat- and water-soluble vitamins; increased drug metabolism; decreased warfarin requirement	Decreased basal metabolic rate; slight positive nitrogen balance; delayed degradation of insulin with increased sensitivity; increased cholesterol and triglycerides; decreased hormone degradation; decreased requirements for fat- and water-soluble vitamins; decreased drug metabolism; increased warfarin requirement

[1]The anemia of hyperthyroidism is usually normochromic and caused by increased red blood cell turnover. The anemia of hypothyroidism may be normochromic, hyperchromic, or hypochromic and may be due to decreased production rate, decreased iron absorption, decreased folic acid absorption, or to autoimmune pernicious anemia. LDH, lactic dehydrogenase; AST, aspartate aminotransferase.

Possible explanations include increased numbers of β receptors or enhanced amplification of the β-receptor signal. Other clinical symptoms reminiscent of excessive epinephrine activity (and partially alleviated by adrenoceptor antagonists) include lid lag and retraction, tremor, excessive sweating, anxiety, and nervousness. The opposite constellation of effects is seen in hypothyroidism (Table 38–4).

Thyroid Preparations

See the Preparations Available section at the end of this chapter for a list of available preparations. These preparations may be synthetic (levothyroxine, liothyronine, liotrix) or of animal origin (desiccated thyroid).

Thyroid hormones are not effective and can be detrimental in the management of obesity, abnormal vaginal bleeding, or depression if thyroid hormone levels are normal. Anecdotal reports of a beneficial effect of T_3 administered with antidepressants were not confirmed in a controlled study.

Synthetic levothyroxine is the preparation of choice for thyroid replacement and suppression therapy because of its stability, content uniformity, low cost, lack of allergenic foreign protein, easy laboratory measurement of serum levels, and long half-life (7 days), which permits once-daily administration. In addition, T_4 is converted to T_3 intracellularly; thus, administration of T_4 produces both hormones. Generic levothyroxine preparations provide comparable efficacy and are more cost-effective than branded preparations.

Although liothyronine (T_3) is three to four times more potent than levothyroxine, it is not recommended for routine replacement therapy because of its shorter half-life (24 hours), which requires multiple daily doses; its higher cost; and the greater difficulty of monitoring its adequacy of replacement by conventional laboratory tests. Furthermore, because of its greater hormone activity and consequent greater risk of cardiotoxicity, T_3 should be avoided in patients with cardiac disease. It is best used for short-term suppression of TSH. Because oral administration of T_3 is unnecessary, use of the more expensive mixture of thyroxine and liothyronine (liotrix) instead of levothyroxine is never required.

The use of desiccated thyroid rather than synthetic preparations is never justified, since the disadvantages of protein antigenicity, product instability, variable hormone concentrations, and difficulty in laboratory monitoring far outweigh the advantage of lower cost. Significant amounts of T_3 found in some thyroid extracts and liotrix may produce significant elevations in T_3 levels and toxicity. Equi-effective doses are 100 mg of desiccated thyroid, 100 mcg of levothyroxine, and 37.5 mcg of liothyronine.

The shelf life of synthetic hormone preparations is about 2 years, particularly if they are stored in dark bottles to minimize spontaneous deiodination. The shelf life of desiccated thyroid is not known with certainty, but its potency is better preserved if it is kept dry.

ANTITHYROID AGENTS

Reduction of thyroid activity and hormone effects can be accomplished by agents that interfere with the production of thyroid hormones, by agents that modify the tissue response to thyroid hormones, or by glandular destruction with radiation or surgery. Goitrogens are agents that suppress secretion of T_3 and T_4 to subnormal levels and thereby increase TSH, which in turn produces glandular enlargement (goiter). The antithyroid compounds used clinically include the thioamides, iodides, and radioactive iodine.

THIOAMIDES

The thioamides methimazole and propylthiouracil are major drugs for treatment of thyrotoxicosis. In the United Kingdom, carbimazole, which is converted to methimazole in vivo, is widely used. Methimazole is about ten times more potent than propylthiouracil and is the drug of choice in adults and children. Due to a black box warning about severe hepatitis, propylthiouracil should be reserved for use during the first trimester of pregnancy, in thyroid storm, and in those experiencing adverse reactions to methimazole (other than agranulocytosis or hepatitis). The chemical structures of these compounds are shown in Figure 38–5. The thiocarbamide group is essential for antithyroid activity.

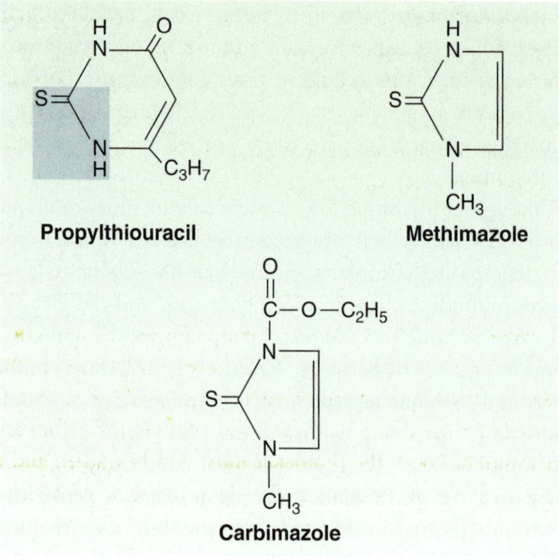

FIGURE 38–5 Structure of thioamides. The thiocarbamide moiety is shaded in color.

Pharmacokinetics

Methimazole is completely absorbed but at variable rates. It is readily accumulated by the thyroid gland and has a volume of distribution similar to that of propylthiouracil. Excretion is slower than with propylthiouracil; 65–70% of a dose is recovered in the urine in 48 hours.

In contrast, propylthiouracil is rapidly absorbed, reaching peak serum levels after 1 hour. The bioavailability of 50–80% may be due to incomplete absorption or a large first-pass effect in the liver. The volume of distribution approximates total body water with accumulation in the thyroid gland. Most of an ingested dose of propylthiouracil is excreted by the kidney as the inactive glucuronide within 24 hours.

The short plasma half-life of these agents (1.5 hours for propylthiouracil and 6 hours for methimazole) has little influence on the duration of the antithyroid action or the dosing interval because both agents are accumulated by the thyroid gland. For propylthiouracil, giving the drug every 6–8 hours is reasonable since a single 100 mg dose can inhibit iodine organification by 60% for 7 hours. Since a single 30 mg dose of methimazole exerts an antithyroid effect for longer than 24 hours, a single daily dose is effective in the management of mild to severe hyperthyroidism.

Both thioamides cross the placental barrier and are concentrated by the fetal thyroid, so that caution must be employed when using these drugs in pregnancy. Because of the risk of fetal hypothyroidism, both thioamides are classified as Food and Drug Administration pregnancy category D (evidence of human fetal risk based on adverse reaction data from investigational or marketing experience, see Chapter 59). Of the two, propylthiouracil is preferable during the first trimester of pregnancy because it is more strongly protein-bound and, therefore, crosses the placenta less readily. In addition, methimazole has been, albeit rarely, associated with congenital malformations. Both thioamides are secreted in low concentrations in breast milk but are considered safe for the nursing infant.

Pharmacodynamics

The thioamides act by multiple mechanisms. The major action is to prevent hormone synthesis by inhibiting the thyroid peroxidase-catalyzed reactions and blocking iodine organification. In addition, they block coupling of the iodotyrosines. They do not block uptake of iodide by the gland. Propylthiouracil and (to a much lesser extent) methimazole inhibit the peripheral deiodination of T_4 and T_3 (Figure 38–1). Since the synthesis rather than the release of hormones is affected, the onset of these agents is slow, often requiring 3–4 weeks before stores of T_4 are depleted.

Toxicity

Adverse reactions to the thioamides occur in 3–12% of treated patients. Most reactions occur early, especially nausea and gastrointestinal distress. An altered sense of taste or smell may occur with methimazole. The most common adverse effect is a maculopapular pruritic rash (4–6%), at times accompanied by systemic signs such as fever. Rare adverse effects include an urticarial rash, vasculitis, a lupus-like reaction, lymphadenopathy, hypopro-thrombinemia, exfoliative dermatitis, polyserositis, and acute arthralgia. An increased risk of severe hepatitis, sometimes result-ing in death, has been reported with propylthiouracil (black box warning), so it should be avoided in children and adults unless no other options are available. Cholestatic jaundice is more common with methimazole than propylthiouracil. Asymptomatic eleva-tions in transaminase levels can also occur.

The most dangerous complication is agranulocytosis (granulo-cyte count < 500 cells/mm^3), an infrequent but potentially fatal adverse reaction. It occurs in 0.1–0.5% of patients taking thioam-ides, but the risk may be increased in older patients and in those receiving more than 40 mg/d of methimazole. The reaction is usu-ally rapidly reversible when the drug is discontinued, but broad-spectrum antibiotic therapy may be necessary for complicating infections. Colony-stimulating factors (eg, G-CSF; see Chapter 33) may hasten recovery of the granulocytes. The cross-sensitivity between propylthiouracil and methimazole is about 50%; there-fore, switching drugs in patients with severe reactions is not recommended.

ANION INHIBITORS

Monovalent anions such as perchlorate (ClO_4^-), pertechnetate (TcO_4^-), and thiocyanate (SCN^-) can block uptake of iodide by the gland through competitive inhibition of the iodide transport mechanism. Since these effects can be overcome by large doses of iodides, their effectiveness is somewhat unpredictable.

The major clinical use for potassium perchlorate is to block thyroidal reuptake of I^- in patients with iodide-induced hyperthy-roidism (eg, amiodarone-induced hyperthyroidism). However, potassium perchlorate is rarely used clinically because it is associ-ated with aplastic anemia.

IODIDES

Prior to the introduction of the thioamides in the 1940s, iodides were the major antithyroid agents; today they are rarely used as sole therapy.

Pharmacodynamics

Iodides have several actions on the thyroid. They inhibit organifi-cation and hormone release and decrease the size and vascularity of the hyperplastic gland. In susceptible individuals, iodides can induce hyperthyroidism (Jod-Basedow phenomenon) or precipi-tate hypothyroidism.

In pharmacologic doses (> 6 mg/d), the major action of iodides is to inhibit hormone release, possibly through inhibition of thyroglobulin proteolysis. Improvement in thyrotoxic symptoms occurs rapidly—within 2–7 days—hence the value of iodide therapy in thyroid storm. In addition, iodides decrease the vascu-larity, size, and fragility of a hyperplastic gland, making the drugs valuable as preoperative preparation for surgery.

Clinical Use of Iodide

Disadvantages of iodide therapy include an increase in intraglan-dular stores of iodine, which may delay onset of thioamide therapy or prevent use of radioactive iodine therapy for several weeks. Thus, iodides should be initiated after onset of thioamide therapy and avoided if treatment with radioactive iodine seems likely. Iodide should not be used alone, because the gland will escape from the iodide block in 2–8 weeks, and its withdrawal may pro-duce severe exacerbation of thyrotoxicosis in an iodine-enriched gland. Chronic use of iodides in pregnancy should be avoided, since they cross the placenta and can cause fetal goiter. In radiation emergencies involving release of radioactive iodine isotopes, the thyroid-blocking effects of potassium iodide can protect the gland from subsequent damage if administered before radiation exposure.

Toxicity

Adverse reactions to iodine (iodism) are uncommon and in most cases reversible upon discontinuance. They include acneiform rash (similar to that of bromism), swollen salivary glands, mucous membrane ulcerations, conjunctivitis, rhinorrhea, drug fever, metal-lic taste, bleeding disorders, and rarely, anaphylactoid reactions.

RADIOACTIVE IODINE

^{131}I is the only isotope used for treatment of thyrotoxicosis (others are used in diagnosis). Administered orally in solution as sodium ^{131}I, it is rapidly absorbed, concentrated by the thyroid, and incor-porated into storage follicles. Its therapeutic effect depends on emission of β rays with an effective half-life of 5 days and a pen-etration range of 400–2000 μm. Within a few weeks after admin-istration, destruction of the thyroid parenchyma is evidenced by epithelial swelling and necrosis, follicular disruption, edema, and leukocyte infiltration. Advantages of radioiodine include easy administration, effectiveness, low expense, and absence of pain. Fears of radiation-induced genetic damage, leukemia, and neoplasia have not been realized after more than 50 years of clinical experi-ence with radioiodine therapy for hyperthyroidism. Radioactive iodine should not be administered to pregnant women or nursing mothers, since it crosses the placenta to destroy the fetal thyroid gland and is excreted in breast milk.

ADRENOCEPTOR-BLOCKING AGENTS

Beta blockers without intrinsic sympathomimetic activity (eg, metoprolol, propranolol, atenolol) are effective therapeutic adjuncts in the management of thyrotoxicosis since many of these symptoms mimic those associated with sympathetic stimulation. Propranolol has been the β blocker most widely studied and used in the therapy of thyrotoxicosis. Beta blockers cause clinical improvement of hyperthyroid symptoms but do not typically alter thyroid hormone levels. Propranolol at doses greater than 160 mg/d may also reduce T_3 levels approximately 20% by inhibiting the peripheral conversion of T_4 to T_3.

TABLE 38–5 Etiology and pathogenesis of hypothyroidism.

Cause	Pathogenesis	Goiter	Degree of Hypothyroidism
Hashimoto's thyroiditis	Autoimmune destruction of thyroid	Present early, absent later	Mild to severe
Drug-induced[1]	Blocked hormone formation[2]	Present	Mild to moderate
Dyshormonogenesis	Impaired synthesis of T_4 due to enzyme deficiency	Present	Mild to severe
Radiation, ^{131}I, x-ray, thyroidectomy	Destruction or removal of gland	Absent	Severe
Congenital (cretinism)	Athyreosis or ectopic thyroid, iodine deficiency; TSH receptor-blocking antibodies	Absent or present	Severe
Secondary (TSH deficit)	Pituitary or hypothalamic disease	Absent	Mild

[1]Iodides, lithium, fluoride, thioamides, aminosalicylic acid, phenylbutazone, amiodarone, perchlorate, ethionamide, thiocyanate, cytokines (interferons, interleukins), bexarotene, tyrosine kinase inhibitors, etc. See Table 38–3.

[2]See Table 38–3 for specific pathogenesis.

■ CLINICAL PHARMACOLOGY OF THYROID & ANTITHYROID DRUGS

HYPOTHYROIDISM

Hypothyroidism is a syndrome resulting from deficiency of thyroid hormones and is manifested largely by a reversible slowing down of all body functions (Table 38–4). In infants and children, there is striking retardation of growth and development that results in dwarfism and irreversible mental retardation.

The etiology and pathogenesis of hypothyroidism are outlined in Table 38–5. Hypothyroidism can occur with or without thyroid enlargement (goiter). The laboratory diagnosis of hypothyroidism in the adult is easily made by the combination of a low free thyroxine and elevated serum TSH (Table 38–2).

The most common cause of hypothyroidism in the USA at this time is probably Hashimoto's thyroiditis, an immunologic disorder in genetically predisposed individuals. In this condition, there is evidence of humoral immunity in the presence of antithyroid antibodies and lymphocyte sensitization to thyroid antigens. Certain medications can also cause hypothyroidism (Table 38–5).

MANAGEMENT OF HYPOTHYROIDISM

Except for hypothyroidism caused by drugs, which can be treated in some cases by simply removing the depressant agent, the general strategy of replacement therapy is appropriate. The most satisfactory preparation is levothyroxine, administered as either a branded or generic preparation. Treatment with combination levothyroxine plus liothyronine has not been found to be superior to levothyroxine alone. Infants and children require more T_4 per kilogram of body weight than adults. The average dosage for an infant 1–6 months of age is 10–15 mcg/kg/d, whereas the average dosage for an adult is about 1.7 mcg/kg/d. Older adults (> 65 years of age) may require less thyroxine for replacement. There is some variability in the absorption of thyroxine, so this dosage will vary from patient to patient. Since interactions with certain foods (eg, bran, soy, coffee) and drugs (Table 38–3) can impair its absorption, thyroxine should be administered on an empty stomach (eg, 30 minutes before meals or 1 hour after meals or at bedtime). Its long half-life of 7 days permits once-daily dosing. Children should be monitored for normal growth and development. Serum TSH and free thyroxine should be measured at regular intervals and TSH maintained within an optimal range of 0.5–2.5 mU/L. It takes 6–8 weeks after starting a given dose of thyroxine to reach steady-state levels in the bloodstream. Thus, dosage changes should be made slowly.

In long-standing hypothyroidism, in older patients, and in patients with underlying cardiac disease, it is imperative to start treatment with reduced dosages. In such adult patients, levothyroxine is given in a dosage of 12.5–25 mcg/d for 2 weeks, increasing the daily dose by 12.5–25 mcg every 2 weeks until euthyroidism or drug toxicity is observed. In older patients, the heart is very sensitive to the level of circulating thyroxine, and if angina pectoris or cardiac arrhythmia develops, it is essential to stop or reduce the dose of thyroxine immediately. In younger patients or those with very mild disease, full replacement therapy may be started immediately.

The toxicity of thyroxine is directly related to the hormone level. In children, restlessness, insomnia, and accelerated bone maturation and growth may be signs of thyroxine toxicity. In adults, increased nervousness, heat intolerance, episodes of palpitation and tachycardia, or unexplained weight loss may be the presenting symptoms. If these symptoms are present, it is important to monitor serum TSH (Table 38–2), which will determine whether the symptoms are due to excess thyroxine blood levels. Chronic overtreatment with T_4, particularly in elderly patients, can increase the risk of atrial fibrillation and accelerated osteoporosis.

Special Problems in Management of Hypothyroidism

A. Myxedema and Coronary Artery Disease

Since myxedema frequently occurs in older persons, it is often associated with underlying coronary artery disease. In this situation, the low levels of circulating thyroid hormone actually protect the heart against increasing demands that could result in angina pectoris or myocardial infarction. Correction of myxedema must be done cautiously to avoid provoking arrhythmia, angina, or acute myocardial infarction. If coronary artery surgery is indicated, it should be done first, prior to correction of the myxedema by thyroxine administration.

B. Myxedema Coma

Myxedema coma is an end state of untreated hypothyroidism. It is associated with progressive weakness, stupor, hypothermia, hypoventilation, hypoglycemia, hyponatremia, water intoxication, shock, and death.

Myxedema coma is a medical emergency. The patient should be treated in the intensive care unit, since tracheal intubation and mechanical ventilation may be required. Associated illnesses such as infection or heart failure must be treated by appropriate therapy. It is important to give all preparations intravenously, because patients with myxedema coma absorb drugs poorly from other routes. Intravenous fluids should be administered with caution to avoid excessive water intake. These patients have large pools of empty T_3 and T_4 binding sites that must be filled before there is adequate free thyroxine to affect tissue metabolism. Accordingly, the treatment of choice in myxedema coma is to give a loading dose of levothyroxine intravenously—usually 300–400 mcg initially, followed by 50–100 mcg daily. Intravenous T_3 can also be used but may be more cardiotoxic and more difficult to monitor. Intravenous hydrocortisone is indicated if the patient has associated adrenal or pituitary insufficiency but is probably not necessary in most patients with primary myxedema. Opioids and sedatives must be used with extreme caution.

C. Hypothyroidism and Pregnancy

Hypothyroid women frequently have anovulatory cycles and are therefore relatively infertile until restoration of the euthyroid state. This has led to the widespread use of thyroid hormone for infertility, although there is no evidence for its usefulness in infertile euthyroid patients. In a pregnant hypothyroid patient receiving thyroxine, it is extremely important that the daily dose of thyroxine be adequate because early development of the fetal brain depends on maternal thyroxine. In many hypothyroid patients, an increase in the thyroxine dose (about 30–50%) is required to normalize the serum TSH level during pregnancy. It is reasonable to counsel women to take an extra 25 mcg thyroxine tablet as soon as they are pregnant and to separate thyroxine from prenatal vitamins by at least 4 hours. Because of the elevated maternal TBG levels and, therefore, elevated total T_4 levels, adequate maternal thyroxine dosages warrant maintenance of TSH between 0.5 and 3.0 mU/L and the total T_4 at or above the upper range of normal.

D. Subclinical Hypothyroidism

Subclinical hypothyroidism, defined as an elevated TSH level and normal thyroid hormone levels, is found in 4–10% of the general population but increases to 20% in women older than age 50.

The consensus of expert thyroid organizations concluded that thyroid hormone therapy should be considered for patients with TSH levels greater than 10 mIU/L while close TSH monitoring is appropriate for those with lower TSH elevations.

E. Drug-Induced Hypothyroidism

Drug-induced hypothyroidism (Table 38–3) can be satisfactorily managed with levothyroxine therapy if the offending agent cannot be stopped. In the case of amiodarone-induced hypothyroidism, levothyroxine therapy may be necessary even after discontinuance because of amiodarone's very long half-life.

HYPERTHYROIDISM

Hyperthyroidism (thyrotoxicosis) is the clinical syndrome that results when tissues are exposed to high levels of thyroid hormone (Table 38–4).

GRAVES' DISEASE

The most common form of hyperthyroidism is Graves' disease, or diffuse toxic goiter. The presenting signs and symptoms of Graves' disease are set forth in Table 38–4.

Pathophysiology

Graves' disease is considered to be an autoimmune disorder in which helper T lymphocytes stimulate B lymphocytes to synthesize antibodies to thyroidal antigens. The antibody described previously (TSH-R Ab [stim]) is directed against the TSH receptor site in the thyroid cell membrane and has the capacity to stimulate growth and biosynthetic activity of the thyroid cell. Spontaneous remission occurs but some patients require years of antithyroid therapy.

Laboratory Diagnosis

In most patients with hyperthyroidism, T_3, T_4, FT_4, and FT_3 are elevated and TSH is suppressed (Table 38–2). Radioiodine uptake is usually markedly elevated as well. Antithyroglobulin, thyroid peroxidase, and TSH-R Ab [stim] antibodies are usually present.

Management of Graves' Disease

The three primary methods for controlling hyperthyroidism are antithyroid drug therapy, surgical thyroidectomy, and destruction of the gland with radioactive iodine.

A. Antithyroid Drug Therapy

Drug therapy is most useful in young patients with small glands and mild disease. Methimazole or propylthiouracil is administered until the disease undergoes spontaneous remission. This is the only therapy that leaves an intact thyroid gland, but it does require a long period of treatment and observation (12–18 months), and there is a 50–70% incidence of relapse.

Methimazole is preferable to propylthiouracil (except in pregnancy and thyroid storm) because it has a lower risk of serious liver injury and can be administered once daily, which may enhance adherence. Antithyroid drug therapy is usually begun with divided doses, shifting to maintenance therapy with single daily doses when the patient becomes clinically euthyroid. However, mild to moderately severe thyrotoxicosis can often be controlled with methimazole given in a single morning dose of 20–40 mg initially for 4–8 weeks to normalize hormone levels. Maintenance therapy requires 5–15 mg once daily. Alternatively, therapy is started with propylthiouracil, 100–150 mg every 6 or 8 hours until the patient is euthyroid, followed by gradual reduction of the dose to the maintenance level of 50–150 mg once daily. In addition to inhibiting iodine organification, propylthiouracil also inhibits the conversion of T_4 to T_3, so it brings the level of activated thyroid hormone down more quickly than does methimazole. The best clinical guide to remission is reduction in the size of the goiter. Laboratory tests most useful in monitoring the course of therapy are serum FT_3, FT_4, and TSH levels.

Reactions to antithyroid drugs have been described above. A minor rash can often be controlled by antihistamine therapy. Because the more severe reaction of agranulocytosis is often heralded by sore throat or high fever, patients receiving antithyroid drugs must be instructed to discontinue the drug and seek immediate medical attention if these symptoms develop. White cell and differential counts and a throat culture are indicated in such cases, followed by appropriate antibiotic therapy. Treatment should also be stopped if significant elevations in transaminases occur.

B. Thyroidectomy

A near-total thyroidectomy is the treatment of choice for patients with very large glands or multinodular goiters. Patients are treated with antithyroid drugs until euthyroid (about 6 weeks). In addition, for 10–14 days prior to surgery, they receive saturated solution of potassium iodide, 5 drops twice daily, to diminish vascularity of the gland and simplify surgery. About 80–90% of patients will require thyroid supplementation following near-total thyroidectomy.

C. Radioactive Iodine

Radioiodine therapy utilizing ^{131}I is the preferred treatment for most patients over 21 years of age. In patients without heart disease, the therapeutic dose may be given immediately in a range of 80–120 μCi/g of estimated thyroid weight corrected for uptake. In patients with underlying heart disease or severe thyrotoxicosis and in elderly patients, it is desirable to treat with antithyroid drugs (preferably methimazole) until the patient is euthyroid. The medication is then stopped for 5–7 days before the appropriate dose of ^{131}I is administered. Iodides should be avoided to ensure maximal ^{131}I uptake. Six to 12 weeks following the administration of radioiodine, the gland will shrink in size and the patient will usually become euthyroid or hypothyroid. A second dose may be required in some patients. Hypothyroidism occurs in about 80% of patients following radioiodine therapy. Serum FT_4 and TSH levels should be monitored regularly. When hypothyroidism develops, prompt replacement with oral levothyroxine, 50–150 mcg daily, should be instituted.

D. Adjuncts to Antithyroid Therapy

During the acute phase of thyrotoxicosis, β-adrenoceptor–blocking agents without intrinsic sympathomimetic activity are extremely helpful. Propranolol, 20–40 mg orally every 6 hours, or metoprolol, 25–50 mg orally every 6–8 hours, will control tachycardia, hypertension, and atrial fibrillation. Beta-adrenoceptor–blocking agents are gradually withdrawn as serum thyroxine levels return to normal. Diltiazem, 90–120 mg three or four times daily, can be used to control tachycardia in patients in whom β blockers are contraindicated, eg, those with asthma. Other calcium channel blockers may not be as effective as diltiazem. Adequate nutrition and vitamin supplements are essential. Barbiturates accelerate T_4 breakdown (by hepatic enzyme induction) and may be helpful both as sedatives and to lower T_4 levels. Bile acid sequestrants (eg, cholestyramine) can also rapidly lower T_4 levels by increasing the fecal excretion of T_4.

TOXIC UNINODULAR GOITER & TOXIC MULTINODULAR GOITER

These forms of hyperthyroidism occur often in older women with nodular goiters. FT_4 is moderately elevated or occasionally normal, but FT_3 or T_3 is strikingly elevated. Single toxic adenomas can be managed with either surgical excision of the adenoma or with radioiodine therapy. Toxic multinodular goiter is usually associated with a large goiter and is best treated by preparation with methimazole (preferable) or propylthiouracil followed by subtotal thyroidectomy.

SUBACUTE THYROIDITIS

During the acute phase of a viral infection of the thyroid gland, there is destruction of thyroid parenchyma with transient release of stored thyroid hormones. A similar state may occur in patients with Hashimoto's thyroiditis. These episodes of transient thyrotoxicosis have been termed *spontaneously resolving hyperthyroidism*. Supportive therapy is usually all that is necessary, such as β-adrenoceptor–blocking agents without intrinsic sympathomimetic activity (eg, propranolol) for tachycardia and aspirin or nonsteroidal anti-inflammatory drugs to control local pain and fever. Corticosteroids may be necessary in severe cases to control the inflammation.

SPECIAL PROBLEMS

Thyroid Storm

Thyroid storm, or thyrotoxic crisis, is sudden acute exacerbation of all of the symptoms of thyrotoxicosis, presenting as a life-threatening syndrome. Vigorous management is mandatory. Propranolol, 1–2 mg slowly intravenously or 40–80 mg orally every 6 hours, is helpful to control the severe cardiovascular manifestations. If propranolol is contraindicated by the presence of severe heart failure or asthma, hypertension and tachycardia may be controlled with diltiazem, 90–120 mg orally three or four times daily or 5–10 mg/h by intravenous infusion (asthmatic patients only). Release of thyroid hormones from the gland is retarded by the administration of saturated solution of potassium iodide, 10 drops orally daily. Hormone synthesis is blocked by the administration of propylthiouracil, 250 mg orally every 6 hours. If the patient is unable to take propylthiouracil by mouth, a rectal formulation* can be prepared and administered in a dosage of 400 mg every 6 hours as a retention enema. Methimazole may also be prepared for rectal administration in a dose of 60 mg daily. Hydrocortisone, 50 mg intravenously every 6 hours, will protect the patient against shock and will block the conversion of T_4 to T_3, rapidly bringing down the level of thyroactive material in the blood.

Supportive therapy is essential to control fever, heart failure, and any underlying disease process that may have precipitated the acute storm. In rare situations, where the above methods are not adequate to control the problem, plasmapheresis or peritoneal dialysis has been used to lower the levels of circulating thyroxine.

Ophthalmopathy

Although severe ophthalmopathy is rare, it is difficult to treat. Management requires effective treatment of the thyroid disease, usually by total surgical excision or ^{131}I ablation of the gland plus oral prednisone therapy (see below). In addition, local therapy may be necessary, eg, elevation of the head to diminish periorbital edema and artificial tears to relieve corneal drying due to exophthalmos. Smoking cessation should be advised to prevent progression of the ophthalmopathy. For the severe, acute inflammatory reaction, a short course of prednisone, 60–100 mg orally daily for about a week and then 60–100 mg every other day, tapering the dose over a period of 6–12 weeks, may be effective. If steroid therapy fails or is contraindicated, irradiation of the posterior orbit, using well-collimated high-energy x-ray therapy, will frequently result in marked improvement of the acute process. Threatened loss of vision is an indication for surgical decompression of the orbit. Eyelid or eye muscle surgery may be necessary to correct residual problems after the acute process has subsided.

Dermopathy

Dermopathy or pretibial myxedema will often respond to topical corticosteroids applied to the involved area and covered with an occlusive dressing.

Thyrotoxicosis during Pregnancy

Ideally, women in the childbearing period with severe disease should have definitive therapy with ^{131}I or subtotal thyroidectomy

prior to pregnancy in order to avoid an acute exacerbation of the disease during pregnancy or following delivery. If thyrotoxicosis does develop during pregnancy, radioiodine is contraindicated because it crosses the placenta and may injure the fetal thyroid. Propylthiouracil (fewer teratogenic risks than methimazole) can be given in the first trimester, and then methimazole can be given for the remainder of the pregnancy in order to avoid potential liver damage. The dosage of propylthiouracil must be kept to the minimum necessary for control of the disease (ie, < 300 mg/d), because it may affect the function of the fetal thyroid gland. Alternatively, a subtotal thyroidectomy can be safely performed during the mid trimester. It is essential to give the patient a thyroid supplement during the balance of the pregnancy.

Neonatal Graves' Disease

Graves' disease may occur in the newborn infant, either due to passage of maternal TSH-R Ab [stim] through the placenta, stimulating the thyroid gland of the neonate, or to genetic transmission of the trait to the fetus. Laboratory studies reveal an elevated free T_4, a markedly elevated T_3, and a low TSH—in contrast to the normal infant, in whom TSH is elevated at birth. TSH-R Ab [stim] is usually found in the serum of both the child and the mother.

If caused by maternal TSH-R Ab [stim], the disease is usually self-limited and subsides over a period of 4–12 weeks, coinciding with the fall in the infant's TSH-R Ab [stim] level. However, treatment is necessary because of the severe metabolic stress the infant experiences. Therapy includes propylthiouracil in a dose of 5–10 mg/kg/d in divided doses at 8-hour intervals; Lugol's solution (8 mg of iodide per drop), 1 drop every 8 hours; and propranolol, 2 mg/kg/d in divided doses. Careful supportive therapy is essential. If the infant is very ill, oral prednisone, 2 mg/kg/d in divided doses, will help block conversion of T_4 to T_3. These medications are gradually reduced as the clinical picture improves and can be discontinued by 6–12 weeks.

SUBCLINICAL HYPERTHYROIDISM

Subclinical hyperthyroidism is defined as a suppressed TSH level (below the normal range) in conjunction with normal thyroid hormone levels. Cardiac toxicity (eg, atrial fibrillation), especially in older persons, is of greatest concern. The consensus of thyroid experts concluded that hyperthyroidism treatment is appropriate in those with TSH less than 0.1 mIU/L, while close monitoring of the TSH level is appropriate for those with less TSH suppression.

Amiodarone-Induced Thyrotoxicosis

In addition to those patients who develop hypothyroidism caused by amiodarone, approximately 3% of patients receiving this drug will develop hyperthyroidism instead. Two types of amiodarone-induced thyrotoxicosis have been reported: iodine-induced (type I), which often occurs in persons with underlying thyroid disease (eg, multinodular goiter); and an inflammatory thyroiditis

---

*To prepare a water suspension propylthiouracil enema, grind eight 50 mg tablets and suspend the powder in 90 mL of sterile water.

(type II) that occurs in patients without thyroid disease due to leakage of thyroid hormone into the circulation. Treatment of type I requires therapy with thioamides, while type II responds best to glucocorticoids. Since it is not always possible to differentiate between the two types, thioamides and glucocorticoids are often administered together. If possible, amiodarone should be discontinued; however, rapid improvement does not occur due to its long half-life.

NONTOXIC GOITER

Nontoxic goiter is a syndrome of thyroid enlargement without excessive thyroid hormone production. Enlargement of the thyroid gland is often due to TSH stimulation from inadequate thyroid hormone synthesis. The most common cause of nontoxic goiter worldwide is iodide deficiency, but in the USA, it is Hashimoto's thyroiditis. Other causes include germ-line or acquired mutations in genes involved in hormone synthesis, dietary goitrogens, and neoplasms (see below).

Goiter due to iodide deficiency is best managed by prophylactic administration of iodide. The optimal daily iodide intake is 150–200 mcg. Iodized salt and iodate used as preservatives in flour and bread are excellent sources of iodine in the diet. In areas where it is difficult to introduce iodized salt or iodate preservatives, a solution of iodized poppy-seed oil has been administered intramuscularly to provide a long-term source of inorganic iodine.

Goiter due to ingestion of goitrogens in the diet is managed by elimination of the goitrogen or by adding sufficient thyroxine to shut off TSH stimulation. Similarly, in Hashimoto's thyroiditis and dyshormonogenesis, adequate thyroxine therapy—150–200 mcg/d orally—will suppress pituitary TSH and result in slow regression of the goiter as well as correction of hypothyroidism.

THYROID NEOPLASMS

Neoplasms of the thyroid gland may be benign (adenomas) or malignant. The primary diagnostic test is a fine needle aspiration biopsy and cytologic examination. Benign lesions may be monitored for growth or symptoms of local obstruction, which would mandate surgical excision. Levothyroxine therapy is not recommended for the suppression of benign nodules, especially in iodine sufficient areas. Management of thyroid carcinoma requires a total thyroidectomy, postoperative radioiodine therapy in selected instances, and lifetime replacement with levothyroxine. The evaluation for recurrence of some thyroid malignancies often involves withdrawal of thyroxine replacement for 4–6 weeks—accompanied by the development of hypothyroidism. Tumor recurrence is likely if there is a rise in serum thyroglobulin (ie, a tumor marker) or a positive ^{131}I scan when TSH is elevated. Alternatively, administration of recombinant human TSH (Thyrogen) can produce comparable TSH elevations without discontinuing thyroxine and avoiding hypothyroidism. Recombinant human TSH is administered intramuscularly once daily for 2 days. A rise in serum thyroglobulin or a positive ^{131}I scan will indicate a recurrence of the thyroid cancer.

SUMMARY Drugs Used in the Management of Thyroid Disease

Class	Mechanism of Action and Effects	Indications	Pharmacokinetics, Toxicities, Interactions
Thyroid Preparations • Levothyroxine (T$_4$) • Liothyronine (T$_3$)	Activation of nuclear receptors results in gene expression with RNA formation and protein synthesis	Hypothyroidism	See Table 38–1• maximum effect seen after 6–8 weeks of therapy • *Toxicity:* See Table 38–4 for symptoms of thyroid excess
Antithyroid Agents **THIOAMIDES** • Methimazole • Propylthiouracil (PTU)	Inhibit thyroid peroxidase reactions • block iodine organification • inhibit peripheral deiodination of T$_4$ and T$_3$ (primarily PTU)	Hyperthyroidism	Oral • duration of action: 24 h (methimazole), 6–8 h (PTU) • delayed onset of action • *Toxicity:* Nausea, gastrointestinal distress, rash, agranulocytosis, hepatitis (PTU black box), hypothyroidism
IODIDES • Lugol solution • Potassium iodide	Inhibit organification and hormone release • reduce the size and vascularity of the gland	Preparation for surgical thyroidectomy	Oral • acute onset within 2–7 days • *Toxicity:* Rare (see text)
BETA BLOCKERS • Propranolol	Inhibition of β adrenoreceptors • inhibit T$_4$ to T$_3$ conversion (only propranolol)	Hyperthyroidism, especially thyroid storm • adjunct to control tachycardia, hypertension, and atrial fibrillation	Onset within hours • duration of 4–6 h (oral propranolol) • *Toxicity:* Asthma, AV blockade, hypotension, bradycardia
RADIOACTIVE IODINE ^{131}I (RAI)	Radiation destruction of thyroid parenchyma	Hyperthyroidism • patients should be euthyroid or on β blockers before RAI • avoid in pregnancy or in nursing mothers	Oral • half-life 5 days • onset of 6–12 weeks • maximum effect in 3–6 months • *Toxicity:* Sore throat, sialitis, hypothyroidism

P R E P A R A T I O N S   A V A I L A B L E

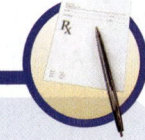

THYROID AGENTS

Levothyroxine [T$_4$] (generic, Levoxyl, Levo-T, Levothroid, Levolet, Novothyrox, Synthroid, Tirosint, Unithroid)
Oral: 25, 50, 75, 88, 100, 112, 125, 137, 150, 175, 200, 300 mcg tablets; 13, 25, 50, 75, 88, 100, 112, 125, 137, 150 mcg capsules
Parenteral: 200, 500 mcg per vial (100 mcg/mL when reconstituted) for injection

Liothyronine [T$_3$] (generic, Cytomel)
Oral: 5, 25, 50 mcg tablets
Parenteral: 10 mcg/mL

Liotrix [a 4:1 ratio of T$_4$: T$_3$] (Thyrolar)
Oral: tablets containing 12.5, 25, 30, 50, 100, 150 mcg T$_4$ and one fourth as much T$_3$

Thyroid desiccated [USP] (generic, Armour, Nature-Throid, Westhroid)
Oral: tablets containing 15, 30, 60, 90, 120, 180, 240, 300 mg; capsules containing 120, 180, 300 mg

ANTITHYROID AGENTS

Radioactive iodine (^{131}I) sodium (Iodotope, Sodium Iodide I 131 Therapeutic)
Oral: available as capsules and solution

Methimazole (generic, Tapazole)
Oral: 5, 10 mg tablets

Potassium iodide
Oral solution (generic, SSKI): 1 g/mL; (Thyroshield) 65 mg/mL
Oral solution (Lugol's solution): 100 mg/mL potassium iodide plus 50 mg/mL iodine
Oral potassium iodide tablets (generic, IOSAT, Thyro-Block, Thyro-Safe): 65, 130 mg

Propylthiouracil [PTU] (generic)
Oral: 50 mg tablets

Thyrotropin; recombinant human TSH (Thyrogen)
Parenteral: 1.1 mg per vial

REFERENCES

General

American Thyroid Association (http://www.thyroid.org).

Biondi B, Cooper DS: The clinical significance of subclinical thyroid dysfunction. Endocr Rev 2008;29:76.

Cooper DS et al: The thyroid gland. In: Gardner DG, Shoback D (editors): *Greenspan's Basic & Clinical Endocrinology*, 9th ed. McGraw-Hill, 2011.

Fitzpatrick DL, Russell MA: Diagnosis and management of thyroid disease in pregnancy. Obstet Gynecol Clin N Am 2010;37:173.

Galli E, Pingitore A, Iervasi G: The role of thyroid hormone in the pathophysiology of heart failure: clinical evidence. Heart Fail Rev 2010;15:155.

Laurberg P et al: Iodine intake as a determinant of thyroid disorders in populations. Best Pract Res Clin Endocrinol Metab 2010;24:13.

Oetting A, Yen PM: New insights into thyroid hormone action. Best Pract Res Clin Endocrinol Metab 2007;21:193.

Williams GR: Neurodevelopment and neurophysiological actions of thyroid hormone. J Neuroendocrinol 2008;20:784.

Guidelines

Anonymous: The Hormone Foundation's patient guide to the management of maternal hypothyroidism before, during and after pregnancy. J Clin Endocrinol Metab 2007;92(8)(Suppl):S1.

Cooper DS et al: Revised American Thyroid Association management guidelines for patients with thyroid nodules and differentiated thyroid cancer. Thyroid 2009;19(11):1167.

Ladenson D et al: American Thyroid Association guidelines for the detection of thyroid dysfunction. Arch Intern Med 2000;160:1573.

US Department of Health and Human Services: Potassium iodide as a thyroid blocking agent in radiation emergencies. December 2001 (http://www.fda.gov/cder/guidance/index.htm).

Hypothyroidism

Dong BJ et al: Bioequivalence of generic and brand-name levothyroxine products in the treatment of hypothyroidism. JAMA 1997;277:1205.

Joffe RT et al: Treatment of clinical hypothyroidism with thyroxine and triiodothyronine: A literature review and meta-analysis. Psychosomatics 2007;48:379.

Jonklaas J et al: Triiodothyronine levels in athyreotic individuals during levothyroxine therapy. JAMA 2008;299:769.

Lania A et al: Central hypothyroidism. Pituitary 2008;11:181.

McDermott MT: In the clinic. Hypothyroidism. Ann Intern Med 2009; 151:ITC61.

Hyperthyroidism

Abraham P et al: Antithyroid drug regimen for treating Graves' hyperthyroidism. Cochrane Database Syst Rev 2010 Jan 20;(1):CD003420. http://onlinelibrary.wiley.com/o/cochrane/clsysrev/articles/CD003420/pdf_fs.html.

Bahn RS: Graves' ophthalmopathy. N Engl J Med 2010;362:726.

Brent GA: Graves' disease. N Engl J Med 2008;358:2594.

Cooper DS, Rivkees SA: Putting propylthiouracil in perspective. J Clin Endocrinol Metab 2009;94:1881.

Silva JE, Bianco SD: Thyroid-adrenergic interactions: Physiological and clinical implications. Thyroid 2008;18:157.

Nodules & Cancer (see Guidelines)

Miller MC: The patient with a thyroid nodule. Med Clin North Am 2010;94:1003.

The Effects of Drugs on Thyroid Function

Barbesino G: Drugs affecting thyroid function. Thyroid 2010;20:763.

Burgi H: Iodine excess. Best Pract Res Clin Endocrinol Metab 2010;24:107.

Eskes SA, Wiersinga WM: Amiodarone and the thyroid. Best Pract Res Clin Endocrinol Metab 2009;23:735.

Haugen BR: Drugs that suppress TSH or cause central hypothyroidism. Best Pract Res Clin Endocrinol Metab 2009;23:793.

Lazarus JH: Lithium and thyroid. Best Pract Res Clin Endocrinol Metab 2009;23:723.

Sherman SI: Tyrosine kinase inhibitors and the thyroid. Best Pract Res Clin Endocrinol Metab 2009;23:713.

Tomer Y, Menconi F: Interferon induced thyroiditis. Best Pract Res Clin Endocrinol Metab 2009;23:703.

CASE STUDY ANSWER

This patient presents with the typical signs and symptoms of hypothyroidism following radioactive iodine therapy. Radioactive iodine therapy and thyroidectomy are reasonable and effective strategies for definitive treatment of her hyperthyroidism, especially before becoming pregnant to avoid an acute exacerbation of the disease during pregnancy or following delivery. This patient's hypothyroid symptoms are easily corrected by the daily administration of levothyroxine, taken orally on an empty stomach. Thyroid function tests should be checked after 6–8 weeks and the dosage adjusted to achieve a normal TSH and resolution of hypothyroid symptoms.

39

Adrenocorticosteroids & Adrenocortical Antagonists

George P. Chrousos, MD

CASE STUDY

A 19-year-old man complains of anorexia, fatigue, dizziness, and weight loss of 8 months' duration. The examining physician discovers postural hypotension and moderate vitiligo (depigmented areas of skin) and obtains routine blood tests. She finds hyponatremia, hyperkalemia, and acidosis and suspects Addison's disease. She performs a standard ACTH 1–24 stimulation test, which reveals an insufficient plasma cortisol response, compatible with primary adrenal insufficiency. The diagnosis of autoimmune Addison's disease is made, and the patient must start replacement of the hormones he cannot produce himself. How should this patient be treated? What precautions should he take?

The natural adrenocortical hormones are steroid molecules produced and released by the adrenal cortex. Both natural and synthetic corticosteroids are used for the diagnosis and treatment of disorders of adrenal function. They are also used—more often and in much larger doses—for treatment of a variety of inflammatory and immunologic disorders.

Secretion of adrenocortical steroids is controlled by the pituitary release of corticotropin (ACTH). Secretion of the salt-retaining hormone aldosterone is primarily under the influence of angiotensin. Corticotropin has some actions that do not depend on its effect on adrenocortical secretion. However, its pharmacologic value as an anti-inflammatory agent and its use in testing adrenal function depend on its secretory action. Its pharmacology is discussed in Chapter 37 and is reviewed only briefly here.

Inhibitors of the synthesis or antagonists of the action of the adrenocortical steroids are important in the treatment of several conditions. These agents are described at the end of this chapter.

■ ADRENOCORTICOSTEROIDS

The adrenal cortex releases a large number of steroids into the circulation. Some have minimal biologic activity and function primarily as precursors, and there are some for which no function has been established. The hormonal steroids may be classified as those having important effects on intermediary metabolism and immune function (**glucocorticoids**), those having principally salt-retaining activity (**mineralocorticoids**), and those having **androgenic** or **estrogenic** activity (see Chapter 40). In humans, the major glucocorticoid is **cortisol** and the most important mineralocorticoid is **aldosterone**. Quantitatively, dehydroepiandrosterone (DHEA) in its sulfated form (DHEAS) is the major adrenal androgen. However, DHEA and two other adrenal androgens, androstenediol and androstenedione, are weak androgens or (by conversion) estrogens. Adrenal androgens constitute the major endogenous precursors of estrogen in women after menopause and in younger patients in whom ovarian function is deficient or absent.

THE NATURALLY OCCURRING GLUCOCORTICOIDS; CORTISOL (HYDROCORTISONE)

Pharmacokinetics

Cortisol (also called hydrocortisone, compound F) exerts a wide range of physiologic effects, including regulation of intermediary metabolism, cardiovascular function, growth, and immunity. Its synthesis and secretion are tightly regulated by the central nervous system, which is very sensitive to negative feedback by the circulating cortisol and exogenous (synthetic) glucocorticoids. Cortisol is synthesized from cholesterol (as shown in Figure 39–1). The mechanisms controlling its secretion are discussed in Chapter 37.

In the normal adult, in the absence of stress, 10–20 mg of cortisol is secreted daily. The rate of secretion follows a circadian rhythm governed by pulses of ACTH that peak in the early morning hours and after meals, especially after lunch (Figure 39–2). In plasma, cortisol is bound to circulating proteins. Corticosteroid-binding globulin (CBG), an α_2 globulin synthesized by the liver, binds about 90% of the circulating hormone under normal circumstances. The remainder is free (about 5–10%) or loosely bound to albumin (about 5%) and is available to exert its effect on target cells. When plasma cortisol levels exceed 20–30 mcg/dL, CBG is saturated, and the concentration of free cortisol rises rapidly. CBG is increased in pregnancy and with estrogen administration and in hyperthyroidism. It is decreased by hypothyroidism, genetic defects in synthesis, and protein deficiency states. Albumin has a large capacity but low affinity for cortisol, and for practical purposes albumin-bound cortisol should be considered free. Synthetic corticosteroids such as dexamethasone are largely bound to albumin rather than CBG.

The half-life of cortisol in the circulation is normally about 60–90 minutes; it may be increased when hydrocortisone (the pharmaceutical preparation of cortisol) is administered in large

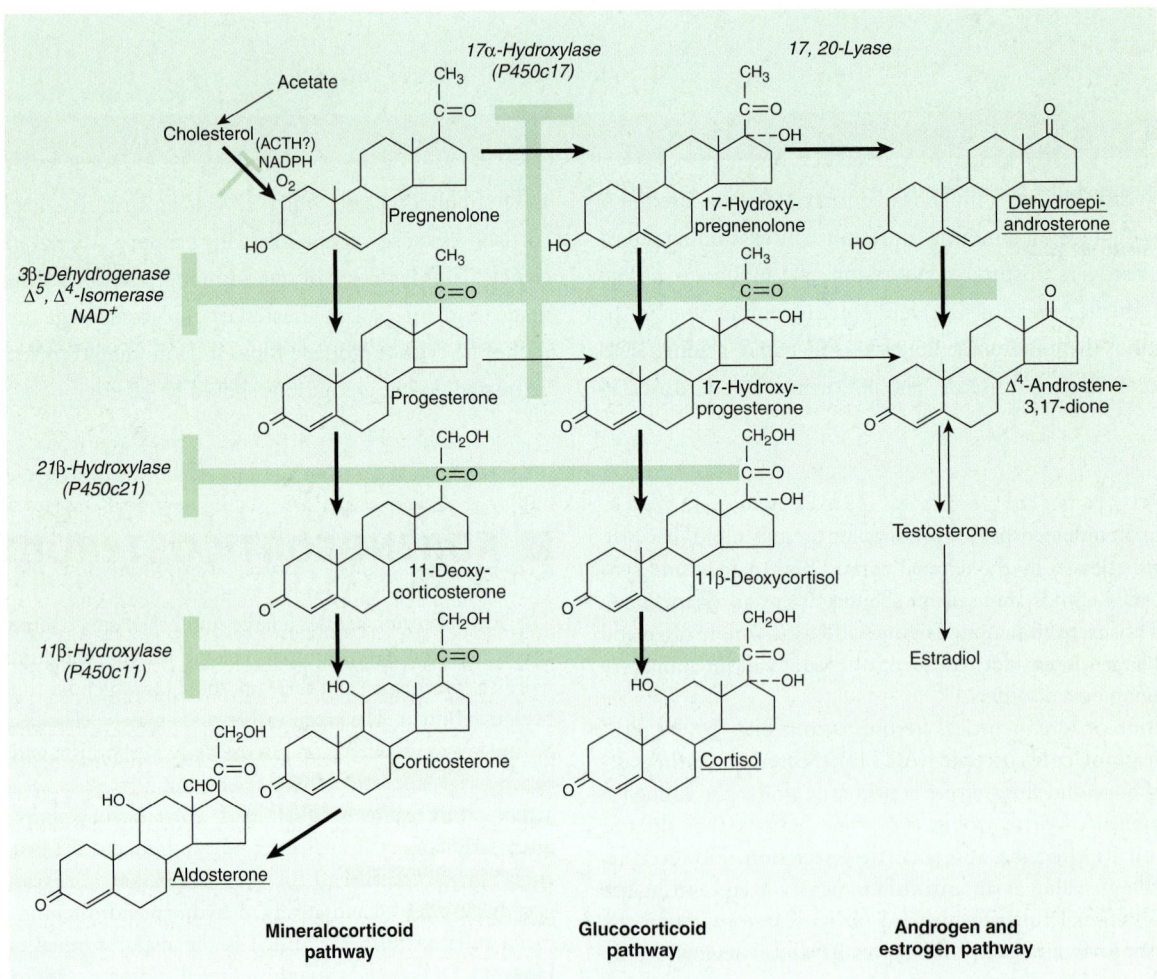

FIGURE 39–1 Outline of major pathways in adrenocortical hormone biosynthesis. The major secretory products are underlined. Pregnenolone is the major precursor of corticosterone and aldosterone, and 17-hydroxypregnenolone is the major precursor of cortisol. The enzymes and cofactors for the reactions progressing down each column are shown on the left and across columns at the top of the figure. When a particular enzyme is deficient, hormone production is blocked at the points indicated by the shaded bars. (Modified after Welikey et al; reproduced, with permission, from Ganong WF: *Review of Medical Physiology*, 17th ed. Originally published by Appleton & Lange. Copyright © 1995 by The McGraw-Hill Companies, Inc.)

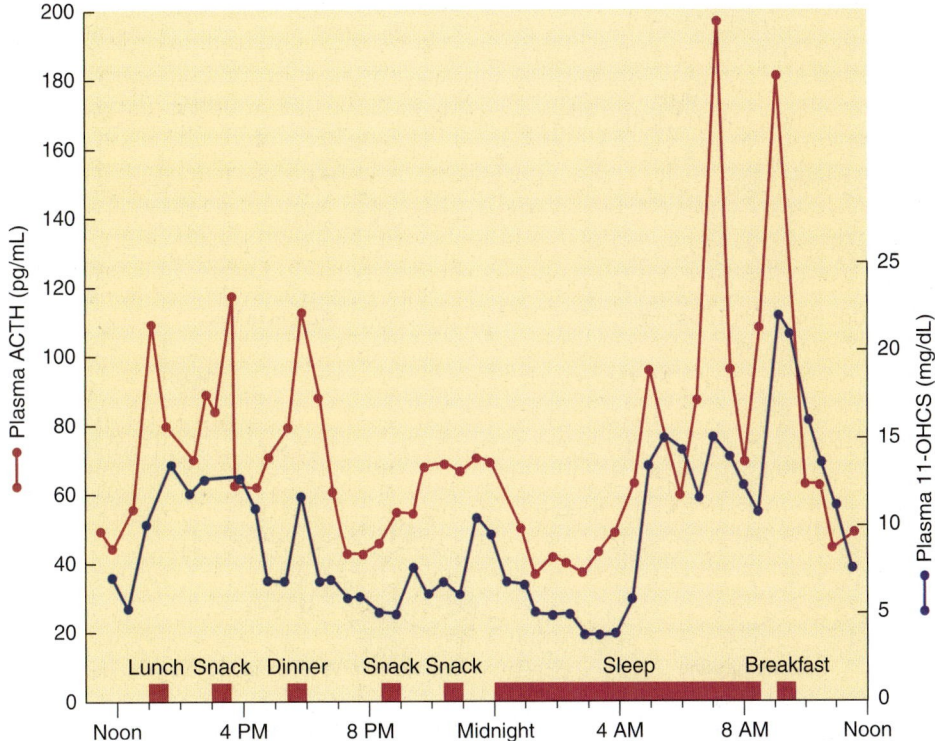

FIGURE 39–2 Fluctuations in plasma ACTH and glucocorticoids throughout the day in a normal girl (age 16). The ACTH was measured by immunoassay and the glucocorticoids as 11-oxysteroids (11-OHCS). Note the marked ACTH and glucocorticoid rises in the morning, before awakening from sleep. (Reproduced, with permission, from Krieger DT et al: Characterization of the normal temporal pattern of plasma corticosteroid levels. J Clin Endocrinol Metab 1971;32:266.)

amounts or when stress, hypothyroidism, or liver disease is present. Only 1% of cortisol is excreted unchanged in the urine as free cortisol; about 20% of cortisol is converted to cortisone by 11-hydroxysteroid dehydrogenase in the kidney and other tissues with mineralocorticoid receptors (see below) before reaching the liver. Most cortisol is metabolized in the liver. About one third of the cortisol produced daily is excreted in the urine as dihydroxy ketone metabolites and is measured as 17-hydroxysteroids (see Figure 39–3 for carbon numbering). Many cortisol metabolites are conjugated with glucuronic acid or sulfate at the C_3 and C_{21} hydroxyls, respectively, in the liver; they are then excreted in the urine.

In some species (eg, the rat), corticosterone is the major glucocorticoid. It is less firmly bound to protein and therefore metabolized more rapidly. The pathways of its degradation are similar to those of cortisol.

Pharmacodynamics

A. Mechanism of Action

Most of the known effects of the glucocorticoids are mediated by widely distributed glucocorticoid receptors. These proteins are members of the superfamily of nuclear receptors, which includes steroid, sterol (vitamin D), thyroid, retinoic acid, and many other receptors with unknown or nonexistent ligands (orphan receptors). All these receptors interact with the promoters of—and regulate the transcription of—target genes (Figure 39–4). In the

absence of the hormonal ligand, glucocorticoid receptors are primarily cytoplasmic, in oligomeric complexes with heat-shock proteins (hsp). The most important of these are two molecules of hsp90, although other proteins are certainly involved. Free hormone from the plasma and interstitial fluid enters the cell and binds to the receptor, inducing conformational changes that allow it to dissociate from the heat shock proteins. The ligand-bound receptor complex then is actively transported into the nucleus, where it interacts with DNA and nuclear proteins. As a homodimer, it binds to **glucocorticoid receptor elements (GREs)** in the promoters of responsive genes. The GRE is composed of two palindromic sequences that bind to the hormone receptor dimer.

In addition to binding to GREs, the ligand-bound receptor also forms complexes with and influences the function of other transcription factors, such as AP1 and NF-κB, which act on non-GRE-containing promoters, to contribute to the regulation of transcription of their responsive genes. These transcription factors have broad actions on the regulation of growth factors, proinflammatory cytokines, etc, and to a great extent mediate the anti-growth, anti-inflammatory, and immunosuppressive effects of glucocorticoids.

Two genes for the corticoid receptor have been identified: one encoding the classic glucocorticoid receptor (**GR**) and the other encoding the mineralocorticoid receptor (**MR**). Alternative splicing of human glucocorticoid receptor pre-mRNA generates two highly homologous isoforms, termed hGR alpha and hGR beta. Human GR alpha is the classic ligand-activated glucocorticoid receptor

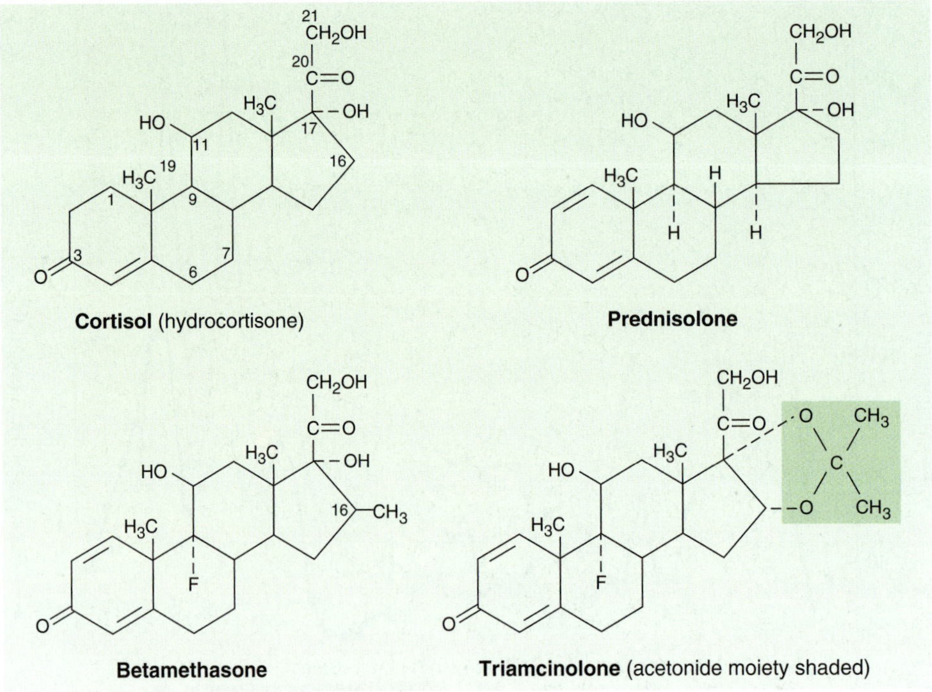

FIGURE 39–3 Chemical structures of several glucocorticoids. The acetonide-substituted derivatives (eg, triamcinolone acetonide) have increased surface activity and are useful in dermatology. Dexamethasone is identical to betamethasone except for the configuration of the methyl group at C_{16}: in betamethasone it is beta (projecting *up* from the plane of the rings); in dexamethasone it is alpha.

which, in the hormone-bound state, modulates the expression of glucocorticoid-responsive genes. In contrast, hGR beta does not bind glucocorticoids and is transcriptionally inactive. However, hGR beta is able to inhibit the effects of hormone-activated hGR alpha on glucocorticoid-responsive genes, playing the role of a physiologically relevant endogenous inhibitor of glucocorticoid action. It was recently shown that the two hGR alternative transcripts have eight distinct translation initiation sites; ie, in a human cell there may be up to 16 GRα and GRβ isoforms, which may form up to 256 homodimers and heterodimers with different transcriptional and possibly non-transcriptional activities. This variability suggests that this important class of steroid receptors has complex stochastic activities.

The prototype glucocorticoid receptor isoform is composed of about 800 amino acids and can be divided into three functional domains (see Figure 2–6). The glucocorticoid-binding domain is located at the carboxyl terminal of the molecule. The DNA-binding domain is located in the middle of the protein and contains nine cysteine residues. This region folds into a "two-finger" structure stabilized by zinc ions connected to cysteines to form two tetrahedrons. This part of the molecule binds to the GREs that regulate glucocorticoid action on glucocorticoid-regulated genes. The zinc fingers represent the basic structure by which the DNA-binding domain recognizes specific nucleic acid sequences. The amino-terminal domain is involved in the transactivation activity of the receptor and increases its specificity.

The interaction of glucocorticoid receptors with GREs or other transcription factors is facilitated or inhibited by several families of proteins called steroid receptor *coregulators*, divided into *coactivators* and *corepressors*. The coregulators do this by serving as bridges between the receptors and other nuclear proteins and by expressing enzymatic activities such as histone acetylase or deacetylase, which alter the conformation of nucleosomes and the transcribability of genes.

Between 10% and 20% of expressed genes in a cell are regulated by glucocorticoids. The number and affinity of receptors for the hormone, the complement of transcription factors and coregulators, and post-transcription events determine the relative specificity of these hormones' actions in various cells. The effects of glucocorticoids are mainly due to proteins synthesized from mRNA transcribed from their target genes.

Some of the effects of glucocorticoids can be attributed to their binding to mineralocorticoid receptors (MRs). Indeed, MRs bind aldosterone and cortisol with similar affinity. A mineralocorticoid effect of cortisol is avoided in some tissues by expression of 11β-hydroxysteroid dehydrogenase type 2, the enzyme responsible for biotransformation to its 11-keto derivative (cortisone), which has minimal affinity for aldosterone receptors.

Recently, the GR was found to interact with CLOCK/BMAL-1, a transcription factor dimer expressed in all tissues and generating the circadian rhythm of cortisol secretion at the suprachiasmatic nucleus of the hypothalamus. CLOCK is an acetyltransferase that acetylates the hinge region of the GR, neutralizing its transcriptional activity and thus rendering target tissues resistant to glucocorticoids. Interestingly, the glucocorticoid target tissue sensitivity rhythm generated is in reverse phase to that of circulating cortisol concentrations, explaining the increased sensitivity of the organism to evening administration of glucocorticoids.

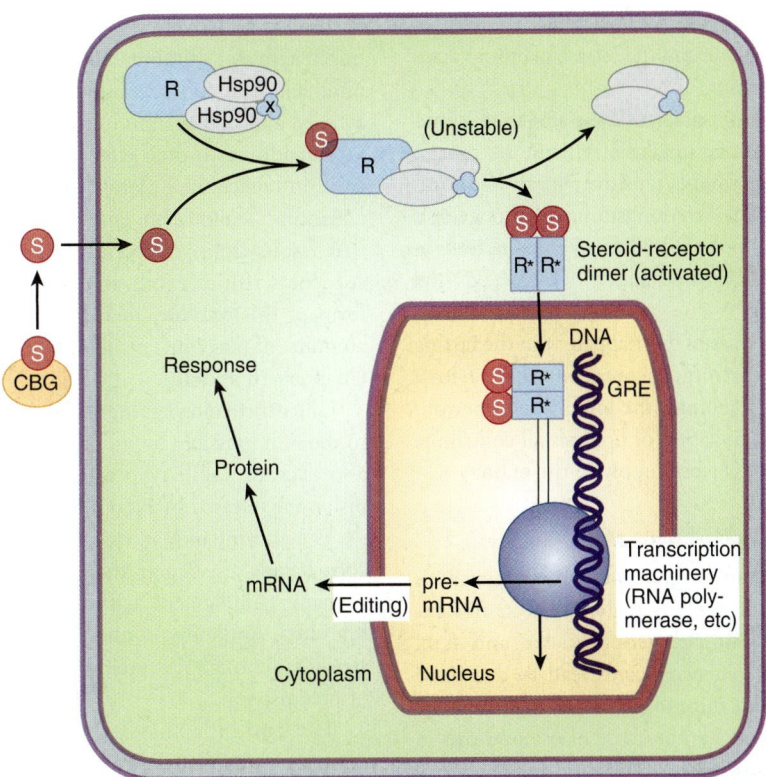

FIGURE 39–4 A model of the interaction of a steroid, S (eg, cortisol), and its receptor, R, and the subsequent events in a target cell. The steroid is present in the blood in bound form on the corticosteroid-binding globulin (CBG) but enters the cell as the free molecule. The intracellular receptor is bound to stabilizing proteins, including two molecules of heat-shock protein 90 (hsp90) and several others, denoted as "X" in the figure. This receptor complex is incapable of activating transcription. When the complex binds a molecule of cortisol, an unstable complex is created and the hsp90 and associated molecules are released. The steroid-receptor complex is now able to dimerize, enter the nucleus, bind to a glucocorticoid response element (GRE) on the regulatory region of the gene, and regulate transcription by RNA polymerase II and associated transcription factors. A variety of regulatory factors (not shown) may participate in facilitating (coactivators) or inhibiting (corepressors) the steroid response. The resulting mRNA is edited and exported to the cytoplasm for the production of protein that brings about the final hormone response. An alternative to the steroid-receptor complex interaction with a GRE is an interaction with and altering the function of other transcription factors, such as NF-κB in the nucleus of cells.

Prompt effects such as initial feedback suppression of pituitary ACTH occur in minutes and are too rapid to be explained on the basis of gene transcription and protein synthesis. It is not known how these effects are mediated. Among the proposed mechanisms are direct effects on cell membrane receptors for the hormone or nongenomic effects of the classic hormone-bound glucocorticoid receptor. The putative membrane receptors might be entirely different from the known intracellular receptors. Recently, all steroid receptors (except the MRs) were shown to have palmitoylation motifs that allow enzymatic addition of palmitate and increased localization of the receptors in the vicinity of plasma membranes. Such receptors are available for direct interactions with and effects on various membrane-associated or cytoplasmic proteins without the need for entry into the nucleus and induction of transcriptional actions.

B. Physiologic Effects

The glucocorticoids have widespread effects because they influence the function of most cells in the body. The major metabolic consequences of glucocorticoid secretion or administration are due to direct actions of these hormones in the cell. However, some important effects are the result of homeostatic responses by insulin and glucagon. Although many of the effects of glucocorticoids are dose-related and become magnified when large amounts are administered for therapeutic purposes, there are also other effects—called *permissive* effects—without which many normal functions become deficient. For example, the response of vascular and bronchial smooth muscle to catecholamines is diminished in the absence of cortisol and restored by physiologic amounts of this glucocorticoid. Similarly, the lipolytic responses of fat cells to catecholamines, ACTH, and growth hormone are attenuated in the absence of glucocorticoids.

C. Metabolic Effects

The glucocorticoids have important dose-related effects on carbohydrate, protein, and fat metabolism. The same effects are responsible for some of the serious adverse effects associated with their use in therapeutic doses. Glucocorticoids stimulate and are required for gluconeogenesis and glycogen synthesis in the fasting state.

They stimulate phosphoenolpyruvate carboxykinase, glucose-6-phosphatase, and glycogen synthase and the release of amino acids in the course of muscle catabolism.

Glucocorticoids increase serum glucose levels and thus stimulate insulin release and inhibit the uptake of glucose by muscle cells, while they stimulate hormone sensitive lipase and thus lipolysis. The increased insulin secretion stimulates lipogenesis and to a lesser degree inhibits lipolysis, leading to a net increase in fat deposition combined with increased release of fatty acids and glycerol into the circulation.

The net results of these actions are most apparent in the fasting state, when the supply of glucose from gluconeogenesis, the release of amino acids from muscle catabolism, the inhibition of peripheral glucose uptake, and the stimulation of lipolysis all contribute to maintenance of an adequate glucose supply to the brain.

D. Catabolic and Antianabolic Effects

Although glucocorticoids stimulate RNA and protein synthesis in the liver, they have catabolic and antianabolic effects in lymphoid and connective tissue, muscle, peripheral fat, and skin. Supraphysiologic amounts of glucocorticoids lead to decreased muscle mass and weakness and thinning of the skin. Catabolic and antianabolic effects on bone are the cause of osteoporosis in Cushing's syndrome and impose a major limitation in the long-term therapeutic use of glucocorticoids. In children, glucocorticoids reduce growth. This effect may be partially prevented by administration of growth hormone in high doses, but this use of growth hormone is not recommended.

E. Anti-Inflammatory and Immunosuppressive Effects

Glucocorticoids dramatically reduce the manifestations of inflammation. This is due to their profound effects on the concentration, distribution, and function of peripheral leukocytes and to their suppressive effects on the inflammatory cytokines and chemokines and on other mediators of inflammation. Inflammation, regardless of its cause, is characterized by the extravasation and infiltration of leukocytes into the affected tissue. These events are mediated by a complex series of interactions of white cell adhesion molecules with those on endothelial cells and are inhibited by glucocorticoids. After a single dose of a short-acting glucocorticoid, the concentration of neutrophils in the circulation increases while the lymphocytes (T and B cells), monocytes, eosinophils, and basophils decrease. The changes are maximal at 6 hours and are dissipated in 24 hours. The increase in neutrophils is due both to the increased influx into the blood from the bone marrow and to the decreased migration from the blood vessels, leading to a reduction in the number of cells at the site of inflammation. The reduction in circulating lymphocytes, monocytes, eosinophils, and basophils is primarily the result of their movement from the vascular bed to lymphoid tissue.

Glucocorticoids also inhibit the functions of tissue macrophages and other antigen-presenting cells. The ability of these cells to respond to antigens and mitogens is reduced. The effect on macrophages is particularly marked and limits their ability to phagocytose and kill microorganisms and to produce tumor necrosis factor-α, interleukin-1, metalloproteinases, and plasminogen activator. Both macrophages and lymphocytes produce less interleukin-12 and interferon-γ, important inducers of TH1 cell activity, and cellular immunity.

In addition to their effects on leukocyte function, glucocorticoids influence the inflammatory response by reducing the prostaglandin, leukotriene, and platelet-activating factor synthesis that results from activation of phospholipase A_2. Finally, glucocorticoids reduce expression of cyclooxygenase-2, the inducible form of this enzyme, in inflammatory cells, thus reducing the amount of enzyme available to produce prostaglandins (see Chapters 18 and 36).

Glucocorticoids cause vasoconstriction when applied directly to the skin, possibly by suppressing mast cell degranulation. They also decrease capillary permeability by reducing the amount of histamine released by basophils and mast cells.

The anti-inflammatory and immunosuppressive effects of glucocorticoids are largely due to the actions described above. In humans, complement activation is unaltered, but its effects are inhibited. Antibody production can be reduced by large doses of steroids, although it is unaffected by moderate doses (eg, 20 mg/d of prednisone).

The anti-inflammatory and immunosuppressive effects of these agents are widely useful therapeutically but are also responsible for some of their most serious adverse effects (see text that follows).

F. Other Effects

Glucocorticoids have important effects on the nervous system. Adrenal insufficiency causes marked slowing of the alpha rhythm of the electroencephalogram and is associated with depression. Increased amounts of glucocorticoids often produce behavioral disturbances in humans: initially insomnia and euphoria and subsequently depression. Large doses of glucocorticoids may increase intracranial pressure (pseudotumor cerebri).

Glucocorticoids given chronically suppress the pituitary release of ACTH, growth hormone, thyroid-stimulating hormone, and luteinizing hormone.

Large doses of glucocorticoids have been associated with the development of peptic ulcer, possibly by suppressing the local immune response against *Helicobacter pylori*. They also promote fat redistribution in the body, with increase of visceral, facial, nuchal, and supraclavicular fat, and they appear to antagonize the effect of vitamin D on calcium absorption. The glucocorticoids also have important effects on the hematopoietic system. In addition to their effects on leukocytes, they increase the number of platelets and red blood cells.

Cortisol deficiency results in impaired renal function (particularly glomerular filtration), augmented vasopressin secretion, and diminished ability to excrete a water load.

Glucocorticoids have important effects on the development of the fetal lungs. Indeed, the structural and functional changes in the lungs near term, including the production of pulmonary surface-active material required for air breathing (surfactant), are stimulated by glucocorticoids.

SYNTHETIC CORTICOSTEROIDS

Glucocorticoids have become important agents for use in the treatment of many inflammatory, immunologic, hematologic, and other disorders. This has stimulated the development of many synthetic steroids with anti-inflammatory and immunosuppressive activity.

Pharmacokinetics

A. Source

Pharmaceutical steroids are usually synthesized from cholic acid obtained from cattle or steroid sapogenins found in plants. Further modifications of these steroids have led to the marketing of a large group of synthetic steroids with special characteristics that are pharmacologically and therapeutically important (Table 39–1; Figure 39–3).

B. Disposition

The metabolism of the naturally occurring adrenal steroids has been discussed above. The synthetic corticosteroids (Table 39–1) are in most cases rapidly and completely absorbed when given by mouth. Although they are transported and metabolized in a fashion similar to that of the endogenous steroids, important differences exist.

Alterations in the glucocorticoid molecule influence its affinity for glucocorticoid and mineralocorticoid receptors as well as its protein-binding affinity, side chain stability, rate of elimination, and metabolic products. Halogenation at the 9 position, unsaturation of the $\Delta 1$–2 bond of the A ring, and methylation at the 2 or 16 position prolong the half-life by more than 50%. The $\Delta 1$ compounds are excreted in the free form. In some cases, the agent given is a prodrug; for example, prednisone is rapidly converted to the active product prednisolone in the body.

Pharmacodynamics

The actions of the synthetic steroids are similar to those of cortisol (see above). They bind to the specific intracellular receptor proteins and produce the same effects but have different ratios of glucocorticoid to mineralocorticoid potency (Table 39–1).

CLINICAL PHARMACOLOGY

A. Diagnosis and Treatment of Disturbed Adrenal Function

1. Adrenocortical insufficiency

a. Chronic (Addison's disease)—Chronic adrenocortical insufficiency is characterized by weakness, fatigue, weight loss, hypotension, hyperpigmentation, and inability to maintain the blood glucose level during fasting. In such individuals, minor noxious,

TABLE 39–1 Some commonly used natural and synthetic corticosteroids for general use.

Agent	Activity[1]			Equivalent Oral Dose (mg)	Forms Available
	Anti-Inflammatory	Topical	Salt-Retaining		
Short- to medium-acting glucocorticoids					
Hydrocortisone (cortisol)	1	1	1	20	Oral, injectable, topical
Cortisone	0.8	0	0.8	25	Oral
Prednisone	4	0	0.3	5	Oral
Prednisolone	5	4	0.3	5	Oral, injectable
Methylprednisolone	5	5	0.25	4	Oral, injectable
Meprednisone[2]	5		0	4	Oral, injectable
Intermediate-acting glucocorticoids					
Triamcinolone	5	5[3]	0	4	Oral, injectable, topical
Paramethasone[2]	10		0	2	Oral, injectable
Fluprednisolone[2]	15	7	0	1.5	Oral
Long-acting glucocorticoids					
Betamethasone	25–40	10	0	0.6	Oral, injectable, topical
Dexamethasone	30	10	0	0.75	Oral, injectable, topical
Mineralocorticoids					
Fludrocortisone	10	0	250	2	Oral
Desoxycorticosterone acetate[2]	0	0	20		Injectable, pellets

[1]Potency relative to hydrocortisone.

[2]Outside USA.

[3]Triamcinolone acetonide: Up to 100.

traumatic, or infectious stimuli may produce acute adrenal insufficiency with circulatory shock and even death.

In primary adrenal insufficiency, about 20–30 mg of hydrocortisone must be given daily, with increased amounts during periods of stress. Although hydrocortisone has some mineralocorticoid activity, this must be supplemented by an appropriate amount of a salt-retaining hormone such as fludrocortisone. Synthetic glucocorticoids that are long-acting and devoid of salt-retaining activity should not be administered to these patients.

b. Acute—When acute adrenocortical insufficiency is suspected, treatment must be instituted immediately. Therapy consists of large amounts of parenteral hydrocortisone in addition to correction of fluid and electrolyte abnormalities and treatment of precipitating factors.

Hydrocortisone sodium succinate or phosphate in doses of 100 mg intravenously is given every 8 hours until the patient is stable. The dose is then gradually reduced, achieving maintenance dosage within 5 days.

The administration of salt-retaining hormone is resumed when the total hydrocortisone dosage has been reduced to 50 mg/d.

2. Adrenocortical hypo- and hyperfunction

a. Congenital adrenal hyperplasia—This group of disorders is characterized by specific defects in the synthesis of cortisol. In pregnancies at high risk for congenital adrenal hyperplasia, fetuses can be protected from genital abnormalities by administration of dexamethasone to the mother. The most common defect is a decrease in or lack of P450c21 (21β-hydroxylase) activity.*

As can be seen in Figure 39–1, this would lead to a reduction in cortisol synthesis and thus produce a compensatory increase in ACTH release. The gland becomes hyperplastic and produces abnormally large amounts of precursors such as 17-hydroxyprogesterone that can be diverted to the androgen pathway, leading to virilization. Metabolism of this compound in the liver leads to pregnanetriol, which is characteristically excreted into the urine in large amounts in this disorder and can be used to make the diagnosis and to monitor efficacy of glucocorticoid substitution. However, the most reliable method of detecting this disorder is the increased response of plasma 17-hydroxyprogesterone to ACTH stimulation.

If the defect is in 11-hydroxylation, large amounts of deoxycorticosterone are produced, and because this steroid has mineralocorticoid activity, hypertension with or without hypokalemic alkalosis ensues. When 17-hydroxylation is defective in the adrenals and gonads, hypogonadism is also present. However, increased amounts of 11-deoxycorticosterone are formed, and the signs and symptoms associated with mineralocorticoid excess—such as hypertension and hypokalemia—are also observed.

---

*Names for the adrenal steroid synthetic enzymes include the following:

P450c11 (11-hydroxylase)

P450c17 (17-hydroxylase)

P450c21 (21-hydroxylase)

When first seen, the infant with congenital adrenal hyperplasia may be in acute adrenal crisis and should be treated as described above, using appropriate electrolyte solutions and an intravenous preparation of hydrocortisone in stress doses.

Once the patient is stabilized, oral hydrocortisone, 12–18 mg/m²/d in two unequally divided doses (two thirds in the morning, one third in late afternoon) is begun. The dosage is adjusted to allow normal growth and bone maturation and to prevent androgen excess. Alternate-day therapy with prednisone has also been used to achieve greater ACTH suppression without increasing growth inhibition. Fludrocortisone, 0.05–0.2 mg/d, should also be administered by mouth, with added salt to maintain normal blood pressure, plasma renin activity, and electrolytes.

b. Cushing's syndrome—Cushing's syndrome is usually the result of bilateral adrenal hyperplasia secondary to an ACTH-secreting pituitary adenoma (Cushing's disease) but occasionally is due to tumors or nodular hyperplasia of the adrenal gland or ectopic production of ACTH by other tumors. The manifestations are those associated with the chronic presence of excessive glucocorticoids. When glucocorticoid hypersecretion is marked and prolonged, a rounded, plethoric face and trunk obesity are striking in appearance. The manifestations of protein loss are often found and include muscle wasting; thinning, purple striae, and easy bruising of the skin; poor wound healing; and osteoporosis. Other serious disturbances include mental disorders, hypertension, and diabetes. This disorder is treated by surgical removal of the tumor producing ACTH or cortisol, irradiation of the pituitary tumor, or resection of one or both adrenals. These patients must receive large doses of cortisol during and after the surgical procedure. Doses of up to 300 mg of soluble hydrocortisone may be given as a continuous intravenous infusion on the day of surgery. The dose must be reduced slowly to normal replacement levels, since rapid reduction in dose may produce withdrawal symptoms, including fever and joint pain. If adrenalectomy has been performed, long-term maintenance is similar to that outlined above for adrenal insufficiency.

c. Primary generalized glucocorticoid resistance (Chrousos) syndrome—This rare sporadic or familial genetic condition is usually due to inactivating mutations of the glucocorticoid receptor gene. In its attempt to compensate for the defect, the hypothalamic-pituitary-adrenal (HPA) axis is hyperfunctioning with the increased production of ACTH leading to high circulating levels of cortisol and cortisol precursors such as corticosterone and 11-deoxycorticosterone with mineralocorticoid activity, as well as of adrenal androgens. These may result in hypertension with or without hypokalemic alkalosis and hyperandrogenism expressed as virilization and precocious puberty in children and acne, hirsutism, male pattern baldness, and menstrual irregularities (mostly oligo-amenorrhea and hypofertility) in women. The therapy of this syndrome is high doses of synthetic glucocorticoids such as dexamethasone with no inherent mineralocorticoid activity. These doses are titrated to normalize the production of cortisol, cortisol precursors, and adrenal androgens.

d. Aldosteronism—Primary aldosteronism usually results from the excessive production of aldosterone by an adrenal adenoma. However, it may also result from abnormal secretion by hyperplastic glands or from a malignant tumor. The clinical findings of hypertension, weakness, and tetany are related to the continued renal loss of potassium, which leads to hypokalemia, alkalosis, and elevation of serum sodium concentrations. This syndrome can also be produced in disorders of adrenal steroid biosynthesis by excessive secretion of deoxycorticosterone, corticosterone, or 18-hydroxycorticosterone—all compounds with inherent mineralocorticoid activity.

In contrast to patients with secondary aldosteronism (see text that follows), these patients have low (suppressed) levels of plasma renin activity and angiotensin II. When treated with fludrocortisone (0.2 mg twice daily orally for 3 days) or deoxycorticosterone acetate (20 mg/d intramuscularly for 3 days—but not available in the USA), patients fail to retain sodium and the secretion of aldosterone is not significantly reduced. When the disorder is mild, it may escape detection if serum potassium levels are used for screening. However, it may be detected by an increased ratio of plasma aldosterone to renin. Patients generally improve when treated with spironolactone, an aldosterone receptor-blocking agent, and the response to this agent is of diagnostic and therapeutic value.

3. Use of glucocorticoids for diagnostic purposes—It is sometimes necessary to suppress the production of ACTH to identify the source of a particular hormone or to establish whether its production is influenced by the secretion of ACTH. In these circumstances, it is advantageous to use a very potent substance such as dexamethasone because the use of small quantities reduces the possibility of confusion in the interpretation of hormone assays in blood or urine. For example, if complete suppression is achieved by the use of 50 mg of cortisol, the urinary 17-hydroxycorticosteroids will be 15–18 mg/24 h, since one third of the dose given will be recovered in urine as 17-hydroxycorticosteroid. If an equivalent dose of 1.5 mg of dexamethasone is used, the urinary excretion will be only 0.5 mg/24 h and blood levels will be low.

The dexamethasone suppression test is used for the diagnosis of Cushing's syndrome and has also been used in the differential diagnosis of depressive psychiatric states. As a screening test, 1 mg dexamethasone is given orally at 11 PM, and a plasma sample is obtained the following morning. In normal individuals, the morning cortisol concentration is usually less than 3 mcg/dL, whereas in Cushing's syndrome the level is usually greater than 5 mcg/dL. The results are not reliable in the patient with depression, anxiety, concurrent illness, and other stressful conditions or in the patient who is receiving a medication that enhances the catabolism of dexamethasone in the liver. To distinguish between hypercortisolism due to anxiety, depression, and alcoholism (pseudo-Cushing syndrome) and bona fide Cushing's syndrome, a combined test is carried out, consisting of dexamethasone (0.5 mg orally every 6 hours for 2 days) followed by a standard corticotropin-releasing hormone (CRH) test (1 mg/kg given as a bolus intravenous infusion 2 hours after the last dose of dexamethasone).

In patients in whom the diagnosis of Cushing's syndrome has been established clinically and confirmed by a finding of elevated free cortisol in the urine, suppression with large doses of dexamethasone will help to distinguish patients with Cushing's disease from those with steroid-producing tumors of the adrenal cortex or with the ectopic ACTH syndrome. Dexamethasone is given in a dosage of 0.5 mg orally every 6 hours for 2 days, followed by 2 mg orally every 6 hours for 2 days, and the urine is then assayed for cortisol or its metabolites (Liddle's test); or dexamethasone is given as a single dose of 8 mg at 11 PM, and the plasma cortisol is measured at 8 AM the following day. In patients with Cushing's disease, the suppressant effect of dexamethasone usually produces a 50% reduction in hormone levels. In patients in whom suppression does not occur, the ACTH level will be low in the presence of a cortisol-producing adrenal tumor and elevated in patients with an ectopic ACTH-producing tumor.

B. Corticosteroids and Stimulation of Lung Maturation in the Fetus

Lung maturation in the fetus is regulated by the fetal secretion of cortisol. Treatment of the mother with large doses of glucocorticoid reduces the incidence of respiratory distress syndrome in infants delivered prematurely. When delivery is anticipated before 34 weeks of gestation, intramuscular betamethasone, 12 mg, followed by an additional dose of 12 mg 18–24 hours later, is commonly used. Betamethasone is chosen because maternal protein binding and placental metabolism of this corticosteroid is less than that of cortisol, allowing increased transfer across the placenta to the fetus.

C. Corticosteroids and Nonadrenal Disorders

The synthetic analogs of cortisol are useful in the treatment of a diverse group of diseases unrelated to any known disturbance of adrenal function (Table 39–2). The usefulness of corticosteroids in these disorders is a function of their ability to suppress inflammatory and immune responses and to alter leukocyte function, as previously described and as described in Chapter 55. These agents are useful in disorders in which host response is the cause of the major manifestations of the disease. In instances in which the inflammatory or immune response is important in controlling the pathologic process, therapy with corticosteroids may be dangerous but justified to prevent irreparable damage from an inflammatory response—if used in conjunction with specific therapy for the disease process.

Since corticosteroids are not usually curative, the pathologic process may progress while clinical manifestations are suppressed. Therefore, chronic therapy with these drugs should be undertaken with great care and only when the seriousness of the disorder warrants their use and when less hazardous measures have been exhausted.

In general, attempts should be made to bring the disease process under control using medium- to intermediate-acting glucocorticoids such as prednisone and prednisolone (Table 39–1), as well as all ancillary measures possible to keep the dose low. Where possible, alternate-day therapy should be used (see the following text). Therapy should not be decreased or stopped abruptly. When prolonged therapy is anticipated, it is helpful to obtain chest x-rays and a tuberculin test, since glucocorticoid therapy can reactivate dormant tuberculosis. The presence of diabetes, peptic ulcer, osteoporosis, and psychological disturbances should be taken into consideration, and cardiovascular function should be assessed.

TABLE 39–2 Some therapeutic indications for the use of glucocorticoids in nonadrenal disorders.

Disorder	Examples
Allergic reactions	Angioneurotic edema, asthma, bee stings, contact dermatitis, drug reactions, allergic rhinitis, serum sickness, urticaria
Collagen-vascular disorders	Giant cell arteritis, lupus erythematosus, mixed connective tissue syndromes, polymyositis, polymyalgia rheumatica, rheumatoid arthritis, temporal arteritis
Eye diseases	Acute uveitis, allergic conjunctivitis, choroiditis, optic neuritis
Gastrointestinal diseases	Inflammatory bowel disease, nontropical sprue, subacute hepatic necrosis
Hematologic disorders	Acquired hemolytic anemia, acute allergic purpura, leukemia, lymphoma, autoimmune hemolytic anemia, idiopathic thrombocytopenic purpura, multiple myeloma
Systemic inflammation	Acute respiratory distress syndrome (sustained therapy with moderate dosage accelerates recovery and decreases mortality)
Infections	Acute respiratory distress syndrome, sepsis
Inflammatory conditions of bones and joints	Arthritis, bursitis, tenosynovitis
Neurologic disorders	Cerebral edema (large doses of dexamethasone are given to patients following brain surgery to minimize cerebral edema in the postoperative period), multiple sclerosis
Organ transplants	Prevention and treatment of rejection (immunosuppression)
Pulmonary diseases	Aspiration pneumonia, bronchial asthma, prevention of infant respiratory distress syndrome, sarcoidosis
Renal disorders	Nephrotic syndrome
Skin diseases	Atopic dermatitis, dermatoses, lichen simplex chronicus (localized neurodermatitis), mycosis fungoides, pemphigus, seborrheic dermatitis, xerosis
Thyroid diseases	Malignant exophthalmos, subacute thyroiditis
Miscellaneous	Hypercalcemia, mountain sickness

Treatment for transplant rejection is a very important application of glucocorticoids. The efficacy of these agents is based on their ability to reduce antigen expression from the grafted tissue, delay revascularization, and interfere with the sensitization of cytotoxic T lymphocytes and the generation of primary antibody-forming cells.

Toxicity

The benefits obtained from glucocorticoids vary considerably. Use of these drugs must be carefully weighed in each patient against

their widespread effects on every part of the organism. The major undesirable effects of glucocorticoids are the result of their hormonal actions, which lead to the clinical picture of iatrogenic Cushing's syndrome (see later in text).

When glucocorticoids are used for short periods (< 2 weeks), it is unusual to see serious adverse effects even with moderately large doses. However, insomnia, behavioral changes (primarily hypomania), and acute peptic ulcers are occasionally observed even after only a few days of treatment. Acute pancreatitis is a rare but serious acute adverse effect of high-dose glucocorticoids.

A. Metabolic Effects

Most patients who are given daily doses of 100 mg of hydrocortisone or more (or the equivalent amount of synthetic steroid) for longer than 2 weeks undergo a series of changes that have been termed iatrogenic Cushing's syndrome. The rate of development is a function of the dosage and the genetic background of the patient. In the face, rounding, puffiness, fat deposition, and plethora usually appear (moon facies). Similarly, fat tends to be redistributed from the extremities to the trunk, the back of the neck, and the supraclavicular fossae. There is an increased growth of fine hair over the face, thighs and trunk. Steroid-induced punctate acne may appear, and insomnia and increased appetite are noted. In the treatment of dangerous or disabling disorders, these changes may not require cessation of therapy. However, the underlying metabolic changes accompanying them can be very serious by the time they become obvious. The continuing breakdown of protein and diversion of amino acids to glucose production increase the need for insulin and over time result in weight gain; visceral fat deposition; myopathy and muscle wasting; thinning of the skin, with striae and bruising; hyperglycemia; and eventually osteoporosis, diabetes, and aseptic necrosis of the hip. Wound healing is also impaired under these circumstances. When diabetes occurs, it is treated with diet and insulin. These patients are often resistant to insulin but rarely develop ketoacidosis. In general, patients treated with corticosteroids should be on high-protein and potassium-enriched diets.

B. Other Complications

Other serious adverse effects of glucocorticoids include peptic ulcers and their consequences. The clinical findings associated with certain disorders, particularly bacterial and mycotic infections, may be masked by the corticosteroids, and patients must be carefully monitored to avoid serious mishap when large doses are used. Severe myopathy is more frequent in patients treated with long-acting glucocorticoids. The administration of such compounds has been associated with nausea, dizziness, and weight loss in some patients. It is treated by changing drugs, reducing dosage, and increasing potassium and protein intake.

Hypomania or acute psychosis may occur, particularly in patients receiving very large doses of corticosteroids. Long-term therapy with intermediate- and long-acting steroids is associated with depression and the development of posterior subcapsular cataracts. Psychiatric follow-up and periodic slit-lamp examination is indicated in such patients. Increased intraocular pressure is common, and glaucoma may be induced. Benign intracranial hypertension also occurs. In dosages of 45 mg/m^2/d or more of hydrocortisone or its equivalent, growth retardation occurs in children. Medium-, intermediate-, and long-acting glucocorticoids have greater growth-suppressing potency than the natural steroid at equivalent doses.

When given in larger than physiologic amounts, steroids such as cortisone and hydrocortisone, which have mineralocorticoid effects in addition to glucocorticoid effects, cause some sodium and fluid retention and loss of potassium. In patients with normal cardiovascular and renal function, this leads to a hypokalemic, hypochloremic alkalosis and eventually to a rise in blood pressure. In patients with hypoproteinemia, renal disease, or liver disease, edema may also occur. In patients with heart disease, even small degrees of sodium retention may lead to heart failure. These effects can be minimized by using synthetic non-salt-retaining steroids, sodium restriction, and judicious amounts of potassium supplements.

C. Adrenal Suppression

When corticosteroids are administered for more than 2 weeks, adrenal suppression may occur. If treatment extends over weeks to months, the patient should be given appropriate supplementary therapy at times of minor stress (two-fold dosage increases for 24–48 hours) or severe stress (up to ten-fold dosage increases for 48–72 hours) such as accidental trauma or major surgery. If corticosteroid dosage is to be reduced, it should be tapered slowly. If therapy is to be stopped, the reduction process should be quite slow when the dose reaches replacement levels. It may take 2–12 months for the hypothalamic-pituitary-adrenal axis to function acceptably, and cortisol levels may not return to normal for another 6–9 months. The glucocorticoid-induced suppression is not a pituitary problem, and treatment with ACTH does not reduce the time required for the return of normal function.

If the dosage is reduced too rapidly in patients receiving glucocorticoids for a certain disorder, the symptoms of the disorder may reappear or increase in intensity. However, patients without an underlying disorder (eg, patients cured surgically of Cushing's disease) also develop symptoms with rapid reductions in corticosteroid levels. These symptoms include anorexia, nausea or vomiting, weight loss, lethargy, headache, fever, joint or muscle pain, and postural hypotension. Although many of these symptoms may reflect true glucocorticoid deficiency, they may also occur in the presence of normal or even elevated plasma cortisol levels, suggesting glucocorticoid dependence.

Contraindications & Cautions

A. Special Precautions

Patients receiving glucocorticoids must be monitored carefully for the development of hyperglycemia, glycosuria, sodium retention with edema or hypertension, hypokalemia, peptic ulcer, osteoporosis, and hidden infections.

The dosage should be kept as low as possible, and intermittent administration (eg, alternate-day) should be used when satisfactory therapeutic results can be obtained on this schedule. Even patients maintained on relatively low doses of corticosteroids may

require supplementary therapy at times of stress, such as when surgical procedures are performed or intercurrent illness or accidents occur.

B. Contraindications

Glucocorticoids must be used with great caution in patients with peptic ulcer, heart disease or hypertension with heart failure, certain infectious illnesses such as varicella and tuberculosis, psychoses, diabetes, osteoporosis, or glaucoma.

Selection of Drug & Dosage Schedule

Glucocorticoid preparations differ with respect to relative anti-inflammatory and mineralocorticoid effect, duration of action, cost, and dosage forms available (Table 39–1), and these factors should be taken into account in selecting the drug to be used.

A. ACTH versus Adrenocortical Steroids

In patients with normal adrenals, ACTH was used in the past to induce the endogenous production of cortisol to obtain similar effects. However, except when an increase in androgens is desirable, the use of ACTH as a therapeutic agent has been abandoned. Instances in which ACTH was claimed to be more effective than glucocorticoids were probably due to the administration of smaller amounts of corticosteroids than were produced by the dosage of ACTH.

B. Dosage

In determining the dosage regimen to be used, the physician must consider the seriousness of the disease, the amount of drug likely to be required to obtain the desired effect, and the duration of therapy. In some diseases, the amount required for maintenance of the desired therapeutic effect is less than the dose needed to obtain the initial effect, and the lowest possible dosage for the needed effect should be determined by gradually lowering the dose until a small increase in signs or symptoms is noted.

When it is necessary to maintain continuously elevated plasma corticosteroid levels to suppress ACTH, a slowly absorbed parenteral preparation or small oral doses at frequent intervals are required. The opposite situation exists with respect to the use of corticosteroids in the treatment of inflammatory and allergic disorders. The same total quantity given in a few doses may be more effective than that given in many smaller doses or in a slowly absorbed parenteral form.

Severe autoimmune conditions involving vital organs must be treated aggressively, and undertreatment is as dangerous as overtreatment. To minimize the deposition of immune complexes and the influx of leukocytes and macrophages, 1 mg/kg/d of prednisone in divided doses is required initially. This dosage is maintained until the serious manifestations respond. The dosage can then be gradually reduced.

When large doses are required for prolonged periods of time, alternate-day administration of the compound may be tried after control is achieved. When used in this manner, very large amounts (eg, 100 mg of prednisone) can sometimes be administered with less marked adverse effects because there is a recovery period between each dose. The transition to an alternate-day schedule can be made after the disease process is under control. It should be done gradually and with additional supportive measures between doses.

When selecting a drug for use in large doses, a medium- or intermediate-acting synthetic steroid with little mineralocorticoid effect is advisable. If possible, it should be given as a single morning dose.

C. Special Dosage Forms

Local therapy, such as topical preparations for skin disease, ophthalmic forms for eye disease, intra-articular injections for joint disease, inhaled steroids for asthma, and hydrocortisone enemas for ulcerative colitis, provides a means of delivering large amounts of steroid to the diseased tissue with reduced systemic effects.

Beclomethasone dipropionate, and several other glucocorticoids—primarily budesonide, flunisolide, and mometasone furoate, administered as aerosols—have been found to be extremely useful in the treatment of asthma (see Chapter 20).

Beclomethasone dipropionate, triamcinolone acetonide, budesonide, flunisolide, and mometasone furoate are available as nasal sprays for the topical treatment of allergic rhinitis. They are effective at doses (one or two sprays one, two, or three times daily) that in most patients result in plasma levels that are too low to influence adrenal function or have any other systemic effects.

Corticosteroids incorporated in ointments, creams, lotions, and sprays are used extensively in dermatology. These preparations are discussed in more detail in Chapter 61.

MINERALOCORTICOIDS (ALDOSTERONE, DEOXYCORTICOSTERONE, FLUDROCORTISONE)

The most important mineralocorticoid in humans is aldosterone. However, small amounts of deoxycorticosterone (DOC) are also formed and released. Although the amount is normally insignificant, DOC was of some importance therapeutically in the past. Its actions, effects, and metabolism are qualitatively similar to those described below for aldosterone.

Fludrocortisone, a synthetic corticosteroid, is the most commonly prescribed salt-retaining hormone.

Aldosterone

Aldosterone is synthesized mainly in the zona glomerulosa of the adrenal cortex. Its structure and synthesis are illustrated in Figure 39–1.

The rate of aldosterone secretion is subject to several influences. ACTH produces a moderate stimulation of its release, but this effect is not sustained for more than a few days in the normal individual. Although aldosterone is no less than one third as effective as cortisol in suppressing ACTH, the quantities of aldosterone produced by the adrenal cortex and its plasma concentrations are insufficient to participate in any significant feedback control of ACTH secretion.

Without ACTH, aldosterone secretion falls to about half the normal rate, indicating that other factors, eg, angiotensin, are able to maintain and perhaps regulate its secretion (see Chapter 17). Independent variations between cortisol and aldosterone secretion can also be demonstrated by means of lesions in the nervous system such as decerebration, which decreases the secretion of cortisol while increasing the secretion of aldosterone.

A. Physiologic and Pharmacologic Effects

Aldosterone and other steroids with mineralocorticoid properties promote the reabsorption of sodium from the distal part of the distal convoluted renal tubule and from the cortical collecting tubules, loosely coupled to the excretion of potassium and hydrogen ion. Sodium reabsorption in the sweat and salivary glands, gastrointestinal mucosa, and across cell membranes in general is also increased. Excessive levels of aldosterone produced by tumors or overdosage with synthetic mineralocorticoids lead to hypokalemia, metabolic alkalosis, increased plasma volume, and hypertension.

Mineralocorticoids act by binding to the mineralocorticoid receptor in the cytoplasm of target cells, especially principal cells of the distal convoluted and collecting tubules of the kidney. The drug-receptor complex activates a series of events similar to those described above for the glucocorticoids and illustrated in Figure 39–4. It is of interest that this receptor has the same affinity for cortisol, which is present in much higher concentrations in the extracellular fluid. The specificity for mineralocorticoids in the kidney appears to be conferred, at least in part, by the presence of the enzyme 11β-hydroxysteroid dehydrogenase type 2, which converts cortisol to cortisone. The latter has low affinity for the receptor and is inactive as a mineralocorticoid or glucocorticoid in the kidney. The major effect of activation of the aldosterone receptor is increased expression of Na^+/K^+-ATPase and the epithelial sodium channel (ENaC).

B. Metabolism

Aldosterone is secreted at the rate of 100–200 mcg/d in normal individuals with a moderate dietary salt intake. The plasma level in men (resting supine) is about 0.007 mcg/dL. The half-life of aldosterone injected in tracer quantities is 15–20 minutes, and it does not appear to be firmly bound to serum proteins.

The metabolism of aldosterone is similar to that of cortisol, about 50 mcg/24 h appearing in the urine as conjugated tetrahydroaldosterone. Approximately 5–15 mcg/24 h is excreted free or as the 3-oxo glucuronide.

Deoxycorticosterone (DOC)

DOC, which also serves as a precursor of aldosterone (Figure 39–1), is normally secreted in amounts of about 200 mcg/d. Its half-life when injected into the human circulation is about 70 minutes. Preliminary estimates of its concentration in plasma are approximately 0.03 mcg/dL. The control of its secretion differs from that of aldosterone in that the secretion of DOC is primarily under the control of ACTH. Although the response to ACTH is enhanced by dietary sodium restriction, a low-salt diet does not increase DOC secretion. The secretion of DOC may be markedly increased in abnormal conditions such as adrenocortical carcinoma and congenital adrenal hyperplasia with reduced P450c11 or P450c17 activity.

Fludrocortisone

This compound, a potent steroid with both glucocorticoid and mineralocorticoid activity, is the most widely used mineralocorticoid. Oral doses of 0.1 mg two to seven times weekly have potent salt-retaining activity and are used in the treatment of adrenocortical insufficiency associated with mineralocorticoid deficiency. These dosages are too small to have important anti-inflammatory or antigrowth effects.

ADRENAL ANDROGENS

The adrenal cortex secretes large amounts of DHEA and smaller amounts of androstenedione and testosterone. Although these androgens are thought to contribute to the normal maturation process, they do not stimulate or support major androgen-dependent pubertal changes in humans. Recent studies suggest that DHEA and its sulfate may have other important physiologic actions. If that is correct, these results are probably due to the peripheral conversion of DHEA to more potent androgens or to estrogens and interaction with androgen and estrogen receptors, respectively. Additional effects may be exerted through an interaction with the GABA$_A$ and glutamate receptors in the brain or with

a nuclear receptor in several central and peripheral sites. The therapeutic use of DHEA in humans has been explored, but the substance has already been adopted with uncritical enthusiasm by members of the sports drug culture and the vitamin and food supplement culture.

The results of a placebo-controlled trial of DHEA in patients with systemic lupus erythematosus have been reported as well as those of a study of DHEA replacement in women with adrenal insufficiency. In both studies a small beneficial effect was seen, with significant improvement of the disease in the former and a clearly added sense of well-being in the latter. The androgenic or estrogenic actions of DHEA could explain the effects of the compound in both situations.

■ ANTAGONISTS OF ADRENOCORTICAL AGENTS

SYNTHESIS INHIBITORS & GLUCOCORTICOID ANTAGONISTS

Inhibitors of steroid synthesis act at several different steps and one glucocorticoid antagonist acts at the receptor level.

Aminoglutethimide

Aminoglutethimide (Figure 39–5) blocks the conversion of cholesterol to pregnenolone (see Figure 39–1) and causes a reduction

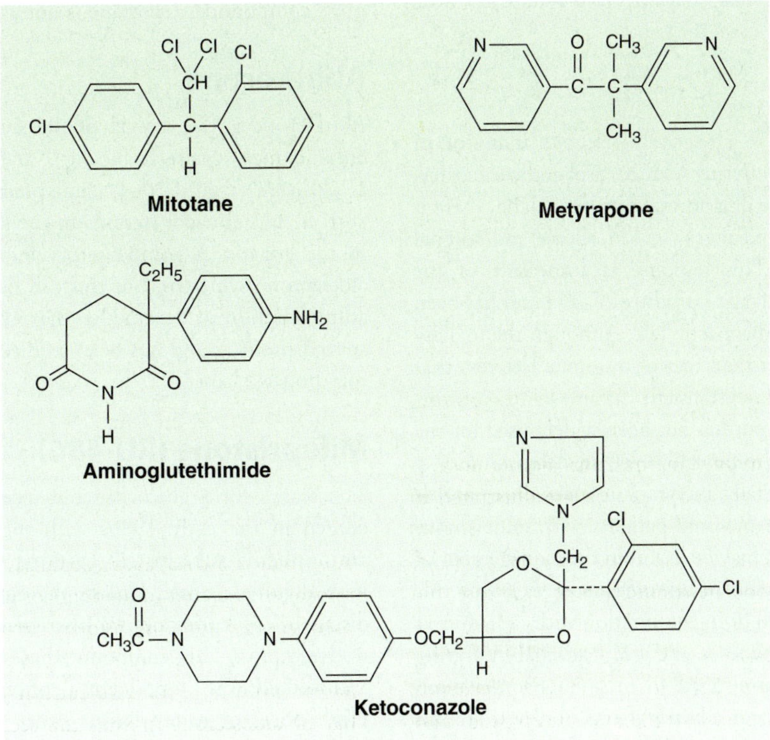

FIGURE 39–5 Some adrenocortical antagonists. Because of their toxicity, some of these compounds are no longer available in the USA.

in the synthesis of all hormonally active steroids. It has been used in conjunction with dexamethasone or hydrocortisone to reduce or eliminate estrogen production in patients with carcinoma of the breast. In a dosage of 1 g/d it was well tolerated; however, with higher dosages, lethargy and skin rash were common effects. The use of aminoglutethimide in breast cancer patients has now been supplanted by tamoxifen or by another class of drugs, the aromatase inhibitors (see Chapters 40 and 54). Aminoglutethimide can be used in conjunction with metyrapone or ketoconazole to reduce steroid secretion in patients with Cushing's syndrome due to adrenocortical cancer who do not respond to mitotane.

Aminoglutethimide also apparently increases the clearance of some steroids. It has been shown to enhance the metabolism of dexamethasone, reducing its half-life from 4–5 hours to 2 hours.

Ketoconazole

Ketoconazole, an antifungal imidazole derivative (see Chapter 48), is a potent and rather nonselective inhibitor of adrenal and gonadal steroid synthesis. This compound inhibits the cholesterol side-chain cleavage, P450c17, C17,20-lyase, 3β-hydroxysteroid dehydrogenase, and P450c11 enzymes required for steroid hormone synthesis. The sensitivity of the P450 enzymes to this compound in mammalian tissues is much lower than that needed to treat fungal infections, so that its inhibitory effects on steroid biosynthesis are seen only at high doses.

Ketoconazole has been used for the treatment of patients with Cushing's syndrome due to several causes. Dosages of 200–1200 mg/d have produced a reduction in hormone levels and clinical improvement in some patients. This drug has some hepatotoxicity and should be started at 200 mg/d and slowly increased by 200 mg/d every 2–3 days up to a total daily dose of 1000 mg.

Metyrapone

Metyrapone (Figure 39–5) is a relatively selective inhibitor of steroid 11-hydroxylation, interfering with cortisol and corticosterone synthesis. In the presence of a normal pituitary gland, there is a compensatory increase in pituitary ACTH release and adrenal 11-deoxycortisol secretion. This response is a measure of the capacity of the anterior pituitary to produce ACTH and has been adapted for clinical use as a diagnostic test. Although the toxicity of metyrapone is much lower than that of mitotane (see text that follows), the drug may produce transient dizziness and gastrointestinal disturbances. This agent has not been widely used for the treatment of Cushing's syndrome. However, in doses of 0.25 g twice daily to 1 g four times daily, metyrapone can reduce cortisol production to normal levels in some patients with endogenous Cushing's syndrome. Thus, it may be useful in the management of severe manifestations of cortisol excess while the cause of this condition is being determined or in conjunction with radiation or surgical treatment. Metyrapone is the only adrenal-inhibiting medication that can be administered to pregnant women with Cushing's syndrome. The major adverse effects observed are salt and water retention and hirsutism resulting from diversion of the 11-deoxycortisol precursor to DOC and androgen synthesis.

Metyrapone is commonly used in tests of adrenal function. The blood levels of 11-deoxycortisol and the urinary excretion of 17-hydroxycorticoids are measured before and after administration of the compound. Normally, there is a twofold or greater increase in the urinary 17-hydroxycorticoid excretion. A dose of 300–500 mg every 4 hours for six doses is often used, and urine collections are made on the day before and the day after treatment. In patients with Cushing's syndrome, a normal response to metyrapone indicates that the cortisol excess is not the result of a cortisol-secreting adrenal carcinoma or adenoma, since secretion by such tumors produces suppression of ACTH and atrophy of normal adrenal cortex.

Pituitary function may also be tested by administering metyrapone, 2–3 g orally at midnight and by measuring the level of ACTH or 11-deoxycortisol in blood drawn at 8 AM or by comparing the excretion of 17-hydroxycorticosteroids in the urine during the 24-hour periods preceding and following administration of the drug. In patients with suspected or known lesions of the pituitary, this procedure is a means of estimating the ability of the gland to produce ACTH. Metyrapone has been withdrawn from the market in the USA but is available on a compassionate basis.

Trilostane

Trilostane is a 3β-17 hydroxysteroid dehydrogenase inhibitor that interferes with the synthesis of adrenal and gonadal hormones and is comparable to aminoglutethimide. Trilostane's adverse effects are predominantly gastrointestinal; adverse effects occur in about 50% of patients with both trilostane and aminoglutethimide. There is no cross-resistance or crossover of side effects between these compounds. Trilostane is not available in the USA.

Abiraterone

Abiraterone is the newest of the steroid synthesis inhibitors to enter clinical trials. It blocks 17α-hydroxylase (P450c17) and 17,20-lyase (Figure 39–1), and predictably reduces synthesis of cortisol and gonadal steroids in the adrenal and gonadal steroids in the gonads. A compensatory increase occurs in ACTH and aldosterone synthesis, but this can be prevented by concomitant administration of dexamethasone. Abiraterone is an orally active steroid prodrug and has been studied in the treatment of refractory prostate cancer.

Mifepristone (RU-486)

The search for a glucocorticoid receptor antagonist finally succeeded in the early 1980s with the development of the 11β-aminophenyl-substituted 19-norsteroid called RU-486, later named mifepristone. Unlike the enzyme inhibitors previously discussed, mifepristone is a pharmacologic antagonist at the steroid receptor. This compound has strong antiprogestin activity and initially was proposed as a contraceptive-contragestive agent. High doses of mifepristone exert antiglucocorticoid activity by blocking the glucocorticoid receptor, since mifepristone binds to it with high affinity, causing (1) some stabilization of the hsp-glucocorticoid receptor complex and inhibition of the dissociation of the RU-486–bound glucocorticoid receptor from the hsp chaperone proteins; and (2) alteration of the interaction of the glucocorticoid receptor with coregulators, favoring the formation of a transcriptionally inactive complex in the cell nucleus. The result is inhibition of glucocorticoid receptor activation.

The mean half-life of mifepristone is 20 hours. This is longer than that of many natural and synthetic glucocorticoid agonists (dexamethasone has a half-life of 4–5 hours). Less than 1% of the daily dose is excreted in the urine, suggesting a minor role of kidneys in the clearance of the compound. The long plasma half-life of mifepristone results from extensive and strong binding to plasma proteins. Less than 5% of the compound is found in the free form when plasma is analyzed by equilibrium dialysis. Mifepristone can bind to albumin and α_1-acid glycoprotein, but it has no affinity for corticosteroid-binding globulin.

In humans, mifepristone causes generalized glucocorticoid resistance. Given orally to several patients with Cushing's syndrome due to ectopic ACTH production or adrenal carcinoma, it was able to reverse the cushingoid phenotype, to eliminate carbohydrate intolerance, normalize blood pressure, to correct thyroid and gonadal hormone suppression, and to ameliorate the psychological sequelae of hypercortisolism in these patients. At present, this use of mifepristone can only be recommended for inoperable patients with ectopic ACTH secretion or adrenal carcinoma who have failed to respond to other therapeutic manipulations. Its pharmacology and use in women as a progesterone antagonist are discussed in Chapter 40.

Mitotane

Mitotane (Figure 39–5), a drug related to the DDT class of insecticides, has a nonselective cytotoxic action on the adrenal cortex in dogs and to a lesser extent in humans. This drug is administered orally in divided doses up to 12 g daily. About one third of patients with adrenal carcinoma show a reduction in tumor mass. In 80% of patients, the toxic effects are sufficiently severe to require dose reduction. These include diarrhea, nausea, vomiting, depression, somnolence, and skin rashes. The drug has been withdrawn from the market in the USA but is available on a compassionate basis.

MINERALOCORTICOID ANTAGONISTS

In addition to agents that interfere with aldosterone synthesis (see above), there are steroids that compete with aldosterone for its receptor and decrease its effect peripherally. Progesterone is mildly active in this respect.

Spironolactone is a 7α-acetylthiospironolactone. Its onset of action is slow, and the effects last for 2–3 days after the drug is discontinued. It is used in the treatment of primary aldosteronism in dosages of 50–100 mg/d. This agent reverses many of the manifestations of aldosteronism. It has been useful in establishing the diagnosis in some patients and in ameliorating the signs and symptoms when surgical removal of an adenoma is delayed. When used diagnostically for the detection of aldosteronism in hypokalemic patients with hypertension, dosages of 400–500 mg/d for 4–8 days—with an adequate intake of sodium and potassium—restore potassium levels to or toward normal. Spironolactone is also useful in preparing these patients for surgery. Dosages of 300–400 mg/d for 2 weeks are used for this purpose and may reduce the incidence of cardiac arrhythmias.

Spironolactone

Spironolactone is also an androgen antagonist and as such is sometimes used in the treatment of hirsutism in women. Dosages of 50–200 mg/d cause a reduction in the density, diameter, and rate of growth of facial hair in patients with idiopathic hirsutism or hirsutism secondary to androgen excess. The effect can usually be seen in 2 months and becomes maximal in about 6 months.

Spironolactone as a diuretic is discussed in Chapter 15. The drug has benefits in heart failure greater than those predicted from its diuretic effects alone (see Chapter 13). Adverse effects reported for spironolactone include hyperkalemia, cardiac arrhythmia, menstrual abnormalities, gynecomastia, sedation, headache, gastrointestinal disturbances, and skin rashes.

Eplerenone, another aldosterone antagonist, is approved for the treatment of hypertension (see Chapters 11 and 15). Like spironolactone, eplerenone has also been found to reduce mortality in heart failure. This aldosterone receptor antagonist is somewhat more selective than spironolactone and has no reported effects on androgen receptors. The standard dosage in hypertension is 50–100 mg/d. The most common toxicity is hyperkalemia, but this is usually mild.

Drospirenone, a progestin in an oral contraceptive (see Chapter 40), also antagonizes the effects of aldosterone.

PREPARATIONS AVAILABLE[1]

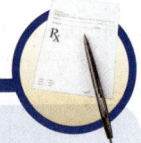

GLUCOCORTICOIDS FOR ORAL & PARENTERAL USE

Betamethasone (Celestone)
Oral: 0.6 mg/5 mL syrup

Betamethasone sodium phosphate (Celestone Phosphate)
Parenteral: 4 mg/mL for IV, IM, intralesional, or intra-articular injection

Cortisone (generic, Cortone Acetate)
Oral: 25 mg tablets

Dexamethasone (generic, Decadron)
Oral: 0.25, 0.5, 0.75, 1, 1.5, 2, 4, 6 mg tablets; 0.5 mg/5 mL elixir; 0.5 mg/5 mL, 1 mg/mL solution

Dexamethasone acetate (generic, Decadron-LA)
Parenteral: 8 mg/mL suspension for IM, intralesional, or intra-articular injection; 16 mg/mL suspension for intralesional injection

Dexamethasone sodium phosphate (generic, Decadron Phosphate)
Parenteral: 4, 10, 20 mg/mL for IV, IM, intralesional, or intra-articular injection; 24 mg/mL for IV use only

Hydrocortisone [cortisol] (generic, Cortef)
Oral: 5, 10, 20 mg tablets

Hydrocortisone acetate (generic)
Parenteral: 25, 50 mg/mL suspension for intralesional, soft tissue, or intra-articular injection

Hydrocortisone cypionate (Cortef)
Oral: 10 mg/5 mL suspension

Hydrocortisone sodium phosphate (Hydrocortone)
Parenteral: 50 mg/mL for IV, IM, or SC injection

Hydrocortisone sodium succinate (generic, SoluCortef)
Parenteral: 100, 250, 500, 1000 mg/vial for IV, IM injection

Methylprednisolone (generic, Medrol)
Oral: 2, 4, 8, 16, 24, 32 mg tablets

Methylprednisolone acetate (generic, DepoMedrol)
Parenteral: 20, 40, 80 mg/mL for IM, intralesional, or intra-articular injection

Methylprednisolone sodium succinate (generic, Solu-Medrol)
Parenteral: 40, 125, 500, 1000, 2000 mg/vial

Prednisolone (generic, Delta-Cortef, Prelone)
Oral: 5 mg tablets; 5, 15 mg/5 mL syrup

Prednisolone acetate (generic)
Parenteral: 25, 50 mg/mL for soft tissue or intra-articular injection

Prednisolone sodium phosphate (generic, Hydeltrasol)
Oral: 5 mg/5 mL solution
Parenteral: 20 mg/mL for IV, IM, intra-articular, or intralesional injection

Prednisone (generic, Meticorten)
Oral: 1, 2.5, 5, 10, 20, 50 mg tablets; 1, 5 mg/mL solution and syrup

Triamcinolone acetonide (generic, Kenalog)
Parenteral: 3, 10, 40 mg/mL for IM, intra-articular, or intralesional injection

Triamcinolone hexacetonide (Aristospan)
Parenteral: 5, 20 mg/mL for intra-articular, intralesional, or sublesional injection

MINERALOCORTICOIDS

Fludrocortisone acetate (generic, Florinef Acetate)
Oral: 0.1 mg tablets

ADRENAL STEROID INHIBITORS

Ketoconazole (generic, Nizoral)
Oral: 200 mg tablets (unlabeled use)

Mifepristone (Mifeprex)
Oral: 200 mg tablets

Mitotane (Lysodren)
Oral: 500 mg tablets

[1]Glucocorticoids for aerosol use: See Chapter 20. Glucocorticoids for dermatologic use: See Chapter 61. Glucocorticoids for gastrointestinal use: See Chapter 62.

REFERENCES

Alesci S et al: Glucocorticoid-induced osteoporosis: From basic mechanisms to clinical aspects. Neuroimmunomodulation 2005;12:1.

Bamberger CM, Schulte HM, Chrousos GP: Molecular determinants of glucocorticoid receptor function and tissue sensitivity to glucocorticoids. Endocr Rev 1996;17:245.

Charmandari E, Kino T: Chrousos syndrome: A seminal report, a phylogenetic enigma and the clinical implications of glucocorticoid signaling changes. Eur J Clin Invest 2010;40:932.

Charmandari E, Tsigos C, Chrousos GP: Neuroendocrinology of stress. Ann Rev Physiol 2005;67:259.

Chrousos GP: Stress and disorders of the stress system. Nat Endocrinol Rev 2009;5:374.

Chrousos GP, Kino T: Glucocorticoid signaling in the cell: Expanding clinical implications to complex human behavioral and somatic disorders. In: Glucocorticoids and mood: Clinical manifestations, risk factors, and molecular mechanisms. Proc NY Acad Sci 2009;1179:153.

Elenkov IJ, Chrousos GP: Stress hormones, TH1/TH2 patterns, pro/anti-inflammatory cytokines and susceptibility to disease. Trends Endocrinol Metab 1999;10:359.

Elenkov IJ et al: Cytokine dysregulation, inflammation, and wellbeing. Neuroimmunomodulation 2005;12:255.

Franchimont D et al: Glucocorticoids and inflammation revisited: The state of the art. Neuroimmunomodulation 2002–03;10:247.

Graber AL et al: Natural history of pituitary-adrenal recovery following long-term suppression with corticosteroids. J Clin Endocrinol Metab 1965;25:11.

Hochberg Z, Pacak K, Chrousos GP: Endocrine withdrawal syndromes. Endocrine Rev 2003;24:523.

Kalantaridou S, Chrousos GP: Clinical review 148: Monogenic disorders of puberty. J Clin Endocrinol Metab 2002;87:2481.

Kino T, Charmandari E, Chrousos G (editors): Glucocorticoid action: Basic and clinical implications. Ann NY Acad Sci 2004;1024 (entire volume).

Kino T et al: The GTP-binding (G) protein β interacts with the activated glucocorticoid receptor and suppresses its transcriptional activity in the nucleus. J Cell Biol 2005;20:885.

Koch CA, Pacak K, Chrousos GP: The molecular pathogenesis of hereditary and sporadic adrenocortical and adrenomedullary tumors. J Clin Endocrinol Metab 2002;87:5367.

Mao J, Regelson W, Kalimi M: Molecular mechanism of RU 486 action: A review. Mol Cellular Biochem 1992;109:1.

Marik PE et al: Clinical practice guidelines for the diagnosis and management of corticosteroid insufficiency in critical illness: Recommendations of an international task force. Crit Care Med 2008;36:1937.

Meduri GU et al: Steroid treatment in ARDS: A critical appraisal of the ARDS network trial and the recent literature. Intens Care Med 2008;34:61.

Meduri GU et al: Activation and regulation of systemic inflammation in ARDS: Rationale for prolonged glucocorticoid therapy. Chest 2009;136:1631.

Merke DP et al: Future directions in the study and management of congenital adrenal hyperplasia due to 21-hydroxylase deficiency. Ann Intern Med 2002;136:320.

Nader N, Chrousos GP, Kino T: Interactions of the circadian CLOCK system and the HPA axis. Trends Endocrinol Metab 2010;21:277.

Pervanidou P, Kanaka-Gantenbein C, Chrousos GP: Assessment of metabolic profile in a clinical setting. Curr Opin Clin Nutr Metab Care 2006;9:589.

Tsigos C, Chrousos GP: Differential diagnosis and management of Cushing's syndrome. Annu Rev Med 1996;47:443.

CASE STUDY ANSWER

The patient should be placed on replacement oral hydrocortisone at 10 mg/m^2/d and fludrocortisone at 75 mcg/d. He should be given a MedicAlert bracelet and instructions for minor and major stress glucocorticoid coverage at 2 times and 10 times replacement of hydrocortisone over 24 and 48 hours, respectively.

The Gonadal Hormones & Inhibitors

George P. Chrousos, MD

CASE STUDY

A 25-year-old woman with menarche at 13 years and menstrual periods until about 1 year ago complains of hot flushes, skin and vaginal dryness, weakness, poor sleep, and scanty and infrequent menstrual periods of a year's duration. She visits her gynecologist, who obtains plasma levels of follicle-stimulating hormone and luteinizing hormone, both of which are moderately elevated. She is diagnosed with premature ovarian failure and recommended estrogen and progesterone replacement therapy. A dual-energy absorptiometry scan (DEXA) reveals a bone density t-score of <2.5 SD, ie, frank osteoporosis. How should the ovarian hormones she lacks be replaced? What extra measures should she take for her osteoporosis while receiving treatment?

■ THE OVARY (ESTROGENS, PROGESTINS, OTHER OVARIAN HORMONES, ORAL CONTRACEPTIVES, INHIBITORS & ANTAGONISTS, & OVULATION-INDUCING AGENTS)

The ovary has important gametogenic functions that are integrated with its hormonal activity. In the human female, the gonad is relatively quiescent during childhood, the period of rapid growth and maturation. At puberty, the ovary begins a 30- to 40-year period of cyclic function called the **menstrual cycle** because of the regular episodes of bleeding that are its most obvious manifestation. It then fails to respond to gonadotropins secreted by the anterior pituitary gland, and the cessation of cyclic bleeding that occurs is called **menopause.**

The mechanism responsible for the onset of ovarian function at the time of puberty is thought to be neural in origin, because the immature gonad can be stimulated by gonadotropins already present in the pituitary and because the pituitary is responsive to exogenous hypothalamic gonadotropin-releasing hormone. The maturation of centers in the brain may withdraw a childhood-related inhibitory effect upon hypothalamic arcuate nucleus neurons, allowing them to produce **gonadotropin-releasing hormone (GnRH)** in pulses with the appropriate amplitude, which stimulates the release of **follicle-stimulating hormone (FSH)** and **luteinizing hormone (LH)** (see Chapter 37). At first, small amounts of the latter two hormones are released during the night, and the limited quantities of ovarian estrogen secreted in response start to cause breast development. Subsequently, FSH and LH are secreted throughout the day and night, causing secretion of higher amounts of estrogen and leading to further breast enlargement, alterations in fat distribution, and a growth spurt that culminates in epiphysial closure in the long bones. The change of ovarian function at puberty is called **gonadarche.**

A year or so after gonadarche, sufficient estrogen is produced to induce endometrial changes and periodic bleeding. After the first few irregular cycles, which may be anovulatory, normal cyclic function is established.

At the beginning of each cycle, a variable number of follicles (vesicular follicles), each containing an ovum, begin to enlarge in response to FSH. After 5 or 6 days, one follicle, called the dominant

ACRONYMS

CBG	Corticosteroid-binding globulin (transcortin)
DHEA	Dehydroepiandrosterone
DHEAS	Dehydroepiandrosterone sulfate
ERE	Estrogen response element
FSH	Follicle-stimulating hormone
GnRH	Gonadotropin-releasing hormone
HDL	High-density lipoprotein
HRT	Hormone replacement therapy (also called HT)
LDL	Low-density lipoprotein
LH	Luteinizing hormone
PRE	Progesterone response element
SERM	Selective estrogen receptor modulator
SHBG	Sex hormone-binding globulin
TBG	Thyroxine-binding globulin

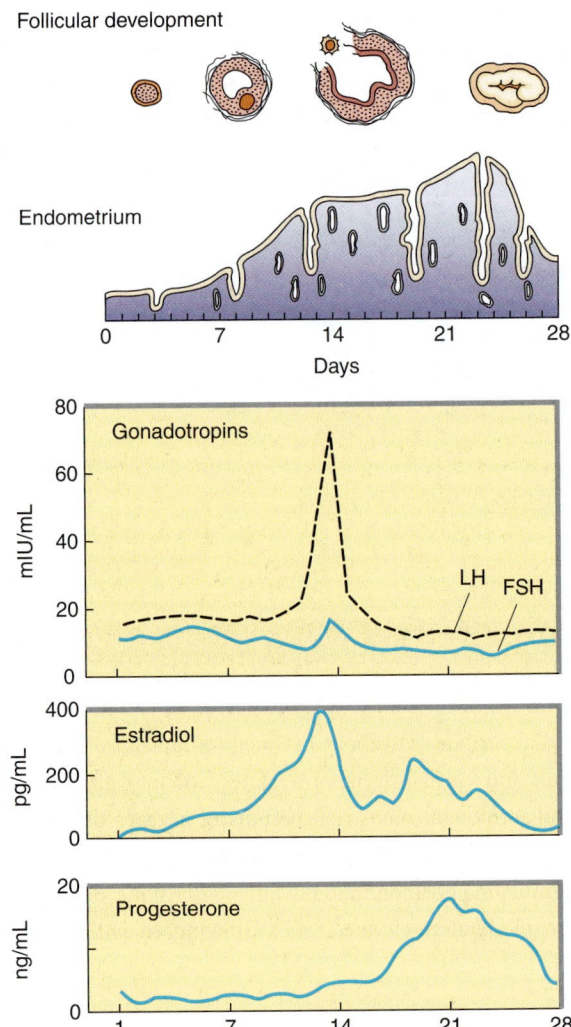

FIGURE 40–1 The menstrual cycle, showing plasma levels of pituitary and ovarian hormones and histologic changes.

follicle, begins to develop more rapidly. The outer theca and inner granulosa cells of this follicle multiply and, under the influence of LH, synthesize and release estrogens at an increasing rate. The estrogens appear to inhibit FSH release and may lead to regression of the smaller, less mature follicles. The mature dominant ovarian follicle consists of an ovum surrounded by a fluid-filled antrum lined by granulosa and theca cells. The estrogen secretion reaches a peak just before midcycle, and the granulosa cells begin to secrete progesterone. These changes stimulate the brief surge in LH and FSH release that precedes and causes ovulation. When the follicle ruptures, the ovum is released into the abdominal cavity near the opening of the uterine tube.

Following the above events, the cavity of the ruptured follicle fills with blood (corpus hemorrhagicum), and the luteinized theca and granulosa cells proliferate and replace the blood to form the corpus luteum. The cells of this structure produce estrogens and progesterone for the remainder of the cycle, or longer if pregnancy occurs.

If pregnancy does not occur, the corpus luteum begins to degenerate and ceases hormone production, eventually becoming a corpus albicans. The endometrium, which proliferated during the follicular phase and developed its glandular function during the luteal phase, is shed in the process of menstruation. These events are summarized in Figure 40–1.

The ovary normally ceases its gametogenic and endocrine function with time. This change is accompanied by a cessation in uterine bleeding (menopause) and occurs at a mean age of 52 years in the USA. Although the ovary ceases to secrete estrogen, significant levels of estrogen persist in many women as a result of conversion of adrenal and ovarian steroids such as androstenedione to estrone and estradiol in adipose and possibly other nonendocrine tissues.

Disturbances in Ovarian Function

Disturbances of cyclic function are common even during the peak years of reproduction. A minority of these result from inflammatory or neoplastic processes that influence the functions of the uterus,

ovaries, or pituitary. Many of the minor disturbances leading to periods of amenorrhea or anovulatory cycles are self-limited. They are often associated with emotional or physical stress and reflect temporary alterations in the stress centers in the brain that control the secretion of GnRH. Anovulatory cycles are also associated with eating disorders (bulimia, anorexia nervosa) and with severe exercise such as distance running and swimming. Among the more common organic causes of persistent ovulatory disturbances are pituitary prolactinomas and syndromes and tumors characterized by excessive ovarian or adrenal androgen production. Normal ovarian function can be modified by androgens produced by the adrenal cortex or tumors arising from it. The ovary also gives rise to androgen-producing neoplasms such as arrhenoblastomas, as well as to estrogen-producing granulosa cell tumors.

THE ESTROGENS

Estrogenic activity is shared by a large number of chemical substances. In addition to the variety of steroidal estrogens derived from animal sources, numerous nonsteroidal estrogens have been synthesized. Many phenols are estrogenic, and estrogenic activity has been identified in such diverse forms of life as those found in ocean sediments. Estrogen-mimetic compounds (flavonoids) are found in many plants, including saw palmetto, and soybeans and other foods. Studies have shown that a diet rich in these plant products may cause slight estrogenic effects. Additionally, some compounds used in the manufacture of plastics (bisphenols, alkylphenols, phthalate phenols) have been found to be estrogenic. It has been proposed that these agents are associated with an increased breast cancer incidence in both women and men in the industrialized world.

Natural Estrogens

The major estrogens produced by women are **estradiol** (estradiol-17β, E_2), **estrone** (E_1), and **estriol** (E_3) (Figure 40–2). Estradiol is the major secretory product of the ovary. Although some estrone is produced in the ovary, most estrone and estriol are formed in the liver from estradiol or in peripheral tissues from androstenedione and other androgens (see Figure 39–1). As noted above, during

the first part of the menstrual cycle estrogens are produced in the ovarian follicle by the theca and granulosa cells. After ovulation, the estrogens as well as progesterone are synthesized by the luteinized granulosa and theca cells of the corpus luteum, and the pathways of biosynthesis are slightly different.

During pregnancy, a large amount of estrogen is synthesized by the fetoplacental unit—consisting of the fetal adrenal zone, secreting androgen precursor, and the placenta, which aromatizes it into estrogen. The estriol synthesized by the fetoplacental unit is released into the maternal circulation and excreted into the urine. Repeated assay of maternal urinary estriol excretion has been used in the assessment of fetal well-being.

One of the most prolific natural sources of estrogenic substances is the stallion, which liberates more of these hormones than the pregnant mare or pregnant woman. The equine estrogens—equilenin and equilin—and their congeners are unsaturated in the B as well as the A ring and are excreted in large quantities in urine, from which they can be recovered and used for medicinal purposes.

In normal women, estradiol is produced at a rate that varies during the menstrual cycle, resulting in plasma levels as low as

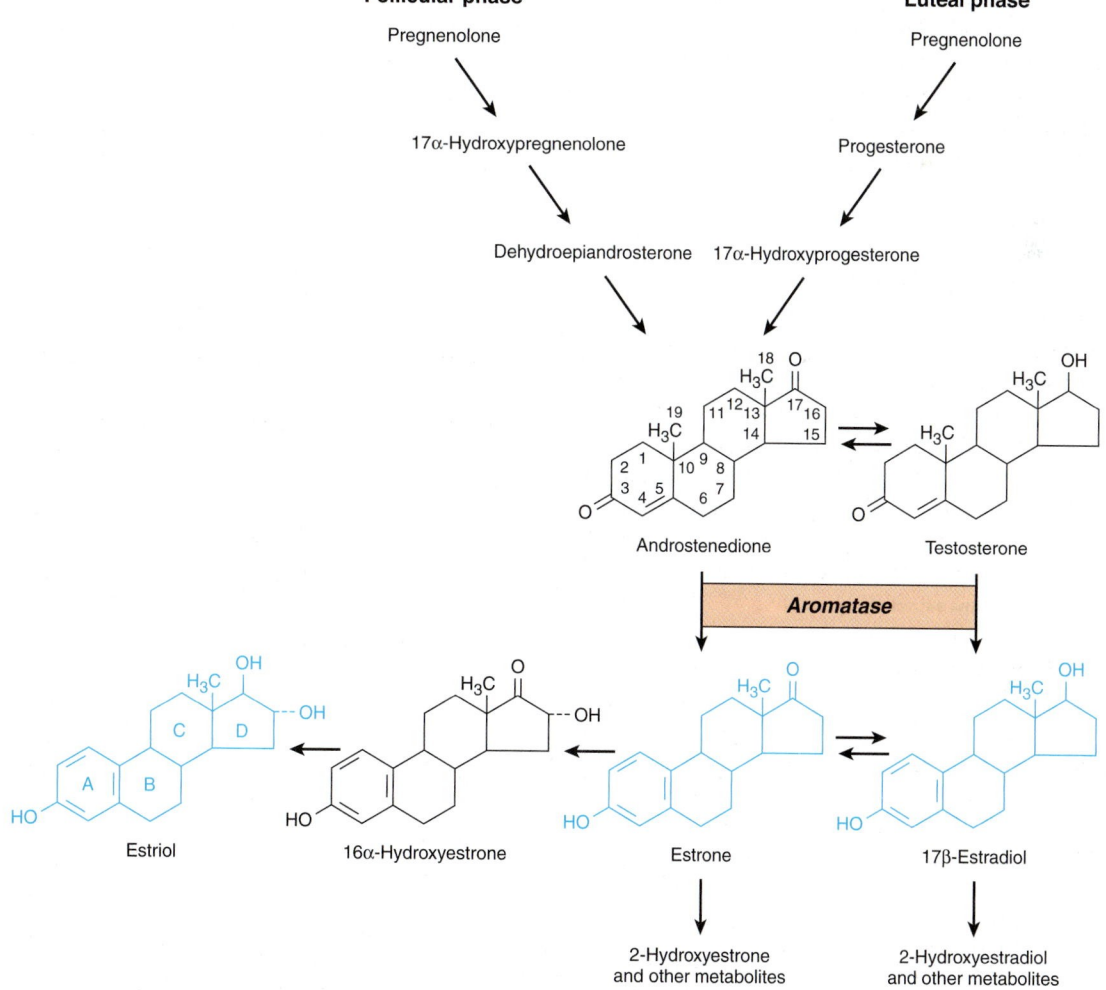

FIGURE 40–2 Biosynthesis and metabolism of estrogens and testosterone.

50 pg/mL in the early follicular phase to as high as 350–850 pg/mL at the time of the preovulatory peak (Figure 40–1).

Synthetic Estrogens

A variety of chemical alterations have been applied to the natural estrogens. The most important effect of these alterations has been to increase their oral effectiveness. Some structures are shown in Figure 40–3. Those with therapeutic use are listed in Table 40–1.

In addition to the steroidal estrogens, a variety of nonsteroidal compounds with estrogenic activity have been synthesized and used clinically. These include dienestrol, diethylstilbestrol, benzestrol, hexestrol, methestrol, methallenestril, and chlorotrianisene (Figure 40–3).

Pharmacokinetics

When released into the circulation, estradiol binds strongly to an α_2 globulin (sex hormone-binding globulin [SHBG]) and with lower affinity to albumin. Bound estrogen is relatively unavailable for diffusion into cells, and it is the free fraction that is physiologically active. Estradiol is converted by the liver and other tissues to estrone and estriol (Figure 40–2) and their 2-hydroxylated derivatives and conjugated metabolites (which are too insoluble in lipid to cross the cell membrane readily) and excreted in the bile. Estrone and estriol have low affinity for the estrogen receptor. However, the conjugates may be hydrolyzed in the intestine to active, reabsorbable compounds. Estrogens are also excreted in small amounts in the breast milk of nursing mothers.

Because significant amounts of estrogens and their active metabolites are excreted in the bile and reabsorbed from the intestine, the resulting enterohepatic circulation ensures that orally administered estrogens will have a high ratio of hepatic to peripheral effects. As noted below, the hepatic effects are thought to be responsible for some undesirable actions such as synthesis of increased clotting factors and plasma renin substrate. The hepatic effects of estrogen can be minimized by routes that avoid first-pass liver exposure, ie, vaginal, transdermal, or by injection.

Physiologic Effects

A. Mechanism

Plasma estrogens in the blood and interstitial fluid are bound to SHBG, from which they dissociate to enter the cell and bind to their receptor. Two genes code for two estrogen receptor isoforms,

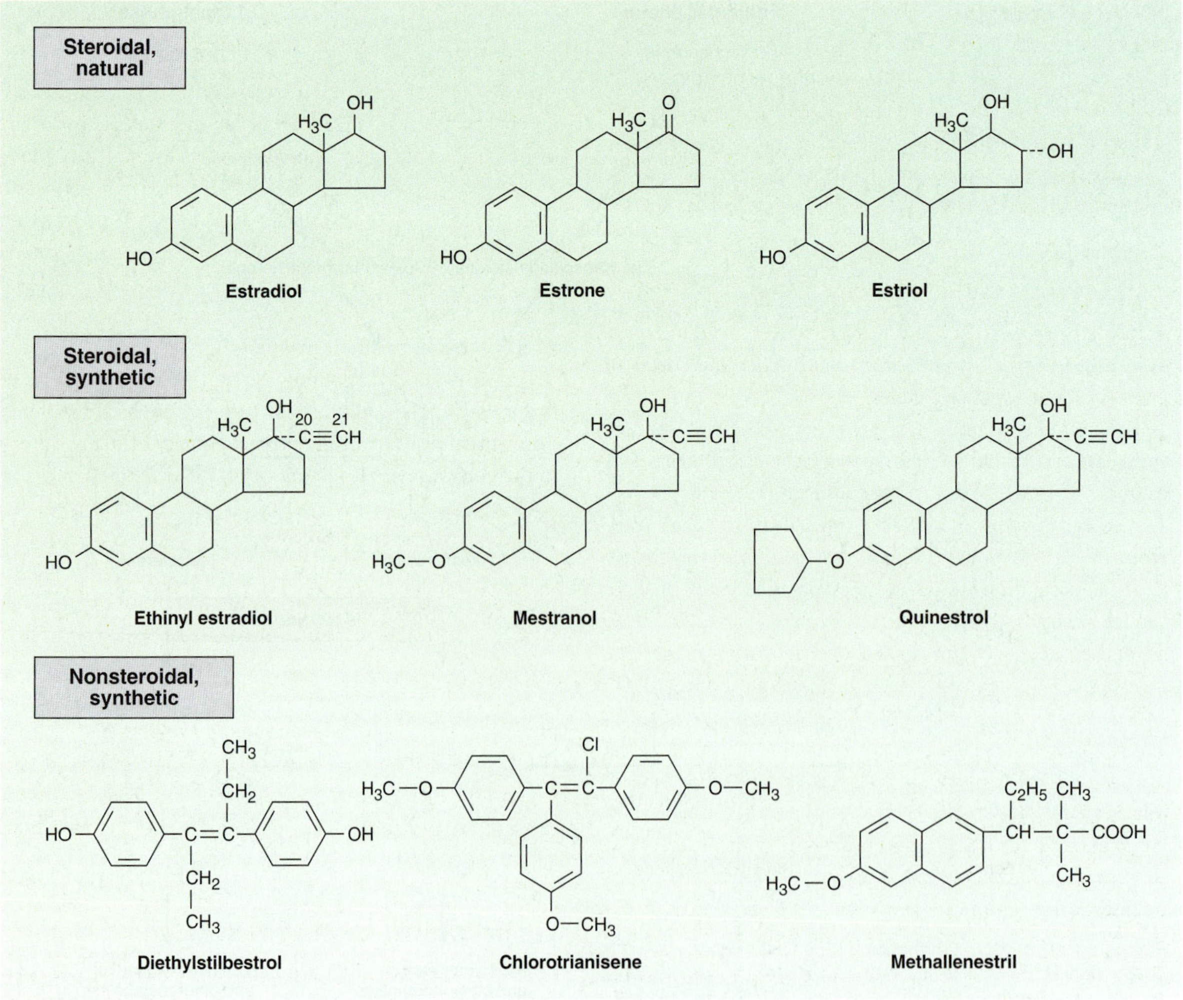

FIGURE 40–3 Compounds with estrogenic activity.

TABLE 40–1 Commonly used estrogens.

Preparation	Average Replacement Dosage
Ethinyl estradiol	0.005–0.02 mg/d
Micronized estradiol	1–2 mg/d
Estradiol cypionate	2–5 mg every 3–4 weeks
Estradiol valerate	2–20 mg every other week
Estropipate	1.25–2.5 mg/d
Conjugated, esterified, or mixed estrogenic substances:	
Oral	0.3–1.25 mg/d
Injectable	0.2–2 mg/d
Transdermal	Patch
Quinestrol	0.1–0.2 mg/week
Chlorotrianisene	12–25 mg/d
Methallenestril	3–9 mg/d

α and β, which are members of the superfamily of steroid, sterol, retinoic acid, and thyroid receptors. The estrogen receptors are found predominantly in the nucleus bound to heat shock proteins that stabilize them (see Figure 39–4).

Binding of the hormone to its receptor alters its conformation and releases it from the stabilizing proteins (predominantly Hsp90). The receptor-hormone complex forms homodimers that bind to a specific sequence of nucleotides called **estrogen response elements (EREs)** in the promoters of various genes and regulate their transcription. The ERE is composed of two half-sites arranged as a palindrome separated by a small group of nucleotides called the spacer. The interaction of a receptor dimer with the ERE also involves a number of nuclear proteins, the coregulators, as well as components of the transcription machinery. The receptor may also bind to other transcription factors to influence the effects of these factors on their responsive genes.

The relative concentrations and types of receptors, receptor coregulators, and transcription factors confer the cell specificity of the hormone's actions. The genomic effects of estrogens are mainly due to proteins synthesized by translation of RNA transcribed from a responsive gene. Some of the effects of estrogens are indirect, mediated by the autocrine and paracrine actions of autacoids such as growth factors, lipids, glycolipids, and cytokines produced by the target cells in response to estrogen.

Rapid estrogen-induced effects such as granulosa cell Ca^{2+} uptake and increased uterine blood flow do not require gene activation. These appear to be mediated by nongenomic effects of the classic estrogen receptor-estrogen complex, influencing several intracellular signaling pathways.

Recently, all steroid receptors except the mineralocorticoid receptors were shown to have palmitoylation motifs that allow enzymatic addition of palmitate and increased localization of the receptors in the vicinity of plasma membranes. Such receptors are available for direct interactions with, and effects on, various membrane-associated or cytoplasmic proteins without the need for entry into the nucleus and induction of transcriptional actions.

B. Female Maturation

Estrogens are required for the normal sexual maturation and growth of the female. They stimulate the development of the vagina, uterus, and uterine tubes as well as the secondary sex characteristics. They stimulate stromal development and ductal growth in the breast and are responsible for the accelerated growth phase and the closing of the epiphyses of the long bones that occur at puberty. They contribute to the growth of axillary and pubic hair and alter the distribution of body fat to produce typical female body contours. Larger quantities also stimulate development of pigmentation in the skin, most prominent in the region of the nipples and areolae and in the genital region.

C. Endometrial Effects

In addition to its growth effects on uterine muscle, estrogen plays an important role in the development of the endometrial lining. When estrogen production is properly coordinated with the production of progesterone during the normal human menstrual cycle, regular periodic bleeding and shedding of the endometrial lining occur. Continuous exposure to estrogens for prolonged periods leads to hyperplasia of the endometrium that is usually associated with abnormal bleeding patterns.

D. Metabolic and Cardiovascular Effects

Estrogens have a number of important metabolic and cardiovascular effects. They seem to be partially responsible for maintenance of the normal structure and function of the skin and blood vessels in women. Estrogens also decrease the rate of resorption of bone by promoting the apoptosis of osteoclasts and by antagonizing the osteoclastogenic and pro-osteoclastic effects of parathyroid hormone and interleukin-6. Estrogens also stimulate adipose tissue production of leptin and are in part responsible for the higher levels of this hormone in women than in men.

In addition to stimulating the synthesis of enzymes and growth factors leading to uterine and breast growth and differentiation, estrogens alter the production and activity of many other proteins in the body. Metabolic alterations in the liver are especially important, so that there is a higher circulating level of proteins such as transcortin (corticosteroid-binding globulin, CBG), thyroxine-binding globulin (TBG), SHBG, transferrin, renin substrate, and fibrinogen. This leads to increased circulating levels of thyroxine, estrogen, testosterone, iron, copper, and other substances.

Alterations in the composition of the plasma lipids caused by estrogens are characterized by an increase in the high-density lipoproteins (HDL), a slight reduction in the low-density lipoproteins (LDL), and a reduction in total plasma cholesterol levels. Plasma triglyceride levels are increased. Estrogens decrease hepatic oxidation of adipose tissue lipid to ketones and increase synthesis of triglycerides.

E. Effects on Blood Coagulation

Estrogens enhance the coagulability of blood. Many changes in factors influencing coagulation have been reported, including increased circulating levels of factors II, VII, IX, and X and decreased antithrombin III, partially as a result of the hepatic effects mentioned above. Increased plasminogen levels and decreased platelet adhesiveness have also been found (see Hormonal Contraception, below).

F. Other Effects

Estrogens induce the synthesis of progesterone receptors. They are responsible for estrous behavior in animals and may influence behavior and libido in humans. Administration of estrogens stimulates central components of the stress system, including the production of corticotropin-releasing hormone and the activity of the sympathetic system, and promotes a sense of well-being when given to women who are estrogen-deficient. They also facilitate the loss of intravascular fluid into the extracellular space, producing edema. The resulting decrease in plasma volume causes a compensatory retention of sodium and water by the kidney. Estrogens also modulate sympathetic nervous system control of smooth muscle function.

Clinical Uses*

A. Primary Hypogonadism

Estrogens have been used extensively for replacement therapy in estrogen-deficient patients. The estrogen deficiency may be due to primary failure of development of the ovaries, premature menopause, castration, or menopause.

Treatment of primary hypogonadism is usually begun at 11–13 years of age in order to stimulate the development of secondary sex characteristics and menses, to stimulate optimal growth, to prevent osteoporosis and to avoid the psychological consequences of delayed puberty and estrogen deficiency. Treatment attempts to mimic the physiology of puberty. It is initiated with small doses of estrogen (0.3 mg conjugated estrogens or 5–10 mcg ethinyl estradiol) on days 1–21 each month and is slowly increased to adult doses and then maintained until the age of menopause (approximately 51 years of age). A progestin is added after the first uterine bleeding. When growth is completed, chronic therapy consists mainly of the administration of adult doses of both estrogens and progestins, as described below.

B. Postmenopausal Hormonal Therapy

In addition to the signs and symptoms that follow closely upon the cessation of normal ovarian function—such as loss of menstrual periods, vasomotor symptoms, sleep disturbances, and genital atrophy—there are longer-lasting changes that influence the health and well-being of postmenopausal women. These include an acceleration of bone loss, which in susceptible women may lead to vertebral, hip, and wrist fractures; and lipid changes, which may contribute to the acceleration of atherosclerotic cardiovascular disease noted in postmenopausal women. The effects of estrogens on bone have been extensively studied, and the effects of hormone withdrawal have been well-characterized. However, the role of estrogens and progestins in the cause and prevention of cardiovascular

disease, which is responsible for 350,000 deaths per year, and breast cancer, which causes 35,000 deaths per year, is less well understood.

When normal ovulatory function ceases and the estrogen levels fall after menopause, oophorectomy, or premature ovarian failure, there is an accelerated rise in plasma cholesterol and LDL concentrations, while LDL receptors decline. HDL is not much affected, and levels remain higher than in men. Very-low-density lipoprotein and triglyceride levels are also relatively unaffected. Since cardiovascular disorders account for most deaths in this age group, the risk for these disorders constitutes a major consideration in deciding whether or not hormonal "replacement" therapy (HRT, also correctly called HT) is indicated and influences the selection of hormones to be administered. Estrogen replacement therapy has a beneficial effect on circulating lipids and lipoproteins, and this was earlier thought to be accompanied by a reduction in myocardial infarction by about 50% and of fatal strokes by as much as 40%. These findings, however, have been disputed by the results of a large study from the Women's Health Initiative (WHI) project showing no cardiovascular benefit from estrogen plus progestin replacement therapy in perimenopausal or older postmenopausal patients. In fact, there may be a small increase in cardiovascular problems as well as breast cancer in women who received the replacement therapy. Interestingly, a small protective effect against colon cancer was observed. Although current clinical guidelines do not recommend routine hormone therapy in postmenopausal women, the validity of the WHI report has been questioned. In any case, there is no increased risk for breast cancer if therapy is given immediately after menopause and for the first 7 years, while the cardiovascular risk depends on the degree of atherosclerosis at the onset of therapy. Transdermal or vaginal administration of estrogen may be associated with decreased cardiovascular risk because it bypasses the liver circulation. Women with premature menopause should definitely receive hormone therapy.

In some studies, a protective effect of estrogen replacement therapy against Alzheimer's disease was observed. However, several other studies have not supported these results.

Progestins antagonize estrogen's effects on LDL and HDL to a variable extent. However, one large study has shown that the addition of a progestin to estrogen replacement therapy does not influence the cardiovascular risk.

Optimal management of the postmenopausal patient requires careful assessment of her symptoms as well as consideration of her age and the presence of (or risks for) cardiovascular disease, osteoporosis, breast cancer, and endometrial cancer. Bearing in mind the effects of the gonadal hormones on each of these disorders, the goals of therapy can then be defined and the risks of therapy assessed and discussed with the patient.

If the main indication for therapy is hot flushes and sleep disturbances, therapy with the lowest dose of estrogen required for symptomatic relief is recommended. Treatment may be required for only a limited period of time and the possible increased risk for breast cancer avoided. In women who have undergone hysterectomy, estrogens alone can be given 5 days per week or continuously, since progestins are not required to reduce the risk for endometrial hyperplasia and cancer. Hot flushes, sweating, insomnia, and atrophic

---

*The use of estrogens in contraception is discussed later in this chapter.

vaginitis are generally relieved by estrogens; many patients experience some increased sense of well-being; and climacteric depression and other psychopathologic states are improved.

The role of estrogens in the prevention and treatment of osteoporosis has been carefully studied (see Chapter 42). The amount of bone present in the body is maximal in the young active adult in the third decade of life and begins to decline more rapidly in middle age in both men and women. The development of osteoporosis also depends on the amount of bone present at the start of this process, on vitamin D and calcium intake, and on the degree of physical activity. The risk of osteoporosis is highest in smokers who are thin, Caucasian, and inactive and have a low calcium intake and a strong family history of osteoporosis. Depression also is a major risk factor for development of osteoporosis in women.

Estrogens should be used in the smallest dosage consistent with relief of symptoms. In women who have not undergone hysterectomy, it is most convenient to prescribe estrogen on the first 21–25 days of each month. The recommended dosages of estrogen are 0.3–1.25 mg/d of conjugated estrogen or 0.01–0.02 mg/d of ethinyl estradiol. Dosages in the middle of these ranges have been shown to be maximally effective in preventing the decrease in bone density occurring at menopause. From this point of view, it is important to begin therapy as soon as possible after the menopause for maximum effect. In these patients and others not taking estrogen, calcium supplements that bring the total daily calcium intake up to 1500 mg are useful.

Patients at low risk of developing osteoporosis who manifest only mild atrophic vaginitis can be treated with topical preparations. The vaginal route of application is also useful in the treatment of urinary tract symptoms in these patients. It is important to realize, however, that although locally administered estrogens escape the first-pass effect (so that some undesirable hepatic effects are reduced), they are almost completely absorbed into the circulation, and these preparations should be given cyclically.

As noted below, the administration of estrogen is associated with an increased risk of endometrial carcinoma. The administration of a progestational agent with the estrogen prevents endometrial hyperplasia and markedly reduces the risk of this cancer. When estrogen is given for the first 25 days of the month and the progestin medroxyprogesterone (10 mg/d) is added during the last 10–14 days, the risk is only half of that in women not receiving hormone replacement therapy. On this regimen, some women will experience a return of symptoms during the period off estrogen administration. In these patients, the estrogen can be given continuously. If the progestin produces sedation or other undesirable effects, its dose can be reduced to 2.5–5 mg for the last 10 days of the cycle with a slight increase in the risk for endometrial hyperplasia. These regimens are usually accompanied by bleeding at the end of each cycle. Some women experience migraine headaches during the last few days of the cycle. The use of a continuous estrogen regimen will often prevent their occurrence. Women who object to the cyclic bleeding associated with sequential therapy can also consider continuous therapy. Daily therapy with 0.625 mg of conjugated equine estrogens and 2.5–5 mg of medroxyprogesterone will eliminate cyclic bleeding, control vasomotor symptoms, prevent genital atrophy, maintain bone density, and show a favorable lipid profile with a small decrease in LDL and an increase in HDL concentrations. These women have endometrial atrophy on biopsy. About half of these patients experience breakthrough bleeding during the first few months of therapy. Seventy to 80 percent become amenorrheic after the first 4 months, and most remain so. The main disadvantage of continuous therapy is the need for uterine biopsy if bleeding occurs after the first few months.

As noted above, estrogens may also be administered vaginally or transdermally. When estrogens are given by these routes, the liver is bypassed on the first circulation, and the ratio of the liver effects to peripheral effects is reduced.

In patients in whom estrogen replacement therapy is contraindicated, such as those with estrogen-sensitive tumors, relief of vasomotor symptoms may be obtained by the use of clonidine.

C. Other Uses

Estrogens combined with progestins can be used to suppress ovulation in patients with intractable dysmenorrhea or when suppression of ovarian function is used in the treatment of hirsutism and amenorrhea due to excessive secretion of androgens by the ovary. Under these circumstances, greater suppression may be needed, and oral contraceptives containing 50 mcg of estrogen or a combination of a low estrogen pill with GnRH suppression may be required.

Adverse Effects

Adverse effects of variable severity have been reported with the therapeutic use of estrogens. Many other effects reported in conjunction with hormonal contraceptives may be related to their estrogen content. These are discussed below.

A. Uterine Bleeding

Estrogen therapy is a major cause of postmenopausal uterine bleeding. Unfortunately, vaginal bleeding at this time of life may also be due to carcinoma of the endometrium. To avoid confusion, patients should be treated with the smallest amount of estrogen possible. It should be given cyclically so that bleeding, if it occurs, will be more likely to occur during the withdrawal period. As noted above, endometrial hyperplasia can be prevented by administration of a progestational agent with estrogen in each cycle.

B. Cancer

The relation of estrogen therapy to cancer continues to be the subject of active investigation. Although no adverse effect of short-term estrogen therapy on the incidence of breast cancer has been demonstrated, a small increase in the incidence of this tumor may occur with prolonged therapy. Although the risk factor is small (1.25), the impact may be great since this tumor occurs in 10% of women, and addition of progesterone does not confer a protective effect. Studies indicate that following unilateral excision of breast cancer, women receiving tamoxifen (an estrogen partial agonist, see below) show a 35% decrease in contralateral breast cancer compared with controls. These studies also demonstrate that tamoxifen is well tolerated by most patients, produces estrogen-like alterations in plasma lipid levels, and stabilizes bone mineral loss. Studies bearing on the possible efficacy of tamoxifen in postmenopausal women at high risk for breast cancer are under way. A recent study shows that postmenopausal hormone replacement therapy with estrogens plus progestins was associated with greater breast epithelial cell proliferation and breast epithelial cell density than estrogens alone or no replacement therapy. Furthermore, with estrogens plus progestins, breast proliferation was localized to the terminal duct-lobular unit of the breast, which is the main site of development of breast cancer. Thus, further studies are needed to conclusively assess the possible association between progestins and breast cancer risk.

Many studies show an increased risk of endometrial carcinoma in patients taking estrogens alone. The risk seems to vary with the dose and duration of treatment: 15 times greater in patients taking large doses of estrogen for 5 or more years, in contrast with two to four times greater in patients receiving lower doses for short periods. However, as noted above, the concomitant use of a progestin prevents this increased risk and may in fact reduce the incidence of endometrial cancer to less than that in the general population.

There have been a number of reports of adenocarcinoma of the vagina in young women whose mothers were treated with large doses of diethylstilbestrol early in pregnancy. These cancers are most common in young women (ages 14–44). The incidence is less than 1 per 1000 women exposed—too low to establish a cause-and-effect relationship with certainty. However, the risks for infertility, ectopic pregnancy, and premature delivery are also increased. It is now recognized that there is no indication for the use of diethylstilbestrol during pregnancy, and it should be avoided. It is not known whether other estrogens have a similar effect or whether the observed phenomena are peculiar to diethylstilbestrol. This agent should be used only in the treatment of cancer (eg, of the prostate) or as a "morning after" contraceptive (see below).

C. Other Effects

Nausea and breast tenderness are common and can be minimized by using the smallest effective dose of estrogen. Hyperpigmentation also occurs. Estrogen therapy is associated with an increase in frequency of migraine headaches as well as cholestasis, gallbladder disease, and hypertension.

Contraindications

Estrogens should not be used in patients with estrogen-dependent neoplasms such as carcinoma of the endometrium or in those with—or at high risk for—carcinoma of the breast. They should be avoided in patients with undiagnosed genital bleeding, liver disease, or a history of thromboembolic disorder. In addition, the use of estrogens should be avoided by heavy smokers.

Preparations & Dosages

The dosages of commonly used natural and synthetic preparations are listed in Table 40–1. Although all of the estrogens produce almost the same hormonal effects, their potencies vary both between agents and depending on the route of administration. As noted above, estradiol is the most active endogenous estrogen, and

it has the highest affinity for the estrogen receptor. However, its metabolites estrone and estriol have weak uterine effects.

For a given level of gonadotropin suppression, oral estrogen preparations have more effect on the circulating levels of CBG, SHBG, and a host of other liver proteins, including angiotensinogen, than do transdermal preparations. The oral route of administration allows greater concentrations of hormone to reach the liver, thus increasing the synthesis of these proteins. Transdermal preparations were developed to avoid this effect. When administered transdermally, 50–100 mcg of estradiol has effects similar to those of 0.625–1.25 mg of conjugated oral estrogens on gonadotropin concentrations, endometrium, and vaginal epithelium. Furthermore, the transdermal estrogen preparations do not significantly increase the concentrations of renin substrate, CBG, and TBG and do not produce the characteristic changes in serum lipids. Combined oral preparations containing 0.625 mg of conjugated estrogens and 2.5 mg of medroxyprogesterone acetate are available for menopausal replacement therapy. Tablets containing 0.625 mg of conjugated estrogens and 5 mg of medroxyprogesterone acetate are available to be used in conjunction with conjugated estrogens in a sequential fashion. Estrogens alone are taken on days 1–14 and the combination on days 15–28.

THE PROGESTINS

Natural Progestins: Progesterone

Progesterone is the most important progestin in humans. In addition to having important hormonal effects, it serves as a precursor to the estrogens, androgens, and adrenocortical steroids. It is synthesized in the ovary, testis, and adrenal cortex from circulating cholesterol. Large amounts are also synthesized and released by the placenta during pregnancy.

In the ovary, progesterone is produced primarily by the corpus luteum. Normal males appear to secrete 1–5 mg of progesterone daily, resulting in plasma levels of about 0.03 mcg/dL. The level is only slightly higher in the female during the follicular phase of the cycle, when only a few milligrams per day of progesterone are secreted. During the luteal phase, plasma levels range from 0.5 mcg/dL to more than 2 mcg/dL (Figure 40–1). Plasma levels of progesterone are further elevated and reach their peak levels in the third trimester of pregnancy.

Synthetic Progestins

A variety of progestational compounds have been synthesized. Some are active when given by mouth. They are not a uniform group of compounds, and all of them differ from progesterone in one or more respects. Table 40–2 lists some of these compounds and their effects. In general, the 21-carbon compounds (hydroxyprogesterone, medroxyprogesterone, megestrol, and dimethisterone) are the most closely related, pharmacologically as well as chemically, to progesterone. A new group of third-generation synthetic progestins has been introduced, principally as components of oral contraceptives. These "19-nor, 13-ethyl" steroid compounds

TABLE 40–2 Properties of some progestational agents.

| | Route | Duration of Action | Activities[1] | | | | |
			Estrogenic	Androgenic	Antiestrogenic	Antiandrogenic	Anabolic
Progesterone and derivatives							
Progesterone	IM	1 day	–	–	+	–	–
Hydroxyprogesterone caproate	IM	8–14 days	sl	sl	–	–	–
Medroxyprogesterone acetate	IM, PO	Tabs: 1–3 days; injection: 4–12 weeks	–	+	+	–	–
Megestrol acetate	PO	1–3 days	–	+	–	+	–
17-Ethinyl testosterone derivatives							
Dimethisterone	PO	1–3 days	–	–	sl	–	–
19-Nortestosterone derivatives							
Desogestrel	PO	1–3 days	–	–	–	–	–
Norethynodrel[2]	PO	1–3 days	+	–	–	–	–
Lynestrenol[3]	PO	1–3 days	+	+	–	–	+
Norethindrone[2]	PO	1–3 days	sl	+	+	–	+
Norethindrone acetate[2]	PO	1–3 days	sl	+	+	–	+
Ethynodiol diacetate[2]	PO	1–3 days	sl	+	+	–	+
L-Norgestrel[2]	PO	1–3 days	–	+	+	–	+

[1]**Interpretation:** + = active; – = inactive; sl = slightly active. Activities have been reported in various species using various end points and may not apply to humans.
[2]See Table 40–3.
[3]Not available in USA.

include desogestrel (Figure 40–4), gestodene, and norgestimate. They are claimed to have lower androgenic activity than older synthetic progestins.

Pharmacokinetics

Progesterone is rapidly absorbed following administration by any route. Its half-life in the plasma is approximately 5 minutes, and small amounts are stored temporarily in body fat. It is almost completely metabolized in one passage through the liver, and for that reason it is quite ineffective when the usual formulation is administered orally. However, high-dose oral micronized progesterone preparations have been developed that provide adequate progestational effect.

In the liver, progesterone is metabolized to pregnanediol and conjugated with glucuronic acid. It is excreted into the urine as pregnanediol glucuronide. The amount of pregnanediol in the urine has been used as an index of progesterone secretion. This measure has been very useful despite the fact that the proportion of secreted progesterone converted to this compound varies from day to day and from individual to individual. In addition to progesterone, 20α- and 20β-hydroxyprogesterone (20α- and 20β-hydroxy-4-pregnene-3-one) are also found. These compounds have about one fifth the progestational activity of progesterone in humans and other species. Little is known of their physiologic

role, but 20α-hydroxyprogesterone is produced in large amounts in some species and may be of some importance biologically.

The usual routes of administration and durations of action of the synthetic progestins are listed in Table 40–2. Most of these agents are extensively metabolized to inactive products that are excreted mainly in the urine.

Physiologic Effects

A. Mechanism

The mechanism of action of progesterone—described in more detail above—is similar to that of other steroid hormones. Progestins enter the cell and bind to progesterone receptors that are distributed between the nucleus and the cytoplasm. The ligand-receptor complex binds to a progesterone response element (PRE) to activate gene transcription. The response element for progesterone appears to be similar to the corticosteroid response element, and the specificity of the response depends upon which receptor is present in the cell as well as upon other cell-specific receptor coregulators and interacting transcription factors. The progesterone-receptor complex forms a dimer before binding to DNA. Like the estrogen receptor, it can form heterodimers as well as homodimers between two isoforms, A and B. These isoforms are produced by alternative splicing of the same gene.

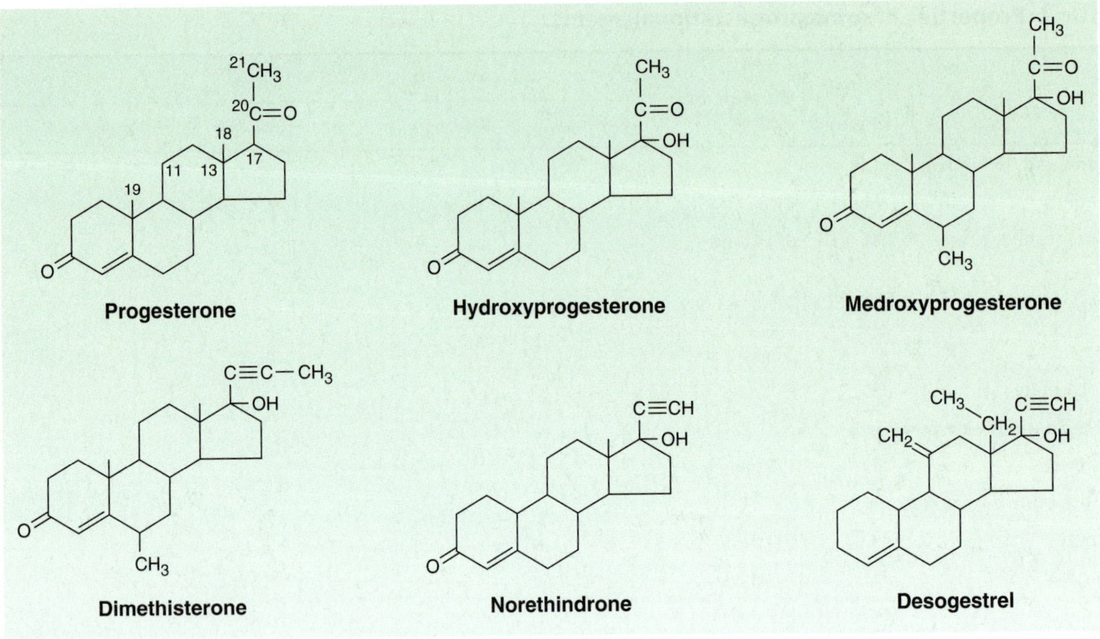

FIGURE 40–4 Progesterone and some progestational agents in clinical use.

B. Effects of Progesterone

Progesterone has little effect on protein metabolism. It stimulates lipoprotein lipase activity and seems to favor fat deposition. The effects on carbohydrate metabolism are more marked. Progesterone increases basal insulin levels and the insulin response to glucose. There is usually no manifest change in carbohydrate tolerance. In the liver, progesterone promotes glycogen storage, possibly by facilitating the effect of insulin. Progesterone also promotes ketogenesis.

Progesterone can compete with aldosterone for the mineralocorticoid receptor of the renal tubule, causing a decrease in Na^+ reabsorption. This leads to an increased secretion of aldosterone by the adrenal cortex (eg, in pregnancy). Progesterone increases body temperature in humans. The mechanism of this effect is not known, but an alteration of the temperature-regulating centers in the hypothalamus has been suggested. Progesterone also alters the function of the respiratory centers. The ventilatory response to CO_2 is increased by progesterone but synthetic progestins with an ethinyl group do not have respiratory effects. This leads to a measurable reduction in arterial and alveolar P_{CO_2} during pregnancy and in the luteal phase of the menstrual cycle. Progesterone and related steroids also have depressant and hypnotic effects on the brain.

Progesterone is responsible for the alveolobular development of the secretory apparatus in the breast. It also participates in the preovulatory LH surge and causes the maturation and secretory changes in the endometrium that are seen following ovulation (Figure 40–1).

Progesterone decreases the plasma levels of many amino acids and leads to increased urinary nitrogen excretion. It induces changes in the structure and function of smooth endoplasmic reticulum in experimental animals.

Other effects of progesterone and its analogs are noted below in the section, Hormonal Contraception.

C. Synthetic Progestins

The 21-carbon progesterone analogs antagonize aldosterone-induced sodium retention (see above). The remaining compounds ("19-nortestosterone" third-generation agents) produce a decidual change in the endometrial stroma, do not support pregnancy in test animals, are more effective gonadotropin inhibitors, and may have minimal estrogenic and androgenic or anabolic activity (Table 40–2; Figure 40–4). They are sometimes referred to as "impeded androgens." Progestins without androgenic activity include desogestrel, norgestimate, and gestodene. The first two of these compounds are dispensed in combination with ethinyl estradiol for oral contraception (Table 40–3) in the USA. Oral contraceptives containing the progestins cyproterone acetate (also an antiandrogen) in combination with ethinyl estradiol are investigational in the USA.

Clinical Uses

A. Therapeutic Applications

The major uses of progestational hormones are for hormone replacement therapy (see above) and hormonal contraception (see below). In addition, they are useful in producing long-term ovarian suppression for other purposes. When used alone in large doses parenterally (eg, medroxyprogesterone acetate, 150 mg intramuscularly every 90 days), prolonged anovulation and amenorrhea result. This therapy has been employed in the treatment of dysmenorrhea, endometriosis, and bleeding disorders when estrogens are contraindicated, and for contraception. The major problem

TABLE 40–3 Some oral and implantable contraceptive agents in use.[1]

	Estrogen (mg)		Progestin (mg)	
Monophasic combination tablets				
Alesse, Aviane, Lessinea, Levlite	Ethinyl estradiol	0.02	L-Norgestrel	0.1
Levlen, Levora, Nordette, Portia	Ethinyl estradiol	0.03	L-Norgestrel	0.15
Crysella, Lo-Ovral, Low-Ogestrel	Ethinyl estradiol	0.03	Norgestrel	0.30
Yasmin	Ethinyl estradiol	0.03	Drospirenone	3.0
Brevicon, Modicon, Necon 0.5/35, Nortrel 0.5/35	Ethinyl estradiol	0.035	Norethindrone	1.0
Ortho-Cyclen, Sprintec	Ethinyl estradiol	0.035	Norgestimate	0.25
Necon 1/35, Norinyl 1+, Nortrel 1/35, Ortho-Novum 1/35	Ethinyl estradiol	0.035	Norethindrone	1.0
Ovcon-35	Ethinyl estradiol	0.035	Norethindrone	0.4
Demulen 1/50, Zovia 1/50E	Ethinyl estradiol	0.05	Ethynodiol diacetate	1.0
Ovcon 50	Ethinyl estradiol	0.05	Norethindrone	1.0
Ovral-28	Ethinyl estradiol	0.05	D,L-Norgestrel	0.5
Norinyl 1/50, Ortho-Novum 1/50	Mestranol	0.05	Norethindrone	1.0
Biphasic combination tablets				
Ortho-Novum 10/11, Necon 10/11				
Days 1–10	Ethinyl estradiol	0.035	Norethindrone	0.5
Days 11–21	Ethinyl estradiol	0.035	Norethindrone	1.0
Triphasic combination tablets				
Enpresse, Triphasil, Tri-Levlen, Trivora				
Days 1–6	Ethinyl estradiol	0.03	L-Norgestrel	0.05
Days 7–11	Ethinyl estradiol	0.04	L-Norgestrel	0.075
Days 12–21	Ethinyl estradiol	0.03	L-Norgestrel	0.125
Ortho-Novum 7/7/7, Necon 7/7/7				
Days 1–7	Ethinyl estradiol	0.035	Norethindrone	0.5
Days 8–14	Ethinyl estradiol	0.035	Norethindrone	0.75
Days 15–21	Ethinyl estradiol	0.035	Norethindrone	1.0
Ortho-Tri-Cyclen				
Days 1–7	Ethinyl estradiol	0.035	Norgestimate	0.18
Days 8–14	Ethinyl estradiol	0.035	Norgestimate	0.215
Days 15–21	Ethinyl estradiol	0.035	Norgestimate	0.25
Daily progestin tablets				
Nora-BE, Nor-QD, Ortho Micronor, Jolivette, Camila, Errin	…		Norethindrone	0.35
Ovrette	…		D,L-Norgestrel	0.075
Implantable progestin preparation				
Implanon	…		Etonogestrel (one tube of 68 mg)	

[1]The estrogen-containing compounds are arranged in order of increasing content of estrogen. Other preparations are available. (Ethinyl estradiol and mestranol have similar potencies.)

with this regimen is the prolonged time required in some patients for ovulatory function to return after cessation of therapy. It should not be used for patients planning a pregnancy in the near future. Similar regimens will relieve hot flushes in some menopausal women and can be used if estrogen therapy is contraindicated.

Medroxyprogesterone acetate, 10–20 mg orally twice weekly—or intramuscularly in doses of 100 mg/m^2 every 1–2 weeks—will prevent menstruation, but it will not arrest accelerated bone maturation in children with precocious puberty.

Progestins do not appear to have any place in the therapy of threatened or habitual abortion. Early reports of the usefulness of these agents resulted from the unwarranted assumption that after several abortions the likelihood of repeated abortions was over 90%. When progestational agents were administered to patients with previous abortions, a salvage rate of 80% was achieved. It is now recognized that similar patients abort only 20% of the time even when untreated. On the other hand, progesterone was given experimentally to delay premature labor with encouraging results.

Progesterone and medroxyprogesterone have been used in the treatment of women who have difficulty in conceiving and who demonstrate a slow rise in basal body temperature. There is no convincing evidence that this treatment is effective.

Preparations of progesterone and medroxyprogesterone have been used to treat premenstrual syndrome. Controlled studies have not confirmed the effectiveness of such therapy except when doses sufficient to suppress ovulation have been used.

B. Diagnostic Uses

Progesterone can be used as a test of estrogen secretion. The administration of progesterone, 150 mg/d, or medroxyprogesterone, 10 mg/d, for 5–7 days, is followed by withdrawal bleeding in amenorrheic patients only when the endometrium has been stimulated by estrogens. A combination of estrogen and progestin can be given to test the responsiveness of the endometrium in patients with amenorrhea.

Contraindications, Cautions, & Adverse Effects

Studies of progestational compounds alone and with combination oral contraceptives indicate that the progestin in these agents may increase blood pressure in some patients. The more androgenic progestins also reduce plasma HDL levels in women. (See Hormonal Contraception, below.) Two recent studies suggest that combined progestin plus estrogen replacement therapy in postmenopausal women may increase breast cancer risk significantly compared with the risk in women taking estrogen alone. These findings require careful examination and if confirmed will lead to important changes in postmenopausal hormone replacement practice.

OTHER OVARIAN HORMONES

The normal ovary produces small amounts of **androgens,** including testosterone, androstenedione, and dehydroepiandrosterone. Of these, only testosterone has a significant amount of biologic activity, although androstenedione can be converted to testosterone or estrone in peripheral tissues. The normal woman produces less than 200 mcg of testosterone in 24 hours, and about one third of this is probably formed in the ovary directly. The physiologic significance of these small amounts of androgens is not established, but they may be partly responsible for normal hair growth at puberty, for stimulation of female libido, and, possibly, for metabolic effects. Androgen production by the ovary may be markedly increased in some abnormal states, usually in association with hirsutism and amenorrhea as noted above.

The ovary also produces **inhibin** and **activin.** These peptides consist of several combinations of α and β subunits and are described in greater detail later. The αβ dimer (inhibin) inhibits FSH secretion while the ββ dimer (activin) increases FSH secretion. Studies in primates indicate that inhibin has no direct effect on ovarian steroidogenesis but that activin modulates the response to LH and FSH. For example, simultaneous treatment with activin and human FSH enhances FSH stimulation of progesterone synthesis and aromatase activity in granulosa cells. When combined with LH, activin suppressed the LH-induced progesterone response by 50% but markedly enhanced basal and LH-stimulated aromatase activity. Activin may also act as a growth factor in other tissues. The physiologic roles of these modulators are not fully understood.

Relaxin is another peptide that can be extracted from the ovary. The three-dimensional structure of relaxin is related to that of growth-promoting peptides and is similar to that of insulin. Although the amino acid sequence differs from that of insulin, this hormone, like insulin, consists of two chains linked by disulfide bonds, cleaved from a prohormone. It is found in the ovary, placenta, uterus, and blood. Relaxin synthesis has been demonstrated in luteinized granulosa cells of the corpus luteum. It has been shown to increase glycogen synthesis and water uptake by the myometrium and decreases uterine contractility. In some species, it changes the mechanical properties of the cervix and pubic ligaments, facilitating delivery.

In women, relaxin has been measured by immunoassay. Levels were highest immediately after the LH surge and during menstruation. A physiologic role for this peptide has not been established.

Clinical trials with relaxin have been conducted in patients with dysmenorrhea. Relaxin has also been administered to patients in premature labor and during prolonged labor. When applied to the cervix of a woman at term, it facilitates dilation and shortens labor.

Several other nonsteroidal substances such as corticotropin-releasing hormone, follistatin, and prostaglandins are produced by the ovary. These probably have paracrine effects within the ovary.

HORMONAL CONTRACEPTION (ORAL, PARENTERAL, & IMPLANTED CONTRACEPTIVES)

A large number of oral contraceptives containing estrogens or progestins (or both) are now available for clinical use (Table 40–3). These preparations vary chemically and pharmacologically and have many properties in common as well as definite differences important for the correct selection of the optimum agent.

Two types of preparations are used for oral contraception: (1) combinations of estrogens and progestins and (2) continuous progestin therapy without concomitant administration of estrogens. The combination agents are further divided into **monophasic** forms (constant dosage of both components during the cycle) and **biphasic** or **triphasic** forms (dosage of one or both components is changed once or twice during the cycle). The preparations for oral use are all adequately absorbed, and in combination preparations the pharmacokinetics of neither drug is significantly altered by the other.

Only one implantable contraceptive preparation is available at present in the USA. Etonogestrel, also used in some oral contraceptives, is available in the subcutaneous implant form listed in Table 40–3. Several hormonal contraceptives are available as vaginal rings or intrauterine devices. Intramuscular injection of large doses of medroxyprogesterone also provides contraception of long duration.

Pharmacologic Effects

A. Mechanism of Action

The combinations of estrogens and progestins exert their contraceptive effect largely through selective inhibition of pituitary function that results in inhibition of ovulation. The combination agents also produce a change in the cervical mucus, in the uterine endometrium, and in motility and secretion in the uterine tubes, all of which decrease the likelihood of conception and implantation. The continuous use of progestins alone does not always inhibit ovulation. The other factors mentioned, therefore, play a major role in the prevention of pregnancy when these agents are used.

B. Effects on the Ovary

Chronic use of combination agents depresses ovarian function. Follicular development is minimal, and corpora lutea, larger follicles, stromal edema, and other morphologic features normally seen in ovulating women are absent. The ovaries usually become smaller even when enlarged before therapy.

The great majority of patients return to normal menstrual patterns when these drugs are discontinued. About 75% will ovulate in the first posttreatment cycle and 97% by the third posttreatment cycle. About 2% of patients remain amenorrheic for periods of up to several years after administration is stopped.

The cytologic findings on vaginal smears vary depending on the preparation used. However, with almost all of the combined drugs, a low maturation index is found because of the presence of progestational agents.

C. Effects on the Uterus

After prolonged use, the cervix may show some hypertrophy and polyp formation. There are also important effects on the cervical mucus, making it more like postovulation mucus, ie, thicker and less copious.

Agents containing both estrogens and progestins produce further morphologic and biochemical changes of the endometrial stroma under the influence of the progestin, which also stimulates glandular secretion throughout the luteal phase. The agents containing "19-nor" progestins—particularly those with the smaller amounts of estrogen—tend to produce more glandular atrophy and usually less bleeding.

D. Effects on the Breast

Stimulation of the breasts occurs in most patients receiving estrogen-containing agents. Some enlargement is generally noted. The administration of estrogens and combinations of estrogens and progestins tends to suppress lactation. When the doses are small, the effects on breast-feeding are not appreciable. Studies of the transport of the oral contraceptives into breast milk suggest that only small amounts of these compounds cross into the milk, and they have not been considered to be of importance.

E. Other Effects of Oral Contraceptives

1. Effects on the central nervous system—The central nervous system effects of the oral contraceptives have not been well studied in humans. A variety of effects of estrogen and progesterone have been noted in animals. Estrogens tend to increase excitability in the brain, whereas progesterone tends to decrease it. The thermogenic action of progesterone and some of the synthetic progestins is also thought to occur in the central nervous system.

It is very difficult to evaluate any behavioral or emotional effects of these compounds in humans. Although the incidence of pronounced changes in mood, affect, and behavior appears to be low, milder changes are commonly reported, and estrogens are being successfully employed in the therapy of premenstrual tension syndrome, postpartum depression, and climacteric depression.

2. Effects on endocrine function—The inhibition of pituitary gonadotropin secretion has been mentioned. Estrogens also alter adrenal structure and function. Estrogens given orally or at high doses increase the plasma concentration of the α_2 globulin that binds cortisol (corticosteroid-binding globulin). Plasma concentrations may be more than double the levels found in untreated individuals, and urinary excretion of free cortisol is elevated.

These preparations cause alterations in the renin-angiotensin-aldosterone system. Plasma renin activity has been found to increase, and there is an increase in aldosterone secretion.

Thyroxine-binding globulin is increased. As a result, total plasma thyroxine (T_4) levels are increased to those commonly seen during pregnancy. Since more of the thyroxine is bound, the free thyroxine level in these patients is normal. Estrogens also increase the plasma level of SHBG and decrease plasma levels of free androgens by increasing their binding; large amounts of estrogen may decrease androgens by gonadotropin suppression.

3. Effects on blood—Serious thromboembolic phenomena occurring in women taking oral contraceptives gave rise to a great many studies of the effects of these compounds on blood coagulation. A clear picture of such effects has not yet emerged. The oral contraceptives do not consistently alter bleeding or clotting times. The changes that have been observed are similar to those reported in pregnancy. There is an increase in factors VII, VIII, IX, and X and a decrease in antithrombin III. Increased amounts of coumarin anticoagulants may be required to prolong prothrombin time in patients taking oral contraceptives.

There is an increase in serum iron and total iron-binding capacity similar to that reported in patients with hepatitis.

Significant alterations in the cellular components of blood have not been reported with any consistency. A number of patients have been reported to develop folic acid deficiency anemias.

4. Effects on the liver—These hormones also have profound effects on the function of the liver. Some of these effects are deleterious and will be considered below in the section on adverse effects. The effects on serum proteins result from the effects of the estrogens on the synthesis of the various α_2 globulins and fibrinogen. Serum haptoglobins produced in the liver are depressed rather than increased by estrogen. Some of the effects on carbohydrate and lipid metabolism are probably influenced by changes in liver metabolism (see below).

Important alterations in hepatic drug excretion and metabolism also occur. Estrogens in the amounts seen during pregnancy or used in oral contraceptive agents delay the clearance of sulfobromophthalein and reduce the flow of bile. The proportion of cholic acid in bile acids is increased while the proportion of chenodeoxycholic acid is decreased. These changes may be responsible for the observed increase in cholelithiasis associated with the use of these agents.

5. Effects on lipid metabolism—As noted above, estrogens increase serum triglycerides and free and esterified cholesterol. Phospholipids are also increased, as are HDL; levels of LDL usually decrease. Although the effects are marked with doses of 100 mcg of mestranol or ethinyl estradiol, doses of 50 mcg or less have minimal effects. The progestins (particularly the "19-nortestosterone" derivatives) tend to antagonize these effects of estrogen. Preparations containing small amounts of estrogen and a progestin may slightly decrease triglycerides and HDL.

6. Effects on carbohydrate metabolism—The administration of oral contraceptives produces alterations in carbohydrate metabolism similar to those observed in pregnancy. There is a reduction in the rate of absorption of carbohydrates from the gastrointestinal tract. Progesterone increases the basal insulin level and the rise in insulin induced by carbohydrate ingestion. Preparations with more potent progestins such as norgestrel may cause progressive decreases in carbohydrate tolerance over several years. However, the changes in glucose tolerance are reversible on discontinuing medication.

7. Effects on the cardiovascular system—These agents cause small increases in cardiac output associated with higher systolic and diastolic blood pressure and heart rate. The pressure returns to normal when treatment is terminated. Although the magnitude of the pressure change is small in most patients, it is marked in a few. It is important that blood pressure be followed in each patient. An increase in blood pressure has been reported to occur in a few postmenopausal women treated with estrogens alone.

8. Effects on the skin—The oral contraceptives have been noted to increase pigmentation of the skin (chloasma). This effect seems to be enhanced in women with dark complexions and by exposure to ultraviolet light. Some of the androgen-like progestins might increase the production of sebum, causing acne in some patients. However, since ovarian androgen is suppressed, many patients note decreased sebum production, acne, and terminal hair growth. The sequential oral contraceptive preparations as well as estrogens alone often decrease sebum production.

Clinical Uses

The most important use of combined estrogens and progestins is for oral contraception. A large number of preparations are available for this specific purpose, some of which are listed in Table 40–3. They are specially packaged for ease of administration. In general, they are very effective; when these agents are taken according to directions, the risk of conception is extremely small. The pregnancy rate with combination agents is estimated to be about 0.5–1 per 100 woman years at risk. Contraceptive failure has been observed in some patients when one or more doses are missed, if phenytoin is also being used (which may increase catabolism of the compounds), or if antibiotics are taken that alter enterohepatic cycling of metabolites.

Progestins and estrogens are also useful in the treatment of endometriosis. When severe dysmenorrhea is the major symptom, the suppression of ovulation with estrogen alone may be followed by painless periods. However, in most patients this approach to therapy is inadequate. The long-term administration of large doses of progestins or combinations of progestins and estrogens prevents the periodic breakdown of the endometrial tissue and in some cases will lead to endometrial fibrosis and prevent the reactivation of implants for prolonged periods.

As is true with most hormonal preparations, many of the undesired effects are physiologic or pharmacologic actions that are objectionable only because they are not pertinent to the situation for which they are being used. Therefore, the product containing the smallest effective amounts of hormones should be selected for use.

Adverse Effects

The incidence of serious known toxicities associated with the use of these drugs is low—far lower than the risks associated with pregnancy. There are a number of reversible changes in intermediary metabolism. Minor adverse effects are frequent, but most are mild and many are transient. Continuing problems may respond to simple changes in pill formulation. Although it is not often necessary to discontinue medication for these reasons, as many as one third of all patients started on oral contraception discontinue use for reasons other than a desire to become pregnant.

A. Mild Adverse Effects

1. Nausea, mastalgia, breakthrough bleeding, and edema are related to the amount of estrogen in the preparation. These effects can often be alleviated by a shift to a preparation containing smaller amounts of estrogen or to agents containing progestins with more androgenic effects.

2. Changes in serum proteins and other effects on endocrine function (see above) must be taken into account when thyroid, adrenal, or pituitary function is being evaluated. Increases in sedimentation rate are thought to be due to increased levels of fibrinogen.

3. Headache is mild and often transient. However, migraine is often made worse and has been reported to be associated with an increased frequency of cerebrovascular accidents. When this occurs or when migraine has its onset during therapy with these agents, treatment should be discontinued.

4. Withdrawal bleeding sometimes fails to occur—most often with combination preparations—and may cause confusion with regard to pregnancy. If this is disturbing to the patient, a different preparation may be tried or other methods of contraception used.

B. Moderate Adverse Effects

Any of the following may require discontinuance of oral contraceptives:

1. Breakthrough bleeding is the most common problem in using progestational agents alone for contraception. It occurs in as many as 25% of patients. It is more frequently encountered in patients taking low-dose preparations than in those taking combination pills with higher levels of progestin and estrogen. The biphasic and triphasic oral contraceptives (Table 40–3) decrease breakthrough bleeding without increasing the total hormone content.

2. Weight gain is more common with the combination agents containing androgen-like progestins. It can usually be controlled by shifting to preparations with less progestin effect or by dieting.

3. Increased skin pigmentation may occur, especially in dark-skinned women. It tends to increase with time, the incidence being about 5% at the end of the first year and about 40% after 8 years. It is thought to be exacerbated by vitamin B deficiency. It is often reversible upon discontinuance of medication but may disappear very slowly.

4. Acne may be exacerbated by agents containing androgen-like progestins (Table 40–2), whereas agents containing large amounts of estrogen usually cause marked improvement in acne.

5. Hirsutism may also be aggravated by the "19-nortestosterone" derivatives, and combinations containing nonandrogenic progestins are preferred in these patients.

6. Ureteral dilation similar to that observed in pregnancy has been reported, and bacteriuria is more frequent.

7. Vaginal infections are more common and more difficult to treat in patients who are using oral contraceptives.

8. Amenorrhea occurs in some patients. Following cessation of administration of oral contraceptives, 95% of patients with normal menstrual histories resume normal periods and all but a few resume normal cycles during the next few months. However, some patients remain amenorrheic for several years. Many of these patients also have galactorrhea. Patients who have had menstrual irregularities before taking oral contraceptives are particularly susceptible to prolonged amenorrhea when the agents are discontinued. Prolactin levels should be measured in these patients, since many have prolactinomas.

C. Severe Adverse Effects

1. Vascular disorders—Thromboembolism was one of the earliest of the serious unanticipated effects to be reported and has been the most thoroughly studied.

a. Venous thromboembolic disease—Superficial or deep thromboembolic disease in women not taking oral contraceptives occurs in about 1 patient per 1000 woman years. The overall incidence of these disorders in patients taking low-dose oral contraceptives is about threefold higher. The risk for this disorder is increased during the first month of contraceptive use and remains constant for several years or more. The risk returns to normal within a month when use is discontinued. The risk of venous thrombosis or pulmonary embolism is increased among women with predisposing conditions such as stasis, altered clotting factors such as antithrombin III, increased levels of homocysteine, or injury. Genetic disorders, including mutations in the genes governing the production of protein C (factor V Leiden), protein S, hepatic cofactor II, and others, markedly increase the risk of venous thromboembolism. The incidence of these disorders is too low for cost-effective screening by current methods, but prior episodes or a family history may be helpful in identifying patients with increased risk.

The incidence of venous thromboembolism appears to be related to the estrogen but not the progestin content of oral contraceptives and is not related to age, parity, mild obesity, or cigarette smoking. Decreased venous blood flow, endothelial proliferation in veins and arteries, and increased coagulability of blood resulting from changes in platelet functions and fibrinolytic systems contribute to the increased incidence of thrombosis. The major plasma inhibitor of thrombin, antithrombin III, is substantially decreased during oral contraceptive use. This change occurs in the first month of treatment and lasts as long as treatment persists, reversing within a month thereafter.

b. Myocardial infarction—The use of oral contraceptives is associated with a slightly higher risk of myocardial infarction in women who are obese, have a history of preeclampsia or hypertension, or have hyperlipoproteinemia or diabetes. There is a much higher risk in women who smoke. The risk attributable to oral contraceptives in women 30–40 years of age who do not smoke is about 4 cases per 100,000 users per year, as compared with 185 cases per 100,000 among women 40–44 who smoke heavily. The association with myocardial infarction is thought to involve acceleration of atherogenesis because of decreased glucose tolerance, decreased levels of HDL, increased levels of LDL, and increased platelet aggregation. In addition, facilitation of coronary arterial spasm may play a role in some of these patients. The progestational component of oral contraceptives decreases HDL cholesterol levels, in proportion to the androgenic activity of the progestin. The net effect, therefore, will depend on the specific composition of the pill used and the patient's susceptibility to the particular effects. Recent studies suggest that risk of infarction is not increased in past users who have discontinued oral contraceptives.

c. Cerebrovascular disease—The risk of stroke is concentrated in women over age 35. It is increased in current users of oral contraceptives but not in past users. However, subarachnoid hemorrhages have been found to be increased among both current and past users and may increase with time. The risk of thrombotic or hemorrhagic stroke attributable to oral contraceptives (based on older, higher-dose preparations) has been estimated to about 37 cases per 100,000 users per year.

In summary, available data indicate that oral contraceptives increase the risk of various cardiovascular disorders at all ages and among both smokers and nonsmokers. However, this risk appears to be concentrated in women 35 years of age or older who are heavy smokers. It is clear that these risk factors must be considered in each individual patient for whom oral contraceptives are being considered. Some experts have suggested that screening for coagulopathy should be performed before starting oral contraception.

2. Gastrointestinal disorders—Many cases of cholestatic jaundice have been reported in patients taking progestin-containing drugs. The differences in incidence of these disorders from one population to another suggest that genetic factors may be involved. The jaundice caused by these agents is similar to that produced by other 17-alkyl-substituted steroids. It is most often observed in the first three cycles and is particularly common in women with a history of cholestatic jaundice during pregnancy. Jaundice and pruritus disappear 1–8 weeks after the drug is discontinued.

These agents have also been found to increase the incidence of symptomatic gallbladder disease, including cholecystitis and cholangitis. This is probably the result of the alterations responsible for jaundice and bile acid changes described above.

It also appears that the incidence of hepatic adenomas is increased in women taking oral contraceptives. Ischemic bowel disease secondary to thrombosis of the celiac and superior and inferior mesenteric arteries and veins has also been reported in women using these drugs.

3. Depression—Depression of sufficient degree to require cessation of therapy occurs in about 6% of patients treated with some preparations.

4. Cancer—The occurrence of malignant tumors in patients taking oral contraceptives has been studied extensively. It is now clear that these compounds *reduce* the risk of endometrial and ovarian cancer. The lifetime risk of breast cancer in the population as a whole does not seem to be affected by oral contraceptive use. Some studies have shown an increased risk in younger women, and it is possible that tumors that develop in younger women become clinically apparent sooner. The relation of risk of cervical cancer to oral contraceptive use is still controversial. It should be noted that a number of recent studies associate the use of oral contraceptives by women who are infected with human papillomavirus with an increased risk of cervical cancer.

5. Other—In addition to the above effects, a number of other adverse reactions have been reported for which a causal relation has not been established. These include alopecia, erythema multiforme, erythema nodosum, and other skin disorders.

Contraindications & Cautions

These drugs are contraindicated in patients with thrombophlebitis, thromboembolic phenomena, and cardiovascular and cerebrovascular disorders or a past history of these conditions. They should not be used to treat vaginal bleeding when the cause is unknown. They should be avoided in patients with known or suspected tumors of the breast or other estrogen-dependent neoplasms. Since these preparations have caused aggravation of preexisting disorders, they should be avoided or used with caution in patients with liver disease, asthma, eczema, migraine, diabetes, hypertension, optic neuritis, retrobulbar neuritis, or convulsive disorders.

The oral contraceptives may produce edema, and for that reason they should be used with great caution in patients in heart failure or in whom edema is otherwise undesirable or dangerous.

Estrogens may increase the rate of growth of fibroids. Therefore, for women with these tumors, agents with the smallest amounts of estrogen and the most androgenic progestins should be selected. The use of progestational agents alone for contraception might be especially useful in such patients (see below).

These agents are contraindicated in adolescents in whom epiphysial closure has not yet been completed.

Women using oral contraceptives must be made aware of an important interaction that occurs with antimicrobial drugs. Because the normal gastrointestinal flora increase the enterohepatic cycling (and bioavailability) of estrogens, antimicrobial drugs that interfere with these organisms may reduce the efficacy of oral contraceptives. Additionally, coadministration with potent inducers of the hepatic microsomal metabolizing enzymes, such as rifampin, may increase liver catabolism of estrogens or progestins and diminish the efficacy of oral contraceptives.

Contraception with Progestins Alone

Small doses of progestins administered orally or by implantation under the skin can be used for contraception. They are particularly suited for use in patients for whom estrogen administration is undesirable. They are about as effective as intrauterine devices or combination pills containing 20–30 mcg of ethinyl estradiol. There is a high incidence of abnormal bleeding.

Effective contraception can also be achieved by injecting 150 mg of depot medroxyprogesterone acetate (DMPA) every 3 months. After a 150 mg dose, ovulation is inhibited for at least 14 weeks. Almost all users experience episodes of unpredictable spotting and bleeding, particularly during the first year of use. Spotting and bleeding decrease with time, and amenorrhea is common. This preparation is not desirable for women planning a pregnancy soon after cessation of therapy because ovulation suppression can sometimes persist for as long as 18 months after the last injection. Long-term DMPA use reduces menstrual blood loss and is associated with a decreased risk of endometrial cancer. Suppression of endogenous estrogen secretion may be associated with a reversible reduction in bone density, and changes in plasma lipids are associated with an increased risk of atherosclerosis.

The progestin implant method utilizes the subcutaneous implantation of capsules containing etonogestrel. These capsules release one fifth to one third as much steroid as oral agents, are extremely effective, and last for 2–4 years. The low levels of hormone have little effect on lipoprotein and carbohydrate metabolism or blood pressure. The disadvantages include the need for surgical insertion and removal of capsules and some irregular bleeding rather than predictable menses. An association of intracranial hypertension with an earlier type of implant utilizing norgestrel was observed in a small number of women. Patients experiencing headache or visual disturbances should be checked for papilledema.

Contraception with progestins is useful in patients with hepatic disease, hypertension, psychosis or mental retardation, or prior thromboembolism. The side effects include headache, dizziness, bloating and weight gain of 1–2 kg, and a reversible reduction of glucose tolerance.

TABLE 40–4 Schedules for use of postcoital contraceptives.

Conjugated estrogens: 10 mg three times daily for 5 days
Ethinyl estradiol: 2.5 mg twice daily for 5 days
Diethylstilbestrol: 50 mg daily for 5 days
Mifepristone: 600 mg once with misoprostol, 400 mcg once[1]
L-Norgestrel: 0.75 mg twice daily for 1 day (eg, Plan B[2])
Norgestrel, 0.5 mg, with ethinyl estradiol, 0.05 mg (eg, Ovral, Preven[2]): Two tablets and then two in 12 hours

[1]Mifepristone given on day 1, misoprostol on day 3.

[2]Sold as emergency contraceptive kits.

Postcoital Contraceptives

Pregnancy can be prevented following coitus by the administration of estrogens alone, progestin alone, or in combination (**"morning after"** contraception). When treatment is begun within 72 hours, it is effective 99% of the time. Some effective schedules are shown in Table 40–4. The hormones are often administered with antiemetics, since 40% of patients have nausea or vomiting. Other adverse effects include headache, dizziness, breast tenderness, and abdominal and leg cramps.

Mifepristone, an antagonist at progesterone and glucocorticoid receptors, has a luteolytic effect and is effective as a postcoital contraceptive. When combined with a prostaglandin it is also an effective abortifacient.

Beneficial Effects of Oral Contraceptives

It has become apparent that reduction in the dose of the constituents of oral contraceptives has markedly reduced mild and severe adverse effects, providing a relatively safe and convenient method of contraception for many young women. Treatment with oral contraceptives has also been shown to be associated with many benefits unrelated to contraception. These include a reduced risk of ovarian cysts, ovarian and endometrial cancer, and benign breast disease. There is a lower incidence of ectopic pregnancy. Iron deficiency and rheumatoid arthritis are less common, and premenstrual symptoms, dysmenorrhea, endometriosis, acne, and hirsutism may be ameliorated with their use.

■ ESTROGEN & PROGESTERONE INHIBITORS & ANTAGONISTS

TAMOXIFEN & RELATED PARTIAL AGONIST ESTROGENS

Tamoxifen, a competitive partial agonist inhibitor of estradiol at the estrogen receptor (Figure 40–5), was the first **selective estrogen receptor modulator (SERM)** to be introduced. It is extensively used in the palliative treatment of breast cancer in postmenopausal women and is approved for chemoprevention of breast cancer in high-risk women (see Chapter 54). It is a nonsteroidal agent (see structure below) that is given orally. Peak plasma levels are reached in a few hours. Tamoxifen has an initial half-life of 7–14 hours in the circulation and is predominantly excreted by the liver. It is used in doses of 10–20 mg twice daily. Hot flushes and nausea and vomiting occur in 25% of patients, and many other minor adverse effects are observed. Studies of patients treated with tamoxifen as adjuvant therapy for early breast cancer have shown a 35% decrease in contralateral breast cancer. However, adjuvant therapy extended beyond 5 years in patients with breast cancer has shown no further improvement in outcome. **Toremifene** is a structurally similar compound with very similar properties, indications, and toxicities.

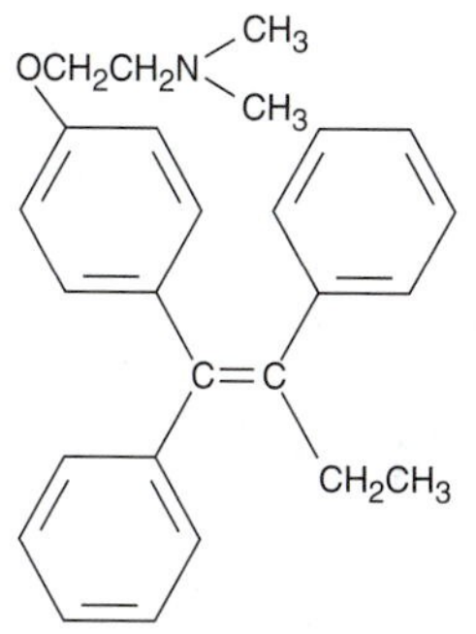

Tamoxifen

Prevention of the expected loss of lumbar spine bone density and plasma lipid changes consistent with a reduction in the risk for atherosclerosis have also been reported in tamoxifen-treated patients following spontaneous or surgical menopause. However, this agonist activity also affects the uterus and may increase the risk of endometrial cancer.

Raloxifene is another partial estrogen agonist-antagonist (SERM) at some but not all target tissues. It has similar effects on lipids and bone but appears not to stimulate the endometrium or breast. Although subject to a high first-pass effect, raloxifene has a very large volume of distribution and a long half-life (>24 hours), so it can be taken once a day. Raloxifene has been approved in the USA for the prevention of postmenopausal osteoporosis and prophylaxis of breast cancer in women with risk factors.

Clomiphene is an older partial agonist, a weak estrogen that also acts as a competitive inhibitor of endogenous estrogens (Figure 40–5). It has found use as an ovulation-inducing agent (see below).

MIFEPRISTONE

Mifepristone is a "19-norsteroid" that binds strongly to the progesterone receptor and inhibits the activity of progesterone. The drug has luteolytic properties in 80% of women when given in the midluteal period. The mechanism of this effect is unknown, but it may provide the basis for using mifepristone as a contraceptive (as opposed to an abortifacient). However, because the compound has a long half-life, large doses may prolong the follicular phase of

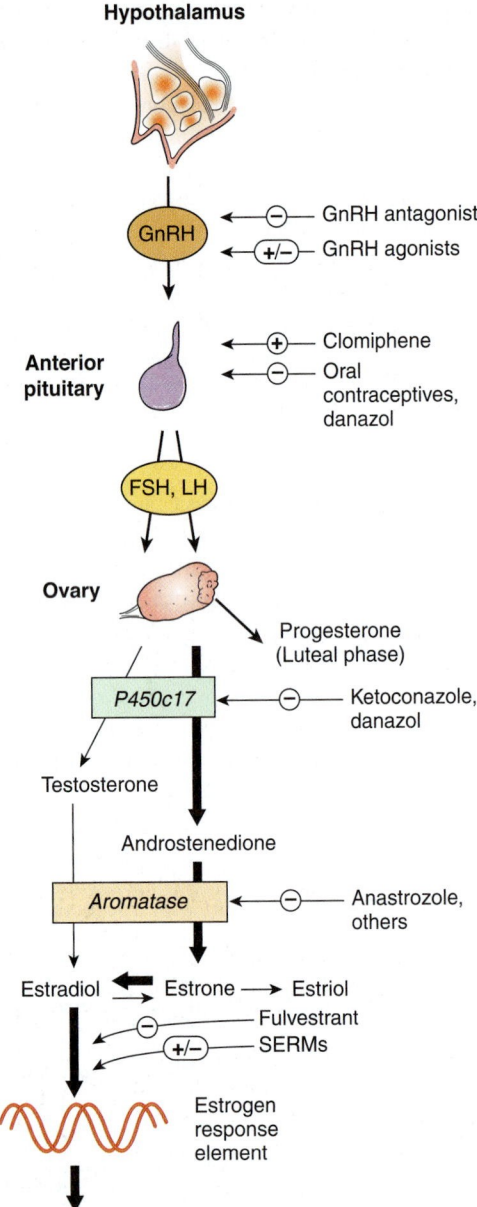

FIGURE 40–5 Control of ovarian secretion and the actions of its hormones. In the follicular phase the ovary produces mainly estrogens; in the luteal phase it produces estrogens and progesterone. SERMs, selective estrogen receptor modulators. See text.

the subsequent cycle and so make it difficult to use continuously for this purpose. A single dose of 600 mg is an effective emergency postcoital contraceptive, though it may result in delayed ovulation in the following cycle. As noted in Chapter 39, the drug also binds to and acts as an antagonist at the glucocorticoid receptor. Limited clinical studies suggest that mifepristone or other analogs with similar properties may be useful in the treatment of endometriosis, Cushing's syndrome, breast cancer, and possibly other neoplasms such as meningiomas that contain glucocorticoid or progesterone receptors.

Mifepristone

Mifepristone's major use thus far has been to terminate early pregnancies. Doses of 400–600 mg/d for 4 days or 800 mg/d for 2 days successfully terminated pregnancy in over 85% of the women studied. The major adverse effect was prolonged bleeding that on most occasions did not require treatment. The combination of a single oral dose of 600 mg of mifepristone and a vaginal pessary containing 1 mg of prostaglandin E_1 or oral misoprostol has been found to effectively terminate pregnancy in over 95% of patients treated during the first 7 weeks after conception. The adverse effects of the medications included vomiting, diarrhea, and abdominal or pelvic pain. As many as 5% of patients have vaginal bleeding requiring intervention. Because of these adverse effects, mifepristone is administered only by physicians at family planning centers. **Note:** In a very small number of cases, use of a vaginal tablet for the prostaglandin dose has been associated with sepsis, so it is recommended that *both* drugs be given by mouth in all patients.

ZK 98734 (lilopristone) is a potent experimental progesterone inhibitor and abortifacient in doses of 25 mg twice daily. Like mifepristone, it also appears to have antiglucocorticoid activity.

DANAZOL

Danazol, an isoxazole derivative of ethisterone (17α-ethinyltestosterone) with weak progestational, androgenic, and glucocorticoid activities, is used to suppress ovarian function. Danazol inhibits the midcycle surge of LH and FSH and can prevent the compensatory increase in LH and FSH following castration in animals, but it does not significantly lower or suppress basal LH or FSH levels in normal women (Figure 40–5). Danazol binds to androgen, progesterone, and glucocorticoid receptors and can translocate the androgen receptor into the nucleus to initiate androgen-specific RNA synthesis. It does not bind to intracellular estrogen receptors, but it does bind to sex hormone-binding and corticosteroid-binding globulins. It inhibits P450scc (the cholesterol side chain-cleaving enzyme), 3β-hydroxysteroid dehydrogenase, 17α-hydroxysteroid dehydrogenase, P450c17 (17α-hydroxylase), P450c11 (11β-hydroxylase), and P450c21 (21β-hydroxylase). However, it does not inhibit aromatase, the enzyme required for estrogen synthesis. It increases the mean clearance of progesterone, probably by competing with the hormone for binding proteins, and may have similar effects on other active steroid hormones. Ethisterone, a major metabolite of danazol, has both progestational and mild androgenic effects.

Danazol is slowly metabolized in humans, having a half-life of over 15 hours. This results in stable circulating levels when the drug is administered twice daily. It is highly concentrated in the liver, adrenals, and kidneys and is excreted in both feces and urine.

Danazol has been employed as an inhibitor of gonadal function and has found its major use in the treatment of endometriosis. For this purpose, it can be given in a dosage of 600 mg/d. The dosage is reduced to 400 mg/d after 1 month and to 200 mg/d in 2 months. About 85% of patients show marked improvement in 3–12 months.

Danazol has also been used in the treatment of fibrocystic disease of the breast and hematologic or allergic disorders, including hemophilia, Christmas disease, idiopathic thrombocytopenic purpura, and angioneurotic edema.

The major adverse effects are weight gain, edema, decreased breast size, acne and oily skin, increased hair growth, deepening of the voice, headache, hot flushes, changes in libido, and muscle cramps. Although mild adverse effects are very common, it is seldom necessary to discontinue the drug because of them. Occasionally, because of its inherent glucocorticoid activity, danazol may cause adrenal suppression.

Danazol should be used with great caution in patients with hepatic dysfunction, since it has been reported to produce mild to moderate hepatocellular damage in some patients, as evidenced by enzyme changes. It is also contraindicated during pregnancy and breast-feeding, as it may produce urogenital abnormalities in the offspring.

OTHER INHIBITORS

Anastrozole, a selective nonsteroidal inhibitor of aromatase (the enzyme required for estrogen synthesis, Figures 40–2 and 40–5), is effective in some women whose breast tumors have become resistant to tamoxifen (see Chapter 54). **Letrozole** is similar. **Exemestane,** a steroid molecule, is an irreversible inhibitor of aromatase. Like anastrozole and letrozole, it is approved for use in women with advanced breast cancer (see Chapter 54).

Several other aromatase inhibitors are undergoing clinical trials in patients with breast cancer. **Fadrozole** is an oral nonsteroidal (triazole) inhibitor of aromatase activity. These compounds appear to be as effective as tamoxifen. In addition to their use in breast cancer, aromatase inhibitors have been successfully employed as adjuncts to androgen antagonists in the treatment of precocious puberty and as primary treatment in the excessive aromatase syndrome.

Fulvestrant is a pure estrogen receptor antagonist that has been somewhat more effective than those with partial agonist effects in some patients who have become resistant to tamoxifen. ICI 164,384 is a newer antagonist; it inhibits dimerization of the occupied estrogen receptor and interferes with its binding to DNA. It has also been used experimentally in breast cancer patients who have become resistant to tamoxifen.

GnRH and its analogs (**nafarelin, buserelin,** etc) have become important in both stimulating and inhibiting ovarian function. They are discussed in Chapter 37.

OVULATION-INDUCING AGENTS

CLOMIPHENE

Clomiphene citrate, a partial estrogen agonist, is closely related to the estrogen chlorotrianisene (Figure 40–3). This compound is well absorbed when taken orally. It has a half-life of 5–7 days and is excreted primarily in the urine. It exhibits significant protein binding and enterohepatic circulation and is distributed to adipose tissues.

Pharmacologic Effects

A. Mechanisms of Action

Clomiphene is a partial agonist at estrogen receptors. The estrogenic agonist effects are best demonstrated in animals with marked gonadal deficiency. Clomiphene has also been shown to effectively inhibit the action of stronger estrogens. In humans it leads to an increase in the secretion of gonadotropins and estrogens by inhibiting estradiol's negative feedback effect on the gonadotropins (Figure 40–5).

B. Effects

The pharmacologic importance of this compound rests on its ability to stimulate ovulation in women with oligomenorrhea or amenorrhea and ovulatory dysfunction. The majority of patients suffer from polycystic ovary syndrome, a common disorder affecting about 7% of women of reproductive age. The syndrome is characterized by gonadotropin-dependent ovarian hyperandrogenism associated with anovulation and infertility. The disorder is frequently accompanied by adrenal hyperandrogenism. Clomiphene probably blocks the feedback inhibitory influence of estrogens on the hypothalamus, causing a surge of gonadotropins, which leads to ovulation.

Clinical Use

Clomiphene is used in the treatment of disorders of ovulation in patients who wish to become pregnant. Usually, a single ovulation is induced by a single course of therapy, and the patient must be treated repeatedly until pregnancy is achieved, since normal ovulatory function does not usually resume. The compound is of no value in patients with ovarian or pituitary failure.

When clomiphene is administered in a dosage of 100 mg/d for 5 days, a rise in plasma LH and FSH is observed after several days. In patients who ovulate, the initial rise is followed by a second rise of gonadotropin levels just prior to ovulation.

Adverse Effects

The most common adverse effects in patients treated with this drug are hot flushes, which resemble those experienced by menopausal patients. They tend to be mild, and disappear when the drug is discontinued. There have been occasional reports of eye symptoms due to intensification and prolongation of afterimages. These are generally of short duration. Headache, constipation, allergic skin reactions, and reversible hair loss have been reported occasionally.

The effective use of clomiphene is associated with some stimulation of the ovaries and usually with ovarian enlargement. The degree of enlargement tends to be greater and its incidence higher in patients who have enlarged ovaries at the beginning of therapy.

A variety of other symptoms such as nausea and vomiting, increased nervous tension, depression, fatigue, breast soreness, weight gain, urinary frequency, and heavy menses have also been reported. However, these appear to result from the hormonal changes associated with an ovulatory menstrual cycle rather than from the medication. The incidence of multiple pregnancy is approximately 10%. Clomiphene has not been shown to have an adverse effect when inadvertently given to women who are already pregnant.

Contraindications & Cautions

Special precautions should be observed in patients with enlarged ovaries. These women are thought to be more sensitive to this drug and should receive small doses. Any patient who complains of abdominal symptoms should be examined carefully. Maximum ovarian enlargement occurs after the 5-day course has been completed, and many patients can be shown to have a palpable increase in ovarian size by the seventh to tenth days. Treatment with clomiphene for more than a year may be associated with an increased risk of low-grade ovarian cancer; however, the evidence for this effect is not conclusive.

Special precautions must also be taken in patients who have visual symptoms associated with clomiphene therapy, since these symptoms may make activities such as driving more hazardous.

OTHER DRUGS USED IN OVULATORY DISORDERS

In addition to clomiphene, a variety of other hormonal and nonhormonal agents are used in treating anovulatory disorders. They are discussed in Chapter 37.

■ THE TESTIS (ANDROGENS & ANABOLIC STEROIDS, ANTIANDROGENS, & MALE CONTRACEPTION)

The testis, like the ovary, has both gametogenic and endocrine functions. The onset of gametogenic function of the testes is controlled largely by the secretion of FSH by the pituitary. High concentrations of testosterone locally are also required for continuing sperm production in the seminiferous tubules. The Sertoli cells in the seminiferous tubules may be the source of the estradiol produced in the testes via aromatization of locally produced

testosterone. With LH stimulation, testosterone is produced by the interstitial or Leydig cells found in the spaces between the seminiferous tubules.

The Sertoli cells in the testis synthesize and secrete a variety of active proteins, including müllerian duct inhibitory factor, inhibin, and activin. As in the ovary, inhibin and activin appear to be the product of three genes that produce a common α subunit and two β subunits, A and B. Activin is composed of the two β subunits $(\beta_A\beta_B)$. There are two inhibins (A and B), which contain the α subunit and one of the β subunits. Activin stimulates pituitary FSH release and is structurally similar to transforming growth factor-β, which also increases FSH. The inhibins in conjunction with testosterone and dihydrotestosterone are responsible for the feedback inhibition of pituitary FSH secretion.

ANDROGENS & ANABOLIC STEROIDS

In humans, the most important androgen secreted by the testis is testosterone. The pathways of synthesis of testosterone in the testes are similar to those previously described for the adrenal gland and ovary (Figures 39–1 and 40–2).

In men, approximately 8 mg of testosterone is produced daily. About 95% is produced by the Leydig cells and only 5% by the adrenals. The testis also secretes small amounts of another potent androgen, dihydrotestosterone, as well as androstenedione and dehydroepiandrosterone, which are weak androgens. Pregnenolone and progesterone and their 17-hydroxylated derivatives are also released in small amounts. Plasma levels of testosterone in males are about 0.6 mcg/dL after puberty and appear to decline after age 50. Testosterone is also present in the plasma of women in concentrations of approximately 0.03 mcg/dL and is derived in approximately equal parts from the ovaries and adrenals and by the peripheral conversion of other hormones.

About 65% of circulating testosterone is bound to sex hormone-binding globulin. SHBG is increased in plasma by estrogen, by thyroid hormone, and in patients with cirrhosis of the liver. It is decreased by androgen and growth hormone and is lower in obese individuals. Most of the remaining testosterone is bound to albumin. Approximately 2% remains free and available to enter cells and bind to intracellular receptors.

METABOLISM

In many target tissues, testosterone is converted to dihydrotestosterone by 5α-reductase. In these tissues, dihydrotestosterone is the major active androgen. The conversion of testosterone to estradiol by P450 aromatase also occurs in some tissues, including adipose tissue, liver, and the hypothalamus, where it may be of importance in regulating gonadal function.

The major pathway for the degradation of testosterone in humans occurs in the liver, with the reduction of the double bond and ketone in the A ring, as is seen in other steroids with a Δ^4-ketone configuration in the A ring. This leads to the production of inactive substances such as androsterone and etiocholanolone that are then conjugated and excreted in the urine.

Androstenedione, dehydroepiandrosterone (DHEA), and dehydroepiandrosterone sulfate (DHEAS) are also produced in significant amounts in humans, although largely in the adrenal gland rather than in the testes. They contribute slightly to the normal maturation process supporting other androgen-dependent pubertal changes in the human, primarily development of pubic and axillary hair and bone maturation. As noted in Chapter 39, some studies suggest that DHEA and DHEAS may have other central nervous system and metabolic effects and may prolong life in rabbits. In men they may improve the sense of well-being and inhibit atherosclerosis. In a placebo-controlled clinical trial in patients with systemic lupus erythematosus, DHEA demonstrated some beneficial effects (see Adrenal Androgens, Chapter 39). Adrenal androgens are to a large extent metabolized in the same fashion as testosterone. Both steroids—but particularly androstenedione—can be converted by peripheral tissues to estrone in very small amounts (1–5%). The P450 aromatase enzyme responsible for this conversion is also found in the brain and is thought to play an important role in development.

Physiologic Effects

In the normal male, testosterone or its active metabolite 5α-dihydrotestosterone is responsible for the many changes that occur in puberty. In addition to the general growth-promoting properties of androgens on body tissues, these hormones are responsible for penile and scrotal growth. Changes in the skin include the appearance of pubic, axillary, and beard hair. The sebaceous glands become more active, and the skin tends to become thicker and oilier. The larynx grows and the vocal cords become thicker, leading to a lower-pitched voice. Skeletal growth is stimulated and epiphysial closure accelerated. Other effects include growth of the prostate and seminal vesicles, darkening of the skin, and increased skin circulation. Androgens play an important role in stimulating and maintaining sexual function in men. Androgens increase lean body mass and stimulate body hair growth and sebum secretion. Metabolic effects include the reduction of hormone binding and other carrier proteins and increased liver synthesis of clotting factors, triglyceride lipase, α_1-antitrypsin, haptoglobin, and sialic acid. They also stimulate renal erythropoietin secretion and decrease HDL levels.

Synthetic Steroids with Androgenic & Anabolic Action

Testosterone, when administered by mouth, is rapidly absorbed. However, it is largely converted to inactive metabolites, and only about one sixth of the dose administered is available in active form. Testosterone can be administered parenterally, but it has a more prolonged absorption time and greater activity in the propionate, enanthate, undecanoate, or cypionate ester forms. These derivatives are hydrolyzed to release free testosterone at the site of injection. Testosterone derivatives alkylated at the 17 position, eg, methyltestosterone and fluoxymesterone, are active when given by mouth.

Testosterone and its derivatives have been used for their anabolic effects as well as in the treatment of testosterone deficiency.

TABLE 40–5 Androgens: Preparations available and relative androgenic:anabolic activity in animals.

Drug	Androgenic Anabolic Activity
Testosterone	1:1
Testosterone cypionate	1:1
Testosterone enanthate	1:1
Methyltestosterone	1:1
Fluoxymesterone	1:2
Oxymetholone	1:3
Oxandrolone	1:3–1:13
Nandrolone decanoate	1:2.5–1:4

Although testosterone and other known active steroids can be isolated in pure form and measured by weight, biologic assays are still used in the investigation of new compounds. In some of these studies in animals, the anabolic effects of the compound as measured by trophic effects on muscles or the reduction of nitrogen excretion may be dissociated from the other androgenic effects. This has led to the marketing of compounds claimed to have anabolic activity associated with only weak androgenic effects. Unfortunately, this dissociation is less marked in humans than in the animals used for testing (Table 40–5), and all are potent androgens.

Pharmacologic Effects

A. Mechanism of Action

Like other steroids, testosterone acts intracellularly in target cells. In skin, prostate, seminal vesicles, and epididymis, it is converted to 5α-dihydrotestosterone by 5α-reductase. In these tissues, dihydrotestosterone is the dominant androgen. The distribution of this enzyme in the fetus is different and has important developmental implications.

Testosterone and dihydrotestosterone bind to the intracellular androgen receptor, initiating a series of events similar to those described above for estradiol and progesterone, leading to growth, differentiation, and synthesis of a variety of enzymes and other functional proteins.

B. Effects

In the male at puberty, androgens cause development of the secondary sex characteristics (see above). In the adult male, large doses of testosterone—when given alone—or its derivatives suppress the secretion of gonadotropins and result in some atrophy of the interstitial tissue and the tubules of the testes. Since fairly large doses of androgens are required to suppress gonadotropin secretion, it has been postulated that inhibin, in combination with androgens, is responsible for the feedback control of secretion. In women, androgens are capable of producing changes similar to those observed in the prepubertal male. These include growth of

TABLE 40–6 Androgen preparations for replacement therapy.

Drug	Route of Administration	Dosage
Methyltestosterone	Oral	25–50 mg/d
	Sublingual (buccal)	5–10 mg/d
Fluoxymesterone	Oral	2–10 mg/d
Testosterone enanthate	Intramuscular	See text
Testosterone cypionate	Intramuscular	See text
Testosterone	Transdermal	2.5–10 mg/d
	Topical gel (1%)	5–10 g/d

facial and body hair, deepening of the voice, enlargement of the clitoris, frontal baldness, and prominent musculature. The natural androgens stimulate erythrocyte production.

The administration of androgens reduces the excretion of nitrogen into the urine, indicating an increase in protein synthesis or a decrease in protein breakdown within the body. This effect is much more pronounced in women and children than in normal men.

Clinical Uses

A. Androgen Replacement Therapy in Men

Androgens are used to replace or augment endogenous androgen secretion in hypogonadal men (Table 40–6). Even in the presence of pituitary deficiency, androgens are used rather than gonadotropin except when normal spermatogenesis is to be achieved. In patients with hypopituitarism, androgens are not added to the treatment regimen until puberty, at which time they are instituted in gradually increasing doses to achieve the growth spurt and the development of secondary sex characteristics. In these patients, therapy should be started with long-acting agents such as testosterone enanthate or cypionate in doses of 50 mg intramuscularly, initially every 4, then every 3, and finally every 2 weeks, with each change taking place at 3-month intervals. The dose is then doubled to 100 mg every 2 weeks until maturation is complete. Finally, it is changed to the adult replacement dose of 200 mg at 2-week intervals.

Testosterone propionate, though potent, has a short duration of action and is not practical for long-term use. Testosterone undecanoate can be given orally, administering large amounts of the steroid twice daily (eg, 40 mg/d); however, this is not recommended because oral testosterone administration has been associated with liver tumors. Testosterone can also be administered transdermally; skin patches or gels are available for scrotal or other skin area application. Two applications daily are usually required for replacement therapy. Implanted pellets and other longer-acting preparations are under study. The development of polycythemia or hypertension may require some reduction in dose.

B. Gynecologic Disorders

Androgens are used occasionally in the treatment of certain gynecologic disorders, but the undesirable effects in women are such that they must be used with great caution. Androgens have been used to reduce breast engorgement during the postpartum period, usually in conjunction with estrogens. The weak androgen danazol is used in the treatment of endometriosis (see above).

Androgens are sometimes given in combination with estrogens for replacement therapy in the postmenopausal period in an attempt to eliminate the endometrial bleeding that may occur when only estrogens are used and to enhance libido. They have been used for chemotherapy of breast tumors in premenopausal women.

C. Use as Protein Anabolic Agents

Androgens and anabolic steroids have been used in conjunction with dietary measures and exercises in an attempt to reverse protein loss after trauma, surgery, or prolonged immobilization and in patients with debilitating diseases.

D. Anemia

In the past, large doses of androgens were employed in the treatment of refractory anemias such as aplastic anemia, Fanconi's anemia, sickle cell anemia, myelofibrosis, and hemolytic anemias. Recombinant erythropoietin has largely replaced androgens for this purpose.

E. Osteoporosis

Androgens and anabolic agents have been used in the treatment of osteoporosis, either alone or in conjunction with estrogens. With the exception of substitution therapy in hypogonadism, bisphosphonates have largely replaced androgen use for this purpose.

F. Use as Growth Stimulators

These agents have been used to stimulate growth in boys with delayed puberty. If the drugs are used carefully, these children will probably achieve their expected adult height. If treatment is too vigorous, the patient may grow rapidly at first but will not achieve full predicted final stature because of the accelerated epiphysial closure that occurs. It is difficult to control this type of therapy adequately even with frequent X-ray examination of the epiphyses, since the action of the hormones on epiphysial centers may continue for many months after therapy is discontinued.

G. Anabolic Steroid and Androgen Abuse in Sports

The use of anabolic steroids by athletes has received worldwide attention. Many athletes and their coaches believe that anabolic steroids—in doses 10–200 times larger than the daily normal physiologic production—increase strength and aggressiveness, thereby improving competitive performance. Such effects have been unequivocally demonstrated only in women. Furthermore, the adverse effects of these drugs clearly make their use inadvisable.

H. Aging

Androgen production falls with age in men and may contribute to the decline in muscle mass, strength, and libido. Preliminary studies of androgen replacement in aging males with low androgen levels show an increase in lean body mass and hematocrit and a decrease in bone turnover. Longer studies will be required to assess the usefulness of this therapy.

Adverse Effects

The adverse effects of these compounds are due largely to their masculinizing actions and are most noticeable in women and pre-pubertal children. In women, the administration of more than 200–300 mg of testosterone per month is usually associated with hirsutism, acne, amenorrhea, clitoral enlargement, and deepening of the voice. These effects may occur with even smaller doses in some women. Some of the androgenic steroids exert progestational activity, leading to endometrial bleeding upon discontinuation. These hormones also alter serum lipids and could conceivably increase susceptibility to atherosclerotic disease in women.

Except under the most unusual circumstances, androgens should not be used in infants. Recent studies in animals suggest that administration of androgens in early life may have profound effects on maturation of central nervous system centers governing sexual development, particularly in the female. Administration of these drugs to pregnant women may lead to masculinization or undermasculinization of the external genitalia in the female and male fetus, respectively. Although the above-mentioned effects may be less marked with the anabolic agents, they do occur.

Sodium retention and edema are not common but must be carefully watched for in patients with heart and kidney disease.

Most of the synthetic androgens and anabolic agents are 17-alkyl-substituted steroids. Administration of drugs with this structure is often associated with evidence of hepatic dysfunction. Hepatic dysfunction usually occurs early in the course of treatment, and the degree is proportionate to the dose. Bilirubin levels may increase until clinical jaundice is apparent. The cholestatic jaundice is reversible upon cessation of therapy, and permanent changes do not occur. In older males, prostatic hyperplasia may develop, causing urinary retention.

Replacement therapy in men may cause acne, sleep apnea, erythrocytosis, gynecomastia, and azoospermia. Supraphysiologic doses of androgens produce azoospermia and decrease in testicular size, both of which may take months to recover after cessation of therapy. The alkylated androgens in high doses can produce peliosis hepatica, cholestasis, and hepatic failure. They lower plasma HDL and may increase LDL. Hepatic adenomas and carcinomas have also been reported. Behavioral effects include psychological dependence, increased aggressiveness, and psychotic symptoms.

Contraindications & Cautions

The use of androgenic steroids is contraindicated in pregnant women or women who may become pregnant during the course of therapy.

Androgens should not be administered to male patients with carcinoma of the prostate or breast. Until more is known about the effects of these hormones on the central nervous system in developing children, they should be avoided in infants and young children.

Special caution is required in giving these drugs to children to produce a growth spurt. In most patients, the use of somatotropin is more appropriate (see Chapter 37).

Care should be exercised in the administration of these drugs to patients with renal or cardiac disease predisposed to edema. If sodium and water retention occurs, it will respond to diuretic therapy.

Methyltestosterone therapy is associated with creatinuria, but the significance of this finding is not known.

Caution: Several cases of hepatocellular carcinoma have been reported in patients with aplastic anemia treated with androgen anabolic therapy. Erythropoietin and colony-stimulating factors (see Chapter 33) should be used instead.

ANDROGEN SUPPRESSION & ANTIANDROGENS

ANDROGEN SUPPRESSION

The treatment of advanced prostatic carcinoma often requires orchiectomy or large doses of estrogens to reduce available endogenous androgen. The psychological effects of the former and gynecomastia produced by the latter make these approaches undesirable. As noted in Chapter 37, the GnRH analogs such as goserelin, nafarelin, buserelin, and leuprolide acetate produce effective gonadal suppression when blood levels are continuous rather than pulsatile (see Chapter 37 and Figure 40–6).

ANTIANDROGENS

The potential usefulness of antiandrogens in the treatment of patients producing excessive amounts of testosterone has led to the search for effective drugs that can be used for this purpose. Several approaches to the problem, especially inhibition of synthesis and receptor antagonism, have met with some success.

Steroid Synthesis Inhibitors

Ketoconazole, used primarily in the treatment of fungal disease, is an inhibitor of adrenal and gonadal steroid synthesis, as described in Chapter 39. It does not affect ovarian aromatase, but it reduces human placental aromatase activity. It displaces estradiol and dihydrotestosterone from sex hormone-binding protein in vitro and increases the estradiol:testosterone ratio in plasma in vivo by a different mechanism. However, it does not appear to be clinically useful in women with increased androgen levels because of the toxicity associated with prolonged use of the 400–800 mg/d required. The drug has also been used experimentally to treat prostatic carcinoma, but the results have not been encouraging. Men treated with ketoconazole often develop reversible gynecomastia during therapy; this may be due to the demonstrated increase in the estradiol:testosterone ratio.

Conversion of Steroid Precursors to Androgens

Several compounds have been developed that inhibit the 17-hydroxylation of progesterone or pregnenolone, thereby preventing the action of the side chain-splitting enzyme and the further transformation of these steroid precursors to active androgens. A few of these compounds have been tested clinically but have been

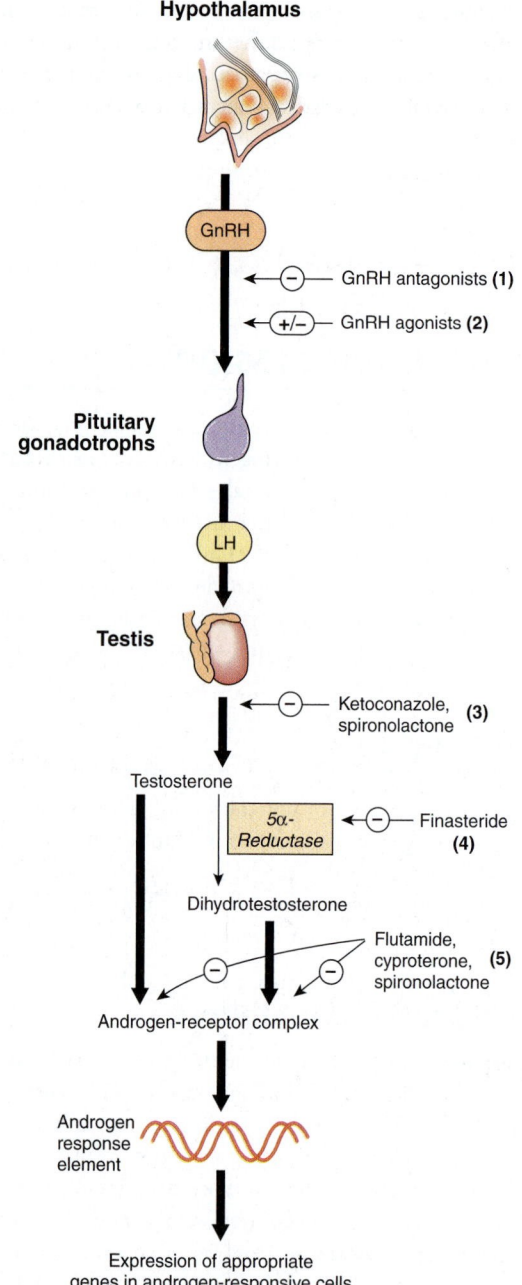

Hypothalamus

GnRH

← ⊖ — GnRH antagonists (1)

← ⊕/⊖ — GnRH agonists (2)

Pituitary gonadotrophs

LH

Testis

← ⊖ — Ketoconazole, spironolactone (3)

Testosterone

5α-Reductase ← ⊖ — Finasteride (4)

Dihydrotestosterone

Flutamide, cyproterone, (5) spironolactone

Androgen-receptor complex

Androgen response element

Expression of appropriate genes in androgen-responsive cells

FIGURE 40–6 Control of androgen secretion and activity and some sites of action of antiandrogens: **(1)** competitive inhibition of GnRH receptors; **(2)** stimulation (+, pulsatile administration) or inhibition via desensitization of GnRH receptors (–, continuous administration); **(3)** decreased synthesis of testosterone in the testis; **(4)** decreased synthesis of dihydrotestosterone by inhibition of 5α-reductase; **(5)** competition for binding to cytosol androgen receptors.

too toxic for prolonged use. As noted in Chapter 39, **abiraterone,** a newer 17-hydroxylase inhibitor, may prove to be clinically successful.

Since dihydrotestosterone—not testosterone—appears to be the essential androgen in the prostate, androgen effects in this and similar dihydrotestosterone-dependent tissues can be reduced by

an inhibitor of 5α-reductase (Figure 40–6). **Finasteride,** a steroid-like inhibitor of this enzyme, is orally active and causes a reduction in dihydrotestosterone levels that begins within 8 hours after administration and lasts for about 24 hours. The half-life is about 8 hours (longer in elderly individuals). Forty to 50 percent of the dose is metabolized; more than half is excreted in the feces. Finasteride has been reported to be moderately effective in reducing prostate size in men with benign prostatic hyperplasia and is approved for this use in the USA. The dosage is 5 mg/d. **Dutasteride** is a similar orally active steroid derivative with a slow onset of action and a much longer half-life than finasteride. The dosage is 0.5 mg daily. These drugs are not approved for use in women or children, although finasteride has been used successfully in the treatment of hirsutism in women and early male pattern baldness in men (1 mg/d).

Finasteride

Receptor Inhibitors

Cyproterone and **cyproterone acetate** are effective antiandrogens that inhibit the action of androgens at the target organ. The acetate form has a marked progestational effect that suppresses the feedback enhancement of LH and FSH, leading to a more effective antiandrogen effect. These compounds have been used in women to treat hirsutism and in men to decrease excessive sexual drive and are being studied in other conditions in which the reduction of androgenic effects would be useful. Cyproterone acetate in a dosage of 2 mg/d administered concurrently with an estrogen is used in the treatment of hirsutism in women, doubling as a contraceptive pill; it has orphan drug status in the USA.

Flutamide, a substituted anilide, is a potent antiandrogen that has been used in the treatment of prostatic carcinoma. Although not a steroid, it behaves like a competitive antagonist at the androgen receptor. It is rapidly metabolized in humans. It frequently causes mild gynecomastia (probably by increasing testicular estrogen production) and occasionally causes mild reversible hepatic toxicity. Administration of this compound causes some improvement in most patients with prostatic carcinoma who have not had prior endocrine therapy. Preliminary studies indicate that flutamide is also useful in the management of excess androgen effect in women.

Flutamide

Bicalutamide and **nilutamide** are potent orally active antiandrogens that can be administered as a single daily dose and are used in patients with metastatic carcinoma of the prostate. Studies in patients with carcinoma of the prostate indicate that these agents are well tolerated. Bicalutamide is recommended for use in combination with a GnRH analog (to reduce tumor flare) and may have fewer gastrointestinal side effects than flutamide. A dosage of 150–200 mg/d (when used alone) is required to reduce prostate-specific antigen levels to those achieved by castration, but, in combination with a GnRH analog, 50 mg/d may be adequate. Nilutamide is approved for use following surgical castration in a dosage of 300 mg/d for 30 days followed by 150 mg/d.

Spironolactone, a competitive inhibitor of aldosterone (see Chapter 15), also competes with dihydrotestosterone for the androgen receptors in target tissues. It also reduces 17α-hydroxylase activity, lowering plasma levels of testosterone and androstenedione. It is used in dosages of 50–200 mg/d in the treatment of hirsutism in women and appears to be as effective as finasteride, flutamide, or cyproterone in this condition.

CHEMICAL CONTRACEPTION IN MEN

Although many studies have been conducted, an effective oral contraceptive for men has not yet been found. For example, various androgens, including testosterone and testosterone enanthate, in a dosage of 400 mg per month, produced azoospermia in less than half the men treated. Minor adverse reactions, including gynecomastia and acne, were encountered. Testosterone in combination with danazol was well tolerated but no more effective than testosterone alone. Androgens in combination with a progestin such as medroxyprogesterone acetate were no more effective. However, preliminary studies indicate that the intramuscular administration of 100 mg of testosterone enanthate weekly together with 500 mg of levonorgestrel daily orally can produce azoospermia in 94% of men.

Cyproterone acetate, a very potent progestin and antiandrogen, also produces oligospermia; however, it does not cause reliable contraception.

At present, pituitary hormones—and potent antagonist analogs of GnRH—are receiving increased attention. A GnRH antagonist in combination with testosterone has been shown to produce reversible azoospermia in nonhuman primates.

GOSSYPOL

Extensive trials of this cottonseed derivative have been conducted in China. This compound destroys elements of the seminiferous epithelium but does not significantly alter the endocrine function of the testis.

In Chinese studies, large numbers of men were treated with 20 mg/d of gossypol or gossypol acetic acid for 2 months, followed by a maintenance dosage of 60 mg/wk. On this regimen, 99% of men developed sperm counts below 4 million/mL. Preliminary data indicate that recovery (return of normal sperm count) following discontinuance of gossypol administration is more apt to occur in men whose counts do not fall to extremely low levels and when administration is not continued for more than 2 years. Hypokalemia is the major adverse effect and may lead to transient paralysis. Because of low efficacy and significant toxicity, gossypol has been abandoned as a candidate male contraceptive.

P R E P A R A T I O N S   A V A I L A B L E [1]

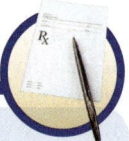

ESTROGENS

Conjugated estrogens (Premarin)
Oral: 0.3, 0.45, 0.625, 0.9, 1.25 mg tablets
Parenteral: 25 mg/5 mL for IM, IV injection
Vaginal: 0.625 mg/g cream base

Diethylstilbestrol (Stilphostrol)
Oral: 50 mg tablets
Parenteral: 0.25 g

Esterified estrogens (Cenestin, Enjuvia, Menest)
Oral: 0.3, 0.45, 0.625, 0.9, 1.25, 2.5 mg tablets

Estradiol cypionate in oil (Depo-Estradiol)
Parenteral: 5 mg/mL for IM injection

Estradiol (generic, Estrace, others)
Oral: 0.45, 0.5, 0.9, 1, 1.5, 1.8, 2 mg tablets
Vaginal: 0.1 mg/g cream, 2 mg ring, 25 mcg tablets

Estradiol transdermal (generic, Estraderm, many others)
Transdermal patch: 0.014, 0.025, 0.0375, 0.05, 0.06, 0.075, 0.1 mg/d release rates
Topical: 2.5 mg/g emulsion (Estrasorb); 0.75 mg/1.25 g unit dose (Estrogel)

Estradiol valerate in oil (generic)
Parenteral: 10, 20, 40 mg/mL for IM injection

Estrone (Menest)
Oral: 0.3, 0.625, 1.25, 2.5 mg tablets

Estropipate (generic, Ogen)
Oral: 0.625, 1.25, 2.5, 5 mg tablets
Vaginal: 1.5 mg/g cream base

PROGESTINS

Levonorgestrel (Norplant)
Kit for subcutaneous implant: 6 capsules of 36 mg each
Intrauterine system: 52 mg

Medroxyprogesterone acetate (generic, Provera)
Oral: 2.5, 5, 10 mg tablets
Parenteral (Depo-Provera): 150, 400 mg/mL for IM injection

Megestrol acetate (generic, Megace)
Oral: 20, 40 mg tablets; 40, 125 mg/mL suspension

Norethindrone acetate (generic, Aygestin)
Oral: 5 mg tablets

Progesterone (generic)
Oral: 100, 200 mg capsules
Topical: 4, 8% vaginal gel, 100 mg insert
Parenteral: 50 mg/mL in oil for IM injection
Intrauterine contraceptive system: 38 mg in silicone

ANDROGENS & ANABOLIC STEROIDS

Fluoxymesterone (generic)
Oral: 10 mg tablets

Methyltestosterone (generic)
Oral: 10, 25 mg tablets; 10 mg capsules; 10 mg buccal tablets

Nandrolone decanoate (generic)
Parenteral: 100, 200 mg/mL in oil for injection

Oxandrolone (Oxandrin)
Oral: 2.5, 10 mg tablets

Oxymetholone (Androl-50)
Oral: 50 mg tablets

Testosterone
Buccal system: 30 mg

Testosterone cypionate in oil (generic, Depo-testosterone)
Parenteral: 100, 200 mg/mL for IM injection

Testosterone enanthate in oil (generic, Delatestryl)
Parenteral: 200 mg/mL for IM injection

Testosterone transdermal system
Patch (Androderm): 2.5, 5 mg/24 h release rate
Gel (AndroGel): 1%

Testosterone pellets (Testopel)
Parenteral: 75 mg/pellet for parenteral injection (not IV)

ANTAGONISTS & INHIBITORS

See also Chapter 37

Anastrozole (Arimidex)
Oral: 1 mg tablets

Bicalutamide (Casodex)
Oral: 50 mg tablets

Clomiphene (generic, Clomid, Serophene, Milophene)
Oral: 50 mg tablets

Danazol (generic, Danocrine)
Oral: 50, 100, 200 mg capsules

Dutasteride (Avodart)
Oral: 0.5 mg tablets

Exemestane (Aromasin)
Oral: 25 mg tablets

Finasteride
Oral: 1 mg tablets (Propecia); 5 mg tablets (Proscar)

Flutamide (Eulexin)
Oral: 125 mg capsules

Fulvestrant (Faslodex)
Parenteral: 50 mg/mL for IM injection

Letrozole (Femara)
Oral: 2.5 mg tablets

Mifepristone (Mifeprex)
Oral: 200 mg tablets

Nilutamide (Nilandron)
Oral: 50, 150 mg tablets

Raloxifene (Evista)
Oral: 60 mg tablets

Tamoxifen (generic, Nolvadex)
Oral: 10, 20 mg tablets; 10 mg/5 mL oral solution

Toremifene (Fareston)
Oral: 60 mg tablets

[1]Oral contraceptives are listed in Table 40–3.

REFERENCES

Acconcia F et al: Palmitoylation-dependent estrogen receptor alpha membrane localization: Regulation by 17beta-estradiol. Mol Biol Cell 2005;16:231.

Anderson GL et al for the Women's Health Initiative Steering Committee: Effects of conjugated equine estrogen in postmenopausal women with hysterectomy. JAMA 2004;291:1701.

Bacopoulou F, Greydanus DE, Chrousos GP: Reproductive and contraceptive issues in chronically ill adolescents. Eur J Contracept Reprod Health Care 2010;15:389.

Bamberger CM, Schulte HM, Chrousos GP: Molecular determinants of glucocorticoid receptor function and tissue sensitivity. Endocr Rev 1996;17:221.

Basaria S et al: Adverse events associated with testosterone administration. N Engl J Med 2010;363:109.

Baulieu E-E: Contragestion and other clinical applications of RU 486, an antiprogesterone at the receptor. Science 1989;245:1351.

Bechlioulis A et al: Endothelial function, but not carotid intima-media thickness, is affected early in menopause and is associated with severity of hot flushes. J Clin Endocrinol Metab 2010;95:1199.

Burkman R, Schlesselman JJ, Zieman M: Safety concerns and health benefits associated with oral contraception. Am J Obstet Gynecol 2004;190 (Suppl 4):S5.

Chlebowski RT et al: Estrogen plus progestin and breast cancer. Incidence and mortality in postmenopausal women. JAMA 2010;304:1684.

Chrousos GP: Perspective: Stress and sex vs. immunity and inflammation. Science Signaling 2010;3:e36.

Chrousos GP, Torpy DJ, Gold PW: Interactions between the hypothalamic-pituitary-adrenal axis and the female reproductive system: Clinical implications. Ann Intern Med 1998;129:229.

Diamanti-Kandarakis E et al: Pathophysiology and types of dyslipidemia in PCOS. Trends Endocrinol Metab 2007;18:280.

Gomes MPV, Deitcher SR: Risk of venous thromboembolic disease associated with hormonal contraceptives and hormone replacement therapy: A clinical review. Arch Intern Med 2004;164:1965.

Hall JM, McDonnell DP, Korach KS: Allosteric regulation of estrogen receptor structure, function, and co-activator recruitment by different estrogen response elements. Mol Endocrinol 2002;16:469.

Harman SM et al: Longitudinal effects of aging on serum total and free testosterone levels in healthy men. Baltimore Longitudinal Study of Aging. J Clin Endocrinol Metab 2001;86:724.

Kalantaridou S, Chrousos GP: Monogenic disorders of puberty. J Clin Endocrinol Metab 2002;87:2481.

Kalantaridou S et al: Premature ovarian failure, endothelial dysfunction, and estrogen-progesterone replacement. Trends Endocrinol Metab 2006;17:101.

Kalantaridou SN et al: Impaired endothelial function in young women with premature ovarian failure: Normalization with hormone therapy. J Clin Endocrinol Metab 2004;89:3907.

Kanaka-Gantenbein C et al: Assisted reproduction and its neuroendocrine impact on the offspring. Prog Brain Res 2010;182C:161.

Manson JE et al: Estrogen plus progestin and the risk of coronary heart disease. N Engl J Med 2003;349:523.

Merke DP et al: Future directions in the study and management of congenital adrenal hyperplasia due to 21-hydroxylase deficiency. Ann Intern Med 2002;136:320.

Mooradian AD, Morley JD, Korenman SG: Biological action of androgens. Endocr Rev 1987;8:1.

Naka KK et al: Effect of the insulin sensitizers metformin and pioglitazone on endothelial function in young women with polycystic ovary syndrome: A prospective randomized study. Fertil Steril 2011;95:203.

Price VH: Treatment of hair loss. N Engl J Med 1999;341:964.

Rossouw JE et al: Risks and benefits of estrogen plus progestin in healthy postmenopausal women: Principal results from the Women's Health Initiative randomized controlled trial. JAMA 2002;288:321.

Smith RE: A review of selective estrogen receptor modulators in national surgical adjuvant breast and bowel project clinical trials. Semin Oncol 2003;30(Suppl 16):4.

Snyder PJ et al: Effect of testosterone replacement in hypogonadal men. J Clin Endocrinol Metab 2000;85:2670.

US Preventive Services Task Force: Hormone therapy for the prevention of chronic conditions in postmenopausal women. Ann Intern Med 2005;142:855.

Wehrmacher WH, Messmore H: Women's Health Initiative is fundamentally flawed. Gend Med 2005;2:4.

Weisberg E: Interactions between oral contraceptives and antifungals/antibacterials. Is contraceptive failure the result? Clin Pharmacokinet 1999;36:309.

Young NR et al: Body composition and muscle strength in healthy men receiving T enanthate for contraception. J Clin Endocrinol Metab 1993;77:1028.

Zandi PP et al: Hormone replacement therapy and incidence of Alzheimer's disease in older women. JAMA 2002;288:2123.

CASE STUDY ANSWER

The patient should be advised to start daily transdermal estradiol therapy (100 mcg/d) along with oral natural progesterone (200 mg/d) for the last 12 days of each 28-day cycle. On this regimen, her symptoms should disappear and normal monthly uterine bleeding resume. She should also be advised to get adequate exercise and increase her calcium and vitamin D intake as treatment for her osteoporosis.

Pancreatic Hormones & Antidiabetic Drugs

Martha S. Nolte Kennedy, MD

CASE STUDY

A 56-year-old Hispanic woman presents to her medical practitioner with symptoms of fatigue, increased thirst, frequent urination, and exercise intolerance with shortness of breath of many months' duration. She does not get regular medical care and is unaware of any medical problems. Her family history is significant for obesity, diabetes, high blood pressure, and coronary artery disease in both parents and several siblings. She is not taking any medications. Five of her six children had a birthweight of over 9 pounds. Physical examination reveals a BMI (body mass index) of 34, blood pressure of 150/90 mm Hg, and evidence of mild peripheral neuropathy. Laboratory tests reveal a random blood sugar of 261 mg/dL; this is confirmed with a fasting plasma glucose of 192 mg/dL. A fasting lipid panel reveals total cholesterol 264 mg/dL, triglycerides 255 mg/dL, high-density lipoproteins 43 mg/dL, and low-density lipoproteins 170 mg/dL. What type of diabetes does this woman have? What further evaluations should be obtained? How would you treat her diabetes?

■ THE ENDOCRINE PANCREAS

The endocrine pancreas in the adult human consists of approximately 1 million islets of Langerhans interspersed throughout the pancreatic gland. Within the islets, at least four hormone-producing cells are present (Table 41–1). Their hormone products include **insulin,** the storage and anabolic hormone of the body; **islet amyloid polypeptide (IAPP, or amylin),** which modulates appetite, gastric emptying, and glucagon and insulin secretion; **glucagon,** the hyperglycemic factor that mobilizes glycogen stores; **somatostatin,** a universal inhibitor of secretory cells; **gastrin,** which stimulates gastric acid secretion; and **pancreatic peptide,** a small protein that facilitates digestive processes by a mechanism not yet clarified.

Diabetes mellitus is defined as an elevated blood glucose associated with absent or inadequate pancreatic insulin secretion, with or without concurrent impairment of insulin action. The disease states underlying the diagnosis of diabetes mellitus are now classified into four categories: type 1, *insulin-dependent diabetes;* type 2, *non–insulin-dependent diabetes;* type 3, *other;* and type 4, *gestational diabetes mellitus* (Expert Committee, 2003).

Type 1 Diabetes Mellitus

The hallmark of type 1 diabetes is selective beta cell (B cell) destruction and *severe* or *absolute* insulin deficiency. Type 1 diabetes is further subdivided into immune and idiopathic causes. The immune form is the most common form of type 1 diabetes. Although most patients are younger than 30 years of age at the time of diagnosis, the onset can occur at any age. Type 1 diabetes is found in all ethnic groups, but the highest incidence is in people from northern Europe and from Sardinia. Susceptibility appears to involve a multifactorial genetic linkage, but only 10–15% of patients have a positive family history.

For persons with type 1 diabetes, insulin replacement therapy is necessary to sustain life. Pharmacologic insulin is administered by injection into the subcutaneous tissue using a manual injection device or an insulin pump that continuously infuses insulin under

TABLE 41–1 Pancreatic islet cells and their secretory products.

Cell Types	Approximate Percent of Islet Mass	Secretory Products
Alpha (A) cell	20	Glucagon, proglucagon
Beta (B) cell	75	Insulin, C-peptide, proinsulin, amylin
Delta (D) cell	3–5	Somatostatin
G cell	1	Gastrin
F cell (PP cell)[1]	1	Pancreatic polypeptide (PP)

[1]Within pancreatic polypeptide-rich lobules of adult islets, located only in the posterior portion of the head of the human pancreas, glucagon cells are scarce (< 0.5%) and F cells make up as much as 80% of the cells.

the skin. Interruption of the insulin replacement therapy can be life-threatening and can result in **diabetic ketoacidosis** or death. Diabetic ketoacidosis is caused by insufficient or absent insulin and results from excess release of fatty acids and subsequent formation of toxic levels of ketoacids.

Type 2 Diabetes Mellitus

Type 2 diabetes is characterized by tissue resistance to the action of insulin combined with a *relative* deficiency in insulin secretion. A given individual may have more resistance or more beta-cell deficiency, and the abnormalities may be mild or severe. Although insulin is produced by the beta cells in these patients, it is inadequate to overcome the resistance, and the blood glucose rises. The impaired insulin action also affects fat metabolism, resulting in increased free fatty acid flux and triglyceride levels and reciprocally low levels of high-density lipoprotein (HDL).

Individuals with type 2 diabetes may not require insulin to survive, but 30% or more will benefit from insulin therapy to control blood glucose. It is likely that 10–20% of individuals in whom type 2 diabetes was initially diagnosed actually have both type 1 and type 2 or a slowly progressing type 1 called latent autoimmune diabetes of adults (LADA), and they ultimately require full insulin replacement. Although persons with type 2 diabetes ordinarily do not

develop ketosis, ketoacidosis may occur as the result of stress such as infection or the use of medication that enhances resistance, eg, corticosteroids. Dehydration in individuals with untreated or poorly controlled type 2 diabetes can lead to a life-threatening condition called **nonketotic hyperosmolar coma**. In this condition, the blood glucose may rise to 6–20 times the normal range and an altered mental state develops or the person loses consciousness. Urgent medical care and rehydration are required.

Type 3 Diabetes Mellitus

The type 3 designation refers to multiple *other* specific causes of an elevated blood glucose: pancreatectomy, pancreatitis, nonpancreatic diseases, drug therapy, etc. For a detailed list the reader is referred to the reference Expert Committee, 2003.

Type 4 Diabetes Mellitus

Gestational diabetes (GDM) is defined as any abnormality in glucose levels noted for the first time during pregnancy. Gestational diabetes is diagnosed in approximately 7% of all pregnancies in the USA. During pregnancy, the placenta and placental hormones create an insulin resistance that is most pronounced in the last trimester. Risk assessment for diabetes is suggested starting at the first prenatal visit. High-risk women should be screened immediately. Screening may be deferred in lower-risk women until the 24th to 28th week of gestation.

■ INSULIN

Chemistry

Insulin is a small protein with a molecular weight in humans of 5808. It contains 51 amino acids arranged in two chains (A and B) linked by disulfide bridges; there are species differences in the amino acids of both chains. Proinsulin, a long single-chain protein molecule, is processed within the Golgi apparatus of beta cells and packaged into granules, where it is hydrolyzed into insulin and a residual connecting segment called C-peptide by removal of four amino acids (Figure 41–1).

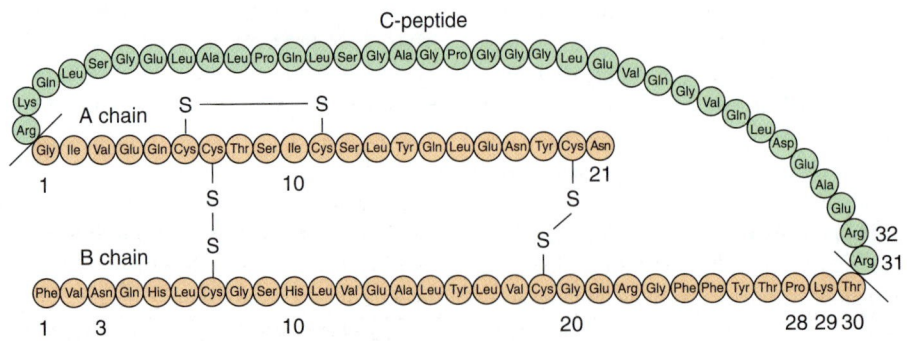

FIGURE 41–1 Structure of human proinsulin (C-peptide plus A and B chains) and insulin. Insulin is shown as the shaded (orange color) peptide chains, A and B. Differences in the A and B chains and amino acid modifications for the rapid-acting insulin analogs (aspart, lispro, and glulisine) and long-acting insulin analogs (glargine and detemir) are discussed in the text.

Insulin and C-peptide are secreted in equimolar amounts in response to all insulin secretagogues; a small quantity of unprocessed or partially hydrolyzed proinsulin is released as well. Although proinsulin may have some mild hypoglycemic action, C-peptide has no known physiologic function. Granules within the beta cells store the insulin in the form of crystals consisting of two atoms of zinc and six molecules of insulin. The entire human pancreas contains up to 8 mg of insulin, representing approximately 200 biologic units. Originally, the unit was defined on the basis of the hypoglycemic activity of insulin in rabbits. With improved purification techniques, the unit is presently defined on the basis of weight, and present insulin standards used for assay purposes contain 28 units per milligram.

Insulin Secretion

Insulin is released from pancreatic beta cells at a low basal rate and at a much higher stimulated rate in response to a variety of stimuli, especially glucose. Other stimulants such as other sugars (eg, mannose), amino acids (especially gluconeogenic amino acids, eg, leucine, arginine), hormones such as glucagon-like polypeptide-1 (GLP-1), glucose-dependent insulinotropic polypeptide (GIP), glucagon, cholecystokinin, high concentrations of fatty acids, and β-adrenergic sympathetic activity are recognized. Stimulatory drugs are sulfonylureas, meglitinide and nateglinide, isoproterenol, and acetylcholine. Inhibitory signals are hormones including insulin itself and leptin, α-adrenergic sympathetic activity, chronically elevated glucose, and low concentrations of fatty acids. Inhibitory drugs include diazoxide, phenytoin, vinblastine, and colchicine.

One mechanism of stimulated insulin release is diagrammed in Figure 41–2. As shown in the figure, hyperglycemia results in increased intracellular ATP levels, which close the ATP-dependent potassium channels. Decreased outward potassium efflux results in depolarization of the beta cell and opening of voltage-gated calcium channels. The resulting increased intracellular calcium triggers secretion of the hormone. The insulin secretagogue drug group (sulfonylureas, meglitinides, and D-phenylalanine) exploits parts of this mechanism.

Insulin Degradation

The liver and kidney are the two main organs that remove insulin from the circulation. The liver normally clears the blood of approximately 60% of the insulin released from the pancreas by virtue of its location as the terminal site of portal vein blood flow, with the kidney removing 35–40% of the endogenous hormone. However, in insulin-treated diabetics receiving subcutaneous insulin injections, this ratio is reversed, with as much as 60% of exogenous insulin being cleared by the kidney and the liver removing no more than 30–40%. The half-life of circulating insulin is 3–5 minutes.

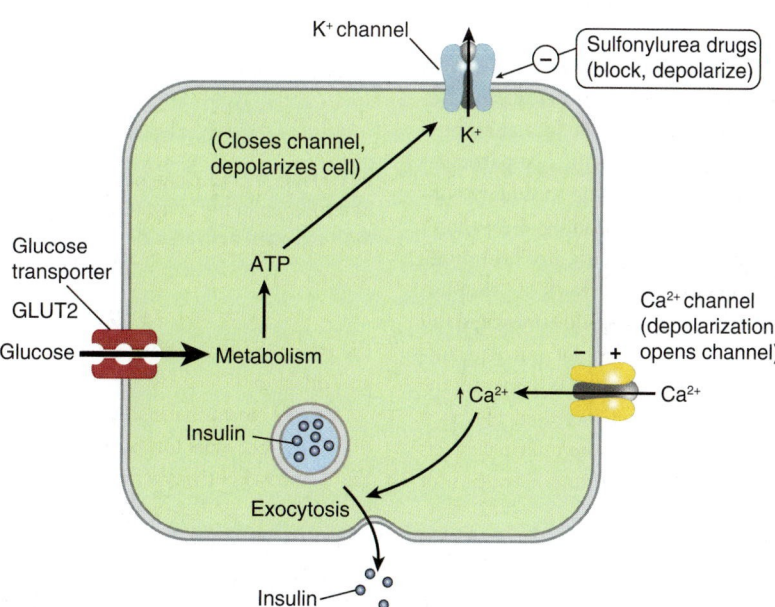

FIGURE 41–2 One model of control of insulin release from the pancreatic beta cell by glucose and by sulfonylurea drugs. In the resting cell with normal (low) ATP levels, potassium diffuses down its concentration gradient through ATP-gated potassium channels, maintaining the intracellular potential at a fully polarized, negative level. Insulin release is minimal. If glucose concentration rises, ATP production increases, potassium channels close, and depolarization of the cell results. As in muscle and nerve, voltage-gated calcium channels open in response to depolarization, allowing more calcium to enter the cell. Increased intracellular calcium results in increased insulin secretion. Insulin secretagogues close the ATP-dependent potassium channel, thereby depolarizing the membrane and causing increased insulin release by the same mechanism. (Modified and reproduced, with permission, from *Basic & Clinical Endocrinology*, 4th ed. Greenspan F, Baxter JD [editors]: Originally published by Appleton & Lange. Copyright © 1994 by The McGraw-Hill Companies, Inc.)

Circulating Insulin

Basal insulin values of 5–15 μU/mL (30–90 pmol/L) are found in normal humans, with a peak rise to 60–90 μU/mL (360–540 pmol/L) during meals.

The Insulin Receptor

After insulin has entered the circulation, it diffuses into tissues, where it is bound by specialized receptors that are found on the membranes of most tissues. The biologic responses promoted by these insulin-receptor complexes have been identified in the primary target tissues, ie, liver, muscle, and adipose tissue. The receptors bind insulin with high specificity and affinity in the picomolar range. The full insulin receptor consists of two covalently linked heterodimers, each containing an α subunit, which is entirely extracellular and constitutes the recognition site, and a β subunit that spans the membrane (Figure 41–3). The β subunit contains a tyrosine kinase. The binding of an insulin molecule to the α subunits at the outside surface of the cell activates the receptor and through a conformational change brings the catalytic loops of the opposing cytoplasmic β subunits into closer proximity. This facilitates mutual phosphorylation of tyrosine residues on the β subunits and tyrosine kinase activity directed at cytoplasmic proteins.

The first proteins to be phosphorylated by the activated receptor tyrosine kinases are the docking proteins, insulin receptor substrates (IRS). After tyrosine phosphorylation at several critical sites, the IRS molecules bind to and activate other kinases—most significantly phosphatidylinositol-3-kinase—which produce further phosphorylations. Alternatively, they may bind to an adaptor protein such as growth factor receptor-binding protein 2, which translates the insulin signal to a guanine nucleotide-releasing factor that ultimately activates the GTP binding protein, ras, and the mitogen-activated protein kinase (MAPK) system. The particular IRS-phosphorylated tyrosine kinases have binding specificity with downstream molecules based on their surrounding 4–5 amino acid sequences or motifs that recognize specific Src homology 2 (SH2) domains on the other protein. This network of phosphorylations within the cell represents insulin's second message and results in multiple effects, including translocation of glucose transporters (especially GLUT 4, Table 41–2) to the cell membrane with a resultant increase in glucose uptake; increased glycogen synthase activity and increased glycogen formation; multiple effects on protein synthesis, lipolysis, and lipogenesis; and activation of

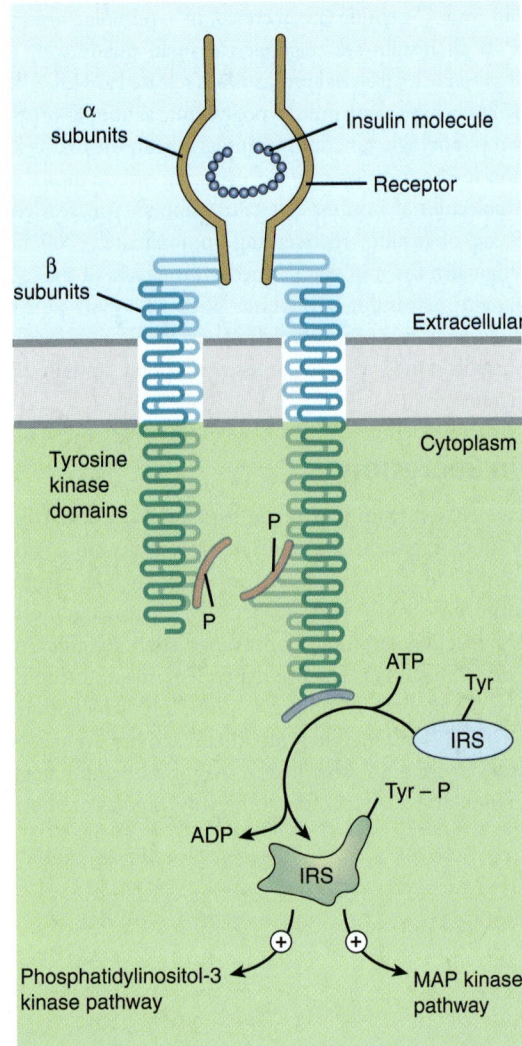

FIGURE 41–3 Schematic diagram of the insulin receptor heterodimer in the activated state. IRS, insulin receptor substrate; MAP, mitogen-activated protein; P, phosphate; Tyr, tyrosine.

transcription factors that enhance DNA synthesis and cell growth and division.

Various hormonal agents (eg, glucocorticoids) lower the affinity of insulin receptors for insulin; growth hormone in excess increases this affinity slightly. Aberrant serine and threonine phosphorylation

TABLE 41–2 Glucose transporters.

Transporter	Tissues	Glucose K$_m$ (mmol/L)	Function
GLUT 1	All tissues, especially red cells, brain	1–2	Basal uptake of glucose; transport across the blood-brain barrier
GLUT 2	Beta cells of pancreas; liver, kidney; gut	15–20	Regulation of insulin release, other aspects of glucose homeostasis
GLUT 3	Brain, placenta	< 1	Uptake into neurons, other tissues
GLUT 4	Muscle, adipose	≈ 5	Insulin-mediated uptake of glucose
GLUT 5	Gut, kidney	1–2	Absorption of fructose

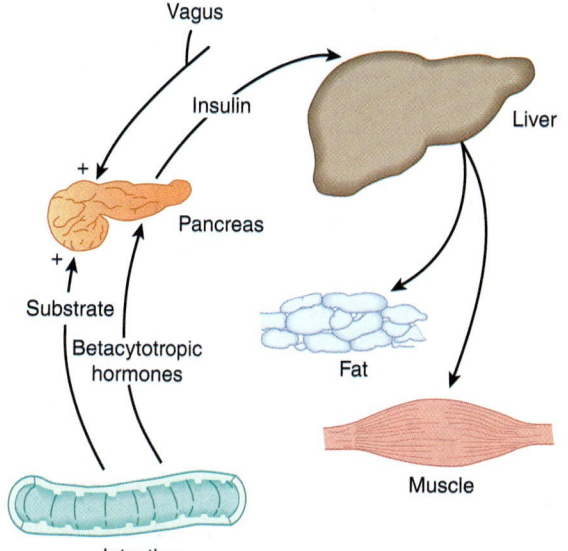

FIGURE 41–4 Insulin promotes synthesis (from circulating nutrients) and storage of glycogen, triglycerides, and protein in its major target tissues: liver, fat, and muscle. The release of insulin from the pancreas is stimulated by increased blood glucose, incretins, vagal nerve stimulation, and other factors (see text).

TABLE 41–3 Endocrine effects of insulin.

Effect on liver:
Reversal of catabolic features of insulin deficiency
Inhibits glycogenolysis
Inhibits conversion of fatty acids and amino acids to keto acids
Inhibits conversion of amino acids to glucose
Anabolic action
Promotes glucose storage as glycogen (induces glucokinase and glycogen synthase, inhibits phosphorylase)
Increases triglyceride synthesis and very-low-density lipoprotein formation
Effect on muscle:
Increased protein synthesis
Increases amino acid transport
Increases ribosomal protein synthesis
Increased glycogen synthesis
Increases glucose transport
Induces glycogen synthase and inhibits phosphorylase
Effect on adipose tissue:
Increased triglyceride storage
Lipoprotein lipase is induced and activated by insulin to hydrolyze triglycerides from lipoproteins
Glucose transport into cell provides glycerol phosphate to permit esterification of fatty acids supplied by lipoprotein transport
Intracellular lipase is inhibited by insulin

of the insulin receptor β subunits or IRS molecules may result in insulin resistance and functional receptor down-regulation.

Effects of Insulin on Its Targets

Insulin promotes the storage of fat as well as glucose (both sources of energy) within specialized target cells (Figure 41–4) and influences cell growth and the metabolic functions of a wide variety of tissues (Table 41–3).

Characteristics of Available Insulin Preparations

Commercial insulin preparations differ in a number of ways, such as differences in the recombinant DNA production techniques, amino acid sequence, concentration, solubility, and the time of onset and duration of their biologic action.

A. Principal Types and Duration of Action of Insulin Preparations

Four principal types of injected insulins are available: (1) rapid-acting, with very fast onset and short duration; (2) short-acting, with rapid onset of action; (3) intermediate-acting; and (4) long-acting, with slow onset of action (Figure 41–5, Table 41–4). Injected rapid-acting and short-acting insulins are dispensed as clear solutions at neutral pH and contain small amounts of zinc to improve their stability and shelf life. Injected intermediate-acting NPH insulins have been modified to provide prolonged action and are dispensed as a turbid suspension at neutral pH with protamine in phosphate buffer (neutral protamine Hagedorn [NPH] insulin). Insulin glargine and insulin detemir are clear, soluble long-acting insulins.

The goal of subcutaneous insulin therapy is to replicate normal physiologic insulin secretion and replace the background or basal (overnight, fasting, and between-meal) as well as bolus or prandial (mealtime) insulin. An exact reproduction of the normal glycemic profile is not technically possible because of the limitations inherent in subcutaneous administration of insulin. Current regimens generally use insulin analogs because of their more predictable action. Intensive therapy ("tight control") attempts to restore near-normal glucose patterns throughout the day while minimizing the risk of hypoglycemia.

Intensive regimens involving multiple daily injections (MDI) use long-acting insulin analogs to provide basal or background coverage, and rapid-acting insulin analogs to meet the mealtime requirements. The latter insulins are given as supplemental doses to correct transient hyperglycemia. The most sophisticated insulin regimen delivers rapid-acting insulin analogs through a continuous subcutaneous insulin infusion device. Conventional therapy consists of split-dose injections of mixtures of rapid- or short-acting and intermediate-acting insulins.

1. Rapid-acting insulin—Three injected rapid-acting insulin analogs—**insulin lispro, insulin aspart,** and **insulin glulisine**—are commercially available. The rapid-acting insulins permit more physiologic prandial insulin replacement because their rapid onset

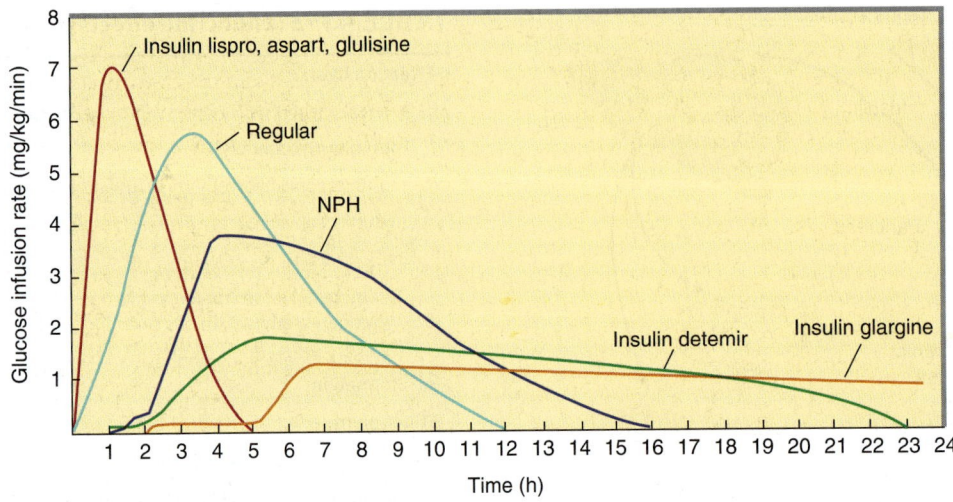

FIGURE 41–5 Extent and duration of action of various types of insulin as indicated by the glucose infusion rates (mg/kg/min) required to maintain a constant glucose concentration. The durations of action shown are typical of an average dose of 0.2–0.3 U/kg. The durations of regular and NPH insulin increase considerably when dosage is increased.

TABLE 41–4 Some insulin preparations available in the USA.[1]

Preparation	Species Source	Concentration
Rapid-acting insulins		
Insulin lispro, Humalog (Lilly)	Human analog	U100
Insulin aspart, Novolog (Novo Nordisk)	Human analog	U100
Insulin glulisine, Apidra (Aventis)	Human analog	U100
Short-acting insulins		
Regular Novolin R (Novo Nordisk)	Human	U100
Regular Humulin R (Lilly)	Human	U100, U500
Intermediate-acting insulins		
NPH Humulin N (Lilly)	Human	U100
NPH Novolin N (Novo Nordisk)	Human	U100
Premixed insulins		
Novolin 70 NPH/30 regular (Novo Nordisk)	Human	U100
Humulin 70 NPH/30 regular (Lilly)	Human	U100
75/25 NPL, Lispro (Lilly)	Human analog	U100
70/30 NPA, Aspart (Novo Nordisk)	Human analog	U100
Long-acting insulins		
Insulin detemir, Levemir (Novo Nordisk)	Human analog	U100
Insulin glargine, Lantus (Aventis/Hoechst Marion Roussel)	Human analog	U100

[1]These agents (except insulin lispro, insulin aspart, insulin detemir, insulin glargine, insulin glulisine, and U500 regular Humulin) are available without a prescription. All insulins should be refrigerated and brought to room temperature just before injection.

NPL, neutral protamine lispro; NPA, neutral protamine aspart.

and early peak action more closely mimic normal endogenous prandial insulin secretion than does regular insulin, and they have the additional benefit of allowing insulin to be taken immediately before the meal without sacrificing glucose control. Their duration of action is rarely more than 4–5 hours, which decreases the risk of late postmeal hypoglycemia. The injected rapid-acting insulins have the lowest variability of absorption (approximately 5%) of all available commercial insulins (compared with 25% for regular insulin and 25% to over 50% for long-acting analog formulations and intermediate insulin, respectively). They are the preferred insulins for use in continuous subcutaneous insulin infusion devices.

Insulin lispro, the first monomeric insulin analog to be marketed, is produced by recombinant technology wherein two amino acids near the carboxyl terminal of the B chain have been reversed in position: Proline at position B28 has been moved to B29, and lysine at position B29 has been moved to B28 (Figure 41–1). Reversing these two amino acids does not interfere in any way with insulin lispro's binding to the insulin receptor, its circulating half-life, or its immunogenicity, which are similar to those of human regular insulin. However, the advantage of this analog is its very low propensity—in contrast to human insulin—to self-associate in antiparallel fashion and form dimers. To enhance the shelf life of insulin in vials, insulin lispro is stabilized into hexamers by a cresol preservative. When injected subcutaneously, the drug quickly dissociates into monomers and is rapidly absorbed with onset of action within 5–15 minutes and peak activity as early as 1 hour. The time to peak action is relatively constant, regardless of the dose.

Insulin aspart is created by the substitution of the B28 proline with a negatively charged aspartic acid (Figure 41–1). This modification reduces the normal ProB28 and GlyB23 monomer-monomer interaction, thereby inhibiting insulin self-aggregation. Its absorption and activity profile are similar to those of insulin lispro, and it is more reproducible than regular insulin, but it has binding properties, activity, and mitogenicity characteristics similar to those of regular insulin in addition to equivalent immunogenicity.

Insulin glulisine is formulated by substituting a lysine for asparagine at B3 and glutamic acid for lysine at B29. Its absorption, action, and immunologic characteristics are similar to those of other injected rapid-acting insulins. After high-dose insulin glulisine interaction with the insulin receptor, there may be downstream differences in IRS-2 pathway activation relative to human insulin. The clinical significance of such differences is unclear.

2. Short-acting insulin—Regular insulin is a short-acting soluble crystalline zinc insulin that is now made by recombinant DNA techniques to produce a molecule identical to that of human insulin. Its effect appears within 30 minutes, peaks between 2 and 3 hours after subcutaneous injection, and generally lasts 5–8 hours. In high concentrations, eg, in the vial, regular insulin molecules self-aggregate in antiparallel fashion to form dimers that stabilize around zinc ions to create insulin hexamers. The hexameric nature of regular insulin causes a delayed onset and prolongs the time to peak action. After subcutaneous injection, the insulin hexamers

are too large and bulky to be transported across the vascular endothelium into the bloodstream. As the insulin depot is diluted by interstitial fluid and the concentration begins to fall, the hexamers break down into dimers and finally monomers. This results in three rates of absorption of the injected insulin, with the final monomeric phase having the fastest uptake out of the injection site.

The clinical consequence is that when regular insulin is administered at mealtime, the blood glucose rises faster than the insulin with resultant early postprandial hyperglycemia and an increased risk of late postprandial hypoglycemia. Therefore, regular insulin should be injected 30–45 or more minutes before the meal to minimize the mismatching. As with all older insulin formulations, the duration of action as well as the time of onset and the intensity of peak action increase with the size of the dose. Clinically, this is a critical issue because the pharmacokinetics and pharmacodynamics of small doses of regular and NPH insulins differ greatly from those of large doses. The delayed absorption, dose-dependent duration of action, and variability of absorption (~ 25%) of regular human insulin frequently results in a mismatching of insulin availability with need, and its use is declining.

However, short-acting, regular soluble insulin is the only type that should be administered intravenously because the dilution causes the hexameric insulin to immediately dissociate into monomers. It is particularly useful for intravenous therapy in the management of diabetic ketoacidosis and when the insulin requirement is changing rapidly, such as after surgery or during acute infections.

3. Intermediate-acting and long-acting insulins

a. NPH (neutral protamine Hagedorn, or isophane) insulin— NPH insulin is an intermediate-acting insulin whose absorption and onset of action are delayed by combining appropriate amounts of insulin and protamine so that neither is present in an uncomplexed form ("isophane"). After subcutaneous injection, proteolytic tissue enzymes degrade the protamine to permit absorption of insulin. NPH insulin has an onset of approximately 2–5 hours and duration of 4–12 hours (Figure 41–5); it is usually mixed with regular, lispro, aspart, or glulisine insulin and given two to four times daily for insulin replacement. The dose regulates the action profile; specifically, small doses have lower, earlier peaks and a short duration of action with the converse true for large doses. The action of NPH is highly unpredictable, and its variability of absorption is over 50%. The clinical use of NPH is waning because of its adverse pharmacokinetics combined with the availability of long-acting insulin analogs that have a more predictable and physiologic action.

b. Insulin glargine—Insulin glargine is a soluble, "peakless" (ie, having a broad plasma concentration plateau), long-acting insulin analog. This product was designed to provide reproducible, convenient, background insulin replacement. The attachment of two arginine molecules to the B-chain carboxyl terminal and substitution of a glycine for asparagine at the A21 position created an analog that is soluble in an acidic solution but precipitates in the more neutral body pH after subcutaneous injection. Individual insulin molecules slowly dissolve away from the crystalline depot and provide a low, continuous level of circulating insulin. Insulin glargine has a slow onset of action (1–1.5 hours) and achieves a maximum effect after 4–6 hours. This maximum activity is maintained for 11–24 hours or longer. Glargine is usually given once daily, although some very insulin-sensitive or insulin-resistant individuals benefit from split (twice a day) dosing. To maintain solubility, the formulation is unusually acidic (pH 4.0), and insulin glargine should not be mixed with other insulins. Separate syringes must be used to minimize the risk of contamination and subsequent loss of efficacy. The absorption pattern of insulin glargine appears to be independent of the anatomic site of injection, and this drug is associated with less immunogenicity than human insulin in animal studies. Glargine's interaction with the insulin receptor is similar to that of native insulin and shows no increase in mitogenic activity in vitro. It has sixfold to sevenfold greater binding than native insulin to the insulin-like growth factor-1 (IGF-1) receptor, but the clinical significance of this is unclear.

c. Insulin detemir—This insulin is the most recently developed long-acting insulin analog. The terminal threonine is dropped from the B30 position and myristic acid (a C-14 fatty acid chain) is attached to the terminal B29 lysine. These modifications prolong the availability of the injected analog by increasing both self-aggregation in subcutaneous tissue and reversible albumin binding. Insulin detemir has the most reproducible effect of the intermediate- and long-acting insulins, and its use is associated with less hypoglycemia than NPH insulin. Insulin detemir has a dose-dependent onset of action of 1–2 hours and duration of action of more than 12 hours. It is given twice daily to obtain a smooth background insulin level.

4. Mixtures of insulins—Because intermediate-acting NPH insulins require several hours to reach adequate therapeutic levels, their use in diabetic patients usually requires supplements of rapid- or short-acting insulin before meals. For convenience, these are often mixed together in the same syringe before injection. Insulin lispro, aspart, and glulisine can be *acutely* mixed (ie, just before injection) with NPH insulin without affecting their rapid absorption. However, *premixed* preparations have thus far been unstable. To remedy this, intermediate insulins composed of isophane complexes of protamine with insulin lispro and insulin aspart have been developed. These intermediate insulins have been designated as "NPL" (neutral protamine lispro) and "NPA" (neutral protamine aspart) and have the same duration of action as NPH insulin. They have the advantage of permitting formulation as premixed combinations of NPL and insulin lispro, and as NPA and insulin aspart, and they have been shown to be safe and effective in clinical trials. The Food and Drug Administration (FDA) has approved 50%/50% and 75%/25% NPL/insulin lispro and 70%/30% NPA/insulin aspart premixed formulations. Additional ratios are available abroad. Insulin glargine and detemir must be given as separate injections. They are not miscible acutely or in a premixed preparation with any other insulin formulation.

Premixed formulations of 70%/30% NPH/regular continue to be available. These preparations have all the limitations of regular

insulin, namely, highly dose dependent pharmacokinetic and pharmacodynamic profiles, and variability in absorption.

B. Insulin Production

Mass production of human insulin and insulin analogs by recombinant DNA techniques is carried out by inserting the human or a modified human proinsulin gene into *Escherichia coli* or yeast and treating the extracted proinsulin to form the insulin or insulin analog molecules.

C. Concentration

All insulins in the USA and Canada are available in a concentration of 100 U/mL (U100). A limited supply of U500 regular human insulin is available for use in rare cases of severe insulin resistance in which larger doses of insulin are required.

Insulin Delivery Systems

A. Standard Delivery

The standard mode of insulin therapy is subcutaneous injection using conventional disposable needles and syringes.

B. Portable Pen Injectors

To facilitate multiple subcutaneous injections of insulin, particularly during intensive insulin therapy, portable pen-sized injectors have been developed. These contain cartridges of insulin and replaceable needles.

Disposable insulin pens are also available for selected formulations. These are regular insulin, insulin lispro, insulin aspart, insulin glulisine, insulin glargine, insulin detemir, and several mixtures of NPH with regular, lispro, or aspart insulin (Table 41–4). They have been well accepted by patients because they eliminate the need to carry syringes and bottles of insulin to the workplace and while traveling.

C. Continuous Subcutaneous Insulin Infusion Devices (CSII, Insulin Pumps)

Continuous subcutaneous insulin infusion devices are external open-loop pumps for insulin delivery. The devices have a user-programmable pump that delivers individualized basal and bolus insulin replacement doses based on blood glucose self-monitoring results.

Normally, the 24-hour background basal rates are preprogrammed and relatively constant from day to day, although temporarily altered rates can be superimposed to adjust for a short-term change in requirement. For example, the basal delivery rate might need to be decreased for several hours because of the increased insulin sensitivity associated with strenuous activity.

Boluses are used to correct high blood glucose levels and to cover mealtime insulin requirements based on the carbohydrate content of the food and concurrent activity. Bolus amounts are either dynamically programmed or use preprogrammed algorithms. When the boluses are dynamically programmed, the user calculates the dose based on the amount of carbohydrate consumed and the current blood glucose level. Alternatively, the meal or snack dose algorithm (grams of carbohydrate covered by a unit of insulin) and insulin sensitivity or blood glucose correction factor (fall in blood glucose level in response to a unit of insulin) can be preprogrammed into the pump. If the user enters the carbohydrate content of the food and current blood glucose value, the insulin pump will calculate the most appropriate dose of insulin. Advanced insulin pumps also have an "insulin on board" feature that adjusts a high blood glucose correction dose to correct for residual activity of previous bolus doses.

The traditional pump—which contains an insulin reservoir, the program chip, the keypad, and the display screen—is about the size of a pager. It is usually placed on a belt or in a pocket, and the insulin is infused through thin plastic tubing that is connected to the subcutaneously inserted infusion set. The abdomen is the favored site for the infusion set, although flanks and thighs are also used. The insulin reservoir, tubing, and infusion set need to be changed using sterile techniques every 2 or 3 days. Currently, only one pump does not require tubing. In this model, the pump is attached directly to the infusion set. Programming is done through a hand-held unit that communicates wirelessly with the pump. CSII delivery is regarded as the most physiologic method of insulin replacement.

Use of these continuous infusion devices is encouraged for people who are unable to obtain target control while on multiple injection regimens and in circumstances in which excellent glycemic control is desired, such as during pregnancy. Optimal use of these devices requires responsible involvement and commitment by the patient. Insulin aspart, lispro, and glulisine all are specifically approved for pump use and are preferred pump insulins because their favorable pharmacokinetic attributes allow glycemic control without increasing the risk of hypoglycemia.

Treatment with Insulin

The current classification of diabetes mellitus identifies a group of patients who have virtually no insulin secretion and whose survival depends on administration of exogenous insulin. This insulin-dependent group (type 1) represents 5–10% of the diabetic population in the USA. Most type 2 diabetics do not require exogenous insulin for survival, but many need exogenous supplementation of their endogenous secretion to achieve optimum health.

Benefit of Glycemic Control in Diabetes Mellitus

The consensus of the American Diabetes Association is that intensive glycemic control and targeting normal or near-normal glucose control associated with comprehensive self-management training should become standard therapy in diabetic patients (see Box: Benefits of Tight Glycemic Control in Diabetes). Exceptions include patients with advanced renal disease and the elderly, because the risks of hypoglycemia may outweigh the benefit of normal or near-normal glycemic control in these groups. In children under 7 years, the extreme susceptibility of the developing brain to incur damage from hypoglycemia contraindicates attempts at intensive glycemic control.

Insulin Regimens

A. Intensive Insulin Therapy

Intensive insulin regimens are prescribed for almost everyone with type 1 diabetes—diabetes associated with a severe deficiency or absence of endogenous insulin production—as well as many with type 2 diabetes.

Generally, the total daily insulin requirement in units is equal to the weight in pounds divided by four, or 0.55 times the person's weight in kilograms. Approximately half the total daily insulin dose covers the background or basal insulin requirements, and the remainder covers meal and snack requirement and high blood sugar corrections. This is an approximate calculation and has to be individualized. Examples of reduced insulin requirement include newly diagnosed persons and those with ongoing endogenous insulin production, longstanding diabetes with insulin sensitivity, significant renal insufficiency, or other endocrine deficiencies. Increased insulin requirements typically occur with obesity, during adolescence, during the latter trimesters of pregnancy, and in individuals with type 2 diabetes.

In intensive insulin regimens, the meal or snack and high blood sugar correction boluses are prescribed by formulas. The patient uses the formulas to calculate the rapid-acting insulin bolus dose by considering how much carbohydrate is in the meal or snack, the current plasma glucose, and the target glucose. The formula for the meal or snack bolus is expressed as an insulin-to-carbohydrate ratio, which refers to how many grams of carbohydrate will be disposed of by 1 unit of rapid-acting insulin. The high blood sugar correction formula is expressed as the predicted fall in plasma glucose (in mg/dL) after 1 unit of rapid-acting insulin. Diurnal variations in insulin sensitivity can be accommodated by prescribing different basal rates and bolus insulin doses throughout the day. Continuous subcutaneous insulin infusion devices provide the most sophisticated and physiologic insulin replacement.

B. Conventional Insulin Therapy

Conventional insulin therapy is usually prescribed only for certain people with type 2 diabetes who are felt not to benefit from intensive glucose control. The insulin regimen ranges from one injection per day to many injections per day, using intermediate- or long-acting insulin alone or with short- or rapid-acting insulin or premixed insulins. Referred to as sliding-scale regimens, conventional insulin regimens customarily fix the dose of the intermediate- or long-acting insulin, but vary the short- or rapid-acting insulin based on the plasma glucose level before the injection.

Insulin Treatment of Special Circumstances

A. Diabetic Ketoacidosis

Diabetic ketoacidosis (DKA) is a life-threatening medical emergency caused by inadequate or absent insulin replacement, which occurs in people with type 1 diabetes and infrequently in those with type 2 diabetes. It typically occurs in newly diagnosed type 1 patients or in those who have experienced interrupted insulin replacement, and rarely in people with type 2 diabetes who have concurrent unusually stressful conditions such as sepsis or

Benefits of Tight Glycemic Control in Diabetes

A long-term randomized prospective study involving 1441 type 1 patients in 29 medical centers reported in 1993 that "near normalization" of blood glucose resulted in a delay in onset and a major slowing of progression of microvascular and neuropathic complications of diabetes during follow-up periods of up to 10 years (Diabetes Control and Complications Trial [DCCT] Research Group, 1993). In the intensively treated group, mean glycated hemoglobin HbA_{1c} of 7.2% (normal < 6%) and mean blood glucose of 155 mg/dL were achieved, whereas in the conventionally treated group, HbA_{1c} averaged 8.9% with mean blood glucose of 225 mg/dL. Over the study period, which averaged 7 years, a reduction of approximately 60% in risk of diabetic retinopathy, nephropathy, and neuropathy was noted in the tight control group compared with the standard control group.

The DCCT study, in addition, introduced the concept of *glycemic memory*, which comprises the long-term benefits of any significant period of glycemic control. During a 6-year follow-up period, both the intensively and the conventionally treated groups had similar levels of glycemic control, and both had progression of carotid intimal-medial thickness. However, the intensively treated cohort had significantly less progression of intimal thickness.

The United Kingdom Prospective Diabetes Study (UKPDS) was a very large randomized prospective study carried out to study the effects of intensive glycemic control with several types of therapies and the effects of blood pressure control in type 2 diabetic patients. A total of 3867 newly diagnosed type 2 diabetic patients were studied over 10 years. A significant fraction of these were overweight and hypertensive. Patients were given dietary treatment alone or intensive therapy with insulin, chlorpropamide, glyburide, or glipizide. Metformin was an option for patients with inadequate response to other therapies. Tight control of blood pressure was added as a variable, with an angiotensin-converting enzyme inhibitor, a β blocker, or in some cases, a calcium channel blocker available for this purpose.

Tight control of diabetes, with reduction of HbA_{1c} from 9.1% to 7%, was shown to reduce the risk of microvascular complications overall compared with that achieved with conventional therapy (mostly diet alone, which decreased HbA_{1c} to 7.9%). Cardiovascular complications were not noted for any particular therapy; metformin treatment alone reduced the risk of macrovascular disease (myocardial infarction, stroke). Epidemiologic analysis of the study suggested that every 1% decrease in the HbA_{1c} achieved an estimated risk reduction of 37% for microvascular complications, 21% for any diabetes-related end point and death related to diabetes, and 14% for myocardial infarction.

Tight control of hypertension also had a surprisingly significant effect on microvascular disease (as well as more conventional hypertension-related sequelae) in these diabetic patients. Epidemiologic analysis of the results suggested that every 10 mm Hg decrease in the systolic pressure achieved an estimated risk reduction of 13% for diabetic microvascular complications, and 12% for any diabetes-related complication, 15% for death related to diabetes, and 11% for myocardial infarction.

Post-study monitoring showed that 5 years after the closure of the UKPDS, the benefits of intensive management on diabetic end points was maintained and the risk reduction for a myocardial infarction became significant. The benefits of metformin therapy were maintained.

These studies show that tight glycemic control benefits both type 1 and type 2 patients.

The STOP-NIDDM trial followed 1429 patients with impaired glucose tolerance who were randomized to treatment with acarbose or placebo over 3 years. This trial demonstrated that normalization of glycemic control in subjects with impaired glucose tolerance significantly diminished cardiovascular risk. The acarbose-treated group had a significant reduction in the development of major cardiovascular events and hypertension. A prospective placebo-controlled subgroup analysis has shown a marked decrease in the progression of intimal-medial thickness.

---

pancreatitis or are on high-dose steroid therapy. Signs and symptoms include nausea, vomiting, abdominal pain, deep slow (Kussmaul) breathing, change in mental status, elevated blood and urinary ketones and glucose, an arterial blood pH lower than 7.3, and low bicarbonate (< 15 mmol/L).

The fundamental treatment for DKA includes aggressive intravenous hydration and insulin therapy and maintenance of potassium and other electrolyte levels. Fluid and insulin therapy is based on the patient's individual needs and requires frequent reevaluation and modification. Close attention has to be given to hydration and renal status, the sodium and potassium levels, and the rate of correction of plasma glucose and plasma osmolality. Fluid therapy generally begins with normal saline. Regular human insulin should be used for intravenous therapy with a usual starting dose of about 0.1 IU/kg/h.

B. Hyperosmolar Hyperglycemic Syndrome

Hyperosmolar hyperglycemic syndrome (HHS) is diagnosed in persons with type 2 diabetes and is characterized by profound hyperglycemia and dehydration. It is associated with inadequate oral hydration, especially in elderly patients, with other illnesses, the use of medication that elevates the blood sugar or causes dehydration, such as phenytoin, steroids, diuretics, and β blockers, and with peritoneal dialysis and hemodialysis. The diagnostic hallmarks are declining mental status and even seizures, a plasma glucose of over 600 mg/dL, and a calculated serum osmolality higher than 320 mmol/L. Persons with HHS are not acidotic unless DKA is also present.

The treatment of HHS centers around aggressive rehydration and restoration of glucose and electrolyte homeostasis; the rate of correction of these variables must be monitored closely. Low-dose insulin therapy may be required.

Complications of Insulin Therapy

A. Hypoglycemia

1. Mechanisms and diagnosis—Hypoglycemic reactions are the most common complication of insulin therapy. They usually result from inadequate carbohydrate consumption, unusual physical exertion, or too large a dose of insulin.

Rapid development of hypoglycemia in persons with intact hypoglycemic awareness causes signs of autonomic hyperactivity—both sympathetic (tachycardia, palpitations, sweating, tremulousness) and parasympathetic (nausea, hunger)—and may progress to convulsions and coma if untreated.

In persons exposed to frequent hypoglycemic episodes during tight glycemic control, autonomic warning signals of hypoglycemia are less common or even absent. This dangerous acquired condition is termed "hypoglycemic unawareness." When patients lack the early warning signs of low blood glucose, they may not take corrective measures in time. In patients with persistent, untreated hypoglycemia, the manifestations of insulin excess may develop—confusion, weakness, bizarre behavior, coma, seizures—at which point they may not be able to procure or safely swallow glucose-containing foods. Hypoglycemic awareness may be restored by preventing frequent hypoglycemic episodes. An identification bracelet, necklace, or card in the wallet or purse, as well as some form of rapidly absorbed glucose, should be carried by every diabetic person who is receiving hypoglycemic drug therapy.

2. Treatment of hypoglycemia—All the manifestations of hypoglycemia are relieved by glucose administration. To expedite absorption, simple sugar or glucose should be given, preferably in liquid form. To treat mild hypoglycemia in a patient who is conscious and able to swallow, dextrose tablets, glucose gel, or any sugar-containing beverage or food may be given. If more severe hypoglycemia has produced unconsciousness or stupor, the treatment of choice is to give 20–50 mL of 50% glucose solution by intravenous infusion over a period of 2–3 minutes. If intravenous therapy is not available, 1 mg of glucagon injected either subcutaneously or intramuscularly may restore consciousness within 15 minutes to permit ingestion of sugar. If the patient is stuporous and glucagon is not available, small amounts of honey or syrup can be inserted into the buccal pouch. In general, however, oral feeding is contraindicated in unconscious patients. Emergency medical services should be called immediately for all episodes of severely impaired consciousness.

B. Immunopathology of Insulin Therapy

At least five molecular classes of insulin antibodies may be produced in diabetics during the course of insulin therapy: IgA, IgD, IgE, IgG, and IgM. There are two major types of immune disorders in these patients:

1. Insulin allergy—Insulin allergy, an immediate type hypersensitivity, is a rare condition in which local or systemic urticaria results from histamine release from tissue mast cells sensitized by anti-insulin IgE antibodies. In severe cases, anaphylaxis results.

Because sensitivity is often to noninsulin protein contaminants, the human and analog insulins have markedly reduced the incidence of insulin allergy, especially local reactions.

2. Immune insulin resistance—A low titer of circulating IgG anti-insulin antibodies that neutralize the action of insulin to a negligible extent develops in most insulin-treated patients. Rarely, the titer of insulin antibodies leads to insulin resistance and may be associated with other systemic autoimmune processes such as lupus erythematosus.

C. Lipodystrophy at Injection Sites

Injection of animal insulin preparations sometimes led to atrophy of subcutaneous fatty tissue at the site of injection. Since the development of human and analog insulin preparations of neutral pH, this type of immune complication is almost never seen. Injection of these newer preparations directly into the atrophic area often results in restoration of normal contours.

Hypertrophy of subcutaneous fatty tissue remains a problem if injected repeatedly at the same site. However, this may be corrected by avoiding the specific injection site or by liposuction.

D. Increased Cancer Risk

An increased risk of cancer attributed to insulin resistance and hyperinsulinemia has been reported in individuals with insulin resistance, prediabetes, and type 2 diabetes. Treatment with insulin and sulfonylureas, which increase circulating insulin levels, but not metformin possibly exacerbates that risk. These epidemiologic observations are preliminary and have not changed prescribing guidelines.

■ ORAL ANTIDIABETIC AGENTS

Seven categories of oral antidiabetic agents are now available in the USA for the treatment of persons with type 2 diabetes: insulin secretagogues (sulfonylureas, meglitinides, D-phenylalanine derivatives), biguanides, thiazolidinediones, α-glucosidase inhibitors, incretin-based therapies, an amylin analog, and a bile acid-binding sequestrant. The sulfonylureas and biguanides have been available the longest and are the traditional treatment choice for type 2 diabetes. Novel classes of rapid-acting insulin secretagogues, the meglitinides and D-phenylalanine derivatives, are alternatives to the short-acting sulfonylureas. Insulin secretagogues increase insulin secretion from beta cells. Biguanides decrease hepatic glucose production. The thiazolidinediones reduce insulin resistance. The incretin-based therapies control post-meal glucose excursions by increasing insulin release and decreasing glucagon secretion. The amylin analog also decreases post-meal glucose levels and reduces appetite. Alpha-glucosidase inhibitors slow the digestion and absorption of starch and disaccharides. Although still speculative, the mechanism of bile acid sequestrant's glucose-lowering effect is presumed to be related to a decrease in hepatic glucose output.

TABLE 41–5 Regulation of insulin release in humans.

Stimulants of insulin release
Humoral: Glucose, mannose, leucine, arginine, other amino acids, fatty acids (high concentrations)
Hormonal: Glucagon, glucagon-like peptide 1(7–37), glucose-dependent insulinotropic polypeptide, cholecystokinin, gastrin
Neural: β-Adrenergic stimulation, vagal stimulation
Drugs: Sulfonylureas, meglitinide, nateglinide, isoproterenol, acetylcholine
Inhibitors of insulin release
Hormonal: Somatostatin, insulin, leptin
Neural: α-Sympathomimetic effect of catecholamines
Drugs: Diazoxide, phenytoin, vinblastine, colchicine

Modified and reproduced, with permission, from Greenspan FS, Strewler GJ (editors): *Basic & Clinical Endocrinology*, 5th ed. Originally published by Appleton & Lange. Copyright © 1997 by The McGraw-Hill Companies, Inc.

INSULIN SECRETAGOGUES: SULFONYLUREAS

Mechanism of Action

The major action of sulfonylureas is to increase insulin release from the pancreas (Table 41–5). Two additional mechanisms of action have been proposed—a reduction of serum glucagon levels and closure of potassium channels in extrapancreatic tissue (which are of unknown but probably minimal significance).

A. Insulin Release from Pancreatic Beta Cells

Sulfonylureas bind to a 140-kDa high-affinity sulfonylurea receptor (Figure 41–2) that is associated with a beta-cell inward rectifier ATP-sensitive potassium channel. Binding of a sulfonylurea inhibits the efflux of potassium ions through the channel and results in depolarization. Depolarization opens a voltage-gated calcium channel and results in calcium influx and the release of preformed insulin.

B. Reduction of Serum Glucagon Concentrations

Long-term administration of sulfonylureas to type 2 diabetics reduces serum glucagon levels, which may contribute to the hypoglycemic effect of the drugs. The mechanism for this suppressive effect of sulfonylureas on glucagon levels is unclear but appears to involve indirect inhibition due to enhanced release of both insulin and somatostatin, which inhibit alpha-cell secretion.

Efficacy & Safety of the Sulfonylureas

In 1970, the University Group Diabetes Program (UGDP) in the USA reported that the number of deaths due to cardiovascular disease in diabetic patients treated with tolbutamide was excessive compared with either insulin-treated patients or those receiving placebos. Owing to design flaws, this study and its conclusions

were not generally accepted. In the United Kingdom, the UKPDS did not find an untoward cardiovascular effect of sulfonylurea usage in their large, long-term study.

The sulfonylureas continue to be widely prescribed, and six are available in the USA (Table 41–6). They are conventionally divided into first-generation and second-generation agents, which differ primarily in their potency and adverse effects. The first-generation sulfonylureas are increasingly difficult to procure, and as the second-generation agents become generic and less expensive, the older compounds probably will be discontinued.

FIRST-GENERATION SULFONYLUREAS

Tolbutamide is well absorbed but rapidly metabolized in the liver. Its duration of effect is relatively short, with an elimination half-life of 4–5 hours, and it is best administered in divided doses. Because of its short half-life, it is the safest sulfonylurea for elderly diabetics. Prolonged hypoglycemia has been reported rarely, mostly in patients receiving certain drugs (eg, dicumarol, phenylbutazone, some sulfonamides) that inhibit the metabolism of tolbutamide.

Chlorpropamide has a half-life of 32 hours and is slowly metabolized in the liver to products that retain some biologic activity; approximately 20–30% is excreted unchanged in the urine. Chlorpropamide also interacts with the drugs mentioned above that depend on hepatic oxidative catabolism, and it is contraindicated in patients with hepatic or renal insufficiency. Dosages higher than 500 mg daily increase the risk of jaundice. The average maintenance dosage is 250 mg daily, given as a single dose in the morning. Prolonged hypoglycemic reactions are more common in elderly patients, and the drug is contraindicated in this group. Other adverse effects include a hyperemic flush after alcohol ingestion in genetically predisposed patients and dilutional hyponatremia. Hematologic toxicity (transient leukopenia, thrombocytopenia) occurs in less than 1% of patients.

Tolazamide is comparable to chlorpropamide in potency but has a shorter duration of action. Tolazamide is more slowly absorbed than the other sulfonylureas, and its effect on blood glucose does not appear for several hours. Its half-life is about 7 hours. Tolazamide is metabolized to several compounds that retain hypoglycemic effects. If more than 500 mg/d are required, the dose should be divided and given twice daily.

SECOND-GENERATION SULFONYLUREAS

The second-generation sulfonylureas are prescribed more frequently in the USA than are the first-generation agents because they have fewer adverse effects and drug interactions. These potent sulfonylurea compounds—glyburide, glipizide, and glimepiride—should be used with caution in patients with cardiovascular disease or in elderly patients, in whom hypoglycemia would be especially dangerous.

Glyburide is metabolized in the liver into products with very low hypoglycemic activity. The usual starting dosage is 2.5 mg/d

TABLE 41–6 Sulfonylureas.

Sulfonylureas	Chemical Structure	Daily Dose	Duration of Action (hours)
Tolbutamide (Orinase)	H_3C—〇—SO_2—NH—C(=O)—NH—$(CH_2)_3$—CH_3	0.5–2 g in divided doses	6–12
Tolazamide (Tolinase)	H_3C—〇—SO_2—NH—C(=O)—NH—N⟨ring⟩	0.1–1 g as single dose or in divided doses	10–14
Chlorpropamide (Diabinese)	Cl—〇—SO_2—NH—C(=O)—NH—$(CH_2)_2$—CH_3	0.1–0.5 g as single dose	Up to 60
Glyburide (glibenclamide[1]) (DiaβEta, Micronase, Glynase PresTab)	Cl, C(=O)—NH—$(CH_2)_2$—〇—SO_2—NH—C(=O)—NH—⟨cyclohexyl⟩, OCH_3	1.25–20 mg	10–24
Glipizide (glydiazinamide[1]) (Glucotrol, Glucotrol XL)	pyrazine—C(=O)—NH—$(CH_2)_2$—〇—SO_2—NH—C(=O)—NH—⟨cyclohexyl⟩, H_3C	5–30 mg (20 mg in Glucotrol XL)	10–24[2]
Glimepiride (Amaryl)	H_3C, H_5C_2 ring—N—$CONHCH_2CH_2$—〇—$SO_2NHCONH$—⟨ring⟩—CH_3	1–4 mg	12–24

[1]Outside USA.

[2]Elimination half-life considerably shorter (see text).

or less, and the average maintenance dosage is 5–10 mg/d given as a single morning dose; maintenance dosages higher than 20 mg/d are not recommended. A formulation of "micronized" glyburide (Glynase PresTab) is available in a variety of tablet sizes. However, there is some question as to its bioequivalence with nonmicronized formulations, and the FDA recommends careful monitoring to re-titrate dosage when switching from standard glyburide doses or from other sulfonylurea drugs.

Glyburide has few adverse effects other than its potential for causing hypoglycemia. Flushing has rarely been reported after ethanol ingestion, and the compound slightly enhances free water clearance. Glyburide is contraindicated in the presence of hepatic impairment and in patients with renal insufficiency.

Glipizide has the shortest half-life (2–4 hours) of the more potent agents. For maximum effect in reducing postprandial hyperglycemia, this agent should be ingested 30 minutes before breakfast because absorption is delayed when the drug is taken with food. The recommended starting dosage is 5 mg/d, with up to 15 mg/d given as a single dose. When higher daily dosages are required, they should be divided and given before meals. The maximum total daily dosage recommended by the manufacturer is 40 mg/d, although some studies indicate that the maximum therapeutic effect is achieved by 15–20 mg of the drug. An extended-release preparation (Glucotrol XL) provides 24-hour action after a once-daily morning dose (maximum of 20 mg/d). However, this formulation appears to have sacrificed its lower propensity for severe hypoglycemia compared with longer-acting glyburide without showing any demonstrable therapeutic advantages over the latter (which can be obtained as a generic drug).

Because of its shorter half-life, the regular formulation of glipizide is much less likely than glyburide to produce serious hypoglycemia. At least 90% of glipizide is metabolized in the liver to inactive products, and 10% is excreted unchanged in the urine. Glipizide therapy is therefore contraindicated in patients with significant hepatic or renal impairment, who would be at high risk for hypoglycemia.

Glimepiride is approved for once-daily use as monotherapy or in combination with insulin. Glimepiride achieves blood glucose lowering with the lowest dose of any sulfonylurea compound. A single daily dose of 1 mg has been shown to be effective, and the recommended maximal daily dose is 8 mg. Glimepiride has a long duration of effect with a half-life of 5 hours, allowing once-daily dosing and thereby improving compliance. It is completely metabolized by the liver to metabolites with weak or no activity.

INSULIN SECRETAGOGUE: MEGLITINIDE

Repaglinide is the first member of the meglitinide group of insulin secretagogues (Table 41–7). These drugs modulate beta-cell insulin release by regulating potassium efflux through the potassium channels previously discussed. There is overlap with the sulfonylureas in their molecular sites of action because the meglitinides have two binding sites in common with the sulfonylureas and one unique binding site.

Repaglinide has a very fast onset of action, with a peak concentration and peak effect within approximately 1 hour after ingestion, but the duration of action is 4–7 hours. It is hepatically cleared by CYP3A4 with a plasma half-life of 1 hour. Because of its rapid onset, repaglinide is indicated for use in controlling postprandial glucose excursions. The drug should be taken just before each meal in doses of 0.25–4 mg (maximum 16 mg/d); hypoglycemia is a risk if the meal is delayed or skipped or contains inadequate carbohydrate. This drug should be used cautiously in individuals with renal and hepatic impairment. Repaglinide is approved as monotherapy or in combination with biguanides.

There is no sulfur in its structure, so repaglinide may be used in type 2 diabetics with sulfur or sulfonylurea allergy.

INSULIN SECRETAGOGUE: D-PHENYLALANINE DERIVATIVE

Nateglinide, a D-phenylalanine derivative, is the latest insulin secretagogue to become clinically available. Nateglinide stimulates very rapid and transient release of insulin from beta cells through closure of the ATP-sensitive K^+ channel. It also partially restores initial insulin release in response to an intravenous glucose tolerance test. This may be a significant advantage of the drug because type 2 diabetes is associated with loss of this initial insulin response. The restoration of more normal insulin secretion may suppress glucagon release early in the meal and result in less endogenous or hepatic glucose production. Nateglinide may have a special role in the treatment of individuals with isolated postprandial hyperglycemia, but it has minimal effect on overnight or fasting glucose levels. Nateglinide is efficacious when given alone or in combination with nonsecretagogue oral agents (such as metformin). In contrast to other insulin secretagogues, dose titration is not required.

Nateglinide is ingested just before meals. It is absorbed within 20 minutes after oral administration with a time to peak concentration of less than 1 hour and is metabolized in the liver by CYP2C9 and CYP3A4 with a half-life of about 1 hour. The overall duration of action is about 4 hours. Nateglinide amplifies the insulin secretory response to a glucose load, but it has a markedly diminished effect in the presence of normoglycemia. The incidence of hypoglycemia with nateglinide may be the lowest of all the secretagogues, and nateglinide has the advantage of being safe in those with very reduced renal function.

TABLE 41–7 Other insulin secretagogues.

Drug	Chemical Structure	Oral Dose	$t_{1/2}$	Duration of Action (hours)
Repaglinide (Prandin)		0.25–4 mg before meals	1 hour	4–7
Nateglinide (Starlix)		60–120 mg before meals	1 hour	4

BIGUANIDES

The structure of **metformin** is shown below. Phenformin (an older biguanide) was discontinued in the USA because of its association with lactic acidosis and because there was no documentation of any long-term benefit from its use.

Metformin

Mechanisms of Action

A full explanation of the mechanism of action of the biguanides remains elusive, but their primary effect is to reduce hepatic glucose production through activation of the enzyme AMP-activated protein kinase (AMPK). Possible minor mechanisms of action include impairment of renal gluconeogenesis, slowing of glucose absorption from the gastrointestinal tract, with increased glucose to lactate conversion by enterocytes, direct stimulation of glycolysis in tissues, increased glucose removal from blood, and reduction of plasma glucagon levels. The biguanide blood glucose-lowering action does not depend on functioning pancreatic beta cells. Patients with type 2 diabetes have considerably less fasting hyperglycemia as well as lower postprandial hyperglycemia after administration of biguanides; however, hypoglycemia during biguanide therapy is essentially unknown. These agents are therefore more appropriately termed "euglycemic" agents.

Metabolism & Excretion

Metformin has a half-life of 1.5–3 hours, is not bound to plasma proteins, is not metabolized, and is excreted by the kidneys as the active compound. As a consequence of metformin's blockade of gluconeogenesis, the drug may impair the hepatic metabolism of lactic acid. In patients with renal insufficiency, biguanides accumulate and thereby increase the risk of lactic acidosis, which appears to be a dose-related complication.

Clinical Use

Biguanides are recommended as first-line therapy for type 2 diabetes. Because metformin is an insulin-sparing agent and does not increase body weight or provoke hypoglycemia, it offers obvious advantages over insulin or sulfonylureas in treating hyperglycemia in such persons. The UKPDS reported that metformin therapy decreases the risk of macrovascular as well as microvascular disease; this is in contrast to the other therapies, which only modified microvascular morbidity. Biguanides are also indicated for use in combination with insulin secretagogues or thiazolidinediones in type 2 diabetics in whom oral monotherapy is inadequate. Metformin is useful in the prevention of type 2 diabetes; the landmark Diabetes Prevention Program concluded that metformin is efficacious in preventing the new onset of type 2 diabetes in middle-aged, obese persons with impaired glucose tolerance and

fasting hyperglycemia. It is interesting that metformin did not prevent diabetes in older, leaner prediabetics.

The dosage of metformin is from 500 mg to a maximum of 2.55 g daily, with the lowest effective dose being recommended. Depending on whether the primary abnormality is fasting hyperglycemia or postprandial hyperglycemia, metformin therapy can be initiated as a once-daily dose at bedtime or before a meal. A common schedule for fasting hyperglycemia would be to begin with a single 500-mg tablet at bedtime for a week or more. If this is tolerated without gastrointestinal discomfort and if hyperglycemia persists, a second 500-mg tablet may be added with the evening meal. If further dose increases are required, an additional 500-mg tablet can be added to be taken with breakfast or the midday meal, or the larger (850-mg) tablet can be prescribed twice daily or even three times daily (the maximum recommended dosage) if needed. Dosage should always be divided because ingestion of more than 1000 mg at any one time usually provokes significant gastrointestinal adverse effects.

Epidemiologic studies suggest that metformin use may dramatically reduce the risk of some cancers. These data are still preliminary, and the speculative mechanism of action is a decrease in insulin (which also functions as a growth factor) levels as well as direct cellular effects mediated by AMPK.

Toxicities

The most common toxic effects of metformin are gastrointestinal (anorexia, nausea, vomiting, abdominal discomfort, and diarrhea), which occur in up to 20% of patients. They are dose related, tend to occur at the onset of therapy, and are often transient. However, metformin may have to be discontinued in 3–5% of patients because of persistent diarrhea. Absorption of vitamin B_{12} appears to be reduced during long-term metformin therapy, and annual screening of serum vitamin B_{12} levels and red blood cell parameters has been encouraged by the manufacturer to determine the need for vitamin B_{12} injections. In the absence of hypoxia or renal or hepatic insufficiency, lactic acidosis is less common with metformin therapy than with phenformin therapy.

Biguanides are contraindicated in patients with renal disease, alcoholism, hepatic disease, or conditions predisposing to tissue anoxia (eg, chronic cardiopulmonary dysfunction) because of the increased risk of lactic acidosis induced by these drugs.

THIAZOLIDINEDIONES

Thiazolidinediones (Tzds) act to decrease insulin resistance. Tzds are ligands of **peroxisome proliferator-activated receptor-gamma (PPAR-γ),** part of the steroid and thyroid superfamily of nuclear receptors. These PPAR receptors are found in muscle, fat, and liver. PPAR-γ receptors modulate the expression of the genes involved in lipid and glucose metabolism, insulin signal transduction, and adipocyte and other tissue differentiation. The available Tzds do not have identical clinical effects, and new drug development will focus on defining PPAR effects and designing ligands that have selective action—much like the selective estrogen receptor modulators (see Chapter 40).

TABLE 41–8 Thiazolidinediones.

Thiazolidinedione	Chemical Structure	Oral Dose
Pioglitazone (Actos)		15–45 mg once daily
Rosiglitazone (Avandia)		2–8 mg once daily

In addition to targeting adipocytes, myocytes, and hepatocytes, Tzds also have significant effects on vascular endothelium, the immune system, the ovaries, and tumor cells. Some of these responses may be independent of the PPAR-γ pathway. The Tzd oncogenic effects are complex and may be both tumorigenic and antitumorigenic.

In persons with diabetes, a major site of Tzd action is adipose tissue, where the drug promotes glucose uptake and utilization and modulates synthesis of lipid hormones or cytokines and other proteins involved in energy regulation. Tzds also regulate adipocyte apoptosis and differentiation. Numerous other effects have been documented in animal studies, but applicability to human tissues has yet to be determined.

Two thiazolidinediones are currently available: pioglitazone and rosiglitazone (Table 41–8). Their distinct side chains create differences in therapeutic action, metabolism, metabolite profile, and adverse effects. An earlier compound, troglitazone, was withdrawn from the market because of hepatic toxicity thought to be related to its side chain.

Pioglitazone has PPAR-α as well as PPAR-γ activity. It is absorbed within 2 hours of ingestion; although food may delay uptake, total bioavailability is not affected. Absorption is decreased with concomitant use of bile acid sequestrants. Pioglitazone is metabolized by CYP2C8 and CYP3A4 to active metabolites. The bioavailability of numerous other drugs also degraded by these enzymes may be affected by pioglitazone therapy, including estrogen-containing oral contraceptives; additional methods of contraception are advised. Pioglitazone may be taken once daily; the usual starting dose is 15–30 mg/d, and the maximum is 45 mg/d. A triglyceride-lowering effect is observed with pioglitazone and is more significant than that of rosiglitazone, presumably because of its PPAR-α-binding characteristics. Pioglitazone is approved as a monotherapy and in combination with metformin, sulfonylureas, and insulin for the treatment of type 2 diabetes. The risk of bladder cancer appears to be cumulatively increased with high doses.

Rosiglitazone is rapidly absorbed and highly protein-bound. It is metabolized in the liver to minimally active metabolites, predominantly by CYP2C8 and to a lesser extent by CYP2C9. It is administered once or twice daily; 2–8 mg is the usual total dose.

Rosiglitazone shares the common Tzd adverse effects but appears to carry more cardiovascular risk than pioglitazone. Concurrent administration of nitrates and insulin putatively enhances the risk of myocardial infarction and is contraindicated; renin-angiotensin system blockers may have a similar risk but are not specifically prohibited. Because of toxicities, the FDA now limits rosiglitazone prescriptions to patients already on treatment with the medication, and to those whose blood sugar cannot be controlled with other antidiabetic medicines and who, after consultation with their provider, do not wish to be on pioglitazone or a pioglitazone-containing drug. *For those restricted populations, rosiglitazone is approved for use in type 2 diabetes as monotherapy, in double combination therapy with a biguanide or sulfonylurea, or in quadruple combination with a biguanide, sulfonylurea, and insulin.*

Tzds are considered euglycemics and are efficacious in about 70% of new users. The overall response is similar to that achieved with sulfonylurea and biguanide monotherapy. Individuals experiencing secondary failure with other oral agents should benefit from the addition (rather than substitution) of a Tzd. Because their mechanism of action involves gene regulation, the Tzds have a slow onset and offset of activity over weeks or even months. Combination therapy with sulfonylureas and insulin can lead to hypoglycemia and may require dosage adjustment.

An adverse effect common to both Tzds is fluid retention, which presents as a mild anemia and peripheral edema, especially when the drugs are used in combination with insulin or insulin secretagogues. Both drugs increase the risk of heart failure. Many users have a dose-related weight gain (average 1–3 kg), which may be fluid related. Rarely, new or worsening macular edema has been reported in association with treatment. Loss of bone mineral density and increased atypical extremity bone fractures in women are described for both compounds, which is postulated to be due to decreased osteoblast formation. Studies are ongoing to determine whether the demineralization and fracture risk is increased in men. Long-term therapy is associated with a drop in triglyceride levels and a slight rise in high-density lipoprotein (HDL) and low-density lipoprotein (LDL) cholesterol values. These agents should not be used during pregnancy or in the presence of significant liver disease (ALT more than 2.5 times upper limit of normal) or with a concurrent diagnosis of heart failure. Because of the hepatotoxicity observed with troglitazone, a discontinued Tzd, the FDA continues to require monitoring of liver function tests before initiation of Tzd therapy and periodically afterward. To date, hepatotoxicity has not been associated with rosiglitazone or pioglitazone. Anovulatory women may resume ovulation and should be counseled on the increased risk of pregnancy.

Thiazolidinediones have benefit in the *prevention* of type 2 diabetes. The Diabetes Prevention Trial reported a 75% reduction in diabetes incidence rate when troglitazone was administered to patients with prediabetes. Another study reported that troglitazone therapy significantly decreased the recurrence of diabetes mellitus in high-risk Hispanic women with a history of gestational diabetes.

Although these medications are highly efficacious, the adverse effects of weight gain, congestive heart failure, demineralization and increased bone fracture in women; possible (for rosiglitazone) worsening of cardiovascular status; and unknown oncogenic risk potentially limit their popularity and future use.

ALPHA-GLUCOSIDASE INHIBITORS

Acarbose and **miglitol** are competitive inhibitors of the intestinal α-glucosidases and reduce postmeal glucose excursions by delaying the digestion and absorption of starch and disaccharides (Table 41–9). Only monosaccharides, such as glucose and fructose, can be transported out of the intestinal lumen and into the bloodstream. Complex starches, oligosaccharides, and disaccharides must be broken down into individual monosaccharides before being absorbed in the duodenum and upper jejunum. This digestion is facilitated by enteric enzymes, including pancreatic α-amylase and α-glucosidases that are attached to the brush border of the intestinal cells. Miglitol differs structurally from acarbose and is six times more potent in inhibiting sucrase. Although the binding affinity of the two compounds differs, acarbose and miglitol both target the α-glucosidases: sucrase, maltase, glucoamylase, and dextranase. Miglitol alone has effects on isomaltase and on β-glucosidases, which split β-linked sugars such as lactose. Acarbose alone has a small effect on α-amylase. The consequence of enzyme inhibition is to minimize upper intestinal digestion and defer digestion (and thus absorption) of the ingested starch and disaccharides to the distal small intestine, thereby lowering postmeal glycemic excursions as much as 45–60 mg/dL and creating an insulin-sparing effect.

Monotherapy with these drugs is associated with a modest drop (0.5–1%) in glycohemoglobin levels and a 20–25 mg/dL fall in fasting glucose levels. They are FDA-approved for persons with type 2 diabetes as monotherapy and in combination with sulfonylureas, in which the glycemic effect is additive. Both acarbose and miglitol are taken in doses of 25–100 mg just before ingesting the first portion of each meal; therapy should be initiated with the lowest dose and slowly titrated upward, and a similar amount of starch and disaccharides should be ingested at each meal.

Prominent adverse effects include flatulence, diarrhea, and abdominal pain and result from the appearance of undigested carbohydrate in the colon that is then fermented into short-chain fatty acids, releasing gas. These adverse effects tend to diminish with ongoing use because chronic exposure to carbohydrate induces the expression of α-glucosidase in the jejunum and ileum, increasing distal small intestine glucose absorption and minimizing the passage of carbohydrate into the colon. Although not a problem with monotherapy or combination therapy with a biguanide, hypoglycemia may occur with concurrent sulfonylurea treatment. Hypoglycemia should be treated with glucose (dextrose) and not sucrose, whose breakdown may be blocked. These drugs are contraindicated in patients with inflammatory bowel disease or any intestinal condition that could be worsened by gas and distention. Because both miglitol and acarbose are excreted by the kidneys, these medications should not be prescribed in individuals with renal impairment. Acarbose has been associated with reversible hepatic enzyme elevation and should be used with caution in the presence of hepatic disease.

The STOP-NIDDM trial demonstrated that α-glucosidase therapy in prediabetic persons successfully prevented a significant number of new cases of type 2 diabetes and helped restore beta-cell function, in addition to reducing cardiovascular disease and hypertension. Intervention with acarbose also reduced cardiovascular events in persons with diabetes. Diabetes and cardiovascular disease prevention may become a further indication for this class of medications.

TABLE 41–9 Alpha-glucosidase inhibitors.

Alpha-Glucosidase Inhibitor	Chemical Structure	Oral Dose
Acarbose (Precose)		25–100 mg before meals
Miglitol (Glyset)		25–100 mg before meals

Alpha-glucosidase inhibitors are infrequently prescribed in the United States because of their prominent gastrointestinal adverse effects and relatively minor glucose-lowering benefit.

BILE ACID SEQUESTRANTS

Initially developed as a bile acid sequestrant and cholesterol-lowering drug, **colesevelam hydrochloride** is now approved as an antihyperglycemic therapy for persons with type 2 diabetes who are taking other medications or have not achieved adequate control with diet and exercise. The exact mechanism of action is unknown but presumed to involve an interruption of the enterohepatic circulation and a decrease in farnesoid X receptor (FXR) activation. FXR is a nuclear receptor with multiple effects on cholesterol, glucose, and bile acid metabolism. Bile acids are natural ligands of the FXR. Additionally, the drug may impair glucose absorption.

Colesevelam is administered as a pill or an oral suspension in a dosage of 1875 mg twice daily or 3750 mg once daily. It is not systemically absorbed or modified and is eliminated intact in the feces. In clinical trials, it lowered the hemoglobin A_{1c} (HbA_{1c}) concentration about 0.5%, and LDL cholesterol by 15% or more. Side effects include gastrointestinal complaints (constipation, indigestion, flatulence). The medication may impair absorption of multiple other medications including fat-soluble vitamins, glyburide, levothyroxine, and oral contraceptives, and should not be used in individuals with hypertriglyceridemia, a history of pancreatitis secondary to hypertriglyceridemia, or esophageal, gastric, or intestinal disorders.

AMYLIN ANALOG

Pramlintide, a synthetic analog of amylin, is an injectable antihyperglycemic agent that modulates postprandial glucose levels and is approved for preprandial use in persons with type 1 and type 2 diabetes. It is administered in addition to insulin in those who are unable to achieve their target postprandial blood sugar levels. Pramlintide suppresses glucagon release via undetermined mechanisms, delays gastric emptying, and has central nervous system–mediated anorectic effects. It is rapidly absorbed after subcutaneous administration; levels peak within 20 minutes, and the duration of action is not more than 150 minutes. Pramlintide is renally metabolized and excreted, but even at low creatinine clearance there is no significant change in bioavailability. It has not been evaluated in dialysis patients. The most reliable absorption is from the abdomen and thigh; arm administration is less reliable.

Pramlintide should be injected immediately before eating; doses range from 15 to 60 mcg subcutaneously for individuals with type 1 diabetes and from 60 to 120 mcg subcutaneously for individuals with type 2 diabetes. Therapy with this agent should be initiated with the lowest dose and titrated upward. Because of the risk of hypoglycemia, concurrent rapid- or short-acting mealtime insulin doses should be decreased by 50% or more. Concurrent insulin secretagogue doses also may need to be decreased in persons with type 2 diabetes. Pramlintide should always be injected by itself with a separate syringe; it cannot be mixed with insulin. The major adverse effects of pramlintide are hypoglycemia and gastrointestinal symptoms, including nausea, vomiting, and anorexia.

GLUCAGON-LIKE POLYPEPTIDE-1 (GLP-1) RECEPTOR AGONISTS

In type 2 diabetes, the release of glucagon-like polypeptide is diminished postprandially, which leads to inadequate glucagon suppression and excessive hepatic glucose output. Two synthetic analogs of glucagon-like polypeptide, **exenatide** and **liraglutide,** are commercially available to help restore GLP-1 activity. These therapies have multiple actions such as potentiation of glucose-mediated insulin secretion, suppression of postprandial glucagon release through as-yet unknown mechanisms, slowed gastric emptying, and a central loss of appetite. The increased insulin secretion is speculated to be due in part to an increase in beta-cell mass. The increased beta-cell mass may result from decreased beta-cell apoptosis, increased beta-cell formation, or both.

Exenatide, a derivative of the exendin-4 peptide in Gila monster venom, was the first incretin therapy to become available for the treatment of diabetes. It has a 53% homology with native GLP-1, and a glycine substitution to reduce degradation by dipeptidyl peptidase-4 (DPP-4). Exenatide is approved as an injectable, adjunctive therapy in persons with type 2 diabetes treated with metformin or metformin plus sulfonylureas who still have suboptimal glycemic control. Exenatide is absorbed equally from arm, abdomen, or thigh injection sites, reaching a peak concentration in approximately 2 hours with a duration of action of up to 10 hours. It undergoes glomerular filtration, and dosage adjustment is required only when the creatinine clearance is less than 30 mL/min.

Exenatide is injected subcutaneously within 60 minutes before a meal; therapy is initiated at 5 mcg twice daily, with a maximum dosage of 10 mcg twice daily. When exenatide is added to preexisting sulfonylurea therapy, the oral hypoglycemic dosage may need to be decreased to prevent hypoglycemia. The major adverse effects are nausea (about 44% of users) and vomiting and diarrhea. The nausea decreases with ongoing exenatide usage. Exenatide mono- and combination therapy results in HbA_{1c} reductions from 0.2% to 1.2%. Weight loss in the range of 2–3 kg is reported in some users, presumably because of the nausea and anorectic effects. A serious and, in some cases, fatal adverse effect of exenatide is necrotizing and hemorrhagic pancreatitis. Antibodies to exenatide are formed with chronic use, the clinical significance of which is unclear.

Liraglutide is a long-acting synthetic GLP-1 analog with 97% homology to native GLP-1 but has a prolonged half-life that permits once-daily dosing. Liraglutide interacts with the GLP-1 receptor and acts to increase insulin and decrease glucagon release.

Liraglutide is approved for the treatment of type 2 diabetes as an injectable therapy in patients who achieve inadequate control with diet and exercise, and are receiving concurrent treatment with metformin, sulfonylureas, or Tzds. It is not recommended as a first-line therapy or for use with insulin. Treatment is initiated at 0.6 mg and is titrated in weekly increments of 0.6 mg as needed, and as tolerated, to achieve glycemic goals. Peak levels are obtained in 8–12 hours, and the elimination half-life is about 13 hours.

Liraglutide therapy results in a reduction of HbA$_{1c}$ from 0.8% to 1.5%; weight loss ranges from nominal to 3.2 kg.. Experience with liraglutide in patients with renal or hepatic impairment is limited and it should be used with caution in these populations.

Common side effects of liraglutide are headache, nausea, and diarrhea; antibody formation, urticaria, and other immune reactions also are observed Hypoglycemia can occur with concomitant sulfonylurea use and may require a dose reduction of the oral hypoglycemic agent. Pancreatitis is another serious adverse effect; liraglutide is contraindicated in individuals with a history of pancreatitis and should be permanently discontinued if pancreatitis develops. Because rodents exposed to liraglutide developed thyroid C-cell tumors, there is an FDA mandated "black box" warning that liraglutide is contraindicated in individuals with a personal or family history of medullary cancer or multiple endocrine neoplasia type 2.

Although they require injection, the GLP-1 receptor ligands have gained popularity because of the improved glucose control and associated anorexia and weight loss in some users. Safety issues, however, may deter future use.

DIPEPTIDYL PEPTIDASE-4 (DPP-4) INHIBITORS

Sitagliptin, saxagliptin, and **linagliptin** are inhibitors of DPP-4, the enzyme that degrades incretin hormones. These drugs increase circulating levels of native GLP-1 and glucose-dependent insulinotropic polypeptide (GIP), which ultimately decreases postprandial glucose excursions by increasing glucose-mediated insulin secretion and decreasing glucagon levels. They are approved as adjunctive therapy to diet and exercise in the treatment of individuals with type 2 diabetes who have failed to achieve glycemic goals.

Sitagliptin has an oral bioavailability of over 85%, achieves peak concentrations within 1–4 hours, and has a half-life of approximately 12 hours. It is primarily (87%) excreted in the urine in part by active tubular secretion of the drug. Hepatic metabolism is limited and mediated largely by the cytochrome CYP3A4 isoform and, to a lesser degree, by CYP2C8. The metabolites have insignificant activity. The usual dosage is 100 mg orally once daily. Sitagliptin has been studied as monotherapy and in combination with metformin, sulfonylureas, and Tzds. Therapy with sitagliptin has resulted in HbA$_{1c}$ reductions of between 0.5% and 1.0%.

Common adverse effects include nasopharyngitis, upper respiratory infections, headaches, and hypoglycemia when the drug is combined with insulin secretagogues or insulin. There are postmarketing reports of acute pancreatitis (fatal and nonfatal) and severe allergic and hypersensitivity reactions. Sitagliptin should be immediately discontinued if pancreatitis or allergic and hypersensitivity reactions occur. Dosage should be reduced in patients with renal impairment and may need to be adjusted to prevent hypoglycemia if there is concurrent insulin secretagogue or insulin therapy.

Saxagliptin is given orally as 2.5–5 mg daily. The drug reaches maximal concentrations within 2 hours (4 hours for its active metabolite). It is minimally protein bound, and undergoes hepatic metabolism by CYP3A4/5. The major metabolite is active, and

excretion is by both renal and hepatic pathways. The terminal plasma half-life is 2.5 hours for saxagliptin and 3.1 hours for its active metabolite. Dosage adjustment is recommended for individuals with renal impairment and concurrent use of strong CYP3A4/5 inhibitors such as antiviral, antifungal, and certain antibacterial agents.

Saxagliptin is approved as monotherapy and in combination with biguanides, sulfonylureas, and Tzds. It has not been studied in combination with insulin. During clinical trials, mono- and combination therapy with sitagliptin resulted in an HbA$_{1c}$ reduction in the range of 0.4–0.9%.

Adverse effects include an increased rate of infections (upper respiratory tract and urinary tract), headaches, peripheral edema (when combined with a Tzd), hypoglycemia (when combined with a sulfonylurea), and hypersensitivity reactions (urticaria, facial edema). The dose of a concurrently administered insulin secretagogue or insulin may need to be lowered to prevent hypoglycemia.

Linagliptin is the most recently introduced drug in this class and appears to have properties similar to sitagliptin and saxagliptin. It is approved for use as monotherapy and in combination with metformin, glimepiride, and pioglitazone.

COMBINATION THERAPY—ORAL ANTIDIABETIC AGENTS & INJECTABLE MEDICATION

Combination Therapy in Type 2 Diabetes Mellitus

Failure to maintain a good response to therapy over the long term owing to a progressive decrease in beta-cell mass, reduction in physical activity, decline in lean body mass, or increase in ectopic fat deposition remains a disconcerting problem in the management of type 2 diabetes. Multiple medications may be required to achieve glycemic control. Unless there is a contraindication, medical therapy should be initiated with a biguanide. If clinical failure occurs with metformin monotherapy, a second agent or insulin is added. The second-line drug can be an insulin secretagogue, Tzd, incretin-based therapy, amylin analog, or a glucosidase inhibitor; preference is given to sulfonylureas or insulin because of cost, adverse effects, and safety concerns. Third-line therapy can include metformin, multiple other oral medications, or a noninsulin injectable and metformin and intensified insulin therapy. Recommended fourth-line therapy is intensified insulin management with or without metformin or Tzd.

A. Combination Therapy with GLP-1 Receptor Agonists

Exenatide and liraglutide are approved for use in individuals who fail to achieve desired glycemic control on metformin, sulfonylureas, metformin plus sulfonylureas, or (for liraglutide) metformin plus sulfonylureas and Tzds. Hypoglycemia is a risk when the GLP-1 receptor agonists are used with an insulin secretagogue or with insulin. The doses of the latter drugs should be reduced at the initiation of therapy and subsequently titrated.

B. Combination Therapy with DPP-4 Inhibitors

Sitagliptin, saxagliptin, and linagliptin are approved for use in individuals who fail to achieve desired glycemic control on metformin, sulfonylureas, or Tzds. Hypoglycemia is a risk when the DPP-4 inhibitors are used with an insulin secretagogue or with insulin, and a dosage adjustment of the latter drugs may be required to prevent hypoglycemia.

C. Combination Therapy with Pramlintide

Pramlintide is approved for concurrent mealtime administration in individuals with type 2 diabetes treated with insulin, metformin, or a sulfonylurea who are unable to achieve their postprandial glucose targets. Combination therapy results in a significant reduction in early postprandial glucose excursions; mealtime insulin or sulfonylurea doses usually have to be reduced to prevent hypoglycemia.

D. Combination Therapy with Insulin

Bedtime insulin has been suggested as an adjunct to oral antidiabetic therapy in patients with type 2 diabetes who have not responded to maximal oral therapy. Although not formally FDA approved, clinical practice has evolved to include sulfonylureas, meglitinides, D-phenylalanine derivatives, biguanides, thiazolidinediones, α-glucosidase inhibitors, GLP-1 receptor agonists, DPP-4 inhibitors, and bile acid sequestrants given in conjunction with insulin. National and international committee practice guidelines, however, recommend avoiding polypharmacy, especially with more expensive agents, and urge early introduction of insulin when an individual is unable to achieve glycemic targets.

Persons unable to achieve glycemic control with bedtime insulin as described generally require full insulin replacement and multiple daily injections of insulin. Insulin secretagogues are redundant when a person is receiving multiple daily insulin injections, but persons with severe insulin resistance may benefit from the addition of metformin. When metformin is added to the regimen of a person already taking insulin, the blood glucose should be closely monitored and the insulin dosage decreased as needed to avoid hypoglycemia.

Combination Therapy in Type 1 Diabetes Mellitus

Insulin secretagogues (sulfonylureas, meglitinides, or D-phenylalanine derivatives), Tzds, metformin, α-glucosidase inhibitors, GLP-1 receptor agonists, DPP-4 inhibitors, or bile acid sequestrants are *not* approved for use in type 1 diabetes.

Combination Therapy with Pramlintide

Pramlintide is approved for concurrent mealtime administration in individuals with type 1 diabetes who have poor glucose control after eating despite optimal insulin therapy. The addition of pramlintide leads to a significant reduction in early postprandial glucose excursions; mealtime insulin doses usually should be reduced to prevent hypoglycemia.

■ GLUCAGON

Chemistry & Metabolism

Glucagon is synthesized in the alpha cells of the pancreatic islets of Langerhans (Table 41–1). Glucagon is a peptide—identical in all mammals—consisting of a single chain of 29 amino acids, with a molecular weight of 3485. Selective proteolytic cleavage converts a large precursor molecule of approximately 18,000 MW to glucagon. One of the precursor intermediates consists of a 69-amino-acid peptide called **glicentin,** which contains the glucagon sequence interposed between peptide extensions.

Glucagon is extensively degraded in the liver and kidney as well as in plasma and at its tissue receptor sites. Because of its rapid inactivation by plasma, chilling of the collecting tubes and addition of inhibitors of proteolytic enzymes are necessary when samples of blood are collected for immunoassay of circulating glucagon. Its half-life in plasma is between 3 and 6 minutes, which is similar to that of insulin.

"Gut Glucagon"

Glicentin immunoreactivity has been found in cells of the small intestine as well as in pancreatic alpha cells and in effluents of perfused pancreas. The intestinal cells secrete **enteroglucagon,** a family of glucagon-like peptides, of which glicentin is a member, along with glucagon-like peptides 1 and 2 (GLP-1 and GLP-2). Unlike the pancreatic alpha cell, these intestinal cells lack the enzymes to convert glucagon precursors to true glucagon by removing the carboxyl terminal extension from the molecule.

Glucagon-like Peptide 1 (GLP-1)

The function of the enteroglucagons has not been clarified, although smaller peptides can bind hepatic glucagon receptors where they exert partial activity. A derivative of the 37-amino-acid form of GLP-1 that lacks the first six amino acids (GLP-1[7–37]) is a potent stimulant of insulin synthesis and release and beta-cell mass. In addition, it inhibits glucagon secretion, slows gastric emptying, and has an anorectic effect. After oral glucose ingestion, GLP-1 along with another gut hormone, GIP, accounts for as much as 70% of the induced insulin secretion. GLP-1 represents the predominant form of GLP in the human intestine and has been termed *insulinotropin*. It has been considered as a potential therapeutic agent in type 2 diabetes. However, GLP-1 requires continuous subcutaneous infusion to produce a sustained lowering of both fasting and postprandial hyperglycemia in type 2 diabetic patients; therefore, its clinical usefulness is limited. Exenatide and liraglutide (see previous text) are GLP-1 receptor agonist analogs with more practical half-lives.

Pharmacologic Effects of Glucagon

A. Metabolic Effects

The first six amino acids at the amino terminal of the glucagon molecule bind to specific G_s protein-coupled receptors on liver

cells. This leads to an increase in cAMP, which facilitates catabolism of stored glycogen and increases gluconeogenesis and ketogenesis. The immediate pharmacologic result of glucagon infusion is to raise blood glucose at the expense of stored hepatic glycogen. There is no effect on skeletal muscle glycogen, presumably because of the lack of glucagon receptors on skeletal muscle. Pharmacologic amounts of glucagon cause release of insulin from normal pancreatic beta cells, catecholamines from pheochromocytoma, and calcitonin from medullary carcinoma cells.

B. Cardiac Effects

Glucagon has a potent inotropic and chronotropic effect on the heart, mediated by the cAMP mechanism described above. Thus, it produces an effect very similar to that of β-adrenoceptor agonists without requiring functioning β receptors.

C. Effects on Smooth Muscle

Large doses of glucagon produce profound relaxation of the intestine. In contrast to the above effects of the peptide, this action on the intestine may be due to mechanisms other than adenylyl cyclase activation.

Clinical Uses

A. Severe Hypoglycemia

The major use of glucagon is for emergency treatment of severe hypoglycemic reactions in patients with type 1 diabetes when unconsciousness precludes oral feedings and intravenous glucose treatment is not possible. Recombinant glucagon is currently available in 1-mg vials for parenteral use (Glucagon Emergency Kit). Nasal sprays have been developed for this purpose but have not yet received FDA approval.

B. Endocrine Diagnosis

Several tests use glucagon to diagnose endocrine disorders. In patients with type 1 diabetes mellitus, a classic research test of pancreatic beta-cell secretory reserve uses 1 mg of glucagon administered as an intravenous bolus. Because insulin-treated patients develop circulating anti-insulin antibodies that interfere with radioimmunoassays of insulin, measurements of C-peptide are used to indicate beta-cell secretion.

C. Beta-Adrenoceptor Blocker Overdose

Glucagon is sometimes useful for reversing the cardiac effects of an overdose of β-blocking agents because of its ability to increase cAMP production in the heart. However, it is not clinically useful in the treatment of cardiac failure.

D. Radiology of the Bowel

Glucagon has been used extensively in radiology as an aid to X-ray visualization of the bowel because of its ability to relax the intestine.

Adverse Reactions

Transient nausea and occasional vomiting can result from glucagon administration. These are generally mild, and glucagon is relatively free of severe adverse reactions. It should not be used in a patient with pheochromocytoma.

■ ISLET AMYLOID POLYPEPTIDE (IAPP, AMYLIN)

Amylin is a 37-amino-acid peptide originally derived from islet amyloid deposits in pancreas material from patients with long-standing type 2 diabetes or insulinomas. It is produced by pancreatic beta cells, packaged within beta-cell granules in a concentration 1–2% that of insulin and co-secreted with insulin in a pulsatile manner and in response to physiologic secretory stimuli. Approximately 1 molecule of amylin is released for every 10 molecules of insulin. It circulates in a glycated (active) and nonglycated (inactive) form with physiologic concentrations ranging from 4 to 25 pmol/L and is primarily excreted by the kidney. Amylin appears to be a member of the superfamily of neuroregulatory peptides, with 46% homology with the calcitonin gene-related peptide CGRP (see Chapter 17). The physiologic effect of amylin may be to modulate insulin release by acting as a negative feedback on insulin secretion. At pharmacologic doses, amylin reduces glucagon secretion, slows gastric emptying by a vagally medicated mechanism, and centrally decreases appetite. An analog of amylin, **pramlintide** (see previous section), differs from amylin by the substitution of proline at positions 25, 28, and 29. These modifications make pramlintide soluble and non–self-aggregating, and suitable for pharmacologic use.

SUMMARY Drugs Used for Diabetes

Subclass	Mechanism of Action	Effects	Clinical Applications	Pharmacokinetics, Toxicities, Interactions
INSULINS • Rapid-acting: Lispro, aspart, glulisine • Short-acting: Regular • Intermediate-acting: NPH • Long-acting: Detemir, glargine	Activate insulin receptor	Reduce circulating glucose • promote glucose transport and oxidation; glycogen, lipid, protein synthesis; and regulation of gene expression	Type 1 and type 2 diabetes	Parenteral (SC or IV) • duration varies (see text) • *Toxicity:* Hypoglycemia, weight gain, lipodystrophy (rare)
SULFONYLUREAS • Glipizide • Glyburide • Glimepiride	Insulin secretagogues: Close K$^+$ channels in beta cells • increase insulin release	In patients with functioning beta cells, reduce circulating glucose • increase glycogen, fat, and protein formation • gene regulation	Type 2 diabetes	Orally active • duration 10–24 h • *Toxicity:* Hypoglycemia, weight gain
• Tolazamide, tolbutamide, chlorpropamide: Older sulfonylureas, lower potency, greater toxicity; rarely used				
GLITINIDES • Repaglinide	Insulin secretagogue: Similar to sulfonylureas with some overlap in binding sites	In patients with functioning beta cells, reduces circulating glucose • increases glycogen, fat, and protein formation • gene regulation	Type 2 diabetes	Oral • very fast onset of action • duration 5–8 h • *Toxicity:* Hypoglycemia
• Nateglinide	Insulin secretagogue: Similar to sulfonylureas with some overlap in binding sites	In patients with functioning beta cells, reduces circulating glucose • increases glycogen, fat, and protein formation • gene regulation	Type 2 diabetes	Oral • very fast onset and short duration (< 4 h) • *Toxicity:* Hypoglycemia
BIGUANIDES • Metformin	Obscure: Reduced hepatic and renal gluconeogenesis	Decreased endogenous glucose production	Type 2 diabetes	Oral • maximal plasma concentration in 2–3 h • *Toxicity:* Gastrointestinal symptoms, lactic acidosis (rare) • cannot use if impaired renal/hepatic function • congestive heart failure (CHF), hypoxic/acidotic states, alcoholism
ALPHA-GLUCOSIDASE INHIBITORS • Acarbose, miglitol	Inhibit intestinal α-glucosidases	Reduce conversion of starch and disaccharides to monosaccharides • reduce postprandial hyperglycemia	Type 2 diabetes	Oral • rapid onset • *Toxicity:* Gastrointestinal symptoms • cannot use if impaired renal/hepatic function, intestinal disorders

(continued)

Subclass	Mechanism of Action	Effects	Clinical Applications	Pharmacokinetics, Toxicities, Interactions
THIAZOLIDINEDIONES				
• Pioglitazone	Regulates gene expression by binding to PPAR-γ and PPAR-α	Reduces insulin resistance	Type 2 diabetes	Oral • long-acting (> 24 h) • *Toxicity:* Fluid retention, edema, anemia, weight gain, macular edema, bone fractures in women • cannot use if CHF, hepatic disease
• Rosiglitazone	Regulates gene expression by binding to PPAR-γ	Reduces insulin resistance	Type 2 diabetes	Oral • long-acting (> 24 h) • *Toxicity:* Fluid retention, edema, anemia, weight gain, macular edema, bone fractures in women • cannot use if CHF, hepatic disease • may worsen heart disease
GLUCAGON-LIKE POLYPEPTIDE-1 (GLP-1) RECEPTOR AGONISTS				
• Exenatide	Analog of GLP-1: Binds to GLP-1 receptors	Reduces post-meal glucose excursions: Increases glucose-mediated insulin release, lowers glucagon levels, slows gastric emptying, decreases appetite	Type 2 diabetes	Parenteral (SC) • half-life ~2.4 h • *Toxicity:* Nausea, headache, vomiting, anorexia, mild weight loss, pancreatitis
• *Liraglutide: Similar to exenatide; duration up to 24 h; immune reactions, possible thyroid carcinoma risk*				
DIPEPTIDYL PEPTIDASE-4 (DPP-4) INHIBITORS				
• Sitagliptin	DPP-4 inhibitor: Blocks degradation of GLP-1, raises circulating GLP-1 levels	Reduces post-meal glucose excursions: Increases glucose-mediated insulin release, lowers glucagon levels, slows gastric emptying, decreases appetite	Type 2 diabetes	Oral • half-life ~12 h • 24-h duration of action • *Toxicity:* Rhinitis, upper respiratory infections, headaches, pancreatitis, rare allergic reactions
• *Saxagliptin, linagliptin: Similar to sitagliptin; longer duration of action*				
AMYLIN ANALOG				
• Pramlintide	Analog of amylin: Binds to amylin receptors	Reduces post-meal glucose excursions: Lowers glucagon levels, slows gastric emptying, decreases appetite	Type 1 and type 2 diabetes	Parenteral (SC) • rapid onset • half-life ~ 48 min • *Toxicity:* Nausea, anorexia, hypoglycemia, headache
BILE ACID SEQUESTRANT				
Colesevelam hydrochloride	Bile acid binder	Lowers glucose through unknown mechanisms	Type 2 diabetes	Oral • 24-h duration of action • *Toxicity:* Constipation, indigestion, flatulence

P R E P A R A T I O N S   A V A I L A B L E[1]

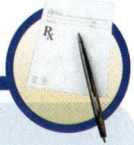

SULFONYLUREAS

Chlorpropamide (generic, Diabinese)
Oral: 100, 250 mg tablets

Glimepiride (generic, Amaryl)
Oral: 1, 2, 4 mg tablets

Glipizide (generic, Glucotrol, Glucotrol XL)
Oral: 5, 10 mg tablets; 2.5, 5, 10 mg extended-release tablets

Glyburide (generic, Diaβeta, Micronase, Glynase PresTab)
Oral: 1.25, 2.5, 5 mg tablets; 1.5, 3, 4.5, 6 mg Glynase PresTab, micronized tablets

Tolazamide (generic, Tolinase)
Oral: 100, 250, 500 mg tablets

Tolbutamide (generic, Orinase)
Oral: 500 mg tablets

MEGLITINIDE & RELATED DRUGS

Nateglinide (Starlix)
Oral: 60, 120 mg tablets

Repaglinide (Prandin)
Oral: 0.5, 1, 2 mg tablets

BIGUANIDE

Metformin (generic, Glucophage, Glucophage XR)
Oral: 500, 850, 1000 mg tablets; extended-release (XR): 500, 750, 1000 mg tablets; 500 mg/5 mL solution

METFORMIN COMBINATIONS[2]

Glipizide plus metformin (generic, Metaglip)
Oral: 2.5/250, 2.5/500, 5/500 mg tablets

Glyburide plus metformin (generic, Glucovance)
Oral: 1.25/250, 2.5/500, 5/500 mg tablets

Pioglitazone plus metformin
Oral: 15/500, 15/850 mg tablets

Repaglinide plus metformin
Oral: 1/500, 2/500 mg tablets

Rosiglitazone plus metformin (Avandamet)
Oral: 1/500, 2/500, 4/500, 2/1000, 4/1000 mg tablets

Saxagliptin plus metformin (Kombiglyze)
Oral: 5/500, 5/1000, 2.5/1000 mg tablets

Sitagliptin plus metformin (Janumet)
Oral: 50/500, 50/1000 mg tablets

THIAZOLIDINEDIONE DERIVATIVES

Pioglitazone (Actos)
Oral: 15, 30, 45 mg tablets

Rosiglitazone (Avandia)
Oral: 2, 4, 8 mg tablets

THIAZOLIDINEDIONE COMBINATION

Pioglitazone plus glimepiride (Duetact)
Oral: 30/2, 30/4 mg tablets

Rosiglitazone plus glimepiride (Avandaryl)
Oral: 4/1, 4/2, 4/4, 8/2, 8/4 mg rosiglitazone/mg glimepiride tablets

ALPHA-GLUCOSIDASE INHIBITORS

Acarbose (Precose)
Oral: 25, 50, 100 mg tablets

Miglitol (Glyset)
Oral: 25, 50, 100 mg tablets

AMYLIN ANALOGS

Pramlintide (Symlin)
Parenteral: vial: 0.6, 1 mg/mL

GLUCAGON-LIKE POLYPEPTIDE-1 RECEPTOR AGONISTS

Exenatide (Byetta)
Parenteral: 250 mcg/mL

Liraglutide (Victoza)
Parenteral: 0.6, 1.2, 1.8 mg

DIPEPTIDYL PEPTIDASE-4 INHIBITOR

Linagliptin (Tradjenta)
Oral: tablets [TK]

Saxagliptin (Onglyza)
Oral: 2.5, 5 mg tablets

Sitagliptin (Januvia)
Oral: 25, 50 100 mg tablets

BILE ACID SEQUESTRANT

Colesevelam hydrochloride
Oral: 625 mg tablets, 1.875, 3.75 g packages for oral suspension

GLUCAGON

Glucagon (generic)
Parenteral: 1 mg lyophilized powder to reconstitute for injection

[1]See Table 41–4 for insulin preparations.

[2]Other combinations are available.

REFERENCES

Action to Control Cardiovascular Risks in Diabetes Study Group: Effects oft intensive glucose lowering in type 2 diabetes. N Engl J Med 2008;358:2545.

Adler AI et al: Association of systolic blood pressure with macrovascular and microvascular complications of type 2 diabetes (UKPDS 36): Prospective observational study. Br Med J 2000;321:412.

ADVANCE Collaborative Group: Intensive blood glucose control and vascular outcomes in patients with type 2 diabetes. N Engl J Med 2008;358:2560.

Baggio LA et al: Biology of incretins: GLP-1 and GIP. Gastroenterology 2007;132:2131.

Bloomgarden ZT: Gut-derived incretin hormones and new therapeutic approaches. Diabetes Care 2004;27:2554.

Bowker SL et al: Increased cancer-related mortality for patients with type 2 diabetes who use sulfonylureas or insulin. Diabetes Care 2006;29:254.

Chaisson JL et al: Acarbose treatment and the risk of cardiovascular disease and hypertension in patients with impaired glucose tolerance: The STOP-NIDDM trial. JAMA 2003;290:486.

Chapman I et al: Effect of pramlintide on satiety and food intake in obese subjects and subjects with type 2 diabetes. Diabetologia 2005;48:838.

Davis TM et al: The continuing legacy of the United Kingdom Prospective Diabetes Study. Med J Aust 2004;180:104.

Diabetes Control and Complications Trial/Epidemiology of Diabetes Interventions and Complications Research Group: Intensive diabetes therapy and carotid intima-media thickness in type 1 diabetes mellitus. N Engl J Med 2003;348:2294.

Diabetes Prevention Program Research Group: Prevention of type 2 diabetes with troglitazone in the diabetes prevention program. Diabetes 2005;54:1150.

Diabetes Prevention Program Research Group: Reduction in the incidence of type 2 diabetes with lifestyle intervention or metformin. N Engl J Med 2002;346:393.

Dormandy JA et al: Secondary prevention of macrovascular events in patients with type 2 diabetes in the PROactive study (PROspective pioglitAzone Clinical Trial in macroVascular Events): A randomized controlled trial. Lancet 2005;366:1279.

Dunning BE et al: Alpha cell function in health and disease: Influence of glucagon-like peptide-1. Diabetologia 2005;48:1700.

Dupre J: Extendin-4 normalized postcibial glycemic excursions in type 1 diabetes. J Clin Endocrinol Metab 2004;89:3469.

Dupre J: Glycemic effects of incretins in type 1 diabetes mellitus: A concise review, with emphasis on studies in humans. Regul Pept 2005;128:149.

Erdmann E et al: Pioglitazone and the risk of cardiovascular events in patients with type 2 diabetes receiving concomitant treatment with nitrates, renin-angiotensin system blockers, or insulin: Results from the PROactive study (PROactive 20). Diabetes 2010;2:212.

Expert Committee on the Diagnosis and Classification of Diabetes Mellitus: Report of the Expert Committee on the Diagnosis and Classification of Diabetes Mellitus. Diabetes Care 2003;26(Suppl 1):S5.

Gaede P et al: Effect of a multifactorial intervention on mortality in type 2 diabetes. N Engl J Med 2008;358:580.

Grossman S: Differentiating incretin therapies based on structure, activity, and metabolism: focus on liraglutide. Pharmacotherapy 2009;29(12 Pt 2):25S.

Hanefeld M et al: Acarbose reduces the risk for myocardial infarction in type 2 diabetic patients: Meta-analysis of seven long term studies. Eur Heart J 2004;25:10.

Heinemann L et al: Time action profile of the long-acting insulin analog insulin glargine (HOE901) in comparison with those of NPH insulin and placebo. Diabetes Care 2000;23:644.

Heptulla RA et al: The role of amylin and glucagon in the dampening of glycemic excursions in children with type 1 diabetes. Diabetes 2005;54:1100.

Home PD et al: Rosiglitazone evaluated for cardiovascular outcomes—an interim analysis. N Engl J Med 2007;357:28.

Houten SM et al: Endocrine functions of bile acids. EMBO J 2006;25:1419.

Kahn SE et al: Glycemic durability of rosiglitazone, metformin, or glyburide monotherapy. N Engl J Med 2006;355:2427.

Kido Y et al: The insulin receptor and its cellular targets. J Clin Endocrinol Metab 2001;86:972.

Kitabchi A et al: Thirty years of personal experience in hyperglycemic crises: Diabetic ketoacidosis and hyperglycemic hyperosmolar state. J Clin Endocrinol Metab 2008;93:1541.

Kolterman O et al: Pharmacokinetics, pharmacodynamics, and safety of exenatide in patients with type 2 diabetes mellitus. Am J Health-Syst Pharm 2005;62:173.

Lefebvre P et al: Role of bile acids and bile acid receptors in metabolic regulation. Physiol Rev 2009;89:147.

Levien TL: Nateglinide therapy for type 2 diabetes mellitus. Ann Pharmacother 2001;35:1426.

Lincoff AM et al: Pioglitazone and risk of cardiovascular events in patients with type 2 diabetes mellitus (a meta-analysis of randomized trials). JAMA 2007;298:1180.

Nathan DM et al: Management of hyperglycemia in type 2 diabetes mellitus: A consensus algorithm for the initiation and adjustment of therapy. Diabetes Care 2006;29:1963.

Nauck MA et al: Glucagon-like peptide 1 and its derivatives in the treatment of diabetes. Regul Pept 2005;128:135.

Neumiller JJ et al: Dipeptidyl peptidase-4 inhibitors for the treatment of type 2 diabetes mellitus. Pharmacotherapy 2010;30:463.

Nissen SE et al: Effect of rosiglitazone on the risk of myocardial infarction and death from cardiovascular causes. N Engl J Med 2007;356:2457.

Ottensmeyer FP et al: Mechanism of transmembrane signalling: Insulin binding and the insulin receptor. Biochemistry 2000;39:12103.

Plank J et al: A double-blind, randomized, dose-response study investigating the pharmacodynamic and pharmacokinetic properties of the long-acting insulin analog detemir. Diabetes Care 2005;28:1107.

Ranganath LR: The entero-insular axis: Implications for human metabolism. Clin Chem Lab Med 2008;46:43.

Ratner RE et al: Amylin replacement with pramlintide as an adjunct to insulin therapy improves long term glycemic and weight control in type 1 diabetes: A 1-year randomized controlled trial. Diabetic Med 2004;21:1204.

Reitman ML et al: Pharmacogenetics of metformin response: A step in the path toward personalized medicine. J Clin Invest 2007;117:1226.

Riche DM et al: Bone loss and fracture risk associated with thiazolidinedione therapy. Pharmacotherapy 2010; posted 10.05.2010 www.medscape.com.

Schmitz O et al: Amylin agonists: A novel approach in the treatment of diabetes. Diabetes 2004;53(Suppl 3):S233.

Singh S et al: Long-term risk of cardiovascular events with rosiglitazone (a meta-analysis). JAMA 2007;298:1189.

United Kingdom Prospective Diabetes Study (UKPDS) Group: Glycemic control with diet, sulfonylurea, metformin, or insulin in patients with type 2 diabetes mellitus: Progressive requirement for multiple therapies: UKPDS 49. JAMA 1999;281:2005.

United Kingdom Prospective Diabetes Study (UKPDS) Group: Tight blood pressure control and risk of macrovascular and microvascular complications in type 2 diabetes: UKPDS 38. Br Med J 1998;317:703.

CASE STUDY ANSWER

This patient has multiple risk factors for type 2 diabetes. Although she does not have a prior history of fasting hyperglycemia, glucose intolerance, or gestational diabetes, other risk factors are present. Further evaluations that should be obtained include HbA_{1c} concentration, dilated retinal examination, baseline laboratory tests, spot urine test for microalbumin/creatinine ratio, plasma creatinine level, and neurologic examination. The patient should be taught how to use a glucose meter and monitor her fingerstick blood glucose level, referred to a nutritionist for dietary instruction, and given diabetes self-management education. Assuming she has no renal or hepatic impairment, hygienic interventions (diet and exercise) and metformin would be the first line of treatment. If she is unable to achieve adequate glycemic control on metformin, an additional agent such an insulin secretagogue (ie, sulfonylureas, meglitinide, or nateglinide), insulin, or another antidiabetic medication could be added.

Agents That Affect Bone Mineral Homeostasis

42

Daniel D. Bikle, MD, PhD

CASE STUDY

A 65-year-old man is referred to you from his primary care physician (PCP) for evaluation and management of possible osteoporosis. He saw his PCP for evaluation of low back pain. X-rays of the spine showed some degenerative changes in the lumbar spine plus several wedge deformities in the thoracic spine. The patient is a long-time smoker (up to two packs per day) and has two to four glasses of wine with dinner, more on the weekends. He has chronic bronchitis, presumably from smoking, and has been treated many times with oral prednisone for exacerbations of bronchitis. He is currently on 10 mg/d prednisone. Examination shows kyphosis of the thoracic spine, with some tenderness to fist percussion over the thoracic spine. The DEXA (dual-energy X-ray absorptiometry) measurement of the lumbar spine is "within the normal limits," but the radiologist noted that the reading may be misleading because of degenerative changes. The hip measurement shows a T score (number of standard deviations by which the patient's measured bone density differs from that of a normal young adult) in the femoral neck of −2.2. What further workup should be considered, and what therapy should be initiated?

■ BASIC PHARMACOLOGY

Calcium and phosphate, the major mineral constituents of bone, are also two of the most important minerals for general cellular function. Accordingly, the body has evolved complex mechanisms to carefully maintain calcium and phosphate homeostasis (Figure 42–1). Approximately 98% of the 1–2 kg of calcium and 85% of the 1 kg of phosphorus in the human adult are found in bone, the principal reservoir for these minerals. This reservoir is dynamic, with constant remodeling of bone and ready exchange of bone mineral with that in the extracellular fluid. Bone also serves as the principal structural support for the body and provides the space for hematopoiesis. This relationship is more than fortuitous as elements of the bone marrow affect skeletal processes just as skeletal elements affect hematopoietic processes. Abnormalities in bone mineral homeostasis can lead to a wide variety of cellular dysfunctions (eg, tetany, coma, muscle weakness), and to disturbances in structural support of the body (eg, osteoporosis with fractures) and loss of hematopoietic capacity (eg, infantile osteopetrosis).

Calcium and phosphate enter the body from the intestine. The average American diet provides 600–1000 mg of calcium per day, of which approximately 100–250 mg is absorbed. This amount represents net absorption, because both absorption (principally in the duodenum and upper jejunum) and secretion (principally in the ileum) occur. The quantity of phosphorus in the American diet is about the same as that of calcium. However, the efficiency of absorption (principally in the jejunum) is greater, ranging from 70% to 90%, depending on intake. In the steady state, renal excretion of calcium and phosphate balances intestinal absorption. In general, over 98% of filtered calcium and 85% of filtered phosphate is reabsorbed by the kidney. The movement of calcium and phosphate across the intestinal and renal epithelia is closely regulated. Dysfunction of the intestine (eg, nontropical sprue) or kidney (eg, chronic renal failure) can disrupt bone mineral homeostasis.

Three hormones serve as the principal regulators of calcium and phosphate homeostasis: **parathyroid hormone (PTH), fibroblast growth factor 23 (FGF23),** and **vitamin D** (Figure 42–2). Vitamin D is a prohormone rather than a true

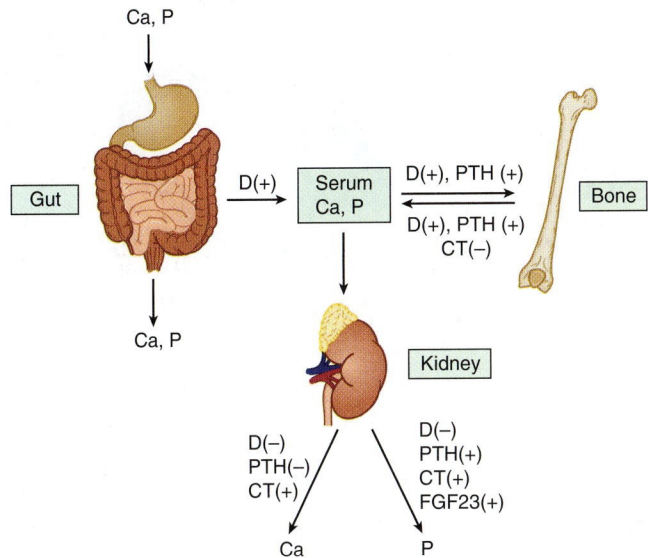

FIGURE 42–1 Mechanisms contributing to bone mineral homeostasis. Serum calcium (Ca) and phosphorus (P) concentrations are controlled principally by three hormones, 1,25-dihydroxyvitamin D (1,25[OH]$_2$D, D), fibroblast growth factor 23 (FGF23), and parathyroid hormone (PTH), through their action on absorption from the gut and from bone and on renal excretion. PTH and 1,25(OH)$_2$D increase the input of calcium and phosphorus from bone into the serum and stimulate bone formation. 1,25(OH)$_2$D also increases calcium and phosphate absorption from the gut. In the kidney, 1,25(OH)$_2$D decreases excretion of both calcium and phosphorus, whereas PTH reduces calcium but increases phosphorus excretion. FGF23 stimulates renal excretion of phosphate. Calcitonin (CT) is a less critical regulator of calcium homeostasis, but in pharmacologic concentrations can reduce serum calcium and phosphorus by inhibiting bone resorption and stimulating their renal excretion. Feedback may alter the effects shown; for example, 1,25(OH)$_2$D increases urinary calcium excretion indirectly through increased calcium absorption from the gut and inhibition of PTH secretion and may increase urinary phosphate excretion because of increased phosphate absorption from the gut and stimulation of FGF23 production.

hormone, because it must be further metabolized to gain biologic activity. PTH stimulates the production of the active metabolite of vitamin D, 1,25-dihydroxyvitamin D (1,25[OH]$_2$D), in the kidney. Other tissues also produce 1,25(OH)$_2$D; the control of this production differs from that in the kidney, as will be discussed subsequently. The complex interplay among PTH, FGF23, and 1,25(OH)$_2$D is discussed in detail later. To summarize briefly: 1,25(OH)$_2$D suppresses the production of PTH as does calcium, whereas phosphate stimulates PTH secretion. 1,25(OH)$_2$D stimulates the intestinal absorption of calcium and phosphate. 1,25(OH)$_2$D and PTH promote both bone formation and resorption in part by stimulating the proliferation and differentiation of osteoblasts and osteoclasts. Both PTH and 1,25(OH)$_2$D enhance renal retention of calcium, but PTH promotes renal phosphate excretion, whereas 1,25(OH)$_2$D promotes renal reabsorption of phosphate. FGF23 is a recently discovered hormone produced primarily by bone that stimulates renal phosphate excretion and

inhibits renal production of 1,25(OH)$_2$D. 1,25(OH)$_2$D and phosphate in turn stimulate the production of FGF23.

Other hormones—calcitonin, prolactin, growth hormone, insulin, thyroid hormone, glucocorticoids, and sex steroids—influence calcium and phosphate homeostasis under certain physiologic circumstances and can be considered secondary regulators. Deficiency or excess of these secondary regulators within a physiologic range does not produce the disturbance of calcium and phosphate homeostasis that is observed in situations of deficiency or excess of PTH, FGF23, and vitamin D. However, certain of these secondary regulators—especially calcitonin, glucocorticoids, and estrogens—are useful therapeutically and discussed in subsequent sections.

In addition to these hormonal regulators, calcium and phosphate themselves, other ions such as sodium and fluoride, and a variety of drugs (bisphosphonates, plicamycin, and diuretics) also alter calcium and phosphate homeostasis.

PRINCIPAL HORMONAL REGULATORS OF BONE MINERAL HOMEOSTASIS

PARATHYROID HORMONE

Parathyroid hormone (PTH) is a single-chain peptide hormone composed of 84 amino acids. It is produced in the parathyroid gland in a precursor form of 115 amino acids, the remaining 31 amino terminal amino acids being cleaved off before secretion. Within the gland is a calcium-sensitive protease capable of cleaving the intact hormone into fragments, thereby providing one mechanism by which calcium limits the production of PTH. A second mechanism involves the calcium-sensing receptor which, when stimulated by calcium, reduces PTH production and secretion. The parathyroid gland also contains the vitamin D receptor and the enzyme, CYP27B1, that produces the active metabolite of vitamin D, 1,25-dihydroxyvitamin D (1,25(OH)2D) thus enabling circulating or endogenously produced 1,25(OH)2D to suppress PTH production. Biologic activity resides in the amino terminal region such that synthetic PTH 1-34 (available as teriparatide) is fully active. Loss of the first two amino terminal amino acids eliminates most biologic activity.

The metabolic clearance of intact PTH is rapid, with a half-time of disappearance measured in minutes. Most of the clearance occurs in the liver and kidney. The inactive carboxyl terminal fragments produced by metabolism of the intact hormone have a much lower clearance, especially in renal failure. In the past, this accounted for the very high PTH values observed in patients with renal failure when the hormone was measured by radioimmunoassays directed against the carboxyl terminal region. Currently, most PTH assays differentiate between intact PTH 1-34 and large inactive fragments, so that it is possible to more accurately evaluate biologically active PTH status in patients with renal failure.

PTH regulates calcium and phosphate flux across cellular membranes in bone and kidney, resulting in increased serum calcium and decreased serum phosphate (Figure 42–1). In bone, PTH increases the activity and number of osteoclasts, the cells

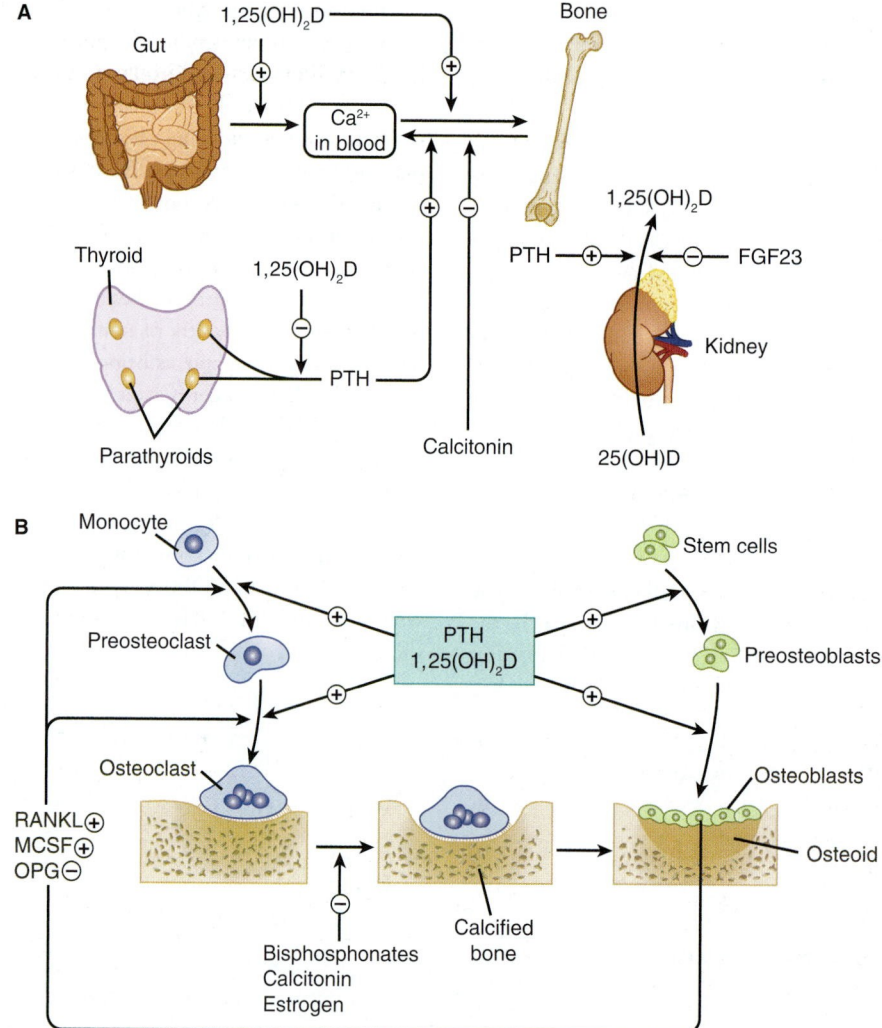

FIGURE 42–2 The hormonal interactions controlling bone mineral homeostasis. In the body **(A)**, 1,25-dihydroxyvitamin D (1,25[OH]$_2$D) is produced by the kidney under the control of parathyroid hormone (PTH), which stimulates its production, and fibroblast growth factor 23 (FGF23), which inhibits its production. 1,25(OH)$_2$D in turn inhibits the production of PTH by the parathyroid glands and stimulates FGF23 release from bone. 1,25(OH)$_2$D is the principal regulator of intestinal calcium and phosphate absorption. At the level of the bone **(B)**, both PTH and 1,25(OH)$_2$D regulate bone formation and resorption, with each capable of stimulating both processes. This is accomplished by their stimulation of preosteoblast proliferation and differentiation into osteoblasts, the bone-forming cell. PTH and 1,25(OH)$_2$D stimulate the expression of RANKL by the osteoblast, which, with MCSF, stimulates the differentiation and subsequent activation of osteoclasts, the bone-resorbing cell. FGF23 in excess leads to osteomalacia by inhibiting 1,25(OH)$_2$D production and lowering phosphate levels. MCSF, macrophage colony-stimulating factor; OPG, osteoprotegerin; RANKL, ligand for receptor for activation of nuclear factor-κB.

responsible for bone resorption (Figure 42–2). However, this stimulation of osteoclasts is not a direct effect. Rather, PTH acts on the osteoblast (the bone-forming cell) to induce membrane-bound and secreted soluble forms of a protein called **RANK ligand (RANKL)**. RANKL acts on osteoclasts and osteoclast precursors to increase both the numbers and activity of osteoclasts. This action increases bone remodeling, a specific sequence of cellular events initiated by osteoclastic bone resorption and followed by osteoblastic bone formation. An antibody that inhibits the action of RANKL has been developed (**denosumab**) for the treatment of excess bone resorption in patients with osteoporosis and certain cancers. Although both bone resorption and bone

formation are enhanced by PTH, the net effect of excess endogenous PTH is to increase bone resorption. However, administration of exogenous PTH in low and intermittent doses increases bone formation without first stimulating bone resorption. This net anabolic action may be indirect, involving other growth factors such as insulin-like growth factor 1 (IGF-1). It has led to the approval of recombinant PTH 1-34 (**teriparatide**) for the treatment of osteoporosis. In the kidney, PTH increases tubular reabsorption of calcium and magnesium but reduces reabsorption of phosphate, amino acids, bicarbonate, sodium, chloride, and sulfate. Another important action of PTH on the kidney is stimulation of 1,25-dihydroxyvitamin D (1,25[OH]$_2$D) production.

VITAMIN D

Vitamin D is a secosteroid produced in the skin from 7-dehydrocholesterol under the influence of ultraviolet radiation. Vitamin D is also found in certain foods and is used to supplement dairy products. Both the natural form (vitamin D_3, cholecalciferol) and the plant-derived form (vitamin D_2, ergocalciferol) are present in the diet. These forms differ in that ergocalciferol contains a double bond (C_{22-23}) and an additional methyl group in the side chain (Figure 42–3). Ergocalciferol and its metabolites bind less well than cholecalciferol and its metabolites to vitamin D-binding protein, the major transport protein of these compounds in blood, and have a different path of catabolism. As a result their half-lives are shorter than those of the cholecalciferol metabolites. This influences treatment strategies, as will be discussed. However, the key steps in metabolism and biologic activities of the active metabolites are comparable, so with this exception the following comments apply equally well to both forms of vitamin D.

Vitamin D is a precursor to a number of biologically active metabolites (Figure 42–3). Vitamin D is first hydroxylated in the liver to form 25-hydroxyvitamin D (25[OH]D, calcifediol). This metabolite is further converted in the kidney to a number of other forms, the best studied of which are 1,25-dihydroxyvitamin D (1,25[OH]$_2$D, calcitriol) and 24,25-dihydroxyvitamin D (24,25[OH]$_2$D). The regulation of vitamin D metabolism is complex, involving calcium, phosphate, and a variety of hormones, the most important of which is PTH, which stimulates, and FGF23, which inhibits the production of 1,25(OH)$_2$D by the kidney. Of the natural metabolites, only vitamin D and 1,25(OH)$_2$D (as calcitriol) are available for clinical use (Table 42–1). A number of analogs of 1,25(OH)$_2$D have been synthesized to extend the usefulness of this metabolite to a variety of nonclassic conditions. Calcipotriene (calcipotriol), for example, is being used to treat psoriasis, a hyperproliferative skin disorder (Chapter 61). Doxercalciferol and paricalcitol are approved for the treatment of secondary hyperparathyroidism in patients with chronic kidney disease. Other analogs are being investigated for the treatment of various malignancies.

Vitamin D and its metabolites circulate in plasma tightly bound to the vitamin D-binding protein. This α-globulin binds 25(OH)D and 24,25(OH)$_2$D with comparable high affinity and vitamin D and 1,25(OH)$_2$D with lower affinity. As noted above the affinity for the D_2 metabolites is less than that for the D_3

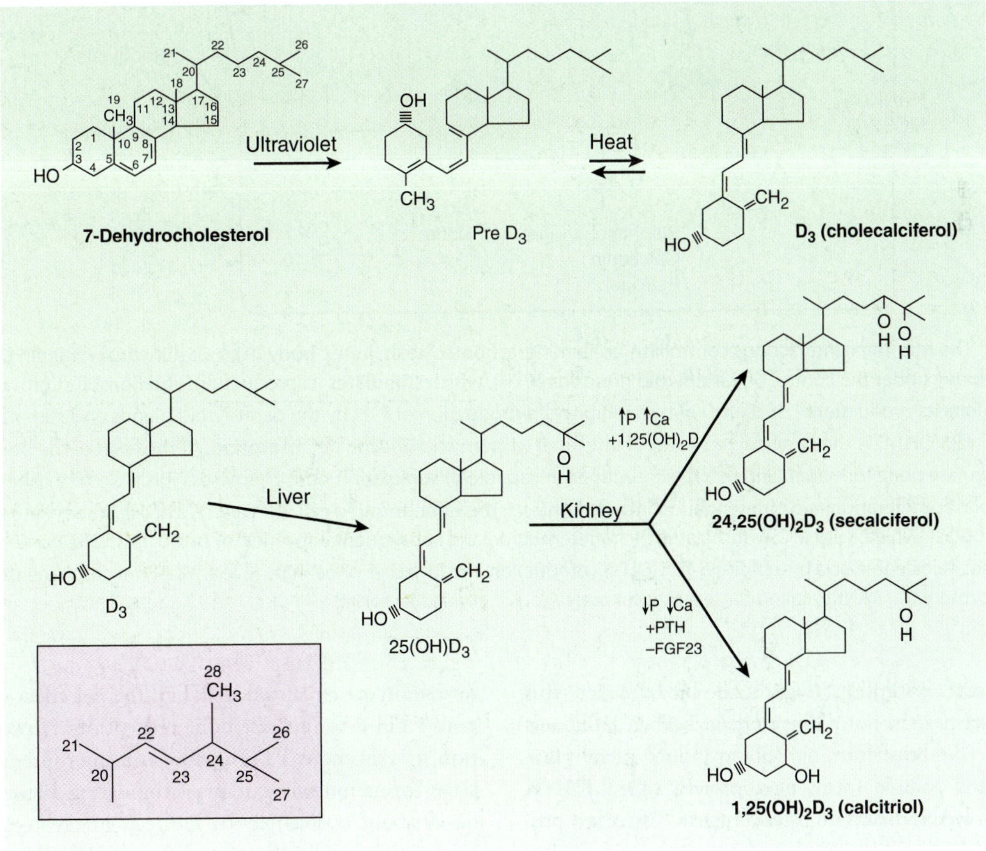

FIGURE 42–3 Conversion of 7-dehydrocholesterol to vitamin D_3 and metabolism of D_3 to 1,25-dihydroxyvitamin D_3 (1,25[OH]$_2$D$_3$) and 24,25-dihydroxyvitamin D_3 (24,25[OH]$_2$D$_3$). Control of the latter step is exerted primarily at the level of the kidney, where low serum phosphorus, low serum calcium, and high parathyroid hormone favor the production of 1,25(OH)$_2$D$_3$, whereas fibroblast growth factor 23 inhibits its production. The inset shows the side chain for ergosterol. Ergosterol undergoes similar transformation to vitamin D_2 (ergocalciferol), which, in turn, is metabolized to 25-hydroxyvitamin D_2, 1,25-dihydroxyvitamin D_2, and 24,25-dihydroxyvitamin D_2. In humans, corresponding D_2 and D_3 derivatives have equivalent effects although they differ in pharmacokinetics.

TABLE 42–1 Vitamin D and its major metabolites and analogs.

Chemical and Generic Names	Abbreviation
Vitamin D_3; cholecalciferol	D_3
Vitamin D_2; ergocalciferol	D_2
25-Hydroxyvitamin D_3; calcifediol	$25(OH)D_3$
1,25-Dihydroxyvitamin D_3; calcitriol	$1,25(OH)_2D_3$
24,25-Dihydroxyvitamin D_3; secalciferol	$24,25(OH)_2D_3$
Dihydrotachysterol	DHT
Calcipotriene (calcipotriol)	None
1α-Hydroxyvitamin D_2; doxercalciferol	$1\alpha(OH)D_2$
19-nor-1,25-Dihydroxyvitamin D_2; paricalcitol	19-nor-$1,25(OH)D_2$

metabolites. In normal subjects, the terminal half-life of injected calcifediol is 23 days, whereas in anephric subjects it is 42 days. The half-life of $24,25(OH)_2D$ is probably similar. Tracer studies with vitamin D have shown a rapid clearance from the blood. The liver appears to be the principal organ for clearance. Excess vitamin D is stored in adipose tissue. The metabolic clearance of calcitriol in humans indicates a rapid turnover, with a terminal half-life measured in hours. Several of the $1,25(OH)_2D$ analogs are bound poorly by the vitamin D-binding protein. As a result, their clearance is very rapid, with a terminal half-life of minutes. Such analogs have less of the hypercalcemic, hypercalciuric effects of calcitriol, an important aspect of their use for the management of conditions such as psoriasis and hyperparathyroidism.

The mechanism of action of the vitamin D metabolites remains under active investigation. However, $1,25(OH)_2D$ is well established as the most potent agent with respect to stimulation of intestinal calcium and phosphate transport and bone resorption. $1,25(OH)_2D$ appears to act on the intestine both by induction of new protein synthesis (eg, calcium-binding protein and TRPV6, an intestinal calcium channel) and by modulation of calcium flux across the brush border and basolateral membranes by a means that does not require new protein synthesis. The molecular action of $1,25(OH)_2D$ on bone has received less attention. However, like PTH, $1,25(OH)_2D$ can induce RANKL in osteoblasts and proteins such as osteocalcin, which may regulate the mineralization process. The metabolites $25(OH)D$ and $24,25(OH)_2D$ are far less potent stimulators of intestinal calcium and phosphate transport or bone resorption. However, $25(OH)D$ appears to be more potent than $1,25(OH)_2D$ in stimulating renal reabsorption of calcium and phosphate and may be the major metabolite regulating calcium flux and contractility in muscle. Specific receptors for $1,25(OH)_2D$ exist in target tissues. However, the role and even the existence of separate receptors for $25(OH)D$ and $24,25(OH)_2D$ remain controversial.

The receptor for $1,25(OH)_2D$ exists in many tissues—not just bone, gut, and kidney. In these "nonclassic" tissues, $1,25(OH)_2D$ exerts a number of actions including regulation of the secretion of PTH, insulin, and renin, dendritic cell as well as T-cell differentiation, and proliferation and differentiation of a number of cancer cells. Thus, the clinical utility of $1,25(OH)_2D$ and its analogs is expanding.

FIBROBLAST GROWTH FACTOR 23

Fibroblast growth factor 23 (FGF23) is a single-chain protein with 251 amino acids including a 24-amino-acid leader sequence. It inhibits $1,25(OH)_2D$ production and phosphate reabsorption (via the sodium phosphate co-transporters NaPi 2a and 2c) in the kidney, leading to both hypophosphatemia and inappropriately low levels of circulating $1,25(OH)_2D$. Whereas FGF23 was originally identified in certain mesenchymal tumors, osteoblasts and osteocytes in bone appear to be its primary site of production. Other tissues can also produce FGF23, though at lower levels. FGF23 requires O-glycosylation for its secretion, a glycosylation mediated by the glycosyl transferase GALNT3. Mutations in GALNT3 result in abnormal deposition of calcium phosphate in periarticular tissues (tumoral calcinosis) with elevated phosphate and $1,25(OH)_2D$. FGF23 is normally inactivated by cleavage at an RXXR site (amino acids 176–179). Mutations in this site lead to excess FGF23, the underlying problem in autosomal dominant hypophosphatemic rickets. A similar disease, X-linked hypophosphatemic rickets, is due to mutations in PHEX, an endopeptidase, which initially was thought to cleave FGF23. However, this concept has been shown to be invalid, and the mechanism by which PHEX mutations lead to increased FGF23 levels remains obscure. FGF23 binds to FGF receptors 1 and 3c in the presence of the accessory receptor Klotho. Both Klotho and the FGF receptor must be present for signaling. Mutations in Klotho disrupt FGF23 signaling, resulting in elevated phosphate and $1,25(OH)_2D$ levels with what has been characterized as premature aging. FGF23 production is stimulated by $1,25(OH)_2D$ and directly or indirectly inhibited by the dentin matrix protein DMP1 found in osteocytes. Mutations in DMP1 lead to increased FGF23 levels and osteomalacia.

INTERACTION OF PTH, FGF23, & VITAMIN D

A summary of the principal actions of PTH, FGF23, and vitamin D on the three main target tissues—intestine, kidney, and bone—is presented in Table 42–2. The net effect of PTH is to raise serum calcium and reduce serum phosphate; the net effect of FGF23 is to decrease serum phosphate; the net effect of vitamin D is to raise both. Regulation of calcium and phosphate homeostasis is achieved through important feedback loops. Calcium is one of two principal regulators of PTH secretion. It binds to a novel ion recognition site that is part of a G_q protein-coupled receptor called the calcium-sensing receptor (CaSR) that employs the phosphoinositide second messenger system to link changes in the extracellular calcium concentration to changes in the intracellular free calcium. As serum calcium levels rise and activate this receptor, intracellular calcium levels increase and inhibit PTH secretion. This inhibition by calcium of PTH secretion, along with inhibition of renin and atrial natriuretic factor secretion, is the opposite of the effect in other tissues such as the beta cell of the pancreas, in which calcium stimulates secretion. Phosphate regulates PTH secretion directly and indirectly by forming complexes with calcium in the serum. Because it is the ionized free concentration of extracellular calcium

TABLE 42–2 Actions of parathyroid hormone (PTH), vitamin D, and FGF23 on gut, bone, and kidney.

	PTH	Vitamin D	FGF23
Intestine	Increased calcium and phosphate absorption (by increased 1,25(OH)$_2$D production)	Increased calcium and phosphate absorption by 1,25(OH)$_2$D	Decreased calcium and phosphate absorption by decreased 1,25(OH)$_2$ production
Kidney	Decreased calcium excretion, increased phosphate excretion	Calcium and phosphate excretion may be decreased by 25(OH)D and 1,25(OH)$_2$D[1]	Increased phosphate excretion
Bone	Calcium and phosphate resorption increased by high doses. Low doses may increase bone formation.	Increased calcium and phosphate resorption by 1,25(OH)$_2$D; bone formation may be increased by 1,25(OH)$_2$D and 24,25(OH)$_2$D	Decreased mineralization due to hypophosphatemia and low 1,25(OH)2D levels, but may have a direct action on bone as well.
Net effect on serum levels	Serum calcium increased, serum phosphate decreased	Serum calcium and phosphate both increased	Decreased serum phosphate

[1]Direct effect. Vitamin D also indirectly increases urine calcium owing to increased calcium absorption from the intestine and decreased PTH.

that is detected by the parathyroid gland, increases in serum phosphate levels reduce the ionized calcium, leading to enhanced PTH secretion. Such feedback regulation is appropriate to the net effect of PTH to raise serum calcium and reduce serum phosphate levels. Likewise, both calcium and phosphate at high levels reduce the amount of 1,25(OH)$_2$D produced by the kidney and increase the amount of 24,25(OH)$_2$D produced.

High serum calcium works directly and indirectly by reducing PTH secretion. High serum phosphate works directly and indirectly by increasing FGF23 levels. Since 1,25(OH)$_2$D raises serum calcium and phosphate, whereas 24,25(OH)$_2$D has less effect, such feedback regulation is again appropriate. 1,25(OH)$_2$D directly inhibits PTH secretion (independent of its effect on serum calcium) by a direct inhibitory effect on PTH gene transcription. This provides yet another negative feedback loop. In patients with chronic renal failure who frequently are deficient in producing 1,25(OH)$_2$D, loss of this 1,25(OH)$_2$D-mediated feedback loop coupled with impaired phosphate excretion and intestinal calcium absorption often leads to secondary hyperparathyroidism. The ability of 1,25(OH)$_2$D to inhibit PTH secretion directly is being exploited with calcitriol analogs that have less effect on serum calcium because of their lesser effect on intestinal calcium absorption. Such drugs are proving useful in the management of secondary hyperparathyroidism accompanying chronic kidney disease and may be useful in selected cases of primary hyperparathyroidism. 1,25(OH)$_2$D also stimulates the production of FGF23. This completes the negative feedback loop in that FGF23 inhibits 1,25(OH)$_2$D production while promoting hypophosphatemia, which in turn inhibits FGF23 production and stimulates 1,25(OH)$_2$D production.

SECONDARY HORMONAL REGULATORS OF BONE MINERAL HOMEOSTASIS

A number of hormones modulate the actions of PTH, FGF23, and vitamin D in regulating bone mineral homeostasis. Compared with that of PTH, FGF23, and vitamin D, the physiologic impact of such secondary regulation on bone mineral homeostasis is minor. However, in pharmacologic amounts, several of these hormones, including cal-

citonin, glucocorticoids, and estrogens, have actions on bone mineral homeostatic mechanisms that can be exploited therapeutically.

CALCITONIN

The calcitonin secreted by the parafollicular cells of the mammalian thyroid is a single-chain peptide hormone with 32 amino acids and a molecular weight of 3600. A disulfide bond between positions 1 and 7 is essential for biologic activity. Calcitonin is produced from a precursor with MW 15,000. The circulating forms of calcitonin are multiple, ranging in size from the monomer (MW 3600) to forms with an apparent MW of 60,000. Whether such heterogeneity includes precursor forms or covalently linked oligomers is not known. Because of its chemical heterogeneity, calcitonin preparations are standardized by bioassay in rats. Activity is compared to a standard maintained by the British Medical Research Council (MRC) and expressed as MRC units.

Human calcitonin monomer has a half-life of about 10 minutes. Salmon calcitonin has a longer half-life, making it more attractive as a therapeutic agent. Much of the clearance occurs in the kidney by metabolism; little intact calcitonin appears in the urine.

The principal effects of calcitonin are to lower serum calcium and phosphate by actions on bone and kidney. Calcitonin inhibits osteoclastic bone resorption. Although bone formation is not impaired at first after calcitonin administration, with time both formation and resorption of bone are reduced. In the kidney, calcitonin reduces both calcium and phosphate reabsorption as well as reabsorption of other ions, including sodium, potassium, and magnesium. Tissues other than bone and kidney are also affected by calcitonin. Calcitonin in pharmacologic amounts decreases gastrin secretion and reduces gastric acid output while increasing secretion of sodium, potassium, chloride, and water in the gut. Pentagastrin is a potent stimulator of calcitonin secretion (as is hypercalcemia), suggesting a possible physiologic relationship between gastrin and calcitonin. In the adult human, no readily demonstrable problem develops in cases of calcitonin deficiency (thyroidectomy) or excess (medullary carcinoma of the thyroid). However, the ability of calcitonin to block bone resorption and lower serum calcium makes it a useful drug for the treatment of Paget's disease, hypercalcemia, and osteoporosis.

GLUCOCORTICOIDS

Glucocorticoid hormones alter bone mineral homeostasis by antagonizing vitamin D-stimulated intestinal calcium transport, stimulating renal calcium excretion, and blocking bone formation. Although these observations underscore the negative impact of glucocorticoids on bone mineral homeostasis, these hormones have proved useful in reversing the hypercalcemia associated with lymphomas and granulomatous diseases such as sarcoidosis (in which unregulated ectopic production of 1,25[OH]$_2$D occurs) or in cases of vitamin D intoxication. Prolonged administration of glucocorticoids is a common cause of osteoporosis in adults and can cause stunted skeletal development in children.

ESTROGENS

Estrogens can prevent accelerated bone loss during the immediate postmenopausal period and at least transiently increase bone in postmenopausal women.

The prevailing hypothesis advanced to explain these observations is that estrogens reduce the bone-resorbing action of PTH. Estrogen administration leads to an increased 1,25(OH)$_2$D level in blood, but estrogens have no direct effect on 1,25(OH)$_2$D production in vitro. The increased 1,25(OH)$_2$D levels in vivo following estrogen treatment may result from decreased serum calcium and phosphate and increased PTH. Estrogen receptors have been found in bone, and estrogen has direct effects on bone remodeling. Case reports of men who lack the estrogen receptor or who are unable to produce estrogen because of aromatase deficiency noted marked osteopenia and failure to close epiphyses. This further substantiates the role of estrogen in bone development, even in men. The principal therapeutic application for estrogen administration in disorders of bone mineral homeostasis is the treatment or prevention of postmenopausal osteoporosis. However, long-term use of estrogen has fallen out of favor due to concern about adverse effects. Selective estrogen receptor modulators (SERMs) have been developed to retain the beneficial effects on bone while minimizing deleterious effects on breast, uterus, and the cardiovascular system (see Box: Newer Therapies for Osteoporosis and Chapter 40).

Newer Therapies for Osteoporosis

Bone undergoes a continuous remodeling process involving resorption and formation. Any process that disrupts this balance by increasing bone resorption relative to formation results in osteoporosis. Inadequate gonadal hormone production is a major cause of osteoporosis in men and women. Estrogen replacement therapy at menopause is a well-established means of preventing osteoporosis in the female, but many women fear its adverse effects, particularly the increased risk of breast cancer from continued estrogen use (the well-demonstrated increased risk of endometrial cancer is prevented by combining the estrogen with a progestin) and do not like the persistence of menstrual bleeding that often accompanies this form of therapy. Medical enthusiasm for this treatment has waned with the demonstration that it does not protect against and may increase the risk of heart disease. Raloxifene is the first of the selective estrogen receptor modulators (SERMs; see Chapter 40) to be approved for the prevention of osteoporosis. Raloxifene shares some of the beneficial effects of estrogen on bone without increasing the risk of breast or endometrial cancer (it may actually reduce the risk of breast cancer). Although not as effective as estrogen in increasing bone density, raloxifene has been shown to reduce vertebral fractures.

Nonhormonal forms of therapy for osteoporosis with proven efficacy in reducing fracture risk have also been developed. Bisphosphonates such as alendronate, risedronate, and ibandronate have been conclusively shown to increase bone density and reduce fractures over at least 5 years when used continuously at a dosage of 10 mg/d or 70 mg/wk for alendronate; 5 mg/d or 35 mg/wk for risedronate; or 2.5 mg/d or 150 mg/month for ibandronate, and more recently intravenous zoledronate, 5 mg annually. Side-by-side trials between alendronate and calcitonin (another approved nonestrogen drug for osteoporosis) indicated a greater efficacy of alendronate. Bisphosphonates are poorly absorbed and must be given on an empty stomach or infused intravenously. At the higher oral doses used in the treatment of Paget's disease, alendronate causes gastric irritation, but this is not a significant problem at the doses recommended for osteoporosis when patients are instructed to take the drug with a glass of water and remain upright. Denosumab is a human monoclonal antibody directed against RANKL, and is very effective in inhibiting osteoclastogenesis and activity. Denosumab is given in 60 mg doses subcutaneously every 6 months. All of these drugs inhibit bone resorption with secondary effects to inhibit bone formation. On the other hand, teriparatide, the recombinant form of PTH 1-34, directly stimulates bone formation. However, teriparatide must be given daily by subcutaneous injection. Its efficacy in preventing fractures appears to be at least as great as that of the bisphosphonates. In all cases, adequate intake of calcium and vitamin D needs to be maintained.

Furthermore, there are several other forms of therapy in the pipeline. In Europe, strontium ranelate, a drug that appears to stimulate bone formation and inhibit bone resorption, has been used for several years with favorable results in large clinical trials; approval for use in the USA is expected. Additional promising new treatments undergoing clinical trials include an antibody against sclerostin (a protein produced by osteocytes that inhibits bone formation), that has been shown to stimulate bone formation, and inhibitors of cathepsin K, an enzyme in osteoclasts that facilitates bone resorption.

NONHORMONAL AGENTS AFFECTING BONE MINERAL HOMEOSTASIS

BISPHOSPHONATES

The bisphosphonates are analogs of pyrophosphate in which the P-O-P bond has been replaced with a nonhydrolyzable P-C-P bond (Figure 42–4). Currently available bisphosphonates include **etidronate, pamidronate, alendronate, risedronate, tiludronate, ibandronate**, and **zoledronate**. With the development of the more potent bisphosphonates, etidronate is seldom used.

Results from animal and clinical studies indicate that less than 10% of an oral dose of these drugs is absorbed. Food reduces absorption even further, necessitating their administration on an empty stomach. A major adverse effect of oral forms of the bisphosphonates (risedronate, alendronate, ibandronate) is esophageal and gastric irritation, which limits the use of this route by patients with upper gastrointestinal disorders. This complication can be circumvented with infusions of pamidronate, zoledronate, and ibandronate. Intravenous dosing also allows a larger amount of drug to enter the body and markedly reduces the frequency of administration (eg, zoledronate is infused once per year). Nearly half of the absorbed drug accumulates in bone; the remainder is excreted unchanged in the urine. Decreased renal function dictates a reduction in dosage. The portion of drug retained in bone depends on the rate of bone turnover; drug in bone often is retained for months if not years.

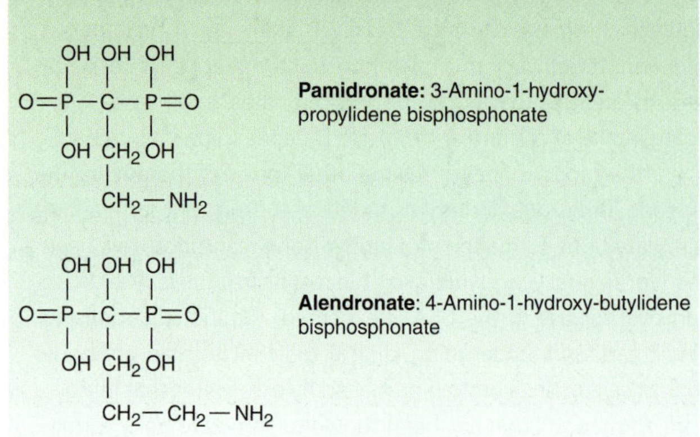

The bisphosphonates exert multiple effects on bone mineral homeostasis, which make them useful for the treatment of hypercalcemia associated with malignancy, for Paget's disease, and for osteoporosis (see Box: Newer Therapies for Osteoporosis). They owe at least part of their clinical usefulness and toxicity to their ability to retard formation and dissolution of hydroxyapatite crystals within and outside the skeletal system. Some of the newer bisphosphonates appear to increase bone mineral density well beyond the 2-year period predicted for a drug whose effects are limited to slowing bone resorption. This may be due to their other cellular effects, which include inhibition of $1,25(OH)_2D$ production, inhibition of intestinal calcium transport, metabolic changes in bone cells such as inhibition of glycolysis, inhibition of cell growth, and changes in acid and alkaline phosphatase activity.

Amino bisphosphonates such as alendronate and risedronate inhibit farnesyl pyrophosphate synthase, an enzyme in the mevalonate pathway that appears to be critical for osteoclast survival. The cholesterol-lowering statin drugs (eg, lovastatin), which block mevalonate synthesis (see Chapter 35), stimulate bone formation, at least in animal studies. Thus, the mevalonate pathway appears to be important in bone cell function and provides new targets for drug development. The mevalonate pathway effects vary depending on the bisphosphonate (ie, only amino bisphosphonates have this property), and may account for some of the clinical differences observed in the effects of the various bisphosphonates on bone mineral homeostasis.

With the exception of the induction of a mineralization defect by higher than approved doses of etidronate and gastric and esophageal irritation by the oral bisphosphonates, these drugs have proved to be remarkably free of adverse effects when used at the doses recommended for the treatment of osteoporosis. Esophageal irritation can be minimized by taking the drug with a full glass of water and remaining upright for 30 minutes or by using the intravenous forms of these compounds. Of the other complications, osteonecrosis of the jaw has received considerable attention but is rare in patients receiving usual doses of bisphosphonates (perhaps 1/100,000 patient-years). This complication is more frequent when high intravenous doses of zoledronate are used to control bone metastases and cancer-induced hypercalcemia. More recently, concern has been raised about over-suppressing bone turnover, and case reports have appeared describing unusual subtrochanteric (femur) fractures in patients on long-term bisphosphonate treatment. This complication appears to be rare, comparable to that of osteonecrosis of the jaw, but has led some authorities to recommend a "drug holiday" after 5 years of treatment if the clinical condition warrants it (ie, if the fracture risk of discontinuing the bisphosphonate is not deemed high).

FIGURE 42–4 The structure of pyrophosphate and of the first three bisphosphonates—etidronate, pamidronate, and alendronate—that were approved for use in the USA.

DENOSUMAB

Denosumab is a fully human monoclonal antibody that binds to and prevents the action of RANKL. As described earlier, RANKL is produced by osteoblasts. It stimulates osteoclastogenesis via RANK, the receptor for RANKL that is present on osteoclasts and osteoclast precursors. By interfering with RANKL function, denosumab inhibits osteoclast formation and activity. It is at least as effective as the potent bisphosphonates in inhibiting bone resorption and has recently been approved for treatment of postmenopausal osteoporosis and some cancers (prostate and breast). The latter application is to limit the development of bone metastases or bone loss resulting from the use of drugs suppressing gonadal function. Denosumab is administered subcutaneously every 6 months, which avoids gastrointestinal side effects. The drug appears to be well tolerated but two concerns remain. First, a number of cells in the immune system also express RANKL, suggesting that there could be an increased risk of infection associated with the use of denosumab. Second, because the suppression of bone turnover with denosumab is similar to that of the potent bisphosphonates, the risk of osteonecrosis of the jaw and subtrochanteric fractures may be increased, although this has not been reported in the clinical trials leading to its approval by the Food and Drug Administration (FDA).

CALCIMIMETICS

Cinacalcet is the first representative of a new class of drugs that activates the calcium-sensing receptor (CaSR). CaSR is widely distributed but has its greatest concentration in the parathyroid gland. By activating the parathyroid gland CaSR, cinacalcet inhibits PTH secretion. Cinacalcet is approved for the treatment of secondary hyperparathyroidism in chronic kidney disease and for the treatment of parathyroid carcinoma. CaSR antagonists are also being developed, and may be useful in conditions of hypoparathyroidism or as a means to stimulate intermittent PTH secretion in the treatment of osteoporosis.

PLICAMYCIN (MITHRAMYCIN)

Plicamycin is a cytotoxic antibiotic (see Chapter 54) that has been used clinically for two disorders of bone mineral metabolism: Paget's disease and hypercalcemia. The cytotoxic properties of the drug appear to involve binding to DNA and interruption of DNA-directed RNA synthesis. The reasons for its usefulness in the treatment of Paget's disease and hypercalcemia are unclear but may relate to the need for protein synthesis to sustain bone resorption. The doses required to treat Paget's disease and hypercalcemia are about one tenth the amount required to achieve cytotoxic effects. With the development of other less toxic drugs for these purposes, the clinical use of plicamycin is seldom indicated.

THIAZIDE DIURETICS

The chemistry and pharmacology of the thiazide family of drugs are discussed in Chapter 15. The principal application of thiazides in the treatment of bone mineral disorders is in reducing renal calcium excretion. Thiazides may increase the effectiveness of PTH in stimulating reabsorption of calcium by the renal tubules or may act on calcium reabsorption secondarily by increasing sodium reabsorption in the proximal tubule. In the distal tubule, thiazides block sodium reabsorption at the luminal surface,

increasing the calcium-sodium exchange at the basolateral membrane and thus enhancing calcium reabsorption into the blood at this site (see Figure 15–4). Thiazides have proved to be useful in reducing the hypercalciuria and incidence of urinary stone formation in subjects with idiopathic hypercalciuria. Part of their efficacy in reducing stone formation may lie in their ability to decrease urine oxalate excretion and increase urine magnesium and zinc levels, both of which inhibit calcium oxalate stone formation.

FLUORIDE

Fluoride is well established as effective for the prophylaxis of dental caries and has previously been investigated for the treatment of osteoporosis. Both therapeutic applications originated from epidemiologic observations that subjects living in areas with naturally fluoridated water (1–2 ppm) had less dental caries and fewer vertebral compression fractures than subjects living in nonfluoridated water areas. Fluoride accumulates in bones and teeth, where it may stabilize the hydroxyapatite crystal. Such a mechanism may explain the effectiveness of fluoride in increasing the resistance of teeth to dental caries, but it does not explain its ability to promote new bone growth.

Fluoride in drinking water appears to be most effective in preventing dental caries if consumed before the eruption of the permanent teeth. The optimum concentration in drinking water supplies is 0.5–1 ppm. Topical application is most effective if done just as the teeth erupt. There is little further benefit to giving fluoride after the permanent teeth are fully formed. Excess fluoride in drinking water leads to mottling of the enamel proportionate to the concentration above 1 ppm.

Because of the paucity of agents that stimulate new bone growth in patients with osteoporosis, fluoride for this disorder has been examined (see Osteoporosis, below). Results of earlier studies indicated that fluoride alone, without adequate calcium supplementation, produced osteomalacia. More recent studies, in which calcium supplementation has been adequate, have demonstrated an improvement in calcium balance, an increase in bone mineral, and an increase in trabecular bone volume. Despite these promising effects of fluoride on bone mass, clinical studies have failed to demonstrate a reliable reduction in fractures, and some studies showed an increase in fracture rate. At present, fluoride is not approved by the FDA for treatment or prevention of osteoporosis, and it is unlikely to be.

Adverse effects observed—at the doses used for testing fluoride's effect on bone—include nausea and vomiting, gastrointestinal blood loss, arthralgias, and arthritis in a substantial proportion of patients. Such effects are usually responsive to reduction of the dose or giving fluoride with meals (or both).

STRONTIUM RANELATE

Strontium ranelate is composed of two atoms of strontium bound to an organic ion, ranelic acid. Although not yet approved for use in the USA, this drug is used in Europe for the treatment of osteoporosis. Strontium ranelate appears to block differentiation of osteoclasts while promoting their apoptosis, thus inhibiting bone resorption. At the same time, strontium ranelate appears to promote bone formation. Unlike bisphosphonates, denosumab, or teriparatide, this drug increases bone formation markers while inhibiting bone resorption markers. Large clinical trials have demonstrated its efficacy in increasing bone mineral density and decreasing fractures in the spine and hip. Toxicities reported thus far are similar to placebo.

■ CLINICAL PHARMACOLOGY

Individuals with disorders of bone mineral homeostasis usually present with abnormalities in serum or urine calcium levels (or both), often accompanied by abnormal serum phosphate levels. These abnormal mineral concentrations may themselves cause symptoms requiring immediate treatment (eg, coma in malignant hypercalcemia, tetany in hypocalcemia). More commonly, they serve as clues to an underlying disorder in hormonal regulators (eg, primary hyperparathyroidism), target tissue response (eg, chronic kidney disease), or drug misuse (eg, vitamin D intoxication). In such cases, treatment of the underlying disorder is of prime importance.

Since bone and kidney play central roles in bone mineral homeostasis, conditions that alter bone mineral homeostasis usually affect one or both of these tissues secondarily. Effects on bone can result in osteoporosis (abnormal loss of bone; remaining bone histologically normal), osteomalacia (abnormal bone formation due to inadequate mineralization), or osteitis fibrosa (excessive bone resorption with fibrotic replacement of resorption cavities and marrow). Biochemical markers of skeletal involvement include changes in serum levels of the skeletal isoenzyme of alkaline phosphatase, osteocalcin, and N- and C- terminal propeptides of type I collagen (reflecting osteoblastic activity), and serum and urine levels of tartrate-resistant acid phosphatase and collagen breakdown products (reflecting osteoclastic activity). The kidney becomes involved when the calcium × phosphate product in serum rises above the point at which ectopic calcification occurs (nephrocalcinosis) or when the calcium × oxalate (or phosphate) product in urine exceeds saturation, leading to nephrolithiasis. Subtle early indicators of such renal involvement include polyuria, nocturia, and hyposthenuria. Radiologic evidence of nephrocalcinosis and stones is not generally observed until later. The degree of the ensuing renal failure is best followed by monitoring the decline in creatinine clearance. On the other hand, chronic kidney disease can be a primary cause of bone disease because of altered handling of calcium and phosphate, decreased $1,25(OH)_2D$ production, and secondary hyperparathyroidism.

ABNORMAL SERUM CALCIUM & PHOSPHATE LEVELS

HYPERCALCEMIA

Hypercalcemia causes central nervous system depression, including coma, and is potentially lethal. Its major causes (other than thiazide therapy) are hyperparathyroidism and cancer, with or without bone metastases. Less common causes are hypervitaminosis D, sarcoidosis, thyrotoxicosis, milk-alkali syndrome, adrenal insufficiency, and immobilization. With the possible exception of hypervitaminosis D, the latter disorders seldom require emergency lowering of serum calcium. A number of approaches are used to manage the hypercalcemic crisis.

Saline Diuresis

In hypercalcemia of sufficient severity to produce symptoms, rapid reduction of serum calcium is required. The first steps include rehydration with saline and diuresis with furosemide, although the efficacy of furosemide in this setting has not been proved and use of the drug for this purpose appears to be falling out of favor. Most patients presenting with severe hypercalcemia have a substantial component of prerenal azotemia owing to dehydration, which prevents the kidney from compensating for the rise in serum calcium by excreting more calcium in the urine. Therefore, the initial infusion of 500–1000 mL/h of saline to reverse the dehydration and restore urine flow can by itself substantially lower serum calcium. The addition of a loop diuretic such as furosemide following rehydration enhances urine flow and also inhibits calcium reabsorption in the ascending limb of the loop of Henle (see Chapter 15). Monitoring of central venous pressure is important to forestall the development of heart failure and pulmonary edema in predisposed subjects. In many subjects, saline diuresis suffices to reduce serum calcium to a point at which more definitive diagnosis and treatment of the underlying condition can be achieved. If this is not the case or if more prolonged medical treatment of hypercalcemia is required, the following agents are available (discussed in order of preference).

Bisphosphonates

Pamidronate, 60–90 mg, infused over 2–4 hours, and zoledronate, 4 mg, infused over at least 15 minutes, have been approved for the treatment of hypercalcemia of malignancy and have largely replaced the less effective etidronate for this indication. The bisphosphonate effects generally persist for weeks, but treatment can be repeated after a 7-day interval if necessary and if renal function is not impaired. Some patients experience a self-limited flu-like syndrome after the initial infusion, but subsequent infusions generally do not have this side effect. Repeated doses of these drugs have been linked to renal deterioration and osteonecrosis of the jaw, but this adverse effect is rare.

Calcitonin

Calcitonin has proved useful as ancillary treatment in some patients. Calcitonin by itself seldom restores serum calcium to normal, and refractoriness frequently develops. However, its lack of toxicity permits frequent administration at high doses (200 MRC units or more). An effect on serum calcium is observed within 4–6 hours and lasts for 6–10 hours. Calcimar (salmon calcitonin) is available for parenteral and nasal administration.

Gallium Nitrate

Gallium nitrate is approved by the FDA for the management of hypercalcemia of malignancy. This drug inhibits bone resorption.

At a dosage of 200 mg/m^2 body surface area per day given as a continuous intravenous infusion in 5% dextrose for 5 days, gallium nitrate proved superior to calcitonin in reducing serum calcium in cancer patients. Because of potential nephrotoxicity, patients should be well hydrated and have good renal output before starting the infusion.

Plicamycin (Mithramycin)

Because of its toxicity, plicamycin (mithramycin) is not the drug of first choice for the treatment of hypercalcemia. However, when other forms of therapy fail, 25–50 mcg/kg of plicamycin given intravenously usually lowers serum calcium substantially within 24–48 hours. This effect can last several days. This dose can be repeated as necessary. The most dangerous toxic effect is sudden thrombocytopenia followed by hemorrhage. Hepatic and renal toxicity can also occur. Hypocalcemia, nausea, and vomiting may limit therapy. Use of this drug must be accompanied by careful monitoring of platelet counts, liver and kidney function, and serum calcium levels.

Phosphate

Intravenous phosphate administration is probably the fastest and surest way to reduce serum calcium, but it is a hazardous procedure if not done properly. Intravenous phosphate should be used only after other methods of treatment (bisphosphonates, calcitonin, and saline diuresis) have failed to control symptomatic hypercalcemia. Phosphate must be given slowly (50 mmol or 1.5 g elemental phosphorus over 6–8 hours) and the patient switched to oral phosphate (1–2 g/d elemental phosphorus, as one of the salts indicated below) as soon as symptoms of hypercalcemia have cleared. The risks of intravenous phosphate therapy include sudden hypocalcemia, ectopic calcification, acute renal failure, and hypotension. Oral phosphate can also lead to ectopic calcification and renal failure if serum calcium and phosphate levels are not carefully monitored, but the risk is less and the time of onset much longer. Phosphate is available in oral and intravenous forms as sodium or potassium salts. Amounts required to provide 1 g of elemental phosphorus are as follows:

Intravenous:

In-Phos: 40 mL
Hyper-Phos-K: 15 mL

Oral:

Fleet Phospho-Soda: 6.2 mL
Neutra-Phos: 300 mL
K-Phos-Neutral: 4 tablets

Glucocorticoids

Glucocorticoids have no clear role in the immediate treatment of hypercalcemia. However, the chronic hypercalcemia of sarcoidosis, vitamin D intoxication, and certain cancers may respond within several days to glucocorticoid therapy. Prednisone in oral doses of 30–60 mg daily is generally used, although equivalent doses of other glucocorticoids are effective. The rationale for the use of glucocorticoids in these diseases differs, however. The hypercalcemia of sarcoidosis is secondary to increased production of 1,25(OH)$_2$D, possibly by the sarcoid tissue itself. Glucocorticoid therapy directed at the reduction of sarcoid tissue results in restoration of normal serum calcium and 1,25(OH)$_2$D levels. The treatment of hypervitaminosis D with glucocorticoids probably does not alter vitamin D metabolism significantly but is thought to reduce vitamin D-mediated intestinal calcium transport. An action of glucocorticoids to reduce vitamin D-mediated bone resorption has not been excluded, however. The effect of glucocorticoids on the hypercalcemia of cancer is probably twofold. The malignancies responding best to glucocorticoids (ie, multiple myeloma and related lymphoproliferative diseases) are sensitive to the lytic action of glucocorticoids. Therefore part of the effect may be related to decreased tumor mass and activity. Glucocorticoids have also been shown to inhibit the secretion or effectiveness of cytokines elaborated by multiple myeloma and related cancers that stimulate osteoclastic bone resorption. Other causes of hypercalcemia—particularly primary hyperparathyroidism—do not respond to glucocorticoid therapy.

HYPOCALCEMIA

The main features of hypocalcemia are neuromuscular—tetany, paresthesias, laryngospasm, muscle cramps, and seizures. The major causes of hypocalcemia in the adult are hypoparathyroidism, vitamin D deficiency, chronic kidney disease, and malabsorption. Hypocalcemia can also accompany the infusion of potent bisphosphonates and denosumab for the treatment of osteoporosis, but this is seldom of clinical significance unless the patient is already hypocalcemic at the onset of the infusion. Neonatal hypocalcemia is a common disorder that usually resolves without therapy. The roles of PTH, vitamin D, and calcitonin in the neonatal syndrome are under investigation. Large infusions of citrated blood can produce hypocalcemia secondary to the formation of citrate-calcium complexes. Calcium and vitamin D (or its metabolites) form the mainstay of treatment of hypocalcemia.

Calcium

A number of calcium preparations are available for intravenous, intramuscular, and oral use. Calcium gluceptate (0.9 mEq calcium/mL), calcium gluconate (0.45 mEq calcium/mL), and calcium chloride (0.68–1.36 mEq calcium/mL) are available for intravenous therapy. Calcium gluconate is preferred because it is less irritating to veins. Oral preparations include calcium carbonate (40% calcium), calcium lactate (13% calcium), calcium phosphate (25% calcium), and calcium citrate (21% calcium). Calcium carbonate is often the preparation of choice because of its high percentage of calcium, ready availability (eg, Tums), low cost, and antacid properties. In achlorhydric patients, calcium carbonate should be given with meals to increase absorption, or the patient should be switched to calcium citrate, which is somewhat better absorbed. Combinations of vitamin D and calcium are available, but treatment must be tailored to the individual patient and the individual disease, a flexibility lost by fixed-dosage combinations.

Treatment of severe symptomatic hypocalcemia can be accomplished with slow infusion of 5–20 mL of 10% calcium gluconate. Rapid infusion can lead to cardiac arrhythmias. Less severe hypocalcemia is best treated with oral forms sufficient to provide approximately 400–1200 mg of elemental calcium (1–3 g calcium carbonate) per day. Dosage must be adjusted to avoid hypercalcemia and hypercalciuria.

Vitamin D

When rapidity of action is required, $1,25(OH)_2D_3$ (calcitriol), 0.25–1 mcg daily, is the vitamin D metabolite of choice because it is capable of raising serum calcium within 24–48 hours. Calcitriol also raises serum phosphate, although this action is usually not observed early in treatment. The combined effects of calcitriol and all other vitamin D metabolites and analogs on both calcium and phosphate make careful monitoring of these mineral levels especially important to prevent ectopic calcification secondary to an abnormally high serum calcium × phosphate product. Since the choice of the appropriate vitamin D metabolite or analog for long-term treatment of hypocalcemia depends on the nature of the underlying disease, further discussion of vitamin D treatment is found under the headings of the specific diseases.

HYPERPHOSPHATEMIA

Hyperphosphatemia is a common complication of renal failure and is also found in all types of hypoparathyroidism (idiopathic, surgical, and pseudohypoparathyroidism), vitamin D intoxication, and the rare syndrome of tumoral calcinosis (usually due to insufficient bioactive FGF23). Emergency treatment of hyperphosphatemia is seldom necessary but can be achieved by dialysis or glucose and insulin infusions. In general, control of hyperphosphatemia involves restriction of dietary phosphate plus phosphate-binding gels such as **sevelamer** and calcium supplements. Because of their potential to induce aluminum-associated bone disease, aluminum-containing antacids should be used sparingly and only when other measures fail to control the hyperphosphatemia. In patients with chronic kidney disease enthusiasm for the use of large doses of calcium to control hyperphosphatemia has waned because of the risk of ectopic calcification.

HYPOPHOSPHATEMIA

Hypophosphatemia is associated with a variety of conditions, including primary hyperparathyroidism, vitamin D deficiency, idiopathic hypercalciuria, conditions associated with increased bioactive FGF23 (eg, X-linked and autosomal dominant hypophosphatemic rickets and tumor-induced osteomalacia), other forms of renal phosphate wasting (eg, Fanconi's syndrome), overzealous use of phosphate binders, and parenteral nutrition with inadequate phosphate content. Acute hypophosphatemia may cause a reduction in the intracellular levels of high-energy organic phosphates (eg, ATP), interfere with normal hemoglobin-to-tissue oxygen transfer by decreasing red cell 2,3-diphosphoglycerate levels, and lead to rhabdomyolysis. However, clinically significant acute effects of hypophosphatemia are seldom seen, and emergency treatment is generally not indicated. The long-term effects of hypophosphatemia include proximal muscle weakness and abnormal bone mineralization (osteomalacia). Therefore, hypophosphatemia should be avoided when using forms of therapy that can lead to hypophosphatemia (eg, phosphate binders, certain types of parenteral nutrition) and treated in conditions that cause hypophosphatemia, such as the various forms of hypophosphatemic rickets. Oral forms of phosphate are listed above.

SPECIFIC DISORDERS INVOLVING BONE MINERAL-REGULATING HORMONES

PRIMARY HYPERPARATHYROIDISM

This rather common disease, if associated with symptoms and significant hypercalcemia, is best treated surgically. Oral phosphate and bisphosphonates have been tried but cannot be recommended. Asymptomatic patients with mild disease often do not get worse and may be left untreated. The calcimimetic agent **cinacalcet**, discussed previously, has been approved for secondary hyperparathyroidism and is in clinical trials for the treatment of primary hyperparathyroidism. If such drugs prove efficacious and cost effective, medical management of this disease will need to be reconsidered.

HYPOPARATHYROIDISM

In PTH deficiency (idiopathic or surgical hypoparathyroidism) or an abnormal target tissue response to PTH (pseudohypoparathyroidism), serum calcium falls and serum phosphate rises. In such patients, $1,25(OH)_2D$ levels are usually low, presumably reflecting the lack of stimulation by PTH of $1,25(OH)_2D$ production. The skeletons of patients with idiopathic or surgical hypoparathyroidism are normal except for a slow turnover rate. A number of patients with pseudohypoparathyroidism appear to have osteitis fibrosa, suggesting that the normal or high PTH levels found in such patients are capable of acting on bone but not on the kidney. The distinction between pseudohypoparathyroidism and idiopathic hypoparathyroidism is made on the basis of normal or high PTH levels but deficient renal response (ie, diminished excretion of cAMP or phosphate) in patients with pseudohypoparathyroidism.

The principal therapeutic concern is to restore normocalcemia and normophosphatemia. Vitamin D (25,000–100,000 units three times per week) and dietary calcium supplements have been used in the past. More rapid increments in serum calcium can be achieved with calcitriol. Many patients treated with vitamin D experience episodes of hypercalcemia. This complication is more rapidly reversible with cessation of therapy using calcitriol than therapy with vitamin D. This would be of importance to the patient in whom such hypercalcemic crises are common. Although teriparatide (PTH 1-34) is not approved for the treatment of hypoparathyroidism, it can be quite effective in patients who respond poorly to calcium and vitamin D and may become the drug of choice for this condition.

NUTRITIONAL VITAMIN D DEFICIENCY OR INSUFFICIENCY

The level of vitamin D thought to be necessary for good health is being reexamined with the appreciation that vitamin D acts on a large number of cell types beyond those responsible for bone and mineral metabolism. A level of 25(OH)D above 10 ng/mL is necessary for preventing rickets or osteomalacia. However, substantial epidemiologic and some prospective trial data indicate that a higher level, such as 30 ng/mL, is required to optimize intestinal calcium absorption, optimize the accrual and maintenance of bone mass, reduce falls and fractures, and prevent a wide variety of diseases including diabetes mellitus, hyperparathyroidism, autoimmune diseases, and cancer. However, an expert panel for the Institute of Medicine (IOM) has recently recommended that a level of 20 ng/mL (50 nM) was sufficient for 97.5% of the population, although up to 50 ng/mL (125 nM) was considered safe. For individuals between the ages of 1–70 yrs 600 iu vitamin was thought to be sufficient to meet these goals, although up to 4000 iu vitamin D was considered safe. These recommendations are based primarily on data from randomized placebo controlled clinical trials (RCT) that evaluated falls and fractures; data supporting the non skeletal effects of vitamin D were considered too preliminary to be used in their recommendations because of lack of RCT for these other actions. The lower end of these recommendations has been considered too low and the upper end too restrictive by a number of vitamin D experts, but the call for better clinical data especially for the non skeletal actions is well taken. These guidelines—at least with respect to the lower recommended levels of vitamin D supplementation—are unlikely to correct vitamin D deficiency in individuals with obesity, dark complexions, limited capacity for sunlight exposure, or malabsorption. Furthermore, a large body of data from animal and cell studies as well and epidemiologic associations support a large range of beneficial actions of vitamin D that with adequate RCT data may alter these IOM recommendations. Vitamin D deficiency or insufficiency can be treated by higher dosages (4000 units per day or 50,000 units per week for several weeks). No other vitamin D metabolite is indicated. Because the half-life of vitamin D$_3$ metabolites in blood is greater than that of vitamin D$_2$, there may be some advantage to using vitamin D$_3$ supplements, although when administered on a daily or weekly schedule these differences may be moot. The diet should also contain adequate amounts of calcium and phosphate.

CHRONIC KIDNEY DISEASE

The major sequelae of chronic kidney disease that impact bone mineral homeostasis are deficient 1,25(OH)$_2$D production, retention of phosphate with an associated reduction in ionized calcium levels, and the secondary hyperparathyroidism that results from the parathyroid gland response to lowered serum ionized calcium

and low 1,25(OH)$_2$D. FGF23 levels are also increased in this disorder in part due to the increased phosphate, and this can further reduce 1,25(OH)$_2$D production by the kidney. With impaired 1,25(OH)$_2$D production, less calcium is absorbed from the intestine and less bone is resorbed under the influence of PTH. As a result hypocalcemia usually develops, furthering the development of secondary hyperparathyroidism. The bones show a mixture of osteomalacia and osteitis fibrosa.

In contrast to the hypocalcemia that is more often associated with chronic kidney disease, some patients may become hypercalcemic from overzealous treatment with calcium. However, the most common cause of hypercalcemia is the development of severe secondary (sometimes referred to as tertiary) hyperparathyroidism. In such cases, the PTH level in blood is very high. Serum alkaline phosphatase levels also tend to be high. Treatment often requires parathyroidectomy. A less common circumstance leading to hypercalcemia is development of a form of bone disease characterized by a profound decrease in bone cell activity and loss of the calcium buffering action of bone (adynamic bone disease). In the absence of kidney function, any calcium absorbed from the intestine accumulates in the blood. Such patients are very sensitive to the hypercalcemic action of 1,25(OH)$_2$D. These individuals generally have a high serum calcium but nearly normal alkaline phosphatase and PTH levels. The bone in such patients may have a high aluminum content, especially in the mineralization front, which blocks normal bone mineralization. These patients do not respond favorably to parathyroidectomy. Deferoxamine, an agent used to chelate iron (see Chapter 57), also binds aluminum and is being used to treat this disorder. However, with the reduction in use of aluminum-containing phosphate binders, most cases of adynamic bone disease are not associated with aluminum deposition but are attributed to overzealous suppression of PTH secretion.

Vitamin D Preparations

The choice of vitamin D preparation to be used in the setting of chronic kidney disease depends on the type and extent of bone disease and hyperparathyroidism. Individuals with vitamin D deficiency or insufficiency should first have their 25(OH)D levels restored to normal (above 30 ng/mL) with vitamin D. 1,25(OH)$_2$D$_3$ (calcitriol) rapidly corrects hypocalcemia and at least partially reverses secondary hyperparathyroidism and osteitis fibrosa. Many patients with muscle weakness and bone pain gain an improved sense of well-being.

Two analogs of calcitriol—doxercalciferol and paricalcitol—are approved for the treatment of secondary hyperparathyroidism of chronic kidney disease. Their principal advantage is that they are less likely than calcitriol to induce hypercalcemia for any given reduction in PTH. Their greatest impact is in patients in whom the use of calcitriol may lead to unacceptably high serum calcium levels.

Regardless of the drug used, careful attention to serum calcium and phosphate levels is required. A calcium × phosphate product (in mg/dL units) less than 55 is desired with both calcium and phosphate in the normal range. Calcium adjustments in the diet and dialysis bath and phosphate restriction (dietary and with oral ingestion of phosphate binders) should be used along with vitamin D metabolites. Monitoring of serum PTH and alkaline phosphatase levels is useful in determining whether therapy is correcting or preventing secondary hyperparathyroidism. In patients on dialysis, a PTH value of approximately twice the upper limits of normal is considered desirable to prevent adynamic bone disease. Although not generally available, percutaneous bone biopsies for quantitative histomorphometry may help in choosing appropriate therapy and following the effectiveness of such therapy, especially in cases suspected of adynamic bone disease. Unlike the rapid changes in serum values, changes in bone morphology require months to years. Monitoring of serum vitamin D metabolite levels is useful for determining adherence, absorption, and metabolism.

INTESTINAL OSTEODYSTROPHY

A number of gastrointestinal and hepatic diseases cause disordered calcium and phosphate homeostasis, which ultimately leads to bone disease. The bones in such patients show a combination of osteoporosis and osteomalacia. Osteitis fibrosa does not occur, in contrast to renal osteodystrophy. The important common feature in this group of diseases appears to be malabsorption of calcium and vitamin D. Liver disease may, in addition, reduce the production of 25(OH)D from vitamin D, although its importance in patients other than those with terminal liver failure remains in dispute. The malabsorption of vitamin D is probably not limited to exogenous vitamin D as the liver secretes into bile a substantial number of vitamin D metabolites and conjugates that are normally reabsorbed in (presumably) the distal jejunum and ileum. Interference with this process could deplete the body of endogenous vitamin D metabolites in addition to limiting absorption of dietary vitamin D.

In mild forms of malabsorption, high doses of vitamin D (25,000–50,000 units three times per week) should suffice to raise serum levels of 25(OH)D into the normal range. Many patients with severe disease do not respond to vitamin D. Clinical experience with the other metabolites is limited, but both calcitriol and

calcifediol have been used successfully in doses similar to those recommended for treatment of renal osteodystrophy. Theoretically, calcifediol should be the drug of choice under these conditions, because no impairment of the renal metabolism of 25(OH)D to 1,25(OH)$_2$D and 24,25(OH)$_2$D exists in these patients. However, calcifediol is no longer available in the USA. Both calcitriol and 24,25(OH)$_2$D may be of importance in reversing the bone disease. Intramuscular injections of vitamin D would be an alternative form of therapy, but there are currently no FDA-approved intramuscular preparations available in the USA.

As in the other diseases discussed, treatment of intestinal osteodystrophy with vitamin D and its metabolites should be accompanied by appropriate dietary calcium supplementation and monitoring of serum calcium and phosphate levels.

OSTEOPOROSIS

Osteoporosis is defined as abnormal loss of bone predisposing to fractures. It is most common in postmenopausal women but also occurs in men. The annual direct medical cost of fractures in older women and men in the USA is estimated to be 17–20 billion dollars per year, and is increasing as our population ages. Osteoporosis is most commonly associated with loss of gonadal function as in menopause but may also occur as an adverse effect of long-term administration of glucocorticoids or other drugs, including those that inhibit sex steroid production; as a manifestation of endocrine disease such as thyrotoxicosis or hyperparathyroidism; as a feature of malabsorption syndrome; as a consequence of alcohol abuse and cigarette smoking; or without obvious cause (idiopathic). The ability of some agents to reverse the bone loss of osteoporosis is shown in Figure 42–5. The postmenopausal form of osteoporosis may be accompanied by lower 1,25(OH)$_2$D levels and reduced intestinal calcium transport. This form of osteoporosis is due to reduced estrogen production and can be treated

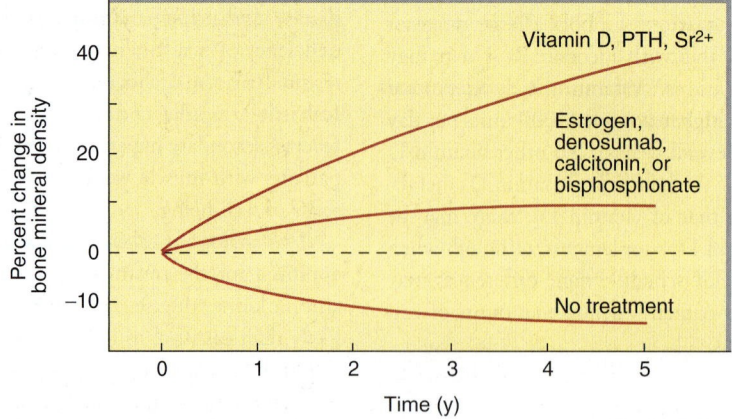

FIGURE 42–5 Typical changes in bone mineral density with time after the onset of menopause, with and without treatment. In the untreated condition, bone is lost during aging in both men and women. Strontium (Sr^{2+}), parathyroid hormone (PTH), and vitamin D promote bone formation and can increase bone mineral density in subjects who respond to them throughout the period of treatment, although PTH and vitamin D in high doses also activate bone resorption. In contrast, estrogen, calcitonin, denosumab, and bisphosphonates block bone resorption. This leads to a transient increase in bone mineral density because bone formation is not initially decreased. However, with time, both bone formation and bone resorption decrease with these pure antiresorptive agents, and bone mineral density reaches a new plateau.

with estrogen (combined with a progestin in women with a uterus to prevent endometrial carcinoma). However, concern that estrogen increases the risk of breast cancer and fails to reduce or may actually increase the development of heart disease has reduced enthusiasm for this form of therapy, at least in older individuals.

Bisphosphonates are potent inhibitors of bone resorption. They increase bone density and reduce the risk of fractures in the hip, spine, and other locations. **Alendronate, risedronate, ibandronate,** and **zoledronate** are approved for the treatment of osteoporosis, using daily dosing schedules of alendronate, 10 mg/d, risedronate, 5 mg/d, or ibandronate, 2.5 mg/d; or weekly schedules of alendronate, 70 mg/wk, or risedronate, 35 mg/wk; or monthly schedules of ibandronate, 150 mg/month; or quarterly (every 3 months) injections of ibandronate, 3 mg; or annual infusions of zoledronate, 5 mg. These drugs are effective in men as well as women and for various causes of osteoporosis.

As previously noted, estrogen-like SERMs (selective estrogen receptor modulators, Chapter 40) have been developed that prevent the increased risk of breast and uterine cancer associated with estrogen while maintaining the benefit to bone. The SERM **raloxifene** is approved for treatment of osteoporosis. Like tamoxifen, raloxifene reduces the risk of breast cancer. It protects against spine fractures but not hip fractures—unlike bisphosphonates, denosumab, and teriparatide, which protect against both. Raloxifene does not prevent hot flushes and imposes the same increased risk of venous thromboembolism as estrogen. To counter the reduced intestinal calcium transport associated with osteoporosis, vitamin D therapy is often used in combination with dietary calcium supplementation. There is no clear evidence that pharmacologic doses of vitamin D are of much additional benefit beyond cyclic estrogens and calcium supplementation. However, in several large studies, vitamin D supplementation (800 IU/d) with calcium has been shown to improve bone density, reduce falls, and prevent fractures. Calcitriol and its analog, $1\alpha(OH)D_3$, have also been shown to increase bone mass and reduce fractures. Use of these agents for osteoporosis is not FDA-approved, although they are used for this purpose in other countries.

Teriparatide, the recombinant form of PTH 1-34, is approved for treatment of osteoporosis. Teriparatide is given in a dosage of 20 mcg subcutaneously daily. Teriparatide stimulates new bone formation, but unlike fluoride, this new bone appears structurally normal and is associated with a substantial reduction in the incidence of fractures. Teriparatide is approved for only 2 years of use. Trials examining the sequential use of teriparatide followed by a bisphosphonate after 1 or 2 years are in progress and look promising. Use of teriparatide with a bisphosphonate has not shown greater efficacy than the bisphosphonate alone.

Calcitonin is approved for use in the treatment of postmenopausal osteoporosis. It has been shown to increase bone mass and reduce fractures, but only in the spine. It does not appear to be as effective as bisphosphonates or teriparatide.

Denosumab, the RANKL inhibitor, has recently been approved for treatment of postmenopausal osteoporosis. It is given subcutaneously every 6 months in 60 mg doses. Like the bisphosphonates it suppresses bone resorption and secondarily bone formation. Denosumab reduces the risk of both vertebral

and nonvertebral fractures with comparable effectiveness to the potent bisphosphonates.

Strontium ranelate has not been approved in the USA for the treatment of osteoporosis but is being used in Europe, generally at a dose of 2 g/d.

X-LINKED & AUTOSOMAL DOMINANT HYPOPHOSPHATEMIA & RELATED DISEASES

These disorders usually manifest in childhood as rickets and hypophosphatemia, although they may first present in adults. In both X-linked and autosomal dominant hypophosphatemia, biologically active FGF23 accumulates, leading to phosphate wasting in the urine and hypophosphatemia. In autosomal dominant hypophosphatemia, mutations in the FGF23 gene replace an arginine required for hydrolysis and result in increased FGF23 stability. X-linked hypophosphatemia is caused by mutations in the gene encoding the PHEX protein, an endopeptidase. Initially, it was thought that FGF23 was a direct substrate for PHEX, but this no longer appears to be the case. Tumor-induced osteomalacia is a similar acquired syndrome in adults that results from overexpression of FGF23 in tumor cells. The current concept for all of these diseases is that FGF23 blocks the renal uptake of phosphate and blocks $1,25(OH)_2D$ production leading to rickets in children and osteomalacia in adults. Phosphate is critical to normal bone mineralization; when phosphate stores are deficient, a clinical and pathologic picture resembling vitamin D–dependent rickets develops. However, affected children fail to respond to the standard doses of vitamin D used in the treatment of nutritional rickets. A defect in $1,25(OH)_2D$ production by the kidney has also been noted, because the serum $1,25(OH)_2D$ levels tend to be low in comparison with the degree of hypophosphatemia observed. This combination of low serum phosphate and low or low-normal serum $1,25(OH)_2D$ provides the rationale for treating these patients with oral phosphate (1–3 g daily) and calcitriol (0.25–2 mcg daily). Reports of such combination therapy are encouraging in this otherwise debilitating disease, although prolonged treatment often leads to secondary hyperparathyroidism.

VITAMIN D–DEPENDENT RICKETS TYPES I & II (PSEUDOVITAMIN D DEFICIENCY RICKETS & HEREDITARY VITAMIN D–RESISTANT RICKETS)

These distinctly different autosomal recessive diseases present as childhood rickets that do not respond to conventional doses of vitamin D. Type I vitamin D–dependent rickets, now known as pseudovitamin D deficiency rickets, is due to an isolated deficiency of $1,25(OH)_2D$ production caused by mutations in 25(OH)-D-1α-hydroxylase (CYP27B1). This condition can be treated with vitamin D (4000 units daily) or calcitriol (0.25–0.5 mcg daily). Type II vitamin D–dependent rickets, now known as hereditary vitamin D resistant rickets, is caused by mutations in the gene for the vitamin D receptor. The serum levels of $1,25(OH)_2D$ are very high in type II but inappropriately low for the level of calcium in type I vitamin D–dependent rickets. Treatment with large doses of calcitriol has been claimed to be effective in restoring normocalcemia in some patients, presumably those with a partially functional vitamin D receptor, although many patients are completely resistant to all forms of vitamin D. Calcium and phosphate infusions have been shown to correct the rickets in some children, similar to studies in mice in which the *VDR* gene has been deleted. These diseases are rare.

NEPHROTIC SYNDROME

Patients with nephrotic syndrome can lose vitamin D metabolites in the urine, presumably by loss of the vitamin D-binding protein. Such patients may have very low 25(OH)D levels. Some of them develop bone disease. It is not yet clear what value vitamin D therapy has in such patients, because therapeutic trials with vitamin D (or any vitamin D metabolite) have not yet been carried out. Because the problem is not related to vitamin D metabolism, one would not anticipate any advantage in using the more expensive vitamin D metabolites in place of vitamin D.

IDIOPATHIC HYPERCALCIURIA

Individuals with idiopathic hypercalciuria, characterized by hypercalciuria and nephrolithiasis with normal serum calcium and PTH levels, have been divided into three groups: (1) hyperabsorbers, patients with increased intestinal absorption of calcium, resulting in high-normal serum calcium, low-normal PTH, and a secondary increase in urine calcium; (2) renal calcium leakers, patients with a primary decrease in renal reabsorption of filtered calcium, leading to low-normal serum calcium and high-normal serum PTH; and (3) renal phosphate leakers, patients with a primary decrease in renal reabsorption of phosphate, leading to increased $1,25(OH)_2D$ production, increased intestinal calcium absorption, increased ionized serum calcium, low-normal PTH levels, and a secondary increase in urine calcium. There is some disagreement about this classification, and many patients are not readily categorized. Many such patients present with mild hypophosphatemia, and oral phosphate has been used with some success in reducing stone formation. However, a clear role for phosphate in the treatment of this disorder has not been established.

Therapy with hydrochlorothiazide, up to 50 mg twice daily, or chlorthalidone, 50–100 mg daily, is recommended. Loop diuretics such as furosemide and ethacrynic acid should not be used because they increase urinary calcium excretion. The major toxicity of thiazide diuretics, besides hypokalemia, hypomagnesemia, and hyperglycemia, is hypercalcemia. This is seldom more than a biochemical observation unless the patient has a disease such as hyperparathyroidism in which bone turnover is accelerated. Accordingly, one should screen patients for such disorders before starting thiazide therapy and monitor serum and urine calcium when therapy has begun.

An alternative to thiazides is allopurinol. Some studies indicate that hyperuricosuria is associated with idiopathic hypercalcemia

and that a small nidus of urate crystals could lead to the calcium oxalate stone formation characteristic of idiopathic hypercalcemia. Allopurinol, 100–300 mg daily, may reduce stone formation by reducing uric acid excretion.

OTHER DISORDERS OF BONE MINERAL HOMEOSTASIS

PAGET'S DISEASE OF BONE

Paget's disease is a localized bone disorder characterized by uncontrolled osteoclastic bone resorption with secondary increases in poorly organized bone formation. The cause of Paget's disease is obscure, although some studies suggest that a slow virus may be involved. The disease is fairly common, although symptomatic bone disease is less common. The biochemical parameters of elevated serum alkaline phosphatase and urinary hydroxyproline are useful for diagnosis. Along with the characteristic radiologic and bone scan findings, these biochemical determinations provide good markers by which to follow therapy.

The goal of treatment is to reduce bone pain and stabilize or prevent other problems such as progressive deformity, hearing loss, high-output cardiac failure, and immobilization hypercalcemia. Calcitonin and bisphosphonates are the first-line agents for this disease. Treatment failures may respond to plicamycin. Calcitonin is administered subcutaneously or intramuscularly in doses of 50–100 MRC (Medical Research Council) units every day or every other day. Nasal inhalation at 200–400 units per day is also effective. Higher or more frequent doses have been advocated when this initial regimen is ineffective. Improvement in bone pain and reduction in serum alkaline phosphatase and urine hydroxyproline levels require weeks to months. Often a patient who responds well initially loses the response to calcitonin. This refractoriness is not correlated with the development of antibodies.

Sodium etidronate, alendronate, risedronate, and tiludronate are the bisphosphonates currently approved for clinical use in Paget's disease of bone in the USA. Other bisphosphonates, including pamidronate, are being used in other countries. The recommended dosages of bisphosphonates are etidronate, 5 mg/kg/d; alendronate, 40 mg/d; risedronate, 30 mg/d; and tiludronate, 400 mg/d. Long-term (months to years) remission may be expected in patients who respond to a bisphosphonate. Treatment should not exceed 6 months per course but can be repeated after 6 months if necessary. The principal toxicity of etidronate is the development of osteomalacia and an increased incidence of fractures when the dosage is raised substantially above 5 mg/kg/d. The newer bisphosphonates such as risedronate and alendronate do not share this adverse effect. Some patients treated with etidronate develop bone pain similar in nature to the bone pain of osteomalacia. This subsides after stopping the drug. The principal adverse effect of alendronate and the newer bisphosphonates is gastric irritation when used at these high doses. This is reversible on cessation of the drug.

The use of a potentially lethal cytotoxic drug such as plicamycin in a generally benign disorder such as Paget's disease is recommended only when other less toxic agents (calcitonin, alendronate) have failed and the symptoms are debilitating. Clinical data on long-term use of plicamycin are insufficient to determine its usefulness for extended therapy. However, short courses involving 15–25 mcg/kg/d intravenously for 5–10 days followed by 15 mcg/kg intravenously each week have been used to control the disease.

ENTERIC OXALURIA

Patients with short bowel syndromes and associated fat malabsorption can present with renal stones composed of calcium and oxalate. Such patients characteristically have normal or low urine calcium levels but elevated urine oxalate levels. The reasons for the development of oxaluria in such patients are thought to be twofold: first, in the intestinal lumen, calcium (which is now bound to fat) fails to bind oxalate and no longer prevents its absorption; second, enteric flora, acting on the increased supply of nutrients reaching the colon, produce larger amounts of oxalate. Although one would ordinarily avoid treating a patient with calcium oxalate stones with calcium supplementation, this is precisely what is done in patients with enteric oxaluria. The increased intestinal calcium binds the excess oxalate and prevents its absorption. One to 2 g of calcium carbonate can be given daily in divided doses, with careful monitoring of urinary calcium and oxalate to be certain that urinary oxalate falls without a dangerous increase in urinary calcium.

SUMMARY Major Drugs Used in Diseases of Bone Mineral Homeostasis

Subclass	Mechanism of Action	Effects	Clinical Applications	Toxicities
VITAMIN D, METABOLITES, ANALOGS				
• Cholecalciferol • Ergocalciferol • Calcitriol • Doxercalciferol • Paricalcitol • Calcipotriene	Regulate gene transcription via the vitamin D receptor	Stimulate intestinal calcium absorption, bone resorption, renal calcium and phosphate reabsorption • decrease parathyroid hormone (PTH) • promote innate immunity • inhibit adaptive immunity	Osteoporosis, osteomalacia, renal failure, malabsorption, psoriasis	Hypercalcemia, hypercalciuria • the vitamin D preparations have much longer half-life than the metabolites and analogs
BISPHOSPHONATES				
• Alendronate • Risedronate • Ibandronate • Pamidronate • Zoledronate	Suppress the activity of osteoclasts in part via inhibition of farnesyl pyrophosphate synthesis	Inhibit bone resorption and secondarily bone formation	Osteoporosis, bone metastases, hypercalcemia	Adynamic bone, possible renal failure, rare osteonecrosis of the jaw, rare subtrochanteric (femur) fractures
HORMONES				
• Teriparatide • Calcitonin	These hormones act via their cognate G protein-coupled receptors	Teriparatide stimulates bone turnover • calcitonin suppresses bone resorption	Both are used in osteoporosis • calcitonin is used for hypercalcemia	Teriparatide may cause hypercalcemia and hypercalciuria
SELECTIVE ESTROGEN RECEPTOR MODULATORS (SERMs)				
• Raloxifene	Interacts selectively with estrogen receptors	Inhibits bone resorption without stimulating breast or endometrial hyperplasia	Osteoporosis	Does not prevent hot flashes • increased risk of venous thromboembolism
RANK LIGAND (RANKL) INHIBITOR				
• Denosumab	Monoclonal antibody • binds to RANKL and prevents it from stimulating osteoclast differentiation and function	Blocks bone resorption	Osteoporosis	May increase risk of infections
CALCIUM RECEPTOR AGONIST				
• Cinacalcet	Activates the calcium-sensing receptor	Inhibits PTH secretion	Hyperparathyroidism	Nausea
MINERALS				
• Calcium • Phosphate • Strontium	Multiple physiologic actions through regulation of multiple enzymatic pathways	Strontium suppresses bone resorption and increases bone formation • calcium and phosphate required for bone mineralization	Osteoporosis • osteomalacia • deficiencies in calcium or phosphate	Ectopic calcification

PREPARATIONS AVAILABLE

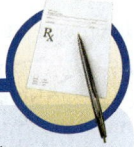

VITAMIN D, METABOLITES, AND ANALOGS

Calcitriol
Oral (generic, Rocaltrol): 0.25, 0.5 mcg capsules, 1 mcg/mL solution
Parenteral (generic, Calcijex): 1, 2 mcg/mL for injection

Cholecalciferol [D$_3$] (vitamin D$_3$, Delta-D)
Oral: numerous forms containing 400–50,000 IU per unit

Doxercalciferol (Hectorol)
Oral: 0.5, 1, 2.5 mcg capsules
Parenteral: 2 mcg/mL

Ergocalciferol [D$_2$] (vitamin D$_2$, Calciferol, Drisdol)
Oral: 50,000 IU capsules; 8000 IU/mL drops

Paricalcitol (Zemplar)
Oral: 1, 2, 4 mcg capsules
Parenteral: 2, 5 mcg/mL for injection

CALCIUM

Calcium acetate [25% calcium] (generic, PhosLo)
Oral: 668 mg (169 mg calcium) tablets or capsules

Calcium carbonate [40% calcium] (generic, Tums, Cal-Sup, Os-Cal 500, others)
Oral: Numerous forms available containing 260–600 mg calcium per unit

Calcium chloride [27% calcium] (generic)
Parenteral: 10% solution for IV injection

Calcium citrate [21% calcium] (generic, Citracal)
Oral: 950 mg (200 mg calcium), 2376 mg (500 mg calcium)

Calcium glubionate [6.5% calcium] (Calcionate, Calciquid)
Oral: 1.8 g (115 mg calcium)/5 mL syrup

Calcium gluceptate [8% calcium] (Calcium Gluceptate)
Parenteral: 1.1 g/5 mL solution for IM or IV injection

Calcium gluconate [9% calcium] (generic)
Oral: 500 mg (45 mg calcium), 650 mg (58.5 mg calcium), 975 mg (87.75 mg calcium), 1 g (90 mg calcium) tablets
Parenteral: 10% solution for IV or IM injection

Calcium lactate [13% calcium] (generic)
Oral: 650 mg (84.5 mg calcium), 770 mg (100 mg calcium) tablets

Tricalcium phosphate [39% calcium] (Posture)
Oral: 1565 mg (600 mg calcium) tablets (as phosphate)

PHOSPHATE AND PHOSPHATE BINDER

Phosphate
Oral (Fleet Phospho-soda): solution containing 2.5 g phosphate/5 mL (816 mg phosphorus/5 mL; 751 mg sodium/5 mL)

Oral (K-Phos-Neutral): tablets containing 250 mg phosphorus, 298 mg sodium, 45 mg phosphorus
Oral (Neutra-Phos): For reconstitution in 75 mL water, packet containing 250 mg phosphorus; 164 mg sodium; 278 mg potassium
Oral (Neutra-Phos-K): For reconstitution in 75 mL water, packet containing 250 mg phosphorus; 556 mg potassium; 0 mg sodium
Parenteral (potassium or sodium phosphate): 3 mmol/mL

Sevelamer carbonate or HCl (Renagel, Renvela)
Oral: 400, 800 mg capsules

BISPHOSPHONATES

Alendronate sodium (generic, Fosamax)
Oral: 5, 10, 35, 40, 70 mg tablets; 70 mg/75 mL oral solution

Etidronate disodium (generic, Didronel)
Oral: 200, 400 mg tablets

Ibandronate sodium (Boniva)
Oral: 2.5, 150 mg tablets
Parenteral: 1 mg/mL for IV injection

Pamidronate disodium (generic, Aredia)
Parenteral: 30, 60, 90 mg/vial for IV injection

Risedronate sodium (Actonel)
Oral: 5, 30, 35, 75, 150 mg tablets

Tiludronate disodium (Skelid)
Oral: 200 mg tablets (as tiludronic acid)

Zoledronic acid (Zometa)
Parenteral: 4 mg/vial for IV injection

OTHER DRUGS

Calcitonin-Salmon
Nasal spray (Miacalcin): 200 IU/puff
Parenteral (Calcimar, Miacalcin, Salmonine): 200 IU/mL for injection

Cinacalcet (Sensipar)
Oral: 30, 60, 90 mg tablets

Denosumab (Prolia)
Parenteral: 60 mg/mL solution for SC injection

Gallium nitrate (Ganite)
Parenteral: 25 mg/mL solution for IV injection

Plicamycin (mithramycin) (Mithracin)
Parenteral: 2.5 mg per vial powder to reconstitute for injection

Sodium fluoride (generic)
Oral: 0.55 mg (0.25 mg F), 1.1 mg (0.5 mg F), 2.2 mg (1.0 mg F) tablets; drops

Teriparatide (Forteo)
Subcutaneous: 250 mcg/mL in prefilled pen for SC injectiont

REFERENCES

Becker DJ, Kilgore ML, Morrisey MA: The societal burden of osteoporosis. Curr Rheumatol Rep 2010;12:186.

Bikle DD: Nonclassic actions of vitamin D. J Clin Endocrinol Metabol 2009;94:26.

Black DM et al: One year of alendronate after one year of parathyroid hormone (1-84) for osteoporosis. N Engl J Med 2005;353:555.

Clines GA, Guise TA: Mechanisms and treatment for bone metastases. Clin Adv Hematol Oncol 2004;2:295.

Cummings SR et al: Denosumab for prevention of fractures in postmenopausal women with osteoporosis. N Engl J Med 2009;361:756.

Favus MJ: Bisphosphonates for osteoporosis. N Engl J Med 2010;363:2027.

Finkelstein JS et al: The effects of parathyroid hormone, alendronate, or both in men with osteoporosis. N Engl J Med 2003;349:1216.

Green J, Lipton A: Anticancer properties of zoledronic acid. Cancer Invest 2010;28:944.

Holick MF: Vitamin D deficiency. N Engl J Med 2007;357:266.

Holick MF et al: Evaluation, treatment, and prevention of vitamin D deficiency: an Endocrine Sociey Clinical Practice Guideline J Clin Endocrinol Metab 2011;96:1911.

Hutton E: Evaluation and management of hypercalcemia. JAAPA 2005;18:30.

Kearns AE, Khosla S, Kostenuik PJ: Receptor activator of nuclear factor kappaB ligand and osteoprotegerin regulation of bone remodeling in health and disease. Endocr Rev 2008;29:155.

Meunier PJ et al: The effects of strontium ranelate on the risk of vertebral fractures in women with postmenopausal osteoporosis. N Engl J Med 2004;350:459.

Neer RM et al: Effect of parathyroid hormone (1-34) on fractures and bone mineral density in postmenopausal women with osteoporosis. N Engl J Med 2001;344:1434.

Orwoll E et al: Alendronate for the treatment of osteoporosis in men. N Engl J Med 2000;343:604.

Pettifor JM: Rickets and vitamin D deficiency in children and adolescents. Endocrinol Metab Clin North Am 2005;34:537.

Qazi RA, Martin KJ: Vitamin D in kidney disease: Pathophysiology and the utility of treatment. Endocrinol Metab Clin North Am 2010;39:355.

Ross AC et al: The 2011 report on dietary reference intakes for calcium and vitamin D from the Institute of Medicine: what clinicians need to know. J Clin Endocrinol Metab 2011;96:53.

Smith MR et al: Denosumab in men receiving androgen-deprivation therapy for prostate cancer. N Engl J Med 2009;361:745.

Stewart AF: Clinical practice. Hypercalcemia associated with cancer. N Engl J Med 2005;352:373.

Strom TM, Juppner H: PHEX, FGF23, DMP1 and beyond. Curr Opin Nephrol Hypertens 2008;17:357.

Tfelt-Hanson J, Brown EM: The calcium-sensing receptor in normal physiology and pathophysiology: A review. Crit Rev Clin Lab Sci 2005;42:35.

Wüthrich RP, Martin D, Bilezikian JP: The role of calcimimetics in the treatment of hyperparathyroidism. Eur J Clin Invest 2007;37:915.

CASE STUDY ANSWER

There are multiple reasons for this patient's osteoporosis, including a heavy smoking history, possible alcoholism, and chronic inflammatory disease treated with glucocorticoids. High levels of cytokines from the chronic inflammation activate osteoclasts. Glucocorticoids increase urinary losses of calcium, suppress bone formation, and inhibit intestinal calcium absorption as well as decreasing gonadotropin production, leading to hypogonadism. Management should include measurement of serum testosterone, serum calcium, and the 24-hour urine calcium level, with treatment as appropriate for these secondary causes, plus initiation of bisphosphonate or denosumab therapy as primary treatment.

INTRODUCTION TO ANTIMICROBIAL AGENTS

Antimicrobial agents provide some of the most dramatic examples of the advances of modern medicine. Many infectious diseases once considered incurable and lethal are now amenable to treatment with a few pills. The remarkably powerful and specific activity of antimicrobial drugs is due to their selectivity for targets that are either unique to prokaryote and fungal microorganisms or much more important in these organisms than in humans. Among these targets are bacterial and fungal cell wall-synthesizing enzymes (Chapters 43 and 48), the bacterial ribosome (Chapters 44 and 45), the enzymes required for nucleotide synthesis and DNA replication (Chapter 46), and the machinery of viral replication (Chapter 49). The special group of drugs used in mycobacterial infections is discussed in Chapter 47. The much older and less selective cytotoxic antiseptics and disinfectants are discussed in Chapter 50. The clinical uses of all these agents are summarized in Chapter 51.

The major problem threatening the continued success of antimicrobial drugs is the development of resistant organisms. Microorganisms can adapt to environmental pressures in a variety of effective ways, and their response to antibiotic pressure is no exception. An inevitable consequence of antimicrobial usage is the selection of resistant microorganisms, perhaps the most obvious example of evolution in action. Overuse and inappropriate use of antibiotics in patients has fueled a major increase in prevalence of multidrug-resistant pathogens. Antibacterial antibiotics are misused by providers in a variety of ways, including use in patients who are unlikely to have bacterial infections, use over unnecessarily prolonged periods, and use of multiple agents or broad-spectrum agents when not needed.

As a result of antibiotic pressure, highly resistant gram-negative organisms with novel mechanisms of resistance are increasingly reported. Some of these strains have spread over vast geographic areas as a result of patients seeking medical care in different countries. Much larger quantities of antibiotics have been used in agriculture to stimulate growth and prevent infection in farm animals and this has added to the selection pressure that results in resistant organisms.

Unfortunately, as the need has grown in recent years, development of novel drugs has slowed. The most vulnerable molecular targets of antimicrobial drugs have been identified and, in many cases, crystallized and characterized. Pending the identification of new targets and compounds, it seems likely that over the next decade we will have to rely on currently available families of drugs. In the face of continuing development of resistance, considerable effort will be required to maintain the effectiveness of these drug groups.

Beta-Lactam & Other Cell Wall- & Membrane-Active Antibiotics

43

Daniel H. Deck, PharmD &
Lisa G. Winston, MD*

C A S E   S T U D Y

A 55-year-old man is brought to the local hospital emergency department by ambulance. His wife reports that he had been in his normal state of health until 3 days ago when he developed a fever and a productive cough. During the last 24 hours he has complained of a headache and is increasingly confused. His wife reports that his medical history is significant only for hypertension, for which he takes hydrochlorothiazide and lisinopril, and that he is allergic to amoxicillin. She says that he developed a rash many years ago when prescribed amoxicillin for bronchitis. In the emergency department, the man is febrile (38.7°C [101.7°F]), hypotensive (90/54 mm Hg), tachypneic (36/min), and tachycardic (110/min). He has no signs of meningismus but is oriented only to person. A stat chest x-ray shows a left lower lung consolidation consistent with pneumonia. The plan is to start empiric antibiotics and perform a lumbar puncture to rule out bacterial meningitis. What antibiotic regimen should be started to treat both pneumonia and meningitis? Does the history of amoxicillin rash affect the antibiotic choice? Why or why not?

■ BETA-LACTAM COMPOUNDS

PENICILLINS

The penicillins share features of chemistry, mechanism of action, pharmacology, and immunologic characteristics with cephalosporins, monobactams, carbapenems, and β-lactamase inhibitors. All are β-lactam compounds, so named because of their four-membered lactam ring.

Chemistry

All penicillins have the basic structure shown in Figure 43–1. A thiazolidine ring (A) is attached to a β-lactam ring (B) that carries a secondary amino group (RNH–). Substituents (R; examples shown in Figure 43–2) can be attached to the amino group. Structural integrity of the 6-aminopenicillanic acid nucleus (rings A plus B) is essential for the biologic activity of these compounds.

Hydrolysis of the β-lactam ring by bacterial β-lactamases yields penicilloic acid, which lacks antibacterial activity.

A. Classification

Substituents of the 6-aminopenicillanic acid moiety determine the essential pharmacologic and antibacterial properties of the resulting molecules. Penicillins can be assigned to one of three groups (below). Within each of these groups are compounds that are relatively stable to gastric acid and suitable for oral administration, eg, penicillin V, dicloxacillin, and amoxicillin. The side chains of some representatives of each group are shown in Figure 43–2, with a few distinguishing characteristics.

1. Penicillins (eg, penicillin G)—These have greatest activity against gram-positive organisms, gram-negative cocci, and non-β-lactamase producing anaerobes. However, they have little activity against gram-negative rods, and they are susceptible to hydrolysis by β-lactamases.

2. Antistaphylococcal penicillins (eg, nafcillin)—These penicillins are resistant to staphylococcal β-lactamases. They are

*The authors thank Dr. Henry F. Chambers for his contributions to this chapter in previous editions.

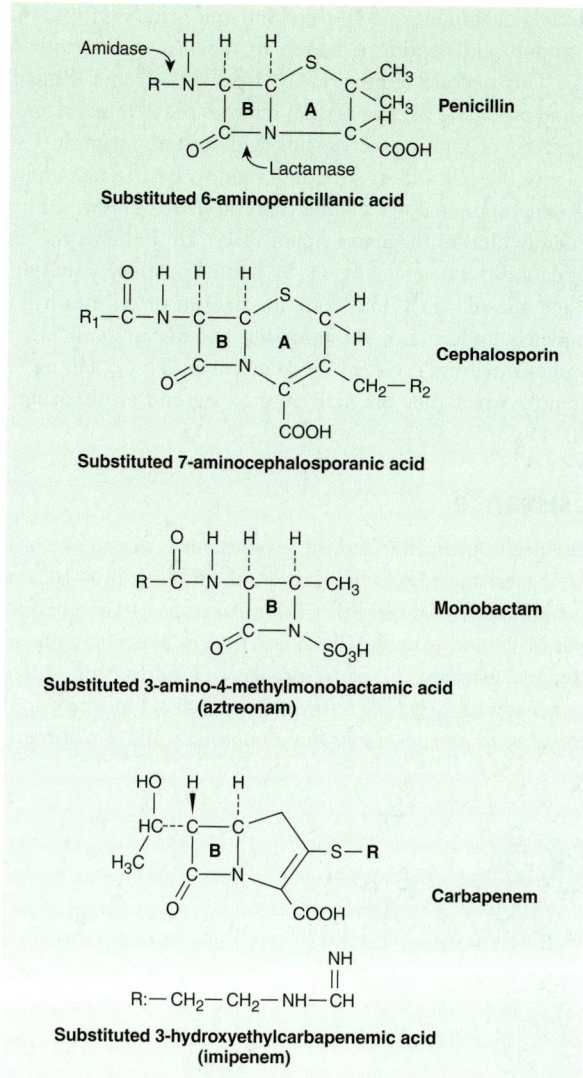

FIGURE 43–1 Core structures of four β-lactam antibiotic families. The ring marked B in each structure is the β-lactam ring. The penicillins are susceptible to bacterial metabolism and inactivation by amidases and lactamases at the points shown. Note that the carbapenems have a different stereochemical configuration in the lactam ring that imparts resistance to most common β lactamases. Substituents for the penicillin and cephalosporin families are shown in Figures 43–2 and 43–6, respectively.

active against staphylococci and streptococci but not against enterococci, anaerobic bacteria, and gram-negative cocci and rods.

3. Extended-spectrum penicillins (ampicillin and the antipseudomonal penicillins)—These drugs retain the antibacterial spectrum of penicillin and have improved activity against gram-negative organisms. Like penicillin, however, they are relatively susceptible to hydrolysis by β-lactamases.

B. Penicillin Units and Formulations

The activity of penicillin G was originally defined in units. Crystalline sodium penicillin G contains approximately

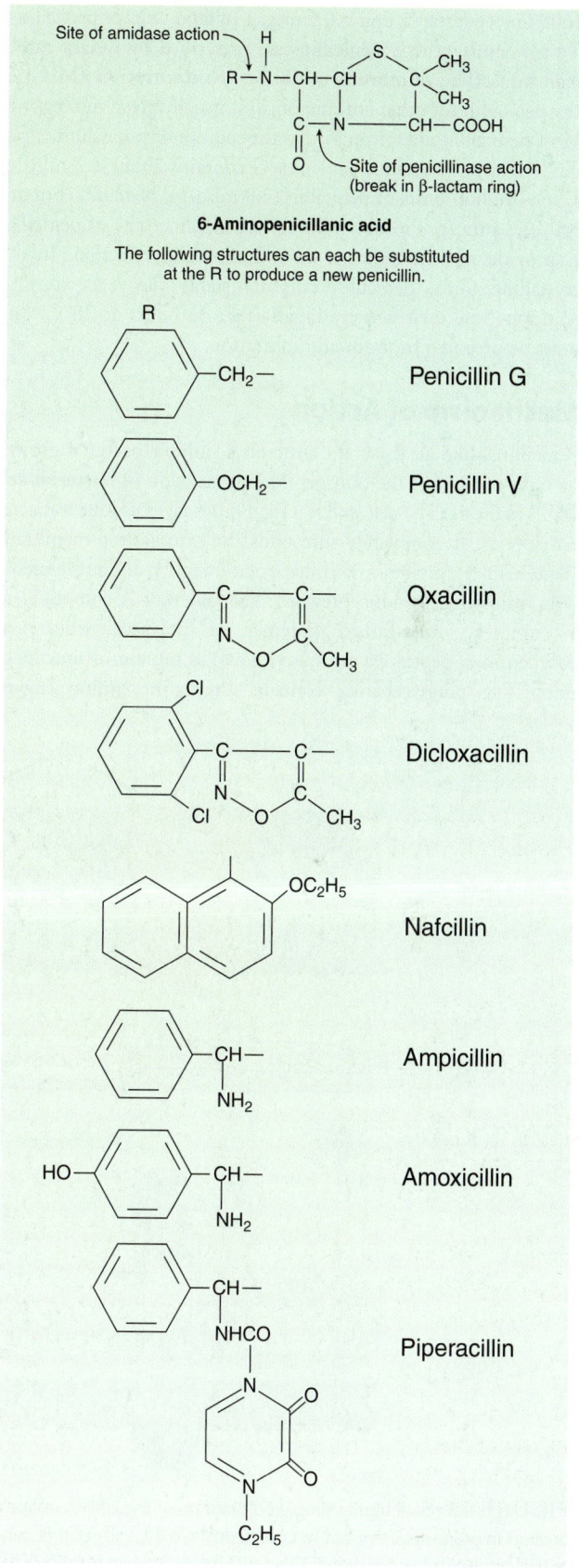

FIGURE 43–2 Side chains of some penicillins (R groups of Figure 43–1).

1600 units per mg (1 unit = 0.6 mcg; 1 million units of penicillin = 0.6 g). Semisynthetic penicillins are prescribed by weight rather than units. The **minimum inhibitory concentration (MIC)** of any penicillin (or other antimicrobial) is usually given in mcg/mL. Most penicillins are formulated as the sodium or potassium salt of the free acid. Potassium penicillin G contains about 1.7 mEq of K^+ per million units of penicillin (2.8 mEq/g). Nafcillin contains Na^+, 2.8 mEq/g. Procaine salts and benzathine salts of penicillin G provide repository forms for intramuscular injection. In dry crystalline form, penicillin salts are stable for years at 4°C. Solutions lose their activity rapidly (eg, 24 hours at 20°C) and must be prepared fresh for administration.

Mechanism of Action

Penicillins, like all β-lactam antibiotics, inhibit bacterial growth by interfering with the transpeptidation reaction of **bacterial cell wall synthesis.** The cell wall is a rigid outer layer unique to bacterial species. It completely surrounds the cytoplasmic membrane (Figure 43–3), maintains cell shape and integrity, and prevents cell lysis from high osmotic pressure. The cell wall is composed of a complex, cross-linked polymer of polysaccharides and polypeptides, peptidoglycan (also known as murein or mucopeptide). The polysaccharide contains alternating amino sugars,

N-acetylglucosamine and N-acetylmuramic acid (Figure 43–4). A five-amino-acid peptide is linked to the N-acetylmuramic acid sugar. This peptide terminates in D-alanyl-D-alanine. Penicillin-binding protein (PBP, an enzyme) removes the terminal alanine in the process of forming a cross-link with a nearby peptide. Cross-links give the cell wall its structural rigidity. Beta-lactam antibiotics, structural analogs of the natural D-Ala-D-Ala substrate, covalently bind to the active site of PBPs. This inhibits the transpeptidation reaction (Figure 43–5), halting peptidoglycan synthesis, and the cell dies. The exact mechanism of cell death is not completely understood, but autolysins and disruption of cell wall morphogenesis are involved. Beta-lactam antibiotics kill bacterial cells only when they are actively growing and synthesizing cell wall.

Resistance

Resistance to penicillins and other β-lactams is due to one of four general mechanisms: (1) inactivation of antibiotic by β-lactamase, (2) modification of target PBPs, (3) impaired penetration of drug to target PBPs, and (4) efflux. Beta-lactamase production is the most common mechanism of resistance. Hundreds of different β-lactamases have been identified. Some, such as those produced by *Staphylococcus aureus*, *Haemophilus influenzae*, and *Escherichia coli*,

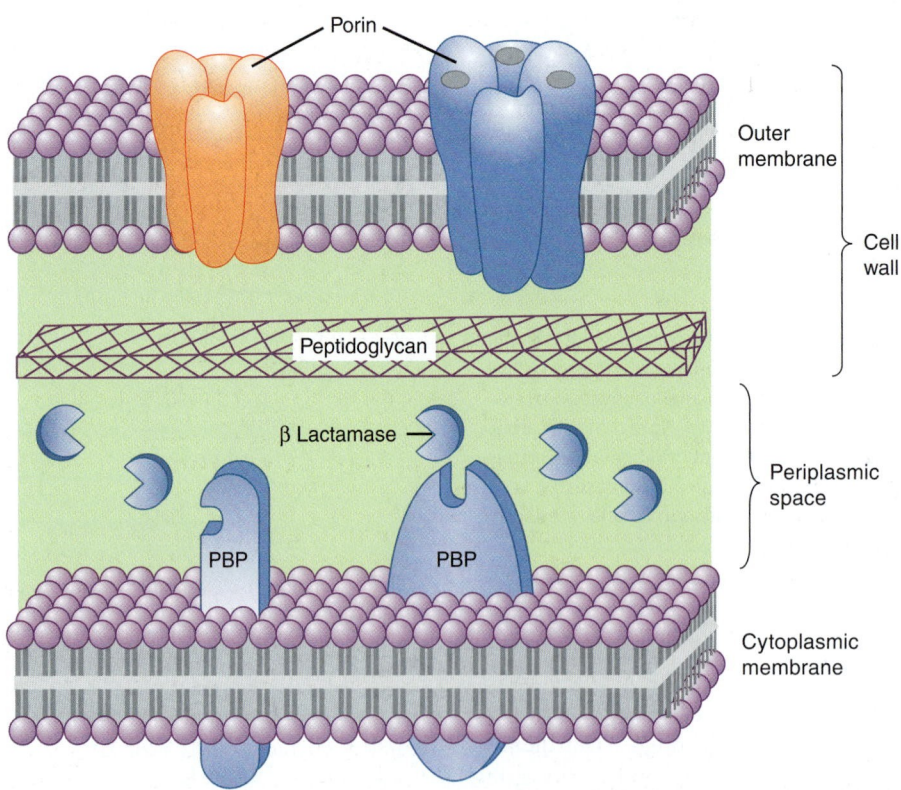

FIGURE 43–3 A highly simplified diagram of the cell envelope of a gram-negative bacterium. The outer membrane, a lipid bilayer, is present in gram-negative but not gram-positive organisms. It is penetrated by porins, proteins that form channels providing hydrophilic access to the cytoplasmic membrane. The peptidoglycan layer is unique to bacteria and is much thicker in gram-positive organisms than in gram-negative ones. Together, the outer membrane and the peptidoglycan layer constitute the cell wall. Penicillin-binding proteins (PBPs) are membrane proteins that cross-link peptidoglycan. Beta lactamases, if present, reside in the periplasmic space or on the outer surface of the cytoplasmic membrane, where they may destroy β-lactam antibiotics that penetrate the outer membrane.

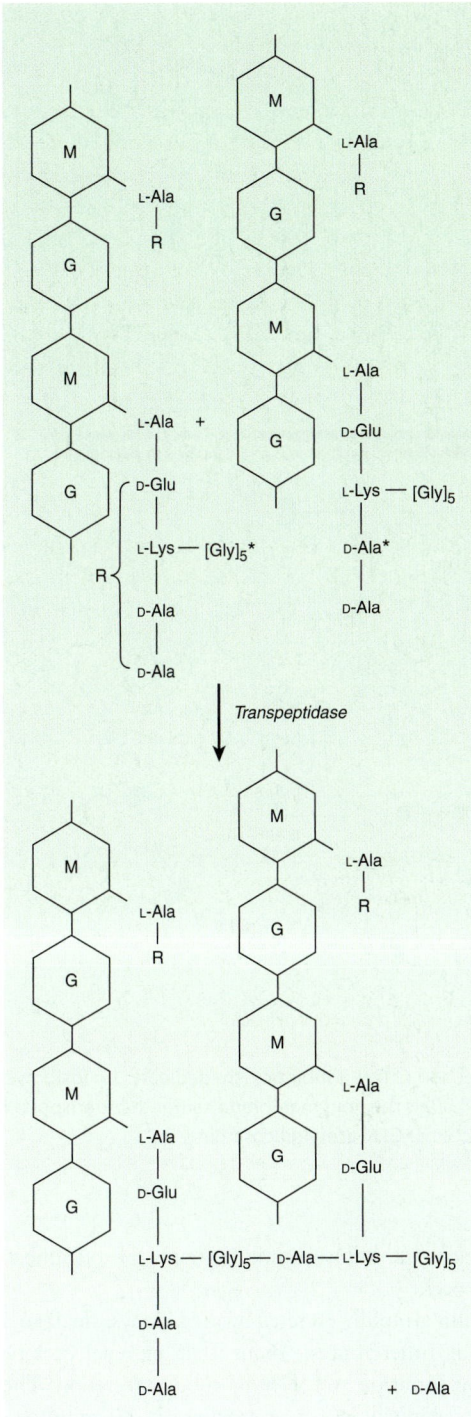

FIGURE 43–4 The transpeptidation reaction in *Staphylococcus aureus* that is inhibited by β-lactam antibiotics. The cell wall of gram-positive bacteria is made up of long peptidoglycan polymer chains consisting of the alternating aminohexoses *N*-acetylglucosamine (G) and *N*-acetylmuramic acid (M) with pentapeptide side chains linked (in *S aureus*) by pentaglycine bridges. The exact composition of the side chains varies among species. The diagram illustrates small segments of two such polymer chains and their amino acid side chains. These linear polymers must be cross-linked by transpeptidation of the side chains at the points indicated by the asterisk to achieve the strength necessary for cell viability.

are relatively narrow in substrate specificity, preferring penicillins to cephalosporins. Other β-lactamases, eg, AmpC β-lactamase produced by *Pseudomonas aeruginosa* and *Enterobacter* sp, and extended-spectrum β-lactamases (ESBLs), hydrolyze both cephalosporins and penicillins. Carbapenems are highly resistant to hydrolysis by penicillinases and cephalosporinases, but they are hydrolyzed by metallo-β lactamase and carbapenemases.

Altered target PBPs are the basis of methicillin resistance in staphylococci and of penicillin resistance in pneumococci and enterococci. These resistant organisms produce PBPs that have low affinity for binding β-lactam antibiotics, and consequently, they are not inhibited except at relatively high, often clinically unachievable, drug concentrations.

Resistance due to impaired penetration of antibiotic to target PBPs occurs only in gram-negative species because of their impermeable outer cell wall membrane, which is absent in gram-positive bacteria. Beta-lactam antibiotics cross the outer membrane and enter gram-negative organisms via outer membrane protein channels called porins. Absence of the proper channel or down-regulation of its production can greatly impair drug entry into the cell. Poor penetration alone is usually not sufficient to confer resistance because enough antibiotic eventually enters the cell to inhibit growth. However, this barrier can become important in the presence of a β-lactamase, even a relatively inactive one, as long as it can hydrolyze drug faster than it enters the cell. Gram-negative organisms also may produce an efflux pump, which consists of cytoplasmic and periplasmic protein components that efficiently transport some β-lactam antibiotics from the periplasm back across the outer membrane.

Pharmacokinetics

Absorption of orally administered drug differs greatly for different penicillins, depending in part on their acid stability and protein binding. Gastrointestinal absorption of nafcillin is erratic, so it is not suitable for oral administration. Dicloxacillin, ampicillin, and amoxicillin are acid-stable and relatively well absorbed, producing serum concentrations in the range of 4–8 mcg/mL after a 500-mg oral dose. Absorption of most oral penicillins (amoxicillin being an exception) is impaired by food, and the drugs should be administered at least 1–2 hours before or after a meal.

Intravenous administration of penicillin G is preferred to the intramuscular route because of irritation and local pain from intramuscular injection of large doses. Serum concentrations 30 minutes after an intravenous injection of 1 g of a penicillin (equivalent to approximately 1.6 million units of penicillin G) are 20–50 mcg/mL. Only a small amount of the total drug in serum is present as free drug, the concentration of which is determined by protein binding. Highly protein-bound penicillins (eg, nafcillin) generally achieve lower free-drug concentrations in serum than less protein-bound penicillins (eg, penicillin G or ampicillin). Protein binding becomes clinically relevant when the protein-bound percentage is approximately 95% or more. Penicillins are widely distributed in body fluids and tissues with a few exceptions. They are polar molecules, so intracellular concentrations are well below those found in extracellular fluids.

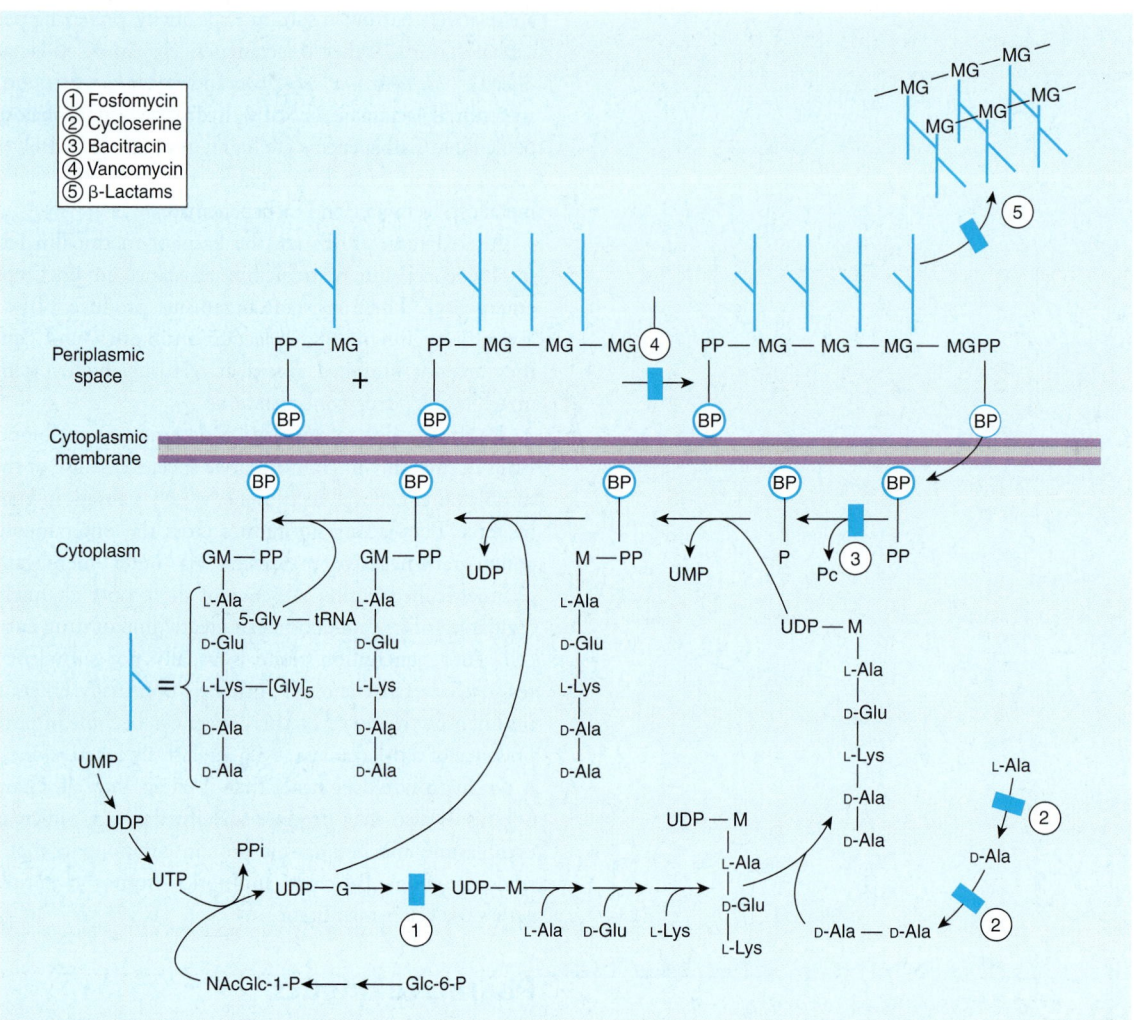

FIGURE 43–5 The biosynthesis of cell wall peptidoglycan, showing the sites of action of five antibiotics (shaded bars; 1 = fosfomycin, 2 = cycloserine, 3 = bacitracin, 4 = vancomycin, 5 = β-lactam antibiotics). Bactoprenol (BP) is the lipid membrane carrier that transports building blocks across the cytoplasmic membrane; M, *N*-acetylmuramic acid; Glc, glucose; NAcGlc or G, *N*-acetylglucosamine.

Benzathine and procaine penicillins are formulated to delay absorption, resulting in prolonged blood and tissue concentrations. A single intramuscular injection of 1.2 million units of benzathine penicillin maintains serum levels above 0.02 mcg/mL for 10 days, sufficient to treat β-hemolytic streptococcal infection. After 3 weeks, levels still exceed 0.003 mcg/mL, which is enough to prevent β-hemolytic streptococcal infection. A 600,000 unit dose of procaine penicillin yields peak concentrations of 1–2 mcg/mL and clinically useful concentrations for 12–24 hours after a single intramuscular injection.

Penicillin concentrations in most tissues are equal to those in serum. Penicillin is also excreted into sputum and milk to levels 3–15% of those in the serum. Penetration into the eye, the prostate, and the central nervous system is poor. However, with active inflammation of the meninges, as in bacterial meningitis, penicillin concentrations of 1–5 mcg/mL can be achieved with a daily parenteral dose of 18–24 million units. These concentrations are sufficient to kill susceptible strains of pneumococci and meningococci.

Penicillin is rapidly excreted by the kidneys; small amounts are excreted by other routes. About 10% of renal excretion is by glomerular filtration and 90% by tubular secretion. The normal half-life of penicillin G is approximately 30 minutes; in renal failure, it may be as long as 10 hours. Ampicillin and the extended-spectrum penicillins are secreted more slowly than penicillin G and have half-lives of 1 hour. For penicillins that are cleared by the kidney, the dose must be adjusted according to renal function, with approximately one fourth to one third the normal dose being administered if creatinine clearance is 10 mL/min or less (Table 43–1).

Nafcillin is primarily cleared by biliary excretion. Oxacillin, dicloxacillin, and cloxacillin are eliminated by both the kidney and biliary excretion; no dosage adjustment is required for these drugs in renal failure. Because clearance of penicillins is less efficient in

TABLE 43–1 Guidelines for dosing of some commonly used penicillins.

Antibiotic (Route of Administration)	Adult Dose	Pediatric Dose[1]	Neonatal Dose[2]	Adjusted Dose as a Percentage of Normal Dose for Renal Failure Based on Creatinine Clearance (Cl_{cr})	
				Cl_{cr} Approx 50 mL/min	Cl_{cr} Approx 10 mL/min
Penicillins					
Penicillin G (IV)	$1–4 \times 10^6$ units q4–6h	25,000–400,000 units/kg/d in 4–6 doses	75,000–150,000 units/kg/d in 2 or 3 doses	50–75%	25%
Penicillin V (PO)	0.25–0.5 g qid	25–50 mg/kg/d in 4 doses		None	None
Antistaphylococcal penicillins					
Cloxacillin, dicloxacillin (PO)	0.25–0.5 g qid	25–50 mg/kg/d in 4 doses		100%	100%
Nafcillin (IV)	1–2 g q4–6h	50–100 mg/kg/d in 4–6 doses	50–75 mg/kg/d in 2 or 3 doses	100%	100%
Oxacillin (IV)	1–2 g q4–6h	50–100 mg/kg/d in 4–6 doses	50–75 mg/kg/d in 2 or 3 doses	100%	100%
Extended-spectrum penicillins					
Amoxicillin (PO)	0.25–0.5 g tid	20–40 mg/kg/d in 3 doses		66%	33%
Amoxicillin/potassium clavulanate (PO)	500/125 tid–875/125 mg bid	20–40 mg/kg/d in 3 doses		66%	33%
Piperacillin (IV)	3–4 g q4–6h	300 mg/kg/d in 4–6 doses	150 mg/kg/d in 2 doses	50–75%	25–33%
Ticarcillin (IV)	3 g q4–6h	200–300 mg/kg/d in 4–6 doses	150–200 mg/kg/d in 2 or 3 doses	50–75%	25–33%

[1]The total dose should not exceed the adult dose.
[2]The dose shown is during the first week of life. The daily dose should be increased by approximately 33–50% after the first week of life. The lower dosage range should be used for neonates weighing less than 2 kg. After the first month of life, pediatric doses may be used.

the newborn, doses adjusted for weight alone result in higher systemic concentrations for longer periods than in the adult.

Clinical Uses

Except for oral amoxicillin, penicillins should be given 1–2 hours before or after a meal; they should not be given with food to minimize binding to food proteins and acid inactivation. Blood levels of all penicillins can be raised by simultaneous administration of probenecid, 0.5 g (10 mg/kg in children) every 6 hours orally, which impairs renal tubular secretion of weak acids such as β-lactam compounds. Penicillins should never be used for viral infections and should be prescribed only when there is reasonable suspicion of, or documented infection with, susceptible organisms.

A. Penicillin

Penicillin G is a drug of choice for infections caused by streptococci, meningococci, some enterococci, penicillin-susceptible pneumococci, non-β-lactamase-producing staphylococci, *Treponema pallidum* and certain other spirochetes, *Clostridium* species,

Actinomyces and certain other gram-positive rods, and non-β-lactamase-producing gram-negative anaerobic organisms. Depending on the organism, the site, and the severity of infection, effective doses range between 4 and 24 million units per day administered intravenously in four to six divided doses. High-dose penicillin G can also be given as a continuous intravenous infusion.

Penicillin V, the oral form of penicillin, is indicated only in minor infections because of its relatively poor bioavailability, the need for dosing four times a day, and its narrow antibacterial spectrum. Amoxicillin (see below) is often used instead.

Benzathine penicillin and procaine penicillin G for intramuscular injection yield low but prolonged drug levels. A single intramuscular injection of benzathine penicillin, 1.2 million units, is effective treatment for β-hemolytic streptococcal pharyngitis; given intramuscularly once every 3–4 weeks, it prevents reinfection. Benzathine penicillin G, 2.4 million units intramuscularly once a week for 1–3 weeks, is effective in the treatment of syphilis. Procaine penicillin G, formerly a work horse for treating uncomplicated pneumococcal pneumonia or gonorrhea, is rarely used now because many strains are penicillin-resistant.

B. Penicillins Resistant to Staphylococcal Beta Lactamase (Methicillin, Nafcillin, and Isoxazolyl Penicillins)

These semisynthetic penicillins are indicated for infection by β-lactamase-producing staphylococci, although penicillin-susceptible strains of streptococci and pneumococci are also susceptible to these agents. *Listeria monocytogenes*, enterococci, and methicillin-resistant strains of staphylococci are resistant. In recent years the empirical use of these drugs has decreased substantially because of increasing rates of methicillin-resistance in staphylococci. However, for infections caused by methicillin-susceptible and penicillin-resistant strains of staphylococci, these are considered the drugs of choice.

An isoxazolyl penicillin such as oxacillin, cloxacillin, or dicloxacillin, 0.25–0.5 g orally every 4–6 hours (15–25 mg/kg/d for children), is suitable for treatment of mild to moderate localized staphylococcal infections. All are relatively acid-stable and have reasonable bioavailability. However, food interferes with absorption, and the drugs should be administered 1 hour before or after meals.

For serious systemic staphylococcal infections, oxacillin or nafcillin, 8–12 g/d, is given by intermittent intravenous infusion of 1–2 g every 4–6 hours (50–100 mg/kg/d for children).

C. Extended-Spectrum Penicillins (Aminopenicillins, Carboxypenicillins, and Ureidopenicillins)

These drugs have greater activity than penicillin against gram-negative bacteria because of their enhanced ability to penetrate the gram-negative outer membrane. Like penicillin G, they are inactivated by many β lactamases.

The aminopenicillins, ampicillin and amoxicillin, have nearly identical spectrums of activity, but amoxicillin is better absorbed orally. Amoxicillin, 250–500 mg three times daily, is equivalent to the same amount of ampicillin given four times daily. Amoxacillin is given orally to treat urinary tract infections, sinusitis, otitis, and lower respiratory tract infections. Ampicillin and amoxicillin are the most active of the oral β-lactam antibiotics against pneumococci with elevated MICs to penicillin and are the preferred β-lactam antibiotics for treating infections suspected to be caused by these strains. Ampicillin (but not amoxicillin) is effective for shigellosis. Its use to treat uncomplicated salmonella gastroenteritis is controversial because it may prolong the carrier state.

Ampicillin, at dosages of 4–12 g/d intravenously, is useful for treating serious infections caused by susceptible organisms, including anaerobes, enterococci, *L monocytogenes*, and β-lactamase-negative strains of gram-negative cocci and bacilli such as *E coli*, and *Salmonella* sp. Non-β-lactamase producing strains of *H influenzae* are generally susceptible, but strains that are resistant because of altered PBPs are emerging. Many gram-negative species produce β lactamases and are resistant, precluding use of ampicillin for empirical therapy of urinary tract infections, meningitis, and typhoid fever. Ampicillin is not active against *Klebsiella* sp, *Enterobacter* sp, *P aeruginosa*, *Citrobacter* sp, *Serratia marcescens*, indole-positive proteus species, and other gram-negative aerobes that are commonly encountered in hospital-acquired infections. These organisms produce β lactamase that inactivates ampicillin.

Carbenicillin, the first antipseudomonal carboxypenicillin, is no longer used in the USA, as there are more active, better tolerated alternatives. A carboxypenicillin with activity similar to that of carbenicillin is ticarcillin. It is less active than ampicillin against enterococci. The ureidopenicillins, piperacillin, mezlocillin, and azlocillin, are also active against selected gram-negative bacilli, such as *Klebsiella pneumoniae*. Although supportive clinical data are lacking for superiority of combination therapy over single-drug therapy, because of the propensity of *P aeruginosa* to develop resistance during treatment, an antipseudomonal penicillin is frequently used in combination with an aminoglycoside or fluoroquinolone for pseudomonal infections outside the urinary tract.

Ampicillin, amoxicillin, ticarcillin, and piperacillin are also available in combination with one of several β-lactamase inhibitors: clavulanic acid, sulbactam, or tazobactam. The addition of a β-lactamase inhibitor extends the activity of these penicillins to include β-lactamase-producing strains of *S aureus* as well as some β-lactamase-producing gram-negative bacteria (see Beta-Lactamase Inhibitors).

Adverse Reactions

The penicillins are generally well tolerated, and unfortunately, this encourages their misuse and inappropriate use. Most of the serious adverse effects are due to hypersensitivity. All penicillins are cross-sensitizing and cross-reacting. The antigenic determinants are degradation products of penicillins, particularly penicilloic acid and products of alkaline hydrolysis bound to host protein. A history of a penicillin reaction is not reliable; about 5–8% of people claim such a history, but only a small number of these will have an allergic reaction when given penicillin. Less than 1% of persons who previously received penicillin without incident will have an allergic reaction when given penicillin. Because of the potential for anaphylaxis, however, penicillin should be administered with caution or a substitute drug given if the person has a history of serious penicillin allergy. The incidence of allergic reactions in young children is negligible.

Allergic reactions include anaphylactic shock (very rare—0.05% of recipients); serum sickness-type reactions (now rare—urticaria, fever, joint swelling, angioneurotic edema, intense pruritus, and respiratory compromise occurring 7–12 days after exposure); and a variety of skin rashes. Oral lesions, fever, interstitial nephritis (an autoimmune reaction to a penicillin-protein complex), eosinophilia, hemolytic anemia and other hematologic disturbances, and vasculitis may also occur. Most patients allergic to penicillins can be treated with alternative drugs. However, if necessary (eg, treatment of enterococcal endocarditis or neurosyphilis in a patient with serious penicillin allergy), desensitization can be accomplished with gradually increasing doses of penicillin.

In patients with renal failure, penicillin in high doses can cause seizures. Nafcillin is associated with neutropenia; oxacillin can cause hepatitis; and methicillin causes interstitial nephritis (and is no longer used for this reason). Large doses of penicillins given orally may lead to gastrointestinal upset, particularly nausea, vomiting, and diarrhea. Ampicillin has been associated with pseudomembranous colitis. Secondary infections such as vaginal candidiasis may occur. Ampicillin and amoxicillin can cause skin rashes that are not allergic in nature. These rashes frequently occur when aminopenicillins are inappropriately prescribed for a viral illness.

■ CEPHALOSPORINS & CEPHAMYCINS

Cephalosporins are similar to penicillins, but more stable to many bacterial β lactamases and therefore have a broader spectrum of activity. However, strains of *E coli* and *Klebsiella* sp expressing extended-spectrum β lactamases that can hydrolyze most cephalosporins are a growing clinical concern. Cephalosporins are not active against enterococci and *L monocytogenes*.

Chemistry

The nucleus of the cephalosporins, 7-aminocephalosporanic acid (Figure 43–6), bears a close resemblance to 6-aminopenicillanic acid (Figure 43–1). The intrinsic antimicrobial activity of natural cephalosporins is low, but the attachment of various R_1 and R_2 groups has yielded hundreds of potent compounds of low toxicity. Cephalosporins can be classified into four major groups or generations, depending mainly on the spectrum of antimicrobial activity.

FIRST-GENERATION CEPHALOSPORINS

First-generation cephalosporins include **cefazolin, cefadroxil, cephalexin, cephalothin, cephapirin,** and **cephradine.** These drugs are very active against gram-positive cocci, such as pneumococci, streptococci, and staphylococci. Traditional cephalosporins are not active against methicillin-resistant strains of staphylococci; however, new compounds have been developed that have activity against methicillin-resistant strains (see below). *E coli, K pneumoniae,* and *Proteus mirabilis* are often sensitive, but activity against *P aeruginosa,* indole-positive proteus species, *Enterobacter* sp, *S marcescens, Citrobacter* sp, and *Acinetobacter* sp is poor. Anaerobic cocci (eg, peptococci, peptostreptococci) are usually sensitive, but *Bacteroides fragilis* is not.

Pharmacokinetics & Dosage

A. Oral

Cephalexin, cephradine, and cefadroxil are absorbed from the gut to a variable extent. After oral doses of 500 mg, serum levels are 15–20 mcg/mL. Urine concentration is usually very high, but in most tissues levels are variable and generally lower than in serum. Cephalexin and cephradine are given orally in dosages of 0.25–0.5 g four times daily (15–30 mg/kg/d) and cefadroxil in dosages of 0.5–1 g twice daily. Excretion is mainly by glomerular filtration and tubular secretion into the urine. Drugs that block tubular secretion, eg, probenecid, may increase serum levels substantially. In patients with impaired renal function, dosage must be reduced (Table 43–2).

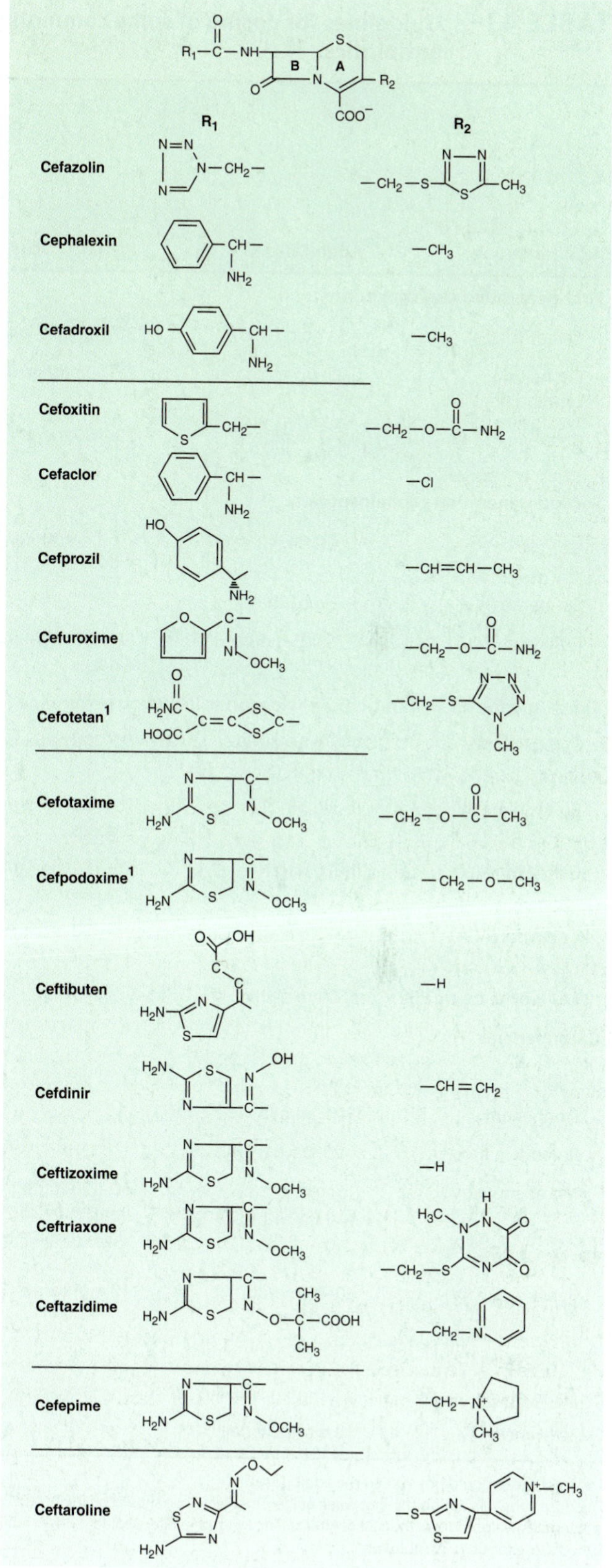

FIGURE 43–6 Structures of some cephalosporins. R_1 and R_2 structures are substituents on the 7-aminocephalosporanic acid nucleus pictured at the top. Other structures (cefoxitin and below) are complete in themselves. [1] Additional substituents not shown.

TABLE 43–2 Guidelines for dosing of some commonly used cephalosporins and other cell-wall inhibitor antibiotics.

Antibiotic (Route of Administration)	Adult Dose	Pediatric Dose[1]	Neonatal Dose[2]	Adjusted Dose as a Percentage of Normal Dose for Renal Failure Based on Creatinine Clearance (Cl_{cr})	
				Cl_{cr} Approx 50 mL/min	Cl_{cr} Approx 10 mL/min
First-generation cephalosporins					
Cefadroxil (PO)	0.5–1 g qd–bid	30 mg/kg/d in 2 doses		50%	25%
Cephalexin, cephradine (PO)	0.25–0.5 g qid	25–50 mg/kg/d in 4 doses		50%	25%
Cefazolin (IV)	0.5–2 g q8h	25–100 mg/kg/d in 3 or 4 doses		50%	25%
Second-generation cephalosporins					
Cefoxitin (IV)	1–2 g q6–8h	75–150 mg/kg/d in 3 or 4 doses		50–75%	25%
Cefotetan (IV)	1–2 g q12h			50%	25%
Cefuroxime (IV)	0.75–1.5 g q8h	50–100 mg/kg/d in 3 or 4 doses		66%	25–33%
Third- and fourth-generation cephalosporins including ceftaroline fosamil					
Cefotaxime (IV)	1–2 g q6–12h	50–200 mg/kg/d in 4–6 doses	100 mg/kg/d in 2 doses	50%	25%
Ceftazidime (IV)	1–2 g q8–12h	75–150 mg/kg/d in 3 doses	100–150 mg/kg/d in 2 or 3 doses	50%	25%
Ceftriaxone (IV)	1–4 g q24h	50–100 mg/kg/d in 1 or 2 doses	50 mg/kg/d qd	None	None
Cefepime (IV)	0.5–2 g q12h	75–120 mg/kg/d in 2 or 3 divided doses		50%	25%
Ceftaroline fosamil (IV)	600 mg q12h			50–66%	33%
Carbapenems					
Ertapenem (IM or IV)	1 g q24h			100%[3]	50%
Doripenem	500 mg q8h			50%	33%
Imipenem (IV)	0.25–0.5 g q6–8h			75%	50%
Meropenem (IV)	1 g q8h (2 g q8h for meningitis)	60–120 mg/kg/d in 3 doses (maximum of 2 g q8h)		66%	50%
Glycopeptides					
Vancomycin (IV)	30–60 mg/kg/d in 2–3 doses	40 mg/kg/d in 3 or 4 doses	15 mg/kg load, then 20 mg/kg/d in 2 doses	40%	10%
Lipopeptides (IV)					
Daptomycin	4-6 mg/kg IV daily			None	50%
Telavancin	10 mg/kg IV daily			75%	50%

[1]The total dose should not exceed the adult dose.
[2]The dose shown is during the first week of life. The daily dose should be increased by approximately 33–50% after the first week of life. The lower dosage range should be used for neonates weighing less than 2 kg. After the first month of life, pediatric doses may be used.
[3]50% of dose for $Cl_{cr} < 30$ mL/min.

B. Parenteral

Cefazolin is the only first-generation parenteral cephalosporin still in general use. After an intravenous infusion of 1 g, the peak level of cefazolin is 90–120 mcg/mL. The usual intravenous dosage of cefazolin for adults is 0.5–2 g intravenously every 8 hours. Cefazolin can also be administered intramuscularly. Excretion is via the kidney, and dose adjustments must be made for impaired renal function.

Clinical Uses

Oral drugs may be used for the treatment of urinary tract infections and staphylococcal or streptococcal infections, including cellulitis or soft tissue abscess. However, oral cephalosporins should not be relied on in serious systemic infections.

Cefazolin penetrates well into most tissues. It is a drug of choice for surgical prophylaxis. Cefazolin may also be a choice in infections for which it is the least toxic drug (eg, penicillinase-producing *E coli* or *K pneumoniae*) and in individuals with staphylococcal or streptococcal infections who have a history of penicillin allergy other than immediate hypersensitivity. Cefazolin does not penetrate the central nervous system and cannot be used to treat meningitis. Cefazolin is an alternative to an antistaphylococcal penicillin for patients who are allergic to penicillin.

SECOND-GENERATION CEPHALOSPORINS

Members of the second-generation cephalosporins include **cefaclor, cefamandole, cefonicid, cefuroxime, cefprozil, loracarbef,** and **ceforanide;** and the structurally related cephamycins **cefoxitin, cefmetazole,** and **cefotetan,** which have activity against anaerobes. This is a heterogeneous group with marked individual differences in activity, pharmacokinetics, and toxicity. In general, they are active against organisms inhibited by first-generation drugs, but in addition they have extended gram-negative coverage. *Klebsiella* sp (including those resistant to cephalothin) are usually sensitive. Cefamandole, cefuroxime, cefonicid, ceforanide, and cefaclor are active against *H influenzae* but not against serratia or *B fragilis.* In contrast, cefoxitin, cefmetazole, and cefotetan are active against *B fragilis* and some serratia strains but are less active against *H influenzae.* As with first-generation agents, none is active against enterococci or *P aeruginosa.* Second-generation cephalosporins may exhibit in vitro activity against *Enterobacter* sp., but resistant mutants that constitutively express a chromosomal β lactamase that hydrolyzes these compounds (and third-generation cephalosporins) are readily selected, and they should not be used to treat enterobacter infections.

Pharmacokinetics & Dosage

A. Oral

Cefaclor, cefuroxime axetil, cefprozil, and loracarbef can be given orally. The usual dosage for adults is 10–15 mg/kg/d in two to four divided doses; children should be given 20–40 mg/kg/d up to

a maximum of 1 g/d. Except for cefuroxime axetil, these drugs are not predictably active against penicillin-non-susceptible pneumococci and should be used cautiously, if at all, to treat suspected or proved pneumococcal infections. Cefaclor is more susceptible to β-lactamase hydrolysis compared with the other agents, and its usefulness is correspondingly diminished.

B. Parenteral

After a 1-g intravenous infusion, serum levels are 75–125 mcg/mL for most second-generation cephalosporins. Intramuscular administration is painful and should be avoided. Doses and dosing intervals vary depending on the specific agent (Table 43–2). There are marked differences in half-life, protein binding, and interval between doses. All are renally cleared and require dosage adjustment in renal failure.

Clinical Uses

The oral second-generation cephalosporins are active against β-lactamase-producing *H influenzae* or *Moraxella catarrhalis* and have been primarily used to treat sinusitis, otitis, and lower respiratory tract infections, in which these organisms have an important role. Because of their activity against anaerobes (including many *B fragilis* strains), cefoxitin, cefotetan, or cefmetazole can be used to treat mixed anaerobic infections such as peritonitis, diverticulitis, and pelvic inflammatory disease. Cefuroxime is used to treat community-acquired pneumonia because it is active against β-lactamase-producing *H influenzae* or *K pneumoniae* and some penicillin-non-susceptible pneumococci. Although cefuroxime crosses the blood-brain barrier, it is less effective in treatment of meningitis than ceftriaxone or cefotaxime and should not be used.

THIRD-GENERATION CEPHALOSPORINS

Third-generation agents include **cefoperazone, cefotaxime, ceftazidime, ceftizoxime, ceftriaxone, cefixime, cefpodoxime proxetil, cefdinir, cefditoren pivoxil, ceftibuten,** and **moxalactam.**

Antimicrobial Activity

Compared with second-generation agents, these drugs have expanded gram-negative coverage, and some are able to cross the blood-brain barrier. Third-generation drugs are active against *Citrobacter, S marcescens,* and *Providencia* (although resistance can emerge during treatment of infections caused by these species due to selection of mutants that constitutively produce cephalosporinase). They are also effective against β-lactamase-producing strains of haemophilus and neisseria. Ceftazidime and cefoperazone are the only two drugs with useful activity against *P aeruginosa.* Like the second-generation drugs, third-generation cephalosporins are hydrolyzed by constitutively produced AmpC β lactamase, and they are not reliably active against *Enterobacter* species. *Serratia, Providencia,* and *Citrobacter* also produce a chromosomally encoded cephalosporinase that, when constitutively expressed, can confer resistance to third-generation cephalosporins. Ceftizoxime and moxalactam are active against *B fragilis.* Cefixime, cefdinir, ceftibuten, and cefpodoxime proxetil are oral agents possessing similar activity except that cefixime and ceftibuten are much less active against pneumococci and have poor activity against *S aureus*.

Pharmacokinetics & Dosage

Intravenous infusion of 1 g of a parenteral cephalosporin produces serum levels of 60–140 mcg/mL. Third-generation cephalosporins penetrate body fluids and tissues well and, with the exception of cefoperazone and all oral cephalosporins, achieve levels in the cerebrospinal fluid sufficient to inhibit most susceptible pathogens.

The half-lives of these drugs and the necessary dosing intervals vary greatly: Ceftriaxone (half-life 7–8 hours) can be injected once every 24 hours at a dosage of 15–50 mg/kg/d. A single daily 1-g dose is sufficient for most serious infections, with 2 g every 12 hours recommended for treatment of meningitis. Cefoperazone (half-life 2 hours) can be infused every 8–12 hours in a dosage of 25–100 mg/kg/d. The remaining drugs in the group (half-life 1–1.7 hours) can be infused every 6–8 hours in dosages between 2 and 12 g/d, depending on the severity of infection. Cefixime can be given orally (200 mg twice daily or 400 mg once daily) for urinary tract infections and as a single 400 mg dose for uncomplicated gonococcal urethritis and cervicitis. The adult dose for cefpodoxime proxetil or cefditoren pivoxil is 200–400 mg twice daily; for ceftibuten, 400 mg once daily; and for cefdinir, 300 mg/12 h. The excretion of cefoperazone and ceftriaxone is mainly through the biliary tract, and no dosage adjustment is required in renal insufficiency. The others are excreted by the kidney and therefore require dosage adjustment in renal insufficiency.

Clinical Uses

Third-generation cephalosporins are used to treat a wide variety of serious infections caused by organisms that are resistant to most other drugs. Strains expressing extended-spectrum β lactamases, however, are not susceptible. Third-generation cephalosporins should be avoided in treatment of enterobacter infections—even if the clinical isolate appears susceptible in vitro—because of emergence of resistance. Ceftriaxone and cefotaxime are approved for treatment of meningitis, including meningitis caused by pneumococci, meningococci, *H influenzae*, and susceptible enteric gram-negative rods, but not by *L monocytogenes*. Ceftriaxone and cefotaxime are the most active cephalosporins against penicillin-non-susceptible strains of pneumococci and are recommended for empirical therapy of serious infections that may be caused by these strains. Meningitis caused by strains of pneumococci with penicillin MICs > 1 mcg/mL may not respond even to these agents, and addition of vancomycin is recommended. Other potential indications include empirical therapy of sepsis of unknown cause in both the immunocompetent and the immunocompromised patient and treatment of infections for which a cephalosporin is the least toxic drug available. In neutropenic, febrile immunocompromised patients, ceftazidime is often used in combination with other antibiotics.

FOURTH-GENERATION CEPHALOSPORINS

Cefepime is an example of a so-called fourth-generation cephalosporin. It is more resistant to hydrolysis by chromosomal β lactamases (eg, those produced by *Enterobacter*). However, like the third-generation compounds, it is hydrolyzed by extended-spectrum β lactamases. Cefepime has good activity against *P aeruginosa*, Enterobacteriaceae, *S aureus*, and *S pneumoniae*. It is highly active against *Haemophilus* and *Neisseria* sp. It penetrates well into cerebrospinal fluid. It is cleared by the kidneys and has a half-life of 2 hours, and its pharmacokinetic properties are very similar to those of ceftazidime. Unlike ceftazidime, however, cefepime has good activity against most penicillin-non-susceptible strains of streptococci, and it is useful in treatment of enterobacter infections.

Cephalosporins Active against Methicillin-Resistant Staphylococci

Beta-lactam antibiotics with activity against methicillin-resistant staphylococci are currently under development. **Ceftaroline** fosamil, the prodrug of the active metabolite ceftaroline, is the first such drug to be approved for clinical use in the USA. Ceftaroline has increased binding to penicillin-binding protein 2a, which mediates methicillin resistance in staphylococci, resulting in bactericidal activity against these strains. It has some activity against enterococci and a broad gram-negative spectrum, although it is not active against extended-spectrum β-lactamase-producing strains. Since clinical experience with this and similar investigational drugs is limited, their role in therapy is not yet defined.

ADVERSE EFFECTS OF CEPHALOSPORINS

A. Allergy

Cephalosporins are sensitizing and may elicit a variety of hypersensitivity reactions that are identical to those of penicillins, including anaphylaxis, fever, skin rashes, nephritis, granulocytopenia, and hemolytic anemia. However, the chemical nucleus of cephalosporins is sufficiently different from that of penicillins so that some individuals with a history of penicillin allergy may tolerate cephalosporins. The frequency of cross-allergenicity between the two groups of drugs is uncertain but is probably around 5–10%. Cross-allergenicity appears to be more common with penicillins and early generation cephalosporins compared with later generation cephalosporins. However, patients with a history of anaphylaxis to penicillins should not receive cephalosporins.

B. Toxicity

Local irritation can produce pain after intramuscular injection and thrombophlebitis after intravenous injection. Renal toxicity, including interstitial nephritis and tubular necrosis, has been demonstrated with several cephalosporins and caused the withdrawal of cephaloridine from clinical use.

Cephalosporins that contain a methylthiotetrazole group (cefamandole, cefmetazole, cefotetan, and cefoperazone) may cause hypoprothrombinemia and bleeding disorders. Oral administration of vitamin K₁, 10 mg twice weekly, can prevent this. Drugs with the methylthiotetrazole ring can also cause severe disulfiram-like reactions; consequently, alcohol and alcohol-containing medications must be avoided.

■ OTHER BETA-LACTAM DRUGS

MONOBACTAMS

Monobactams are drugs with a monocyclic β-lactam ring (Figure 43–1). Their spectrum of activity is limited to aerobic gram-negative rods (including *P aeruginosa*). Unlike other β-lactam antibiotics, they have no activity against gram-positive bacteria or anaerobes. **Aztreonam** is the only monobactam available in the USA. It has structural similarities to ceftazidime; hence, its gram-negative spectrum is similar to that of the third-generation cephalosporins. It is stable to many β lactamases with the notable exceptions being AmpC β lactamases and extended-spectrum β lactamases. It penetrates well into the cerebrospinal fluid. Aztreonam is given intravenously every 8 hours in a dose of 1–2 g, providing peak serum levels of 100 mcg/mL. The half-life is 1–2 hours and is greatly prolonged in renal failure.

Penicillin-allergic patients tolerate aztreonam without reaction. Occasional skin rashes and elevations of serum aminotransferases occur during administration of aztreonam, but major toxicity is uncommon. In patients with a history of penicillin anaphylaxis, aztreonam may be used to treat serious infections such as pneumonia, meningitis, and sepsis caused by susceptible gram-negative pathogens.

BETA-LACTAMASE INHIBITORS (CLAVULANIC ACID, SULBACTAM, & TAZOBACTAM)

These substances resemble β-lactam molecules (Figure 43–7), but they have very weak antibacterial action. They are potent inhibitors of many but not all bacterial β lactamases and can protect hydrolyzable penicillins from inactivation by these enzymes. Beta-lactamase

inhibitors are most active against Ambler class A β lactamases (plasmid-encoded transposable element [TEM] β lactamases in particular), such as those produced by staphylococci, *H influenzae*, *N gonorrhoeae*, salmonella, shigella, *E coli*, and *K pneumoniae*. They are not good inhibitors of class C β lactamases, which typically are chromosomally encoded and inducible, produced by *Enterobacter* sp, *Citrobacter* sp, *S marcescens*, and *P aeruginosa*, but they do inhibit chromosomal β lactamases of *B fragilis* and *M catarrhalis*.

The three inhibitors differ slightly with respect to pharmacology, stability, potency, and activity, but these differences usually are of little therapeutic significance. Beta-lactamase inhibitors are available only in fixed combinations with specific penicillins. The antibacterial spectrum of the combination is determined by the companion penicillin, not the β-lactamase inhibitor. (The fixed combinations available in the USA are listed in Preparations Available.) An inhibitor extends the spectrum of a penicillin provided that the inactivity of the penicillin is due to destruction by β lactamase and that the inhibitor is active against the β lactamase that is produced. Thus, ampicillin-sulbactam is active against β-lactamase-producing *S aureus* and *H influenzae* but not against serratia, which produces a β lactamase that is not inhibited by sulbactam. Similarly, if a strain of *P aeruginosa* is resistant to piperacillin, it is also resistant to piperacillin-tazobactam because tazobactam does not inhibit the chromosomal β lactamase produced by *P aeruginosa*.

The indications for penicillin-β-lactamase inhibitor combinations are empirical therapy for infections caused by a wide range of potential pathogens in both immunocompromised and immunocompetent patients and treatment of mixed aerobic and anaerobic infections, such as intra-abdominal infections. Doses are the same as those used for the single agents except that the recommended dosage of piperacillin in the piperacillin-tazobactam combination is 3–4 g every 6 hours. Adjustments for renal insufficiency are made based on the penicillin component.

CARBAPENEMS

The carbapenems are structurally related to β-lactam antibiotics (Figure 43–1). **Doripenem, ertapenem, imipenem,** and **meropenem** are licensed for use in the USA. Imipenem, the first drug of this class, has a wide spectrum with good activity against many gram-negative rods, including *P aeruginosa*, gram-positive

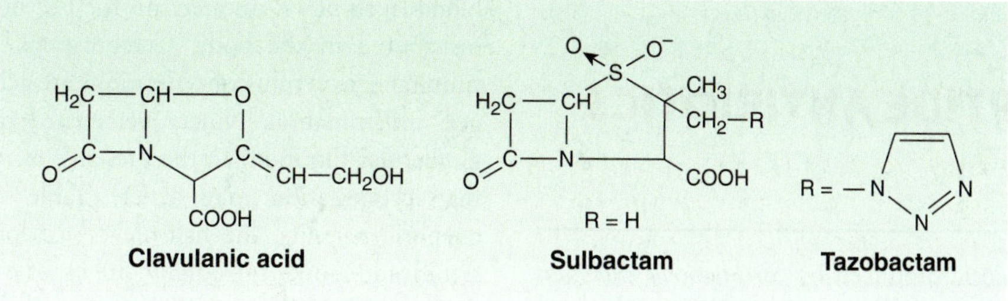

FIGURE 43–7 Beta-lactamase inhibitors.

organisms, and anaerobes. It is resistant to most β lactamases but not carbapenemases or metallo-β lactamases. *Enterococcus faecium*, methicillin-resistant strains of staphylococci, *Clostridium difficile*, *Burkholderia cepacia*, and *Stenotrophomonas maltophilia* are resistant. Imipenem is inactivated by dehydropeptidases in renal tubules, resulting in low urinary concentrations. Consequently, it is administered together with an inhibitor of renal dehydropeptidase, **cilastatin,** for clinical use. Doripenem and meropenem are similar to imipenem but have slightly greater activity against gram-negative aerobes and slightly less activity against gram-positives. They are not significantly degraded by renal dehydropeptidase and do not require an inhibitor. Ertapenem is less active than the other carbapenems against *P aeruginosa* and *Acinetobacter* species. It is not degraded by renal dehydropeptidase.

Carbapenems penetrate body tissues and fluids well, including the cerebrospinal fluid. All are cleared renally, and the dose must be reduced in patients with renal insufficiency. The usual dosage of imipenem is 0.25–0.5 g given intravenously every 6–8 hours (half-life 1 hour). The usual adult dosage of meropenem is 0.5–1 g intravenously every 8 hours. The usual adult dosage of doripenem is 0.5 g administered as a 1- or 4-hour infusion every 8 hours. Ertapenem has the longest half-life (4 hours) and is administered as a once-daily dose of 1 g intravenously or intramuscularly. Intramuscular ertapenem is irritating, and for that reason the drug is formulated with 1% lidocaine for administration by this route.

A carbapenem is indicated for infections caused by susceptible organisms that are resistant to other available drugs, eg, *P aeruginosa*, and for treatment of mixed aerobic and anaerobic infections. Carbapenems are active against many penicillin-non-susceptible strains of pneumococci. Carbapenems are highly active in the treatment of enterobacter infections because they are resistant to destruction by the β lactamase produced by these organisms. Clinical experience suggests that carbapenems are also the treatment of choice for infections caused by extended-spectrum β-lactamase-producing gram-negative bacteria. Ertapenem is insufficiently active against *P aeruginosa* and should not be used to treat infections caused by that organism. Imipenem, meropenem, or doripenem, with or without an aminoglycoside, may be effective treatment for febrile neutropenic patients.

The most common adverse effects of carbapenems—which tend to be more common with imipenem—are nausea, vomiting, diarrhea, skin rashes, and reactions at the infusion sites. Excessive levels of imipenem in patients with renal failure may lead to seizures. Meropenem, doripenem, and ertapenem are much less likely to cause seizures than imipenem. Patients allergic to penicillins may be allergic to carbapenems as well.

■ GLYCOPEPTIDE ANTIBIOTICS

VANCOMYCIN

Vancomycin is an antibiotic produced by *Streptococcus orientalis* and *Amycolatopsis orientalis*. With the exception of *Flavobacterium*, it is active only against gram-positive bacteria. Vancomycin is a

glycopeptide of molecular weight 1500. It is water soluble and quite stable.

Mechanisms of Action & Basis of Resistance

Vancomycin inhibits cell wall synthesis by binding firmly to the D-Ala-D-Ala terminus of nascent peptidoglycan pentapeptide (Figure 43–5). This inhibits the transglycosylase, preventing further elongation of peptidoglycan and cross-linking. The peptidoglycan is thus weakened, and the cell becomes susceptible to lysis. The cell membrane is also damaged, which contributes to the antibacterial effect.

Resistance to vancomycin in enterococci is due to modification of the D-Ala-D-Ala binding site of the peptidoglycan building block in which the terminal D-Ala is replaced by D-lactate. This results in the loss of a critical hydrogen bond that facilitates high-affinity binding of vancomycin to its target and loss of activity. This mechanism is also present in vancomycin-resistant *S aureus* strains (MIC ≥ 16 mcg/mL), which have acquired the enterococcal resistance determinants. The underlying mechanism for reduced vancomycin susceptibility in vancomycin-intermediate strains (MICs = 4–8 mcg/mL) of *S aureus* is not fully known. However these strains have altered cell wall metabolism that results in a thickened cell wall with increased numbers of D-Ala-D-Ala residues, which serve as dead-end binding sites for vancomycin. Vancomycin is sequestered within the cell wall by these false targets and may be unable to reach its site of action.

Antibacterial Activity

Vancomycin is bactericidal for gram-positive bacteria in concentrations of 0.5–10 mcg/mL. Most pathogenic staphylococci, including those producing β lactamase and those resistant to nafcillin and methicillin, are killed by 2 mcg/mL or less. Vancomycin kills staphylococci relatively slowly and only if cells are actively dividing; the rate is less than that of the penicillins both in vitro and in vivo. Vancomycin is synergistic in vitro with gentamicin and streptomycin against *Enterococcus faecium* and *Enterococcus faecalis* strains that do not exhibit high levels of aminoglycoside resistance.

Pharmacokinetics

Vancomycin is poorly absorbed from the intestinal tract and is administered orally only for the treatment of antibiotic-associated colitis caused by *C difficile*. Parenteral doses must be administered intravenously. A 1-hour intravenous infusion of 1 g produces blood levels of 15–30 mcg/mL for 1–2 hours. The drug is widely distributed in the body. Cerebrospinal fluid levels 7–30% of simultaneous serum concentrations are achieved if there is meningeal inflammation. Ninety percent of the drug is excreted by glomerular filtration. In the presence of renal insufficiency, striking accumulation may occur (Table 43–2). In functionally anephric patients, the half-life of vancomycin is 6–10 days. A significant amount (roughly 50%) of vancomycin is removed during a standard hemodialysis run when a modern, high-flux membrane is used.

Clinical Uses

Important indications for parenteral vancomycin are bloodstream infections and endocarditis caused by methicillin-resistant staphylococci. However, vancomycin is not as effective as an antistaphylococcal penicillin for treatment of serious infections such as endocarditis caused by methicillin-susceptible strains. Vancomycin in combination with gentamicin is an alternative regimen for treatment of enterococcal endocarditis in a patient with serious penicillin allergy. Vancomycin (in combination with cefotaxime, ceftriaxone, or rifampin) is also recommended for treatment of meningitis suspected or known to be caused by a penicillin-resistant strain of pneumococcus (ie, penicillin MIC > 1 mcg/mL). The recommended dosage in a patient with normal renal function is 30–60 mg/kg/d in two or three divided doses. The traditional dosing regimen in adults with normal renal function is 1 g every 12 hours (~ 30 mg/kg/d); however, this dose will not typically achieve the trough concentrations (15–20 mcg/mL) recommended for serious infections. For serious infections (see below), a starting dose of 45–60 mg/kg/d should be given with titration of the dose to achieve trough levels of 15–20 mcg/mL. The dosage in children is 40 mg/kg/d in three or four divided doses. Clearance of vancomycin is directly proportional to creatinine clearance, and the dosage is reduced accordingly in patients with renal insufficiency. For functionally anephric adult patients, a 1-g dose administered once a week may be sufficient. For patients receiving hemodialysis, a common dosing regimen is a 1-g loading dose followed by 500 mg after each dialysis session. Patients receiving a prolonged course of therapy should have serum concentrations checked. Recommended trough concentrations are 10–15 mcg/mL for mild to moderate infections such as cellulitis and 15–20 mcg/mL for more serious infections such as endocarditis, meningitis, and necrotizing pneumonia.

Oral vancomycin, 0.125–0.25 g every 6 hours, is used to treat antibiotic-associated colitis caused by *C difficile*. Because of the emergence of vancomycin-resistant enterococci and the potential selective pressure of oral vancomycin for these resistant organisms, metronidazole had been preferred as initial therapy over the last two decades. However, receipt of oral vancomycin does not appear to be a significant risk factor for acquisition of vancomycin-resistant enterococci. Additionally, recent clinical data suggest that vancomycin is associated with a better clinical response than metronidazole for more severe cases of *C difficile* colitis. Therefore, oral vancomycin may be used as a first line treatment for severe cases or for cases that fail to respond to metronidazole.

Adverse Reactions

Adverse reactions are encountered in about 10% of cases. Most reactions are minor. Vancomycin is irritating to tissue, resulting in phlebitis at the site of injection. Chills and fever may occur. Ototoxicity is rare and nephrotoxicity uncommon with current preparations. However, administration with another ototoxic or nephrotoxic drug, such as an aminoglycoside, increases the risk of these toxicities. Ototoxicity can be minimized by maintaining peak serum concentrations below 60 mcg/mL. Among the more common reactions is the so-called "red man" or "red neck" syndrome. This infusion-related flushing is caused by release of histamine. It can be largely prevented by prolonging the infusion period to 1–2 hours or pretreatment with an antihistamine such as diphenhydramine.

TEICOPLANIN

Teicoplanin is a glycopeptide antibiotic that is very similar to vancomycin in mechanism of action and antibacterial spectrum. Unlike vancomycin, it can be given intramuscularly as well as intravenously. Teicoplanin has a long half-life (45–70 hours), permitting once-daily dosing. This drug is available in Europe but has not been approved for use in the United States.

TELAVANCIN

Telavancin is a semisynthetic lipoglycopeptide derived from vancomycin. Telavancin is active versus gram-positive bacteria, including strains with reduced susceptibility to vancomycin. Telavancin has two mechanisms of action. Like vancomycin, telavancin inhibits cell wall synthesis by binding to the D-Ala-D-Ala terminus of peptidoglycan in the growing cell wall. In addition, it disrupts the bacterial cell membrane potential and increases membrane permeability. The half-life of telavancin is approximately 8 hours, which supports once-daily intravenous dosing. Telavancin is approved for treatment of complicated skin and soft tissue infections at a dose of 10 mg/kg IV daily. Unlike vancomycin therapy, monitoring of serum telavancin levels is not required. Telavancin is potentially teratogenic, so administration to pregnant women must be avoided.

DALBAVANCIN

Dalbavancin is a semisynthetic lipoglycopeptide derived from teicoplanin. Dalbavancin shares the same mechanism of action as vancomycin and teicoplanin but has improved activity against many gram-positive bacteria including methicillin-resistant and vancomycin-intermediate *S aureus*. It is not active against most strains of vancomycin-resistant enterococci. Dalbavancin has an extremely long half-life of 6–11 days, which allows for once-weekly intravenous administration. Development of dalbavancin has been put on hold pending additional clinical trials.

■ OTHER CELL WALL- OR MEMBRANE-ACTIVE AGENTS

DAPTOMYCIN

Daptomycin is a novel cyclic lipopeptide fermentation product of *Streptomyces roseosporus* (Figure 43–8). It was discovered decades ago but has only recently been developed as the need for drugs

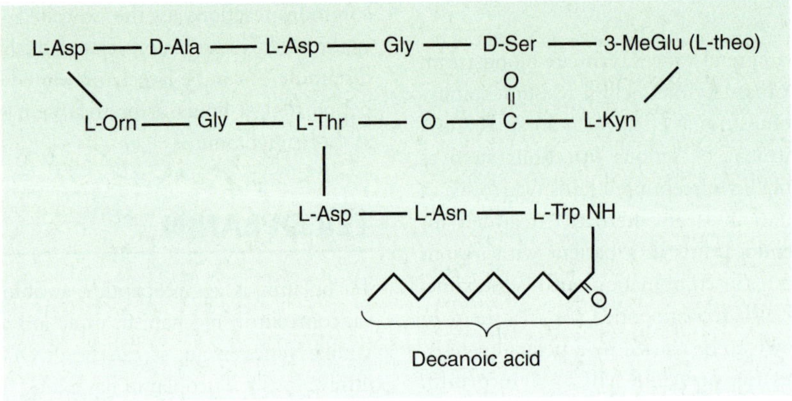

L-Asp —— D-Ala —— L-Asp —— Gly —— D-Ser —— 3-MeGlu (L-theo)

L-Orn —— Gly —— L-Thr —— O —— C —— L-Kyn

L-Asp —— L-Asn —— L-Trp NH

Decanoic acid

FIGURE 43–8 Structure of daptomycin. (Kyn, deaminated tryptophan.)

active against resistant organisms has become more acute. Its spectrum of activity is similar to that of vancomycin except that it is more rapidly bactericidal in vitro and may be active against vancomycin-resistant strains of enterococci and *S aureus*. The precise mechanism of action is not fully understood, but it is known to bind to the cell membrane via calcium-dependent insertion of its lipid tail. This results in depolarization of the cell membrane with potassium efflux and rapid cell death (Figure 43–9). Daptomycin is cleared renally. The approved doses are 4 mg/kg/dose for treatment of skin and soft tissue infections and 6 mg/kg/dose for treatment of bacteremia and endocarditis once daily in patients with normal renal function and every other day in patients with creatinine clearance of less than 30 mL/min. For

serious infections, many experts recommend using doses of daptomycin higher than 6 mg/kg/dose. In clinical trials powered for noninferiority, daptomycin was equivalent in efficacy to vancomycin. It can cause myopathy, and creatine phosphokinase levels should be monitored weekly. Pulmonary surfactant antagonizes daptomycin, and it should not be used to treat pneumonia. Daptomycin can also cause an allergic pneumonitis in patients receiving prolonged therapy (> 2 weeks). Treatment failures have been reported in association with an increase in daptomycin MIC for clinical isolates obtained during therapy, but the relation between the increase in MIC and treatment failure is unclear at this point. Daptomycin is an effective alternative to vancomycin, and its ultimate role continues to unfold.

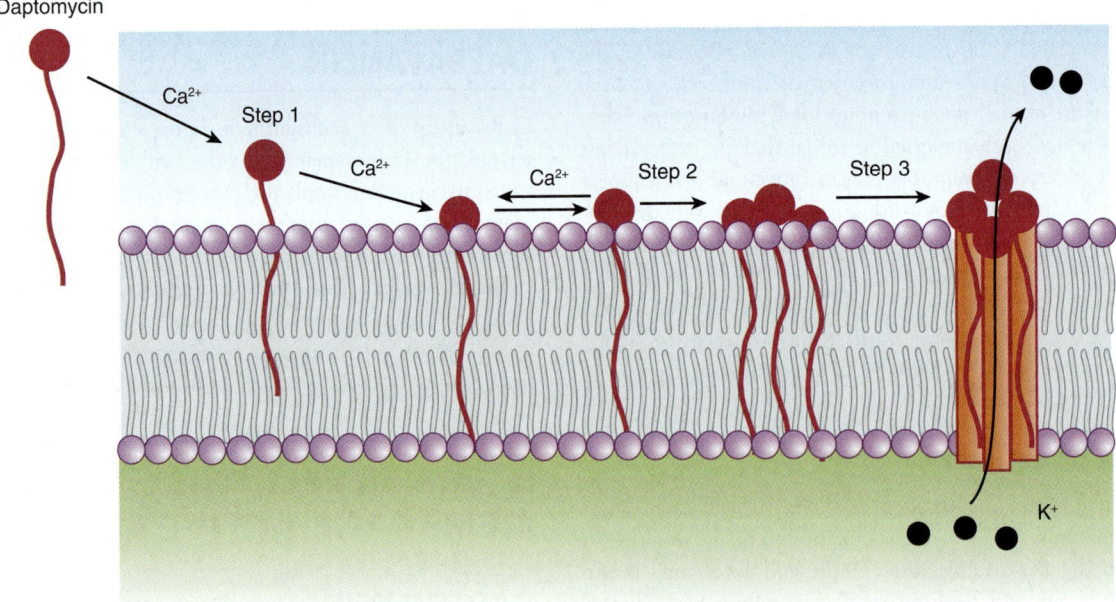

FIGURE 43–9 Proposed mechanism of action of daptomycin. Daptomycin first binds to the cytoplasmic membrane (step 1) and then forms complexes in a calcium-dependent manner (steps 2 and 3). Complex formation causes a rapid loss of cellular potassium, possibly by pore formation, and membrane depolarization. This is followed by arrest of DNA, RNA, and protein synthesis resulting in cell death. Cell lysis does not occur.

FOSFOMYCIN

Fosfomycin trometamol, a stable salt of fosfomycin (phosphonomycin), inhibits a very early stage of bacterial cell wall synthesis (Figure 43–5). An analog of phosphoenolpyruvate, it is structurally unrelated to any other antimicrobial agent. It inhibits the cytoplasmic enzyme enolpyruvate transferase by covalently binding to the cysteine residue of the active site and blocking the addition of phosphoenolpyruvate to UDP-*N*-acetylglucosamine. This reaction is the first step in the formation of UDP-*N*-acetylmuramic acid, the precursor of *N*-acetylmuramic acid, which is found only in bacterial cell walls. The drug is transported into the bacterial cell by glycerophosphate or glucose 6-phosphate transport systems. Resistance is due to inadequate transport of drug into the cell.

Fosfomycin is active against both gram-positive and gram-negative organisms at concentrations ≥ 125 mcg/mL. Susceptibility tests should be performed in growth medium supplemented with glucose 6-phosphate to minimize false-positive indications of resistance. In vitro synergism occurs when fosfomycin is combined with β-lactam antibiotics, aminoglycosides, or fluoroquinolones.

Fosfomycin trometamol is available in both oral and parenteral formulations, although only the oral preparation is approved for use in the USA. Oral bioavailability is approximately 40%. Peak serum concentrations are 10 mcg/mL and 30 mcg/mL following a 2-g or 4-g oral dose, respectively. The half-life is approximately 4 hours. The active drug is excreted by the kidney, with urinary concentrations exceeding MICs for most urinary tract pathogens.

Fosfomycin is approved for use as a single 3-g dose for treatment of uncomplicated lower urinary tract infections in women. The drug appears to be safe for use in pregnancy.

BACITRACIN

Bacitracin is a cyclic peptide mixture first obtained from the Tracy strain of *Bacillus subtilis* in 1943. It is active against gram-positive microorganisms. Bacitracin inhibits cell wall formation by interfering with dephosphorylation in cycling of the lipid carrier that transfers peptidoglycan subunits to the growing cell wall (Figure 43–5). There is no cross-resistance between bacitracin and other antimicrobial drugs.

Bacitracin is highly nephrotoxic when administered systemically and is only used topically (Chapter 61). Bacitracin is poorly absorbed. Topical application results in local antibacterial activity without systemic toxicity. Bacitracin, 500 units/g in an ointment base (often combined with polymyxin or neomycin), is indicated for the suppression of mixed bacterial flora in surface lesions of the skin, in wounds, or on mucous membranes. Solutions of bacitracin containing 100–200 units/mL in saline can be used for irrigation of joints, wounds, or the pleural cavity.

CYCLOSERINE

Cycloserine is an antibiotic produced by *Streptomyces orchidaceous*. It is water soluble and very unstable at acid pH. Cycloserine inhibits many gram-positive and gram-negative organisms, but it is used almost exclusively to treat tuberculosis caused by strains of *Mycobacterium tuberculosis* resistant to first-line agents. Cycloserine is a structural analog of D-alanine and inhibits the incorporation of D-alanine into peptidoglycan pentapeptide by inhibiting alanine racemase, which converts L-alanine to D-alanine, and D-alanyl- D-alanine ligase (Figure 43–5). After ingestion of 0.25 g of cycloserine blood levels reach 20–30 mcg/mL—sufficient to inhibit many strains of mycobacteria and gram-negative bacteria. The drug is widely distributed in tissues. Most of the drug is excreted in active form into the urine. The dosage for treating tuberculosis is 0.5 to 1 g/d in two or three divided doses.

Cycloserine causes serious dose-related central nervous system toxicity with headaches, tremors, acute psychosis, and convulsions. If oral dosages are maintained below 0.75 g/d, such effects can usually be avoided.

SUMMARY Beta-Lactam & Other Cell Wall- & Membrane-Active Antibiotics

Subclass	Mechanism of Action	Effects	Clinical Applications	Pharmacokinetics, Toxicities, Interactions
PENICILLINS				
• Penicillin G	Prevents bacterial cell wall synthesis by binding to and inhibiting cell wall transpeptidases	Rapid bactericidal activity against susceptible bacteria	Streptococcal infections, meningococcal infections, neurosyphilis	IV administration • rapid renal clearance (half-life 30 min, so requires frequent dosing (every 4 h) • *Toxicity:* Immediate hypersensitivity, rash, seizures
• Penicillin V: Oral, low systemic levels limit widespread use				
• Benzathine penicillin, procaine penicillin: Intramuscular, long-acting formulations				
• Nafcillin, oxacillin: Intravenous, added stability to staphylococcal β lactamase, biliary clearance				
• Ampicillin, amoxicillin, ticarcillin, piperacillin: Greater activity versus gram-negative bacteria; addition of β-lactamase inhibitor restores activity against many β-lactamase-producing bacteria				

(continued)

Subclass	Mechanism of Action	Effects	Clinical Applications	Pharmacokinetics, Toxicities, Interactions
CEPHALOSPORINS				
• Cefazolin	Prevents bacterial cell wall synthesis by binding to and inhibiting cell wall transpeptidases	Rapid bactericidal activity against susceptible bacteria	Skin and soft tissue infections, urinary tract infections, surgical prophylaxis	IV administration • renal clearance (half-life 1.5 h) • dosed every 8 h • poor penetration into the central nervous system (CNS) • *Toxicity:* Rash, drug fever

• *Cephalexin: Oral, first-generation drug, used for treating skin and soft tissue infections and urinary tract infections*

• *Cefuroxime: Oral and intravenous, second-generation drug, improved activity versus pneumococcus and* Haemophilus influenzae

• *Cefotetan, cefoxitin: Intravenous, second-generation drugs, activity versus* Bacteroides fragilis *allows for use in abdominal/pelvic infections*

• *Ceftriaxone: Intravenous, third-generation drug, mixed clearance with long half-life (6 hours), good CNS penetration, many uses including pneumonia, meningitis, pyelonephritis, and gonorrhea*

• *Cefotaxime: Intravenous, third-generation, similar to ceftriaxone; however, clearance is renal and half-life is 1 hour*

• *Ceftazidime: Intravenous, third-generation drug, poor gram-positive activity, good activity versus* Pseudomonas

• *Cefepime: Intravenous, fourth-generation drug, broad activity with improved stability to chromosomal β lactamase*

• *Ceftaroline: Intravenous, active against methicillin-resistant staphylococci, broad gram-negative activity*

CARBAPENEMS				
• Imipenem-cilastatin	Prevents bacterial cell wall synthesis by binding to and inhibiting cell wall transpeptidases	Rapid bactericidal activity against susceptible bacteria	Serious infections such as pneumonia and sepsis	IV administration • renal clearance (half-life 1 h), dosed every 6–8 h, cilastatin added to prevent hydrolysis by renal dehydropeptidase • *Toxicity:* Seizures especially in renal failure or with high doses (> 2 g/d)

• *Meropenem, doripenem: Intravenous, similar activity to imipenem; stable to renal dehydropeptidase, lower incidence of seizures*

• *Ertapenem: Intravenous, longer half-life allows for once-daily dosing, lacks activity versus* Pseudomonas *and* Acinetobacter

MONOBACTAMS				
• Aztreonam	Prevents bacterial cell wall synthesis by binding to and inhibiting cell wall transpeptidases	Rapid bactericidal activity against susceptible bacteria	Infections caused by aerobic, gram-negative bacteria in patients with immediate hypersensitivity to penicillins	IV administration • renal clearance half-life 1.5 h • dosed every 8 h • *Toxicity:* No cross-allergenicity with penicillins
GLYCOPEPTIDE				
• Vancomycin	Inhibits cell wall synthesis by binding to the D-Ala-D-Ala terminus of nascent peptidoglycan	Bactericidal activity against susceptible bacteria, slower kill than β-lactam antibiotics	Infections caused by gram-positive bacteria including sepsis, endocarditis, and meningitis • *C difficile* colitis (oral formulation)	Oral, IV administration • renal clearance (half-life 6 h) • starting dose of 30 mg/kg/d in two or three divided doses in patients with normal renal function • trough concentrations of 10–15 mcg/mL sufficient for most infections • *Toxicity:* "Red man" syndrome • nephrotoxicity uncommon

• *Teicoplanin: Intravenous, similar to vancomycin except that long half-life (45–75 h) permits once-daily dosing*

• *Dalbavancin: Intravenous, very long half-life (6–11 days) permits once-weekly dosing, more active than vancomycin*

• *Telavancin: Intravenous, dual mechanism of action results in improved activity against bacteria with reduced susceptibility to vancomycin, once-daily dosing*

LIPOPEPTIDE				
• Daptomycin	Binds to cell membrane, causing depolarization and rapid cell death	Bactericidal activity against susceptible bacteria • more rapidly bactericidal than vancomycin	Infections caused by gram-positive bacteria including sepsis and endocarditis	IV administration • renal clearance (half-life 8 h) • dosed once daily • inactivated by pulmonary surfactant so cannot be used to treat pneumonia • *Toxicity:* Myopathy • monitoring of weekly creatine phosphokinase levels recommended

PREPARATIONS AVAILABLE

PENICILLINS

Amoxicillin (generic, Amoxil, others)
Oral: 125, 200, 250, 400 mg chewable tablets; 500, 875 mg tablets; 250, 500 mg capsules; powder to reconstitute for 50, 125, 200, 250, 400 mg/mL solution

Amoxicillin/potassium clavulanate (generic, Augmentin)[1]
Oral: 250, 500, 875 mg tablets; 125, 200, 250, 400 mg chewable tablets; 1000 mg extended-release tablet; powder to reconstitute for 125, 200, 250 mg/5 mL suspension

Ampicillin (generic)
Oral: 250, 500 mg capsules; powder to reconstitute for 125, 250 mg suspensions
Parenteral: powder to reconstitute for injection (125, 250, 500 mg, 1, 2 g per vial)

Ampicillin/sulbactam sodium (generic, Unasyn)[2]
Parenteral: 1, 2 g ampicillin powder to reconstitute for IV or IM injection

Carbenicillin (Geocillin)
Oral: 382 mg tablets

Dicloxacillin (generic)
Oral: 250, 500 mg capsules

Nafcillin (generic)
Parenteral: 1, 2 g per IV piggyback units

Oxacillin (generic)
Parenteral: powder to reconstitute for injection (0.5, 1, 2, 10 g per vial)

Penicillin G (generic, Pentids, Pfizerpen)
Parenteral: powder to reconstitute for injection (1, 2, 3, 5, 10, 20 million units)

Penicillin G benzathine (Permapen, Bicillin)
Parenteral: 0.6, 1.2, 2.4 million units per dose

Penicillin G procaine (generic)
Parenteral: 0.6, 1.2 million units/mL for IM injection only

Penicillin V (generic, V-Cillin, Pen-Vee K, others)
Oral: 250, 500 mg tablets; powder to reconstitute for 125, 250 mg/5 mL solution

Piperacillin (Pipracil)
Parenteral: powder to reconstitute for injection (2, 3, 4 g per vial)

Piperacillin and tazobactam sodium (Zosyn)[3]
Parenteral: 2, 3, 4 g powder to reconstitute for IV injection

Ticarcillin (Ticar)
Parenteral: powder to reconstitute for injection (1, 3, 6 g per vial)

Ticarcillin/clavulanate potassium (Timentin)[4]
Parenteral: 3 g powder to reconstitute for injection

CEPHALOSPORINS & OTHER BETA-LACTAM DRUGS

Narrow-Spectrum (First-Generation) Cephalosporins
Cefadroxil (generic, Duricef)
Oral: 500 mg capsules; 1 g tablets; 125, 250, 500 mg/5 mL suspension

Cefazolin (generic, Ancef, Kefzol)
Parenteral: powder to reconstitute for injection (0.25, 0.5, 1 g per vial or IV piggyback unit)

Cephalexin (generic, Keflex, others)
Oral: 250, 500 mg capsules and tablets; 1 g tablets; 125, 250 mg/5 mL suspension

Intermediate-Spectrum (Second-Generation) Cephalosporins
Cefaclor (generic, Ceclor)
Oral: 250, 500 mg capsules; 375, 500 mg extended-release tablets; powder to reconstitute for 125, 187, 250, 375 mg/5 mL suspension

Cefmetazole (Zefazone)
Parenteral: 1, 2 g powder for IV injection

Cefotetan (Cefotan)
Parenteral: powder to reconstitute for injection (1, 2, 10 g per vial)

Cefoxitin (Mefoxin)
Parenteral: powder to reconstitute for injection (1, 2, 10 g per vial)

Cefprozil (Cefzil)
Oral: 250, 500 mg tablets; powder to reconstitute 125, 250 mg/5 mL suspension

Cefuroxime (generic, Ceftin, Kefurox, Zinacef)
Oral: 125, 250, 500 mg tablets; 125, 250 mg/5 mL suspension
Parenteral: powder to reconstitute for injection (0.75, 1.5, 7.5 g per vial or infusion pack)

Loracarbef (Lorabid)
Oral: 200, 400 mg capsules; powder for 100, 200 mg/5 mL suspension

Broad-Spectrum (Third- & Fourth-Generation) Cephalosporins
Cefdinir (Omnicef)
Oral: 300 mg capsules; 125 mg/5 mL suspension

Cefditoren (Spectracef)
Oral: 200 mg tablets

Cefepime (Maxipime)
Parenteral: powder for injection 0.5, 1, 2 g

Cefixime (Suprax)
Oral: 200, 400 mg tablets; powder for oral suspension, 100 mg/5 mL

Cefotaxime (Claforan)
Parenteral: powder to reconstitute for injection (0.5, 1, 2 g per vial)

Cefpodoxime proxetil (Vantin)
Oral: 100, 200 mg tablets; 50, 100 mg granules for suspension in 5 mL

Ceftaroline fosamil (Teflaro)
Parenteral: powder to reconstitute for injection (0.6 g per vial)

Ceftazidime (generic, Fortaz, Tazidime)
Parenteral: powder to reconstitute for injection (0.5, 1, 2 g per vial)

Ceftibuten (Cedax)
Oral: 400 mg capsules; 90, 180 mg/5 mL powder for oral suspension

Ceftizoxime (Cefizox)
Parenteral: powder to reconstitute for injection and solution for injection (0.5, 1, 2 g per vial)

Ceftriaxone (Rocephin)
Parenteral: powder to reconstitute for injection (0.25, 0.5, 1, 2, 10 g per vial)

Carbapenems & Monobactam

Aztreonam (Azactam)
Parenteral: powder to reconstitute for injection (0.5, 1, 2 g)

Doripenem (Doribax)
Parenteral: powder to reconstitute for injection (500 mg per vial)

Ertapenem (Invanz)
Parenteral: 1 g powder to reconstitute for IV (0.9% diluent) or IM (1% lidocaine diluent) injection

Imipenem/cilastatin (Primaxin)
Parenteral: powder to reconstitute for injection (250, 500, 750 mg imipenem per vial)

Meropenem (Merrem IV)
Parenteral: powder for injection (0.5, 1 g per vial)

OTHER DRUGS DISCUSSED IN THIS CHAPTER

Cycloserine (Seromycin Pulvules)
Oral: 250 mg capsules

Daptomycin (Cubicin)
Parenteral: 0.25 or 0.5 g lyophilized powder to reconstitute for IV injection

Fosfomycin (Monurol)
Oral: 3 g packet

Telavancin (Vibativ)
Parenteral: 0.25 and 0.75 g powder to reconstitute for IV injection

Vancomycin (generic, Vancocin, Vancoled)
Oral: 125, 250 mg pulvules; powder to reconstitute for 250 mg/5 mL, 500 mg/6 mL solution
Parenteral: 0.5, 1, 5, 10 g powder to reconstitute for IV injection

[1]Clavulanate content varies with the formulation; see package insert.
[2]Sulbactam content is half the ampicillin content.
[3]Tazobactam content is 12.5% of the piperacillin content.
[4]Clavulanate content 0.1 g.

REFERENCES

Biek D et al: Ceftaroline fosamil: A novel broad-spectrum cephalosporin with expanded Gram-positive activity. J Antimicrob Chemother 2010;65(Suppl 4):iv9.

Billeter M et al: Dalbavancin: A novel once-weekly lipoglycopeptide antibiotic. Clin Infect Dis 2008;46:577.

Bush K et al: Anti-MRSA beta-lactams in development, with a focus on ceftobiprole: The first anti-MRSA beta-lactam to demonstrate clinical efficacy. Expert Opin Investig Drugs 2007;16:419.

Carpenter CF, Chambers HF: Daptomycin: Another novel agent for treating infections due to drug-resistant gram-positive pathogens. Clin Infect Dis 2004;38:994.

Centers for Disease Control and Prevention: Vancomycin-resistant *Staphylococcus aureus*—Pennsylvania, 2002. JAMA 2002;288:2116.

Chow JW et al: *Enterobacter* bacteremia: Clinical features and emergence of antibiotic resistance during therapy. Ann Intern Med 1991;115:585.

Fowler VG et al: Daptomycin versus standard therapy for bacteremia and endocarditis caused by *Staphylococcus aureus*. N Engl J Med 2006;355:653.

Hiramatsu K et al: Methicillin resistant *Staphylococcus aureus* clinical strain with reduced vancomycin susceptibility. J Antimicrob Chemother 1997;40:135.

Hiramatsu K: Vancomycin-resistant *Staphylococcus aureus*: A new model of antibiotic resistance. Lancet Infect Dis 2001;1:147.

Jacoby GA, Munoz-Price LS: The new beta-lactamases. N Engl J Med 2005;352:380.

Keating GM, Perry CM: Ertapenem: A review of its use in the treatment of bacterial infections. Drugs 2005;65:2151.

Leonard SN, Rybak MJ: Telavancin: An antimicrobial with a multifunctional mechanism of action for the treatment of serious gram-positive infections. Pharmacotherapy 2008;28:458.

Mandell L: Doripenem: A new carbapenem in the treatment of nosocomial infections. Clin Infect Dis 2009;49(Suppl 1):S1.

Noskin GA et al: National trends in *Staphylococcus aureus* infection rates: Impact on economic burden and mortality over a 6-year period. Clin Infect Dis 2007;45:1132.

Park MA, Li JT: Diagnosis and management of penicillin allergy. Mayo Clin Proc 2005;80:405.

Rybak M et al: Therapeutic monitoring of vancomycin in adults patients: A consensus review of the American Society of Health-System Pharmacists, the Infectious Diseases Society of America, and the Society of Infectious Diseases Pharmacists. Am J Health Syst Pharm 2009;66:82.

Sanders EW Jr, Tenny JH, Kessler RE: Efficacy of cefepime in the treatment of infections due to multiply resistant Enterobacter species. Clin Infect Dis 1996;23:454.

Wexler HM: In vitro activity of ertapenem: Review of recent studies. J Antimicrob Chemother 2004;53(Suppl 2):ii11.

Zar FA et al: A comparison of vancomycin and metronidazole for the treatment of *Clostridium difficile*-associated diarrhea. Clin Infect Dis 2007;45:302.

CASE STUDY ANSWER

An intravenous third-generation cephalosporin (ceftriaxone or cefotaxime) with adequate penetration into inflamed meninges that is active against the common bacteria that cause community-acquired pneumonia and meningitis (pneumococcus, meningococcus, *Haemophilus*) should be ordered. Vancomycin should also be administered until culture and sensitivity results are available in case the patient is infected with a resistant pneumococcus. Although the patient has a history of rash to amoxicillin, the presentation is not consistent with an anaphylactic reaction. The aminopenicillins are frequently associated with rashes that are not allergic in nature. In this instance, cross-reactivity with a cephalosporin is unlikely.

Tetracyclines, Macrolides, Clindamycin, Chloramphenicol, Streptogramins, & Oxazolidinones

Daniel H. Deck, PharmD
& Lisa G. Winston, MD

CASE STUDY

A 19-year-old woman with no significant past medical history presents to her college medical clinic complaining of a 2-week history of foul-smelling vaginal discharge. She denies any fever or abdominal pain but does report vaginal bleeding after sexual intercourse. When questioned about her sexual activity, she reports having vaginal intercourse, at times unprotected, with two men in the last 6 months. A pelvic examination is performed and is positive for mucopurulent discharge from the endocervical canal. No cervical motion tenderness is present. A first-catch urine specimen is obtained to be tested for chlamydia and gonococcus. A pregnancy test is also ordered as the patient reports she "missed her last period." Pending these results, the decision is made to treat her empirically for gonococcal and chlamydial cervicitis. What are two potential treatment options for her possible chlamydial infection? How does her potential pregnancy affect the treatment decision?

The drugs described in this chapter inhibit bacterial protein synthesis by binding to and interfering with ribosomes. Most are bacteriostatic, but a few are bactericidal against certain organisms.

Because of overuse, tetracycline and macrolide resistance is common. Except for tigecycline and the streptogramins, these antibiotics are usually administered orally.

■ TETRACYCLINES

All of the tetracyclines have the basic structure shown below:

| | R₇ | R₆ | R₅ | Renal Clearance (mL/min) |

	R₇	**R₆**	**R₅**	**Renal Clearance (mL/min)**
Chlortetracycline	—Cl	—CH₃	—H	35
Oxytetracycline	—H	—CH₃	—OH	90
Tetracycline	—H	—CH3	—H	65
Demeclocycline	—Cl	—H	—H	35
Methacycline	—H	=CH₂*	—OH	31
Doxycycline	—H	—CH₃*	—OH	16
Minocycline	—N(CH₃)₂	—H	—H	10

*There is no — OH at position 6 on methacycline and doxycycline.

Free tetracyclines are crystalline amphoteric substances of low solubility. They are available as hydrochlorides, which are more soluble. Such solutions are acid and, with the exception of chlortetracycline, fairly stable. Tetracyclines chelate divalent metal ions, which can interfere with their absorption and activity. A newly approved tetracycline analog, tigecycline, is a glycylcycline and a semisynthetic derivative of minocycline.

Tigecycline

Mechanism of Action & Antimicrobial Activity

Tetracyclines are broad-spectrum bacteriostatic antibiotics that inhibit protein synthesis. Tetracyclines enter microorganisms in part by passive diffusion and in part by an energy-dependent process of active transport. Susceptible organisms concentrate the drug intracellularly. Once inside the cell, tetracyclines bind reversibly to the 30S subunit of the bacterial ribosome, blocking the binding of aminoacyl-tRNA to the acceptor site on the mRNA-ribosome complex (Figure 44–1). This prevents addition of amino acids to the growing peptide.

Tetracyclines are active against many gram-positive and gram-negative bacteria, including certain anaerobes, rickettsiae, chlamydiae, and mycoplasmas. The antibacterial activities of most tetracyclines are similar except that tetracycline-resistant strains may be susceptible to doxycycline, minocycline, and tigecycline, all of which are poor substrates for the efflux pump that mediates resistance. Differences in clinical efficacy for susceptible organisms are minor and attributable largely to features of absorption, distribution, and excretion of individual drugs.

Resistance

Three mechanisms of resistance to tetracycline analogs have been described: (1) impaired influx or increased efflux by an active transport protein pump; (2) ribosome protection due to production of proteins that interfere with tetracycline binding to the ribosome; and (3) enzymatic inactivation. The most important of these are production of an efflux pump and ribosomal protection. Tet(AE) efflux pump-expressing gram-negative species are resistant to the older tetracyclines, doxycycline, and minocycline. They are susceptible, however, to tigecycline, which is not a substrate of these pumps. Similarly, the Tet(K) efflux pump of staphylococci confers resistance to tetracycline, but not to doxycycline, minocycline, or tigecycline, none of which are pump substrates. The Tet(M) ribosomal protection protein expressed by gram-positives produces resistance to tetracycline, doxycycline, and minocycline, but not to tigecycline, which because of its bulky t-butylglycylamido substituent, has a steric hindrance effect on Tet(M) binding to the ribosome. Tigecycline is a substrate of the chromosomally encoded multidrug efflux pumps of *Proteus* sp and *Pseudomonas aeruginosa*, accounting for their intrinsic resistance to all tetracyclines including tigecycline.

Pharmacokinetics

Tetracyclines differ in their absorption after oral administration and in their elimination. Absorption after oral administration is approximately 30% for chlortetracycline; 60–70% for tetracycline, oxytetracycline, demeclocycline, and methacycline; and 95–100% for doxycycline and minocycline. Tigecycline is poorly absorbed orally and must be administered intravenously. A portion of an orally administered dose of tetracycline remains in the gut lumen, alters intestinal flora, and is excreted in the feces. Absorption occurs mainly in the upper small intestine and is impaired by food (except doxycycline and minocycline); by divalent cations (Ca²⁺, Mg²⁺, Fe²⁺) or Al³⁺; by dairy products and antacids, which contain multivalent cations; and by alkaline pH. Specially buffered tetracycline solutions are formulated for intravenous administration.

Tetracyclines are 40–80% bound by serum proteins. Oral dosages of 500 mg every 6 hours of tetracycline hydrochloride or oxytetracycline produce peak blood levels of 4–6 mcg/mL. Intravenously injected tetracyclines give somewhat higher levels, but only temporarily. Peak levels of 2–4 mcg/mL are achieved with a 200-mg dose of doxycycline or minocycline. Steady-state peak serum concentrations of tigecycline are 0.6 mcg/mL at the standard dosage. Tetracyclines are distributed widely to tissues and body fluids except for cerebrospinal fluid, where concentrations are 10–25% of those in serum. Minocycline reaches very high concentrations in tears and saliva, which makes it useful for eradication of the meningococcal carrier state. Tetracyclines cross the placenta to reach the fetus and are also excreted in milk. As a result of chelation with calcium, tetracyclines are bound to—and damage—growing bones and teeth. Carbamazepine, phenytoin, barbiturates, and chronic alcohol ingestion may shorten the half-life of doxycycline 50% by induction of hepatic enzymes that metabolize the drug.

Tetracyclines are excreted mainly in bile and urine. Concentrations in bile exceed those in serum tenfold. Some of the drug excreted in

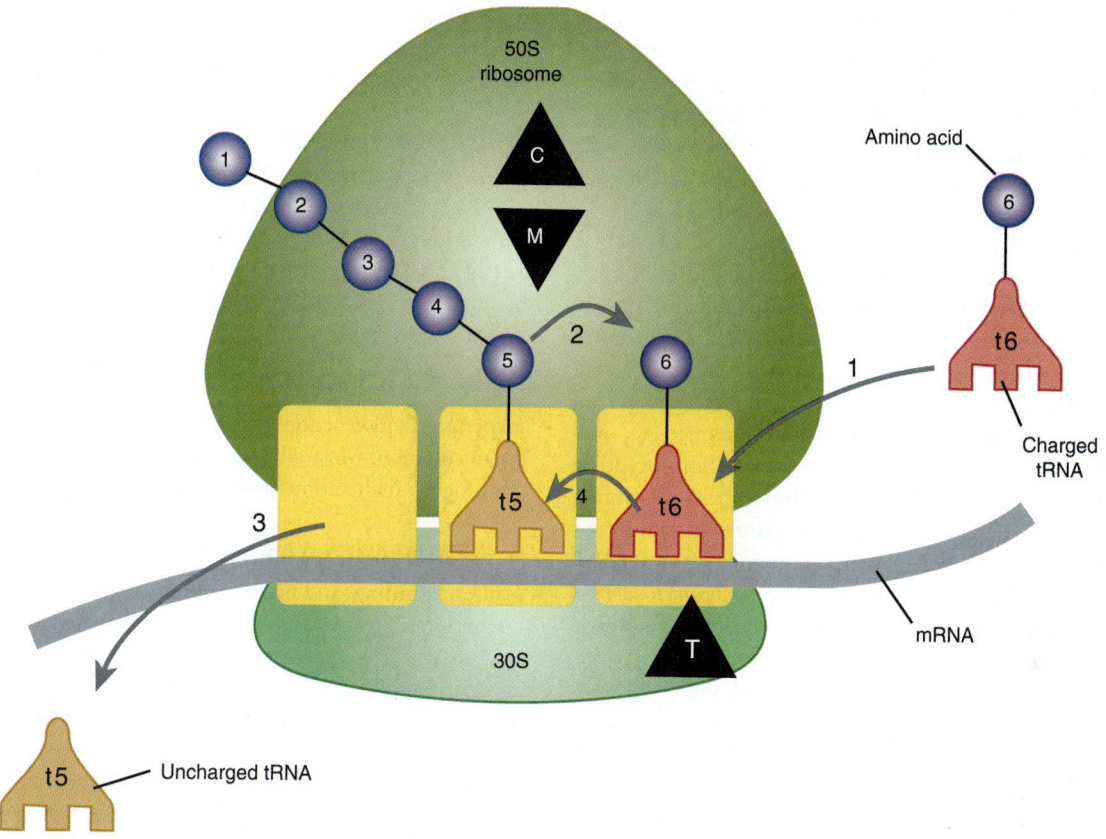

FIGURE 44–1 Steps in bacterial protein synthesis and targets of several antibiotics. Amino acids are shown as numbered circles. The 70S ribosomal mRNA complex is shown with its 50S and 30S subunits. In step 1, the charged tRNA unit carrying amino acid 6 binds to the acceptor site on the 70S ribosome. The peptidyl tRNA at the donor site, with amino acids 1 through 5, then binds the growing amino acid chain to amino acid 6 (peptide bond formation, step 2). The uncharged tRNA left at the donor site is released (step 3), and the new 6-amino acid chain with its tRNA shifts to the peptidyl site (translocation, step 4). The antibiotic binding sites are shown schematically as triangles. Chloramphenicol (C) and macrolides (M) bind to the 50S subunit and block peptide bond formation (step 2). The tetracyclines (T) bind to the 30S subunit and prevent binding of the incoming charged tRNA unit (step 1).

bile is reabsorbed from the intestine (enterohepatic circulation) and may contribute to maintenance of serum levels. Ten to fifty percent of various tetracyclines is excreted into the urine, mainly by glomerular filtration. Ten to forty percent of the drug is excreted in feces. Doxycycline and tigecycline, in contrast to other tetracyclines, are eliminated by nonrenal mechanisms, do not accumulate significantly, and require no dosage adjustment in renal failure.

Tetracyclines are classified as short-acting (chlortetracycline, tetracycline, oxytetracycline), intermediate-acting (demeclocycline and methacycline), or long-acting (doxycycline and minocycline) based on serum half-lives of 6–8 hours, 12 hours, and 16–18 hours, respectively. Tigecycline has a half-life of 36 hours. The almost complete absorption and slow excretion of doxycycline and minocycline allow for once-daily dosing for certain indications, but by convention these two drugs are usually dosed twice daily.

Clinical Uses

A tetracycline is the drug of choice in the treatment of infections caused by rickettsiae. Tetracyclines are also excellent drugs for the treatment of *Mycoplasma pneumonia*, chlamydiae, and some spirochetes. They are used in combination regimens to treat gastric and duodenal ulcer disease caused by *Helicobacter pylori*. They may be used in various gram-positive and gram-negative bacterial infections, including vibrio infections, provided the organism is not resistant. In cholera, tetracyclines rapidly stop the shedding of vibrios, but tetracycline resistance has appeared during epidemics. Tetracyclines remain effective in most chlamydial infections, including sexually transmitted infections. Tetracyclines are no longer recommended for treatment of gonococcal disease because of resistance. A tetracycline—in combination with other antibiotics—is indicated for plague, tularemia, and brucellosis. Tetracyclines are sometimes used in the treatment or prophylaxis of protozoal infections, eg, those due to *Plasmodium falciparum* (see Chapter 52). Other uses include treatment of acne, exacerbations of bronchitis, community-acquired pneumonia, Lyme disease, relapsing fever, leptospirosis, and some nontuberculous mycobacterial infections (eg, *Mycobacterium marinum*). Tetracyclines formerly were used for a variety of common infections, including bacterial gastroenteritis and urinary tract infections. However, many strains of bacteria causing these infections are now resistant, and other agents have largely supplanted tetracyclines.

Minocycline, 200 mg orally daily for 5 days, can eradicate the meningococcal carrier state, but because of side effects and resistance of many meningococcal strains, rifampin is preferred. **Demeclocycline** inhibits the action of antidiuretic hormone in the renal tubule and has been used in the treatment of inappropriate secretion of antidiuretic hormone or similar peptides by certain tumors (see Chapter 15).

Tigecycline, the first glycylcycline to reach clinical practice, has several unique features that warrant its consideration apart from the older tetracyclines. Many tetracycline-resistant strains are susceptible to tigecycline because the common resistance determinants have no activity against it. Its spectrum is very broad. Coagulase-negative staphylococci and *Staphylococcus aureus,* including methicillin-resistant, vancomycin-intermediate, and vancomycin-resistant strains; streptococci, penicillin-susceptible and resistant; enterococci, including vancomycin-resistant strains; gram-positive rods; Enterobacteriaceae; multidrug-resistant strains of *Acinetobacter* sp; anaerobes, both gram-positive and gram-negative; rickettsiae, *Chlamydia* sp, and *Legionella pneumophila;* and rapidly growing mycobacteria all are susceptible. *Proteus* sp and *P aeruginosa,* however, are intrinsically resistant.

Tigecycline, formulated for intravenous administration only, is given as a 100-mg loading dose, then 50 mg every 12 hours. As with all tetracyclines, tissue and intracellular penetration is excellent; consequently, the volume of distribution is quite large and peak serum concentrations are low. Elimination is primarily biliary, and no dosage adjustment is needed for patients with renal insufficiency. In addition to the tetracycline class effects, the chief adverse effect of tigecycline is nausea, which occurs in up to one third of patients, and occasionally vomiting. Neither nausea nor vomiting usually requires discontinuation of the drug.

Tigecycline is Food and Drug Administration (FDA)-approved for treatment of skin and skin-structure infection, intra-abdominal infections, and community-acquired pneumonia. Because active drug concentrations in the urine are relatively low, tigecycline may not be effective for urinary tract infections and has no indication for this use. Because it is active against a wide variety of multidrug-resistant nosocomial pathogens (eg, methicillin-resistant *S aureus,* extended-spectrum β-lactamase-producing gram-negatives, and *Acinetobacter* sp, tigecycline is a welcome addition to the antimicrobial drug group. However, its clinical efficacy in infections with multidrug-resistant organisms, compared with other agents, is largely unknown.

A. Oral Dosage

The oral dosage for rapidly excreted tetracyclines, equivalent to tetracycline hydrochloride, is 0.25–0.5 g four times daily for adults and 20–40 mg/kg/d for children (8 years of age and older). For severe systemic infections, the higher dosage is indicated, at least for the first few days. The daily dose is 600 mg for demeclocycline or methacycline, 100 mg once or twice daily for doxycycline, and 100 mg twice daily for minocycline. Doxycycline is the oral tetracycline of choice because it can be given twice daily, and its absorption is not significantly affected by food. All tetracyclines chelate with metals, and none should be orally administered with milk, antacids, or ferrous sulfate. To avoid deposition in growing bones or teeth, tetracyclines should be avoided in pregnant women and children younger than 8 years.

B. Parenteral Dosage

Several tetracyclines are available for intravenous injection in doses of 0.1–0.5 g every 6–12 hours (similar to oral doses) but doxycycline is the usual preferred agent, at a dosage of 100 mg every 12–24 hours. Intramuscular injection is not recommended because of pain and inflammation at the injection site.

Adverse Reactions

Hypersensitivity reactions (drug fever, skin rashes) to tetracyclines are uncommon. Most adverse effects are due to direct toxicity of the drug or to alteration of microbial flora.

A. Gastrointestinal Adverse Effects

Nausea, vomiting, and diarrhea are the most common reasons for discontinuing tetracycline medication. These effects are attributable to direct local irritation of the intestinal tract. Nausea, anorexia, and diarrhea can usually be controlled by administering the drug with food or carboxymethylcellulose, reducing drug dosage, or discontinuing the drug.

Tetracyclines alter the normal gastrointestinal flora, with suppression of susceptible coliform organisms and overgrowth of pseudomonas, proteus, staphylococci, resistant coliforms, clostridia, and candida. This can result in intestinal functional disturbances, anal pruritus, vaginal or oral candidiasis, or *Clostridium difficile*-associated colitis.

B. Bony Structures and Teeth

Tetracyclines are readily bound to calcium deposited in newly formed bone or teeth in young children. When a tetracycline is given during pregnancy, it can be deposited in the fetal teeth, leading to fluorescence, discoloration, and enamel dysplasia; it can also be deposited in bone, where it may cause deformity or growth inhibition. Because of these effects, tetracyclines are generally avoided in pregnancy. If the drug is given for long periods to children younger than 8 years, similar changes can result.

C. Other Toxicities

Tetracyclines can impair hepatic function, especially during pregnancy, in patients with preexisting hepatic insufficiency and when high doses are given intravenously. Hepatic necrosis has been reported with daily doses of 4 g or more intravenously.

Renal tubular acidosis and other renal injury resulting in nitrogen retention have been attributed to the administration of outdated tetracycline preparations. Tetracyclines given along with diuretics may produce nitrogen retention. Tetracyclines other than doxycycline may accumulate to toxic levels in patients with impaired kidney function.

Intravenous injection can lead to venous thrombosis. Intramuscular injection produces painful local irritation and should be avoided.

Systemically administered tetracycline, especially demeclocycline, can induce sensitivity to sunlight or ultraviolet light, particularly in fair-skinned persons.

Dizziness, vertigo, nausea, and vomiting have been noted particularly with doxycycline at doses above 100 mg. With dosages of 200–400 mg/d of minocycline, 35–70% of patients will have these reactions.

■ MACROLIDES

The macrolides are a group of closely related compounds characterized by a macrocyclic lactone ring (usually containing 14 or 16 atoms) to which deoxy sugars are attached. The prototype drug, erythromycin, which consists of two sugar moieties attached to a 14-atom lactone ring, was obtained in 1952 from *Streptomyces erytheus*. Clarithromycin and azithromycin are semisynthetic derivatives of erythromycin.

Erythromycin ($R_1 = CH_3$, $R_2 = H$)
Clarithromycin ($R_1, R_2 = CH_3$)

ERYTHROMYCIN

Chemistry

The general structure of erythromycin is shown with the macrolide ring and the sugars desosamine and cladinose. It is poorly soluble in water (0.1%) but dissolves readily in organic solvents. Solutions are fairly stable at 4°C but lose activity rapidly at 20°C and at acid pH. Erythromycins are usually dispensed as various esters and salts.

Mechanism of Action & Antimicrobial Activity

The antibacterial action of erythromycin and other macrolides may be inhibitory or bactericidal, particularly at higher concentrations, for susceptible organisms. Activity is enhanced at alkaline pH. Inhibition of protein synthesis occurs via binding to the 50S ribosomal RNA. The binding site is near the peptidyltransferase center, and peptide chain elongation (ie, transpeptidation) is prevented by blocking of the polypeptide exit tunnel. As a result, peptidyl-tRNA is dissociated from the ribosome. Erythromycin also inhibits the formation of the 50S ribosomal subunit (Figure 44–1).

Erythromycin is active against susceptible strains of gram-positive organisms, especially pneumococci, streptococci, staphylococci, and corynebacteria. *Mycoplasma pneumoniae, L pneumophila, Chlamydia trachomatis, Chlamydia psittaci, Chlamydia pneumoniae, H pylori, Listeria monocytogenes,* and certain mycobacteria *(Mycobacterium kansasii, Mycobacterium scrofulaceum)* are also susceptible. Gram-negative organisms such as *Neisseria* sp, *Bordetella pertussis, Bartonella henselae,* and *Bartonella quintana* as well as some *Rickettsia* species, *Treponema pallidum,* and *Campylobacter* species are susceptible. *Haemophilus influenzae* is somewhat less susceptible.

Resistance to erythromycin is usually plasmid-encoded. Three mechanisms have been identified: (1) reduced permeability of the cell membrane or active efflux; (2) production (by Enterobacteriaceae) of esterases that hydrolyze macrolides; and (3) modification of the ribosomal binding site (so-called ribosomal protection) by chromosomal mutation or by a macrolide-inducible or constitutive methylase. Efflux and methylase production are the most important resistance mechanisms in gram-positive organisms. Cross-resistance is complete between erythromycin and the other macrolides. Constitutive methylase production also confers resistance to structurally unrelated but mechanistically similar compounds such as clindamycin and streptogramin B (so-called macrolide-lincosamide-streptogramin, or MLS-type B, resistance), which share the same ribosomal binding site. Because nonmacrolides are poor inducers of the methylase, strains expressing an inducible methylase will appear susceptible in vitro. However, constitutive mutants that are resistant can be selected out and emerge during therapy with clindamycin.

Pharmacokinetics

Erythromycin base is destroyed by stomach acid and must be administered with enteric coating. Food interferes with absorption. Stearates and esters are fairly acid-resistant and somewhat better absorbed. The lauryl salt of the propionyl ester of erythromycin (erythromycin estolate) is the best-absorbed oral preparation. Oral dosage of 2 g/d results in serum erythromycin base and ester concentrations of approximately 2 mcg/mL. However, only the base is microbiologically active, and its concentration tends to be similar regardless of the formulation. A 500-mg intravenous dose of erythromycin lactobionate produces serum concentrations of 10 mcg/mL 1 hour after dosing. The serum half-life is approximately 1.5 hours normally and 5 hours in patients with anuria. Adjustment for renal failure is not necessary. Erythromycin is not removed by dialysis. Large amounts of an administered dose are excreted in the bile and lost in feces, and only 5% is excreted in the urine. Absorbed drug is distributed widely except to the brain and cerebrospinal fluid. Erythromycin is taken up by polymorphonuclear leukocytes and macrophages. It traverses the placenta and reaches the fetus.

Clinical Uses

Erythromycin is a drug of choice in corynebacterial infections (diphtheria, corynebacterial sepsis, erythrasma); in respiratory, neonatal, ocular, or genital chlamydial infections; and in treatment of community-acquired pneumonia because its spectrum of activity includes pneumococcus, *M pneumoniae*, and *L pneumophila*. Erythromycin is also useful as a penicillin substitute in penicillin-allergic individuals with infections caused by staphylococci (assuming that the isolate is susceptible), streptococci, or pneumococci. Emergence of erythromycin resistance in strains of group A streptococci and pneumococci (penicillin-non-susceptible pneumococci in particular) has made macrolides less attractive as first-line agents for treatment of pharyngitis, skin and soft tissue infections, and pneumonia. Erythromycin has been recommended as prophylaxis against endocarditis during dental procedures in individuals with valvular heart disease, although clindamycin, which is better tolerated, has largely replaced it. Although erythromycin estolate is the best-absorbed salt, it imposes the greatest risk of adverse reactions. Therefore, the stearate or succinate salt may be preferred.

The oral dosage of erythromycin base, stearate, or estolate is 0.25–0.5 g every 6 hours (for children, 40 mg/kg/d). The dosage of erythromycin ethylsuccinate is 0.4–0.6 g every 6 hours. Oral erythromycin base (1 g) is sometimes combined with oral neomycin or kanamycin for preoperative preparation of the colon. The intravenous dosage of erythromycin gluceptate or lactobionate is 0.5–1.0 g every 6 hours for adults and 20–40 mg/kg/d for children. The higher dosage is recommended when treating pneumonia caused by *L pneumophila*.

Adverse Reactions

Anorexia, nausea, vomiting, and diarrhea are common. Gastrointestinal intolerance, which is due to a direct stimulation of gut motility, is the most common reason for discontinuing erythromycin and substituting another antibiotic.

Erythromycins, particularly the estolate, can produce acute cholestatic hepatitis (fever, jaundice, impaired liver function), probably as a hypersensitivity reaction. Most patients recover from this, but hepatitis recurs if the drug is readministered. Other allergic reactions include fever, eosinophilia, and rashes.

Erythromycin metabolites inhibit cytochrome P450 enzymes and, thus, increase the serum concentrations of numerous drugs, including theophylline, warfarin, cyclosporine, and methylprednisolone. Erythromycin increases serum concentrations of oral digoxin by increasing its bioavailability.

CLARITHROMYCIN

Clarithromycin is derived from erythromycin by addition of a methyl group and has improved acid stability and oral absorption compared with erythromycin. Its mechanism of action is the same as that of erythromycin. Clarithromycin and erythromycin are similar with respect to antibacterial activity except that clarithromycin is more active against *Mycobacterium avium* complex (see Chapter 47). Clarithromycin also has activity against *Mycobacterium leprae, Toxoplasma gondii,* and *H influenzae*. Erythromycin-resistant streptococci and staphylococci are also resistant to clarithromycin.

A 500-mg dose of clarithromycin produces serum concentrations of 2–3 mcg/mL. The longer half-life of clarithromycin (6 hours) compared with erythromycin permits twice-daily dosing. The recommended dosage is 250–500 mg twice daily or 1000 mg of the extended-release formulation once daily. Clarithromycin penetrates most tissues well, with concentrations equal to or exceeding serum concentrations.

Clarithromycin is metabolized in the liver. The major metabolite is 14-hydroxyclarithromycin, which also has antibacterial activity. Portions of active drug and this major metabolite are eliminated in the urine, and dosage reduction (eg, a 500-mg loading dose, then 250 mg once or twice daily) is recommended for patients with creatinine clearances less than 30 mL/min. Clarithromycin has drug interactions similar to those described for erythromycin.

The advantages of clarithromycin compared with erythromycin are lower incidence of gastrointestinal intolerance and less frequent dosing.

AZITHROMYCIN

Azithromycin, a 15-atom lactone macrolide ring compound, is derived from erythromycin by addition of a methylated nitrogen into the lactone ring. Its spectrum of activity, mechanism of action, and clinical uses are similar to those of clarithromycin. Azithromycin is active against *M avium* complex and *T gondii*. Azithromycin is slightly less active than erythromycin and clarithromycin against staphylococci and streptococci and slightly more active against *H influenzae*. Azithromycin is highly active against *Chlamydia* sp.

Azithromycin differs from erythromycin and clarithromycin mainly in pharmacokinetic properties. A 500-mg dose of azithromycin produces relatively low serum concentrations of approximately 0.4 mcg/mL. However, azithromycin penetrates into most tissues (except cerebrospinal fluid) and phagocytic cells extremely well, with tissue concentrations exceeding serum concentrations by 10- to 100-fold. The drug is slowly released from tissues (tissue half-life of 2–4 days) to produce an elimination half-life approaching 3 days. These unique properties permit once-daily dosing and shortening of the duration of treatment in many cases. For example, a single 1-g dose of azithromycin is as effective as a 7-day course of doxycycline for chlamydial cervicitis and urethritis. Community-acquired pneumonia can be treated with azithromycin given as a 500-mg loading dose, followed by a 250-mg single daily dose for the next 4 days.

Azithromycin is rapidly absorbed and well tolerated orally. It should be administered 1 hour before or 2 hours after meals. Aluminum and magnesium antacids do not alter bioavailability but delay absorption and reduce peak serum concentrations. Because it has a 15-member (not 14-member) lactone ring, azithromycin does not inactivate cytochrome P450 enzymes and, therefore, is free of the drug interactions that occur with erythromycin and clarithromycin.

KETOLIDES

Ketolides are semisynthetic 14-membered-ring macrolides, differing from erythromycin by substitution of a 3-keto group for the neutral sugar l-cladinose. **Telithromycin** is approved for limited clinical use. It is active in vitro against *Streptococcus pyogenes*, *S pneumoniae*, *S aureus*, *H influenzae*, *Moraxella catarrhalis*, *Mycoplasma* sp, *L pneumophila*, *Chlamydia* sp, *H pylori*, *Neisseria gonorrhoeae*, *B fragilis*, *T gondii*, and certain nontuberculosis mycobacteria. Many macrolide-resistant strains are susceptible to ketolides because the structural modification of these compounds renders them poor substrates for efflux pump-mediated resistance, and they bind to ribosomes of some bacterial species with higher affinity than macrolides.

Oral bioavailability of telithromycin is 57%, and tissue and intracellular penetration is generally good. Telithromycin is metabolized in the liver and eliminated by a combination of biliary and urinary routes of excretion. It is administered as a once-daily dose of 800 mg, which results in peak serum concentrations of approximately 2 mcg/mL. It is a reversible inhibitor of the CYP3A4 enzyme system and may slightly prolong the QT_c interval. In the USA, telithromycin is now indicated only for treatment of community-acquired bacterial pneumonia. Other respiratory tract infections were removed as indications when it was recognized that use of telithromycin can result in hepatitis and liver failure.

■ CLINDAMYCIN

Clindamycin is a chlorine-substituted derivative of **lincomycin**, an antibiotic that is elaborated by *Streptomyces lincolnensis*.

Clindamycin

Mechanism of Action & Antibacterial Activity

Clindamycin, like erythromycin, inhibits protein synthesis by interfering with the formation of initiation complexes and with aminoacyl translocation reactions. The binding site for clindamycin on the 50S subunit of the bacterial ribosome is identical with that for erythromycin. Streptococci, staphylococci, and pneumococci are inhibited by clindamycin, 0.5–5 mcg/mL. Enterococci and gram-negative aerobic organisms are resistant. *Bacteroides* sp and other anaerobes, both gram-positive and gram-negative, are usually susceptible. Resistance to clindamycin, which generally confers cross-resistance to macrolides, is due to (1) mutation of the ribosomal receptor site; (2) modification of the receptor by a constitutively expressed methylase (see section on erythromycin resistance, above); and (3) enzymatic inactivation of clindamycin. Gram-negative aerobic species are intrinsically resistant because of poor permeability of the outer membrane.

Pharmacokinetics

Oral dosages of clindamycin, 0.15–0.3 g every 8 hours (10–20 mg/kg/d for children), yield serum levels of 2–3 mcg/mL. When administered intravenously, 600 mg of clindamycin every 8 hours gives levels of 5–15 mcg/mL. The drug is about 90% protein-bound. Clindamycin penetrates well into most tissues, with brain and cerebrospinal fluid being important exceptions. It penetrates well into abscesses and is actively taken up and concentrated by phagocytic cells. Clindamycin is metabolized by the liver, and both active drug and active metabolites are excreted in bile and urine. The half-life is about 2.5 hours in normal individuals, increasing to 6 hours in patients with anuria. No dosage adjustment is required for renal failure.

Clinical Uses

Clindamycin is indicated for the treatment of skin and soft-tissue infections caused by streptococci and staphylococci. It is often active against community-acquired strains of methicillin-resistant *S aureus*, an increasingly common cause of skin and soft tissue infections. Clindamycin is also indicated for treatment of anaerobic infections caused by *Bacteroides* sp and other anaerobes that often participate in mixed infections. Clindamycin, sometimes in combination with an aminoglycoside or cephalosporin, is used to treat penetrating wounds of the abdomen and the gut; infections originating in the female genital tract, eg, septic abortion, pelvic abscesses, or pelvic inflammatory disease; and lung abscesses. Clindamycin is now recommended rather than erythromycin for prophylaxis of endocarditis in patients with valvular heart disease who are undergoing certain dental procedures and have significant penicillin allergies. Clindamycin plus primaquine is an effective alternative to trimethoprim-sulfamethoxazole for moderate to moderately severe *Pneumocystis jiroveci* pneumonia in AIDS patients. It is also used in combination with pyrimethamine for AIDS-related toxoplasmosis of the brain.

Adverse Effects

Common adverse effects are diarrhea, nausea, and skin rashes. Impaired liver function (with or without jaundice) and neutropenia sometimes occur. Administration of clindamycin is a risk factor for diarrhea and colitis due to *C difficile*.

■ STREPTOGRAMINS

Mechanism of Action & Antibacterial Activity

Quinupristin-dalfopristin is a combination of two streptogramins—quinupristin, a streptogramin B, and dalfopristin, a streptogramin A—in a 30:70 ratio. The streptogramins share the same ribosomal binding site as the macrolides and clindamycin and thus inhibit protein synthesis in an identical manner. It is rapidly bactericidal for most susceptible organisms except *Enterococcus faecium*, which is killed slowly. Quinupristin-dalfopristin is active against gram-positive cocci, including multidrug-resistant strains of streptococci, penicillin-resistant strains of *S pneumoniae*, methicillin-susceptible and -resistant strains of staphylococci, and *E faecium* (but not *Enterococcus faecalis*). Resistance is due to modification of the quinupristin binding site (MLS-B type resistance), enzymatic inactivation of dalfopristin, or efflux.

Pharmacokinetics

Quinupristin-dalfopristin is administered intravenously at a dosage of 7.5 mg/kg every 8–12 hours. Peak serum concentrations following an infusion of 7.5 mg/kg over 60 minutes are 3 mcg/mL for quinupristin and 7 mcg/mL for dalfopristin. Quinupristin and dalfopristin are rapidly metabolized, with half-lives of 0.85 and 0.7 hours, respectively. Elimination is principally by the fecal route. Dose adjustment is not necessary for renal failure, peritoneal dialysis, or hemodialysis. Patients with hepatic insufficiency may not tolerate the drug at usual doses, however, because of increased area under the concentration curve of both parent drugs and metabolites. This may necessitate a dose reduction to 7.5 mg/kg every 12 hours or 5 mg/kg every 8 hours. Quinupristin and dalfopristin significantly inhibit CYP3A4, which metabolizes warfarin, diazepam, astemizole, terfenadine, cisapride, nonnucleoside reverse transcriptase inhibitors, and cyclosporine, among others. Dosage reduction of cyclosporine may be necessary.

Clinical Uses & Adverse Effects

Quinupristin-dalfopristin is approved for treatment of infections caused by staphylococci or by vancomycin-resistant strains of *E faecium*, but not *E faecalis*, which is intrinsically resistant, probably because of an efflux-type resistance mechanism. The principal toxicities are infusion-related events, such as pain at the infusion site, and an arthralgia-myalgia syndrome.

■ CHLORAMPHENICOL

Crystalline chloramphenicol is a neutral, stable compound with the following structure:

Chloramphenicol

It is soluble in alcohol but poorly soluble in water. Chloramphenicol succinate, which is used for parenteral administration, is highly water-soluble. It is hydrolyzed in vivo with liberation of free chloramphenicol.

Mechanism of Action & Antimicrobial Activity

Chloramphenicol is a potent inhibitor of microbial protein synthesis. It binds reversibly to the 50S subunit of the bacterial ribosome

(Figure 44–1) and inhibits peptide bond formation (step 2). Chloramphenicol is a bacteriostatic broad-spectrum antibiotic that is active against both aerobic and anaerobic gram-positive and gram-negative organisms. It is active also against *Rickettsiae* but not *Chlamydiae*. Most gram-positive bacteria are inhibited at concentrations of 1–10 mcg/mL, and many gram-negative bacteria are inhibited by concentrations of 0.2–5 mcg/mL. *H influenzae, Neisseria meningitidis*, and some strains of bacteroides are highly susceptible, and for these organisms, chloramphenicol may be bactericidal.

Low-level resistance to chloramphenicol may emerge from large populations of chloramphenicol-susceptible cells by selection of mutants that are less permeable to the drug. Clinically significant resistance is due to production of chloramphenicol acetyltransferase, a plasmid-encoded enzyme that inactivates the drug.

Pharmacokinetics

The usual dosage of chloramphenicol is 50–100 mg/kg/d. After oral administration, crystalline chloramphenicol is rapidly and completely absorbed. A 1-g oral dose produces blood levels between 10 and 15 mcg/mL. Chloramphenicol palmitate is a prodrug that is hydrolyzed in the intestine to yield free chloramphenicol. The parenteral formulation is a prodrug, chloramphenicol succinate, which hydrolyzes to yield free chloramphenicol, giving blood levels somewhat lower than those achieved with orally administered drug. Chloramphenicol is widely distributed to virtually all tissues and body fluids, including the central nervous system and cerebrospinal fluid, such that the concentration of chloramphenicol in brain tissue may be equal to that in serum. The drug penetrates cell membranes readily.

Most of the drug is inactivated either by conjugation with glucuronic acid (principally in the liver) or by reduction to inactive aryl amines. Active chloramphenicol (about 10% of the total dose administered) and its inactive degradation products (about 90% of the total) are eliminated in the urine. A small amount of active drug is excreted into bile and feces. The systemic dosage of chloramphenicol need not be altered in renal insufficiency, but it must be reduced markedly in hepatic failure. Newborns less than a week old and premature infants also clear chloramphenicol less well, and the dosage should be reduced to 25 mg/kg/d.

Clinical Uses

Because of potential toxicity, bacterial resistance, and the availability of many other effective alternatives, chloramphenicol is rarely used in the United States. It may be considered for treatment of serious rickettsial infections such as typhus and Rocky Mountain spotted fever. It is an alternative to a β-lactam antibiotic for treatment of bacterial meningitis occurring in patients who have major hypersensitivity reactions to penicillin. The dosage is 50–100 mg/kg/d in four divided doses.

Chloramphenicol is used topically in the treatment of eye infections because of its broad spectrum and its penetration of ocular tissues and the aqueous humor. It is ineffective for chlamydial infections.

Adverse Reactions

Adults occasionally develop gastrointestinal disturbances, including nausea, vomiting, and diarrhea. This is rare in children. Oral or vaginal candidiasis may occur as a result of alteration of normal microbial flora.

Chloramphenicol commonly causes a dose-related reversible suppression of red cell production at dosages exceeding 50 mg/kg/d after 1–2 weeks. Aplastic anemia, a rare consequence (1 in 24,000 to 40,000 courses of therapy) of chloramphenicol administration by any route, is an idiosyncratic reaction unrelated to dose, although it occurs more frequently with prolonged use. It tends to be irreversible and can be fatal.

Newborn infants lack an effective glucuronic acid conjugation mechanism for the degradation and detoxification of chloramphenicol. Consequently, when infants are given dosages above 50 mg/kg/d, the drug may accumulate, resulting in the **gray baby syndrome,** with vomiting, flaccidity, hypothermia, gray color, shock, and vascular collapse. To avoid this toxic effect, chloramphenicol should be used with caution in infants and the dosage limited to 50 mg/kg/d (or less during the first week of life) in full-term infants more than 1 week old and 25 mg/kg/d in premature infants.

Chloramphenicol inhibits hepatic microsomal enzymes that metabolize several drugs. Half-lives of these drugs are prolonged, and the serum concentrations of phenytoin, tolbutamide, chlorpropamide, and warfarin are increased. Like other bacteriostatic inhibitors of microbial protein synthesis, chloramphenicol can antagonize bactericidal drugs such as penicillins or aminoglycosides.

■ OXAZOLIDINONES

Mechanism of Action & Antimicrobial Activity

Linezolid is a member of the oxazolidinones, a new class of synthetic antimicrobials. It is active against gram-positive organisms including staphylococci, streptococci, enterococci, gram-positive anaerobic cocci, and gram-positive rods such as corynebacteria, *Nocardia* sp, and *L monocytogenes*. It is primarily a bacteriostatic agent but is bactericidal against streptococci. It is also active against *Mycobacterium tuberculosis*.

Linezolid inhibits protein synthesis by preventing formation of the ribosome complex that initiates protein synthesis. Its unique binding site, located on 23S ribosomal RNA of the 50S subunit, results in no cross-resistance with other drug classes. Resistance is caused by mutation of the linezolid binding site on 23S ribosomal RNA.

Pharmacokinetics

Linezolid is 100% bioavailable after oral administration and has a half-life of 4–6 hours. It is metabolized by oxidative metabolism, yielding two inactive metabolites. It is neither an inducer nor an inhibitor of cytochrome P450 enzymes. Peak serum concentrations average 18 mcg/mL following a 600-mg oral dose. The recommended dosage for most indications is 600 mg twice daily, either orally or intravenously.

Clinical Uses

Linezolid is approved for vancomycin-resistant *E faecium* infections; nosocomial pneumonia; community-acquired pneumonia; and both complicated and uncomplicated skin and soft tissue infections caused by susceptible gram-positive bacteria. Off-label uses of linezolid include treatment of multidrug-resistant tuberculosis and *Nocardia* infections.

Adverse Effects

The principal toxicity of linezolid is hematologic; the effects are reversible and generally mild. Thrombocytopenia is the most common manifestation (seen in approximately 3% of treatment courses), particularly when the drug is administered for longer than 2 weeks. Anemia and neutropenia may also occur, most commonly in patients with a predisposition to or underlying bone marrow suppression. Cases of optic and peripheral neuropathy and lactic acidosis have been reported with prolonged courses of linezolid. These side effects are thought to be related to linezolid-induced inhibition of mitochondrial protein synthesis. There are case reports of serotonin syndrome occurring when linezolid is co-administered with serotonergic drugs, most frequently selective serotonin reuptake inhibitor antidepressants. The FDA issued a warning regarding the use of the drug with serotonergic agents in 2011.

SUMMARY Tetracyclines, Macrolides, Clindamycin, Chloramphenicol, Streptogramins, & Oxazolidinones

Subclass	Mechanism of Action	Effects	Clinical Applications	Pharmacokinetics, Toxicities, Interactions
TETRACYCLINES				
• Tetracycline	Prevents bacterial protein synthesis by binding to the 30S ribosomal subunit	Bacteriostatic activity against susceptible bacteria	Infections caused by mycoplasma, chlamydiae, rickettsiae, some spirochetes • malaria • *H pylori* • acne	Oral • mixed clearance (half-life 8 h) • dosed every 6 h • divalent cations impair oral absorption • *Toxicity:* Gastrointestinal upset, hepatotoxicity, photosensitivity, deposition in bone and teeth

- *Doxycycline: Oral and IV; longer half-life (18 h) so dosed twice daily; nonrenal elimination; absorption is minimally affected by divalent cations; used to treat community-acquired pneumonia and exacerbations of bronchitis*
- *Minocycline: Oral; longer half-life (16 h) so dosed twice daily; frequently causes reversible vestibular toxicity*
- *Tigecycline: IV; unaffected by common tetracycline resistance mechanisms; very broad spectrum of activity against gram-positive, gram-negative, and anaerobic bacteria; nausea and vomiting are the primary toxicities*

Subclass	Mechanism of Action	Effects	Clinical Applications	Pharmacokinetics, Toxicities, Interactions
MACROLIDES				
• Erythromycin	Prevents bacterial protein synthesis by binding to the 50S ribosomal subunit	Bacteriostatic activity against susceptible bacteria	Community-acquired pneumonia • pertussis • corynebacterial and chlamydial infections	Oral, IV • hepatic clearance (half-life 1.5 h) • dosed every 6 h • cytochrome P450 inhibitor • *Toxicity:* Gastrointestinal upset, hepatotoxicity, QT_c prolongation

- *Clarithromycin: Oral; longer half-life (4 h) so dosed twice daily; added activity versus M avium complex, toxoplasma, and M leprae*
- *Azithromycin: Oral, IV; very long half-life (68 h) allows for once-daily dosing and 5-day course of therapy of community-acquired pneumonia; does not inhibit cytochrome P450 enzymes*
- *Telithromycin: Oral; unaffected by efflux-mediated resistance so is active versus many erythromycin-resistant strains of pneumococci; rare cases of fulminant hepatic failure*

Subclass	Mechanism of Action	Effects	Clinical Applications	Pharmacokinetics, Toxicities, Interactions
LINCOSAMIDE				
• Clindamycin	Prevents bacterial protein synthesis by binding to the 50S ribosomal subunit	Bacteriostatic activity against susceptible bacteria	Skin and soft tissue infections • anaerobic infections	Oral, IV • hepatic clearance (half-life 2.5 h) • dosed every 6–8 hours • *Toxicity:* Gastrointestinal upset, *C difficile* colitis
STREPTOGRAMINS				
• Quinupristin-dalfopristin	Prevents bacterial protein synthesis by binding to the 50S ribosomal subunit	Rapid bactericidal activity against most susceptible bacteria	Infections caused by staphylococci or vancomycin-resistant strains of *E faecium*	IV • hepatic clearance • dosed every 8–12 h • cytochrome P450 inhibitor • *Toxicity:* Severe infusion-related myalgias and arthralgias
CHLORAMPHENICOL	Prevents bacterial protein synthesis by binding to the 50S ribosomal subunit	Bacteriostatic activity against susceptible bacteria	Use is rare in the developed world because of serious toxicities	Oral, IV • hepatic clearance (half-life 2.5 h) • dosage is 50–100 mg/kg/d in four divided doses • *Toxicity:* Dose-related anemia, idiosyncratic aplastic anemia, gray baby syndrome
OXAZOLIDINONES				
• Linezolid	Prevents bacterial protein synthesis by binding to the 23S ribosomal RNA of 50S subunit	Bacteriostatic activity against susceptible bacteria	Infections caused by methicillin-resistant staphylococci and vancomycin-resistant enterococci	Oral, IV • hepatic clearance (half-life 6 h) • dosed twice-daily • *Toxicity:* Duration-dependent bone marrow suppression, neuropathy, and optic neuritis • serotonin syndrome may occur when coadministered with other serotonergic drugs (eg, selective serotonin reuptake inhibitors)

PREPARATIONS AVAILABLE

CHLORAMPHENICOL

Chloramphenicol (generic, Chloromycetin)
Parenteral: 100 mg powder to reconstitute for injection

TETRACYCLINES

Demeclocycline (Declomycin)
Oral: 150, 300 mg tablets

Doxycycline (generic, Vibramycin, others)
Oral: 20, 50, 75, 100 mg tablets and capsules; powder to reconstitute for 25 mg/5 mL suspension; 50 mg/5 mL syrup
Parenteral: 100, 200 mg powder to reconstitute for injection

Minocycline (generic, Minocin, various)
Oral: 20, 50, 75, 100 mg tablets and capsules; 50 mg/5 mL suspension

Tetracycline (generic, others)
Oral: 250, 500 mg capsules; 125 mg/5 mL suspension

Tigecycline (Tygacil)
Parenteral: 50 mg powder to reconstitute for IV administration

MACROLIDES

Azithromycin (Zithromax)
Oral: 250, 500, 600 mg capsules; powder for 100, 200 mg/5 mL oral suspension
Parenteral: 500 mg powder for injection

Clarithromycin (generic, Biaxin)
Oral: 250, 500 mg tablets, 500, 1000 mg extended-release tablets; granules for 125, 250 mg/5 mL oral suspension

Erythromycin (generic, others)
Oral (base): 250, 333, 500 mg enteric-coated tablets
Oral (base) delayed-release: 250 mg capsules, 500 mg tablets
Oral (estolate): 125, 250 mg/5 mL suspension
Oral (ethylsuccinate): 400 mg tablets; 200, 400 mg/5 mL suspension
Oral (stearate): 250, 500 mg film-coated tablets
Parenteral: lactobionate, 0.5, 1 g powder to reconstitute for IV injection

KETOLIDES

Telithromycin (Ketek)
Oral: 300, 400 mg tablets

LINCOMYCIN

Clindamycin (generic, Cleocin)
Oral: 75, 150, 300 mg capsules; 75 mg/5 mL granules to reconstitute for solution
Parenteral: 150 mg/mL in 2, 4, 6, 60 mL vials for injection

STREPTOGRAMINS

Quinupristin and dalfopristin (Synercid)
Parenteral: 30:70 formulation in 500 mg vial for reconstitution for IV injection

OXAZOLIDINONE

Linezolid (Zyvox)
Oral: 600 mg tablets; 100 mg powder for 5 mL suspension
Parenteral: 2 mg/mL for IV infusion

REFERENCES

De Vriese AS et al: Linezolid-induced inhibition of mitochondrial protein synthesis. Clin Infect Dis 2006;42:1111.

Fortun J et al: Linezolid for the treatment of multidrug-resistant tuberculosis. J Antimicrob Chemother 2005;56:180.

Gee T et al: Pharmacokinetics and tissue penetration of linezolid following multiple oral doses. Antimicrob Agents Chemother 2001;45:1843.

Hancock RE: Mechanisms of action of newer antibiotics for gram-positive pathogens. Lancet Infect Dis 2005;5:209.

Lawrence KR et al: Serotonin toxicity associated with the use of linezolid: A review of postmarketing data. Clin Infect Dis 2006;42:1578.

Livermore DM. Tigecycline: What is it, and where should it be used? J Antimicrob Chemother 2005;56:611.

Moran GJ et al: Methicillin-resistant *S aureus* infections among patients in the emergency department. N Engl J Med 2006;355:666.

Noskin GA: Tigecycline: A new glycylcycline for treatment of serious infections. Clin Infect Dis 2005;41(Suppl 5):S303.

Schlossberg D: Azithromycin and clarithromycin. Med Clin North Am 1995;79:803.

Speer BS, Shoemaker MB, Salyers AA: Bacterial resistance to tetracycline: Mechanism, transfer, and clinical significance. Clin Microbiol Rev 1992;5:387.

Zhanel GG et al: The ketolides: A critical review. Drugs 2002;62:1771.

Zuckerman JM: Macrolides and ketolides: Azithromycin, clarithromycin, telithromycin. Infect Dis Clin North Am 2004;18:621.

CASE STUDY ANSWER

A tetracycline or a macrolide is effective in the treatment of chlamydial cervicitis. Doxycycline at a dose of 100 mg PO bid for 7 days is the preferred tetracycline, while azithromycin as a single 1 g dose is the preferred macrolide. If the patient is pregnant, then tetracyclines would be contraindicated and she should receive azithromycin, which is safe in pregnancy.

Aminoglycosides & Spectinomycin

Daniel H. Deck, PharmD & Lisa G. Winston, MD[*]

C A S E   S T U D Y

A 45-year-old man with no medical history was admitted to the intensive care unit (ICU) 10 days ago after suffering third-degree burns over 40% of his body. He had been relatively stable until the last 24 hours. Now he is febrile (39.5°C [103.1°F]), and his white blood cell count has risen from 8,500 to 20,000/mm^3. He has also had an episode of hypotension (86/50 mm Hg) that responded to a fluid bolus. Blood cultures were obtained at the time of his fever and results are pending. The ICU attending physician is concerned about sepsis and decides to treat with empiric combination therapy directed against *Pseudomonas*. The combination therapy includes tobramycin. The patient weighs 70 kg (154 lb) and has an estimated creatinine clearance of 90 mL/min. How should tobramycin be dosed using once-daily and conventional dosing strategies? How should each regimen be monitored for efficacy and toxicity?

The drugs described in this chapter are bactericidal inhibitors of protein synthesis that interfere with ribosomal function. These agents are useful mainly against aerobic gram-negative microorganisms.

■ AMINOGLYCOSIDES

The aminoglycosides include **streptomycin, neomycin, kanamycin, amikacin, gentamicin, tobramycin, sisomicin, netilmicin,** and others. They are used most widely in combination with a β-lactam antibiotic in serious infections with gram-negative bacteria, in combination with vancomycin or a β-lactam antibiotic for gram-positive endocarditis, and for treatment of tuberculosis.

General Properties of Aminoglycosides

A. Physical and Chemical Properties

Aminoglycosides have a hexose ring, either streptidine (in streptomycin) or 2-deoxystreptamine (in other aminoglycosides), to which

various amino sugars are attached by glycosidic linkages (Figures 45–1 and 45–2). They are water-soluble, stable in solution, and more active at alkaline than at acid pH.

B. Mechanism of Action

The mode of action of streptomycin has been studied far more closely than that of other aminoglycosides, but they probably all act similarly. Aminoglycosides are irreversible inhibitors of protein synthesis, but the precise mechanism for bactericidal activity is not known. The initial event is passive diffusion via porin channels across the outer membrane (see Figure 43–3). Drug is then actively transported across the cell membrane into the cytoplasm by an oxygen-dependent process. The transmembrane electrochemical gradient supplies the energy for this process, and transport is coupled to a proton pump. Low extracellular pH and anaerobic conditions inhibit transport by reducing the gradient. Transport may be enhanced by cell wall-active drugs such as penicillin or vancomycin; this enhancement may be the basis of the synergism of these antibiotics with aminoglycosides.

Inside the cell, aminoglycosides bind to specific 30S-subunit ribosomal proteins (S12 in the case of streptomycin). Protein synthesis is inhibited by aminoglycosides in at least three ways (Figure 45–3): (1) interference with the initiation complex of peptide

---

[*]The authors thank Dr. Henry F. Chambers for his contributions to previous editions.

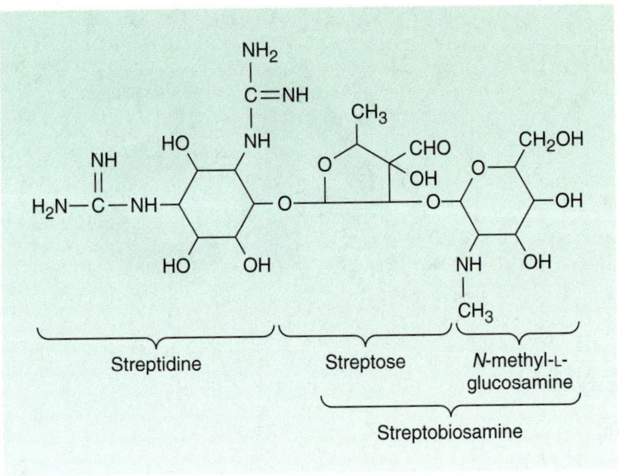

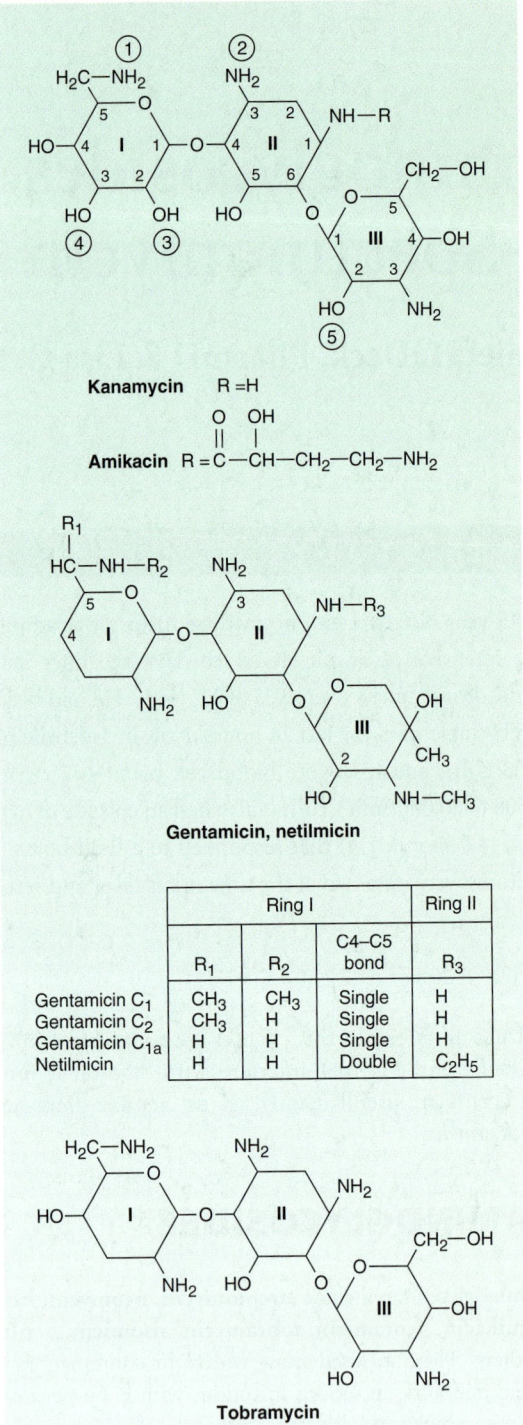

FIGURE 45–1   Structure of streptomycin.

formation; (2) misreading of mRNA, which causes incorporation of incorrect amino acids into the peptide and results in a nonfunctional or toxic protein; and (3) breakup of polysomes into nonfunctional monosomes. These activities occur more or less simultaneously, and the overall effect is irreversible and lethal for the cell.

C. Mechanisms of Resistance

Three principal mechanisms have been established: (1) production of a transferase enzyme or enzymes inactivates the aminoglycoside by adenylylation, acetylation, or phosphorylation. This is the principal type of resistance encountered clinically. (Specific transferase enzymes are discussed below.) (2) There is impaired entry of aminoglycoside into the cell. This may be genotypic, resulting from mutation or deletion of a porin protein or proteins involved in transport and maintenance of the electrochemical gradient; or phenotypic, eg, resulting from growth conditions under which the oxygen-dependent transport process described above is not functional. (3) The receptor protein on the 30S ribosomal subunit may be deleted or altered as a result of a mutation.

D. Pharmacokinetics and Once-Daily Dosing

Aminoglycosides are absorbed very poorly from the intact gastrointestinal tract, and almost the entire oral dose is excreted in feces after oral administration. However, the drugs may be absorbed if ulcerations are present. After intramuscular injection, aminoglycosides are well absorbed, giving peak concentrations in blood within 30–90 minutes. Aminoglycosides are usually administered intravenously as a 30- to 60-minute infusion; after a brief distribution phase, this results in serum concentrations that are identical with those following intramuscular injection. The normal half-life of aminoglycosides in serum is 2–3 hours, increasing to 24–48 hours in patients with significant impairment of renal function. Aminoglycosides are only partially and irregularly removed by hemodialysis—eg, 40–60% for gentamicin—and even less effectively by peritoneal dialysis. Aminoglycosides are highly polar compounds that do not enter cells readily. They are largely excluded from the central nervous system and the eye. In the

	Ring I			Ring II
	R_1	R_2	C4–C5 bond	R_3
Gentamicin C_1	CH_3	CH_3	Single	H
Gentamicin C_2	CH_3	H	Single	H
Gentamicin C_{1a}	H	H	Single	H
Netilmicin	H	H	Double	C_2H_5

FIGURE 45–2   Structures of several important aminoglycoside antibiotics. Ring II is 2-deoxystreptamine. The resemblance between kanamycin and amikacin and between gentamicin, netilmicin, and tobramycin can be seen. The circled numerals on the kanamycin molecule indicate points of attack of plasmid-mediated bacterial transferase enzymes that can inactivate this drug. ①, ②, and ③, acetyltransferase; ④, phosphotransferase; ⑤, adenylyltransferase. Amikacin is resistant to modification at ②, ③, ④, and ⑤.

Normal bacterial cell

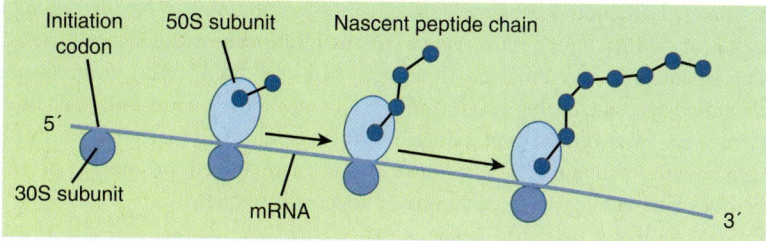

Aminoglycoside-treated bacterial cell

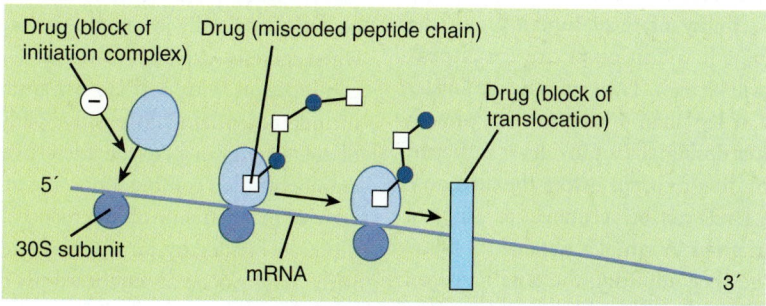

FIGURE 45–3 Putative mechanisms of action of the aminoglycosides in bacteria. Normal protein synthesis is shown in the top panel. At least three aminoglycoside effects have been described, as shown in the bottom panel: block of formation of the initiation complex; miscoding of amino acids in the emerging peptide chain due to misreading of the mRNA; and block of translocation on mRNA. Block of movement of the ribosome may occur after the formation of a single initiation complex, resulting in an mRNA chain with only a single ribosome on it, a so-called monosome. (Reproduced, with permission, from Trevor AT, Katzung BG, Masters SB: *Pharmacology: Examination & Board Review,* 6th ed. McGraw-Hill, 2002.)

presence of active inflammation, however, cerebrospinal fluid levels reach 20% of plasma levels, and in neonatal meningitis, the levels may be higher. Intrathecal or intraventricular injection is required for high levels in cerebrospinal fluid. Even after parenteral administration, concentrations of aminoglycosides are not high in most tissues except the renal cortex. Concentration in most secretions is also modest; in the bile, it may reach 30% of the blood level. With prolonged therapy, diffusion into pleural or synovial fluid may result in concentrations 50–90% of that of plasma.

Traditionally, aminoglycosides have been administered in two or three equally divided doses per day in patients with normal renal function. However, administration of the entire daily dose in a single injection may be preferred in many clinical situations. Aminoglycosides have **concentration-dependent killing;** that is, increasing concentrations kill an increasing proportion of bacteria and at a more rapid rate. They also have a significant **postantibiotic effect,** such that the antibacterial activity persists beyond the time during which measurable drug is present. The postantibiotic effect of aminoglycosides can last several hours. Because of these properties, a given total amount of aminoglycoside may have better efficacy when administered as a single large dose than when administered as multiple smaller doses. When administered with a cell wall-active antibiotic (a β lactam or vancomycin), aminoglycosides exhibit **synergistic killing** against certain bacteria. The effect of the drugs in combination is greater than the anticipated effect of each individual drug, ie, the killing effect of the combination is more than additive.

Adverse effects from aminoglycosides are both time- and concentration-dependent. Toxicity is unlikely to occur until a certain threshold concentration is reached, but once that concentration is achieved, the time beyond this threshold becomes critical. This threshold is not precisely defined, but a trough concentration above 2 mcg/mL is predictive of toxicity. At clinically relevant doses, the total time above this threshold is greater with multiple smaller doses of drug than with a single large dose.

Numerous clinical studies demonstrate that a single daily dose of aminoglycoside is just as effective—and probably less toxic—than multiple smaller doses. Therefore, many authorities now recommend that aminoglycosides be administered as a single daily dose in many clinical situations. However, the efficacy of once-daily aminoglycoside dosing in combination therapy of enterococcal and staphylococcal endocarditis remains to be defined, and the standard low-dose, thrice-daily administration is still recommended. In contrast, there are limited data supporting once-daily dosing in streptococcal endocarditis. The role of once-daily dosing in pregnancy and in neonates also is not well defined.

Once-daily dosing has potential practical advantages. For example, repeated determinations of serum concentrations are probably unnecessary unless aminoglycoside is given for more than 3 days. A drug administered once a day rather than three times a day is less labor intensive. And once-a-day dosing is more feasible for outpatient therapy.

Aminoglycosides are cleared by the kidney, and excretion is directly proportional to creatinine clearance. To avoid accumulation and toxic levels, once-daily dosing of aminoglycosides is generally avoided if renal function is impaired. Rapidly changing renal function, which may occur with acute kidney injury, must also be monitored to avoid overdosing or underdosing. Provided these pitfalls are avoided, once-daily aminoglycoside dosing is safe and effective. If the creatinine clearance is > 60 mL/min, then a single daily dose of 5–7 mg/kg of gentamicin or tobramycin is recommended (15 mg/kg for amikacin). For patients with creatinine clearance < 60 mL/min, traditional dosing as described below is recommended. With once-daily dosing, serum concentrations need not be routinely checked until the second or third day of therapy, depending on the stability of renal function and the anticipated duration of therapy. It is unnecessary to check peak concentrations because they will be high. The goal is to administer drug so that concentrations of less than 1 mcg/mL are present between 18 and 24 hours after dosing. This provides a sufficient period of time for washout of drug to occur before the next dose is given. Appropriate trough levels can be accurately determined by measuring serum concentrations in samples obtained 2 hours and 12 hours after dosing and then adjusting the dose based on the actual clearance of drug or by measuring the concentration in a sample obtained 8 hours after a dose. If the 8-hour concentration is between 1.5 mcg/mL and 6 mcg/mL, the target trough can be achieved at 18 hours.

With traditional dosing, adjustments must be made to prevent accumulation of drug and toxicity in patients with renal insufficiency. Either the dose of drug is kept constant and the interval between doses is increased, or the interval is kept constant and the dose is reduced. Nomograms and formulas have been constructed relating serum creatinine levels to adjustments in treatment regimens. Because aminoglycoside clearance is directly proportional to the creatinine clearance, a method for determining the aminoglycoside dose is to estimate creatinine clearance using the Cockcroft-Gault formula described in Chapter 60. For a traditional twice- or thrice-daily dosing regimen, peak serum concentrations should be determined from a blood sample obtained 30–60 minutes after a dose, and trough concentrations from a sample obtained just before the next dose. Doses of gentamicin and tobramycin should be adjusted to maintain peak levels between 5 and 10 mcg/mL and trough levels < 2 mcg/mL (< 1 mcg/mL is optimal).

E. Adverse Effects

All aminoglycosides are ototoxic and nephrotoxic. Ototoxicity and nephrotoxicity are more likely to be encountered when therapy is continued for more than 5 days, at higher doses, in the elderly, and in the setting of renal insufficiency. Concurrent use with loop diuretics (eg, furosemide, ethacrynic acid) or other nephrotoxic antimicrobial agents (eg, vancomycin or amphotericin) can potentiate nephrotoxicity and should be avoided if possible. Ototoxicity can manifest either as auditory damage, resulting in tinnitus and high-frequency hearing loss initially, or as vestibular damage, evident by vertigo, ataxia, and loss of balance. Nephrotoxicity results in rising serum creatinine levels or reduced creatinine clearance, although the earliest indication often is an increase in trough serum aminoglycoside concentrations. Neomycin, kanamycin, and amikacin

are the most ototoxic agents. Streptomycin and gentamicin are the most vestibulotoxic. Neomycin, tobramycin, and gentamicin are the most nephrotoxic.

In very high doses, aminoglycosides can produce a curare-like effect with neuromuscular blockade that results in respiratory paralysis. This paralysis is usually reversible by calcium gluconate (given promptly) or neostigmine. Hypersensitivity occurs infrequently.

F. Clinical Uses

Aminoglycosides are mostly used against gram-negative enteric bacteria, especially when the isolate may be drug-resistant and when there is suspicion of sepsis. They are almost always used in combination with a β-lactam antibiotic to extend coverage to include potential gram-positive pathogens and to take advantage of the synergism between these two classes of drugs. Penicillin-aminoglycoside combinations also are used to achieve bactericidal activity in treatment of enterococcal endocarditis and to shorten duration of therapy for viridans streptococcal and some patients with staphylococcal endocarditis. Which aminoglycoside and what dose should be used depend on the infection being treated and the susceptibility of the isolate.

STREPTOMYCIN

Streptomycin (Figure 45–1) was isolated from a strain of *Streptomyces griseus*. The antimicrobial activity of streptomycin is typical of that of other aminoglycosides, as are the mechanisms of resistance. Resistance has emerged in most species, severely limiting the current usefulness of streptomycin, with the exceptions listed below. Ribosomal resistance to streptomycin develops readily, limiting its role as a single agent.

Clinical Uses

A. Mycobacterial Infections

Streptomycin is mainly used as a second-line agent for treatment of tuberculosis. The dosage is 0.5–1 g/d (7.5–15 mg/kg/d for children), which is given intramuscularly or intravenously. It should be used only in combination with other agents to prevent emergence of resistance. See Chapter 47 for additional information regarding the use of streptomycin in mycobacterial infections.

B. Nontuberculous Infections

In plague, tularemia, and sometimes brucellosis, streptomycin, 1 g/d (15 mg/kg/d for children), is given intramuscularly in combination with an oral tetracycline.

Penicillin plus streptomycin is effective for enterococcal endocarditis and 2-week therapy of viridans streptococcal endocarditis. Gentamicin has largely replaced streptomycin for these indications. Streptomycin remains a useful agent for treating enterococcal infections, however, because approximately 15% of enterococcal isolates that are resistant to gentamicin (and therefore resistant to netilmicin, tobramycin, and amikacin) will be susceptible to streptomycin.

Adverse Reactions

Fever, skin rashes, and other allergic manifestations may result from hypersensitivity to streptomycin. This occurs most frequently with prolonged contact with the drug either in patients who receive a prolonged course of treatment (eg, for tuberculosis) or in medical personnel who handle the drug. Desensitization is occasionally successful.

Pain at the injection site is common but usually not severe. The most serious toxic effect with streptomycin is disturbance of vestibular function—vertigo and loss of balance. The frequency and severity of this disturbance are in proportion to the age of the patient, the blood levels of the drug, and the duration of administration. Vestibular dysfunction may follow a few weeks of unusually high blood levels (eg, in individuals with impaired renal function) or months of relatively low blood levels. Vestibular toxicity tends to be irreversible. Streptomycin given during pregnancy can cause deafness in the newborn and, therefore, is relatively contraindicated.

GENTAMICIN

Gentamicin is an aminoglycoside (Figure 45–2) isolated from *Micromonospora purpurea*. It is effective against both gram-positive and gram-negative organisms, and many of its properties resemble those of other aminoglycosides. **Sisomicin** is very similar to the C_{1a} component of gentamicin.

Antimicrobial Activity

Gentamicin sulfate, 2–10 mcg/mL, inhibits in vitro many strains of staphylococci and coliforms and other gram-negative bacteria. It is active alone, but also as a synergistic companion with β-lactam antibiotics, against *Escherichia coli*, *Proteus*, *Klebsiella pneumoniae*, *Enterobacter*, *Serratia*, *Stenotrophomonas*, and other gram-negative rods that may be resistant to multiple other antibiotics. Like all aminoglycosides, it has no activity against anaerobes.

Resistance

Streptococci and enterococci are relatively resistant to gentamicin owing to failure of the drug to penetrate into the cell. However, gentamicin in combination with vancomycin or a penicillin produces a potent bactericidal effect, which in part is due to enhanced uptake of drug that occurs with inhibition of cell wall synthesis. Resistance to gentamicin rapidly emerges in staphylococci during monotherapy owing to selection of permeability mutants. Ribosomal resistance is rare. Among gram-negative bacteria, resistance is most commonly due to plasmid-encoded aminoglycoside-modifying enzymes. Gram-negative bacteria that are gentamicin-resistant usually are susceptible to amikacin, which is much more resistant to modifying enzyme activity. The enterococcal enzyme that modifies gentamicin is a bifunctional enzyme that also inactivates amikacin, netilmicin, and tobramycin, but not streptomycin; the latter is modified by a different enzyme. This is why some gentamicin-resistant enterococci are susceptible to streptomycin.

Clinical Uses

A. Intramuscular or Intravenous Administration

Gentamicin is used mainly in severe infections (eg, sepsis and pneumonia) caused by gram-negative bacteria that are likely to be resistant to other drugs, especially *P aeruginosa*, *Enterobacter* sp, *Serratia marcescens*, *Proteus* sp, *Acinetobacter* sp, and *Klebsiella* sp. It usually is used in combination with a second agent because an aminoglycoside alone may not be effective for infections outside the urinary tract. For example, gentamicin should not be used as a single agent to treat staphylococcal infections because resistance develops rapidly. Aminoglycosides also should not be used for single-agent therapy of pneumonia because penetration of infected lung tissue is poor and local conditions of low pH and low oxygen tension contribute to poor activity. Gentamicin 5–6 mg/kg/d traditionally is given intravenously in three equal doses, but once-daily administration is just as effective for some organisms and less toxic (see above).

Gentamicin, in combination with a cell wall-active antibiotic, is also indicated in the treatment of endocarditis caused by gram-positive bacteria (streptococci, staphylococci, and enterococci). The synergistic killing achieved by combination therapy may achieve bactericidal activity necessary for cure or allow for the shortening of the duration of therapy. The doses of gentamicin used for synergy against gram-positive bacteria are lower than traditional doses. Typically the drug is administered at a dose of 3 mg/kg/day in three divided doses. Peak levels should be approximately 3 mcg/mL, while trough levels should be < 1 mcg/mL. There are limited data to support administering the 3-mg/kg dose as a single daily injection in the treatment of streptococcal endocarditis.

B. Topical and Ocular Administration

Creams, ointments, and solutions containing 0.1–0.3% gentamicin sulfate have been used for the treatment of infected burns, wounds, or skin lesions and in attempts to prevent intravenous catheter infections. The effectiveness of topical preparations for these indications is unclear. Topical gentamicin is partly inactivated by purulent exudates. Ten mg can be injected subconjunctivally for treatment of ocular infections.

C. Intrathecal Administration

Meningitis caused by gram-negative bacteria has been treated by the intrathecal injection of gentamicin sulfate, 1–10 mg/d. However, neither intrathecal nor intraventricular gentamicin was beneficial in neonates with meningitis, and intraventricular gentamicin was toxic, raising questions about the usefulness of this form of therapy. Moreover, the availability of third-generation cephalosporins for gram-negative meningitis has rendered this therapy obsolete in most cases.

Adverse Reactions

Nephrotoxicity is usually reversible and mild. It occurs in 5–25% of patients receiving gentamicin for longer than 3–5 days. Such toxicity requires, at the very least, adjustment of the dosing regimen and should prompt reconsideration of the need for the drug, particularly if there is a less toxic alternative agent. Measurement of gentamicin serum levels is essential. Ototoxicity, which tends to be irreversible, manifests itself mainly as vestibular dysfunction. Loss of hearing can also occur. The incidence of ototoxicity is in part genetically determined, having been linked to point mutations in mitochondrial DNA, and occurs in 1–5% for patients receiving gentamicin for more than 5 days. Hypersensitivity reactions to gentamicin are uncommon.

TOBRAMYCIN

This aminoglycoside (Figure 45–2) has an antibacterial spectrum similar to that of gentamicin. Although there is some cross-resistance between gentamicin and tobramycin, it is unpredictable in individual strains. Separate laboratory susceptibility tests are therefore necessary.

The pharmacokinetic properties of tobramycin are virtually identical with those of gentamicin. The daily dose of tobramycin is 5–6 mg/kg intramuscularly or intravenously, traditionally divided into three equal amounts and given every 8 hours. Monitoring blood levels in renal insufficiency is an essential guide to proper dosing.

Tobramycin has almost the same antibacterial spectrum as gentamicin with a few exceptions. Gentamicin is slightly more active against *S marcescens*, whereas tobramycin is slightly more active against *P aeruginosa*; *Enterococcus faecalis* is susceptible to both gentamicin and tobramycin, but *E faecium* is resistant to tobramycin. Gentamicin and tobramycin are otherwise interchangeable clinically.

Like other aminoglycosides, tobramycin is ototoxic and nephrotoxic. Nephrotoxicity of tobramycin may be slightly less than that of gentamicin, but the difference is clinically inconsequential.

Tobramycin is also formulated in solution (300 mg in 5 mL) for inhalation for treatment of *P aeruginosa* lower respiratory tract infections complicating cystic fibrosis. The drug is recommended as a 300-mg dose regardless of the patient's age or weight for administration twice daily in repeated cycles of 28 days on therapy, followed by 28 days off therapy. Serum concentrations 1 hour after inhalation average 1 mcg/mL; consequently, nephrotoxicity and ototoxicity rarely occur. Caution should be used when administering tobramycin to patients with preexisting renal, vestibular, or hearing disorders.

AMIKACIN

Amikacin is a semisynthetic derivative of kanamycin; it is less toxic than the parent molecule (Figure 45–2). It is resistant to many enzymes that inactivate gentamicin and tobramycin, and it therefore can be used against some microorganisms resistant to the latter drugs. Many gram-negative bacteria, including many strains of *Proteus*, *Pseudomonas*, *Enterobacter*, and *Serratia*, are inhibited by 1–20 mcg/mL amikacin in vitro. After injection of 500 mg of amikacin every 12 hours (15 mg/kg/d) intramuscularly, peak levels in serum are 10–30 mcg/mL.

Strains of multidrug-resistant *Mycobacterium tuberculosis*, including streptomycin-resistant strains, are usually susceptible to amikacin. Kanamycin-resistant strains may be cross-resistant to amikacin. The dosage of amikacin for tuberculosis is 7.5–15 mg/kg/d as a once-daily or two to three times weekly injection and always in combination with other drugs to which the isolate is susceptible.

Like all aminoglycosides, amikacin is nephrotoxic and ototoxic (particularly for the auditory portion of the eighth nerve). Serum concentrations should be monitored. Target peak serum concentrations for an every-12-hours dosing regimen are 20–40 mcg/mL, and troughs should be maintained between 4 and 8 mcg/mL.

NETILMICIN

Netilmicin shares many characteristics with gentamicin and tobramycin. However, the addition of an ethyl group to the 1-amino position of the 2-deoxystreptamine ring (ring II, Figure 45–2) sterically protects the netilmicin molecule from enzymatic degradation at the 3-amino (ring II) and 2-hydroxyl (ring III) positions. Consequently, netilmicin may be active against some gentamicin-resistant and tobramycin-resistant bacteria.

The dosage (5–7 mg/kg/d) and the routes of administration are the same as for gentamicin. Netilmicin is largely interchangeable with gentamicin or tobramycin but is no longer available in the United States.

NEOMYCIN & KANAMYCIN

Neomycin and kanamycin are closely related. **Paromomycin** is also a member of this group. All have similar properties.

Antimicrobial Activity & Resistance

Drugs of the neomycin group are active against gram-positive and gram-negative bacteria and some mycobacteria. *P aeruginosa* and streptococci are generally resistant. Mechanisms of antibacterial action and resistance are the same as with other aminoglycosides. The widespread use of these drugs in bowel preparation for elective surgery has resulted in the selection of resistant organisms and some outbreaks of enterocolitis in hospitals. Cross-resistance between kanamycin and neomycin is complete.

Pharmacokinetics

Drugs of the neomycin group are poorly absorbed from the gastrointestinal tract. After oral administration, the intestinal flora is suppressed or modified, and the drug is excreted in the feces. Excretion of any absorbed drug is mainly through glomerular filtration into the urine.

Clinical Uses

Neomycin and kanamycin are now limited to topical and oral use. Neomycin is too toxic for parenteral use. With the advent of more potent and less toxic aminoglycosides, parenteral administration of kanamycin has also been largely abandoned. Paromomycin has recently been shown to be effective against visceral leishmaniasis when given parenterally (see Chapter 52), and this serious infection may represent an important new use for this drug.

A. Topical Administration

Solutions containing 1–5 mg/mL are used on infected surfaces or injected into joints, the pleural cavity, tissue spaces, or abscess cavities where infection is present. The total amount of drug given in this fashion must be limited to 15 mg/kg/d because at higher doses enough drug may be absorbed to produce systemic toxicity. Whether topical application for active infection adds anything to appropriate systemic therapy is questionable. Ointments, often formulated as a neomycin-polymyxin-bacitracin combination, can be applied to infected skin lesions or in the nares for suppression of staphylococci but they are largely ineffective.

B. Oral Administration

In preparation for elective bowel surgery, 1 g of neomycin is given orally every 6–8 hours for 1–2 days, often combined with 1 g of erythromycin base. This reduces the aerobic bowel flora with little effect on anaerobes. In hepatic encephalopathy, coliform flora can be suppressed by giving 1 g every 6–8 hours together with reduced protein intake, thus reducing ammonia production. Use of neomycin for hepatic encephalopathy has been largely supplanted by lactulose and other medications that are less toxic. Use of paromomycin in the treatment of protozoal infections is discussed in Chapter 52.

Adverse Reactions

All members of the neomycin group have significant nephrotoxicity and ototoxicity. Auditory function is affected more than vestibular function. Deafness has occurred, especially in adults with impaired renal function and prolonged elevation of drug levels.

The sudden absorption of postoperatively instilled kanamycin from the peritoneal cavity (3–5 g) has resulted in curare-like neuromuscular blockade and respiratory arrest. Calcium gluconate and neostigmine can act as antidotes.

Although hypersensitivity is not common, prolonged application of neomycin-containing ointments to skin and eyes has resulted in severe allergic reactions.

■ SPECTINOMYCIN

Spectinomycin is an aminocyclitol antibiotic that is structurally related to aminoglycosides. It lacks amino sugars and glycosidic bonds.

Spectinomycin

Spectinomycin is active in vitro against many gram-positive and gram-negative organisms, but it is used almost solely as an alternative treatment for drug-resistant gonorrhea or gonorrhea in penicillin-allergic patients. The majority of gonococcal isolates are inhibited by 6 mcg/mL of spectinomycin. Strains of gonococci may be resistant to spectinomycin, but there is no cross-resistance with other drugs used in gonorrhea. Spectinomycin is rapidly absorbed after intramuscular injection. A single dose of 40 mg/kg up to a maximum of 2 g is given. There is pain at the injection site and, occasionally, fever and nausea. Nephrotoxicity and anemia have been observed rarely. Spectinomycin is no longer available for use in the United States but may be available elsewhere.

SUMMARY Aminoglycosides

Subclass	Mechanism of Action	Effects	Clinical Applications	Pharmacokinetics, Toxicities, Interactions
AMINOGLYCOSIDES & SPECTINOMYCIN				
• Gentamicin	Prevents bacterial protein synthesis by binding to the 30S ribosomal subunit	Bactericidal activity against susceptible bacteria • synergistic effects against gram-positive bacteria when combined with β lactams or vancomycin • concentration-dependent killing and a significant post-antibiotic effect	Sepsis caused by aerobic gram-negative bacteria • synergistic activity in endocarditis caused by streptococci, staphylococci, and enterococci	IV • renal clearance (half-life 2.5 h) • conventional dosing 1.3–1.7 mg/kg q8h with goal peak levels 5–8 mcg/mL • trough levels < 2 mcg/mL • once-daily dosing at 5–7 mg/kg as effective and may have less toxicity than conventional dosing • *Toxicity:* Nephrotoxicity (reversible), ototoxicity (irreversible), neuromuscular blockade

- *Tobramycin: Intravenous; more active than gentamicin versus* Pseudomonas; *may also have less nephrotoxicity*
- *Amikacin: Intravenous; resistant to many enzymes that inactivate gentamicin and tobramycin; higher doses and target peaks and troughs than gentamicin and tobramycin*
- *Streptomycin: Intramuscular, widespread resistance limits use to specific indications such as tuberculosis and enterococcal endocarditis*
- *Neomycin: Oral or topical, poor bioavailability; used before bowel surgery to decrease aerobic flora; also used to treat hepatic encephalopathy*
- *Spectinomycin: Intramuscular; sole use is for treatment of antibiotic-resistant gonococcal infections or gonococcal infections in penicillin-allergic patients*

P R E P A R A T I O N S   A V A I L A B L E

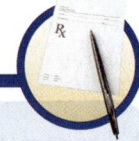

Amikacin (generic, Amikin)
    Parenteral: 50, 250 mg (in vials) for IM, IV injection

Gentamicin (generic, Garamycin)
    Parenteral: 10, 40 mg/mL vials for IM, IV injection

Kanamycin (Kantrex)
    Parenteral: 500, 1000 mg for IM, IV injection; 75 mg for pediatric injection

Neomycin (generic, Mycifradin)
    Oral: 500 mg tablets

Paromomycin (Humatin)
    Oral: 250 mg capsules

Streptomycin (generic)
    Parenteral: 400 mg/mL for IM injection

Tobramycin (generic, Nebcin)
    Parenteral: 10, 40 mg/mL for IM, IV injection; powder to reconstitute for injection
    Solution for inhalation (TOBI): 300 mg in 5 mL sodium chloride solution

REFERENCES

Busse H-J, Wöstmann C, Bakker EP: The bactericidal action of streptomycin: Membrane permeabilization caused by the insertion of mistranslated proteins into the cytoplasmic membrane of *Escherichia coli* and subsequent caging of the antibiotic inside the cells due to degradation of these proteins. J Gen Microbiol 1992;138:551.

Cheer SM, Waugh J, Noble S: Inhaled tobramycin (TOBI): A review of its use in the management of *Pseudomonas aeruginosa* infections in patients with cystic fibrosis. Drugs 2003;63:2501.

Contopoulos-Ioannidis DG et al: Extended-interval aminoglycoside administration for children: A meta-analysis. Pediatrics 2004;114:111.

Kaye D: Current use for old antibacterial agents: Polymyxins, rifampin, and aminoglycosides. Infect Dis Clin North Am 2004;18:669.

Le T, Bayer AS: Combination antibiotic therapy for infective endocarditis. Clin Infect Dis 2003;36:615.

Olsen KM et al: Effect of once-daily dosing vs. multiple daily dosing of tobramycin on enzyme markers of nephrotoxicity. Crit Care Med 2004;32:1678.

Pappas G et al: Brucellosis. N Engl J Med 2005;352:2325.

Paul M et al: Beta lactam monotherapy versus beta lactam-aminoglycoside combination therapy for sepsis in immunocompetent patients: Systematic review and meta-analysis of randomised trials. BMJ 2004;328:668.

Paul M, Soares-Weiser K, Leibovici L: Beta lactam monotherapy versus beta lactam-aminoglycoside combination therapy for fever with neutropenia: Systematic review and meta-analysis. BMJ 2003;326:1111.

Poole K: Aminoglycoside resistance in *Pseudomonas aeruginosa*. Antimicrob Agents Chemother 2005;49:479.

CASE STUDY ANSWER

The patient has normal renal function and thus qualifies for once-daily dosing. Tobramycin could be administered as a single once-daily injection at a dose of 350–490 mg (5–7 mg/kg). A serum level between 1.5 and 6 mcg/mL measured 8 hours after infusion correlates with an appropriate trough level. Alternatively, the same total daily dose could be divided and administered every 8 hours, as a conventional dosing strategy. With conventional dosing, peak and trough concentrations should be monitored with the target peak concentration of 5–10 mcg/mL and the target trough concentration of < 2 mcg/mL.

Sulfonamides, Trimethoprim, & Quinolones

Daniel H. Deck, PharmD, & Lisa G. Winston, MD[*]

C A S E   S T U D Y

A 59-year-old woman presents to an urgent care clinic with a 4-day history of frequent and painful urination. She has had fevers, chills, and flank pain for the past 2 days. Her physician advised her to come immediately to the clinic for evaluation. In the clinic she is febrile (38.5°C [101.3°F]) but otherwise stable and states she is not experiencing any nausea or vomiting. Her urine dipstick test is positive for leukocyte esterase. Urinalysis and urine culture are ordered. Her past medical history is significant for three urinary tract infections in the past year. Each episode was uncomplicated, treated with trimethoprim-sulfamethoxazole, and promptly resolved. She also has osteoporosis for which she takes a daily calcium supplement. The decision is made to treat her with oral antibiotics for a complicated urinary tract infection with close follow-up. Given her history, what would be a reasonable empiric antibiotic choice? Depending on the antibiotic choice are there potential drug interactions?

■ ANTIFOLATE DRUGS

SULFONAMIDES

Chemistry

The basic formulas of the sulfonamides and their structural similarity to *p*-aminobenzoic acid (PABA) are shown in Figure 46–1. Sulfonamides with varying physical, chemical, pharmacologic, and antibacterial properties are produced by attaching substituents to the amido group ($-SO_2-NH-R$) or the amino group ($-NH_2$) of the sulfanilamide nucleus. Sulfonamides tend to be much more soluble at alkaline than at acid pH. Most can be prepared as sodium salts, which are used for intravenous administration.

Mechanism of Action & Antimicrobial Activity

Sulfonamide-susceptible organisms, unlike mammals, cannot use exogenous folate but must synthesize it from PABA. This pathway (Figure 46–2) is thus essential for production of purines and nucleic acid synthesis. As structural analogs of PABA, sulfonamides inhibit dihydropteroate synthase and folate production. Sulfonamides inhibit both gram-positive and gram-negative bacteria, *Nocardia* sp, *Chlamydia trachomatis,* and some protozoa. Some enteric bacteria, such as *Escherichia coli, Klebsiella pneumoniae, Salmonella, Shigella,* and *Enterobacter* sp are also inhibited. It is interesting that rickettsiae are not inhibited by sulfonamides but are instead stimulated in their growth. Activity is poor against anaerobes. *Pseudomonas aeruginosa* is intrinsically resistant to sulfonamide antibiotics.

Combination of a sulfonamide with an inhibitor of dihydrofolate reductase (trimethoprim or pyrimethamine) provides synergistic activity because of sequential inhibition of folate synthesis (Figure 46–2).

---

[*]The authors thank Henry F. Chambers, MD, for his contributions to previous editions.

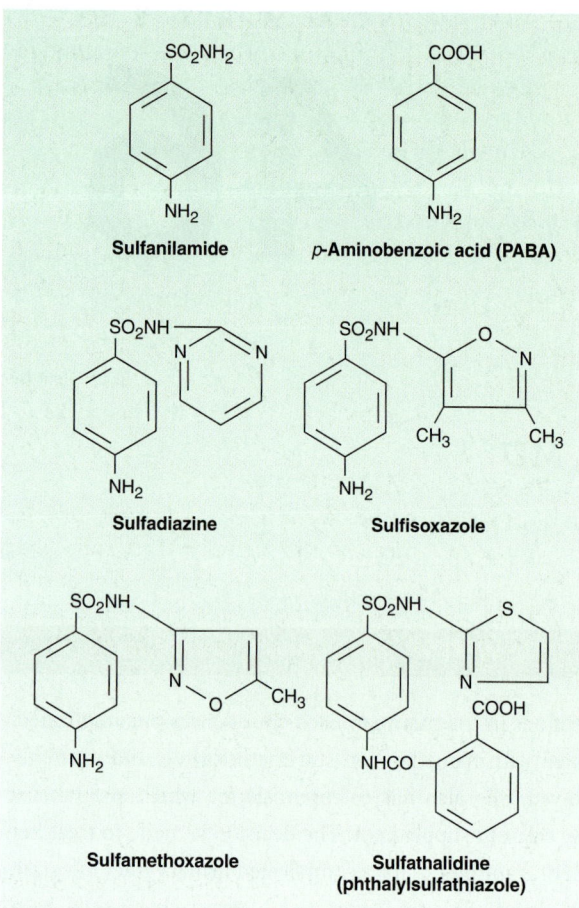

FIGURE 46–1 Structures of some sulfonamides and *p*-aminobenzoic acid.

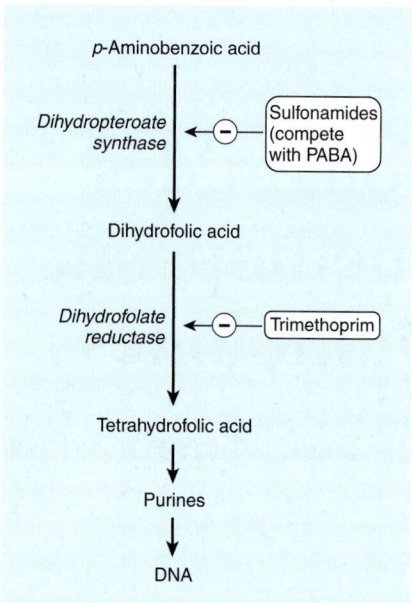

FIGURE 46–2 Actions of sulfonamides and trimethoprim.

system and cerebrospinal fluid), placenta, and fetus. Protein binding varies from 20% to over 90%. Therapeutic concentrations are in the range of 40–100 mcg/mL of blood. Blood levels generally peak 2–6 hours after oral administration.

A portion of absorbed drug is acetylated or glucuronidated in the liver. Sulfonamides and inactive metabolites are then excreted into the urine, mainly by glomerular filtration. In significant renal failure, the dosage of sulfonamide must be reduced.

Resistance

Mammalian cells (and some bacteria) lack the enzymes required for folate synthesis from PABA and depend on exogenous sources of folate; therefore, they are not susceptible to sulfonamides. Sulfonamide resistance may occur as a result of mutations that (1) cause overproduction of PABA, (2) cause production of a folic acid-synthesizing enzyme that has low affinity for sulfonamides, or (3) impair permeability to the sulfonamide. Dihydropteroate synthase with low sulfonamide affinity is often encoded on a plasmid that is transmissible and can disseminate rapidly and widely. Sulfonamide-resistant dihydropteroate synthase mutants also can emerge under selective pressure.

Pharmacokinetics

Sulfonamides can be divided into three major groups: (1) oral, absorbable; (2) oral, nonabsorbable; and (3) topical. The oral, absorbable sulfonamides can be classified as short-, intermediate-, or long-acting on the basis of their half-lives (Table 46–1). They are absorbed from the stomach and small intestine and distributed widely to tissues and body fluids (including the central nervous

TABLE 46–1 Pharmacokinetic properties of some sulfonamides and pyrimidines.

Drug	Half-Life	Oral Absorption
Sulfonamides		
Sulfacytine	Short	Prompt (peak levels in 1–4 hours)
Sulfisoxazole	Short (6 hours)	Prompt
Sulfamethizole	Short (9 hours)	Prompt
Sulfadiazine	Intermediate (10–17 hours)	Slow (peak levels in 4–8 hours)
Sulfamethoxazole	Intermediate (10–12 hours)	Slow
Sulfapyridine	Intermediate (17 hours)	Slow
Sulfadoxine	Long (7–9 days)	Intermediate
Pyrimidines		
Trimethoprim	Intermediate (11 hours)	Prompt
Pyrimethamine	Long (4–6 days)	Prompt

Clinical Uses

Sulfonamides are infrequently used as single agents. Many strains of formerly susceptible species, including meningococci, pneumococci, streptococci, staphylococci, and gonococci, are now resistant. The fixed-drug combination of trimethoprim-sulfamethoxazole is the drug of choice for infections such as *Pneumocystis jiroveci* (formerly *P carinii*) pneumonia, toxoplasmosis, nocardiosis, and occasionally other bacterial infections.

A. Oral Absorbable Agents

Sulfisoxazole and sulfamethoxazole are short- to medium-acting agents used almost exclusively to treat urinary tract infections. The usual adult dosage is 1 g of sulfisoxazole four times daily or 1 g of sulfamethoxazole two or three times daily.

Sulfadiazine in combination with pyrimethamine is first-line therapy for treatment of acute toxoplasmosis. The combination of sulfadiazine with pyrimethamine, a potent inhibitor of dihydrofolate reductase, is synergistic because these drugs block sequential steps in the folate synthetic pathway blockade (Figure 46–2). The dosage of sulfadiazine is 1 g four times daily, with pyrimethamine given as a 75-mg loading dose followed by a 25-mg once-daily dose. Folinic acid, 10 mg orally each day, should also be administered to minimize bone marrow suppression.

Sulfadoxine is the only long-acting sulfonamide currently available in the USA and only as a combination formulation with pyrimethamine (Fansidar), a second-line agent in the treatment of malaria (see Chapter 52).

B. Oral Nonabsorbable Agents

Sulfasalazine (salicylazosulfapyridine) is widely used in ulcerative colitis, enteritis, and other inflammatory bowel disease (see Chapter 62).

C. Topical Agents

Sodium sulfacetamide ophthalmic solution or ointment is effective in the treatment of bacterial conjunctivitis and as adjunctive therapy for trachoma. Another sulfonamide, mafenide acetate, is used topically but can be absorbed from burn sites. The drug and its primary metabolite inhibit carbonic anhydrase and can cause metabolic acidosis, a side effect that limits its usefulness. Silver sulfadiazine is a much less toxic topical sulfonamide and is preferred to mafenide for prevention of infection of burn wounds.

Adverse Reactions

All sulfonamides, including antimicrobial sulfas, diuretics, diazoxide, and the sulfonylurea hypoglycemic agents, have been considered to be partially cross-allergenic. However, evidence for this is not extensive. The most common adverse effects are fever, skin rashes, exfoliative dermatitis, photosensitivity, urticaria, nausea, vomiting, diarrhea, and difficulties referable to the urinary tract (see below). Stevens-Johnson syndrome, although relatively uncommon (< 1% of treatment courses), is a particularly serious and potentially fatal type of skin and mucous membrane eruption

associated with sulfonamide use. Other unwanted effects include stomatitis, conjunctivitis, arthritis, hematopoietic disturbances (see below), hepatitis, and, rarely, polyarteritis nodosa and psychosis.

A. Urinary Tract Disturbances

Sulfonamides may precipitate in urine, especially at neutral or acid pH, producing crystalluria, hematuria, or even obstruction. This is rarely a problem with the more soluble sulfonamides (eg, sulfisoxazole). Sulfadiazine when given in large doses, particularly if fluid intake is poor, can cause crystalluria. Crystalluria is treated by administration of sodium bicarbonate to alkalinize the urine and fluids to increase urine flow. Sulfonamides have also been implicated in various types of nephrosis and in allergic nephritis.

B. Hematopoietic Disturbances

Sulfonamides can cause hemolytic or aplastic anemia, granulocytopenia, thrombocytopenia, or leukemoid reactions. Sulfonamides may provoke hemolytic reactions in patients with glucose-6-phosphate dehydrogenase deficiency. Sulfonamides taken near the end of pregnancy increase the risk of kernicterus in newborns.

TRIMETHOPRIM & TRIMETHOPRIM-SULFAMETHOXAZOLE MIXTURES

Mechanism of Action

Trimethoprim, a trimethoxybenzylpyrimidine, selectively inhibits bacterial dihydrofolic acid reductase, which converts dihydrofolic acid to tetrahydrofolic acid, a step leading to the synthesis of purines and ultimately to DNA (Figure 46–2). Trimethoprim is about 50,000 times less efficient in inhibition of mammalian dihydrofolic acid reductase. Pyrimethamine, another benzylpyrimidine, selectively inhibits dihydrofolic acid reductase of protozoa compared with that of mammalian cells. As noted above, trimethoprim or pyrimethamine in combination with a sulfonamide blocks sequential steps in folate synthesis, resulting in marked enhancement (synergism) of the activity of both drugs. The combination often is bactericidal, compared with the bacteriostatic activity of a sulfonamide alone.

Trimethoprim

Pyrimethamine

Resistance

Resistance to trimethoprim can result from reduced cell permeability, overproduction of dihydrofolate reductase, or production of an altered reductase with reduced drug binding. Resistance can emerge by mutation, although more commonly it is due to plasmid-encoded trimethoprim-resistant dihydrofolate reductases. These resistant enzymes may be coded within transposons on conjugative plasmids that exhibit a broad host range, accounting for rapid and widespread dissemination of trimethoprim resistance among numerous bacterial species.

Pharmacokinetics

Trimethoprim is usually given orally, alone or in combination with sulfamethoxazole, which has a similar half-life. Trimethoprim-sulfamethoxazole can also be given intravenously. Trimethoprim is well absorbed from the gut and distributed widely in body fluids and tissues, including cerebrospinal fluid.

Because trimethoprim is more lipid-soluble than sulfamethoxazole, it has a larger volume of distribution than the latter drug. Therefore, when 1 part of trimethoprim is given with 5 parts of sulfamethoxazole (the ratio in the formulation), the peak plasma concentrations are in the ratio of 1:20, which is optimal for the combined effects of these drugs in vitro. About 30–50% of the sulfonamide and 50–60% of the trimethoprim (or their respective metabolites) are excreted in the urine within 24 hours. The dose should be reduced by half for patients with creatinine clearances of 15–30 mL/min.

Trimethoprim (a weak base) concentrates in prostatic fluid and in vaginal fluid, which are more acidic than plasma. Therefore, it has more antibacterial activity in prostatic and vaginal fluids than many other antimicrobial drugs.

Clinical Uses

A. Oral Trimethoprim

Trimethoprim can be given alone (100 mg twice daily) in acute urinary tract infections. Many community-acquired organisms are susceptible to the high concentrations that are found in the urine (200–600 mcg/mL).

B. Oral Trimethoprim-Sulfamethoxazole (TMP-SMZ)

A combination of trimethoprim-sulfamethoxazole is effective treatment for a wide variety of infections including *P jiroveci* pneumonia, shigellosis, systemic salmonella infections, urinary tract infections, prostatitis, and some nontuberculous mycobacterial infections. It is active against most *Staphylococcus aureus* strains, both methicillin-susceptible and methicillin-resistant, and against respiratory tract pathogens such as pneumococcus, *Haemophilus* sp, *Moraxella catarrhalis,* and *K pneumoniae* (but not *Mycoplasma pneumoniae*). However, the increasing prevalence of strains of *E coli* (up to 30% or more) and pneumococci that are resistant to trimethoprim-sulfamethoxazole must be considered before using this combination for empiric therapy of upper urinary tract infections or pneumonia.

One double-strength tablet (each tablet contains trimethoprim 160 mg plus sulfamethoxazole 800 mg) given every 12 hours is effective treatment for urinary tract infections and prostatitis. One half of the regular (single-strength) tablet given three times weekly for many months may serve as prophylaxis in recurrent urinary tract infections of some women. One double-strength tablet every 12 hours is effective treatment for infections caused by susceptible strains of shigella and salmonella. The dosage for children treated for shigellosis, urinary tract infection, or otitis media is 8 mg/kg trimethoprim and 40 mg/kg sulfamethoxazole every 12 hours.

Infections with *P jiroveci* and some other pathogens can be treated orally with high doses of the combination (dosed on the basis of the trimethoprim component at 15–20 mg/kg/d) or can be prevented in immunosuppressed patients by one double-strength tablet daily or three times weekly.

C. Intravenous Trimethoprim-Sulfamethoxazole

A solution of the mixture containing 80 mg trimethoprim plus 400 mg sulfamethoxazole per 5 mL diluted in 125 mL of 5% dextrose in water can be administered by intravenous infusion over 60–90 minutes. It is the agent of choice for moderately severe to severe pneumocystis pneumonia. It may be used for gram-negative bacterial sepsis, including that caused by some multidrug-resistant species such as enterobacter and serratia; shigellosis; typhoid fever; or urinary tract infection caused by a susceptible organism when the patient is unable to take the drug by mouth. The dosage is 10–20 mg/kg/d of the trimethoprim component.

D. Oral Pyrimethamine with Sulfonamide

Pyrimethamine and sulfadiazine have been used for treatment of leishmaniasis and toxoplasmosis. In falciparum malaria, the combination of pyrimethamine with sulfadoxine (Fansidar) has been used (see Chapter 52).

Adverse Effects

Trimethoprim produces the predictable adverse effects of an antifolate drug, especially megaloblastic anemia, leukopenia, and granulocytopenia. The combination trimethoprim-sulfamethoxazole may cause all of the untoward reactions associated with sulfonamides. Nausea and vomiting, drug fever, vasculitis, renal damage, and central nervous system disturbances occasionally occur also. Patients with AIDS and pneumocystis pneumonia have a particularly high frequency of untoward reactions to trimethoprim-sulfamethoxazole, especially fever, rashes, leukopenia, diarrhea, elevations of hepatic aminotransferases, hyperkalemia, and hyponatremia.

■ DNA GYRASE INHIBITORS

FLUOROQUINOLONES

The important quinolones are synthetic fluorinated analogs of nalidixic acid (Figure 46–3). They are active against a variety of gram-positive and gram-negative bacteria.

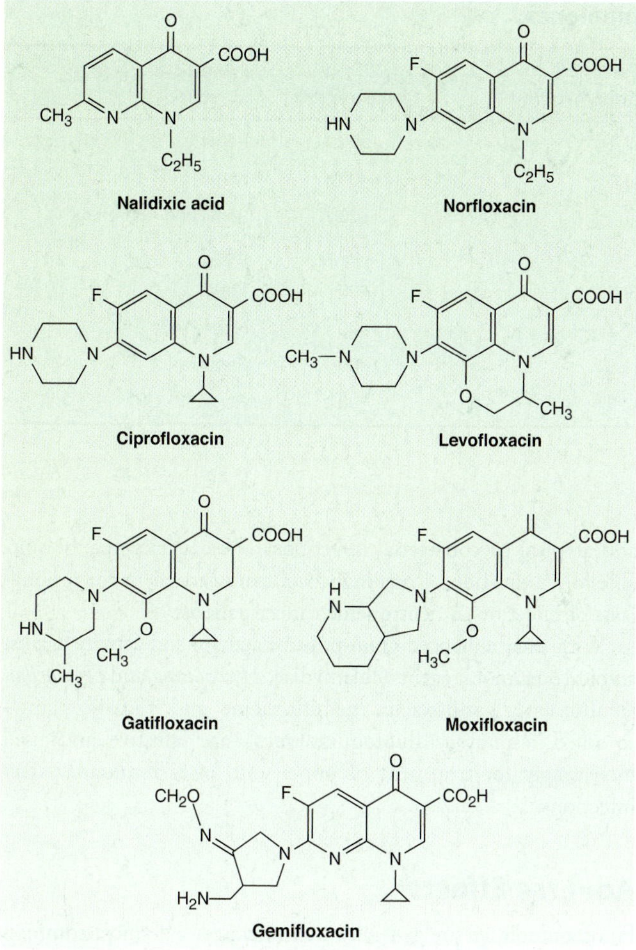

FIGURE 46–3 Structures of nalidixic acid and some fluoroquinolones.

Mechanism of Action

Quinolones block bacterial DNA synthesis by inhibiting bacterial topoisomerase II (DNA gyrase) and topoisomerase IV. Inhibition of DNA gyrase prevents the relaxation of positively supercoiled DNA that is required for normal transcription and replication. Inhibition of topoisomerase IV interferes with separation of replicated chromosomal DNA into the respective daughter cells during cell division.

Antibacterial Activity

Earlier quinolones such as nalidixic acid did not achieve systemic antibacterial levels and were useful only in the treatment of lower urinary tract infections. Fluorinated derivatives (ciprofloxacin, levofloxacin, and others; Figure 46–3 and Table 46–2) have greatly improved antibacterial activity compared with nalidixic acid and achieve bactericidal levels in blood and tissues.

Fluoroquinolones were originally developed because of their excellent activity against gram-negative aerobic bacteria; they had limited activity against gram-positive organisms. Several newer agents have improved activity against gram-positive cocci. This relative activity against gram-negative versus gram-positive species is useful for classification of these agents. Norfloxacin is the least active of the fluoroquinolones against both gram-negative and gram-positive organisms, with minimum inhibitory concentrations (MICs) fourfold to eightfold higher than those of ciprofloxacin. Ciprofloxacin, enoxacin, lomefloxacin, levofloxacin, ofloxacin, and pefloxacin comprise a second group of similar agents possessing excellent gram-negative activity and moderate to good activity against gram-positive bacteria. MICs for gram-negative cocci and bacilli, including *Enterobacter* sp, *P aeruginosa*, *Neisseria meningitidis*, *Haemophilus* sp, and *Campylobacter jejuni*, are 1–2 mcg/mL and often less. Methicillin-susceptible strains of *S aureus* are generally susceptible to these fluoroquinolones, but methicillin-resistant strains of staphylococci are often resistant. Streptococci and enterococci tend to be less susceptible than staphylococci, and efficacy in infections caused by these organisms is limited. Ciprofloxacin is the most active agent of this group against gram-negative organisms, *P aeruginosa* in particular. Levofloxacin, the L-isomer of ofloxacin, has superior activity against gram-positive organisms, including *Streptococcus pneumoniae.*

Gatifloxacin, gemifloxacin, and moxifloxacin make up a third group of fluoroquinolones with improved activity against gram-positive organisms, particularly *S pneumoniae* and some staphylococci. Gemifloxacin is active in vitro against ciprofloxacin-resistant strains of *S pneumoniae,* but in vivo efficacy is unproven. Although MICs of these agents for staphylococci are lower than those of ciprofloxacin (and the other compounds mentioned in the paragraph above), it is not known whether the enhanced activity is sufficient to permit use of these agents for treatment of infections caused by ciprofloxacin-resistant strains. In general, none of these agents is as active as ciprofloxacin against gram-negative organisms. Fluoroquinolones also are active against agents of atypical pneumonia (eg, mycoplasmas and chlamydiae) and against intracellular pathogens such as *Legionella pneumophila* and some mycobacteria, including *Mycobacterium tuberculosis* and *Mycobacterium avium* complex. Moxifloxacin also has modest activity against anaerobic bacteria. Because of toxicity, gatifloxacin is no longer available in the United States.

Resistance

During fluoroquinolone therapy, resistant organisms emerge in about one of every 10^7–10^9 organisms, especially among staphylococci, *P aeruginosa*, and *Serratia marcescens*. Resistance is due to one or more point mutations in the quinolone binding region of the target enzyme or to a change in the permeability of the organism. However, this does not account for the relative ease with which resistance develops in exquisitely susceptible bacteria. More recently two types of plasmid-mediated resistance have been described. The first type utilizes Qnr proteins, which protect DNA gyrase from the fluoroquinolones. The second is a variant of an aminoglycoside acetyltransferase capable of modifying ciprofloxacin. Both mechanisms confer low-level resistance that may facilitate the point mutations that confer high-level resistance. Resistance to one fluoroquinolone, particularly if it is of high level, generally confers cross-resistance to all other members of this class.

TABLE 46–2 Pharmacokinetic properties of some fluoroquinolones.

Drug	Half-Life (h)	Oral Bioavailability (%)	Peak Serum Concentration (mcg/mL)	Oral Dose (mg)	Primary Route of Excretion
Ciprofloxacin	3–5	70	2.4	500	Renal
Gatifloxacin	8	98	3.4	400	Renal
Gemifloxacin	8	70	1.6	320	Renal and nonrenal
Levofloxacin	5–7	95	5.7	500	Renal
Lomefloxacin	8	95	2.8	400	Renal
Moxifloxacin	9–10	> 85	3.1	400	Nonrenal
Norfloxacin	3.5–5	80	1.5	400	Renal
Ofloxacin	5–7	95	2.9	400	Renal

Pharmacokinetics

After oral administration, the fluoroquinolones are well absorbed (bioavailability of 80–95%) and distributed widely in body fluids and tissues (Table 46–2). Serum half-lives range from 3 to 10 hours. The relatively long half-lives of levofloxacin, gemifloxacin, gatifloxacin, and moxifloxacin permit once-daily dosing. Oral absorption is impaired by divalent and trivalent cations, including those in antacids. Therefore, oral fluoroquinolones should be taken 2 hours before or 4 hours after any products containing these cations. Serum concentrations of intravenously administered drug are similar to those of orally administered drug. Most fluoroquinolones are eliminated by renal mechanisms, either tubular secretion or glomerular filtration (Table 46–2). Dosage adjustment is required for patients with creatinine clearances less than 50 mL/min, the exact adjustment depending on the degree of renal impairment and the specific fluoroquinolone being used. Dosage adjustment for renal failure is not necessary for moxifloxacin. Nonrenally cleared fluoroquinolones are relatively contraindicated in patients with hepatic failure.

Clinical Uses

Fluoroquinolones (other than moxifloxacin, which achieves relatively low urinary levels) are effective in urinary tract infections caused by many organisms, including *P aeruginosa*. These agents are also effective for bacterial diarrhea caused by *Shigella, Salmonella,* toxigenic *E coli,* and *Campylobacter.* Fluoroquinolones (except norfloxacin, which does not achieve adequate systemic concentrations) have been used in infections of soft tissues, bones, and joints and in intra-abdominal and respiratory tract infections, including those caused by multidrug-resistant organisms such as *Pseudomonas* and *Enterobacter.* Ciprofloxacin is a drug of choice for prophylaxis and treatment of anthrax, although the newer fluoroquinolones are active in vitro and very likely in vivo as well.

Ciprofloxacin and levofloxacin are no longer recommended for the treatment of gonococcal infection in the United States as resistance is now common. However, both drugs are effective in treating chlamydial urethritis or cervicitis. Ciprofloxacin, levofloxacin, or moxifloxacin is occasionally used for treatment of tuberculosis

and atypical mycobacterial infections. These agents may be suitable for eradication of meningococci from carriers or for prophylaxis of infection in neutropenic cancer patients.

With their enhanced gram-positive activity and activity against atypical pneumonia agents (chlamydiae, *Mycoplasma,* and *Legionella*), levofloxacin, gatifloxacin, gemifloxacin, and moxifloxacin—so-called respiratory fluoroquinolones—are effective and used increasingly for treatment of upper and lower respiratory tract infections.

Adverse Effects

Fluoroquinolones are generally well tolerated. The most common effects are nausea, vomiting, and diarrhea. Occasionally, headache, dizziness, insomnia, skin rash, or abnormal liver function tests develop. Photosensitivity has been reported with lomefloxacin and pefloxacin. QT_c prolongation may occur with gatifloxacin, levofloxacin, gemifloxacin, and moxifloxacin, which should be avoided or used with caution in patients with known QT_c interval prolongation or uncorrected hypokalemia; in those receiving class IA (eg, quinidine or procainamide) or class III antiarrhythmic agents (sotalol, ibutilide, amiodarone); and in patients receiving other agents known to increase the QT_c interval (eg, erythromycin, tricyclic antidepressants). Gatifloxacin has been associated with hyperglycemia in diabetic patients and with hypoglycemia in patients also receiving oral hypoglycemic agents. Because of these serious effects (including some fatalities), gatifloxacin was withdrawn from sales in the United States in 2006; it may be available elsewhere.

Fluoroquinolones may damage growing cartilage and cause an arthropathy. Thus, these drugs are not routinely recommended for patients under 18 years of age. However, the arthropathy is reversible, and there is a growing consensus that fluoroquinolones may be used in children in some cases (eg, for treatment of pseudomonal infections in patients with cystic fibrosis). Tendonitis, a rare complication that has been reported in adults, is potentially more serious because of the risk of tendon rupture. Risk factors for tendonitis include advanced age, renal insufficiency, and concurrent steroid use. Fluoroquinolones should be avoided during pregnancy in the absence of specific data documenting their safety.

SUMMARY Sulfonamides, Trimethoprim, and Fluoroquinolones

Subclass	Mechanism of Action	Effects	Clinical Applications	Pharmacokinetics, Toxicities, Interactions
FOLATE ANTAGONISTS				
• Trimethoprim-sulfamethoxazole	Synergistic combination of folate antagonists blocks purine production and nucleic acid synthesis	Bactericidal activity against susceptible bacteria	Urinary tract infections • *P jiroveci* pneumonia • toxoplasmosis • nocardiosis	Oral, IV • renal clearance (half-life 8 h) • dosed every 8–12 h • formulated in a 5:1 ratio of sulfamethoxazole to trimethoprim • *Toxicity:* Rash, fever, bone marrow suppression, hyperkalemia

- *Sulfisoxazole: Oral; used only for lower urinary tract infections*
- *Sulfadiazine: Oral; first-line therapy for toxoplasmosis when combined with pyrimethamine*
- *Trimethoprim: Oral; used only for lower urinary tract infections; may be safely prescribed to patients with sulfonamide allergy*
- *Pyrimethamine: Oral; first-line therapy for toxoplasmosis when combined with sulfadiazine; coadminister with leucovorin to limit bone marrow toxicity*
- *Pyrimethamine-sulfadoxine: Oral; second-line malaria treatment*

FLUOROQUINOLONES				
• Ciprofloxacin	Inhibits DNA replication by binding to DNA gyrase and topoisomerase IV	Bactericidal activity against susceptible bacteria	Urinary tract infections • gastroenteritis • osteomyelitis • anthrax	Oral, IV • mixed clearance (half-life 4 h) • dosed every 12 h • divalent and trivalent cations impair oral absorption • *Toxicity:* Gastrointestinal upset, neurotoxicity, tendonitis

- *Ofloxacin: Oral; has improved pharmacokinetics and pharmacodynamics; use is limited to urinary tract infections and nongonococcal urethritis and cervicitis*
- *Levofloxacin: Oral, IV; L-isomer of ofloxacin; once-daily dosing; renal clearance; "respiratory" fluoroquinolone with improved activity versus pneumococcus*
- *Moxifloxacin: Oral, IV; "respiratory" fluoroquinolone; once-daily dosing; improved activity versus anaerobes and M tuberculosis; hepatic clearance results in lower urinary levels so use in urinary tract infections is not recommended*
- *Gemifloxacin: Oral; "respiratory" fluoroquinolone*

PREPARATIONS AVAILABLE

GENERAL-PURPOSE SULFONAMIDES

Sulfadiazine (generic)
Oral: 500 mg tablets

Sulfisoxazole (generic)
Oral: 500 mg tablets; 500 mg/5 mL syrup

SULFONAMIDES FOR SPECIAL APPLICATIONS

Mafenide (Sulfamylon)
Topical: 85 mg/g cream; 5% solution

Silver sulfadiazine (generic, Silvadene)
Topical: 10 mg/g cream

Sulfacetamide sodium (generic)
Ophthalmic: 1, 10, 15, 30% solutions; 10% ointment

TRIMETHOPRIM

Trimethoprim (generic, Proloprim, Trimpex)
Oral: 100, 200 mg tablets

Trimethoprim-sulfamethoxazole [co-trimoxazole, TMP-SMZ] (generic, Bactrim, Septra, others)
Oral: 80 mg trimethoprim + 400 mg sulfamethoxazole per single-strength tablet; 160 mg trimethoprim + 800 mg sulfamethoxazole per double-strength tablet; 40 mg trimethoprim + 200 mg sulfamethoxazole per 5 mL suspension
Parenteral: 80 mg trimethoprim + 400 mg sulfamethoxazole per 5 mL for infusion (in 5 mL ampules and 5, 10, 20 mL vials)

PYRIMETHAMINE

Pyrimethamine (generic, Daraprim)
Oral: 25 mg tablets

Pyrimethamine-sulfadoxine (Fansidar)
Oral: 25 mg pyrimethamine + 500 mg sulfadoxine per tablet

QUINOLONES & FLUOROQUINOLONES

Ciprofloxacin (generic, Cipro, Cipro I.V.)
Oral: 100, 250, 500, 750 mg tablets; 500, 1000 mg extended-release tablet; 50, 100 mg/mL suspension
Parenteral: 10 mg/mL for IV infusion
Ophthalmic (Ciloxan): 3 mg/mL solution; 3.3 mg/g ointment

Gemifloxacin (Factive)
Oral: 320 mg tablet

Levofloxacin (Levaquin)
Oral: 250, 500, 750 mg tablets; 25 mg/mL solution
Parenteral: 5, 25 mg/mL for IV injection
Ophthalmic (Quixin): 5 mg/mL solution

Lomefloxacin (Maxaquin)
Oral: 400 mg tablets

Moxifloxacin (Avelox, Avelox I.V.)
Oral: 400 mg tablets
Parenteral: 400 mg in IV bag

Norfloxacin (Noroxin)
Oral: 400 mg tablets

Ofloxacin (Floxin)
Oral: 200, 300, 400 mg tablets
Ophthalmic (Ocuflox): 3 mg/mL solution
Otic (Floxin Otic): 0.3% solution

REFERENCES

Davidson R et al: Resistance to levofloxacin and failure of treatment of pneumococcal pneumonia. N Engl J Med 2002;346:747.

Frothingham R: Rates of torsades de pointes associated with ciprofloxacin, ofloxacin, levofloxacin, gatifloxacin, and moxifloxacin. Pharmacotherapy 2001;21:1468.

Keating GM, Scott LJ: Moxifloxacin: A review of its use in the management of bacterial infections. Drugs 2004;64:2347.

Mandell LA et al: Update of practice guidelines for the management of community-acquired pneumonia in immunocompetent adults. Clin Infect Dis 2003;37:1405.

Mwenya DM et al: Impact of cotrimoxazole on carriage and antibiotic resistance of Streptococcus pneumoniae and Haemophilus influenzae in HIV-infected children in Zambia. Antimicrob Agents Chemother 2010;54:3756

Nouira S et al: Standard versus newer antibacterial agents in the treatment of severe acute exacerbation of chronic obstructive pulmonary disease: A randomized trial of trimethoprim-sulfamethoxazole versus ciprofloxacin. Clin Infect Dis 2010;51:143.

Robicsek A et al: The worldwide emergence of plasmid-mediated quinolone resistance. Lancet ID 2006;6:629.

Scheld WM: Maintaining fluoroquinolone class efficacy: Review of influencing factors. Emerg Infect Dis 2003;9:1.

Schmitz GR et al: Randomized controlled trial of trimethoprim-sulfamethoxazole for uncomplicated skin abscesses in patients at risk for community-associated methicillin-resistant Staphylococcus aureus infection. Ann Emerg Med 2010;56:283.

Strom BL et al: Absence of cross-reactivity between sulfonamide antibiotics and sulfonamide nonantibiotics. N Engl J Med 2003;349:1628.

Talan DA et al: Prevalence of and risk factor analysis of trimethoprim-sulfamethoxazole- and fluoroquinolone-resistant E. coli infection among emergency department patients with pyelonephritis. Clin Infect Dis 2008; 47:1150.

Yoo BK et al: Gemifloxacin: A new fluoroquinolone approved for treatment of respiratory infections. Ann Pharmacother 2004;38:1226.

CASE STUDY ANSWER

A fluoroquinolone that achieves good urinary levels (ciprofloxacin or levofloxacin) would be a reasonable choice for empiric treatment of this patient's complicated urinary tract infection. Her recent exposure to multiple courses of trimethoprim-sulfamethoxazole increases her chances of having a urinary tract infection with an isolate that is resistant to this antibiotic, making trimethoprim-sulfamethoxazole a poor choice. The patient should be told to take the oral fluoroquinolone 2 hours before or 4 hours after her calcium supplement as divalent and trivalent cations can significantly impair the absorption of oral fluoroquinolones.

47

Antimycobacterial Drugs

Daniel H. Deck, PharmD, & Lisa G. Winston, MD*

C A S E   S T U D Y

A 45-year-old homeless man presents to the emergency department complaining of a 2-month history of fatigue, weight loss (10 kg), fevers, night sweats, and a productive cough. He is currently living on the street but has spent time in homeless shelters and prison in the last several years. He reports drinking 2–3 pints of hard alcohol per day for the last 15 years, and also reports a history of intravenous drug use. In the emergency department, a chest x-ray shows a right

apical infiltrate. Given the high suspicion for pulmonary tuberculosis, the patient is placed in respiratory isolation. His first sputum smear shows many acid-fast bacilli, and a rapid HIV antibody test returns with a positive result. What drugs should be started for treatment of presumptive pulmonary tuberculosis? Does the patient have a heightened risk of developing medication toxicity? If so, which medication(s) would be likely to cause toxicity?

Mycobacteria are intrinsically resistant to most antibiotics. Because they grow more slowly than other bacteria, antibiotics that are most active against rapidly growing cells are relatively ineffective. Mycobacterial cells can also be dormant and thus completely resistant to many drugs or killed only very slowly. The lipid-rich mycobacterial cell wall is impermeable to many agents. Mycobacterial species are intracellular pathogens, and organisms residing within macrophages are inaccessible to drugs that penetrate these cells poorly. Finally, mycobacteria are notorious for their ability to develop resistance. Combinations of two or more drugs are required to overcome these obstacles and to prevent emergence of resistance during the course of therapy. The response of mycobacterial infections to chemotherapy is slow, and treatment must be administered for months to years, depending on which drugs are used. The drugs used to treat tuberculosis, atypical mycobacterial infections, and leprosy are described in this chapter.

■ DRUGS USED IN TUBERCULOSIS

Isoniazid (INH), rifampin (or other rifamycin), pyrazinamide, ethambutol, and **streptomycin** are the five first-line agents for treatment of tuberculosis (Table 47–1). Isoniazid and rifampin are the most active drugs. An isoniazid-rifampin combination administered for 9 months will cure 95–98% of cases of tuberculosis caused by susceptible strains. The addition of pyrazinamide to an isoniazid-rifampin combination for the first 2 months allows the total duration of therapy to be reduced to 6 months without loss of efficacy (Table 47–2). In practice, therapy is initiated with a four-drug regimen of isoniazid, rifampin, and pyrazinamide plus either ethambutol or streptomycin until susceptibility of the clinical isolate has been determined. Neither ethambutol nor streptomycin adds substantially to the overall activity of the regimen (ie, the duration of treatment cannot be further reduced if either drug is used), but they provide additional coverage if the isolate proves to be resistant to isoniazid, rifampin, or both. The prevalence of isoniazid resistance among clinical isolates in the United States is approximately 10%. Prevalence of resistance to both isoniazid and rifampin (ie, multidrug resistance) is about 3%.

---

*The authors thank Henry F. Chambers, MD, for his contributions to previous editions.

TABLE 47–1 Antimicrobials used in the treatment of tuberculosis.

Drug	Typical Adult Dosage[1]
First-line agents (in approximate order of preference)	
Isoniazid	300 mg/d
Rifampin	600 mg/d
Pyrazinamide	25 mg/kg/d
Ethambutol	15–25 mg/kg/d
Streptomycin	15 mg/kg/d
Second-line agents	
Amikacin	15 mg/kg/d
Aminosalicylic acid	8–12 g/d
Capreomycin	15 mg/kg/d
Ciprofloxacin	1500 mg/d, divided
Clofazimine	200 mg/d
Cycloserine	500–1000 mg/d, divided
Ethionamide	500–750 mg/d
Levofloxacin	500 mg/d
Rifabutin	300 mg/d[2]
Rifapentine	600 mg once or twice weekly

[1]Assuming normal renal function.

[2]150 mg/d if used concurrently with a protease inhibitor.

TABLE 47–2 Recommended duration of therapy for tuberculosis.

Regimen (in Approximate Order of Preference)	Duration in Months
Isoniazid, rifampin, pyrazinamide	6
Isoniazid, rifampin	9
Rifampin, ethambutol, pyrazinamide	6
Rifampin, ethambutol	12
Isoniazid, ethambutol	18
All others	≥ 24

ISONIAZID

Isoniazid is the most active drug for the treatment of tuberculosis caused by susceptible strains. It is a small molecule (MW 137) that is freely soluble in water. The structural similarity to pyridoxine is shown below.

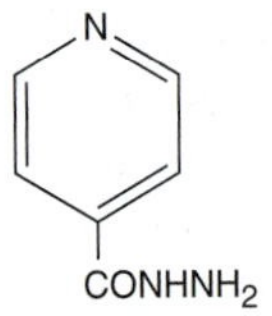

Isoniazid

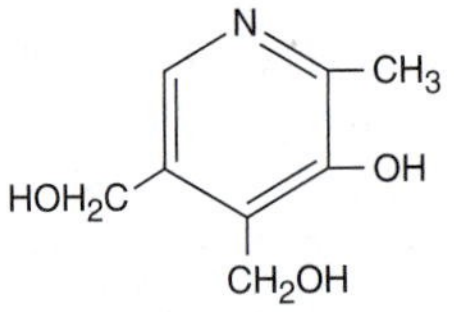

Pyridoxine

In vitro, isoniazid inhibits most tubercle bacilli at a concentration of 0.2 mcg/mL or less and is bactericidal for actively growing tubercle bacilli. It is less effective against atypical mycobacterial species. Isoniazid penetrates into macrophages and is active against both extracellular and intracellular organisms.

Mechanism of Action & Basis of Resistance

Isoniazid inhibits synthesis of mycolic acids, which are essential components of mycobacterial cell walls. Isoniazid is a prodrug that is activated by KatG, the mycobacterial catalase-peroxidase. The activated form of isoniazid forms a covalent complex with an acyl carrier protein (AcpM) and KasA, a beta-ketoacyl carrier protein synthetase, which blocks mycolic acid synthesis and kills the cell. Resistance to isoniazid is associated with mutations resulting in overexpression of *inhA*, which encodes an NADH-dependent acyl carrier protein reductase; mutation or deletion of the *katG* gene; promoter mutations resulting in overexpression of *ahpC*, a putative virulence gene involved in protection of the cell from oxidative stress; and mutations in *kasA*. Overproducers of *inhA* express low-level isoniazid resistance and cross-resistance to ethionamide. *KatG* mutants express high-level isoniazid resistance and often are not cross-resistant to ethionamide.

Drug-resistant mutants are normally present in susceptible mycobacterial populations at about 1 bacillus in 10^6. Since tuberculous lesions often contain more than 10^8 tubercle bacilli, resistant mutants are readily selected if isoniazid or any other drug is given as a single agent. The use of two independently acting drugs in combination is much more effective. The probability that a bacillus is initially resistant to both drugs is approximately 1 in $10^6 \times 10^6$, or 1 in 10^{12}, several orders of magnitude greater than the number of infecting organisms. Thus, at least two (or more in certain cases) active agents should always be used to treat active tuberculosis to prevent emergence of resistance during therapy.

Pharmacokinetics

Isoniazid is readily absorbed from the gastrointestinal tract. A 300-mg oral dose (5 mg/kg in children) achieves peak plasma concentrations of 3–5 mcg/mL within 1–2 hours. Isoniazid diffuses readily into all body fluids and tissues. The concentration in the central nervous system and cerebrospinal fluid ranges between 20% and 100% of simultaneous serum concentrations.

Metabolism of isoniazid, especially acetylation by liver *N*-acetyltransferase, is genetically determined (see Chapter 4).

The average plasma concentration of isoniazid in rapid acetylators is about one third to one half of that in slow acetylators, and average half-lives are less than 1 hour and 3 hours, respectively. More rapid clearance of isoniazid by rapid acetylators is usually of no therapeutic consequence when appropriate doses are administered daily, but subtherapeutic concentrations may occur if drug is administered as a once-weekly dose or if there is malabsorption.

Isoniazid metabolites and a small amount of unchanged drug are excreted, mainly in the urine. The dose need not be adjusted in renal failure. Dose adjustment is not well defined in patients with severe preexisting hepatic insufficiency (isoniazid is contraindicated if it is the cause of the hepatitis) and should be guided by serum concentrations if a reduction in dose is contemplated.

Clinical Uses

The typical dosage of isoniazid is 5 mg/kg/d; a typical adult dose is 300 mg given once daily. Up to 10 mg/kg/d may be used for serious infections or if malabsorption is a problem. A 15 mg/kg dose, or 900 mg, may be used in a twice-weekly dosing regimen in combination with a second antituberculous agent (eg, rifampin 600 mg). Pyridoxine, 25–50 mg/d, is recommended for those with conditions predisposing to neuropathy, an adverse effect of isoniazid. Isoniazid is usually given by mouth but can be given parenterally in the same dosage.

Isoniazid as a single agent is also indicated for treatment of latent tuberculosis. The dosage is 300 mg/d (5 mg/kg/d) or 900 mg twice weekly for 9 months.

Adverse Reactions

The incidence and severity of untoward reactions to isoniazid are related to dosage and duration of administration.

A. Immunologic Reactions

Fever and skin rashes are occasionally seen. Drug-induced systemic lupus erythematosus has been reported.

B. Direct Toxicity

Isoniazid-induced hepatitis is the most common major toxic effect. This is distinct from the minor increases in liver aminotransferases (up to three or four times normal), which do not require cessation of the drug and which are seen in 10–20% of patients, who usually are asymptomatic. Clinical hepatitis with loss of appetite, nausea, vomiting, jaundice, and right upper quadrant pain occurs in 1% of isoniazid recipients and can be fatal, particularly if the drug is not discontinued promptly. There is histologic evidence of hepatocellular damage and necrosis. The risk of hepatitis depends on age. It occurs rarely under age 20, in 0.3% of those aged 21–35, 1.2% of those aged 36–50, and 2.3% for those aged 50 and above. The risk of hepatitis is greater in individuals with alcohol dependence and possibly during pregnancy and the postpartum period. Development of isoniazid hepatitis contraindicates further use of the drug.

Peripheral neuropathy is observed in 10–20% of patients given dosages greater than 5 mg/kg/d, but it is infrequently seen with the standard 300-mg adult dose. Peripheral neuropathy is more likely to occur in slow acetylators and patients with predisposing conditions such as malnutrition, alcoholism, diabetes, AIDS, and uremia. Neuropathy is due to a relative pyridoxine deficiency. Isoniazid promotes excretion of pyridoxine, and this toxicity is readily reversed by administration of pyridoxine in a dosage as low as 10 mg/d. Central nervous system toxicity, which is less common, includes memory loss, psychosis, and seizures. These effects may also respond to pyridoxine.

Miscellaneous other reactions include hematologic abnormalities, provocation of pyridoxine deficiency anemia, tinnitus, and gastrointestinal discomfort. Isoniazid can reduce the metabolism of phenytoin, increasing its blood level and toxicity.

RIFAMPIN

Rifampin is a semisynthetic derivative of rifamycin, an antibiotic produced by *Streptomyces mediterranei*. It is active in vitro against gram-positive and gram-negative cocci, some enteric bacteria, mycobacteria, and chlamydiae. Susceptible organisms are inhibited by less than 1 mcg/mL. Resistant mutants are present in all microbial populations at approximately 1 in 10^6 organisms and are rapidly selected out if rifampin is used as a single drug, especially in a patient with active infection. There is no cross-resistance to other classes of antimicrobial drugs, but there is cross-resistance to other rifamycin derivatives, eg, rifabutin and rifapentine.

Mechanism of Action, Resistance, & Pharmacokinetics

Rifampin binds to the β subunit of bacterial DNA-dependent RNA polymerase and thereby inhibits RNA synthesis. Resistance results from any one of several possible point mutations in *rpoB*, the gene for the β subunit of RNA polymerase. These mutations result in reduced binding of rifampin to RNA polymerase. Human RNA polymerase does not bind rifampin and is not inhibited by it. Rifampin is bactericidal for mycobacteria. It readily penetrates most tissues and penetrates into phagocytic cells. It can kill organisms that are poorly accessible to many other drugs, such as intracellular organisms and those sequestered in abscesses and lung cavities.

Rifampin is well absorbed after oral administration and excreted mainly through the liver into bile. It then undergoes enterohepatic recirculation, with the bulk excreted as a deacylated metabolite in feces and a small amount excreted in the urine. Dosage adjustment for renal or hepatic insufficiency is not necessary. Usual doses result in serum levels of 5–7 mcg/mL. Rifampin is distributed widely in body fluids and tissues. The drug is relatively highly protein-bound, and adequate cerebrospinal fluid concentrations are achieved only in the presence of meningeal inflammation.

Clinical Uses

A. Mycobacterial Infections

Rifampin, usually 600 mg/d (10 mg/kg/d) orally, must be administered with isoniazid or other antituberculous drugs to patients with active tuberculosis to prevent emergence of drug-resistant mycobacteria. In some short-course therapies, 600 mg of rifampin is given twice weekly. Rifampin, 600 mg daily or twice weekly for 6 months, also is effective in combination with other agents in some atypical mycobacterial infections and in leprosy. Rifampin, 600 mg daily for 4 months as a single drug, is an alternative to isoniazid for patients with latent tuberculosis who are unable to take isoniazid or who have had exposure to a case of active tuberculosis caused by an isoniazid-resistant, rifampin-susceptible strain.

B. Other Indications

Rifampin has other uses in bacterial infections. An oral dosage of 600 mg twice daily for 2 days can eliminate meningococcal carriage. Rifampin, 20 mg/kg/d for 4 days, is used as prophylaxis in contacts of children with *Haemophilus influenzae* type b disease. Rifampin combined with a second agent is used to eradicate staphylococcal carriage. Rifampin combination therapy is also indicated for treatment of serious staphylococcal infections such as osteomyelitis and prosthetic valve endocarditis.

Adverse Reactions

Rifampin imparts a harmless orange color to urine, sweat, and tears (soft contact lenses may be permanently stained). Occasional adverse effects include rashes, thrombocytopenia, and nephritis. Rifampin may cause cholestatic jaundice and occasionally hepatitis, and it commonly causes light-chain proteinuria. If administered less often than twice weekly, rifampin may cause a flu-like syndrome characterized by fever, chills, myalgias, anemia, and thrombocytopenia. Its use has been associated with acute tubular necrosis. Rifampin strongly induces most cytochrome P450 isoforms (1A2, 2C9, 2C19, 2D6, and 3A4), which increases the elimination of numerous other drugs including methadone, anticoagulants, cyclosporine, some anticonvulsants, protease inhibitors, some nonnucleoside reverse transcriptase inhibitors, contraceptives, and a host of others (see Chapters 4 and 66). Co-administration of rifampin results in significantly lower serum levels of these drugs.

ETHAMBUTOL

Ethambutol is a synthetic, water-soluble, heat-stable compound, the dextro-isomer of the structure shown below, dispensed as the dihydrochloride salt.

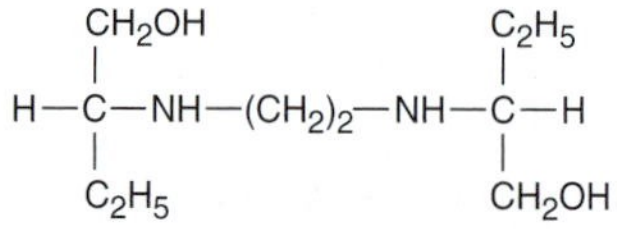

Ethambutol

Mechanism of Action & Clinical Uses

Susceptible strains of *Mycobacterium tuberculosis* and other mycobacteria are inhibited in vitro by ethambutol, 1–5 mcg/mL. Ethambutol inhibits mycobacterial arabinosyl transferases, which

are encoded by the *embCAB* operon. Arabinosyl transferases are involved in the polymerization reaction of arabinoglycan, an essential component of the mycobacterial cell wall. Resistance to ethambutol is due to mutations resulting in overexpression of *emb* gene products or within the *embB* structural gene.

Ethambutol is well absorbed from the gut. After ingestion of 25 mg/kg, a blood level peak of 2–5 mcg/mL is reached in 2–4 hours. About 20% of the drug is excreted in feces and 50% in urine in unchanged form. Ethambutol accumulates in renal failure, and the dose should be reduced by half if creatinine clearance is less than 10 mL/min. Ethambutol crosses the blood-brain barrier only when the meninges are inflamed. Concentrations in cerebrospinal fluid are highly variable, ranging from 4% to 64% of serum levels in the setting of meningeal inflammation.

As with all antituberculous drugs, resistance to ethambutol emerges rapidly when the drug is used alone. Therefore, ethambutol is always given in combination with other antituberculous drugs.

Ethambutol hydrochloride, 15–25 mg/kg, is usually given as a single daily dose in combination with isoniazid or rifampin. The higher dose is recommended for treatment of tuberculous meningitis. The dose of ethambutol is 50 mg/kg when a twice-weekly dosing schedule is used.

Adverse Reactions

Hypersensitivity to ethambutol is rare. The most common serious adverse event is retrobulbar neuritis, resulting in loss of visual acuity and red-green color blindness. This dose-related adverse effect is more likely to occur at dosages of 25 mg/kg/d continued for several months. At 15 mg/kg/d or less, visual disturbances are very rare. Periodic visual acuity testing is desirable if the 25 mg/kg/d dosage is used. Ethambutol is relatively contraindicated in children too young to permit assessment of visual acuity and red-green color discrimination.

PYRAZINAMIDE

Pyrazinamide (PZA) is a relative of nicotinamide. It is stable and slightly soluble in water. It is inactive at neutral pH, but at pH 5.5 it inhibits tubercle bacilli at concentrations of approximately 20 mcg/mL. The drug is taken up by macrophages and exerts its activity against mycobacteria residing within the acidic environment of lysosomes.

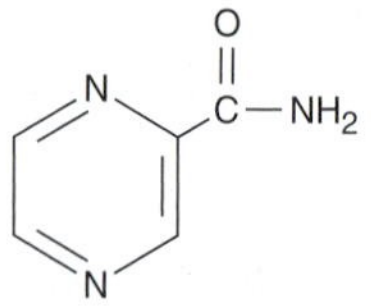

Pyrazinamide (PZA)

Mechanism of Action & Clinical Uses

Pyrazinamide is converted to pyrazinoic acid—the active form of the drug—by mycobacterial pyrazinamidase, which is encoded by *pncA*. The specific drug target is unknown, but pyrazinoic acid disrupts mycobacterial cell membrane metabolism and transport functions. Resistance may be due to impaired uptake of pyrazinamide or mutations in *pncA* that impair conversion of pyrazinamide to its active form.

Serum concentrations of 30–50 mcg/mL at 1–2 hours after oral administration are achieved with dosages of 25 mg/kg/d. Pyrazinamide is well absorbed from the gastrointestinal tract and widely distributed in body tissues, including inflamed meninges. The half-life is 8–11 hours. The parent compound is metabolized by the liver, but metabolites are renally cleared; therefore, pyrazinamide should be administered at 25–35 mg/kg three times weekly (not daily) in hemodialysis patients and those in whom the creatinine clearance is less than 30 mL/min. In patients with normal renal function, a dose of 40–50 mg/kg is used for thrice-weekly or twice-weekly treatment regimens.

Pyrazinamide is an important front-line drug used in conjunction with isoniazid and rifampin in short-course (ie, 6-month) regimens as a "sterilizing" agent active against residual intracellular organisms that may cause relapse. Tubercle bacilli develop resistance to pyrazinamide fairly readily, but there is no cross-resistance with isoniazid or other antimycobacterial drugs.

Adverse Reactions

Major adverse effects of pyrazinamide include hepatotoxicity (in 1–5% of patients), nausea, vomiting, drug fever, and hyperuricemia. The latter occurs uniformly and is not a reason to halt therapy. Hyperuricemia may provoke acute gouty arthritis.

STREPTOMYCIN

The mechanism of action and other pharmacologic features of streptomycin are discussed in Chapter 45. The typical adult dose is 1 g/d (15 mg/kg/d). If the creatinine clearance is less than 30 mL/min or the patient is on hemodialysis, the dose is 15 mg/kg two or three times per week. Most tubercle bacilli are inhibited by streptomycin, 1–10 mcg/mL, in vitro. Nontuberculosis species of mycobacteria other than *Mycobacterium avium* complex (MAC) and *Mycobacterium kansasii* are resistant. All large populations of tubercle bacilli contain some streptomycin-resistant mutants. On average, 1 in 10^8 tubercle bacilli can be expected to be resistant to streptomycin at levels of 10–100 mcg/mL. Resistance is due to a point mutation in either the *rpsL* gene encoding the S12 ribosomal protein gene or the *rrs* gene encoding 16S ribosomal rRNA, which alters the ribosomal binding site.

Streptomycin penetrates into cells poorly and is active mainly against extracellular tubercle bacilli. Streptomycin crosses the blood-brain barrier and achieves therapeutic concentrations with inflamed meninges.

Clinical Use in Tuberculosis

Streptomycin sulfate is used when an injectable drug is needed or desirable and in the treatment of infections resistant to other drugs. The usual dosage is 15 mg/kg/d intramuscularly or intravenously daily for adults (20–40 mg/kg/d, not to exceed 1–1.5 g for children) for several weeks, followed by 1–1.5 g two or three times weekly for several months. Serum concentrations of approximately 40 mcg/mL are achieved 30–60 minutes after intramuscular injection of a 15 mg/kg dose. Other drugs are always given in combination to prevent emergence of resistance.

Adverse Reactions

Streptomycin is ototoxic and nephrotoxic. Vertigo and hearing loss are the most common adverse effects and may be permanent. Toxicity is dose-related, and the risk is increased in the elderly. As with all aminoglycosides, the dose must be adjusted according to renal function (see Chapter 45). Toxicity can be reduced by limiting therapy to no more than 6 months whenever possible.

SECOND-LINE DRUGS FOR TUBERCULOSIS

The alternative drugs listed below are usually considered only (1) in case of resistance to first-line agents; (2) in case of failure of clinical response to conventional therapy; and (3) in case of serious treatment-limiting adverse drug reactions. Expert guidance to deal with the toxic effects of these second-line drugs is desirable. For many drugs listed in the following text, the dosage, emergence of resistance, and long-term toxicity have not been fully established.

Ethionamide

Ethionamide is chemically related to isoniazid and similarly blocks the synthesis of mycolic acids. It is poorly water soluble and available only in oral form. It is metabolized by the liver.

Ethionamide

Most tubercle bacilli are inhibited in vitro by ethionamide, 2.5 mcg/mL or less. Some other species of mycobacteria also are inhibited by ethionamide, 10 mcg/mL. Serum concentrations in plasma and tissues of approximately 20 mcg/mL are achieved by a dosage of 1 g/d. Cerebrospinal fluid concentrations are equal to those in serum.

Ethionamide is administered at an initial dose of 250 mg once daily, which is increased in 250-mg increments to the recommended dosage of 1 g/d (or 15 mg/kg/d), if possible. The 1 g/d dosage, though theoretically desirable, is poorly tolerated because of the intense gastric irritation and neurologic symptoms that commonly occur, and one often must settle for a total daily dose of 500–750 mg. Ethionamide is also hepatotoxic. Neurologic symptoms may be alleviated by pyridoxine.

Resistance to ethionamide as a single agent develops rapidly in vitro and in vivo. There can be low-level cross-resistance between isoniazid and ethionamide.

Capreomycin

Capreomycin is a peptide protein synthesis inhibitor antibiotic obtained from *Streptomyces capreolus*. Daily injection of 1 g intramuscularly results in blood levels of 10 mcg/mL or more. Such concentrations in vitro are inhibitory for many mycobacteria, including multidrug-resistant strains of *M tuberculosis*.

Capreomycin (15 mg/kg/d) is an important injectable agent for treatment of drug-resistant tuberculosis. Strains of *M tuberculosis* that are resistant to streptomycin or amikacin usually are susceptible to capreomycin. Resistance to capreomycin, when it occurs, may be due to an *rrs* mutation.

Capreomycin is nephrotoxic and ototoxic. Tinnitus, deafness, and vestibular disturbances occur. The injection causes significant local pain, and sterile abscesses may occur.

Dosing of capreomycin is the same as that of streptomycin. Toxicity is reduced if 1 g is given two or three times weekly after an initial response has been achieved with a daily dosing schedule.

Cycloserine

Cycloserine is an inhibitor of cell wall synthesis and is discussed in Chapter 43. Concentrations of 15–20 mcg/mL inhibit many strains of *M tuberculosis*. The dosage of cycloserine in tuberculosis is 0.5–1 g/d in two divided oral doses. Cycloserine is cleared renally, and the dose should be reduced by half if creatinine clearance is less than 50 mL/min.

The most serious toxic effects are peripheral neuropathy and central nervous system dysfunction, including depression and psychotic reactions. Pyridoxine, 150 mg/d, should be given with cycloserine because this ameliorates neurologic toxicity. Adverse effects, which are most common during the first 2 weeks of therapy, occur in 25% or more of patients, especially at higher doses. Adverse effects can be minimized by monitoring peak serum concentrations. The peak concentration is reached 2–4 hours after dosing. The recommended range of peak concentrations is 20–40 mcg/mL.

Aminosalicylic Acid (PAS)

Aminosalicylic acid is a folate synthesis antagonist that is active almost exclusively against *M tuberculosis*. It is structurally similar to *p*-aminobenzoic acid (PABA) and to the sulfonamides (see Chapter 46).

Aminosalicylic acid (PAS)

Tubercle bacilli are usually inhibited in vitro by aminosalicylic acid, 1–5 mcg/mL. Aminosalicylic acid is readily absorbed from the gastrointestinal tract. Serum levels are 50 mcg/mL or more after a 4-g oral dose. The dosage is 8–12 g/d orally for adults and 300 mg/kg/d for children. The drug is widely distributed in tissues and body fluids except the cerebrospinal fluid. Aminosalicylic acid is rapidly excreted in the urine, in part as active aminosalicylic acid and in part as the acetylated compound and other metabolic products. Very high concentrations of aminosalicylic acid are reached in the urine, which can result in crystalluria.

Aminosalicylic acid is used infrequently because other oral drugs are better tolerated. Gastrointestinal symptoms are common and may be diminished by giving the drug with meals and with antacids. Peptic ulceration and hemorrhage may occur. Hypersensitivity reactions manifested by fever, joint pains, skin rashes, hepatosplenomegaly, hepatitis, adenopathy, and granulocytopenia often occur after 3–8 weeks of aminosalicylic acid therapy, making it necessary to stop aminosalicylic acid administration temporarily or permanently.

Kanamycin & Amikacin

The aminoglycoside antibiotics are discussed in Chapter 45. Kanamycin has been used for treatment of tuberculosis caused by streptomycin-resistant strains, but the availability of less toxic alternatives (eg, capreomycin and amikacin) has rendered it obsolete.

The role of amikacin in treatment of tuberculosis has increased with the increasing incidence and prevalence of multidrug-resistant tuberculosis. Prevalence of amikacin-resistant strains is low (< 5%), and most multidrug-resistant strains remain amikacin-susceptible. *M tuberculosis* is inhibited at concentrations of 1 mcg/mL or less. Amikacin is also active against atypical mycobacteria. There is no cross-resistance between streptomycin and amikacin, but kanamycin resistance often indicates resistance to amikacin as well. Serum concentrations of 30–50 mcg/mL are achieved 30–60 minutes after a 15 mg/kg intravenous infusion. Amikacin is indicated for treatment of tuberculosis suspected or known to be caused by streptomycin-resistant or multidrug-resistant strains. Amikacin must be used in combination with at least one and preferably two or three other drugs to which the isolate is susceptible for treatment of drug-resistant cases. The recommended dosages are the same as those for streptomycin.

Fluoroquinolones

In addition to their activity against many gram-positive and gram-negative bacteria (discussed in Chapter 46), ciprofloxacin, levofloxacin, gatifloxacin, and moxifloxacin inhibit strains of *M tuberculosis* at concentrations less than 2 mcg/mL. They are also active against atypical mycobacteria. Moxifloxacin is the most active against *M tuberculosis* by weight in vitro. Levofloxacin tends to be slightly more active than ciprofloxacin against *M tuberculosis*, whereas ciprofloxacin is slightly more active against atypical mycobacteria.

Fluoroquinolones are an important addition to the drugs available for tuberculosis, especially for strains that are resistant to first-line agents. Resistance, which may result from any one of several single point mutations in the gyrase A subunit, develops rapidly if a fluoroquinolone is used as a single agent; thus, the drug must be used in combination with two or more other active

agents. The standard dosage of ciprofloxacin is 750 mg orally twice a day. The dosage of levofloxacin is 500–750 mg once a day. The dosage of moxifloxacin is 400 mg once a day.

Linezolid

Linezolid (discussed in Chapter 44) inhibits strains of *M tuberculosis* in vitro at concentrations of 4–8 mcg/mL. It achieves good intracellular concentrations, and it is active in murine models of tuberculosis. Linezolid has been used in combination with other second- and third-line drugs to treat patients with tuberculosis caused by multidrug-resistant strains. Conversion of sputum cultures to negative was associated with linezolid use in these cases, and some may have been cured. Significant and at times treatment-limiting adverse effects, including bone marrow suppression and irreversible peripheral and optic neuropathy, have been reported with the prolonged courses of therapy that are necessary for treatment of tuberculosis. A 600-mg (adult) dose administered once a day (half of that used for treatment of other bacterial infections) seems to be sufficient and may limit the occurrence of these adverse effects. Although linezolid may eventually prove to be an important new agent for treatment of tuberculosis, at this point it should be considered a drug of last resort for infection caused by multidrug-resistant strains that also are resistant to several other first- and second-line agents.

Rifabutin

Rifabutin is derived from rifamycin and is related to rifampin. It has significant activity against *M tuberculosis*, MAC, and *Mycobacterium fortuitum* (see below). Its activity is similar to that of rifampin, and cross-resistance with rifampin is virtually complete. Some rifampin-resistant strains may appear susceptible to rifabutin in vitro, but a clinical response is unlikely because the molecular basis of resistance, *rpoB* mutation, is the same. Rifabutin is both substrate and inducer of cytochrome P450 enzymes. Because it is a less potent inducer, rifabutin is indicated in place of rifampin for treatment of tuberculosis in patients with HIV infection who are receiving antiretroviral therapy with a protease inhibitor or with a nonnucleoside reverse transcriptase inhibitor (eg, efavirenz), drugs that also are cytochrome P450 substrates.

The typical dosage of rifabutin is 300 mg/d unless the patient is receiving a protease inhibitor, in which case the dosage should be reduced to 150 mg/d. If efavirenz (also a cytochrome P450 inducer) is used, the recommended dosage of rifabutin is 450 mg/d.

Rifabutin is effective in prevention and treatment of disseminated atypical mycobacterial infection in AIDS patients with CD4 counts below 50/μL. It is also effective for preventive therapy of tuberculosis, either alone in a 3–4 month regimen or with pyrazinamide in a 2-month regimen.

Rifapentine

Rifapentine is an analog of rifampin. It is active against both *M tuberculosis* and MAC. As with all rifamycins, it is a bacterial RNA polymerase inhibitor, and cross-resistance between rifampin and rifapentine is complete. Like rifampin, rifapentine is a potent inducer of cytochrome P450 enzymes, and it has the same drug interaction profile. Toxicity is similar to that of rifampin. Rifapentine and its microbiologically active metabolite, 25-desacetylrifapentine, have an elimination half-life of 13 hours. Rifapentine, 600 mg (10 mg/kg) once weekly, is indicated for treatment of tuberculosis caused by rifampin-susceptible strains during the continuation phase only (ie, after the first 2 months of therapy and ideally after conversion of sputum cultures to negative). Rifapentine should not be used to treat patients with HIV infection because of an unacceptably high relapse rate with rifampin-resistant organisms.

■ RIFAXIMIN

Rifaximin is a rifampin derivative that is not absorbed from the gastrointestinal tract. It is approved for oral administration in the prevention of hepatic encephalopathy and for the treatment of travelers' diarrhea caused by noninvasive strains of *Escherichia coli* in patients 12 years of age and older. It has also been used off label for irritable bowel syndrome and for *Clostridium difficile* colitis not responsive to other drugs.

■ DRUGS ACTIVE AGAINST ATYPICAL MYCOBACTERIA

About 10% of mycobacterial infections seen in clinical practice in the United States are caused by nontuberculous or "atypical" mycobacteria. These organisms have distinctive laboratory characteristics, are present in the environment, and are generally not communicable from person to person. As a rule, these mycobacterial species are less susceptible than *M tuberculosis* to antituberculous drugs. On the other hand, agents such as erythromycin, sulfonamides, or tetracycline, which are not active against *M tuberculosis*, may be effective for infections caused by atypical mycobacteria. Emergence of resistance during therapy is also a problem with these mycobacterial species, and active infection should be treated with combinations of drugs. *M kansasii* is susceptible to rifampin and ethambutol, partially resistant to isoniazid, and completely resistant to pyrazinamide. A three-drug combination of isoniazid, rifampin, and ethambutol is the conventional treatment for *M kansasii* infection. A few representative pathogens, with the clinical presentation and the drugs to which they are often susceptible, are given in Table 47–3.

M avium complex (MAC), which includes both *M avium* and *M intracellulare*, is an important and common cause of disseminated disease in late stages of AIDS (CD4 counts < 50/μL). MAC is much less susceptible than *M tuberculosis* to most antituberculous drugs. Combinations of agents are required to suppress the infection. Azithromycin, 500 mg once daily, or clarithromycin, 500 mg twice daily, plus ethambutol, 15–25 mg/kg/d, is an effective and well-tolerated regimen for treatment of disseminated disease. Some authorities recommend use of a third agent, such as ciprofloxacin, 750 mg twice daily, or rifabutin, 300 mg once daily. Other agents that may be useful are listed in Table 47–3. Azithromycin and clarithromycin are the drugs of choice for reducing the incidence of MAC

TABLE 47–3 Clinical features and treatment options for infections with atypical mycobacteria.

Species	Clinical Features	Treatment Options
M kansasii	Resembles tuberculosis	Ciprofloxacin, clarithromycin, ethambutol, isoniazid, rifampin, trimethoprim-sulfamethoxazole
M marinum	Granulomatous cutaneous disease	Amikacin, clarithromycin, ethambutol, doxycycline, minocycline, rifampin, trimethoprim-sulfamethoxazole
M scrofulaceum	Cervical adenitis in children	Amikacin, erythromycin (or other macrolide), rifampin, streptomycin (Surgical excision is often curative and the treatment of choice.)
M avium complex	Pulmonary disease in patients with chronic lung disease; disseminated infection in AIDS	Amikacin, azithromycin, clarithromycin, ciprofloxacin, ethambutol, rifabutin
M chelonae	Abscess, sinus tract, ulcer; bone, joint, tendon infection	Amikacin, doxycycline, imipenem, macrolides, tobramycin
M fortuitum	Abscess, sinus tract, ulcer; bone, joint, tendon infection	Amikacin, cefoxitin, ciprofloxacin, doxycycline, ofloxacin, trimethoprim-sulfamethoxazole
M ulcerans	Skin ulcers	Isoniazid, streptomycin, rifampin, minocycline (Surgical excision may be effective.)

bacteremia in AIDS patients with CD4 cell counts less than 100/μL. Rifabutin in a single daily dose of 300 mg has been shown to reduce the incidence of MAC bacteremia but is less effective than macrolides.

■ DRUGS USED IN LEPROSY

Mycobacterium leprae has never been grown in vitro, but animal models, such as growth in injected mouse footpads, have permitted laboratory evaluation of drugs. Only those drugs with the widest clinical use are presented here. Because of increasing reports of dapsone resistance, treatment of leprosy with combinations of the drugs listed below is recommended.

DAPSONE & OTHER SULFONES

Several drugs closely related to the sulfonamides have been used effectively in the long-term treatment of leprosy. The most widely used is dapsone (diaminodiphenylsulfone). Like the sulfonamides, it inhibits folate synthesis. Resistance can emerge in large populations of *M leprae*, eg, in lepromatous leprosy, if very low doses are given. Therefore, the combination of dapsone, rifampin, and clofazimine is recommended for initial therapy. Dapsone may also be used to prevent and treat *Pneumocystis jiroveci* pneumonia in AIDS patients.

Sulfones are well absorbed from the gut and widely distributed throughout body fluids and tissues. Dapsone's half-life is 1–2 days, and drug tends to be retained in skin, muscle, liver, and kidney. Skin heavily infected with *M leprae* may contain several times more drug than normal skin. Sulfones are excreted into bile and reabsorbed in the intestine. Excretion into urine is variable, and most excreted drug is acetylated. In renal failure, the dose may have to be adjusted. The usual adult dosage in leprosy is 100 mg daily. For children, the dose is proportionately less, depending on weight.

Dapsone is usually well tolerated. Many patients develop some hemolysis, particularly if they have glucose-6-phosphate dehydrogenase deficiency. Methemoglobinemia is common, but usually is not a problem clinically. Gastrointestinal intolerance, fever, pruritus, and various rashes occur. During dapsone therapy of lepromatous leprosy, erythema nodosum leprosum often develops. It is sometimes difficult to distinguish reactions to dapsone from manifestations of the underlying illness. Erythema nodosum leprosum may be suppressed by **corticosteroids** or by **thalidomide**.

RIFAMPIN

Rifampin (see earlier discussion) in a dosage of 600 mg daily is highly effective in lepromatous leprosy. Because of the probable risk of emergence of rifampin-resistant *M leprae*, the drug is given in combination with dapsone or another antileprosy drug. A single monthly dose of 600 mg may be beneficial in combination therapy.

CLOFAZIMINE

Clofazimine is a phenazine dye that can be used as an alternative to dapsone. Its mechanism of action is unknown but may involve DNA binding.

Absorption of clofazimine from the gut is variable, and a major portion of the drug is excreted in feces. Clofazimine is stored widely in reticuloendothelial tissues and skin, and its crystals can be seen inside phagocytic reticuloendothelial cells. It is slowly released from these deposits, so that the serum half-life may be 2 months.

Clofazimine is given for sulfone-resistant leprosy or when patients are intolerant to sulfones. A common dosage is 100 mg/d orally. The most prominent untoward effect is skin discoloration ranging from red-brown to nearly black. Gastrointestinal intolerance occurs occasionally.

SUMMARY First-Line Antimycobacterial Drugs

Subclass	Mechanism of Action	Effects	Clinical Applications	Pharmacokinetics, Toxicities, Interactions
ISONIAZID	Inhibits synthesis of mycolic acids, an essential component of mycobacterial cell walls	Bactericidal activity against susceptible strains of *M tuberculosis*	First-line agent for tuberculosis • treatment of latent infection • less active against other mycobacteria	Oral, IV • hepatic clearance (half-life 1 h) • reduces levels of phenytoin • *Toxicity:* Hepatotoxic, peripheral neuropathy (give pyridoxine to prevent)
RIFAMYCINS • Rifampin	Inhibits DNA-dependent RNA polymerase, thereby blocking production of RNA	Bactericidal activity against susceptible bacteria and mycobacteria • resistance rapidly emerges when used as a single drug in the treatment of active infection	First-line agent for tuberculosis • atypical mycobacterial infections • eradication of meningococcal colonization, staphylococcal infections	Oral, IV • hepatic clearance (half-life 3.5 h) • potent cytochrome P450 inducer • turns body fluids orange color • *Toxicity:* Rash, nephritis, thrombocytopenia, cholestasis, flu-like syndrome with intermittent dosing
• *Rifabutin: Oral; similar to rifampin but less cytochrome P450 induction and fewer drug interactions*				
• *Rifapentine: Oral; long-acting analog of rifampin that may be given once weekly in the continuation phase of tuberculosis treatment*				
PYRAZINAMIDE	Not fully understood • pyrazinamide is converted to the active pyrazinoic acid under acidic conditions in macrophage lysosomes	Bacteriostatic activity against susceptible strains of *M tuberculosis* • may be bactericidal against actively dividing organisms	"Sterilizing" agent used during first 2 months of therapy • allows total duration of therapy to be shortened to 6 months	Oral • hepatic clearance (half-life 9 h), but metabolites are renally cleared so use doses 3 × weekly if creatinine clearance < 30 mL/min • *Toxicity:* Hepatotoxic, hyperuricemia
ETHAMBUTOL	Inhibits mycobacterial arabinosyl transferases, which are involved in the polymerization reaction of arabinoglycan, an essential component of the mycobacterial cell wall	Bacteriostatic activity against susceptible mycobacteria	Given in four-drug initial combination therapy for tuberculosis until drug sensitivities are known • also used for atypical mycobacterial infections	Oral • mixed clearance (half-life 4 h) • dose must be reduced in renal failure • *Toxicity:* Retrobulbar neuritis
STREPTOMYCIN	Prevents bacterial protein synthesis by binding to the S12 ribosomal subunit (see also Chapter 45)	Bactericidal activity against susceptible mycobacteria	Used in tuberculosis when an injectable drug is needed or desirable and in treatment of drug-resistant strains	IM, IV • renal clearance (half-life 2.5 h) • administered daily initially, then 2 × week • *Toxicity:* Nephrotoxic, ototoxic

PREPARATIONS AVAILABLE[1]

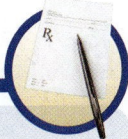

DRUGS USED IN TUBERCULOSIS

Aminosalicylate sodium (Paser)
   Oral: 4 g delayed-release granules

Capreomycin (Capastat Sulfate)
   Parenteral: 1 g powder to reconstitute for injection

Cycloserine (Seromycin Pulvules)
   Oral: 250 mg capsules

Ethambutol (Myambutol)
   Oral: 100, 400 mg tablets

Ethionamide (Trecator-SC)
   Oral: 250 mg tablets

Isoniazid (generic)
   Oral: 100, 300 mg tablets; syrup, 50 mg/5 mL
   Parenteral: 100 mg/mL for injection

Pyrazinamide (generic)
   Oral: 500 mg tablets

Rifabutin (Mycobutin)
   Oral: 150 mg capsules

Rifampin (generic, Rifadin, Rimactane)
   Oral: 150, 300 mg capsules
   Parenteral: 600 mg powder for IV injection

Rifapentine (Priftin)
   Oral: 150 mg tablets

Rifaximin (Xifaxan)
   Oral: 200, 550 mg tablets

Streptomycin (generic)
   Parenteral: 1 g lyophilized for IM injection

DRUGS USED IN LEPROSY

Clofazimine (Lamprene)
   Oral: 50 mg capsules

Dapsone (generic)
   Oral: 25, 100 mg tablets

[1]Drugs used against atypical mycobacteria are listed in Chapters 43–46.

REFERENCES

Diagnosis and treatment of disease caused by nontuberculous mycobacteria. Am J Respir Crit Care Med 1997;156 (2 Part 2):S1.

Gillespie SH et al: Early bactericidal activity of a moxifloxacin and isoniazid combination in smear-positive pulmonary tuberculosis. J Antimicrob Chemother 2005;56:1169.

Hugonnet J-E et al: Meropenem-clavulanate is effective against extensively drug-resistant *Mycobacterium tuberculosis*. Science 2009;323:1215.

Jasmer RM, Nahid P, Hopewell PC: Latent tuberculosis infection. N Engl J Med 2002;347:1860.

Kinzig-Schippers M et al: Should we use N-acetyltransferase type 2 genotyping to personalize isoniazid doses? Antimicrob Agents Chemother 2005;49:1733.

Mitnick CD et al: Comprehensive treatment of extensively drug-resistant tuberculosis. N Engl J Med 2008;359:563.

Sulochana S, Rahman F, Paramasivan CN: In vitro activity of fluoroquinolones against *Mycobacterium tuberculosis*. J Chemother 2005;17:169.

Targeted tuberculin testing and treatment of latent tuberculosis infection. Am J Respir Crit Care Med 2000;161(4 Part 2):S221.

Update: Adverse event data and revised American Thoracic Society/CDC recommendations against the use of rifampin and pyrazinamide for treatment of latent tuberculosis infection—United States, 2003. MMWR Morb Mortal Wkly Rep 2003;52:735.

von der Lippe B, Sandven P, Brubakk O: Efficacy and safety of linezolid in multidrug resistant tuberculosis (MDR-TB)—a report of ten cases. J Infect 2006;52:92.

Zhang Y, Yew WW: Mechanisms of drug resistance in *Mycobacterium tuberculosis*. Int J Tuberc Lung Dis 2009;13:1320.

CASE STUDY ANSWER

The patient should be started on four-drug therapy with rifampin, isoniazid, pyrazinamide, and ethambutol. If a protease-inhibitor-based antiretroviral regimen is used to treat his HIV, rifabutin should replace rifampin because of the serious drug-drug interaction between rifampin and protease inhibitors. The patient is at increased risk of developing hepatotoxicity from both isoniazid and pyrazinamide given his history of chronic alcohol dependence.

Antifungal Agents

Don Sheppard, MD, & Harry W. Lampiris, MD

48

CASE STUDY

A 55-year-old man presents to the emergency department with a 2-week history of an expanding ulcer on his left lower leg. He has a history of chronic neutropenia and transfusion-dependent anemia secondary to myelodysplastic syndrome requiring chronic therapy with deferoxamine for hepatic iron overload. He first noticed a red bump on his leg while fishing at his cabin in the woods and thought it was a bug bite. It rapidly enlarged, first as a red swollen area, and then began to ulcerate. He was given dicloxacillin orally, but with no improvement. In the emergency department he is febrile to 39°C (102.2°F), and looks unwell. On his left leg he has a 6 by 12 cm black ulcer with surrounding swelling and erythema that is quite tender. His complete blood count demonstrates an absolute neutrophil count of 300 and a total white blood cell count of 1000. An immediate operative debridement yields pathologic specimens demonstrating broad club-like nonseptate hyphae and extensive tissue necrosis. What initial medical therapy would be most appropriate?

Human fungal infections have increased dramatically in incidence and severity in recent years, owing mainly to advances in surgery, cancer treatment, treatment of patients with solid organ and bone marrow transplantation, the HIV epidemic, and increasing use of broad-spectrum antimicrobial therapy in critically ill patients. These changes have resulted in increased numbers of patients at risk for fungal infections.

For many years, **amphotericin B** was the only efficacious antifungal drug available for systemic use. While highly effective in many serious infections, it is also quite toxic. In the last several decades, pharmacotherapy of fungal disease has been revolutionized by the introduction of the relatively nontoxic **azole** drugs (both oral and parenteral formulations) and the **echinocandins** (only available for parenteral administration). The new agents in these classes offer more targeted, less toxic therapy than older agents such as amphotericin B for patients with serious systemic fungal infections. Combination therapy is being reconsidered, and new formulations of old agents are becoming available. Unfortunately, the appearance of azole-resistant organisms, as well as the rise in the number of patients at risk for mycotic infections, has created new challenges.

The antifungal drugs presently available fall into the following categories: systemic drugs (oral or parenteral) for systemic infections, oral systemic drugs for mucocutaneous infections, and topical drugs for mucocutaneous infections.

■ SYSTEMIC ANTIFUNGAL DRUGS FOR SYSTEMIC INFECTIONS

AMPHOTERICIN B

Amphotericin A and B are antifungal antibiotics produced by *Streptomyces nodosus*. Amphotericin A is not in clinical use.

Chemistry & Pharmacokinetics

Amphotericin B is an amphoteric polyene macrolide (polyene = containing many double bonds; macrolide = containing a large lactone ring of 12 or more atoms). It is nearly insoluble in water and is therefore prepared as a colloidal suspension of amphotericin B and sodium desoxycholate for intravenous injection. Several formulations have been developed in which amphotericin B is

TABLE 48–1 Properties of conventional amphotericin B and some lipid formulations.[1]

Drug	Physical Form	Dosing (mg/kg/d)	C_{max}	Clearance	Nephrotoxicity	Infusional Toxicity	Daily Cost ($)
Conventional formulation							
Fungizone	Micelles	1	…	…	…	…	24
Lipid formulations							
AmBisome	Spheres	3–5	↑	↓	↓	↓	1300
Amphotec	Disks	5	↓	↑	↓	↑(?)	660
Abelcet	Ribbons	5	↓	↑	↓	↓(?)	570

[1]Changes in C_{max} (peak plasma concentration), clearance, nephrotoxicity, and infusional toxicity are relative to conventional amphotericin B.

packaged in a lipid-associated delivery system (Table 48–1 and Box: Liposomal Amphotericin B).

Amphotericin B

Amphotericin B is poorly absorbed from the gastrointestinal tract. Oral amphotericin B is thus effective only on fungi within the lumen of the tract and cannot be used for treatment of systemic disease. The intravenous injection of 0.6 mg/kg/d of amphotericin B results in average blood levels of 0.3–1 mcg/mL; the drug is more than 90% bound by serum proteins. Although it is mostly metabolized, some amphotericin B is excreted slowly in the urine over a period of several days. The serum half-life is approximately 15 days. Hepatic impairment, renal impairment, and dialysis have little impact on drug concentrations, and therefore no dose adjustment is required. The drug is widely distributed in most tissues, but only 2–3% of the blood level is reached in cerebrospinal fluid, thus occasionally necessitating intrathecal therapy for certain types of fungal meningitis.

Mechanisms of Action & Resistance

Amphotericin B is selective in its fungicidal effect because it exploits the difference in lipid composition of fungal and mammalian cell membranes. **Ergosterol,** a cell membrane sterol, is found in the cell membrane of fungi, whereas the predominant sterol of bacteria and human cells is **cholesterol.** Amphotericin B binds to ergosterol and alters the permeability of the cell by forming amphotericin B-associated pores in the cell membrane (Figure 48–1). As suggested by its chemistry, amphotericin B combines avidly with

Liposomal Amphotericin B

Therapy with amphotericin B is often limited by toxicity, especially drug-induced renal impairment. This has led to the development of lipid drug formulations on the assumption that lipid-packaged drug binds to the mammalian membrane less readily, permitting the use of effective doses of the drug with lower toxicity. Liposomal amphotericin preparations package the active drug in lipid delivery vehicles, in contrast to the colloidal suspensions, which were previously the only available forms. Amphotericin binds to the lipids in these vehicles with an affinity between that for fungal ergosterol and that for human cholesterol. The lipid vehicle then serves as an amphotericin reservoir, reducing nonspecific binding to human cell membranes. This preferential binding allows for a reduction of toxicity without sacrificing efficacy and permits use of larger doses. Furthermore, some fungi contain lipases that may liberate free amphotericin B directly at the site of infection.

Three such formulations are now available and have differing pharmacologic properties as summarized in Table 48–1. Although clinical trials have demonstrated different renal and infusion-related toxicities for these preparations compared with regular amphotericin B, there are no trials comparing the different formulations with each other. Limited studies have suggested at best a moderate improvement in the clinical efficacy of the lipid formulations compared with conventional amphotericin B. Because the lipid preparations are much more expensive, their use is usually restricted to patients intolerant to, or not responding to, conventional amphotericin treatment.

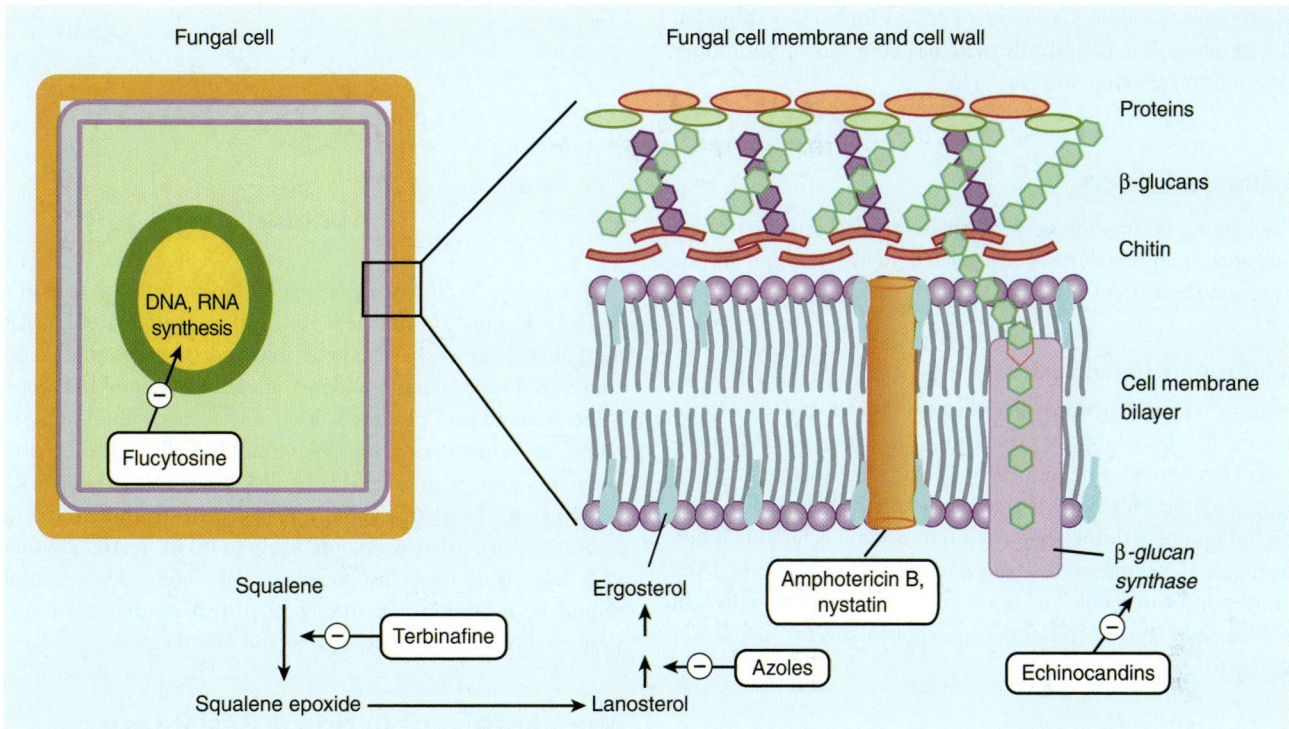

FIGURE 48–1 Targets of antifungal drugs. Except for flucytosine (and possibly griseofulvin, not shown), all currently available antifungals target the fungal cell membrane or cell wall.

lipids (ergosterol) along the double bond-rich side of its structure and associates with water molecules along the hydroxyl-rich side. This amphipathic characteristic facilitates pore formation by multiple amphotericin molecules, with the lipophilic portions around the outside of the pore and the hydrophilic regions lining the inside. The pore allows the leakage of intracellular ions and macromolecules, eventually leading to cell death. Some binding to human membrane sterols does occur, probably accounting for the drug's prominent toxicity.

Resistance to amphotericin B occurs if ergosterol binding is impaired, either by decreasing the membrane concentration of ergosterol or by modifying the sterol target molecule to reduce its affinity for the drug.

Antifungal Activity & Clinical Uses

Amphotericin B remains the antifungal agent with the broadest spectrum of action. It has activity against the clinically significant yeasts, including *Candida albicans* and *Cryptococcus neoformans*; the organisms causing endemic mycoses, including *Histoplasma capsulatum*, *Blastomyces dermatitidis*, and *Coccidioides immitis*; and the pathogenic molds, such as *Aspergillus fumigatus* and the agents of mucormycosis. Some fungal organisms such as *Candida lusitaniae* and *Pseudallescheria boydii* display intrinsic amphotericin B resistance.

Owing to its broad spectrum of activity and fungicidal action, amphotericin B remains a useful agent for nearly all life-threatening mycotic infections, although newer, less toxic agents have largely replaced it for most conditions. Amphotericin B is often used as the initial induction regimen to rapidly reduce fungal burden and then replaced by one of the newer azole drugs (described below) for chronic therapy or prevention of relapse. Such induction therapy is especially important for immunosuppressed patients and those with severe fungal pneumonia, severe cryptococcal meningitis, or disseminated infections with one of the endemic mycoses such as histoplasmosis or coccidioidomycosis. Once a clinical response has been elicited, these patients then often continue maintenance therapy with an azole; therapy may be lifelong in patients at high risk for disease relapse. For treatment of systemic fungal disease, amphotericin B is given by slow intravenous infusion at a dosage of 0.5–1 mg/kg/d. It is usually continued to a defined total dose (eg, 1–2 g), rather than a defined time span, as used with other antimicrobial drugs.

Intrathecal therapy for fungal meningitis is poorly tolerated and fraught with difficulties related to maintaining cerebrospinal fluid access. Thus, intrathecal therapy with amphotericin B is being increasingly supplanted by other therapies but remains an option in cases of fungal central nervous system infections that have not responded to other agents.

Local or topical administration of amphotericin B has been used with success. Mycotic corneal ulcers and keratitis can be cured with topical drops as well as by direct subconjunctival injection. Fungal arthritis has been treated with adjunctive local injection directly into the joint. Candiduria responds to bladder irrigation with amphotericin B, and this route has been shown to produce no significant systemic toxicity.

Adverse Effects

The toxicity of amphotericin B can be divided into two broad categories: immediate reactions, related to the infusion of the drug, and those occurring more slowly.

A. Infusion-Related Toxicity

Infusion-related reactions are nearly universal and consist of fever, chills, muscle spasms, vomiting, headache, and hypotension. They can be ameliorated by slowing the infusion rate or decreasing the daily dose. Premedication with antipyretics, antihistamines, meperidine, or corticosteroids can be helpful. When starting therapy, many clinicians administer a test dose of 1 mg intravenously to gauge the severity of the reaction. This can serve as a guide to an initial dosing regimen and premedication strategy.

B. Cumulative Toxicity

Renal damage is the most significant toxic reaction. Renal impairment occurs in nearly all patients treated with clinically significant doses of amphotericin. The degree of azotemia is variable and often stabilizes during therapy, but it can be serious enough to necessitate dialysis. A reversible component is associated with decreased renal perfusion and represents a form of prerenal renal failure. An irreversible component results from renal tubular injury and subsequent dysfunction. The irreversible form of amphotericin nephrotoxicity usually occurs in the setting of prolonged administration (> 4 g cumulative dose). Renal toxicity commonly manifests as renal tubular acidosis and severe potassium and magnesium wasting. There is some evidence that the prerenal component can be attenuated with sodium loading, and it is common practice to administer normal saline infusions with the daily doses of amphotericin B.

Abnormalities of liver function tests are occasionally seen, as is a varying degree of anemia due to reduced erythropoietin production by damaged renal tubular cells. After intrathecal therapy with amphotericin, seizures and a chemical arachnoiditis may develop, often with serious neurologic sequelae.

FLUCYTOSINE

Chemistry & Pharmacokinetics

Flucytosine (5-FC) was discovered in 1957 during a search for novel antineoplastic agents. Though devoid of anticancer properties, it became apparent that it was a potent antifungal agent. Flucytosine is a water-soluble pyrimidine analog related to the chemotherapeutic agent 5-fluorouracil (5-FU). Its spectrum of action is much narrower than that of amphotericin B.

Flucytosine

Flucytosine is currently available in North America only in an oral formulation. The dosage is 100–150 mg/kg/d in patients with normal renal function. It is well absorbed (> 90%), with serum concentrations peaking 1–2 hours after an oral dose. It is poorly protein-bound and penetrates well into all body fluid compartments, including the cerebrospinal fluid. It is eliminated by glomerular filtration with a half-life of 3–4 hours and is removed by hemodialysis. Levels rise rapidly with renal impairment and can lead to toxicity. Toxicity is more likely to occur in AIDS patients and those with renal insufficiency. Peak serum concentrations should be measured periodically in patients with renal insufficiency and maintained between 50 and 100 mcg/mL.

Mechanisms of Action & Resistance

Flucytosine is taken up by fungal cells via the enzyme cytosine permease. It is converted intracellularly first to 5-FU and then to 5-fluorodeoxyuridine monophosphate (FdUMP) and fluorouridine triphosphate (FUTP), which inhibit DNA and RNA synthesis, respectively (Figure 48–1). Human cells are unable to convert the parent drug to its active metabolites, resulting in selective toxicity.

Synergy with amphotericin B has been demonstrated in vitro and in vivo. It may be related to enhanced penetration of the flucytosine through amphotericin-damaged fungal cell membranes. In vitro synergy with azole drugs has also been seen, although the mechanism is unclear.

Resistance is thought to be mediated through altered metabolism of flucytosine, and, though uncommon in primary isolates, it develops rapidly in the course of flucytosine monotherapy.

Clinical Uses & Adverse Effects

The spectrum of activity of flucytosine is restricted to *C neoformans*, some *Candida* sp, and the dematiaceous molds that cause chromoblastomycosis. Flucytosine is not used as a single agent because of its demonstrated synergy with other agents and to avoid the development of secondary resistance. Clinical use at present is confined to combination therapy, either with amphotericin B for cryptococcal meningitis or with itraconazole for chromoblastomycosis.

The adverse effects of flucytosine result from metabolism (possibly by intestinal flora) to the toxic antineoplastic compound fluorouracil. Bone marrow toxicity with anemia, leukopenia, and thrombocytopenia are the most common adverse effects, with derangement of liver enzymes occurring less frequently. A form of toxic enterocolitis can occur. There seems to be a narrow therapeutic window, with an increased risk of toxicity at higher drug levels and resistance developing rapidly at subtherapeutic concentrations. The use of drug concentration measurements may be helpful in reducing the incidence of toxic reactions, especially when flucytosine is combined with nephrotoxic agents such as amphotericin B.

AZOLES

Chemistry & Pharmacokinetics

Azoles are synthetic compounds that can be classified as either imidazoles or triazoles according to the number of nitrogen atoms in the five-membered azole ring, as indicated below. The imidazoles consist of ketoconazole, miconazole, and clotrimazole (Figure 48–2). The latter two drugs are now used only in topical therapy. The triazoles include itraconazole, fluconazole, voriconazole, and posaconazole.

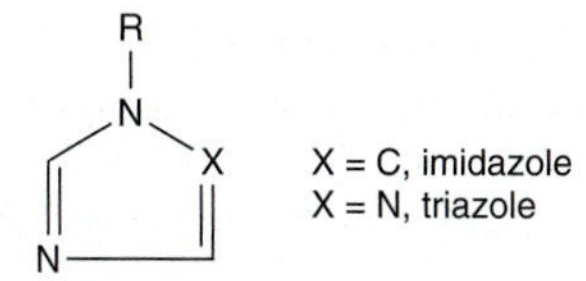

X = C, imidazole
X = N, triazole

Azole nucleus

The pharmacology of each of the azoles is unique and accounts for some of the variations in clinical use. Table 48–2 summarizes the differences among five of the azoles.

Mechanisms of Action & Resistance

The antifungal activity of azole drugs results from the reduction of ergosterol synthesis by inhibition of fungal cytochrome P450 enzymes (Figure 48–1). The selective toxicity of azole drugs results

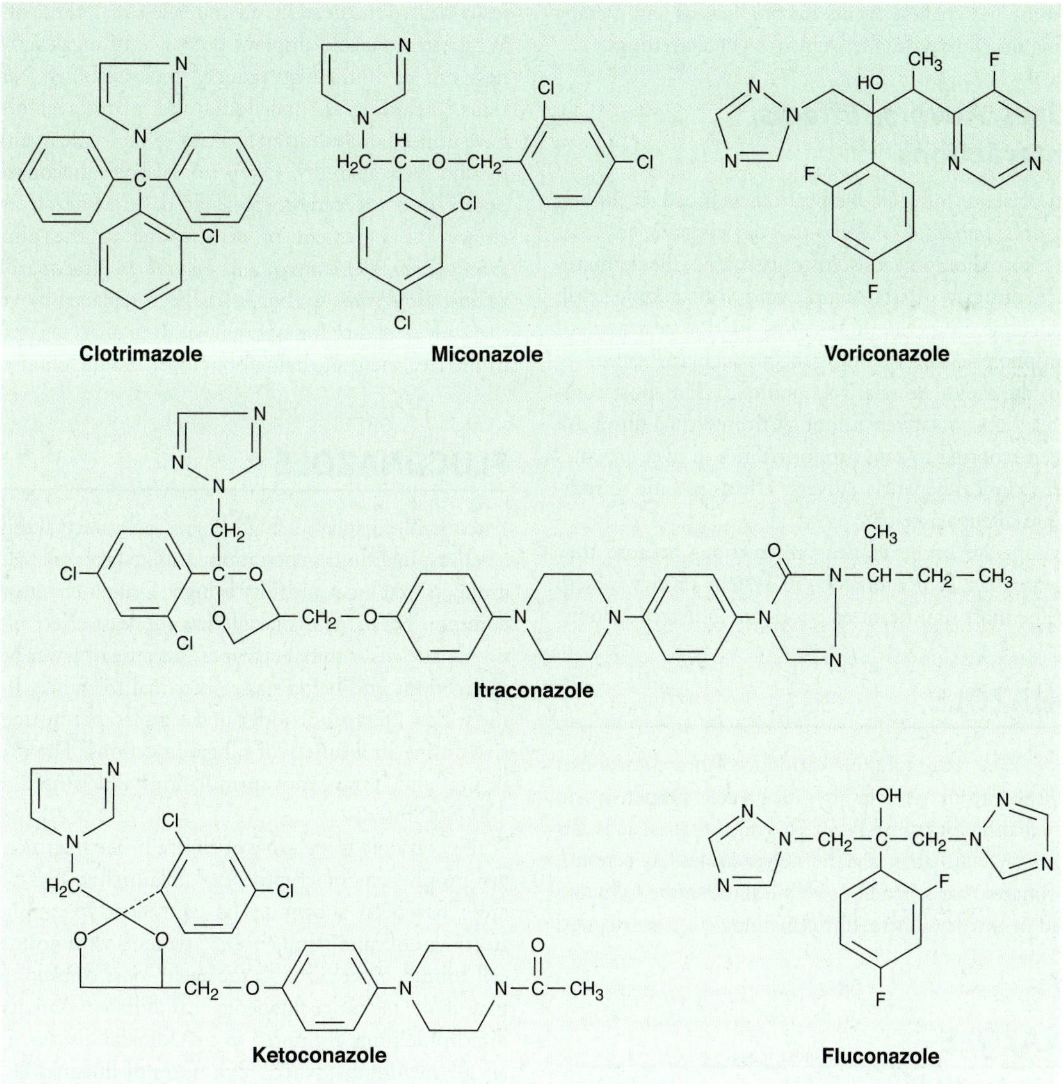

FIGURE 48–2 Structural formulas of some antifungal azoles.

TABLE 48–2 Pharmacologic properties of five systemic azole drugs.

	Water Solubility	Absorption	CSF: Serum Concentration Ratio	$t_{1/2}$ (hours)	Elimination	Formulations
Ketoconazole	Low	Variable	< 0.1	7–10	Hepatic	Oral
Itraconazole	Low	Variable	< 0.01	24–42	Hepatic	Oral, IV
Fluconazole	High	High	> 0.7	22–31	Renal	Oral, IV
Voriconazole	High	High	…	6	Hepatic	Oral, IV
Posaconazole	Low	High	…	25	Hepatic	Oral

from their greater affinity for fungal than for human cytochrome P450 enzymes. Imidazoles exhibit a lesser degree of selectivity than the triazoles, accounting for their higher incidence of drug interactions and adverse effects.

Resistance to azoles occurs via multiple mechanisms. Once rare, increasing numbers of resistant strains are being reported, suggesting that increasing use of these agents for prophylaxis and therapy may be selecting for clinical drug resistance in certain settings.

Clinical Uses, Adverse Effects, & Drug Interactions

The spectrum of action of azole medications is broad, including many species of *Candida, C neoformans*, the endemic mycoses (blastomycosis, coccidioidomycosis, histoplasmosis), the dermatophytes, and, in the case of itraconazole and voriconazole, even *Aspergillus* infections. They are also useful in the treatment of intrinsically amphotericin-resistant organisms such as *P boydii*.

As a group, the azoles are relatively nontoxic. The most common adverse reaction is relatively minor gastrointestinal upset. All azoles have been reported to cause abnormalities in liver enzymes and, very rarely, clinical hepatitis. Adverse effects specific to individual agents are discussed below.

All azole drugs are prone to drug interactions because they affect the mammalian cytochrome P450 system of enzymes to some extent. The most significant reactions are indicated below.

KETOCONAZOLE

Ketoconazole was the first oral azole introduced into clinical use. It is distinguished from triazoles by its greater propensity to inhibit mammalian cytochrome P450 enzymes; that is, it is less selective for fungal P450 than are the newer azoles. As a result, systemic ketoconazole has fallen out of clinical use in the USA and is not discussed in any detail here. Its dermatologic use is discussed in Chapter 61.

ITRACONAZOLE

Itraconazole is available in oral and intravenous formulations and is used at a dosage of 100–400 mg/d. Drug absorption is increased

by food and by low gastric pH. Like other lipid-soluble azoles, it interacts with hepatic microsomal enzymes, though to a lesser degree than ketoconazole. An important drug interaction is reduced bioavailability of itraconazole when taken with rifamycins (rifampin, rifabutin, rifapentine). It does not affect mammalian steroid synthesis, and its effects on the metabolism of other hepatically cleared medications are much less than those of ketoconazole. While itraconazole displays potent antifungal activity, effectiveness can be limited by reduced bioavailability. Newer formulations, including an oral liquid and an intravenous preparation, have utilized cyclodextran as a carrier molecule to enhance solubility and bioavailability. Like ketoconazole, itraconazole penetrates poorly into the cerebrospinal fluid. Itraconazole is the azole of choice for treatment of disease due to the dimorphic fungi *Histoplasma, Blastomyces*, and *Sporothrix*. Itraconazole has activity against *Aspergillus* sp, but it has been replaced by voriconazole as the azole of choice for aspergillosis. Itraconazole is used extensively in the treatment of dermatophytoses and onychomycosis.

FLUCONAZOLE

Fluconazole displays a high degree of water solubility and good cerebrospinal fluid penetration. Unlike ketoconazole and itraconazole, its oral bioavailability is high. Drug interactions are also less common because fluconazole has the least effect of all the azoles on hepatic microsomal enzymes. Because of fewer hepatic enzyme interactions and better gastrointestinal tolerance, fluconazole has the widest therapeutic index of the azoles, permitting more aggressive dosing in a variety of fungal infections. The drug is available in oral and intravenous formulations and is used at a dosage of 100–800 mg/d.

Fluconazole is the azole of choice in the treatment and secondary prophylaxis of cryptococcal meningitis. Intravenous fluconazole has been shown to be equivalent to amphotericin B in treatment of candidemia in ICU patients with normal white blood cell counts. Fluconazole is the agent most commonly used for the treatment of mucocutaneous candidiasis. Activity against the dimorphic fungi is limited to coccidioidal disease, and in particular for meningitis, where high doses of fluconazole often obviate the need for intrathecal amphotericin B. Fluconazole displays no activity against *Aspergillus* or other filamentous fungi.

Prophylactic use of fluconazole has been demonstrated to reduce fungal disease in bone marrow transplant recipients and AIDS patients, but the emergence of fluconazole-resistant fungi has raised concerns about this indication.

VORICONAZOLE

Voriconazole is available in intravenous and oral formulations. The recommended dosage is 400 mg/d. The drug is well absorbed orally, with a bioavailability exceeding 90%, and it exhibits less protein binding than itraconazole. Metabolism is predominantly hepatic. Voriconazole is a clinically relevant inhibitor of mammalian CYP3A4, and dose reduction of a number of medications is required when voriconazole is started. These include cyclosporine, tacrolimus, and HMG-CoA reductase inhibitors. Observed toxicities include rash and elevated hepatic enzymes. Visual disturbances are common, occurring in up to 30% of patients receiving intravenous voriconazole, and include blurring and changes in color vision or brightness. These visual changes usually occur immediately after a dose of voriconazole and resolve within 30 minutes. Photosensitivity dermatitis is commonly observed in patients receiving chronic oral therapy.

Voriconazole is similar to itraconazole in its spectrum of action, having excellent activity against Candida sp (including fluconazole-resistant species such as Candida krusei) and the dimorphic fungi. Voriconazole is less toxic than amphotericin B and is the treatment of choice for invasive aspergillosis.

POSACONAZOLE

Posaconazole is the newest triazole to be licensed in the USA. It is available only in a liquid oral formulation and is used at a dosage of 800 mg/d, divided into two or three doses. Absorption is improved when taken with meals high in fat. Posaconazole is rapidly distributed to the tissues, resulting in high tissue levels but relatively low blood levels. Visual changes have not been reported, but drug interactions with increased levels of CYP3A4 substrates such as tacrolimus and cyclosporine have been documented.

Posaconazole is the broadest spectrum member of the azole family, with activity against most species of Candida and Aspergillus. It is the only azole with significant activity against the agents of mucormycosis. It is currently licensed for salvage therapy in invasive aspergillosis, as well as prophylaxis of fungal infections during induction chemotherapy for leukemia, and for allogeneic bone marrow transplant patients with graft-versus-host disease.

ECHINOCANDINS

Chemistry & Pharmacokinetics

Echinocandins are the newest class of antifungal agents to be developed. They are large cyclic peptides linked to a long-chain fatty acid. **Caspofungin, micafungin,** and **anidulafungin** are the only licensed agents in this category of antifungals, although other drugs are under active investigation. These agents are active against Candida and Aspergillus, but not C neoformans or the agents of zygomycosis and mucormycosis.

Echinocandins are available only in intravenous formulations. Caspofungin is administered as a single loading dose of 70 mg, followed by a daily dose of 50 mg. Caspofungin is water soluble and highly protein-bound. The half-life is 9–11 hours, and the metabolites are excreted by the kidneys and gastrointestinal tract. Dosage adjustments are required only in the presence of severe hepatic insufficiency. Micafungin displays similar properties with a half-life of 11–15 hours and is used at a dose of 150 mg/d for treatment of esophageal candidiasis, 100 mg/d for treatment of candidemia, and 50 mg/d for prophylaxis of fungal infections. Anidulafungin has a half-life of 24–48 hours. For esophageal candidiasis, it is administered intravenously at 100 mg on the first day and 50 mg/d thereafter for 14 days. For candidemia, a loading dose of 200 mg is recommended with 100 mg/d thereafter for at least 14 days after the last positive blood culture.

Mechanism of Action

Echinocandins act at the level of the fungal cell wall by inhibiting the synthesis of β(1–3)-glucan (Figure 48–1). This results in disruption of the fungal cell wall and cell death.

Clinical Uses & Adverse Effects

Caspofungin is currently licensed for disseminated and mucocutaneous candidal infections, as well as for empiric antifungal therapy during febrile neutropenia, and has largely replaced amphotericin B for the latter indication. Of note, caspofungin is licensed for use in invasive aspergillosis only as salvage therapy in patients who have failed to respond to amphotericin B, and not as primary therapy. Micafungin is licensed for mucocutaneous candidiasis, candidemia, and prophylaxis of candidal infections in bone marrow transplant patients. Anidulafungin is approved for use in esophageal candidiasis and invasive candidiasis, including candidemia.

Echinocandin agents are extremely well tolerated, with minor gastrointestinal side effects and flushing reported infrequently. Elevated liver enzymes have been noted in several patients receiving caspofungin in combination with cyclosporine, and this combination should be avoided. Micafungin has been shown to increase levels of nifedipine, cyclosporine, and sirolimus. Anidulafungin does not seem to have significant drug interactions, but histamine release may occur during intravenous infusion.

■ ORAL SYSTEMIC ANTIFUNGAL DRUGS FOR MUCOCUTANEOUS INFECTIONS

GRISEOFULVIN

Griseofulvin is a very insoluble fungistatic drug derived from a species of penicillium. Its only use is in the systemic treatment of dermatophytosis (see Chapter 61). It is administered in a microcrystalline form at a dosage of 1 g/d. Absorption is improved when it is given with fatty foods. Griseofulvin's mechanism of action at the cellular level is unclear, but it is deposited in newly forming skin where it binds to keratin, protecting the skin from new infection. Because its action is to prevent infection of these new skin structures, griseofulvin must be administered for 2–6 weeks for skin and hair infections to allow the replacement of infected keratin by the resistant structures. Nail infections may require therapy for months to allow regrowth of the new protected nail and is often followed by relapse. Adverse effects include an allergic syndrome much like serum sickness, hepatitis, and drug interactions with warfarin and phenobarbital. Griseofulvin has been largely replaced by newer antifungal medications such as itraconazole and terbinafine.

TERBINAFINE

Terbinafine is a synthetic allylamine that is available in an oral formulation and is used at a dosage of 250 mg/d. It is used in the treatment of dermatophytoses, especially onychomycosis (see Chapter 61). Like griseofulvin, terbinafine is a keratophilic medication, but unlike griseofulvin, it is fungicidal. Like the azole drugs, it interferes with ergosterol biosynthesis, but rather than interacting with the P450 system, terbinafine inhibits the fungal enzyme squalene epoxidase (Figure 48–1). This leads to the accumulation of the sterol squalene, which is toxic to the organism. One tablet given daily for 12 weeks achieves a cure rate of up to 90% for onychomycosis and is more effective than griseofulvin or itraconazole. Adverse effects are rare, consisting primarily of gastrointestinal upset and headache. Terbinafine does not seem to affect the P450 system and has demonstrated no significant drug interactions to date.

■ TOPICAL ANTIFUNGAL THERAPY

NYSTATIN

Nystatin is a polyene macrolide much like amphotericin B. It is too toxic for parenteral administration and is only used topically.

Nystatin is currently available in creams, ointments, suppositories, and other forms for application to skin and mucous membranes. It is not absorbed to a significant degree from skin, mucous membranes, or the gastrointestinal tract. As a result, nystatin has little toxicity, although oral use is often limited by the unpleasant taste.

Nystatin is active against most *Candida* sp and is most commonly used for suppression of local candidal infections. Some common indications include oropharyngeal thrush, vaginal candidiasis, and intertriginous candidal infections.

TOPICAL AZOLES

The two azoles most commonly used topically are clotrimazole and miconazole; several others are available (see Preparations Available). Both are available over-the-counter and are often used for vulvovaginal candidiasis. Oral clotrimazole troches are available for treatment of oral thrush and are a pleasant-tasting alternative to nystatin. In cream form, both agents are useful for dermatophytic infections, including tinea corporis, tinea pedis, and tinea cruris. Absorption is negligible, and adverse effects are rare.

Topical and shampoo forms of ketoconazole are also available and useful in the treatment of seborrheic dermatitis and pityriasis versicolor. Several other azoles are available for topical use (see Preparations Available).

TOPICAL ALLYLAMINES

Terbinafine and naftifine are allylamines available as topical creams (see Chapter 61). Both are effective for treatment of tinea cruris and tinea corporis. These are prescription drugs in the USA.

SUMMARY Antifungal Drugs

Subclass	Mechanism of Action	Effects	Clinical Applications	Pharmacokinetics, Toxicities, Interactions
POLYENE MACROLIDE				
• Amphotericin B	Forms pores in fungal membranes (which contain ergosterol) but not in mammalian (cholesterol-containing) membranes	Loss of intracellular contents through pores is fungicidal • broad spectrum of action	Localized and systemic candidemia • *Cryptococcus* • *Histoplasma* • *Blastomyces* • *Coccidioides* • *Aspergillus*	Oral but not absorbed • IV for systemic use • intrathecal for fungal meningitis • topical for ocular and bladder infections • duration, days • *Toxicity:* Infusion reactions • renal impairment • *Interactions:* Additive with other renal toxic drugs
• *Lipid formulations: Lower toxicity, higher doses can be used*				
PYRIMIDINE ANALOG				
• Flucytosine	Interferes with DNA and RNA synthesis selectively in fungi	Synergistic with amphotericin • systemic toxicity in host due to DNA and RNA effects	*Cryptococcus* and chromoblastomycosis infections	Oral • duration, hours • renal excretion • *Toxicity:* Myelosuppression
AZOLES				
• Ketoconazole	Blocks fungal P450 enzymes and interferes with ergosterol synthesis	Poorly selective • interferes with mammalian P450 function	Broad spectrum but toxicity restricts use to topical therapy	Oral, topical • *Toxicity and interactions:* Interferes with steroid hormone synthesis and phase I drug metabolism
• Itraconazole	Same as for ketoconazole	Much more selective than ketoconazole	Broad spectrum: *Candida, Cryptococcus,* blastomycosis, coccidioidomycosis, histoplasmosis	Oral and IV • duration, 1–2 d • poor entry into central nervous system (CNS) • *Toxicity and interactions:* Low toxicity
• *Fluconazole, voriconazole, posaconazole: Fluconazole has excellent CNS penetration, used in fungal meningitis*				
ECHINOCANDINS				
• Caspofungin	Blocks β-glucan synthase	Prevents synthesis of fungal cell wall	Fungicidal *Candida sp* • also used in aspergillosis	IV only • duration, 11–15 h • *Toxicity:* Minor gastrointestinal effects, flushing • *Interactions:* Increases cyclosporine levels (avoid combination)
• *Micafungin, anidulafungin: Micafungin increases levels of nifedipine, cyclosporine, sirolimus; anidulafungin is relatively free of this interaction*				
ALLYLAMINE				
• Terbinafine	Inhibits epoxidation of squalene in fungi • increased levels are toxic to them	Reduces ergosterol • prevents synthesis of fungal cell membrane	Mucocutaneous fungal infections	Oral • duration, days • *Toxicity:* Gastrointestinal upset, headache, hepatotoxicity • *Interactions:* None reported

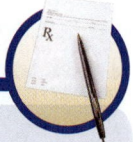

PREPARATIONS AVAILABLE

Amphotericin B
Parenteral:
Conventional formulation (Amphotericin B, Fungizone): 50 mg powder for injection
Lipid formulations:
(Abelcet): 100 mg/20 mL suspension for injection
(AmBisome): 50 mg powder for injection
(Amphotec): 50, 100 mg powder for injection
Topical: 3% cream, lotion, ointment

Anidulafungin (Eraxis)
Parenteral: 50 mg powder for injection

Butenafine (Lotrimin Ultra, Mentax)
Topical: 1% cream

Butoconazole (Gynazole-1, Mycelex-3)
Topical: 2% vaginal cream

Caspofungin (Cancidas)
Parenteral: 50, 70 mg powder for injection

Clotrimazole (generic, Lotrimin)
Topical: 1% cream, solution, lotion; 100, 200 mg vaginal suppositories

Econazole (generic, Spectazole)
Topical: 1% cream

Fluconazole (Diflucan)
Oral: 50, 100, 150, 200 mg tablets; powder for 10, 40 mg/mL suspension
Parenteral: 2 mg/mL in 100 and 200 mL vials

Flucytosine (Ancobon)
Oral: 250, 500 mg capsules

Griseofulvin (Grifulvin, Grisactin, Fulvicin P/G)
Oral microsize: 125, 250 mg tablets; 250 mg capsule, 125 mg/5 mL suspension
Oral ultramicrosize:[1] 125, 165, 250, 330 mg tablets

Itraconazole (Sporanox)
Oral: 100 mg capsules; 10 mg/mL solution
Parenteral: 10 mg/mL for IV infusion

Ketoconazole (generic, Nizoral)
Oral: 200 mg tablets
Topical: 2% cream, shampoo

Micafungin (Mycamine)
Parenteral: 50 mg powder for injection

Miconazole (generic, Micatin)
Topical: 2% cream, powder, spray; 100, 200 mg vaginal suppositories

Naftifine (Naftin)
Topical: 1% cream, gel

Natamycin (Natacyn)
Topical: 5% ophthalmic suspension

Nystatin (generic, Mycostatin)
Oral: 500,000 unit tablets
Topical: 100,000 units/g cream, ointment, powder; 100,000 units vaginal tablets

Oxiconazole (Oxistat)
Topical: 1% cream, lotion

Posaconazole (Noxafil)
Oral: suspension 40 mg/mL

Sulconazole (Exelderm)
Topical: 1% cream, solution

Terbinafine (Lamisil)
Oral: 250 mg tablets
Topical: 1% cream, gel

Terconazole (Terazol 3, Terazol 7)
Topical: 0.4%, 0.8% vaginal cream; 80 mg vaginal suppositories

Tioconazole (Vagistat-1, Monistat 1)
Topical: 6.5% vaginal ointment

Tolnaftate (generic, Aftate, Tinactin)
Topical: 1% cream, gel, solution, aerosol powder

Voriconazole (Vfend)
Oral: 50, 200 mg tablets; oral suspension 40 mg/mL
Parenteral: 200 mg vials, reconstituted to a 5 mg/mL solution

[1]Ultramicrosize formulations of griseofulvin are approximately 1.5 times more potent, milligram for milligram, than the microsize preparations.

REFERENCES

Brüggemann RJ et al: Clinical relevance of the pharmacokinetic interactions of azole antifungal drugs with other coadministered agents. Clin Infect Dis 2009;48:1441.

Cornely OA et al: Posazonacole vs. fluconazole or itraconazole prophylaxis in patients with neutropenia. N Engl J Med 2007;356:348.

Diekema DJ et al: Activities of caspofungin, itraconazole, posaconazole, ravuconazole, voriconazole, and amphotericin B against 448 recent clinical isolates of filamentous fungi. J Clin Microbiol 2003;41:3623.

Groll A, Piscitelli SC, Walsh TJ: Clinical pharmacology of systemic antifungal agents: A comprehensive review of agents in clinical use, current investigational compounds, and putative targets for antifungal drug development. Adv Pharmacol 1998;44:343.

Herbrecht R et al: Voriconazole versus amphotericin B for primary therapy of invasive aspergillosis. N Engl J Med 2002;347:408.

Kim R, Khachikian D, Reboli AC: A comparative evaluation of properties and clinical efficacy of the echinocandins. Expert Opin Pharmacother 2007;8:1479.

Pasqualotto AC, Denning DW: New and emerging treatments for fungal infection. J Antimicrob Chemoth 2008;61(Suppl 1):i19.

Rogers TR: Treatment of zygomycosis: Current and new options. J Antimicrob Chemother 2008;61(Suppl 1):i35.

Wong-Beringer A, Jacobs RA, Guglielmo BJ: Lipid formulations of amphotericin B. Clinical efficacy and toxicities. Clin Infect Dis 1998;27:603.

The club-like nonseptate hyphae observed in cultures of intraoperative specimens from this patient are characteristic of *Rhizopus*, one of the agents of mucormycosis. This patient should be treated with an initial, prolonged course of therapy with liposomal amphotericin B and caspofungin and subsequent chronic suppressive therapy with posaconazole.

Antiviral Agents

Sharon Safrin, MD

CASE STUDY

A 35-year-old white woman who recently tested seropositive for both HIV and hepatitis B virus surface antigen is referred for evaluation. She is feeling well overall but reports a 25-pack-year smoking history. She drinks 3–4 beers per week and has no known medication allergies. She has a history of heroin use and is currently receiving methadone. Physical examination reveals normal vital signs and no abnormalities. White blood cell count is 5800 cells/mm^3 with a normal differential, hemoglobin is 11.8 g/dL, all liver function tests are within normal limits, CD4 cell count is 278 cells/mm^3, and viral load (HIV RNA) is 110,000 copies/mL. What other laboratory tests should be ordered? Which antiretroviral medications would you begin?

Viruses are obligate intracellular parasites; their replication depends primarily on synthetic processes of the host cell. Therefore, to be effective, antiviral agents must either block viral entry into or exit from the cell or be active inside the host cell. As a corollary, non-selective inhibitors of virus replication may interfere with host cell function and result in toxicity.

Progress in antiviral chemotherapy began in the early 1950s, when the search for anticancer drugs generated several new compounds capable of inhibiting viral DNA synthesis. The two first-generation antiviral agents, 5-iododeoxyuridine and trifluorothymidine, had poor specificity (ie, they inhibited host cell DNA as well as viral DNA) that rendered them too toxic for systemic use. However, both agents are effective when used topically for the treatment of herpes keratitis.

Knowledge of the mechanisms of viral replication has provided insights into critical steps in the viral life cycle that can serve as potential targets for antiviral therapy. Recent research has focused on identifying agents with greater selectivity, higher potency, in vivo stability, and reduced toxicity. Antiviral therapy is now available for herpesviruses, hepatitis C virus (HCV), hepatitis B virus (HBV), papillomavirus, influenza, and human immunodeficiency virus (HIV). Antiviral drugs share the common property of being virustatic; they are active only against replicating viruses and do not affect latent virus. Whereas some infections require monotherapy for brief periods of time (eg, acyclovir for herpes simplex virus), others require dual therapy for prolonged periods of time (interferon alfa/ribavirin for HCV), whereas still others require multiple drug therapy for indefinite periods (HIV). In chronic illnesses such

ACRONYMS & OTHER NAMES

3TC	Lamivudine
AZT	Zidovudine (previously azidothymidine)
CMV	Cytomegalovirus
CYP	Cytochrome P450
d4T	Stavudine
ddC	Zalcitabine
ddl	Didanosine
EBV	Epstein-Barr virus
FTC	Emtricitabine
HBeAg	Hepatitis e antigen
HBV	Hepatitis B virus
HCV	Hepatitis C virus
HHV-6	Human herpesvirus-6
HIV	Human immunodeficiency virus
HSV	Herpes simplex virus
NNRTI	Nonnucleoside reverse transcriptase inhibitor
NRTI	Nucleoside/nucleotide reverse transcriptase inhibitor
PI	Protease inhibitor
RSV	Respiratory syncytial virus
SVR	Sustained viral response
UGT1A1	UDP-glucuronosyl transferase 1A1
VZV	Varicella-zoster virus

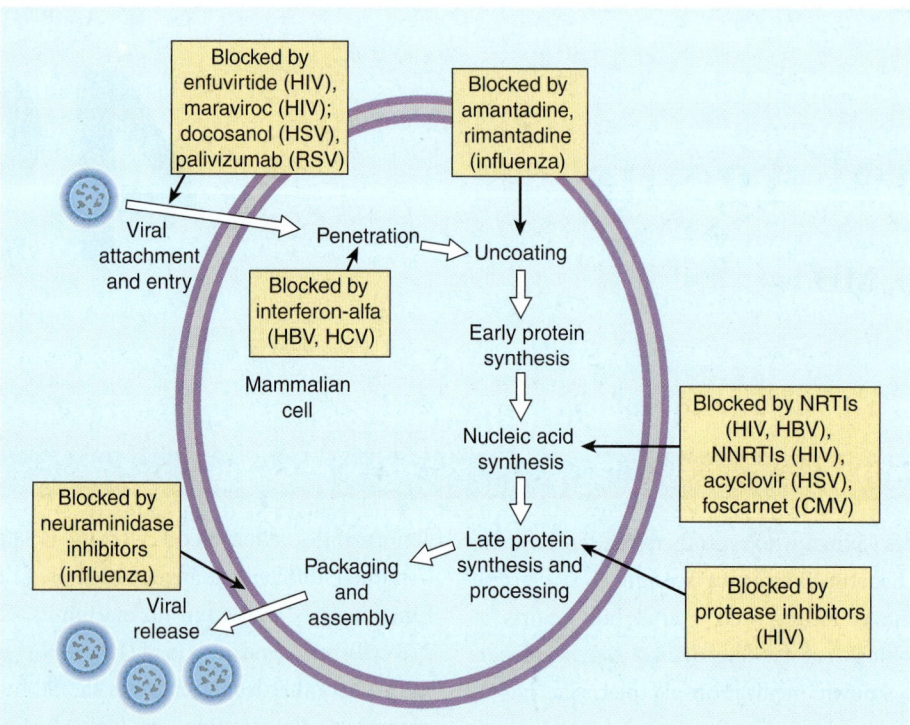

FIGURE 49–1 The major sites of antiviral drug action. Note: Interferon alfas are speculated to have multiple sites of action. (Modified and reproduced, with permission, from Trevor AJ, Katzung BG, Masters SB: *Pharmacology: Examination & Board Review,* 9th ed. McGraw-Hill, 2010.)

as viral hepatitis and HIV infection, potent inhibition of viral replication is crucial in limiting the extent of systemic damage.

Viral replication requires several steps (Figure 49–1): (1) attachment of the virus to receptors on the host cell surface; (2) entry of the virus through the host cell membrane; (3) uncoating of viral nucleic acid; (4) synthesis of early regulatory proteins, eg, nucleic acid polymerases; (5) synthesis of new viral RNA or DNA; (6) synthesis of late, structural proteins; (7) assembly (maturation) of viral particles; and (8) release from the cell. Antiviral agents can potentially target any of these steps.

■ AGENTS TO TREAT HERPES SIMPLEX VIRUS (HSV) & VARICELLA-ZOSTER VIRUS (VZV) INFECTIONS

Three oral nucleoside analogs are licensed for the treatment of HSV and VZV infections: acyclovir, valacyclovir, and famciclovir. They have similar mechanisms of action and comparable indications for clinical use; all are well tolerated. Acyclovir has been the most extensively studied; it was licensed first and is the only one of the three that is available for intravenous use in the United States. Comparative trials have demonstrated similar efficacies of these three agents for the treatment of HSV but modest superiority of famciclovir and valacyclovir for the treatment of herpes zoster infections.

ACYCLOVIR

Acyclovir (Figure 49–2) is an acyclic guanosine derivative with clinical activity against HSV-1, HSV-2, and VZV, but it is approximately 10 times more potent against HSV-1 and HSV-2 than against VZV. In vitro activity against Epstein-Barr virus (EBV), cytomegalovirus (CMV), and human herpesvirus-6 (HHV-6) is present but weaker.

Acyclovir requires three phosphorylation steps for activation. It is converted first to the monophosphate derivative by the virus-specified thymidine kinase and then to the di- and triphosphate compounds by host cell enzymes (Figure 49–3). Because it requires the viral kinase for initial phosphorylation, acyclovir is selectively activated—and the active metabolite accumulates—only in infected cells. Acyclovir triphosphate inhibits viral DNA synthesis by two mechanisms: competition with deoxyGTP for the viral DNA polymerase, resulting in binding to the DNA template as an irreversible complex; and chain termination following incorporation into the viral DNA.

The bioavailability of oral acyclovir is low (15–20%) and is unaffected by food. An intravenous formulation is available. Topical formulations produce high concentrations in herpetic lesions, but systemic concentrations are undetectable by this route.

Acyclovir is cleared primarily by glomerular filtration and tubular secretion. The half-life is 2.5–3 hours in patients with normal renal function and 20 hours in patients with anuria.

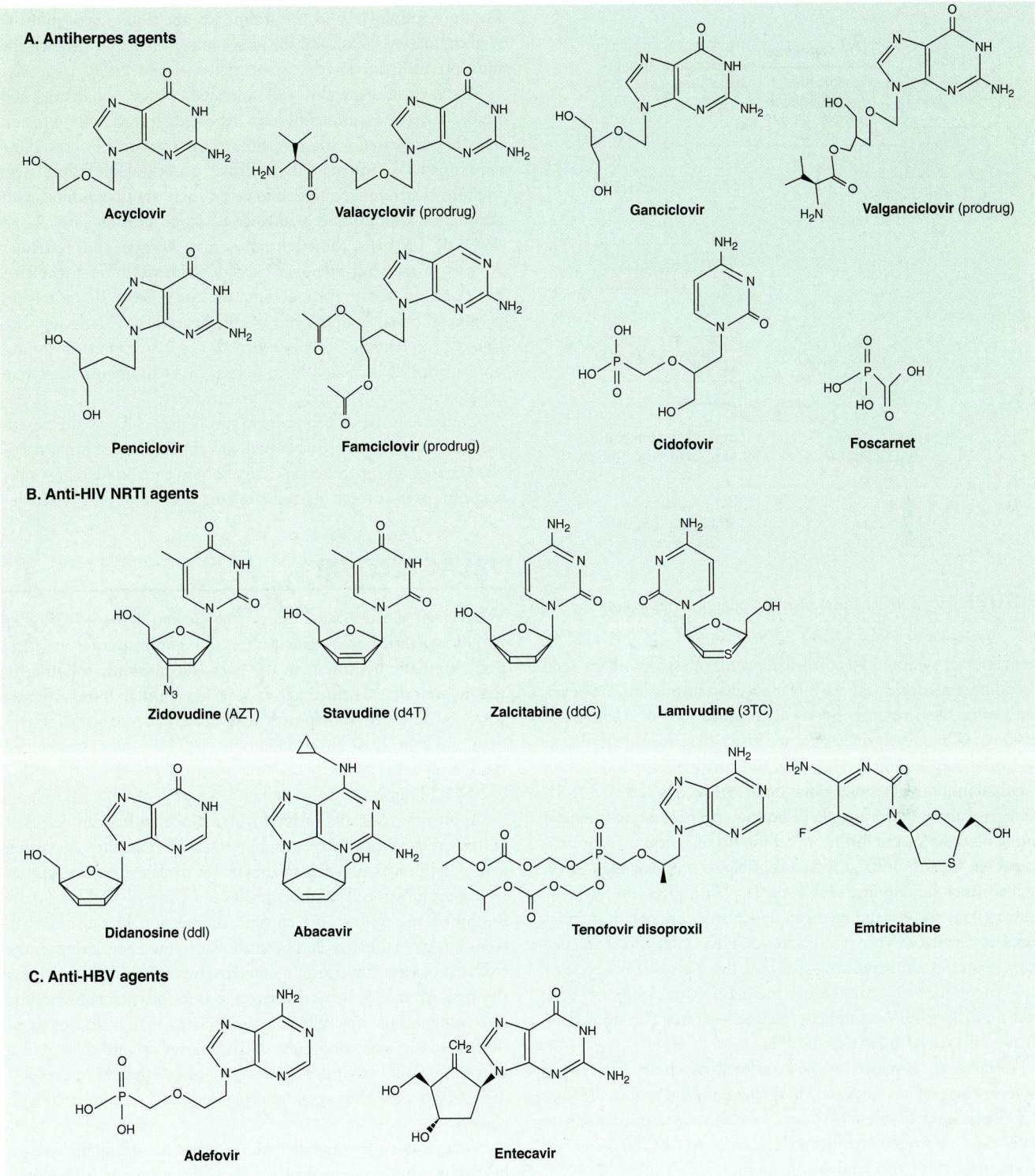

A. Antiherpes agents

Acyclovir   Valacyclovir (prodrug)   Ganciclovir   Valganciclovir (prodrug)

Penciclovir   Famciclovir (prodrug)   Cidofovir   Foscarnet

B. Anti-HIV NRTI agents

Zidovudine (AZT)   Stavudine (d4T)   Zalcitabine (ddC)   Lamivudine (3TC)

Didanosine (ddI)   Abacavir   Tenofovir disoproxil   Emtricitabine

C. Anti-HBV agents

Adefovir   Entecavir

FIGURE 49–2 Chemical structures of some antiviral nucleoside and nucleotide analogs.

Acyclovir diffuses readily into most tissues and body fluids. Cerebrospinal fluid concentrations are 20–50% of serum values.

Oral acyclovir has multiple uses. In first episodes of genital herpes, oral acyclovir shortens the duration of symptoms by approximately 2 days, the time to lesion healing by 4 days, and the duration of viral shedding by 7 days. In recurrent genital herpes, the time course is shortened by 1–2 days. Treatment of first-episode genital herpes does not alter the frequency or severity of recurrent outbreaks. Long-term suppression with oral acyclovir in patients with frequent recurrences of genital herpes decreases the

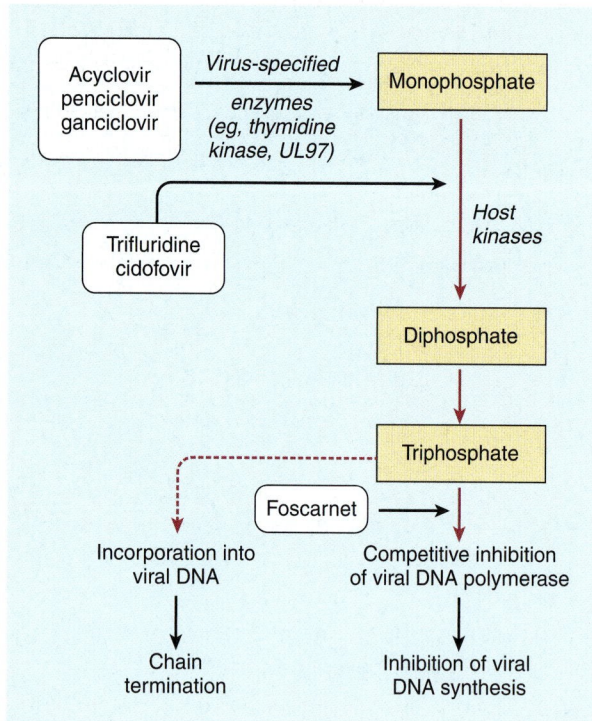

FIGURE 49–3 Mechanism of action of antiherpes agents.

frequency of symptomatic recurrences and of asymptomatic viral shedding, thus decreasing the rate of sexual transmission. However, outbreaks may resume upon discontinuation of suppressive acyclovir. Oral acyclovir is only modestly beneficial in recurrent herpes labialis. In contrast, acyclovir therapy significantly decreases the total number of lesions, duration of symptoms, and viral shedding in patients with varicella (if begun within 24 hours after the onset of rash) or cutaneous zoster (if begun within 72 hours). However, because VZV is less susceptible to acyclovir than HSV, higher doses are required (Table 49–1). When given prophylactically to patients undergoing organ transplantation, oral or intravenous acyclovir prevents reactivation of HSV infection. Evidence from recent clinical trials suggests that the use of daily acyclovir (400 mg twice daily) may reduce the plasma viral load of HIV-1 and the risk of HIV-associated disease progression in individuals dually infected with HSV-2 and HIV-1.

Intravenous acyclovir is the treatment of choice for herpes simplex encephalitis, neonatal HSV infection, and serious HSV or VZV infections (Table 49–1). In immunocompromised patients with VZV infection, intravenous acyclovir reduces the incidence of cutaneous and visceral dissemination.

Topical acyclovir cream is substantially less effective than oral therapy for primary HSV infection. It is of no benefit in treating recurrent genital herpes.

Resistance to acyclovir can develop in HSV or VZV through alteration in either the viral thymidine kinase or the DNA polymerase, and clinically resistant infections have been reported in immunocompromised hosts. Most clinical isolates are resistant on the basis of deficient thymidine kinase activity and thus are cross-resistant to valacyclovir, famciclovir, and ganciclovir. Agents such as

foscarnet, cidofovir, and trifluridine do not require activation by viral thymidine kinase and thus have preserved activity against the most prevalent acyclovir-resistant strains (Figure 49–3).

Acyclovir is generally well tolerated. Nausea, diarrhea, and headache have occasionally been reported. Intravenous infusion may be associated with reversible renal toxicity (ie, crystalline nephropathy or interstitial nephritis) or neurologic effects (eg, tremors, delirium, seizures). However, these are uncommon with adequate hydration and avoidance of rapid infusion rates. High doses of acyclovir cause chromosomal damage and testicular atrophy in rats, but there has been no evidence of teratogenicity, reduction in sperm production, or cytogenetic alterations in peripheral blood lymphocytes in patients receiving daily suppression of genital herpes for more than 10 years. A recent study found no evidence of increased birth defects in 1150 infants who were exposed to acyclovir during the first trimester.

Concurrent use of nephrotoxic agents may enhance the potential for nephrotoxicity. Probenecid and cimetidine decrease acyclovir clearance and increase exposure. Somnolence and lethargy may occur in patients receiving concomitant zidovudine and acyclovir.

VALACYCLOVIR

Valacyclovir is the L-valyl ester of acyclovir (Figure 49–2). It is rapidly converted to acyclovir after oral administration via first-pass enzymatic hydrolysis in the liver and intestine, resulting in serum levels that are three to five times greater than those achieved with oral acyclovir and approximate those achieved with intravenous acyclovir. Oral bioavailability is 54–70%, and cerebrospinal fluid levels are about 50% of those in serum. Elimination half-life is 2.5–3.3 hours.

Approved uses of valacyclovir include treatment of first or recurrent genital herpes, suppression of frequently recurring genital herpes, as a 1-day treatment for orolabial herpes, and as treatment for varicella and herpes zoster (Table 49–1). Once-daily dosing of valacyclovir for chronic suppression in persons with recurrent genital herpes has been shown to markedly decrease the risk of sexual transmission. In comparative trials with acyclovir for the treatment of patients with zoster, rates of cutaneous healing were similar, but valacyclovir was associated with a shorter duration of zoster-associated pain. Higher doses of valacyclovir (2 g four times daily) have also been shown to be effective in preventing CMV disease after organ transplantation when compared with placebo.

Valacyclovir is generally well tolerated, although nausea, headache, vomiting, or rash occasionally occur. At high doses, confusion, hallucinations, and seizures have been reported. AIDS patients who received high-dosage valacyclovir chronically (ie, 8 g/d) had an increased incidence of gastrointestinal intolerance as well as thrombotic thrombocytopenic purpura and hemolytic-uremic syndrome; this dose has also been associated with confusion and hallucinations in transplant patients. In a recent study, there was no evidence of increased birth defects in 181 infants who were exposed to valacyclovir during the first trimester.

TABLE 49–1 Agents to treat or prevent herpes simplex virus (HSV) and varicella-zoster virus (VZV) infections.

	Route of Administration	Use	Recommended Adult Dosage and Regimen
Acyclovir[1]	Oral	First episode genital herpes treatment	400 mg tid or 200 mg 5 times daily × 7–10 days
		Recurrent genital herpes treatment	400 mg tid or 200 mg 5 times daily or 800 mg bid × 3–5 days or 800 mg tid × 2 days
		Genital herpes in the HIV-infected host treatment	400 mg 3–5 times daily × 5–10 days
		Genital herpes suppression in the HIV-infected host	400–800 mg bid–tid
		Herpes proctitis treatment	400 mg 5 times daily until healed
		Orolabial herpes treatment	400 mg 5 times daily × 5 days
		Varicella treatment (age ≥ 2 years)	800 mg qid × 5 days
		Zoster treatment	800 mg 5 times daily × 7–10 days
	Intravenous	Severe HSV treatment	5 mg/kg q8h × 7–10 days
		Mucocutaneous herpes in the immunocompromised host treatment	10 mg/kg q8h × 7–14 days
		Herpes encephalitis treatment	10–15 mg/kg q8h × 14–21 days
		Neonatal HSV infection treatment	10–20 mg/kg q8h × 14–21 days
		Varicella or zoster in the immunosuppressed host treatment	10 mg/kg q8h × 7 days
	Topical (5% cream)	Herpes labialis treatment	Thin film covering lesion 5 times daily × 4 days
Famciclovir[1]	Oral	First episode genital herpes treatment	500 mg tid × 5–10 days
		Recurrent genital herpes treatment	1000 mg bid × 1 day
		Genital herpes in the HIV-infected host treatment	500 mg bid × 5–10 days
		Genital herpes suppression	250 mg bid
		Genital herpes suppression in the HIV-infected host	500 mg bid
		Orolabial herpes treatment	1500 mg once
		Orolabial or genital herpes suppression	250-500 mg bid
		Zoster	500 mg tid × 7 days
Valacyclovir[1]	Oral	First episode genital herpes treatment	1000 mg bid × 10 days
		Recurrent genital herpes treatment	500 mg bid × 3 days
		Genital herpes in the HIV-infected host treatment	500–1000 mg bid × 5–10 days
		Genital herpes suppression	500–1000 mg once daily
		Genital herpes suppression in the HIV-infected host	500 mg bid
		Orolabial herpes	2000 mg bid × 1 day
		Varicella (age ≥ 12 years)	20 mg/d tid × 5 days (maximum, 1 g tid)
		Zoster	1 g tid × 7 days
Foscarnet[1]	Intravenous	Acyclovir-resistant HSV and VZV infections	40 mg/kg q8h until healed
Docosanol	Topical (10% cream)	Recurrent herpes labialis	Thin film covering lesion q2h × 4 days
Penciclovir	Topical (1% cream)	Herpes labialis or herpes genitalis	Thin film covering lesions q2h × 4 days
Trifluridine	Topical (1% solution)	Acyclovir-resistant HSV infection	Thin film covering lesion 5 times daily until healed

[1]Dosage must be reduced in patients with renal insufficiency.

HSV, herpes simplex virus; VZV, varicella-zoster virus.

FAMCICLOVIR

Famciclovir is the diacetyl ester prodrug of 6-deoxypenciclovir, an acyclic guanosine analog (Figure 49–2). After oral administration, famciclovir is rapidly deacetylated and oxidized by first-pass metabolism to penciclovir. It is active in vitro against HSV-1, HSV-2, VZV, EBV, and HBV. As with acyclovir, activation by phosphorylation is catalyzed by the virus-specified thymidine kinase in infected cells, followed by competitive inhibition of the viral DNA polymerase to block DNA synthesis. Unlike acyclovir, however, penciclovir does not cause chain termination. Penciclovir triphosphate has lower affinity for the viral DNA polymerase than acyclovir triphosphate, but it achieves higher intracellular concentrations. The most commonly encountered clinical mutants of HSV are thymidine kinase-deficient; these are cross-resistant to acyclovir and famciclovir.

The bioavailability of penciclovir from orally administered famciclovir is 70%. The intracellular half-life of penciclovir triphosphate is prolonged, at 7–20 hours. Penciclovir is excreted primarily in the urine.

Oral famciclovir is effective for the treatment of first and recurrent genital herpes, for chronic daily suppression of genital herpes, for treatment of herpes labialis, and for the treatment of acute zoster (Table 49–1). One-day usage of famciclovir significantly accelerates time to healing of recurrent genital herpes and of herpes labialis. Comparison of famciclovir to valacyclovir for treatment of herpes zoster in immunocompetent patients showed similar rates of cutaneous healing and pain resolution; both agents shortened the duration of zoster-associated pain compared with acyclovir.

Oral famciclovir is generally well tolerated, although headache, nausea, or diarrhea may occur. As with acyclovir, testicular toxicity has been demonstrated in animals receiving repeated doses. However, men receiving daily famciclovir (250 mg every 12 hours) for 18 weeks had no changes in sperm morphology or motility. In a recent study, there was no evidence of increased birth defects in 32 infants who were exposed to famciclovir during the first trimester. The incidence of mammary adenocarcinoma was increased in female rats receiving famciclovir for 2 years.

PENCICLOVIR

The guanosine analog penciclovir, the active metabolite of famciclovir, is available for topical use. Penciclovir cream (1%) shortens the duration of recurrent herpes labialis or genitalis (Table 49–1). When applied within 1 hour of the onset of prodromal symptoms and continued every 2 hours during waking hours for 4 days, median time until healing was shortened by 17 hours compared with placebo. Adverse effects are uncommon, although application site reactions occur in about 1% of patients.

DOCOSANOL

Docosanol is a saturated 22-carbon aliphatic alcohol that inhibits fusion between the plasma membrane and the HSV envelope, thereby preventing viral entry into cells and subsequent viral replication. Topical docosanol 10% cream is available without a prescription; application site reactions occur in approximately 2% of patients. When applied within 12 hours of the onset of prodromal symptoms, five times daily, median healing time was shortened by 18 hours compared with placebo in recurrent orolabial herpes.

TRIFLURIDINE

Trifluridine (trifluorothymidine) is a fluorinated pyrimidine nucleoside that inhibits viral DNA synthesis in HSV-1, HSV-2, CMV, vaccinia, and some adenoviruses. It is phosphorylated intracellularly by host cell enzymes, and then competes with thymidine triphosphate for incorporation by the viral DNA polymerase (Figure 49–3). Incorporation of trifluridine triphosphate into both viral and host DNA prevents its systemic use. Application of a 1% solution is effective in treating keratoconjunctivitis and recurrent epithelial keratitis due to HSV-1 or HSV-2. Cutaneous application of trifluridine solution, alone or in combination with interferon alfa, has been used successfully in the treatment of acyclovir-resistant HSV infections.

INVESTIGATIONAL AGENTS

Valomaciclovir is an inhibitor of the viral DNA polymerase; it is currently under clinical evaluation for the treatment of patients with acute VZV infection (shingles) and acute EBV infection (infectious mononucleosis).

■ AGENTS TO TREAT CYTOMEGALOVIRUS (CMV) INFECTIONS

CMV infections occur primarily in the setting of advanced immunosuppression and are typically due to reactivation of latent infection. Dissemination of infection results in end-organ disease, including retinitis, colitis, esophagitis, central nervous system disease, and pneumonitis. Although the incidence in HIV-infected patients has markedly decreased with the advent of potent antiretroviral therapy, clinical reactivation of CMV infection after organ transplantation is still prevalent.

The availability of oral valganciclovir and the ganciclovir intraocular implant has decreased the use of intravenous ganciclovir, intravenous foscarnet, and intravenous cidofovir for the treatment of end-organ CMV disease (Table 49–2). Oral valganciclovir has largely replaced oral ganciclovir because of its lower pill burden.

GANCICLOVIR

Ganciclovir is an acyclic guanosine analog (Figure 49–2) that requires activation by triphosphorylation before inhibiting the viral DNA polymerase. Initial phosphorylation is catalyzed by the virus-specified protein kinase phosphotransferase UL97 in

TABLE 49–2 Agents to treat cytomegalovirus (CMV) infection.

Agent	Route of Administration	Use	Recommended Adult Dosage[1]
Valganciclovir	Oral	CMV retinitis treatment	Induction: 900 mg bid × 21 days
			Maintenance: 900 mg daily
	Oral	CMV prophylaxis (transplant patients)	900 mg daily
Ganciclovir	Intravenous	CMV retinitis treatment	Induction: 5 mg/kg q12h × 14–21 days
			Maintenance: 5 mg/kg/d or 6 mg/kg five times per week
	Oral	CMV prophylaxis	1 g tid
		CMV retinitis treatment	1 g tid
	Intraocular implant	CMV retinitis treatment	4.5 mg every 5–8 months
Foscarnet	Intravenous	CMV retinitis treatment	Induction: 60 mg/kg q8h or 90 mg/kg q12h × 14–21 days
			Maintenance: 90–120 mg/kg/d
Cidofovir	Intravenous	CMV retinitis treatment	Induction: 5 mg/kg/wk × 2 weeks
			Maintenance: 5 mg/kg every week

[1]Dosage must be reduced in patients with renal insufficiency.

CMV-infected cells. The activated compound competitively inhibits viral DNA polymerase and causes termination of viral DNA elongation (Figure 49–3). Ganciclovir has in vitro activity against CMV, HSV, VZV, EBV, HHV-6, and HHV-8. Its activity against CMV is up to 100 times greater than that of acyclovir.

Ganciclovir may be administered intravenously, orally, or via intraocular implant. The bioavailability of oral ganciclovir is poor. Cerebrospinal fluid concentrations are approximately 50% of serum concentrations. The elimination half-life is 4 hours, and the intracellular half-life is prolonged at 16–24 hours. Clearance of the drug is linearly related to creatinine clearance. Ganciclovir is readily cleared by hemodialysis.

Intravenous ganciclovir has been shown to delay progression of CMV retinitis in patients with AIDS. Dual therapy with foscarnet and ganciclovir is more effective in delaying progression of retinitis than either drug alone (see Foscarnet), although adverse effects are compounded. Intravenous ganciclovir is also used to treat CMV colitis, esophagitis, and pneumonitis (the latter often treated with a combination of ganciclovir and intravenous cytomegalovirus immunoglobulin) in immunocompromised patients. Intravenous ganciclovir, followed by either oral ganciclovir or high-dose oral acyclovir, reduces the risk of CMV infection in transplant recipients. Oral ganciclovir is indicated for prevention of end-organ CMV disease in AIDS patients and as maintenance therapy of CMV retinitis after induction. Although less effective than intravenous ganciclovir, the oral form carries a diminished risk of myelosuppression and of catheter-related complications. The risk of Kaposi's sarcoma is reduced in AIDS patients receiving long-term ganciclovir, presumably because of activity against HHV-8.

Ganciclovir may also be administered intraocularly to treat CMV retinitis, either by direct intravitreal injection or by intraocular implant. The implant has been shown to delay progression of retinitis to a greater degree than systemic ganciclovir therapy. Surgical replacement of the implant is required at intervals of 5–8 months. Concurrent therapy with a systemic anti-CMV agent is recommended to prevent other sites of end-organ CMV disease.

Resistance to ganciclovir increases with duration of usage. The more common mutation, in UL97, results in decreased levels of the triphosphorylated (ie, active) form of ganciclovir. The less common UL54 mutation in DNA polymerase results in higher levels of resistance and potential cross-resistance with cidofovir and foscarnet. Antiviral susceptibility testing is recommended in patients in whom resistance is suspected clinically, as is the substitution of alternative therapies and concomitant reduction in immunosuppressive therapies, if possible. The addition of CMV hyperimmune globulin may also be considered.

The most common adverse effect of systemic ganciclovir treatment, particularly after intravenous administration, is myelosuppression. Myelosuppression may be additive in patients receiving concurrent zidovudine, azathioprine, or mycophenolate mofetil. Other potential adverse effects are nausea, diarrhea, fever, rash, headache, insomnia, and peripheral neuropathy. Central nervous system toxicity (confusion, seizures, psychiatric disturbance) and hepatotoxicity have been rarely reported. Ganciclovir is mutagenic in mammalian cells and carcinogenic and embryotoxic at high doses in animals and causes aspermatogenesis; the clinical significance of these preclinical data is unclear.

Levels of ganciclovir may rise in patients concurrently taking probenecid or trimethoprim. Concurrent use of ganciclovir with didanosine may result in increased levels of didanosine.

VALGANCICLOVIR

Valganciclovir is an L-valyl ester prodrug of ganciclovir that exists as a mixture of two diastereomers (Figure 49–2). After oral administration, both diastereomers are rapidly hydrolyzed to ganciclovir by esterases in the intestinal wall and liver.

Valganciclovir is well absorbed and rapidly metabolized in the intestinal wall and liver to ganciclovir; no other metabolites have been detected. The bioavailability of oral valganciclovir is 60%; it is recommended that the drug be taken with food. The AUC_{0-24h} resulting from valganciclovir (900 mg once daily) is similar to that after 5 mg/kg once daily of intravenous ganciclovir and approximately 1.65 times that of oral ganciclovir. The major route of elimination is renal, through glomerular filtration and active tubular secretion. Plasma concentrations of valganciclovir are reduced approximately 50% by hemodialysis.

Valganciclovir is indicated for the treatment of CMV retinitis in patients with AIDS and for the prevention of CMV disease in high-risk kidney, heart, and kidney-pancreas transplant patients. Adverse effects, drug interactions, and resistance patterns are the same as those associated with ganciclovir.

FOSCARNET

Foscarnet (phosphonoformic acid) is an inorganic pyrophosphate analog (Figure 49–2) that inhibits herpesvirus DNA polymerase, RNA polymerase, and HIV reverse transcriptase directly without requiring activation by phosphorylation. Foscarnet blocks the pyrophosphate binding site of these enzymes and inhibits cleavage of pyrophosphate from deoxynucleotide triphosphates. It has in vitro activity against HSV, VZV, CMV, EBV, HHV-6, HHV-8, HIV-1, and HIV-2.

Foscarnet is available in an intravenous formulation only; poor oral bioavailability and gastrointestinal intolerance preclude oral use. Cerebrospinal fluid concentrations are 43–67% of steady-state serum concentrations. Although the mean plasma half-life is 3–7 hours, up to 30% of foscarnet may be deposited in bone, with a half-life of several months. The clinical repercussions of this are unknown. Clearance of foscarnet is primarily renal and is directly proportional to creatinine clearance. Serum drug concentrations are reduced approximately 50% by hemodialysis.

Foscarnet is effective in the treatment of CMV retinitis, CMV colitis, CMV esophagitis, acyclovir-resistant HSV infection, and acyclovir-resistant VZV infection. The dosage of foscarnet must be titrated according to the patient's calculated creatinine clearance before each infusion. Use of an infusion pump to control the rate of infusion is important to prevent toxicity, and large volumes of fluid are required because of the drug's poor solubility. The combination of ganciclovir and foscarnet is synergistic in vitro against CMV and has been shown to be superior to either agent alone in delaying progression of retinitis; however, toxicity is also increased when these agents are administered concurrently. As with ganciclovir, a decrease in the incidence of Kaposi's sarcoma has been observed in patients who have received long-term foscarnet.

Foscarnet has been administered intravitreally for the treatment of CMV retinitis in patients with AIDS, but data regarding efficacy and safety are incomplete.

Resistance to foscarnet in HSV and CMV isolates is due to point mutations in the DNA polymerase gene and is typically associated with prolonged or repeated exposure to the drug. Mutations in the HIV-1 reverse transcriptase gene have also been described. Although foscarnet-resistant CMV isolates are typically cross-resistant to ganciclovir, foscarnet activity is usually maintained against ganciclovir- and cidofovir-resistant isolates of CMV.

Potential adverse effects of foscarnet include renal impairment, hypo- or hypercalcemia, hypo- or hyperphosphatemia, hypokalemia, and hypomagnesemia. Saline preloading helps prevent nephrotoxicity, as does avoidance of concomitant administration of drugs with nephrotoxic potential (eg, amphotericin B, pentamidine, aminoglycosides). The risk of severe hypocalcemia, caused by chelation of divalent cations, is increased with concomitant use of pentamidine. Genital ulcerations associated with foscarnet therapy may be due to high levels of ionized drug in the urine. Nausea, vomiting, anemia, elevation of liver enzymes, and fatigue have been reported; the risk of anemia may be additive in patients receiving concurrent zidovudine. Central nervous system toxicity includes headache, hallucinations, and seizures; the risk of seizures may be increased with concurrent use of imipenem. Foscarnet caused chromosomal damage in preclinical studies.

CIDOFOVIR

Cidofovir (Figure 49–2) is a cytosine nucleotide analog with in vitro activity against CMV, HSV-1, HSV-2, VZV, EBV, HHV-6, HHV-8, adenovirus, poxviruses, polyomaviruses, and human papillomavirus. In contrast to ganciclovir, phosphorylation of cidofovir to the active diphosphate is independent of viral enzymes (Figure 49–3); thus activity is maintained against thymidine kinase-deficient or -altered strains of CMV or HSV. Cidofovir diphosphate acts both as a potent inhibitor of and as an alternative substrate for viral DNA polymerase, competitively inhibiting DNA synthesis and becoming incorporated into the viral DNA chain. Cidofovir-resistant isolates tend to be cross-resistant with ganciclovir but retain susceptibility to foscarnet.

Although the terminal half-life of cidofovir is approximately 2.6 hours, the active metabolite cidofovir diphosphate, has a prolonged intracellular half-life of 17–65 hours, thus allowing infrequent dosing. A separate metabolite, cidofovir phosphocholine, has a half-life of at least 87 hours and may serve as an intracellular reservoir of active drug. Cerebrospinal fluid penetration is poor. Elimination is by active renal tubular secretion. High-flux hemodialysis reduces serum levels of cidofovir by approximately 75%.

Intravenous cidofovir is effective for the treatment of CMV retinitis and is used experimentally to treat adenovirus, human papillomavirus, and poxvirus infections. Intravenous cidofovir must be administered with high-dose probenecid (2 g at 3 hours before the infusion and 1 g at 2 and 8 hours after), which blocks active tubular secretion and decreases nephrotoxicity. Before each infusion, cidofovir dosage must be adjusted for alterations in the calculated creatinine clearance or for the presence of urine protein, and aggressive adjunctive hydration is required. Initiation of cidofovir therapy is contraindicated in patients with existing renal insufficiency. Direct intravitreal administration of cidofovir is not recommended because of ocular toxicity.

The primary adverse effect of intravenous cidofovir is a dose-dependent proximal tubular nephrotoxicity, which may be reduced with prehydration using normal saline. Proteinuria, azotemia, metabolic acidosis, and Fanconi's syndrome may occur. Concurrent administration of other potentially nephrotoxic agents (eg, amphotericin B, aminoglycosides, nonsteroidal anti-inflammatory drugs, pentamidine, foscarnet) should be avoided. Prior administration of foscarnet may increase the risk of nephrotoxicity. Other potential adverse effects include uveitis, ocular hypotony, and neutropenia (15–24%). Concurrent probenecid use may result in other toxicities or drug-drug interactions (see Chapter 36). Cidofovir is mutagenic, gonadotoxic, and embryotoxic, and caused mammary adenocarcinomas in rats.

■ ANTIRETROVIRAL AGENTS

Substantial advances have been made in antiretroviral therapy since the introduction of the first agent, zidovudine, in 1987 (Table 49–3). Greater knowledge of viral dynamics through the use of viral load and resistance testing has made it clear that combination therapy with maximally potent agents will reduce viral replication to the lowest possible level and decrease the likelihood of emergence of resistance. Thus, administration of combination antiretroviral therapy, typically comprising at least three antiretroviral agents, has become the standard of care. Viral susceptibility to specific agents varies among patients and may change with time, owing to development of resistance. Therefore, such combinations must be chosen with care and tailored to the individual, as must changes to a given regimen. In addition to potency and susceptibility, important factors in the selection of agents for any given patient are tolerability, convenience, and optimization of adherence.

The retroviral genomic RNA serves as the template for synthesis of a double-stranded DNA copy, the provirus (Figure 49–4). Synthesis of the provirus is mediated by a virus-encoded RNA-dependent DNA polymerase, or "reverse transcriptase." The provirus is translocated to the nucleus and integrated into host DNA. Transcription of this integrated DNA is regulated primarily by cellular machinery.

Six classes of antiretroviral agents are currently available for use: nucleoside/nucleotide reverse transcriptase inhibitors (NRTIs), nonnucleoside reverse transcriptase inhibitors (NNRTIs), protease inhibitors (PIs), fusion inhibitors, CCR5 receptor antagonists, and integrase inhibitors. As new agents have become available, several older ones have had diminished usage, because of either suboptimal safety profile or inferior antiviral potency. It is important to recognize that the high rate of mutation of HIV-1 per replication cycle results in a great potential for genotypic variation. Genotypic resistance has been reported for each of the antiretroviral agents currently in use. Treatment that slows or stops replication is critical in reducing the number of cumulative mutations, as is the use of combinations of agents with differing susceptibility patterns.

Discussion of antiretroviral agents in this chapter is specific to HIV-1. It should be noted that in vitro susceptibility of HIV-2 to the NRTIs is similar to that of HIV-1, albeit with a lower genetic barrier to resistance. There is innate resistance of HIV-2 to the NNRTIs, due to a different structure of the reverse transcriptases' NNRTI binding pockets; enfuvirtide (see below) has no activity against HIV-2. Data on the activity of PI agents and maraviroc against HIV-2 are sparse and inconclusive.

NUCLEOSIDE & NUCLEOTIDE REVERSE TRANSCRIPTASE INHIBITORS

The NRTIs act by competitive inhibition of HIV-1 reverse transcriptase; incorporation into the growing viral DNA chain causes premature chain termination due to inhibition of binding with the incoming nucleotide (Figure 49–4). Each agent requires intracytoplasmic activation via phosphorylation by cellular enzymes to the triphosphate form.

Typical resistance mutations include M184V, L74V, D67N, and M41L. Lamivudine or emtricitabine therapy tends to select rapidly for the M184V mutation in regimens that are not fully suppressive. While the M184V mutation confers reduced susceptibility to abacavir, didanosine, and zalcitabine, its presence may restore phenotypic susceptibility to zidovudine. The K65R mutation is associated with reduced susceptibility to tenofovir, abacavir, lamivudine, and emtricitabine.

All NRTIs may be associated with mitochondrial toxicity, probably owing to inhibition of mitochondrial DNA polymerase gamma. Less commonly, lactic acidosis with hepatic steatosis may occur, which can be fatal. NRTI treatment should be suspended in the setting of rapidly rising aminotransferase levels, progressive hepatomegaly, or metabolic acidosis of unknown cause. The thymidine analogs zidovudine and stavudine may be particularly associated with dyslipidemia and insulin resistance. Also, some evidence suggests an increased risk of myocardial infarction in patients receiving abacavir or didanosine; this bears further investigation.

ABACAVIR

Abacavir is a guanosine analog (Figure 49–2) that is well absorbed following oral administration (83%) and is unaffected by food. The serum half-life is 1.5 hours. The drug undergoes hepatic glucuronidation and carboxylation. Cerebrospinal fluid levels are approximately one third those of plasma.

Abacavir is often co-administered with lamivudine, and a once-daily, fixed-dose combination formulation is available. Abacavir is also available in a fixed-dose combination with lamivudine and zidovudine.

High-level resistance to abacavir appears to require at least two or three concomitant mutations and thus tends to develop slowly.

Hypersensitivity reactions, occasionally fatal, have been reported in up to 8% of patients receiving abacavir and may be more severe in association with once-daily dosing. Symptoms, which generally occur within the first 6 weeks of therapy, include fever, fatigue, nausea, vomiting, diarrhea, and abdominal pain.

TABLE 49–3 Currently available antiretroviral agents.

Agent	Class of Agent	Recommended Adult Dosage	Administration Recommendation	Characteristic Adverse Effects	Comments
Abacavir	NRTI[1]	300 mg bid or 600 mg qd	Testing to rule out the presence of the HLA-B5701 allele is recommended prior to the initiation of therapy	Rash, hypersensitivity reaction, nausea. Possible increase in myocardial infarction	Avoid alcohol
Atazanavir	PI[2]	400 mg qd or 300 mg qd with ritonavir 100 mg qd. Adjust dose in hepatic insufficiency	Take with food. Separate dosing from ddl or antacids by 1 h. Separate dosing from cimetidine and other acid-reducing agents by 12 h	Nausea, vomiting, diarrhea, abdominal pain, headache, peripheral neuropathy, skin rash, indirect hyperbilirubinemia, prolonged PR and/or QT$_c$ interval	See footnote 4 for contraindicated medications. Also avoid etravirine, fosamprenavir, nevirapine, and proton pump inhibitors. Avoid in severe hepatic insufficiency
Darunavir	PI[2]	Treatment-experienced: 600 mg bid with ritonavir 100 mg bid. Treatment-naïve: 800 mg qd with ritonavir 100 mg qd. Tablets can be dissolved in water	Take with food	Diarrhea, headache, nausea, rash, hyperlipidemia, ↑ liver enzymes, ↑ serum amylase	Avoid in patients with sulfa allergy. See footnote 4 for contraindicated medications
Delavirdine	NNRTI	400 mg tid	Separate dosing from ddl or antacids by 1 h	Rash, ↑ liver enzymes, headache, nausea, diarrhea	See footnote 4 for contraindicated medications. Also avoid concurrent fosamprenavir and rifabutin. Teratogenic in rats
Didanosine (ddl)	NRTI[1]	Tablets, 400 mg qd or 200 mg bid,[3] adjusted for weight. Buffered powder, 250 mg bid[3]	30 min before or 2 h after meals. Separate dosing from fluoroquinolones and tetracyclines by 2 h	Peripheral neuropathy, pancreatitis, diarrhea, nausea, hyperuricemia. Possible increase in myocardial infarction	Avoid concurrent neuropathic drugs (eg, stavudine, zalcitabine, isoniazid), ribavirin, and alcohol. Do not administer with tenofovir
Efavirenz	NNRTI	600 mg qd	Take on an empty stomach. Bedtime dosing recommended initially to minimize central nervous system side effects	Central nervous system effects, rash, ↑ liver enzymes, headache, nausea	See footnote 4 for contraindicated medications. Teratogenic in primates
Emtricitabine	NRTI[1]	200 mg qd.[3] Tablets can be dissolved in water	Oral solution should be refrigerated	Headache, diarrhea, nausea, asthenia, skin hyperpigmentation	Do not administer concurrent lamivudine. Avoid disulfiram and metronidazole with oral solution
Enfuvirtide	Fusion inhibitor	90 mg subcutaneously bid	Store at room temperature as a powder; refrigerate once reconstituted	Local injection site reactions, hypersensitivity reaction	
Etravirine	NNRTI	200 mg bid	Take after a meal; do not take on an empty stomach	Rash, nausea, diarrhea	See footnote 4 for contraindicated medications. Do not administer with other NNRTIs, indinavir, atazanavir-ritonavir, fosamprenavir-ritonavir, tipranavir-ritonavir, or any unboosted PI
Fosamprenavir	PI[2]	1400 mg bid or 700 mg bid with ritonavir 100 mg bid or 1400 mg daily with ritonavir 100–200 mg qd. Adjust dose in hepatic insufficiency	Separate dosing from antacids or didanosine by ≥ 1 h. Avoid concurrent high-fat meals	Diarrhea, nausea, vomiting, hypertriglyceridemia, rash, headache, perioral paresthesias, ↑ liver enzymes	See footnote 4 for contraindicated medications. Do not administer with etravirine; do not administer with lopinavir/ritonavir or in severe hepatic insufficiency. Also avoid cimetidine, disulfiram, metronidazole, vitamin E, ritonavir oral solution, and alcohol when using the oral solution

(continued)

TABLE 49–3 **Currently available antiretroviral agents. (Continued)**

Agent	Class of Agent	Recommended Adult Dosage	Administration Recommendation	Characteristic Adverse Effects	Comments
Indinavir	PI[2]	800 mg tid or 800 mg bid with ritonavir 100–200 mg bid. Adjust dose in hepatic insufficiency	Best on an empty stomach. Drink at least 48 oz liquid daily. Separate dosing from ddI by 1 h. Store in original container, which contains desiccant	Nephrolithiasis, nausea, indirect hyperbilirubinemia, headache, asthenia, blurred vision	See footnote 4 for contraindicated medications. Do not administer with etravirine
Lamivudine	NRTI[1]	150 mg bid or 300 mg qd[3]		Nausea, headache, dizziness, fatigue	Do not administer with zalcitabine
Lopinavir/ritonavir	PI/PI[2]	Treatment-experienced: 400 mg/100 mg bid. Treatment-naïve: 800 mg/200 mg qd. May need dose adjustment in hepatic insufficiency	Take with food. Separate dosing from ddI by 1 h. Store capsules and solution in refrigerator	Diarrhea, abdominal pain, nausea, hypertriglyceridemia, headache, ↑ liver enzymes	See footnote 4 for contraindicated medications. Also avoid fosamprenavir. Avoid disulfiram and metronidazole with oral solution
Maraviroc	CCR5 inhibitor	300 mg bid; 150 bid with CYP3A inhibitors; 600 mg bid with CYP3A inducers[3]		Muscle and joint pain, diarrhea, sleep disturbance, ↑ liver enzymes	See footnote 4 for medications that must be co-administered with caution. Avoid rifampin
Nelfinavir	PI[2]	750 mg tid or 1250 mg bid	Take with food	Diarrhea, nausea, flatulence	See footnote 4 for contraindicated medications. Do not administer with etravirine
Nevirapine	NNRTI	200 mg bid. Adjust dose in hepatic insufficiency	Dose-escalate from 200 mg daily over 14 days to decrease frequency of rash	Rash, hepatitis (occasionally fulminant), nausea, headache	See footnote 4 for contraindicated medications. Do not administer with atazanavir
Raltegravir	Integrase inhibitor	400 mg bid. Increase dose to 800 mg bid if administered with rifampin	Separate dosing from antacids by ≥ 4 h	Diarrhea, nausea, fatigue, headache, dizziness, muscle aches, ↑ creatine kinase	Avoid rifampin
Ritonavir	PI[2]	600 mg bid	Take with food. Separate dosing with ddI by 2 h. Dose-escalate from 300 mg bid over 1–2 weeks to improve tolerance. Refrigerate capsules but not oral solution	Nausea, diarrhea, paresthesias, hepatitis	See footnote 4 for contraindicated medications. Avoid disulfiram and metronidazole with oral solution
Saquinavir	PI[2]	1000 mg bid with ritonavir 100 mg bid	Take within 2 h of a full meal. Refrigeration recommended	Nausea, diarrhea, rhinitis, abdominal pain, dyspepsia, rash	See footnote 4 for contraindicated medications. Avoid in severe hepatic insufficiency. Use sunscreen owing to an increase in photosensitivity. Avoid concomitant garlic capsules
Stavudine	NRTI[1]	30–40 mg bid, depending on weight[3]		Peripheral neuropathy, lipodystrophy, hyperlipidemia, rapidly progressive ascending neuromuscular weakness (rare), pancreatitis	Avoid concurrent zidovudine and neuropathic drugs (eg, ddI, zalcitabine, isoniazid)
Tenofovir	NRTI[1]	300 mg qd[3]	Take with food	Nausea, diarrhea, vomiting, flatulence, headache, renal insufficiency	Avoid concurrent atazanavir, probenecid, didanosine
Tipranavir	PI[2]	500 mg bid with ritonavir 200 mg bid. Avoid use in hepatic insufficiency	Take with food. Separate from ddI by at least 2 h. Avoid antacids. Avoid in patients with sulfa allergy. Refrigeration required	Diarrhea, nausea, vomiting, abdominal pain, rash, ↑ liver enzymes, hypercholesterolemia, hypertriglyceridemia	See footnote 4 for contraindicated medications. Avoid concurrent fosamprenavir, saquinavir, etravirine. Do not administer to patients at risk for bleeding

(continued)

TABLE 49–3 Currently available antiretroviral agents. (Continued)

Agent	Class of Agent	Recommended Adult Dosage	Administration Recommendation	Characteristic Adverse Effects	Comments
Zalcitabine	NRTI[1]	0.75 mg tid[3]	Administer 1 h before or 2 h after an antacid	Peripheral neuropathy; oral ulcerations, pancreatitis, headache, nausea, rash, arthralgias	Avoid concurrent cimetidine; avoid concurrent neuropathic drugs (eg, ddI, stavudine, isoniazid). Do not administer with lamivudine
Zidovudine	NRTI[1]	200 mg tid or 300 mg bid[3]		Macrocytic anemia, neutropenia, nausea, headache, insomnia, asthenia	Avoid concurrent stavudine and myelosuppressive drugs (eg, ganciclovir, ribavirin)

[1] All NRTI agents, including tenofovir, carry the risk of lactic acidosis with hepatic steatosis as a potential adverse event.

[2] All PI agents, with the possible exception of fosamprenavir, carry the risk of hyperlipidemia, fat maldistribution, hyperglycemia, and insulin resistance as potential adverse events.

[3] Adjust dose in renal insufficiency.

[4] Because of altered systemic exposures, contraindicated concurrent drugs generally include antiarrhythmics (flecainide, propafenone), antihistamines (astemizole, terfenadine), sedative-hypnotics (alprazolam, diazepam, flurazepam, midazolam, triazolam, trazodone, clorazepate), neuroleptics (pimozide), ergot alkaloid derivatives, HMG-CoA reductase inhibitors (atorvastatin, simvastatin, lovastatin, rosuvastatin), anticonvulsants (phenobarbital, phenytoin), oral contraceptives (ethinyl estradiol/norethindrone acetate), cisapride, rifampin, rifapentine, and St. John's wort. Drugs that should be used with caution owing to altered levels include amiodarone, bepridil, quinidine, lidocaine, nifedipine, nicardipine, felodipine, sildenafil, vardenafil, tadalafil, warfarin, levodopa, tacrolimus, cyclosporine, rapamycin, voriconazole, itraconazole, ketoconazole, carbamazepine, desipramine, bupropion, dofetilide, fluticasone, atovaquone, dapsone, dexamethasone, methadone, omeprazole, and lansoprazole. The dosages of rifabutin and clarithromycin should be decreased when administered concurrently.

NNRTI, nonnucleoside reverse transcriptase inhibitor; NRTI, nucleoside/nucleotide reverse transcriptase inhibitor; PI, protease inhibitor.

Respiratory symptoms such as dyspnea, pharyngitis, and cough may also be present, and skin rash occurs in about 50% of patients. The laboratory abnormalities of a mildly elevated serum aminotransferase or creatine kinase level may be present but are nonspecific. Although the syndrome tends to resolve quickly with discontinuation of medication, rechallenge with abacavir results in return of symptoms within hours and may be fatal. Testing for the HLA-B5701 allele before initiation of abacavir therapy is recommended to identify patients with an increased risk for an abacavir-associated hypersensitivity reaction. Although the positive predictive value of this test is only about 50%, it has a negative predictive value of approximately 100%.

Other potential adverse events are rash, fever, nausea, vomiting, diarrhea, headache, dyspnea, fatigue, and pancreatitis (rare). Abacavir should be used cautiously in patients with existing cardiac risk factors due to a possible increased risk of myocardial events. Since abacavir may lower methadone levels, patients receiving these two agents concurrently should be monitored for signs of opioid withdrawal and may require an increased dose of methadone.

DIDANOSINE

Didanosine (ddI) is a synthetic analog of deoxyadenosine (Figure 49–2). Oral bioavailability is approximately 40%; dosing on an empty stomach is optimal, but buffered formulations are necessary to prevent inactivation by gastric acid (Table 49–3). Cerebrospinal fluid concentrations of the drug are approximately 20% of serum concentrations. Serum half-life is 1.5 hours, but the intracellular half-life of the activated compound is as long as 20–24 hours. The drug is eliminated by both cellular metabolism and renal excretion.

The major clinical toxicity associated with didanosine therapy is dose-dependent pancreatitis. Other risk factors for pancreatitis (eg, alcohol abuse, hypertriglyceridemia) are relative contraindications, and concurrent drugs with the potential to cause pancreatitis, including zalcitabine, stavudine, ribavirin, and hydroxyurea, should be avoided (Table 49–3). The risk of peripheral distal sensory neuropathy, another potential toxicity, may be increased with concurrent use of stavudine, isoniazid, vincristine, or ribavirin. Other reported adverse effects include diarrhea (particularly with the buffered formulation), hepatitis, esophageal ulceration, cardiomyopathy, central nervous system toxicity (headache, irritability, insomnia), and hypertriglyceridemia. Previously asymptomatic hyperuricemia may precipitate attacks of gout in susceptible individuals; concurrent use of allopurinol may increase levels of didanosine. Reports of retinal changes and optic neuritis in patients receiving didanosine, particularly in adults receiving high doses and in children, mandate periodic retinal examinations. Lipoatrophy appears to be more common in patients receiving didanosine or other thymidine analogs. As with abacavir, didanosine should be used cautiously in patients with cardiac risk factors due to a possibly increased risk of myocardial infarction.

The buffer in didanosine tablets and powder interferes with absorption of indinavir, delavirdine, atazanavir, dapsone, itraconazole, and fluoroquinolone agents; therefore, administration should be separated in time. Serum levels of didanosine are increased when co-administered with tenofovir or ganciclovir, and are decreased by atazanavir, delavirdine, ritonavir, tipranavir, and methadone (Table 49–4).

EMTRICITABINE

Emtricitabine (FTC) is a fluorinated analog of lamivudine with a long intracellular half-life (> 24 hours), allowing for once-daily dosing (Figure 49–2). Oral bioavailability of the capsules is 93% and is unaffected by food, but penetration into the cerebrospinal

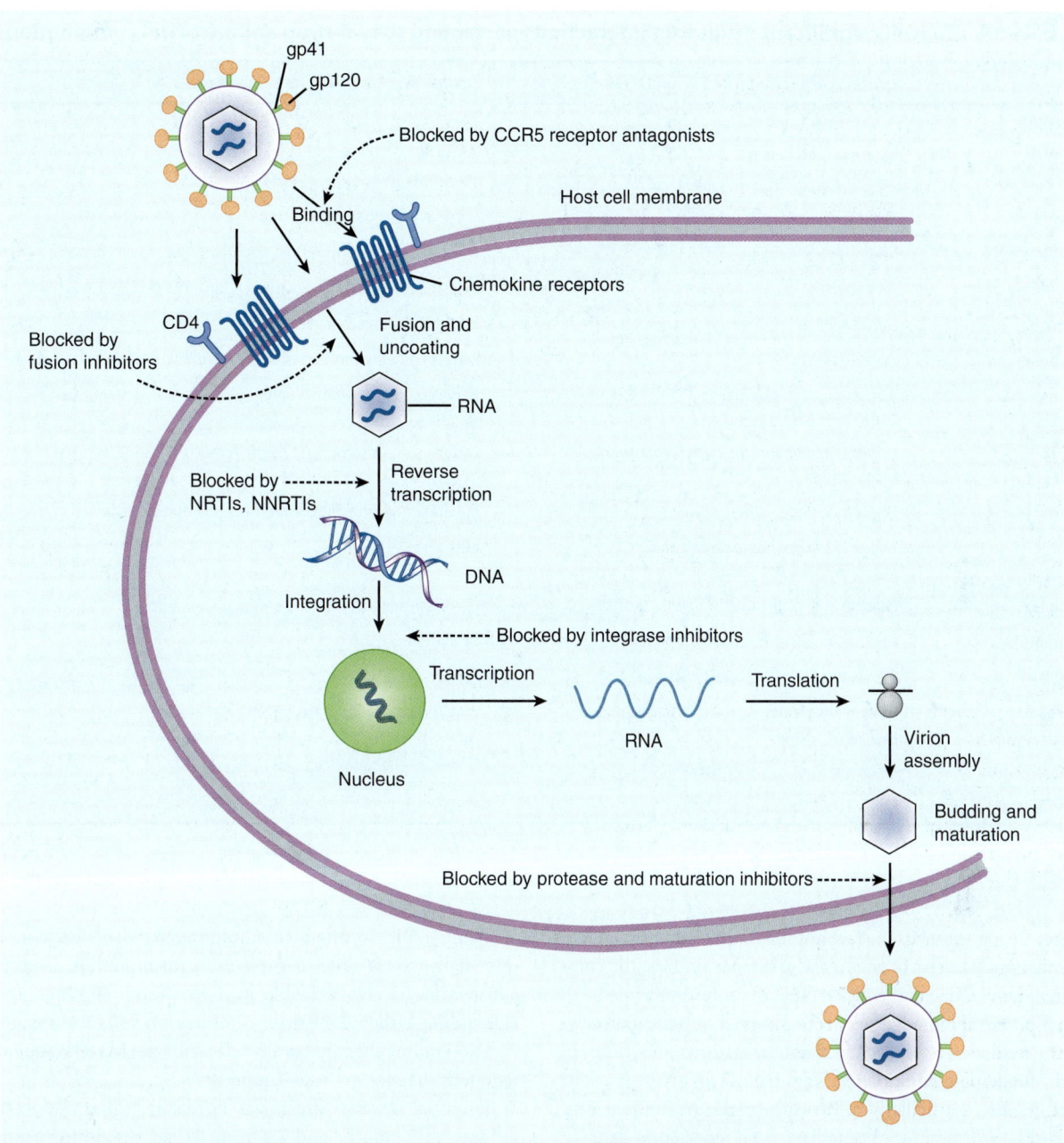

FIGURE 49–4 Life cycle of HIV. Binding of viral glycoproteins to host cell CD4 and chemokine receptors leads to fusion of the viral and host cell membranes via gp41 and entry of the virion into the cell. After uncoating, reverse transcription copies the single-stranded HIV RNA genome into double-stranded DNA, which is integrated into the host cell genome. Gene transcription by host cell enzymes produces messenger RNA, which is translated into proteins that assemble into immature noninfectious virions that bud from the host cell membrane. Maturation into fully infectious virions is through proteolytic cleavage. NNRTIs, nonnucleoside reverse transcriptase inhibitors; NRTIs, nucleoside/nucleotide reverse transcriptase inhibitors.

fluid is low. Elimination is by both glomerular filtration and active tubular secretion. The serum half-life is about 10 hours.

The oral solution, which contains propylene glycol, is contraindicated in young children, pregnant women, patients with renal or hepatic failure, and those using metronidazole or disulfiram. Also, because of its activity against HBV, patients co-infected with HIV and HBV should be closely monitored if treatment with emtricitabine is interrupted or discontinued, owing to the likelihood of hepatitis flare.

Emtricitabine is often co-administered with tenofovir, and a once-daily, fixed-dose combination formulation is available, both alone and in combination with efavirenz. In a recent placebo-controlled study, use of emtricitabine and tenofovir was effective as preexposure prophylaxis, reducing HIV acquisition in men who have sex with men.

Like lamivudine, the M184V/I mutation is most frequently associated with emtricitabine use and may emerge rapidly in

TABLE 49–4 Clinically significant drug-drug interactions pertaining to two-drug antiretroviral combinations.[1]

Agent	Drugs That Increase Its Serum Levels	Drugs That Decrease Its Serum Levels
Abacavir		Tipranavir
Atazanavir	Ritonavir	Didanosine, efavirenz, etravirine, nevirapine, ritonavir, stavudine, tenofovir, tipranavir
Darunavir	Indinavir	Lopinavir/ritonavir, saquinavir
Delavirdine	Etravirine	Didanosine, fosamprenavir, lopinavir, nelfinavir, ritonavir
Didanosine	Tenofovir	Atazanavir, delavirdine, ritonavir, tipranavir
Efavirenz	Darunavir	Etravirine, nelfinavir, nevirapine
Etravirine	Delavirdine	Darunavir, efavirenz, nevirapine, ritonavir, saquinavir, tipranavir
Fosamprenavir	Atazanavir, delavirdine, etravirine, indinavir, nelfinavir	Efavirenz, lopinavir/ritonavir, nevirapine, tipranavir
Indinavir	Darunavir, delavirdine, nelfinavir, tipranavir, zidovudine	Didanosine, fosamprenavir, efavirenz, etravirine, nevirapine
Lopinavir/ritonavir	Darunavir, delavirdine, indinavir, ritonavir	Efavirenz, nelfinavir, nevirapine, tenofovir, tipranavir
Maraviroc	Atazanavir, darunavir, delavirdine, lopinavir/ritonavir, nevirapine	Efavirenz, etravirine
Nelfinavir	Delavirdine, etravirine, indinavir, ritonavir	Nevirapine
Nevirapine	Atazanavir, fosamprenavir, lopinavir	Etravirine
Ritonavir	Delavirdine	Tenofovir
Saquinavir	Atazanavir, delavirdine, indinavir, lopinavir, nelfinavir, ritonavir	Efavirenz, etravirine, nevirapine, tipranavir
Tenofovir	Atazanavir, lopinavir/ritonavir	
Tipranavir	Enfuvirtide	Efavirenz

[1]Dose adjustment may be necessary if co-administered.

patients receiving regimens that are not fully suppressive. Because of their similar mechanisms of action and resistance profiles, the combination of lamivudine and emtricitabine is not recommended.

The most common adverse effects observed in patients receiving emtricitabine are headache, diarrhea, nausea, and rash. In addition, hyperpigmentation of the palms or soles may be observed (~ 3%), particularly in African-Americans (up to 13%). No drug-drug interactions of note have been reported to date.

LAMIVUDINE

Lamivudine (3TC) is a cytosine analog (Figure 49–2) with in vitro activity against HIV-1 that is synergistic with a variety of antiretroviral nucleoside analogs—including zidovudine and stavudine—against both zidovudine-sensitive and zidovudine-resistant HIV-1 strains. As with emtricitabine, lamivudine has activity against HBV; therefore, discontinuation in patients that are co-infected with HIV and HBV may be associated with a flare of hepatitis.

Oral bioavailability exceeds 80% and is not food-dependent. In children, the average cerebrospinal fluid:plasma ratio of lamivudine was 0.2. Serum half-life is 2.5 hours, whereas the intracellular half-life of the triphosphorylated compound is 11–14 hours. Most of the drug is eliminated unchanged in the urine.

Lamivudine is often co-administered with abacavir, and a once-daily, fixed-dose combination formulation is available. Lamivudine is also available in a fixed-dose combination with zidovudine, either alone or in combination with abacavir.

Lamivudine therapy rapidly selects for the M184V mutation in regimens that are not fully suppressive.

Potential adverse effects are headache, dizziness, insomnia, fatigue, dry mouth, and gastrointestinal discomfort, although these are typically mild and infrequent. Lamivudine's bioavailability increases when it is co-administered with trimethoprim-sulfamethoxazole. Lamivudine and zalcitabine may inhibit the intracellular phosphorylation of one another; therefore, their concurrent use should be avoided if possible. Short-term safety of lamivudine has been demonstrated for both mother and infant.

STAVUDINE

The thymidine analog stavudine (d4T) (Figure 49–2) has high oral bioavailability (86%) that is not food-dependent. The serum half-life is 1.1 hours, the intracellular half-life is 3.0–3.5 hours, and mean cerebrospinal fluid concentrations are 55% of those of plasma. Excretion is by active tubular secretion and glomerular filtration.

The major toxicity is a dose-related peripheral sensory neuropathy. The incidence of neuropathy may be increased when stavudine is administered with other neuropathy-inducing drugs such as didanosine, zalcitabine, vincristine, isoniazid, or ribavirin, or in patients with advanced immunosuppression. Symptoms typically resolve upon discontinuation of stavudine; in such cases, a reduced dosage may be cautiously restarted. Other potential adverse effects are pancreatitis, arthralgias, and elevation in serum aminotransferases. Lactic acidosis with hepatic steatosis, as well as lipodystrophy, appear to occur more frequently in patients receiving stavudine than in those receiving other NRTI agents. Moreover, because the co-administration of stavudine and didanosine may increase the incidence of lactic acidosis and pancreatitis, concurrent use should be avoided. This combination has been implicated in several deaths in HIV-infected pregnant women. A rare adverse effect is a rapidly progressive ascending neuromuscular weakness. Since zidovudine may reduce the phosphorylation of stavudine, these two drugs should not be used together. There is no evidence of human teratogenicity in those taking stavudine.

TENOFOVIR

Tenofovir is an acyclic nucleoside phosphonate (ie, nucleotide) analog of adenosine (Figure 49–2). Like the nucleoside analogs, tenofovir competitively inhibits HIV reverse transcriptase and causes chain termination after incorporation into DNA. However, only two rather than three intracellular phosphorylations are required for active inhibition of DNA synthesis. Tenofovir is also approved for the treatment of patients with HBV infection.

Tenofovir disoproxil fumarate is a water-soluble prodrug of active tenofovir. The oral bioavailability in fasted patients is approximately 25% and increases to 39% after a high-fat meal. The prolonged serum (12–17 hours) and intracellular half-lives allow once-daily dosing. Elimination occurs by both glomerular filtration and active tubular secretion.

Tenofovir is often co-administered with emtricitabine, and a once-daily, fixed-dose combination formulation is available, either alone or in combination with efavirenz. A recent placebo-controlled study found that use of emtricitabine and tenofovir was effective as preexposure prophylaxis, reducing HIV acquisition in men who have sex with men. In another placebo-controlled study, use of the experimental 1% tenofovir gel as a vaginal microbicide was effective in decreasing the incidence of heterosexual HIV acquisition.

The primary mutation associated with resistance to tenofovir is K65R.

Gastrointestinal complaints (eg, nausea, diarrhea, vomiting, flatulence) are the most common adverse effects but rarely require discontinuation of therapy. Since tenofovir is formulated with lactose, these may occur more frequently in patients with lactose intolerance. Other potential adverse effects include headache and asthenia. Tenofovir-associated proximal renal tubulopathy causes excessive renal phosphate and calcium losses and 1-hydroxylation defects of vitamin D, and preclinical studies in several animal species have demonstrated bone toxicity (eg, osteomalacia). Monitoring of bone mineral density should be considered with long-term use in those with risk factors for or with known osteoporosis, as well as in children. Reduction of renal function over time, as well as cases of acute renal failure and Fanconi's syndrome, have been reported in patients receiving tenofovir alone or in combination with emtricitabine. For this reason, tenofovir should be used with caution in patients at risk for renal dysfunction. Tenofovir may compete with other drugs that are actively secreted by the kidneys, such as cidofovir, acyclovir, and ganciclovir. Concurrent use of atazanavir or lopinavir/ritonavir may increase serum levels of tenofovir (Table 49–4).

Tenofovir is associated with decreased fetal growth and reduction in fetal bone porosity in monkeys. There is significant placental passage in humans.

ZALCITABINE

Zalcitabine (ddC) is a cytosine analog with high oral bioavailability (87%) and a serum half-life of 1–2 hours (Figure 49–2). An intracellular half-life of 2.6 hours necessitates thrice-daily dosing, which limits its usefulness. Plasma levels decrease by 25–39% when the drug is administered with food or antacids. The drug is excreted renally. Cerebrospinal fluid concentrations are approximately 20% of those in the plasma.

Although a variety of mutations associated with in vitro resistance to zalcitabine have been described, phenotypic resistance appears to be rare.

Zalcitabine therapy is associated with a dose-dependent peripheral neuropathy that can be treatment-limiting in 10–20% of patients but appears to be slowly reversible if treatment is stopped promptly. The potential for causing peripheral neuropathy constitutes a relative contraindication to use with other drugs that may cause neuropathy, including stavudine, didanosine, isoniazid, vincristine, and ribavirin. Decreased creatinine clearance or concurrent use of potential nephrotoxins (eg, amphotericin B, foscarnet, and aminoglycosides) may increase the risk of zalcitabine neuropathy, as does more advanced immunosuppression. The other major reported toxicity is oral and esophageal ulceration. Pancreatitis occurs less frequently than with didanosine administration, but co-administration of other drugs that cause pancreatitis may increase the frequency of this adverse effect. Headache, nausea, rash, and arthralgias may occur but tend to be mild or to resolve during therapy. Zalcitabine causes thymic lymphoma in rodents, as well as hydrocephalus at high doses; clinical relevance is unclear. The AUC of zalcitabine increases when co-administered with probenecid or cimetidine, and bioavailability decreases with concurrent antacids or metoclopramide. Lamivudine inhibits the phosphorylation of zalcitabine in vitro, potentially interfering with its efficacy.

ZIDOVUDINE

Zidovudine (**azidothymidine; AZT**) is a deoxythymidine analog (Figure 49–2) that is well absorbed (63%) and distributed to most body tissues and fluids, including the cerebrospinal fluid, where drug levels are 60–65% of those in serum. Although the serum half-life averages 1 hour, the intracellular half-life of the phosphorylated compound is 3–4 hours, allowing twice-daily dosing. Zidovudine is eliminated primarily by renal excretion following glucuronidation in the liver.

Zidovudine is available in a fixed-dose combination formulation with lamivudine, either alone or in combination with abacavir.

Zidovudine was the first antiretroviral agent to be approved and has been well studied. The drug has been shown to decrease the rate of clinical disease progression and prolong survival in HIV-infected individuals. Efficacy has also been demonstrated in the treatment of HIV-associated dementia and thrombocytopenia. In pregnancy (Table 49–5), a regimen of oral zidovudine beginning between 14 and 34 weeks of gestation, intravenous zidovudine during labor, and zidovudine syrup to the neonate from birth through 6 weeks of age has been shown to reduce the rate of vertical (mother-to-newborn) transmission of HIV by up to 23%.

High-level zidovudine resistance is generally seen in strains with three or more of the five most common mutations: M41L, D67N, K70R, T215F, and K219Q. However, the emergence of certain mutations that confer decreased susceptibility to one drug (eg, L74V for didanosine and M184V for lamivudine) may enhance zidovudine susceptibility in previously zidovudine-resistant strains. Withdrawal of zidovudine may permit the reversion of zidovudine-resistant HIV-1 isolates to the susceptible wild-type phenotype.

The most common adverse effect of zidovudine is myelosuppression, resulting in macrocytic anemia (1–4%) or neutropenia (2–8%). Gastrointestinal intolerance, headaches, and insomnia may occur but tend to resolve during therapy. Lipoatrophy appears to be more common in patients receiving zidovudine or other thymidine analogs. Less common toxicities include thrombocytopenia, hyperpigmentation of the nails, and myopathy. High doses can cause anxiety, confusion, and tremulousness. Zidovudine causes vaginal neoplasms in mice; however, no human cases of genital neoplasms have been reported to date. Short-term safety has been demonstrated for both mother and infant.

TABLE 49–5 The use of antiretroviral agents in pregnancy.[1]

Recommended Agents	Alternate Agents
Nucleoside/nucleotide reverse transcriptase inhibitors (NRTIs)	
Lamivudine, zidovudine	Abacavir, didanosine, emtricitabine, stavudine
Nonnucleoside reverse transcriptase inhibitors (NNRTIs)	
Nevirapine	
Protease inhibitors (PIs)	
Lopinavir/ritonavir	Atazanavir/ritonavir, indinavir/ritonavir, nelfinavir, ritonavir, saquinavir

[1]Data are insufficient to recommend the use of entry inhibitors or integrase inhibitors in pregnancy at the present time.

Increased serum levels of zidovudine may occur with concomitant administration of probenecid, phenytoin, methadone, fluconazole, atovaquone, valproic acid, and lamivudine, either through inhibition of first-pass metabolism or through decreased clearance. Zidovudine may decrease phenytoin levels. Hematologic toxicity may be increased during co-administration of other myelosuppressive drugs such as ganciclovir, ribavirin, and cytotoxic agents. Combination regimens containing zidovudine and stavudine should be avoided due to in vitro antagonism.

NONNUCLEOSIDE REVERSE TRANSCRIPTASE INHIBITORS

The NNRTIs bind directly to HIV-1 reverse transcriptase (Figure 49–4), resulting in allosteric inhibition of RNA- and DNA-dependent DNA polymerase activity. The binding site of NNRTIs is near to but distinct from that of NRTIs. Unlike the NRTI agents, NNRTIs neither compete with nucleoside triphosphates nor require phosphorylation to be active.

Baseline genotypic testing is recommended prior to initiating NNRTI treatment because primary resistance rates range from approximately 2% to 8%. NNRTI resistance occurs rapidly with monotherapy and can result from a single mutation. The K103N and Y181C mutations confer resistance across the entire class of NNRTIs, with the exception of the newest agent, etravirine. Other mutations (eg, L100I, Y188C, G190A) may confer cross-resistance among the NNRTI class. However, there is no cross-resistance between the NNRTIs and the NRTIs; in fact, some nucleoside-resistant viruses display hypersusceptibility to NNRTIs.

As a class, NNRTI agents tend to be associated with varying levels of gastrointestinal intolerance and skin rash, the latter of which may infrequently be serious (eg, Stevens-Johnson syndrome). A further limitation to use of NNRTI agents as a component of antiretroviral therapy is their metabolism by the CYP450 system, leading to innumerable potential drug-drug interactions (Tables 49–3 and 49–4). All NNRTI agents are substrates for CYP3A4 and can act as inducers (nevirapine), inhibitors (delavirdine), or mixed inducers and inhibitors (efavirenz, etravirine). Given the large number of non-HIV medications that are also metabolized by this pathway (see Chapter 4), drug-drug interactions must be expected and looked for; dosage adjustments are frequently required and some combinations are contraindicated.

DELAVIRDINE

Delavirdine has an oral bioavailability of about 85%, but this is reduced by antacids or H$_2$-blockers. It is extensively bound (~ 98%) to plasma proteins and has correspondingly low cerebrospinal fluid levels. Serum half-life is approximately 6 hours.

Skin rash occurs in up to 38% of patients receiving delavirdine; it typically occurs during the first 1–3 weeks of therapy and does not preclude rechallenge. However, severe rash such as erythema multiforme and Stevens-Johnson syndrome have rarely been reported. Other possible adverse effects are headache, fatigue, nausea, diarrhea, and increased serum aminotransferase levels.

Delavirdine has been shown to be teratogenic in rats, causing ventricular septal defects and other malformations at dosages not unlike those achieved in humans. Thus, pregnancy should be avoided when taking delavirdine.

Delavirdine is extensively metabolized by the CYP3A and CYP2D6 enzymes and also inhibits CYP3A4 and 2C9. Therefore, there are numerous potential drug-drug interactions to consider (Tables 49–3 and 49–4). The concurrent use of delavirdine with fosamprenavir and rifabutin is not recommended because of decreased delavirdine levels. Other medications likely to alter delavirdine levels include didanosine, lopinavir, nelfinavir, and ritonavir. Co-administration of delavirdine with indinavir or saquinavir prolongs the elimination half-life of these protease inhibitors, thus allowing them to be dosed twice rather than thrice daily.

EFAVIRENZ

Efavirenz can be given once daily because of its long half-life (40–55 hours). It is moderately well absorbed following oral administration (45%). Since toxicity may increase owing to increased bioavailability after a high-fat meal, efavirenz should be taken on an empty stomach. Efavirenz is principally metabolized by CYP3A4 and CYP2B6 to inactive hydroxylated metabolites; the remainder is eliminated in the feces as unchanged drug. It is highly bound to albumin (~ 99%), and cerebrospinal fluid levels range from 0.3% to 1.2% of plasma levels.

The principal adverse effects of efavirenz involve the central nervous system. Dizziness, drowsiness, insomnia, nightmares, and headache tend to diminish with continued therapy; dosing at bedtime may also be helpful. Psychiatric symptoms such as depression, mania, and psychosis have been observed and may necessitate discontinuation. Skin rash has also been reported early in therapy in up to 28% of patients; the rash is usually mild to moderate in severity and typically resolves despite continuation. Rarely, rash has been severe or life-threatening. Other potential adverse reactions are nausea, vomiting, diarrhea, crystalluria, elevated liver enzymes, and an increase in total serum cholesterol by 10–20%. High rates of fetal abnormalities occurred in pregnant monkeys exposed to efavirenz in doses roughly equivalent to the human dosage; several cases of congenital anomalies have been reported in humans. Therefore, efavirenz should be avoided in pregnant women, particularly in the first trimester.

As both an inducer and an inhibitor of CYP3A4, efavirenz induces its own metabolism and interacts with the metabolism of many other drugs (Tables 49–3 and 49–4). Since efavirenz may lower methadone levels, patients receiving these two agents concurrently should be monitored for signs of opioid withdrawal and may require an increased dose of methadone.

ETRAVIRINE

In 2008, etravirine was approved in the United States for use in treatment-experienced patients with HIV infection. Etravirine

may be effective against strains of HIV that have developed resistance to first-generation NNRTIs, depending on the number of mutations present. Although etravirine has a higher genetic barrier to resistance than the other NNRTIs, mutations selected by etravirine usually are associated with resistance to efavirenz, nevirapine, and delavirdine.

The most common adverse effects of etravirine are rash, nausea, and diarrhea. The rash is typically mild and usually resolves after 1–2 weeks without discontinuation of therapy. Rarely, rash has been severe or life-threatening. Laboratory abnormalities include elevations in serum cholesterol, triglyceride, glucose, and hepatic transaminase levels. Transaminase elevations are more common in patients with HBV or HCV co-infection.

Etravirine is a substrate as well as an inducer of CYP3A4 and an inhibitor of CYP2C9 and CYP2C19; it has many therapeutically significant drug-drug interactions (Tables 49–3 and 49–4). Some of the interactions are difficult to predict. For example, etravirine may decrease itraconazole and ketoconazole concentrations but increase voriconazole concentrations.

NEVIRAPINE

The oral bioavailability of nevirapine is excellent (> 90%) and is not food-dependent. The drug is highly lipophilic and achieves cerebrospinal fluid levels that are 45% of those in plasma. Serum half-life is 25–30 hours. It is extensively metabolized by the CYP3A isoform to hydroxylated metabolites and then excreted, primarily in the urine.

A single dose of nevirapine (200 mg) is effective in the prevention of transmission of HIV from mother to newborn when administered to women at the onset of labor and followed by a 2 mg/kg oral dose to the neonate within 3 days after delivery. There is no evidence of human teratogenicity. However, resistance has been documented after this single dose.

Rash, usually a maculopapular eruption that spares the palms and soles, occurs in up to 20% of patients, usually in the first 4–6 weeks of therapy. Although typically mild and self-limited, rash is dose-limiting in about 7% of patients. Women appear to have an increased incidence of rash. When initiating therapy, gradual dose escalation over 14 days is recommended to decrease the incidence of rash. Severe and life-threatening skin rashes have been rarely reported, including Stevens-Johnson syndrome and toxic epidermal necrolysis. Nevirapine therapy should be immediately discontinued in patients with severe rash and in those with accompanying constitutional symptoms; since rash may accompany hepatotoxicity, liver function tests should be assessed. Symptomatic liver toxicity may occur in up to 4% of patients and is more frequent in those with higher pretherapy CD4 cell counts (ie, > 250 cells/mm^3 in women and > 400 cells/mm^3 in men), in women, and in those with HBV or HCV co-infection. Fulminant, life-threatening hepatitis has been reported, typically within the first 18 weeks of therapy. Other adverse effects include fever, nausea, headache, and somnolence.

Nevirapine is a moderate inducer of CYP3A metabolism, resulting in decreased levels of amprenavir, indinavir, lopinavir, saquinavir, efavirenz, and methadone. Drugs that induce the CYP3A system, such as rifampin, rifabutin, and St. John's wort, can decrease levels of nevirapine, whereas those that inhibit CYP3A activity, such as fluconazole, ketoconazole, and clarithromycin, can increase nevirapine levels. Since nevirapine may lower methadone levels, patients receiving these two agents concurrently should be monitored for signs of opioid withdrawal and may require an increased dose of methadone.

PROTEASE INHIBITORS

During the later stages of the HIV growth cycle, the *gag* and *gag-pol* gene products are translated into polyproteins, and these become immature budding particles. The HIV protease is responsible for cleaving these precursor molecules to produce the final structural proteins of the mature virion core. By preventing posttranslational cleavage of the Gag-Pol polyprotein, protease inhibitors (PIs) prevent the processing of viral proteins into functional conformations, resulting in the production of immature, noninfectious viral particles (Figure 49–4). Unlike the NRTIs, PIs do not need intracellular activation.

Specific genotypic alterations that confer phenotypic resistance are fairly common with these agents, thus contraindicating monotherapy. Some of the most common mutations conferring broad resistance to PIs are substitutions at the 10, 46, 54, 82, 84, and 90 codons; the number of mutations may predict the level of phenotypic resistance. The I50L substitution emerging during atazanavir therapy has been associated with *increased* susceptibility to other PIs. Darunavir and tipranavir appear to have improved virologic activity in patients harboring HIV-1 resistant to other PIs.

A syndrome of redistribution and accumulation of body fat that results in central obesity, dorsocervical fat enlargement (buffalo hump), peripheral and facial wasting, breast enlargement, and a cushingoid appearance has been observed in patients receiving antiretroviral therapy. These abnormalities may be particularly associated with the use of PIs, although the recently licensed atazanavir appears to be an exception (see below). Concurrent increases in triglyceride and low-density lipoprotein levels, along with hyperglycemia and insulin resistance, have also been noted. The cause is not yet known.

Whether PI agents are associated with bone loss and osteoporosis after long-term use is controversial and under investigation. PIs have been associated with increased spontaneous bleeding in patients with hemophilia A or B; an increased risk of intracranial hemorrhage has been reported in patients receiving tipranavir with ritonavir.

The concurrent use of saquinavir and ritonavir has recently been found to be associated with QT and PR interval prolongation, and is contraindicated. QT prolongation may result in life-threatening torsades de pointes arrhythmia.

All of the antiretroviral PIs are extensively metabolized by CYP3A4, with ritonavir having the most pronounced inhibitory effect and saquinavir the least. Some PI agents, such as amprenavir and ritonavir, are also inducers of specific CYP isoforms. As a result, there is enormous potential for drug-drug interactions with other antiretroviral agents and other commonly used medications

(Tables 49–3 and 49–4). Expert resources about drug-drug interactions should be consulted, as dosage adjustments are frequently required and some combinations are contraindicated. It is noteworthy that the potent CYP3A4 inhibitory properties of ritonavir are used to clinical advantage by having it "boost" the levels of other PI agents when given in combination, thus acting as a pharmacokinetic enhancer rather than an antiretroviral agent. Ritonavir boosting increases drug exposure, thereby prolonging the drug's half-life and allowing reduction in frequency; in addition, the genetic barrier to resistance is raised.

ATAZANAVIR

Atazanavir is an azapeptide PI with a pharmacokinetic profile that allows once-daily dosing. It should be taken with a light meal to enhance bioavailability. Atazanavir requires an acidic medium for absorption and exhibits pH-dependent aqueous solubility; therefore, separation of ingestion from acid-reducing agents by at least 12 hours is recommended and concurrent proton pump inhibitors are contraindicated. Atazanavir is able to penetrate both the cerebrospinal and seminal fluids. The plasma half-life is 6–7 hours, which increases to approximately 11 hours when co-administered with ritonavir. The primary route of elimination is biliary; atazanavir should not be given to patients with severe hepatic insufficiency.

Resistance to atazanavir has been associated with various known PI mutations as well as with the novel I50L substitution. Whereas some atazanavir resistance mutations have been associated in vitro with decreased susceptibility to other PIs, the I50L mutation has been associated with increased susceptibility to other PIs.

The most common adverse effects in patients receiving atazanavir are diarrhea and nausea; vomiting, abdominal pain, headache, peripheral neuropathy, and skin rash may also occur. As with indinavir, indirect hyperbilirubinemia with overt jaundice may occur in approximately 10% of patients, owing to inhibition of the UGT1A1 glucuronidation enzyme. Elevation of hepatic enzymes has also been observed, usually in patients with underlying HBV or HCV co-infection. Nephrolithiasis has recently been described in association with atazanavir use. In contrast to the other PIs, atazanavir does not appear to be associated with dyslipidemia, fat redistribution, or the metabolic syndrome. Atazanavir may be associated with prolongation of the electrocardiographic PR interval, which is usually inconsequential but may be exacerbated by other causative agents such as calcium channel blockers and may result in AV block QT prolongation is another potential electrocardiographic effect of atazanavir but is rarely clinically significant.

As an inhibitor of CYP3A4 and CYP2C9, the potential for drug-drug interactions with atazanavir is great (Tables 49–3 and 49–4). Atazanavir AUC is reduced by up to 76% when combined with a proton pump inhibitor; thus, these combinations are to be avoided. In addition, co-administration of atazanavir with other drugs that inhibit UGT1A1, such as irinotecan, may increase its levels. Tenofovir and efavirenz should not be co-administered with atazanavir unless ritonavir is added to boost levels.

DARUNAVIR

Darunavir is licensed as a PI that must be co-administered with ritonavir. It was initially licensed for use in treatment-experienced patients only; thus there is less clinical experience with its use in treatment-naïve patients. Darunavir may be administered once daily in treatment-naïve patients.

Symptomatic adverse effects of darunavir include diarrhea, nausea, headache, and rash. Laboratory abnormalities include dyslipidemia (though possibly less frequent than with other boosted PI regimens) and increases in amylase and hepatic transaminase levels. Liver toxicity, including severe hepatitis, has been reported in some patients taking darunavir; the risk of hepatotoxicity may be higher for persons with HBV, HCV, or other chronic liver disease.

Darunavir contains a sulfonamide moiety and should be used cautiously in patients with sulfonamide allergy.

Darunavir both inhibits and is metabolized by the CYP3A enzyme system, conferring many possible drug-drug interactions (Tables 49–3 and 49–4). In addition, the co-administered ritonavir is a potent inhibitor of CYP3A and CYP2D6, and an inducer of other hepatic enzyme systems.

FOSAMPRENAVIR

Fosamprenavir is a prodrug of amprenavir that is rapidly hydrolyzed by enzymes in the intestinal epithelium. Because of its significantly lower daily pill burden, fosamprenavir tablets have replaced amprenavir capsules for adults. Fosamprenavir is most often administered in combination with low-dose ritonavir.

Amprenavir is rapidly absorbed from the gastrointestinal tract, and its prodrug can be taken with or without food. However, high-fat meals decrease absorption and thus should be avoided. The plasma half-life is relatively long (7–11 hours). Amprenavir is metabolized in the liver by CYP3A4 and should be used with caution in the setting of hepatic insufficiency.

The most common adverse effects of fosamprenavir are headache, nausea, diarrhea, perioral paresthesias, depression, and rash. Up to 3% of patients may experience rashes (including Stevens-Johnson syndrome) severe enough to warrant drug discontinuation.

Amprenavir is both an inducer and an inhibitor of CYP3A4 and is contraindicated with numerous drugs (Tables 49–3 and 49–4). The oral solution, which contains propylene glycol, is contraindicated in young children, pregnant women, patients with renal or hepatic failure, and those using metronidazole or disulfiram. Also, the oral solutions of amprenavir and ritonavir should not be co-administered because the propylene glycol in one and the ethanol in the other may compete for the same metabolic pathway, leading to accumulation of either. Because the oral solution also contains vitamin E at several times the recommended daily dosage, supplemental vitamin E should be avoided. Amprenavir, a sulfonamide, is contraindicated in patients with a history of sulfa allergy. Lopinavir/ritonavir should not be co-administered with amprenavir owing to decreased amprenavir and

altered lopinavir exposures. An increased dosage of amprenavir is recommended when co-administered with efavirenz (with or without the addition of ritonavir to boost levels).

INDINAVIR

Indinavir requires an acidic environment for optimum solubility and therefore must be consumed on an empty stomach or with a small, low-fat, low-protein meal for maximal absorption (60–65%). The serum half-life is 1.5–2 hours, protein binding is approximately 60%, and the drug has a high level of cerebrospinal fluid penetration (up to 76% of serum levels). Excretion is primarily fecal. An increase in AUC by 60% and in half-life to 2.8 hours in the setting of hepatic insufficiency necessitates dose reduction.

The most common adverse effects of indinavir are indirect hyperbilirubinemia and nephrolithiasis due to urinary crystallization of the drug. Nephrolithiasis can occur within days after initiating therapy, with an estimated incidence of approximately 10%. Consumption of at least 48 ounces of water daily is important to maintain adequate hydration. Thrombocytopenia, elevations of serum aminotransferase levels, nausea, diarrhea, insomnia, dry throat, dry skin, and indirect hyperbilirubinemia have also been reported. Insulin resistance may be more common with indinavir than with the other PIs, occurring in 3–5% of patients. There have also been rare cases of acute hemolytic anemia. In rats, high doses of indinavir are associated with development of thyroid adenomas.

Since indinavir is an inhibitor of CYP3A4, numerous and complex drug interactions can occur (Tables 49–3 and 49–4). Combination with ritonavir (boosting) allows for twice-daily rather than thrice-daily dosing and eliminates the food restriction associated with use of indinavir. However, there is potential for an increase in nephrolithiasis with this combination compared with indinavir alone; thus, a high fluid intake (1.5–2 L/d) is advised.

LOPINAVIR

Lopinavir is currently formulated only in combination with ritonavir, which inhibits the CYP3A-mediated metabolism of lopinavir, thereby resulting in increased exposure to lopinavir. In addition to improved patient compliance due to reduced pill burden, lopinavir/ritonavir is generally well tolerated.

Lopinavir should be taken with food to enhance bioavailability. The drug is highly protein bound (98–99%), and its half-life is 5–6 hours. Lopinavir is extensively metabolized by CYP3A, which is inhibited by ritonavir. Serum levels of lopinavir may be increased in patients with hepatic impairment.

The most common adverse effects of lopinavir are diarrhea, abdominal pain, nausea, vomiting, and asthenia. Elevations in serum cholesterol and triglycerides are common. Potential drug-drug interactions are extensive (Tables 49–3 and 49–4). Increased dosage of lopinavir/ritonavir is recommended when co-administered with efavirenz or nevirapine, which induce lopinavir metabolism. Concurrent use of fosamprenavir should be avoided owing to altered exposure to lopinavir with decreased levels of amprenavir. Also, concomitant use of lopinavir/ritonavir and rifampin is contraindicated due to an increased risk for hepatotoxicity. Since the oral solution of lopinavir/ritonavir contains alcohol, concurrent disulfiram and metronidazole are contraindicated. There is no evidence of human teratogenicity of lopinavir/ritonavir; short-term safety in pregnant women has been demonstrated for mother and infant.

NELFINAVIR

Nelfinavir has high absorption in the fed state (70–80%), undergoes metabolism by CYP3A, and is excreted primarily in the feces. The plasma half-life in humans is 3.5–5 hours, and the drug is more than 98% protein-bound.

The most common adverse effects associated with nelfinavir are diarrhea and flatulence. Diarrhea often responds to antidiarrheal medications but can be dose-limiting. Nelfinavir is an inhibitor of the CYP3A system, and multiple drug interactions may occur (Tables 49–3 and 49–4). An increased dosage of nelfinavir is recommended when co-administered with rifabutin (with a decreased dose of rifabutin), whereas a decrease in saquinavir dose is suggested with concurrent nelfinavir. Co-administration with efavirenz should be avoided due to decreased nelfinavir levels. Nelfinavir has a favorable safety and pharmacokinetic profile for pregnant women compared with that of other PIs (Table 49–5); there is no evidence of human teratogenicity.

RITONAVIR

Ritonavir has a high bioavailability (about 75%) that increases with food. It is 98% protein-bound and has a serum half-life of 3–5 hours. Metabolism to an active metabolite occurs via the CYP3A and CYP2D6 isoforms; excretion is primarily in the feces. Caution is advised when administering the drug to persons with impaired hepatic function.

Potential adverse effects of ritonavir, particularly when administered at full dosage, are gastrointestinal disturbances, paresthesias (circumoral or peripheral), elevated serum aminotransferase levels, altered taste, headache, and elevations in serum creatine kinase. Nausea, vomiting, diarrhea, or abdominal pain typically occur during the first few weeks of therapy but may diminish over time or if the drug is taken with meals. Dose escalation over 1–2 weeks is recommended to decrease the dose-limiting side effects. Liver adenomas and carcinomas have been induced in male mice receiving ritonavir; no similar effects have been observed to date in humans.

Ritonavir is a potent inhibitor of CYP3A4, resulting in many potential drug interactions (Tables 49–3 and 49–4). However, this characteristic has been used to great advantage when ritonavir is administered in low doses (100–200 mg twice daily) in combination with any of the other PI agents, in that increased blood levels of the latter agents permit lower or less frequent dosing (or both) with greater tolerability as well as the potential for greater efficacy against resistant virus. Therapeutic levels of digoxin and theophylline should be monitored when co-administered with ritonavir

owing to a likely increase in their concentrations. The concurrent use of saquinavir and ritonavir is contraindicated due to an increased risk of QT prolongation (with torsades de pointes arrhythmia) and PR interval prolongation. There is limited experience with full-dose ritonavir during pregnancy to date; however, low-dose ritonavir as a "booster" has appeared to be well tolerated in mother and infant.

SAQUINAVIR

In its original formulation as a hard gel capsule (saquinavir-H; Invirase), oral saquinavir was poorly bioavailable (only about 4% after food). However, reformulation of saquinavir-H for once-daily dosing in combination with low-dose ritonavir has both improved antiviral efficacy and decreased gastrointestinal adverse effects.

Saquinavir should be taken within 2 hours after a fatty meal for enhanced absorption. Saquinavir is 97% protein-bound, and serum half-life is approximately 2 hours. Saquinavir has a large volume of distribution, but penetration into the cerebrospinal fluid is negligible. Excretion is primarily in the feces. Reported adverse effects include gastrointestinal discomfort (nausea, diarrhea, abdominal discomfort, dyspepsia) and rhinitis. When administered in combination with low-dose ritonavir, there appears to be less dyslipidemia or gastrointestinal toxicity than with some of the other boosted PI regimens. However, the concurrent use of saquinavir and ritonavir is newly recognized to confer an increased risk of QT prolongation (with torsades de pointes arrhythmia) and PR interval prolongation.

Saquinavir is subject to extensive first-pass metabolism by CYP3A4 and functions as a CYP3A4 inhibitor as well as a substrate; thus, there are many potential drug-drug interactions (Tables 49–3 and 49–4). A decreased dose of saquinavir is recommended when co-administered with nelfinavir. Increased saquinavir levels when co-administered with omeprazole necessitate close monitoring for toxicities. Digoxin levels may increase if co-administered with saquinavir and should therefore be monitored. Liver function tests should be monitored if saquinavir is co-administered with delavirdine or rifampin. There is no evidence of human teratogenicity from saquinavir; there is short-term safety data for both mother and infant.

TIPRANAVIR

Tipranavir is a newer PI indicated for use in treatment-experienced HIV-1-infected patients who harbor strains resistant to other PI agents. It is used in combination with ritonavir to achieve effective serum levels and is not approved for treatment-naïve patients.

Bioavailability is poor but is increased when taken with a high-fat meal. The drug is metabolized by the liver microsomal system and is contraindicated in patients with hepatic insufficiency. Tipranavir contains a sulfonamide moiety and should not be administered to patients with known sulfa allergy.

The most common adverse effects from tipranavir are diarrhea, nausea, vomiting, and abdominal pain. An urticarial or maculopapular rash is more common in women and may be accompanied by systemic symptoms or desquamation. Liver toxicity, including life-threatening hepatic decompensation, has been observed and is more common in patients with chronic HBV or HCV infection. Tipranavir should be discontinued in patients who have increased serum transaminase levels that are more than 10 times the upper limit of normal or more than 5 times normal in combination with increased serum bilirubin. Because of an increased risk for intracranial hemorrhage in patients receiving tipranavir/ritonavir, the drug should be avoided in patients with head trauma or bleeding diathesis. Other potential adverse effects include depression, elevation in amylase, and decreased white blood cell count.

Tipranavir both inhibits and induces the CYP3A4 system. When used in combination with ritonavir, its net effect is inhibition. Tipranavir also induces P-glycoprotein transporter and thus may alter the disposition of many other drugs (Table 49–4). Concurrent administration of tipranavir with fosamprenavir or saquinavir should be avoided owing to decreased blood levels of the latter drugs. Tipranavir/ritonavir may also decrease serum levels of valproic acid and omeprazole. Levels of lovastatin, simvastatin, atorvastatin, and rosuvastatin may be increased, increasing the risk for rhabdomyolysis and myopathy. Tipranavir contains a sulfonamide moiety and should be used cautiously in patients with sulfonamide allergy.

ENTRY INHIBITORS

The process of HIV-1 entry into host cells is complex; each step presents a potential target for inhibition. Viral attachment to the host cell entails binding of the viral envelope glycoprotein complex gp160 (consisting of gp120 and gp41) to its cellular receptor CD4. This binding induces conformational changes in gp120 that enable access to the chemokine receptors CCR5 or CXCR4. Chemokine receptor binding induces further conformational changes in gp120, allowing exposure to gp41 and leading to fusion of the viral envelope with the host cell membrane and subsequent entry of the viral core into the cellular cytoplasm.

ENFUVIRTIDE

Enfuvirtide is a synthetic 36-amino-acid peptide fusion inhibitor that blocks HIV entry into the cell (Figure 49–4). Enfuvirtide binds to the gp41 subunit of the viral envelope glycoprotein, preventing the conformational changes required for the fusion of the viral and cellular membranes. Enfuvirtide, which must be administered by subcutaneous injection, is the only parenterally administered antiretroviral agent. Metabolism appears to be by proteolytic hydrolysis without involvement of the CYP450 system. Elimination half-life is 3.8 hours.

Resistance to enfuvirtide can result from mutations in gp41; the frequency and significance of this phenomenon are being investigated. However, enfuvirtide lacks cross-resistance with the other currently approved antiretroviral drug classes.

The most common adverse effects associated with enfuvirtide therapy are local injection site reactions, consisting of painful erythematous nodules. Although frequent, these are typically mild

to moderate and rarely lead to discontinuation. Other symptomatic side effects may include insomnia, headache, dizziness, and nausea. Hypersensitivity reactions may rarely occur, are of varying severity, and may recur on rechallenge. Eosinophilia is the primary laboratory abnormality seen with enfuvirtide administration. In prospective clinical trials, an increased rate of bacterial pneumonia was noted in patients receiving enfuvirtide. No drug-drug interactions have been identified that would require the alteration of the dosage of concomitant antiretroviral or other drugs.

MARAVIROC

Maraviroc binds specifically and selectively to the host protein CCR5, one of two chemokine receptors necessary for entrance of HIV into CD4+ cells. Maraviroc is approved for adults with CCR5-tropic (also known as R5) HIV-1 infection who are experiencing virologic failure due to resistance to other antiretroviral agents. Studies have shown that 52–60% of patients in whom at least two antiviral regimens had failed were infected with R5 HIV. Since maraviroc is active against HIV that uses the CCR5 co-receptor exclusively, and not against HIV strains with CXCR4, dual, or mixed tropism, tropism testing should be performed before initiating treatment with maraviroc. Clinical experience with the use of maraviroc in treatment-naïve patients is limited.

The absorption of maraviroc is rapid but variable, with the time to maximum absorption generally being 1–4 hours after ingestion of the drug. Most of the drug (≥ 75%) is excreted in the feces, whereas approximately 20% is excreted in urine. The recommended dose of maraviroc varies according to renal function and the concomitant use of CYP3A inducers or inhibitors. Maraviroc is contraindicated in patients with severe or end-stage renal impairment who are taking concurrent CYP3A inhibitors or inducers, and caution is advised when used in patients with preexisting hepatic impairment and in those co-infected with HBV or HCV. Maraviroc has been shown to have excellent penetration into the cervicovaginal fluid, with levels almost four times higher than the corresponding concentrations in blood plasma.

Resistance to maraviroc is associated with one or more mutations in the V3 loop of gp120. There appears to be no cross-resistance with drugs from any other class, including the fusion inhibitor enfuvirtide. However, virologic failure of regimens containing maraviroc may potentially be caused by emergence of non–CCR5-tropic virus (eg, CXCR4-tropic virus) or by changes in viral tropism, owing to the development of multiple mutations throughout gp160.

Maraviroc is a substrate for CYP3A4 and therefore requires adjustment in the presence of drugs that interact with these enzymes (Tables 49–3 and 49–4). It is also a substrate for P-glycoprotein, which limits intracellular concentrations of the drug. The dosage of maraviroc must be decreased if it is co-administered with strong CYP3A inhibitors (eg, delavirdine, ketoconazole, itraconazole, clarithromycin, or any protease inhibitor other than tipranavir) and must be increased if co-administered with CYP3A inducers (eg, efavirenz, etravirine, rifampin, carbamazepine, phenytoin, or St. John's wort).

Potential adverse effects include cough, upper respiratory tract infections, postural hypotension (particularly in the setting of renal insufficiency), muscle and joint pain, abdominal pain, diarrhea, and sleep disturbance. Due to reports of hepatotoxicity, which may be preceded by evidence of a systemic allergic reaction (ie, pruritic rash, eosinophilia, or elevated IgE), discontinuation of maraviroc should be considered promptly if this constellation of signs occurs. Myocardial ischemia and infarction have been observed in patients receiving maraviroc; therefore caution is advised in patients at increased cardiovascular risk.

There has been some concern that blockade of the chemokine CCR5 receptor—a human protein—may result in decreased immune surveillance, with a subsequent increased risk of malignancy (eg, lymphoma) or infection. To date, however, there has been no evidence of an increased risk of either malignancy or infection in patients receiving maraviroc.

INTEGRASE STRAND TRANSFER INHIBITORS

RALTEGRAVIR

Raltegravir is a pyrimidinone analog that binds integrase, a viral enzyme essential to the replication of both HIV-1 and HIV-2. By doing so, it inhibits strand transfer, the third and final step of provirus integration, thus interfering with the integration of reverse-transcribed HIV DNA into the chromosomes of host cells (Figure 49–4). It was initially licensed for use in treatment-experienced adult patients infected with strains of HIV-1 resistant to multiple other agents, but more recently has received approval for use in initial therapy as well. However, clinical experience is limited in treatment-naïve patients.

Absolute bioavailability of raltegravir has not been established but does not appear to be food-dependent. The drug is metabolized by glucuronidation and does not interact with the cytochrome P450 system; therefore, it is expected to have fewer drug-drug interactions than many of the other antiretroviral agents. However, in combination with rifampin, a strong inducer of UDP-glucuronosyl transferase 1A1 (UGT1A1), the dose of raltegravir should be increased from 400 mg twice daily to 800 mg twice daily. Since polyvalent cations (eg, magnesium, calcium, and iron) may bind integrase inhibitors and interfere with their activity, antacids should be used cautiously and taken separately from raltegravir.

Although virologic failure has been uncommon in clinical trials of raltegravir to date, in vitro resistance requires only a single point mutation (eg, at codons 148 or 155). The low genetic barrier to resistance emphasizes the importance of combination therapies and of adherence. Integrase mutations are not expected to affect sensitivity to other classes of antiretroviral agents.

Potential adverse effects of raltegravir include insomnia, headache, diarrhea, nausea, dizziness, and fatigue. Increases in creatine kinase may occur, with potential myopathy or rhabdomyolysis; there is minimal effect on serum lipids.

NEW & INVESTIGATIONAL ANTIRETROVIRAL AGENTS

New therapies are continually being sought that exploit other HIV targets, have activity against resistant viral strains, have a lower incidence of adverse effects, and offer convenient dosing. Newly approved agents and those currently in advanced stages of clinical development include the NRTI agents **elvucitabine, racivir,** and **apricitabine;** the NNRTI agent **rilpivirine;** entry inhibitors such as the CCR5 receptor antagonists **vicriviroc** and **PRO 140,** the fusion inhibitor **TNX-355 (ibalizumab);** and integrase inhibitors such as **elvitegravir.** In addition, new drug classes such as maturation inhibitors **(bevirimat)** are under investigation.

■ ANTIHEPATITIS AGENTS

Several agents effective against HBV and HCV are now available (Table 49–6). Current treatment is suppressive rather than curative and the high prevalence of these infections worldwide, with their concomitant morbidity and mortality, reflect a critical need for improved therapeutics.

INTERFERON ALFA

Interferons are host cytokines that exert complex antiviral, immunomodulatory, and antiproliferative actions (see Chapter 55). Interferon alfa appears to function by induction of intracellular signals following binding to specific cell membrane receptors, resulting in inhibition of viral penetration, translation, transcription, protein processing, maturation, and release, as well as increased host expression of major histocompatibility complex antigens, enhanced phagocytic activity of macrophages, and augmentation of the proliferation and survival of cytotoxic T cells.

Injectable preparations of interferon alfa are available for treatment of both HBV and HCV infections (Table 49–6). Interferon alfa-2a and interferon alfa-2b may be administered either subcutaneously or intramuscularly; interferon alfacon-1 is administered subcutaneously. Elimination half-life is 2–5 hours for interferon alfa-2a and -2b, depending on the route of administration. The half-life of interferon alfacon-1 in patients with chronic HCV ranges from 6 to 10 hours. Alfa interferons are filtered at the glomerulus and undergo rapid proteolytic degradation during tubular reabsorption, such that detection in the systemic circulation is negligible. Liver metabolism and subsequent biliary excretion are considered minor pathways.

A meta-analysis of clinical trials in patients with chronic HBV infection showed that treatment with interferon alfa is associated with a higher incidence of hepatitis e antigen (HBeAg) seroconversion and undetectable HBV DNA levels compared with placebo. The addition of the pegylated moiety results in further increases in the proportion of patients with HBeAg seroconversion (~ 30%) and a decline by approximately 4 log copies/mL (a 99.99% reduction) in HBV DNA after 1 year.

TABLE 49–6 Drugs used to treat viral hepatitis.

Agent	Indication	Recommended Adult Dosage	Route of Administration
Hepatitis B			
Lamivudine[1]	Chronic hepatitis B	100 mg once daily (150 mg once daily if co-infection with HIV is present)	Oral
Adefovir[1]	Chronic hepatitis B	10 mg once daily	Oral
Entecavir[1]	Chronic hepatitis B	0.5–1 mg once daily	Oral
Tenofovir[1]	Chronic hepatitis B	300 mg once daily	Oral
Telbivudine[1]	Chronic hepatitis B	600 mg once daily	Oral
Interferon alfa-2b	Chronic hepatitis B	5 million units once daily or 10 million units three times weekly	Subcutaneous or intramuscular
Pegylated interferon alfa-2a[1]	Chronic hepatitis B	180 mcg once weekly	Subcutaneous
Hepatitis C			
Pegylated interferon alfa-2a[1]	Chronic hepatitis C	180 mcg once weekly plus ribavirin (800–1200 mg/d)	Subcutaneous
Pegylated interferon alfa-2b[1]	Chronic hepatitis C	1.5 mcg/kg once weekly with ribavirin (800–1200 mg/d)	Subcutaneous
Interferon alfa-2b[1]	Acute hepatitis C	5 million units once daily for 3–4 weeks, then 5 million units three times weekly	Subcutaneous or intramuscular

[1]Dose must be reduced in patients with renal insufficiency.

The use of pegylated (polyethylene glycol-complexed) interferon alfa-2a and pegylated interferon alfa-2b results in slower clearance and longer terminal half-lives and steadier concentrations, which allows for less frequent dosing in patients with chronic HCV infection. Renal elimination accounts for about 30% of clearance, and clearance is approximately halved in subjects with impaired renal function; dosage must therefore be adjusted.

The adverse effects of interferon alfa include a flu-like syndrome (ie, headache, fevers, chills, myalgias, and malaise) that typically occurs within 6 hours after dosing; this syndrome occurs in more than 30% of patients during the first week of therapy and tends to resolve upon continued administration. Transient hepatic enzyme elevations may occur in the first 8–12 weeks of therapy and appear to be more common in responders. Potential adverse effects during chronic therapy include neurotoxicities (mood disorders, depression, somnolence, confusion, seizures), myelosuppression, profound fatigue, weight loss, rash, cough, myalgia, alopecia, tinnitus, reversible hearing loss, retinopathy, pneumonitis, and possibly cardiotoxicity. Induction of autoantibodies may occur, causing exacerbation or unmasking of autoimmune disease (particularly thyroiditis). The polyethylene glycol molecule is a nontoxic polymer that is readily excreted in the urine.

Contraindications to interferon alfa therapy include hepatic decompensation, autoimmune disease, and history of cardiac arrhythmia. Caution is advised in the setting of psychiatric disease, epilepsy, thyroid disease, ischemic cardiac disease, severe renal insufficiency, and cytopenia. Alfa interferons are abortifacient in primates and should not be administered in pregnancy. Potential drug-drug interactions include increased theophylline and methadone levels. Co-administration with didanosine is not recommended because of a risk of hepatic failure, and co-administration with zidovudine may exacerbate cytopenias.

TREATMENT OF HEPATITIS B VIRUS INFECTION

The goals of chronic HBV therapy are to sustain suppression of HBV replication, resulting in slowing of progression of hepatic disease (with retardation of hepatic fibrosis and even reversal of cirrhosis), prevention of complications (ie, cirrhosis, hepatic failure, and hepatocellular carcinoma), and reduction of the need for liver transplantation. This translates into suppression of HBV DNA to undetectable levels, seroconversion of HBeAg (or more rarely, HBsAg) from positive to negative, and reduction in elevated hepatic transaminase levels. These end points are correlated with improvement in necroinflammatory disease, a decreased risk of hepatocellular carcinoma and cirrhosis, and a decreased need for liver transplantation. All the currently licensed therapies achieve these goals. However, because current therapies suppress HBV replication without eradicating the virus, initial responses may not be durable. The covalently closed circular (ccc) viral DNA exists in stable form indefinitely within the cell, serving as a reservoir for HBV throughout the life of the cell and resulting in the capacity to reactivate. Relapse is more common in patients co-infected with HBV and hepatitis D virus.

As of 2010 seven drugs were approved for treatment of chronic HBV infection in the United States: five oral nucleoside/nucleotide analogs (lamivudine, adefovir dipivoxil, tenofovir, entecavir, telbivudine) and two injectable interferon drugs (interferon alfa-2b, pegylated interferon alfa-2a) (Table 49–6). The use of interferon has been supplanted by long-acting pegylated interferon, allowing

REFERENCES

Centers for Disease Control and Prevention: Sexually transmitted diseases treatment guidelines, 2006. MMWR 2006;55(RR-11):16.

Drugs for non-HIV viral infections. Med Lett Drugs Ther 2010;98:71.

Ghany MG et al: Diagnosis, management, and treatment of hepatitis C: An update. Hepatology 2009;49:1335.

Hirsch MS: Antiviral drug resistance testing in adult HIV-1 infection: 2008 recommendations of an international AIDS society-USA panel. Clin Infect Dis 2008;47:266.

Lok ASF, McMahon BJ: Chronic hepatitis B: Update 2009. Hepatology 2009;50:1.

Moss RB et al: Targeting pandemic influenza: A primer on influenza antivirals and drug resistance. J Anitimicrob Chemother 2010;5:1086.

Panel on Treatment of HIV-Infected Pregnant Women and Prevention of Perinatal Transmission: *Recommendations for Use of Antiretroviral Drugs in Pregnant HIV-1-Infected Women for Maternal Health and Interventions to Reduce Perinatal HIV Transmission in the United States.* May 24, 2010;1. Available at http://aidsinfo.nih.gov/ContentFiles/PerinatalGL.pdf.

Thompson MA et al: Antiretroviral treatment of adult HIV infection: 2010 recommendations of the International AIDS Society USA panel. JAMA 2010;304:321.

RELEVANT WEB SITES

http://www.aidsinfo.nih.gov
http://www.hiv-druginteractions.org
http://www.hivinsite.com
http://www.iasusa.org

CASE STUDY ANSWER

Combination antiviral therapy against both HIV and hepatitis B virus (HBV) is indicated in this patient, given the high viral load and low CD4 cell count. However, the use of methadone and possibly excessive alcohol consumption necessitate caution. Tenofovir and emtricitabine (two nucleoside/nucleotide reverse transcriptase inhibitors) would be a potentially excellent choice as components of an initial regimen, since both are active against HIV-1 and HBV, do not interact with methadone, and are available in a once-daily, fixed-dose combination. Efavirenz, a nonnucleoside reverse transcriptase inhibitor, could be added and still maintain a once-daily regimen. Prior to initiation of this regimen, renal function should be checked, and a bone mineral density test should be considered. Pregnancy should be ruled out, and the patient should be counseled that efavirenz should not be taken during pregnancy. The potential for lowered methadone levels with efavirenz necessitates close monitoring and possibly an increased dose of methadone.

Etravirine (Intelence)
Oral: 100 mg tablets

Famciclovir (Famvir)
Oral: 125, 250, 500 mg tablets

Fosamprenavir (Lexiva)
Oral: 700 mg tablets

Foscarnet (Foscavir)
Parenteral: 24 mg/mL for IV injection

Ganciclovir (Cytovene)
Oral: 250, 500 mg capsules
Parenteral: 500 mg/vial for IV injection
Intraocular implant (Vitrasert): 4.5 mg ganciclovir/implant

Imiquimod (Aldara)
Topical: 5% cream

Indinavir (Crixivan)
Oral: 100, 200, 333, 400 mg capsules

Interferon alfa-2a (Roferon-A)
Parenteral: 3, 6, 9, 36 million IU vials

Interferon alfa-2b (Intron A)
Parenteral: 3, 5, 10, 18, 25, and 50 million IU vials

Interferon alfa-2b (Rebetron)
Parenteral: 3 million IU vials (supplied with oral ribavirin, 200 mg capsules)

Interferon alfa-n3 (Alferon N)
Parenteral: 5 million IU/vial

Interferon alfacon-1 (Infergen)
Parenteral: 9 and 15 mcg vials

Lamivudine
Oral (Epivir): 150, 300 mg tablets; 10 mg/mL oral solution
Oral (Epivir-HBV): 100 mg tablets; 5 mg/mL solution
Oral (Combivir): 150 mg tablets in combination with 300 mg zidovudine
Oral (Trizivir): 150 mg tablets in combination with 300 mg abacavir and 300 mg zidovudine

Lopinavir/ritonavir (Kaletra)
Oral: 133.3 mg/33.3 mg capsules; 80 mg/20 mg per mL solution

Maraviroc (Selzentry)
Oral: 150, 300 mg tablets

Nelfinavir (Viracept)
Oral: 250, 625 mg tablets; 50 mg/g powder

Nevirapine (Viramune)
Oral: 200 mg tablets; 50 mg/5 mL suspension

Oseltamivir (Tamiflu)
Oral: 75 mg capsules; powder to reconstitute as suspension (12 mg/mL)

Palivizumab (Synagis)
Parenteral: 50, 100 mg/vial

Peginterferon alfa-2a (pegylated interferon alfa-2a, Pegasys)
Parenteral: 180 mcg/mL

Peginterferon alfa-2b (pegylated interferon alfa-2b, PEG-Intron)
Parenteral: powder to reconstitute as 100, 160, 240, 300 mcg/mL injection

Penciclovir (Denavir)
Topical: 1% cream

Raltegravir (Isentress)
Oral: 400 mg tablets

Ribavirin
Aerosol (Virazole): powder to reconstitute for aerosol; 6 g/100 mL vial
Oral (Rebetol, generic): 200 mg capsules, tablets; 40 mg/mL oral solution
Oral (Rebetron): 200 mg in combination with 3 million units interferon alfa-2b (Intron-A)

Rilpivirine
Oral (Edurant): 25 mg tablets
Oral (Complera): 200 mg emtricitabine, 25 mg rilpivirine, 300 mg tenofovir) tablets

Rimantadine (Flumadine)
Oral: 100 mg tablets; 50 mg/5 mL syrup

Ritonavir (Norvir)
Oral: 100 mg capsules; 80 mg/mL oral solution

Saquinavir
Oral (Invirase): 200 mg hard gel capsules, 500 mg tablets

Stavudine
Oral (Zerit): 15, 20, 30, 40 mg capsules; powder for 1 mg/mL oral solution
Oral extended-release (Zerit XR): 37.5, 50, 75, 100 mg capsules

Telaprivir (Incivik)
Oral: 200 mg capsules

Telbivudine (Tyzeka)
Oral: 600 mg tablets

Tenofovir (Viread)
Oral: 300 mg tablets

Tipranavir (Aptivus)
Oral: 250 mg capsules

Trifluridine (Viroptic)
Topical: 1% ophthalmic solution

Valacyclovir (Valtrex)
Oral: 500, 1000 mg tablets

Valganciclovir (Valcyte)
Oral: 450 mg capsules

Zalcitabine (dideoxycytidine, ddC) (Hivid)
Oral: 0.375, 0.75 mg tablets

Zanamivir (Relenza)
Inhalational: 5 mg/blister

Zidovudine (azidothymidine, AZT) (Retrovir)
Oral: 100 mg capsules, 300 mg tablets, 50 mg/5 mL syrup
Oral (Combivir): 300 mg tablets in combination with 150 mg lamivudine
Oral (Trizivir): 300 mg tablets in combination with 150 mg lamivudine and 300 mg zidovudine
Parenteral: 10 mg/mL

REFERENCES

Centers for Disease Control and Prevention: Sexually transmitted diseases treatment guidelines, 2006. MMWR 2006;55(RR-11):16.

Drugs for non-HIV viral infections. Med Lett Drugs Ther 2010;98:71.

Ghany MG et al: Diagnosis, management, and treatment of hepatitis C: An update. Hepatology 2009;49:1335.

Hirsch MS: Antiviral drug resistance testing in adult HIV-1 infection: 2008 recommendations of an international AIDS society-USA panel. Clin Infect Dis 2008;47:266.

Lok ASF, McMahon BJ: Chronic hepatitis B: Update 2009. Hepatology 2009;50:1.

Moss RB et al: Targeting pandemic influenza: A primer on influenza antivirals and drug resistance. J Anitimicrob Chemother 2010;5:1086.

Panel on Treatment of HIV-Infected Pregnant Women and Prevention of Perinatal Transmission: *Recommendations for Use of Antiretroviral Drugs in Pregnant HIV-1-Infected Women for Maternal Health and Interventions to Reduce Perinatal HIV Transmission in the United States.* May 24, 2010;1. Available at http://aidsinfo.nih.gov/ContentFiles/PerinatalGL.pdf.

Thompson MA et al: Antiretroviral treatment of adult HIV infection: 2010 recommendations of the International AIDS Society USA panel. JAMA 2010;304:321.

RELEVANT WEB SITES

http://www.aidsinfo.nih.gov
http://www.hiv-druginteractions.org
http://www.hivinsite.com
http://www.iasusa.org

CASE STUDY ANSWER

Combination antiviral therapy against both HIV and hepatitis B virus (HBV) is indicated in this patient, given the high viral load and low CD4 cell count. However, the use of methadone and possibly excessive alcohol consumption necessitate caution. Tenofovir and emtricitabine (two nucleoside/nucleotide reverse transcriptase inhibitors) would be a potentially excellent choice as components of an initial regimen, since both are active against HIV-1 and HBV, do not interact with methadone, and are available in a once-daily, fixed-dose combination. Efavirenz, a nonnucleoside reverse transcriptase inhibitor, could be added and still maintain a once-daily regimen. Prior to initiation of this regimen, renal function should be checked, and a bone mineral density test should be considered. Pregnancy should be ruled out, and the patient should be counseled that efavirenz should not be taken during pregnancy. The potential for lowered methadone levels with efavirenz necessitates close monitoring and possibly an increased dose of methadone.

RIBAVIRIN

In addition to oral administration for HCV infection in combination with interferon alfa (see Antihepatitis Agents), aerosolized ribavirin is administered by nebulizer (20 mg/mL for 12–18 hours per day) to children and infants with severe respiratory syncytial virus (RSV) bronchiolitis or pneumonia to reduce the severity and duration of illness. Aerosolized ribavirin has also been used to treat influenza A and B infections but has not gained widespread use. Systemic absorption is low (< 1%). Aerosolized ribavirin is generally well tolerated but may cause conjunctival or bronchial irritation. Health care workers should be protected against extended inhalation exposure. The aerosolized drug may precipitate on contact lenses.

Intravenous ribavirin decreases mortality in patients with Lassa fever and other viral hemorrhagic fevers if started early. High concentrations inhibit West Nile virus in vitro, but clinical data are lacking. Clinical benefit has been reported in cases of severe measles pneumonitis and certain encephalitides, and continuous infusion of ribavirin has decreased virus shedding in several patients with severe lower respiratory tract influenza or parainfluenza infections. At steady state, cerebrospinal fluid levels are about 70% of those in plasma.

PALIVIZUMAB

Palivizumab is a humanized monoclonal antibody directed against an epitope in the A antigen site on the F surface protein of RSV. It is licensed for the prevention of RSV infection in high-risk infants and children, such as premature infants and those with bronchopulmonary dysplasia or congenital heart disease. A placebo-controlled trial using once-monthly intramuscular injections (15 mg/kg) for 5 months beginning at the start of the RSV season demonstrated a 55% reduction in the risk of hospitalization for RSV in treated patients, as well as decreases in the need for supplemental oxygen, the illness severity score, and the need for intensive care. Although resistant strains have been isolated in the laboratory, no resistant clinical isolates have yet been identified. Potential adverse effects include upper respiratory tract infection, fever, rhinitis, rash, diarrhea, vomiting, cough, otitis media, and elevation in serum aminotransferase levels.

A number of other agents are under investigation for the treatment or prophylaxis of patients with RSV infection, including the RNA interference (RNAi) therapeutic ALN-RSV01, the humanized monoclonal antibody motavizumab, and the benzodiazepine RSV604.

IMIQUIMOD

Imiquimod is an immune response modifier shown to be effective in the topical treatment of external genital and perianal warts (ie, condyloma acuminatum; see Chapter 61). The 5% cream is applied three times weekly and washed off 6–10 hours after each application. Recurrences appear to be less common than after ablative therapies. Imiquimod may also be effective against molluscum contagiosum but is not licensed in the United States for this indication. Local skin reactions are the most common adverse effect; these tend to resolve within weeks after therapy. However, pigmentary skin changes may persist. Systemic adverse effects such as fatigue and influenza-like syndrome have occasionally been reported.

PREPARATIONS AVAILABLE

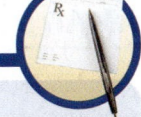

Abacavir
Oral (Ziagen): 300 mg tablets; 20 mg/mL solution
Oral (Epzicom): 600 mg plus 300 mg lamivudine
Oral (Trizivir): 300 mg tablets in combination with 150 mg
lamivudine and 300 mg zidovudine

Acyclovir (generic, Zovirax)
Oral: 200 mg capsules; 400, 800 mg tablets; 200 mg/5 mL suspension
Parenteral: 50 mg/mL; powder to reconstitute for injection (500, 1000 mg/vial)
Topical: 5% ointment

Adefovir (Hepsera)
Oral: 10 mg tablets

Amantadine (generic, Symmetrel)
Oral: 100 mg capsules, tablets; 50 mg/5 mL syrup

Atazanavir (Reyataz)
Oral: 100, 150, 200 mg capsules

Boceprivir (Victrelis)
Oral: 375 mg tablets

Cidofovir (Vistide)
Parenteral: 375 mg/vial (75 mg/mL) for IV injection

Darunavir (Prezista)
Oral: 300 mg tablets (must be taken with ritonavir)

Delavirdine (Rescriptor)
Oral: 100, 200 mg tablets

Didanosine (dideoxyinosine, ddI)
Oral (Videx): 25, 50, 100, 150, 200 mg tablets; 100, 167, 250 mg
powder for oral solution; 2, 4 g powder for pediatric solution
Oral (Videx-EC): 125, 200, 250, 400 mg delayed-release capsules

Docosanol (Abreva) (over-the-counter)
Topical: 10% cream

Efavirenz (Sustiva)
Oral: 50, 100, 200 mg capsules; 600 mg tablets

Emtricitabine
Oral (Emtriva): 200 mg tablets
Oral (Truvada): 200 mg plus 300 mg tenofovir tablets
Oral (Atripla): 200 mg plus 300 mg tenofovir plus 600 mg efavirenz

Enfuvirtide (Fuzeon)
Parenteral: 90 mg/mL for injection

Entecavir (Baraclude)
Oral: 0.5, 1 mg tablets; 0.05 mg/mL oral solution

adjusted in such patients. Potential adverse effects include nausea, vomiting, and abdominal pain, which occur in 5–10% of patients early in therapy but tend to resolve spontaneously. Taking oseltamivir with food does not interfere with absorption and may decrease nausea and vomiting. Headache, fatigue, and diarrhea have also been reported and appear to be more common with prophylactic use. Rash is rare. Transient neuropsychiatric events (self-injury or delirium) have been reported, particularly in adolescents and adults living in Japan.

Zanamivir is delivered directly to the respiratory tract via inhalation. Ten to twenty percent of the active compound reaches the lungs, and the remainder is deposited in the oropharynx. The concentration of the drug in the respiratory tract is estimated to be more than 1000 times the 50% inhibitory concentration for neuraminidase, and the pulmonary half-life is 2.8 hours. Five to fifteen percent of the total dose (10 mg twice daily for 5 days for treatment and 10 mg once daily for prevention) is absorbed and excreted in the urine with minimal metabolism. Potential adverse effects include cough, bronchospasm (occasionally severe), reversible decrease in pulmonary function, and transient nasal and throat discomfort. Zanamivir administration is not recommended for patients with underlying airway disease.

Resistance to oseltamivir may be associated with point mutations in the viral hemagglutinin or neuraminidase (eg, the H275Y mutation) genes. Rates of resistance to oseltamivir among seasonal H1N1 viruses have risen abruptly and dramatically worldwide, reaching 97.4% in tested strains in the United States from 2008 to 2009. Resistance to oseltamivir in pandemic H1N1 viruses and resistance to zanamivir in seasonal and pandemic H1N1 viruses are rare. All influenza A (H3N2) and influenza B viruses were susceptible to both oseltamivir and zanamivir. Swine-origin influenza A (H1N1) viruses are nearly always susceptible to both oseltamivir and zanamivir.

AMANTADINE & RIMANTADINE

Amantadine (1-aminoadamantane hydrochloride) and its α-methyl derivative, rimantadine, are tricyclic amines of the adamantane family that block the M2 proton ion channel of the virus particle and inhibit uncoating of the viral RNA within infected host cells, thus preventing its replication. They are active against influenza A only. Rimantadine is four to ten times more active than amantadine in vitro. Amantadine is well absorbed and 67% protein-bound. Its plasma half-life is 12–18 hours and varies by creatinine clearance. Rimantadine is about 40% protein-bound and has a half-life of 24–36 hours. Nasal secretion and salivary levels approximate those in the serum, and cerebrospinal fluid levels are 52–96% of those in the serum; nasal mucus concentrations of rimantadine average 50% higher than those in plasma. Amantadine is excreted unchanged in the urine, whereas rimantadine undergoes extensive metabolism by hydroxylation, conjugation, and glucuronidation before urinary excretion. Dose reductions are required for both agents in the elderly and in patients with renal insufficiency, and for rimantadine in patients with marked hepatic insufficiency.

In the absence of resistance, both amantadine and rimantadine, at 100 mg twice daily or 200 mg once daily, are 70–90% protective in the prevention of clinical illness when initiated before exposure. When begun within 1–2 days after the onset of illness, the duration of fever and systemic symptoms is reduced by 1–2 days.

The primary target for both agents is the M2 protein within the viral membrane, incurring both influenza A specificity and a mutation-prone site that results in the rapid development of resistance in up to 50% of treated individuals. Resistant isolates with single-point mutations are genetically stable, retain pathogenicity, can be transmitted to close contacts, and may be shed chronically by immunocompromised patients. The marked increase in the prevalence of resistance to both agents in clinical isolates over the last decade, in influenza A H1N1 as well as H3N2, has limited the usefulness of these agents for either the treatment or the prevention of influenza. Cross-resistance to zanamivir and oseltamivir does not occur.

The most common adverse effects are gastrointestinal (nausea, anorexia) and central nervous system (nervousness, difficulty in concentrating, insomnia, light-headedness); side effects are dose-related and may diminish or disappear after the first week of treatment despite continued drug ingestion. More serious side effects (eg, marked behavioral changes, delirium, hallucinations, agitation, and seizures) may be due to alteration of dopamine neurotransmission (see Chapter 28); are less frequent with rimantadine than with amantadine; are associated with high plasma concentrations; may occur more frequently in patients with renal insufficiency, seizure disorders, or advanced age; and may increase with concomitant antihistamines, anticholinergic drugs, hydrochlorothiazide, and trimethoprim-sulfamethoxazole. Clinical manifestations of anticholinergic activity tend to be present in acute amantadine overdose. Both agents are teratogenic and embryotoxic in rodents, and birth defects have been reported after exposure during pregnancy.

INVESTIGATIONAL AGENTS

The neuraminidase inhibitor **peramivir,** a cyclopentane analog, has activity against both influenza A and B viruses. Peramivir received temporary emergency use authorization by FDA for intravenous administration in November 2009 due to the H1N1 pandemic. The drug is marketed in South Korea but has not yet been licensed in the United States. Clinical data on cross-resistance to oseltamivir and zanamivir are not yet available. Reported side effects include diarrhea, nausea, vomiting, and neutropenia.

■ OTHER ANTIVIRAL AGENTS

INTERFERONS

Interferons have been studied for numerous clinical indications. In addition to HBV and HCV infections (see Antihepatitis Agents), intralesional injection of interferon alfa-2b or alfa-n3 may be used for treatment of condylomata acuminata (see Chapter 61).

RIBAVIRIN

Ribavirin is a guanosine analog that is phosphorylated intracellularly by host cell enzymes. Although its mechanism of action has not been fully elucidated, it appears to interfere with the synthesis of guanosine triphosphate, to inhibit capping of viral messenger RNA, and to inhibit the viral RNA-dependent polymerase of certain viruses. Ribavirin triphosphate inhibits the replication of a wide range of DNA and RNA viruses, including influenza A and B, parainfluenza, respiratory syncytial virus, paramyxoviruses, HCV, and HIV-1.

The absolute oral bioavailability of ribavirin is 45–64%, increases with high-fat meals, and decreases with co-administration of antacids. Plasma protein binding is negligible, volume of distribution is large, and cerebrospinal fluid levels are about 70% of those in plasma. Ribavirin elimination is primarily through the urine; therefore, clearance is decreased in patients with creatinine clearances less than 30 mL/min.

Higher doses of ribavirin (ie, 1000–1200 mg/d, according to weight, rather than 800 mg/d) or a longer duration of therapy or both may be more efficacious in those with a lower likelihood of response to therapy (eg, those with genotype 1 or 4) or in those who have relapsed. This must be balanced with an increased likelihood of toxicity. A dose-dependent hemolytic anemia occurs in 10–20% of patients. Other potential adverse effects are depression, fatigue, irritability, rash, cough, insomnia, nausea, and pruritus. Contraindications to ribavirin therapy include anemia, end-stage renal failure, ischemic vascular disease, and pregnancy. Ribavirin is teratogenic and embryotoxic in animals as well as mutagenic in mammalian cells. Patients exposed to the drug should not conceive children for at least 6 months thereafter.

NEW & INVESTIGATIONAL AGENTS

Among the agents for the treatment of HCV infection, those holding the greatest promise currently are the HCV NS3 protease inhibitors **telaprevir** and **boceprevir**. These highly potent agents are likely to decrease the overall duration of therapy, with possibly greater tolerability than current regimens. Another class of promising agents is the HCV NS5B polymerase inhibitors, including both nucleoside and nonnucleoside analogs.

■ ANTI-INFLUENZA AGENTS

Influenza virus strains are classified by their core proteins (ie, A, B, or C), species of origin (eg, avian, swine), and geographic site of isolation. Influenza A, the only strain that causes pandemics, is classified into 16 H (hemagglutinin) and 9 N (neuraminidase) known subtypes based on surface proteins. Although influenza B viruses usually infect only people, influenza A viruses can infect a variety of animal hosts. Current influenza A subtypes that are circulating among worldwide populations include H1N1, H1N2, and H3N2. Fifteen subtypes are known to infect birds, providing an extensive reservoir. Although avian influenza subtypes are typically highly species-specific, they have on rare occasions crossed the species barrier to infect humans and cats. Viruses of the H5 and H7 subtypes (eg, H5N1, H7N7, and H7N3) may rapidly mutate within poultry flocks from a low to high pathogenic form and have recently expanded their host range to cause both avian and human disease. Of particular concern is the avian H5N1 virus, which first caused human infection (including severe disease and death) in 1997 and has become endemic in Southeast Asian poultry since 2003. To date, the spread of H5N1 virus from person to person has been rare, limited, and unsustained. However, the emergence of the 2009 H1N1 influenza virus (previously called "swine flu") in 2009–2010 caused the first influenza pandemic (ie, global outbreak of disease caused by a new flu virus) in more than 40 years.

Although antiviral drugs available for influenza have activity against influenza A, many or most of the circulating strains of avian H5N1, as well as H1 and H3 strains causing seasonal influenza in the United States, are resistant to amantadine and rimantadine. Resistance to oseltamivir has also increased dramatically.

OSELTAMIVIR & ZANAMIVIR

The neuraminidase inhibitors oseltamivir and zanamivir, analogs of sialic acid, interfere with release of progeny influenza virus from infected host cells, thus halting the spread of infection within the respiratory tract. These agents competitively and reversibly interact with the active enzyme site to inhibit viral neuraminidase activity at low nanomolar concentrations. Inhibition of viral neuraminidase results in clumping of newly released influenza virions to each other and to the membrane of the infected cell. Unlike amantadine and rimantadine, oseltamivir and zanamivir have activity against both influenza A and influenza B viruses. Early administration is crucial because replication of influenza virus peaks at 24–72 hours after the onset of illness. When a 5-day course of therapy is initiated within 36–48 hours after the onset of symptoms, the duration of illness is decreased by 1–2 days compared with those on placebo, severity is diminished, and the incidence of secondary complications in children and adults decreases. Once-daily prophylaxis is 70–90% effective in preventing disease after exposure. Oseltamivir is approved by the Food and Drug Administration (FDA) for patients 1 year and older, whereas zanamivir is approved in patients 7 years or older.

Oseltamivir is an orally administered prodrug that is activated by hepatic esterases and widely distributed throughout the body. The dosage is 75 mg twice daily for 5 days for treatment and 75 mg once daily for prevention; dosage must be modified in patients with renal insufficiency. Oral bioavailability is approximately 80%, plasma protein binding is low, and concentrations in the middle ear and sinus fluid are similar to those in plasma. The half-life of oseltamivir is 6–10 hours, and excretion is by glomerular filtration and tubular secretion in the urine. Probenecid reduces renal clearance of oseltamivir by 50%. Serum concentrations of oseltamivir carboxylate, the active metabolite of oseltamivir, increase with declining renal function; therefore, dosage should be negative occurs in about 17% of patients and is durable at 3 years in about 70% of responders. Continuation of treatment for 4–8 months after seroconversion may improve the durability of response. Response in HBeAg-negative patients is initially high but less durable.

Although lamivudine initially results in rapid and potent virus suppression, chronic therapy may ultimately be limited by the emergence of lamivudine-resistant HBV isolates (eg, L180M or M204I/V), estimated to occur in 15–30% of patients at 1 year and 70% at 5 years of therapy. Resistance has been associated with flares of hepatitis and progressive liver disease. Cross-resistance between lamivudine and emtricitabine or entecavir may occur; however, adefovir maintains activity against lamivudine-resistant strains of HBV.

In the doses used for HBV infection, lamivudine has an excellent safety profile. Headache, nausea, and dizziness are rare. Co-infection with HIV may increase the risk of pancreatitis. No evidence of mitochondrial toxicity has been reported.

TELBIVUDINE

Telbivudine is a thymidine nucleoside analog with activity against HBV DNA polymerase. It is phosphorylated by cellular kinases to the active triphosphate form, which has an intracellular half-life of 14 hours. The phosphorylated compound competitively inhibits HBV DNA polymerase, resulting in incorporation into viral DNA and chain termination. It is not active in vitro against HIV-1.

Oral bioavailability is unaffected by food. Plasma protein-binding is low (3%) and distribution wide. The serum half-life is approximately 15 hours and excretion is renal. There are no known metabolites and no known interactions with the CYP450 system or other drugs.

In a comparative trial against lamivudine in patients with chronic HBV infection, significantly more patients receiving telbivudine achieved the combined end point of suppression of HBV DNA to less than 5 log copies/mL plus loss of serum HBeAg. The mean reduction in HBV DNA from baseline, the proportion with ALT normalization, and HBeAg seroconversion all were greater in those receiving telbivudine. Liver biopsies performed 1 year later showed less scarring. However, emergence of resistance, typically due to the M204I mutation, may occur in up to 22% of patients with durations of therapy exceeding 1 year, and may result in virologic rebound.

Adverse effects are mild; they include fatigue, headache, abdominal pain, upper respiratory infection, increased creatine kinase levels, and nausea and vomiting. Both uncomplicated myalgia and myopathy have been reported, as has peripheral neuropathy. As with other nucleoside analogs, lactic acidosis and severe hepatomegaly with steatosis may occur during therapy as well as flares of hepatitis after discontinuation.

TENOFOVIR

Tenofovir, a nucleotide analog of adenosine in use as an antiretroviral agent, has recently gained licensure for the treatment of patients with chronic HBV infection. The characteristics of tenofovir are described earlier in this chapter. Tenofovir maintains activity against lamivudine- and entecavir-resistant hepatitis virus isolates but has reduced activity against adefovir-resistant strains. Although similar in structure to adefovir dipivoxil, comparative trials showed a significantly higher rate of complete response, defined as serum HBV DNA levels less than 400 copies/mL, as well as of histologic improvement, in patients with chronic HBV infection receiving tenofovir than in those receiving adefovir dipivoxil. The emergence of resistance appears to be substantially less frequent during therapy with tenofovir than with adefovir.

INVESTIGATIONAL AGENTS

Compounds in clinical development for the treatment of patients with HBV infection include the nucleoside analogs **emtricitabine** and **clevudine,** as well as the immunologic modulator **thymosin alpha-1,** agents that facilitate uptake by the liver using conjugation to ligands, and RNA interference compounds.

TREATMENT OF HEPATITIS C INFECTION

In contrast to the treatment of patients with chronic HBV infection, the primary goal of treatment in patients with HCV infection is viral eradication. In clinical trials, the primary efficacy end point is typically achievement of sustained viral response (SVR), defined as the absence of detectable viremia for 6 months after completion of therapy. SVR is associated with improvement in liver histology, reduction in risk of hepatocellular carcinoma, and, occasionally, with regression of cirrhosis as well. Late relapse occurs in less than 5% of patients who achieve SVR.

In acute hepatitis C, the rate of clearance of the virus without therapy is estimated at 15–30%. In one (uncontrolled) study, treatment of acute infection with interferon alfa-2b, in doses higher than those used for chronic hepatitis C, resulted in a sustained rate of clearance of 95% at 6 months. Therefore, if HCV RNA testing documents persistent viremia 12 weeks after initial seroconversion, antiviral therapy is recommended.

Treatment of patients with chronic HCV infection is recommended for those with an increased risk for progression to cirrhosis. The parameters for selection are complex. In those who are to be treated, the current standard of treatment is once-weekly pegylated interferon alfa in combination with daily oral ribavirin. Pegylated interferon alfa-2a and -2b have replaced their unmodified interferon alfa counterparts because of superior efficacy in combination with ribavirin, regardless of genotype. It is also clear that combination therapy with oral ribavirin is more effective than monotherapy with either interferon or ribavirin alone. Therefore, monotherapy with pegylated interferon alfa is recommended only in patients who cannot tolerate ribavirin. Factors associated with a favorable therapeutic response include HCV genotype 2 or 3, absence of cirrhosis on liver biopsy, and low pretreatment HCV RNA levels.

TABLE 49–6 Drugs used to treat viral hepatitis.

Agent	Indication	Recommended Adult Dosage	Route of Administration
Hepatitis B			
Lamivudine[1]	Chronic hepatitis B	100 mg once daily (150 mg once daily if co-infection with HIV is present)	Oral
Adefovir[1]	Chronic hepatitis B	10 mg once daily	Oral
Entecavir[1]	Chronic hepatitis B	0.5–1 mg once daily	Oral
Tenofovir[1]	Chronic hepatitis B	300 mg once daily	Oral
Telbivudine[1]	Chronic hepatitis B	600 mg once daily	Oral
Interferon alfa-2b	Chronic hepatitis B	5 million units once daily or 10 million units three times weekly	Subcutaneous or intramuscular
Pegylated interferon alfa-2a[1]	Chronic hepatitis B	180 mcg once weekly	Subcutaneous
Hepatitis C			
Pegylated interferon alfa-2a[1]	Chronic hepatitis C	180 mcg once weekly plus ribavirin (800–1200 mg/d)	Subcutaneous
Pegylated interferon alfa-2b[1]	Chronic hepatitis C	1.5 mcg/kg once weekly with ribavirin (800–1200 mg/d)	Subcutaneous
Interferon alfa-2b[1]	Acute hepatitis C	5 million units once daily for 3–4 weeks, then 5 million units three times weekly	Subcutaneous or intramuscular

[1]Dose must be reduced in patients with renal insufficiency.

The use of pegylated (polyethylene glycol-complexed) interferon alfa-2a and pegylated interferon alfa-2b results in slower clearance and longer terminal half-lives and steadier concentrations, which allows for less frequent dosing in patients with chronic HCV infection. Renal elimination accounts for about 30% of clearance, and clearance is approximately halved in subjects with impaired renal function; dosage must therefore be adjusted.

The adverse effects of interferon alfa include a flu-like syndrome (ie, headache, fevers, chills, myalgias, and malaise) that typically occurs within 6 hours after dosing; this syndrome occurs in more than 30% of patients during the first week of therapy and tends to resolve upon continued administration. Transient hepatic enzyme elevations may occur in the first 8–12 weeks of therapy and appear to be more common in responders. Potential adverse effects during chronic therapy include neurotoxicities (mood disorders, depression, somnolence, confusion, seizures), myelosuppression, profound fatigue, weight loss, rash, cough, myalgia, alopecia, tinnitus, reversible hearing loss, retinopathy, pneumonitis, and possibly cardiotoxicity. Induction of autoantibodies may occur, causing exacerbation or unmasking of autoimmune disease (particularly thyroiditis). The polyethylene glycol molecule is a nontoxic polymer that is readily excreted in the urine.

Contraindications to interferon alfa therapy include hepatic decompensation, autoimmune disease, and history of cardiac arrhythmia. Caution is advised in the setting of psychiatric disease, epilepsy, thyroid disease, ischemic cardiac disease, severe renal insufficiency, and cytopenia. Alfa interferons are abortifacient in primates and should not be administered in pregnancy. Potential drug-drug interactions include increased theophylline and methadone levels. Co-administration with didanosine is not recommended because of a risk of hepatic failure, and co-administration with zidovudine may exacerbate cytopenias.

TREATMENT OF HEPATITIS B VIRUS INFECTION

The goals of chronic HBV therapy are to sustain suppression of HBV replication, resulting in slowing of progression of hepatic disease (with retardation of hepatic fibrosis and even reversal of cirrhosis), prevention of complications (ie, cirrhosis, hepatic failure, and hepatocellular carcinoma), and reduction of the need for liver transplantation. This translates into suppression of HBV DNA to undetectable levels, seroconversion of HBeAg (or more rarely, HBsAg) from positive to negative, and reduction in elevated hepatic transaminase levels. These end points are correlated with improvement in necroinflammatory disease, a decreased risk of hepatocellular carcinoma and cirrhosis, and a decreased need for liver transplantation. All the currently licensed therapies achieve these goals. However, because current therapies suppress HBV replication without eradicating the virus, initial responses may not be durable. The covalently closed circular (ccc) viral DNA exists in stable form indefinitely within the cell, serving as a reservoir for HBV throughout the life of the cell and resulting in the capacity to reactivate. Relapse is more common in patients co-infected with HBV and hepatitis D virus.

As of 2010 seven drugs were approved for treatment of chronic HBV infection in the United States: five oral nucleoside/nucleotide analogs (lamivudine, adefovir dipivoxil, tenofovir, entecavir, telbivudine) and two injectable interferon drugs (interferon alfa-2b, pegylated interferon alfa-2a) (Table 49–6). The use of interferon has been supplanted by long-acting pegylated interferon, allowing once-weekly rather than daily or thrice-weekly dosing. In general, nucleoside/nucleotide analog therapies have better tolerability and ultimately produce a higher response rate than the interferons (though less rapid); however, response may be less sustained after discontinuation of the nucleoside/nucleotide therapies, and emergence of resistance may be problematic. The nucleotides are effective in nucleoside resistance and vice versa. In addition, oral agents may be used in patients with decompensated liver disease, and the therapy is chronic rather than finite as with interferon therapy.

Several anti-HBV agents have anti-HIV activity as well, including lamivudine, adefovir dipivoxil, and tenofovir. Emtricitabine, an antiretroviral NRTI, is under clinical evaluation for HBV treatment in combination with tenofovir, which may be particularly suited to individuals co-infected with HIV and HBV. Because NRTI agents may be used in patients co-infected with HBV and HIV, it is important to note that acute exacerbation of hepatitis may occur upon discontinuation or interruption of these agents.

ADEFOVIR DIPIVOXIL

Although initially and abortively developed for treatment of HIV infection, adefovir dipivoxil gained approval, at lower and less toxic doses, for treatment of HBV infection. Adefovir dipivoxil is the diester prodrug of adefovir, an acyclic phosphonated adenine nucleotide analog (Figure 49–2). It is phosphorylated by cellular kinases to the active diphosphate metabolite and then competitively inhibits HBV DNA polymerase and causes chain termination after incorporation into viral DNA. Adefovir is active in vitro against a wide range of DNA and RNA viruses, including HBV, HIV, and herpesviruses.

Oral bioavailability of adefovir dipivoxil is about 59% and is unaffected by meals; it is rapidly and completely hydrolyzed to the parent compound by intestinal and blood esterases. Protein binding is low (< 5%). The intracellular half-life of the diphosphate is prolonged, ranging from 5 to 18 hours in various cells; this makes once-daily dosing feasible. Adefovir is excreted by a combination of glomerular filtration and active tubular secretion and requires dose adjustment for renal dysfunction; however, it may be administered to patients with decompensated liver disease.

Of the oral agents, adefovir may be slower to suppress HBV DNA levels and the least likely to induce HBeAg seroconversion. Although emergence of resistance is rare during the first year of therapy, it approaches 30% at the end of 4 years. Naturally occurring (ie, primary) adefovir-resistant rt233 HBV mutants have recently been described. There is no cross-resistance between adefovir and lamivudine.

Adefovir dipivoxil is well tolerated. A dose-dependent nephrotoxicity has been observed in clinical trials, manifested by increased serum creatinine with decreased serum phosphorous and more common in patients with baseline renal insufficiency and those receiving high doses (60 mg/d). Other potential adverse effects are headache, diarrhea, asthenia, and abdominal pain. As with other NRTI agents, lactic acidosis and hepatic steatosis are considered a risk owing to mitochondrial dysfunction. No clinically important drug-drug interactions have been recognized to date; however, co-administration with drugs that reduce renal function or compete for active tubular secretion may increase serum concentrations of adefovir or the co-administered drug. Pivalic acid, a by-product of adefovir dipivoxil metabolism, can esterify free carnitine and result in decreased carnitine levels. However, it is not felt necessary to administer carnitine supplementation with the low doses used to treat patients with HBV (10 mg/d). Adefovir is embryotoxic in rats at high doses and is genotoxic in preclinical studies.

ENTECAVIR

Entecavir is an orally administered guanosine nucleoside analog (Figure 49–2) that competitively inhibits all three functions of HBV DNA polymerase, including base priming, reverse transcription of the negative strand, and synthesis of the positive strand of HBV DNA. Oral bioavailability approaches 100% but is decreased by food; therefore, entecavir should be taken on an empty stomach. The intracellular half-life of the active phosphorylated compound is 15 hours. It is excreted by the kidney, undergoing both glomerular filtration and net tubular secretion.

Comparison with lamivudine in patients with chronic HBV infection demonstrated similar rates of HBeAg seroconversion but significantly higher rates of HBV DNA viral suppression with entecavir, normalization of serum alanine aminotransferase levels, and histologic improvement in the liver. Entecavir appears to have a higher barrier to the emergence of resistance than lamivudine. Although selection of resistant isolates with the S202G mutation has been documented during therapy, clinical resistance is rare (< 1% at 4 years). Also, decreased susceptibility to entecavir may occur in association with lamivudine resistance.

Entecavir is well tolerated. The most frequent adverse events are headache, fatigue, dizziness, and nausea. Lung adenomas and carcinomas in mice, hepatic adenomas and carcinomas in rats and mice, vascular tumors in mice, and brain gliomas and skin fibromas in rats have been observed at varying exposures. Co-administration of entecavir with drugs that reduce renal function or compete for active tubular secretion may increase serum concentrations of either entecavir or the co-administered drug.

LAMIVUDINE

The pharmacokinetics of lamivudine are described earlier in this chapter (see section, Nucleoside and Nucleotide Reverse Transcriptase Inhibitors). The more prolonged intracellular half-life in HBV cell lines (17–19 hours) than in HIV-infected cell lines (10.5–15.5 hours) allows for lower doses and less frequent administration. Lamivudine can be safely administered to patients with decompensated liver disease.

Lamivudine inhibits HBV DNA polymerase and HIV reverse transcriptase by competing with deoxycytidine triphosphate for incorporation into the viral DNA, resulting in chain termination. Lamivudine achieves 3–4 log decreases in viral replication in most patients and suppression of HBV DNA to undetectable levels in about 44% of patients. Seroconversion of HBeAg from positive to

Miscellaneous Antimicrobial Agents; Disinfectants, Antiseptics, & Sterilants

Daniel H. Deck, PharmD, & Lisa G. Winston, MD[*]

C A S E   S T U D Y

A 66-year-old man is admitted to the intensive care unit of a hospital for treatment of community-acquired pneumonia. He receives ceftriaxone and azithromycin upon admission, rapidly improves, and is transferred to a semiprivate ward room. On day 7 of his hospitalization, he develops copious diarrhea with eight bowel movements that day but is otherwise clinically stable. *Clostridium difficile*-associated colitis is suspected and a toxin assay is sent to confirm this diagnosis. What is an acceptable treatment for the patient's diarrhea? The patient is transferred to a single-bed room the following day. The housekeeping staff asks if the old room should be cleaned with alcohol or bleach. Which product should be chosen? Why?

■ METRONIDAZOLE, MUPIROCIN, POLYMYXINS, & URINARY ANTISEPTICS

METRONIDAZOLE

Metronidazole is a nitroimidazole antiprotozoal drug (see Chapter 52) that also has potent antibacterial activity against anaerobes, including *Bacteroides* and *Clostridium* species. Metronidazole is selectively absorbed by anaerobic bacteria and sensitive protozoa. Once taken up by anaerobes, it is nonenzymatically reduced by reacting with reduced ferredoxin. This reduction results in products that are toxic to anaerobic cells, and allows for their selective accumulation in anaerobes. The metabolites of metronidazole are taken up into bacterial DNA, forming unstable molecules. This action only occurs when metronidazole is partially reduced, and because this reduction usually happens only in anaerobic cells, it has relatively little effect on human cells or aerobic bacteria.

Metronidazole is well absorbed after oral administration, is widely distributed in tissues, and reaches serum levels of 4–6 mcg/mL after a 250-mg oral dose. It can also be given intravenously or by rectal suppository. The drug penetrates well into the cerebrospinal fluid and brain, reaching levels similar to those in serum. Metronidazole is metabolized in the liver and may accumulate in hepatic insufficiency.

Metronidazole is indicated for treatment of anaerobic or mixed intra-abdominal infections (in combination with other agents with activity against aerobic organisms), vaginitis (trichomonas infection, bacterial vaginosis), *Clostridium difficile* colitis, and brain abscess. The typical dosage is 500 mg three times daily orally or intravenously (30 mg/kg/d). Vaginitis may respond to a single 2 g dose. A vaginal gel is available for topical use.

Adverse effects include nausea, diarrhea, stomatitis, and peripheral neuropathy with prolonged use. Metronidazole has a disulfiram-like effect, and patients should be instructed to avoid

[*]The authors thank Henry F. Chambers, MD, the author of this chapter in previous editions, for his contributions.

alcohol. Although teratogenic in some animals, metronidazole has not been associated with this effect in humans. Other properties of metronidazole are discussed in Chapter 52.

A structurally similar agent, **tinidazole,** is a once-daily drug approved for treatment of trichomonas infection, giardiasis, and amebiasis. It also is active against anaerobic bacteria, but is not approved by the Food and Drug Administration (FDA) for treatment of anaerobic infections.

MUPIROCIN

Mupirocin (pseudomonic acid) is a natural substance produced by *Pseudomonas fluorescens.* It is rapidly inactivated after absorption, and systemic levels are undetectable. It is available as an ointment for topical application.

Mupirocin is active against gram-positive cocci, including methicillin-susceptible and methicillin-resistant strains of *Staphylococcus aureus.* Mupirocin inhibits staphylococcal isoleucyl tRNA synthetase. Low-level resistance, defined as a minimum inhibitory concentration (MIC) of up to 100 mcg/mL, is due to point mutation in the gene of the target enzyme. Low-level resistance has been observed after prolonged use. However, local concentrations achieved with topical application are well above this MIC, and this level of resistance does not lead to clinical failure. High-level resistance, with MICs exceeding 1000 mcg/mL, is due to the presence of a second isoleucyl tRNA synthetase gene, which is plasmid-encoded. High-level resistance results in complete loss of activity. Strains with high-level resistance have caused hospital-associated (nosocomial) outbreaks of staphylococcal infection and colonization. Although higher rates of resistance are encountered with intensive use of mupirocin, more than 95% of staphylococcal isolates are still susceptible.

Mupirocin is indicated for topical treatment of minor skin infections, such as impetigo (see Chapter 61). Topical application over large infected areas, such as decubitus ulcers or open surgical wounds, is an important factor leading to emergence of mupirocin-resistant strains and is not recommended. Mupirocin effectively eliminates *S aureus* nasal carriage by patients or health care workers, but results are mixed with respect to its ability to prevent subsequent staphylococcal infection.

POLYMYXINS

The polymyxins are a group of basic peptides active against gram-negative bacteria and include **polymyxin B** and **polymyxin E (colistin).** Polymyxins act as cationic detergents. They attach to and disrupt bacterial cell membranes. They also bind and inactivate endotoxin. Gram-positive organisms, *Proteus* sp, and *Neisseria* sp are resistant.

Owing to their significant toxicity with systemic administration, polymyxins are largely restricted to topical use. Ointments containing polymyxin B, 0.5 mg/g, in mixtures with bacitracin or neomycin (or both) are commonly applied to infected superficial skin lesions. Emergence of strains of *Acinetobacter baumannii, Pseudomonas aeruginosa,* and Enterobacteriaceae that are resistant to all other agents has renewed interest in polymyxins as a parenteral agents for salvage therapy of infections caused by these organisms.

FIDAXOMICIN

Fidaxomicin is a narrow-spectrum, macrocyclic antibiotic that is active against gram-positive aerobes and anaerobes but lacks activity against gram-negative bacteria. Fidaxomicin inhibits bacterial protein synthesis by binding to the sigma subunit of RNA polymerase. When administered orally, systemic absorption is negligible but fecal concentrations are high. Fidaxomicin has been approved by the FDA for the treatment for *C difficile* colitis in adults. Preliminary data have demonstrated it is as effective as oral vancomycin and may be associated with lower rates of relapsing disease. The FDA has granted orphan drug designation to all formulations of fidaxomicin for the treatment of *C difficile* infection in pediatric patients aged 16 years and younger. Fidaxomicin is administered as 200 mg orally twice daily.

URINARY ANTISEPTICS

Urinary antiseptics are oral agents that exert antibacterial activity in the urine but have little or no systemic antibacterial effect. Their usefulness is limited to lower urinary tract infections. Prolonged suppression of bacteriuria with urinary antiseptics may be desirable in chronic or recurrent urinary tract infections in which eradication of infection by short-term systemic therapy has not been possible.

Nitrofurantoin

At therapeutic doses, **nitrofurantoin** is bactericidal for many gram-positive and gram-negative bacteria; however, *P aeruginosa* and many strains of *Proteus* are inherently resistant. Nitrofurantoin has a complex mechanism of action that is not fully understood. Antibacterial activity appears to correlate with rapid intracellular conversion of nitrofurantoin to highly reactive intermediates by bacterial reductases. These intermediates react nonspecifically with many ribosomal proteins and disrupt the synthesis of proteins, RNA, DNA, and metabolic processes. It is not known which of the multiple actions of nitrofurantoin is primarily responsible for its bactericidal activity.

There is no cross-resistance between nitrofurantoin and other antimicrobial agents, and resistance emerges slowly. As resistance to trimethoprim-sulfamethoxazole and fluoroquinolones has become more common in *Escherichia coli,* nitrofurantoin has become an important alternative oral agent for treatment of uncomplicated urinary tract infection.

Nitrofurantoin is well absorbed after ingestion. It is metabolized and excreted so rapidly that no systemic antibacterial action is achieved. The drug is excreted into the urine by both glomerular filtration and tubular secretion. With average daily doses, concentrations of 200 mcg/mL are reached in urine. In renal failure, urine levels are insufficient for antibacterial action, but high blood levels may cause toxicity. Nitrofurantoin is contraindicated in patients with significant renal insufficiency (creatinine clearance < 60 mL/min).

The dosage for urinary tract infection in adults is 100 mg orally taken four times daily. The drug should not be used to treat upper urinary tract infection. Oral nitrofurantoin can be given for months for the suppression of chronic urinary tract infection. It is desirable to keep urinary pH below 5.5, which greatly enhances drug activity. A single daily dose of nitrofurantoin, 100 mg, can prevent recurrent urinary tract infections in some women.

Anorexia, nausea, and vomiting are the principal side effects of nitrofurantoin. Neuropathies and hemolytic anemia occur in patients with glucose-6-phosphate dehydrogenase deficiency. Nitrofurantoin antagonizes the action of nalidixic acid. Rashes, pulmonary infiltration and fibrosis, and other hypersensitivity reactions have been reported.

Methenamine Mandelate & Methenamine Hippurate

Methenamine mandelate is the salt of mandelic acid and methenamine and possesses properties of both of these urinary antiseptics. Methenamine hippurate is the salt of hippuric acid and methenamine. Below pH 5.5, methenamine releases formaldehyde, which is antibacterial (see Aldehydes, below). Mandelic acid or hippuric acid taken orally is excreted unchanged in the urine, in which these drugs are bactericidal for some gram-negative bacteria when pH is less than 5.5.

Methenamine mandelate, 1 g four times daily, or methenamine hippurate, 1 g twice daily by mouth (children, 50 mg/kg/d or 30 mg/kg/d, respectively), is used only as a urinary antiseptic to suppress, not treat, urinary tract infection. Acidifying agents (eg, ascorbic acid, 4–12 g/d) may be given to lower urinary pH below 5.5. Sulfonamides should not be given at the same time because they may form an insoluble compound with the formaldehyde released by methenamine. Persons taking methenamine mandelate may exhibit falsely elevated tests for catecholamine metabolites.

■ DISINFECTANTS, ANTISEPTICS, & STERILANTS

Disinfectants are strong chemical agents that inhibit or kill microorganisms (Table 50–1). Antiseptics are disinfecting agents with sufficiently low toxicity for host cells that they can be used directly on skin, mucous membranes, or wounds. Sterilants kill both vegetative cells and spores when applied to materials for appropriate times and temperatures. Some of the terms used in this context are defined in Table 50–2.

Disinfection prevents infection by reducing the number of potentially infective organisms by killing, removing, or diluting them. Disinfection can be accomplished by application of chemical agents or use of physical agents such as ionizing radiation, dry or moist heat, or superheated steam (autoclave, 120°C) to kill microorganisms. Often a combination of agents is used, eg, water and moderate heat over time (pasteurization); ethylene oxide and moist heat (a sterilant); or addition of disinfectant to a detergent. Prevention of infection also can be achieved by washing, which dilutes the potentially infectious organism, or by establishing a

TABLE 50–1 Activities of disinfectants.

	Bacteria			Viruses			Other		
	Gram-Positive	Gram-Negative	Acid-Fast	Spores	Lipophilic	Hydrophilic	Fungi	Amebic Cysts	Prions
Alcohols (isopropanol, ethanol)	HS	HS	S	R	S	V	...	...	R
Aldehydes (glutaraldehyde, formaldehyde)	HS	HS	MS	S (slow)	S	MS	S	...	R
Chlorhexidine gluconate	HS	MS	R	R	V	R	...	...	R
Sodium hypochlorite, chlorine dioxide	HS	HS	MS	S (pH 7.6)	S	S (at high conc)	MS	S	MS (at high conc)
Hexachlorophene	S (slow)	R	R	R	R	R	R	R	R
Povidone, iodine	HS	HS	S	S (at high conc)	S	R	S	S	R
Phenols, quaternary ammonium compounds	HS	HS	MS	R	S	R	S	...	R

HS, highly susceptible; S, susceptible; MS, moderately susceptible; R, resistant; V, variable; ..., no data.

TABLE 50–2   Commonly used terms related to chemical and physical killing of microorganisms.

Antisepsis	Application of an agent to living tissue for the purpose of preventing infection
Decontamination	Destruction or marked reduction in number or activity of microorganisms
Disinfection	Chemical or physical treatment that destroys most vegetative microbes or viruses, but not spores, in or on inanimate surfaces
Sanitization	Reduction of microbial load on an inanimate surface to a level considered acceptable for public health purposes
Sterilization	A process intended to kill or remove all types of microorganisms, including spores, and usually including viruses, with an acceptably low probability of survival
Pasteurization	A process that kills nonsporulating microorganisms by hot water or steam at 65–100°C

barrier, eg, gloves, condom, or respirator, which prevents the pathogen from gaining entry to the host.

Hand hygiene is the most important means of preventing transmission of infectious agents from person to person or from regions of high microbial load, eg, mouth, nose, or gut, to potential sites of infection. Soap and warm water efficiently and effectively remove bacteria. Skin disinfectants along with detergent and water are usually used preoperatively as a surgical scrub for surgeons' hands and the patient's surgical incision.

Evaluation of effectiveness of antiseptics, disinfectants, and sterilants, although seemingly simple in principle, is very complex. Factors in any evaluation include the intrinsic resistance of the microorganism, the number of microorganisms present, mixed populations of organisms, amount of organic material present (eg, blood, feces, tissue), concentration and stability of disinfectant or sterilant, time and temperature of exposure, pH, and hydration and binding of the agent to surfaces. Specific, standardized assays of activity are defined for each use. Toxicity for humans also must be evaluated. In the United States, the Environmental Protection Agency (EPA) regulates disinfectants and sterilants and the FDA regulates antiseptics.

Users of antiseptics, disinfectants, and sterilants need to consider their short-term and long-term toxicity because they may have general biocidal activity and may accumulate in the environment or in the body of the patient or caregiver using the agent. Disinfectants and antiseptics may also become contaminated by resistant microorganisms—eg, spores, *P aeruginosa*, or *Serratia marcescens*—and actually transmit infection. Most topical antiseptics interfere with wound healing to some degree. Simple cleansing of wounds with soap and water is less damaging than the application of antiseptics. Topical antibiotics with a narrow spectrum of action and low toxicity (eg, bacitracin and mupirocin) can be used for temporary control of bacterial growth and are generally preferred to antiseptics. Methenamine-containing agents release

formaldehyde in a low antibacterial concentration at acid pH and can be an effective urinary antiseptic for long-term control of urinary tract infections.

Some of the chemical classes of antiseptics, disinfectants, and sterilants are described briefly in the text that follows. The reader is referred to the general references for descriptions of physical disinfection and sterilization methods.

ALCOHOLS

The two alcohols most frequently used for antisepsis and disinfection are **ethanol** and **isopropyl alcohol (isopropanol)**. They are rapidly active, killing vegetative bacteria, *Mycobacterium tuberculosis*, and many fungi, and inactivating lipophilic viruses. The optimum bactericidal concentration is 60–90% by volume in water. They probably act by denaturation of proteins. They are not used as sterilants because they are not sporicidal, do not penetrate protein-containing organic material, may not be active against hydrophilic viruses, and lack residual action because they evaporate completely. The alcohols are useful in situations in which sinks with running water are not available for washing with soap and water. Their skin-drying effect can be partially alleviated by addition of emollients to the formulation. Use of alcohol-based hand rubs has been shown to reduce transmission of health care-associated bacterial pathogens and is recommended by the Centers for Disease Control and Prevention (CDC) as the preferred method of hand decontamination. Alcohol-based hand rubs are ineffective against spores of *C difficile,* and assiduous handwashing with soap and water is still required for decontamination after caring for a patient with infection from this organism.

Alcohols are flammable and must be stored in cool, well-ventilated areas. They must be allowed to evaporate before cautery, electrosurgery, or laser surgery. Alcohols may be damaging if applied directly to corneal tissue. Therefore, instruments such as tonometers that have been disinfected in alcohol should be rinsed with sterile water, or the alcohol should be allowed to evaporate before they are used.

CHLORHEXIDINE

Chlorhexidine is a cationic biguanide with very low water solubility. Water-soluble chlorhexidine digluconate is used in water-based formulations as an antiseptic. It is active against vegetative bacteria and mycobacteria and has moderate activity against fungi and viruses. It strongly adsorbs to bacterial membranes, causing leakage of small molecules and precipitation of cytoplasmic proteins. It is active at pH 5.5–7.0. Chlorhexidine gluconate is slower in its action than alcohols, but, because of its persistence, it has residual activity when used repeatedly, producing bactericidal action equivalent to alcohols. It is most effective against gram-positive cocci and less active against gram-positive and gram-negative rods. Spore germination is inhibited by chlorhexidine. Chlorhexidine digluconate is resistant to inhibition by blood and organic materials. However, anionic and nonionic agents in moisturizers, neutral soaps, and surfactants may neutralize its action. Chlorhexidine digluconate formulations of 4% concentration have slightly greater antibacterial activity than newer 2% formulations. The combination of chlorhexidine gluconate in 70% alcohol, available in some countries including the United States, is the preferred agent for skin antisepsis in many surgical and percutaneous procedures. The advantage of this combination over povidone-iodine may derive from its more rapid action after application, its retained activity after exposure to body fluids, and its persistent activity on the skin. Chlorhexidine has a very low skin-sensitizing or irritating capacity. Oral toxicity is low because it is poorly absorbed from the alimentary tract. Chlorhexidine must not be used during surgery on the middle ear because it causes sensorineural deafness. Similar neural toxicity may be encountered during neurosurgery.

HALOGENS

Iodine

Iodine in a 1:20,000 solution is bactericidal in 1 minute and kills spores in 15 minutes. Tincture of iodine USP contains 2% iodine and 2.4% sodium iodide in alcohol. It is the most active antiseptic for intact skin. It is not commonly used because of serious hypersensitivity reactions that may occur and because of its staining of clothing and dressings.

Iodophors

Iodophors are complexes of iodine with a surface-active agent such as **polyvinyl pyrrolidone (PVP; povidone-iodine).** Iodophors retain the activity of iodine. They kill vegetative bacteria, mycobacteria, fungi, and lipid-containing viruses. They may be sporicidal upon prolonged exposure. Iodophors can be used as antiseptics or disinfectants, the latter containing more iodine. The amount of free iodine is low, but it is released as the solution is diluted. An iodophor solution must be diluted according to the manufacturer's directions to obtain full activity.

Iodophors are less irritating and less likely to produce skin hypersensitivity than tincture of iodine. They require drying time on skin before becoming active, which can be a disadvantage. Although iodophors have a somewhat broader spectrum of activity than chlorhexidine, including sporicidal action, they lack its persistent activity on skin.

Chlorine

Chlorine is a strong oxidizing agent and universal disinfectant that is most commonly provided as a 5.25% **sodium hypochlorite** solution, a typical formulation for **household bleach.** Because formulations may vary, the exact concentration should be verified on the label. A 1:10 dilution of household bleach provides 5000 ppm of available chlorine. The CDC recommends this concentration for disinfection of blood spills. Less than 5 ppm kills vegetative bacteria, whereas up to 5000 ppm is necessary to kill spores. A concentration of 1000–10,000 ppm is tuberculocidal. One hundred ppm kills vegetative fungal cells in 1 hour, but fungal spores require 500 ppm. Viruses are inactivated by 200–500 ppm. Dilutions of 5.25% sodium hypochlorite made up in pH 7.5–8.0 tap water retain their activity for months when kept in tightly closed, opaque containers. Frequent opening and closing of the container reduces the activity markedly.

Because chlorine is inactivated by blood, serum, feces, and protein-containing materials, surfaces should be cleaned before chlorine disinfectant is applied. Undissociated hypochlorous acid (HOCl) is the active biocidal agent. When pH is increased, the less active hypochlorite ion, OCl^-, is formed. When hypochlorite solutions contact formaldehyde, the carcinogen bischloromethyl is formed. Rapid evolution of irritating chlorine gas occurs when hypochlorite solutions are mixed with acid and urine. Solutions are corrosive to aluminum, silver, and stainless steel.

Alternative chlorine-releasing compounds include **chlorine dioxide** and **chloramine T.** These agents retain chlorine longer and have a prolonged bactericidal action.

PHENOLICS

Phenol itself (perhaps the oldest of the surgical antiseptics) is no longer used even as a disinfectant because of its corrosive effect on tissues, its toxicity when absorbed, and its carcinogenic effect. These adverse actions are diminished by forming derivatives in which a functional group replaces a hydrogen atom in the aromatic ring. The phenolic agents most commonly used are **o-phenylphenol, o-benzyl-p-chlorophenol,** and **p-tertiary amylphenol.** Mixtures of phenolic derivatives are often used. Some of these are derived from coal tar distillates, eg, cresols and xylenols. Skin absorption and skin irritation still occur with these derivatives, and appropriate care is necessary in their use. Detergents are often added to formulations to clean and remove organic material that may decrease the activity of a phenolic compound.

Phenolic compounds disrupt cell walls and membranes, precipitate proteins, and inactivate enzymes. They are bactericidal (including mycobacteria) and fungicidal and are capable of inactivating lipophilic viruses. They are not sporicidal. Dilution and time of exposure recommendations of the manufacturer must be followed.

Phenolic disinfectants are used for hard surface decontamination in hospitals and laboratories, eg, floors, beds, and counter or bench tops. They are not recommended for use in nurseries and especially in bassinets, where their use has been associated with hyperbilirubinemia. Use of **hexachlorophene** as a skin disinfectant has caused cerebral edema and convulsions in premature infants and, occasionally, in adults.

QUATERNARY AMMONIUM COMPOUNDS

The quaternary ammonium compounds ("quats") are cationic surface-active detergents. The active cation has at least one long water-repellent hydrocarbon chain, which causes the molecules to concentrate as an oriented layer on the surface of solutions and colloidal or suspended particles. The charged nitrogen portion of the cation has high affinity for water and prevents separation out of solution. The bactericidal action of quaternary compounds has been attributed to inactivation of energy-producing enzymes, denaturation of proteins, and disruption of the cell membrane. These agents are fungistatic and sporistatic and also inhibit algae. They are bactericidal for gram-positive bacteria and moderately active against gram-negative bacteria. Lipophilic viruses are inactivated. They are not tuberculocidal or sporicidal, and they do not inactivate hydrophilic viruses. Quaternary ammonium compounds bind to the surface of colloidal protein in blood, serum, and milk and to the fibers in cotton, mops, cloths, and paper towels used to apply them, which can cause inactivation of the agent by removing it from solution. They are inactivated by anionic detergents (soaps), by many nonionic detergents, and by calcium, magnesium, ferric, and aluminum ions.

Quaternary compounds are used for sanitation of noncritical surfaces (floors, bench tops, etc). Their low toxicity has led to their use as sanitizers in food production facilities. The CDC recommends that quaternary ammonium compounds such as **benzalkonium chloride** *not* be used as antiseptics because several outbreaks of infections have occurred that were due to growth of *Pseudomonas* and other gram-negative bacteria in quaternary ammonium antiseptic solutions.

ALDEHYDES

Formaldehyde and **glutaraldehyde** are used for disinfection or sterilization of instruments such as fiberoptic endoscopes, respiratory therapy equipment, hemodialyzers, and dental handpieces that cannot withstand exposure to the high temperatures of steam sterilization. They are not corrosive for metal, plastic, or rubber. These agents have a broad spectrum of activity against microorganisms and viruses. They act by alkylation of chemical groups in proteins and nucleic acids. Failures of disinfection or sterilization can occur as a result of dilution below the known effective concentration, the presence of organic material, and the failure of liquid to penetrate into small channels in the instruments. Automatic circulating baths are available that increase penetration of aldehyde solution into the instrument while decreasing exposure of the operator to irritating fumes.

Formaldehyde is available as a 40% weight per volume solution in water (100% **formalin**). An 8% formaldehyde solution in water has a broad spectrum of activity against bacteria, fungi, and viruses. Sporicidal activity may take as long as 18 hours. Its rapidity of action is increased by solution in 70% isopropanol. Formaldehyde solutions are used for high-level disinfection of hemodialyzers, preparation of vaccines, and preservation and embalming of tissues. The 4% formaldehyde (10% formalin) solutions used for fixation of tissues and embalming may not be mycobactericidal.

Glutaraldehyde is a dialdehyde (1,5-pentanedial). Solutions of 2% weight per volume glutaraldehyde are most commonly used. The solution must be alkalinized to pH 7.4–8.5 for activation.

Activated solutions are bactericidal, sporicidal, fungicidal, and virucidal for both lipophilic and hydrophilic viruses. Glutaraldehyde has greater sporicidal activity than formaldehyde, but its tuberculocidal activity may be less. Lethal action against mycobacteria and spores may require prolonged exposure. Once activated, solutions have a shelf life of 14 days, after which polymerization reduces activity. Other means of activation and stabilization can increase the shelf life. Because glutaraldehyde solutions are frequently reused, the most common reason for loss of activity is dilution and exposure to organic material. Test strips to measure residual activity are recommended.

Formaldehyde has a characteristic pungent odor and is highly irritating to respiratory mucous membranes and eyes at concentrations of 2–5 ppm. The United States Occupational Safety and Health Administration (OSHA) has declared that formaldehyde is a potential carcinogen and has established an employee exposure standard that limits the 8-hour time-weighted average (TWA) exposure to 0.75 ppm. Protection of health care workers from exposure to glutaraldehyde concentrations greater than 0.2 ppm is advisable. Increased air exchange, enclosure in hoods with exhausts, tight-fitting lids on exposure devices, and use of protective personal equipment such as goggles, respirators, and gloves may be necessary to achieve these exposure limits.

Ortho-phthalaldehyde (OPA) is a phenolic dialdehyde chemical sterilant with a spectrum of activity comparable to glutaraldehyde, although it is several times more rapidly bactericidal. OPA solution typically contains 0.55% OPA. Its label claim is that high-level disinfection can be achieved in 12 minutes at room temperature compared with 45 minutes for 2.4% glutaraldehyde. Unlike glutaraldehyde, OPA requires no activation, is less irritating to mucous membranes, and does not require exposure monitoring. It has good materials compatibility and an acceptable environmental safety profile. OPA is useful for disinfection or sterilization of endoscopes, surgical instruments, and other medical devices.

SUPEROXIDIZED WATER

Electrolysis of saline yields a mixture of oxidants, primarily hypochlorous acid and chlorine, with potent disinfectant and sterilant properties. The solution generated by the process, which has been commercialized and marketed as Sterilox for disinfection of endoscopes and dental materials, is rapidly bactericidal, fungicidal, tuberculocidal, and sporicidal. High-level disinfection is achieved with a contact time of 10 minutes. The solution is nontoxic and nonirritating and requires no special disposal precautions.

PEROXYGEN COMPOUNDS

The peroxygen compounds, **hydrogen peroxide** and **peracetic acid,** have high killing activity and a broad spectrum against bacteria, spores, viruses, and fungi when used in appropriate concentration. They have the advantage that their decomposition products are not toxic and do not injure the environment. They are powerful oxidizers that are used primarily as disinfectants and sterilants.

Hydrogen peroxide is a very effective disinfectant when used for inanimate objects or materials with low organic content such as water. Organisms with the enzymes catalase and peroxidase rapidly degrade hydrogen peroxide. The innocuous degradation products are oxygen and water. Concentrated solutions containing 90% weight per volume H_2O_2 are prepared electrochemically. When diluted in high-quality deionized water to 6% and 3% and put into clean containers, they remain stable. Hydrogen peroxide has been proposed for disinfection of respirators, acrylic resin implants, plastic eating utensils, soft contact lenses, and cartons intended to contain milk or juice products. Concentrations of 10–25% hydrogen peroxide are sporicidal. Vapor phase hydrogen peroxide (VPHP) is a cold gaseous sterilant that has the potential to replace the toxic or carcinogenic gases ethylene oxide and formaldehyde. VPHP does not require a pressurized chamber and is active at temperatures as low as 4°C and concentrations as low as 4 mg/L. It is incompatible with liquids and cellulose products. It penetrates the surface of some plastics. Automated equipment using vaporized hydrogen peroxide (eg, Sterrad) or hydrogen peroxide mixed with formic acid (Endoclens) is available for sterilizing endoscopes.

Peracetic acid (CH_3COOOH) is prepared commercially from 90% hydrogen peroxide, acetic acid, and sulfuric acid as a catalyst. It is explosive in the pure form. It is usually used in dilute solution and transported in containers with vented caps to prevent increased pressure as oxygen is released. Peracetic acid is more active than hydrogen peroxide as a bactericidal and sporicidal agent. Concentrations of 250–500 ppm are effective against a broad range of bacteria in 5 minutes at pH 7.0 at 20°C. Bacterial spores are inactivated by 500–30,000 ppm peracetic acid. Only slightly increased concentrations are necessary in the presence of organic matter. Viruses require variable exposures. Enteroviruses require 2000 ppm for 15–30 minutes for inactivation.

An automated machine (Steris) that uses buffered peracetic acid liquid of 0.1–0.5% concentration has been developed for sterilization of medical, surgical, and dental instruments. Peracetic acid sterilization systems have also been adopted for hemodialyzers. The food processing and beverage industries use peracetic acid extensively because the breakdown products in high dilution do not produce objectionable odor, taste, or toxicity. Because rinsing is not necessary in this use, time and money are saved.

Peracetic acid is a potent tumor promoter but a weak carcinogen. It is not mutagenic in the Ames test.

HEAVY METALS

Heavy metals, principally mercury and silver, are now rarely used as disinfectants. Mercury is an environmental hazard, and some pathogenic bacteria have developed plasmid-mediated resistance to mercurials. Hypersensitivity to thimerosal is common, possibly in up to 40% of the population. These compounds are absorbed from solution by rubber and plastic closures. Nevertheless, **thimerosal** 0.001–0.004% is still used safely as a preservative of vaccines, antitoxins, and immune sera. Although a causative link to autism has never been established, thimerosal-free vaccines are available for use in children and pregnant woman.

Inorganic silver salts are strongly bactericidal. **Silver nitrate,** 1:1000, has been most commonly used, particularly as a preventive for gonococcal ophthalmitis in newborns. Antibiotic ointments have replaced silver nitrate for this indication. **Silver sulfadiazine** slowly releases silver and is used to suppress bacterial growth in burn wounds (see Chapter 46).

STERILANTS

For many years, pressurized **steam (autoclaving)** at 120°C for 30 minutes has been the basic method for sterilizing instruments and other heat-resistant materials. When autoclaving is not possible, as with lensed instruments and materials containing plastic and rubber, **ethylene oxide**—diluted with either fluorocarbon or carbon dioxide to diminish explosive hazard—is used at 440–1200 mg/L at 45–60°C with 30–60% relative humidity. The higher concentrations have been used to increase penetration.

Ethylene oxide is classified as a mutagen and carcinogen. The OSHA permissible exposure limit (PEL) for ethylene oxide is 1 ppm calculated as a time-weighted average. Alternative sterilants now being used increasingly include vapor phase hydrogen peroxide, peracetic acid, ozone, gas plasma, chlorine dioxide, formaldehyde, and propylene oxide. Each of these sterilants has potential advantages and problems. Automated peracetic acid systems are being used increasingly for high-level decontamination and sterilization of endoscopes and hemodialyzers because of their effectiveness, automated features, and the low toxicity of the residual products of sterilization.

PRESERVATIVES

Disinfectants are used as preservatives to prevent the overgrowth of bacteria and fungi in pharmaceutical products, laboratory sera and reagents, cosmetic products, and contact lenses. Multi-use vials of medication that may be reentered through a rubber diaphragm, and eye and nose drops, require preservatives. Preservatives should not be irritating or toxic to tissues to which they will be applied, they must be effective in preventing growth of microorganisms likely to contaminate them, and they must have sufficient solubility and stability to remain active.

Commonly used preservative agents include organic acids such as **benzoic acid** and salts, the **parabens,** (alkyl esters of *p*-hydroxybenzoic acid), sorbic acid and salts, phenolic compounds, quaternary ammonium compounds, alcohols, and mercurials such as thimerosal in 0.001–0.004% concentration.

SUMMARY Miscellaneous Antimicrobials

Subclass	Mechanism of Action	Effects	Clinical Applications	Pharmacokinetics, Toxicities, Interactions
NITROIMIDAZOLE				
• Metronidazole	Disruption of electron transport chain	Bactericidal activity against susceptible anaerobic bacteria and protozoa	Anaerobic infections • vaginitis • *C difficile* colitis	Oral or IV • hepatic clearance (half-life = 8 h) • disulfiram-like reaction when given with alcohol • *Toxicity:* Gastrointestinal upset • metallic taste • neuropathy • seizures
• *Tinidazole: Oral; similar to metronidazole but dosed once daily; approved for trichomonas, giardiasis, and amebiasis*				
URINARY ANTISEPTICS				
• Nitrofurantoin	Not fully understood • disrupts protein synthesis and inhibits multiple bacterial enzyme systems	Bacteriostatic or bactericidal activity against susceptible bacteria	Uncomplicated urinary tract infections • long-term prophylaxis	Oral • rapid renal clearance (half-life = 0.5 h) • blood levels are negligible • contraindicated in renal failure • *Toxicity:* Gastrointestinal upset • neuropathies • hypersensitivity in patients with pulmonary fibrosis
• *Methenamine hippurate and methenamine mandelate: Oral; release formaldehyde at acidic pH in the urine; used only for suppression, not treatment, of urinary tract infections*				
MACROLIDE				
• Fidaxomicin	Inhibits bacterial RNA polymerase	Bactericidal in gram positive bacteria	*C difficile* colitis	Oral • blood levels negligible

PREPARATIONS AVAILABLE

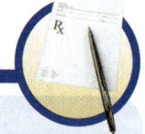

MISCELLANEOUS ANTIMICROBIAL DRUGS

Colistimethate sodium (Coly-Mycin M)
Parenteral: 150 mg for injection

Fidaxomicin (Dificid)
Oral: 200 mg tablets

Methenamine hippurate (Hiprex, Urex)
Oral: 1.0 g tablets

Methenamine mandelate (generic)
Oral: 0.5, 1 g tablets; 0.5 g/5 mL suspension

Metronidazole (generic, Flagyl)
Oral: 250, 500 mg tablets; 375 mg capsules; 750 mg extended-release tablets
Topical: 0.75% gel
Parenteral: 5 mg/mL; 500 mg for injection

Mupirocin (Bactroban)
Topical: 2% ointment, cream

Nitrofurantoin (generic, Macrodantin)
Oral: 25, 50, 100 mg capsules, 25 mg/5 mL suspension

Polymyxin B (Polymyxin B Sulfate)
Parenteral: 500,000 units per vial for injection
Ophthalmic: 500,000 units per vial

DISINFECTANTS, ANTISEPTICS, & STERILANTS

Benzalkonium (generic, Zephiran)
Topical: 17% concentrate; 50% solution; 1:750 solution

Benzoyl peroxide (generic)
Topical: 2.5%, 5%, 10% liquid; 5%, 5.5%, 10% lotion; 5%, 10% cream; 2.5%, 4%, 5%, 6%, 10%, 20% gel

Chlorhexidine gluconate (Hibiclens, Hibistat, others)
Topical: 2%, 4% cleanser, sponge; 0.5% rinse in 70% alcohol
Oral rinse (Peridex, Periogard): 0.12%

Glutaraldehyde (Cidex)
Instruments: 2%, 3.2% solution

Hexachlorophene (pHisoHex)
Topical: 3% liquid; 0.23% foam

Iodine aqueous (generic, Lugol's Solution)
Topical: 2–5% in water with 2.4% sodium iodide or 10% potassium iodide

Iodine tincture (generic)
Topical: 2% iodine or 2.4% sodium iodide in 47% alcohol, in 15, 30, 120 mL and in larger quantities

Nitrofurazone (generic, Furacin)
Topical: 0.2% solution, ointment, and cream

Ortho-phthalaldehyde (Cidex OPA)
Instruments: 0.55% solution

Povidone-iodine (generic, Betadine)
Topical: available in many forms, including aerosol, ointment, antiseptic gauze pads, skin cleanser (liquid or foam), solution, and swabsticks

Silver nitrate (generic)
Topical: 10, 25, 50% solution

Thimerosal (generic, Mersol)
Topical: 1:1000 tincture and solution

REFERENCES

Bischoff WE et al: Handwashing compliance by health care workers: The impact of introducing an accessible, alcohol-based hand antiseptic. Arch Intern Med 2000;160:1017.

Chambers HF, Winston LG: Mupirocin prophylaxis misses by a nose. Ann Intern Med 2004;140:484.

Humphreys PN: Testing standards for sporicides. J Hosp Infect 2011;77:193.

Louie TJ et al. Fidaxomicin versus vancomycin for Clostridium difficile infection. N Engl J Med 2011;364:422.

Gordin FM et al: Reduction in nosocomial transmission of drug-resistant bacteria after introduction of an alcohol-based hand-rub. Infect Control Hosp Epidemiol 2005;26:650.

Noorani A et al: Systematic review and meta-analysis of preoperative antisepsis with chlorhexidine versus povidone-iodine in clean-contaminated surgery. Br J Surg 2010;97:1614.

Rutala WA, Weber DJ: New disinfection and sterilization methods. Emerg Infect Dis 2001;7:348.

Tinidazole. Med Lett Drugs Ther 2004;46:70.

Widmer AF, Frei R: Decontamination, disinfection, and sterilization. In: Murray PR et al (editors). Manual of Clinical Microbiology, 7th ed. American Society for Microbiology, 1999.

CASE STUDY ANSWER

The patient should be treated with oral metronidazole, which is considered the preferred drug for mild to moderate cases of *C difficile*-associated colitis. The room should not be cleaned with alcohol since it does not kill *C difficile* spores. A concentrated bleach solution (5000 ppm) would be preferred because it is sporicidal.

Clinical Use of Antimicrobial Agents

Harry W. Lampiris, MD, &
Daniel S. Maddix, PharmD

CASE STUDY

A 51-year-old alcoholic patient presents to the emergency department with fever, headache, neck stiffness, and altered mental status for 12 hours. Vital signs are blood pressure 90/55 mm Hg, pulse 120/min, respirations 30/min, temperature 40°C [104°F] rectal. The patient is minimally responsive to voice and does not follow commands. Examination is significant for a right third cranial nerve palsy and nuchal rigidity. Laboratory results show a white blood cell count of 24,000/mm^3 with left shift, but other hematologic and chemistry values are within normal limits. An emergency CT scan of the head is normal. Blood cultures are obtained, and a lumbar puncture reveals the following cerebrospinal fluid (CSF) values: white blood cells 5000/mm^3, red blood cells 10/mm^3, protein 200 mg/dL, glucose 15 mg/dL (serum glucose 96 taken at same time). CSF Gram stain reveals gram-positive cocci in pairs. What is the most likely diagnosis in this patient? What organisms should be treated empirically? Are there other pharmacologic interventions to consider before initiating antimicrobial therapy?

The development of antimicrobial drugs represents one of the most important advances in therapeutics, both in the control or cure of serious infections and in the prevention and treatment of infectious complications of other therapeutic modalities such as cancer chemotherapy, immunosuppression, and surgery. However, evidence is overwhelming that antimicrobial agents are vastly overprescribed in outpatient settings in the United States, and the availability of antimicrobial agents without prescription in many developing countries has—by facilitating the development of resistance—already severely limited therapeutic options in the treatment of life-threatening infections. Therefore, the clinician should first determine whether antimicrobial therapy is warranted for a given patient. The specific questions one should ask include the following:

1. Is an antimicrobial agent indicated on the basis of clinical findings? Or is it prudent to wait until such clinical findings become apparent?

2. Have appropriate clinical specimens been obtained to establish a microbiologic diagnosis?

3. What are the likely etiologic agents for the patient's illness?

4. What measures should be taken to protect individuals exposed to the index case to prevent secondary cases, and what measures should be implemented to prevent further exposure?

5. Is there clinical evidence (eg, from well-executed clinical trials) that antimicrobial therapy will confer clinical benefit for the patient?

Once a specific cause is identified based on specific microbiologic tests, the following further questions should be considered:

1. If a specific microbial pathogen is identified, can a narrower-spectrum agent be substituted for the initial empiric drug?

2. Is one agent or a combination of agents necessary?

3. What are the optimal dose, route of administration, and duration of therapy?

4. What specific tests (eg, susceptibility testing) should be undertaken to identify patients who will not respond to treatment?

5. What adjunctive measures can be undertaken to eradicate the infection? For example, is surgery feasible for removal of devitalized tissue or foreign bodies—or drainage of an abscess—into which antimicrobial agents may be unable to penetrate?

Is it possible to decrease the dosage of immunosuppressive therapy in patients who have undergone organ transplantation? Is it possible to reduce morbidity or mortality due to the infection by reducing host immunologic response to the infection (eg, by the use of corticosteroids for the treatment of severe *Pneumocystis jiroveci* pneumonia or meningitis due to *Streptococcus pneumoniae*)?

■ EMPIRIC ANTIMICROBIAL THERAPY

Antimicrobial agents are frequently used before the pathogen responsible for a particular illness or the susceptibility to a particular antimicrobial agent is known. This use of antimicrobial agents is called empiric (or presumptive) therapy and is based on experience with a particular clinical entity. The usual justification for empiric therapy is the hope that early intervention will improve the outcome; in the best cases, this has been established by placebo-controlled, double-blind prospective clinical trials. For example, treatment of febrile episodes in neutropenic cancer patients with empiric antimicrobial therapy has been demonstrated to have impressive morbidity and mortality benefits even though the specific bacterial agent responsible for fever is determined for only a minority of such episodes.

Finally, there are many clinical entities, such as certain episodes of community-acquired pneumonia, in which it is difficult to identify a specific pathogen. In such cases, a clinical response to empiric therapy may be an important clue to the likely pathogen.

Frequently, the signs and symptoms of infection diminish as a result of empiric therapy, and microbiologic test results become available that establish a specific microbiologic diagnosis. At the time that the pathogenic organism responsible for the illness is identified, empiric therapy is optimally modified to **definitive therapy,** which is typically narrower in coverage and is given for an appropriate duration based on the results of clinical trials or experience when clinical trial data are not available.

Approach to Empiric Therapy

Initiation of empiric therapy should follow a specific and systematic approach.

A. Formulate a Clinical Diagnosis of Microbial Infection

Using all available data, the clinician should determine that there is anatomic evidence of infection (eg, pneumonia, cellulitis, sinusitis).

B. Obtain Specimens for Laboratory Examination

Examination of stained specimens by microscopy or simple examination of an uncentrifuged sample of urine for white blood cells and bacteria may provide important etiologic clues in a very short time. Cultures of selected anatomic sites (blood, sputum, urine, cerebrospinal fluid, and stool) and nonculture methods (antigen testing, polymerase chain reaction, and serology) may also confirm specific etiologic agents.

C. Formulate a Microbiologic Diagnosis

The history, physical examination, and immediately available laboratory results (eg, Gram stain of urine or sputum) may provide highly specific information. For example, in a young man with urethritis and a Gram-stained smear from the urethral meatus demonstrating intracellular gram-negative diplococci, the most likely pathogen is *Neisseria gonorrhoeae*. In the latter instance, however, the clinician should be aware that a significant number of patients with gonococcal urethritis have uninformative Gram stains for the organism and that a significant number of patients with gonococcal urethritis harbor concurrent chlamydial infection that is not demonstrated on the Gram-stained smear.

D. Determine the Necessity for Empiric Therapy

Whether or not to initiate empiric therapy is an important clinical decision based partly on experience and partly on data from clinical trials. Empiric therapy is indicated when there is a significant risk of serious morbidity if therapy is withheld until a specific pathogen is detected by the clinical laboratory.

In other settings, empiric therapy may be indicated for public health reasons rather than for demonstrated superior outcome of therapy in a specific patient. For example, urethritis in a young sexually active man usually requires treatment for *N gonorrhoeae* and *Chlamydia trachomatis* despite the absence of microbiologic confirmation at the time of diagnosis. Because the risk of noncompliance with follow-up visits in this patient population may lead to further transmission of these sexually transmitted pathogens, empiric therapy is warranted.

E. Institute Treatment

Selection of empiric therapy may be based on the microbiologic diagnosis or a clinical diagnosis without available microbiologic clues. If no microbiologic information is available, the antimicrobial spectrum of the agent or agents chosen must necessarily be broader, taking into account the most likely pathogens responsible for the patient's illness.

Choice of Antimicrobial Agent

Selection from among several drugs depends on **host factors** that include the following: (1) concomitant disease states (eg, AIDS, neutropenia due to the use of cytotoxic chemotherapy, organ transplantation, severe chronic liver or kidney disease) or the use of immunosuppressive medications; (2) prior adverse drug effects; (3) impaired elimination or detoxification of the drug (may be genetically predetermined but more frequently is associated with impaired renal or hepatic function due to underlying disease); (4) age of the patient; (5) pregnancy status; and (6) epidemiologic exposure (eg, exposure to a sick family member or pet, recent hospitalization, recent travel, occupational exposure, or new sexual partner).

Pharmacologic factors include (1) the kinetics of absorption, distribution, and elimination; (2) the ability of the drug to be delivered to the site of infection; (3) the potential toxicity of an agent; and (4) pharmacokinetic or pharmacodynamic interactions with other drugs.

Knowledge of the **susceptibility** of an organism to a specific agent in a hospital or community setting is important in the selection of empiric therapy. Pharmacokinetic differences among agents with similar antimicrobial spectrums may be exploited to reduce the frequency of dosing (eg, ceftriaxone may be conveniently given once every 24 hours). Finally, increasing consideration is being given to the cost of antimicrobial therapy, especially when multiple agents with comparable efficacy and toxicity are available for a specific infection. Changing from intravenous to oral antibiotics for prolonged administration can be particularly cost-effective.

Brief guides to empiric therapy based on presumptive microbial diagnosis and site of infection are given in Tables 51–1 and 51–2.

ANTIMICROBIAL THERAPY OF INFECTIONS WITH KNOWN ETIOLOGY

INTERPRETATION OF CULTURE RESULTS

Properly obtained and processed specimens for culture frequently yield reliable information about the cause of infection. The lack of a confirmatory microbiologic diagnosis may be due to the following:

1. Sample error, eg, obtaining cultures after antimicrobial agents have been administered, or contamination of specimens sent for culture

2. Noncultivable or slow-growing organisms (*Histoplasma capsulatum*, *Bartonella* or *Brucella* species), in which cultures are often discarded before sufficient growth has occurred for detection

3. Requesting *bacterial* cultures when infection is due to other organisms

4. Not recognizing the need for special media or isolation techniques (eg, charcoal yeast extract agar for isolation of legionella species, shell-vial tissue culture system for rapid isolation of cytomegalovirus)

Even in the setting of a classic infectious disease for which isolation techniques have been established for decades (eg, pneumococcal pneumonia, pulmonary tuberculosis, streptococcal pharyngitis), the sensitivity of the culture technique may be inadequate to identify all cases of the disease.

GUIDING ANTIMICROBIAL THERAPY OF ESTABLISHED INFECTIONS

Susceptibility Testing

Testing bacterial pathogens in vitro for their susceptibility to antimicrobial agents is extremely valuable in confirming susceptibility, ideally to a narrow-spectrum nontoxic antimicrobial drug. Tests measure the concentration of drug required to inhibit growth of the organism (**minimal inhibitory concentration [MIC]**) or to kill the organism (**minimal bactericidal concentration [MBC]**). The results of these tests can then be correlated with known drug concentrations in various body compartments. Only MICs are

routinely measured in most infections, whereas in infections in which bactericidal therapy is required for eradication of infection (eg, meningitis, endocarditis, sepsis in the granulocytopenic host), MBC measurements occasionally may be useful.

Specialized Assay Methods

A. Beta-Lactamase Assay

For some bacteria (eg, *Haemophilus* species), the susceptibility patterns of strains are similar except for the production of β lactamase. In these cases, extensive susceptibility testing may not be required, and a direct test for β lactamase using a chromogenic β-lactam substrate (nitrocephin disk) may be substituted.

B. Synergy Studies

Synergy studies are in vitro tests that attempt to measure synergistic, additive, indifferent, or antagonistic drug interactions. In general, these tests have not been standardized and have not correlated well with clinical outcome. (See section on Antimicrobial Drug Combinations for details.)

MONITORING THERAPEUTIC RESPONSE: DURATION OF THERAPY

The therapeutic response may be monitored microbiologically or clinically. Cultures of specimens taken from infected sites should eventually become sterile or demonstrate eradication of the pathogen and are useful for documenting recurrence or relapse. Follow-up cultures may also be useful for detecting superinfections or the development of resistance. Clinically, the patient's systemic manifestations of infection (malaise, fever, leukocytosis) should abate, and the clinical findings should improve (eg, as shown by clearing of radiographic infiltrates or lessening hypoxemia in pneumonia).

The duration of definitive therapy required for cure depends on the pathogen, the site of infection, and host factors (immunocompromised patients generally require longer courses of treatment). Precise data on duration of therapy exist for some infections (eg, streptococcal pharyngitis, syphilis, gonorrhea, tuberculosis, and cryptococcal meningitis). In many other situations, duration of therapy is determined empirically. For recurrent infections (eg, sinusitis, urinary tract infections), longer courses of antimicrobial therapy or surgical intervention are frequently necessary for eradication.

Clinical Failure of Antimicrobial Therapy

When the patient has an inadequate clinical or microbiologic response to antimicrobial therapy selected by in vitro susceptibility testing, systematic investigation should be undertaken to determine the cause of failure. Errors in susceptibility testing are rare, but the original results should be confirmed by repeat testing. Drug dosing and absorption should be scrutinized and tested directly using serum measurements, pill counting, or directly observed therapy.

The clinical data should be reviewed to determine whether the patient's immune function is adequate and, if not, what can be

TABLE 51–1 **Empiric antimicrobial therapy based on microbiologic etiology.**

Suspected or Proven Disease or Pathogen	Drugs of First Choice	Alternative Drugs
Gram-negative cocci (aerobic)		
Moraxella (Branhamella) catarrhalis	TMP-SMZ,[1] cephalosporin (second- or third-generation)[2]	Quinolone,[3] macrolide[4]
Neisseria gonorrhoeae	Ceftriaxone, cefixime	Spectinomycin, azithromycin
Neisseria meningitides	Penicillin G	Chloramphenicol, ceftriaxone, cefotaxime
Gram-negative rods (aerobic)		
E coli, Klebsiella, Proteus	Cephalosporin (first- or second-generation),[2] TMP-SMZ[1]	Quinolone,[3] aminoglycoside[5]
Enterobacter, Citrobacter, Serratia	TMP-SMZ,[1] quinolone,[3] carbapenem[6]	Antipseudomonal penicillin,[7] aminoglycoside,[5] cefepime
Shigella	Quinolone[3]	TMP-SMZ,[1] ampicillin, azithromycin, ceftriaxone
Salmonella	Quinolone,[3] ceftriaxone	Chloramphenicol, ampicillin, TMP-SMZ[1]
Campylobacter jejuni	Erythromycin or azithromycin	Tetracycline, quinolone[3]
Brucella species	Doxycycline + rifampin or aminoglycoside[5]	Chloramphenicol + aminoglycoside[5] or TMP-SMZ[1]
Helicobacter pylori	Proton pump inhibitor + amoxicillin + clarithromycin	Bismuth + metronidazole + tetracycline + proton pump inhibitor
Vibrio species	Tetracycline	Quinolone,[3] TMP-SMZ[1]
Pseudomonas aeruginosa	Antipseudomonal penicillin ± aminoglycoside[5]	Antipseudomonal penicillin ± quinolone,[3] cefepime, ceftazidime, antipseudomonal carbapenem,[6] or aztreonam ± aminoglycoside[5]
Burkholderia cepacia (formerly *Pseudomonas cepacia*)	TMP-SMZ[1]	Ceftazidime, chloramphenicol
Stenotrophomonas maltophilia (formerly *Xanthomonas maltophilia*)	TMP-SMZ[1]	Minocycline, ticarcillin-clavulanate, tigecycline, ceftazidime, quinolone[3]
Legionella species	Azithromycin or quinolone[3]	Clarithromycin, erythromycin
Gram-positive cocci (aerobic)		
Streptococcus pneumoniae	Penicillin[8]	Doxycycline, ceftriaxone, antipneumococcal quinolone,[3] macrolide,[4] linezolid
Streptococcus pyogenes (group A)	Penicillin, clindamycin	Erythromycin, cephalosporin (first-generation)[2]
Streptococcus agalactiae (group B)	Penicillin (± aminoglycoside[5])	Vancomycin
Viridans streptococci	Penicillin	Cephalosporin (first- or third-generation),[2] vancomycin
Staphylococcus aureus		
β-Lactamase negative	Penicillin	Cephalosporin (first-generation),[2] vancomycin
β-Lactamase positive	Penicillinase-resistant penicillin[9]	As above
Methicillin-resistant	Vancomycin	TMP-SMZ,[1] minocycline, linezolid, daptomycin, tigecycline
Enterococcus species[10]	Penicillin ± aminoglycoside[5]	Vancomycin ± aminoglycoside[5]
Gram-positive rods (aerobic)		
Bacillus species (non-*anthracis*)	Vancomycin	Imipenem, quinolone,[3] clindamycin
Listeria species	Ampicillin (± aminoglycoside[5])	TMP-SMZ[1]
Nocardia species	Sulfadiazine, TMP-SMZ[1]	Minocycline, imipenem, amikacin, linezolid
Anaerobic bacteria		
Gram-positive (clostridia, *Peptococcus*, *Actinomyces*, *Peptostreptococcus*)	Penicillin, clindamycin	Vancomycin, carbapenem,[6] chloramphenicol
Clostridium difficile	Metronidazole	Vancomycin, bacitracin
Bacteroides fragilis	Metronidazole	Chloramphenicol, carbapenem,[6] β-lactam–β-lactamase-inhibitor combinations, clindamycin

(continued)

TABLE 51–1 Empiric antimicrobial therapy based on microbiologic etiology. (Continued)

Suspected or Proven Disease or Pathogen	Drugs of First Choice	Alternative Drugs
Fusobacterium, Prevotella, Porphyromonas	Metronidazole, clindamycin, penicillin	As for *B fragilis*
Mycobacteria		
Mycobacterium tuberculosis	Isoniazid + rifampin + ethambutol + pyrazinamide	Streptomycin, moxifloxacin, amikacin, ethionamide, cycloserine, PAS, linezolid
Mycobacterium leprae		
Multibacillary	Dapsone + rifampin + clofazimine	
Paucibacillary	Dapsone + rifampin	
Mycoplasma pneumoniae	Tetracycline, erythromycin	Azithromycin, clarithromycin, quinolone[3]
Chlamydia		
C trachomatis	Tetracycline, azithromycin	Clindamycin, ofloxacin
C pneumoniae	Tetracycline, erythromycin	Clarithromycin, azithromycin
C psittaci	Tetracycline	Chloramphenicol
Spirochetes		
Borrelia recurrentis	Doxycycline	Erythromycin, chloramphenicol, penicillin
Borrelia burgdorferi		
Early	Doxycycline, amoxicillin	Cefuroxime axetil, penicillin
Late	Ceftriaxone	
Leptospira species	Penicillin	Tetracycline
Treponema species	Penicillin	Tetracycline, azithromycin, ceftriaxone
Fungi		
Aspergillus species	Voriconazole	Amphotericin B, itraconazole, caspofungin
Blastomyces species	Amphotericin B	Itraconazole, fluconazole
Candida species	Amphotericin B, echinocandin[11]	Fluconazole, itraconazole, voriconazole
Cryptococcus	Amphotericin B ± flucytosine (5-FC)	Fluconazole, voriconazole
Coccidioides immitis	Amphotericin B	Fluconazole, itraconazole, voriconazole, posaconazole
Histoplasma capsulatum	Amphotericin B	Itraconazole
Mucoraceae (Rhizopus, Absidia)	Amphotericin B	Posaconazole
Sporothrix schenckii	Amphotericin B	Itraconazole

[1]Trimethoprim-sulfamethoxazole (TMP-SMZ) is a mixture of one part trimethoprim plus five parts sulfamethoxazole.

[2]First-generation cephalosporins: cefazolin for parenteral administration; cefadroxil or cephalexin for oral administration. Second-generation cephalosporins: cefuroxime for parenteral administration; cefaclor, cefuroxime axetil, cefprozil for oral administration. Third-generation cephalosporins: ceftazidime, cefotaxime, ceftriaxone for parenteral administration; cefixime, cefpodoxime, ceftibuten, cefdinir, cefditoren for oral administration. Fourth-generation cephalosporin: cefepime for parenteral administration. Cephamycins: cefoxitin and cefotetan for parenteral administration.

[3]Quinolones: ciprofloxacin, gemifloxacin, levofloxacin, moxifloxacin, norfloxacin, ofloxacin. Norfloxacin is not effective for the treatment of systemic infections. Gemifloxacin, levofloxacin, and moxifloxacin have excellent activity against pneumococci. Ciprofloxacin and levofloxacin have good activity against *Pseudomonas aeruginosa.*

[4]Macrolides: azithromycin, clarithromycin, dirithromycin, erythromycin.

[5]Generally, streptomycin and gentamicin are used to treat infections with gram-positive organisms, whereas gentamicin, tobramycin, and amikacin are used to treat infections with gram-negatives.

[6]Carbapenems: doripenem, ertapenem, imipenem, meropenem. Ertapenem lacks activity against enterococci, *Acinetobacter,* and *P aeruginosa.*

[7]Antipseudomonal penicillin: piperacillin, piperacillin/tazobactam, ticarcillin/clavulanic acid.

[8]See footnote 3 in Table 51–2 for guidelines on the treatment of penicillin-resistant pneumococcal meningitis.

[9]Parenteral nafcillin or oxacillin; oral dicloxacillin.

[10]There is no regimen that is reliably bactericidal for vancomycin-resistant enterococcus for which there is extensive clinical experience; daptomycin has bactericidal activity in vitro. Regimens that have been reported to be efficacious include nitrofurantoin (for urinary tract infection); potential regimens for bacteremia include daptomycin, linezolid, and dalfopristin/quinupristin.

[11]Echinocandins: anidulafungin, caspofungin, micafungin.

TABLE 51–2 Empiric antimicrobial therapy based on site of infection.

Presumed Site of Infection	Common Pathogens	Drugs of First Choice	Alternative Drugs
Bacterial endocarditis			
Acute	*Staphylococcus aureus*	Vancomycin + gentamicin	Penicillinase-resistant penicillin[1] + gentamicin
Subacute	*Viridans* streptococci, enterococci	Penicillin + gentamicin	Vancomycin + gentamicin
Septic arthritis			
Child	*H influenzae, S aureus,* β-hemolytic streptococci	Ceftriaxone	Ampicillin-sulbactam
Adult	*S aureus,* Enterobacteriaceae	Cefazolin	Vancomycin, quinolone
Acute otitis media, sinusitis	*H influenzae, S pneumoniae, M catarrhalis*	Amoxicillin	Amoxicillin-clavulanate, cefuroxime axetil, TMP-SMZ
Cellulitis	*S aureus,* group A streptococcus	Penicillinase-resistant penicillin, cephalosporin (first-generation)[2]	Vancomycin, clindamycin, linezolid, daptomycin
Meningitis			
Neonate	Group B streptococcus, *E coli, Listeria*	Ampicillin + cephalosporin (third-generation)	Ampicillin + aminoglycoside, chloramphenicol, meropenem
Child	*H influenzae,* pneumococcus, meningococcus	Ceftriaxone or cefotaxime ± vancomycin[3]	Chloramphenicol, meropenem
Adult	Pneumococcus, meningococcus	Ceftriaxone, cefotaxime	Vancomycin + ceftriaxone or cefotaxime[3]
Peritonitis due to ruptured viscus	Coliforms, *B fragilis*	Metronidazole + cephalosporin (third-generation), piperacillin/tazobactam	Carbapenem, tigecycline
Pneumonia			
Neonate	As in neonatal meningitis		
Child	Pneumococcus, *S aureus, H influenzae*	Ceftriaxone, cefuroxime, cefotaxime	Ampicillin-sulbactam
Adult (community-acquired)	Pneumococcus, *Mycoplasma, Legionella, H influenzae, S aureus, C pneumonia,* coliforms	**Outpatient:** Macrolide,[4] amoxicillin, tetracycline	**Outpatient:** Quinolone
		Inpatient: Macrolide[4] + cefotaxime, ceftriaxone, ertapenem, or ampicillin	**Inpatient:** Doxycycline + cefotaxime, ceftriaxone, ertapenem, or ampicillin; respiratory quinolone[5]
Septicemia[6]	Any	Vancomycin + cephalosporin (third-generation) or piperacillin/tazobactam or imipenem or meropenem	
Septicemia with granulocytopenia	Any	Antipseudomonal penicillin + aminoglycoside; ceftazidime; cefepime; imipenem or meropenem; consider addition of systemic antifungal therapy if fever persists beyond 5 days of empiric therapy	

[1]See footnote 9, Table 51–1.

[2]See footnote 2, Table 51–1.

[3]When meningitis with penicillin-resistant pneumococcus is suspected, empiric therapy with this regimen is recommended.

[4]Erythromycin, clarithromycin, or azithromycin (an azalide) may be used.

[5]Quinolones used to treat pneumonococcal infections include levofloxacin, moxifloxacin, and gemifloxacin.

[6]Adjunctive immunomodulatory drugs such as drotrecogin-alfa can also be considered for patients with severe sepsis.

done to maximize it. For example, are adequate numbers of granulocytes present and are HIV infection, malnutrition, or underlying malignancy present? The presence of abscesses or foreign bodies should also be considered. Finally, culture and susceptibility testing should be repeated to determine whether superinfection has occurred with another organism or whether the original pathogen has developed drug resistance.

ANTIMICROBIAL PHARMACODYNAMICS

The time course of drug concentration is closely related to the antimicrobial effect at the site of infection and to any toxic effects. Pharmacodynamic factors include pathogen susceptibility testing, drug bactericidal versus bacteriostatic activity, drug synergism, antagonism, and postantibiotic effects. Together with pharmacokinetics, pharmacodynamic information permits the selection of optimal antimicrobial dosage regimens.

Bacteriostatic versus Bactericidal Activity

Antibacterial agents may be classified as bacteriostatic or bactericidal (Table 51–3). For agents that are primarily bacteriostatic, inhibitory drug concentrations are much lower than bactericidal drug concentrations. In general, cell wall-active agents are bactericidal, and drugs that inhibit protein synthesis are bacteriostatic.

The classification of antibacterial agents as bactericidal or bacteriostatic has limitations. Some agents that are considered to be bacteriostatic may be bactericidal against selected organisms. On the other hand, enterococci are inhibited but not killed by vancomycin, penicillin, or ampicillin used as single agents.

Bacteriostatic and bactericidal agents are equivalent for the treatment of most infectious diseases in immunocompetent hosts. Bactericidal agents should be selected over bacteriostatic ones in circumstances in which local or systemic host defenses are impaired. Bactericidal agents are required for treatment of endocarditis and other endovascular infections, meningitis, and infections in neutropenic cancer patients.

Bactericidal agents can be divided into two groups: agents that exhibit **concentration-dependent killing** (eg, aminoglycosides and quinolones) and agents that exhibit **time-dependent killing** (eg, β lactams and vancomycin). For drugs whose killing action is concentration-dependent, the rate and extent of killing increase with increasing drug concentrations. Concentration-dependent killing is one of the pharmacodynamic factors responsible for the efficacy of once-daily dosing of aminoglycosides.

For drugs whose killing action is time-dependent, bactericidal activity continues as long as serum concentrations are greater than the MBC. Drug concentrations of time-dependent killing agents that lack a postantibiotic effect should be maintained above the MIC for the entire interval between doses.

Postantibiotic Effect

Persistent suppression of bacterial growth after limited exposure to an antimicrobial agent is known as the postantibiotic effect (PAE). The PAE can be expressed mathematically as follows:

$$PAE = T - C$$

where T is the time required for the viable count in the test (in vitro) culture to increase tenfold above the count observed immediately before drug removal and C is the time required for the count in an untreated culture to increase tenfold above the count observed immediately after completion of the same procedure used on the test culture. The PAE reflects the time required for bacteria to return to logarithmic growth.

Proposed mechanisms include (1) slow recovery after reversible nonlethal damage to cell structures; (2) persistence of the drug at a binding site or within the periplasmic space; and (3) the need to synthesize new enzymes before growth can resume. Most antimicrobials possess significant in vitro PAEs (≥ 1.5 hours) against susceptible gram-positive cocci (Table 51–4). Antimicrobials with significant PAEs against susceptible gram-negative bacilli are limited to carbapenems and agents that inhibit protein or DNA synthesis.

In vivo PAEs are usually much longer than in vitro PAEs. This is thought to be due to **postantibiotic leukocyte enhancement (PALE)** and exposure of bacteria to subinhibitory antibiotic concentrations. The efficacy of once-daily dosing regimens is in part due to the PAE. Aminoglycosides and quinolones possess concentration-dependent PAEs; thus, high doses of aminoglycosides given once daily result in enhanced bactericidal activity and extended PAEs. This combination of pharmacodynamic effects allows aminoglycoside serum concentrations that are below the MICs of target organisms to remain effective for extended periods of time.

PHARMACOKINETIC CONSIDERATIONS

Route of Administration

Many antimicrobial agents have similar pharmacokinetic properties when given orally or parenterally (ie, tetracyclines, trimethoprim-sulfamethoxazole, quinolones, chloramphenicol, metronidazole, clindamycin, rifampin, linezolid, and fluconazole). In most cases, oral therapy with these drugs is equally effective, is less costly, and results in fewer complications than parenteral therapy.

The intravenous route is preferred in the following situations: (1) for critically ill patients; (2) for patients with bacterial meningitis or endocarditis; (3) for patients with nausea, vomiting, gastrectomy, or diseases that may impair oral absorption; and (4) when giving antimicrobials that are poorly absorbed following oral administration.

TABLE 51–3 Bactericidal and bacteriostatic antibacterial agents.

Bactericidal Agents	Bacteriostatic Agents
Aminoglycosides	Chloramphenicol
Bacitracin	Clindamycin
β-Lactam antibiotics	Ethambutol
Daptomycin	Macrolides
Glycopeptide antibiotics	Nitrofurantoin
Isoniazid	Novobiocin
Ketolides	Oxazolidinones
Metronidazole	Sulfonamides
Polymyxins	Tetracyclines
Pyrazinamide	Tigecycline
Quinolones	Trimethoprim
Rifampin	
Streptogramins	

TABLE 51–4 Antibacterial agents with in vitro postantibiotic effects ≥ 1.5 hours.

Against Gram-Positive Cocci	Against Gram-Negative Bacilli
Aminoglycosides	Aminoglycosides
Carbapenems	Carbapenems
Cephalosporins	Chloramphenicol
Chloramphenicol	Quinolones
Clindamycin	Rifampin
Daptomycin	Tetracyclines
Glycopeptide antibiotics	Tigecycline
Ketolides	
Macrolides	
Oxazolidinones	
Penicillins	
Quinolones	
Rifampin	
Streptogramins	
Sulfonamides	
Tetracyclines	
Tigecycline	
Trimethoprim	

Conditions That Alter Antimicrobial Pharmacokinetics

Various diseases and physiologic states alter the pharmacokinetics of antimicrobial agents. Impairment of renal or hepatic function may result in decreased elimination. Table 51–5 lists drugs that require dosage reduction in patients with renal or hepatic insufficiency. Failure to reduce antimicrobial agent dosage in such patients may cause toxic effects. Conversely, patients with burns, cystic fibrosis, or trauma may have increased dosage requirements for selected agents. The pharmacokinetics of antimicrobials is also altered in the elderly, in neonates, and in pregnancy.

Drug Concentrations in Body Fluids

Most antimicrobial agents are well distributed to most body tissues and fluids. Penetration into the cerebrospinal fluid is an exception. Most do not penetrate uninflamed meninges to an appreciable extent. In the presence of meningitis, however, the cerebrospinal fluid concentrations of many antimicrobials increase (Table 51–6).

Monitoring Serum Concentrations of Antimicrobial Agents

For most antimicrobial agents, the relation between dose and therapeutic outcome is well established, and serum concentration monitoring is unnecessary for these drugs. To justify routine serum concentration monitoring, it should be established (1) that a direct relationship exists between drug concentrations and efficacy or toxicity; (2) that substantial interpatient variability exists in serum concentrations on standard doses; (3) that a small difference exists between therapeutic and toxic serum concentrations; (4) that the clinical efficacy or toxicity of the drug is delayed or difficult to measure; and (5) that an accurate assay is available.

In clinical practice, serum concentration monitoring is routinely performed on patients receiving aminoglycosides. Despite the lack of supporting evidence for its usefulness or need, serum vancomycin concentration monitoring is also widespread. Flucytosine serum concentration monitoring has been shown to reduce toxicity when doses are adjusted to maintain peak concentrations below 100 mcg/mL.

■ MANAGEMENT OF ANTIMICROBIAL DRUG TOXICITY

Owing to the large number of antimicrobials available, it is usually possible to select an effective alternative in patients who develop serious drug toxicity (Table 51–1). However, for some infections there are no effective alternatives to the drug of choice. For example, in patients with neurosyphilis who have a history of

TABLE 51–5 Antimicrobial agents that require dosage adjustment or are contraindicated in patients with renal or hepatic impairment.

Dosage Adjustment Needed in Renal Impairment	Contraindicated in Renal Impairment	Dosage Adjustment Needed in Hepatic Impairment
Acyclovir, amantadine, aminoglycosides, aztreonam, carbapenems, cephalosporins,[1] clarithromycin, colistin, cycloserine, daptomycin, didanosine, emtricitabine, ethambutol, ethionamide, famciclovir, fluconazole, flucytosine, foscarnet, ganciclovir, lamivudine, penicillins,[3] pyrazinamide, quinolones,[4] rimantadine, stavudine, telavancin, telbivudine, telithromycin, tenofovir, terbinafine, trimethoprim-sulfamethoxazole, valacyclovir, vancomycin, zidovudine	Cidofovir, methenamine, nalidixic acid, nitrofurantoin, sulfonamides (long-acting), tetracyclines[2]	Amprenavir, atazanavir, chloramphenicol, clindamycin, erythromycin, fosamprenavir, indinavir, metronidazole, rimantadine, tigecycline

[1]Except ceftriaxone.

[2]Except doxycycline and possibly minocycline.

[3]Except antistaphylococcal penicillins (eg, nafcillin and dicloxacillin).

[4]Except moxifloxacin.

TABLE 51–6 Cerebrospinal fluid (CSF) penetration of selected antimicrobials.

Antimicrobial Agent	CSF Concentration (Uninflamed Meninges) as % of Serum Concentration	CSF Concentration (Inflamed Meninges) as % of Serum Concentration
Ampicillin	2–3	2–100
Aztreonam	2	5
Cefepime	0–2	4–12
Cefotaxime	22.5	27–36
Ceftazidime	0.7	20–40
Ceftriaxone	0.8–1.6	16
Cefuroxime	20	17–88
Ciprofloxacin	6–27	26–37
Imipenem	3.1	11–41
Meropenem	0–7	1–52
Nafcillin	2–15	5–27
Penicillin G	1–2	8–18
Sulfamethoxazole	40	12–47
Trimethoprim	< 41	12–69
Vancomycin	0	1–53

anaphylaxis to penicillin, it is necessary to perform skin testing and desensitization to penicillin. It is important to obtain a clear history of drug allergy and other adverse drug reactions. A patient with a documented antimicrobial allergy should carry a card with the name of the drug and a description of the reaction. Cross-reactivity between penicillins and cephalosporins is less than 10%. Cephalosporins may be administered to patients with penicillin-induced maculopapular rashes but should be avoided in patients with a history of penicillin-induced immediate hypersensitivity reactions. On the other hand, aztreonam does not cross-react with penicillins and can be safely administered to patients with a history of penicillin-induced anaphylaxis. For mild reactions, it may be possible to continue therapy with use of adjunctive agents or dosage reduction.

Adverse reactions to antimicrobials occur with increased frequency in several groups, including neonates, geriatric patients, renal failure patients, and AIDS patients. Dosage adjustment of the drugs listed in Table 51–5 is essential for the prevention of adverse effects in patients with renal failure. In addition, several agents are contraindicated in patients with renal impairment because of increased rates of serious toxicity (Table 51–5). See the preceding chapters for discussions of specific drugs.

Polypharmacy also predisposes to drug interactions. Although the mechanism is not known, AIDS patients have an unusually high incidence of toxicity to a number of drugs, including clindamycin, aminopenicillins, and sulfonamides. Many of these reactions, including rash and fever, may respond to dosage reduction or

treatment with corticosteroids and antihistamines. Other examples are discussed in the preceding chapters and in Chapter 66.

■ ANTIMICROBIAL DRUG COMBINATIONS

RATIONALE FOR COMBINATION ANTIMICROBIAL THERAPY

Most infections should be treated with a single antimicrobial agent. Although indications for combination therapy exist, antimicrobial combinations are often overused in clinical practice. The unnecessary use of antimicrobial combinations increases toxicity and costs and may occasionally result in reduced efficacy due to antagonism of one drug by another. Antimicrobial combinations should be selected for one or more of the following reasons:

1. To provide broad-spectrum empiric therapy in seriously ill patients.

2. To treat polymicrobial infections (such as intra-abdominal abscesses, which typically are due to a combination of anaerobic and aerobic gram-negative organisms, and enterococci). The antimicrobial combination chosen should cover the most common known or suspected pathogens but need not cover all possible pathogens. The availability of antimicrobials with excellent polymicrobial coverage (eg, β-lactamase inhibitor combinations or carbapenems) may reduce the need for combination therapy in the setting of polymicrobial infections.

3. To decrease the emergence of resistant strains. The value of combination therapy in this setting has been clearly demonstrated for tuberculosis.

4. To decrease dose-related toxicity by using reduced doses of one or more components of the drug regimen. The use of flucytosine in combination with amphotericin B for the treatment of cryptococcal meningitis in non–HIV-infected patients allows for a reduction in amphotericin B dosage with decreased amphotericin B-induced nephrotoxicity.

5. To obtain enhanced inhibition or killing. This use of antimicrobial combinations is discussed in the paragraphs that follow.

SYNERGISM & ANTAGONISM

When the inhibitory or killing effects of two or more antimicrobials used together are significantly greater than expected from their effects when used individually, synergism is said to result. Synergism is marked by a fourfold or greater reduction in the MIC or MBC of each drug when used in combination versus when used alone. Antagonism occurs when the combined inhibitory or killing effects of two or more antimicrobial drugs are significantly less than observed when the drugs are used individually.

Mechanisms of Synergistic Action

The need for synergistic combinations of antimicrobials has been clearly established for the treatment of enterococcal endocarditis. Bactericidal activity is essential for the optimal management of bacterial endocarditis. Penicillin or ampicillin in combination with gentamicin or streptomycin is superior to monotherapy with a penicillin or vancomycin. When tested alone, penicillins and vancomycin are only bacteriostatic against susceptible enterococcal isolates. When these agents are combined with an aminoglycoside, however, bactericidal activity results. The addition of gentamicin or streptomycin to penicillin allows for a reduction in the duration of therapy for selected patients with viridans streptococcal endocarditis. Some evidence exists that synergistic combinations of antimicrobials may be of benefit in the treatment of gram-negative bacillary infections in febrile neutropenic cancer patients and in systemic infections caused by *Pseudomonas aeruginosa.*

Other synergistic antimicrobial combinations have been shown to be more effective than monotherapy with individual components. Trimethoprim-sulfamethoxazole has been successfully used for the treatment of bacterial infections and *P jiroveci* (*carinii*) pneumonia.[*] β-Lactamase inhibitors restore the activity of intrinsically active but hydrolyzable β lactams against organisms such as *Staphylococcus aureus* and *Bacteroides fragilis.* Three major mechanisms of antimicrobial synergism have been established:

1. **Blockade of sequential steps in a metabolic sequence:** Trimethoprim-sulfamethoxazole is the best-known example of this mechanism of synergy (see Chapter 46). Blockade of the two sequential steps in the folic acid pathway by trimethoprim-sulfamethoxazole results in a much more complete inhibition of growth than achieved by either component alone.

2. **Inhibition of enzymatic inactivation:** Enzymatic inactivation of β-lactam antibiotics is a major mechanism of antibiotic resistance. Inhibition of β lactamase by β-lactamase inhibitor drugs (eg, sulbactam) results in synergism.

3. **Enhancement of antimicrobial agent uptake:** Penicillins and other cell wall-active agents can increase the uptake of aminoglycosides by a number of bacteria, including staphylococci, enterococci, streptococci, and *P aeruginosa.* Enterococci are thought to be intrinsically resistant to aminoglycosides because of permeability barriers. Similarly, amphotericin B is thought to enhance the uptake of flucytosine by fungi.

Mechanisms of Antagonistic Action

There are few clinically relevant examples of antimicrobial antagonism. The most striking example was reported in a study of patients with pneumococcal meningitis. Patients who were treated with the combination of penicillin and chlortetracycline had a mortality rate of 79% compared with a mortality rate of 21% in patients who received penicillin monotherapy (illustrating the first mechanism set forth below).

The use of an antagonistic antimicrobial combination does not preclude other potential beneficial interactions. For example, rifampin may antagonize the action of anti-staphylococcal penicillins or vancomycin against staphylococci. However, the aforementioned antimicrobials may prevent the emergence of resistance to rifampin.

Two major mechanisms of antimicrobial antagonism have been established:

1. **Inhibition of cidal activity by static agents:** Bacteriostatic agents such as tetracyclines and chloramphenicol can antagonize the action of bactericidal cell wall-active agents because cell wall-active agents require that the bacteria be actively growing and dividing.

2. **Induction of enzymatic inactivation:** Some gram-negative bacilli, including enterobacter species, *P aeruginosa, Serratia marcescens,* and *Citrobacter freundii,* possess inducible β lactamases. β-Lactam antibiotics such as imipenem, cefoxitin, and ampicillin are potent inducers of β-lactamase production. If an inducing agent is combined with an intrinsically active but hydrolyzable β lactam such as piperacillin, antagonism may result.

■ ANTIMICROBIAL PROPHYLAXIS

Antimicrobial agents are effective in preventing infections in many settings. Antimicrobial prophylaxis should be used in circumstances in which efficacy has been demonstrated and benefits outweigh the risks of prophylaxis. Antimicrobial prophylaxis may be divided into surgical prophylaxis and nonsurgical prophylaxis.

Surgical Prophylaxis

Surgical wound infections are a major category of nosocomial infections. The estimated annual cost of surgical wound infections in the United States is $1.5 billion.

The National Research Council (NRC) Wound Classification Criteria have served as the basis for recommending antimicrobial prophylaxis. NRC criteria consist of four classes [see Box: National Research Council (NRC) Wound Classification Criteria].

The Study of the Efficacy of Nosocomial Infection Control (SENIC) identified four independent risk factors for postoperative wound infections: operations on the abdomen, operations lasting more than 2 hours, contaminated or dirty wound classification, and at least three medical diagnoses. Patients with at least two SENIC risk factors who undergo clean surgical procedures have an increased risk of developing surgical wound infections and should receive antimicrobial prophylaxis.

Surgical procedures that necessitate the use of antimicrobial prophylaxis include contaminated and clean-contaminated operations, selected operations in which postoperative infection may be catastrophic such as open heart surgery, clean procedures that involve placement of prosthetic materials, and any procedure in an immunocompromised host. The operation should carry a significant risk of postoperative site infection or cause significant bacterial contamination.

General principles of antimicrobial surgical prophylaxis include the following:

1. The antibiotic should be active against common surgical wound pathogens; unnecessarily broad coverage should be avoided.

2. The antibiotic should have proved efficacy in clinical trials.

---

[*]*Pneumocystis jiroveci* is a fungal organism found in humans (*P carinii* infects animals) that responds to antiprotozoal drugs. See Chapter 52.

National Research Council (NRC) Wound Classification Criteria

Clean: Elective, primarily closed procedure; respiratory, gastrointestinal, biliary, genitourinary, or oropharyngeal tract not entered; no acute inflammation and no break in technique; expected infection rate ≤ 2%.

Clean contaminated: Urgent or emergency case that is otherwise clean; elective, controlled opening of respiratory, gastrointestinal, biliary, or oropharyngeal tract; minimal spillage or minor break in technique; expected infection rate ≤ 10%.

Contaminated: Acute nonpurulent inflammation; major technique break or major spill from hollow organ; penetrating trauma less than 4 hours old; chronic open wounds to be grafted or covered; expected infection rate about 20%.

Dirty: Purulence or abscess; preoperative perforation of respiratory, gastrointestinal, biliary, or oropharyngeal tract; penetrating trauma more than 4 hours old; expected infection rate about 40%.

3. The antibiotic must achieve concentrations greater than the MIC of suspected pathogens, and these concentrations must be present at the time of incision.
4. The shortest possible course—ideally a single dose—of the most effective and least toxic antibiotic should be used.

5. The newer broad-spectrum antibiotics should be reserved for therapy of resistant infections.
6. If all other factors are equal, the least expensive agent should be used.

The proper selection and administration of antimicrobial prophylaxis are of utmost importance. Common indications for surgical prophylaxis are shown in Table 51–7. Cefazolin is the prophylactic agent of choice for head and neck, gastroduodenal, biliary tract, gynecologic, and clean procedures. Local wound infection patterns should be considered when selecting antimicrobial prophylaxis. The selection of vancomycin over cefazolin may be necessary in hospitals with high rates of methicillin-resistant *S aureus* or *S epidermidis* infections. The antibiotic should be present in adequate concentrations at the operative site before incision and throughout the procedure; initial dosing is dependent on the volume of distribution, peak levels, clearance, protein binding, and bioavailability. Parenteral agents should be administered during the interval beginning 60 minutes before incision; administration up to the time of incision is preferred. In cesarean section, the antibiotic is administered after umbilical cord clamping. If short-acting agents such as cefoxitin are used, doses should be repeated if the procedure exceeds 3–4 hours in duration. Single-dose prophylaxis is effective for most procedures and results in decreased toxicity and antimicrobial resistance.

Improper administration of antimicrobial prophylaxis leads to excessive surgical wound infection rates. Common errors in antibiotic prophylaxis include selection of the wrong antibiotic,

TABLE 51–7 Recommendations for surgical antimicrobial prophylaxis.

Type of Operation	Common Pathogens	Drug of Choice
Cardiac (with median sternotomy)	Staphylococci, enteric gram-negative rods	Cefazolin
Noncardiac, thoracic	Staphylococci, streptococci, enteric gram-negative rods	Cefazolin
Vascular (abdominal and lower extremity)	Staphylococci, enteric gram-negative rods	Cefazolin
Neurosurgical (craniotomy)	Staphylococci	Cefazolin
Orthopedic (with hardware insertion)	Staphylococci	Cefazolin
Head and neck (with entry into the oropharynx)	*S aureus*, oral flora	Cefazolin + metronidazole
Gastroduodenal (high-risk patients[1])	*S aureus*, oral flora, enteric gram-negative rods	Cefazolin
Biliary tract (high-risk patients[2])	*S aureus*, enterococci, enteric gram-negative rods	Cefazolin
Colorectal (elective surgery)	Enteric gram-negative rods, anaerobes	Oral erythromycin plus neomycin[3]
Colorectal (emergency surgery or obstruction)	Enteric gram-negative rods, anaerobes	Cefoxitin, cefotetan, or cefazolin + metronidazole
Appendectomy, nonperforated	Enteric gram-negative rods, anaerobes	Cefoxitin or cefazolin + metronidazole
Hysterectomy	Enteric gram-negative rods, anaerobes, enterococci, group B streptococci	Cefazolin or cefoxitin
Cesarean section	Enteric gram-negative rods, anaerobes, enterococci, group B streptococci	Cefazolin[4]

[1]Gastric procedures for cancer, ulcer, bleeding, or obstruction; morbid obesity; suppression of gastric acid secretion.

[2]Age > 60, acute cholecystitis, prior biliary tract surgery, common duct stones, jaundice, or diabetes mellitus.

[3]In conjunction with mechanical bowel preparation.

[4]Administer immediately following cord clamping.

TABLE 51–8 Recommendations for nonsurgical antimicrobial prophylaxis.

Infection to Be Prevented	Indication(s)	Drug of Choice	Efficacy
Anthrax	Suspected exposure	Ciprofloxacin or doxycycline	Proposed effective
Cholera	Close contacts of a case	Tetracycline	Proposed effective
Diphtheria	Unimmunized contacts	Penicillin or erythromycin	Proposed effective
Endocarditis	Dental, oral, or upper respiratory tract procedures[1] in at-risk patients[2]	Amoxicillin or clindamycin	Proposed effective
Genital herpes simplex	Recurrent infection (≥ 4 episodes per year)	Acyclovir	Excellent
Perinatal herpes simplex type 2 infection	Mothers with primary HSV or frequent recurrent genital HSV	Acyclovir	Proposed effective
Group B streptococcal (GBS) infection	Mothers with cervical or vaginal GBS colonization and their newborns with one or more of the following: (a) onset of labor or membrane rupture before 37 weeks' gestation, (b) prolonged rupture of membranes (> 12 hours), (c) maternal intrapartum fever, (d) history of GBS bacteriuria during pregnancy, (e) mothers who have given birth to infants who had early GBS disease or with a history of streptococcal bacteriuria during pregnancy	Ampicillin or penicillin	Excellent
Haemophilus influenzae type B infection	Close contacts of a case in incompletely immunized children (> 48 months old)	Rifampin	Excellent
HIV infection	Health care workers exposed to blood after needle-stick injury	Tenofovir/emtricitabine ± lopinavir/ritonavir	Good
	Pregnant HIV-infected women who are at ≥ 14 weeks of gestation; newborns of HIV-infected women for the first 6 weeks of life, beginning 8–12 hours after birth	HAART[3]	Excellent
Influenza A and B	Unvaccinated geriatric patients, immunocompromised hosts, and health care workers during outbreaks	Oseltamivir	Good
Malaria	Travelers to areas endemic for chloroquine-susceptible disease	Chloroquine	Excellent
	Travelers to areas endemic for chloroquine-resistant disease	Mefloquine, doxycycline, or atovaquone/proguanil	Excellent
Meningococcal infection	Close contacts of a case	Rifampin, ciprofloxacin, or ceftriaxone	Excellent
Mycobacterium avium complex	HIV-infected patients with CD4 count < 75/μL	Azithromycin, clarithromycin, or rifabutin	Excellent
Otitis media	Recurrent infection	Amoxicillin	Good
Pertussis	Close contacts of a case	Azithromycin	Excellent
Plague	Close contacts of a case	Tetracycline	Proposed effective
Pneumococcemia	Children with sickle cell disease or asplenia	Penicillin	Excellent
Pneumocystis jiroveci pneumonia (PCP)	High-risk patients (eg, AIDS, leukemia, transplant)	Trimethoprim-sulfamethoxazole, dapsone, or atovaquone	Excellent
Rheumatic fever	History of rheumatic fever or known rheumatic heart disease	Benzathine penicillin	Excellent
Toxoplasmosis	HIV-infected patients with IgG antibody to *Toxoplasma* and CD4 count < 100/μL	Trimethoprim-sulfamethoxazole	Good
Tuberculosis	Persons with positive tuberculin skin tests and one or more of the following: (a) HIV infection, (b) close contacts with newly diagnosed disease, (c) recent skin test conversion, (d) medical conditions that increase the risk of developing tuberculosis, (e) age < 35	Isoniazid, rifampin, or pyrazinamide	Excellent
Urinary tract infections (UTI)	Recurrent infection	Trimethoprim-sulfamethoxazole	Excellent

[1]Prophylaxis is recommended for the following: dental procedures that involve manipulation of gingival tissue or the periapical region of teeth or perforation of the oral mucosa, and invasive procedure of the respiratory tract that involves incision or biopsy of the respiratory mucosa, such as tonsillectomy and adenoidectomy.

[2]Prophylaxis should be targeted to those with the following risk factors: prosthetic heart valves, previous bacterial endocarditis, congenital cardiac malformations, cardiac transplantation patients who develop cardiac valvulopathy.

[3]Highly active antiretroviral therapy. See http://www.hivatis.org/ for updated guidelines.

administering the first dose too early or too late, failure to repeat doses during prolonged procedures, excessive duration of prophylaxis, and inappropriate use of broad-spectrum antibiotics.

Nonsurgical Prophylaxis

Nonsurgical prophylaxis includes the administration of antimicrobials to prevent colonization or asymptomatic infection as well as the administration of drugs following colonization by or inoculation of pathogens but before the development of disease. Nonsurgical prophylaxis is indicated in individuals who are at high risk for temporary exposure to selected virulent pathogens and in patients who are at increased risk for developing infection because of underlying disease (eg, immunocompromised hosts). Prophylaxis is most effective when directed against organisms that are predictably susceptible to antimicrobial agents. Common indications and drugs for nonsurgical prophylaxis are listed in Table 51–8.

REFERENCES

American Thoracic Society: Guidelines for the management of adults with hospital-acquired, ventilator-associated, and healthcare-associated pneumonia. Am J Respir Crit Care Med 2005;171:388.

Antimicrobial prophylaxis for surgery. Treat Guidel Med Lett 2009;7:47.

Baddour LM et al: Infective endocarditis: Diagnosis, antimicrobial therapy, and management of complications. Circulation 2005;111:3167.

Blumberg HM et al: American Thoracic Society/Centers for Disease Control and Prevention/Infectious Diseases Society of America: Treatment of tuberculosis. Am J Respir Crit Care Med 2003;167:603.

Bochner BS et al: Anaphylaxis. N Engl J Med 1991;324:1785.

Bratzler DW et al: Antimicrobial prophylaxis for surgery: An advisory statement from the National Surgical Infection Prevention Project. Clin Infect Dis 2004;38:1706.

Gonzales R et al: Principles of appropriate antibiotic use for treatment of acute respiratory tract infections in adults: Background, specific aims, and methods. Ann Intern Med 2001;134:479.

Guidelines for prevention and treatment of opportunistic infections in HIV-infected adults and adolescents. Recommendations of the National Institutes of Health (NIH), the Centers for Disease Control and Prevention (CDC), and the HIV Medicine Association of the Infectious Diseases Society of America (HIVMA/IDSA). AIDSinfo April 10, 2009. http://AIDSinfo.nih.gov

Jones RN, Pfaller MA: Bacterial resistance: A worldwide problem. Diagn Microbiol Infect Dis 1998;31:379.

Kaye KS, Kaye D: Antibacterial therapy and newer agents. Infect Dis Clin North Am 2009;23:757.

Mandell LA et al: Infectious Diseases Society of America/American Thoracic Society Consensus guidelines on the management of community-acquired pneumonia in adults. Clin Infect Dis 2007;44:S27.

Mazuski JE: Surgical infections. Surg Clin North Am 2009;89:295.

National Nosocomial Infections Surveillance (NNIS) System Report, Data Summary from January 1992–June 2004, issued October 2004. Am J Infect Control 2004;32:470.

Sexually transmitted diseases treatment guidelines 2006. Centers for Disease Control and Prevention. MMWR Morb Mortal Wkly Rep 2006;54(RR-11):1.

Tunkel AR et al: Practice guidelines for the management of bacterial meningitis. Clin Infect Dis 2004;39:1267.

Wilson W et al: Prevention of infective endocarditis: Guidelines from the American Heart Association. Circulation 2007;116:1736.

CASE STUDY ANSWER

The most likely diagnosis for this patient is *Streptococcus pneumoniae* meningitis, the most common bacterial cause of meningitis in adults. Other possible microbiologic etiologies include *Neisseria meningitidis, Listeria monocytogenes,* and enteric gram-negative bacilli. Intravenous antimicrobials to which local strains of these organisms are sensitive should be started while awaiting culture and sensitivity results. In addition, the use of dexamethasone has also been demonstrated to reduce mortality in adults with pneumococcal meningitis in conjunction with appropriate antimicrobial therapy.

Antiprotozoal Drugs

Philip J. Rosenthal, MD

CASE STUDY

A 5-year-old American girl presents with a 1-week history of intermittent chills, fever, and sweats. She had returned home 2 weeks earlier after leaving the United States for the first time to spend 3 weeks with her grandparents in Nigeria. She received all standard childhood immunizations, but no additional treatment before travel, since her parents have returned to their native Nigeria frequently without medical consequences. Three days ago, the child was seen in an outpatient clinic and diagnosed with a viral syndrome. Examination reveals a lethargic child, with a temperature of 39.8°C (103.6°F) and splenomegaly. She has no skin rash or lymphadenopathy. Initial laboratory studies are remarkable for hematocrit 29.8%, platelets 45,000/mm^3, creatinine 2.5 mg/dL (220 μmol/L), and mildly elevated bilirubin and transaminases. A blood smear shows ring forms of *Plasmodium falciparum* at 1.5% parasitemia. What treatment should be started?

■ MALARIA

Malaria is the most important parasitic disease of humans and causes hundreds of millions of illnesses per year. Four species of plasmodium typically cause human malaria: *Plasmodium falciparum, P vivax, P malariae,* and *P ovale.* A fifth species, *P knowlesi,* is primarily a pathogen of monkeys, but has recently been recognized to cause illness, including severe disease, in humans in Asia. Although all of the latter species may cause significant illness, *P falciparum* is responsible for the majority of serious complications and deaths. Drug resistance is an important therapeutic problem, most notably with *P falciparum.*

PARASITE LIFE CYCLE

An anopheline mosquito inoculates plasmodium sporozoites to initiate human infection (Figure 52–1). Circulating sporozoites rapidly invade liver cells, and exoerythrocytic stage tissue schizonts mature in the liver. Merozoites are subsequently released from the liver and invade erythrocytes. Only erythrocytic parasites cause clinical illness. Repeated cycles of infection can lead to the infection of many erythrocytes and serious disease. Sexual stage gametocytes also develop in erythrocytes before being taken up by mosquitoes, where they develop into infective sporozoites.

In *P falciparum* and *P malariae* infection, only one cycle of liver cell invasion and multiplication occurs, and liver infection ceases spontaneously in less than 4 weeks. Thus, treatment that eliminates erythrocytic parasites will cure these infections. In *P vivax* and *P ovale* infections, a dormant hepatic stage, the hypnozoite, is not eradicated by most drugs, and subsequent relapses can therefore occur after therapy directed against erythrocytic parasites. Eradication of both erythrocytic and hepatic parasites is required to cure these infections and usually requires two or more drugs.

DRUG CLASSIFICATION

Several classes of antimalarial drugs are available (Table 52–1 and Figure 52–2). Drugs that eliminate developing or dormant liver forms are called **tissue schizonticides;** those that act on erythrocytic parasites are **blood schizonticides;** and those that kill sexual stages and prevent transmission to mosquitoes are **gametocides.** No single available agent can reliably effect a **radical cure,** ie, eliminate both hepatic and erythrocytic stages. Few available agents are **causal prophylactic drugs,** ie, capable of preventing erythrocytic infection. However, all effective chemoprophylactic agents kill erythrocytic parasites before they increase sufficiently in number to cause clinical disease.

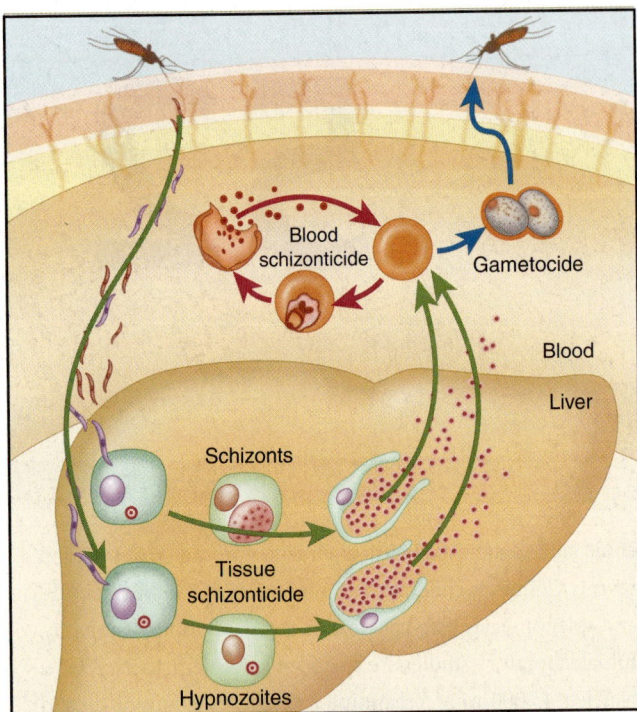

FIGURE 52–1 Life cycle of malaria parasites. Only the asexual erythrocytic stage of infection causes clinical malaria. All effective antimalarial treatments are blood schizonticides that kill this stage. (Reproduced, with permission, from Baird JK: Effectiveness of antimalarial drugs. N Engl J M 2005;352:1565.)

CHEMOPROPHYLAXIS & TREATMENT

When patients are counseled on the prevention of malaria, it is imperative to emphasize measures to prevent mosquito bites (eg, with insect repellents, insecticides, and bed nets), because parasites are increasingly resistant to multiple drugs and no chemoprophylactic regimen is fully protective. Current recommendations from the Centers for Disease Control and Prevention (CDC) include the use of chloroquine for chemoprophylaxis in the few areas infested by only chloroquine-sensitive malaria parasites (principally the Caribbean and Central America west of the Panama Canal), mefloquine or Malarone* for most other malarious areas, and doxycycline for areas with a very high prevalence of multidrug-resistant falciparum malaria (principally border areas of Thailand) (Table 52–2). CDC recommendations should be checked regularly (Phone: 770-488-7788; Internet: http://www.cdc.gov/malaria), because these may change in response to changing resistance patterns and increasing experience with new drugs. In some circumstances, it may be appropriate for travelers to carry supplies of drugs with them in case they develop a febrile illness when medical attention is unavailable. Regimens for self-treatment include new artemisinin-based combination therapies (see below),

which are widely available internationally (and, in the case of Coartem**, in the USA); Malarone; mefloquine; and quinine. Most authorities do not recommend routine terminal chemoprophylaxis with primaquine to eradicate dormant hepatic stages of *P vivax* and *P ovale* after travel, but this may be appropriate in some circumstances, especially for travelers with major exposure to these parasites.

Multiple drugs are available for the treatment of malaria that presents in the USA (Table 52–3). Most nonfalciparum infections and falciparum malaria from areas without known resistance should be treated with chloroquine. For vivax malaria from areas with suspected chloroquine resistance, including Indonesia and Papua New Guinea, other therapies effective against falciparum malaria may be used. Vivax and ovale malaria should subsequently be treated with primaquine to eradicate liver forms. Uncomplicated falciparum malaria from most areas is typically treated with Malarone or oral quinine, but new artemisinin-based combinations are increasingly the international standard of care, and one combination, Coartem, is now available in the USA. Other agents that are generally effective against resistant falciparum malaria include mefloquine and halofantrine, both of which have toxicity concerns at treatment dosages. Severe falciparum malaria is treated with intravenous artesunate, quinidine, or quinine (intravenous quinine is not available in the USA).

CHLOROQUINE

Chloroquine has been the drug of choice for both treatment and chemoprophylaxis of malaria since the 1940s, but its usefulness against *P falciparum* has been seriously compromised by drug resistance. It remains the drug of choice in the treatment of sensitive *P falciparum* and other species of human malaria parasites.

Chemistry & Pharmacokinetics

Chloroquine is a synthetic 4-aminoquinoline (Figure 52–2) formulated as the phosphate salt for oral use. It is rapidly and almost completely absorbed from the gastrointestinal tract, reaches maximum plasma concentrations in about 3 hours, and is rapidly distributed to the tissues. It has a very large apparent volume of distribution of 100–1000 L/kg and is slowly released from tissues and metabolized. Chloroquine is principally excreted in the urine with an initial half-life of 3–5 days but a much longer terminal elimination half-life of 1–2 months.

Antimalarial Action & Resistance

When not limited by resistance, chloroquine is a highly effective blood schizonticide. It is also moderately effective against gametocytes of *P vivax, P ovale,* and *P malariae* but not against those of *P falciparum.* Chloroquine is not active against liver stage parasites. Chloroquine probably acts by concentrating in parasite food

---

*Malarone is a proprietary formulation of atovaquone plus proguanil.

**Coartem is a proprietary formulation of artemether and lumefantrine.

TABLE 52–1 Major antimalarial drugs.

Drug	Class	Use
Chloroquine	4-Aminoquinoline	Treatment and chemoprophylaxis of infection with sensitive parasites
Amodiaquine[1]	4-Aminoquinoline	Treatment of infection with some chloroquine-resistant *P falciparum* strains and in fixed combination with artesunate
Piperaquine[1]	Bisquinoline	Treatment of *P falciparum* infection in fixed combination with dihydroartemisinin
Quinine	Quinoline methanol	Oral and intravenous[1] treatment of *P falciparum* infections
Quinidine	Quinoline methanol	Intravenous therapy of severe infections with *P falciparum*
Mefloquine	Quinoline methanol	Chemoprophylaxis and treatment of infections with *P falciparum*
Primaquine	8-Aminoquinoline	Radical cure and terminal prophylaxis of infections with *P vivax* and *P ovale*; alternative chemoprophylaxis for all species
Sulfadoxine-pyrimethamine (Fansidar)	Folate antagonist combination	Treatment of infections with some chloroquine-resistant *P falciparum*, including combination with artesunate; intermittent preventive therapy in endemic areas
Atovaquone-proguanil (Malarone)	Quinone-folate antagonist combination	Treatment and chemoprophylaxis of *P falciparum* infection
Doxycycline	Tetracycline	Treatment (with quinine) of infections with *P falciparum*; chemoprophylaxis
Halofantrine[1]	Phenanthrene methanol	Treatment of *P falciparum* infections
Lumefantrine[2]	Amyl alcohol	Treatment of *P falciparum* malaria in fixed combination with artemether (Coartem)
Artemisinins (artesunate, artemether,[2] dihydro-artemisinin[1])	Sesquiterpene lactone endoperoxides	Treatment of *P falciparum* infections; oral combination therapies for uncomplicated disease; intravenous artesunate for severe disease

[1]Not available in the USA.

[2]Available in the USA only as the fixed combination Coartem.

vacuoles, preventing the biocrystallization of the hemoglobin breakdown product, heme, into hemozoin, and thus eliciting parasite toxicity due to the buildup of free heme.

Resistance to chloroquine is now very common among strains of *P falciparum* and uncommon but increasing for *P vivax*. In *P falciparum*, mutations in a putative transporter, PfCRT, have been correlated with resistance. Chloroquine resistance can be reversed by certain agents, including verapamil, desipramine, and chlorpheniramine, but the clinical value of resistance-reversing drugs is not established.

Clinical Uses

A. Treatment

Chloroquine is the drug of choice in the treatment of nonfalciparum and sensitive falciparum malaria. It rapidly terminates fever (in 24–48 hours) and clears parasitemia (in 48–72 hours) caused by sensitive parasites. It is still used to treat falciparum malaria in some areas with widespread resistance, in particular much of Africa, owing to its safety, low cost, antipyretic properties, and partial activity, but continued use of chloroquine for this purpose is discouraged, especially in nonimmune individuals. Chloroquine has been replaced by other drugs, principally artemisinin-based combination therapies, as the standard therapy to treat falciparum malaria in most endemic countries.

Chloroquine does not eliminate dormant liver forms of *P vivax* and *P ovale*, and for that reason primaquine must be added for the radical cure of these species.

B. Chemoprophylaxis

Chloroquine is the preferred chemoprophylactic agent in malarious regions without resistant falciparum malaria. Eradication of *P vivax* and *P ovale* requires a course of primaquine to clear hepatic stages.

C. Amebic Liver Abscess

Chloroquine reaches high liver concentrations and may be used for amebic abscesses that fail initial therapy with metronidazole (see below).

Adverse Effects

Chloroquine is usually very well tolerated, even with prolonged use. Pruritus is common, primarily in Africans. Nausea, vomiting, abdominal pain, headache, anorexia, malaise, blurring of vision, and urticaria are uncommon. Dosing after meals may reduce some adverse effects. Rare reactions include hemolysis in glucose-6-phosphate dehydrogenase (G6PD)-deficient persons, impaired hearing, confusion, psychosis, seizures, agranulocytosis, exfoliative dermatitis, alopecia, bleaching of hair, hypotension,

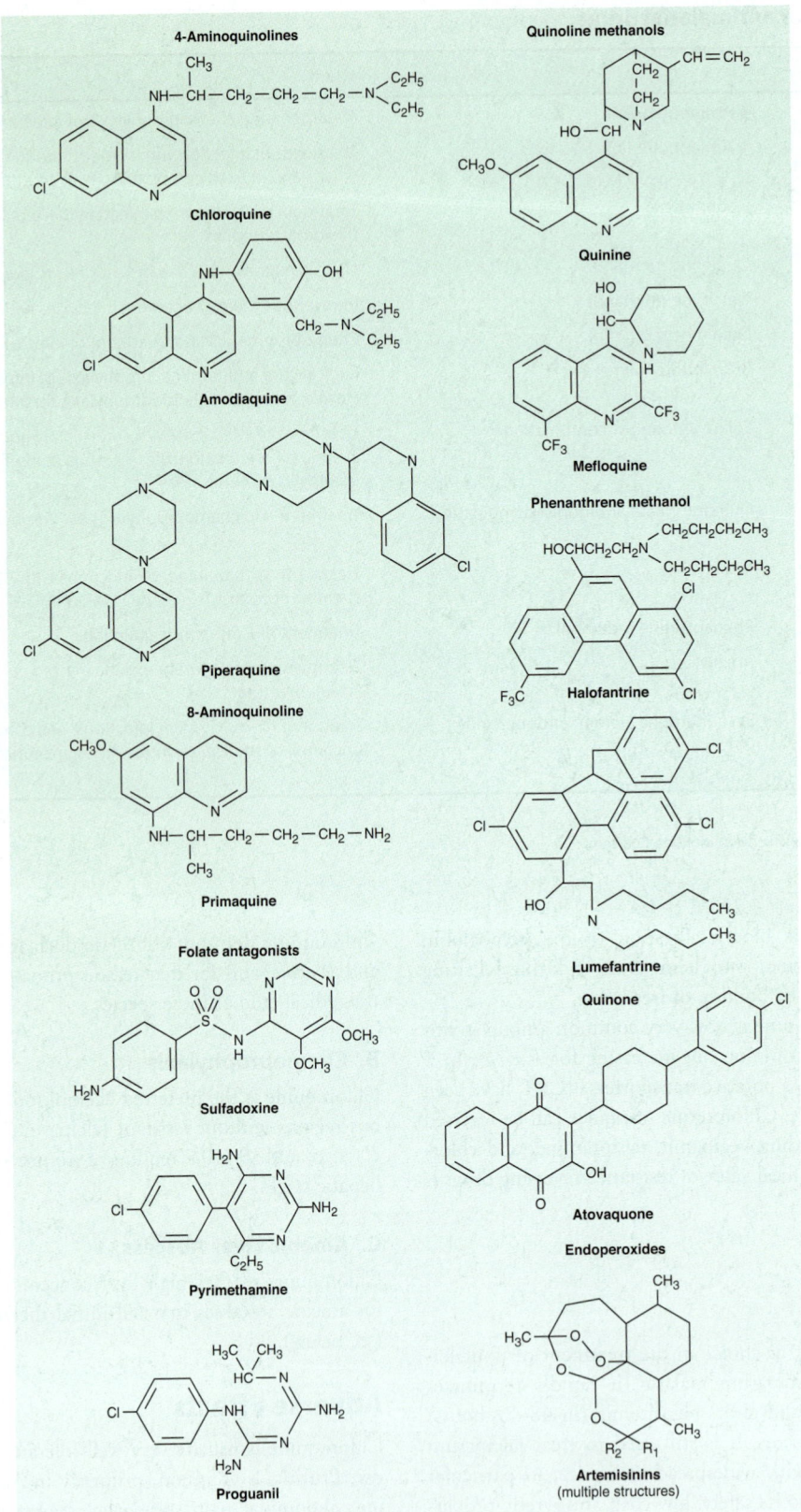

FIGURE 52–2 Structural formulas of antimalarial drugs.

TABLE 52–2 Drugs for the prevention of malaria in travelers.[1]

Drug	Use[2]	Adult Dosage[3]
Chloroquine	Areas without resistant *P falciparum*	500 mg weekly
Malarone	Areas with chloroquine-resistant *P falciparum*	1 tablet (250 mg atovaquone/100 mg proguanil) daily
Mefloquine	Areas with chloroquine-resistant *P falciparum*	250 mg weekly
Doxycycline	Areas with multidrug-resistant *P falciparum*	100 mg daily
Primaquine[4]	Terminal prophylaxis of *P vivax* and *P ovale* infections; alternative for primary prevention	52.6 mg (30 mg base) daily for 14 days after travel; for primary prevention 52.6 mg (30 mg base) daily

[1]Recommendations may change, as resistance to all available drugs is increasing. See text for additional information on toxicities and cautions. For additional details and pediatric dosing, see CDC guidelines (phone: 877-FYI-TRIP; http://www.cdc.gov). Travelers to remote areas should consider carrying effective therapy (see text) for use if they develop a febrile illness and cannot reach medical attention quickly.

[2]Areas without known chloroquine-resistant *P falciparum* are Central America west of the Panama Canal, Haiti, Dominican Republic, Egypt, and most malarious countries of the Middle East. Malarone or mefloquine are currently recommended for other malarious areas except for border areas of Thailand, where doxycycline is recommended.

[3]For drugs other than primaquine, begin 1–2 weeks before departure (except 2 days before for doxycycline and Malarone) and continue for 4 weeks after leaving the endemic area (except 1 week for Malarone). All dosages refer to salts.

[4]Screen for glucose-6-phosphate dehydrogenase (G6PD) deficiency before using primaquine.

TABLE 52–3 Treatment of malaria.

Clinical Setting	Drug Therapy[1]	Alternative Drugs
Chloroquine-sensitive *P falciparum* and *P malariae* infections	Chloroquine phosphate, 1 g, followed by 500 mg at 6, 24, and 48 hours *or* Chloroquine phosphate, 1 g at 0 and 24 hours, then 0.5 g at 48 hours	
P vivax and *P ovale* infections	Chloroquine (as above), then (if G6PD normal) primaquine, 52.6 (30 mg base) for 14 days	For infections from Indonesia, Papua New Guinea, and other areas with suspected resistance: therapies listed for uncomplicated chloroquine-resistant *P falciparum* plus primaquine
Uncomplicated infections with chloroquine-resistant *P falciparum*	Coartem (artemether, 20 mg, plus lumefantrine, 120 mg), four tablets twice daily for 3 days	Malarone, four tablets (total of 1 g atovaquone, 400 mg proguanil) daily for 3 days *or* Mefloquine, 15 mg/kg once or 750 mg, then 500 mg in 6–8 hours *or* Quinine sulfate, 650 mg 3 times daily for 3 days, plus doxycycline, 100 mg twice daily for 7 days, or clindamycin, 600 mg twice daily for 7 days *or* Other artemisinin-based combination regimens (see Table 52–4)
Severe or complicated infections with *P falciparum*	Artesunate,[2] 2.4 mg/kg IV, every 12 hours for 1 day, then daily for 2 additional days; follow with 7-day oral course of doxycycline or clindamycin or full treatment course of Coartem, Malarone, or mefloquine *or* Quinidine gluconate,[4,5] 10 mg/kg IV over 1–2 hours, then 0.02 mg/kg IV/min *or* Quinidine gluconate[4,5] 15 mg/kg IV over 4 hours, then 7.5 mg/kg IV over 4 hours every 8 hours	Artemether,[3] 3.2 mg/kg IM, then 1.6 mg/kg/d IM; follow with oral therapy as for artesunate *or* Quinine dihydrochloride,[3–5] 20 mg/kg IV, then 10 mg/kg every 8 hours

[1]All dosages are oral and refer to salts unless otherwise indicated. See text for additional information on all agents, including toxicities and cautions. See CDC guidelines (phone: 770-488-7788; http://www.cdc.gov) for additional information and pediatric dosing.

[2]Available in the United States only on an investigational basis through the CDC (phone: 770-488-7788).

[3]Not available in the USA.

[4]Cardiac monitoring should be in place during intravenous administration of intravenous quinidine or quinine. Change to an oral regimen as soon as the patient can tolerate it.

[5]Avoid loading doses in persons who have received quinine, quinidine, or mefloquine in the prior 24 hours.

G6PD, glucose-6-phosphate dehydrogenase.

and electrocardiographic changes (QRS widening, T-wave abnormalities). The long-term administration of high doses of chloroquine for rheumatologic diseases (see Chapter 36) can result in irreversible ototoxicity, retinopathy, myopathy, and peripheral neuropathy. These abnormalities are rarely if ever seen with standard-dose weekly chemoprophylaxis, even when given for prolonged periods. Large intramuscular injections or rapid intravenous infusions of chloroquine hydrochloride can result in severe hypotension and respiratory and cardiac arrest. Parenteral administration of chloroquine is best avoided, but if other drugs are not available for parenteral use, it should be infused slowly.

Contraindications & Cautions

Chloroquine is contraindicated in patients with psoriasis or porphyria, in whom it may precipitate acute attacks of these diseases. It should generally not be used in those with retinal or visual field abnormalities or myopathy. Chloroquine should be used with caution in patients with a history of liver disease or neurologic or hematologic disorders. The antidiarrheal agent kaolin and calcium- and magnesium-containing antacids interfere with the absorption of chloroquine and should not be co-administered with the drug. Chloroquine is considered safe in pregnancy and for young children.

OTHER QUINOLINES

Amodiaquine is closely related to chloroquine, and it probably shares mechanisms of action and resistance with that drug. Amodiaquine has been widely used to treat malaria because of its low cost, limited toxicity, and, in some areas, effectiveness against chloroquine-resistant strains of *P falciparum*. Reports of toxicities of amodiaquine, including agranulocytosis, aplastic anemia, and hepatotoxicity, have limited use of the drug in recent years. However, recent reevaluation has shown that serious toxicity from amodiaquine is rare, and it may be used as a replacement for chloroquine in areas with high rates of resistance but limited resources. The most important current use of amodiaquine is in combination therapy. The World Health Organization (WHO) lists amodiaquine plus artesunate as a recommended therapy for falciparum malaria in areas with resistance to older drugs (Table 52–4). This combination is now available as a single tablet (ASAQ, Arsucam, Coarsucam) and is the first-line therapy for the treatment of uncomplicated falciparum malaria in many countries in Africa. Another combination, amodiaquine plus sulfadoxine-pyrimethamine, remains reasonably effective for the treatment of falciparum malaria in many areas with some resistance to the individual drugs, and it is a preferred alternative treatment if artemisinin-containing therapies are unavailable. Chemoprophylaxis with amodiaquine is best avoided because of its apparent increased toxicity with long-term use.

Piperaquine is a bisquinoline that was used widely to treat chloroquine-resistant falciparum malaria in China in the 1970s through the 1980s, but its use waned after resistance became widespread. Recently, piperaquine has been combined with

TABLE 52–4 WHO recommendations for the treatment of falciparum malaria.

Regimen	Notes
Artemether-lumefantrine (Coartem, Riamet)	Co-formulated; first-line therapy in many countries; approved in the USA
Artesunate-amodiaquine (ASAQ, Arsucam, Coarsucam)	Co-formulated; first-line therapy in many African countries
Artesunate-mefloquine	Co-formulated; first-line therapy in parts of Southeast Asia and South America
Dihydroartemisinin-piperaquine (Artekin, Duocotecxin)	Co-formulated; first-line therapy in some countries in Southeast Asia
Artesunate-sulfadoxine-pyrimethamine	First-line therapy in some countries, but efficacy lower than other regimens in most areas

World Health Organization: Guidelines for the Treatment of Malaria. World Health Organization. Geneva, 2010.

dihydroartemisinin in co-formulated tablets (Artekin, Duocotecxin) that have shown excellent efficacy and safety for the treatment of falciparum malaria, without apparent drug resistance. Piperaquine has a longer half-life (~ 28 days) than amodiaquine (~ 14 days), mefloquine (~ 14 days), or lumefantrine (~ 4 days), leading to a longer period of post-treatment prophylaxis with dihydroartemisinin-piperaquine than with the other leading artemisinin-based combinations; this feature should be particularly advantageous in high transmission areas. Dihydroartemisinin-piperaquine is now the first-line therapy for the treatment of uncomplicated malaria in Vietnam.

ARTEMISININ & ITS DERIVATIVES

Artemisinin (**qinghaosu**) is a sesquiterpene lactone endoperoxide (Figure 52–2), the active component of an herbal medicine that has been used as an antipyretic in China for over 2000 years. Artemisinin is insoluble and can only be used orally. Analogs have been synthesized to increase solubility and improve antimalarial efficacy. The most important of these analogs are **artesunate** (water-soluble; useful for oral, intravenous, intramuscular, and rectal administration), **artemether** (lipid-soluble; useful for oral, intramuscular, and rectal administration), and **dihydroartemisinin** (water-soluble; useful for oral administration).

Chemistry & Pharmacokinetics

Artemisinin and its analogs are rapidly absorbed, with peak plasma levels occurring in 1–2 hours and half-lives of 1–3 hours after oral administration. Artemisinin, artesunate, and artemether are rapidly metabolized to the active metabolite dihydroartemisinin. Drug levels appear to decrease after a number of days of therapy.

Antimalarial Action & Resistance

The artemisinins are now widely available around the world. However, artemisinin monotherapy for the treatment of uncomplicated malaria is now strongly discouraged. Rather, co-formulated artemisinin-based combination therapies are recommended to improve efficacy and prevent the selection of artemisinin-resistant parasites. The oral combination regimen Coartem (artemether-lumefantrine) was approved by the Food and Drug Administration (FDA) in 2009, and may be considered the new first-line therapy in the USA for uncomplicated falciparum malaria, although the drug may not be widely available. Intravenous artesunate was made available by the CDC in 2007; use of the drug can be initiated by contact with the CDC, which will release the drug for appropriate indications (falciparum malaria with signs of severe disease or inability to take oral medications) from stocks stored around the USA.

Artemisinin and its analogs are very rapidly acting blood schizonticides against all human malaria parasites. Artemisinins have no effect on hepatic stages. The antimalarial activity of artemisinins may result from the production of free radicals that follows the iron-catalyzed cleavage of the artemisinin endoperoxide bridge in the parasite food vacuole or from inhibition of a parasite calcium ATPase. Artemisinin resistance is not yet an important problem, but *P falciparum* isolates with diminished in vitro susceptibility to artemether have recently been described. In addition, increasing rates of treatment failure and increases in parasite clearance times after use of artesunate or artesunate-mefloquine in parts of Cambodia may be early signs of a worrisome decrease in artesunate efficacy.

Clinical Uses

Artemisinin-based combination therapy is now the standard for treatment of uncomplicated falciparum malaria in nearly all areas endemic for falciparum malaria. These regimens were developed because the short plasma half-lives of the artemisinins led to unacceptably high recrudescence rates after short-course therapy, which were reversed by inclusion of longer-acting drugs. Combination therapy also helps to protect against the selection of artemisinin resistance. However, with completion of dosing after 3 days, the artemisinin components are rapidly eliminated, and so selection of resistance to partner drugs is of concern.

The WHO recommends five artemisinin-based combinations for the treatment of uncomplicated falciparum malaria (Table 52–4). One of these, artesunate-sulfadoxine-pyrimethamine is not recommended in many areas owing to unacceptable levels of resistance to sulfadoxine-pyrimethamine, but it is the first-line therapy in some countries in Asia, South America, and North Africa. The other four recommended regimens are now all available as combination formulations, although manufacturing standards may vary. Artesunate-mefloquine is highly effective in Southeast Asia, where resistance to many antimalarials is common; it is the first-line therapy in some countries in Southeast Asia and South America. This regimen is less practical for other areas, particularly Africa, because of its relatively high cost and poor tolerability. Either artesunate-amodiaquine or artemether-lumefantrine is now the standard treatment for uncomplicated falciparum malaria in most countries in Africa and some additional endemic countries on other continents. Dihydroartemisinin-piperaquine is a newer regimen that has shown excellent efficacy; it is the first-line therapy for falciparum malaria in Vietnam.

The relative efficacy and safety of artemisinin-based combination therapies are now under active investigation. In general, the leading regimens are highly efficacious, safe, and well tolerated, and they are the new standard of care for the treatment of uncomplicated falciparum malaria.

Artemisinins are also proving to have outstanding efficacy in the treatment of complicated falciparum malaria. Large randomized trials and meta-analyses have shown that intramuscular artemether has an efficacy equivalent to that of quinine and that intravenous artesunate is superior to intravenous quinine in terms of parasite clearance time and—most important—patient survival. Intravenous artesunate also has a superior side-effect profile compared with that of intravenous quinine or quinidine. Thus, intravenous artesunate will likely replace quinine as the standard of care for the treatment of severe falciparum malaria, although it is not yet widely available in most areas. Artesunate and artemether have also been effective in the treatment of severe malaria when administered rectally, offering a valuable treatment modality when parenteral therapy is not available.

Adverse Effects & Cautions

Artemisinins are generally very well tolerated. The most commonly reported adverse effects are nausea, vomiting, diarrhea, and dizziness, and these may often be due to underlying malaria rather than the medications. Rare serious toxicities include neutropenia, anemia, hemolysis, elevated liver enzymes, and allergic reactions. Irreversible neurotoxicity has been seen in animals, but only after doses much higher than those used to treat malaria. Artemisinins have been embryotoxic in animal studies, but rates of congenital abnormalities, stillbirths, and abortions were not elevated, compared with those of controls, in women who received artemisinins during pregnancy. Based on this information and the significant risk of malaria during pregnancy, the WHO recommends artemisinin-based combination therapies for the treatment of uncomplicated falciparum malaria during the second and third trimesters of pregnancy, intravenous artesunate or quinine for the treatment of severe malaria during the first trimester, and intravenous artesunate for treatment of severe malaria during the second and third trimesters.

QUININE & QUINIDINE

Quinine and quinidine remain important therapies for falciparum malaria—especially severe disease—although toxicity may complicate therapy. Resistance to quinine is uncommon but may be increasing.

Chemistry & Pharmacokinetics

Quinine is derived from the bark of the cinchona tree, a traditional remedy for intermittent fevers from South America. The alkaloid quinine was purified from the bark in 1820, and it has been used in the treatment and prevention of malaria since that time. Quinidine, the dextrorotatory stereoisomer of quinine, is at least as effective as parenteral quinine in the treatment of severe falciparum malaria. After oral administration, quinine is rapidly absorbed, reaches peak plasma levels in 1–3 hours, and is widely distributed in body tissues. The use of a loading dose in severe malaria allows the achievement of peak levels within a few hours. The pharmacokinetics of quinine varies among populations. Individuals with malaria develop higher plasma levels of the drug than healthy controls, but toxicity is not increased, apparently because of increased protein binding. The half-life of quinine also is longer in those with severe malaria (18 hours) than in healthy controls (11 hours). Quinidine has a shorter half-life than quinine, mostly as a result of decreased protein binding. Quinine is primarily metabolized in the liver and excreted in the urine.

Antimalarial Action & Resistance

Quinine is a rapid-acting, highly effective blood schizonticide against the four species of human malaria parasites. The drug is gametocidal against *P vivax* and *P ovale* but not *P falciparum*. It is not active against liver stage parasites. The mechanism of action of quinine is unknown.

Increasing in vitro resistance of parasites from a number of areas suggests that quinine resistance will be an increasing problem. Resistance to quinine is already common in some areas of Southeast Asia, especially border areas of Thailand, where the drug may fail if used alone to treat falciparum malaria. However, quinine still provides at least a partial therapeutic effect in most patients.

Clinical Uses

A. Parenteral Treatment of Severe Falciparum Malaria

For many years, quinine dihydrochloride or quinidine gluconate have been the treatments of choice for severe falciparum malaria, although intravenous artesunate now provides an alternative for this indication. Quinine can be administered slowly intravenously or, in a dilute solution, intramuscularly, but parenteral preparations of this drug are not available in the USA. Quinidine has been the standard therapy in the USA for the parenteral treatment of severe falciparum malaria. The drug can be administered in divided doses or by continuous intravenous infusion; treatment should begin with a loading dose to rapidly achieve effective plasma concentrations. Because of its cardiac toxicity and the relative unpredictability of its pharmacokinetics, intravenous quinidine should be administered slowly with cardiac monitoring. Therapy should be changed to an effective oral agent as soon as the patient has improved and can tolerate oral medications.

B. Oral Treatment of Falciparum Malaria

Quinine sulfate is appropriate therapy for uncomplicated falciparum malaria except when the infection was transmitted in an area without documented chloroquine-resistant malaria. Quinine is commonly used with a second drug (most often doxycycline or, in children, clindamycin) to shorten quinine's duration of use (usually to 3 days) and limit toxicity. Quinine is less effective than chloroquine against other human malarias and is more toxic. Therefore, it is not used to treat infections with these parasites.

C. Malarial Chemoprophylaxis

Quinine is not generally used in chemoprophylaxis owing to its toxicity, although a daily dose of 325 mg is effective.

D. Babesiosis

Quinine is first-line therapy, in combination with clindamycin, in the treatment of infection with *Babesia microti* or other human babesial infections.

Adverse Effects

Therapeutic dosages of quinine and quinidine commonly cause tinnitus, headache, nausea, dizziness, flushing, and visual disturbances, a constellation of symptoms termed **cinchonism.** Mild symptoms of cinchonism do not warrant the discontinuation of therapy. More severe findings, often after prolonged therapy, include more marked visual and auditory abnormalities, vomiting, diarrhea, and abdominal pain. Hypersensitivity reactions include skin rashes, urticaria, angioedema, and bronchospasm. Hematologic abnormalities include hemolysis (especially with G6PD deficiency), leukopenia, agranulocytosis, and thrombocytopenia. Therapeutic doses may cause hypoglycemia through stimulation of insulin release; this is a particular problem in severe infections and in pregnant patients, who have increased sensitivity to insulin. Quinine can stimulate uterine contractions, especially in the third trimester. However, this effect is mild, and quinine and quinidine remain drugs of choice for severe falciparum malaria even during pregnancy. Intravenous infusions of the drugs may cause thrombophlebitis.

Severe hypotension can follow too-rapid intravenous infusions of quinine or quinidine. Electrocardiographic abnormalities (QT interval prolongation) are fairly common with intravenous quinidine, but dangerous arrhythmias are uncommon when the drug is administered appropriately in a monitored setting.

Blackwater fever is a rare severe illness that includes marked hemolysis and hemoglobinuria in the setting of quinine therapy for malaria. It appears to be due to a hypersensitivity reaction to the drug, although its pathogenesis is uncertain.

Contraindications & Cautions

Quinine (or quinidine) should be discontinued if signs of severe cinchonism, hemolysis, or hypersensitivity occur. It should be avoided if possible in patients with underlying visual or auditory problems. It must be used with great caution in those with underlying cardiac abnormalities. Quinine should not be given concurrently with mefloquine and should be used with caution in a patient with malaria who has previously received mefloquine chemoprophylaxis. Absorption may be blocked by aluminum-containing antacids. Quinine can raise plasma levels of warfarin and digoxin. Dosage must be reduced in renal insufficiency.

MEFLOQUINE

Mefloquine is effective therapy for many chloroquine-resistant strains of *P falciparum* and against other species. Although toxicity is a concern, mefloquine is one of the recommended chemoprophylactic drugs for use in most malaria-endemic regions with chloroquine-resistant strains.

Chemistry & Pharmacokinetics

Mefloquine hydrochloride is a synthetic 4-quinoline methanol that is chemically related to quinine. It can only be given orally because severe local irritation occurs with parenteral use. It is well absorbed, and peak plasma concentrations are reached in about 18 hours. Mefloquine is highly protein-bound, extensively distributed in tissues, and eliminated slowly, allowing a single-dose treatment regimen. The terminal elimination half-life is about 20 days, allowing weekly dosing for chemoprophylaxis. With weekly dosing, steady-state drug levels are reached over a number of weeks; this interval can be shortened to 4 days by beginning a course with three consecutive daily doses of 250 mg, although this is not standard practice. Mefloquine and acid metabolites of the drug are slowly excreted, mainly in the feces. The drug can be detected in the blood for months after the completion of therapy.

Antimalarial Action & Resistance

Mefloquine has strong blood schizonticidal activity against *P falciparum* and *P vivax*, but it is not active against hepatic stages or gametocytes. The mechanism of action of mefloquine is unknown. Sporadic resistance to mefloquine has been reported from many areas. At present, resistance appears to be uncommon except in regions of Southeast Asia with high rates of multidrug resistance (especially border areas of Thailand). Mefloquine resistance appears to be associated with resistance to quinine and halofantrine but not with resistance to chloroquine.

Clinical Uses

A. Chemoprophylaxis

Mefloquine is effective in prophylaxis against most strains of *P falciparum* and probably all other human malarial species. Mefloquine is therefore among the drugs recommended by the CDC for chemoprophylaxis in all malarious areas except for those with no chloroquine resistance (where chloroquine is preferred) and some rural areas of Southeast Asia with a high prevalence of mefloquine resistance. As with chloroquine, eradication of *P vivax* and *P ovale* requires a course of primaquine.

B. Treatment

Mefloquine is effective in treating most falciparum malaria. The drug is not appropriate for treating individuals with severe or complicated malaria, since quinine, quinidine, and artemisinins are more rapidly active, and since drug resistance is less likely with those agents. The combination of artesunate plus mefloquine showed excellent antimalarial efficacy in regions of Southeast Asia with some resistance to mefloquine, and this regimen is now one of the combination therapies recommended by the WHO for the treatment of uncomplicated falciparum malaria (Table 52–4). Artesunate-mefloquine is the first-line therapy for uncomplicated malaria in a number of countries in Asia and South America.

Adverse Effects

Weekly dosing with mefloquine for chemoprophylaxis may cause nausea, vomiting, dizziness, sleep and behavioral disturbances, epigastric pain, diarrhea, abdominal pain, headache, rash, and dizziness. Neuropsychiatric toxicities have received a good deal of publicity, but despite frequent anecdotal reports of seizures and psychosis, a number of controlled studies have found the frequency of serious adverse effects from mefloquine to be no higher than that with other common antimalarial chemoprophylactic regimens. Leukocytosis, thrombocytopenia, and aminotransferase elevations have been reported.

The latter adverse effects are more common with the higher dosages required for treatment. These effects may be lessened by administering the drug in two doses separated by 6–8 hours. The incidence of neuropsychiatric symptoms appears to be about ten times more common than with chemoprophylactic dosing, with widely varying frequencies of up to about 50% being reported. Serious neuropsychiatric toxicities (depression, confusion, acute psychosis, or seizures) have been reported in less than 1 in 1000 treatments, but some authorities believe that these toxicities are actually more common. Mefloquine can also alter cardiac conduction, and arrhythmias and bradycardia have been reported.

Contraindications & Cautions

Mefloquine is contraindicated in a patient with a history of epilepsy, psychiatric disorders, arrhythmia, cardiac conduction defects, or sensitivity to related drugs. It should not be co-administered with quinine, quinidine, or halofantrine, and caution is required if quinine or quinidine is used to treat malaria after mefloquine chemoprophylaxis. Theoretical risks of mefloquine must be balanced with the risk of contracting falciparum malaria. The CDC no longer advises against mefloquine use in patients receiving β-adrenoceptor antagonists. Mefloquine is also now considered safe in young children. Available data suggest that mefloquine is safe throughout pregnancy, although experience in the first trimester is limited. An older recommendation to avoid mefloquine use in those requiring fine motor skills (eg, airline pilots) is controversial. Mefloquine chemoprophylaxis should be discontinued if significant neuropsychiatric symptoms develop.

PRIMAQUINE

Primaquine is the drug of choice for the eradication of dormant liver forms of *P vivax* and *P ovale* and can also be used for chemoprophylaxis against all malarial species.

Chemistry & Pharmacokinetics

Primaquine phosphate is a synthetic 8-aminoquinoline (Figure 52–2). The drug is well absorbed orally, reaching peak plasma levels in

1–2 hours. The plasma half-life is 3–8 hours. Primaquine is widely distributed to the tissues, but only a small amount is bound there. It is rapidly metabolized and excreted in the urine. Its three major metabolites appear to have less antimalarial activity but more potential for inducing hemolysis than the parent compound.

Antimalarial Action & Resistance

Primaquine is active against hepatic stages of all human malaria parasites. It is the only available agent active against the dormant hypnozoite stages of *P vivax* and *P ovale*. Primaquine is also gametocidal against the four human malaria species. Primaquine acts against erythrocytic stage parasites, but this activity is too weak to play an important role. The mechanism of antimalarial action is unknown.

Some strains of *P vivax* in New Guinea, Southeast Asia, Central and South America, and other areas are relatively resistant to primaquine. Liver forms of these strains may not be eradicated by a single standard treatment with primaquine and may require repeated therapy. Because of decreasing efficacy, the standard dosage of primaquine for radical cure of *P vivax* infection was recently doubled to 30 mg base daily for 14 days.

Clinical Uses

A. Therapy (Radical Cure) of Acute Vivax and Ovale Malaria

Standard therapy for these infections includes chloroquine to eradicate erythrocytic forms and primaquine to eradicate liver hypnozoites and prevent a subsequent relapse. Chloroquine is given acutely, and therapy with primaquine is withheld until the G6PD status of the patient is known. If the G6PD level is normal, a 14-day course of primaquine is given. Prompt evaluation of the G6PD level is helpful, since primaquine appears to be most effective when instituted before completion of dosing with chloroquine.

B. Terminal Prophylaxis of Vivax and Ovale Malaria

Standard chemoprophylaxis does not prevent a relapse of vivax or ovale malaria, because the hypnozoite forms of these parasites are not eradicated by chloroquine or other available blood schizonticide agents. To markedly diminish the likelihood of relapse, some authorities advocate the use of primaquine after the completion of travel to an endemic area.

C. Chemoprophylaxis of Malaria

Primaquine has been studied as a daily chemoprophylactic agent. Daily treatment with 30 mg (0.5 mg/kg) of base provided good levels of protection against falciparum and vivax malaria. However, potential toxicities of long-term use remain a concern, and primaquine is generally recommended for this purpose only when mefloquine, Malarone, and doxycycline cannot be used.

D. Gametocidal Action

A single dose of primaquine (45 mg base) can be used as a control measure to render *P falciparum* gametocytes noninfective to mosquitoes. This therapy is of no clinical benefit to the patient but will disrupt transmission.

E. *Pneumocystis jiroveci* Infection

The combination of clindamycin and primaquine is an alternative regimen in the treatment of pneumocystosis, particularly mild to moderate disease. This regimen offers improved tolerance compared with high-dose trimethoprim-sulfamethoxazole or pentamidine, although its efficacy against severe pneumocystis pneumonia is not well studied.

Adverse Effects

Primaquine in recommended doses is generally well tolerated. It infrequently causes nausea, epigastric pain, abdominal cramps, and headache, and these symptoms are more common with higher dosages and when the drug is taken on an empty stomach. More serious but rare adverse effects are leukopenia, agranulocytosis, leukocytosis, and cardiac arrhythmias. Standard doses of primaquine may cause hemolysis or methemoglobinemia (manifested by cyanosis), especially in persons with G6PD deficiency or other hereditary metabolic defects.

Contraindications & Cautions

Primaquine should be avoided in patients with a history of granulocytopenia or methemoglobinemia, in those receiving potentially myelosuppressive drugs (eg, quinidine), and in those with disorders that commonly include myelosuppression. It is never given parenterally because it may induce marked hypotension.

Patients should be tested for G6PD deficiency before primaquine is prescribed. When a patient is deficient in G6PD, treatment strategies may consist of withholding therapy and treating subsequent relapses, if they occur, with chloroquine; treating patients with standard dosing, paying close attention to their hematologic status; or treating with weekly primaquine (45 mg base) for 8 weeks. G6PD-deficient individuals of Mediterranean and Asian ancestry are most likely to have severe deficiency, whereas those of African ancestry usually have a milder biochemical defect. This difference can be taken into consideration in choosing a treatment strategy. In any event, primaquine should be discontinued if there is evidence of hemolysis or anemia. Primaquine should be avoided in pregnancy because the fetus is relatively G6PD-deficient and thus at risk of hemolysis.

ATOVAQUONE

Atovaquone, a hydroxynaphthoquinone (Figure 52–2), was initially developed as an antimalarial agent, and as a component of **Malarone** is recommended for treatment and prevention of malaria. Atovaquone has also been approved by the FDA for the treatment of mild to moderate *P jiroveci* pneumonia.

The drug is only administered orally. Its bioavailability is low and erratic, but absorption is increased by fatty food. The drug is heavily protein-bound and has a half-life of 2–3 days. Most of the drug is eliminated unchanged in the feces. Atovaquone acts against plasmodia by disrupting mitochondrial electron transport. It is active against tissue and erythrocytic schizonts, allowing chemoprophylaxis to be discontinued only 1 week after the end of exposure (compared with 4 weeks for mefloquine or doxycycline, which lack activity against tissue schizonts).

Initial use of atovaquone to treat malaria led to disappointing results, with frequent failures, apparently due to the selection of resistant parasites during therapy. In contrast, Malarone, a fixed combination of atovaquone (250 mg) and proguanil (100 mg), is highly effective for both the treatment and chemoprophylaxis of falciparum malaria, and it is now approved for both indications in the USA. For chemoprophylaxis, Malarone must be taken daily (Table 52–2). It has an advantage over mefloquine and doxycycline in requiring shorter periods of treatment before and after the period at risk for malaria transmission, but it is more expensive than the other agents. It should be taken with food.

Atovaquone is an alternative therapy for *P jiroveci* infection, although its efficacy is lower than that of trimethoprim-sulfamethoxazole. Standard dosing is 750 mg taken with food twice daily for 21 days. Adverse effects include fever, rash, nausea, vomiting, diarrhea, headache, and insomnia. Serious adverse effects appear to be minimal, although experience with the drug remains limited. Atovaquone has also been effective in small numbers of immunocompromised patients with toxoplasmosis unresponsive to other agents, although its role in this disease is not yet defined.

Malarone is generally well tolerated. Adverse effects include abdominal pain, nausea, vomiting, diarrhea, headache, and rash, and these are more common with the higher dosage required for treatment. Reversible elevations in liver enzymes have been reported. The safety of atovaquone in pregnancy is unknown. Plasma concentrations of atovaquone are decreased about 50% by co-administration of tetracycline or rifampin.

INHIBITORS OF FOLATE SYNTHESIS

Inhibitors of enzymes involved in folate metabolism are used, generally in combination regimens, in the treatment and prevention of malaria.

Chemistry & Pharmacokinetics

Pyrimethamine is a 2,4-diaminopyrimidine related to trimethoprim (see Chapter 46). **Proguanil** is a biguanide derivative (Figure 52–2). Both drugs are slowly but adequately absorbed from the gastrointestinal tract. Pyrimethamine reaches peak plasma levels 2–6 hours after an oral dose, is bound to plasma proteins, and has an elimination half-life of about 3.5 days. Proguanil reaches peak plasma levels about 5 hours after an oral dose and has an elimination half-life of about 16 hours. Therefore, proguanil must be administered daily for chemoprophylaxis, whereas pyrimethamine can be given once a week. Pyrimethamine is extensively metabolized before excretion. Proguanil is a prodrug; only its triazine metabolite, cycloguanil, is active. **Fansidar,** a fixed combination of the sulfonamide **sulfadoxine** (500 mg per tablet) and **pyrimethamine** (25 mg per tablet), is well absorbed. Its components display peak plasma levels within 2–8 hours and are excreted mainly by the kidneys. The average half-life of sulfadoxine is about 170 hours.

Antimalarial Action & Resistance

Pyrimethamine and proguanil act slowly against erythrocytic forms of susceptible strains of all four human malaria species. Proguanil also has some activity against hepatic forms. Neither drug is adequately gametocidal or effective against the persistent liver stages of *P vivax* or *P ovale*. Sulfonamides and sulfones are weakly active against erythrocytic schizonts but not against liver stages or gametocytes. They are not used alone as antimalarials but are effective in combination with other agents.

The mechanism of action of pyrimethamine and proguanil involves selective inhibition of plasmodial dihydrofolate reductase, a key enzyme in the pathway for synthesis of folate. Sulfonamides and sulfones inhibit another enzyme in the folate pathway, dihydropteroate synthase. As described in Chapter 46 and shown in Figure 46–2, combinations of inhibitors of these two enzymes provide synergistic activity.

Resistance to folate antagonists and sulfonamides is common in many areas for *P falciparum* and less common for *P vivax*. Resistance is due primarily to mutations in dihydrofolate reductase and dihydropteroate synthase, with increasing numbers of mutations leading to increasing levels of resistance. At present, resistance seriously limits the efficacy of sulfadoxine-pyrimethamine (Fansidar) for the treatment of malaria in most areas, but in Africa most parasites exhibit an intermediate level of resistance, such that antifolates may continue to offer some preventive efficacy against malaria. Because different mutations may mediate resistance to different agents, cross-resistance is not uniformly seen.

Clinical Uses

A. Chemoprophylaxis

Chemoprophylaxis with single folate antagonists is no longer recommended because of frequent resistance, but a number of agents are used in combination regimens. The combination of chloroquine (500 mg weekly) and proguanil (200 mg daily) was previously widely used, but with increasing resistance to both agents it is no longer recommended. Fansidar and Maloprim (the latter is a combination of pyrimethamine and the sulfone dapsone) are both effective against sensitive parasites with weekly dosing, but they are no longer recommended because of resistance and toxicity. Considering protection of populations in endemic regions, trimethoprim-sulfamethoxazole, an antifolate combination that is more active against bacteria than malaria parasites, is increasingly used as a daily prophylactic therapy for HIV-infected patients in developing countries. Although it is administered primarily to prevent typical HIV opportunistic and bacterial infections, this regimen offers partial preventive efficacy against malaria in Africa.

B. Intermittent Preventive Therapy

A new strategy for malaria control is intermittent preventive therapy, in which high-risk patients receive intermittent treatment for malaria, regardless of their infection status, typically with Fansidar, which benefits from simple dosing and prolonged activity. Considering the two highest risk groups for severe malaria in

Africa, this strategy is best validated in pregnant women and is increasingly studied in young children. Typical schedules include single doses of Fansidar during the second and third trimesters of pregnancy and monthly doses whenever children present for scheduled immunizations or, in areas with seasonal malaria, monthly doses during the transmission season. However, optimal preventive dosing schedules have not been established.

C. Treatment of Chloroquine-Resistant Falciparum Malaria

Fansidar is commonly used to treat uncomplicated falciparum malaria and until recently it was a first-line therapy for this indication in some tropical countries. Advantages of Fansidar are ease of administration (a single oral dose) and low cost. However, rates of resistance are increasing, and Fansidar is no longer a recommended therapy. In particular, Fansidar should not be used for severe malaria, since it is slower-acting than other available agents. Fansidar is also not reliably effective in vivax malaria, and its usefulness against *P ovale* and *P malariae* has not been adequately studied. A new antifolate-sulfone combination, chlorproguanil-dapsone (Lapdap), was until recently available in some African countries for the treatment of uncomplicated falciparum malaria, and the combination of chlorproguanil-dapsone and artesunate (Dacart) was under development. However, this project was discontinued in 2008 as a result of concerns about hematologic toxicity in those with G6PD deficiency, and chlorproguanil-dapsone will no longer be marketed.

D. Toxoplasmosis

Pyrimethamine, in combination with sulfadiazine, is first-line therapy in the treatment of toxoplasmosis, including acute infection, congenital infection, and disease in immunocompromised patients. For immunocompromised patients, high-dose therapy is required followed by chronic suppressive therapy. Folinic acid is included to limit myelosuppression. Toxicity from the combination is usually due primarily to sulfadiazine. The replacement of sulfadiazine with clindamycin provides an effective alternative regimen.

E. Pneumocystosis

P jiroveci is the cause of human pneumocystosis and is now recognized to be a fungus, but this organism is discussed in this chapter because it responds to antiprotozoal drugs, not antifungals. (The related species *P carinii* is now recognized to be the cause of animal infections.) First-line therapy of pneumocystosis is trimethoprim plus sulfamethoxazole (see also Chapter 46). Standard treatment includes high-dose intravenous or oral therapy (15 mg trimethoprim and 75 mg sulfamethoxazole per day in three or four divided doses) for 21 days. High-dose therapy entails significant toxicity, especially in patients with AIDS. Important toxicities include nausea, vomiting, fever, rash, leukopenia, hyponatremia, elevated hepatic enzymes, azotemia, anemia, and thrombocytopenia. Less common effects include severe skin reactions, mental status changes, pancreatitis, and hypocalcemia. Trimethoprim-sulfamethoxazole is also the standard chemoprophylactic drug for

the prevention of *P jiroveci* infection in immunocompromised individuals. Dosing is one double-strength tablet daily or three times per week. The chemoprophylactic dosing schedule is much better tolerated than high-dose therapy in immunocompromised patients, but rash, fever, leukopenia, or hepatitis may necessitate changing to another drug.

Adverse Effects & Cautions

Most patients tolerate pyrimethamine and proguanil well. Gastrointestinal symptoms, skin rashes, and itching are rare. Mouth ulcers and alopecia have been described with proguanil. Fansidar is no longer recommended for chemoprophylaxis because of uncommon but severe cutaneous reactions, including erythema multiforme, Stevens-Johnson syndrome, and toxic epidermal necrolysis. Severe reactions appear to be much less common with single-dose or intermittent therapy, and use of the drug has been justified by the risks associated with falciparum malaria.

Rare adverse effects with a single dose of Fansidar are those associated with other sulfonamides, including hematologic, gastrointestinal, central nervous system, dermatologic, and renal toxicity. Maloprim is no longer recommended for chemoprophylaxis because of unacceptably high rates of agranulocytosis. Folate antagonists should be used cautiously in the presence of renal or hepatic dysfunction. Although pyrimethamine is teratogenic in animals, Fansidar has been safely used in pregnancy for therapy and as an intermittent chemoprophylactic regimen to improve pregnancy outcomes. Proguanil is considered safe in pregnancy. Folate supplements should be routinely administered during pregnancy, but in women receiving Fansidar preventive therapy, high-dose folate supplementation (eg, 5 mg daily) should probably be avoided because it may limit preventive efficacy. The standard recommended dosage of 0.4–0.6 mg daily is less likely to affect Fansidar's protective efficacy.

ANTIBIOTICS

A number of antibiotics in addition to the folate antagonists and sulfonamides are modestly active antimalarials. The antibiotics that are bacterial protein synthesis inhibitors appear to act against malaria parasites by inhibiting protein synthesis in a plasmodial prokaryote-like organelle, the apicoplast. None of the antibiotics should be used as single agents in the treatment of malaria because their action is much slower than that of standard antimalarials.

Tetracycline and doxycycline (see Chapter 44) are active against erythrocytic schizonts of all human malaria parasites. They are not active against liver stages. Doxycycline is used in the treatment of falciparum malaria in conjunction with quinine, allowing a shorter and better-tolerated course of that drug. Doxycycline is also used to complete treatment courses after initial treatment of severe malaria with intravenous quinine, quinidine, or artesunate. In all of these cases a 1-week treatment course of doxycycline is carried out. Doxycycline has also become a standard chemoprophylactic drug, especially for use in areas of Southeast Asia with high rates of resistance to other antimalarials, including mefloquine.

Doxycycline adverse effects include gastrointestinal symptoms, candidal vaginitis, and photosensitivity. Its safety in long-term chemoprophylaxis has not been extensively evaluated.

Clindamycin (see Chapter 44) is slowly active against erythrocytic schizonts and can be used after treatment courses of quinine, quinidine, or artesunate in those for whom doxycycline is not recommended, such as children and pregnant women. Azithromycin (see Chapter 44) also has antimalarial activity and is now under study as an alternative chemoprophylactic drug. Antimalarial activity of fluoroquinolones has been demonstrated, but efficacy for the therapy or chemoprophylaxis of malaria has been suboptimal.

Antibiotics also are active against other protozoans. Tetracycline and erythromycin are alternative therapies for the treatment of intestinal amebiasis. Clindamycin, in combination with other agents, is effective therapy for toxoplasmosis, pneumocystosis, and babesiosis. Spiramycin is a macrolide antibiotic that is used to treat primary toxoplasmosis acquired during pregnancy. Treatment lowers the risk of the development of congenital toxoplasmosis.

HALOFANTRINE & LUMEFANTRINE

Halofantrine hydrochloride, a phenanthrene-methanol, is effective against erythrocytic (but not other) stages of all four human malaria species. Oral absorption is variable and is enhanced with food. Because of toxicity concerns, it should not be taken with meals. Plasma levels peak 16 hours after dosing, and the half-life is about 4 days. Excretion is mainly in the feces. The mechanism of action of halofantrine is unknown. The drug is not available in the USA (although it has been approved by the FDA), but it is widely available in malaria-endemic countries.

Halofantrine (three 500-mg doses at 6-hour intervals, repeated in 1 week for nonimmune individuals) is rapidly effective against most strains of *P falciparum,* but its use is limited by irregular absorption and cardiac toxicity. It should not be used for chemoprophylaxis. Halofantrine is generally well tolerated. The most common adverse effects are abdominal pain, diarrhea, vomiting, cough, rash, headache, pruritus, and elevated liver enzymes. Of greater concern, the drug alters cardiac conduction, with dose-related prolongation of QT and PR intervals. This effect is seen with standard doses and is worsened by prior mefloquine therapy. Rare instances of dangerous arrhythmias and deaths have been reported. The drug is contraindicated in patients who have cardiac conduction defects or who have recently taken mefloquine. Halofantrine is embryotoxic in animals and therefore contraindicated in pregnancy.

Lumefantrine, an aryl alcohol related to halofantrine, is available only as a fixed-dose combination with artemether (Coartem), which is now the first-line therapy for uncomplicated falciparum malaria in many countries. In addition, Coartem is approved in many nonendemic countries, including the USA. The half-life of lumefantrine, when used in combination, is approximately 4 days. Drug levels may be altered by interactions with other drugs, including those that affect CYP3A4 metabolism, but this area has not been well studied. As with halofantrine, oral absorption is highly variable and improved when the drug is taken with food.

Since lumefantrine does not engender the dangerous toxicity concerns of halofantrine, Coartem should be administered with fatty food to maximize antimalarial efficacy. Coartem is highly effective in the treatment of falciparum malaria when administered twice daily for 3 days. Coartem can cause minor prolongation of the QT interval, but this appears to be clinically insignificant, and the drug does not carry the risk of dangerous arrhythmias seen with halofantrine and quinidine. Indeed, Coartem is very well tolerated. The most commonly reported adverse events in drug trials have been gastrointestinal disturbances, headache, dizziness, rash, and pruritus, and in many cases these toxicities may have been due to underlying malaria or concomitant medications rather than to Coartem.

■ AMEBIASIS

Amebiasis is infection with *Entamoeba histolytica.* This organism can cause asymptomatic intestinal infection, mild to moderate colitis, severe intestinal infection (dysentery), ameboma, liver abscess, and other extraintestinal infections. The choice of drugs for amebiasis depends on the clinical presentation (Table 52–5).

Treatment of Specific Forms of Amebiasis

A. Asymptomatic Intestinal Infection

Asymptomatic carriers generally are not treated in endemic areas, but in nonendemic areas they are treated with a luminal amebicide. A tissue amebicidal drug is unnecessary. Standard luminal amebicides are diloxanide furoate, iodoquinol, and paromomycin. Each drug eradicates carriage in about 80–90% of patients with a single course of treatment. Therapy with a luminal amebicide is also required in the treatment of all other forms of amebiasis.

B. Amebic Colitis

Metronidazole plus a luminal amebicide is the treatment of choice for amebic colitis and dysentery. Tetracyclines and erythromycin are alternative drugs for moderate colitis but are not effective against extraintestinal disease. Dehydroemetine or emetine can also be used, but are best avoided because of toxicity.

C. Extraintestinal Infections

The treatment of choice for extraintestinal infections is metronidazole plus a luminal amebicide. A 10-day course of metronidazole cures over 95% of uncomplicated liver abscesses. For unusual cases in which initial therapy with metronidazole has failed, aspiration of the abscess and the addition of chloroquine to a repeat course of metronidazole should be considered. Dehydroemetine and emetine are toxic alternative drugs.

METRONIDAZOLE & TINIDAZOLE

Metronidazole, a nitroimidazole (Figure 52–3), is the drug of choice in the treatment of extraluminal amebiasis. It kills trophozoites but not cysts of *E histolytica* and effectively eradicates

TABLE 52–5 Treatment of amebiasis. Not all preparations are available in the USA.[1]

Clinical Setting	Drugs of Choice and Adult Dosage	Alternative Drugs and Adult Dosage
Asymptomatic intestinal infection	Luminal agent: Diloxanide furoate,[2] 500 mg 3 times daily for 10 days *or* Iodoquinol, 650 mg 3 times daily for 21 days *or* Paromomycin, 10 mg/kg 3 times daily for 7 days	
Mild to moderate intestinal infection	Metronidazole, 750 mg 3 times daily (or 500 mg IV every 6 hours) for 10 days *or* Tinidazole, 2 g daily for 3 days *plus* Luminal agent (see above)	Luminal agent (see above) *plus either* Tetracycline, 250 mg 3 times daily for 10 days *or* Erythromycin, 500 mg 4 times daily for 10 days
Severe intestinal infection	Metronidazole, 750 mg 3 times daily (or 500 mg IV every 6 hours) for 10 days *or* Tinidazole, 2 g daily for 3 days *plus* Luminal agent (see above)	Luminal agent (see above) *plus either* Tetracycline, 250 mg 3 times daily for 10 days *or* Dehydroemetine[2] or emetine,[2] 1 mg/kg SC or IM for 3–5 days
Hepatic abscess, ameboma, and other extraintestinal disease	Metronidazole, 750 mg 3 times daily (or 500 mg IV every 6 hours) for 10 days *or* Tinidazole, 2 g daily for 5 days *plus* Luminal agent (see above)	Dehydroemetine[2] or emetine,[2] 1 mg/kg SC or IM for 8–10 days, followed by (liver abscess only) chloroquine, 500 mg twice daily for 2 days, then 500 mg daily for 21 days *plus* Luminal agent (see above)

[1]Route is oral unless otherwise indicated. See text for additional details and cautions.

[2]Not available in the USA.

intestinal and extraintestinal tissue infections. Tinidazole, a related nitroimidazole available in the USA since 2004, appears to have similar activity and a better toxicity profile than metronidazole. It offers simpler dosing regimens and can be substituted for the indications listed below.

Pharmacokinetics & Mechanism of Action

Oral metronidazole and tinidazole are readily absorbed and permeate all tissues by simple diffusion. Intracellular concentrations rapidly approach extracellular levels. Peak plasma concentrations are reached in 1–3 hours. Protein binding of both drugs is low (10–20%); the half-life of unchanged drug is 7.5 hours for metronidazole and 12–14 hours for tinidazole. Metronidazole and its metabolites are excreted mainly in the urine. Plasma clearance of metronidazole is decreased in patients with impaired liver function.

The nitro group of metronidazole is chemically reduced in anaerobic bacteria and sensitive protozoans. Reactive reduction products appear to be responsible for antimicrobial activity. The mechanism of tinidazole is assumed to be the same.

Clinical Uses

A. Amebiasis

Metronidazole or tinidazole is the drug of choice in the treatment of all tissue infections with *E histolytica*. Neither drug is reliably effective against luminal parasites and so must be used with a luminal amebicide to ensure eradication of the infection.

B. Giardiasis

Metronidazole is the treatment of choice for giardiasis. The dosage for giardiasis is much lower—and the drug thus better tolerated—than that for amebiasis. Efficacy after a single treatment is about 90%. Tinidazole is at least equally effective.

C. Trichomoniasis

Metronidazole is the treatment of choice. A single dose of 2 g is effective. Metronidazole-resistant organisms can lead to treatment failures. Tinidazole may be effective against some of these resistant organisms.

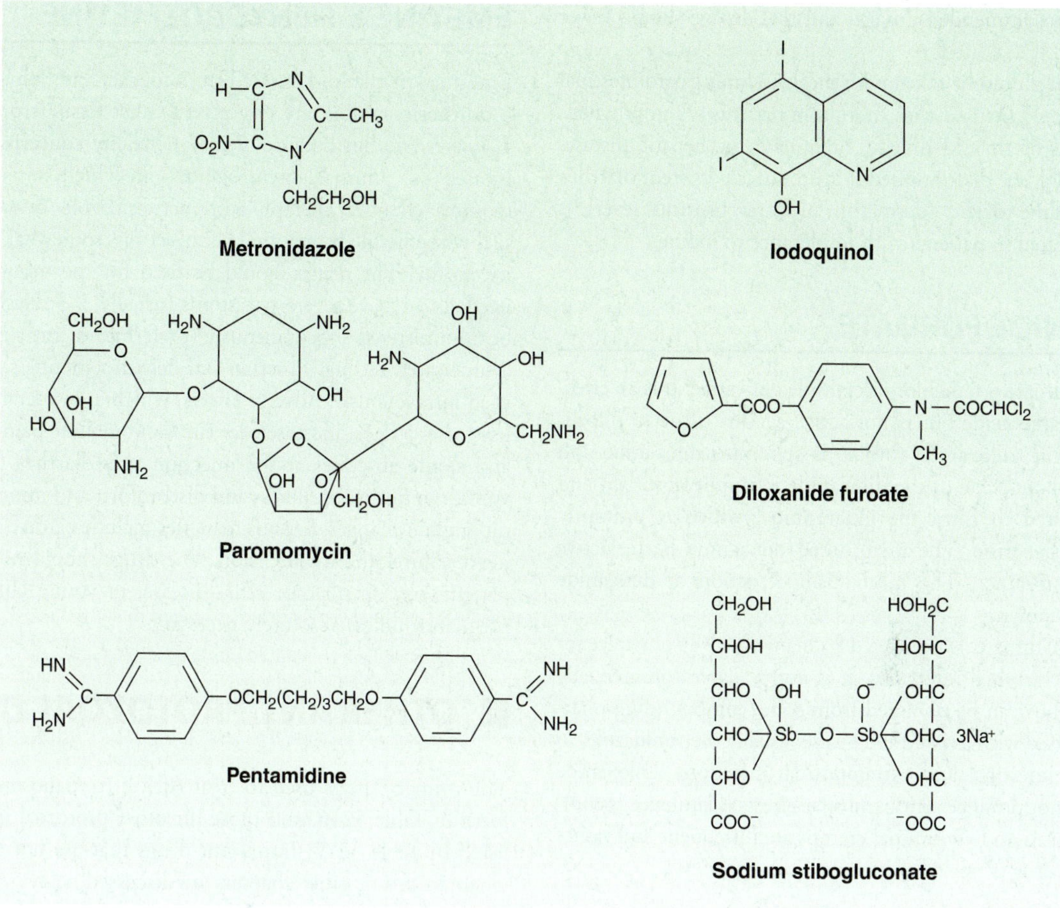

FIGURE 52–3 Structural formulas of other antiprotozoal drugs.

Adverse Effects & Cautions

Nausea, headache, dry mouth, or a metallic taste in the mouth occurs commonly. Infrequent adverse effects include vomiting, diarrhea, insomnia, weakness, dizziness, thrush, rash, dysuria, dark urine, vertigo, paresthesias, and neutropenia. Taking the drug with meals lessens gastrointestinal irritation. Pancreatitis and severe central nervous system toxicity (ataxia, encephalopathy, seizures) are rare. Metronidazole has a disulfiram-like effect, so that nausea and vomiting can occur if alcohol is ingested during therapy. The drug should be used with caution in patients with central nervous system disease. Intravenous infusions have rarely caused seizures or peripheral neuropathy. The dosage should be adjusted for patients with severe liver or renal disease. Tinidazole has a similar adverse-effect profile, although it appears to be somewhat better tolerated than metronidazole.

Metronidazole has been reported to potentiate the anticoagulant effect of coumarin-type anticoagulants. Phenytoin and phenobarbital may accelerate elimination of the drug, whereas cimetidine may decrease plasma clearance. Lithium toxicity may occur when the drug is used with metronidazole.

Metronidazole and its metabolites are mutagenic in bacteria. Chronic administration of large doses led to tumorigenicity in mice. Data on teratogenicity are inconsistent. Metronidazole is thus best avoided in pregnant or nursing women, although congenital abnormalities have not clearly been associated with use in humans.

IODOQUINOL

Iodoquinol (diiodohydroxyquin) is a halogenated hydroxyquinoline. It is an effective luminal amebicide that is commonly used with metronidazole to treat amebic infections. Pharmacokinetic data are incomplete but 90% of the drug is retained in the intestine and excreted in the feces. The remainder enters the circulation, has a half-life of 11–14 hours, and is excreted in the urine as glucuronides.

The mechanism of action of iodoquinol against trophozoites is unknown. It is effective against organisms in the bowel lumen but not against trophozoites in the intestinal wall or extraintestinal tissues.

Infrequent adverse effects include diarrhea—which usually stops after several days—anorexia, nausea, vomiting, abdominal pain, headache, rash, and pruritus. The drug may increase protein-bound serum iodine, leading to a decrease in measured ^{131}I uptake that persists for months. Some halogenated hydroxyquinolines can produce severe neurotoxicity with prolonged use at greater than recommended doses. Iodoquinol is not known to produce these effects at its recommended dosage, and this dosage should never be exceeded.

Iodoquinol should be taken with meals to limit gastrointestinal toxicity. It should be used with caution in patients with optic neuropathy, renal or thyroid disease, or nonamebic hepatic disease. The drug should be discontinued if it produces persistent diarrhea or signs of iodine toxicity (dermatitis, urticaria, pruritus, fever). It is contraindicated in patients with intolerance to iodine.

DILOXANIDE FUROATE

Diloxanide furoate is a dichloroacetamide derivative. It is an effective luminal amebicide but is not active against tissue trophozoites. In the gut, diloxanide furoate is split into diloxanide and furoic acid; about 90% of the diloxanide is rapidly absorbed and then conjugated to form the glucuronide, which is promptly excreted in the urine. The unabsorbed diloxanide is the active antiamebic substance. The mechanism of action of diloxanide furoate is unknown.

Diloxanide furoate is considered by many the drug of choice for asymptomatic luminal infections. It is not available commercially in the USA, but can be obtained from some compounding pharmacies. It is used with a tissue amebicide, usually metronidazole, to treat serious intestinal and extraintestinal infections. Diloxanide furoate does not produce serious adverse effects. Flatulence is common, but nausea and abdominal cramps are infrequent and rashes are rare. The drug is not recommended in pregnancy.

PAROMOMYCIN SULFATE

Paromomycin sulfate is an aminoglycoside antibiotic (see also Chapter 45) that is not significantly absorbed from the gastrointestinal tract. It is used only as a luminal amebicide and has no effect against extraintestinal amebic infections. The small amount absorbed is slowly excreted unchanged, mainly by glomerular filtration. However, the drug may accumulate with renal insufficiency and contribute to renal toxicity. Paromomycin is an effective luminal amebicide that appears to have similar efficacy and probably less toxicity than other agents; in a recent study, it was superior to diloxanide furoate in clearing asymptomatic infections. Adverse effects include occasional abdominal distress and diarrhea. Parenteral paromomycin is now used to treat visceral leishmaniasis and is discussed separately in the text that follows.

EMETINE & DEHYDROEMETINE

Emetine, an alkaloid derived from ipecac, and dehydroemetine, a synthetic analog, are effective against tissue trophozoites of *E histolytica,* but because of major toxicity concerns their use is limited to unusual circumstances in which severe amebiasis requires effective therapy and metronidazole cannot be used. Dehydroemetine is preferred because of its somewhat better toxicity profile. The drugs should be used for the minimum period needed to relieve severe symptoms (usually 3–5 days) and should be administered subcutaneously (preferred) or intramuscularly in a supervised setting. Emetine and dehydroemetine should not be used intravenously. Adverse effects, which are generally mild with use for 3–5 days, increase over time and include pain, tenderness, and sterile abscesses at the injection site; diarrhea, nausea, and vomiting; muscle weakness and discomfort; and minor electrocardiographic changes. Serious toxicities include cardiac arrhythmias, heart failure, and hypotension. The drugs should not be used in patients with cardiac or renal disease, in young children, or in pregnancy unless absolutely necessary.

■ OTHER ANTIPROTOZOAL DRUGS

The primary drugs used to treat African trypanosomiasis are set forth in Table 52–6, and those for other protozoal infections are listed in Table 52–7. Important drugs that are not covered elsewhere in this or other chapters are discussed below.

PENTAMIDINE

Pentamidine has activity against trypanosomatid protozoans and against *P jiroveci,* but toxicity is significant.

Chemistry & Pharmacokinetics

Pentamidine is an aromatic diamidine (Figure 52–3) formulated as an isethionate salt. Pentamidine is only administered parenterally. The drug leaves the circulation rapidly, with an initial half-life of about 6 hours, but it is bound avidly by tissues. Pentamidine thus accumulates and is eliminated very slowly, with a terminal elimination half-life of about 12 days. The drug can be detected in urine 6 or more weeks after treatment. Only trace amounts of pentamidine appear in the central nervous system, so it is not

TABLE 52–6 Treatment of African trypanosomiasis.

Disease	Stage	First-Line Drugs	Alternative Drugs
West African	Early	Pentamidine	Suramin, eflornithine
	CNS involvement	Eflornithine	Melarsoprol,[1] eflornithine-nifurtimox[1]
East African	Early	Suramin[1]	Pentamidine
	CNS involvement	Melarsoprol[1]	

[1]Available in the USA from the Drug Service, CDC, Atlanta, Georgia (phone: 404-639-3670; http://www.cdc.gov/laboratory/drugservice/index.html).

TABLE 52–7 Treatment of other protozoal infections. Not all preparations are available in the USA.[1]

Organism or Clinical Setting	Drugs of Choice[2]	Alternative Drugs
Babesia species	Clindamycin, 600 mg 3 times daily for 7 days plus Quinine, 650 mg for 7 days	Atovaquone or azithromycin
Balantidium coli	Tetracycline, 500 mg 4 times daily for 10 days	Metronidazole, 750 mg 3 times daily for 5 days
Cryptosporidium species	Paromomycin, 500–750 mg 3 or 4 times daily for 10 days	Azithromycin, 500 mg daily for 21 days
Cyclospora cayetanensis	Trimethoprim-sulfamethoxazole, one double-strength tablet 4 times daily for 7–14 days	
Dientamoeba fragilis	Iodoquinol, 650 mg 3 times daily for 20 days	Tetracycline, 500 mg 4 times daily for 10 days or Paromomycin, 500 mg 3 times daily for 7 days
Giardia lamblia	Metronidazole, 250 mg 3 times daily for 5 days or Tinidazole, 2 g once	Furazolidone, 100 mg 4 times daily for 7 days or Albendazole, 400 mg daily for 5 days
Isospora belli	Trimethoprim-sulfamethoxazole, one double-strength tablet 4 times daily for 10 days, then twice daily for 21 days	Pyrimethamine, 75 mg daily for 14 days plus Folinic acid, 10 mg daily for 14 days
Microsporidia	Albendazole, 400 mg twice daily for 20–30 days	
Leishmaniasis		
Visceral (L donovani, L chagasi, L infantum) or mucosal (L braziliensis)	Sodium stibogluconate, 20 mg/kg/d IV or IM for 28 days	Meglumine antimoniate or Pentamidine or Amphotericin or Miltefosine or Paromomycin
Cutaneous (L major, L tropica, L mexicana, L braziliensis)	Sodium stibogluconate, 20 mg/kg/d IV or IM for 20 days	Meglumine antimoniate or Amphotericin or Pentamidine or Topical or intralesional therapies
Pneumocystis jiroveci, P carinii[3]	Trimethoprim-sulfamethoxazole, 15–20 mg trimethoprim component/kg/d IV, or two double-strength tablets every 8 hours for 21 days	Pentamidine or Trimethoprim-dapsone or Clindamycin plus primaquine or Atovaquone
Toxoplasma gondii		

(continued)

TABLE 52–7 **Treatment of other protozoal infections. Not all preparations are available in the USA.**[1] **(Continued)**

Organism or Clinical Setting	Drugs of Choice[2]	Alternative Drugs
Acute, congenital, immunocompromised	Pyrimethamine *plus* clindamycin *plus* folinic acid	Pyrimethamine *plus* sulfadiazine *plus* folinic acid
Pregnancy	Spiramycin, 3 g daily until delivery	
Trichomonas vaginalis	Metronidazole, 2 g once or 250 mg 3 times daily for 7 days *or* Tinidazole, 2 g once	
Trypanosoma cruzi	Nifurtimox *or* Benznidazole	

[1]Additional information may be obtained from the Parasitic Disease Drug Service, Parasitic Diseases Branch, CDC, Atlanta, Georgia (phone: 404-639-3670; http://www.cdc.gov/laboratory/drugservice/index.html).

[2]Established, relatively simple dosing regimens are provided. Route is oral unless otherwise indicated. See text for additional information, toxicities, cautions, and discussions of dosing for the more rarely used drugs, many of which are highly toxic.

[3]*P jiroveci* (*carinii* in animals) has traditionally been considered a protozoan because of its morphology and drug sensitivity, but recent molecular analyses have shown it to be most closely related to fungi.

effective against central nervous system African trypanosomiasis. Pentamidine can also be inhaled as a nebulized powder for the prevention of pneumocystosis. Absorption into the systemic circulation after inhalation appears to be minimal. The mechanism of action of pentamidine is unknown.

Clinical Uses

A. Pneumocystosis

Pentamidine is a well-established alternative therapy for pulmonary and extrapulmonary disease caused by *P jiroveci*. The drug has somewhat lower efficacy and greater toxicity than trimethoprim-sulfamethoxazole. The standard dosage is 3 mg/kg/d intravenously for 21 days. Significant adverse reactions are common, and with multiple regimens now available to treat *P jiroveci* infection, pentamidine is best reserved for patients with severe disease who cannot tolerate or fail other drugs.

Pentamidine is also an alternative agent for primary or secondary prophylaxis against pneumocystosis in immunocompromised individuals, including patients with advanced AIDS. For this indication, pentamidine is administered as an inhaled aerosol (300 mg inhaled monthly). The drug is well tolerated in this form. Its efficacy is very good but clearly less than that of daily trimethoprim-sulfamethoxazole. Because of its cost and ineffectiveness against nonpulmonary disease, it is best reserved for patients who cannot tolerate oral chemoprophylaxis with other drugs.

B. African Trypanosomiasis (Sleeping Sickness)

Pentamidine has been used since 1940 and is the drug of choice to treat the early hemolymphatic stage of disease caused by *Trypanosoma brucei gambiense* (West African sleeping sickness). The drug is inferior to suramin for the treatment of early East African sleeping sickness. Pentamidine should not be used to treat late trypanosomiasis

with central nervous system involvement. A number of dosing regimens have been described, generally providing 2–4 mg/kg daily or on alternate days for a total of 10–15 doses. Pentamidine has also been used for chemoprophylaxis against African trypanosomiasis, with dosing of 4 mg/kg every 3–6 months.

C. Leishmaniasis

Pentamidine is an alternative to sodium stibogluconate in the treatment of visceral leishmaniasis, with similar efficacy, although resistance has been reported. The drug has been successful in some cases that have failed therapy with antimonials. The dosage is 2–4 mg/kg intramuscularly daily or every other day for up to 15 doses, and a second course may be necessary. Pentamidine has also shown success against cutaneous leishmaniasis, but it is not routinely used for this purpose.

Adverse Effects & Cautions

Pentamidine is a highly toxic drug, with adverse effects noted in about 50% of patients receiving 4 mg/kg/d. Rapid intravenous administration can lead to severe hypotension, tachycardia, dizziness, and dyspnea, so the drug should be administered slowly (over 2 hours), and patients should be recumbent and monitored closely during treatment. With intramuscular administration, pain at the injection site is common, and sterile abscesses may develop.

Pancreatic toxicity is common. Hypoglycemia due to inappropriate insulin release often appears 5–7 days after onset of treatment, can persist for days to several weeks, and may be followed by hyperglycemia. Reversible renal insufficiency is also common. Other adverse effects include rash, metallic taste, fever, gastrointestinal symptoms, abnormal liver function tests, acute pancreatitis, hypocalcemia, thrombocytopenia, hallucinations, and cardiac arrhythmias. Inhaled pentamidine is generally well tolerated but may cause cough, dyspnea, and bronchospasm.

SODIUM STIBOGLUCONATE

Pentavalent antimonials, including sodium stibogluconate (pentostam; Figure 52–3) and meglumine antimoniate, are generally considered first-line agents for cutaneous and visceral leishmaniasis except in parts of India, where the efficacy of these drugs has diminished greatly. The drugs are rapidly absorbed and distributed after intravenous (preferred) or intramuscular administration and eliminated in two phases, with short initial (about 2-hour) half-life and much longer terminal (> 24-hour) half-life. Treatment is given once daily at a dosage of 20 mg/kg/d intravenously or intramuscularly for 20 days in cutaneous leishmaniasis and 28 days in visceral and mucocutaneous disease.

The mechanism of action of the antimonials is unknown. Their efficacy against different species may vary, possibly based on local drug resistance patterns. Cure rates are generally quite good, but resistance to sodium stibogluconate is increasing in some endemic areas, notably in India where other agents (eg, amphotericin or miltefosine) are generally recommended.

Few adverse effects occur initially, but the toxicity of stibogluconate increases over the course of therapy. Most common are gastrointestinal symptoms, fever, headache, myalgias, arthralgias, and rash. Intramuscular injections can be very painful and lead to sterile abscesses. Electrocardiographic changes may occur, most commonly T-wave changes and QT prolongation. These changes are generally reversible, but continued therapy may lead to dangerous arrhythmias. Thus, the electrocardiogram should be monitored during therapy. Hemolytic anemia and serious liver, renal, and cardiac effects are rare.

NITAZOXANIDE

Nitazoxanide is a nitrothiazolyl-salicylamide prodrug. Nitazoxanide was recently approved in the USA for use against *Giardia lamblia* and *Cryptosporidium parvum*. It is rapidly absorbed and converted to tizoxanide and tizoxanide conjugates, which are subsequently excreted in both urine and feces. The active metabolite, tizoxanide, inhibits the pyruvate-ferredoxin oxidoreductase pathway. Nitazoxanide appears to have activity against metronidazole-resistant protozoal strains and is well tolerated. Unlike metronidazole, nitazoxanide and its metabolites appear to be free of mutagenic effects. Other organisms that may be susceptible to nitazoxanide include *E histolytica*, *Helicobacter pylori*, *Ascaris lumbricoides*, several tapeworms, and *Fasciola hepatica*. The recommended adult dosage is 500 mg twice daily for 3 days.

OTHER DRUGS FOR TRYPANOSOMIASIS & LEISHMANIASIS

Available therapies for all forms of trypanosomiasis are seriously deficient in efficacy, safety, or both. Availability of these therapies is also a concern, since they are supplied mainly through donation or nonprofit production by pharmaceutical companies. For visceral leishmaniasis, three new promising therapies are liposomal amphotericin, miltefosine, and paromomycin.

A. Suramin

Suramin is a sulfated naphthylamine that was introduced in the 1920s. It is the first-line therapy for early hemolymphatic East African trypanosomiasis (*T brucei rhodesiense* infection), but because it does not enter the central nervous system, it is not effective against advanced disease. Suramin is less effective than pentamidine for early West African trypanosomiasis. The drug's mechanism of action is unknown. It is administered intravenously and displays complex pharmacokinetics with very tight protein binding. Suramin has a short initial half-life but a terminal elimination half-life of about 50 days. The drug is slowly cleared by renal excretion.

Suramin is administered after a 200-mg intravenous test dose. Regimens that have been used include 1 g on days 1, 3, 7, 14, and 21 or 1 g each week for 5 weeks. Combination therapy with pentamidine may improve efficacy. Suramin can also be used for chemoprophylaxis against African trypanosomiasis. Adverse effects are common. Immediate reactions can include fatigue, nausea, vomiting, and, more rarely, seizures, shock, and death. Later reactions include fever, rash, headache, paresthesias, neuropathies, renal abnormalities including proteinuria, chronic diarrhea, hemolytic anemia, and agranulocytosis.

B. Melarsoprol

Melarsoprol is a trivalent arsenical that has been available since 1949 and is first-line therapy for advanced central nervous system East African trypanosomiasis, and second-line therapy (after eflornithine) for advanced West African trypanosomiasis. After intravenous administration it is excreted rapidly, but clinically relevant concentrations accumulate in the central nervous system within 4 days. Melarsoprol is administered in propylene glycol by slow intravenous infusion at a dosage of 3.6 mg/kg/d for 3–4 days, with repeated courses at weekly intervals, if needed. A new regimen of 2.2 mg/kg daily for 10 days had efficacy and toxicity similar to what was observed with three courses over 26 days. Melarsoprol is extremely toxic. The use of such a toxic drug is justified only by the severity of advanced trypanosomiasis and the lack of available alternatives. Immediate adverse effects include fever, vomiting, abdominal pain, and arthralgias. The most important toxicity is a reactive encephalopathy that generally appears within the first week of therapy (in 5–10% of patients) and is probably due to disruption of trypanosomes in the central nervous system. Common consequences of the encephalopathy include cerebral edema, seizures, coma, and death. Other serious toxicities include renal and cardiac disease and hypersensitivity reactions. Failure rates with melarsoprol appear to have increased recently in parts of Africa, suggesting the possibility of drug resistance.

C. Eflornithine

Eflornithine (difluoromethylornithine), an inhibitor of ornithine decarboxylase, is the only new drug registered to treat African trypanosomiasis in the last half-century. It is now the first-line drug for advanced West African trypanosomiasis, but is not effective for East African disease. Eflornithine is less toxic than melarsoprol but not as widely available. The drug had very limited

availability until recently, when it was developed for use as a topical depilatory cream, leading to donation of the drug for the treatment of trypanosomiasis. Eflornithine is administered intravenously, and good central nervous system drug levels are achieved. The elimination half-life is about 3 hours. The usual regimen is 100 mg/kg intravenously every 6 hours for 7–14 days (14 days was superior for a newly diagnosed infection). Eflornithine appears to be as effective as melarsoprol against advanced *T brucei gambiense* infection, but its efficacy against *T brucei rhodesiense* is limited by drug resistance. Toxicity from eflornithine is significant, but considerably less than that from melarsoprol. Adverse effects include diarrhea, vomiting, anemia, thrombocytopenia, leukopenia, and seizures. These effects are generally reversible. Increased experience with eflornithine and increased availability of the compound in endemic areas may lead to its replacement of suramin, pentamidine, and melarsoprol in the treatment of *T brucei gambiense* infection.

D. Nifurtimox

Nifurtimox, a nitrofuran, is the most commonly used drug for American trypanosomiasis (Chagas' disease). Nifurtimox is also under study in the treatment of African trypanosomiasis, particularly in combination with eflornithine. Nifurtimox is well absorbed after oral administration and eliminated with a plasma half-life of about 3 hours. The drug is administered at a dosage of 8–10 mg/kg/d (divided into three to four doses) orally for 3–4 months in the treatment of acute Chagas' disease. Nifurtimox decreases the severity of acute disease and usually eliminates detectable parasites, but it is often ineffective in fully eradicating infection. Thus, it often fails to prevent progression to the gastrointestinal and cardiac syndromes associated with chronic infection that are the most important clinical consequences of *Trypanosoma cruzi* infection. Efficacy may vary in different parts of South America, possibly related to drug resistance in some areas. Nifurtimox has not been proved effective in the treatment of chronic Chagas' disease. Toxicity related to nifurtimox is common. Adverse effects include nausea, vomiting, abdominal pain, fever, rash, restlessness, insomnia, neuropathies, and seizures. These effects are generally reversible but often lead to cessation of therapy before completion of a standard course.

E. Benznidazole

Benznidazole is an orally administered nitroimidazole that appears to have efficacy similar to that of nifurtimox in the treatment of acute Chagas' disease. Availability of the drug is currently limited. Important toxicities include peripheral neuropathy, rash, gastrointestinal symptoms, and myelosuppression.

F. Amphotericin

This important antifungal drug (see Chapter 48) is an alternative therapy for visceral leishmaniasis, especially in parts of India with high-level resistance to sodium stibogluconate. Liposomal amphotericin has shown excellent efficacy at a dosage of 3 mg/kg/d intravenously on days 1–5, 14, and 21. Nonliposomal amphotericin (1 mg/kg intravenously every other day for 30 days) is much less expensive, also efficacious, and widely used in India. Amphotericin is also used for cutaneous leishmaniasis in some areas. The use of amphotericin, and especially liposomal preparations, is limited in developing countries by difficulty of administration, cost, and toxicity.

G. Miltefosine

Miltefosine is an alkylphosphocholine analog that is the first effective oral drug for visceral leishmaniasis. It has recently shown excellent efficacy in the treatment of visceral leishmaniasis in India, where it is administered orally (2.5 mg/kg/d with varied dosing schedules) for 28 days. It was also recently shown to be effective in regimens including a single dose of liposomal amphotericin followed by 7–14 days of miltefosine. A 28-day course of miltefosine (2.5 mg/kg/d) was also effective for the treatment of New World cutaneous leishmaniasis. Vomiting and diarrhea are common but generally short-lived toxicities. Transient elevations in liver enzymes and nephrotoxicity are also seen. The drug should be avoided in pregnancy (or in women who may become pregnant within 2 months of treatment) because of its teratogenic effects. Miltefosine is registered for the treatment of visceral leishmaniasis in India and some other countries, and—considering the serious limitations of other drugs, including parenteral administration, toxicity, and resistance—it may become the treatment of choice for that disease. Resistance to miltefosine develops readily in vitro. To circumvent this problem, various drug combinations, including miltefosine with antimonials, amphotericin, or paromomycin, are under study.

H. Paromomycin

Paromomycin sulfate is an aminoglycoside antibiotic that until recently was used in parasitology only for oral therapy of intestinal parasitic infections (see previous text). It has recently been developed for the treatment of visceral leishmaniasis. A phase 3 trial in India showed excellent efficacy for this disease, with a daily intramuscular dosage of 11 mg/kg for 21 days yielding a 95% cure rate, and noninferiority compared with amphotericin. The drug was registered for the treatment of visceral leishmaniasis in India in 2006. However, a recent trial showed poorer efficacy in Africa, with the cure rate for paromomycin significantly inferior to that with sodium stibogluconate. In initial studies, paromomycin was well tolerated, with common mild injection pain, uncommon ototoxicity and reversible liver enzyme elevations, and no nephrotoxicity. Paromomycin is much less expensive than liposomal amphotericin or miltefosine, the other promising new therapies for visceral leishmaniasis.

P R E P A R A T I O N S   A V A I L A B L E

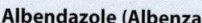

Albendazole (Albenza)
Oral: 200 mg tablets

Artemether/lumefantrine (Coartem)
Oral: 20 mg artemether/120 mg lumefantrine tablets

Artesunate*

Atovaquone (Mepron)
Oral: 750 mg/5 mL suspension

Atovaquone-proguanil (Malarone)
Oral: 250 mg atovaquone + 100 mg proguanil tablets; pediatric 62.5 mg atovaquone + 25 mg proguanil tablets

Chloroquine (generic, Aralen)
Oral: 250, 500 mg tablets (equivalent to 150, 300 mg base, respectively)
Parenteral: 50 mg/mL (equivalent to 40 mg/mL base) for injection

Clindamycin (generic, Cleocin)
Oral: 75, 150, 300 mg capsules; 75 mg/5 mL suspension
Parenteral: 150 mg/mL for injection

Doxycycline (generic, Vibramycin)
Oral: 20, 50, 100 mg capsules; 50, 100 mg tablets; 25 mg/5 mL suspension; 50 mg/5 mL syrup
Parenteral: 100, 200 mg for injection

Eflornithine (Ornidyl)
Parenteral: 200 mg/mL for injection

Iodoquinol (Yodoxin)
Oral: 210, 650 mg tablets

Mefloquine (generic, Lariam)
Oral: 250 mg tablets

Melarsoprol (Mel B)*

Metronidazole (generic, Flagyl)
Oral: 250, 500 mg tablets; 375 mg capsules; extended-release 750 mg tablets
Parenteral: 5 mg/mL

Nifurtimox*

Nitazoxanide (Alinia)
Oral: 500 mg tablets, powder for 100 mg/5 mL oral solution

Paromomycin (Humatin)
Oral: 250 mg capsules

Pentamidine (Pentam 300, Pentacarinat, pentamidine isethionate)
Parenteral: 300 mg powder for injection
Aerosol (Nebupent): 300 mg powder

Primaquine (generic)
Oral: 26.3 mg (equivalent to 15 mg base) tablet

Pyrimethamine (Daraprim)
Oral: 25 mg tablets

Quinidine gluconate (generic)
Parenteral: 80 mg/mL (equivalent to 50 mg/mL base) for injection

Quinine (generic)
Oral: 260 mg tablets; 200, 260, 325 mg capsules

Sodium stibogluconate*

Sulfadoxine and pyrimethamine (Fansidar)
Oral: 500 mg sulfadoxine plus 25 mg pyrimethamine tablets

Suramin*

Tinidazole (Tindamax)
Oral: 250, 500 mg tablets

*Available in the USA only from the Drug Service, CDC, Atlanta, Georgia (phone: 404-639-3670; http://www.cdc.gov/laboratory/drugservice/index.html).

REFERENCES

General

Drugs for parasitic infections. Med Lett Drugs Ther 2010;Supplement.

Malaria

Baird JK: Effectiveness of antimalarial drugs. N Engl J Med 2005;352:1565.

Baird JK: Resistance to therapies for infection by *Plasmodium vivax*. Clin Microbiol Rev 2009;22:508.

Barnes KI et al: Efficacy of rectal artesunate compared with parenteral quinine in initial treatment of moderately severe malaria in African children and adults: A randomised study. Lancet 2004;363:1598.

Boggild AK et al: Atovaquone-proguanil: Report from the CDC expert meeting on malaria chemoprophylaxis (II). Am J Trop Med Hyg 2007;76:208.

Dondorp AM et al: Artemisinin resistance in *Plasmodium falciparum* malaria. N Engl J Med 2009;361:455.

Dondorp A et al: Artesunate versus quinine for treatment of severe falciparum malaria: A randomised trial. Lancet 2005;366:717.

Dondorp AM et al: Artesunate versus quinine in the treatment of severe falciparum malaria in African children (AQUAMAT): An open-label, randomised trial. Lancet 2010;376:1647.

Dorsey G et al: Combination therapy for uncomplicated falciparum malaria in Ugandan children: A randomized trial. JAMA 2007;297:2210.

Efferth T, Kaina B: Toxicity of the antimalarial artemisinin and its derivatives. Crit Rev Toxicol 2010;40:405.

Freedman DO: Malaria prevention in short-term travelers. N Engl J Med 2008;359:603.

Greenwood BM et al: Malaria. Lancet 2005;365:1487.

Hill DR et al: Primaquine: Report from CDC expert meeting on malaria chemoprophylaxis I. Am J Trop Med Hyg 2006;75:402.

Nosten F, White NJ: Artemisinin-based combination treatment of falciparum malaria. Am J Trop Med Hyg 2007;77(Suppl 6):181.

Nosten F et al: Antimalarial drugs in pregnancy: A review. Curr Drug Saf 2006;1:1.

Rosenthal PJ: Artesunate for the treatment of severe falciparum malaria. N Engl J Med 2008;358:1829.

Stepniewska K, White NJ: Pharmacokinetic determinants of the window of selection for antimalarial drug resistance. Antimicrob Agents Chemother 2008;52:1589.

Taylor WR, White NJ: Antimalarial drug toxicity: A review. Drug Saf 2004;27:25.

White NJ: Cardiotoxicity of antimalarial drugs. Lancet Infect Dis 2007;7:549.

White NJ: Qinghaosu (artemisinin): The price of success. Science 2008;320:330.

Whitty CJ, et al: Malaria: An update on treatment of adults in non-endemic countries. Br Med J 2006;333:241.

World Health Organization: Guidelines for the treatment of malaria. Geneva. 2010. http://www.who.int/malaria/publications/atoz/9789241547925/en/index.html

Intestinal Protozoal Infections

Blessmann J et al: Treatment of amoebic liver abscess with metronidazole alone or in combination with ultrasound-guided needle aspiration: A comparative, prospective and randomized study. Trop Med Int Health 2003;8:1030.

Fox LM, Saravolatz LD: Nitazoxanide: A new thiazolide antiparasitic agent. Clin Infect Dis 2005;40:1173.

Haque R et al: Amebiasis. N Engl J Med 2003;348:1565.

Petri WA: Therapy of intestinal protozoa. Trends Parasitol 2003;19:523.

Pierce KK et al: Update on human infections caused by intestinal protozoa. Curr Opin Gastroenterol 2009;25:12.

Pritt BS, Clark DG: Amebiasis. Mayo Clin Proc 2008;83:1154.

Rossignol JF: *Cryptosporidium* and *Giardia*: Treatment options and prospects for new drugs. Exp Parasitol 2010;124:45.

Other Protozoal Infections

Amato VS et al: Treatment of mucosal leishmaniasis in Latin America: Systematic review. Am J Trop Med Hyg 2007;77:266.

Aronson NE et al: A randomized controlled trial of local heat therapy versus intravenous sodium stibogluconate for the treatment of cutaneous Leishmania major infection. PLoS Negl Trop Dis 2010;4:e628.

Bhattacharya SK et al: Phase 4 trial of miltefosine for the treatment of Indian visceral leishmaniasis. J Infect Dis 2007;196:591.

Bisser S et al: Equivalence trial of melarsoprol and nifurtimox monotherapy and combination therapy for the treatment of second-stage *Trypanosoma brucei gambiense* sleeping sickness. J Infect Dis 2007;195:322.

Brun R et al: Human African trypanosomiasis. Lancet 2010;375:148.

Chappuis F et al: Visceral leishmaniasis: What are the needs for diagnosis, treatment and control? Nat Rev Microbiol 2007;5:873.

Croft SL, Barrett MP, Urbina JA: Chemotherapy of trypanosomiases and leishmaniasis. Trends Parasitol 2005;21:508.

Hailu A et al: Geographical variation in the response of visceral leishmaniasis to paromomycin in East Africa: A multicentre, open-label, randomized trial. PLoS Negl Trop Dis 2010;4:e709.

Jackson Y et al: Tolerance and safety of nifurtimox in patients with chronic Chagas disease. Clin Infect Dis 2010;51:e69.

Lescure FX et al: Chagas disease: Changes in knowledge and management. Lancet Infect Dis 2010;10:556.

Murray HW et al: Advances in leishmaniasis. Lancet 2005;366:1561.

Priotto G et al: Nifurtimox-eflornithine combination therapy for second-stage African *Trypanosoma brucei gambiense* trypanosomiasis: A multicentre, randomised, phase III, non-inferiority trial. Lancet 2009;374:56.

Rassi A et al: Chagas disease. Lancet. 2010;375:1388.

Reithinger R et al: Cutaneous leishmaniasis. Lancet Infect Dis 2007;7:581.

Schmid C et al: Effectiveness of a 10-day melarsoprol schedule for the treatment of late-stage human African trypanosomiasis: Confirmation from a multinational study (IMPAMEL II). J Infect Dis 2005;191:1922.

Soto J et al: Efficacy of miltefosine for Bolivian cutaneous leishmaniasis. Am J Trop Med Hyg 2008;78:210.

Sundar S et al: Injectable paromomycin for visceral leishmaniasis in India. N Engl J Med 2007;356:2571.

Sundar S et al: New treatment approach in Indian visceral leishmaniasis: Single-dose liposomal amphotericin B followed by short-course oral miltefosine. Clin Infect Dis 2008;47:1000.

Sundar S et al: Oral miltefosine for Indian visceral leishmaniasis. N Engl J Med 2002;347:1739.

Tuon FF et al: Treatment of New World cutaneous leishmaniasis—a systematic review with a meta-analysis. Int J Dermatol 2008;47:109.

van Griensven J, et al: Combination therapy for visceral leishmaniasis. Lancet Infect Dis 2010;10:184.

Vélez I et al: Efficacy of miltefosine for the treatment of American cutaneous leishmaniasis. Am J Trop Med Hyg 2010;83:351.

Wortmann G et al: Liposomal amphotericin B for treatment of cutaneous leishmaniasis. Am J Trop Med Hyg 2010;83:1028.

CASE STUDY ANSWER

This child has acute falciparum malaria, and her lethargy and abnormal laboratory tests are consistent with progression to severe disease. She should be hospitalized and treated urgently with intravenous artesunate or, if this is unavailable, intravenous quinine or quinidine. She should be followed closely for progression of severe malaria, in particular neurologic, renal, or pulmonary complications, and if treated with quinine or quinidine should have cardiac monitoring for potential toxicities.

Clinical Pharmacology of the Antihelminthic Drugs

Philip J. Rosenthal, MD

CASE STUDY

A 29-year-old Peruvian man presents with the incidental finding of a 10 by 8 by 8 cm liver cyst on an abdominal computed tomography (CT) scan. The patient had noted 2 days of abdominal pain and fever, and his clinical evaluation and CT scan were consistent with appendicitis. His clinical findings resolved after laparoscopic appendectomy. Ten years ago, the patient emigrated to the United States from a rural area of Peru where his family trades in sheepskins. His father and sister have undergone resection of abdominal masses, but details of their diagnoses are unavailable. What is your differential diagnosis? What are your diagnostic and therapeutic plans?

■ CHEMOTHERAPY OF HELMINTHIC INFECTIONS

Helminths (worms) are multicellular organisms that infect very large numbers of humans and cause a broad range of diseases. Over 1 billion people are infected with intestinal nematodes, and many millions are infected with filarial nematodes, flukes, and tapeworms. They are an even greater problem in domestic animals. Many drugs, which are directed against a number of different targets, are available to treat helminthic infections. In many cases, especially in the developing world, the goal is control of infection, with elimination of most parasites controlling disease symptoms and decreasing the transmission of infection. In other cases, complete elimination of parasites is the goal of therapy, although this goal can be challenging with certain helminthic infections, because of both limited efficacy of drugs and frequent reinfection after therapy in endemic areas.

Table 53–1 lists the major helminthic infections and provides a guide to the drug of choice and alternative drugs for each infection. In the text that follows, these drugs are arranged alphabetically. In general, parasites should be identified before treatment is started.

ALBENDAZOLE

Albendazole, a broad-spectrum oral antihelminthic, is the drug of choice and is approved in the USA for treatment of hydatid disease and cysticercosis. It is also used in the treatment of pinworm and hookworm infections, ascariasis, trichuriasis, and strongyloidiasis.

Basic Pharmacology

Albendazole is a benzimidazole carbamate. After oral administration, it is erratically absorbed (increased with a fatty meal) and then rapidly undergoes first-pass metabolism in the liver to the active metabolite albendazole sulfoxide. It reaches variable maximum plasma concentrations about 3 hours after a 400-mg oral dose, and its plasma half-life is 8–12 hours. The sulfoxide is mostly protein-bound, distributes well to tissues, and enters bile, cerebrospinal fluid, and hydatid cysts. Albendazole metabolites are excreted in the urine.

Benzimidazoles are thought to act against nematodes by inhibiting microtubule synthesis. Albendazole also has larvicidal effects in hydatid disease, cysticercosis, ascariasis, and hookworm infection and ovicidal effects in ascariasis, ancylostomiasis, and trichuriasis.

TABLE 53–1 Drugs for the treatment of helminthic infections.[1]

Infecting Organism	Drug of Choice	Alternative Drugs
Roundworms (nematodes)		
Ascaris lumbricoides (roundworm)	Albendazole or pyrantel pamoate or mebendazole	Ivermectin, piperazine
Trichuris trichiura (whipworm)	Mebendazole or albendazole	Ivermectin
Necator americanus (hookworm); *Ancylostoma duodenale* (hookworm)	Albendazole or mebendazole or pyrantel pamoate	
Strongyloides stercoralis (threadworm)	Ivermectin	Albendazole or thiabendazole
Enterobius vermicularis (pinworm)	Mebendazole or pyrantel pamoate	Albendazole
Trichinella spiralis (trichinosis)	Mebendazole or albendazole; add corticosteroids for severe infection	
Trichostrongylus species	Pyrantel pamoate or mebendazole	Albendazole
Cutaneous larva migrans (creeping eruption)	Albendazole or ivermectin	Thiabendazole (topical)
Visceral larva migrans	Albendazole	Mebendazole
Angiostrongylus cantonensis	Albendazole or mebendazole	
Wuchereria bancrofti (filariasis); *Brugia malayi* (filariasis); tropical eosinophilia; *Loa loa* (loiasis)	Diethylcarbamazine	Ivermectin
Onchocerca volvulus (onchocerciasis)	Ivermectin	
Dracunculus medinensis (guinea worm)	Metronidazole	Thiabendazole or mebendazole
Capillaria philippinensis (intestinal capillariasis)	Albendazole	Mebendazole
Flukes (trematodes)		
Schistosoma haematobium (bilharziasis)	Praziquantel	Metrifonate
Schistosoma mansoni	Praziquantel	Oxamniquine
Schistosoma japonicum	Praziquantel	
Clonorchis sinensis (liver fluke); *Opisthorchis* species	Praziquantel	Albendazole
Paragonimus westermani (lung fluke)	Praziquantel	Bithionol
Fasciola hepatica (sheep liver fluke)	Bithionol or triclabendazole	
Fasciolopsis buski (large intestinal fluke)	Praziquantel or niclosamide	
Heterophyes heterophyes; *Metagonimus yokogawai* (small intestinal flukes)	Praziquantel or niclosamide	
Tapeworms (cestodes)		
Taenia saginata (beef tapeworm)	Praziquantel or niclosamide	Mebendazole
Diphyllobothrium latum (fish tapeworm)	Praziquantel or niclosamide	
Taenia solium (pork tapeworm)	Praziquantel or niclosamide	
Cysticercosis (pork tapeworm larval stage)	Albendazole	Praziquantel
Hymenolepis nana (dwarf tapeworm)	Praziquantel	Niclosamide, nitazoxanide
Echinococcus granulosus (hydatid disease); *Echinococcus multilocularis*	Albendazole	

[1]Additional information may be obtained from the Parasitic Disease Drug Service, Parasitic Diseases Branch, Centers for Disease Control and Prevention, Atlanta, Georgia, 30333. Telephone: (404) 639-3670. Some of the drugs listed are not generally available in the USA.

Clinical Uses

Albendazole is administered on an empty stomach when used against intraluminal parasites but with a fatty meal when used against tissue parasites.

A. Ascariasis, Trichuriasis, and Hookworm and Pinworm Infections

For adults and children older than 2 years of age with ascariasis and hookworm infections, the treatment is a single dose of 400 mg

orally (repeated for 2–3 days for heavy ascaris infections and in 2 weeks for pinworm infections). These treatments typically achieve good cure rates and marked reduction in egg counts in those not cured. For trichuriasis, three daily 400-mg oral doses of albendazole are now recommended. A recent meta-analysis showed albendazole to be superior to mebendazole or pyrantel pamoate for treatment of hookworm infection; other studies showed that three doses of mebendazole and albendazole increased stool clearance of eggs compared with single treatments, with albendazole superior to mebendazole. Cure rates for trichuriasis with single-dose albendazole or mebendazole were less than 30%, which suggests that the three-dose regimen just noted, or other drugs (eg, ivermectin), might be superior.

B. Hydatid Disease

Albendazole is the treatment of choice for medical therapy and is a useful adjunct to surgical removal or aspiration of cysts. It is more active against *Echinococcus granulosus* than against *E multilocularis*. Dosing is 400 mg twice daily with meals for 1 month or longer. Daily therapy for up to 6 months has been well tolerated. One reported therapeutic strategy is to treat with albendazole and praziquantel, to assess response after 1 month or more, and, depending on the response, to then manage the patient with continued chemotherapy or combined surgical and drug therapy.

C. Neurocysticercosis

Indications for medical therapy for neurocysticercosis are controversial, since antihelminthic therapy is not clearly superior to therapy with corticosteroids alone and may exacerbate neurologic disease. Therapy is probably most appropriate for symptomatic parenchymal or intraventricular cysts. Corticosteroids are usually given with the antihelminthic drug to decrease inflammation caused by dying organisms. Albendazole is now generally considered the drug of choice over praziquantel because of its shorter course, lower cost, improved penetration into the subarachnoid space, and increased drug levels (as opposed to decreased levels of praziquantel) when administered with corticosteroids. Albendazole is given in a dosage of 400 mg twice daily for up to 21 days.

D. Other Infections

Albendazole is the drug of choice in the treatment of cutaneous larva migrans (400 mg daily for 3 days), visceral larva migrans (400 mg twice daily for 5 days), intestinal capillariasis (400 mg daily for 10 days), microsporidial infections (400 mg twice daily for 2 weeks or longer), and gnathostomiasis (400 mg twice daily for 3 weeks). It also has activity against trichinosis (400 mg twice daily for 1–2 weeks) and clonorchiasis (400 mg twice daily for 1 week). There have been reports of some effectiveness in treatment of opisthorchiasis, toxocariasis, and loiasis, and conflicting reports of effectiveness in giardiasis and taeniasis. Albendazole is included in programs to control lymphatic filariasis, but it appears to be less active than diethylcarbamazine or ivermectin for this purpose. Albendazole has been recommended as empiric therapy to treat those who return from the tropics with persistent unexplained eosinophilia.

Adverse Reactions, Contraindications, & Cautions

When used for 1–3 days, albendazole is nearly free of significant adverse effects. Mild and transient epigastric distress, diarrhea, headache, nausea, dizziness, lassitude, and insomnia can occur. In long-term use for hydatid disease, albendazole is well tolerated, but it can cause abdominal distress, headaches, fever, fatigue, alopecia, increases in liver enzymes, and pancytopenia.

Blood counts and liver function studies should be monitored during long-term therapy. The drug should not be given to patients with known hypersensitivity to other benzimidazole drugs or to those with cirrhosis. The safety of albendazole in pregnancy and in children younger than 2 years of age has not been established.

BITHIONOL

Bithionol is an alternative to triclabendazole for the treatment of fascioliasis (sheep liver fluke). Bithionol is also an alternative drug in the treatment of pulmonary paragonimiasis.

Basic Pharmacology

After ingestion, bithionol reaches peak blood levels in 4–8 hours. Excretion appears to be mainly via the kidney.

Clinical Uses

For treatment of paragonimiasis and fascioliasis, the dosage of bithionol is 30–50 mg/kg in two or three divided doses, given orally after meals on alternate days for 10–15 doses. For pulmonary paragonimiasis, cure rates are over 90%. For cerebral paragonimiasis, repeat courses of therapy may be necessary.

Adverse Reactions, Contraindications, & Cautions

Adverse effects, which occur in up to 40% of patients, are generally mild and transient, but occasionally their severity requires interruption of therapy. These problems include diarrhea, abdominal cramps, anorexia, nausea, vomiting, dizziness, and headache. Skin rashes may occur after a week or more of therapy, suggesting a reaction to antigens released from dying worms.

Bithionol should be used with caution in children younger than 8 years of age because there has been limited experience in this age group.

DIETHYLCARBAMAZINE CITRATE

Diethylcarbamazine is a drug of choice in the treatment of filariasis, loiasis, and tropical eosinophilia. It has been replaced by ivermectin for the treatment of onchocerciasis.

Basic Pharmacology

Diethylcarbamazine, a synthetic piperazine derivative, is marketed as a citrate salt. It is rapidly absorbed from the gastrointestinal tract; after a 0.5 mg/kg dose, peak plasma levels are reached within 1–2 hours. The plasma half-life is 2–3 hours in the presence of acidic urine but about 10 hours if the urine is alkaline, a Henderson-Hasselbalch trapping effect (see Chapter 1). The drug rapidly equilibrates with all tissues except fat. It is excreted, principally in the urine, as unchanged drug and the N-oxide metabolite. Dosage may have to be reduced in patients with persistent urinary alkalosis or renal impairment.

Diethylcarbamazine immobilizes microfilariae and alters their surface structure, displacing them from tissues and making them more susceptible to destruction by host defense mechanisms. The mode of action against adult worms is unknown.

Clinical Uses

The drug should be taken after meals.

A. *Wuchereria bancrofti, Brugia malayi, Brugia timori,* and *Loa loa*

Diethylcarbamazine is the drug of choice for treatment of infections with these parasites because of its efficacy and lack of serious toxicity. Microfilariae of all species are rapidly killed; adult parasites are killed more slowly, often requiring several courses of treatment. The drug is highly effective against adult *L loa*. The extent to which *W bancrofti* and *B malayi* adults are killed is not known, but after appropriate therapy microfilariae do not reappear in the majority of patients.

These infections are treated for 2 or (for *L loa*) 3 weeks, with initial low doses to reduce the incidence of allergic reactions to dying microfilariae. This regimen is 50 mg (1 mg/kg in children) on day 1, three 50 mg doses on day 2, three 100 mg doses (2 mg/kg in children) on day 3, and then 2 mg/kg three times daily to complete the 2–3 week course.

Antihistamines may be given for the first few days of therapy to limit allergic reactions, and corticosteroids should be started and doses of diethylcarbamazine lowered or interrupted if severe reactions occur. Cures may require several courses of treatment. For patients with high *L loa* worm burdens (more than 2500 circulating parasites/mL), strategies to decrease risks of severe toxicity include apheresis, if available, to remove microfilariae before treatment with diethylcarbamazine or therapy with albendazole, which is slower acting and better tolerated, before therapy with diethylcarbamazine or ivermectin.

Diethylcarbamazine may also be used for chemoprophylaxis (300 mg weekly or 300 mg on 3 successive days each month for loiasis; 50 mg monthly for bancroftian and Malayan filariasis).

B. Other Uses

For tropical eosinophilia, diethylcarbamazine is given orally at a dosage of 2 mg/kg three times daily for 7 days. Diethylcarbamazine is effective in *Mansonella streptocerca* infections, since it kills both adults and microfilariae. Limited information suggests that the drug is not effective, however, against adult *M ozzardi* or *M perstans* and that it has limited activity against microfilariae of these parasites. An important application of diethylcarbamazine has been mass treatment to reduce the prevalence of *W bancrofti* infection, generally in combination with ivermectin or albendazole.

This strategy has led to excellent progress in disease control in a number of countries.

Adverse Reactions, Contraindications, & Cautions

Reactions to diethylcarbamazine, which are generally mild and transient, include headache, malaise, anorexia, weakness, nausea, vomiting, and dizziness. Adverse effects also occur as a result of the release of proteins from dying microfilariae or adult worms. Reactions are particularly severe with onchocerciasis, but diethylcarbamazine is no longer commonly used for this infection, because ivermectin is equally efficacious and less toxic. Reactions to dying microfilariae are usually mild in *W bancrofti*, more intense in *B malayi*, and occasionally severe in *L loa* infections. Reactions include fever, malaise, papular rash, headache, gastrointestinal symptoms, cough, chest pain, and muscle or joint pain. Leukocytosis is common. Eosinophilia may increase with treatment. Proteinuria may also occur. Symptoms are most likely to occur in patients with heavy loads of microfilariae. Retinal hemorrhages and, rarely, encephalopathy have been described.

Between the third and twelfth days of treatment, local reactions may occur in the vicinity of dying adult or immature worms. These include lymphangitis with localized swellings in *W bancrofti* and *B malayi*, small wheals in the skin in *L loa*, and flat papules in *M streptocerca* infections. Patients with attacks of lymphangitis due to *W bancrofti* or *B malayi* should be treated during a quiescent period between attacks.

Caution is advised when using diethylcarbamazine in patients with hypertension or renal disease.

DOXYCYCLINE

This tetracycline antibiotic is described in more detail in Chapter 44. Doxycycline has recently been shown to have significant macrofilaricidal activity against *W bancrofti*, suggesting better activity than any other available drug against adult worms. Activity is also seen against onchocerciasis. Doxycycline acts indirectly, by killing *Wolbachia,* an intracellular bacterial symbiont of filarial parasites. It may prove to be an important drug for filariasis, both for treatment of active disease and in mass chemotherapy campaigns.

IVERMECTIN

Ivermectin is the drug of choice in strongyloidiasis and onchocerciasis. It is also an alternative drug for a number of other helminthic infections.

Basic Pharmacology

Ivermectin, a semisynthetic macrocyclic lactone, is a mixture of avermectin B_{1a} and B_{1b}. It is derived from the soil actinomycete *Streptomyces avermitilis.*

Ivermectin is used only orally in humans. The drug is rapidly absorbed, reaching maximum plasma concentrations 4 hours after a

12 mg dose. The drug has a wide tissue distribution and a volume of distribution of about 50 L. Its half-life is about 16 hours. Excretion of the drug and its metabolites is almost exclusively in the feces.

Ivermectin appears to paralyze nematodes and arthropods by intensifying γ-aminobutyric acid (GABA)–mediated transmission of signals in peripheral nerves. In onchocerciasis, ivermectin is microfilaricidal. It does not effectively kill adult worms but blocks the release of microfilariae for some months after therapy. After a single standard dose, microfilariae in the skin diminish rapidly within 2–3 days, remain low for months, and then gradually increase; microfilariae in the anterior chamber of the eye decrease slowly over months, eventually clear, and then gradually return. With repeated doses of ivermectin, the drug appears to have a low-level macrofilaricidal action and to permanently reduce microfilarial production.

Clinical Uses

A. Onchocerciasis

Treatment is with a single oral dose of ivermectin, 150 mcg/kg, with water on an empty stomach. Doses are repeated; regimens vary from monthly to less frequent (every 6–12 months) dosing schedules. After acute therapy, treatment is repeated at 12-month intervals until the adult worms die, which may take 10 years or longer. With the first treatment only, patients with microfilariae in the cornea or anterior chamber may be treated with corticosteroids to avoid inflammatory eye reactions.

Ivermectin also now plays a key role in onchocerciasis control. Annual mass treatments have led to major reductions in disease transmission. However, evidence of diminished responsiveness after mass administration of ivermectin has raised concern regarding selection of drug-resistant parasites.

B. Strongyloidiasis

Treatment consists of two daily doses of 200 mcg/kg. In immuno-suppressed patients with disseminated infection, repeated treatment is often needed, and cure may not be possible. In this case, suppressive therapy—ie, once monthly—may be helpful.

C. Other Parasites

Ivermectin reduces microfilariae in *B malayi* and *M ozzardi* infections but not in *M perstans* infections. It has been used with diethylcarbamazine and albendazole for the control of *W bancrofti*, but it does not kill adult worms. In loiasis, although the drug reduces microfilaria concentrations, it can occasionally induce severe reactions and appears to be more dangerous in this regard than diethylcarbamazine. Ivermectin is also effective in controlling scabies, lice, and cutaneous larva migrans and in eliminating a large proportion of ascarid worms.

Adverse Reactions, Contraindications, & Cautions

In strongyloidiasis treatment, infrequent adverse effects include fatigue, dizziness, nausea, vomiting, abdominal pain, and rashes. In onchocerciasis treatment, adverse effects are principally from the killing of microfilariae and can include fever, headache, dizziness, somnolence, weakness, rash, increased pruritus, diarrhea, joint and muscle pains, hypotension, tachycardia, lymphadenitis, lymphangitis, and peripheral edema. This reaction starts on the first day and peaks on the second day after treatment. This reaction occurs in 5–30% of persons and is generally mild, but it may be more frequent and more severe in individuals who are not long-term residents of onchocerciasis-endemic areas. A more intense reaction occurs in 1–3% of persons and a severe reaction in 0.1%, including high fever, hypotension, and bronchospasm. Corticosteroids are indicated in these cases, at times for several days. Toxicity diminishes with repeated dosing. Swellings and abscesses occasionally occur at 1–3 weeks, presumably at sites of adult worms.

Some patients develop corneal opacities and other eye lesions several days after treatment. These are rarely severe and generally resolve without corticosteroid treatment.

It is best to avoid concomitant use of ivermectin with other drugs that enhance GABA activity, eg, barbiturates, benzodiazepines, and valproic acid. Ivermectin should not be used during pregnancy. Safety in children younger than 5 years has not been established.

MEBENDAZOLE

Mebendazole is a synthetic benzimidazole that has a wide spectrum of antihelminthic activity and a low incidence of adverse effects.

Basic Pharmacology

Less than 10% of orally administered mebendazole is absorbed. The absorbed drug is protein-bound (> 90%), is rapidly converted to inactive metabolites (primarily during its first pass in the liver), and has a half-life of 2–6 hours. It is excreted mostly in the urine, principally as decarboxylated derivatives. In addition, a portion of absorbed drug and its derivatives are excreted in the bile. Absorption is increased if the drug is ingested with a fatty meal.

Mebendazole probably acts by inhibiting microtubule synthesis; the parent drug appears to be the active form. Efficacy of the drug varies with gastrointestinal transit time, with intensity of infection, and perhaps with the strain of parasite. The drug kills hookworm, ascaris, and trichuris eggs.

Clinical Uses

Mebendazole is indicated for use in ascariasis, trichuriasis, hookworm and pinworm infections, and certain other helminthic infections. It can be taken before or after meals; the tablets should be chewed before swallowing. For pinworm infection, the dose is 100 mg once, repeated at 2 weeks. For ascariasis, trichuriasis, hookworm, and trichostrongylus infections, a dosage of 100 mg twice daily for 3 days is used for adults and for children older than 2 years of age. Cure rates are good for pinworm infections and ascariasis, but have been disappointing in recent studies of trichuriasis. Cure rates are also lower for hookworm infections, but a marked reduction in the worm burden occurs in those not cured. For intestinal capillariasis, mebendazole is used at a dosage of 200 mg twice daily for 21 or more days. In trichinosis, limited reports suggest efficacy against adult worms in the intestinal tract and tissue larvae. Treatment is three times daily, with fatty foods, at 200–400 mg per dose for 3 days and then 400–500 mg per dose for 10 days; corticosteroids should be coadministered for severe infections.

Adverse Reactions, Contraindications, & Cautions

Short-term mebendazole therapy for intestinal nematodes is nearly free of adverse effects. Mild nausea, vomiting, diarrhea, and abdominal pain have been reported infrequently. Rare side effects, usually with high-dose therapy, are hypersensitivity reactions (rash, urticaria), agranulocytosis, alopecia, and elevation of liver enzymes.

Mebendazole is teratogenic in animals and therefore contraindicated in pregnancy. It should be used with caution in children younger than 2 years of age because of limited experience and rare reports of convulsions in this age group. Plasma levels may be decreased by concomitant use of carbamazepine or phenytoin and increased by cimetidine. Mebendazole should be used with caution in patients with cirrhosis.

METRIFONATE (TRICHLORFON)

Metrifonate is a safe, low-cost alternative drug for the treatment of *Schistosoma haematobium* infections. It is not active against *S mansoni* or *S japonicum*. It is not available in the USA.

Basic Pharmacology

Metrifonate, an organophosphate compound, is rapidly absorbed after oral administration. After the standard oral dose, peak blood levels are reached in 1–2 hours; the half-life is about 1.5 hours. Clearance appears to be through nonenzymatic transformation to dichlorvos, its active metabolite. Metrifonate and dichlorvos are well distributed to the tissues and are completely eliminated in 24–48 hours.

The mode of action is thought to be related to cholinesterase inhibition. This inhibition temporarily paralyzes the adult worms, resulting in their shift from the bladder venous plexus to small arterioles of the lungs, where they are trapped, encased by the immune system, and die. The drug is not effective against *S haematobium* eggs; live eggs continue to pass in the urine for several months after all adult worms have been killed.

Clinical Uses

In the treatment of *S haematobium*, an oral dose of 7.5–10 mg/kg is given three times at 14-day intervals. Cure rates on this schedule are 44–93%, with marked reductions in egg counts in those not cured. Metrifonate was also effective as a prophylactic agent when given monthly to children in a highly endemic area, and it has been used in mass treatment programs. In mixed infections with *S haematobium* and *S mansoni*, metrifonate has been successfully combined with oxamniquine.

Adverse Reactions, Contraindications, & Cautions

Some studies note mild and transient cholinergic symptoms, including nausea and vomiting, diarrhea, abdominal pain, bronchospasm, headache, sweating, fatigue, weakness, dizziness, and vertigo. These symptoms may begin within 30 minutes and persist up to 12 hours.

Metrifonate should not be used after recent exposure to insecticides or drugs that might potentiate cholinesterase inhibition. Metrifonate is contraindicated in pregnancy.

NICLOSAMIDE

Niclosamide is a second-line drug for the treatment of most tapeworm infections, but it is not available in the USA.

Basic Pharmacology

Niclosamide is a salicylamide derivative. It appears to be minimally absorbed from the gastrointestinal tract—neither the drug nor its metabolites have been recovered from the blood or urine.

Adult worms (but not ova) are rapidly killed, presumably due to inhibition of oxidative phosphorylation or stimulation of ATPase activity.

Clinical Uses

The adult dose of niclosamide is 2 g once, given in the morning on an empty stomach. The tablets must be chewed thoroughly and then swallowed with water.

A. *Taenia saginata* (Beef Tapeworm), *T solium* (Pork Tapeworm), and *Diphyllobothrium latum* (Fish Tapeworm)

A single 2 g dose of niclosamide results in cure rates of over 85% for *D latum* and about 95% for *T saginata*. It is probably equally effective against *T solium*. Cysticercosis can theoretically occur after treatment of *T solium* infections, because viable ova are released into the gut lumen after digestion of segments, but no such cases have been reported.

B. Other Tapeworms

Most patients treated with niclosamide for *Hymenolepis diminuta* and *Dipylidium caninum* infections are cured with a 7-day course of treatment; a few require a second course. Praziquantel is superior for *Hymenolepis nana* (dwarf tapeworm) infection. Niclosamide is not effective against cysticercosis or hydatid disease.

C. Intestinal Fluke Infections

Niclosamide can be used as an alternative drug in the treatment of *Fasciolopsis buski*, *Heterophyes heterophyes*, and *Metagonimus yokogawai* infections. The standard dose is given every other day for three doses.

Adverse Reactions, Contraindications, & Cautions

Infrequent, mild, and transitory adverse events include nausea, vomiting, diarrhea, and abdominal discomfort. The consumption of alcohol should be avoided on the day of treatment and for 1 day afterward. The safety of the drug has not been established in pregnancy or for children younger than 2 years of age.

OXAMNIQUINE

Oxamniquine is an alternative to praziquantel for the treatment of *S mansoni* infections. It has also been used extensively for mass treatment. It is not effective against *S haematobium* or *S japonicum*. It is not available in the USA.

Basic Pharmacology

Oxamniquine, a semisynthetic tetrahydroquinoline, is readily absorbed orally; it should be taken with food. Its plasma half-life is about 2.5 hours. The drug is extensively metabolized to inactive metabolites and excreted in the urine—up to 75% in the first 24 hours. Intersubject variations in serum concentration have been noted, which may explain some treatment failures.

Oxamniquine is active against both mature and immature stages of *S mansoni* but does not appear to be cercaricidal. The mechanism of action is unknown. Contraction and paralysis of the worms results in detachment from terminal venules in the mesentery and transit to the liver, where many die; surviving females return to the mesenteric vessels but cease to lay eggs. Strains of *S mansoni* in different parts of the world vary in susceptibility. Oxamniquine has been effective in instances of praziquantel resistance.

Clinical Uses

Oxamniquine is safe and effective in all stages of *S mansoni* disease, including advanced hepatosplenomegaly. In the acute (Katayama) syndrome, treatment results in disappearance of acute symptoms and clearance of the infection. The drug is generally less effective in children, who require higher doses than adults. It is better tolerated with food.

Optimal dosage schedules vary for different regions of the world. In the western hemisphere and western Africa, the adult oxamniquine dosage is 12–15 mg/kg given once. In northern and southern Africa, standard schedules are 15 mg/kg twice daily for 2 days. In eastern Africa and the Arabian peninsula, standard dosage is 15–20 mg/kg twice in 1 day. Cure rates are 70–95%, with marked reduction in egg excretion in those not cured. In mixed schistosome infections, oxamniquine has been successfully used in combination with metrifonate.

Adverse Reactions, Contraindications, & Cautions

Mild symptoms, starting about 3 hours after a dose and lasting for several hours, occur in more than one third of patients. Central nervous system symptoms (dizziness, headache, drowsiness) are most common; nausea and vomiting, diarrhea, colic, pruritus, and urticaria also occur. Infrequent adverse effects are low-grade fever, an orange to red discoloration of the urine, proteinuria, microscopic hematuria, and a transient decrease in leukocytes. Seizures have been reported rarely.

Since the drug makes many patients dizzy or drowsy, it should be used with caution in patients whose work or activity requires mental alertness (eg, no driving for 24 hours). It should be used with caution in those with a history of epilepsy. Oxamniquine is contraindicated in pregnancy.

PIPERAZINE

Piperazine is an alternative for the treatment of ascariasis, with cure rates over 90% when taken for 2 days, but it is not recommended for other helminth infections. Piperazine is available as the hexahydrate and as a variety of salts. It is readily absorbed, and maximum plasma levels are reached in 2–4 hours. Most of the drug is excreted unchanged in the urine in 2–6 hours, and excretion is complete within 24 hours.

Piperazine causes paralysis of ascaris by blocking acetylcholine at the myoneural junction; unable to maintain their position in the host, live worms are expelled by normal peristalsis.

For ascariasis, the dosage of piperazine (as the hexahydrate) is 75 mg/kg (maximum dose, 3.5 g) orally once daily for 2 days. For heavy infections, treatment should be continued for 3–4 days or repeated after 1 week.

Occasional mild adverse effects include nausea, vomiting, diarrhea, abdominal pain, dizziness, and headache. Neurotoxicity and allergic reactions are rare. Piperazine compounds should not be given to women during pregnancy, to patients with impaired renal or hepatic function, or to those with a history of epilepsy or chronic neurologic disease.

PRAZIQUANTEL

Praziquantel is effective in the treatment of schistosome infections of all species and most other trematode and cestode infections, including cysticercosis. The drug's safety and effectiveness as a single oral dose have also made it useful in mass treatment of several infections.

Basic Pharmacology

Praziquantel is a synthetic isoquinoline-pyrazine derivative. It is rapidly absorbed, with a bioavailability of about 80% after oral administration. Peak serum concentrations are reached 1–3 hours after a therapeutic dose. Cerebrospinal fluid concentrations of praziquantel reach 14–20% of the drug's plasma concentration. About 80% of the drug is bound to plasma proteins. Most of the drug is rapidly metabolized to inactive mono- and polyhydroxylated products after a first pass in the liver. The half-life is 0.8–1.5 hours. Excretion is mainly via the kidneys (60–80%) and bile (15–35%). Plasma concentrations of praziquantel increase when the drug is taken with a high-carbohydrate meal or with cimetidine; bioavailability is markedly reduced with some antiepileptics (phenytoin, carbamazepine) or with corticosteroids.

Praziquantel appears to increase the permeability of trematode and cestode cell membranes to calcium, resulting in paralysis, dislodgement, and death. In schistosome infections of experimental animals, praziquantel is effective against adult worms and immature stages, and it has a prophylactic effect against cercarial infection.

Clinical Uses

Praziquantel tablets are taken with liquid after a meal; they should be swallowed without chewing because their bitter taste can induce retching and vomiting.

A. Schistosomiasis

Praziquantel is the drug of choice for all forms of schistosomiasis. The dosage is 20 mg/kg per dose for two (*S mansoni* and *S haematobium*) or three (*S japonicum* and *S mekongi*) doses at intervals of 4–6 hours. High cure rates (75–95%) are achieved when patients are evaluated at 3–6 months; there is marked reduction in egg counts in those not cured. The drug is effective in adults and children and is generally well tolerated by patients in the hepatosplenic stage of advanced disease. There is no standard regimen for acute schistosomiasis (Katayama syndrome), but standard doses as described above, often with corticosteroids to limit inflammation from the acute immune response and dying worms, are recommended. Increasing evidence indicates rare *S mansoni* drug resistance, which may be countered with extended courses of therapy (eg, 3–6 days at standard dosing) or treatment with oxamniquine. Effectiveness of praziquantel for chemoprophylaxis has not been established.

B. Clonorchiasis, Opisthorchiasis, and Paragonimiasis

Standard dosing is 25 mg/kg three times daily for 2 days for each of these fluke infections.

C. Taeniasis and Diphyllobothriasis

A single dose of praziquantel, 5–10 mg/kg, results in nearly 100% cure rates for *T saginata*, *T solium*, and *D latum* infections. Because praziquantel does not kill eggs, it is theoretically possible that larvae of *T solium* released from eggs in the large bowel could penetrate the intestinal wall and give rise to cysticercosis, but this hazard is probably minimal.

D. Neurocysticercosis

Albendazole is now the preferred drug, but when it is not appropriate or available, praziquantel has similar efficacy. Indications for praziquantel are similar to those for albendazole. The praziquantel dosage is 100 mg/kg/d in three divided doses for 1 day, then 50 mg/kg/d to complete a 2- to 4-week course. Clinical responses to therapy vary from dramatic improvements of seizures and other neurologic findings to no response and even progression of the disease. Praziquantel—but not albendazole—has diminished bioavailability when taken concurrently with a corticosteroid. Recommendations on use of both antihelminthics and corticosteroids in neurocysticercosis vary.

E. *Hymenolepis nana*

Praziquantel is the drug of choice for *H nana* infections and the first drug to be highly effective. A single dose of 25 mg/kg is taken initially and repeated in 1 week.

F. Hydatid Disease

In hydatid disease, praziquantel kills protoscoleces but does not affect the germinal membrane. Praziquantel is being evaluated as an adjunct with albendazole pre- and postsurgery. In addition to its direct action, praziquantel enhances the plasma concentration of albendazole.

G. Other Parasites

Limited trials at a dosage of 25 mg/kg three times daily for 1–2 days indicate effectiveness of praziquantel against fasciolopsiasis, metagonimiasis, and other forms of heterophyiasis. Praziquantel was not effective for fascioliasis, however, even at dosages as high as 25 mg/kg three times daily for 3–7 days.

Adverse Reactions, Contraindications, & Cautions

Mild and transient adverse effects are common. They begin within several hours after ingestion of praziquantel and may persist for about 1 day. Most common are headache, dizziness, drowsiness, and lassitude; others include nausea, vomiting, abdominal pain, loose stools, pruritus, urticaria, arthralgia, myalgia, and low-grade fever. Mild and transient elevations of liver enzymes have been reported. Several days after starting praziquantel, low-grade fever, pruritus, and skin rashes (macular and urticarial), sometimes associated with worsened eosinophilia, may occur, probably due to the release of proteins from dying worms rather than direct drug toxicity. The intensity and frequency of adverse effects increase with dosage such that they occur in up to 50% of patients who receive 25 mg/kg three times in 1 day.

In neurocysticercosis, neurologic abnormalities may be exacerbated by inflammatory reactions around dying parasites. Common findings in patients who do not receive corticosteroids, usually presenting during or shortly after therapy, are headache, meningismus, nausea, vomiting, mental changes, and seizures (often accompanied by increased cerebrospinal fluid pleocytosis). More serious findings, including arachnoiditis, hyperthermia, and intracranial hypertension, may also occur. Corticosteroids are commonly used with praziquantel in the treatment of neurocysticercosis to decrease the inflammatory reaction, but this is controversial and complicated by knowledge that corticosteroids decrease the plasma level of praziquantel up to 50%. Praziquantel is contraindicated in ocular cysticercosis, because parasite destruction in the eye may cause irreparable damage. Some workers also caution against use of the drug in spinal neurocysticercosis.

The safety of praziquantel in children younger than age 4 years is not established, but no specific problems in young children have been documented. Indeed, the drug appears to be better tolerated in children than in adults. Praziquantel increased abortion rates in rats and therefore should be avoided in pregnancy if possible. Because the drug induces dizziness and drowsiness, patients should not drive during therapy and should be warned regarding activities requiring particular physical coordination or alertness.

PYRANTEL PAMOATE

Pyrantel pamoate is a broad-spectrum antihelminthic highly effective for the treatment of pinworm, ascaris, and *Trichostrongylus orientalis* infections. It is moderately effective against both species of hookworm. It is not effective in trichuriasis or strongyloidiasis. Oxantel pamoate, an analog of pyrantel not available in the USA, has been used successfully in the treatment of trichuriasis; the two drugs have been combined for their broad-spectrum antihelminthic activity.

Basic Pharmacology

Pyrantel pamoate is a tetrahydropyrimidine derivative. It is poorly absorbed from the gastrointestinal tract and active mainly against luminal organisms. Peak plasma levels are reached in 1–3 hours. Over half of the administered dose is recovered unchanged in the feces.

Pyrantel is effective against mature and immature forms of susceptible helminths within the intestinal tract but not against migratory stages in the tissues or against ova. The drug is a neuromuscular blocking agent that causes release of acetylcholine and inhibition of cholinesterase; this results in paralysis of worms, which is followed by expulsion.

Clinical Uses

The standard dose is 11 mg (base)/kg (maximum, 1 g), given orally once with or without food. For pinworm, the dose is repeated in 2 weeks, and cure rates are greater than 95%. The drug is available in the USA without prescription for this indication.

For ascariasis, a single dose yields cure rates of 85–100%. Treatment should be repeated if eggs are found 2 weeks after treatment. For hookworm infections, a single dose is effective against light infections; but for heavy infections, especially with *Necator americanus*, a 3-day course is necessary to reach 90% cure rates. A course of treatment can be repeated in 2 weeks.

Adverse Reactions, Contraindications, & Cautions

Adverse effects are infrequent, mild, and transient. They include nausea, vomiting, diarrhea, abdominal cramps, dizziness, drowsiness, headache, insomnia, rash, fever, and weakness. Pyrantel should be used with caution in patients with liver dysfunction, because low, transient aminotransferase elevations have been noted in a small number of patients. Experience with the drug in pregnant women and children younger than 2 years of age is limited.

THIABENDAZOLE

Thiabendazole is an alternative to ivermectin or albendazole for the treatment of strongyloidiasis and cutaneous larva migrans.

Basic Pharmacology

Thiabendazole is a benzimidazole compound. Although it is a chelating agent that forms stable complexes with a number of metals, including iron, it does not bind calcium.

Thiabendazole is rapidly absorbed after ingestion. With a standard dose, drug concentrations in plasma peak within 1–2 hours; the half-life is 1.2 hours. The drug is almost completely metabolized in the liver to the 5-hydroxy form; 90% is excreted in the urine in 48 hours, largely as the glucuronide or sulfonate conjugate. Thiabendazole can also be absorbed from the skin.

The mechanism of action of thiabendazole is probably the same as that of other benzimidazoles (see above). The drug has ovicidal effects against some parasites.

Clinical Uses

The standard dosage, 25 mg/kg (maximum 1.5 g) twice daily, should be given after meals. Tablets should be chewed. For strongyloides infection, treatment is for 2 days. Cure rates are reportedly 93%. A course can be repeated in 1 week if indicated. In patients with hyperinfection syndrome, the standard dose is continued twice daily for 5–7 days. For cutaneous larva migrans, thiabendazole cream can be applied topically, or the oral drug can be given for 2 days (although albendazole is less toxic and therefore preferred).

Adverse Reactions, Contraindications, & Cautions

Thiabendazole is much more toxic than other benzimidazoles and more toxic than ivermectin, so other agents are now preferred for most indications. Common adverse effects include dizziness, anorexia, nausea, and vomiting. Less common problems are epigastric pain, abdominal cramps, diarrhea, pruritus, headache, drowsiness, and neuropsychiatric symptoms. Irreversible liver failure and fatal Stevens-Johnson syndrome have been reported.

Experience with thiabendazole is limited in children weighing less than 15 kg. The drug should not be used in pregnancy or in the presence of hepatic or renal disease

PREPARATIONS AVAILABLE [1]

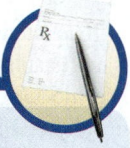

Albendazole (Albenza)

Oral: 200 mg tablets; 100 mg/5 mL suspension

Note: Albendazole is approved in the USA for the treatment of cysticercosis and hydatid disease.

Bithionol (Bitin)[1]

Diethylcarbamazine (Hetrazan)

Oral: 50 mg tablets

Ivermectin (Mectizan, Stromectol)

Oral: 3, 6 mg tablets

Note: Ivermectin is approved for use in the USA for the treatment of onchocerciasis and strongyloidiasis. See Chapter 65 for comment on the unlabeled use of drugs.

Mebendazole (generic, Vermox)

Oral: 100 mg chewable tablets; outside the USA, 100 mg/5 mL suspension

Metrifonate (trichlorfon, Bilarcil)[1]

Niclosamide (Niclocide)[1]

Oxamniquine (Vansil, Mansil)[1]

Oxantel pamoate (Quantrel); oxantel/pyrantel pamoate (Telopar)

Oral: tablets containing 100 mg (base) of each drug; suspensions containing 20 or 50 mg (base) per mL

Note: Oxantel pamoate and oxantel/pyrantel pamoate are not available in the USA.

Piperazine (generic, Vermizine)[1]

Praziquantel (Biltricide; others outside the USA)

Oral: 600 mg tablets (other strengths outside the USA)

Pyrantel pamoate (Antiminth, Combantrin, Pin-rid, Pin-X)

Oral: 50 mg (base)/mL suspension; 180 mg; 62.5 mg (base) capsules (available without prescription in the USA)

Suramin (Bayer 205, others)[1]

Thiabendazole (Mintezol)

Oral: 500 mg chewable tablets; suspension, 500 mg/mL

[1]Additional information may be obtained from the Parasitic Disease Drug Service, Parasitic Diseases Branch, Centers for Disease Control and Prevention, Atlanta, Georgia, 30333. Telephone: (404) 639-3670.

REFERENCES

Bagheri H et al: Adverse drug reactions to anthelmintics. Ann Pharmacother 2004;38:383.

Basáñez MG et al: Effect of single-dose ivermectin on *Onchocerca volvulus*: A systematic review and meta-analysis. Lancet Infect Dis 2008;8:310.

Bethony J et al: Soil-transmitted helminth infections: Ascariasis, trichuriasis, and hookworm. Lancet 2006;367:1521.

Bockarie MJ et al: Efficacy of single-dose diethylcarbamazine compared with diethylcarbamazine combined with albendazole against *Wuchereria bancrofti* infection in Papua New Guinea. Am J Trop Med Hyg 2007;76:62.

Bockarie MJ et al: Mass treatment to eliminate filariasis in Papua New Guinea. N Engl J Med 2002;347:1841.

Craig P, Ito A: Intestinal cestodes. Curr Opin Infect Dis 2007;20:524.

Danso-Appiah A et al: Drugs for treating urinary schistosomiasis. Cochrane Database Syst Rev 2008:CD000053

Dayan AD: Albendazole, mebendazole and praziquantel. Review of non-clinical toxicity and pharmacokinetics. Acta Trop 2003;86:141.

Drugs for parasitic infections. Med Lett Drugs Ther 2007;(Suppl 1).

Flohr C et al: Low efficacy of mebendazole against hookworm in Vietnam: Two randomized controlled trials. Am J Trop Med Hyg 2007;76:732.

Fox LM: Ivermectin: Uses and impact 20 years on. Curr Opin Infect Dis 2006;19:588.

Garcia HH et al: Current consensus guidelines for treatment of neurocysticercosis. Clin Microbiol Rev 2002;15:747.

Garcia HH et al: A trial of antiparasitic treatment to reduce the rate of seizures due to cerebral cysticercosis. N Engl J Med 2004;350:249.

Horton J: Albendazole: A broad spectrum anthelminthic for treatment of individuals and populations. Curr Opin Infect Dis 2002;15:599.

Keiser J, Utzinger J: Efficacy of current drugs against soil-transmitted helminth infections: Systematic review and meta-analysis. JAMA 2008; 299:1937.

Matthaiou DK et al: Albendazole versus praziquantel in the treatment of neurocysticercosis: A meta-analysis of comparative trials. PLoS Negl Trop Dis 2008;2:e194.

Meltzer E et al: Eosinophilia among returning travelers: A practical approach. Am J Trop Med Hyg 2008;78:702.

Osei-Atweneboana MY: Prevalence and intensity of *Onchocerca volvulus* infection and efficacy of ivermectin in endemic communities in Ghana: A two-phase epidemiological study. Lancet 2007;369:2021.

Ramzy RM et al: Effect of yearly mass drug administration with diethylcarbamazine and albendazole on bancroftian filariasis in Egypt: A comprehensive assessment. Lancet 2006;367:992.

Reddy M et al: Oral drug therapy for multiple neglected tropical diseases: A systematic review. JAMA 2007;298:1911.

Smego RA Jr, Sebanego P: Treatment options for hepatic cystic echinococcosis. Int J Infect Dis 2005;9:69.

Supali T et al: Doxycycline treatment of *Brugia malayi*-infected persons reduces microfilaremia and adverse reactions after diethylcarbamazine and albendazole treatment. Clin Infect Dis 2008;46:1385.

Taylor MJ et al: Macrofilaricidal activity after doxycycline treatment of *Wuchereria bancrofti*: A double-blind, randomised placebo-controlled trial. Lancet 2005;365:2116.

Tisch DJ, Michael E, Kazura JW: Mass chemotherapy options to control lymphatic filariasis: A systematic review. Lancet Infect Dis 2005;5:514.

Udall DN: Recent updates on onchocerciasis: Diagnosis and treatment. Clin Infect Dis 2007;44:53.

CASE STUDY ANSWER

The presentation is highly suggestive of cystic hydatid disease (infection with *Echinococcus granulosis*), which is transmitted by eggs from the feces of dogs in contact with livestock. Other causes of liver fluid collections include amebic and pyogenic abscesses, but these are usually not cystic in appearance. For echinococcosis, a typical cystic lesion and positive serology support the diagnosis, and treatment generally entails albendazole in conjunction with cautious surgery or percutaneous aspiration. One approach entails treatment with albendazole followed by aspiration to confirm the diagnosis and, if it is confirmed, to remove most of the infecting worms.

Cancer Chemotherapy

54

Edward Chu, MD, &
Alan C. Sartorelli, PhD

CASE STUDY

A 55-year-old man presents with increasing fatigue, 15-pound weight loss, and a microcytic anemia. Colonoscopy identifies a mass in the ascending colon, and biopsy specimens reveal well-differentiated colorectal cancer (CRC). He undergoes surgical resection and is found to have high-risk stage III CRC with five positive lymph nodes. After surgery, he feels entirely well with no symptoms. Of note, he has no other comorbid illnesses. What is this patient's prognosis? Should he receive adjuvant chemotherapy? The patient receives a combination of 5-fluorouracil (5-FU), leucovorin, and oxaliplatin as adjuvant therapy. One week after receiving the first cycle of therapy, he experiences significant toxicity in the form of myelosuppression, diarrhea, and altered mental status. What is the most likely explanation for this increased toxicity? Is there any role for genetic testing to determine the etiology of this level of toxicity?

Cancer continues to be the second leading cause of mortality from disease in the USA, accounting for nearly 500,000 deaths in 2008. Cancer is a disease characterized by a loss in the normal control mechanisms that govern cell survival, proliferation, and differentiation. Cells that have undergone neoplastic transformation usually express cell surface antigens that may be of normal fetal type, may display other signs of apparent immaturity, and may exhibit qualitative or quantitative chromosomal abnormalities, including various translocations and the appearance of amplified gene sequences. It is now well established that a small subpopulation of cells, referred to as tumor stem cells, reside within a tumor mass. They retain the ability to undergo repeated cycles of proliferation as well as to migrate to distant sites in the body to colonize various organs in the process called metastasis. Such tumor stem cells thus can express clonogenic (colony-forming) capability, and they are characterized by chromosome abnormalities reflecting their genetic instability, which leads to progressive selection of subclones that can survive more readily in the multicellular environment of the host. This genetic instability also allows them to become resistant to chemotherapy and radiotherapy. The invasive and metastatic processes as well as a series of metabolic abnormalities associated with the cancer result in tumor-related symptoms and eventual death of the patient unless the neoplasm can be eradicated with treatment.

CAUSES OF CANCER

The incidence, geographic distribution, and behavior of specific types of cancer are related to multiple factors, including sex, age, race, genetic predisposition, and exposure to environmental carcinogens. Of these factors, **environmental exposure** is probably most important. Exposure to ionizing radiation has been well documented as a significant risk factor for a number of cancers, including acute leukemias, thyroid cancer, breast cancer, lung cancer, soft tissue sarcoma, and basal cell and squamous cell skin cancers. Chemical carcinogens (particularly those in tobacco smoke) as well as azo dyes, aflatoxins, asbestos, benzene, and radon have all been well documented as leading to a wide range of human cancers.

Several **viruses** have been implicated in the etiology of various human cancers. For example, hepatitis B and hepatitis C are associated with the development of hepatocellular cancer; HIV is associated with Hodgkin's and non-Hodgkin's lymphomas; human papillomavirus is associated with cervical cancer and head and neck cancer; and Ebstein-Barr virus is associated with nasopharyngeal cancer. Expression of virus-induced neoplasia may also depend on additional host and environmental factors that modulate the transformation process. Cellular genes are known that are homologous to the transforming genes of the retroviruses, a family

ACRONYMS

ABVD	Doxorubicin (Adriamycin, hydroxydaunorubicin), bleomycin, vinblastine, dacarbazine
CHOP	Cyclophosphamide, doxorubicin (hydroxydaunorubicin, Adriamycin), vincristine (Oncovin), prednisone
CMF	Cyclophosphamide, methotrexate, fluorouracil
COP	Cyclophosphamide, vincristine (Oncovin), prednisone
FAC	5-Fluorouracil, doxorubicin (Adriamycin, hydroxydaunorubicin), cyclophosphamide
FEC	5-Fluorouracil, epirubicin, cyclophosphamide
5-FU	5-Fluorouracil
FOLFIRI	5-Fluorouracil, leucovorin, irinotecan
FOLFOX	5-Fluorouracil, leucovorin, oxaliplatin
MP	Melphalan, prednisone
6-MP	6-Mercaptopurine
MOPP	Mechlorethamine, vincristine (Oncovin), procarbazine, prednisone
MTX	Methotrexate
PCV	Procarbazine, lomustine, vincristine
PEB	Cisplatin (platinum), etoposide, bleomycin
6-TG	6-Thioguanine
VAD	Vincristine, doxorubicin (Adriamycin), dexamethasone
XELOX	Capecitabine, oxaliplatin

of RNA viruses, and induce oncogenic transformation. These mammalian cellular genes, known as **oncogenes,** have been shown to code for specific growth factors and their corresponding receptors. These genes may be amplified (increased number of gene copies) or mutated, both of which can lead to constitutive overexpression in malignant cells. The *bcl-2* family of genes represents a series of pro-survival genes that promotes survival by directly inhibiting apoptosis, a key pathway of programmed cell death.

Another class of genes, known as **tumor suppressor genes,** may be deleted or mutated, which gives rise to the neoplastic phenotype. The *p53* gene is the best-established tumor suppressor gene identified to date, and the normal wild-type gene appears to play an important role in suppressing neoplastic transformation. Of note, *p53* is mutated in up to 50% of all human solid tumors, including liver, breast, colon, lung, cervix, bladder, prostate, and skin.

CANCER TREATMENT MODALITIES

With present methods of treatment, about one third of patients are cured with local treatment strategies, such as surgery or radiotherapy, when the tumor remains localized at the time of diagnosis. Earlier diagnosis might lead to increased cure rates with such local treatment. In the remaining cases, however, early micrometastasis is a characteristic feature, indicating that a systemic approach with chemotherapy is required for effective cancer management. In patients with locally advanced disease, chemotherapy

is often combined with radiotherapy to allow for surgical resection to take place, and such a combined modality approach has led to improved clinical outcomes. At present, about 50% of patients who are initially diagnosed with cancer can be cured. In contrast, chemotherapy alone is able to cure less than 10% of all cancer patients when the tumor is diagnosed at an advanced stage.

Chemotherapy is presently used in three main clinical settings: (1) primary induction treatment for advanced disease or for cancers for which there are no other effective treatment approaches, (2) neoadjuvant treatment for patients who present with localized disease, for whom local forms of therapy such as surgery or radiation, or both, are inadequate by themselves, (3) adjuvant treatment to local methods of treatment, including surgery, radiation therapy, or both.

Primary induction chemotherapy refers to chemotherapy administered as the primary treatment in patients who present with advanced cancer for which no alternative treatment exists. This has been the main approach in treating patients with advanced metastatic disease, and in most cases, the goals of therapy are to relieve tumor-related symptoms, improve overall quality of life, and prolong time to tumor progression. Studies in a wide range of solid tumors have shown that chemotherapy in patients with advanced disease confers survival benefit when compared with supportive care, providing sound rationale for the early initiation of drug treatment. However, cancer chemotherapy can be curative in only a small subset of patients who present with advanced disease. In adults, these curable cancers include Hodgkin's and non-Hodgkin's lymphoma, acute myelogenous leukemia, germ cell cancer, and choriocarcinoma, while the curable childhood cancers include acute lymphoblastic leukemia, Burkitt's lymphoma, Wilms' tumor, and embryonal rhabdomyosarcoma.

Neoadjuvant chemotherapy refers to the use of chemotherapy in patients who present with localized cancer for which alternative local therapies, such as surgery, exist but which are less than completely effective. At present, neoadjuvant therapy is most often administered in the treatment of anal cancer, bladder cancer, breast cancer, esophageal cancer, laryngeal cancer, locally advanced non-small cell lung cancer, and osteogenic sarcoma. For some of these diseases, such as anal cancer, gastroesophageal cancer, laryngeal cancer, and non-small cell lung cancer, optimal clinical benefit is derived when chemotherapy is administered with radiation therapy either concurrently or sequentially.

One of the most important roles for cancer chemotherapy is as an adjuvant to local treatment modalities such as surgery or radiation therapy, and this has been termed **adjuvant chemotherapy.** The goal of chemotherapy in this setting is to reduce the incidence of both local and systemic recurrence and to improve the overall survival of patients. In general, chemotherapy regimens with clinical activity against advanced disease may have curative potential following surgical resection of the primary tumor, provided the appropriate dose and schedule are administered. Adjuvant chemotherapy is effective in prolonging both disease-free survival (DFS) and overall survival (OS) in patients with breast cancer, colon cancer, gastric cancer, non-small cell lung cancer, Wilms' tumor, anaplastic astrocytoma, and osteogenic sarcoma. Patients with primary malignant melanoma at high risk of local recurrence or systemic metastases derive clinical benefit from adjuvant treatment with the biologic agent α-interferon, although this treatment must be given for 1 year's duration for maximal clinical efficacy. Finally, the antihormonal agents tamoxifen, anastrozole, and letrozole are effective in the adjuvant therapy of postmenopausal women with early-stage breast cancer whose breast tumors express the estrogen receptor (see Chapter 40 for additional detail). However, because these agents are cytostatic rather than cytocidal, they must be administered on a long-term basis, with the standard recommendation being 5 years' duration.

ROLE OF CELL CYCLE KINETICS & ANTICANCER EFFECT

The key principles of cell cycle kinetics were initially developed using the murine L1210 leukemia as the experimental model system (Figure 54–1). However, drug treatment of human cancers requires a clear understanding of the differences between the characteristics of this rodent leukemia and of human cancers, as well as an understanding of the differences in growth rates of normal target tissues between mice and humans. For example, L1210 is a rapidly growing leukemia with a high percentage of cells synthesizing DNA, as measured by the uptake of tritiated thymidine (the labeling index). Because L1210 leukemia has a growth fraction of 100% (ie, all its cells are actively progressing through the cell cycle), its life cycle is consistent and predictable. Based on the murine L1210 model, the cytotoxic effects of anticancer drugs follow log cell-kill kinetics. As such, a given agent would be predicted to kill a constant fraction of cells as opposed to a constant number.

Thus, if a particular dose of an individual drug leads to a 3 log kill of cancer cells and reduces the tumor burden from 10^{10} to 10^{7} cells, the same dose used at a tumor burden of 10^{5} cells reduces the tumor mass to 10^{2} cells. Cell kill is, therefore, proportional, regardless of tumor burden. The cardinal rule of chemotherapy—the invariable inverse relation between cell number and curability—was established with this model, and this relationship is applicable to other hematologic malignancies.

Although growth of murine leukemias simulates exponential cell kinetics, mathematical modeling data suggest that most human solid tumors do not grow in such an exponential manner. Taken together, the experimental data in human solid cancers support a Gompertzian model of tumor growth and regression. The critical distinction between Gompertzian and exponential growth is that the growth fraction of the tumor is not constant with Gompertzian kinetics but instead decreases exponentially with time (exponential growth is matched by exponential retardation of growth, due to blood supply limitations and other factors). The growth fraction peaks when the tumor is approximately one third its maximum size. Under the Gompertzian model, when a patient with advanced cancer is treated, the tumor mass is larger, its growth fraction is low, and the fraction of cells killed is, therefore, small. An important feature of Gompertzian growth is that response to chemotherapy in drug-sensitive tumors depends, in large measure, on where the tumor is in its particular growth curve.

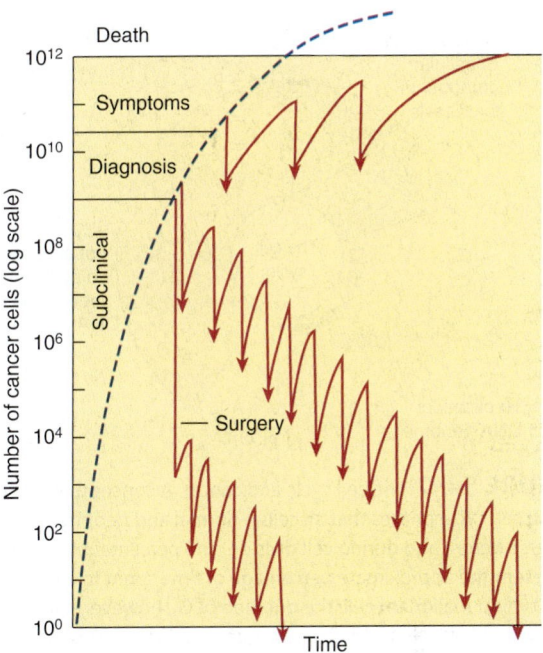

FIGURE 54–1 The log-kill hypothesis. Relationship of tumor cell number to time of diagnosis, symptoms, treatment, and survival. Three alternative approaches to drug treatment are shown for comparison with the course of tumor growth when no treatment is given *(dashed line)*. In the protocol diagrammed at top, treatment (indicated by the arrows) is given infrequently, and the result is manifested as prolongation of survival but with recurrence of symptoms between courses of treatment and eventual death of the patient. The combination chemotherapy treatment diagrammed in the middle section is begun earlier and is more intensive. Tumor cell kill exceeds regrowth, drug resistance does not develop, and "cure" results. In this example, treatment has been continued long after all clinical evidence of cancer has disappeared (1–3 years). This approach has been established as effective in the treatment of childhood acute leukemia, testicular cancers, and Hodgkin's lymphoma. In the treatment diagrammed near the bottom of the graph, early surgery has been employed to remove the primary tumor and intensive adjuvant chemotherapy has been administered long enough (up to 1 year) to eradicate the remaining tumor cells that comprise the occult micrometastases.

Information on cell and population kinetics of cancer cells explains, in part, the limited effectiveness of most available anticancer drugs. A schematic summary of cell cycle kinetics is presented in Figure 54–2. This information is relevant to the mode of action, indications, and scheduling of cell cycle-specific (CCS) and cell cycle-nonspecific (CCNS) drugs. Agents falling into these two major classes are summarized in Table 54–1.

The Role of Drug Combinations

With rare exceptions (eg, choriocarcinoma and Burkitt's lymphoma), single drugs at clinically tolerable doses have been unable to cure cancer. In the 1960s and early 1970s, drug combination regimens were developed based on the known biochemical actions

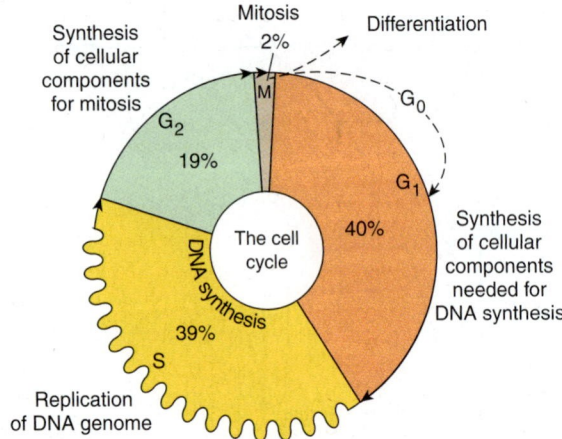

FIGURE 54–2 The cell cycle and cancer. A conceptual depiction of the cell cycle phases that all cells—normal and neoplastic—must traverse before and during cell division. The percentages given represent the approximate percentage of time spent in each phase by a typical malignant cell; the duration of G_1, however, can vary markedly. Many of the effective anticancer drugs exert their action on cells traversing the cell cycle and are called cell cycle-specific (CCS) drugs (see Table 54–1). A second group of agents called cell cycle-nonspecific (CCNS) drugs can sterilize tumor cells whether they are cycling or resting in the G_0 compartment. CCNS drugs can kill both G_0 and cycling cells (although cycling cells are more sensitive).

TABLE 54–1 Cell cycle effects of major classes of anticancer drugs.

Cell Cycle-Specific (CCS) Agents	Cell Cycle-Nonspecific (CCNS) Agents
Antimetabolites (S phase)	**Alkylating agents**
Capecitabine	Altretamine
Cladribine	Bendamustine
Clofarabine	Busulfan
Cytarabine (ara-C)	Carmustine
Fludarabine	Chlorambucil
5-Fluorouracil (5-FU)	Cyclophosphamide
Gemcitabine	Dacarbazine
6-Mercaptopurine (6-MP)	Lomustine
Methotrexate (MTX)	Mechlorethamine
Nelarabine	Melphalan
Pralatrexate	Temozolomide
6-Thioguanine (6-TG)	Thiotepa
Epipodophyllotoxin (topoisomerase II inhibitor) (G_1–S phase)	**Antitumor antibiotics**
Etoposide	Dactinomycin
	Mitomycin
Taxanes (M phase)	**Camptothecins (topoisomerase I inhibitors)**
Albumin-bound paclitaxel	Irinotecan
Cabazitaxel	Topotecan
Paclitaxel	
Vinca alkaloids (M phase)	**Platinum analogs**
Vinblastine	Carboplatin
Vincristine	Cisplatin
Vinorelbine	Oxaliplatin
Antimicrotubule inhibitor (M phase)	**Anthracyclines**
Ixabepilone	Daunorubicin
Antitumor antibiotics (G_2–M phase)	Doxorubicin
Bleomycin	Epirubicin
	Idarubicin
	Mitoxantrone

of available anticancer drugs rather than on their clinical efficacy. Such regimens were, however, largely ineffective. The era of effective combination chemotherapy began when a number of active drugs from different classes became available for use in combination in the treatment of the acute leukemias and lymphomas. Following this initial success with hematologic malignancies, combination chemotherapy was extended to the treatment of solid tumors.

The use of combination chemotherapy is important for several reasons. First, it provides maximal cell kill within the range of toxicity tolerated by the host for each drug as long as dosing is not compromised. Second, it provides a broader range of interaction between drugs and tumor cells with different genetic abnormalities in a heterogeneous tumor population. Finally, it may prevent or slow the subsequent development of cellular drug resistance. The same principles apply to the therapy of chronic infections, such as HIV and tuberculosis.

Certain principles have guided the selection of drugs in the most effective drug combinations, and they provide a paradigm for the development of new drug therapeutic programs.

1. **Efficacy:** Only drugs known to be somewhat effective when used alone against a given tumor should be selected for use in combination. If available, drugs that produce complete remission in some fraction of patients are preferred to those that produce only partial responses.

2. **Toxicity:** When several drugs of a given class are available and are equally effective, a drug should be selected on the basis of toxicity that does not overlap with the toxicity of other drugs in the combination. Although such selection leads to a wider range of adverse effects, it minimizes the risk of a lethal effect caused by multiple insults to the same organ system by different drugs and allows dose intensity to be maximized.

3. **Optimum scheduling:** Drugs should be used in their optimal dose and schedule, and drug combinations should be given at consistent intervals. Because long intervals between cycles negatively affect dose intensity, the treatment-free interval between cycles should be the shortest time necessary for recovery of the most sensitive normal target tissue, which is usually the bone marrow.

4. **Mechanism of interaction:** There should be a clear understanding of the biochemical, molecular, and pharmacokinetic mechanisms of interaction between the individual drugs in a given combination, to allow for maximal effect. Omission of a drug from a combination may allow overgrowth by a tumor clone sensitive to that drug alone and resistant to other drugs in the combination.

5. **Avoidance of arbitrary dose changes:** An arbitrary reduction in the dose of an effective drug in order to add other less effective drugs may reduce the dose of the most effective agent below the threshold of effectiveness and destroy the ability of the combination to cure disease in a given patient.

Dosage Factors

Dose intensity is one of the main factors limiting the ability of chemotherapy or radiation therapy to achieve cure. The dose-response curve in biologic systems is usually sigmoidal in shape, with a threshold, a linear phase, and a plateau phase. For chemotherapy, therapeutic selectivity is dependent on the difference between the dose-response curves of normal and tumor tissues. In experimental animal models, the dose-response curve is usually steep in the linear phase, and a reduction in dose when the tumor is in the linear phase of the dose-response curve almost always results in a loss in the capacity to cure the tumor effectively before a reduction in the antitumor activity is observed. Although complete remissions continue to be observed with dose reduction as low as 20%, residual tumor cells may not be entirely eliminated, thereby allowing for eventual relapse. Because anticancer drugs are associated with toxicity, it is often appealing for clinicians to avoid acute toxicity by simply reducing the dose or by increasing the time interval between each cycle of treatment. However, such empiric modifications in dose represent a major cause of treatment failure in patients with drug-sensitive tumors.

A positive relationship between dose intensity and clinical efficacy has been documented in several solid tumors, including advanced ovarian, breast, lung, and colon cancers, as well as in hematologic malignancies, such as the lymphomas. At present, there are three main approaches to dose-intense delivery of chemotherapy. The first approach, **dose escalation,** involves increasing the doses of the respective anticancer agents. The second strategy is administration of anticancer agents in a dose-intense manner by **reducing the interval** between treatment cycles, while the third approach involves **sequential scheduling** of either single agents or of combination regimens. Each of these strategies is presently being applied to a wide range of solid cancers, including breast, colorectal, and non-small cell lung, and in general, such dose-intense regimens have significantly improved clinical outcomes.

DRUG RESISTANCE

A fundamental issue in cancer chemotherapy is the development of cellular drug resistance. Some tumor types, eg, malignant melanoma, renal cell cancer, and brain cancer, exhibit *primary* resistance, ie, absence of response on the first exposure, to currently available agents. The presence of inherent drug resistance was first proposed by Goldie and Coleman in the early 1980s and was thought to result from the genomic instability associated with the development of most cancers. For example, mutations in the *p53* tumor suppressor gene occur in up to 50% of all human tumors. Preclinical and clinical studies have shown that loss of *p53* function leads to resistance to radiation therapy as well as resistance to

a wide range of anticancer agents. Defects in the mismatch repair enzyme family, which are tightly linked to the development of familial and sporadic colorectal cancer, lead to resistance to several unrelated anticancer agents, including the fluoropyrimidines, the thiopurines, and cisplatin/carboplatin. In contrast to *primary* resistance, *acquired* resistance develops in response to exposure to a given anticancer agent. Experimentally, drug resistance can be highly specific to a single drug and is usually based on a specific change in the genetic machinery of a given tumor cell with amplification or increased expression of one or more genes. In other instances, a multidrug-resistant phenotype occurs, associated with increased expression of the *MDR1* gene, which encodes a cell surface transporter glycoprotein (P-glycoprotein, see Chapter 1). This form of drug resistance leads to enhanced drug efflux and reduced intracellular accumulation of a broad range of structurally unrelated anticancer agents, including the anthracyclines, vinca alkaloids, taxanes, camptothecins, epipodophyllotoxins, and even small molecule inhibitors, such as imatinib.

■ BASIC PHARMACOLOGY OF CANCER CHEMOTHERAPEUTIC DRUGS

ALKYLATING AGENTS

The major clinically useful alkylating agents (Figure 54–3) have a structure containing a bis(chloroethyl)amine, ethyleneimine, or nitrosourea moiety, and they are classified in several different groups. Among the bis(chloroethyl)amines, cyclophosphamide, mechlorethamine, melphalan, and chlorambucil are the most useful. Ifosfamide is closely related to cyclophosphamide but has a somewhat different spectrum of activity and toxicity. Thiotepa and busulfan are used to treat breast and ovarian cancer, and chronic myeloid leukemia, respectively. The major nitrosoureas are carmustine (BCNU) and lomustine (CCNU).

Mechanism of Action

As a class, the alkylating agents exert their cytotoxic effects via transfer of their alkyl groups to various cellular constituents. Alkylations of DNA within the nucleus probably represent the major interactions that lead to cell death. However, these drugs react chemically with sulfhydryl, amino, hydroxyl, carboxyl, and phosphate groups of other cellular nucleophiles as well. The general mechanism of action of these drugs involves intramolecular cyclization to form an ethyleneimonium ion that may directly or through formation of a carbonium ion transfer an alkyl group to a cellular constituent (Figure 54–4). In addition to alkylation, a secondary mechanism that occurs with nitrosoureas involves carbamoylation of lysine residues of proteins through formation of isocyanates.

The major site of alkylation within DNA is the N7 position of guanine; however, other bases are also alkylated albeit to lesser degrees, including N1 and N3 of adenine, N3 of cytosine, and O6 of guanine, as well as phosphate atoms and proteins associated with DNA. These interactions can occur on a single strand or on

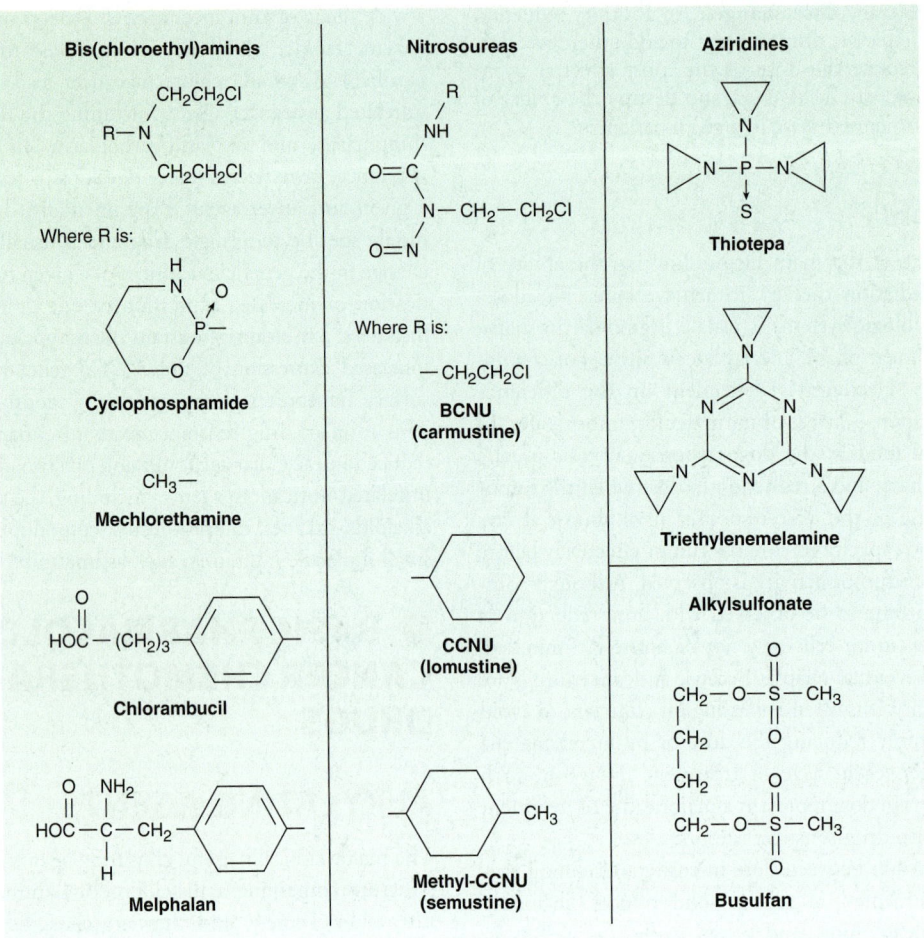

FIGURE 54–3 Structures of major classes of alkylating agents.

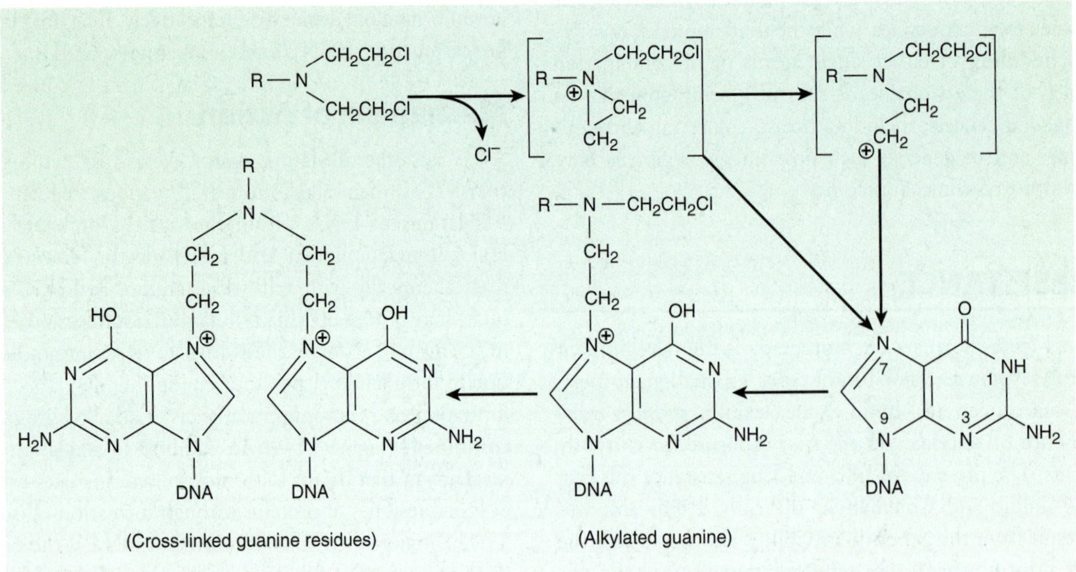

FIGURE 54–4 Mechanism of alkylation of DNA guanine. A bis(chloroethyl)amine forms an ethyleneimonium ion that reacts with a base such as N7 of guanine in DNA, producing an alkylated purine. Alkylation of a second guanine residue, through the illustrated mechanism, results in cross-linking of DNA strands.

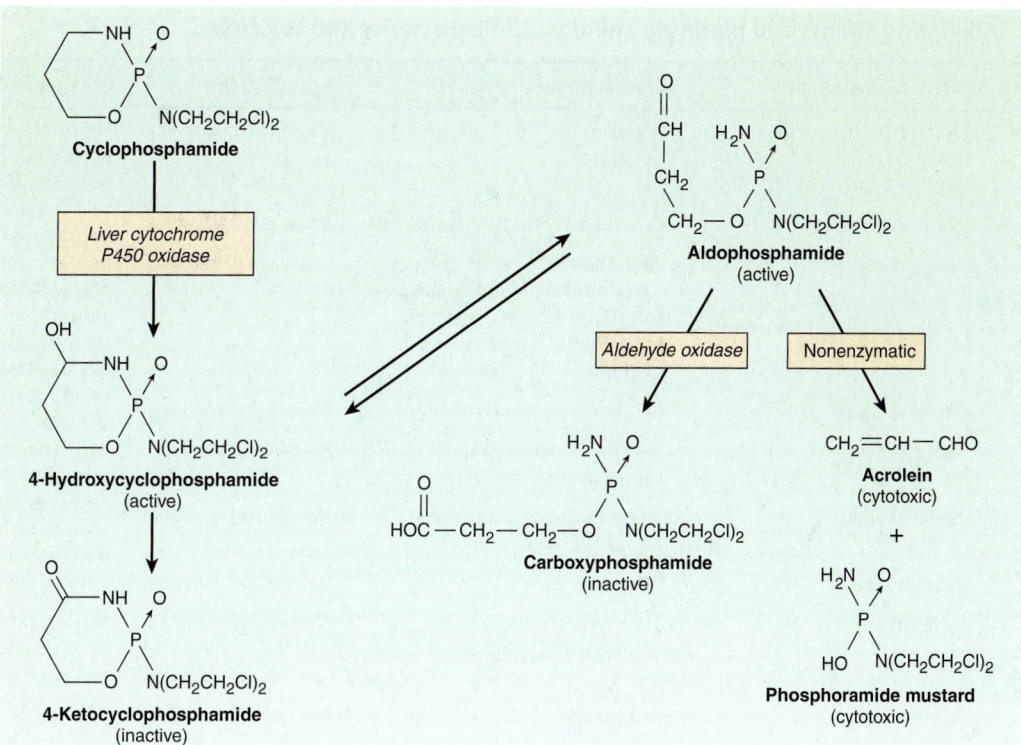

FIGURE 54–5 Cyclophosphamide metabolism.

both strands of DNA through cross-linking, as most major alkylating agents are bifunctional, with two reactive groups. Alkylation of guanine can result in miscoding through abnormal base pairing with thymine or in depurination by excision of guanine residues. The latter effect leads to DNA strand breakage through scission of the sugar-phosphate backbone of DNA. Cross-linking of DNA appears to be of major importance to the cytotoxic action of alkylating agents, and replicating cells are most susceptible to these drugs. Thus, although alkylating agents are not cell cycle specific, cells are most susceptible to alkylation in late G_1 and S phases of the cell cycle.

Resistance

The mechanism of acquired resistance to alkylating agents may involve increased capability to repair DNA lesions, decreased transport of the alkylating drug into the cell, and increased expression or activity of glutathione and glutathione-associated proteins, which are needed to conjugate the alkylating agent, or increased glutathione S-transferase activity, which catalyzes the conjugation.

Adverse Effects

The adverse effects usually associated with alkylating agents are generally dose-related and occur primarily in rapidly growing tissues such as bone marrow, gastrointestinal tract, and reproductive system. Nausea and vomiting can be a serious issue with a number of these agents. In addition, they are potent vesicants and can damage tissues at the site of administration as well as produce systemic toxicity. As a class, alkylating agents are carcinogenic in nature, and there is an increased risk of secondary malignancies, especially acute myelogenous leukemia.

Cyclophosphamide is one of the most widely used alkylating agents. One of the potential advantages of this compound relates to its high oral bioavailability. As a result, it can be administered via the oral and intravenous routes with equal clinical efficacy. It is inactive in its parent form, and must be activated to cytotoxic forms by liver microsomal enzymes (Figure 54–5). The cytochrome P450 mixed-function oxidase system converts cyclophosphamide to 4-hydroxycyclophosphamide, which is in equilibrium with aldophosphamide. These active metabolites are delivered to both tumor and normal tissue, where nonenzymatic cleavage of aldophosphamide to the cytotoxic forms—phosphoramide mustard and acrolein—occurs. The liver appears to be protected through the enzymatic formation of the inactive metabolites 4-ketocyclophosphamide and carboxyphosphamide.

The major toxicities of the individual alkylating agents are outlined in Table 54–2 and discussed below.

NITROSOUREAS

These drugs appear to be non-cross-resistant with other alkylating agents; all require biotransformation, which occurs by nonenzymatic decomposition, to metabolites with both alkylating and carbamoylating activities. The nitrosoureas are highly lipid-soluble and are able to cross the blood-brain barrier, making them effective

TABLE 54–2 Alkylating agents and platinum analogs: Clinical activity and toxicities.

Alkylating Agent	Mechanism of Action	Clinical Applications	Acute Toxicity	Delayed Toxicity
Mechlorethamine	Forms DNA cross-links, resulting in inhibition of DNA synthesis and function	Hodgkin's and non-Hodgkin's lymphoma	Nausea and vomiting	Moderate depression of peripheral blood count; excessive doses produce severe bone marrow depression with leukopenia, thrombocytopenia, and bleeding; alopecia and hemorrhagic cystitis occasionally occur with cyclophosphamide; cystitis can be prevented with adequate hydration; busulfan is associated with skin pigmentation, pulmonary fibrosis, and adrenal insufficiency
Chlorambucil	Same as above	CLL and non-Hodgkin's lymphoma	Nausea and vomiting	
Cyclophosphamide	Same as above	Breast cancer, ovarian cancer, non-Hodgkin's lymphoma, CLL, soft tissue sarcoma, neuroblastoma, Wilms' tumor, rhabdomyosarcoma	Nausea and vomiting	
Bendamustine	Same as above	CLL, non-Hodgkin's lymphoma	Nausea and vomiting	
Melphalan	Same as above	Multiple myeloma, breast cancer, ovarian cancer	Nausea and vomiting	
Thiotepa	Same as above	Breast cancer, ovarian cancer, superficial bladder cancer	Nausea and vomiting	
Busulfan	Same as above	CML	Nausea and vomiting	
Carmustine	Same as above	Brain cancer, Hodgkin's and non-Hodgkin's lymphoma	Nausea and vomiting	Myelosuppression; rarely interstitial lung disease and interstitial nephritis
Lomustine	Same as above	Brain cancer	Nausea and vomiting	
Altretamine	Same as above	Ovarian cancer	Nausea and vomiting	Myelosuppression, peripheral neuropathy, flu-like syndrome
Temozolomide	Methylates DNA and inhibits DNA synthesis and function	Brain cancer, melanoma	Nausea and vomiting, headache and fatigue	Myelosuppression, mild elevation in liver function tests, photosensitivity
Procarbazine	Methylates DNA and inhibits DNA synthesis and function	Hodgkin's and non-Hodgkin's lymphoma, brain tumors	Central nervous system depression	Myelosuppression, hypersensitivity reactions
Dacarbazine	Methylates DNA and inhibits DNA synthesis and function	Hodgkin's lymphoma, melanoma, soft tissue sarcoma	Nausea and vomiting	Myelosuppression, central nervous system toxicity with neuropathy, ataxia, lethargy, and confusion
Cisplatin	Forms intrastrand and interstrand DNA cross-links; binding to nuclear and cytoplasmic proteins	Non-small cell and small cell lung cancer, breast cancer, bladder cancer, cholangiocarcinoma, gastroesophageal cancer, head and neck cancer, ovarian cancer, germ cell cancer	Nausea and vomiting	Nephrotoxicity, peripheral sensory neuropathy, ototoxicity, nerve dysfunction
Carboplatin	Same as cisplatin	Non-small cell and small cell lung cancer, breast cancer, bladder cancer, head and neck cancer, ovarian cancer	Nausea and vomiting	Myelosuppression; rarely peripheral neuropathy, renal toxicity, hepatic dysfunction
Oxaliplatin	Same as cisplatin	Colorectal cancer, gastroesophageal cancer, pancreatic cancer	Nausea and vomiting, laryngopharyngeal dysesthesias	Myelosuppression, peripheral sensory neuropathy, diarrhea

CLL, chronic lymphocytic leukemia; CML, chronic myelogenous leukemia.

in the treatment of brain tumors. Although the majority of alkylations by the nitrosoureas are on the N7 position of guanine in DNA, the critical alkylation responsible for cytotoxicity appears to be on the O6 position of guanine, which leads to G-C crosslinks in DNA. After oral administration of lomustine, peak plasma levels of metabolites appear within 1–4 hours; central nervous system concentrations reach 30–40% of the activity present in the plasma. Urinary excretion appears to be the major route of elimination from the body. One naturally occurring sugar-containing nitrosourea, streptozocin, is interesting because it has minimal bone marrow toxicity. This agent has activity in the treatment of insulin-secreting islet cell carcinoma of the pancreas.

NONCLASSIC ALKYLATING AGENTS

Several other compounds have mechanisms of action that involve DNA alkylation as their cytotoxic mechanism of action. These agents include procarbazine, dacarbazine, and bendamustine. Their respective clinical activities and associated toxicities are listed in Table 54–2.

Procarbazine

Procarbazine is an orally active methylhydrazine derivative, and in the clinical setting, it is used in combination regimens for Hodgkin's and non-Hodgkin's lymphoma as well as brain tumors.

The precise mechanism of action of procarbazine is uncertain; however, it inhibits DNA, RNA, and protein biosynthesis; prolongs interphase; and produces chromosome breaks. Oxidative metabolism of this drug by microsomal enzymes generates azoprocarbazine and H_2O_2, which may be responsible for DNA strand scission. A variety of other drug metabolites are formed that may be cytotoxic. One metabolite is a weak monoamine oxidase (MAO) inhibitor, and adverse events can occur when procarbazine is given with other MAO inhibitors as well as with sympathomimetic agents, tricyclic antidepressants, antihistamines, central nervous system depressants, antidiabetic agents, alcohol, and tyramine-containing foods.

There is an increased risk of secondary cancers in the form of acute leukemia, and its carcinogenic potential is thought to be higher than that of most other alkylating agents.

Dacarbazine

Dacarbazine is a synthetic compound that functions as an alkylating agent following metabolic activation in the liver by oxidative N-demethylation to the monomethyl derivative. This metabolite spontaneously decomposes to diazomethane, which generates a methyl carbonium ion that is believed to be the key cytotoxic species. Dacarbazine is administered parenterally and is used in the treatment of malignant melanoma, Hodgkin's lymphoma, soft tissue sarcomas, and neuroblastoma. In terms of safety profile, the main dose-limiting toxicity is myelosuppression, but nausea and vomiting can be severe in some cases. This agent is a potent vesicant, and care must be taken to avoid extravasation during drug administration.

Bendamustine

Bendamustine is a bifunctional alkylating agent consisting of a purine benzimidazole ring and a nitrogen mustard moiety. As with other alkylating agents, it forms cross-links with DNA resulting in single- and double-stranded breaks, leading to inhibition of DNA synthesis and function. This molecule also inhibits mitotic checkpoints and induces mitotic catastrophe, which leads to cell death. Of note, the cross-resistance between bendamustine and other alkylating agents is only partial, thereby providing a rationale for its clinical activity despite the development of resistance to other alkylating agents. This agent is approved for use in chronic lymphocytic leukemia, with activity also observed in Hodgkin's and non-Hodgkin's lymphoma, multiple myeloma, and breast cancer. The main dose-limiting toxicities include myelosuppression and mild nausea and vomiting. Hypersensitivity infusion reactions, skin rash, and other skin reactions occur rarely.

PLATINUM ANALOGS

Three platinum analogs are currently used in clinical practice: cisplatin, carboplatin, and oxaliplatin. Cisplatin (cis-diamminedichloroplatinum [II]) is an inorganic metal complex that was initially discovered through a serendipitous observation that neutral platinum complexes inhibited division and filamentous growth of *Escherichia coli*. Several platinum analogs were subsequently synthesized. Although the precise mechanism of action of the platinum analogs is unclear, they are thought to exert their cytotoxic effects in the same manner as alkylating agents. As such, they kill tumor cells in all stages of the cell cycle and bind DNA through the formation of intrastrand and interstrand cross-links, thereby leading to inhibition of DNA synthesis and function. The primary binding site is the N7 position of guanine, but covalent interaction with the N3 position of adenine and O6 position of cytosine can also occur. In addition to targeting DNA, the platinum analogs have been shown to bind to both cytoplasmic and nuclear proteins, which may also contribute to their cytotoxic and antitumor effects. The platinum complexes appear to synergize with certain other anticancer drugs, including alkylating agents, fluoropyrimidines, and taxanes.

$$H_3N \quad \diagdown \quad Cl$$
$$Pt$$
$$H_3N \quad \diagup \quad Cl$$

Cisplatin

Cisplatin has major antitumor activity in a broad range of solid tumors, including non-small cell and small cell lung cancer, esophageal and gastric cancer, cholangiocarcinoma, head and neck cancer, and genitourinary cancers, particularly testicular, ovarian, and bladder cancer. When used in combination regimens, cisplatin-based therapy has led to the cure of nonseminomatous testicular cancer. Cisplatin and the other platinum analogs are extensively cleared by the kidneys and excreted in the urine. As a result, dose modification is required in patients with renal dysfunction.

Carboplatin is a second-generation platinum analog whose mechanisms of cytotoxic action, mechanisms of resistance, and clinical pharmacology are identical to those described for cisplatin.

As with cisplatin, carboplatin has broad-spectrum activity against a wide range of solid tumors. However, in contrast to cisplatin, it exhibits significantly less renal toxicity and gastrointestinal toxicity. Its main dose-limiting toxicity is myelosuppression. It has therefore been widely used in transplant regimens to treat refractory hematologic malignancies. Moreover, since vigorous intravenous hydration is not required for carboplatin therapy, carboplatin is viewed as an easier agent to administer to patients, and as such, it has replaced cisplatin in various combination chemotherapy regimens.

Oxaliplatin is a third-generation diaminocyclohexane platinum analog. Its mechanism of action and clinical pharmacology are identical to those of cisplatin and carboplatin. However, tumors that are resistant to cisplatin or carboplatin on the basis of mismatch repair defects are not cross-resistant to oxaliplatin, and this finding may explain the activity of this platinum compound in colorectal cancer. Oxaliplatin was initially approved for use as second-line therapy in combination with the fluoropyrimidine 5-fluorouracil (5-FU) and leucovorin, termed the FOLFOX regimen, for metastatic colorectal cancer. The FOLFOX regimen was subsequently (2005) approved for the first-line treatment of metastatic colorectal cancer. At this time, oxaliplatin-based chemotherapy has also been approved in the adjuvant therapy of high-risk stage II and stage III colon cancer. Clinical activity has been observed in other gastrointestinal cancers, such as pancreatic, gastroesophageal, and hepatocellular cancer. In the side effect profile, neurotoxicity is the main dose-limiting toxicity, and is manifested by a peripheral sensory neuropathy. There are two forms of neurotoxicity, an acute form that is often triggered and worsened by exposure to cold, and a chronic form that is dose-dependent. Although this chronic form is dependent on the cumulative dose of drug administered, it tends to be reversible, in contrast to cisplatin-induced neurotoxicity.

The major toxicities of the individual platinum analogs are outlined in Table 54–2.

ANTIMETABOLITES

The development of drugs with actions on intermediary metabolism of proliferating cells has been important both conceptually and clinically. While biochemical properties unique to all cancer cells have yet to be discovered, there are a number of quantitative differences in metabolism between cancer cells and normal cells that render cancer cells more sensitive to the antimetabolites. Many of these agents have been rationally designed and synthesized based on knowledge of critical cellular processes involved in DNA biosynthesis.

The individual antimetabolites and their respective clinical spectrum and toxicities are presented in Table 54–3 and are discussed below.

ANTIFOLATES

Methotrexate

Methotrexate (MTX) is a folic acid analog that binds with high affinity to the active catalytic site of dihydrofolate reductase (DHFR). This results in inhibition of the synthesis of tetrahydrofolate (THF),

the key one-carbon carrier for enzymatic processes involved in de novo synthesis of thymidylate, purine nucleotides, and the amino acids serine and methionine. Inhibition of these various metabolic processes thereby interferes with the formation of DNA, RNA, and key cellular proteins (see Figure 33–3). Intracellular formation of polyglutamate metabolites, with the addition of up to 5–7 glutamate residues, is critically important for the therapeutic action of MTX, and this process is catalyzed by the enzyme folylpolyglutamate synthase (FPGS). MTX polyglutamates are selectively retained within cancer cells, and they display increased inhibitory effects on enzymes involved in de novo purine nucleotide and thymidylate biosynthesis, making them important determinants of MTX's cytotoxic action.

Folic acid

Methotrexate

Resistance to MTX has been attributed to (1) decreased drug transport via the reduced folate carrier or folate receptor protein, (2) decreased formation of cytotoxic MTX polyglutamates, (3) increased levels of the target enzyme DHFR through gene amplification and other genetic mechanisms, and (4) altered DHFR protein with reduced affinity for MTX. Recent studies have suggested that decreased accumulation of drug through activation of the multidrug resistance transporter P170 glycoprotein may also result in drug resistance.

MTX is administered by the intravenous, intrathecal, or oral route. However, oral bioavailability is saturable and erratic at doses greater than 25 mg/m^2. Renal excretion is the main route of elimination and is mediated by glomerular filtration and tubular secretion. As a result, dose modification is required in the setting of renal dysfunction. Care must also be taken when MTX is used in the presence of drugs such as aspirin, nonsteroidal anti-inflammatory agents, penicillin, and cephalosporins, as these agents inhibit the renal excretion of MTX. The biologic effects of MTX can be reversed by administration of the reduced folate leucovorin (5-formyltetrahydrofolate) or by L-leucovorin, which is the active enantiomer. Leucovorin rescue is used in conjunction with high-dose MTX therapy to rescue normal cells from undue toxicity, and it has also been used in cases of accidental drug overdose. The main adverse effects are listed in Table 54–3.

TABLE 54–3 Antimetabolites: Clinical activity and toxicities.

Drug	Mechanism of Action	Clinical Applications	Toxicity
Capecitabine	Inhibits TS; incorporation of FUTP into RNA resulting in alteration in RNA processing; incorporation of FdUTP into DNA resulting in inhibition of DNA synthesis and function	Breast cancer, colorectal cancer, gastroesophageal cancer, hepatocellular cancer, pancreatic cancer	Diarrhea, hand-foot syndrome, myelosuppression, nausea and vomiting
5-Fluorouracil	Inhibits TS; incorporation of FUTP into RNA resulting in alteration in RNA processing; incorporation of FdUTP into DNA resulting in inhibition of DNA synthesis and function	Colorectal cancer, anal cancer, breast cancer, gastroesophageal cancer, head and neck cancer, hepatocellular cancer	Nausea, mucositis, diarrhea, bone marrow depression, neurotoxicity
Methotrexate	Inhibits DHFR; inhibits TS; inhibits de novo purine nucleotide synthesis	Breast cancer, head and neck cancer, osteogenic sarcoma, primary central nervous system lymphoma, non-Hodgkin's lymphoma, bladder cancer, choriocarcinoma	Mucositis, diarrhea, myelosuppression with neutropenia and thrombocytopenia
Pemetrexed	Inhibits TS, DHFR, and purine nucleotide synthesis	Mesothelioma, non-small cell lung cancer	Myelosuppression, skin rash, mucositis, diarrhea, fatigue, hand-foot syndrome
Cytarabine	Inhibits DNA chain elongation, DNA synthesis and repair; inhibits ribonucleotide reductase with reduced formation of dNTPs; incorporation of cytarabine triphosphate into DNA	AML, ALL, CML in blast crisis	Nausea and vomiting, myelosuppression with neutropenia and thrombocytopenia, cerebellar ataxia
Gemcitabine	Inhibits DNA synthesis and repair; inhibits ribonucleotide reductase with reduced formation of dNTPs; incorporation of gemcitabine triphosphate into DNA resulting in inhibition of DNA synthesis and function	Pancreatic cancer, bladder cancer, breast cancer, non-small cell lung cancer, ovarian cancer, non-Hodgkin's lymphoma, soft tissue sarcoma	Nausea, vomiting, diarrhea, myelosuppression
Fludarabine	Inhibits DNA synthesis and repair; inhibits ribonucleotide reductase; incorporation of fludarabine triphosphate into DNA; induction of apoptosis	Non-Hodgkin's lymphoma, CLL	Myelosuppression, immunosuppression, fever, myalgias, arthralgias
Cladribine	Inhibits DNA synthesis and repair; inhibits ribonucleotide reductase; incorporation of cladribine triphosphate into DNA; induction of apoptosis	Hairy cell leukemia, CLL, non-Hodgkin's lymphoma	Myelosuppression, nausea and vomiting, and immunosuppression
6-Mercaptopurine (6-MP)	Inhibits de novo purine nucleotide synthesis; incorporation of triphosphate into RNA; incorporation of triphosphate into DNA	AML	Myelosuppression, immunosuppression, and hepatotoxicity
6-Thioguanine	Same as 6-MP	ALL, AML	Same as above

ALL, acute lymphoblastic leukemia; AML, acute myelogenous leukemia; CLL, chronic lymphocytic leukemia; CML, chronic myelogenous leukemia; DHFR, dihydrofolate reductase; dNTP, deoxyribonucleotide triphosphate; FdUTP, 5-fluorodeoxyuridine-5′-triphosphate; FUTP, 5-fluorouridine-5′-triphosphate; TS, thymidine synthase.

Pemetrexed

Pemetrexed is a pyrrolopyrimidine antifolate analog with activity in the S phase of the cell cycle. As in the case of MTX, it is transported into the cell via the reduced folate carrier and requires activation by FPGS to yield higher polyglutamate forms. While this agent targets DHFR and enzymes involved in de novo purine nucleotide biosynthesis, its main mechanism of action is inhibition of thymidylate synthase. At present, this antifolate is approved for use in combination with cisplatin in the treatment of mesothelioma, as a single agent in the second-line therapy of non-small cell lung cancer, and in combination with cisplatin for the first-line treatment of non-small cell lung cancer. As with MTX, pemetrexed is mainly excreted in the urine, and dose modification is required in the setting of renal dysfunction. The main adverse effects include myelosuppression, skin rash, mucositis, diarrhea, fatigue, and hand-foot syndrome. Of note, vitamin supplementation with folic acid and vitamin B_{12} appear to reduce the toxicities associated with pemetrexed, while not interfering with clinical efficacy. The hand-foot syndrome is manifested by painful erythema and swelling of the hands and feet, and dexamethasone treatment has been shown to be effective in reducing the incidence and severity of this toxicity.

Pralatrexate

Pralatrexate is a 10-deaza-aminopterin antifolate analog, and as in the case of MTX, it is transported into the cell via the reduced folate carrier (RFC) and requires activation by FPGS to yield higher polyglutamate forms. However, this molecule was designed to be a more potent substrate for the RFC-1 carrier protein as well as an improved substrate for FPGS. It inhibits DHFR, inhibits enzymes involved in de novo purine nucleotide biosynthesis, and also inhibits thymidylate synthase. Although pralatrexate was originally developed for non-small lung cancer, it is presently approved for use in the treatment of relapsed or refractory peripheral T-cell lymphoma. As with the other antifolate analogs, pralatrexate is mainly excreted in the urine, and dose modification is required in the setting of renal dysfunction. The main adverse effects include myelosuppression, skin rash, mucositis, diarrhea, and fatigue. Vitamin supplementation with folic acid and vitamin B_{12} appear to reduce the toxicities associated with pralatrexate, while not interfering with clinical efficacy.

FLUOROPYRIMIDINES

5-Fluorouracil

5-Fluorouracil (5-FU) is inactive in its parent form and requires activation via a complex series of enzymatic reactions to ribosyl and deoxyribosyl nucleotide metabolites. One of these metabolites, 5-fluoro-2'-deoxyuridine-5'-monophosphate (FdUMP), forms a covalently bound ternary complex with the enzyme thymidylate synthase and the reduced folate 5,10-methylenetetrahydrofolate, a reaction critical for the de novo synthesis of thymidylate. This results in inhibition of DNA synthesis through "thymineless death." 5-FU is converted to 5-fluorouridine-5'-triphosphate (FUTP), which is then incorporated into RNA, where it interferes with RNA processing and mRNA translation. 5-FU is also converted to 5-fluorodeoxyuridine-5'-triphosphate (FdUTP), which can be incorporated into cellular DNA, resulting in inhibition of DNA synthesis and function. Thus, the cytotoxicity of 5-FU is thought to be the result of combined effects on both DNA- and RNA-mediated events.

5-FU is administered intravenously, and the clinical activity of this drug is highly schedule-dependent. Because of its extremely short half-life, on the order of 10–15 minutes, infusional schedules of administration have been generally favored over bolus schedules. Up to 80–85% of an administered dose of 5-FU is catabolized by the enzyme dihydropyrimidine dehydrogenase (DPD). Of note, a pharmacogenetic syndrome involving partial or complete deficiency of the DPD enzyme is seen in up to 5% of cancer patients; in this setting, severe toxicity in the form of myelosuppression, diarrhea, nausea and vomiting, and neurotoxicity is observed.

Uracil   5-FU

5-FU remains the most widely used agent in the treatment of colorectal cancer, both as adjuvant therapy and for advanced disease. It also has activity against a wide variety of solid tumors, including cancers of the breast, stomach, pancreas, esophagus, liver, head and neck, and anus. Major toxicities include myelosuppression, gastrointestinal toxicity in the form of mucositis and diarrhea, skin toxicity manifested by the hand-foot syndrome, and neurotoxicity.

Capecitabine

Capecitabine is a fluoropyrimidine carbamate prodrug with 70–80% oral bioavailability. It undergoes extensive metabolism in the liver by the enzyme carboxylesterase to an intermediate, 5'-deoxy-5-fluorocytidine. This metabolite is then converted to 5'-deoxy-5-fluorouridine by the enzyme cytidine deaminase. These two initial steps occur mainly in the liver. The 5'-deoxy-5-fluorouridine metabolite is finally hydrolyzed by thymidine phosphorylase to 5-FU directly in the tumor. The expression of thymidine phosphorylase has been shown to be significantly higher in a broad range of solid tumors than in corresponding normal tissue, particularly in breast cancer and colorectal cancer.

This oral fluoropyrimidine is used in the treatment of metastatic breast cancer either as a single agent or in combination with other anticancer agents, including docetaxel, paclitaxel, lapatinib, ixabepilone, and trastuzumab. It is also approved for use in the adjuvant therapy of stage III and high-risk stage II colon cancer as well as for treatment of metastatic colorectal cancer as monotherapy. At this time, significant efforts are directed at combining this agent with other active cytotoxic agents, including irinotecan and oxaliplatin. In Europe and Asia, the capecitabine/oxaliplatin (XELOX) regimen is approved for the first-line treatment of metastatic colorectal cancer, and this regimen is now widely used in the USA. The main toxicities of capecitabine include diarrhea and the hand-foot syndrome. While myelosuppression, nausea and vomiting, and mucositis are also observed with this agent, their incidence is significantly less than that observed with intravenous 5-FU.

DEOXYCYTIDINE ANALOGS

Cytarabine

Cytarabine (ara-C) is an S phase-specific antimetabolite that is converted by deoxycytidine kinase to the 5'-mononucleotide (ara-CMP). Ara-CMP is further metabolized to the diphosphate and triphosphate metabolites, and the ara-CTP triphosphate is felt to be the main cytotoxic metabolite. Ara-CTP competitively inhibits DNA polymerase-α and DNA polymerase-β, thereby resulting in blockade of DNA synthesis and DNA repair, respectively. This metabolite is also incorporated into RNA and DNA. Incorporation into DNA leads to interference with chain elongation and defective ligation of fragments of newly synthesized DNA. The cellular retention of ara-CTP appears to correlate with its lethality to malignant cells.

Cytosine
deoxyriboside

Cytosine
arabinoside
(cytarabine)

After intravenous administration, the drug is cleared rapidly, with most of an administered dose being deaminated to inactive forms. The stoichiometric balance between the level of activation and catabolism of cytarabine is important in determining its eventual cytotoxicity.

The clinical activity of cytarabine is highly schedule-dependent and because of its rapid degradation, it is usually administered via continuous infusion over a 5–7 day period. Its activity is limited exclusively to hematologic malignancies, including acute myelogenous leukemia and non-Hodgkin's lymphoma. This agent has absolutely no activity in solid tumors. The main adverse effects associated with cytarabine therapy include myelosuppression, mucositis, nausea and vomiting, and neurotoxicity when high-dose therapy is administered.

Gemcitabine

Gemcitabine is a fluorine-substituted deoxycytidine analog that is phosphorylated initially by the enzyme deoxycytidine kinase to the monophosphate form and then by other nucleoside kinases to the diphosphate and triphosphate nucleotide forms. The antitumor effect is considered to result from several mechanisms: inhibition of ribonucleotide reductase by gemcitabine diphosphate, which reduces the level of deoxyribonucleoside triphosphates required for DNA synthesis; inhibition by gemcitabine triphosphate of DNA polymerase-α and DNA polymerase-β, thereby resulting in blockade of DNA synthesis and DNA repair; and incorporation of gemcitabine triphosphate into DNA, leading to inhibition of DNA synthesis and function. Following incorporation of the gemcitabine triphosphate into DNA, only one additional nucleotide can be added to the growing DNA strand, resulting in chain termination.

Gemcitabine

This nucleoside analog was initially approved for use in advanced pancreatic cancer but is now widely used to treat a broad range of malignancies, including non-small cell lung cancer, bladder cancer, ovarian cancer, soft tissue sarcoma, and non-Hodgkin's lymphoma. Myelosuppression in the form of neutropenia is the principal dose-limiting toxicity. Nausea and vomiting occur in 70% of patients and a flu-like syndrome has also been observed. In rare cases, renal microangiopathy syndromes, including hemolytic-uremic syndrome and thrombotic thrombocytopenic purpura have been reported.

PURINE ANTAGONISTS

6-Thiopurines

6-Mercaptopurine (6-MP) was the first of the thiopurine analogs found to be effective in cancer therapy. This agent is used primarily in the treatment of childhood acute leukemia, and a closely related analog, azathioprine, is used as an immunosuppressive agent (see Chapter 55). As with other thiopurines, 6-MP is inactive in its parent form and must be metabolized by hypoxanthine-guanine phosphoribosyl transferase (HGPRT) to form the monophosphate nucleotide 6-thioinosinic acid, which in turn inhibits several enzymes of de novo purine nucleotide synthesis (Figure 54–6). The monophosphate form is eventually metabolized to the triphosphate form, which can then be incorporated into both RNA and DNA. Significant levels of thioguanylic acid and 6-methylmercaptopurine ribotide (MMPR) are also formed from 6-MP. These metabolites may contribute to its cytotoxic action.

6-Thioguanine (6-TG) also inhibits several enzymes in the de novo purine nucleotide biosynthetic pathway (Figure 54–6). Various metabolic lesions result, including inhibition of purine nucleotide interconversion; decrease in intracellular levels of guanine nucleotides, which leads to inhibition of glycoprotein synthesis; interference with the formation of DNA and RNA; and incorporation of thiopurine nucleotides into both DNA and RNA. 6-TG has a synergistic action when used together with cytarabine in the treatment of adult acute leukemia.

6-MP is converted to an inactive metabolite (6-thiouric acid) by an oxidation reaction catalyzed by xanthine oxidase, whereas 6-TG undergoes deamination. This is an important issue because the purine analog allopurinol, a potent xanthine oxidase inhibitor, is frequently used as a supportive care measure in the treatment of acute leukemias to prevent the development of hyperuricemia that often occurs with tumor cell lysis. Because allopurinol inhibits xanthine oxidase, simultaneous therapy with allopurinol and 6-MP would result in increased levels of 6-MP, thereby leading to excessive

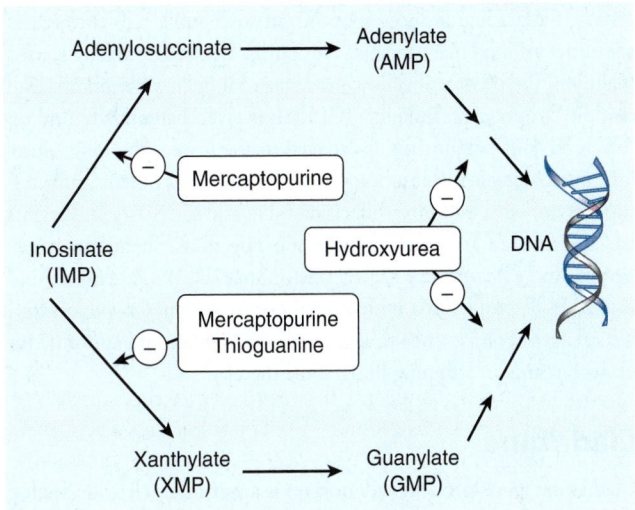

FIGURE 54–6 Mechanism of action of 6-mercaptopurine and 6-thioguanine.

toxicity. In this setting, the dose of mercaptopurine must be reduced by 50–75%. In contrast, such an interaction does not occur with 6-TG, which can be used in full doses with allopurinol.

Hypoxanthine   6-Mercaptopurine   Allopurinol

Guanine   6-Thioguanine

The thiopurines are also metabolized by the enzyme thiopurine methyltransferase (TPMT), in which a methyl group is attached to the thiopurine ring. Patients who have a pharmacogenetic syndrome involving partial or complete deficiency of this enzyme are at increased risk for developing severe toxicities in the form of myelosuppression and gastrointestinal toxicity with mucositis and diarrhea.

Fludarabine

Fludarabine phosphate is rapidly dephosphorylated to 2-fluoro-arab-inofuranosyladenosine and then phosphorylated intracellularly by deoxycytidine kinase to the triphosphate. The triphosphate metabolite interferes with the processes of DNA synthesis and DNA repair through inhibition of DNA polymerase-α and DNA polymerase-β. The triphosphate form can also be directly incorporated into DNA, resulting in inhibition of DNA synthesis and function. The diphosphate metabolite of fludarabine inhibits ribonucleotide reductase, leading to inhibition of essential deoxyribonucleotide triphosphates. Finally, fludarabine induces apoptosis in susceptible cells through as yet undetermined mechanisms. This purine nucleotide analog is used mainly in the treatment of low-grade non-Hodgkin's lymphoma and chronic lymphocytic leukemia (CLL). It is given parenterally, and up to 25–30% of parent drug is excreted in the urine. The main dose-limiting toxicity is myelosuppression. This agent is a potent immunosuppressant with inhibitory effects on CD4 and CD8 T cells. Patients are at increased risk for opportunistic infections, including fungi, herpes, and *Pneumocystis jiroveci* pneumonia (PCP). Patients should receive PCP prophylaxis with trimethoprim-sulfamethoxazole (double strength) at least three times a week, and this should continue for up to 1 year after stopping fludarabine therapy.

Cladribine

Cladribine (2-chlorodeoxyadenosine) is a purine nucleoside analog with high specificity for lymphoid cells. Inactive in its parent form, it is initially phosphorylated by deoxycytidine kinase to the monophosphate form and eventually metabolized to the triphosphate

form, which can then be incorporated into DNA. The triphosphate metabolite can also interfere with DNA synthesis and DNA repair by inhibiting DNA polymerase-α and DNA polymerase-β, respectively. Cladribine is indicated for the treatment of hairy cell leukemia, with activity in other low-grade lymphoid malignancies such as CLL and low-grade non-Hodgkin's lymphoma. It is normally administered as a single continuous 7-day infusion; under these conditions, it has a very manageable safety profile with the main toxicity consisting of transient myelosuppression. As with other purine nucleoside analogs, it has immunosuppressive effects, and a decrease in CD4 and CD8 T cells, lasting for over 1 year, is observed in patients.

NATURAL PRODUCT CANCER CHEMOTHERAPY DRUGS

VINCA ALKALOIDS

Vinblastine

Vinblastine is an alkaloid derived from the periwinkle plant *Vinca rosea*. Its mechanism of action involves inhibition of tubulin polymerization, which disrupts assembly of microtubules, an important part of the cytoskeleton and the mitotic spindle. This inhibitory effect results in mitotic arrest in metaphase, bringing cell division to a halt, which then leads to cell death. Vinblastine and other vinca alkaloids are metabolized by the liver P450 system, and the majority of the drug is excreted in feces via the hepatobiliary system. As such, dose modification is required in the setting of liver dysfunction. The main adverse effects are outlined in Table 54–4, and they include nausea and vomiting, bone marrow suppression, and alopecia. This agent is also a potent vesicant, and care must be taken in its administration. It has clinical activity in the treatment of Hodgkin's and non-Hodgkin's lymphomas, breast cancer, and germ cell cancer.

Vincristine

Vincristine is another alkaloid derivative of *V rosea* and is closely related in structure to vinblastine. Its mechanism of action, mechanism of resistance, and clinical pharmacology are identical to those of vinblastine. Despite these similarities to vinblastine, vincristine has a strikingly different spectrum of clinical activity and safety profile.

R: O=C—H
Vincristine

R: CH₃
Vinblastine

TABLE 54–4 Natural product cancer chemotherapy drugs: Clinical activity and toxicities.

Drug	Mechanism of Action	Clinical Applications[1]	Acute Toxicity	Delayed Toxicity
Bleomycin	Oxygen free radicals bind to DNA causing single- and double-strand DNA breaks	Hodgkin's and non-Hodgkin's lymphoma, germ cell cancer, head and neck cancer	Allergic reactions, fever, hypotension	Skin toxicity, pulmonary fibrosis, mucositis, alopecia
Daunorubicin	Oxygen free radicals bind to DNA causing single- and double-strand DNA breaks; inhibits topoisomerase II; intercalates into DNA	AML, ALL	Nausea, fever, red urine (not hematuria)	Cardiotoxicity (see text), alopecia, myelosuppression
Docetaxel	Inhibits mitosis	Breast cancer, non-small cell lung cancer, prostate cancer, gastric cancer, head and neck cancer, ovarian cancer, bladder cancer	Hypersensitivity	Neurotoxicity, fluid retention, myelosuppression with neutropenia
Doxorubicin	Oxygen free radicals bind to DNA causing single- and double-strand DNA breaks; inhibits topoisomerase II; intercalates into DNA	Breast cancer, Hodgkin's and non-Hodgkin's lymphoma, soft tissue sarcoma, ovarian cancer, non-small cell and small cell lung cancer, thyroid cancer, Wilms' tumor, neuroblastoma	Nausea, red urine (not hematuria)	Cardiotoxicity (see text), alopecia, myelosuppression, stomatitis
Etoposide	Inhibits topoisomerase II	Non-small cell and small cell lung cancer; non-Hodgkin's lymphoma, gastric cancer	Nausea, vomiting, hypotension	Alopecia, myelosuppression
Idarubicin	Oxygen free radicals bind to DNA causing single- and double-strand DNA breaks; inhibits topoisomerase II; intercalates into DNA	AML, ALL, CML in blast crisis	Nausea and vomiting	Myelosuppression, mucositis, cardiotoxicity
Irinotecan	Inhibits topoisomerase I	Colorectal cancer, gastroesophageal cancer, non-small cell and small cell lung cancer	Diarrhea, nausea, vomiting	Diarrhea, myelosuppression, nausea and vomiting
Mitomycin	Acts as an alkylating agent and forms cross-links with DNA; formation of oxygen free radicals, which target DNA	Superficial bladder cancer, gastric cancer, breast cancer, non-small cell lung cancer, head and neck cancer (in combination with radiotherapy)	Nausea and vomiting	Myelosuppression, mucositis, anorexia and fatigue, hemolytic-uremic syndrome
Paclitaxel	Inhibits mitosis	Breast cancer, non-small cell and small cell lung cancer, ovarian cancer, gastroesophageal cancer, prostate cancer, bladder cancer, head and neck cancer	Nausea, vomiting, hypotension, arrhythmias, hypersensitivity	Myelosuppression, peripheral sensory neuropathy
Topotecan	Inhibits topoisomerase I	Small cell lung cancer, ovarian cancer	Nausea and vomiting	Myelosuppression
Vinblastine	Inhibits mitosis	Hodgkin's and non-Hodgkin's lymphoma, germ cell cancer, breast cancer, Kaposi's sarcoma	Nausea and vomiting	Myelosuppression, mucositis, alopecia, syndrome of inappropriate secretion of antidiuretic hormone (SIADH), vascular events
Vincristine	Inhibits mitosis	ALL, Hodgkin's and non-Hodgkin's lymphoma, rhabdomyosarcoma, neuroblastoma, Wilms' tumor	None	Neurotoxicity with peripheral neuropathy, paralytic ileus, myelosuppression, alopecia, SIADH
Vinorelbine	Inhibits mitosis	Non-small cell lung cancer, breast cancer, ovarian cancer	Nausea and vomiting	Myelosuppression, constipation, SIADH

[1]See Table 54–3 for acronyms.

Vincristine has been effectively combined with prednisone for remission induction in acute lymphoblastic leukemia in children. It is also active in various hematologic malignancies such as Hodgkin's and non-Hodgkin's lymphomas, and multiple myeloma, and in several pediatric tumors including rhabdomyosarcoma, neuroblastoma, Ewing's sarcoma, and Wilms' tumor.

The main dose-limiting toxicity is neurotoxicity, usually expressed as a peripheral sensory neuropathy, although autonomic nervous system dysfunction with orthostatic hypotension, urinary retention, and paralytic ileus or constipation, cranial nerve palsies, ataxia, seizures, and coma have been observed. While myelosuppression occurs, it is generally milder and much less significant than with vinblastine.

The other adverse effect that may develop is the syndrome of inappropriate secretion of antidiuretic hormone (SIADH).

Vinorelbine

Vinorelbine is a semisynthetic derivative of vinblastine whose mechanism of action is identical to that of vinblastine and vincristine, ie, inhibition of mitosis of cells in the M phase through inhibition of tubulin polymerization. This agent has activity in non-small cell lung cancer, breast cancer, and ovarian cancer. Myelosuppression with neutropenia is the dose-limiting toxicity, but other adverse effects include nausea and vomiting, transient elevations in liver function tests, neurotoxicity, and SIADH.

TAXANES & RELATED DRUGS

Paclitaxel is an alkaloid ester derived from the Pacific yew (*Taxus brevifolia*) and the European yew (*Taxus baccata*). The drug functions as a mitotic spindle poison through high-affinity binding to microtubules with *enhancement* of tubulin polymerization. This promotion of microtubule assembly by paclitaxel occurs in the absence of microtubule-associated proteins and guanosine triphosphate and results in inhibition of mitosis and cell division.

Paclitaxel has significant activity in a broad range of solid tumors, including ovarian, advanced breast, non-small cell and small cell lung, head and neck, esophageal, prostate, and bladder cancers and AIDS-related Kaposi's sarcoma. It is metabolized extensively by the liver P450 system, and nearly 80% of the drug is excreted in feces via the hepatobiliary route. Dose reduction is required in patients with liver dysfunction. The primary dose-limiting toxicities are listed in Table 54–4. Hypersensitivity reactions may be observed in up to 5% of patients, but the incidence is significantly reduced by premedication with dexamethasone, diphenhydramine, and an H_2 blocker.

A novel albumin-bound paclitaxel formulation (Abraxane) is approved for use in metastatic breast cancer. In contrast to paclitaxel, this formulation is not associated with hypersensitivity reactions, and premedication to prevent such reactions is not required. Moreover, this agent has significantly reduced myelosuppressive effects compared with paclitaxel, and the neurotoxicity that results appears to be more readily reversible than is typically observed with paclitaxel.

Docetaxel is a semisynthetic taxane derived from the European yew tree. Its mechanism of action, metabolism, and elimination are identical to those of paclitaxel. It is approved for use as second-line therapy in advanced breast cancer and non-small cell lung cancer, and it also has major activity in head and neck cancer, small cell lung cancer, gastric cancer, advanced platinum-refractory ovarian cancer, and bladder cancer. Its major toxicities are listed in Table 54–4.

Cabazitaxel is a semisynthetic taxane produced from a precursor extracted from the yew tree. Its mechanism of action, metabolism, and elimination are identical to those of the other taxanes. However, unlike other taxanes, cabazitaxel is a poor substrate for the multidrug resistance P-glycoprotein efflux pump and may therefore be useful for treating multidrug-resistant tumors. It is approved for use

in combination with prednisone in the second-line therapy of hormone-refractory metastatic prostate cancer previously treated with a docetaxel-containing regimen. Its major toxicities include myelosuppression, neurotoxicity, and allergic reactions.

Although not strictly a taxane, **ixabepilone** is a semisynthetic epothilone B analog that functions as a microtubule inhibitor and binds directly to β-tubulin subunits on microtubules, leading to inhibition of normal microtubule dynamics. As such, it is active in the M phase of the cell cycle. This agent is presently approved for metastatic breast cancer in combination with the oral fluoropyrimidine capecitabine or as monotherapy. Of note, this agent continues to have activity in drug-resistant tumors that overexpress P-glycoprotein or tubulin mutations. The main adverse effects include myelosuppression, hypersensitivity reactions, and neurotoxicity in the form of peripheral sensory neuropathy.

EPIPODOPHYLLOTOXINS

Etoposide is a semisynthetic derivative of podophyllotoxin, which is extracted from the mayapple root (*Podophyllum peltatum*). Intravenous and oral formulations of etoposide are approved for clinical use in the USA. The oral bioavailability is about 50%, requiring the oral dose to be twice that of an intravenous dose. Up to 30–50% of drug is excreted in the urine, and dose reduction is required in the setting of renal dysfunction. The main site of action is inhibition of the DNA enzyme topoisomerase II. Etoposide has clinical activity in germ cell cancer, small cell and non-small cell lung cancer, Hodgkin's and non-Hodgkin's lymphomas, and gastric cancer. In addition, it is effective in high-dose regimens in the transplant setting for breast cancer and lymphomas. Major toxicities are listed in Table 54–4.

CAMPTOTHECINS

The camptothecins are natural products derived from the *Camptotheca acuminata* tree originally found in China; they inhibit the activity of topoisomerase I, the key enzyme responsible for cutting and religating single DNA strands. Inhibition of this enzyme results in DNA damage. **Topotecan** and **irinotecan** are the two camptothecin analogs used in clinical practice in the USA. Although they both inhibit the same molecular target, their spectrum of clinical activity is quite different. Topotecan is indicated in the treatment of advanced ovarian cancer as second-line therapy following initial treatment with platinum-based chemotherapy. It is also approved as second-line therapy of small cell lung cancer. The main route of elimination is renal excretion, and dosage must be adjusted in patients with renal impairment.

Irinotecan is a prodrug that is converted mainly in the liver by the carboxylesterase enzyme to the SN-38 metabolite, which is 1000-fold more potent as an inhibitor of topoisomerase I than the parent compound. In contrast to topotecan, irinotecan and SN-38 are mainly eliminated in bile and feces, and dose reduction is required in the setting of liver dysfunction. Irinotecan was originally approved as second-line monotherapy in patients with metastatic colorectal cancer who had failed fluorouracil-based therapy. It is now approved as first-line therapy when used in combination with 5-FU and leucovorin. Myelosuppression and diarrhea are the two most common adverse events (Table 54–4). There are two forms of diarrhea: an early form that occurs within 24 hours after administration and is thought to be a cholinergic event effectively treated with atropine, and a late form that usually occurs 2–10 days after treatment. The late diarrhea can be severe, leading to significant electrolyte imbalance and dehydration in some cases.

ANTITUMOR ANTIBIOTICS

Screening of microbial products has led to the discovery of a number of growth-inhibiting compounds that have proved to be clinically useful in cancer chemotherapy. Many of these antibiotics bind to DNA through intercalation between specific bases and block the synthesis of RNA, DNA, or both; cause DNA strand scission; and interfere with cell replication. All of the anticancer antibiotics now being used in clinical practice are products of various strains of the soil microbe *Streptomyces*. These include the anthracyclines, bleomycin, and mitomycin.

ANTHRACYCLINES

The anthracycline antibiotics, isolated from *Streptomyces peucetius* var *caesius*, are among the most widely used cytotoxic anticancer drugs. The structures of two congeners, doxorubicin and daunorubicin, are shown below. Several other anthracycline analogs have entered clinical practice, including idarubicin, epirubicin, and mitoxantrone. The anthracyclines exert their cytotoxic action through four major mechanisms: (1) inhibition of topoisomerase II; (2) high-affinity binding to DNA through intercalation, with consequent blockade of the synthesis of DNA and RNA, and DNA strand scission; (3) generation of semiquinone free radicals and oxygen free radicals through an iron-dependent, enzyme-mediated reductive process; and (4) binding to cellular membranes to alter fluidity and ion transport. While the precise mechanisms by which the anthracyclines exert their cytotoxic effects remain to be defined (and may depend upon the specific tumor type), it is now well-established that the free radical mechanism is the cause of the cardiotoxicity associated with the anthracyclines (Table 54–4).

R: —C—CH₃   R: —C—CH₂OH

Daunorubicin   **Doxorubicin**

In the clinical setting, anthracyclines are administered via the intravenous route. The anthracyclines are metabolized extensively in the liver, with reduction and hydrolysis of the ring substituents. The hydroxylated metabolite is an active species, whereas the aglycone is inactive. Up to 50% of drug is eliminated in the feces via biliary excretion, and dose reduction is required in the setting of liver dysfunction. Although anthracyclines are usually administered on an every-3-week schedule, alternative schedules such as low-dose weekly or 72- to 96-hour continuous infusions have been shown to yield equivalent clinical efficacy with reduced toxicity.

Doxorubicin is one of the most important anticancer drugs in clinical practice, with major clinical activity in cancers of the breast, endometrium, ovary, testicle, thyroid, stomach, bladder, liver, and lung; in soft tissue sarcomas; and in several childhood cancers, including neuroblastoma, Ewing's sarcoma, osteosarcoma, and rhabdomyosarcoma. It also has clinical activity in hematologic malignancies, including acute lymphoblastic leukemia, multiple myeloma, and Hodgkin's and non-Hodgkin's lymphomas. It is generally used in combination with other anticancer agents (eg, cyclophosphamide, cisplatin, and 5-FU), and clinical activity is improved with combination regimens as opposed to single-agent therapy.

Daunorubicin was the first agent in this class to be isolated, and it is still used in the treatment of acute myeloid leukemia. In contrast to doxorubicin, its efficacy in solid tumors is limited.

Idarubicin is a semisynthetic anthracycline glycoside analog of daunorubicin, and it is approved for use in combination with cytarabine for induction therapy of acute myeloid leukemia. When combined with cytarabine, idarubicin appears to be more active than daunorubicin in producing complete remissions and in improving survival in patients with acute myelogenous leukemia.

Epirubicin is an anthracycline analog whose mechanism of action and clinical pharmacology are identical to those of all other anthracyclines. It was initially approved for use as a component of adjuvant therapy in early-stage, node-positive breast cancer but is also used in the treatment of metastatic breast cancer and gastroesophageal cancer.

Mitoxantrone (dihydroxyanthracenedione) is an anthracene compound whose structure resembles the anthracycline ring. It binds to DNA to produce strand breakage and inhibits both DNA and RNA synthesis. It is currently used in the treatment of advanced, hormone-refractory prostate cancer and low-grade non-Hodgkin's lymphoma. It is also indicated in breast cancer and in pediatric and adult acute myeloid leukemias. Myelosuppression with leukopenia is the dose-limiting toxicity, and mild nausea and vomiting, mucositis, and alopecia also occur. Although the drug is thought to be less cardiotoxic than doxorubicin, both acute and chronic cardiac toxicity are reported. A blue discoloration of the fingernails, sclera, and urine is observed 1–2 days after drug administration.

The main dose-limiting toxicity of all anthracyclines is myelosuppression, with neutropenia more commonly observed than thrombocytopenia. In some cases, mucositis is dose-limiting. Two forms of cardiotoxicity are observed. The acute form occurs within the first 2–3 days and presents as arrhythmias and conduction abnormalities, other electrocardiographic changes, pericarditis, and myocarditis. This form is usually transient and in most cases is asymptomatic. The chronic form results in a dose-dependent, dilated cardiomyopathy associated with heart failure. The chronic cardiac toxicity appears to result from increased production of free radicals within the myocardium. This effect is rarely seen at total doxorubicin dosages below 500–550 mg/m^2. Use of lower weekly doses or continuous infusions of doxorubicin appear to reduce the incidence of cardiac toxicity. In addition, treatment with the iron-chelating agent **dexrazoxane** (ICRF-187) is currently approved to prevent or reduce anthracycline-induced cardiotoxicity in women with metastatic breast cancer who have received a total cumulative dose of doxorubicin of 300 mg/m^2. The anthracyclines can also produce a "radiation recall reaction," with erythema and desquamation of the skin observed at sites of prior radiation therapy.

MITOMYCIN

Mitomycin (mitomycin C) is an antibiotic isolated from *Streptomyces caespitosus*. It undergoes metabolic activation through an enzyme-mediated reduction to generate an alkylating agent that cross-links DNA. Hypoxic tumor stem cells of solid tumors exist in an environment conducive to reductive reactions and are more sensitive to the cytotoxic effects of mitomycin than normal cells and oxygenated tumor cells. It is active in all phases of the cell cycle, and is the best available drug for use in combination with radiation therapy to attack hypoxic tumor cells. Its main clinical use is in the treatment of squamous cell cancer of the anus in combination with 5-FU and radiation therapy. In addition, it is used in combination chemotherapy for squamous cell carcinoma of the cervix and for breast, gastric, and pancreatic cancer. One special application of mitomycin has been in the intravesical treatment of superficial bladder cancer. Because virtually none of the agent is absorbed systemically, there is little to no systemic toxicity when used in this setting.

The common toxicities of mitomycin are outlined in Table 54–4. Hemolytic-uremic syndrome, manifested as microangiopathic hemolytic anemia, thrombocytopenia, and renal failure, as well as occasional instances of interstitial pneumonitis have been reported.

BLEOMYCIN

Bleomycin is a small peptide that contains a DNA-binding region and an iron-binding domain at opposite ends of the molecule. It acts by binding to DNA, which results in single- and double-strand breaks following free radical formation, and inhibition of DNA biosynthesis. The fragmentation of DNA is due to oxidation of a DNA-bleomycin-Fe(II) complex and leads to chromosomal aberrations. Bleomycin is a cell cycle-specific drug that causes accumulation of cells in the G$_2$ phase of the cell cycle.

Bleomycin is indicated for the treatment of Hodgkin's and non-Hodgkin's lymphomas, germ cell tumor, head and neck cancer, and squamous cell cancer of the skin, cervix, and vulva. One advantage of this agent is that it can be given subcutaneously, intramuscularly, or intravenously. Elimination of bleomycin is mainly via renal excretion, and dose modification is recommended in patients with renal dysfunction.

Pulmonary toxicity is dose-limiting for bleomycin and usually presents as pneumonitis with cough, dyspnea, dry inspiratory crackles on physical examination, and infiltrates on chest X-ray. The incidence of pulmonary toxicity is increased in patients older than 70 years of age, in those who receive cumulative doses greater than 400 units, in those with underlying pulmonary disease, and in those who have received prior mediastinal or chest irradiation. In rare cases, pulmonary toxicity can be fatal. Other toxicities are listed in Table 54–4.

MISCELLANEOUS ANTICANCER DRUGS

A large number of anticancer drugs that do not fit traditional categories have been approved for clinical use by the Food and Drug Administration (FDA); they are listed in Table 54–5.

IMATINIB, DASATINIB, & NILOTINIB

Imatinib is an inhibitor of the tyrosine kinase domain of the Bcr-Abl oncoprotein and prevents phosphorylation of the kinase substrate by ATP. It is indicated for the treatment of chronic myelogenous leukemia (CML), a pluripotent hematopoietic stem cell disorder characterized by the t(9:22) Philadelphia chromosomal translocation. This translocation results in the Bcr-Abl fusion protein, the causative agent in CML, and is present in up to 95% of patients with this disease. This agent also inhibits other receptor tyrosine kinases for platelet-derived growth factor receptor (PDGFR), stem cell factor, and c-kit.

Imatinib is well absorbed orally, and it is metabolized in the liver, with elimination of metabolites occurring mainly in feces via biliary excretion. This agent is approved for use as first-line therapy in chronic phase CML, in blast crisis, and as second-line therapy for chronic phase CML that has progressed on prior interferon-alfa therapy. Imatinib is also effective in the treatment of gastrointestinal stromal tumors expressing the c-kit tyrosine kinase. The main adverse effects are listed in Table 54–5.

Dasatinib is an oral inhibitor of several tyrosine kinases, including Bcr-Abl, Src, c-kit, and PDGFR-α. It differs from imatinib in that it binds to the active and inactive conformations of the Abl kinase domain and overcomes imatinib resistance resulting from mutations in the Bcr-Abl kinase. It is approved for use in CML and Philadelphia chromosome-positive acute lymphoblastic leukemia (ALL) with resistance or intolerance to imatinib therapy.

Nilotinib is a second-generation phenylamino-pyrimidine molecule that inhibits Bcr-Abl, c-kit, and PDGFR-β tyrosine kinases. It has a higher binding affinity (up to 20- to 50-fold) for the Abl kinase when compared with imatinib, and it overcomes imatinib resistance resulting from Bcr-Abl mutations. It was originally approved for chronic phase and accelerated phase CML with resistance or intolerance to prior therapy that included imatinib and was recently approved as first-line therapy of chronic phase CML.

TABLE 54–5 Miscellaneous anticancer drugs: Clinical activity and toxicities.

Drug	Mechanism of Action[1]	Clinical Applications[1]	Acute Toxicity	Delayed Toxicity
Asparaginase	Hydrolyzes circulating L-asparagine, resulting in rapid inhibition of protein synthesis	ALL	Nausea, fever, allergic reactions	Hepatotoxicity, increased risk of bleeding and clotting, mental depression, pancreatitis, renal toxicity
Erlotinib	Inhibits EGFR tyrosine kinase leading to inhibition of EGFR signaling	Non-small cell lung cancer, pancreatic cancer	Diarrhea	Skin rash, diarrhea, anorexia, interstitial lung disease
Gefitinib	Same as erlotinib	Non-small cell lung cancer	Hypertension, diarrhea	Same as above
Imatinib	Inhibits Bcr-Abl tyrosine kinase and other receptor tyrosine kinases, including PDGFR, stem cell factor, and c-kit	CML, gastrointestinal stromal tumor (GIST), Philadelphia chromosome-positive ALL	Nausea and vomiting	Fluid retention with ankle and periorbital edema, diarrhea, myalgias, congestive heart failure
Cetuximab	Binds to EGFR and inhibits downstream EGFR signaling; enhances response to chemotherapy and radiotherapy	Colorectal cancer, head and neck cancer (used in combination with radiotherapy), non-small cell lung cancer	Infusion reaction	Skin rash, hypomagnesemia, fatigue, interstitial lung disease
Panitumumab	Binds to EGFR and inhibits downstream EGFR signaling; enhances response to chemotherapy and radiotherapy	Colorectal cancer	Infusion reaction (rarely)	Skin rash, hypomagnesemia, fatigue, interstitial lung disease
Bevacizumab	Inhibits binding of VEGF to VEGFR leading to inhibition of VEGF signaling; inhibits tumor vascular permeability; enhances tumor blood flow and drug delivery	Colorectal cancer, breast cancer, non-small cell lung cancer, renal cell cancer	Hypertension, infusion reaction	Arterial thromboembolic events, gastrointestinal perforations, wound healing complications, proteinuria
Sorafenib	Inhibits multiple RTKs, including raf kinase, VEGF-R2, VEGF-R3, and PDGFR-β leading to inhibition of angiogenesis, invasion, and metastasis	Renal cell cancer, hepatocellular cancer	Nausea, hypertension	Skin rash, fatigue and asthenia, bleeding complications, hypophosphatemia
Sunitinib	Inhibits multiple RTKs, including VEGF-R1, VEGF-R2, VEGF-R3, PDGFR-α and PDGFR-β leading to inhibition of angiogenesis, invasion, and metastasis	Renal cell cancer, GIST	Hypertension	Skin rash, fatigue and asthenia, bleeding complications, cardiac toxicity leading to congestive heart failure in rare cases

[1]See text for acronyms.

Imatinib, dasatinib, and nilotinib are all metabolized in the liver, mainly by the CYP3A4 liver microsomal enzyme. A large fraction of each drug is eliminated in feces via the hepatobiliary route. It is important to review the patient's current list of prescription and nonprescription drugs because these agents have potential drug-drug interactions, especially with those that are also metabolized by the CYP3A4 system. In addition, patients should avoid grapefruit products and the use of St. John's wort, as they may alter the metabolism of these small molecule inhibitors (see Chapter 4).

GROWTH FACTOR RECEPTOR INHIBITORS

Cetuximab & Panitumumab

The epidermal growth factor receptor (EGFR) is a member of the erb-B family of growth factor receptors, and it is overexpressed in a number of solid tumors, including colorectal cancer, head and neck cancer, non-small cell lung cancer, and pancreatic cancer. Activation of the EGFR signaling pathway results in downstream activation of several key cellular events involved in cellular growth and proliferation, invasion and metastasis, and angiogenesis. In addition, this pathway inhibits the cytotoxic activity of various anticancer agents and radiation therapy, presumably through suppression of key apoptotic mechanisms, thereby leading to the development of cellular drug resistance.

Cetuximab is a chimeric monoclonal antibody directed against the extracellular domain of the EGFR, and it is presently approved for use in combination with irinotecan for metastatic colon cancer in the refractory setting or as monotherapy in patients who are deemed to be irinotecan-refractory. Because cetuximab is of the G_1 isotype, its antitumor activity may also be mediated, in part, by immunologic-mediated mechanisms. There is growing evidence that cetuximab can be effectively and safely combined with irinotecan- and oxaliplatin-based chemotherapy in the first-line treatment of metastatic colorectal cancer as well. Of note, the efficacy of cetuximab is restricted to only those patients whose tumors express wild-type *KRAS*. Regimens combining cetuximab with cytotoxic chemotherapy may be of particular benefit in the neoadjuvant therapy of patients with liver-limited disease. Although this antibody was initially approved to be administered on a weekly schedule, pharmacokinetic studies have shown that an every-2-week schedule provides the same level of clinical activity as the weekly schedule. This agent is also approved for use in combination with radiation therapy in patients with locally advanced head and neck cancer. Cetuximab is well tolerated, with the main adverse effects being an acneiform skin rash, hypersensitivity infusion reaction, and hypomagnesemia.

Panitumumab is a fully human monoclonal antibody directed against the EGFR and works through inhibition of the EGFR signaling pathway. In contrast to cetuximab, this antibody is of the G_2 isotype, and as such, it would not be expected to exert any immunologic-mediated effects. Presently, panitumumab is approved for patients with refractory metastatic colorectal cancer who have been treated with all other active agents, and as with cetuximab, this antibody is only effective in patients whose tumors express wild-type *KRAS*. Recent clinical studies have shown that this antibody is effectively and safely combined with oxaliplatin- and irinotecan-based chemotherapy in the first- and second-line treatment of metastatic colorectal cancer. Acneiform skin rash and hypomagnesemia are the two main adverse effects associated with its use. Because this is a fully human antibody, infusion-related reactions are rarely observed.

Gefitinib & Erlotinib

Gefitinib and erlotinib are small molecule inhibitors of the tyrosine kinase domain associated with the EGFR, and both are used in the treatment of non-small cell lung cancer that is refractory to at least one prior chemotherapy regimen. Patients who are nonsmokers and who have a bronchoalveolar histologic subtype appear to be more responsive to these agents. In addition, erlotinib has been approved for use in combination with gemcitabine for the treatment of advanced pancreatic cancer. Both agents are metabolized in the liver by the CYP3A4 enzyme system, and elimination is mainly hepatic with excretion in feces. Caution must be taken when using these agents with drugs that are also metabolized by the liver CYP3A4 system, such as phenytoin and warfarin, and the use of grapefruit products should be avoided. An acneiform skin rash, diarrhea, and anorexia and fatigue are the most common adverse effects observed with these small molecules (Table 54-5).

Bevacizumab, Sorafenib, Sunitinib, & Pazopanib

The vascular endothelial growth factor (VEGF) is one of the most important angiogenic growth factors. The growth of both primary and metastatic tumors requires an intact vasculature. As a result, the VEGF-signaling pathway represents an attractive target for chemotherapy. Several approaches have been taken to inhibit VEGF signaling; they include inhibition of VEGF interactions with its receptor by targeting either the VEGF ligand with antibodies or soluble chimeric decoy receptors, or by direct inhibition of the VEGF receptor-associated tyrosine kinase activity by small molecule inhibitors.

Bevacizumab is a recombinant humanized monoclonal antibody that targets all forms of VEGF-A. This antibody binds to and prevents VEGF-A from interacting with the target VEGF receptors. Bevacizumab can be safely and effectively combined with 5-FU-, irinotecan-, and oxaliplatin-based chemotherapy in the treatment of metastatic colorectal cancer. Bevacizumab is FDA approved as a first-line treatment for metastatic colorectal cancer in combination with any intravenous fluoropyrimidine-containing regimen and is now also approved in combination with chemotherapy for metastatic non-small lung cancer and breast cancer. One potential advantage of this antibody is that it does not appear to exacerbate the toxicities typically observed with cytotoxic chemotherapy. The main safety concerns associated with bevacizumab include hypertension, an increased incidence of arterial thromboembolic events (transient ischemic attack, stroke, angina, and myocardial infarction), wound healing complications, gastrointestinal perforations, and proteinuria.

Sorafenib is a small molecule that inhibits multiple receptor tyrosine kinases (RTKs), especially VEGF-R2 and VEGF-R3, platelet-derived growth factor-β (PDGFR-β), and raf kinase. It was initially approved for advanced renal cell cancer and is also approved for advanced hepatocellular cancer.

Sunitinib is similar to sorafenib in that it inhibits multiple RTKs, although the specific types are somewhat different. They include PDGFR-α and PDGFR-β, VEGF-R1, VEGF-R2, VEGF-R3, and c-kit. It is approved for the treatment of advanced renal cell cancer and for the treatment of gastrointestinal stromal tumors (GIST) after disease progression on or with intolerance to imatinib.

Pazopanib is a small molecule that inhibits multiple RTKs, especially VEGF-R2 and VEGF-R3, PDGFR-β, and raf kinase. This oral agent is approved for the treatment of advanced renal cell cancer.

Sorafenib, sunitinib, and pazopanib are metabolized in the liver by the CYP3A4 system, and elimination is primarily hepatic with excretion in feces. Each of these agents has potential interactions with drugs that are also metabolized by the CYP3A4 system, especially warfarin. In addition, patients should avoid grapefruit products and the use of St. John's wort, as they may alter the clinical activity of these agents. Hypertension, bleeding complications, and fatigue are the most common adverse effects seen with both agents. With respect to sorafenib, skin rash and the hand-foot syndrome are observed in up to 30–50% of patients. For sunitinib, there is also an increased risk of cardiac dysfunction, which in some cases can lead to congestive heart failure.

ASPARAGINASE

Asparaginase (L-asparagine amidohydrolase) is an enzyme used to treat childhood ALL. The drug is isolated and purified from *Escherichia coli* or *Erwinia chrysanthemi* for clinical use. It hydrolyzes circulating L-asparagine to aspartic acid and ammonia. Because tumor cells in ALL lack asparagine synthetase, they require an exogenous source of L-asparagine. Thus, depletion of L-asparagine results in effective inhibition of protein synthesis. In contrast, normal cells can synthesize L-asparagine and thus are less susceptible to the cytotoxic action of asparaginase. The main adverse effect of this agent is a hypersensitivity reaction manifested by fever, chills, nausea and vomiting, skin rash, and urticaria. Severe cases can present with bronchospasm, respiratory failure, and hypotension. Other side effects include an increased risk of both clotting and bleeding as a result of alterations in various clotting factors, pancreatitis, and neurologic toxicity with lethargy, confusion, hallucinations, and in severe cases, coma.

CLINICAL PHARMACOLOGY OF CANCER CHEMOTHERAPEUTIC DRUGS

A thorough knowledge of the kinetics of tumor cell proliferation along with an understanding of the pharmacology and mechanism of action of cancer chemotherapeutic agents is important in designing optimal regimens for patients with cancer. The strategy for developing drug regimens also requires knowledge of the specific characteristics of individual tumors. For example, is there a high growth fraction? Is there a high spontaneous cell death rate? Are most of the cells in G_0? Is a significant fraction of the tumor composed of hypoxic stem cells? Are their normal counterparts under hormonal control? Similarly, an understanding of the pharmacology of specific drugs is important. Are the tumor cells sensitive to the drug? Is the drug cell cycle specific? Does the drug require activation in certain normal tissue such as the liver (cyclophosphamide), or is it activated in the tumor tissue itself (capecitabine)? Knowledge of specific pathway abnormalities (eg, EGFR mutations, *KRAS* mutations) for intracellular signaling may prove important for the next generation of anticancer drugs.

For some tumor types, knowledge of receptor expression is important. In patients with breast cancer, analysis of the tumor for expression of estrogen or progesterone receptors is important in guiding therapy with selective estrogen receptor modulators. In addition, analysis of breast cancer for expression of the HER-2/*neu* growth factor receptor can determine whether the humanized monoclonal anti-HER-2/*neu* antibody, trastuzumab, would be appropriate therapy. In the case of prostate cancer, chemical suppression of androgen secretion with gonadotropin-releasing hormone agonists or antagonists is important. The basic pharmacology of hormonal therapy is discussed in Chapter 40. The use of specific cytotoxic and biologic agents for each of the main cancers is discussed in this section.

THE LEUKEMIAS

ACUTE LEUKEMIA

Childhood Leukemia

Acute lymphoblastic leukemia (ALL) is the main form of leukemia in childhood, and it is the most common form of cancer in children. Children with this disease have a relatively good prognosis.

A subset of patients with neoplastic lymphocytes expressing surface antigenic features of T lymphocytes has a poor prognosis (see Chapter 55). A cytoplasmic enzyme expressed by normal thymocytes, terminal deoxycytidyl transferase (terminal transferase), is also expressed in many cases of ALL. T-cell ALL also expresses high levels of the enzyme adenosine deaminase (ADA). This led to interest in the use of the ADA inhibitor pentostatin (deoxycoformycin) for treatment of such T-cell cases. Until 1948, the median length of survival in ALL was 3 months. With the advent of methotrexate, the length of survival was greatly increased. Subsequently, corticosteroids, 6-mercaptopurine, cyclophosphamide, vincristine, daunorubicin, and asparaginase have all been found to be active against this disease. A combination of vincristine and prednisone plus other agents is currently used to induce remission. Over 90% of children enter complete remission with this therapy with only minimal toxicity. However, circulating leukemic cells often migrate to sanctuary sites located in the brain and testes. The value of prophylactic intrathecal methotrexate therapy for prevention of central nervous system leukemia (a major mechanism of relapse) has been clearly demonstrated. Intrathecal therapy with methotrexate should therefore be considered as a standard component of the induction regimen for children with ALL.

Adult Leukemia

Acute myelogenous leukemia (AML) is the most common leukemia in adults. The single most active agent for AML is cytarabine; however, it is best used in combination with an anthracycline, which leads to complete remissions in about 70% of patients. While there are several anthracyclines that can be effectively combined with cytarabine, idarubicin is preferred.

Patients often require intensive supportive care during the period of induction chemotherapy. Such care includes platelet transfusions to prevent bleeding, the granulocyte colony-stimulating factor filgrastim to shorten periods of neutropenia, and antibiotics to combat infections. Younger patients (eg, age < 55) who are in complete remission and have an HLA-matched donor are candidates for allogeneic bone marrow transplantation. The transplant procedure is preceded by high-dose chemotherapy and total body irradiation followed by immunosuppression. This approach may cure up to 35–40% of eligible patients. Patients over age 60 respond less well to chemotherapy, primarily because their tolerance for aggressive therapy and resistance to infection are lower.

Once remission of AML is achieved, consolidation chemotherapy is required to maintain a durable remission and to induce cure.

CHRONIC MYELOGENOUS LEUKEMIA

Chronic myelogenous leukemia (CML) arises from a chromosomally abnormal hematopoietic stem cell in which a balanced translocation between the long arms of chromosomes 9 and 22, t(9:22), is observed in 90–95% of cases. This translocation results in constitutive expression of the Bcr-Abl fusion oncoprotein with a molecular weight of 210 kDa. The clinical symptoms and course are related to the white blood cell count and its rate of increase. Most patients with white cell counts over 50,000/μL should be treated. The goals of treatment are to reduce the granulocytes to normal levels, to raise the hemoglobin concentration to normal, and to relieve disease-related symptoms. The tyrosine kinase inhibitor imatinib is considered as standard first-line therapy in previously untreated patients with chronic phase CML. Nearly all patients treated with imatinib exhibit a complete hematologic response, and up to 40–50% of patients show a complete cytogenetic response. As described previously, this drug is generally well tolerated and is associated with relatively minor adverse effects. Initially, dasatinib and nilotinib were approved for patients who were intolerant or resistant to imatinib; each shows clinical activity, but both are now also indicated as first-line treatment of chronic phase CML. In addition to these tyrosine kinase inhibitors, other treatment options include interferon-α, busulfan, other oral alkylating agents, and hydroxyurea.

CHRONIC LYMPHOCYTIC LEUKEMIA

Patients with early-stage chronic lymphocytic leukemia (CLL) have a relatively good prognosis, and therapy has not changed the course of the disease. However, in the setting of high-risk disease or in the presence of disease-related symptoms, treatment is indicated.

Chlorambucil and cyclophosphamide are the two most widely used alkylating agents for this disease. Chlorambucil is frequently combined with prednisone, although there is no clear evidence that the combination yields better response rates or survival compared with chlorambucil alone. In most cases, cyclophosphamide is combined with vincristine and prednisone (COP), or it can also be given with these same drugs along with doxorubicin (CHOP). Bendamustine is the newest alkylating agent to be approved for use in this disease, either as monotherapy or in combination with prednisone. The purine nucleoside analog fludarabine is also effective in treating CLL. This agent can be given alone, in combination with cyclophosphamide and with mitoxantrone and dexamethasone, or combined with the anti-CD20 antibody rituximab.

Monoclonal antibody-targeted therapies are being widely used in CLL, especially in relapsed or refractory disease. Rituximab is an anti-CD20 antibody that has documented clinical activity in this setting. This chimeric antibody appears to enhance the antitumor effects of cytotoxic chemotherapy and is also effective in settings in which resistance to chemotherapy has developed. Alemtuzumab is a humanized monoclonal antibody directed against the CD52 antigen and is approved for use in CLL that is refractory to alkylating agent or fludarabine therapy. Response rates up to 30–35% are observed, with disease stabilization in another 30% of patients.

HODGKIN'S & NON-HODGKIN'S LYMPHOMAS

HODGKIN'S LYMPHOMA

The treatment of Hodgkin's lymphoma has undergone dramatic evolution over the last 30 years. This lymphoma is now widely recognized as a B-cell neoplasm in which the malignant Reed-Sternberg

cells have rearranged *VH* genes. In addition, the Epstein-Barr virus genome has been identified in up to 80% of tumor specimens.

Complete staging evaluation is required before a definitive treatment plan can be made. For patients with stage I and stage IIA disease, there has been a significant change in the treatment approach. Initially, these patients were treated with extended-field radiation therapy. However, given the well-documented late effects of radiation therapy, which include hypothyroidism, an increased risk of secondary cancers, and coronary artery disease, combined-modality therapy with a brief course of combination chemotherapy and involved field radiation therapy is now the recommended approach. The main advance for patients with advanced stage III and IV Hodgkin's lymphoma came with the development of MOPP (mechlorethamine, vincristine, procarbazine, and prednisone) chemotherapy in the 1960s. This regimen resulted initially in high complete response rates, on the order of 80–90%, with cures in up to 60% of patients. More recently, the anthracycline-containing regimen termed ABVD (doxorubicin, bleomycin, vinblastine, and dacarbazine) has been shown to be more effective and less toxic than MOPP, especially with regard to the incidence of infertility and secondary malignancies. In general, four cycles of ABVD are given to patients. An alternative regimen, termed Stanford V, utilizes a 12-week course of combination chemotherapy (doxorubicin, vinblastine, mechlorethamine, vincristine, bleomycin, etoposide, and prednisone), followed by involved radiation therapy.

With all of these regimens, over 80% of previously untreated patients with advanced Hodgkin's lymphoma (stages III and IV) are expected to go into complete remission, with disappearance of all disease-related symptoms and objective evidence of disease. In general, approximately 50–60% of all patients with Hodgkin's lymphoma are cured of their disease.

NON-HODGKIN'S LYMPHOMA

Non-Hodgkin's lymphoma is a heterogeneous disease, and the clinical characteristics of non-Hodgkin's lymphoma subsets are related to the underlying histopathologic features and the extent of disease involvement. In general, the nodular (or follicular) lymphomas have a far better prognosis, with a median survival up to 7 years, compared with the diffuse lymphomas, which have a median survival of about 1–2 years.

Combination chemotherapy is the treatment standard for patients with diffuse non-Hodgkin's lymphoma. The anthracycline-containing regimen CHOP (cyclophosphamide, doxorubicin, vincristine, and prednisone) has been considered the best treatment in terms of initial therapy. Randomized phase III clinical studies have now shown that the combination of CHOP with the anti-CD20 monoclonal antibody rituximab results in improved response rates, disease-free survival, and overall survival compared with CHOP chemotherapy alone.

The nodular follicular lymphomas are low-grade, relatively slow-growing tumors that tend to present in an advanced stage and are usually confined to lymph nodes, bone marrow, and spleen. This form of non-Hodgkin's lymphomas, when presenting at an advanced stage, is considered incurable, and treatment is generally palliative. To date, there is no evidence that immediate treatment with combination chemotherapy offers clinical benefit over close observation and "watchful waiting" with initiation of chemotherapy at the onset of disease symptoms.

MULTIPLE MYELOMA

This plasma cell malignancy is one of the models of neoplastic disease in humans as it arises from a single tumor stem cell. Moreover, the tumor cells produce a marker protein (myeloma immunoglobulin) that allows the total body burden of tumor cells to be quantified. Multiple myeloma principally involves the bone marrow and bone, causing bone pain, lytic lesions, bone fractures, and anemia as well as an increased susceptibility to infection.

Most patients with multiple myeloma are symptomatic at the time of initial diagnosis and require treatment with cytotoxic chemotherapy. Treatment with the combination of the alkylating agent melphalan and prednisone (MP protocol) has been a standard regimen for nearly 30 years. About 40% of patients respond to the MP combination, and the median remission is on the order of 2–2.5 years. Recently, combination regimens incorporating **lenalidomide** plus dexamethasone or the proteosome inhibitor **bortezomib** plus melphalan and prednisone have been shown to be more effective as first-line therapy.

In patients who are considered candidates for high-dose therapy with stem cell transplantation, melphalan and other alkylating agents are to be avoided, as they can affect the success of stem cell harvesting.

Thalidomide is a well-established agent for treating refractory or relapsed disease, and about 30% of patients will achieve a response to this therapy. More recently, thalidomide has been used in combination with dexamethasone, and response rates on the order of 65% have been observed. Studies are now under way to directly compare the combination of vincristine, doxorubicin, and dexamethasone (VAD protocol) with the combination of thalidomide and dexamethasone. In some patients, especially those with poor performance status, single-agent pulse dexamethasone administered on a weekly basis can be effective in palliating symptoms. Bortezomib was first approved for use in relapsing or refractory multiple myeloma and is now widely used in the first-line treatment of multiple myeloma. This agent is thought to exert its main cytotoxic effects through inhibition of the 26 S proteosome, which results in down-regulation of the nuclear factor kappa B (NF-κB) signaling pathway. Of note, inhibition of NF-κB has been shown to restore chemosensitivity. Based on this site of action, further efforts are focused on developing bortezomib in various combination regimens.

BREAST CANCER

STAGE I & STAGE II DISEASE

The management of primary breast cancer has undergone a remarkable evolution as a result of major efforts at early diagnosis (through encouragement of self-examination as well as through the use of cancer detection centers) and the implementation of combined modality approaches incorporating systemic chemotherapy as an adjuvant to surgery and radiation therapy. Women with stage I disease (small primary tumors and negative axillary lymph node dissections) are currently treated with surgery alone, and they have an 80% chance of cure.

Women with node-positive disease have a high risk of both local and systemic recurrence. Thus, lymph node status directly indicates the risk of occult distant micrometastasis. In this situation, postoperative use of systemic adjuvant chemotherapy with six cycles of cyclophosphamide, methotrexate, and fluorouracil (CMF protocol) or of fluorouracil, doxorubicin, and cyclophosphamide (FAC) has been shown to significantly reduce the relapse rate and prolong survival. Alternative regimens with equivalent clinical benefit include four cycles of doxorubicin and cyclophosphamide and six cycles of fluorouracil, epirubicin, and cyclophosphamide (FEC). Each of these chemotherapy regimens has benefited women with stage II breast cancer with one to three involved lymph nodes. Women with four or more involved nodes have had limited benefit thus far from adjuvant chemotherapy. Long-term analysis has clearly shown improved survival rates in node-positive premenopausal women who have been treated aggressively with multiagent combination chemotherapy. The results from three randomized clinical trials clearly show that the addition of trastuzumab, a monoclonal antibody directed against the HER-2/*neu* receptor, to anthracycline- and taxane-containing adjuvant chemotherapy benefits women with HER-2-overexpressing breast cancer with respect to disease-free and overall survival.

Breast cancer was the first neoplasm shown to be responsive to hormonal manipulation. Tamoxifen is beneficial in postmenopausal women when used alone or in combination with cytotoxic chemotherapy. The present recommendation is to administer tamoxifen for 5 years of continuous therapy after surgical resection. Longer durations of tamoxifen therapy do not appear to add additional clinical benefit. Postmenopausal women who complete 5 years of tamoxifen therapy should be placed on an aromatase inhibitor such as anastrozole for at least 2.5 years, although the optimal duration is unknown. In women who have completed 2–3 years of tamoxifen therapy, treatment with an aromatase inhibitor for a total of 5 years of hormonal therapy is now recommended (see Chapter 40).

Results from several randomized trials for breast cancer have established that adjuvant chemotherapy for premenopausal women and adjuvant tamoxifen for postmenopausal women are of benefit to women with stage I (node-negative) breast cancer. While this group of patients has the lowest overall risk of recurrence after surgery alone (about 35–50% over 15 years), this risk can be further reduced with adjuvant therapy.

STAGE III & STAGE IV DISEASE

The approach to women with advanced breast cancer remains a major challenge, as current treatment options are only palliative. Combination chemotherapy, endocrine therapy, or a combination of both results in overall response rates of 40–50%, but only a

10–20% complete response rate. Breast cancers expressing estrogen receptors (ER) or progesterone receptors (PR), retain the intrinsic hormonal sensitivities of the normal breast—including the growth-stimulatory response to ovarian, adrenal, and pituitary hormones. Patients who show improvement with hormonal ablative procedures also respond to the addition of tamoxifen. The aromatase inhibitors anastrozole and letrozole are now approved as first-line therapy in women with advanced breast cancer whose tumors are hormone-receptor positive. In addition, these agents and exemestane are approved as second-line therapy following treatment with tamoxifen.

Patients with significant involvement of the lung, liver, or brain and those with rapidly progressive disease rarely benefit from hormonal maneuvers, and initial systemic chemotherapy is indicated in such cases. For the 25–30% of breast cancer patients whose tumors express the HER-2/*neu* cell surface receptor, the humanized monoclonal anti-HER-2/*neu* antibody, trastuzumab, is available for therapeutic use alone or in combination with cytotoxic chemotherapy.

About 50–60% of patients with metastatic disease respond to initial chemotherapy. A broad range of anticancer agents have activity in this disease, including the anthracyclines (doxorubicin, mitoxantrone, and epirubicin), the taxanes (docetaxel, paclitaxel, and albumin-bound paclitaxel) along with the microtubule inhibitor ixabepilone, navelbine, capecitabine, gemcitabine, cyclophosphamide, methotrexate, and cisplatin. The anthracyclines and the taxanes are two of the most active classes of cytotoxic drugs. Combination chemotherapy has been found to induce higher and more durable remissions in up to 50–80% of patients, and anthracycline-containing regimens are now considered the standard of care in first-line therapy. With most combination regimens, partial remissions have a median duration of about 10 months and complete remissions have a duration of about 15 months. Unfortunately, only 10–20% of patients achieve complete remissions with any of these regimens, and as noted, complete remissions are usually not long-lasting.

PROSTATE CANCER

Prostate cancer was the second cancer shown to be responsive to hormonal manipulation. The treatment of choice for patients with advanced prostate cancer is elimination of testosterone production by the testes through either surgical or chemical castration. Bilateral orchiectomy or estrogen therapy in the form of diethylstilbestrol was previously used as first-line therapy. Presently, the use of luteinizing hormone-releasing hormone (LHRH) agonists—including leuprolide and goserelin agonists, alone or in combination with an antiandrogen (eg, flutamide, bicalutamide, or nilutamide)—is the preferred approach. There appears to be no survival advantage of total androgen blockade using a combination of LHRH agonist and antiandrogen agent compared with single-agent therapy. Hormonal treatment reduces symptoms—especially bone pain—in 70–80% of patients and may cause a significant reduction in the prostate-specific antigen (PSA) level, which is now widely accepted as a surrogate marker for response to treatment in

prostate cancer. Although initial hormonal manipulation is able to control symptoms for up to 2 years, patients usually develop progressive disease. Second-line hormonal therapies include aminoglutethimide plus hydrocortisone, the antifungal agent ketoconazole plus hydrocortisone, or hydrocortisone alone.

Unfortunately, nearly all patients with advanced prostate cancer eventually become refractory to hormone therapy. A regimen of mitoxantrone and prednisone is approved in patients with hormone-refractory prostate cancer because it provides effective palliation in those who experience significant bone pain. Estramustine is an antimicrotubule agent that produces an almost 20% response rate as a single agent. However, when used in combination with either etoposide or a taxane such as docetaxel or paclitaxel, response rates are more than doubled to 40–50%. The combination of docetaxel and prednisone was recently shown to confer survival advantage when compared with the mitoxantrone-prednisone regimen, and this combination has now become the standard of care for hormone-refractory prostate cancer.

GASTROINTESTINAL CANCERS

Colorectal cancer (CRC) is the most common type of gastrointestinal malignancy. Nearly 145,000 new cases are diagnosed each year in the USA; worldwide, nearly one million cases are diagnosed each year. At the time of initial presentation, only about 40–45% of patients are potentially curable with surgery. Patients presenting with high-risk stage II disease and stage III disease are candidates for adjuvant chemotherapy with an oxaliplatin-based regimen in combination with 5-FU plus leucovorin (FOLFOX or FLOX) or with oral capecitabine (XELOX) and are generally treated for 6 months following surgical resection. Treatment with this combination regimen reduces the recurrence rate after surgery by 35% and clearly improves overall patient survival compared with surgery alone.

Significant advances have been made over the past 10 years with respect to treatment of metastatic CRC. There are four active cytotoxic agents—5-FU, the oral fluoropyrimidine capecitabine, oxaliplatin, and irinotecan; and three active biologic agents—the anti-VEGF antibody bevacizumab and the anti-EGFR antibodies cetuximab and panitumumab. In general, a fluoropyrimidine with either intravenous 5-FU or oral capecitabine serves as the main foundation of cytotoxic chemotherapy regimens. Recent clinical studies have shown that FOLFOX/FOLFIRI regimens in combination with the anti-VEGF antibody bevacizumab or with the anti-EGFR antibody cetuximab result in significantly improved clinical efficacy with no worsening of the toxicities normally observed with chemotherapy. In order for patients to derive maximal benefit, they should be treated with each of these active agents in a continuum of care approach. Using this strategy, median survivals now are in the 24–28 month range, and in some cases, approach 3 years. One of the main challenges facing clinicians at present is to begin to identify which patients would benefit from these various cytotoxic and biologic agents as well as identify those who might experience increased toxicity.

The incidence of gastric cancer, esophageal cancer, and pancreatic cancer is much lower than for CRC, but these malignancies tend to be more aggressive and result in greater tumor-related symptoms. In most cases, they cannot be completely resected surgically, as most patients present with either locally advanced or metastatic disease at the time of their initial diagnosis. 5-FU-based chemotherapy, using either intravenous 5-FU or oral capecitabine, is generally considered the main backbone for regimens targeting gastroesophageal cancers. In addition, cisplatin-based regimens in combination with either irinotecan or one of the taxanes (paclitaxel or docetaxel) also exhibit clinical activity. Response rates in the 40–50% range are now being reported. Recent studies have shown that the addition of the biologic agent trastuzumab to cisplatin-containing chemotherapy regimens provides significant clinical benefit in gastric cancer patients whose tumors overexpress the HER-2/*neu* receptor. In addition, neoadjuvant approaches with combination chemotherapy and radiation therapy prior to surgery appear to have promise in selected patients.

Although gemcitabine is approved for use as a single agent in metastatic pancreatic cancer, the overall response rate is less than 10%, with complete responses being quite rare. Intense efforts continue to be placed on incorporating gemcitabine into various combination regimens and on identifying novel agents that target signal transduction pathways thought to be critical for the growth of pancreatic cancer. One such agent is the small molecule inhibitor erlotinib, which targets the EGFR-associated tyrosine kinase. This agent is now approved for use in combination with gemcitabine in locally advanced or metastatic pancreatic cancer although the improvement in clinical benefit is relatively small. There is also evidence to support the use of adjuvant chemotherapy with either single-agent gemcitabine or 5-FU/leucovorin in patients with early-stage pancreatic cancer who have undergone successful surgical resection.

LUNG CANCER

Lung cancer is divided into two main histopathologic subtypes, non-small cell and small cell. Non-small cell lung cancer (NSCLC) makes up about 75–80% of all cases of lung cancer, and this group includes adenocarcinoma, squamous cell cancer, and large cell cancer, while small cell lung cancer (SCLC) makes up the remaining 20–25%. When NSCLC is diagnosed in an advanced stage with metastatic disease, the prognosis is extremely poor, with a median survival of about 8 months. It is clear that prevention (primarily through avoidance of cigarette smoking) and early detection remain the most important means of control. When diagnosed at an early stage, surgical resection results in patient cure. Moreover, recent studies have shown that adjuvant platinum-based chemotherapy provides a survival benefit in patients with pathologic stage IB, II, and IIIA disease. However, in most cases, distant metastases have occurred at the time of diagnosis. In certain instances, radiation therapy can be offered for palliation of pain, airway obstruction, or bleeding and to treat patients whose performance status would not allow for more aggressive treatments.

In patients with advanced disease, systemic chemotherapy is generally recommended. Combination regimens that include a platinum agent ("platinum doublets") appear superior to non-platinum doublets, and either cisplatin or carboplatin are appropriate platinum agents for such regimens. For the second drug, paclitaxel and vinorelbine appear to have activity independent of histology, while the

antifolate pemetrexed should be used for non-squamous cell cancer, and gemcitabine for squamous cell cancer. For patients with good performance status and those with non-squamous histology, the combination of the anti-VEGF antibody bevacizumab with carboplatin and paclitaxel is a standard treatment option. In patients deemed not to be appropriate candidates for bevacizumab therapy and those with squamous cell histology, a platinum-based chemotherapy regimen in combination with the anti-EGFR antibody cetuximab is a reasonable treatment strategy. Maintenance chemotherapy with pemetrexed is now used in patients with non-squamous NSCLC whose disease has not progressed after four cycles of platinum-based first-line chemotherapy. Finally, first-line therapy with an EGFR tyrosine kinase inhibitor, such as erlotinib or gefitinib, significantly improves outcomes in NSCLC patients with sensitizing EGFR mutations.

Small cell lung cancer is the most aggressive form of lung cancer, and it is exquisitely sensitive, at least initially, to platinum-based combination regimens, including cisplatin and etoposide or cisplatin and irinotecan. When diagnosed at an early stage, this disease is potentially curable using a combined modality approach of chemotherapy and radiation therapy. Unfortunately, drug resistance eventually develops in nearly all patients with extensive disease. The topoisomerase I inhibitor topotecan is used as second-line monotherapy in patients who have failed a platinum-based regimen.

OVARIAN CANCER

In the majority of patients, ovarian cancer remains occult and becomes symptomatic only after it has already metastasized to the peritoneal cavity. At this stage, it usually presents with malignant ascites. It is important to accurately stage this cancer with laparoscopy, ultrasound, and CT scanning. Patients with stage I disease appear to benefit from whole-abdomen radiotherapy and may receive additional benefit from combination chemotherapy with cisplatin and cyclophosphamide.

Combination chemotherapy is the standard approach to stage III and stage IV disease. Randomized clinical studies have shown that the combination of paclitaxel and cisplatin provides survival benefit compared with the previous standard combination of cisplatin plus cyclophosphamide. More recently, carboplatin plus paclitaxel has become the treatment of choice. In patients who present with recurrent disease, the topoisomerase I inhibitor topotecan, the alkylating agent altretamine, and liposomal doxorubicin are used as single agent monotherapy.

TESTICULAR CANCER

The introduction of platinum-based combination chemotherapy has made an impressive change in the treatment of patients with advanced testicular cancer. Presently, chemotherapy is recommended for patients with stage IIC or stage III seminomas and nonseminomatous disease. Over 90% of patients respond to chemotherapy and, depending upon the extent and severity of disease, complete remissions are observed in up to 70–80% of patents. Over 50% of patients achieving complete remission are cured with chemotherapy. In patients with good risk features, three cycles of cisplatin, etoposide, and bleomycin (PEB protocol) or four cycles of cisplatin and etoposide yield virtually identical results. In patients with high-risk disease, the combination of cisplatin, etoposide, and ifosfamide can be used as well as etoposide and bleomycin with high-dose cisplatin.

MALIGNANT MELANOMA

Malignant melanoma is curable when it presents locally, with surgical resection being the main treatment approach. However, once spread to metastatic sites has been diagnosed, it is one of the most difficult cancers to treat because it is a relatively drug-resistant tumor. While dacarbazine, temozolomide, and cisplatin are the most active cytotoxic agents for this disease, the overall response rates to these agents remain low. Biologic agents, including interferon-α and interleukin-2 (IL-2), have greater activity than traditional cytotoxic agents, and treatment with high-dose IL-2 has led to cures, albeit in a relatively small subset of patients. Significant efforts have focused on utilizing biologic therapy with combination chemotherapy in what have been labeled biochemotherapy regimens. Although overall response rates as well as complete response rates appear to be much higher with biochemotherapy regimens compared with chemotherapy alone, treatment toxicity also seems to be increased. As such, this approach remains investigational.

The BRAFV600E mutation has been identified in the large majority of melanomas. This mutation results in constitutive activation of BRAF kinase, which then leads to activation of downstream signaling pathways involved in cell growth and proliferation. In August 2011, the FDA approved a novel, oral, and highly selective small molecule inhibitor of BRAFV600E (**vemurafenib**) with highly promising activity in metastatic melanoma. Further studies are ongoing to confirm its activity as a single agent as well as in combination with other cytotoxic and biologic agents.

BRAIN CANCER

Chemotherapy has only limited efficacy in the treatment of malignant gliomas. In general, the nitrosoureas, because of their ability to cross the blood-brain barrier, are the most active agents in this disease. Carmustine (BCNU) can be used as a single agent, or lomustine (CCNU) can be used in combination with procarbazine and vincristine (PCV regimen). In addition, the newer alkylating agent temozolomide is active when combined with radiotherapy and used in patients with newly diagnosed glioblastoma multiforme (GBM) as well as in those with recurrent disease. The histopathologic subtype oligodendroglioma has been shown to be especially chemosensitive, and the PCV regimen is the treatment of choice for this disease. There is growing evidence that the anti-VEGF antibody bevacizumab alone or in combination with chemotherapy has promising activity in adult GBM, and bevacizumab was recently approved as a single agent for GBM in the setting of progressive disease following first-line chemotherapy. Of note, small molecule inhibitors of VEGFR-TKs are also undergoing active clinical development because they show interesting activity in adult brain tumors.

SECONDARY MALIGNANCIES & CANCER CHEMOTHERAPY

The development of secondary malignancies is a late complication of the alkylating agents and the epipodophyllotoxin etoposide. The most frequent secondary malignancy is acute myelogenous leukemia (AML). In general, AML develops in up to 15% of patients with Hodgkin's lymphoma who have received radiotherapy plus MOPP chemotherapy and in patients with multiple myeloma, ovarian carcinoma, or breast carcinoma treated with melphalan. The increased risk of AML is observed as early as 2–4 years after the initiation of chemotherapy and typically peaks at 5 and 9 years. With improvements in the clinical efficacy of various combination chemotherapy regimens resulting in prolonged survival and in some cases actual cure of cancer, the issue of how second cancers may affect long-term survival assumes greater importance. There is already evidence that certain alkylating agents (eg, cyclophosphamide) may be less carcinogenic than others (eg, melphalan). In addition to AML, other secondary malignancies have been well-described, including non-Hodgkin's lymphoma and bladder cancer, the latter most typically associated with cyclophosphamide therapy.

SUMMARY Anticancer Drugs

See Tables 54-2, -3, -4, -5

PREPARATIONS AVAILABLE

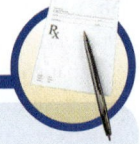

The reader is referred to the manufacturer's literature for the most recent information on preparations available.

REFERENCES

Books & Monographs

Abeloff MD et al: *Clinical Oncology,* 4th ed. Elsevier, 2008.

Chabner BA, Longo DL: *Cancer Chemotherapy and Biotherapy: Principles and Practice,* 4th ed. Lippincott Williams & Wilkins, 2006.

Chu E, DeVita VT Jr: *Cancer Chemotherapy Drug Manual 2011,* 11th ed. Jones & Bartlett, 2010.

DeVita VT Jr, Hellman S, Rosenberg SA: *Cancer: Principles and Practice of Oncology,* 9th ed. Lippincott Williams & Wilkins, 2011.

Harris JR et al: *Diseases of the Breast,* 4th ed. Lippincott Williams & Wilkins, 2009.

Hoppe R et al: *Textbook of Radiation Oncology,* 3rd ed. Elsevier, 2010.

Hoskins WJ, Perez CA, Young RC: *Principles and Practice of Gynecologic Oncology,* 4th ed. Lippincott Williams & Wilkins, 2004.

Kantoff PW et al: *Prostate Cancer: Principles and Practice.* Lippincott Williams & Wilkins, 2001.

Kelsen DP et al: *Gastrointestinal Oncology: Principles and Practices,* 2nd ed. Lippincott Williams & Wilkins, 2007.

Kufe D et al: *Cancer Medicine,* 7th ed. BC Decker, 2006.

Mendelsohn J et al: *The Molecular Basis of Cancer.* WB Saunders, 2008.

Pass HI et al: *Principles and Practice of Lung Cancer: The Official Reference Text of the International Association for the Study of Lung Cancer (IASLC),* 4th ed. Lippincott Williams & Wilkins, 2010.

Pizzo PA, Poplack AG: *Principles and Practice of Pediatric Oncology,* 6th ed. Lippincott Williams & Wilkins, 2010.

Weinberg RA: *Biology of Cancer.* Taylor & Francis, 2006.

Articles & Reviews

DeVita VT, Chu E: The history of cancer chemotherapy. Cancer Res 2008;68:8643.

Redmond KM et al: Resistance mechanisms to cancer chemotherapy. Front Biosci 2008;13:5138.

CASE STUDY ANSWER

The 5-year survival rate for patients with high-risk stage III CRC is on the order of 25–30%. Because the patient has no symptoms after surgery and has no comorbid illnesses, he would be an appropriate candidate to receive aggressive adjuvant chemotherapy. The usual recommendation would be to administer 6 months of oxaliplatin-based chemotherapy using either infusional 5-FU or oral capecitabine as the fluoropyrimidine base in combination with oxaliplatin. Adjuvant chemotherapy is usually begun 4–6 weeks after surgery to allow sufficient time for surgical wound to heal.

Patients with partial or complete deficiency in the enzyme dihydropyrimidine dehydrogenase (DPD) experience an increased incidence of severe toxicity to fluoropyrimidines in the form of myelosuppression, gastrointestinal toxicity, and neurotoxicity. Although mutations in DPD can be identified in peripheral blood mononuclear cells, nearly 50% of patients who exhibit severe 5-FU toxicity do not have a defined mutation in the *DPD* gene. In addition, such mutations may not result in reduced expression of the DPD protein or in altered enzymatic activity. For this reason, genetic testing is not recommended at this time as part of routine clinical practice.

55

Immunopharmacology

Douglas F. Lake, PhD, Adrienne D. Briggs, MD, &
Emmanuel T. Akporiaye, PhD

CASE STUDY

A 30-year-old woman has one living child, age 6. Her child and her husband are Rh positive and she is $Rh_o(D)$ and D^u negative. She is now in her ninth month of pregnancy and is in the labor room having frequent contractions. Her Rh antibody test taken earlier in the pregnancy was negative. What immunotherapy is appropriate for this patient? When and how should it be administered?

Agents that suppress the immune system play an important role in preventing the rejection of organ or tissue grafts and in the treatment of certain diseases that arise from dysregulation of the immune response. While precise details of the mechanisms of action of a number of these agents are still obscure, knowledge of the elements of the immune system is useful in understanding their effects. Agents that augment the immune response or selectively alter the balance of various components of the immune system are also becoming important in the management of certain diseases such as cancer, AIDS, and autoimmune or inflammatory diseases. A growing number of other conditions (infections, cardiovascular diseases, organ transplantation) may also be candidates for immune manipulation.

■ ELEMENTS OF THE IMMUNE SYSTEM

NORMAL IMMUNE RESPONSES

The immune system has evolved to protect the host from invading pathogens and to eliminate disease. At its functioning best, the immune system is exquisitely responsive to invading pathogens while retaining the capacity to recognize self tissues and antigens to which it is tolerant. Protection from infection and disease is provided by the collaborative efforts of the innate and adaptive immune systems.

The Innate Immune System

The innate immune system is the first line of defense against invading pathogens (eg, bacteria, viruses, fungi, parasites) and consists of mechanical, biochemical, and cellular components. Mechanical components include skin/epidermis and mucus; biochemical components include antimicrobial peptides and proteins (eg, defensins), complement, enzymes (eg, lysozyme, acid hydrolases), interferons, acidic pH, and free radicals (eg, hydrogen peroxide, superoxide anions); cellular components include neutrophils, monocytes, macrophages, natural killer (NK), and natural killer-T (NKT) cells. Unlike adaptive immunity, the innate immune response exists prior to infection, is not enhanced by repeated infection, and is generally not antigen-specific. An intact skin or mucosa is the first barrier to infection. When this barrier is breached, an immediate innate immune response, referred to as "inflammation" is provoked that ultimately leads to destruction of the pathogen. The process of pathogen destruction can be accomplished, for example, by biochemical components such as lysozyme (which breaks down the protective peptidoglycan cell wall) and the split products arising from complement activation. Complement components (Figure 55–1) enhance macrophage and neutrophil phagocytosis by acting as opsonins (C3b) and chemoattractants (C3a, C5a), which recruit immune cells from the bloodstream to the site of infection. The activation of complement eventually leads to pathogen lysis via the generation of a membrane attack complex that creates holes in the membrane and results in leakage of cellular components.

During the inflammatory response triggered by infection, neutrophils and monocytes enter the tissue sites from peripheral circulation. This cellular influx is mediated by the action of **chemoattractant cytokines (chemokines)** (eg, interleukin-8 [IL-8; CXCL8], macrophage chemotactic protein-1 [MCP-1; CCL2],

ACRONYMS

ADA	Adenosine deaminase
ALG	Antilymphocyte globulin
APC	Antigen-presenting cell
ATG	Antithymocyte globulin
CD	Cluster of differentiation
CSF	Colony-stimulating factor
CTL	Cytotoxic T lymphocyte
DC	Dendritic cell
DTH	Delayed-type hypersensitivity
FKBP	FK-binding protein
HAMA	Human antimouse antibody
HLA	Human leukocyte antigen
IFN	Interferon
IGIV	Immune globulin intravenous
IL	Interleukin
LFA	Leukocyte function-associated antigen
MAB	Monoclonal antibody
MHC	Major histocompatibility complex
NK cell	Natural killer cell
SCID	Severe combined immunodeficiency disease
TCR	T-cell receptor
TGF-β	Transforming growth factor-β
Tн1, Tн2	T helper cell types 1 and 2
TNF	Tumor necrosis factor

and macrophage inflammatory protein-1α [MIP-1α; CCL3]) released from activated endothelial cells and immune cells (mostly tissue macrophages) at the inflammatory site. Egress of the immune cells from blood vessels into the inflammatory site is mediated by adhesive interactions between cell surface receptors (eg, L-selectin, integrins) on the immune cells and ligands (eg, sialyl-Lewis x, intercellular adhesion molecule-1 [ICAM-1]) on the activated endothelial cell surface. The tissue macrophages as well as dendritic cells express pattern recognition receptors (PRRs) that include Toll-like receptors (TLRs), nucleotide-binding oligomerization domain (NOD)-like receptors (NLRs), scavenger receptors, mannose receptors, and lipopolysaccharide (LPS)-binding protein, which recognize key evolutionarily conserved pathogen components referred to as pathogen-associated molecular patterns (PAMPs). Examples of PAMPs include microbe-derived unmethylated CpG DNA, flagellin, double-stranded RNA, peptidoglycan, and LPS. The PRRs recognize PAMPs in various components of pathogens and stimulate the release of proinflammatory cytokines, chemokines, and interferons. If the innate immune response is successfully executed, the invading pathogen is ingested, degraded, and eliminated, and disease is either prevented or is of short duration.

In addition to monocytes and neutrophils, **natural killer (NK), natural killer-T (NKT),** and **gamma-delta T (γδ T)** cells recruited to the inflammatory site contribute to the innate response by secreting interferon-gamma (IFN-γ) and IL-17, which activate resident tissue macrophages and dendritic cells and recruit neutrophils respectively to successfully eliminate invading pathogens. NK cells are so called because they are able to recognize and destroy virus-infected normal cells as well as tumor cells without prior stimulation. This activity is regulated by "killer cell immunoglobulin-like receptors" (KIRs) on the NK cell surface that are specific for major histocompatibility complex (MHC) class I molecules. When NK cells bind self MHC class I proteins (expressed on all nucleated cells), these receptors deliver inhibitory signals, preventing them from killing normal host cells. Tumor cells or virus-infected cells that have down-regulated MHC class I expression do not engage these KIRs, resulting in activation of NK cells and subsequent destruction of the target cell. NK cells kill target cells by releasing cytotoxic granules such as perforins and granzymes that induce programmed cell death.

NKT cells express T-cell receptors as well as receptors commonly found on NK cells. NKT cells recognize microbial lipid antigens presented by a unique class of MHC-like molecules known as CD1 and have been implicated in host defense against microbial agents, autoimmune diseases, and tumors.

The Adaptive Immune System

The adaptive immune system is mobilized by cues from the innate response when the innate processes are incapable of coping with an infection. The adaptive immune system has a number of characteristics that contribute to its success in eliminating pathogens. These include the ability to (1) respond to a variety of antigens, each in a specific manner; (2) discriminate between foreign ("nonself") antigens (pathogens) and self antigens of the host; and (3) respond to a previously encountered antigen in a learned way by initiating a vigorous memory response. This adaptive response culminates in the production of **antibodies,** which are the effectors of **humoral immunity;** and the activation of **T lymphocytes,** which are the effectors of **cell-mediated immunity.**

The induction of specific adaptive immunity requires the participation of professional **antigen-presenting cells (APCs),** which include dendritic cells (DCs), macrophages, and B lymphocytes. These cells play pivotal roles in the induction of an adaptive immune response because of their capacity to phagocytize particulate antigens (eg, pathogens) or endocytose protein antigens, and enzymatically digest them to generate peptides, which are then loaded onto class I or class II MHC proteins and "presented" to the cell surface T-cell receptor (TCR) (Figure 55–2). CD8 T cells recognize class I-MHC peptide complexes while CD4 T cells recognize class II-MHC peptide complexes. At least two signals are necessary for the activation of T cells. The first signal is delivered following engagement of the TCR with peptide-bound MHC molecules. In the absence of a second signal, the T cells become unresponsive (anergic) or undergo apoptosis. The second signal involves ligation of costimulatory molecules (CD40, CD80 [also known as B7-1], and CD86 [also known as B7-2]) on the APC to

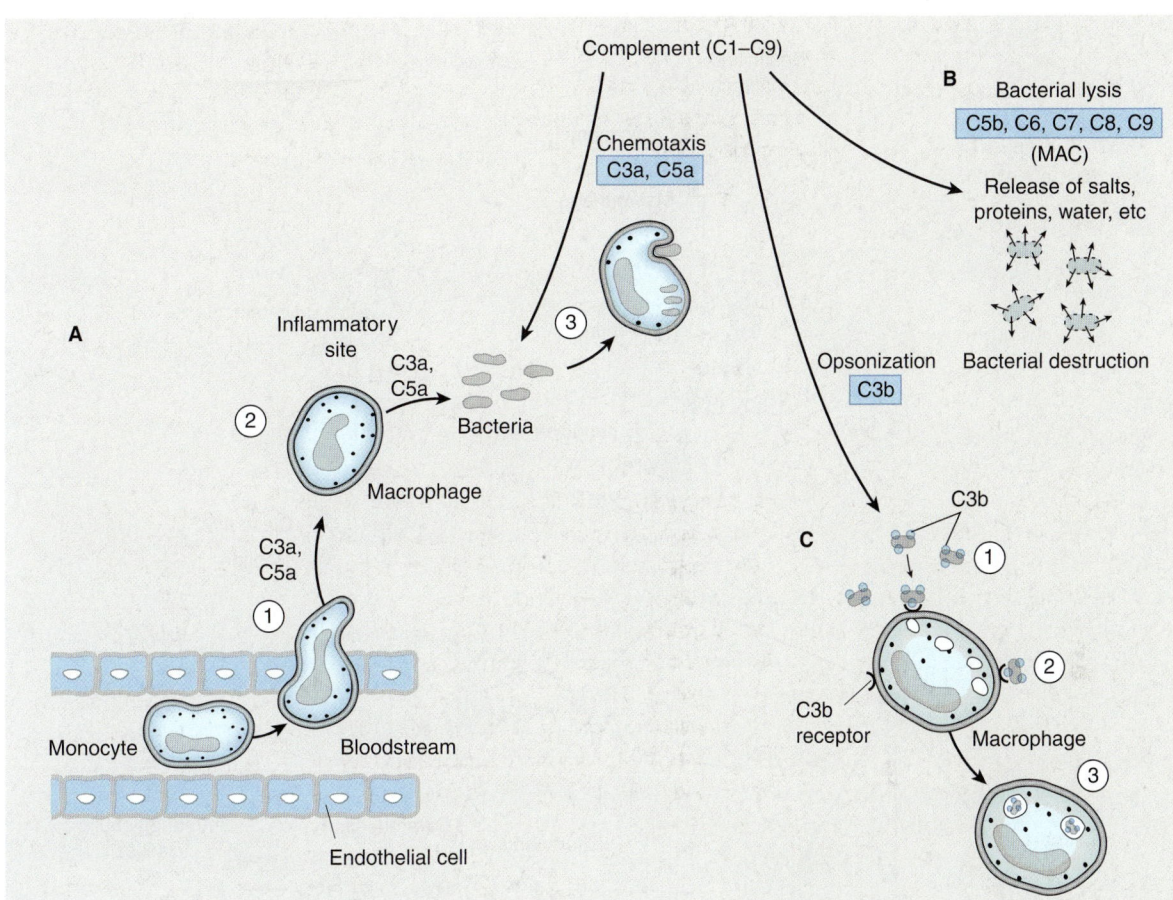

FIGURE 55–1 Role of complement in innate immunity. Complement is made up of nine proteins (C1–C9), which are split into fragments during activation. **A:** Complement components (C3a, C5a) attract phagocytes (1) to inflammatory sites (2), where they ingest and degrade pathogens (3). **B:** Complement components C5b, C6, C7, C8, and C9 associate to form a membrane attack complex (MAC) that lyses bacteria, causing their destruction. **C:** Complement component C3b is an opsonin that coats bacteria (1) and facilitates their ingestion (2) and digestion (3) by phagocytes.

their respective ligands (CD40L for CD40, CD28 for CD80 or CD86). Activation of T cells is regulated via a negative feedback loop involving another molecule known as T-lymphocyte-associated antigen 4 (CTLA-4). Following engagement of CD28 with CD80 or CD86, CTLA-4 in the cytoplasm is mobilized to the cell surface where, because of its higher affinity of binding to CD80 and CD86, it outcompetes or displaces CD28 resulting in suppression of T-cell activation and proliferation. This property of CTLA-4 has been exploited as a strategy for sustaining a desirable immune response such as that directed against cancer. A recombinant humanized antibody that binds CTLA-4 (ipilimumab) prevents its association with CD80/CD86. In so doing, the activated state of T cells is sustained. Recently completed vaccine trials in metastatic melanoma patients receiving anti-CTLA-4 antibody reported objective and durable clinical responses in a few patients. Unfortunately, these beneficial responses were associated with the development of autoimmune toxicity in some patients, raising concern about this approach.

T lymphocytes develop and learn to recognize self and non-self antigens in the thymus; those T cells that bind with high affinity to self antigens in the thymus undergo apoptosis (negative selection),

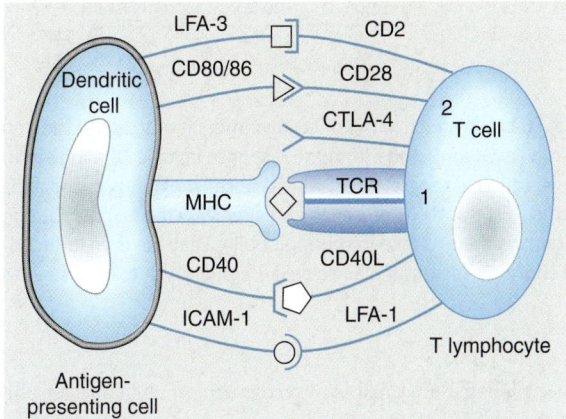

FIGURE 55–2 T-cell activation by an antigen-presenting cell requires engagement of the T-cell receptor by the MHC-peptide complex (signal 1) and binding of the costimulatory molecules (CD80, CD86) on the dendritic cell to CD28 on the T cell (signal 2). The activation signals are strengthened by CD40/CD40L and ICAM-1/LFA-1 interactions. In a normal immune response, T-cell activation is regulated by T-cell-derived CTLA-4, which binds to CD80 or CD86 with higher affinity than CD28 and sends inhibitory signals to the nucleus of the T cell.

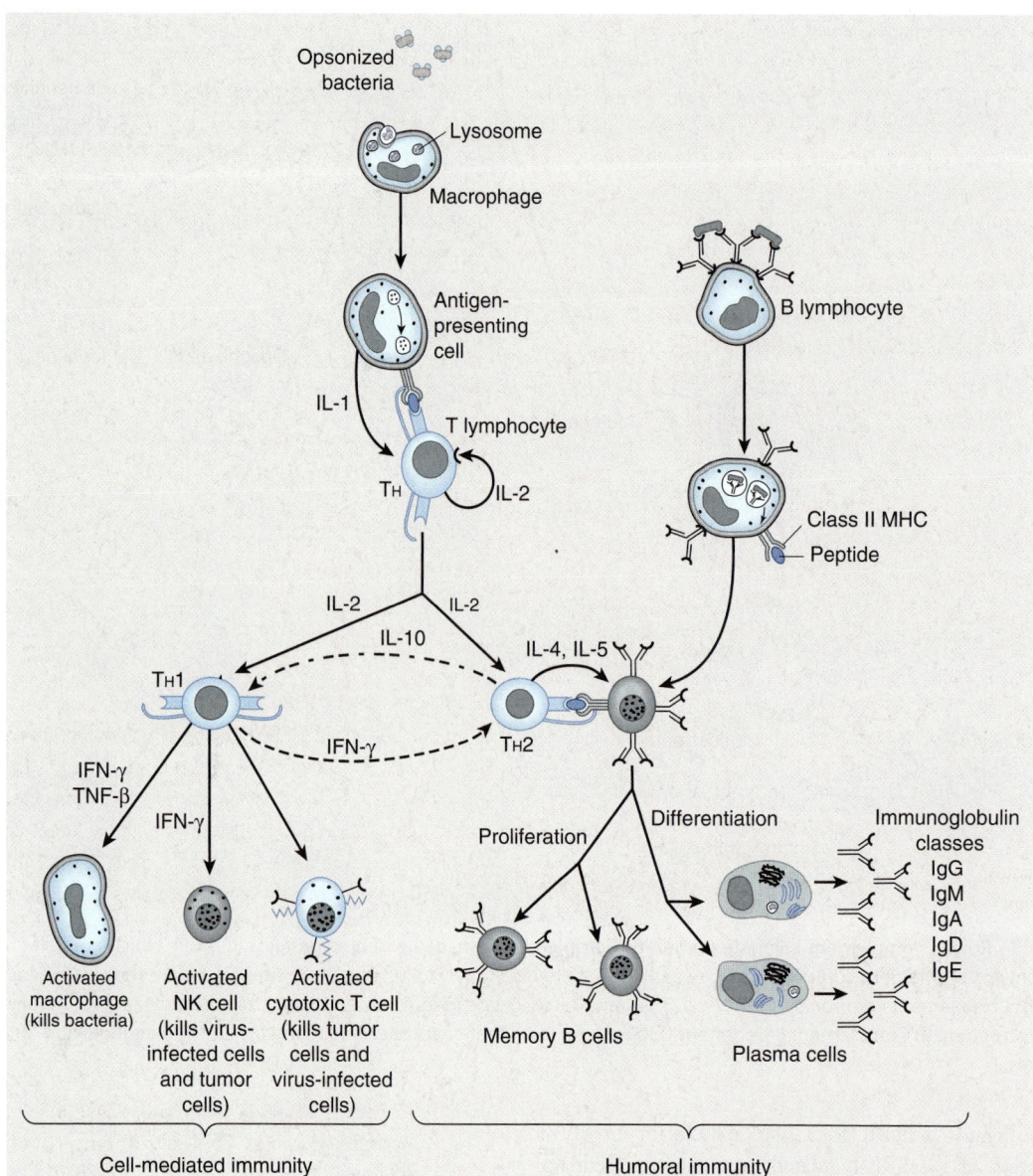

FIGURE 55–3 Scheme of cellular interactions during the generation of cell-mediated and humoral immune responses (see text). The cell-mediated arm of the immune response involves the ingestion and digestion of antigen by antigen-presenting cells such as macrophages. Activated TH cells secrete IL-2, which causes proliferation and activation of cytotoxic T lymphocytes, and TH1 and TH2 cell subsets. TH1 cells also produce IFN-γ and TNF-β, which can directly activate macrophages and NK cells. The humoral response is triggered when B lymphocytes bind antigen via their surface immunoglobulin. They are then induced by TH2-derived IL-4 and IL-5 to proliferate and differentiate into memory cells and antibody-secreting plasma cells. Regulatory cytokines such as IFN-γ and IL-10 down-regulate TH2 and TH1 responses, respectively.

while those that are capable of recognizing foreign antigens in the presence of self MHC molecules are retained and expanded (positive selection) for export to the periphery (lymph nodes, spleen, mucosa-associated lymphoid tissue, peripheral blood), where they become activated after encountering MHC-presented peptides (Figures 55–2 and 55–3).

Studies using murine T-cell clones have demonstrated the presence of two subsets of T helper lymphocytes (**TH1** and **TH2**) based on the cytokines they secrete after activation. This demarcation is not so clear-cut in humans. The TH1 subset characteristically

produces IFN-γ, IL-2, and IL-12 and induces cell-mediated immunity by activation of macrophages, cytotoxic T cells (CTLs), and NK cells. The TH2 subset produces IL-4, IL-5, IL-6, and IL-10 (and sometimes IL-13), which induce B-cell proliferation and differentiation into antibody-secreting plasma cells. IL-10 produced by TH2 cells inhibits cytokine production by TH1 cells via the down-regulation of MHC expression by APCs. Conversely, IFN-γ produced by TH1 cells inhibits the proliferation of TH2 cells (Figure 55–3). Although these subsets have been well described in vitro, the nature of the antigenic challenge that elicits a TH1 or TH2 phenotype is less clear. Extracellular bacteria typically cause the elaboration of TH2 cytokines, culminating in the production of neutralizing or opsonic antibodies. In contrast, intracellular organisms (eg, mycobacteria) elicit the production of TH1 cytokines, which lead to the activation of effector cells such as macrophages. A less well-defined T-cell subset (TH3) has been described that produces transforming growth factor-β (TGF-β), whose numerous functions include down-regulation of proliferation and differentiation of T lymphocytes.

Recently, a subset of CD4 T cells that secrete IL-17 (TH17) has been implicated in neutrophil recruitment to sites of inflammation. A population of CD4 T cells that is essential for preventing autoimmunity and allergy as well as maintaining homeostasis and tolerance to self antigens is the regulatory (Treg) T cell. In the mouse, this cell population exists as natural Treg (nTreg), derived directly from the thymus, and induced (adaptive) Treg (iTreg), generated from naïve CD4 T cells in the periphery. Both populations have also been shown to inhibit antitumor immune responses and are implicated in fostering tumor growth and progression. Recent attempts to distinguish both populations have resulted in the discovery of a transcription factor, Helios, in nTreg but not in iTreg cells.

CD8 T lymphocytes recognize endogenously processed peptides presented by virus-infected cells or tumor cells. These peptides are usually nine-amino-acid fragments derived from virus or protein tumor antigens in the cytoplasm and are loaded onto MHC class I molecules (Figure 55–2) in the endoplasmic reticulum. In contrast, class II MHC molecules present peptides (usually 11–22 amino acids) derived from extracellular (exogenous) pathogens to CD4 T helper cells. In some instances, exogenous antigens, upon ingestion by APCs, can be presented on class I MHC molecules to CD8 T cells. This phenomenon, referred to as "cross-presentation," involves retro-translocation of antigens from the endosome to the cytosol for peptide generation in the proteosome and is thought to be useful in generating effective immune responses against infected host cells that are incapable of priming T lymphocytes. Upon activation, CD8 T cells induce target cell death via lytic granule enzymes ("granzymes"), perforin, and the Fas-Fas ligand (Fas-FasL) apoptosis pathways.

B lymphocytes undergo selection in the bone marrow, during which self-reactive B lymphocytes are clonally deleted while B-cell clones specific for foreign antigens are retained and expanded. The repertoire of antigen specificities by T cells is genetically determined and arises from T-cell *receptor* gene rearrangement while the specificities of B cells arise from *immunoglobulin* gene rearrangement; for both types of cells, these determinations occur prior to encounters with antigen. Upon an encounter with antigen, a mature B cell binds the antigen, internalizes and processes it, and presents its peptide—bound to class II MHC—to CD4 helper cells, which in turn secrete IL-4 and IL-5. These interleukins stimulate B-cell proliferation and differentiation into memory B cells and antibody-secreting plasma cells. The primary antibody response consists mostly of IgM-class immunoglobulins. Subsequent antigenic stimulation results in a vigorous "booster" response accompanied by class (isotype) switching to produce IgG, IgA, and IgE antibodies with diverse effector functions (Figure 55–3). These antibodies also undergo affinity maturation, which allows them to bind more efficiently to the antigen. With the passage of time, this results in accelerated elimination of microorganisms in subsequent infections. Antibodies mediate their functions by acting as opsonins to enhance phagocytosis and cellular cytotoxicity and by activating complement to elicit an inflammatory response and induce bacterial lysis (Figure 55–4).

ABNORMAL IMMUNE RESPONSES

Whereas the normally functioning immune response can successfully neutralize toxins, inactivate viruses, destroy transformed cells, and eliminate pathogens, inappropriate responses can lead to extensive tissue damage (hypersensitivity) or reactivity against self antigens (autoimmunity); conversely, impaired reactivity to appropriate targets (immunodeficiency) may occur and abrogate essential defense mechanisms.

Hypersensitivity

Hypersensitivity can be classified as antibody-mediated or cell-mediated. Three types of hypersensitivity are antibody-mediated (types I–III), while the fourth is cell-mediated (type IV). Hypersensitivity occurs in two phases: the sensitization phase and the effector phase. Sensitization occurs upon initial encounter with an antigen; the effector phase involves immunologic memory and results in tissue pathology upon a subsequent encounter with that antigen.

1. Type I—Immediate, or type I, hypersensitivity is IgE-mediated, with symptoms usually occurring within minutes following the patient's reencounter with antigen. Type I hypersensitivity results from cross-linking of membrane-bound IgE on blood basophils or tissue mast cells by antigen. This cross-linking causes cells to degranulate, releasing substances such as histamine, leukotrienes, and eosinophil chemotactic factor, which induce anaphylaxis, asthma, hay fever, or urticaria (hives) in affected individuals (Figure 55–5). A severe type I hypersensitivity reaction such as systemic anaphylaxis (eg, from insect envenomation, ingestion of certain foods, or drug hypersensitivity) requires immediate medical intervention.

2. Type II—Type II hypersensitivity results from the formation of antigen-antibody complexes between foreign antigen and IgM or IgG immunoglobulins. One example of this type of hypersensitivity is a blood transfusion reaction that can occur if blood is not cross-matched properly. Preformed antibodies bind to red blood cell membrane antigens that activate the complement cascade, generating a membrane attack complex that lyses the transfused red blood cells. In hemolytic disease of the newborn, anti-Rh IgG antibodies produced by an Rh-negative mother cross the placenta, bind to red blood cells of an Rh-positive fetus, and damage them. The disease is prevented in subsequent pregnancies by the administration of anti-Rh antibodies to the mother 24–48 hours after delivery (see Immunosuppressive Antibodies, below).

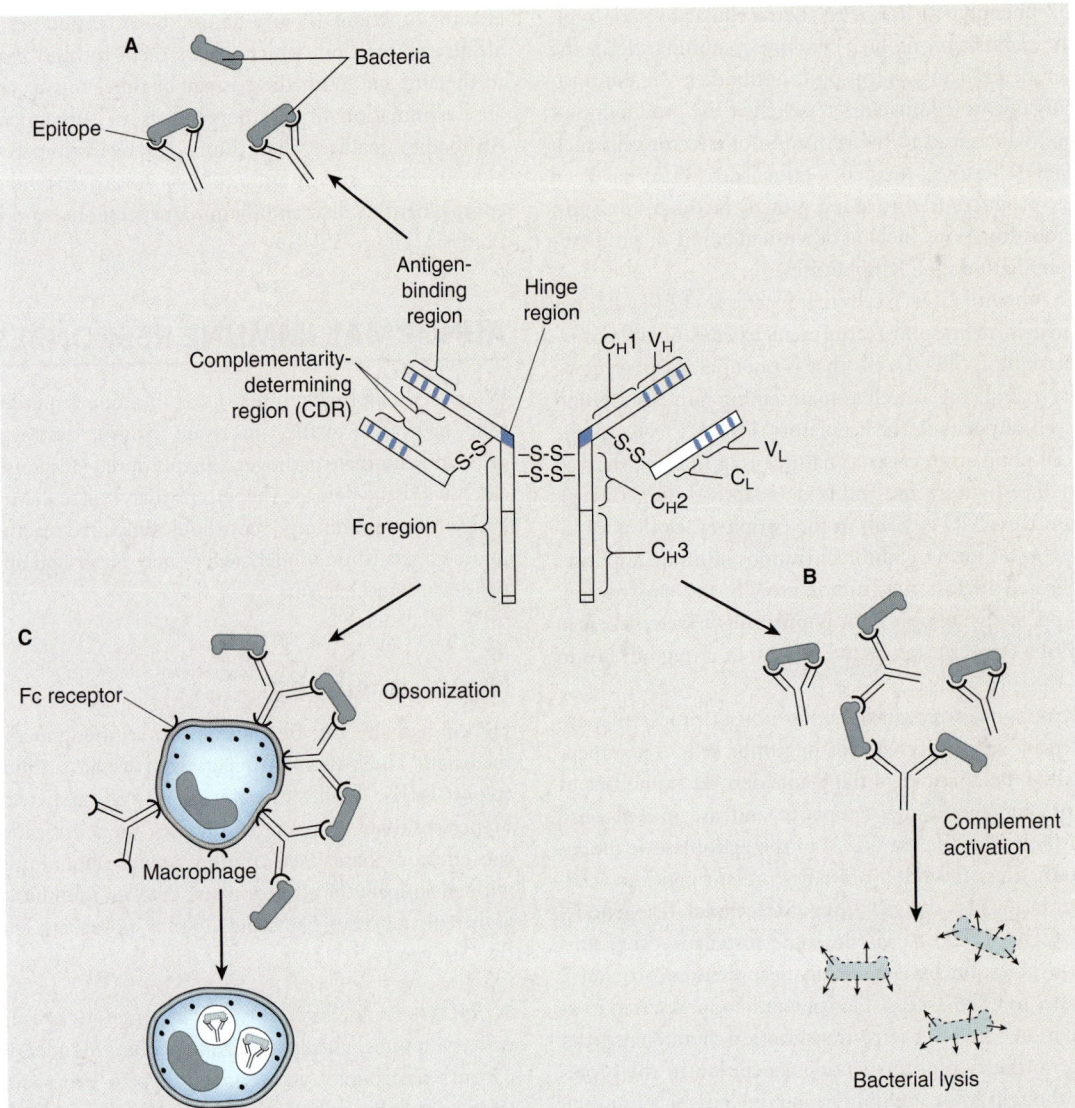

FIGURE 55–4   Antibody has multiple functions. The prototypical antibody consists of two heavy (H) and two light (L) chains, each sub-divided into constant (C_L, C_H) and variable (V_L, V_H) domains. The structure is held together by intra- and interchain disulfide bridges. **A:** The complementarity-determining region (CDR) of the antigen-binding portion of the antibody engages the antigenic determinant (epitope) in a lock and key fashion. **B:** Antigen-antibody complexes activate complement to produce split complement components that cause bacterial lysis. **C:** The Fc portion of antibodies binds to Fc receptors on phagocytes (eg, macrophages, neutrophils) and facilitates uptake of bacteria (opsonization).

Type II hypersensitivity can also be drug-induced and may occur during the administration of penicillin (for example) to allergic patients. In these patients, penicillin binds to red blood cells or other host tissue to form a neoantigen that evokes production of antibodies capable of inducing complement-mediated red cell lysis. In some circumstances, subsequent administration of the drug can lead to systemic anaphylaxis (type I hypersensitivity).

3. Type III—Type III hypersensitivity is due to the presence of elevated levels of antigen-antibody complexes in the circulation that ultimately deposit on basement membranes in tissues and vessels. Immune complex deposition activates complement to produce components with anaphylatoxic and chemotactic activities (C5a, C3a, C4a) that increase vascular permeability and

recruit neutrophils to the site of complex deposition. Complex deposition and the action of lytic enzymes released by neutrophils can cause skin rashes, glomerulonephritis, and arthritis in these individuals. If patients have type III hypersensitivity against a particular antigen, clinical symptoms usually occur 3–4 days after exposure to the antigen.

4. Type IV: Delayed-type hypersensitivity—Unlike type I, II, and III hypersensitivities, delayed-type hypersensitivity (DTH) is cell-mediated, and responses occur 2–3 days after exposure to the sensitizing antigen. DTH is caused by antigen-specific DTH T_H1 cells and induces a local inflammatory response that causes tissue damage characterized by the influx of antigen-*non*specific inflammatory cells, especially macrophages. These cells are

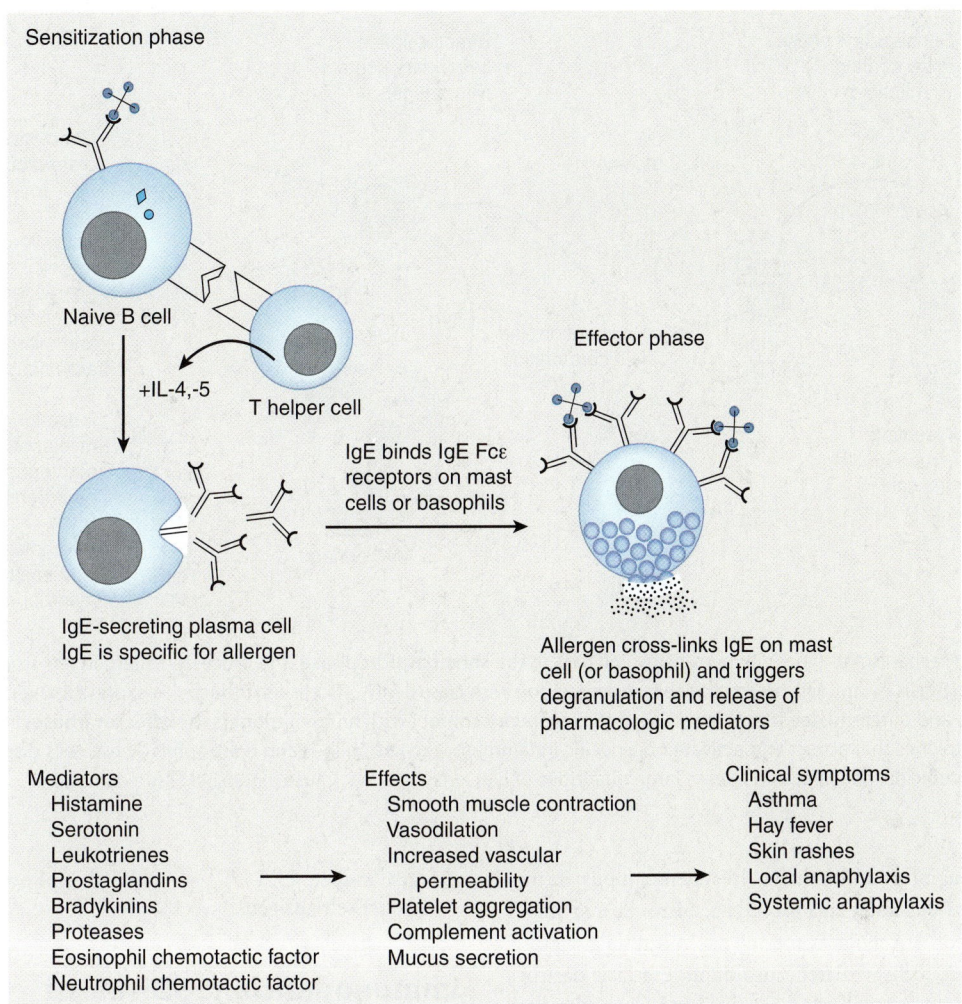

FIGURE 55–5 Mechanism of type I hypersensitivity. Initial exposure to allergen **(sensitization phase)** leads to production of IgE by plasma cells differentiated from allergen-specific B cells (not shown). The secreted IgE binds IgE-specific receptors (FcεR) on blood basophils and tissue mast cells. Reexposure to allergen leads to cross-linking of membrane-bound IgE **(effector phase).** This cross-linking causes degranulation of cytoplasmic granules and release of mediators that induce vasodilation, smooth muscle contraction, and increased vascular permeability. These effects lead to the clinical symptoms characteristic of type I hypersensitivity.

recruited under the influence of T_H1-produced cytokines (Figure 55–6), which chemoattract circulating monocytes and neutrophils, induce myelopoiesis, and activate macrophages. The activated macrophages are primarily responsible for the tissue damage associated with DTH. Although widely considered to be deleterious, DTH responses are very effective in eliminating infections caused by intracellular pathogens such as *Mycobacterium tuberculosis* and *Leishmania* species. Clinical manifestations of DTH include **tuberculin** and **contact hypersensitivities.** Tuberculosis exposure is determined using a DTH skin test. Positive responses show erythema and induration caused by accumulation of macrophages and DTH T (T_{DTH}) cells at the site of the tuberculin injection. **Poison ivy** is the most common cause of contact hypersensitivity, in which pentadecacatechol, the lipophilic chemical in poison ivy, modifies cellular tissue and results in a DTH T-cell response.

Autoimmunity

Autoimmune disease arises when the body mounts an immune response against itself due to failure to distinguish self tissues and cells from foreign (nonself) antigens or loss of tolerance to self. This phenomenon derives from the activation of self-reactive T and B lymphocytes that generate cell-mediated or humoral immune responses directed against self antigens. The pathologic consequences of this reactivity constitute several types of autoimmune diseases. Autoimmune diseases are highly complex due to MHC genetics, environmental conditions, infectious entities, and dysfunctional immune regulation. Examples of such diseases include rheumatoid arthritis, systemic lupus erythematosus, multiple sclerosis, and insulin-dependent diabetes mellitus (type 1 diabetes). In rheumatoid arthritis, IgM antibodies (rheumatoid factors) are produced that react with the Fc portion of IgG and may form immune complexes that activate the complement cascade, causing chronic

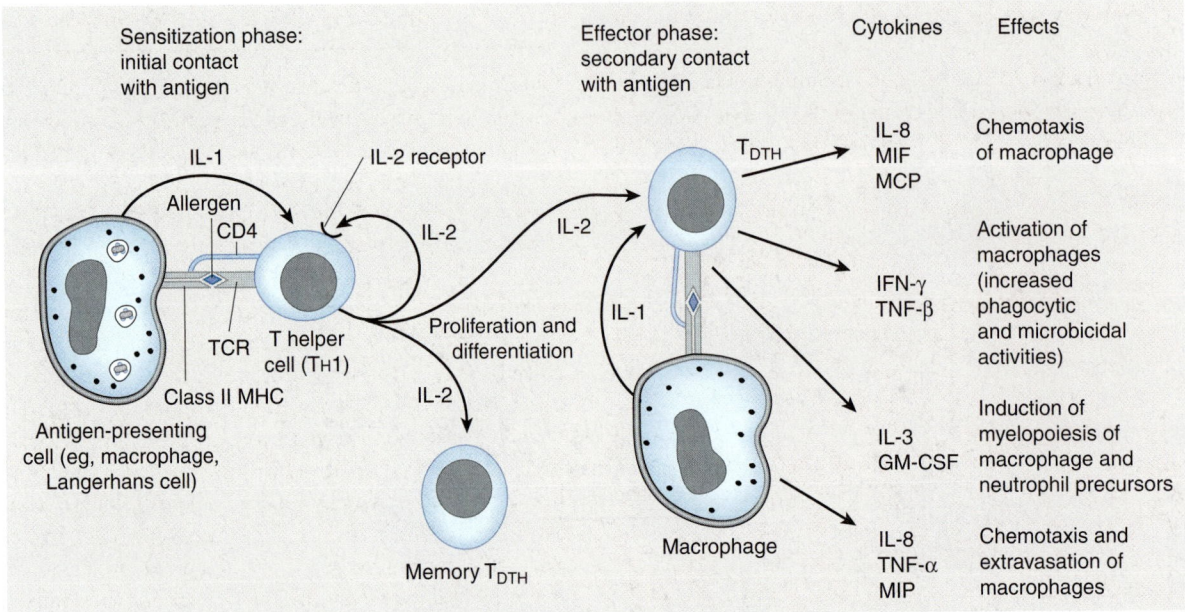

FIGURE 55–6 Mechanism of type IV hypersensitivity (DTH). In the **sensitization phase,** the processed allergen (eg, from poison oak) is presented to CD4 TH1 cells by antigen-presenting cells in association with class II MHC. T cells are induced to express IL-2 receptors and are stimulated to proliferate and differentiate into memory T$_{DTH}$ cells. Secondary contact with antigen triggers the **effector phase,** in which memory T$_{DTH}$ cells release cytokines that attract and activate nonspecific inflammatory macrophages and neutrophils. These cells display increased phagocytic and microbicidal activities and release large quantities of lytic enzymes that cause extensive tissue damage.

inflammation of the joints and kidneys. In systemic lupus erythematosus, antibodies are made against DNA, histones, red blood cells, platelets, and other cellular components. In multiple sclerosis and type 1 diabetes, cell-mediated autoimmune attack destroys myelin surrounding nerve cells and insulin-producing islet beta cells of the pancreas, respectively. In type 1 diabetes, activated CD4 T$_{DTH}$ cells that infiltrate the islets of Langerhans and recognize self islet beta cell peptides are thought to produce cytokines that stimulate macrophages to produce lytic enzymes, which destroy islet beta cells. Autoantibodies directed against the islet beta cell antigens are produced, but do not contribute significantly to disease.

A number of mechanisms have been proposed to explain autoimmunity:

1. Exposure of antigens previously sequestered from the immune system (eg, lens protein, myelin basic protein) to self-reactive T lymphocytes.

2. Molecular mimicry by invading pathogens, in which immune responses are directed at antigenic determinants on pathogens that share identical or similar epitopes with normal host tissue. This phenomenon occurs in rheumatic fever following *Streptococcus pyogenes* infection, in which heart damage is thought to arise from an immune response directed against streptococcal antigens shared with heart muscle. The suggested viral etiology of autoimmune diseases has been ascribed to immune responses (both cell-mediated and humoral) directed against virus epitopes that mimic self antigens.

3. Inappropriate expression of class II MHC molecules on the membranes of cells that normally do not express class II MHC (eg, islet beta cells). Increased expression of MHC II may increase presentation of self peptides to T helper cells, which in turn induce CTL, T$_{DTH}$, and B-lymphocyte cells that react against self antigens.

Immunodeficiency Diseases

Immunodeficiency diseases result from inadequate function in the immune system; the consequences include increased susceptibility to infections and prolonged duration and severity of disease. Immunodeficiency diseases are either congenital or arise from extrinsic factors such as bacterial or viral infections or drug treatment. Affected individuals frequently succumb to infections caused by opportunistic organisms of low pathogenicity for the immunocompetent host. Examples of congenitally acquired immunodeficiency diseases include X-linked agammaglobulinemia, DiGeorge's syndrome, and severe combined immunodeficiency disease (SCID) due to adenosine deaminase (ADA) deficiency.

X-linked agammaglobulinemia is a disease affecting males that is characterized by a failure of immature B lymphocytes to mature into antibody-producing plasma cells. These individuals are susceptible to recurrent bacterial infections, although the cell-mediated responses directed against viruses and fungi are preserved. DiGeorge's syndrome is due to failure of the thymus to develop, resulting in diminished T-cell responses (T$_{DTH}$, CTL), while the humoral response remains functional, but does not benefit from T-cell help.

The ADA enzyme normally prevents the accumulation of toxic deoxy-ATP in cells. Deoxy-ATP is particularly toxic to lymphocytes, and leads to death of T and B cells. Absence of the enzyme therefore results in SCID. Infusion of the purified enzyme (**pegademase,** from bovine sources) and transfer of ADA gene-modified lymphocytes have both been used successfully to treat this disease.

AIDS represents the classic example of immunodeficiency disease caused by extrinsic viral infection, in this instance the human immunodeficiency virus (HIV). This virus exhibits a strong tropism for CD4 T helper cells; these become depleted, giving rise to increased frequency of opportunistic infections and malignancies in infected individuals. AIDS is also characterized by an imbalance in TH1 and TH2 cells, and the ratios of cells and their functions are skewed toward TH2. This results in loss of cytotoxic T-lymphocyte activity, loss of delayed hypersensitivity, and hypergammaglobulinemia.

■ IMMUNOSUPPRESSIVE AGENTS

Immunosuppressive agents have proved very useful in minimizing the occurrence or impact of deleterious effects of exaggerated or inappropriate immune responses. Unfortunately, these agents also have the potential to cause disease and to increase the risk of infection and malignancies.

GLUCOCORTICOIDS

Glucocorticoids (corticosteroids) were the first hormonal agents recognized as having lympholytic properties. Administration of any glucocorticoid reduces the size and lymphoid content of the lymph nodes and spleen, although it has no toxic effect on proliferating myeloid or erythroid stem cells in the bone marrow.

Glucocorticoids are thought to interfere with the cell cycle of activated lymphoid cells. The mechanism of their action is described in Chapter 39. Glucocorticoids are quite cytotoxic to certain subsets of T cells, but their immunologic effects are probably due to their ability to modify cellular functions rather than to direct cytotoxicity. Although cellular immunity is more affected than humoral immunity, the primary antibody response can be diminished, and with continued use, previously established antibody responses are also decreased. Additionally, continuous administration of corticosteroid increases the fractional catabolic rate of IgG, the major class of antibody immunoglobulins, thus lowering the effective concentration of specific antibodies. Contact hypersensitivity mediated by T_{DTH} cells, for example, is usually abrogated by glucocorticoid therapy.

Glucocorticoids are used in a wide variety of conditions (Table 55–1). It is thought that the immunosuppressive and anti-

TABLE 55–1   Clinical uses of immunosuppressive agents.

Source	Immunopharmacologic Agents Used	Response
Autoimmune diseases		
Idiopathic thrombocytopenic purpura (ITP)	Prednisone,[1] vincristine, occasionally cyclophosphamide, mercaptopurine, or azathioprine; commonly high-dose gamma globulin, plasma immunoadsorption or plasma exchange	Usually good
Autoimmune hemolytic anemia	Prednisone,[1] cyclophosphamide, chlorambucil, mercaptopurine, azathioprine, high-dose gamma globulin	Usually good
Acute glomerulonephritis	Prednisone,[1] mercaptopurine, cyclophosphamide	Usually good
Acquired factor XIII antibodies	Cyclophosphamide plus factor XIII	Usually good
Autoreactive tissue disorders (autoimmune diseases)[2]	Prednisone, cyclophosphamide, methotrexate, interferon-α and -β, azathioprine, cyclosporine, infliximab, etanercept, adalimumab	Often good, variable
Isoimmune disease		
Hemolytic disease of the newborn	Rh$_o$(D) immune globulin	Excellent
Organ transplantation		
Renal	Cyclosporine, azathioprine, prednisone, ALG, OKT3, tacrolimus, basiliximab,[3] daclizumab,[3] sirolimus	Very good
Heart	Cyclosporine, azathioprine, prednisone, ALG, OKT3, tacrolimus, basiliximab,[3] daclizumab,[3] sirolimus	Good
Liver	Cyclosporine, prednisone, azathioprine, tacrolimus, sirolimus	Fair
Bone marrow	Cyclosporine, cyclophosphamide, prednisone, methotrexate, ALG	Good
Prevention of cell proliferation		
Coronary stents	Sirolimus (impregnated stent)	Good
Neovascular macular degeneration	Ranibizumab (labeled), bevacizumab (off-label)	Fair

[1]Drug of choice.

[2]Including systemic lupus erythematosus, rheumatoid arthritis, scleroderma, dermatomyositis, mixed tissue disorder, multiple sclerosis, Wegener's granulomatosis, chronic active hepatitis, lipoid nephrosis, and inflammatory bowel disease.

[3]Basiliximab and daclizumab are approved for renal transplant only.

inflammatory properties of corticosteroids account for their beneficial effects in diseases like idiopathic thrombocytopenic purpura and rheumatoid arthritis. Glucocorticoids modulate allergic reactions and are useful in the treatment of diseases like asthma or as premedication for other agents (eg, blood products, chemotherapy) that might cause undesirable immune responses. Glucocorticoids are first-line immunosuppressive therapy for both solid organ and hematopoietic stem cell transplant recipients, with variable results. The toxicities of long-term glucocorticoid therapy can be severe and are discussed in Chapter 39.

CALCINEURIN INHIBITORS

Cyclosporine

Cyclosporine (cyclosporin A, CSA) is an immunosuppressive agent with efficacy in human organ transplantation, in the treatment of graft-versus-host disease after hematopoietic stem cell transplantation, and in the treatment of selected autoimmune disorders. Cyclosporine is a peptide antibiotic that appears to act at an early stage in the antigen receptor-induced differentiation of T cells and blocks their activation. Cyclosporine binds to **cyclophilin,** a member of a class of intracellular proteins called immunophilins. Cyclosporine and cyclophilin form a complex that inhibits the cytoplasmic phosphatase, calcineurin, which is necessary for the activation of a T-cell-specific transcription factor. This transcription factor, NF-AT, is involved in the synthesis of interleukins (eg, IL-2) by activated T cells. In vitro studies have indicated that cyclosporine inhibits the gene transcription of IL-2, IL-3, IFN-γ, and other factors produced by antigen-stimulated T cells, but it does not block the effect of such factors on primed T cells nor does it block interaction with antigen.

Cyclosporine may be given intravenously or orally, though it is slowly and incompletely absorbed (20–50%). The absorbed drug is primarily metabolized by the P450 3A enzyme system in the liver with resultant multiple drug interactions. This propensity for drug interaction contributes to significant interpatient variability in bioavailability, such that cyclosporine requires individual patient dosage adjustments based on steady-state blood levels and the desired therapeutic ranges for the drug. Cyclosporine ophthalmic solution is now available for severe dry eye syndrome, as well as ocular graft-versus-host disease. Inhaled cyclosporine is being investigated for use in lung transplantation.

Toxicities are numerous and include nephrotoxicity, hypertension, hyperglycemia, liver dysfunction, hyperkalemia, altered mental status, seizures, and hirsutism. However, cyclosporine causes very little bone marrow toxicity. While an increased incidence of lymphoma and other cancers (Kaposi's sarcoma, skin cancer) have been observed in transplant recipients receiving cyclosporine, other immunosuppressive agents may also predispose recipients to cancer. Some evidence suggests that tumors may arise after cyclosporine treatment because the drug induces TGF-β, which promotes tumor invasion and metastasis.

Cyclosporine may be used alone or in combination with other immunosuppressants, particularly glucocorticoids. It has been used successfully as the sole immunosuppressant for cadaveric transplantation of the kidney, pancreas, and liver, and it has proved extremely useful in cardiac transplantation as well. In combination with methotrexate, cyclosporine is a standard prophylactic regimen to prevent graft-versus-host disease after allogeneic stem cell transplantation. Cyclosporine has also proved useful in a variety of autoimmune disorders, including uveitis, rheumatoid arthritis, psoriasis, and asthma. Its combination with newer agents is showing considerable efficacy in clinical and experimental settings where effective and less toxic immunosuppression is needed. Newer formulations of cyclosporine have been developed that are improving patient compliance (smaller, better tasting pills) and increasing bioavailability.

Tacrolimus

Tacrolimus (FK 506) is an immunosuppressant macrolide antibiotic produced by *Streptomyces tsukubaensis.* It is not chemically related to cyclosporine, but their mechanisms of action are similar. Both drugs bind to cytoplasmic peptidylprolyl isomerases that are abundant in all tissues. While cyclosporine binds to cyclophilin, tacrolimus binds to the immunophilin **FK-binding protein (FKBP).** Both complexes inhibit calcineurin, which is necessary for the activation of the T-cell-specific transcription factor NF-AT.

On a weight basis, tacrolimus is 10–100 times more potent than cyclosporine in inhibiting immune responses. Tacrolimus is utilized for the same indications as cyclosporine, particularly in organ and stem cell transplantation. Multicenter studies in the USA and in Europe indicate that both graft and patient survival are similar for the two drugs. Tacrolimus has proved to be effective therapy for preventing rejection in solid-organ transplant patients even after failure of standard rejection therapy, including anti-T-cell antibodies. It is now considered a standard prophylactic agent (usually in combination with methotrexate or mycophenolate mofetil) for graft-versus-host disease.

Tacrolimus can be administered orally or intravenously. The half-life of the intravenous form is approximately 9–12 hours. Like cyclosporine, tacrolimus is metabolized primarily by P450 enzymes in the liver, and there is potential for drug interactions. The dosage is determined by trough blood level at steady state. Its toxic effects are similar to those of cyclosporine and include nephrotoxicity, neurotoxicity, hyperglycemia, hypertension, hyperkalemia, and gastrointestinal complaints.

Because of the effectiveness of systemic tacrolimus in some dermatologic diseases, a topical preparation is now available. Tacrolimus ointment is currently used in the therapy of atopic dermatitis and psoriasis.

MAMMALIAN TARGET OF RAPAMYCIN (mTOR) INHIBITORS

The mTOR inhibitors include **sirolimus** (rapamycin) as well as its analogs (called "rapalogs") such as **everolimus** and **temsirolimus.**

Sirolimus is an immunosuppressant macrolide antibiotic produced by *Streptomyces hygroscopicus* and is structurally similar to tacrolimus. Sirolimus binds the circulating immunophilin FK506-binding protein 12, resulting in an active complex that inhibits the kinase activity of mammalian target of rapamycin (mTOR). The mTOR is a key component of a complex intracellular signaling pathway involved in cellular processes such as cell growth and proliferation, angiogenesis, and metabolism. Thus, blockade of mTOR ultimately can, for example, lead to inhibition of interleukin-driven T-cell proliferation. The signaling pathways involved in mTor are an active area of investigation in immunotherapy and targeted cancer therapy. Sirolimus is available only as an oral drug. Its half-life is about 60 hours, while that of everolimus is about 43 hours. Both drugs are rapidly absorbed and elimination is similar to that of cyclosporine and tacrolimus, being substrates for both cytochrome P450 3A and P-glycoprotein. Hence, significant drug interactions can occur. For example, use with cyclosporine can increase the plasma levels of both sirolimus and everolimus such that drug levels need to be monitored. The target dose-range of these drugs will vary depending on clinical use.

Sirolimus has been used effectively alone and in combination with other immunosuppressants (corticosteroids, cyclosporine, tacrolimus, and mycophenolate mofetil) to prevent rejection of solid organ allografts. It is used as prophylaxis and as therapy for steroid-refractory acute and chronic graft-versus-host disease in hematopoietic stem cell transplant recipients. Topical sirolimus is also used in some dermatologic disorders and, in combination with cyclosporine, in the management of uveoretinitis. Recently, sirolimus-eluting coronary stents have been shown to reduce restenosis and other adverse cardiac events in patients with severe coronary artery disease. These benefits appear to be due to its antiproliferative effects. Everolimus is a rapalog with better bioavailability than sirolimus, but it appears that its clinical efficacy is similar to sirolimus in solid organ transplant recipients. Temsirolimus is not currently used as an immunosuppressant. Both temsirolimus and everolimus are used and being investigated as targeted therapy for various cancers.

Toxicities of the mTOR inhibitors can include profound myelosuppression (especially thrombocytopenia), hepatotoxicity, diarrhea, hypertriglyceridemia, pneumonitis, and headache. Because nephrotoxicity is of major concern when administering calcineurin inhibitors, sirolimus is frequently employed as first-line immunosuppressant therapy in both solid organ and stem cell transplantation because renal toxicity is usually not seen. However, increased use in stem cell transplantation regimens as graft-versus-host disease prophylaxis, particularly when combined with tacrolimus, has revealed an increased incidence of hemolytic-uremic syndrome.

MYCOPHENOLATE MOFETIL

Mycophenolate mofetil (MMF) is a semisynthetic derivative of mycophenolic acid, isolated from the mold *Penicillium glaucus*. In vitro, it inhibits T- and B-lymphocyte responses, including mitogen and mixed lymphocyte responses, probably by inhibition of de novo synthesis of purines. Mycophenolate mofetil is hydrolyzed to mycophenolic acid, the active immunosuppressive moiety; it is synthesized and administered as MMF to enhance bioavailability.

Mycophenolate mofetil is available in both oral and intravenous forms. The oral form is rapidly metabolized to mycophenolic acid. Although the cytochrome P450 3A system is not involved, some drug interactions still occur. Plasma drug levels are frequently monitored, similar to the calcineurin inhibitors and PSIs.

Mycophenolate mofetil is used in solid organ transplant patients for refractory rejection and, in combination with prednisone, as an alternative to cyclosporine or tacrolimus in patients who do not tolerate those drugs. Its antiproliferative properties make it the first-line drug for preventing or reducing chronic allograft vasculopathy in cardiac transplant recipients. Mycophenolate mofetil is used as prophylaxis for and treatment of both acute and chronic graft-versus-host disease in hematopoietic stem cell transplant patients. Newer immunosuppressant applications for MMF include lupus nephritis, rheumatoid arthritis, inflammatory bowel disease, and some dermatologic disorders.

Toxicities include gastrointestinal disturbances (nausea and vomiting, diarrhea, abdominal pain) headache, hypertension, and reversible myelosuppression (primarily neutropenia).

IMMUNOMODULATORY DERIVATIVES OF THALIDOMIDE (IMiDs)

Thalidomide is a sedative drug that was withdrawn from the market in the 1960s because of its disastrous teratogenic effects when used during pregnancy. Nevertheless, it has significant immunomodulatory actions and is currently in active use or in clinical trials for over 40 different illnesses. Thalidomide inhibits angiogenesis and has anti-inflammatory and immunomodulatory effects. It inhibits tumor necrosis factor-alpha (TNF-α), reduces phagocytosis by neutrophils, increases production of IL-10, alters adhesion molecule expression, and enhances cell-mediated immunity via interactions with T cells. The complex actions of thalidomide continue to be studied as its clinical use evolves. Owing to thalidomide's serious toxicity profile, considerable effort has been expended in the development of analogs. Immunomodulatory derivatives of thalidomide are termed **IMiDs.** Some IMiDs are much more potent than thalidomide in regulating cytokines and affecting T-cell proliferation.

Thalidomide is currently used in the treatment of multiple myeloma at initial diagnosis and for relapsed-refractory disease. Patients generally show signs of response within 2–3 months of starting the drug, with response rates from 20% to 70%. When combined with dexamethasone, the response rates in myeloma are 90% or more in some studies. Many patients have durable responses—up to 12–18 months in refractory disease and even longer in some patients treated at diagnosis. The success of thalidomide in myeloma has led to numerous clinical trials in other diseases such as myelodysplastic syndrome, acute myelogenous leukemia, and graft-versus-host disease, as well as in solid tumors like colon cancer, renal cell carcinoma, melanoma, and prostate cancer, with variable results to date. Thalidomide has been used for many years in the treatment of some manifestations of leprosy and has been reintroduced in the USA for erythema nodosum leprosum; it is also useful in management of the skin manifestations of lupus erythematosus.

The adverse effect profile of thalidomide is extensive. The most important toxicity is teratogenesis. Because of this effect, thalidomide prescription and use are closely regulated by the manufacturer. Other adverse effects of thalidomide include peripheral neuropathy, constipation, rash, fatigue, hypothyroidism, and increased risk of deep vein thrombosis. Thrombosis is sufficiently frequent, particularly in the hematologic malignancy population, that most patients are placed on some type of anticoagulant when thalidomide treatment is initiated. **Lenalidomide** is an IMiD that in animal and in vitro studies has been shown to be similar to thalidomide in action, but with less toxicity, especially teratogenicity. Lenalidomide was approved by the Food and Drug Administration (FDA) in late 2005 as a consequence of trials that showed its effectiveness in the treatment of the myelodysplastic syndrome with the chromosome 5q31 deletion. Clinical trials using lenalidomide to treat newly diagnosed as well as relapsed or refractory multiple myeloma showed similar efficacy, leading to FDA approval for myeloma as well. Its side effect profile is similar to that of thalidomide, although with less teratogenic effect and fewer thromboembolic events. Pomalidomide (CC4047) is another oral IMiD that is being investigated for the treatment of multiple myeloma and myelodysplasia. The only IMiD currently used as an immunosuppressive medication (ie, in transplant recipients) is thalidomide.

CYTOTOXIC AGENTS

Azathioprine

Azathioprine is a prodrug of mercaptopurine and, like mercaptopurine, functions as an antimetabolite (see Chapter 54). Although its action is presumably mediated by conversion to mercaptopurine and further metabolites, it has been more widely used than mercaptopurine for immunosuppression in humans. These agents represent prototypes of the antimetabolite group of cytotoxic immunosuppressive drugs, and many other agents that kill proliferative cells appear to work at a similar level in the immune response.

Azathioprine is well absorbed from the gastrointestinal tract and is metabolized primarily to mercaptopurine. Xanthine oxidase splits much of the active material to 6-thiouric acid prior to excretion in the urine. After administration of azathioprine, small amounts of unchanged drug and mercaptopurine are also excreted by the kidney, and as much as a twofold increase in toxicity may occur in anephric or anuric patients. Since much of the drug's inactivation depends on xanthine oxidase, patients who are also receiving allopurinol (see Chapters 36 and 54) for control of hyperuricemia should have the dose of azathioprine reduced to one-fourth to one-third the usual amount to prevent excessive toxicity.

Azathioprine and mercaptopurine appear to produce immunosuppression by interfering with purine nucleic acid metabolism at steps that are required for the wave of lymphoid cell proliferation that follows antigenic stimulation. The purine analogs are thus cytotoxic agents that destroy stimulated lymphoid cells. Although continued messenger RNA synthesis is necessary for sustained antibody synthesis by plasma cells, these analogs appear to have less effect on this process than on nucleic acid synthesis in proliferating cells. Cellular immunity as well as primary and secondary serum antibody responses can be blocked by these cytotoxic agents.

Azathioprine and mercaptopurine appear to be of definite benefit in maintaining renal allografts and may be of value in transplantation of other tissues. These antimetabolites have been used with some success in the management of acute glomerulonephritis and in the renal component of systemic lupus erythematosus. They have also proved useful in some cases of rheumatoid arthritis, Crohn's disease, and multiple sclerosis. The drugs have been of occasional use in prednisone-resistant antibody-mediated idiopathic thrombocytopenic purpura and autoimmune hemolytic anemias.

The chief toxic effect of azathioprine and mercaptopurine is bone marrow suppression, usually manifested as leukopenia, although anemia and thrombocytopenia may occur. Skin rashes, fever, nausea and vomiting, and sometimes diarrhea occur, with the gastrointestinal symptoms seen mainly at higher dosages. Hepatic dysfunction, manifested by very high serum alkaline phosphatase levels and mild jaundice, occurs occasionally, particularly in patients with preexisting hepatic dysfunction.

Cyclophosphamide

The alkylating agent cyclophosphamide is one of the most efficacious immunosuppressive drugs available. Cyclophosphamide destroys proliferating lymphoid cells (see Chapter 54) but also appears to alkylate DNA and other molecules in some resting cells. It has been observed that very large doses (eg, > 120 mg/kg intravenously over several days) may induce an apparent specific tolerance to a new antigen if the drug is administered simultaneously with, or shortly after, the antigen. In smaller doses, it has been effective against autoimmune disorders (including systemic lupus erythematosus) and in patients with acquired factor XIII antibodies and bleeding syndromes, autoimmune hemolytic anemia, antibody-induced pure red cell aplasia, and Wegener's granulomatosis.

Treatment with large doses of cyclophosphamide carries considerable risk of pancytopenia and hemorrhagic cystitis and therefore is generally combined with stem cell rescue (transplant) procedures. Although cyclophosphamide appears to induce tolerance for marrow or immune cell grafting, its use does not prevent the subsequent graft-versus-host disease syndrome, which may be serious or lethal if the donor is a poor histocompatibility match (despite the severe immunosuppression induced by high doses of cyclophosphamide). Other adverse effects of cyclophosphamide include nausea, vomiting, cardiac toxicity, and electrolyte disturbances.

Leflunomide

Leflunomide is a prodrug of an inhibitor of pyrimidine synthesis (rather than purine synthesis). It is orally active, and the active metabolite has a long half-life of several weeks. Thus, the drug should be started with a loading dose, but it can be taken once daily after reaching steady state. It is approved only for rheumatoid arthritis at present, although studies are underway combining leflunomide with mycophenolate mofetil for a variety of autoimmune and inflammatory skin disorders, as well as preservation of allografts in solid organ transplantation. Leflunomide also appears (from murine data) to have antiviral activity.

Toxicities include elevation of liver enzymes with some risk of liver damage, renal impairment, and teratogenic effects. A low frequency of cardiovascular effects (angina, tachycardia) was reported in clinical trials of leflunomide.

Hydroxychloroquine

Hydroxychloroquine is an antimalarial agent with immunosuppressant properties. It is thought to suppress intracellular antigen processing and loading of peptides onto MHC class II molecules by increasing the pH of lysosomal and endosomal compartments, thereby decreasing T-cell activation.

Because of these immunosuppressant activities, hydroxychloroquine is used to treat some autoimmune disorders, eg, rheumatoid arthritis and systemic lupus erythematosus. It has also been used to both treat and prevent graft-versus-host disease after allogeneic stem cell transplantation.

Other Cytotoxic Agents

Other cytotoxic agents, including **vincristine, methotrexate,** and **cytarabine** (see Chapter 54), also have immunosuppressive properties. Methotrexate has been used extensively in rheumatoid arthritis (see Chapter 36) and in the treatment of graft-versus-host disease. Although the other agents can be used for immunosuppression, their use has not been as widespread as the purine antagonists, and their indications for immunosuppression are less certain. The use of methotrexate (which can be given orally) appears reasonable in patients with idiosyncratic reactions to purine antagonists. The antibiotic dactinomycin has also been used with some success at the time of impending renal transplant rejection. Vincristine appears to be quite useful in idiopathic thrombocytopenic purpura refractory to prednisone. The related vinca alkaloid **vinblastine** has been shown to prevent mast cell degranulation in vitro by binding to microtubule units within the cell and to prevent release of histamine and other vasoactive compounds.

Pentostatin is an adenosine deaminase inhibitor primarily used as an antineoplastic agent for lymphoid malignancies, and produces a profound lymphopenia. It is now frequently used for steroid-resistant graft-versus-host disease after allogeneic stem cell transplantation, as well as in preparative regimens prior to those transplants to provide severe immunosuppression to prevent allograft rejection.

IMMUNOSUPPRESSIVE ANTIBODIES

The development of hybridoma technology by Milstein and Kohler in 1975 revolutionized the antibody field and radically increased the purity and specificity of antibodies used in the clinic and for diagnostic tests in the laboratory. Hybridomas consist of antibody-forming cells fused to immortal plasmacytoma cells. Hybrid cells that are stable and produce the required antibody can be subcloned for mass culture for antibody production. Large-scale fermentation facilities are now used for this purpose in the pharmaceutical industry.

More recently, molecular biology has been used to develop monoclonal antibodies. Combinatorial libraries of cDNAs encoding immunoglobulin heavy and light chains expressed on bacteriophage surfaces are screened against purified antigens. The result is an antibody fragment with specificity and high affinity for the antigen of interest. This technique has been used to develop antibodies specific for viruses (eg, HIV), bacterial proteins, tumor antigens, and even cytokines. Several antibodies developed in this manner are FDA-approved for use in humans.

Other genetic engineering techniques involve production of chimeric and humanized versions of murine monoclonal antibodies in order to reduce their antigenicity and increase the half-life of the antibody in the patient. Murine antibodies administered as such to human patients elicit production of human antimouse antibodies (HAMAs), which clear the original murine proteins very rapidly. Humanization involves replacing most of the murine antibody with equivalent human regions while keeping only the variable, antigen-specific regions intact. Chimeric mouse-human antibodies have similar properties with less complete replacement of the murine components. The current naming convention for these engineered substances uses the suffix "-umab" or "-zumab" for humanized antibodies, and "-imab" or "-ximab" for chimeric products. These procedures have been successful in reducing or preventing HAMA production for many of the antibodies discussed below.

Antilymphocyte & Antithymocyte Antibodies

Antisera directed against lymphocytes have been prepared sporadically for over 100 years. With the advent of human organ transplantation as a therapeutic option, heterologous antilymphocyte globulin (ALG) took on new importance. ALG and antithymocyte globulin (ATG) are now in clinical use in many medical centers, especially in transplantation programs. The antiserum is usually obtained by immunization of horses, sheep, or rabbits with human lymphoid cells.

ALG acts primarily on the small, long-lived peripheral lymphocytes that circulate between the blood and lymph. With continued administration, "thymus-dependent" (T) lymphocytes from lymphoid follicles are also depleted, as they normally participate in the recirculating pool. As a result of the destruction or inactivation of T cells, an impairment of delayed hypersensitivity and cellular immunity occurs while humoral antibody formation remains relatively intact. ALG and ATG are useful for suppressing certain major compartments (ie, T cells) of the immune system and play a definite role in the management of solid organ and bone marrow transplantation.

Monoclonal antibodies directed against specific cell surface and soluble proteins such as CD3, CD4, CD25, CD40, IL-2 receptor, and TNF-α (discussed below) much more selectively influence T-cell subset function. The high specificity of these antibodies improves selectivity and reduces toxicity of the therapy and alters the disease course in several different autoimmune disorders.

In the management of transplants, ALG and monoclonal antibodies can be used in the induction of immunosuppression, in the treatment of initial rejection, and in the treatment of steroid-resistant rejection. There has been some success in the use of ALG and ATG plus cyclosporine to prepare recipients for bone marrow transplantation. In this procedure, the recipient is treated with ALG or ATG in large doses for 7–10 days prior to transplantation of bone marrow cells from the donor. ALG appears to destroy the T cells in the donor marrow graft, and the probability of severe graft-versus-host syndrome is reduced.

The adverse effects of ALG are mostly those associated with injection of a foreign protein. Local pain and erythema often occur at the injection site (type III hypersensitivity). Since the humoral antibody mechanism remains active, skin-reactive and precipitating antibodies may be formed against the foreign IgG. Similar reactions occur with monoclonal antibodies of murine origin, and reactions thought to be caused by the release of cytokines by T cells and monocytes have also been described.

Anaphylactic and serum sickness reactions to ALG and murine monoclonal antibodies have been observed and usually require cessation of therapy. Complexes of host antibodies with horse ALG may precipitate and localize in the glomeruli of the kidneys. The incidence of lymphoma as well as other forms of cancer is increased in kidney transplant patients. It appears likely that part of the increased risk of cancer is related to the suppression of a normally potent defense system against oncogenic viruses or transformed cells. The preponderance of lymphoma in these cancer cases is thought to be related to the concurrence of chronic immune suppression with chronic low-level lymphocyte proliferation.

Muromonab-CD3

Monoclonal antibodies against T-cell surface proteins are increasingly being used in the clinic for autoimmune disorders and in transplantation settings. Clinical studies have shown that the murine monoclonal antibody muromonab-CD3 (OKT3) directed against the CD3 molecule on the surface of human T cells can be useful in the treatment of renal transplant rejection. In vitro, muromonab CD3 blocks killing by cytotoxic human T cells and several other T-cell functions. In a prospective randomized multicenter trial with cadaveric renal transplants, use of muromonab-CD3 (along with lower doses of steroids or other immunosuppressive drugs) proved more effective at reversing acute rejection than did conventional steroid treatment. Muromonab-CD3 is approved for the treatment of acute renal allograft rejection and steroid-resistant acute cardiac and hepatic transplant rejection. Many other monoclonal antibodies directed against surface markers on lymphocytes

are approved for certain indications (see monoclonal antibody section below), while others are in various stages of development.

Immune Globulin Intravenous (IGIV)

A different approach to immunomodulation is the intravenous use of polyclonal human immunoglobulin. This immunoglobulin preparation (usually IgG) is prepared from pools of thousands of healthy donors, and no single, specific antigen is the target of the "therapeutic antibody." Rather, one expects that the pool of different antibodies will have a normalizing effect upon the patient's immune networks.

IGIV in high doses (2 g/kg) has proved effective in a variety of different applications ranging from immunoglobulin deficiencies to autoimmune disorders to HIV disease to bone marrow transplantation. In patients with Kawasaki's disease, it has been shown to be safe and effective, reducing systemic inflammation and preventing coronary artery aneurysms. It has also brought about good clinical responses in systemic lupus erythematosus and refractory idiopathic thrombocytopenic purpura. Possible mechanisms of action of IGIV include a reduction of T helper cells, increase of regulatory T cells, decreased spontaneous immunoglobulin production, Fc receptor blockade, increased antibody catabolism, and idiotypic-anti-idiotypic interactions with "pathologic antibodies." Although its precise mechanism of action is still unknown, IGIV brings undeniable clinical benefit to many patients with a variety of immune syndromes.

Rh_o(D) Immune Globulin Micro-Dose

One of the earliest major advances in immunopharmacology was the development of a technique for preventing Rh hemolytic disease of the newborn. The technique is based on the observation that a *primary* antibody response to a foreign antigen can be blocked if specific antibody to that antigen is administered passively at the time of exposure to antigen. $Rh_o(D)$ immune globulin is a concentrated (15%) solution of human IgG containing a higher titer of antibodies against the $Rh_o(D)$ antigen of the red cell.

Sensitization of Rh-negative mothers to the D antigen occurs usually at the time of birth of an $Rh_o(D)$-positive or D^u-positive infant, when fetal red cells leak into the mother's bloodstream. Sensitization might also occur occasionally with miscarriages or ectopic pregnancies. In subsequent pregnancies, maternal antibody against Rh-positive cells is transferred to the fetus during the third trimester, leading to the development of erythroblastosis fetalis (hemolytic disease of the newborn).

If an injection of $Rh_o(D)$ antibody is administered to the mother within 24–72 hours after the birth of an Rh-positive infant, the mother's own antibody response to the foreign $Rh_o(D)$-positive cells is suppressed because the infant's red cells are cleared from circulation before the mother can generate a B-cell response against $Rh_o(D)$. Therefore she has no memory B cells that can activate upon subsequent pregnancies with an $Rh_o(D)$-positive fetus.

When the mother has been treated in this fashion, Rh hemolytic disease of the newborn has not been observed in subsequent pregnancies. For this prophylactic treatment to be successful, the mother must be $Rh_o(D)$-negative and D^u-negative and must not already be immunized to the $Rh_o(D)$ factor. Treatment is also often advised for Rh-negative mothers antepartum at 26–28 weeks' gestation who have had miscarriages, ectopic pregnancies, or abortions, when the blood type of the fetus is unknown. ***Note:*** *$Rh_o(D)$ immune globulin is administered to the mother and must not be given to the infant.*

The usual dose of $Rh_o(D)$ immune globulin is 2 mL intramuscularly, containing approximately 300 mcg anti-$Rh_o(D)$ IgG. Adverse reactions are infrequent and consist of local discomfort at the injection site or, rarely, a slight temperature elevation.

Hyperimmune Immunoglobulins

Hyperimmune immunoglobulins are IGIV preparations made from pools of selected human or animal donors with high titers of antibodies against particular agents of interest such as viruses or toxins (see also Appendix I). Various hyperimmune IGIVs are available for treatment of respiratory syncytial virus, cytomegalovirus, varicella zoster, human herpesvirus 3, hepatitis B virus, rabies, tetanus, and digoxin overdose. Intravenous administration of the hyperimmune globulins is a passive transfer of high titer antibodies that either reduces risk or reduces the severity of infection. Rabies hyperimmune globulin is injected around the wound and given intravenously. Tetanus hyperimmune globulin is administered intravenously when indicated for prophylaxis. Rattlesnake and coral snake hyperimmune globulins (antivenoms) are of equine or ovine origin and are effective for North and South American rattlesnakes and some coral snakes (but not Arizona coral snake). Equine and ovine antivenoms are available for rattlesnake envenomations, but only equine antivenom is available for coral snake bite. The ovine antivenom is a Fab preparation and is less immunogenic than whole equine IgG antivenoms, but retains the ability to neutralize the rattlesnake venom.

MONOCLONAL ANTIBODIES (MABs)

Recent advances in the ability to manipulate the genes of immunoglobulins have resulted in development of a wide array of humanized and chimeric monoclonal antibodies directed against therapeutic targets. The only murine elements of humanized monoclonal antibodies are the complementarity-determining regions in the variable domains of immunoglobulin heavy and light chains. Complementarity-determining regions are primarily responsible for the antigen-binding capacity of antibodies. Chimeric antibodies typically contain antigen-binding murine variable regions and human constant regions. The following are brief descriptions of the engineered antibodies that have been approved by the FDA.

Antitumor MABs

Alemtuzumab is a humanized IgG_1 with a kappa chain that binds to CD52 found on normal and malignant B and T lymphocytes, NK cells, monocytes, macrophages, and a small population of granulocytes. Currently, alemtuzumab is approved for the treatment of B-cell chronic lymphocytic leukemia in patients who have been treated with alkylating agents and have failed fludarabine therapy. Alemtuzumab appears to deplete leukemic and normal cells by direct antibody-dependent lysis. Patients receiving this antibody become lymphopenic and may also become neutropenic, anemic, and thrombocytopenic. As a result patients should be closely monitored for opportunistic infections and hematologic toxicity.

Bevacizumab is a humanized IgG_1 monoclonal antibody that binds to vascular endothelial growth factor (VEGF) and inhibits VEGF from binding to its receptor, especially on endothelial cells. It is an antiangiogenic drug that has been shown to inhibit growth of blood vessels (angiogenesis) in tumors. It is approved for first-line treatment of patients with metastatic colorectal cancer alone or in combination with 5-FU-based chemotherapy. It is also approved for treatment of non-small cell lung cancer, glioblastoma multiforme that has progressed after prior treatment, and metastatic kidney cancer when used with interferon-alpha. Since bevacizumab is antiangiogenic, it should not be administered until patients heal from surgery. Patients taking the drug should be watched for hemorrhage, gastrointestinal perforations, and wound healing problems. Bevacizumab has also been used off label by intravitreal injection to slow progression of neovascular macular degeneration (see ranibizumab under Other MABs, below).

Cetuximab is a human-mouse chimeric monoclonal antibody that targets epidermal growth factor receptor (EGFR). Binding of cetuximab to EGFR inhibits tumor cell growth by a variety of mechanisms, including decreases in kinase activity, matrix metalloproteinase activity, and growth factor production, and increased apoptosis. It is indicated for use in patients with EGFR-positive metastatic colorectal cancer and, along with radiation therapy, in patients with head and neck cancer. Cetuximab may be administered in combination with irinotecan or alone in patients who cannot tolerate irinotecan. HAMAs are generated by about 4% of patients being treated with cetuximab.

Ofatumumab is a human IgG_1 monoclonal antibody directed against a different epitope on CD20 than rituximab. It is approved for patients with chronic lymphocytic leukemia (CLL) who are refractory to fludarabine and alemtuzumab. Ofatumumab binds to all B cells including B-CLL. It is thought to lyse B-CLL cells in the presence of complement and to mediate antibody-dependent cellular cytotoxicity. There is a slight risk of hepatitis B virus reactivation in patients taking ofatumumab.

Panitumumab is a fully human IgG_2 kappa light chain monoclonal antibody. It is approved for the treatment of EGFR-expressing metastatic colorectal carcinoma with disease progression on or following fluoropyrimidine-, oxaliplatin-, and irinotecan-containing chemotherapy regimens. Panitumumab binds to EGFR (similar to cetuximab), inhibiting epidermal growth factor from binding to its receptor, and prevents ligand-induced receptor autophosphorylation and activation of receptor-associated kinases. It inhibits cell growth, induces apoptosis, decreases vascular growth factor production, and suppresses internalization of the EGFR. Although some dermatologic and infusion-related toxicities have been observed following infusion of panitumumab, the distinct advantage over cetuximab is that it is fully human, and therefore does not elicit HAMAs. This is the first FDA-approved monoclonal antibody produced from transgenic mice expressing the human immunoglobulin gene loci.

Rituximab is a chimeric murine-human monoclonal IgG_1 (human Fc) that binds to the CD20 molecule on normal and malignant B lymphocytes and is approved for the therapy of patients with relapsed or refractory low-grade or follicular B-cell non-Hodgkin's lymphoma and chronic lymphocytic leukemia. It is also approved for the treatment of rheumatoid arthritis in combination with methotrexate in patients for whom anti-TNF-α therapy has failed. The mechanism of action includes complement-mediated lysis, antibody-dependent cellular cyto-toxicity, and induction of apoptosis in the malignant lymphoma cells. In lymphoma this drug appears to be synergistic with che-motherapy (eg, fludarabine, CHOP, see Chapter 54). Recent reports indicate that rituximab may also be very useful in auto-immune diseases such as multiple sclerosis and systemic lupus erythematosus.

Trastuzumab is a recombinant DNA-derived, humanized monoclonal antibody that binds to the extracellular domain of the human epidermal growth factor receptor HER-2/neu. This anti-body blocks the natural ligand from binding and down-regulates the receptor. Trastuzumab is approved for the treatment of HER-2/neu-positive tumors in patients with breast cancer and patients with metastatic gastric or gastroesophageal junction ade-nocarcinoma. As a single agent it induces remission in about 15–20% of breast cancer patients; in combination with chemo-therapy, it increases response rates and duration as well as 1-year survival. Trastuzumab is under investigation for other tumors that express HER-2/neu (see Chapter 54).

MABs Used to Deliver Isotopes to Tumors

Arcitumomab is a murine Fab fragment from an anti-carcinoembryonic antigen (CEA) antibody labeled with techne-tium 99m (^{99m}Tc) that is used for imaging patients with metastatic colorectal carcinoma (immunoscintigraphy) to determine extent of disease. CEA is often upregulated on tumor in patients with gastrointestinal carcinomas. The use of the Fab fragment decreases the immunogenicity of the agent so that it can be given more than once; intact murine monoclonal antibodies would elicit stronger HAMA.

Capromab pendetide is a murine monoclonal antibody spe-cific for prostate specific membrane antigen. It is coupled to isoto-pic indium (^{111}In) and is used in immunoscintigraphy for patients with biopsy-confirmed prostate cancer and post-prostatectomy in patients with rising prostate specific antibody level to determine extent of disease.

Ibritumomab tiuxetan is an anti-CD20 murine monoclonal antibody labeled with isotopic yttrium (^{90}Y) or ^{111}In. The radia-tion of the isotope coupled to the antibody provides the major antitumor activity. Ibritumomab is approved for use in patients with relapsed or refractory low-grade, follicular, or B-cell non-Hodgkin's lymphoma, including patients with rituximab-refrac-tory follicular disease. It is used in conjunction with rituximab in a two-step therapeutic regimen.

Tositumomab is another anti-CD20 monoclonal antibody and is complexed with iodine 131 (^{131}I). Tositumomab is used in two-step therapy in patients with CD20-positive, follicular non-Hodgkin's lymphoma whose disease is refractory to rituximab and standard chemotherapy. Toxicities are similar to those for ibritu-momab and include severe cytopenias such as thrombocytopenia and neutropenia. Tositumomab should not be administered to patients with greater than 25% bone marrow involvement.

MABs Used as Immunosuppressants and Anti-Inflammatory Agents

A. Anti-TNF-Alpha MABs

Adalimumab, certolizumab pegol, etanercept, golimumab, and infliximab are antibodies that bind TNF-α, a proinflammatory cytokine that is important in rheumatoid arthritis and similar inflammatory diseases (see Chapter 36). Blocking TNF-α from binding to TNF receptors on inflammatory cells results in suppres-sion of downstream inflammatory cytokines such as IL-1 and IL-6 and adhesion molecules involved in leukocyte activation and migration. An increased risk of infection or reactivation of *M tuber-culosis,* hepatitis B virus, and invasive systemic fungi is common to each of these anti-TNF monoclonal antibodies. Patients may also be at increased risk for malignancies including lymphoma.

Adalimumab is a completely human IgG_1 approved for use in patients with rheumatoid arthritis, juvenile idiopathic arthritis, psoriatic arthritis, ankylosing spondylitis, Crohn's disease, and plaque psoriasis. Like the other anti-TNF-α biologicals, adali-mumab blocks the interaction of TNF-α with TNF receptors on cell surfaces; it does not bind TNF-β. Adalimumab lyses cells expressing TNF-α in the presence of complement. Pharmacodynamic studies showed that administration of adalimumab reduced levels of C-reactive protein, erythrocyte sedimentation rate, serum IL-6, and matrix metalloproteinases MMP-1 and MMP-3.

Certolizumab pegol is a recombinant humanized Fab frag-ment that binds to TNF-α. It is coupled to a 40-kDa polyethylene glycol. It neutralizes the activity of membrane-associated and sol-uble TNF-α without lysing cells. Certolizumab is indicated for patients with Crohn's disease and rheumatoid arthritis.

Etanercept is a dimeric fusion protein composed of human IgG_1 constant regions fused to the TNF receptor. Etanercept binds to both TNF-α and TNF-β and appears to have effects similar to those of adalimumab and infliximab, ie, inhibition of TNF-α-mediated inflammation, but its half-life is shorter due to its physical form (fusion protein) and the route of injection (subcutaneously, twice weekly). Etanercept is approved for adult rheumatoid arthritis, polyarticular juvenile idiopathic arthritis, ankylosing spondylitis and psoriatic arthritis. It may be used in combination with meth-otrexate in some patients with arthritis.

Golimumab is a human IgG monoclonal antibody that also binds to soluble and membrane-associated TNF-α. It is an intact human IgG_1 and, like certolizumab pegol, it does not lyse cells expressing membrane-associated TNF-α. It is indicated for patients with rheumatoid arthritis, ankylosing spondylitis, and psoriatic arthritis. It has the advantage of increased half-life such that subcu-taneous injections may be self-administered only once per month.

Infliximab is a human-mouse chimeric IgG$_1$ monoclonal antibody possessing human constant (Fc) regions and murine variable regions. It is administered intravenously but has the same anti-TNF-α activity as adalimumab and etanercept. Infliximab is currently approved for use in Crohn's disease, ulcerative colitis, rheumatoid arthritis, ankylosing spondylitis, plaque psoriasis, and psoriatic arthritis.

B. Abatacept

Abatacept is a recombinant fusion protein composed of the extracellular domain of cytotoxic T-lymphocyte-associated antigen 4 (CTLA-4) fused to hinge, CH$_2$, and CH$_3$ domains of human IgG$_1$. CTLA-4 delivers an inhibitory signal to T cells. It binds more tightly to CD80/86 than CD28 (Figure 55–7). This fusion protein blocks activation of T cells by binding to CD80 or CD86 so that CD28 on T cells cannot bind and stimulate the T cell and lead to cytokine release. Abatacept is approved for patients with rheumatoid arthritis and juvenile idiopathic arthritis. Patients should not take other anti-TNF drugs or anakinra while taking abatacept. As with anti-TNF monoclonal agents, patients should be screened and treated for latent tuberculosis infection before starting abatacept.

C. Alefacept

Alefacept is an engineered protein consisting of the CD2-binding portion of leukocyte-function-associated antigen-3 (LFA-3) fused to a human IgG$_1$ Fc region (hinge, CH$_2$, and CH$_3$). It is approved for the treatment of plaque psoriasis. It inhibits activation of T cells by binding to cell surface CD2, inhibiting the normal CD2/LFA-3 interaction (Figure 55–7). Treatment of patients with alefacept also results in a dose-dependent reduction of the total number of circulating T cells, especially CD4 and CD8 memory effector subsets that predominate in psoriatic plaques. Peripheral T-cell counts of patients receiving alefacept must be monitored and the drug discontinued if CD4 lymphocyte levels fall below 250 cells/μL.

D. Basiliximab and Daclizumab

Basiliximab is a chimeric mouse-human IgG$_1$ that binds to CD25, the IL-2 receptor alpha chain on activated lymphocytes. Daclizumab is a humanized IgG$_1$ that also binds to the alpha subunit of the IL-2 receptor. Both agents function as IL-2 antagonists, blocking IL-2 from binding to activated lymphocytes, and are therefore immunosuppressive. They are indicated for prophylaxis of acute organ rejection in renal transplant patients and either may be used as part of an immunosuppressive regimen that also includes glucocorticoids and cyclosporine A.

E. Natalizumab

Natalizumab is a humanized IgG4 monoclonal antibody that binds to the α4-subunit of α4β1 and α4β7 integrins expressed on the surfaces of all leukocytes except neutrophils, and inhibits the α4-mediated adhesion of leukocytes to their cognate receptor. It is indicated for patients with multiple sclerosis and Crohn's disease who have not tolerated or had inadequate responses to conventional treatments.

F. Omalizumab

Omalizumab is an anti-IgE recombinant humanized monoclonal antibody that is approved for the treatment of allergic asthma in adult and adolescent patients whose symptoms are refractory to inhaled corticosteroids (see Chapter 20). The antibody blocks the binding of IgE to the high-affinity Fcε receptor on basophils and mast cells, which suppresses IgE-mediated release of type I allergy mediators such as histamine and leukotrienes. Total serum IgE levels may remain elevated in patients for up to 1 year after administration of this antibody.

G. Tocilizumab

Tocilizumab is recombinant humanized IgG$_1$ that binds to soluble and membrane-associated IL-6 receptors. It inhibits IL-6-mediated signaling on lymphocytes, suppressing inflammatory processes. It is indicated for treatment of patients with rheumatoid arthritis who are refractory to other anti-TNF-α biologicals. It may be used alone or in combination with methotrexate or other disease-modifying antirheumatic drugs. Patients taking tocilizumab have the same increased risk of infection as those taking anti-TNF-α monoclonal antibodies.

H. Ustekinumab

Ustekinumab is a human IgG$_1$ monoclonal antibody that binds to the p40 subunit of IL-12 and IL-23 cytokines. It blocks IL-12 and IL-23 from binding to their receptors, therefore inhibiting receptor-mediated signaling in lymphocytes. Ustekinumab is indicated for patients with moderate to severe plaque psoriasis. The advantage

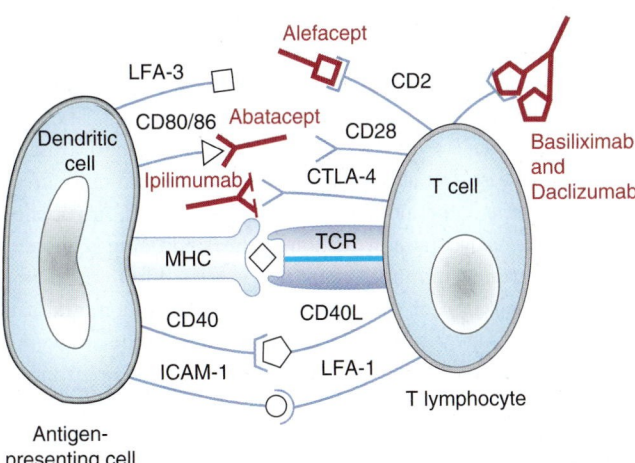

FIGURE 55–7 Actions of some monoclonal antibodies (*shown in red*). CTLA-4-IgFc fusion protein (CTLA-4-Ig, abatacept) binds to CD80/86 on DC and inhibits T-cell costimulation. Alefacept inhibits activation of T cells by blocking the interaction of LFA-3 and CD2. Basiliximab and daclizumab block IL-2 from binding to the IL-2 receptor (CD25) on T cells, preventing activation; CD25 is also important for the survival of T regulatory cells. T-cell activation can be maintained or restored if CTLA-4 interaction with CD80/86 is blocked using an anti-CTLA-4 antibody (ipilimumab, currently in phase 3 clinical trials); ipilimumab inhibits CTLA-4 signaling and prolongs activation.

of ustekinumab over anti-TNF-α drugs for psoriasis is faster and longer term improvement in symptoms along with very infrequent dosing.

Other MABs

Abciximab is a Fab fragment of a murine-human monoclonal antibody that binds to the integrin GPIIb/IIIa receptor on activated platelets and inhibits fibrinogen, von Willebrand factor, and other adhesion molecules from binding to activated platelets, thus preventing their aggregation. It is indicated as an adjunct to percutaneous coronary intervention for the prevention of cardiac ischemic complications. See Chapter 34 for additional details.

Denosumab is a human IgG$_2$ monoclonal antibody specific for human RANKL (receptor activator of nuclear factor kappa-B ligand). By binding RANKL it inhibits the maturation of osteoclasts, the cells responsible for bone resorption. Denosumab is indicated for treatment of postmenopausal women with osteoporosis at high risk for fracture. Before starting denosumab, patients must be evaluated to be sure they are not hypocalcemic. During treatment, patients should receive supplements of calcium and vitamin D.

Eculizumab is a humanized IgG monoclonal antibody that binds the C5 complement component, inhibiting its cleavage into C5a and C5b thereby inhibiting the terminal pore-forming lytic activity of complement. Eculizumab is approved for patients with paroxysmal nocturnal hemoglobinuria (PNH) and dramatically reduces the need for red blood cell transfusions. It prevents PNH symptoms of anemia, fatigue, thrombosis, and hemoglobinemia by inhibiting intravascular hemolysis due to red cell lysis. Clinicians must be aware of increased risk of meningococcal infection in patients receiving this anti-C5 monoclonal antibody.

Palivizumab is a monoclonal antibody that binds to the fusion protein of respiratory syncytial virus, preventing infection in susceptible cells in the airways. It is used in neonates at risk for this viral infection and reduces the frequency of infection and hospitalization by about 50% (see Chapter 49).

Ranibizumab is a recombinant human IgG$_1$ Fab that binds to VEGF-A. It also prevents new blood vessel formation by blocking VEGF from binding to its receptor. Ranibizumab is labeled for intravitreal injection in patients with neovascular age-related macular degeneration and sudden blurring or vision loss secondary to macular edema following retinal vein occlusion. **Pegaptanib** is a pegylated oligonucleotide that binds extracellular VEGF and is also given by intravitreous injection to slow macular degeneration.

■ CLINICAL USES OF IMMUNOSUPPRESSIVE DRUGS

Immunosuppressive agents are commonly used in two clinical circumstances: transplantation and autoimmune disorders. The agents used differ somewhat for the specific disorders treated (see specific agents and Table 55–1), as do administration schedules. Because autoimmune disorders are very complex, optimal treatment schedules have yet to be established in many clinical situations.

SOLID ORGAN & BONE MARROW TRANSPLANTATION

In organ transplantation, tissue typing—based on donor and recipient histocompatibility matching with the human leukocyte antigen (HLA) haplotype system—is required. Close histocompatibility matching reduces the likelihood of graft rejection and may also reduce the requirements for intensive immunosuppressive therapy. Prior to transplant, patients may receive an immunosuppressive regimen, including antithymocyte globulin, muromonab-CD3, daclizumab, or basiliximab. Four types of rejection can occur in a solid organ transplant recipient: **hyperacute, accelerated, acute,** and **chronic.** Hyperacute rejection is due to preformed antibodies against the donor organ, such as anti-blood group antibodies. Hyperacute rejection occurs within hours of the transplant and cannot be stopped with immunosuppressive drugs. It results in rapid necrosis and failure of the transplanted organ. Accelerated rejection is mediated by both antibodies and T cells, and it also cannot be stopped by immunosuppressive drugs. Acute rejection of an organ occurs within days to months and involves mainly cellular immunity. Reversal of acute rejection is usually possible with general immunosuppressive drugs such as azathioprine, mycophenolate mofetil, cyclosporine, tacrolimus, glucocorticoids, cyclophosphamide, methotrexate, and sirolimus. Recently, biologic agents such as anti-CD3 monoclonal antibodies have been used to stem acute rejection. Chronic rejection usually occurs months or even years after transplantation. It is characterized by thickening and fibrosis of the vasculature of the transplanted organ, involving both cellular and humoral immunity. Chronic rejection is treated with the same drugs as those used for acute rejection.

Allogeneic hematopoietic stem cell transplantation is a well-established treatment for many malignant and nonmalignant diseases. An HLA-matched donor, usually a family member, is located, patients are conditioned with high-dose chemotherapy or radiation therapy, and then donor stem cells are infused. The conditioning regimen is used not only to kill cancer cells in the case of malignant disease, but also to totally suppress the immune system so that the patient does not reject the donor stem cells. As patients' blood counts recover (after reduction by the conditioning regimen) they develop a new immune system that is created from the donor stem cells. Rejection of donor stem cells is uncommon, and can only be treated by infusion of more stem cells from the donor.

Graft-versus-host disease, however, is very common, occurring in the majority of patients who receive an allogeneic transplant. Graft-versus-host disease occurs as donor T cells fail to recognize the patient's skin, liver, and gut (usually) as self and attack those tissues. Although patients are given immunosuppressive therapy (cyclosporine, methotrexate, and others) early in the transplant course to help prevent this development, it usually occurs despite these medications. Acute graft-versus-host disease occurs within the first 100 days, and is usually manifested as a skin rash, severe diarrhea, or hepatotoxicity. Additional medications are added, invariably starting with high-dose corticosteroids, and adding drugs such as mycophenolate mofetil, sirolimus, tacrolimus, daclizumab, and others, with variable success rates. Patients generally progress to chronic graft-versus-host disease (after 100 days) and require therapy for variable periods thereafter. Unlike solid organ transplant patients, however, most stem cell transplant patients are able to eventually discontinue immunosuppressive drugs as graft-versus-host disease resolves (usually 1–2 years after their transplant).

AUTOIMMUNE DISORDERS

The effectiveness of immunosuppressive drugs in autoimmune disorders varies widely. Nonetheless, with immunosuppressive therapy, remissions can be obtained in many instances of autoimmune hemolytic anemia, idiopathic thrombocytopenic purpura, type 1 diabetes, Hashimoto's thyroiditis, and temporal arteritis. Improvement is also often seen in patients with systemic lupus erythematosus, acute glomerulonephritis, acquired factor VIII inhibitors (antibodies), rheumatoid arthritis, inflammatory myopathy, scleroderma, and certain other autoimmune states.

Immunosuppressive therapy is utilized in chronic severe asthma, where cyclosporine is often effective and sirolimus is another alternative. Omalizumab (anti-IgE antibody) has been approved for the treatment of severe asthma (see previous section). Tacrolimus is currently under clinical investigation for the management of autoimmune chronic active hepatitis and of multiple sclerosis, where IFN-β has a definitive role.

IMMUNOMODULATION THERAPY

The development of agents that modulate the immune response rather than suppress it has become an important area of pharmacology. The rationale underlying this approach is that such drugs may increase the immune responsiveness of patients who have either selective or generalized immunodeficiency. The major potential uses are in immunodeficiency disorders, chronic infectious diseases, and cancer. The AIDS epidemic has greatly increased interest in developing more effective immunomodulating drugs.

Cytokines

The cytokines are a large and heterogeneous group of proteins with diverse functions. Some are immunoregulatory proteins synthesized within lymphoreticular cells and play numerous interacting roles in the function of the immune system and in the control of hematopoiesis. The cytokines that have been clearly identified are summarized in Table 55–2. In most instances, cytokines mediate their effects through receptors on relevant target cells and appear to act in a manner similar to the mechanism of action of hormones. In other instances, cytokines may have antiproliferative, antimicrobial, and antitumor effects.

The first group of cytokines discovered, the interferons (IFNs), were followed by the colony-stimulating factors (CSFs, discussed in Chapter 33). The latter regulate the proliferation and differentiation of bone marrow progenitor cells. Most of the more recently discovered cytokines have been classified as interleukins (ILs) and numbered in the order of their discovery. Cytokines are produced using gene cloning techniques.

TABLE 55–2 The cytokines.

Cytokine	Properties
Interferon-α (IFN-α)	Antiviral, oncostatic, activates NK cells
Interferon-β (IFN-β)	Antiviral, oncostatic, activates NK cells
Interferon-γ (IFN-γ)	Antiviral, oncostatic, secreted by and activates or up-regulates TH1 cells, NK cells, CTLs, and macrophages
Interleukin-1 (IL-1)	T-cell activation, B-cell proliferation and differentiation
Interleukin-2 (IL-2)	T-cell proliferation, TH1, NK, and LAK cell activation
Interleukin-3 (IL-3)	Hematopoietic precursor proliferation and differentiation
Interleukin-4 (IL-4)	TH2 and CTL activation, B-cell proliferation
Interleukin-5 (IL-5)	Eosinophil proliferation, B-cell proliferation and differentiation
Interleukin-6 (IL-6)	HCF, TH2, CTL, and B-cell proliferation
Interleukin- 7 (IL-7)	CTL, NK, LAK, and B-cell proliferation, thymic precursor stimulation
Interleukin-8 (IL-8)	Neutrophil chemotaxis, proinflammatory
Interleukin-9 (IL-9)	T-cell proliferation
Interleukin-10 (IL-10)	TH1 suppression, CTL activation, B-cell proliferation
Interleukin-11 (IL-11)	Megakaryocyte proliferation, B-cell differentiation
Interleukin-12 (IL-12)	TH1 and CTL proliferation and activation
Interleukin-13 (IL-13)	Macrophage function modulation, B cell proliferation
Interleukin-14 (IL-14)	B-cell proliferation and differentiation
Interleukin-15 (IL-15)	TH1, CTL, and NK/LAK activation, expansion of T-cell memory pools
Interleukin-16 (IL-16)	T-lymphocyte chemotaxis, suppresses HIV replication
Interleukin-17 (IL-17)	Stromal cell cytokine production
Interleukin-18 (IL-18)	Induces TH1 responses
Interleukin-19 (IL-19)	Proinflammatory
Interleukin-20 (IL-20)	Promotes skin differentiation
Interleukin-21 (IL-21)	Promotes proliferation of activated T cells, maturation of NK cells
Interleukin-22 (IL-22)	Regulator of TH2 cells
Interleukin-23 (IL-23)	Promotes proliferation of TH1 memory cells
Interleukin-24 (IL-24)	Induces tumor apoptosis, induces TH1 responses
Interleukin-27 (IL-27)	Stimulates naive CD4 cells to produce IFN-γ
Interleukin-28 and -29 (IL-28, IL-29)	Antiviral, interferon-like properties
Interleukin-30 (IL-30)	p28 subunit of IL-27
Interleukin-31 (IL-31)	Contributes to type I hypersensitivities and TH2 responses

(continued)

TABLE 55–2 The cytokines. (Continued)

Cytokine	Properties
Interleukin-32 (IL-32)	Involved in inflammation
Interleukin-34 (IL-34)	Stimulates monocyte proliferation via the CSF-1 receptor (CSF-1R)
Interleukin-35 (IL-35)	Induces regulatory T cells (iT$_R$35)
Tumor necrosis factor-α (TNF-α)	Oncostatic, macrophage activation, proinflammatory
Tumor necrosis factor-β (TNF-β)	Oncostatic, proinflammatory, chemotactic
Granulocyte colony-stimulating factor	Granulocyte production
Granulocyte-macrophage colony-stimulating factor	Granulocyte, monocyte, eosinophil production
Macrophage colony-stimulating factor	Monocyte production, activation
Erythropoietin (epoetin, EPO)	Red blood cell production
Thrombopoietin (TPO)	Platelet production

HCF, hematopoietic cofactor; LAK, lymphokine-activated killer cell.

Note: Many interleukin activities overlap and are influenced by each other.

Most cytokines (including TNF-α, IFN-γ, IL-2, granulocyte colony-stimulating factor [G-CSF], and granulocyte-macrophage colony-stimulating factor [GM-CSF]) have very short serum half-lives (minutes). The usual subcutaneous route of administration provides slower release into the circulation and a longer duration of action. Each cytokine has its own unique toxicity, but some toxicities are shared. For example, IFN-α, IFN-β, IFN-γ, IL-2, and TNF-α all induce fever, flu-like symptoms, anorexia, fatigue, and malaise.

Interferons are proteins that are currently grouped into three families: **IFN-α**, **IFN-β**, and **IFN-γ**. The IFN-α and IFN-β families comprise type I IFNs, ie, acid-stable proteins that act on the same receptor on target cells. IFN-γ, a type II IFN, is acid-labile and acts on a separate receptor on target cells. Type I IFNs are usually induced by virus infections, with leukocytes producing IFN-α. Fibroblasts and epithelial cells produce IFN-β. IFN-γ is usually the product of activated T lymphocytes.

IFNs interact with cell receptors to produce a wide variety of effects that depend on the cell and IFN types. IFNs, particularly IFN-γ, display immune-enhancing properties, which include increased antigen presentation and macrophage, NK cell, and cytotoxic T-lymphocyte activation. IFNs also inhibit cell proliferation. In this respect, IFN-α and IFN-β are more potent than IFN-γ. Another striking IFN action is increased expression of MHC molecules on cell surfaces. While all three types of IFN induce MHC class I molecules, only IFN-γ induces class II expression. In glial cells, IFN-β antagonizes this effect and may, in fact, decrease antigen presentation within the nervous system.

IFN-α is approved for the treatment of several neoplasms, including hairy cell leukemia, chronic myelogenous leukemia,

malignant melanoma, and Kaposi's sarcoma, and for use in hepatitis B and C infections. It has also shown activity as an anticancer agent in renal cell carcinoma, carcinoid syndrome, and T-cell leukemia. IFN-β is approved for use in relapsing-type multiple sclerosis. IFN-γ is approved for the treatment of chronic granulomatous disease and IL-2, for metastatic renal cell carcinoma and malignant melanoma. Clinical investigations of other cytokines, including IL-1, -3, -4, -6, -10, -11, and -12, are ongoing. Toxicities of IFNs, which include fever, chills, malaise, myalgias, myelosuppression, headache, and depression, can severely restrict their clinical use.

TNF-α has been extensively tested in the therapy of various malignancies, but results have been disappointing due to dose-limiting toxicities. One exception is the use of intra-arterial high-dose TNF-α for malignant melanoma and soft tissue sarcoma of the extremities. In these settings, response rates greater than 80% have been noted.

Cytokines have been under clinical investigation as adjuvants to vaccines, and IFNs and IL-2 have shown some positive effects in the response of human subjects to hepatitis B vaccine. Denileukin diftitox is IL-2 fused to diphtheria toxin, used for the treatment of patients with CD25+ cutaneous T-cell lymphomas. IL-12 and GM-CSF have also shown adjuvant effects with vaccines. GM-CSF is of particular interest because it promotes recruitment of professional antigen-presenting cells such as the dendritic cells required for priming naive antigen-specific T-lymphocyte responses. There are some claims that GM-CSF can itself stimulate an antitumor immune response, resulting in tumor regression in melanoma and prostate cancer.

It is important to emphasize that cytokine interactions with target cells often result in the release of a cascade of different endogenous cytokines, which exert their effects sequentially or simultaneously. For example, IFN-γ exposure increases the number of cell-surface receptors on target cells for TNF-α. Therapy with IL-2 induces the production of TNF-α, while therapy with IL-12 induces the production of IFN-γ.

Cytokine Inhibitors

A more recent application of immunomodulation therapy involves the use of cytokine inhibitors for inflammatory diseases and septic shock, conditions in which cytokines such as IL-1 and TNF-α (see above) are involved in the pathogenesis. Drugs now in use or under investigation include anticytokine antibodies and soluble cytokine receptors. **Anakinra** is a recombinant form of the naturally occurring IL-1 receptor antagonist that prevents IL-1 from binding to its receptor, stemming the cascade of cytokines that would otherwise be released. Anakinra is approved for use in adult rheumatoid arthritis patients who have failed treatment with one or more disease-modifying antirheumatic drugs. **Canakinumab** is a recombinant human anti-IL-1β monoclonal antibody. It binds to human IL-1β and prevents it from binding to IL-1 receptors. **Rilonacept** is a dimeric fusion protein consisting of the ligand-binding domains of the extracellular portions of the human interleukin-1 receptor component (IL-1RI) and IL-1 receptor accessory protein (IL-1RAcP) fused to the Fc portion of human IgG1. These molecules are indicated for treatment of cryopyrin-associated periodic syndromes.

Patients must be carefully monitored for serious infections or malignancies if they are also taking an anti-TNF-α drug, have chronic infections, or are otherwise immunosuppressed.

■ IMMUNOLOGIC REACTIONS TO DRUGS & DRUG ALLERGY

The basic immune mechanism and the ways in which it can be suppressed or stimulated by drugs have been discussed in previous sections of this chapter. Drugs also activate the immune system in undesirable ways that are manifested as adverse drug reactions. These reactions are generally grouped in a broad classification as "drug allergy." Indeed, many drug reactions such as those to penicillin, iodides, phenytoin, and sulfonamides are allergic in nature. These drug reactions are manifested as skin eruptions, edema, anaphylactoid reactions, glomerulonephritis, fever, and eosinophilia.

Drug reactions mediated by immune responses can have several different mechanisms. Thus, any of the four major types of hypersensitivity discussed earlier in this chapter (pages 981-982) can be associated with allergic drug reactions:

- **Type I:** IgE-mediated acute allergic reactions to stings, pollens, and drugs, including anaphylaxis, urticaria, and angioedema. IgE is fixed to tissue mast cells and blood basophils, and after interaction with antigen the cells release potent mediators.

- **Type II:** Drugs often modify host proteins, thereby eliciting antibody responses to the modified protein. These allergic responses involve IgG or IgM in which the antibody becomes fixed to a host cell, which is then subject to complement-dependent lysis or to antibody-dependent cellular cytotoxicity.

- **Type III:** Drugs may cause serum sickness, which involves immune complexes containing IgG complexed with a foreign antigen and is a multisystem complement-dependent vasculitis that may also result in urticaria.

- **Type IV:** Cell-mediated allergy is the mechanism involved in allergic contact dermatitis from topically applied drugs or induration of the skin at the site of an antigen injected intradermally.

In some drug reactions, several of these hypersensitivity responses may occur simultaneously. Some adverse reactions to drugs may be mistakenly classified as allergic or immune when they are actually genetic deficiency states or are idiosyncratic and not mediated by immune mechanisms (eg, hemolysis due to primaquine in glucose-6-phosphate dehydrogenase deficiency, or aplastic anemia caused by chloramphenicol).

IMMEDIATE (TYPE I) DRUG ALLERGY

Type I (immediate) sensitivity allergy to certain drugs occurs when the drug, not capable of inducing an immune response by itself, covalently links to a host carrier protein (hapten). When this happens, the immune system detects the drug-hapten conjugate as "modified self" and responds by generating IgE antibodies specific for the drug-hapten. It is not known why some people mount an IgE response to a drug, while others mount IgG responses. Under the influence of IL-4, IL-5, and IL-13 secreted by TH2 cells, B cells specific for the drug

secrete IgE antibody. The mechanism for IgE-mediated immediate hypersensitivity is diagrammed in Figure 55–5.

Fixation of the IgE antibody to high-affinity Fc receptors (FcεRs) on blood basophils or their tissue equivalent (mast cells) sets the stage for an acute allergic reaction. The most important sites for mast cell distribution are skin, nasal epithelium, lung, and gastrointestinal tract. When the offending drug is reintroduced into the body, it binds and cross-links basophil and mast cell-surface IgE to signal release of the mediators (eg, histamine, leukotrienes; see Chapters 16 and 18) from granules. Mediator release is associated with calcium influx and a fall in intracellular cAMP within the mast cell. Many of the drugs that block mediator release appear to act through the cAMP mechanism (eg, catecholamines, glucocorticoids, theophylline), others block histamine release, and still others block histamine receptors. Other vasoactive substances such as kinins may also be generated during histamine release. These mediators initiate immediate vascular smooth muscle relaxation, increased vascular permeability, hypotension, edema, and bronchoconstriction.

Drug Treatment of Immediate Allergy

One can test an individual for possible sensitivity to a drug by a simple scratch test, ie, by applying an extremely dilute solution of the drug to the skin and making a scratch with the tip of a needle. If allergy is present, an immediate (within 10–15 minutes) wheal (edema) and flare (increased blood flow) will occur. However, skin tests may be negative in spite of IgE hypersensitivity to a hapten or to a metabolic product of the drug, especially if the patient is taking steroids or antihistamines.

Drugs that modify allergic responses act at several links in this chain of events. Prednisone, often used in severe allergic reactions, is immunosuppressive; it blocks proliferation of the IgE-producing clones and inhibits IL-4 production by T helper cells in the IgE response, since glucocorticoids are generally toxic to lymphocytes. In the efferent limb of the allergic response, isoproterenol, epinephrine, and theophylline reduce the release of mediators from mast cells and basophils and produce bronchodilation. Epinephrine opposes histamine; it relaxes bronchiolar smooth muscle and contracts vascular muscle, relieving both bronchospasm and hypotension. The antihistamines competitively inhibit histamine, which would otherwise produce bronchoconstriction and increased capillary permeability in the end organ. Glucocorticoids may also act to reduce tissue injury and edema in the inflamed tissue, as well as facilitating the actions of catecholamines in cells that may have become refractory to epinephrine or isoproterenol. Several agents directed toward the inhibition of leukotrienes may be useful in acute allergic and inflammatory disorders (see Chapter 20).

Desensitization to Drugs

When reasonable alternatives are not available, certain drugs (eg, penicillin, insulin) must be used for life-threatening illnesses even in the presence of known allergic sensitivity. In such cases, desensitization (also called hyposensitization) can sometimes be accomplished by starting with very small doses of the drug and gradually increasing the dose over a period of hours to the full therapeutic range (see Chapter 43). This practice is hazardous and must be performed under direct medical supervision, as anaphylaxis may occur before desensitization has been achieved. It is thought that slow and progressive administration of the drug gradually binds all available IgE on mast cells, triggering a gradual release of granules. Once all of the IgE on the mast cell surfaces has been bound and the cells have been degranulated, therapeutic doses of the offending drug may be given with minimal further immune reaction. Therefore, a patient is only desensitized during administration of the drug.

AUTOIMMUNE (TYPE II) REACTIONS TO DRUGS

Certain autoimmune syndromes can be induced by drugs. Examples include systemic lupus erythematosus following hydralazine or procainamide therapy, "lupoid hepatitis" due to cathartic sensitivity, autoimmune hemolytic anemia resulting from methyldopa administration, thrombocytopenic purpura due to quinidine, and agranulocytosis due to a variety of drugs. As indicated in other chapters of this book, a number of drugs are associated with type I and type II reactions. In these drug-induced autoimmune states, IgG antibodies bind to drug-modified tissue and are destroyed by the complement system or by phagocytic cells with Fc receptors. Fortunately, autoimmune reactions to drugs usually subside within several months after the offending drug is withdrawn. Immunosuppressive therapy is warranted only when the autoimmune response is unusually severe.

SERUM SICKNESS & VASCULITIC (TYPE III) REACTIONS

Immunologic reactions to drugs resulting in serum sickness are more common than immediate anaphylactic responses, but type II and type III hypersensitivities often overlap. The clinical features of serum sickness include urticarial and erythematous skin eruptions, arthralgia or arthritis, lymphadenopathy, glomerulonephritis, peripheral edema, and fever. The reactions generally last 6–12 days and usually subside once the offending drug is eliminated. Antibodies of the IgM or IgG class are usually involved. The mechanism of tissue injury is immune complex formation and deposition on basement membranes (eg, lung, kidney), followed by complement activation and infiltration of leukocytes, causing tissue destruction. Glucocorticoids are useful in attenuating severe serum sickness reactions to drugs. In severe cases plasmapheresis can be used to remove the offending drug and immune complexes from circulation.

Immune vasculitis can also be induced by drugs. The sulfonamides, penicillin, thiouracil, anticonvulsants, and iodides have all been implicated in the initiation of hypersensitivity angiitis. Erythema multiforme is a relatively mild vasculitic skin disorder that may be secondary to drug hypersensitivity. Stevens-Johnson syndrome is probably a more severe form of this hypersensitivity reaction and consists of erythema multiforme, arthritis, nephritis, central nervous system abnormalities, and myocarditis. It has frequently been associated with sulfonamide therapy. Administration of nonhuman monoclonal or polyclonal antibodies such as rattlesnake antivenin may cause serum sickness.

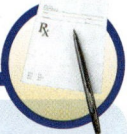

PREPARATIONS AVAILABLE *

Abatacept (Orencia)
Parenteral: 250 mg/vial lyophilized powder

Abciximab (ReoPro)
Parenteral: 2 mg/mL solution for IV injection

Adalimumab (Humira)
Parenteral: 20, 40 mg/vial for SC injection

Alefacept (Amevive)
Parenteral: 15 mg for IV injection

Alemtuzumab (Campath)
Parenteral: 30 mg/mL vial for IV injection

Anakinra (Kineret)
Parenteral: 100 mg/mL prefilled glass syringes for SC injection

Antithymocyte globulin (Thymoglobulin)
Parenteral: 25 mg/vial for IV injection

Azathioprine (generic, Imuran)
Oral: 50 mg tablets
Parenteral: 100 mg/vial for IV injection

Basiliximab (Simulect)
Parenteral: 20 mg powder; reconstitute for IV injection

Bevacizumab (Avastin)
Parenteral: 25 mg/mL for injection

Canakinumab (Ilaris)
Parenteral: 180 mg lyophilized powder for SC injection

Certolizumab (Cimzia)
Parenteral: 200 mg powder for SC injection

Cetuximab (Erbitux)
Parenteral: 2 mg/mL in 50 mL vials

Cyclosporine (Sandimmune, Neoral, SangCya)
Oral: 25, 100 mg capsules; 100 mg/mL solution
Parenteral: 50 mg/mL for IV administration

Daclizumab (Zenapax)
Parenteral: 25 mg/5 mL vial for IV infusion

Denileukin dititox (Ontak)
Parenteral: 150 mcg/mL for SC injection

Denosumab (Prolia)
Parenteral: 60 mg/mL for SC injection

Etanercept (Enbrel)
Parenteral: 25, 50 mg lyophilized powder for SC injection

Golimumab (Simponi)
Parenteral: 50 mg/0.5 mL prefilled syringes for SC injection

Ibritumomab tiuxetan (Zevalin)
Parenteral: 3.2 mg/2 mL for injection

Immune globulin intravenous [IGIV] (various)
Parenteral: 5, 10% solutions; 2.5, 5, 6, 10, 12 g powder for injection

Infliximab (Remicade)
Parenteral: 100 mg lyophilized powder for IV injection

Interferon alfa-2a (Roferon)
Parenteral: 3, 6, 9 million IU

Interferon alfa-2b (Intron-A)
Parenteral: 3–50 million units/vial

Interferon beta-1a (Avonex, Rebif)
Parenteral: 22, 33, 44 mcg powder for IV injection

Interferon beta-1b (Betaseron, Extavia)
Parenteral: 0.3 mg powder for SC injection

Interferon gamma-1b (Actimmune)
Parenteral: 100 mcg vials

Interleukin-2 [IL-2, aldesleukin] (Proleukin)
Parenteral: 22 million unit vials

Leflunomide (Arava)
Oral: 10, 20, 100 mg tablets

Lenalidomide (Revlimid)
Oral: 5, 10, 15, mg capsules

Lymphocyte immune globulin (Atgam)
Parenteral: 50 mg/mL for injection (in 5 mL ampules)

Muromonab-CD3 [OKT3] (Orthoclone OKT3)
Parenteral: 5 mg/5 mL ampule for injection

Mycophenolate mofetil (CellCept, Myfortic)
Oral: 250 mg capsules; 500 mg tablets; 200 mg powder for suspension; 180, 360 mg delayed-release tablets
Parenteral: 500 mg powder; reconstitute for injection

Natalizumab (Tysabri)
Parenteral: 300 mg/15 mL for dilution and IV infusion

Ofatumumab (Arzerra)
Parenteral: 100 mg/5 mL vial; dilute for IV infusion

Omalizumab (Xolair)
Parenteral: 150 mg powder for SC injection

Panitumumab (Vectibix)
Parenteral: single-use 20 mg/mL vials

Pegademase bovine (Adagen)
Parenteral: 250 units/mL for IM injection
Note: Pegademase is bovine adenosine deaminase.

Pegaptanib (Macugen)
Parenteral: 0.3 mL for intravitreal injection

Peginterferon alfa-2a (Pegasys)
Parenteral: 180 mcg/mL

Peginterferon alfa-2b (PEG-Intron)
Parenteral: 50, 80, 120, 150 mcg/0.5 mL

Ranibizumab (Lucentis)
Parenteral: 10 mg/mL for intravitreal injection

Rh$_o$(D) immune globulin micro-dose (RhoGam, others)
Parenteral: in single-dose and micro-dose vials

Rilonacept (Arcalyst)
Parenteral: 220 mg lyophilized powder for SC injection

Rituximab (Rituxan)
Parenteral: 10 mg/mL for IV infusion

Sirolimus (Rapamune)
Oral: 1, 2 mg tablets; 1 mg/mL solution

Tacrolimus [FK 506] (Prograf)
Oral: 0.5, 1, 5 mg capsules
Parenteral: 5 mg/mL
Topical (Protopic): 0.03%, 0.1% ointment

Thalidomide (Thalomid)
Oral: 50, 100, 200 mg capsules
Note: Thalidomide is labeled for use only in erythema nodosum leprosum in the USA.

Tocilizumab (Actemra)
Parenteral: 20 mg/mL vials for dilution and IV infusion

Trastuzumab (Herceptin)
Parenteral: 440 mg powder; reconstitute for IV infusion

Ustekinumab (Stelara)
Parenteral: 45 mg/0.5 mL, 90 mg/mL in prefilled syringes for SC injection

*Several drugs discussed in this chapter are available as orphan drugs but are not listed here. Other drugs not listed here will be found in other chapters (see Index).

REFERENCES

General Immunology

Bonneville M et al: γδ T cell effector functions: A blend of innate programming and acquired plasticity. Nat Rev Immunol 2010;10:467.

Kumar H, Kawai T, Akira S: Toll-like receptors and innate immunity. Biochem Biophys Res Comm 2009;388:621.

Levinson WE, Jawetz E: *Medical Microbiology and Immunology,* 7th ed. McGraw-Hill, 2008.

Murphy KM, Travers P, Walport M (editors): *Janeway's Immunobiology,* 7th ed. Garland Science, 2008.

Thornton AM et al: Expression of helios, an ikaros transcription factor family member, differentiates thymic-derived from peripherally induced Foxp3+ T regulatory cells. J Immunol 2010;184:3433.

Hypersensitivity

Hausmann O: Drug hypersensitivity reactions involving skin. Handbk Exper Pharmacol 2010;196:29.

Phillips EJ: Pharmacogenetics of drug hypersensitivity. Pharmacogenomics 2010;11:973.

Autoimmunity

Bousvaros A: Use of immunomodulators and biologic therapies in children with inflammatory bowel disease. Expert Rev Clin Immunol 2010;6:659.

Carroll WM: Clinical trials of multiple sclerosis therapies: Improvements to demonstrate long-term patient benefit. Mult Scler 2009;15:951.

Kircik LH et al: How and when to use biologics in psoriasis. J Drugs Dermatol 2010;9:s106.

La Cava A: Anticytokine therapies in systemic lupus erythematosus. Immunotherapy 2010;2:575.

Ma MH et al: Remission in early rheumatoid arthritis. J Rheumatol 2010;37:1444.

Immunodeficiency Diseases

Wood PM: Primary antibody deficiency syndromes. Curr Opin Hematol 2010;17:356.

Immunosuppressive Agents

Braun J: Optimal administration and dosage of methotrexate. Clin Exp Rheumatol 2010;28:S46.

Galustian C: The anticancer agents lenalidomide and pomalidomide inhibit the proliferation and function of T regulatory cells. Cancer Immunol Immunother 2009;58:1033.

Li S, Gill N, Lentzch S: Recent advances of IMiDs in cancer therapy. Curr Opin Oncol 2010;22:579.

Ponticelli C: Calcineurin inhibitors in renal transplantation still needed but in reduced doses: A review. Transplant Proc 2010;42:2205.

Vicari-Christensen M: Tacrolimus: Review of pharmacokinetics, pharmacodynamics, and pharmacogenetics to facilitate practitioners' understanding and offer strategies for educating patients and promoting adherence. Prog Transplant 2009;19:277.

Zhou H: Updates of mTOR inhibitors. Anticancer Agents Med Chem 2010;10:571.

Antilymphocyte Globulin & Monoclonal Antibodies

Cummings SR: Denosumab for prevention of fractures in postmenopausal women with osteoporosis. N Engl J Med 2009;361:756.

Gürcan HM: Information for healthcare providers on general features of IGIV with emphasis on differences between commercially available products. Autoimmunity Rev 2010;9:553.

Nelson AL: Development trends for human monoclonal antibody therapeutics. Nat Rev Drug Discov 2010;9:767.

Taylor PC: Pharmacology of TNF blockade in rheumatoid arthritis and other chronic inflammatory diseases. Curr Opin Pharmacol 2010;10:308.

Weiner LM: Monoclonal antibodies: Versatile platforms for cancer immunotherapy. Nat Rev Immunol 2010;10:317.

Cytokines

Foster GR: Pegylated interferons for the treatment of chronic hepatitis C: Pharmacological and clinical differences between peginterferon-alpha-2a and peginterferon-alpha-2b. Drugs 2010;70:147.

Gabay C: IL-1 pathways in inflammation and human diseases. Nat Rev Rheumatol 2010;6:232.

Drug Allergy

Hamilton RG: Human IgE antibody serology: A primer for the practicing North American allergist/immunologist. J Allergy Clin Immunol 2010;126:33.

Khan DA: Drug allergy. J Allergy Clin Immunol 2010;125:S126.

CASE STUDY ANSWER

Within 24–72 hours postpartum, the woman should be given a 2-mL intramuscular injection of 300 mcg anti-Rh_o(D) immune globulin. This will clear any fetal Rh-positive red cells from her circulation so she does not generate anti-Rh_o(D) B cells that might jeopardize any future pregnancy.

C H A P T E R

56

Introduction to Toxicology: Occupational & Environmental

Daniel T. Teitelbaum, MD[*]

Humans live in a chemical environment and inhale, ingest, or absorb from the skin many of these chemicals. Toxicology is concerned with the deleterious effects of these chemical agents on all living systems. In the biomedical area, however, the toxicologist is primarily concerned with adverse effects in humans resulting from exposure to drugs and other chemicals as well as the demonstration of safety or hazard associated with their use.

Occupational Toxicology

Occupational toxicology deals with the chemicals found in the workplace. The major emphasis of occupational toxicology is to identify the agents of concern, identify the acute and chronic diseases that they cause, define the conditions under which they may be used safely, and prevent absorption of harmful amounts of these chemicals. Occupational toxicologists may also define and carry out programs for the surveillance of exposed workers and the environment in which they work. Regulatory limits and voluntary guidelines have been elaborated to establish safe ambient air concentrations for many chemicals found in the workplace.

Governmental and supragovernmental bodies throughout the world have generated workplace health and safety rules, including short-and long-term exposure limits for workers. These permissible exposure limits (PELS) have the power of law. Copies of the United States Occupational Safety and Health Administration (OSHA) standards may be found on OSHA's website at http://www.osha.gov. Copies of the United States Mine Safety and Health Administration (MSHA) standards may be found at http://www.msha.gov.

Voluntary organizations, such as the American Conference of Governmental Industrial Hygienists (ACGIH), periodically prepare lists of recommended **threshold limit values (TLVs)** for many chemicals. These guidelines are periodically updated, but regulatory imperatives in the United States are not updated except under certain extraordinary circumstances. These TLV guidelines are useful as reference points in the evaluation of potential workplace exposures. Copies of current TLV lists may be obtained from the ACGIH at http://www.acgih.org.

Environmental Toxicology

Environmental toxicology deals with the potentially deleterious impact of chemicals, present as pollutants of the environment, on

[*]The author thanks Gabriel L. Plaa, PhD, the previous author of this chapter, for his contributions.

living organisms. The term environment includes all the surroundings of an individual organism, but particularly the air, soil, and water. Although humans are considered a target species of particular interest, other species are of considerable importance as potential biologic targets.

Air pollution is a product of industrialization, technologic development, and increased urbanization. Humans may also be exposed to chemicals used in the agricultural environment as pesticides or in food processing that may persist as residues or ingredients in food products. Air contaminants are regulated in the United States by the Environmental Protection Agency (EPA) based on both health and esthetic considerations. Tables of regulated air contaminants and other regulatory issues that relate to air contaminants in the United States may be found at http://www.epa.gov. Many states also have individual air contaminant regulations that may be more rigorous than those of the EPA. Many other nations and some supragovernmental organizations regulate air contaminants.

The United Nations Food and Agriculture Organization and the World Health Organization (FAO/WHO) Joint Expert Commission on Food Additives adopted the term **acceptable daily intake (ADI)** to denote the daily intake of a chemical from food that, during an entire lifetime, appears to be without appreciable risk. These guidelines are reevaluated as new information becomes available. In the United States, the Food and Drug Administration (FDA) and the Department of Agriculture are responsible for the regulation of contaminants such as pesticides, drugs, and chemicals in foods. Major international problems have occurred because of traffic among nations in contaminated or adulterated foods from countries whose regulations and enforcement of pure food and drug laws are lax or nonexistent.

Ecotoxicology

Ecotoxicology is concerned with the toxic effects of chemical and physical agents on populations and communities of living organisms within defined ecosystems; it includes the transfer pathways of those agents and their interactions with the environment. Traditional toxicology is concerned with toxic effects on individual organisms; ecotoxicology is concerned with the impact on populations of living organisms or on ecosystems.

TOXICOLOGIC TERMS & DEFINITIONS

Hazard & Risk

Hazard is the ability of a chemical agent to cause injury in a given situation or setting; the conditions of use and exposure are primary considerations. To assess hazard, one needs to have knowledge about both the inherent toxicity of the substance and the amounts to which individuals are liable to be exposed. Humans may be able to use potentially toxic substances when the necessary conditions minimizing absorption are established and respected. However, hazard is often a description based on subjective estimates rather than objective evaluation.

Risk is defined as the expected frequency of the occurrence of an undesirable effect arising from exposure to a chemical or physical agent. Estimation of risk makes use of dose-response data and extrapolation from the observed relationships to the expected responses at doses occurring in actual exposure situations. The quality and suitability of the biologic data used in such estimates are major limiting factors.

Routes of Exposure

The route of entry for chemicals into the body differs in different exposure situations. In the industrial setting, inhalation is the major route of entry. The transdermal route is also quite important, but oral ingestion is a relatively minor route. Consequently, primary prevention should be designed to reduce or eliminate absorption by inhalation or by topical contact. Atmospheric pollutants gain entry by inhalation and by dermal contact. Water and soil pollutants are absorbed through inhalation, ingestion, and dermal contact.

Duration of Exposure

Toxic reactions may differ qualitatively depending on the duration of the exposure. A single exposure—or multiple exposures occurring over a brief period from seconds to 1 or 2 days—represents acute exposure. Multiple exposures continuing over a longer period of time represent chronic exposure. In the occupational setting, both acute (eg, accidental discharge) and chronic (eg, repetitive handling of a chemical) exposures occur. Exposures to chemicals found in the environment such as air and water pollutants often cause chronic exposure, but sudden large chemical releases may result in acute massive population exposure with serious or lethal consequences.

ENVIRONMENTAL CONSIDERATIONS

Certain chemical and physical characteristics are important for estimating the potential hazard involved for environmental toxicants. In addition to information regarding effects on different organisms, knowledge about the following properties is essential to predict the environmental impact: the degradability of the substance; its mobility through air, water, and soil; whether or not bioaccumulation occurs; and its transport and biomagnification through food chains. (See Box: Bioaccumulation & Biomagnification.) Chemicals that are poorly degraded (by abiotic or biotic pathways) exhibit environmental persistence and thus can accumulate. Typical examples of such chemicals include the persistent organic pollutants (POP) such as polychlorinated biphenyls and similar substances. Lipophilic substances such as the once-widespread organochlorine pesticides (eg, DDT) tend to bioaccumulate in body fat, resulting in tissue residues. Slowly released over time, these residues and their metabolites may have chronic adverse effects such as endocrine disruption. When the toxicant is incorporated into the food chain, biomagnification occurs as one species feeds on others and concentrates the chemical. Humans stand at the apex of the food chain. They may be

Bioaccumulation & Biomagnification

If the intake of a long-lasting contaminant by an organism exceeds the latter's ability to metabolize or excrete the substance, the chemical accumulates within the tissues of the organism. This is called **bioaccumulation.**

Although the concentration of a contaminant may be virtually undetectable in water, it may be magnified hundreds or thousands of times as the contaminant passes up the food chain. This is called **biomagnification.**

The biomagnification of polychlorinated biphenyls (PCBs) in the Great Lakes of North America is illustrated by the following residue values available from *Environment Canada,* a report published by the Canadian government, and other sources.

Thus, the biomagnification for this substance in the food chain, beginning with phytoplankton and ending with the herring gull, is nearly 50,000-fold. Domestic animals and humans may eat fish from the Great Lakes, resulting in PCB residues in these species as well.

Source	PCB Concentration (ppm)[1]	Concentration Relative to Phytoplankton
Phytoplankton	0.0025	1
Zooplankton	0.123	49.2
Rainbow smelt	1.04	416
Lake trout	4.83	1,932
Herring gull	124	49,600

[1]Sources: *Environment Canada, The State of Canada's Environment,* 1991, Government of Canada, Ottawa; and other publications.

exposed to highly concentrated pollutant loads as bioaccumulation and biomagnification occur. The pollutants that have the widest environmental impact are poorly degradable; are relatively mobile in air, water, and soil; exhibit bioaccumulation; and also exhibit biomagnification.

■ SPECIFIC CHEMICALS

AIR POLLUTANTS

Five major substances account for about 98% of air pollution: carbon monoxide (CO, about 52%), sulfur oxides (about 14%), hydrocarbons (about 14%), nitrogen oxides (about 14%), and particulate matter (about 4%). The sources of these chemicals include transportation, industry, generation of electric power, space heating, and refuse disposal. Sulfur dioxide and smoke resulting from incomplete combustion of coal have been associated with acute adverse effects, particularly among the elderly and individuals with preexisting cardiac or respiratory disease. Ambient air pollution has been implicated as a contributing factor in bronchitis, obstructive ventilatory disease, pulmonary emphysema, bronchial asthma, and lung cancer. EPA standards for these substances apply to the general environment, and OSHA standards apply to workplace exposure.

Carbon Monoxide

Carbon monoxide (CO) is a colorless, tasteless, odorless, and nonirritating gas, a byproduct of incomplete combustion. The average concentration of CO in the atmosphere is about 0.1 ppm; in heavy traffic, the concentration may exceed 100 ppm. The recommended 2008 threshold limit values (TLV-TWA and TLV-STEL) are shown in Table 56–1.

A. Mechanism of Action

CO combines reversibly with the oxygen-binding sites of hemoglobin and has an affinity for hemoglobin that is about 220 times that of oxygen. The product formed—carboxyhemoglobin—cannot transport oxygen. Furthermore, the presence of carboxyhemoglobin interferes with the dissociation of oxygen from the remaining oxyhemoglobin, thus reducing the transfer of oxygen to tissues. The brain and the heart are the organs most affected. Normal nonsmoking adults have carboxyhemoglobin levels of less than 1% saturation (1% of total hemoglobin is in the form of carboxyhemoglobin); this level has been attributed to the endogenous formation of CO from heme catabolism. Smokers may exhibit 5–10% saturation, depending on their smoking habits. A person breathing air containing 0.1% CO (1000 ppm) would have a carboxyhemoglobin level of about 50%.

B. Clinical Effects

The principal signs of CO intoxication are those of hypoxia and progress in the following sequence: (1) psychomotor impairment; (2) headache and tightness in the temporal area; (3) confusion and loss of visual acuity; (4) tachycardia, tachypnea, syncope, and coma; and (5) deep coma, convulsions, shock, and respiratory failure. There is great variability in individual responses to a given carboxyhemoglobin concentration. Carboxyhemoglobin levels below 15% may produce headache and malaise; at 25% many workers complain of headache, fatigue, decreased attention span, and loss of fine motor coordination. Collapse and syncope may appear at around 40%; with levels above 60%, death may ensue as a result of irreversible damage to the brain and myocardium. The clinical effects may be aggravated by heavy labor, high altitudes, and high ambient temperatures. Although CO intoxication is usually thought of as a form of acute toxicity, there is some evidence that chronic exposure to low levels may lead to undesirable effects, including the development of atherosclerotic coronary disease in cigarette smokers. The fetus may be quite susceptible to the effects of CO exposure.

C. Treatment

In cases of acute intoxication, removal of the individual from the exposure source and maintenance of respiration are essential, followed by administration of oxygen—the specific antagonist to CO—within the limits of oxygen toxicity. With room air at 1 atm, the elimination half-time of CO is about 320 minutes; with 100% oxygen, the half-time is about 80 minutes; and with hyperbaric oxygen (2–3 atm), the half-time can be reduced to about 20 minutes. If a hyperbaric oxygen chamber is readily available, it should be used in the treatment of CO poisoning for severely poisoned patients; however, there remain questions about its effectiveness. Progressive recovery from effectively treated CO poisoning, even of a severe degree, is often complete, although some patients demonstrate persistent impairment for a prolonged period of time.

Sulfur Dioxide

Sulfur dioxide (SO_2) is a colorless, irritant gas generated primarily by the combustion of sulfur-containing fossil fuels. The 2008 TLVs are given in Table 56–1.

A. Mechanism of Action

On contact with moist membranes, SO_2 forms sulfurous acid, which is responsible for its severe irritant effects on the eyes, mucous membranes, and skin. Approximately 90% of inhaled SO_2 is absorbed in the upper respiratory tract, the site of its principal effect. The inhalation of SO_2 causes bronchial constriction; parasympathetic reflexes and altered smooth muscle tone appear to be involved. Exposure to 5 ppm SO_2 for 10 minutes leads to increased resistance to airflow in

most humans. Exposures of 5–10 ppm are reported to cause severe bronchospasm; 10–20% of the healthy young adult population is estimated to be reactive to even lower concentrations. The phenomenon of adaptation to irritating concentrations has been reported in workers. However, current studies have not confirmed this phenomenon. Asthmatic individuals are especially sensitive to SO_2.

B. Clinical Effects and Treatment

The signs and symptoms of intoxication include irritation of the eyes, nose, and throat and reflex bronchoconstriction. In asthmatic subjects, exposure to SO_2 may result in an acute asthmatic episode. If severe exposure has occurred, delayed-onset pulmonary edema may be observed. Cumulative effects from chronic low-level exposure to SO_2 are not striking, particularly in humans but these effects have been associated with aggravation of chronic cardiopulmonary disease. When combined exposure to high respirable particulate loads and SO_2 occurs, the mixed irritant load may increase the toxic respiratory response. Treatment is not specific for SO_2 but depends on therapeutic maneuvers used in the treatment of irritation of the respiratory tract and asthma.

Nitrogen Oxides

Nitrogen dioxide (NO_2) is a brownish irritant gas sometimes associated with fires. It is formed also from fresh silage; exposure of farmers to NO_2 in the confines of a silo can lead to silo-filler's disease. The 2008 TLVs are shown in Table 56–1.

A. Mechanism of Action

NO_2 is a relatively insoluble deep lung irritant capable of producing pulmonary edema. The type I cells of the alveoli appear to be the cells chiefly affected on acute exposure. At higher exposure, both type I and type II alveolar cells are damaged. Exposure to 25 ppm of NO_2 is irritating to some individuals; 50 ppm is moderately irritating to the eyes and nose. Exposure for 1 hour to 50 ppm can cause pulmonary edema and perhaps subacute or chronic pulmonary lesions; 100 ppm can cause pulmonary edema and death.

B. Clinical Effects and Treatment

The signs and symptoms of acute exposure to NO_2 include irritation of the eyes and nose, cough, mucoid or frothy sputum production, dyspnea, and chest pain. Pulmonary edema may appear within 1–2 hours. In some individuals, the clinical signs may subside in about 2 weeks; the patient may then pass into a second stage of abruptly increasing severity, including recurring pulmonary edema and fibrotic destruction of terminal bronchioles (bronchiolitis obliterans). Chronic exposure of laboratory animals to 10–25 ppm NO_2 has resulted in emphysematous changes; thus, chronic effects in humans are of concern. There is no specific treatment for acute intoxication by NO_2; therapeutic measures for the management of deep lung irritation and noncardiogenic pulmonary edema are used. These measures include maintenance of gas exchange with adequate oxygenation and alveolar ventilation. Drug therapy may include bronchodilators, sedatives, and antibiotics.

TABLE 56–1 Threshold limit values (TLVs) of some common air pollutants and solvents.

Compound	TLV (ppm)	
	TWA[1]	STEL[2]
Benzene	0.5	2.5
Carbon monoxide	25	NA
Carbon tetrachloride	5	10
Chloroform	10	NA
Nitrogen dioxide	3	5
Ozone	0.05	NA
Sulfur dioxide	2	5
Tetrachloroethylene	25	100
Toluene	50	NA
1,1,1-Trichloroethane	350	450
Trichloroethylene	50	100

[1]TLV-TWA (time weighted average) is the concentration for a normal 8-hour workday or 40-hour workweek to which workers may be repeatedly exposed without adverse effects.

[2]TLV-STEL (short-term exposure limit) is the maximum concentration that should not be exceeded at any time during a 15-minute exposure period.

NA, none assigned.

Ozone

Ozone (O_3) is a bluish irritant gas that occurs normally in the earth's atmosphere, where it is an important absorbent of ultraviolet light. In the workplace, it can occur around high-voltage electrical equipment and around ozone-producing devices used for air and water purification. It is also an important oxidant found in polluted urban air. There is a near-linear gradient between exposure (1-hour level, 20–100 ppb) and response. See Table 56–1 for 2008 TLVs.

A. Clinical Effects and Treatment

O_3 is an irritant of mucous membranes. Mild exposure produces upper respiratory tract irritation. Severe exposure can cause deep lung irritation, with pulmonary edema when inhaled at sufficient concentrations. Ozone penetration in the lung depends on tidal volume; consequently, exercise can increase the amount of ozone reaching the distal lung. Some of the effects of O_3 resemble those seen with radiation, suggesting that O_3 toxicity may result from the formation of reactive free radicals. The gas causes shallow, rapid breathing and a decrease in pulmonary compliance. Enhanced sensitivity of the lung to bronchoconstrictors is also observed.

Exposure around 0.1 ppm O_3 for 10–30 minutes causes irritation and dryness of the throat; above 0.1 ppm, one finds changes in visual acuity, substernal pain, and dyspnea. Pulmonary function is impaired at concentrations exceeding 0.8 ppm. Airway hyperresponsiveness and airway inflammation have been observed in humans.

The response of the lung to O_3 is a dynamic one. The morphologic and biochemical changes are the result of both direct injury and secondary responses to the initial damage. Long-term exposure in animals results in morphologic and functional pulmonary changes. Chronic bronchitis, bronchiolitis, fibrosis, and emphysematous changes have been reported in a variety of species, including humans, exposed to concentrations above 1 ppm. There is no specific treatment for acute O_3 intoxication. Management depends on therapeutic measures used for deep lung irritation and noncardiogenic pulmonary edema (see Nitrogen Oxides, above).

SOLVENTS

Halogenated Aliphatic Hydrocarbons

These agents once found wide use as industrial solvents, degreasing agents, and cleaning agents. The substances include carbon tetrachloride, chloroform, trichloroethylene, tetrachloroethylene (perchloroethylene), and 1,1,1-trichloroethane (methyl chloroform). However, because of the likelihood that halogenated aliphatic hydrocarbons are carcinogenic to humans, carbon tetrachloride and trichloroethylene have largely been removed from the workplace. Perchloroethylene and trichloroethane are still in use for dry cleaning and solvent degreasing, but it is likely that their use will be very limited in the future. Dry cleaning as an occupation is listed as a class 2B carcinogenic activity by the International Agency for Research Against Cancer (IARC). Fluorinated aliphatics such as the freons and closely related compounds have also been used in the workplace and in consumer goods, but because of the severe environmental damage they cause, their use has been limited or eliminated by international treaty agreements. The common halogenated aliphatic solvents also create serious problems as persistent water pollutants. They are widely found in both groundwater and drinking water as a result of poor disposal practices.

See Table 56–1 for recommended TLVs.

A. Mechanism of Action and Clinical Effects

In laboratory animals, the halogenated hydrocarbons cause central nervous system depression, liver injury, kidney injury, and some degree of cardiotoxicity. Several are also carcinogenic in animals and are considered probable carcinogens in humans. Trichloroethylene and tetrachloroethylene are listed as "reasonably anticipated to be a human carcinogen" by the US National Toxicology Program, and as class 2A probable human carcinogens by IARC. These substances are depressants of the central nervous system in humans; chloroform is the most potent. Chronic exposure to tetrachloroethylene and possibly 1,1,1-trichloroethane can cause impaired memory and peripheral neuropathy. Hepatotoxicity is also a common toxic effect that can occur in humans after acute or chronic exposures; carbon tetrachloride is the most potent of the series. Nephrotoxicity can occur in humans exposed to carbon tetrachloride, chloroform, and trichloroethylene. With chloroform, carbon tetrachloride, trichloroethylene, and tetrachloroethylene, carcinogenicity has been observed in lifetime exposure studies performed in rats and mice and in some human epidemiologic studies. Reviews of the epidemiologic literature on the occupational exposure of workers to various halogenated aliphatic hydrocarbon solvents including trichloroethylene and tetrachloroethylene have found significant associations between exposure to the agent and renal, prostate, and testicular cancer. Other cancers have been found to be increased but their incidence has not reached statistical significance.

B. Treatment

There is no specific treatment for acute intoxication resulting from exposure to halogenated hydrocarbons. Management depends on the organ system involved.

Aromatic Hydrocarbons

Benzene is used for its solvent properties and as an intermediate in the synthesis of other chemicals. The 2008 recommended TLVs are given in Table 56–1. Benzene remains an important component of gasoline and may be found in premium gasolines at concentrations as high as 2%. In cold climates such as Alaska, benzene concentrations in gasoline may reach 5%. The PEL promulgated by OSHA is 1 ppm in the air and a 5 ppm limit for skin exposure. The National Institute for Occupational Safety and Health (NIOSH) and others have recommended that the exposure limits for benzene be further reduced to 0.1 ppm because excess blood cancers occur at the current PEL. The acute toxic effect of benzene is depression of the central nervous system. Exposure to 7500 ppm for 30 minutes can be fatal. Exposure to concentrations larger than 3000 ppm may cause euphoria, nausea, locomotor problems, and coma; vertigo, drowsiness, headache, and nausea may occur at concentrations ranging from 250 to 500 ppm. No specific treatment exists for the acute toxic effect of benzene.

Chronic exposure to benzene can result in very serious toxic effects, the most significant of which is bone marrow injury. Aplastic anemia, leukopenia, pancytopenia, and thrombocytopenia occur at higher levels of exposure, as does leukemia. Chronic exposure to much lower levels has been associated with leukemia of several types as well as lymphomas, myeloma, and myelodysplastic syndrome. Recent studies have shown the occurrence of leukemia following exposures as low as 2 ppm-years. The pluri-potent bone marrow stem cells appear to be a target of benzene or its metabolites and other stem cells may also be targets. Epidemiologic data confirm a causal association between benzene exposure and an increased incidence of leukemia in workers. Most organizations now classify benzene as a known human carcinogen.

Toluene (methylbenzene) does not possess the myelotoxic properties of benzene, nor has it been associated with leukemia. It is, however, a central nervous system depressant and a skin and eye irritant. It is also fetotoxic. See Table 56–1 for the TLVs. Exposure to 800 ppm can lead to severe fatigue and ataxia; 10,000 ppm can produce rapid loss of consciousness. Chronic effects of long-term toluene exposure are unclear because human studies indicating behavioral effects usually concern exposures to several solvents. In limited occupational studies, however, metabolic interactions and modification of toluene's effects have not been observed in workers also exposed to other solvents. Less refined grades of toluene contain benzene.

Xylene (dimethylbenzene) has been substituted for benzene in many solvent degreasing operations. Like toluene, the three xylenes do not possess the myelotoxic properties of benzene, nor have they been associated with leukemia. Xylene is a central nervous system depressant and a skin irritant. Less refined grades of xylene contain benzene. Estimated TLV-TWA and TLV-STEL are 100 and 150 ppm, respectively.

PESTICIDES

Organochlorine Pesticides

These agents are usually classified into four groups: DDT (chlorophenothane) and its analogs, benzene hexachlorides, cyclodienes, and toxaphenes (Table 56–2). They are aryl, carbocyclic, or heterocyclic compounds containing chlorine substituents. The individual compounds differ widely in their biotransformation and capacity for storage in tissues; toxicity and storage are not always correlated. They can be absorbed through the skin as well as by inhalation or oral ingestion. There are, however, important quantitative differences between the various derivatives; DDT in solution is poorly absorbed through the skin, whereas dieldrin absorption from the skin is very efficient. Organochlorine pesticides have largely been abandoned because they cause severe environmental damage. DDT continues to have very restricted use for domestic mosquito elimination in malaria-infested areas of Africa. This use is controversial, but it is very effective and is likely to remain in place for the foreseeable future. Organochlorine pesticide residues in humans, animals, and the environment present long-term problems that are not yet fully understood.

A. Human Toxicology

The acute toxic properties of all the organochlorine pesticides in humans are qualitatively similar. These agents interfere with inactivation of the sodium channel in excitable membranes and

TABLE 56–2 Organochlorine pesticides.

Chemical Class	Compounds	Toxicity Rating[1]	ADI
DDT and analogs	Dichlorodiphenyltrichloroethane (DDT)	4	0.005
	Methoxychlor	3	0.1
	Tetrachlorodiphenylethane (TDE)	3	…
Benzene hexachlorides	Benzene hexachloride (BHC; hexachlorocyclohexane)	4	0.008
	Lindane	4	0.008
Cyclodienes	Aldrin	5	0.0001
	Chlordane	4	0.0005
	Dieldrin	5	0.0001
	Heptachlor	4	0.0001
Toxaphenes	Toxaphene (camphechlor)	4	…

[1]Toxicity rating: Probable human oral lethal dosage for class 3 = 500–5000 mg/kg, class 4 = 50–500 mg/kg, and class 5 = 5–50 mg/kg. (See Gosselin et al, 1984.)

ADI, acceptable daily intake (mg/kg/d).

cause rapid repetitive firing in most neurons. Calcium ion transport is inhibited. These events affect repolarization and enhance the excitability of neurons. The major effect is central nervous system stimulation. With DDT, tremor may be the first manifestation, possibly continuing to convulsions, whereas with the other compounds convulsions often appear as the first sign of intoxication. There is no specific treatment for the acute intoxicated state, and management is symptomatic.

The potential carcinogenic properties of organochlorine pesticides have been extensively studied, and results indicate that chronic administration to laboratory animals over long periods results in enhanced oncogenesis. Endocrine pathway disruption is the postulated mechanism. Extrapolation of the animal observations to humans is controversial. However, several large epidemiologic studies found no significant association between the risk of breast cancer and serum levels of DDE, the major metabolite of DDT. Similarly, the results of a case-control study conducted to investigate the relation between DDE and DDT breast adipose tissue levels and breast cancer risk did not support a positive association. In contrast, recent work supports an association between prepubertal exposure to DDT and brain cancer. In addition, recent studies suggest that the risk of testicular cancer is increased in persons with elevated DDE levels. The risk of non-Hodgkin's lymphoma (NHL) also seems to be increased in persons with elevated oxychlordane residues. Therefore, increased cancer risk in people exposed to the halogenated hydrocarbon pesticides is of concern.

B. Environmental Toxicology

The organochlorine pesticides are considered persistent chemicals. Degradation is quite slow when compared with other pesticides, and bioaccumulation, particularly in aquatic ecosystems, is well documented. Their mobility in soil depends on the composition of the soil; the presence of organic matter favors the adsorption of these chemicals onto the soil particles, whereas adsorption is poor in sandy soils. Once adsorbed, they do not readily desorb. These compounds induce significant abnormalities in the endocrine balance of sensitive animal and bird species, in addition to their adverse impact on humans. Their use is appropriately banned in most areas.

Organophosphorus Pesticides

These agents, some of which are listed in Table 56–3, are used to combat a large variety of pests. They are useful pesticides when in direct contact with insects or when used as **plant systemics,** where the agent is translocated within the plant and exerts its effects on insects that feed on the plant. These agents are based on compounds such as soman, sarin, and tabun, which were developed for use as war gases. Some of the less toxic organophosphorus compounds are used in human and veterinary medicine as local or systemic antiparasitics (see Chapters 7 and 53). The compounds are absorbed by the skin as well as by the respiratory and gastrointestinal tracts. Biotransformation is rapid, particularly when compared with the rates observed with the chlorinated hydrocarbon

TABLE 56–3 Organophosphorus pesticides.

Compound	Toxicity Rating[1]	ADI
Azinphos-methyl	5	0.005
Chlorfenvinphos	…	0.002
Diazinon	4	0.002
Dichlorvos	…	0.004
Dimethoate	4	0.01
Fenitrothion	…	0.005
Malathion	4	0.02
Parathion	6	0.005
Parathion-methyl	5	0.02
Trichlorfon	4	0.01

[1]Toxicity rating: Probable human oral lethal dosage for class 4 = 50-500 mg/kg, class 5 = 5-50 mg/kg, and class 6 = ≤ 5 mg/kg. (See Gosselin et al, 1984.)

ADI, acceptable daily intake (mg/kg/d).

pesticides. Storm and collaborators reviewed current and suggested human inhalation occupational exposure limits for 30 organophosphate pesticides (see References).

A. Human Toxicology

In mammals as well as insects, the major effect of these agents is inhibition of acetylcholinesterase through phosphorylation of the esteratic site. The signs and symptoms that characterize acute intoxication are due to inhibition of this enzyme and accumulation of acetylcholine; some of the agents also possess direct cholinergic activity. These effects and their treatment are described in Chapters 7 and 8 of this book. Altered neurologic and cognitive functions, as well as psychological symptoms of variable duration, have been associated with exposure to these pesticides. Furthermore, there is some indication of an association of low arylesterase activity with neurologic symptom complexes in Gulf War veterans.

In addition to—and independently of—inhibition of acetylcholinesterase, some of these agents are capable of phosphorylating another enzyme present in neural tissue, the so-called **neuropathy target esterase.** This results in progressive demyelination of the longest nerves. Associated with paralysis and axonal degeneration, this lesion is sometimes called organophosphorus ester-induced delayed polyneuropathy (OPIDP). Delayed central and autonomic neuropathy may occur in some poisoned patients. Hens are particularly sensitive to these properties and have proved very useful for studying the pathogenesis of the lesion and for identifying potentially neurotoxic organophosphorus derivatives. In humans, neurotoxicity has been observed with **triorthocresyl phosphate (TOCP),** a noninsecticidal organophosphorus compound. It is also thought to occur with the pesticides dichlorvos, trichlorfon, leptophos, methamidophos, mipafox, trichloronat, and others. The polyneuropathy usually begins with burning and tingling sensations, particularly in the feet, with motor weakness a few days later. Sensory and motor difficulties may extend to the

legs and hands. Gait is affected, and ataxia may be present. Central nervous system and autonomic changes may develop even later. There is no specific treatment for this form of delayed neurotoxicity. The long-term prognosis of neuropathy target esterase inhibition is highly variable. Reports of this type of neuropathy (and other toxicities) in pesticide manufacturing workers and in agricultural pesticide applicators have been published.

B. Environmental Toxicology

Organophosphorus pesticides are not considered to be persistent pesticides. They are relatively unstable and break down in the environment as a result of hydrolysis and photolysis. As a class they are considered to have a small impact on the environment in spite of their acute effects on organisms.

Carbamate Pesticides

These compounds (Table 56–4) inhibit acetylcholinesterase by carbamoylation of the esteratic site. Thus, they possess the toxic properties associated with inhibition of this enzyme as described for the organophosphorus pesticides. The effects and treatment are described in Chapters 7 and 8. The clinical effects due to carbamates are of shorter duration than those observed with organophosphorus compounds. The range between the doses that cause minor intoxication and those that result in lethality is larger with carbamates than with the organophosphorus agents. Spontaneous reactivation of cholinesterase is more rapid after inhibition by the carbamates. Although the clinical approach to carbamate poisoning is similar to that for organophosphates, the use of pralidoxime is not recommended.

The carbamates are considered to be nonpersistent pesticides. They exert only a small impact on the environment.

TABLE 56–4 Carbamate pesticides.

Compound	Toxicity Rating[1]	ADI
Aldicarb	6	0.005
Aminocarb	5	...
Carbaryl	4	0.01
Carbofuran	5	0.01
Dimetan	4	...
Dimetilan	4	...
Isolan	5	...
Methomyl	5	...
Propoxur	4	0.02
Pyramat	4	...
Pyrolan	5	...
Zectran	5	...

[1]Toxicity rating: Probable human oral lethal dosage for class 4 = 50–500 mg/kg, class 5 = 5–50 mg/kg, and class 6 = ≤ 5 mg/kg. (See Gosselin et al, 1984.)

ADI, acceptable daily intake (mg/kg/d).

Botanical Pesticides

Pesticides derived from natural sources include **nicotine, rotenone,** and **pyrethrum.** Nicotine is obtained from the dried leaves of *Nicotiana tabacum* and *N rustica*. It is rapidly absorbed from mucosal surfaces; the free alkaloid, but not the salt, is readily absorbed from the skin. Nicotine reacts with the acetylcholine receptor of the postsynaptic membrane (sympathetic and parasympathetic ganglia, neuromuscular junction), resulting in depolarization of the membrane. Toxic doses cause stimulation rapidly followed by blockade of transmission. These actions are described in Chapter 7. Treatment is directed toward maintenance of vital signs and suppression of convulsions.

Rotenone (Figure 56–1) is obtained from *Derris elliptica, D mallaccensis, Lonchocarpus utilis,* and *L urucu.* The oral ingestion of rotenone produces gastrointestinal irritation. Conjunctivitis, dermatitis, pharyngitis, and rhinitis can also occur. Treatment is symptomatic.

Pyrethrum consists of six known insecticidal esters: pyrethrin I (Figure 56–1), pyrethrin II, cinerin I, cinerin II, jasmolin I, and jasmolin II. Synthetic pyrethroids account for an increasing percentage of worldwide pesticide usage. Pyrethrum may be absorbed after inhalation or ingestion; absorption from the skin is not significant. The esters are extensively biotransformed. Pyrethrum pesticides are not highly toxic to mammals. When absorbed in sufficient quantities, the major site of toxic action is the central nervous system; excitation, convulsions, and tetanic paralysis can occur. Voltage-gated sodium, calcium, and chloride channels are considered targets, as well as peripheral-type benzodiazepine receptors. Treatment of exposure is usually directed at management of symptoms. Anticonvulsants are not consistently effective. The chloride channel agonist, ivermectin, is of use, as are pentobarbital and mephenesin. The pyrethroids are highly irritating to the eyes, skin, and respiratory tree. They may cause irritant asthma and, potentially, reactive airways dysfunction syndrome (RADS) and even anaphylaxis. The most common injuries reported in humans result from their allergenic and irritant effects on the airways and skin. Cutaneous paresthesias have been observed in workers spraying synthetic pyrethroids. The use of persistent synthetic pyrethroids for aircraft disinfection to comply with international rules regarding prevention of transfer of insect vectors has resulted in respiratory and skin problems, as well as some neurologic complaints in flight attendants and other aircraft workers. Severe occupational exposures to synthetic pyrethroids in China resulted in marked effects on the central nervous system, including convulsions.

HERBICIDES

Chlorophenoxy Herbicides

2,4-Dichlorophenoxyacetic acid (2,4-D), 2,4,5-trichlorophenoxyacetic acid (2,4,5-T), and their salts and esters are compounds of interest as herbicides used for the destruction of weeds (Figure 56–1). They have been assigned toxicity ratings of 4 or 3, respectively, which place the probable human lethal dosages at 50–500 or 500–5000 mg/kg, respectively.

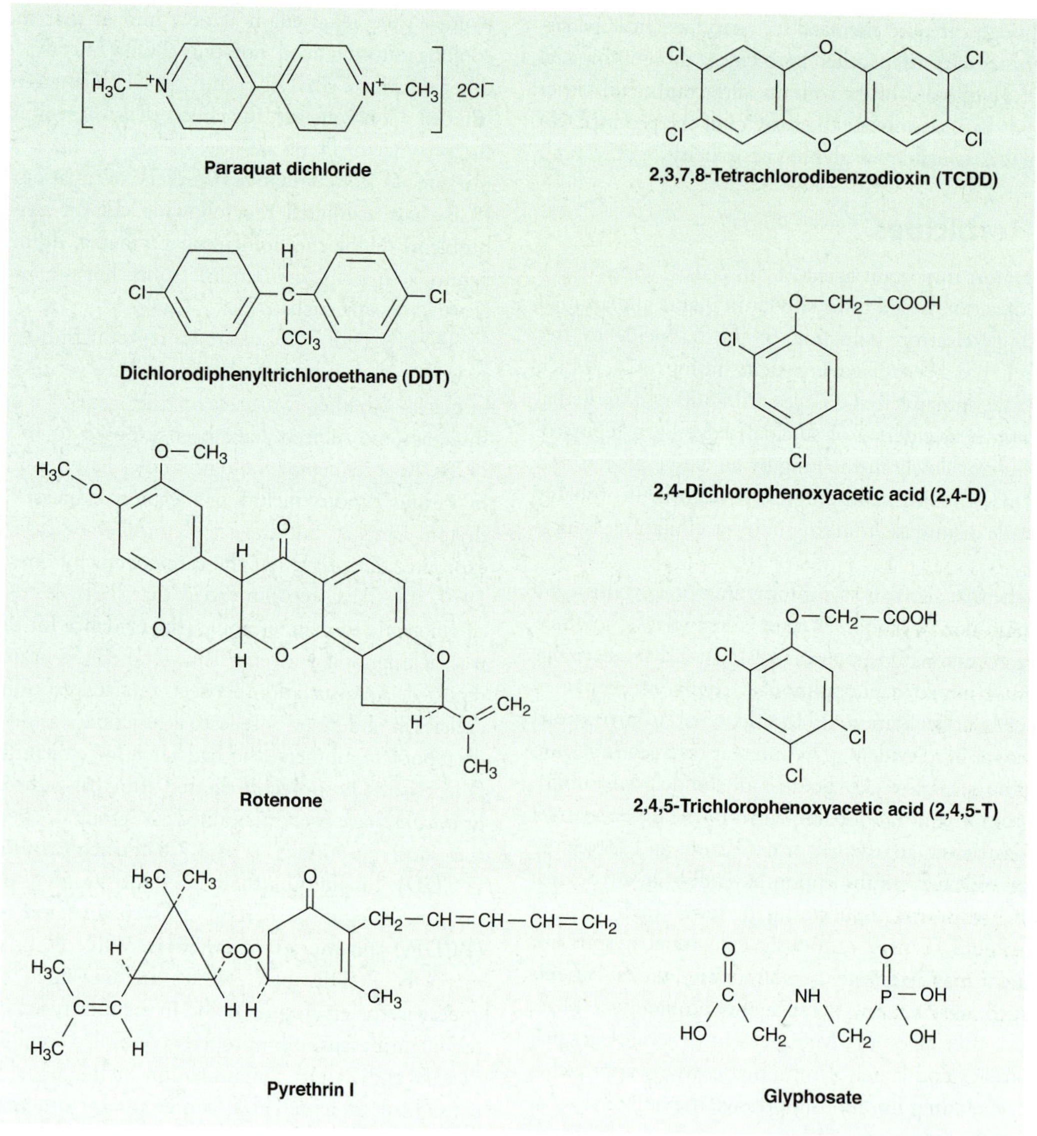

FIGURE 56–1 Chemical structures of selected herbicides and pesticides.

Because 2,4,5-T is often contaminated with dioxins and other polychlorinated compounds, it is no longer used. It was the compound used in "Agent Orange" and caused severe agricultural damage and social disruption.

In humans, 2,4-D in large doses can cause coma and generalized muscle hypotonia. Rarely, muscle weakness and marked hypotonia may persist for several weeks. In laboratory animals, signs of liver and kidney dysfunction have also been reported with chlorphenoxy herbicides. Several epidemiologic studies performed by the US National Cancer Institute confirmed the causal link between 2,4-D and non-Hodgkin's lymphoma. Evidence for a causal link to soft tissue sarcoma, however, is considered equivocal.

The toxicologic profile for these agents, particularly that of 2,4,5-T, is complicated by the presence of chemical contaminants (**dioxins**) produced during the manufacturing process (see below). 2,3,7,8-Tetrachlorodibenzo-*p*-dioxin (dioxin, TCDD) is the most

important of these contaminants. Dioxin is a potent animal carcinogen and a likely human carcinogen.

Glyphosate

Glyphosate (*N*-[phosphonomethyl] glycine, Figure 56–1) is now the most widely used herbicide in the world. It functions as a contact herbicide and is absorbed through the leaves and roots of plants. Because it is nonselective, it may damage important crops even when used as directed. Therefore, genetically modified plants such as soybean, corn, and cotton that are glyphosate-resistant have been developed and patented. They are widely grown throughout the world.

Glyphosate-related poisoning incidents are commonly reported. Most injuries are minor, although some lethal outcomes have been reported.

Glyphosate is a significant eye and skin irritant. It has caused lethal outcomes, although it is far less potent than the bipyridyl

herbicides. Although the pure chemical seems to have little persistence and lower toxicity than other herbicides, the commercial formulations of glyphosate often contain surfactants and other active compounds that complicate the toxicity of the product. No specific treatment is available for glyphosate toxicity.

Bipyridyl Herbicides

Paraquat is the most important agent of this class (Figure 56–1). Its mechanism of action is said to be similar in plants and animals and involves single-electron reduction of the herbicide to free radical species. It has been given a toxicity rating of 4, which places the probable human lethal dosage at 50–500 mg/kg. Lethal human intoxications (accidental or suicidal) have been reported. Paraquat accumulates slowly in the lung by an active process and causes lung edema, alveolitis, and progressive fibrosis. It probably inhibits superoxide dismutase, resulting in intracellular free radical oxygen toxicity.

In humans, the first signs and symptoms after oral exposure are hematemesis and bloody stools. Within a few days, however, delayed toxicity occurs, with respiratory distress and the development of congestive hemorrhagic pulmonary edema accompanied by widespread cellular proliferation. Hepatic, renal, or myocardial involvement may also be evident. The interval between ingestion and death may be several weeks. Because of the delayed pulmonary toxicity, prompt removal of paraquat from the digestive tract is important. Gastric lavage, the use of cathartics, and the use of adsorbents to prevent further absorption have all been advocated; after absorption, treatment is successful in fewer than 50% of cases. Oxygen should be used cautiously to combat dyspnea or cyanosis, because it may aggravate the pulmonary lesions. Patients require prolonged observation, because the proliferative phase begins 1–2 weeks after ingestion. Management of severe paraquat poisoning is complex and largely symptomatic. Many approaches have been used, including immunosuppressive therapy to slow or stop the progressive pulmonary fibrosis. None of the currently proposed methods of treatment is universally successful.

ENVIRONMENTAL POLLUTANTS

Polychlorinated Biphenyls

The **polychlorinated biphenyls (PCBs, coplanar biphenyls)** have been used in a large variety of applications as dielectric and heat transfer fluids, lubricating oils, plasticizers, wax extenders, and flame retardants. Unfortunately, PCBs persist in the environment. Their industrial use and manufacture in the USA were terminated by 1977. The products used commercially were actually mixtures of PCB isomers and homologs containing 12–68% chlorine. These chemicals are highly stable and highly lipophilic, poorly metabolized, and very resistant to environmental degradation; they bioaccumulate in food chains. Food is the major source of PCB residues in humans.

A serious exposure to PCBs—lasting several months—occurred in Japan in 1968 as a result of cooking oil contamination with PCB-containing transfer medium (Yusho disease). Possible effects on the fetus and on the development of the offspring of poisoned women were reported. It is now known that the contaminated cooking oil contained not only PCBs but also polychlorinated dibenzofurans (PCDFs) and polychlorinated quaterphenyls (PCQs). Consequently, the effects that were initially attributed to the presence of PCBs are now thought to have been caused by a mixture of contaminants. Workers occupationally exposed to PCBs have exhibited the following clinical signs: dermatologic problems (chloracne, folliculitis, erythema, dryness, rash, hyperkeratosis, hyperpigmentation), some hepatic involvement, and elevated plasma triglycerides.

The effects of PCBs alone on reproduction and development, as well as their carcinogenic effects, have yet to be established in humans—whether workers or the general population—even though some subjects have been exposed to very high levels of PCBs. Repeated epidemiologic studies have found some increases in various cancers including melanoma, breast, pancreatic, and thyroid cancers, but the small number of cases and uncertain exposure status have left the carcinogenicity question unclear. In 1977, the IARC recommended that PCBs be regarded as likely carcinogenic to man, although the evidence for this classification was lacking. Some adverse behavioral effects in infants have been reported. An association between prenatal exposure to PCBs and deficits in childhood intellectual function was described for children born to mothers who had eaten large quantities of contaminated fish. The **polychlorinated dibenzo-*p*-dioxins (PCDDs),** or *dioxins*, have been mentioned as a group of congeners of which the most important is **2,3,7,8-tetrachlorodibenzo-*p*-dioxin (TCDD)**. In addition, there is a larger group of dioxin-like compounds, including certain **polychlorinated dibenzofurans (PCDFs)** and **coplanar biphenyls.** While PCBs were used commercially, PCDDs and PCDFs are unwanted byproducts that appear in the environment and in manufactured products as contaminants because of improperly controlled combustion processes. PCDD and PCDF contamination of the global environment is considered to represent a contemporary problem produced by human activities. Like PCBs, these chemicals are very stable and highly lipophilic. They are poorly metabolized and very resistant to environmental degradation.

In laboratory animals, TCDD administered in suitable doses has produced a wide variety of toxic effects, including a wasting syndrome (severe weight loss accompanied by reduction of muscle mass and adipose tissue), thymic atrophy, epidermal changes, hepatotoxicity, immunotoxicity, effects on reproduction and development, teratogenicity, and carcinogenicity. The effects observed in workers involved in the manufacture of 2,4,5-T (and therefore presumably exposed to TCDD) consisted of contact dermatitis and chloracne. In severely TCDD-intoxicated patients, discrete chloracne may be the only manifestation.

The presence of TCDD in 2,4,5-T is believed to be largely responsible for other human toxicities associated with the herbicide. There is epidemiologic evidence indicating an association between occupational exposure to the phenoxy herbicides and an excess incidence of non-Hodgkin's lymphoma. The TCDD contaminant in these herbicides seems to play a role in a number of cancers such as soft tissue sarcomas, lung cancer, Hodgkin's lymphomas, and others.

Endocrine Disruptors

The potential hazardous effects of some chemicals in the environment are receiving considerable attention because of their estrogen-like or antiandrogenic properties. Compounds that affect thyroid function are also of concern. Since 1998, the process of prioritization, screening, and testing of chemicals for such actions has been undergoing worldwide development. These chemicals mimic, enhance, or inhibit a hormonal action. They include a number of plant constituents (phytoestrogens) and some mycoestrogens as well as industrial chemicals, particularly persistent organochlorine agents such as DDT and PCBs. Some brominated flame retardants are now being investigated as possible endocrine disrupters. Concerns exist because of their increasing contamination of the environment, the appearance of bioaccumulation, and their potential for toxicity. In vitro assays alone are unreliable for regulatory purposes, and animal studies are considered indispensable. Modified endocrine responses in some reptiles and marine invertebrates have been observed. In humans, however, a causal relation between exposure to a specific environmental agent and an adverse health effect due to endocrine modulation has not been established. Epidemiologic studies of populations exposed to higher concentrations of endocrine disrupting environmental chemicals are underway. There are indications that breast and other reproductive cancers are increased in these patients. Prudence dictates that exposure to environmental chemicals that disrupt endocrine function should be reduced.

Asbestos

Asbestos in many of its forms has been widely used in industry for over 100 years. All forms of asbestos that have been used in industry have been shown to cause progressive lung disease that is characterized by a fibrotic process. Higher levels of exposure produce the process called asbestosis. Lung damage develops even at low concentrations of shorter fibers, whereas higher concentrations of longer fibers are required to cause lung damage. Every form of asbestos, including chrysotile asbestos, causes an increase in lung cancer. Lung cancer occurs in people exposed at fiber concentrations well below concentrations that produce asbestosis. Cigarette smoking and exposure to radon daughters increase the incidence of asbestos-caused lung cancer in a synergistic fashion.

All forms of asbestos also cause mesothelioma of the pleura or peritoneum at very low doses. Other cancers including colon cancer, laryngeal cancer, stomach cancer, and perhaps even lymphoma are increased in asbestos-exposed patients. The mechanism for asbestos-caused cancer is not yet delineated. Arguments that chrysotile asbestos does not cause mesothelioma are contradicted by many epidemiologic studies of worker populations. Recognition that all forms of asbestos are dangerous and carcinogenic has led many countries to ban all uses of asbestos. Countries such as Canada, Zimbabwe, and others that still produce asbestos argue that asbestos can be used safely with careful workplace environmental controls. However, studies of industrial practice make the "safe use" of asbestos highly improbable.

METALS

Occupational and environmental poisoning with metals, metalloids, and metal compounds is a major health problem. Exposure in the workplace is found in many industries, and exposure in the home and elsewhere in the nonoccupational environment is widespread. The classic metal poisons (arsenic, lead, and mercury) continue to be widely used. (Treatment of their toxicities is discussed in Chapter 57.) Occupational exposure and poisoning due to beryllium, cadmium, manganese, and uranium are relatively new occupational problems, which present new and previously unaddressed problems.

Beryllium

Beryllium (Be) is a light alkaline metal that confers special properties on the alloys and ceramics in which it is incorporated. One attractive property of beryllium is its nonsparking quality, which makes it useful in such diverse applications as the manufacture of dental appliances and of nuclear weapons. Beryllium-copper alloys find use as components of computers, in the encasement of the first stage of nuclear weapons, in devices that require hardening such as missile ceramic nose cones, and in the space shuttle heat shield tiles. Because of the use of beryllium in dental appliances, dentists and dental appliance makers are often exposed to beryllium dust in toxic concentrations.

Beryllium is highly toxic by inhalation and is classified by IARC as a class 1, known human carcinogen. Inhalation of beryllium particles produces progressive pulmonary fibrosis and may lead to cancer. Skin disease also develops in workers overexposed to beryllium. The pulmonary disease is called chronic beryllium disease (CBD) and is a chronic granulomatous pulmonary fibrosis. In the 5–15% of the population that is sensitive to beryllium, chronic beryllium disease is the result of activation of an autoimmune attack on the skin and lungs. The disease is progressive and may lead to severe disability and death. Although some treatment approaches to the management of chronic beryllium disease show promise, the prognosis is poor in most cases.

The current permissible exposure levels for beryllium of 0.01 mcg/m^3 averaged over a 30-day period or 2 mcg/m^3 over an 8-hour period are insufficiently protective to prevent chronic beryllium disease. Both NIOSH and the ACGIH have recommended that the PEL and TLV be reduced to 0.05 mcg/m^3. These recommendations have not yet been implemented.

Environmental beryllium exposure is not generally thought to be a hazard to human health except in the vicinity of industrial sites where air, water and soil pollution have occurred.

Cadmium

Cadmium (Cd) is a transition metal widely used in industry. Workers are exposed to cadmium in the manufacture of nickel cadmium batteries, pigments, low-melting-point eutectic materials; in solder; in television phosphors; and in plating operations. It is also used extensively in semiconductors and in plastics as a stabilizer. Cadmium smelting is often done from residual dust from lead smelting operations, and cadmium smelter workers often face both lead and cadmium toxicity.

Cadmium is toxic by inhalation and by ingestion. When metals that have been plated with cadmium or welded with cadmium-containing materials are vaporized by the heat of torches or cutting implements, the fine dust and fumes released produce an acute respiratory disorder called **cadmium fume fever.** This disorder, common in welders, is usually characterized by shaking chills, cough, fever, and malaise. Although it may produce pneumonia, it is usually transient. However, chronic exposure to cadmium dust produces a far more serious progressive pulmonary fibrosis. Cadmium also causes severe kidney damage, including renal failure if exposure continues. Cadmium is a human carcinogen and is listed as a group 1, known human carcinogen by the IARC.

The current OSHA PEL for cadmium is 5 mcg/m^3. This PEL, considered by OSHA to be the lowest feasible limit for the dust, is insufficiently protective of worker health.

REFERENCES

Birnbaum LS, Staska DF: Brominated flame retardants: Cause for concern? Environ Health Perspect 2004;112:9.

Buckley A et al: Hyperbaric oxygen for carbon monoxide poisoning: A systematic review and critical analysis of the evidence. Toxicol Rev 2005;24:75.

Casals-Casas C, Desvergne B: Endocrine disruptors: from endocrine to metabolic disruption. Annu Rev Physiol 2011;73:135.

Crisp TM et al: Environmental endocrine disruption: An effects assessment and analysis. Environ Health Perspect 1998;106(Suppl 1):11.

Degen GH, Bolt HM: Endocrine disruptors: Update on xenoestrogens. Int Arch Occup Environ Health 2000;73:433.

Ecobichon DJ: Our changing perspectives on benefits and risks of pesticides: A historical overview. Neurotoxicology 2000;21:211.

Geusau A et al: Severe 2,3,7,8-tetrachlorodibenzo-*p*-dioxin (TCDD) intoxication: Clinical and laboratory effects. Environ Health Perspect 2001;109:865.

Gosselin RE, Smith RP, Hodge HC: *Clinical Toxicology of Commercial Products,* 5th ed. Williams & Wilkins, 1984.

Haley RW et al: Association of low PON1 type Q (type A) arylesterase activity with neurologic symptom complexes in Gulf War veterans. Toxicol Appl Pharmacol 1999;157:227.

Hamm JI, Chen CY, Birnbaum LS: A mixture of dioxin, furans, and non-ortho PCBs based upon consensus toxic equivalency factors produces dioxin-like reproductive effects. Toxicol Sci 2003;74:182.

Jacobson JL, Jacobson SW: Association of prenatal exposure to an environmental contaminant with intellectual function in childhood. J Toxicol Clin Toxicol 2002;40:467.

Kao JW, Nanagas KA: Carbon monoxide poisoning. Emerg Med Clin North Am 2004;22:985.

Klaassen CD (editor): *Casarett and Doull's Toxicology,* 7th ed. McGraw-Hill, 2007.

Lavin AL, Jacobson OF, DeSesso JM: An assessment of the carcinogenic potential of trichloroethylene in humans. Human Ecol Risk Assess 2000;6:575.

Lévesque B et al: Cancer risk associated with household exposure to chloroform. J Toxicol Environ Health A 2002;65:489.

Lotti M, Moretto A: Organophosphate-induced delayed polyneuropathy. Toxicol Rev 2005;24:37.

MacMahon B: Pesticide residues and breast cancer? J Natl Cancer Inst 1994;86:572.

Mundt KA, Birk T, Burch MT: Critical review of the epidemiological literature on occupational exposure to perchloroethylene and cancer. Int Arch Occup Environ Health 2003;76:473.

Olson KR et al (editors): *Poisoning & Drug Overdose,* 5th ed. McGraw-Hill, 2006.

Raub JA et al: Carbon monoxide poisoning—a public health perspective. Toxicology 2000;145:1.

Ray DE, Fry JR: A reassessment of the neurotoxicity of pyrethroid insecticides. Pharmacol Ther 2006;111:174.

Safe SH: Endocrine disruptors and human health—is there a problem? An update. Environ Health Perspect 2000;108:487.

Soderlund DM et al: Mechanisms of pyrethroid neurotoxicity: Implications for cumulative risk assessment. Toxicology 2002;171:3.

St Hilaire S et al: Estrogen receptor positive breast cancers and their association with environmental factors. Int J Health Geogr 2011;10:10.

Storm JE, Rozman KK, Doull J: Occupational exposure limits for 30 organophosphate pesticides based on inhibition of red blood cell acetylcholinesterase. Toxicology 2000;150:1.

57

Heavy Metal Intoxication & Chelators

Michael J. Kosnett, MD, MPH

CASE STUDY

A 48-year-old painter is referred for evaluation of recent onset of severe abdominal pains, headaches, and myalgias. For the last week, he has been removing old paint from an iron bridge using grinding tools and a blow torch. His employer states that all the bridge workers are provided with the equivalent of "haz-mat" (hazardous materials) suits. What tests should be carried out? Assuming positive test results, what therapy would be appropriate?

Some metals such as iron are essential for life, whereas others such as lead are present in all organisms but serve no useful biologic purpose. Some of the oldest diseases of humans can be traced to heavy metal poisoning associated with metal mining, refining, and use. Even with the present recognition of the hazards of heavy metals, the incidence of intoxication remains significant, and the need for preventive strategies and effective therapy remains high. Toxic heavy metals interfere with the function of essential cations, cause enzyme inhibition, generate oxidative stress, and alter gene expression. As a result, multisystem signs and symptoms are a hallmark of heavy metal intoxication.

When intoxication occurs, chelator molecules (from *chela* "claw"), or their in vivo biotransformation products, may be used to bind the metal and facilitate its excretion from the body. Chelator drugs are discussed in the second part of this chapter.

■ TOXICOLOGY OF HEAVY METALS

LEAD

Lead poisoning is one of the oldest occupational and environmental diseases in the world. Despite its recognized hazards, lead continues to have widespread commercial application, including production of storage batteries (nearly 90% of US consumption), ammunition, metal alloys, solder, glass, plastics, pigments, and ceramics. Corrosion of lead plumbing in older buildings or supply lines may increase the lead concentration of tap water. Environmental lead exposure, ubiquitous by virtue of the anthropogenic distribution of lead to air, water, and food, has declined considerably in the last three decades as a result of the elimination of lead as an additive in gasoline, as well as diminished contact with lead-based paint and other lead-containing consumer products, such as lead solder in canned food. Although these public health measures, together with improved workplace conditions, have decreased the incidence of serious overt lead poisoning, there remains considerable concern over the effects of low-level lead exposure. Extensive evidence indicates that lead may have subtle subclinical adverse effects on neurocognitive function and on blood pressure at low blood lead concentrations formerly not recognized as harmful. Lead serves no useful purpose in the human body. In key target organs such as the developing central nervous system, no level of lead exposure has been shown to be without deleterious effects.

Pharmacokinetics

Inorganic lead is slowly but consistently absorbed via the respiratory and gastrointestinal tracts. Inorganic lead is poorly absorbed through the skin. Absorption of lead dust via the respiratory tract is the most common cause of industrial poisoning. The intestinal tract is the primary route of entry in nonindustrial exposure (Table 57–1). Absorption via the gastrointestinal tract varies with the nature of the lead compound, but in general, adults absorb about 10–15% of the ingested amount, whereas young children absorb up to 50%. Low dietary calcium, iron deficiency, and ingestion on an empty stomach all have been associated with increased lead absorption.

TABLE 57–1 Toxicology of selected arsenic, lead, and mercury compounds.

	Form Entering Body	Major Route of Absorption	Distribution	Major Clinical Effects	Key Aspects of Mechanism	Metabolism and Elimination
Arsenic	Inorganic arsenic salts	Gastrointestinal, respiratory (all mucosal surfaces)	Predominantly soft tissues (highest in liver, kidney). Avidly bound in skin, hair, nails	Cardiovascular: shock, arrhythmias. CNS: encephalopathy, peripheral neuropathy. Gastroenteritis; pancytopenia; cancer (many sites)	Inhibits enzymes; interferes with oxidative phosphorylation; alters cell signaling, gene expression	Methylation. Renal (major); sweat and feces (minor)
Lead	Inorganic lead oxides and salts	Gastrointestinal, respiratory	Soft tissues; redistributed to skeleton (> 90% of adult body burden)	CNS deficits; peripheral neuropathy; anemia; nephropathy; hypertension; reproductive toxicity	Inhibits enzymes; interferes with essential cations; alters membrane structure	Renal (major); feces and breast milk (minor)
	Organic (tetraethyl lead)	Skin, gastrointestinal, respiratory	Soft tissues, especially liver, CNS	Encephalopathy	Hepatic dealkylation (fast) → trialkyme-tabolites (slow) → dissociation to lead	Urine and feces (major); sweat (minor)
Mercury	Elemental mercury	Respiratory tract	Soft tissues, especially kidney, CNS	CNS: tremor, behavioral (erethism); gingivo-stomatitis; peripheral neuropathy; acrodynia; pneumonitis (high-dose)	Inhibits enzymes; alters membranes	Elemental Hg converted to Hg^{2+}. Urine (major); feces (minor)
	Inorganic: Hg^+ (less toxic); Hg^{2+} (more toxic)	Gastrointestinal, skin (minor)	Soft tissues, especially kidney	Acute tubular necrosis; gastroenteritis; CNS effects (rare)	Inhibits enzymes; alters membranes	Urine
	Organic: alkyl, aryl	Gastrointestinal, skin, respiratory (minor)	Soft tissues	CNS effects, birth defects	Inhibits enzymes; alters microtubules, neuronal structure	Deacylation. Fecal (alkyl, major); urine (Hg^{2+} after deacylation, minor)

Once absorbed from the respiratory or gastrointestinal tract, lead enters the bloodstream, where approximately 99% is bound to erythrocytes and 1% is present in the plasma. Lead is subsequently distributed to soft tissues such as the bone marrow, brain, kidney, liver, muscle, and gonads; then to the subperiosteal surface of bone; and later to bone matrix. Lead also crosses the placenta and poses a potential hazard to the fetus. The kinetics of lead clearance from the body follows a multicompartment model, composed predominantly of the blood and soft tissues, with a half-life of 1–2 months; and the skeleton, with a half-life of years to decades. Approximately 70% of the lead that is eliminated appears in the urine, with lesser amounts excreted through the bile, skin, hair, nails, sweat, and breast milk. The fraction not undergoing prompt excretion, approximately half of the absorbed lead, may be incorporated into the skeleton, the repository of more than 90% of the body lead burden in most adults. In patients with high bone lead burdens, slow release from the skeleton may elevate blood lead concentrations for years after exposure ceases, and pathologic high bone turnover states such as hyperthyroidism or prolonged immobilization may result in frank lead intoxication. Migration of retained lead bullet fragments into a joint space or adjacent to bone has been associated with the development of lead poisoning signs and symptoms years or decades after an initial gunshot injury.

Pharmacodynamics

Lead exerts multisystemic toxic effects that are mediated by multiple modes of action, including inhibition of enzymatic function; interference with the action of essential cations, particularly calcium, iron, and zinc; generation of oxidative stress; changes in gene expression; alterations in cell signaling; and disruption of the integrity of membranes in cells and organelles.

A. Nervous System

The developing central nervous system of the fetus and young child is the most sensitive target organ for lead's toxic effect. Epidemiologic studies suggest that blood lead concentrations even less than 5 mcg/dL may result in subclinical deficits in neurocognitive function in lead-exposed young children, with no demonstrable threshold for a "no effect" level. The dose response between low blood lead concentrations and cognitive function in young children is nonlinear, such that the decrement in intelligence associated with an increase in blood lead from less than 1 to 10 mcg/dL (6.2 IQ points) exceeds that associated with a change from 10 to 30 mcg/dL (3.0 IQ points).

Adults are less sensitive to the central nervous system effects of lead, but long-term exposure to blood lead concentrations in the range of 10–30 mcg/dL may be associated with subtle, subclinical effects on neurocognitive function. At blood lead concentrations higher than 30 mcg/dL, behavioral and neurocognitive signs or symptoms may gradually emerge, including irritability, fatigue, decreased libido, anorexia, sleep disturbance, impaired visual-motor coordination, and slowed reaction time. Headache, arthralgias, and myalgias are also common complaints. Tremor occurs but is less common. Lead encephalopathy, usually occurring at blood lead concentrations higher than 100 mcg/dL, is typically accompanied by increased intracranial pressure and may cause ataxia, stupor, coma, convulsions, and death. Recent epidemiological studies suggest that lead may accentuate an age-related decline in cognitive function in older adults. In experimental animals, developmental lead exposure has been associated with increased expression of beta-amyloid, oxidative DNA damage, and Alzheimer's-type pathology in the aging brain. There is wide inter-individual variation in the magnitude of lead exposure required to cause overt lead-related signs and symptoms.

Overt peripheral neuropathy may appear after chronic high-dose lead exposure, usually following months to years of blood lead concentrations higher than 100 mcg/dL. Predominantly motor in character, the neuropathy may present clinically with painless weakness of the extensors, particularly in the upper extremity, resulting in classic wrist-drop. Preclinical signs of lead-induced peripheral nerve dysfunction may be detectable by electrodiagnostic testing.

B. Blood

Lead can induce an anemia that may be either normocytic or microcytic and hypochromic. Lead interferes with heme synthesis by blocking the incorporation of iron into protoporphyrin IX and by inhibiting the function of enzymes in the heme synthesis pathway, including aminolevulinic acid dehydratase and ferrochelatase. Within 2–8 weeks after an elevation in blood lead concentration (generally to 30–50 mcg/dL or greater), increases in heme precursors, notably free erythrocyte protoporphyrin or its zinc chelate, zinc protoporphyrin, may be detectable in whole blood. Lead also contributes to anemia by increasing erythrocyte membrane fragility and decreasing red cell survival time. Frank hemolysis may occur with high exposure. Basophilic stippling on the peripheral blood smear, thought to be a consequence of lead inhibition of the enzyme 3',5'-pyrimidine nucleotidase, is sometimes a suggestive—albeit insensitive and nonspecific—diagnostic clue to the presence of lead intoxication.

C. Kidneys

Chronic high-dose lead exposure, usually associated with months to years of blood lead concentrations greater than 80 mcg/dL, may result in renal interstitial fibrosis and nephrosclerosis. Lead nephropathy may have a latency period of years. Lead may alter uric acid excretion by the kidney, resulting in recurrent bouts of gouty arthritis ("saturnine gout"). Acute high-dose lead exposure sometimes produces transient azotemia, possibly as a consequence of intrarenal vasoconstriction. Studies conducted in general population samples have documented an association between blood lead concentration and measures of renal function, including serum creatinine and creatinine clearance. The presence of other risk factors for renal insufficiency, including hypertension and diabetes, may increase susceptibility to lead-induced renal dysfunction.

D. Reproductive Organs

High-dose lead exposure is a recognized risk factor for stillbirth or spontaneous abortion. Epidemiologic studies of the impact of low-level lead exposure on reproductive outcome such as low birth weight, preterm delivery, or spontaneous abortion have yielded mixed results. However, a well-designed nested case-control study detected an odds ratio for spontaneous abortion of 1.8 (95% CI 1.1–3.1) for every 5 mcg/dL increase in maternal blood lead across an approximate range of 5–20 mcg/dL. Recent studies have linked prenatal exposure to low levels of lead (eg, maternal blood lead concentrations of 5–15 mcg/dL) to decrements in physical and cognitive development assessed during the neonatal period and early childhood. In males, blood lead concentrations higher than 40 mcg/dL have been associated with diminished or aberrant sperm production.

E. Gastrointestinal Tract

Moderate lead poisoning may cause loss of appetite, constipation, and, less commonly, diarrhea. At high dosage, intermittent bouts of severe colicky abdominal pain ("lead colic") may occur. The mechanism of lead colic is unclear but is believed to involve spasmodic contraction of the smooth muscles of the intestinal wall, mediated by alteration in synaptic transmission at the smooth muscle-neuro-muscular junction. In heavily exposed individuals with poor dental hygiene, the reaction of circulating lead with sulfur ions released by microbial action may produce dark deposits of lead sulfide at the gingival margin ("gingival lead lines"). Although frequently mentioned as a diagnostic clue in the past, in recent times this has been a relatively rare sign of lead exposure.

F. Cardiovascular System

Epidemiologic, experimental, and in vitro mechanistic data indicate that lead exposure elevates blood pressure in susceptible individuals. In populations with environmental or occupational lead exposure, blood lead concentration is linked with increases in systolic and diastolic blood pressure. Studies of middle-aged and elderly men and women have identified relatively low levels of lead exposure sustained by the general population to be an independent risk factor for hypertension. In addition, epidemiologic studies suggest that low to moderate levels of lead exposure are risk factors for increased cardiovascular mortality. Lead can also elevate blood pressure in experimental animals. The pressor effect of lead may be mediated by an interaction with calcium mediated contraction of vascular smooth muscle, as well as generation of oxidative stress and an associated interference in nitric oxide signaling pathways.

Major Forms of Lead Intoxication

A. Inorganic Lead Poisoning (Table 57–1)

1. Acute—Acute inorganic lead poisoning is uncommon today. It usually results from industrial inhalation of large quantities of lead oxide fumes or, in small children, from ingestion of a large oral dose of lead in the form of lead-based paint chips; small objects, eg, toys coated or fabricated from lead; or contaminated food or drink. The onset of severe symptoms usually requires several days or weeks of recurrent exposure and manifests as signs and symptoms of encephalopathy or colic. Evidence of hemolytic anemia (or anemia with basophilic stippling if exposure has been subacute) and elevated hepatic aminotransferases may be present.

The diagnosis of acute inorganic lead poisoning may be difficult, and depending on the presenting symptoms, the condition has sometimes been mistaken for appendicitis, peptic ulcer, biliary colic, pancreatitis, or infectious meningitis. Subacute presentation, featuring headache, fatigue, intermittent abdominal cramps, myalgias, and arthralgias, has often been mistaken for a flu-like viral illness. When there has been recent ingestion of lead-containing paint chips, glazes, or weights, radiopacities may be visible on abdominal radiographs.

2. Chronic—The patient with chronic lead intoxication usually presents with multisystemic findings, including complaints of anorexia, fatigue, and malaise; neurologic complaints, including headache, difficulty in concentrating, and irritability or depressed mood; weakness, arthralgias, or myalgias; and gastrointestinal symptoms. Lead poisoning should be strongly suspected in any patient presenting with headache, abdominal pain, and anemia; and less commonly with motor neuropathy, gout, and renal insufficiency. Chronic lead intoxication should be considered in any child with neurocognitive deficits, growth retardation, or developmental delay. It is important to recognize that adverse effects of lead that are of considerable public health significance, such as subclinical decrements in neurodevelopment in children and hypertension in adults, are usually nonspecific and may not come to medical attention.

The diagnosis of lead intoxication is best confirmed by measuring lead in whole blood. Although this test reflects lead currently circulating in blood and soft tissues and is not a reliable marker of either recent or cumulative lead exposure, most patients with lead-related disease have blood lead concentrations higher than the normal range. Average background blood lead concentrations in North America and Europe have declined by 90% in recent decades, and the geometric mean blood lead concentration in the United States in 2005–2006 was estimated to be 1.29 mcg/dL. Though predominantly a research tool, the concentration of lead in bone assessed by noninvasive K X-ray fluorescence measurement of lead has been correlated with long-term cumulative lead exposure, and its relationship to numerous lead-related disorders is a subject of ongoing investigation. Measurement of lead excretion in the urine after a single dose of a chelating agent (sometimes called a "chelation challenge test") primarily reflects the lead content of soft tissues and may not be a reliable marker of long-term lead exposure, remote past exposure, or skeletal lead burden. Because of the lag time associated with lead-induced elevations in circulating heme precursors, the finding of a blood lead concentration of 30 mcg/dL or more with no concurrent increase in zinc protoporphyrin suggests that the lead exposure was of recent onset.

B. Organolead Poisoning

Poisoning from organolead compounds is now very rare, in large part because of the worldwide phase-out of tetraethyl and tetramethyl lead as antiknock additives in gasoline. However, organolead compounds such as lead stearate or lead naphthenate are still used in certain commercial processes. Because of their volatility or lipid solubility, organolead compounds tend to be well absorbed through either the respiratory tract or the skin. Organolead compounds predominantly target the central nervous system, producing dose-dependent effects that may include neurocognitive deficits, insomnia, delirium, hallucinations, tremor, convulsions, and death.

Treatment

A. Inorganic Lead Poisoning

Treatment of inorganic lead poisoning involves immediate termination of exposure, supportive care, and the judicious use of chelation therapy. (Chelation is discussed later in this chapter.) Lead encephalopathy is a medical emergency that requires intensive supportive care. Cerebral edema may improve with corticosteroids and mannitol, and anticonvulsants may be required to treat seizures. Radiopacities on abdominal radiographs may suggest the presence of retained lead objects requiring gastrointestinal decontamination. Adequate urine flow should be maintained, but overhydration should be avoided. Intravenous **edetate calcium disodium (CaNa$_2$EDTA)** is administered at a dosage of 1000–1500 mg/m^2/d (approximately 30–50 mg/kg/d) by continuous infusion for up to 5 days. Some clinicians advocate that chelation treatment for lead encephalopathy be initiated with an intramuscular injection of **dimercaprol**, followed in 4 hours by concurrent administration of dimercaprol and EDTA. Parenteral chelation is limited to 5 or fewer days, at which time oral treatment with another chelator, **succimer**, may be instituted. In symptomatic lead intoxication without encephalopathy, treatment may sometimes be initiated with succimer. The end point for chelation is usually resolution of symptoms or return of the blood lead concentration to the premorbid range. In patients with chronic exposure, cessation of chelation may be followed by an upward rebound in blood lead concentration as the lead re-equilibrates from bone lead stores.

Although most clinicians support chelation for symptomatic patients with elevated blood lead concentrations, the decision to chelate asymptomatic subjects is more controversial. Since 1991, the Centers for Disease Control and Prevention (CDC) has recommended chelation for all children with blood lead concentrations of 45 mcg/dL or greater. However, a recent randomized, double-blind, placebo-controlled clinical trial of succimer in children with blood lead concentrations between 25 mcg/dL and 44 mcg/dL found no benefit on neurocognitive function or long-term blood lead reduction. Prophylactic use of chelating agents in the workplace should never be a substitute for reduction or prevention of excessive exposure.

Management of elevated blood lead levels in children and adults should include a conscientious effort to identify and reduce all potential sources of future lead exposure. Many local, state, or national governmental agencies maintain lead poisoning prevention programs that can assist in case management. Blood lead screening of family members or coworkers of a lead poisoning patient is often indicated to assess the scope of the exposure. Although the CDC blood lead level of concern for childhood lead poisoning of 10 mcg/dL has not been revised since 1991, the adverse impact of lower levels on children is widely acknowledged, and primary prevention of lead exposure is receiving increased emphasis. Although the US Occupational Safety and Health Administration (OSHA) lead regulations introduced in the late 1970s mandate that workers be removed from lead exposure for blood lead levels higher than 50–60 mcg/dL, an expert panel in 2007 recommended that removal be initiated for a single blood lead level greater than 30 mcg/dL, or when two successive blood lead levels measured over a 4-week interval are 20 mcg/dL or more. The longer-term goal should be for workers to maintain blood lead levels at lower than 10 mcg/dL, and for pregnant women to avoid occupational or avocational exposure that would result in blood lead levels higher than 5 mcg/dL. Environmental Protection Agency (EPA) regulations effective since 2010 require that contractors who perform renovation, repair, and painting projects that disturb lead-based paint in pre-1978 residences and child-occupied facilities must be certified and must follow specific work practices to prevent lead contamination.

B. Organic Lead Poisoning

Initial treatment consists of decontaminating the skin and preventing further exposure. Treatment of seizures requires appropriate use of anticonvulsants. Empiric chelation may be attempted if high blood lead concentrations are present.

Arsenic

Arsenic is a naturally occurring element in the earth's crust with a long history of use as a constituent of commercial and industrial products, as a component in pharmaceuticals, and as an agent of deliberate poisoning. Recent commercial applications of arsenic include its use in the manufacture of semiconductors, wood preservatives for industrial applications (eg, marine timbers or utility poles), nonferrous alloys, glass, gel-based insecticidal ant baits, and veterinary pharmaceuticals. In some regions of the world, groundwater may contain high levels of arsenic that has leached from natural mineral deposits. Arsenic in drinking water in the Ganges delta of India and Bangladesh is now recognized as one of the world's most pressing environmental health problems. Arsine, an arsenous hydride (AsH_3) gas with potent hemolytic effects, is manufactured predominantly for use in the semiconductor industry but

may also be generated accidentally when arsenic-containing ores come in contact with acidic solutions.

It is of historical interest that Fowler's solution, which contains 1% potassium arsenite, was widely used as a medicine for many conditions from the eighteenth century through the mid-twentieth century. Organic arsenicals were the first pharmaceutical antimicrobials* and were widely used for the first half of the twentieth century until supplanted by sulfonamides and other more effective and less toxic agents.

Other organoarsenicals, most notably lewisite (dichloro-[2-chlorovinyl]arsine), were developed in the early twentieth century as chemical warfare agents. Arsenic trioxide was reintroduced into the United States Pharmacopeia in 2000 as an orphan drug for the treatment of relapsed acute promyelocytic leukemia and is finding expanded use in experimental cancer treatment protocols (see Chapter 54). Melarsoprol, another trivalent arsenical, is used in the treatment of advanced African trypanosomiasis (see Chapter 52).

Pharmacokinetics

Soluble arsenic compounds are well absorbed through the respiratory and gastrointestinal tracts (Table 57–1). Percutaneous absorption is limited but may be clinically significant after heavy exposure to concentrated arsenic reagents. Most of the absorbed inorganic arsenic undergoes methylation, mainly in the liver, to monomethylarsonic acid and dimethylarsinic acid, which are excreted, along with residual inorganic arsenic, in the urine. When chronic daily absorption is less than 1000 mcg of soluble inorganic arsenic, approximately two thirds of the absorbed dose is excreted in the urine within 2–3 days. After massive ingestions, the elimination half-life is prolonged. Inhalation of arsenic compounds of low solubility may result in prolonged retention in the lung and may not be reflected by urinary arsenic excretion. Arsenic binds to sulfhydryl groups present in keratinized tissue, and following cessation of exposure, hair, nails, and skin may contain elevated levels after urine values have returned to normal. However, arsenic in hair and nails as a result of external deposition may be indistinguishable from that incorporated after internal absorption.

Pharmacodynamics

Arsenic compounds are thought to exert their toxic effects by several modes of action. Interference with enzyme function may result from sulfhydryl group binding by trivalent arsenic or by substitution for phosphate. Inorganic arsenic or its metabolites may induce oxidative stress, alter gene expression, and interfere with cell signal transduction. Although on a molar basis, inorganic trivalent arsenic (As^{3+}, arsenite) is generally two to ten times more acutely toxic than inorganic pentavalent arsenic (As^{5+}, arsenate), in vivo interconversion is known to occur, and the full spectrum of arsenic toxicity has occurred after sufficient exposure to either form. Recent studies suggest that the trivalent form of the methylated metabolites (eg, monomethylarsonous acid [MMA^{III}])

---

*Paul Ehrlich's "magic bullet" for syphilis (arsphenamine, Salvarsan) was an arsenical.

may be more toxic than the inorganic parent compounds. Reduced efficiency in the methylation of MMA to DMA, resulting in an elevated percentage of MMA in the urine, has been associated with an increased risk of chronic adverse effects. Arsenic methylation requires *S*-adenosylmethionine, a universal methyl donor in the body, and arsenic-associated perturbations in one-carbon metabolism may underlie some arsenic-induced epigenetic effects such as altered gene expression.

Arsine gas is oxidized in vivo and exerts a potent hemolytic effect associated with alteration of ion flux across the erythrocyte membrane; it also disrupts cellular respiration in other tissues. Arsenic is a recognized human carcinogen and has been associated with cancer of the lung, skin, and bladder. Marine organisms may contain large amounts of a well-absorbed trimethylated organo-arsenic, arsenobetaine, as well as a variety of arsenosugars and arsenolipids. Arsenobetaine exerts no known toxic effects when ingested by mammals and is excreted in the urine unchanged; arsenosugars are partially metabolized to dimethylarsinic acid. Thio-dimethylarsinic acid has recently been identified as a common but minor human arsenic metabolite of uncertain toxicological significance.

Major Forms of Arsenic Intoxication

A. Acute Inorganic Arsenic Poisoning

Within minutes to hours after exposure to high doses (tens to hundreds of milligrams) of soluble inorganic arsenic compounds, many systems are affected. Initial gastrointestinal signs and symptoms include nausea, vomiting, diarrhea, and abdominal pain. Diffuse capillary leak, combined with gastrointestinal fluid loss, may result in hypotension, shock, and death. Cardiopulmonary toxicity, including congestive cardiomyopathy, cardiogenic or noncardiogenic pulmonary edema, and ventricular arrhythmias, may occur promptly or after a delay of several days. Pancytopenia usually develops within 1 week, and basophilic stippling of erythrocytes may be present soon after. Central nervous system effects, including delirium, encephalopathy, and coma, may occur within the first few days of intoxication. An ascending sensorimotor peripheral neuropathy may begin to develop after a delay of 2–6 weeks. This neuropathy may ultimately involve the proximal musculature and result in neuromuscular respiratory failure. Months after an acute poisoning, transverse white striae (Aldrich-Mees lines) may be visible in the nails.

Acute inorganic arsenic poisoning should be considered in an individual presenting with abrupt onset of gastroenteritis in combination with hypotension and metabolic acidosis. Suspicion should be further heightened when these initial findings are followed by cardiac dysfunction, pancytopenia, and peripheral neuropathy. The diagnosis may be confirmed by demonstration of elevated amounts of inorganic arsenic and its metabolites in the urine (typically in the range of several thousand micrograms in the first 2–3 days after acute symptomatic poisoning). Arsenic disappears rapidly from the blood, and except in anuric patients, blood arsenic levels should not be used for diagnostic purposes. Treatment is based on appropriate gut decontamination, intensive

supportive care, and prompt chelation with **unithiol,** 3–5 mg/kg intravenously every 4–6 hours, or **dimercaprol,** 3–5 mg/kg intramuscularly every 4–6 hours. In animal studies, the efficacy of chelation has been highest when it is administered within minutes to hours after arsenic exposure; therefore, if diagnostic suspicion is high, treatment should not be withheld for the several days to weeks often required to obtain laboratory confirmation.

Succimer has also been effective in animal models and has a higher therapeutic index than dimercaprol. However, because it is available in the United States only for oral administration, its use may not be advisable in the initial treatment of acute arsenic poisoning, when severe gastroenteritis and splanchnic edema may limit absorption by this route.

B. Chronic Inorganic Arsenic Poisoning

Chronic inorganic arsenic poisoning also results in multisystemic signs and symptoms. Overt noncarcinogenic effects may be evident after chronic absorption of more than 0.01 mg/kg/d (~ 500–1000 mcg/d in adults). The time to appearance of symptoms varies with dose and interindividual tolerance. Constitutional symptoms of fatigue, weight loss, and weakness may be present, along with anemia, nonspecific gastrointestinal complaints, and a sensorimotor peripheral neuropathy, particularly featuring a stocking glove pattern of dysesthesia. Skin changes—among the most characteristic effects—typically develop after years of exposure and include a "raindrop" pattern of hyperpigmentation, and hyperkeratoses involving the hands and feet (Figure 57–1). Peripheral vascular disease and noncirrhotic portal hypertension may also occur. Epidemiologic studies suggest a possible link to hypertension, diabetes, chronic nonmalignant respiratory disease, and adverse reproductive outcomes. Cancer of the lung, skin, bladder, and possibly other sites, may appear years after exposure to doses of arsenic that are not high enough to elicit other acute or chronic effects.

Administration of arsenite in cancer chemotherapy regimens, often at a daily dose of 10–20 mg for weeks to a few months, has been associated with prolongation of the QT interval on the electrocardiogram and occasionally has resulted in malignant ventricular arrhythmias such as torsades de pointes.

The diagnosis of chronic arsenic poisoning involves integration of the clinical findings with confirmation of exposure. The urine concentration of the sum of inorganic arsenic and its primary metabolites MMA and DMA is less than 20 mcg/L in the general population. High urine levels associated with overt adverse effects may return to normal within days to weeks after exposure ceases. Because it may contain large amounts of nontoxic organoarsenic, all seafood should be avoided for at least 3 days before submission of a urine sample for diagnostic purposes. The arsenic content of hair and nails (normally less than 1 ppm) may sometimes reveal past elevated exposure, but results should be interpreted cautiously in view of the potential for external contamination.

Management of chronic arsenic poisoning consists primarily of termination of exposure and nonspecific supportive care. Although

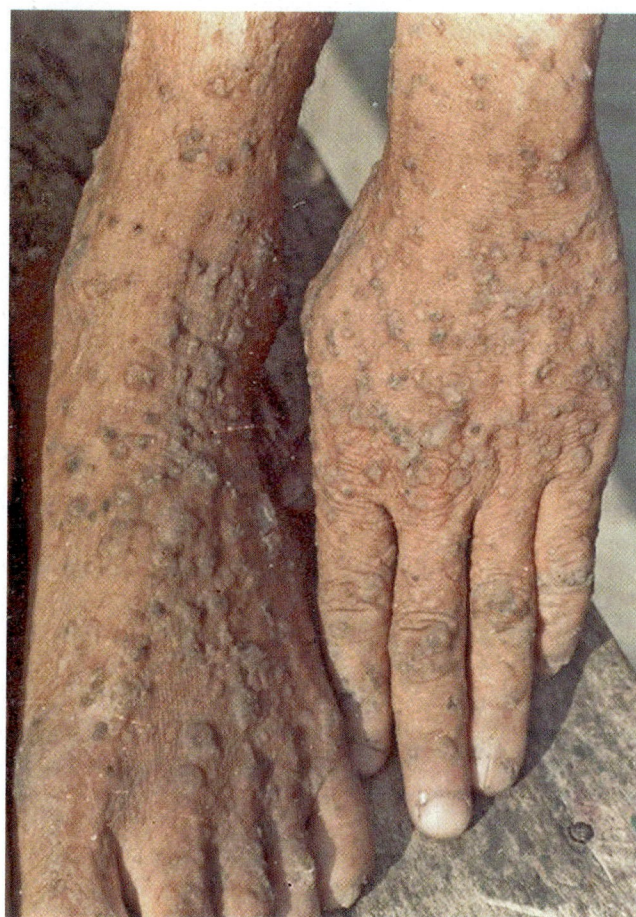

FIGURE 57–1 Dermatologic lesions associated with chronic ingestion of arsenic in drinking water. (Photo courtesy of Dipankar Chakraborti, PhD.)

empiric short-term oral chelation with **unithiol** or **succimer** for symptomatic individuals with elevated urine arsenic concentrations may be considered, it has no proven benefit beyond removal from exposure alone. Preliminary studies suggest that dietary supplementation of folate—thought to be a cofactor in arsenic methylation—might be of value in arsenic-exposed individuals, particularly men, who are also deficient in folate.

C. Arsine Gas Poisoning

Arsine gas poisoning produces a distinctive pattern of intoxication dominated by profound hemolytic effects. After a latent period that may range from 2 hours to 24 hours postinhalation (depending on the magnitude of exposure), massive intravascular hemolysis may occur. Initial symptoms may include malaise, headache, dyspnea, weakness, nausea, vomiting, abdominal pain, jaundice, and hemoglobinuria. Oliguric renal failure, a consequence of hemoglobin deposition in the renal tubules, often appears within 1–3 days. In massive exposures, lethal effects on cellular respiration may occur before renal failure develops. Urinary arsenic levels are elevated but are seldom available to confirm the diagnosis during the critical period of illness. Intensive supportive care—including exchange transfusion, vigorous hydration, and, in the case of acute renal failure, hemodialysis—is the mainstay of therapy.

Currently available chelating agents have not been demonstrated to be of clinical value in arsine poisoning.

MERCURY

Metallic mercury as "quicksilver"—the only metal that is liquid under ordinary conditions—has attracted scholarly and scientific interest from antiquity. The mining of mercury was early recognized as being hazardous to health. As industrial use of mercury became common during the last 200 years, new forms of toxicity were recognized that were found to be associated with various transformations of the metal. In the early 1950s, a mysterious epidemic of birth defects and neurologic disease occurred in the Japanese fishing village of Minamata. The causative agent was determined to be methylmercury in contaminated seafood, traced to industrial discharges into the bay from a nearby factory. In addition to elemental mercury and alkylmercury (including methylmercury), other key mercurials include inorganic mercury salts and aryl mercury compounds, each of which exerts a relatively unique pattern of clinical toxicity.

Mercury is mined predominantly as HgS in cinnabar ore and is then converted commercially to a variety of chemical forms. Key industrial and commercial applications of mercury are found in the electrolytic production of chlorine and caustic soda; the manufacture of electrical equipment, thermometers, and other instruments; fluorescent lamps; and dental amalgam. The widespread use of elemental mercury in artisanal gold production is a growing problem in many developing countries. Mercury use in pharmaceuticals and in biocides has declined substantially in recent years, but occasional use in antiseptics and folk medicines is still encountered. Thimerosal, an organomercurial preservative that is metabolized in part to ethylmercury, has been removed from almost all the vaccines in which it was formerly present. Environmental exposure to mercury from the burning of fossil fuels, or the bioaccumulation of methylmercury in fish, remains a concern in some regions of the world. Low-level exposure to mercury released from dental amalgam fillings occurs, but systemic toxicity from this source has not been established.

Pharmacokinetics

The absorption of mercury varies considerably depending on the chemical form of the metal. Elemental mercury is quite volatile and can be absorbed from the lungs (Table 57–1). It is poorly absorbed from the intact gastrointestinal tract. Inhaled mercury is the primary source of occupational exposure. Organic short-chain alkylmercury compounds are volatile and potentially harmful by inhalation as well as by ingestion. Percutaneous absorption of metallic mercury and inorganic mercury can be of clinical concern following massive acute or long-term chronic exposure. Alkylmercury compounds appear to be well absorbed through the skin, and acute contact with a few drops of dimethylmercury has resulted in severe, delayed toxicity. After absorption, mercury is distributed to the tissues within a few hours, with the highest concentration occurring in the kidney. Inorganic mercury is excreted through the urine and feces. Excretion of inorganic mercury follows a multicompartment model: most is excreted within weeks to months, but a fraction may be retained in the kidneys and brain for years. After inhalation of elemental mercury vapor, urinary mercury levels decline with a half-life of approximately 1–3 months. Methylmercury, which has a blood and whole body half-life of approximately 50 days, undergoes biliary excretion and enterohepatic circulation, with more than two thirds eventually excreted in the feces. Mercury binds to sulfhydryl groups in keratinized tissue, and as with lead and arsenic, traces appear in the hair and nails.

Major Forms of Mercury Intoxication

Mercury interacts with sulfhydryl groups in vivo, inhibiting enzymes and altering cell membranes. The pattern of clinical intoxication from mercury depends to a great extent on the chemical form of the metal and the route and severity of exposure.

A. Acute

Acute inhalation of elemental mercury vapors may cause chemical pneumonitis and noncardiogenic pulmonary edema. Acute gingivostomatitis may occur, and neurologic sequelae (see following text) may also ensue. Acute ingestion of inorganic mercury salts, such as mercuric chloride, can result in a corrosive, potentially life-threatening hemorrhagic gastroenteritis followed within hours to days by acute tubular necrosis and oliguric renal failure.

B. Chronic

Chronic poisoning from inhalation of mercury vapor results in a classic triad of tremor, neuropsychiatric disturbance, and gingivostomatitis. The tremor usually begins as a fine intention tremor of the hands, but the face may also be involved, and progression to choreiform movements of the limbs may occur. Neuropsychiatric manifestations, including memory loss, fatigue, insomnia, and anorexia, are common. There may be an insidious change in mood to shyness, withdrawal, and depression along with explosive anger or blushing (a behavioral pattern referred to as **erethism**). Recent studies suggest that low-dose exposure may produce subclinical neurologic effects. Gingivostomatitis, sometimes accompanied by loosening of the teeth, may be reported after high-dose exposure. Evidence of peripheral nerve damage may be detected on electrodiagnostic testing, but overt peripheral neuropathy is rare. Acrodynia is an uncommon idiosyncratic reaction to subacute or chronic mercury exposure and occurs mainly in children. It is characterized by painful erythema of the extremities and may be associated with hypertension, diaphoresis, anorexia, insomnia, irritability or apathy, and a miliary rash. Chronic exposure to inorganic mercury salts, sometimes via topical application in cosmetic creams, has been associated with neurological symptoms and renal toxicity in case reports and case series.

Methylmercury intoxication affects mainly the central nervous system and results in paresthesias, ataxia, hearing impairment, dysarthria, and progressive constriction of the visual fields. Signs and symptoms of methylmercury intoxication may first appear several weeks or months after exposure begins. Methylmercury is a reproductive toxin. High-dose prenatal exposure to methylmercury may produce mental retardation and a cerebral palsy-like syndrome in the offspring. Low-level prenatal exposures to methylmercury have been associated with a risk of subclinical neurodevelopmental deficits.

A 2004 report by the Institute of Medicine's Immunization Safety Review Committee concluded that available evidence favored rejection of a causal relation between thimerosal-containing vaccines and autism. In like manner, a recent retrospective cohort study conducted by the CDC did not support a causal association between early prenatal or postnatal exposure to mercury from thimerosal-containing vaccines and neuropsychological functioning later in childhood.

Dimethylmercury is a rarely encountered but extremely neurotoxic form of organomercury that may be lethal in small quantities.

The diagnosis of mercury intoxication involves integration of the history and physical findings with confirmatory laboratory testing or other evidence of exposure. In the absence of occupational exposure, the urine mercury concentration is usually less than 5 mcg/L, and whole blood mercury is less than 5 mcg/L. In 1990, the Biological Exposure Index (BEI) Committee of the American Conference of Governmental Industrial Hygienists (ACGIH) recommended that workplace exposures should result in urinary mercury concentrations less than 35 mcg per gram of creatinine and end-of-work-week whole blood mercury concentrations less than 15 mcg/L. To minimize the risk of developmental neurotoxicity from methylmercury, the US Environmental Protection Agency and the Food and Drug Administration (FDA) have advised pregnant women, women who might become pregnant, nursing mothers, and young children to avoid consumption of fish with high mercury levels (eg, swordfish) and to limit consumption of fish with lower levels of mercury to no more than 12 ounces (340 g, or two average meals) per week.

Treatment

A. Acute Exposure

In addition to intensive supportive care, prompt chelation with oral or intravenous **unithiol**, intramuscular **dimercaprol**, or oral **succimer** may be of value in diminishing nephrotoxicity after acute exposure to inorganic mercury salts. Vigorous hydration may help to maintain urine output, but if acute renal failure ensues, days to weeks of hemodialysis or hemodiafiltration in conjunction with chelation may be necessary. Because the efficacy of chelation declines with time since exposure, treatment should not be delayed until the onset of oliguria or other major systemic effects.

B. Chronic Exposure

Unithiol and **succimer** increase urine mercury excretion following acute or chronic elemental mercury inhalation, but the impact of such treatment on clinical outcome is unknown. Dimercaprol has been shown to redistribute mercury to the central nervous system from other tissue sites, and since the brain is a key target organ, dimercaprol should not be used in treatment of exposure to elemental or organic mercury. Limited data suggest that succimer, unithiol, and *N*-acetyl-L-cysteine (NAC) may enhance body clearance of methylmercury.

■ PHARMACOLOGY OF CHELATORS

Chelating agents are drugs used to prevent or reverse the toxic effects of a heavy metal on an enzyme or other cellular target, or to accelerate the elimination of the metal from the body. By forming a complex with the heavy metal, the chelating agent renders the metal unavailable for toxic interactions with functional groups of enzymes or other proteins, coenzymes, cellular nucleophiles, and membranes. Chelating agents contain one or more coordinating atoms, usually oxygen, sulfur, or nitrogen, which donate a pair of electrons to a cationic metal ion to form one or more coordinate-covalent bonds. Depending on the number of metal-ligand bonds, the complex may be referred to as mono-, bi-, or polydentate. Figure 57–2 depicts the hexadentate chelate formed by interaction of edetate (ethylenediaminetetraacetate) with a metal atom, such as lead.

In some cases, the metal-mobilizing effect of a therapeutic chelating agent may not only enhance that metal's excretion—a desired effect—but may also redistribute some of the metal to other vital organs. This has been demonstrated for dimercaprol, which redistributes mercury and arsenic to the brain while also enhancing urinary mercury and arsenic excretion. Although several chelating agents have the capacity to mobilize cadmium, their tendency to redistribute cadmium to the kidney and increase nephrotoxicity has negated their therapeutic value in cadmium intoxication.

In addition to removing the target metal that is exerting toxic effects on the body, some chelating agents may enhance excretion of essential cations, such as zinc in the case of calcium EDTA and diethylenetriaminepentaacetic acid (DTPA), and zinc and copper in the case of succimer. No clinical significance of this effect has been demonstrated, although some animal data suggest the possibility of adverse developmental impact. If prolonged chelation during the prenatal period or early childhood period is necessary, judicious supplementation of the diet with zinc might be considered.

The longer the half-life of a metal in a particular organ, the less effectively it will be removed by chelation. For example, in the case of lead chelation with calcium EDTA or succimer, or of plutonium chelation with DTPA, the metal is more effectively removed from soft tissues than from bone, where incorporation into bone matrix results in prolonged retention.

In most cases, the capacity of chelating agents to prevent or reduce the adverse effects of toxic metals appears to be greatest when such agents are administered very soon after an acute metal exposure. Use of chelating agents days to weeks after an acute metal exposure ends—or their use in the treatment of chronic metal intoxication—may still be associated with increased metal excretion. However, at that point, the capacity of such enhanced

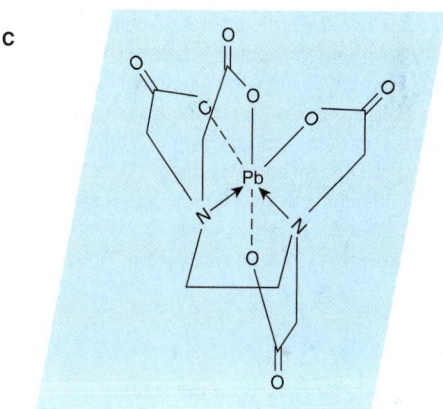

FIGURE 57–2 Salt and chelate formation with edetate (ethylenediaminetetraacetate, EDTA). **A:** In a solution of calcium disodium salt of EDTA, the sodium and hydrogen ions are chemically and biologically available. **B:** In solutions of calcium disodium edetate, calcium is bound by coordinate-covalent bonds with nitrogens as well as by the usual ionic bonds. **C:** In the lead–edetate chelate, lead is incorporated into five heterocyclic rings. (Modified and reproduced, with permission, from Meyers FH, Jawetz E, Goldfien A: *Review of Medical Pharmacology,* 7th ed. Originally published by Lange Medical Publications. McGraw-Hill, 1980.)

excretion to mitigate the pathologic effect of the metal exposure may be reduced.

The most important chelating agents currently in use in the USA are described below.

DIMERCAPROL (2,3-DIMERCAPTOPROPANOL, BAL)

Dimercaprol (Figure 57–3), an oily, colorless liquid with a strong mercaptan-like odor, was developed in Great Britain during

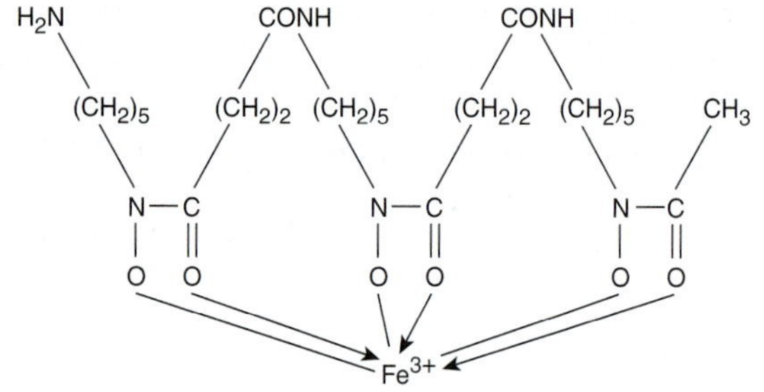

Ferroxamine

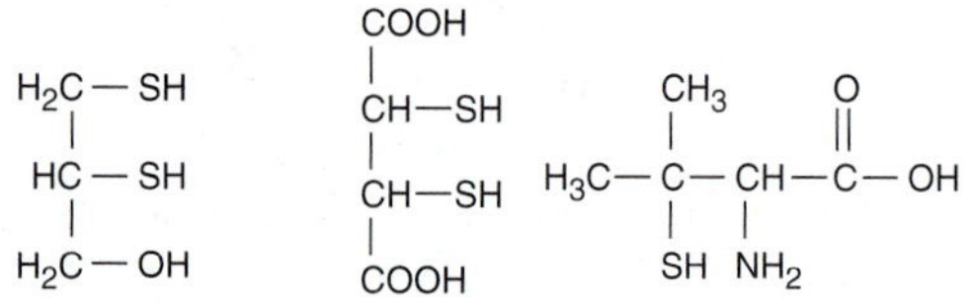

FIGURE 57–3 Chemical structures of several chelators. Ferroxamine (ferrioxamine) without the chelated iron is deferoxamine. It is represented here to show the functional groups; the iron is actually held in a caged system. The structures of the in vivo metal-chelator complexes for dimercaprol, succimer, penicillamine, and unithiol (see text) are not known and may involve the formation of mixed disulfides with amino acids. (Modified and reproduced, with permission from Meyers FH, Jawetz E, and Goldfien A: *Review of Medical Pharmacology,* 7th ed. Originally published by Lange Medical Publications. McGraw-Hill, 1980.)

World War II as a therapeutic antidote against poisoning by the arsenic-containing warfare agent lewisite. It thus became known as British anti-Lewisite, or BAL. Because aqueous solutions of dimercaprol are unstable and oxidize readily, it is dispensed in 10% solution in peanut oil and must be administered by intramuscular injection, which is often painful.

In animal models, dimercaprol prevents and reverses arsenic-induced inhibition of sulfhydryl-containing enzymes and, if given soon after exposure, may protect against the lethal effects of inorganic and organic arsenicals. Human data indicate that it can increase the rate of excretion of arsenic and lead and may offer therapeutic benefit in the treatment of acute intoxication by arsenic, lead, and mercury.

Indications & Toxicity

Dimercaprol is FDA-approved as single-agent treatment of acute poisoning by arsenic and inorganic mercury and for the treatment of severe lead poisoning when used in conjunction with edetate calcium disodium (EDTA; see below). Although studies of its metabolism in humans are limited, intramuscularly administered dimercaprol appears to be readily absorbed, metabolized, and excreted by the kidney within 4–8 hours. Animal models indicate that it may also undergo biliary excretion, but the role of this excretory route in humans and other details of its biotransformation are uncertain.

When used in therapeutic doses, dimercaprol is associated with a high incidence of adverse effects, including hypertension, tachycardia, nausea, vomiting, lacrimation, salivation, fever (particularly in children), and pain at the injection site. Its use has also been associated with thrombocytopenia and increased prothrombin time—factors that may limit intramuscular injection because of the risk of hematoma formation at the injection site. Despite its protective effects in acutely intoxicated animals, dimercaprol may redistribute arsenic and mercury to the central nervous system, and it is not advocated for treatment of chronic poisoning. Water-soluble analogs of dimercaprol—unithiol and succimer—have higher therapeutic indices and have replaced dimercaprol in many settings.

SUCCIMER (DIMERCAPTOSUCCINIC ACID, DMSA)

Succimer is a water-soluble analog of dimercaprol, and like that agent it has been shown in animal studies to prevent and reverse metal-induced inhibition of sulfhydryl-containing enzymes and to protect against the acute lethal effects of arsenic. In humans, treatment with succimer is associated with an increase in urinary lead excretion and a decrease in blood lead concentration. It may also decrease the mercury content of the kidney, a key target organ of inorganic mercury salts. In the USA, succimer is formulated exclusively for oral use, but intravenous formulations have been used successfully elsewhere. It is absorbed rapidly but somewhat variably after oral administration. Peak blood levels of succimer occur at approximately 3 hours. The drug binds in vivo to the amino acid cysteine to form 1:1 and 1:2 mixed disulfides, possibly in the kidney, and it may be these complexes that are the active chelating moieties. Experimental data suggest that multidrug-resistance protein 2 (Mrp2), one of a group of transporter proteins involved in the cellular excretion of xenobiotics, facilitates the renal excretion of mercury compounds that are bound to the transformed succimer and to unithiol. The elimination half-time of transformed succimer is approximately 2–4 hours.

Indications & Toxicity

Succimer is currently FDA-approved for the treatment of children with blood lead concentrations greater than 45 mcg/dL, but it is also commonly used in adults. The typical dosage is 10 mg/kg orally three times a day. Oral administration of succimer is comparable to parenteral EDTA in reducing blood lead concentration and has supplanted EDTA in outpatient treatment of patients who are capable of absorbing the oral drug. However, despite the demonstrated capacity of both succimer and EDTA to enhance lead elimination, their value in reversing established lead toxicity or in otherwise improving therapeutic outcome has yet to be established by a placebo-controlled clinical trial. In a recent study in lead-exposed juvenile rats, high-dose succimer did reduce lead-induced neurocognitive impairment when administered to animals with moderate- and high-dose lead exposure. Conversely, when administered to the control group that was not lead exposed, succimer was associated with a decrement in neurocognitive performance. Based on its protective effects against arsenic in animals and its ability to mobilize mercury from the kidney, succimer has also been used in the treatment of arsenic and mercury poisoning.

In limited clinical trials, succimer has been well tolerated. It has a negligible impact on body stores of calcium, iron, and magnesium. It induces a mild increase in urinary excretion of zinc and, less consistently, copper. This effect on trace metal balance has not been associated with overt adverse effects, but its long-term impact on neurodevelopment is uncertain. Gastrointestinal disturbances, including anorexia, nausea, vomiting, and diarrhea, are the most common side effects, occurring in less than 10% of patients. Rashes, sometimes requiring discontinuation of the medication, have been reported in less than 5% of patients. Mild, reversible increases in liver aminotransferases have been noted in 6–10% of patients, and isolated cases of mild to moderate neutropenia have been reported.

EDETATE CALCIUM DISODIUM (ETHYLENEDIAMINETETRAACETIC ACID, EDTA)

Ethylenediaminetetraacetic acid (Figure 57–2) is an efficient chelator of many divalent and trivalent metals in vitro. To prevent potentially life-threatening depletion of calcium, the drug should be administered only as the calcium disodium salt.

EDTA penetrates cell membranes relatively poorly and therefore chelates extracellular metal ions much more effectively than intracellular ions.

The highly polar ionic character of EDTA limits its oral absorption. Moreover, oral administration may increase lead absorption from the gut. Consequently, EDTA should be administered by intravenous infusion. In patients with normal renal function, EDTA is rapidly excreted by glomerular filtration, with 50% of an injected dose appearing in the urine within 1 hour. EDTA mobilizes lead from soft tissues, causing a marked increase in urinary lead excretion and a corresponding decline in blood lead concentration. In patients with renal insufficiency, excretion of the drug—and its metal-mobilizing effects—may be delayed.

Indications & Toxicity

Edetate calcium disodium is indicated chiefly for the chelation of lead, but it may also have usefulness in poisoning by zinc, manganese, and certain heavy radionuclides. In spite of repeated claims in the alternative medicine literature, EDTA has no demonstrated usefulness in the treatment of atherosclerotic cardiovascular disease.

Because the drug and the mobilized metals are excreted via the urine, the drug is relatively contraindicated in anuric patients. In such instances, the use of low doses of EDTA in combination with high-flux hemodialysis or hemofiltration has been described. Nephrotoxicity from EDTA has been reported, but in most cases can be prevented by maintenance of adequate urine flow, avoidance of excessive doses, and limitation of a treatment course to

5 or fewer consecutive days. EDTA may result in temporary zinc depletion that is of uncertain clinical significance. Analogs of EDTA, the calcium and zinc disodium salts of DTPA, pentetate, have been used for removal ("decorporation") of certain transuranic, rare earth, and transition metal radioisotopes, and in 2004 were approved by the FDA for treatment of contamination with plutonium, americium, and curium.

UNITHIOL (DIMERCAPTOPROPANESULFONIC ACID, DMPS)

Unithiol, a dimercapto chelating agent that is a water-soluble analog of dimercaprol, has been available in the official formularies of Russia and other former Soviet countries since 1958 and in Germany since 1976. It has been legally available from compounding pharmacies in the USA since 1999. Unithiol can be administered orally and intravenously. Bioavailability by the oral route is approximately 50%, with peak blood levels occurring in approximately 3.7 hours. Over 80% of an intravenous dose is excreted in the urine, mainly as cyclic DMPS sulfides. The elimination half-time of total unithiol (parent drug and its transformation products) is approximately 20 hours. Unithiol exhibits protective effects against the toxic action of mercury and arsenic in animal models, and it increases the excretion of mercury, arsenic, and lead in humans. Animal studies and a few case reports suggest that unithiol may also have usefulness in the treatment of poisoning by bismuth compounds.

$$\begin{array}{ccc} \text{SH} & \text{SH} & \text{SO}_2\text{H} \\ | & | & | \\ \text{CH}_2- & \text{CH} - & \text{CH}_2 \end{array}$$

Unithiol

Indications & Toxicity

Unithiol has no FDA-approved indications, but experimental studies and its pharmacologic and pharmacodynamic profile suggest that intravenous unithiol offers advantages over intramuscular dimercaprol or oral succimer in the initial treatment of severe acute poisoning by inorganic mercury or arsenic. Aqueous preparations of unithiol (usually 50 mg/mL in sterile water) can be administered at a dosage of 3–5 mg/kg every 4 hours by slow intravenous infusion over 20 minutes. If a few days of treatment are accompanied by stabilization of the patient's cardiovascular and gastrointestinal status, it may be possible to change to oral administration of 4–8 mg/kg every 6–8 hours. Oral unithiol may also be considered as an alternative to oral succimer in the treatment of lead intoxication.

Unithiol has been reported to have a low overall incidence of adverse effects (< 4%). Self-limited dermatologic reactions (drug exanthems or urticaria) are the most commonly reported adverse effects, although isolated cases of major allergic reactions, including erythema multiforme and Stevens-Johnson syndrome, have been reported. Because rapid intravenous infusion may cause vasodilation and hypotension, unithiol should be infused slowly over an interval of 15–20 minutes.

PENICILLAMINE (D-DIMETHLCYSTEINE)

Penicillamine (Figure 57–3) is a white crystalline, water-soluble derivative of penicillin. D-Penicillamine is less toxic than the L isomer and consequently is the preferred therapeutic form. Penicillamine is readily absorbed from the gut and is resistant to metabolic degradation.

Indications & Toxicity

Penicillamine is used chiefly for treatment of poisoning with copper or to prevent copper accumulation, as in Wilson's disease (hepatolenticular degeneration). It is also used occasionally in the treatment of severe rheumatoid arthritis (see Chapter 36). Its ability to increase urinary excretion of lead and mercury had occasioned its use in outpatient treatment for intoxication with these metals, but succimer, with its stronger metal-mobilizing capacity and lower adverse-effect profile, has generally replaced penicillamine for these purposes.

Adverse effects have been seen in up to one third of patients receiving penicillamine. Hypersensitivity reactions include rash, pruritus, and drug fever, and the drug should be used with extreme caution, if at all, in patients with a history of penicillin allergy. Nephrotoxicity with proteinuria has also been reported, and protracted use of the drug may result in renal insufficiency. Pancytopenia has been associated with prolonged drug intake. Pyridoxine deficiency is a frequent toxic effect of other forms of the drug but is rarely seen with the D form. An acetylated derivative, N-acetylpenicillamine, has been used experimentally in mercury poisoning and may have superior metal-mobilizing capacity, but it is not commercially available.

DEFEROXAMINE

Deferoxamine is isolated from *Streptomyces pilosus*. It binds iron avidly (Figure 57–3) but binds essential trace metals poorly. Furthermore, though competing for loosely bound iron in iron-carrying proteins (hemosiderin and ferritin), it fails to compete for biologically chelated iron, as in microsomal and mitochondrial cytochromes and hemoproteins. Consequently, it is the parenteral chelator of choice for iron poisoning (see Chapters 33 and 58). Deferoxamine plus hemodialysis may also be useful in the treatment of aluminum toxicity in renal failure. Deferoxamine is poorly absorbed when administered orally and may increase iron absorption when given by this route. It should therefore be administered intramuscularly or, preferably, intravenously. It is believed to be metabolized, but the pathways are unknown. The iron-chelator complex is excreted in the urine, often turning the urine an orange-red color.

Rapid intravenous administration may result in hypotension. Adverse idiosyncratic responses such as flushing, abdominal

discomfort, and rash have also been observed. Pulmonary complications (eg, acute respiratory distress syndrome) have been reported in some patients undergoing deferoxamine infusions lasting longer than 24 hours, and neurotoxicity and increased susceptibility to certain infections (eg, with *Yersinia enterocolitica*) have been described after long-term therapy of iron overload conditions (eg, thalassemia major).

DEFERASIROX

Deferasirox is a tridentate chelator with a high affinity for iron and low affinity for other metals, eg, zinc and copper. It is orally active and well absorbed. In the circulation, it binds iron, and the complex is excreted in the bile. Deferasirox was approved by the FDA in 2005 for the oral treatment of iron overload caused by blood transfusions, a problem in the treatment of thalassemia and myelodysplastic syndrome. More than five years of clinical experience suggest that daily long-term usage is generally well tolerated, with the most common adverse effects consisting of mild to moderate gastrointestinal disturbances (<15% of patients) and skin rash ($\approx$ 5% of patients).

PRUSSIAN BLUE (FERRIC HEXACYANOFERRATE)

Ferric hexacyanoferrate (insoluble Prussian blue) is a hydrated crystalline compound in which Fe^{2+} and Fe^{3+} atoms are coordinated with cyanide groups in a cubic lattice structure. Although used as a dark blue commercial pigment for nearly 300 years, it was only three decades ago that its potential usefulness as a pharmaceutical chelator was recognized. Primarily by ion exchange, and secondarily by mechanical trapping or adsorption, the compound has high affinity for certain univalent cations, particularly cesium and thallium. Used as an oral drug, insoluble Prussian blue undergoes minimal gastrointestinal absorption (<1%). Because the complexes it forms with cesium or thallium are nonabsorbable, oral administration of the chelator diminishes intestinal absorption or interrupts enterohepatic and enteroenteric circulation of these cations, thereby accelerating their elimination in the feces. In clinical case series, the use of Prussian blue has been associated with a decline in the biologic half-life (ie, in vivo retention) of radioactive cesium and thallium.

Indications & Toxicity

In 2003, the FDA approved Prussian blue for the treatment of contamination with radioactive cesium (^{137}Cs) and intoxication with thallium salts. Approval was prompted by concern over potential widespread human contamination with radioactive cesium caused by terrorist use of a radioactive dispersal device ("dirty bomb"). The drug is part of the Strategic National Stockpile of pharmaceuticals and medical material maintained by the CDC (http://www.bt.cdc.gov/stockpile/#material). (***Note:*** Although soluble forms of Prussian blue, such as potassium ferric hexacyanoferrate, may have better utility in thallium poisoning, only the insoluble form is currently available as a pharmaceutical.)

After exposure to ^{137}Cs or thallium salts, the approved adult dosage is 3 g orally three times a day; the corresponding pediatric dosage (2–12 years of age) is 1 g orally three times a day. Serial monitoring of urine and fecal radioactivity (^{137}Cs) and urinary

thallium concentrations can guide the recommended duration of therapy. Adjunctive supportive care for possible acute radiation illness (^{137}Cs) or systemic thallium toxicity should be instituted as needed.

Prussian blue has not been associated with significant adverse effects. Constipation, which may occur in some cases, should be treated with laxatives or increased dietary fiber.

PREPARATIONS AVAILABLE

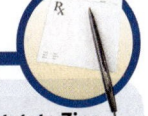

Deferasirox (Exjade)
  Oral: 125, 250, 500 mg tablets
Deferoxamine (Desferal)
  Parenteral: Powder to reconstitute, 500, 2000 mg/vial
Dimercaprol (BAL in Oil)
  Parenteral: 100 mg/mL for IM injection
Edetate calcium [calcium EDTA] (Calcium Disodium Versenate)
  Parenteral: 200 mg/mL for injection
Penicillamine (Cuprimine, Depen)
  Oral: 125, 250 mg capsules; 250 mg tablets

Pentetate Calcium Trisodium ([calcium DTPA] and Pentetate Zinc Trisodium [zinc DTPA])
  Parenteral: 200 mg/mL for injection
Prussian Blue (Radiogardase)
  Oral: 500 mg capsules
Succimer (Chemet)
  Oral: 100 mg capsules
Unithiol (Dimaval)
  Bulk powder available for compounding as oral capsules, or for infusion (50 mg/mL)

REFERENCES

Lead

Brubaker CJ et al: The influence of age of lead exposure on adult gray matter volume. Neurotoxicology 2010;31:259.

Carlisle JC et al: A blood lead benchmark for assessing risks from childhood lead exposure. J Environ Sci Health Part A 2009;44:1200.

Centers for Disease Control and Prevention (CDC): Guidelines for the Identification and Management of Lead Exposure in Pregnant and Lactating Women. CDC, 2010. http://www.cdc.gov/nceh/lead/publications/LeadandPregnancy2010.pdf

Kosnett MJ et al: Recommendations for medical management of adult lead exposure. Environ Health Perspect 2007;115:463.

Lanphear BP et al: Low-level environmental lead exposure and children's intellectual development: An international pooled analysis. Environ Health Perspect 2005;113:894.

U.S. Environmental Protection Agency. Air Quality Criteria for Lead (Final). EPA: Washington, DC, 2006. http://cfpub.epa.gov/ncea/cfm/recordisplay.cfm?deid=158823

Weisskopf MG et al: A prospective study of bone lead concentration and death from all causes, cardiovascular diseases, and cancer in the Department of Veterans Affairs Normative Aging Study. Circulation 2009;120:1056.

Weuve J et al: Cumulative exposure to lead in relation to cognitive function in older women. Environ Health Perspect 2009;117:574.

Arsenic

Caldwell KL et al: Levels of urinary total and speciated arsenic in the US population: National Health and Nutrition Examination Survey 2003–2004. J Exp Sci Environ Epid 2009;19:59.

Chen CJ et al: Arsenic and diabetes and hypertension in human populations. Toxicol Appl Pharmacol 2007;222:298.

Gamble MV: Folate and arsenic metabolism: A double-blind, placebo-controlled folic acid supplementation trial in Bangladesh. Am J Clin Nutr 2006;84:1093.

Lindberg AL et al: The risk of arsenic induced skin lesions in Bangladeshi men and women is affected by arsenic metabolism and the age at first exposure. Tox Appl Pharmacol 2008;230:9.

Parvez F et al: A prospective study of respiratory symptoms associated with chronic arsenic exposure in Bangladesh: findings from the Health Effects of Arsenic Longitudinal Study (HEALS). Thorax 2010;65:528.

Vahter M: Effects of arsenic on maternal and fetal health. Annu Rev Nutr 2009;29:381.

Mercury

Bellinger DC et al: Dental amalgam restorations and children's neuropsychological function: The New England Children's Amalgam Trial. Environ Health Perspect 2007;115:440.

Caldwell KL et al: Total blood mercury concentrations in the U.S. population: 1999–2006. Int J Hyg Environ Health 2009;212:588.

Clarkson TW, Magos L: The toxicology of mercury and its chemical compounds. Crit Rev Toxicol 2006;36:609.

EPA website: What You Need to Know about Mercury in Fish and Shellfish. http://water.epa.gov/scitech/swguidance/fishshellfish/outreach/advice_index.cfm

Hertz-Picciotto I et al: Blood mercury concentrations in CHARGE study children with and without autism. Environ Health Perspect 2010;118:161.

Lederman SA et al: Relation between cord blood mercury levels and early child development in a World Trade Center cohort. Environ Health Perspect 2008;116:1085.

Yorifuji T et al: Long-term exposure to methylmercury and neurologic signs in Minamata and neighboring communities. Epidemiology 2008;19:3.

Chelating Agents

Agarwal MB: Deferasirox: Oral, once daily iron chelator—an expert opinion. Indian J Pediatr 2010;77:185.

Bradberry S, Vale A: A comparison of sodium calcium edetate (edetate calcium disodium) and succimer (DMSA) in the treatment of inorganic lead poisoning. Clin Toxicol 2009;47:841.

Dargan PI et al: Case report: Severe mercuric sulphate poisoning treated with 2,3-dimercaptopropane-1-sulphonate and haemodiafiltration. Crit Care 2003;7:R1.

Gong Z et al: Determination of arsenic metabolic complex excreted in human urine after administration of sodium 2,3-dimercapto-1-propane sulfonate. Chem Res Toxicol 2002;15:1318.

Kosnett MJ: Chelation for heavy metals (arsenic, lead, and mercury): Protective or perilous? Clin Pharmacol Ther 2010;88:412.

Stangle DE et al: Succimer chelation improves learning, attention, and arousal regulation in lead-exposed rats but produces lasting cognitive impairment in the absence of lead exposure. Environ Health Perspect 2007;115:201.

Thompson DF, Called ED: Soluble or insoluble prussian blue for radiocesium and thallium poisoning? Ann Pharmacother 2004;38:1509.

CASE STUDY ANSWER

This scenario is highly suspicious for acute lead intoxication. Lead-based paints have been commonly used as anticorrosion coatings on iron and steel structures, and grinding and torch cutting can result in high-dose exposure to inhaled lead dust and fumes. Measurement of a whole blood lead concentration would be a key diagnostic test. If an elevated blood lead concentration is confirmed, the primary therapeutic intervention will be removal of the individual from further work exposure until blood lead concentration has declined and symptoms resolved. If the blood lead concentration is in excess of 80 mcg/dL (~ 4 μmol/L), treatment with a chelating agent, such as oral succimer or parenteral edetate calcium disodium, should be strongly considered. Upon return to work, use of proper respiratory protection and adherence to protective work practices are essential.

Management of the Poisoned Patient

Kent R. Olson, MD

CASE STUDY

A 62-year-old woman with a history of depression is found in her apartment in a lethargic state. An empty bottle of bupropion is on the bedside table. In the emergency department, she is unresponsive to verbal and painful stimuli. She has a brief generalized seizure, followed by a respiratory arrest. The emergency physician performs endotracheal intubation and administers a drug intravenously, followed by another substance via a nasogastric tube. The patient is admitted to the intensive care unit for continued supportive care and recovers the next morning. What drug might be used intravenously to prevent further seizures? What substance is commonly used to adsorb drugs still present in the gastrointestinal tract?

Over 1 million cases of acute poisoning occur in the USA each year, although only a small number are fatal. Most deaths are due to intentional suicidal overdose by an adolescent or adult. Childhood deaths due to accidental ingestion of a drug or toxic household product have been markedly reduced in the last 40 years as a result of safety packaging and effective poisoning prevention education.

Even with a serious exposure, poisoning is rarely fatal if the victim receives prompt medical attention and good supportive care. Careful management of respiratory failure, hypotension, seizures, and thermoregulatory disturbances has resulted in improved survival of patients who reach the hospital alive.

This chapter reviews the basic principles of poisoning, initial management, and specialized treatment of poisoning, including methods of increasing the elimination of drugs and toxins.

■ TOXICOKINETICS & TOXICODYNAMICS

The term **toxicokinetics** denotes the absorption, distribution, excretion, and metabolism of toxins, toxic doses of therapeutic agents, and their metabolites. The term **toxicodynamics** is used to denote the injurious effects of these substances on body functions. Although many similarities exist between the pharmacokinetics and toxicokinetics of most substances, there are also important differences. The same caution applies to pharmacodynamics and toxicodynamics.

SPECIAL ASPECTS OF TOXICOKINETICS

Volume of Distribution

The volume of distribution (V_d) is defined as the apparent volume into which a substance is distributed in the body (see Chapter 3). A large V_d implies that the drug is not readily accessible to measures aimed at purifying the blood, such as hemodialysis. Examples of drugs with large volumes of distribution (> 5 L/kg) include antidepressants, antipsychotics, antimalarials, opioids, propranolol, and verapamil. Drugs with a relatively small V_d (< 1 L/kg) include salicylate, ethanol, phenobarbital, lithium, valproic acid, and phenytoin (see Table 3–1).

Clearance

Clearance is a measure of the volume of plasma that is cleared of drug per unit time (see Chapter 3). The total clearance for most drugs is the sum of clearances via excretion by the kidneys and metabolism by the liver. In planning a detoxification strategy, it is important to know the contribution of each organ to total clearance. For example, if a drug is 95% cleared by liver metabolism and only 5% cleared by renal excretion, even a dramatic increase in urinary concentration of the drug will have little effect on overall elimination.

Overdosage of a drug can alter the usual pharmacokinetic processes, and this must be considered when applying kinetics to poisoned patients. For example, dissolution of tablets or gastric emptying time may be slowed so that absorption and peak toxic effects are delayed. Drugs may injure the epithelial barrier of the gastrointestinal tract and thereby increase absorption. If the capacity of the liver to metabolize a drug is exceeded, the first-pass effect will be reduced and more drug will be delivered to the circulation. With a dramatic increase in the concentration of drug in the blood, protein-binding capacity may be exceeded, resulting in an increased fraction of free drug and greater toxic effect. At normal dosage, most drugs are eliminated at a rate proportional to the plasma concentration (first-order kinetics). If the plasma concentration is very high and normal metabolism is saturated, the rate of elimination may become fixed (zero-order kinetics). This change in kinetics may markedly prolong the apparent serum half-life and increase toxicity.

SPECIAL ASPECTS OF TOXICODYNAMICS

The general dose-response principles described in Chapter 2 are relevant when estimating the potential severity of an intoxication. When considering quantal dose-response data, both the therapeutic index and the overlap of therapeutic and toxic response curves must be considered. For instance, two drugs may have the same therapeutic index but unequal safe dosing ranges if the slopes of their dose-response curves are not the same. For some drugs, eg, sedative-hypnotics, the major toxic effect is a direct extension of the therapeutic action, as shown by their graded dose-response curve (see Figure 22–1). In the case of a drug with a linear dose-response curve (drug A), lethal effects may occur at 10 times the normal therapeutic dose. In contrast, a drug with a curve that reaches a plateau (drug B) may not be lethal at 100 times the normal dose.

For many drugs, at least part of the toxic effect may be different from the therapeutic action. For example, intoxication with drugs that have atropine-like effects (eg, tricyclic antidepressants) reduces sweating, making it more difficult to dissipate heat. In tricyclic antidepressant intoxication, there may also be increased muscular activity or seizures; the body's production of heat is thus enhanced, and lethal hyperpyrexia may result. Overdoses of drugs that depress the cardiovascular system, eg, β blockers or calcium channel blockers, can profoundly alter not only cardiac function but all functions that are dependent on blood flow. These include renal and hepatic elimination of the toxin and that of any other drugs that may be given.

■ APPROACH TO THE POISONED PATIENT

HOW DOES THE POISONED PATIENT DIE?

An understanding of common mechanisms of death due to poisoning can help prepare the caregiver to treat patients effectively. Many toxins depress the central nervous system (CNS), resulting in obtundation or coma. Comatose patients frequently lose their airway protective

reflexes and their respiratory drive. Thus, they may die as a result of airway obstruction by the flaccid tongue, aspiration of gastric contents into the tracheobronchial tree, or respiratory arrest. These are the most common causes of death due to overdoses of narcotics and sedative-hypnotic drugs (eg, barbiturates and alcohol).

Cardiovascular toxicity is also frequently encountered in poisoning. Hypotension may be due to depression of cardiac contractility; hypovolemia resulting from vomiting, diarrhea, or fluid sequestration; peripheral vascular collapse due to blockade of α-adrenoceptor-mediated vascular tone; or cardiac arrhythmias. Hypothermia or hyperthermia due to exposure as well as the temperature-dysregulating effects of many drugs can also produce hypotension. Lethal arrhythmias such as ventricular tachycardia and fibrillation can occur with overdoses of many cardioactive drugs such as ephedrine, amphetamines, cocaine, digitalis, and theophylline; and drugs not usually considered cardioactive, such as tricyclic antidepressants, antihistamines, and some opioid analogs.

Cellular hypoxia may occur in spite of adequate ventilation and oxygen administration when poisoning is due to cyanide, hydrogen sulfide, carbon monoxide, and other poisons that interfere with transport or utilization of oxygen. Such patients may not be cyanotic, but cellular hypoxia is evident by the development of tachycardia, hypotension, severe lactic acidosis, and signs of ischemia on the electrocardiogram.

Seizures, muscular hyperactivity, and rigidity may result in death. Seizures may cause pulmonary aspiration, hypoxia, and brain damage. Hyperthermia may result from sustained muscular hyperactivity and can lead to muscle breakdown and myoglobinuria, renal failure, lactic acidosis, and hyperkalemia. Drugs and poisons that often cause seizures include antidepressants, isoniazid (INH), diphenhydramine, cocaine, and amphetamines.

Other organ system damage may occur after poisoning and is sometimes delayed in onset. Paraquat attacks lung tissue, resulting in pulmonary fibrosis, beginning several days after ingestion. Massive hepatic necrosis due to poisoning by acetaminophen or certain mushrooms results in hepatic encephalopathy and death 48–72 hours or longer after ingestion.

Finally, some patients may die before hospitalization because the behavioral effects of the ingested drug may result in traumatic injury. Intoxication with alcohol and other sedative-hypnotic drugs is a common contributing factor to motor vehicle accidents. Patients under the influence of hallucinogens such as phencyclidine (PCP) or lysergic acid diethylamide (LSD) may suffer trauma when they become combative or fall from a height.

■ INITIAL MANAGEMENT OF THE POISONED PATIENT

The initial management of a patient with coma, seizures, or otherwise altered mental status should follow the same approach regardless of the poison involved: supportive measures are the basics ("ABCDs") of poisoning treatment.

First, the **airway** should be cleared of vomitus or any other obstruction and an oral airway or endotracheal tube inserted if needed. For many patients, simple positioning in the lateral, left-side-down position is sufficient to move the flaccid tongue out of the airway. **Breathing** should be assessed by observation and pulse oximetry and, if in doubt, by measuring arterial blood gases. Patients with respiratory insufficiency should be intubated and mechanically ventilated. The **circulation** should be assessed by continuous monitoring of pulse rate, blood pressure, urinary output, and evaluation of peripheral perfusion. An intravenous line should be placed and blood drawn for serum glucose and other routine determinations.

At this point, every patient with altered mental status should receive a challenge with concentrated **dextrose,** unless a rapid bedside blood glucose test demonstrates that the patient is not hypoglycemic. Adults are given 25 g (50 mL of 50% dextrose solution) intravenously, children 0.5 g/kg (2 mL/kg of 25% dextrose). Hypoglycemic patients may appear to be intoxicated, and there is no rapid and reliable way to distinguish them from poisoned patients. Alcoholic or malnourished patients should also receive 100 mg of thiamine intramuscularly or in the intravenous infusion solution at this time to prevent Wernicke's syndrome.

The opioid antagonist **naloxone** may be given in a dose of 0.4–2 mg intravenously. Naloxone reverses respiratory and CNS depression due to all varieties of opioid drugs (see Chapter 31). It is useful to remember that these drugs cause death primarily by respiratory depression; therefore, if airway and breathing assistance have already been instituted, naloxone may not be necessary. Larger doses of naloxone may be needed for patients with overdose involving propoxyphene, codeine, and some other opioids. The benzodiazepine antagonist **flumazenil** (see Chapter 22) may be of value in patients with suspected benzodiazepine overdose, but it should not be used if there is a history of tricyclic antidepressant overdose or a seizure disorder, as it can induce convulsions in such patients.

History & Physical Examination

Once the essential initial ABCD interventions have been instituted, one can begin a more detailed evaluation to make a specific diagnosis. This includes gathering any available history and performing a toxicologically oriented physical examination. Other causes of coma or seizures such as head trauma, meningitis, or metabolic abnormalities should be sought and treated. Some common intoxications are described under Common Toxic Syndromes.

A. History

Oral statements about the amount and even the type of drug ingested in toxic emergencies may be unreliable. Even so, family members, police, and fire department or paramedical personnel should be asked to describe the environment in which the toxic emergency occurred and should bring to the emergency department any syringes, empty bottles, household products, or over-the-counter medications in the immediate vicinity of the possibly poisoned patient.

B. Physical Examination

A brief examination should be performed, emphasizing those areas most likely to give clues to the toxicologic diagnosis. These include vital signs, eyes and mouth, skin, abdomen, and nervous system.

1. Vital signs—Careful evaluation of vital signs (blood pressure, pulse, respirations, and temperature) is essential in all toxicologic emergencies. Hypertension and tachycardia are typical with amphetamines, cocaine, and antimuscarinic (anticholinergic) drugs. Hypotension and bradycardia are characteristic features of overdose with calcium channel blockers, β blockers, clonidine, and sedative hypnotics. Hypotension with tachycardia is common with tricyclic antidepressants, trazodone, quetiapine, vasodilators, and β agonists. Rapid respirations are typical of salicylates, carbon monoxide, and other toxins that produce metabolic acidosis or cellular asphyxia. Hyperthermia may be associated with sympathomimetics, anticholinergics, salicylates, and drugs producing seizures or muscular rigidity. Hypothermia can be caused by any CNS-depressant drug, especially when accompanied by exposure to a cold environment.

2. Eyes—The eyes are a valuable source of toxicologic information. Constriction of the pupils (miosis) is typical of opioids, clonidine, phenothiazines, and cholinesterase inhibitors (eg, organophosphate insecticides), and deep coma due to sedative drugs. Dilation of the pupils (mydriasis) is common with amphetamines, cocaine, LSD, and atropine and other anticholinergic drugs. Horizontal nystagmus is characteristic of intoxication with phenytoin, alcohol, barbiturates, and other sedative drugs. The presence of both vertical and horizontal nystagmus is strongly suggestive of phencyclidine poisoning. Ptosis and ophthalmoplegia are characteristic features of botulism.

3. Mouth—The mouth may show signs of burns due to corrosive substances, or soot from smoke inhalation. Typical odors of alcohol, hydrocarbon solvents, or ammonia may be noted. Poisoning due to cyanide can be recognized by some examiners as an odor like bitter almonds.

4. Skin—The skin often appears flushed, hot, and dry in poisoning with atropine and other antimuscarinics. Excessive sweating occurs with organophosphates, nicotine, and sympathomimetic drugs. Cyanosis may be caused by hypoxemia or by methemoglobinemia. Icterus may suggest hepatic necrosis due to acetaminophen or *Amanita phalloides* mushroom poisoning.

5. Abdomen—Abdominal examination may reveal ileus, which is typical of poisoning with antimuscarinic, opioid, and sedative drugs. Hyperactive bowel sounds, abdominal cramping, and diarrhea are common in poisoning with organophosphates, iron, arsenic, theophylline, *A phalloides*, and *A muscaria*.

6. Nervous system—A careful neurologic examination is essential. Focal seizures or motor deficits suggest a structural lesion (eg, intracranial hemorrhage due to trauma) rather than toxic or metabolic encephalopathy. Nystagmus, dysarthria, and ataxia are typical of phenytoin, carbamazepine, alcohol, and other sedative intoxication. Twitching and muscular hyperactivity are common with atropine and other anticholinergic agents, and cocaine and other sympathomimetic drugs. Muscular rigidity can be caused by haloperidol and other antipsychotic agents, and by strychnine or by tetanus. Generalized hypertonicity of muscles and lower extremity clonus are typical of serotonin syndrome. Seizures are often caused by overdose with antidepressants (especially tricyclic antidepressants and bupropion [as in the case study]), cocaine, amphetamines, theophylline, isoniazid, and diphenhydramine. Flaccid coma with absent reflexes and even an isoelectric electroencephalogram may be seen with deep coma due to sedative-hypnotic or other CNS depressant intoxication and may be mistaken for brain death.

Laboratory & Imaging Procedures

A. Arterial Blood Gases

Hypoventilation results in an elevated P_{CO_2} (hypercapnia) and a low P_{O_2} (hypoxia). The P_{O_2} may also be low in a patient with aspiration pneumonia or drug-induced pulmonary edema. Poor tissue oxygenation due to hypoxia, hypotension, or cyanide poisoning will result in metabolic acidosis. The P_{O_2} measures only oxygen dissolved in the plasma and not total blood oxygen content or oxyhemoglobin saturation and may appear normal in patients with severe carbon monoxide poisoning. Pulse oximetry may also give falsely normal results in carbon monoxide intoxication.

B. Electrolytes

Sodium, potassium, chloride, and bicarbonate should be measured. The anion gap is then calculated by subtracting the measured anions from cations:

$$\text{Anion gap} = (Na^+ + K^+) - (HCO_3^- + Cl^-)$$

Normally, the sum of the cations exceeds the sum of the anions by no more than 12–16 mEq/L (or 8–12 mEq/L if the formula used for estimating the anion gap omits the potassium level). A larger-than expected anion gap is caused by the presence of unmeasured anions (lactate, etc) accompanying metabolic acidosis. This may occur with numerous conditions, such as diabetic ketoacidosis, renal failure, or shock-induced lactic acidosis. Drugs that may induce an elevated anion gap metabolic acidosis (Table 58–1) include aspirin, metformin, methanol, ethylene glycol, isoniazid, and iron.

Alterations in the serum potassium level are hazardous because they can result in cardiac arrhythmias. Drugs that may cause hyperkalemia despite normal renal function include potassium itself, β

blockers, digitalis glycosides, potassium-sparing diuretics, and fluoride. Drugs associated with hypokalemia include barium, β agonists, caffeine, theophylline, and thiazide and loop diuretics.

C. Renal Function Tests

Some toxins have direct nephrotoxic effects; in other cases, renal failure is due to shock or myoglobinuria. Blood urea nitrogen and creatinine levels should be measured and urinalysis performed. Elevated serum creatine kinase (CK) and myoglobin in the urine suggest muscle necrosis due to seizures or muscular rigidity. Oxalate crystals in large numbers in the urine suggest ethylene glycol poisoning.

D. Serum Osmolality

The calculated serum osmolality is dependent mainly on the serum sodium and glucose and the blood urea nitrogen and can be estimated from the following formula:

$$2 \times Na^+ \text{ (mEq/L)} + \frac{\text{Glucose (mg/dL)}}{18} + \frac{\text{BUN (mg/dL)}}{3}$$

This calculated value is normally 280–290 mOsm/L. Ethanol and other alcohols may contribute significantly to the measured serum osmolality but, since they are not included in the calculation, cause an osmol gap:

$$\frac{\text{Osmolar}}{\text{gap}} = \frac{\text{Measured}}{\text{osmolality}} - \frac{\text{Calculated}}{\text{osmolality}}$$

Table 58–2 lists the concentration and expected contribution to the serum osmolality in ethanol, methanol, ethylene glycol, and isopropanol poisonings.

E. Electrocardiogram

Widening of the QRS complex duration (to more than 100 milliseconds) is typical of tricyclic antidepressant and quinidine overdoses (Figure 58–1). The QT_c interval may be prolonged (to more than 440 milliseconds) in many poisonings, including quinidine, antidepressants and antipsychotics, lithium, and arsenic (see also http://www.torsades.org/). Variable atrioventricular (AV) block and

TABLE 58–1 Examples of drug-induced anion gap acidosis.

Type of Elevation of the Anion Gap	Agents
Organic acid metabolites	Methanol, ethylene glycol, diethylene glycol
Lactic acidosis	Cyanide, carbon monoxide, ibuprofen, isoniazid, metformin, salicylates, valproic acid; any drug-induced seizures, hypoxia, or hypotension

Note: The normal anion gap calculated from $(Na^+ + K^+) - (HCO_3^- + Cl^-)$ is 12–16 mEq/L; calculated from $(Na^+) - (HCO_3^- + Cl^-)$, it is 8–12 mEq/L.

TABLE 58–2 Some substances that can cause an osmol gap.

Substance[1]	Serum Level (mg/dL)	Corresponding Osmol Gap (mOsm/kg)
Ethanol	350	75
Methanol	80	25
Ethylene glycol	200	35
Isopropanol	350	60

[1]Other substances that can increase the osmol gap include propylene glycol and other glycols, acetone, mannitol, and magnesium.

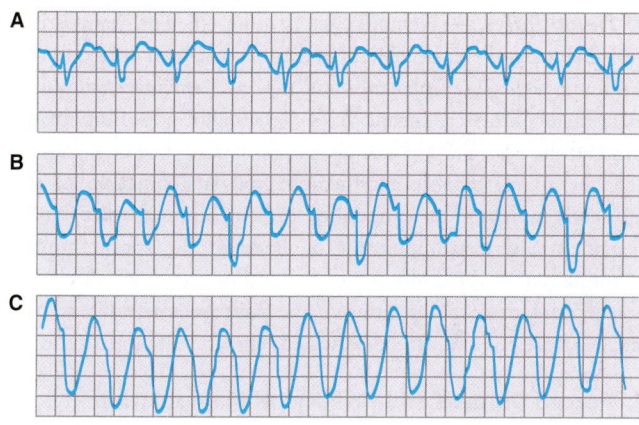

FIGURE 58–1 Changes in the electrocardiogram in tricyclic antidepressant overdosage. **A:** Slowed intraventricular conduction results in prolonged QRS interval (0.18 s; normal, 0.08 s). **B** and **C:** Supraventricular tachycardia with progressive widening of QRS complexes mimics ventricular tachycardia. (Reproduced, with permission, from Benowitz NL, Goldschlager N: Cardiac disturbances in the toxicologic patient. In: Haddad LM, Winchester JF [editors]. *Clinical Management of Poisoning and Drug Overdose.* WB Saunders, 1983.)

a variety of atrial and ventricular arrhythmias are common with poisoning by digoxin and other cardiac glycosides. Hypoxemia due to carbon monoxide poisoning may result in ischemic changes on the electrocardiogram.

F. Imaging Findings

A plain film of the abdomen may be useful because some tablets, particularly iron and potassium, may be radiopaque. Chest radiographs may reveal aspiration pneumonia, hydrocarbon pneumonia, or pulmonary edema. When head trauma is suspected, a computed tomography (CT) scan is recommended.

Toxicology Screening Tests

It is a common misconception that a broad toxicology "screen" is the best way to diagnose and manage an acute poisoning. Unfortunately, comprehensive toxicology screening is time-consuming and expensive and results of tests may not be available for days. Moreover, many highly toxic drugs such as calcium channel blockers, β blockers, and isoniazid are not included in the screening process. The clinical examination of the patient and selected routine laboratory tests are usually sufficient to generate a tentative diagnosis and an appropriate treatment plan. Although screening tests may be helpful in confirming a suspected intoxication or for ruling out intoxication as a cause of apparent brain death, they should not delay needed treatment.

When a specific antidote or other treatment is under consideration, quantitative laboratory testing may be indicated. For example, determination of the acetaminophen level is useful in assessing the need for antidotal therapy with acetylcysteine. Serum levels of salicylate (aspirin), ethylene glycol, methanol, theophylline, carbamazepine, lithium, valproic acid, and other drugs and poisons may indicate the need for hemodialysis (Table 58–3).

TABLE 58–3 Hemodialysis in drug overdose and poisoning.[1]

Hemodialysis may be indicated depending on the severity of poisoning or the blood concentration:
Carbamazepine
Ethylene glycol
Lithium
Methanol
Metformin
Phenobarbital
Salicylate
Theophylline
Valproic acid
Hemodialysis is ineffective or is not useful:
Amphetamines
Antidepressants
Antipsychotic drugs
Benzodiazepines
Calcium channel blockers
Digoxin
Metoprolol and propranolol
Opioids

[1]This listing is not comprehensive.

Decontamination

Decontamination procedures should be undertaken simultaneously with initial stabilization, diagnostic assessment, and laboratory evaluation. Decontamination involves removing toxins from the skin or gastrointestinal tract.

A. Skin

Contaminated clothing should be completely removed and double-bagged to prevent illness in health care providers and for possible laboratory analysis. Wash contaminated skin with soap and water.

B. Gastrointestinal Tract

Controversy remains regarding the efficacy of gut emptying by emesis or gastric lavage, especially when treatment is initiated more than 1 hour after ingestion. For most ingestions, clinical toxicologists recommend simple administration of activated charcoal to bind ingested poisons in the gut before they can be absorbed (as in the case study). In unusual circumstances, induced emesis or gastric lavage may also be used.

1. Emesis—Emesis can be induced with ipecac *syrup* (never *extract* of ipecac), and this method was previously used to treat some childhood ingestions at home under telephone supervision of a physician or poison control center personnel. However, the risks involved with inappropriate use outweighed the unproven benefits, and this treatment is rarely used in the home or hospital. Ipecac should not be used if the suspected intoxicant is a corrosive agent, a petroleum distillate, or a rapid-acting convulsant. Previously popular methods of inducing emesis such as fingertip stimulation of the pharynx, salt water, and apomorphine are ineffective or dangerous and should not be used.

2. Gastric lavage—If the patient is awake or if the airway is protected by an endotracheal tube, gastric lavage may be performed using an orogastric or nasogastric tube—as large a tube as possible. Lavage solutions (usually 0.9% saline) should be at body temperature to prevent hypothermia.

3. Activated charcoal—Owing to its large surface area, activated charcoal can adsorb many drugs and poisons. It is most effective if given in a ratio of at least 10:1 of charcoal to estimated dose of toxin by weight. Charcoal does not bind iron, lithium, or potassium, and it binds alcohols and cyanide only poorly. It does not appear to be useful in poisoning due to corrosive mineral acids and alkali. Studies suggest that oral activated charcoal given alone may be just as effective as gut emptying (eg, ipecac-induced emesis or gastric lavage) followed by charcoal. Repeated doses of oral activated charcoal may enhance systemic elimination of some drugs (including carbamazepine, dapsone, and theophylline) by a mechanism referred to as "gut dialysis," although the clinical benefit is unproved.

4. Cathartics—Administration of a cathartic (laxative) agent may hasten removal of toxins from the gastrointestinal tract and reduce absorption, although no controlled studies have been done. Whole bowel irrigation with a balanced polyethylene glycol-electrolyte solution (GoLYTELY, CoLyte) can enhance gut decontamination after ingestion of iron tablets, enteric-coated medicines, illicit drug-filled packets, and foreign bodies. The solution is administered orally at 1–2 L/h (500 mL/h in children) for several hours until the rectal effluent is clear.

Specific Antidotes

There is a popular misconception that there is an antidote for every poison. Actually, selective antidotes are available for only a few classes of toxins. The major antidotes and their characteristics are listed in Table 58–4.

Methods of Enhancing Elimination of Toxins

After appropriate diagnostic and decontamination procedures and administration of antidotes, it is important to consider whether measures for enhancing elimination, such as hemodialysis or urinary alkalinization, can improve the clinical outcome. Table 58–3 lists intoxications for which dialysis may be beneficial.

A. Dialysis Procedures

1. Peritoneal dialysis—Although it is a relatively simple and available technique, peritoneal dialysis is inefficient in removing most drugs.

2. Hemodialysis—Hemodialysis is more efficient than peritoneal dialysis and has been well studied. It assists in correction of fluid and electrolyte imbalance and may also enhance removal of toxic metabolites (eg, formic acid in methanol poisoning; oxalic and glycolic acids in ethylene glycol poisoning). The efficiency of both peritoneal dialysis and hemodialysis is a function of the molecular weight, water solubility, protein binding, endogenous clearance, and distribution in the body of the specific toxin. Hemodialysis is especially useful in overdose cases in which the precipitating drug can be removed and fluid and electrolyte imbalances are present and can be corrected (eg, salicylate intoxication).

B. Forced Diuresis and Urinary pH Manipulation

Previously popular but of unproved value, forced diuresis may cause volume overload and electrolyte abnormalities and is not recommended. Renal elimination of a few toxins can be enhanced by alteration of urinary pH. For example, urinary alkalinization is useful in cases of salicylate overdose. Acidification may increase the urine concentration of drugs such as phencyclidine and amphetamines but is not advised because it may worsen renal complications from rhabdomyolysis, which often accompanies the intoxication.

■ COMMON TOXIC SYNDROMES

ACETAMINOPHEN

Acetaminophen is one of the drugs commonly involved in suicide attempts and accidental poisonings, both as the sole agent and in combination with other drugs. Acute ingestion of more than 150–200 mg/kg (children) or 7 g total (adults) is considered potentially toxic. A highly toxic metabolite is produced in the liver (see Figure 4–5).

Initially, the patient is asymptomatic or has mild gastrointestinal upset (nausea, vomiting). After 24–36 hours, evidence of liver injury appears, with elevated aminotransferase levels and hypoprothrombinemia. In severe cases, fulminant liver failure occurs, leading to hepatic encephalopathy and death. Renal failure may also occur.

The severity of poisoning is estimated from a serum acetaminophen concentration measurement. If the level is greater than 150–200 mg/L approximately 4 hours after ingestion, the patient is at risk for liver injury. (Chronic alcoholics or patients taking drugs that enhance P450 production of toxic metabolites are at risk with lower levels.) The antidote acetylcysteine acts as a glutathione substitute, binding the toxic metabolite as it is produced. It is most effective when given early and should be started within 8–10 hours if possible. Liver transplantation may be required for patients with fulminant hepatic failure.

AMPHETAMINES & OTHER STIMULANTS

Stimulant drugs commonly abused in the USA include methamphetamine ("crank," "crystal"), methylenedioxymethamphetamine (MDMA, "ecstasy"), and cocaine ("crack") as well as pharmaceuticals such as pseudoephedrine (Sudafed) and ephedrine (as such

TABLE 58–4 Examples of specific antidotes.

Antidote	Poison(s)	Comments
Acetylcysteine (Acetadote, Mucomyst)	Acetaminophen	Best results if given within 8–10 hours of overdose. Follow liver function tests and acetaminophen blood levels. Acetadote is given intravenously; Mucomyst is given orally.
Atropine	Anticholinesterase intoxication: organophosphates, carbamates	An initial dose of 1–2 mg (for children, 0.05 mg/kg) is given IV, and if there is no response, the dose is doubled every 10–15 minutes, with decreased wheezing and pulmonary secretions as therapeutic end points.
Bicarbonate, sodium	Membrane-depressant cardiotoxic drugs (tricyclic antidepressants, quinidine, etc)	1–2 mEq/kg IV bolus usually reverses cardiotoxic effects (wide QRS, hypotension). Give cautiously in heart failure (avoid sodium overload).
Calcium	Fluoride; calcium channel blockers	Large doses may be needed in severe calcium channel blocker overdose. Start with 15 mg/kg IV.
Deferoxamine	Iron salts	If poisoning is severe, give 15 mg/kg/h IV. 100 mg of deferoxamine binds 8.5 mg of iron.
Digoxin antibodies	Digoxin and related cardiac glycosides	One vial binds 0.5 mg digoxin; indications include serious arrhythmias, hyperkalemia.
Esmolol	Theophylline, caffeine, metaproterenol	Short-acting β blocker. Infuse 25–50 mcg/kg/min IV.
Ethanol	Methanol, ethylene glycol	A loading dose is calculated so as to give a blood level of at least 100 mg/dL (42 g/70 kg in adults). Fomepizole (see below) is easier to use.
Flumazenil	Benzodiazepines	Adult dose is 0.2 mg IV, repeated as necessary to a maximum of 3 mg. *Do not give to patients with seizures, benzodiazepine dependence, or tricyclic overdose.*
Fomepizole	Methanol, ethylene glycol	More convenient than ethanol. Give 15 mg/kg; repeat every 12 hours.
Glucagon	β blockers	5–10 mg IV bolus may reverse hypotension and bradycardia.
Hydroxocobalamin	Cyanide	Adult dose is 5 g IV over 15 minutes. Converts cyanide to cyanocobalamin (vitamin B_{12}).
Naloxone	Narcotic drugs, other opioid derivatives	A specific antagonist of opioids; give 0.4–2 mg initially by IV, IM, or SC injection. Larger doses may be needed to reverse the effects of overdose with propoxyphene, codeine, or fentanyl derivatives. Duration of action (2–3 hours) may be significantly shorter than that of the opioid being antagonized.
Oxygen	Carbon monoxide	Give 100% by high-flow nonrebreathing mask; use of hyperbaric chamber is controversial but often recommended for severe poisoning.
Physostigmine	Suggested for delirium caused by anticholinergic agents	Adult dose is 0.5–1 mg IV slowly. The effects are transient (30–60 minutes), and the lowest effective dose may be repeated when symptoms return. May cause bradycardia, increased bronchial secretions, seizures. Have atropine ready to reverse excess effects. *Do not use for tricyclic antidepressant overdose.*
Pralidoxime (2-PAM)	Organophosphate (OP) cholinesterase inhibitors	Adult dose is 1 g IV, which should be repeated every 3–4 hours as needed or preferably as a constant infusion of 250–400 mg/h. Pediatric dose is approximately 250 mg. No proved benefit in carbamate poisoning; uncertain benefit in established OP poisoning.

and in the herbal agent *Ma-huang*) (see Chapter 32). Caffeine is often added to dietary supplements sold as "metabolic enhancers" or "fat-burners." Newer synthetic analogs of amphetamines such as 3,4-methylenedioxypyrovalerone (MDPV) and various derivatives of methcathinone are becoming popular drugs of abuse, often sold on the street as "bath salts" with names like "Ivory Wave," "Bounce," "Bubbles," "Mad Cow," and "Meow Meow."

At the doses usually used by stimulant abusers, euphoria and wakefulness are accompanied by a sense of power and well-being. At higher doses, restlessness, agitation, and acute psychosis may occur, accompanied by hypertension and tachycardia. Prolonged muscular hyperactivity or seizures may contribute to hyperthermia and rhabdomyolysis. Body temperatures as high as 42°C (107.6°F) have been recorded. Hyperthermia can cause brain damage, hypotension, coagulopathy, and renal failure.

Treatment for stimulant toxicity includes general supportive measures as outlined earlier. There is no specific antidote. Seizures and hyperthermia are the most dangerous manifestations and must be treated aggressively. Seizures are usually managed with intravenous benzodiazepines (eg, lorazepam). Temperature is reduced by removing clothing, spraying with tepid water, and encouraging evaporative cooling with fanning. For very high body temperatures (eg, > 40–41°C [104–105.8°F]), neuromuscular paralysis is used to abolish muscle activity quickly.

ANTICHOLINERGIC AGENTS

A large number of prescription and nonprescription drugs, as well as a variety of plants and mushrooms, can inhibit the effects of acetylcholine at muscarinic receptors. Some drugs used for other purposes (eg, antihistamines) also have anticholinergic effects, in addition to other potentially toxic actions. For example, antihistamines such as diphenhydramine can cause seizures; tricyclic antidepressants, which have anticholinergic, quinidine-like, and α-blocking effects, can cause severe cardiovascular toxicity.

The classic anticholinergic (technically, "antimuscarinic") syndrome is remembered as "red as a beet" (skin flushed), "hot as a hare" (hyperthermia), "dry as a bone" (dry mucous membranes, no sweating), "blind as a bat" (blurred vision, cycloplegia), and "mad as a hatter" (confusion, delirium). Patients usually have sinus tachycardia, and the pupils are usually dilated (see Chapter 8). Agitated delirium or coma may be present. Muscle twitching is common, but seizures are unusual unless the patient has ingested an antihistamine or a tricyclic antidepressant. Urinary retention is common, especially in older men.

Treatment for anticholinergic syndrome is largely supportive. Agitated patients may require sedation with a benzodiazepine or an antipsychotic agent (eg, haloperidol). The specific antidote for peripheral and central anticholinergic syndrome is physostigmine, which has a prompt and dramatic effect and is especially useful for patients who are very agitated. Physostigmine is given in small intravenous doses (0.5–1 mg) with careful monitoring, because it can cause bradycardia and seizures if given too rapidly. Physostigmine should not be given to a patient with suspected tricyclic antidepressant overdose because it can aggravate cardiotoxicity, resulting in heart block or asystole. Catheterization may be needed to prevent excessive distention of the bladder.

ANTIDEPRESSANTS

Tricyclic antidepressants (eg, amitriptyline, desipramine, doxepin, many others; see Chapter 30) are among the most common prescription drugs involved in life-threatening drug overdose. Ingestion of more than 1 g of a tricyclic (or about 15–20 mg/kg) is considered potentially lethal.

Tricyclic antidepressants are competitive antagonists at muscarinic cholinergic receptors, and anticholinergic findings (tachycardia, dilated pupils, dry mouth) are common even at moderate doses. Some tricyclics are also strong α blockers, which can lead to vasodilation. Centrally mediated agitation and seizures may be followed by depression and hypotension. Most important is the fact that tricyclics have quinidine-like cardiac depressant effects on the sodium channel that cause slowed conduction with a wide QRS interval and depressed cardiac contractility. This cardiac toxicity may result in serious arrhythmias (Figure 58–1), including ventricular conduction block and ventricular tachycardia.

Treatment of tricyclic antidepressant overdose includes general supportive care as outlined earlier. Endotracheal intubation and assisted ventilation may be needed. Intravenous fluids are given for hypotension, and dopamine or norepinephrine is added if necessary. Many toxicologists recommend norepinephrine as the initial drug of choice for tricyclic-induced hypotension. The antidote for quinidine-like cardiac toxicity (manifested by a wide QRS complex) is sodium bicarbonate: a bolus of 50–100 mEq (or 1–2 mEq/kg) provides a rapid increase in extracellular sodium that helps overcome sodium channel blockade. *Do not use physostigmine!* Although this agent does effectively reverse anticholinergic symptoms, it can aggravate depression of cardiac conduction and cause seizures.

Monoamine oxidase inhibitors (eg, tranylcypromine, phenelzine) are older antidepressants that are occasionally used for resistant depression. They can cause severe hypertensive reactions when interacting foods or drugs are taken (see Chapters 9 and 30), and they can interact with the selective serotonin reuptake inhibitors (SSRIs).

Newer antidepressants (eg, fluoxetine, paroxetine, citalopram, venlafaxine) are mostly SSRIs and are generally safer than the tricyclic antidepressants and monoamine oxidase inhibitors, although they can cause seizures. **Bupropion** (not an SSRI) has caused seizures even in therapeutic doses. Some antidepressants have been associated with QT prolongation and torsades de pointes arrhythmia. SSRIs may interact with each other or especially with monoamine oxidase inhibitors to cause the **serotonin syndrome,** characterized by agitation, muscle hyperactivity, and hyperthermia (see Chapter 16).

ANTIPSYCHOTICS

Antipsychotic drugs include the older phenothiazines and butyrophenones, as well as newer atypical drugs. All of these can cause CNS depression, seizures, and hypotension. Some can cause QT prolongation. The potent dopamine D_2 blockers are also associated with parkinsonian movement disorders (dystonic reactions) and in rare cases with the neuroleptic malignant syndrome, characterized by "lead-pipe" rigidity, hyperthermia, and autonomic instability (see Chapters 16 and 29).

ASPIRIN (SALICYLATE)

Salicylate poisoning (see Chapter 36) is a much less common cause of childhood poisoning deaths since the introduction of child-resistant containers and the reduced use of children's aspirin. It still accounts for numerous suicidal and accidental poisonings. Acute ingestion of more than 200 mg/kg is likely to produce intoxication. Poisoning can also result from chronic overmedication; this occurs most commonly in elderly patients using salicylates for chronic pain who become confused about their dosing. Poisoning causes uncoupling of oxidative phosphorylation and disruption of normal cellular metabolism.

The first sign of salicylate toxicity is often hyperventilation and respiratory alkalosis due to medullary stimulation. Metabolic acidosis follows, and an increased anion gap results from accumulation of lactate as well as excretion of bicarbonate by the kidney to compensate for respiratory alkalosis. Arterial blood gas testing often reveals a mixed respiratory alkalosis and metabolic acidosis. Body temperature may be elevated owing to uncoupling of oxidative phosphorylation. Severe hyperthermia may occur in serious cases. Vomiting and hyperpnea as well as hyperthermia contribute to fluid loss and dehydration. With very severe poisoning, profound metabolic acidosis, seizures, coma, pulmonary edema, and cardiovascular collapse may occur. Absorption of salicylate and signs of toxicity may be delayed after very large overdoses or ingestion of enteric coated tablets.

General supportive care is essential. After massive aspirin ingestions (eg, more than 100 tablets), aggressive gut decontamination is advisable, including gastric lavage, repeated doses of activated charcoal, and consideration of whole bowel irrigation. Intravenous fluids are used to replace fluid losses caused by tachypnea, vomiting, and fever. For moderate intoxications, intravenous sodium bicarbonate is given to alkalinize the urine and promote salicylate excretion by trapping the salicylate in its ionized, polar form. For severe poisoning (eg, patients with severe acidosis, coma, and serum salicylate level > 100 mg/dL), emergency hemodialysis is performed to remove the salicylate more quickly and restore acid-base balance and fluid status.

BETA BLOCKERS

In overdose, β blockers inhibit both $β_1$ and $β_2$ adrenoceptors; selectivity, if any, is lost at high dosage. The most toxic β blocker is propranolol. As little as two to three times the therapeutic dose can cause serious toxicity. This may be because propranolol in high doses may cause sodium channel blocking effects similar to those seen with quinidine-like drugs, and it is lipophilic, allowing it to enter the CNS (see Chapter 10).

Bradycardia and hypotension are the most common manifestations of toxicity. Agents with partial agonist activity (eg, pindolol) can cause tachycardia and hypertension. Seizures and cardiac conduction block (wide QRS complex) may be seen with propranolol overdose.

General supportive care should be provided as outlined earlier. The usual measures used to raise the blood pressure and heart rate, such as intravenous fluids, β-agonist drugs, and atropine, are generally ineffective. Glucagon is a useful antidote that—like β agonists—acts on cardiac cells to raise intracellular cAMP but does so independent of β adrenoceptors. It can improve heart rate and blood pressure when given in high doses (5–20 mg intravenously).

CALCIUM CHANNEL BLOCKERS

Calcium antagonists can cause serious toxicity or death with relatively small overdoses. These channel blockers depress sinus node automaticity and slow AV node conduction (see Chapter 12). They also reduce cardiac output and blood pressure. Serious hypotension is mainly seen with nifedipine and related dihydropyridines, but in severe overdose all of the listed cardiovascular effects can occur with any of the calcium channel blockers.

Treatment requires general supportive care. Since most ingested calcium antagonists are in sustained-release form, it may be possible to expel them before they are completely absorbed; initiate whole bowel irrigation and oral activated charcoal as soon as possible, before calcium antagonist-induced ileus intervenes. Calcium, given intravenously in doses of 2–10 g, is a useful antidote for depressed cardiac contractility but less effective for nodal block or peripheral vascular collapse. Other treatments reported to be helpful in managing hypotension associated with calcium channel blocker poisoning include glucagon and high-dose insulin (0.5–1 unit/kg/h) plus glucose supplementation to maintain euglycemia. Recently case reports have suggested benefit from administration of lipid emulsion (Intralipid, normally used as an intravenous dietary fat supplement) for severe verapamil overdose.

CARBON MONOXIDE & OTHER TOXIC GASES

Carbon monoxide (CO) is a colorless, odorless gas that is ubiquitous because it is created whenever carbon-containing materials are burned. Carbon monoxide poisoning is the leading cause of death due to poisoning in the USA. Most cases occur in victims of fires, but accidental and suicidal exposures are also common. The diagnosis and treatment of carbon monoxide poisoning are described in Chapter 56. Many other toxic gases are produced in fires or released in industrial accidents (Table 58–5).

CHOLINESTERASE INHIBITORS

Organophosphate and carbamate cholinesterase inhibitors (see Chapter 7) are widely used to kill insects and other pests. Most cases of serious organophosphate or carbamate poisoning result from intentional ingestion by a suicidal person, but poisoning has also occurred at work (pesticide application or packaging) or, rarely, as a result of food contamination or terrorist attack (eg, release of the chemical warfare nerve agent sarin in the Tokyo subway system in 1995).

Stimulation of muscarinic receptors causes abdominal cramps, diarrhea, excessive salivation, sweating, urinary frequency, and increased bronchial secretions (see Chapters 6 and 7). Stimulation of nicotinic receptors causes generalized ganglionic activation, which can lead to hypertension and either tachycardia or bradycardia. Muscle twitching and fasciculations may progress to weakness and respiratory muscle paralysis. CNS effects include agitation, confusion, and seizures. The mnemonic DUMBELS (diarrhea, urination, miosis and muscle weakness, bronchospasm, excitation, lacrimation, and seizures, sweating, and salivation) helps recall the common findings. Blood testing may be used to document depressed activity of red blood cell (acetylcholinesterase) and plasma (butyrylcholinesterase) enzymes, which provide an indirect estimate of synaptic cholinesterase activity.

TABLE 58-5 Characteristics of poisoning with some gases.

Gas	Mechanism of Toxicity	Clinical Features and Treatment
Irritant gases (eg, chlorine, ammonia, sulfur dioxide, nitrogen oxides)	Corrosive effect on upper and lower airways	Cough, stridor, wheezing, pneumonia *Treatment:* Humidified oxygen, bronchodilators
Carbon monoxide	Binds to hemoglobin, reducing oxygen delivery to tissues	Headache, dizziness, nausea, vomiting, seizures, coma *Treatment:* 100% oxygen; consider hyperbaric oxygen
Cyanide	Binds to cytochrome, blocks cellular oxygen use	Headache, nausea, vomiting, syncope, seizures, coma *Treatment:* Conventional antidote kit consists of nitrites to induce methemoglobinemia (which binds cyanide) and thiosulfate (which hastens conversion of cyanide to less toxic thiocyanate); a newer antidote kit (Cyanokit) consists of concentrated hydroxocobalamin, which directly converts cyanide into cyanocobalamin
Hydrogen sulfide	Similar to cyanide	Similar to cyanide. Smell of rotten eggs *Treatment:* No specific antidote; some authorities recommend the nitrite portion of the conventional cyanide antidote kit.
Oxidizing agents (eg, nitrogen oxides)	Can cause methemoglobinemia	Dyspnea, cyanosis (due to brown color of methemoglobin), syncope, seizures, coma *Treatment:* Methylene blue (which hastens conversion back to normal hemoglobin)

General supportive care should be provided as outlined above. Precautions should be taken to ensure that rescuers and health care providers are not poisoned themselves by exposure to contaminated clothing or skin. This is especially critical for the most potent substances such as parathion or nerve gas agents. Antidotal treatment consists of atropine and pralidoxime (see Table 58–4). Atropine is an effective competitive inhibitor at muscarinic sites but has no effect at nicotinic sites. Pralidoxime given early enough may be capable of restoring the cholinesterase activity and is active at both muscarinic and nicotinic sites.

CYANIDE

Cyanide (CN⁻) salts and hydrogen cyanide (HCN) are highly toxic chemicals used in chemical synthesis, as rodenticides (eg, "gopher getter"), formerly as a method of execution, and as agents of suicide or homicide. Hydrogen cyanide is formed from the burning of plastics, wool, and many other synthetic and natural products. Cyanide is also released after ingestion of various plants (eg, cassava) and seeds (eg, apple, peach, and apricot).

Cyanide binds readily to cytochrome oxidase, inhibiting oxygen utilization within the cell and leading to cellular hypoxia and lactic acidosis. Symptoms of cyanide poisoning include shortness of breath, agitation, and tachycardia followed by seizures, coma, hypotension, and death. Severe metabolic acidosis is characteristic. The venous oxygen content may be elevated because oxygen is not being taken up by cells.

Treatment of cyanide poisoning includes rapid administration of activated charcoal (although charcoal binds cyanide poorly, it can reduce absorption) and general supportive care. The conventional antidote kit available in the USA includes two forms of nitrite (amyl nitrite and sodium nitrite) and sodium thiosulfate. The nitrites induce methemoglobinemia, which binds to free CN⁻

creating the less toxic cyanomethemoglobin; thiosulfate is a cofactor in the enzymatic conversion of CN⁻ to the much less toxic thiocyanate (SCN⁻).

In 2006 the FDA approved a new cyanide antidote, a concentrated form of hydroxocobalamin, which is now available as the Cyanokit (EMD Pharmaceuticals, Durham, North Carolina). Hydroxocobalamin (one form of vitamin B$_{12}$) combines rapidly with CN⁻ to form cyanocobalamin (another form of vitamin B$_{12}$).

DIGOXIN

Digitalis and other cardiac glycosides and cardenolides are found in many plants (see Chapter 13) and in the skin of some toads. Toxicity may occur as a result of acute overdose or from accumulation of digoxin in a patient with renal insufficiency or from taking a drug that interferes with digoxin elimination. Patients receiving long-term digoxin treatment are often also taking diuretics, which can lead to electrolyte depletion (especially potassium).

Vomiting is common in patients with digitalis overdose. Hyperkalemia may be caused by acute digitalis overdose or severe poisoning, whereas hypokalemia may be present in patients as a result of long-term diuretic treatment. (Digitalis does not cause hypokalemia.) A variety of cardiac rhythm disturbances may occur, including sinus bradycardia, AV block, atrial tachycardia with block, accelerated junctional rhythm, premature ventricular beats, bidirectional ventricular tachycardia, and other ventricular arrhythmias.

General supportive care should be provided. Atropine is often effective for bradycardia or AV block. The use of digoxin antibodies (see Chapter 13) has revolutionized the treatment of digoxin toxicity; they should be administered intravenously in the dosage indicated in the package insert. Symptoms usually improve within

30–60 minutes after antibody administration. Digoxin antibodies may also be tried in cases of poisoning by other cardiac glycosides (eg, digitoxin, oleander), although larger doses may be needed due to incomplete cross-reactivity.

ETHANOL & SEDATIVE-HYPNOTIC DRUGS

Overdosage with ethanol and sedative-hypnotic drugs (eg, benzodiazepines, barbiturates, γ-hydroxybutyrate [GHB], carisoprodol [Soma]; see Chapters 22 and 23) occurs frequently because of their common availability and use.

Patients with ethanol or other sedative-hypnotic overdose may be euphoric and rowdy ("drunk") or in a state of stupor or coma ("dead drunk"). Comatose patients often have depressed respiratory drive. Depression of protective airway reflexes may result in pulmonary aspiration of gastric contents leading to pneumonia. Hypothermia may be present because of environmental exposure and depressed shivering. Ethanol blood levels greater than 300 mg/dL usually cause deep coma, but regular users are often tolerant to the effects of ethanol and may be ambulatory despite even higher levels. Patients with GHB overdose are often deeply comatose for 3–4 hours and then awaken fully in a matter of minutes.

General supportive care should be provided. With careful attention to protecting the airway (including endotracheal intubation) and assisting ventilation, most patients recover as the drug effects wear off. Hypotension usually responds to intravenous fluids, body warming if cold, and, if needed, dopamine. Patients with isolated benzodiazepine overdose may awaken after intravenous flumazenil, a benzodiazepine antagonist. However, this drug is not widely used as empiric therapy for drug overdose because it may precipitate seizures in patients who are addicted to benzodiazepines or who have ingested a convulsant drug (eg, a tricyclic antidepressant). There are no antidotes for ethanol, barbiturates, or most other sedative-hypnotics.

ETHYLENE GLYCOL & METHANOL

Ethylene glycol and methanol are alcohols that are important toxins because of their metabolism to highly toxic organic acids (see Chapter 23). They are capable of causing CNS depression and a drunken state similar to ethanol overdose. In addition, their products of metabolism—formic acid (from methanol) or hippuric, oxalic, and glycolic acids (from ethylene glycol)—cause a severe metabolic acidosis and can lead to coma and blindness (in the case of formic acid) or renal failure (from oxalic acid and glycolic acid). Initially, the patient appears drunk, but after a delay of up to several hours, a severe anion gap metabolic acidosis becomes apparent, accompanied by hyperventilation and altered mental status. Patients with methanol poisoning may have visual disturbances ranging from blurred vision to blindness.

Metabolism of ethylene glycol and methanol to their toxic products can be blocked by inhibiting the enzyme alcohol dehydrogenase

with a competing drug, such as fomepizole (4-methylpyrazole). Ethanol is also an effective antidote, but it can be difficult to achieve a safe and effective blood level.

IRON & OTHER METALS

Iron is widely used in over-the-counter vitamin preparations and is a leading cause of childhood poisoning deaths. As few as 10–12 prenatal multivitamins with iron may cause serious illness in a small child. Poisoning with other metals (lead, mercury, arsenic) is also important, especially in industry. See Chapters 33, 56, and 57 for detailed discussions of poisoning by iron and other metals.

OPIOIDS

Opioids (opium, morphine, heroin, meperidine, methadone, etc) are common drugs of abuse (see Chapters 31 and 32), and overdose is a common result of using the poorly standardized preparations sold on the street. See Chapter 31 for a detailed discussion of opioid overdose and its treatment.

RATTLESNAKE ENVENOMATION

In the USA, rattlesnakes are the most common venomous reptiles. Bites are rarely fatal, and 20% do not involve envenomation. However, about 60% of bites cause significant morbidity due to the destructive digestive enzymes found in the venom. Evidence of rattlesnake envenomation includes severe pain, swelling, bruising, hemorrhagic bleb formation, and obvious fang marks. Systemic effects include nausea, vomiting, muscle fasciculations, tingling and metallic taste in the mouth, shock, and systemic coagulopathy with prolonged clotting time and reduced platelet count.

Studies have shown that emergency field remedies such as incision and suction, tourniquets, and ice packs are far more damaging than useful. Avoidance of unnecessary motion, on the other hand, does help to limit the spread of the venom. Definitive therapy relies on intravenous antivenom (also known as antivenin) and this should be started as soon as possible.

THEOPHYLLINE

Although it has been largely replaced by inhaled β agonists, theophylline continues to be used for the treatment of bronchospasm by some patients with asthma and bronchitis (see Chapter 20). A dose of 20–30 tablets can cause serious or fatal poisoning. Chronic or subacute theophylline poisoning can also occur as a result of accidental overmedication or use of a drug that interferes with theophylline metabolism (eg, cimetidine, ciprofloxacin, erythromycin; see Chapter 4).

In addition to sinus tachycardia and tremor, vomiting is common after overdose. Hypotension, tachycardia, hypokalemia, and hyperglycemia may occur, probably owing to β_2-adrenergic activation. The cause of this activation is not fully understood, but the effects can be ameliorated by β blockers (see below). Cardiac arrhythmias include atrial tachycardias, premature ventricular contractions, and ventricular tachycardia. In severe poisoning (eg, acute overdose with serum level > 100 mg/L), seizures often occur and are usually resistant to common anticonvulsants. Toxicity may be delayed in onset for many hours after ingestion of sustained-release tablet formulations.

General supportive care should be provided. Aggressive gut decontamination should be carried out using repeated doses of activated charcoal and whole bowel irrigation. Propranolol or other β blockers (eg, esmolol) are useful antidotes for β-mediated hypotension and tachycardia. Phenobarbital is preferred over phenytoin for convulsions; most anticonvulsants are ineffective. Hemodialysis is indicated for serum concentrations greater than 100 mg/L and for intractable seizures in patients with lower levels.

REFERENCES

Dart RD (editor): *Medical Toxicology*, 3rd ed. Lippincott Williams & Wilkins, 2004.

Goldfrank LR et al (editors): *Goldfrank's Toxicologic Emergencies*, 9th ed. McGraw-Hill, 2010.

Olson KR et al (editors): *Poisoning & Drug Overdose*, 6th ed. McGraw-Hill, 2011.

POISINDEX. (Revised Quarterly.) Thomson/Micromedex.

CASE STUDY ANSWER

Overdose of bupropion can cause seizures that are often recurrent or prolonged. Drug-induced seizures are treated with an intravenous benzodiazepine such as lorazepam or diazepam. If this is not effective, phenobarbital or another more efficacious central nervous system depressant may be used. To prevent ingested drugs and poisons from being absorbed systemically, a slurry of activated charcoal is often given orally or by nasogastric tube.

C H A P T E R

59

Special Aspects of Perinatal & Pediatric Pharmacology

Gideon Koren, MD[*]

The effects of drugs on the fetus and newborn infant are based on the general principles set forth in Chapters 1–4 of this book. However, the physiologic contexts in which these pharmacologic laws operate are different in pregnant women and in rapidly maturing infants. At present, the special pharmacokinetic factors operative in these patients are beginning to be understood, whereas information regarding pharmacodynamic differences (eg, receptor characteristics and responses) is still incomplete.

DRUG THERAPY IN PREGNANCY

Pharmacokinetics

Most drugs taken by pregnant women can cross the placenta and expose the developing embryo and fetus to their pharmacologic and teratogenic effects. Critical factors affecting placental drug transfer and drug effects on the fetus include the following: (1) the physicochemical properties of the drug; (2) the rate at which the

drug crosses the placenta and the amount of drug reaching the fetus; (3) the duration of exposure to the drug; (4) distribution characteristics in different fetal tissues; (5) the stage of placental and fetal development at the time of exposure to the drug; and (6) the effects of drugs used in combination.

A. Lipid Solubility

As is true also of other biologic membranes, drug passage across the placenta is dependent on lipid solubility and the degree of drug ionization. Lipophilic drugs tend to diffuse readily across the placenta and enter the fetal circulation. For example, thiopental, a drug commonly used for cesarean sections, crosses the placenta almost immediately and can produce sedation or apnea in the newborn infant. Highly ionized drugs such as succinylcholine and tubocurarine, also used for cesarean sections, cross the placenta slowly and achieve very low concentrations in the fetus. Impermeability of the placenta to polar compounds is relative rather than absolute. If high enough maternal-fetal concentration gradients are achieved, polar compounds cross the placenta in measurable amounts. Salicylate, which is almost completely ionized at physiologic pH, crosses the placenta rapidly. This occurs because the small amount of salicylate that is not ionized is highly lipid-soluble.

[*]Supported by a grant from the Canadian Institutes for Health Research, and by the Research Leadership for Better Pharmacotherapy During Pregnancy and Lactation.

1039

B. Molecular Size and pH

The molecular weight of the drug also influences the rate of transfer and the amount of drug transferred across the placenta. Drugs with molecular weights of 250–500 can cross the placenta easily, depending upon their lipid solubility and degree of ionization; those with molecular weights of 500–1000 cross the placenta with more difficulty; and those with molecular weights greater than 1000 cross very poorly. An important clinical application of this property is the choice of heparin as an anticoagulant in pregnant women. Because it is a very large (and polar) molecule, heparin is unable to cross the placenta. Unlike warfarin, which is teratogenic and should be avoided during the first trimester and even beyond (as the brain continues to develop), heparin may be safely given to pregnant women who need anticoagulation. Yet the placenta contains drug transporters, which can carry larger molecules to the fetus. For example, a variety of maternal antibodies cross the placenta and may cause fetal morbidity, as in Rh incompatibility.

Because maternal blood has a pH of 7.4 and that of the fetal blood is 7.3, weakly basic drugs with pK_a above 7.4 will be more ionized in the fetal compartment, leading to ion trapping and, hence, to higher fetal levels (see Chapter 1).

C. Placental Transporters

During the last decade, many drug transporters have been identified in the placenta, with increasing recognition of their effects on drug transfer to the fetus. For example, the P-glycoprotein transporter encoded by the *MDR1* gene pumps back into the maternal circulation a variety of drugs, including cancer drugs (eg, vinblastine, doxorubicin) and other agents. Similarly, viral protease inhibitors, which are substrates of P-glycoprotein, achieve only low fetal concentrations—an effect that may increase the risk of vertical HIV infection from the mother to the fetus. The hypoglycemic drug glyburide shows much lower concentrations in the fetus as compared to the mother. Recent work has documented that this agent is effluxed from the fetal circulation by the BCRP transporter as well as by the MRP3 transporter located in the placental brush border membrane.

D. Protein Binding

The degree to which a drug is bound to plasma proteins (particularly albumin) may also affect the rate of transfer and the amount transferred. However, if a compound is very lipid-soluble (eg, some anesthetic gases), it will not be affected greatly by protein binding. Transfer of these more lipid-soluble drugs and their overall rates of equilibration are more dependent on (and proportionate to) placental blood flow. This is because very lipid-soluble drugs diffuse across placental membranes so rapidly that their overall rates of equilibration do not depend on the free drug concentrations becoming equal on both sides. If a drug is poorly lipid-soluble and is ionized, its transfer is slow and will probably be impeded by its binding to maternal plasma proteins. Differential protein binding is also important since some drugs exhibit greater protein binding in maternal plasma than in fetal plasma because of a lower binding affinity of fetal proteins. This has been shown for sulfonamides, barbiturates, phenytoin, and local anesthetic agents. In addition, very high maternal protein binding of glyburide

(> 98.8%) also contributes to lower fetal levels as compared to maternal concentrations, as mentioned above.

E. Placental and Fetal Drug Metabolism

Two mechanisms help protect the fetus from drugs in the maternal circulation: (1) The placenta itself plays a role both as a semipermeable barrier and as a site of metabolism of some drugs passing through it. Several different types of aromatic oxidation reactions (eg, hydroxylation, *N*-dealkylation, demethylation) have been shown to occur in placental tissue. Pentobarbital is oxidized in this way. Conversely, it is possible that the metabolic capacity of the placenta may lead to creation of toxic metabolites, and the placenta may therefore augment toxicity (eg, ethanol, benzpyrenes). (2) Drugs that have crossed the placenta enter the fetal circulation via the umbilical vein. Approximately 40–60% of umbilical venous blood flow enters the fetal liver; the remainder bypasses the liver and enters the general fetal circulation. A drug that enters the liver may be partially metabolized there before it enters the fetal circulation. In addition, a large proportion of drug present in the umbilical artery (returning to the placenta) may be shunted through the placenta back to the umbilical vein and into the liver again. It should be noted that metabolites of some drugs may be more active than the parent compound and may affect the fetus adversely.

Pharmacodynamics

A. Maternal Drug Actions

The effects of drugs on the reproductive tissues (breast, uterus, etc) of the pregnant woman are sometimes altered by the endocrine environment appropriate for the stage of pregnancy. Drug effects on other maternal tissues (heart, lungs, kidneys, central nervous system, etc) are not changed significantly by pregnancy, although the physiologic context (cardiac output, renal blood flow, etc) may be altered, requiring the use of drugs that are not needed by the same woman when she is not pregnant. For example, cardiac glycosides and diuretics may be needed for heart failure precipitated by the increased cardiac workload of pregnancy, or insulin may be required for control of blood glucose in pregnancy-induced diabetes.

B. Therapeutic Drug Actions in the Fetus

Fetal therapeutics is an emerging area in perinatal pharmacology. This involves drug administration to the pregnant woman with the fetus as the target of the drug. At present, corticosteroids are used to stimulate fetal lung maturation when preterm birth is expected. Phenobarbital, when given to pregnant women near term, can induce fetal hepatic enzymes responsible for the glucuronidation of bilirubin, and the incidence of jaundice is lower in newborns when mothers are given phenobarbital than when phenobarbital is not used. Before phototherapy became the preferred mode of therapy for neonatal indirect hyperbilirubinemia, phenobarbital was used for this indication. Administration of phenobarbital to the mother was suggested recently as a means of decreasing the risk of intracranial bleeding in preterm infants. However, large randomized studies failed to confirm this effect. Antiarrhythmic drugs have also been given to mothers for treatment of fetal cardiac arrhythmias. Although their efficacy has not yet been established by controlled studies, digoxin, flecainide, procainamide, verapamil, and other antiarrhythmic agents have been shown to be effective in case series. During the last two decades it has been shown that maternal use of zidovudine decreases by two thirds transmission of HIV from the mother to the fetus, and use of combinations of three antiretroviral agents can eliminate fetal infection almost entirely (see Chapter 49).

C. Predictable Toxic Drug Actions in the Fetus

Chronic use of opioids by the mother may produce dependence in the fetus and newborn. This dependence may be manifested after delivery as a neonatal withdrawal syndrome. A less well understood fetal drug toxicity is caused by the use of angiotensin-converting enzyme inhibitors during pregnancy. These drugs can result in significant and irreversible renal damage in the fetus and are therefore contraindicated in pregnant women. Adverse effects may also be delayed, as in the case of female fetuses exposed to diethylstilbestrol, who may be at increased risk for adenocarcinoma of the vagina after puberty.

D. Teratogenic Drug Actions

A single intrauterine exposure to a drug can affect the fetal structures undergoing rapid development at the time of exposure.

Thalidomide is an example of a drug that may profoundly affect the development of the limbs after only brief exposure. This exposure, however, must be at a critical time in the development of the limbs. The thalidomide phocomelia risk occurs during the fourth through the seventh weeks of gestation because it is during this time that the arms and legs develop (Figure 59–1).

1. Teratogenic mechanisms—The mechanisms by which different drugs produce teratogenic effects are poorly understood and are probably multifactorial. For example, drugs may have a direct effect on maternal tissues with secondary or indirect effects on fetal tissues. Drugs may interfere with the passage of oxygen or nutrients through the placenta and therefore have effects on the most rapidly metabolizing tissues of the fetus. Finally, drugs may have important direct actions on the processes of differentiation in developing tissues. For example, vitamin A (retinol) has been shown to have important differentiation-directing actions in normal tissues. Several vitamin A analogs (isotretinoin, etretinate) are powerful teratogens, suggesting that they alter the normal processes of differentiation. Finally, deficiency of a critical substance appears to play a role in some types of abnormalities. For example, folic acid supplementation during pregnancy appears to reduce the incidence of neural tube defects (eg, spina bifida).

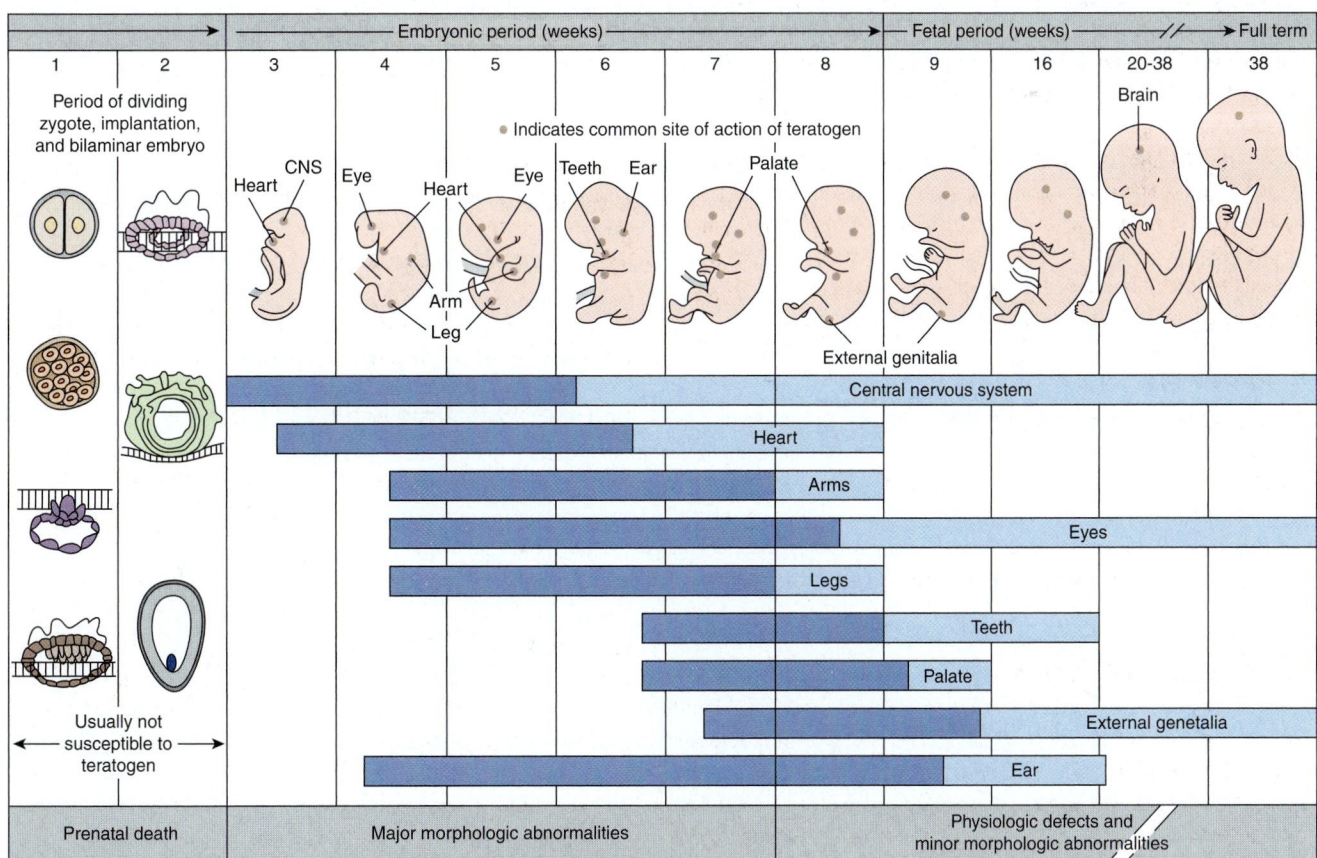

FIGURE 59–1 Schematic diagram of critical periods of human development. (Reproduced, with permission, from Moore KL: *The Developing Human: Clinically Oriented Embryology*, 4th ed. Saunders, 1988.)

Continued exposure to a teratogen may produce cumulative effects or may affect several organs going through varying stages of development. Chronic consumption of high doses of ethanol during pregnancy, particularly during the first and second trimesters, may result in the fetal alcohol syndrome (see Chapter 23). In this syndrome, the central nervous system, growth, and facial development may be affected.

2. Defining a teratogen—To be considered teratogenic, a candidate substance or process should (1) result in a characteristic set of malformations, indicating selectivity for certain target organs; (2) exert its effects at a particular stage of fetal development, eg, during the limited time period of organogenesis of the target organs (Figure 59–1); and (3) show a dose-dependent incidence. Some drugs with known teratogenic or other adverse effects in pregnancy are listed in Table 59–1. Teratogenic effects are not limited only to major malformations, but also include intrauterine growth restriction (eg, cigarette smoking), miscarriage (eg, alcohol), stillbirth (eg, cigarette smoke), and neurocognitive delay (eg, alcohol).

The widely cited Food and Drug Administration (FDA) system for teratogenic potential (Table 59–2) is an attempt to quantify teratogenic risk from A (safe) to X (definite human teratogenic risk). This system has been criticized as inaccurate and impractical. For example, several drugs have been labeled "X" despite extensive opposite human safety data (eg, oral contraceptives). Diazepam and other benzodiazepines are labeled as "D" despite lack of positive evidence of human fetal risk. Presently the FDA is changing its system from the A, B, C grading system to narrative statements that will summarize evidence-based knowledge about each drug in terms of fetal risk and safety.

3. Counseling women about teratogenic risk—Since the thalidomide disaster, medicine has been practiced as if every drug were a potential human teratogen when, in fact, fewer than 30 such drugs have been identified, with hundreds of agents proved safe for the unborn. Owing to high levels of anxiety among pregnant women—and because half of the pregnancies in North America are unplanned—every year many thousands of women need counseling about fetal exposure to drugs, chemicals, and

TABLE 59–1 Drugs with significant teratogenic or other adverse effects on the fetus.

Drug	Trimester	Effect
ACE inhibitors	All, especially second and third	Renal damage
Aminopterin	First	Multiple gross anomalies
Amphetamines	All	Suspected abnormal developmental patterns, decreased school performance
Androgens	Second, third	Masculinization of female fetus
Antidepressants, tricyclic	Third	Neonatal withdrawal symptoms have been reported in a few cases with clomipramine, desipramine, and imipramine
Barbiturates	All	Chronic use can lead to neonatal dependence
Busulfan	All	Various congenital malformations; low birth weight
Carbamazepine	First	Neural tube defects
Chlorpropamide	All	Prolonged symptomatic neonatal hypoglycemia
Clomipramine	Third	Neonatal lethargy, hypotonia, cyanosis, hypothermia
Cocaine	All	Increased risk of spontaneous abortion, abruptio placentae, and premature labor; neonatal cerebral infarction, abnormal development, and decreased school performance
Cyclophosphamide	First	Various congenital malformations
Cytarabine	First, second	Various congenital malformations
Diazepam	All	Chronic use may lead to neonatal dependence
Diethylstilbestrol	All	Vaginal adenosis, clear cell vaginal adenocarcinoma
Ethanol	All	Risk of fetal alcohol syndrome and alcohol-related neurodevelopmental defects
Etretinate	All	High risk of multiple congenital malformations
Heroin	All	Chronic use leads to neonatal dependence
Iodide	All	Congenital goiter, hypothyroidism
Isotretinoin	All	Extremely high risk of CNS, face, ear, and other malformations
Lithium	First, third	Ebstein's anomaly, neonatal toxicity after third trimester
Methadone	All	Chronic use may lead to neonatal abstinence

(continued)

TABLE 59–1 Drugs with significant teratogenic or other adverse effects on the fetus. (Continued)

Drug	Trimester	Effect
Methotrexate	First	Multiple congenital malformations
Methylthiouracil	All	Hypothyroidism
Metronidazole	First	May be mutagenic (from animal studies; there is no evidence for mutagenic or teratogenic effects in humans)
Misoprostol	First	Möbius sequence
Mycophenolate mofetil	First	Major malformations of the face, limbs, and other organs
Organic solvents	First	Multiple malformations
Penicillamine	First	Cutis laxa, other congenital malformations
Phencyclidine	All	Abnormal neurologic examination, poor suck reflex and feeding
Phenytoin	All	Fetal hydantoin syndrome
Propylthiouracil	All	Congenital goiter
Smoking (constituents of tobacco smoke)	All	Intrauterine growth retardation; prematurity; sudden infant death syndrome; perinatal complications
Selective serotonin reuptake inhibitors (SSRIs)	Third	Neonatal abstinence syndrome, persistent pulmonary hypertension of the newborn
Tamoxifen	All	Increased risk of spontaneous abortion or fetal damage
Tetracycline	All	Discoloration and defects of teeth and altered bone growth
Thalidomide	First	Phocomelia (shortened or absent long bones of the limbs) and many internal malformations
Trimethadione	All	Multiple congenital anomalies
Valproic acid	All	Neural tube defects, cardiac and limb malformations
Warfarin	First	Hypoplastic nasal bridge, chondrodysplasia
	Second	CNS malformations
	Third	Risk of bleeding. Discontinue use 1 month before delivery.

radiation. In the Motherisk program in Toronto, thousands of women are counseled every month, and the ability of appropriate counseling to prevent unnecessary abortions has been documented. Clinicians who wish to provide such counsel to pregnant women must ensure that their information is up-to-date and evidence-based and that the woman understands that the baseline teratogenic risk in pregnancy (ie, the risk of a neonatal abnormality in the absence of any known teratogenic exposure) is about 3%. It is also critical to address the maternal-fetal risks of the untreated condition if a medication is avoided. Recent studies show serious morbidity in women who discontinued selective serotonin reuptake inhibitor therapy for depression in pregnancy.

TABLE 59–2 FDA teratogenic risk categories.

Category	Description
A	Controlled studies in women fail to demonstrate a risk to the fetus in the first trimester (and there is no evidence of a risk in late trimesters), and the possibility of fetal harm appears remote.
B	Either animal-reproduction studies have not demonstrated a fetal risk, but there are no controlled studies in pregnant women, or animal-reproduction studies have shown an adverse effect (other than a decrease in fertility) that was not confirmed in controlled studies in women in the first trimester (and there is no evidence of a risk in later trimesters).
C	Either studies in animals have revealed adverse effects on the fetus (teratogenic or embryocidal or other) and there are no controlled studies in women or studies in women or animals are not available. Drugs should be given only if the potential benefit justifies the potential risk to the fetus.
D	There is positive evidence of human fetal risk, but the benefits from use in pregnant women may be acceptable despite the risk (eg, if the drug is needed in a life-threatening situation or for a serious disease for which safer drugs cannot be used or are ineffective).
X	Studies in animals or human beings have demonstrated fetal abnormalities or there is evidence of fetal risk based on human experience or both, and the risk of the use of the drug in pregnant women clearly outweighs any possible benefit. The drug is contraindicated in women who are or may become pregnant.

DRUG THERAPY IN INFANTS & CHILDREN

Physiologic processes that influence pharmacokinetic variables in the infant change significantly in the first year of life, particularly during the first few months. Therefore, special attention must be paid to pharmacokinetics in this age group. Pharmacodynamic differences between pediatric and other patients have not been explored in great detail and are probably small except for those specific target tissues that mature at birth or immediately thereafter (eg, the ductus arteriosus).

Drug Absorption

Drug absorption in infants and children follows the same general principles as in adults. Unique factors that influence drug absorption include blood flow at the site of administration, as determined by the physiologic status of the infant or child; and, for orally administered drugs, gastrointestinal function, which changes rapidly during the first few days after birth. Age after birth also influences the regulation of drug absorption.

A. Blood Flow at the Site of Administration

Absorption after intramuscular or subcutaneous injection depends mainly, in neonates as in adults, on the rate of blood flow to the muscle or subcutaneous area injected. Physiologic conditions that might reduce blood flow to these areas are cardiovascular shock, vasoconstriction due to sympathomimetic agents, and heart failure. However, sick preterm infants requiring intramuscular injections may have very little muscle mass. This is further complicated by diminished peripheral perfusion to these areas. In such cases, absorption becomes irregular and difficult to predict, because the drug may remain in the muscle and be absorbed more slowly than expected. If perfusion suddenly improves, there can be a sudden and unpredictable increase in the amount of drug entering the circulation, resulting in high and potentially toxic concentrations of drug. Examples of drugs especially hazardous in such situations are cardiac glycosides, aminoglycoside antibiotics, and anticonvulsants.

B. Gastrointestinal Function

Significant biochemical and physiologic changes occur in the neonatal gastrointestinal tract shortly after birth. In full-term infants, gastric acid secretion begins soon after birth and increases gradually over several hours. In preterm infants, the secretion of gastric acid occurs more slowly, with the highest concentrations appearing on the fourth day of life. Therefore, drugs that are usually partially or totally inactivated by the low pH of gastric contents should not be administered orally.

Gastric emptying time is prolonged (up to 6 or 8 hours) in the first day or so after delivery. Therefore, drugs that are absorbed primarily in the stomach may be absorbed more completely than anticipated. In the case of drugs absorbed in the small intestine, therapeutic effect may be delayed. Peristalsis in the neonate is irregular and may be slow. The amount of drug absorbed in the small intestine may therefore be unpredictable; more than the usual amount of drug may be absorbed if peristalsis is slowed, and this could result in potential toxicity from an otherwise standard dose.

Table 59–3 summarizes data on oral bioavailability of various drugs in neonates compared with older children and adults. An increase in peristalsis, as in diarrheal conditions, tends to decrease the extent of absorption, because contact time with the large absorptive surface of the intestine is decreased.

Gastrointestinal enzyme activities tend to be lower in the newborn than in the adult. Activities of α-amylase and other pancreatic enzymes in the duodenum are low in infants up to 4 months of age. Neonates also have low concentrations of bile acids and lipase, which may decrease the absorption of lipid-soluble drugs.

Drug Distribution

As body composition changes with development, the distribution volumes of drugs are also changed. The neonate has a higher percentage of its body weight in the form of water (70–75%) than does the adult (50–60%). Differences can also be observed between the full-term neonate (70% of body weight as water) and the small preterm neonate (85% of body weight as water). Similarly, extracellular water is 40% of body weight in the neonate, compared with 20% in the adult. Most neonates will experience diuresis in the first 24–48 hours of life. Since many drugs are distributed throughout the extracellular water space, the size (volume) of the extracellular water compartment may be important in determining the concentration of drug at receptor sites. This is especially important for water-soluble drugs (such as aminoglycosides) and less crucial for lipid-soluble agents.

Preterm infants have much less fat than full-term infants. Total body fat in preterm infants is about 1% of total body weight, compared with 15% in full-term neonates. Therefore, organs that generally accumulate high concentrations of lipid-soluble drugs in adults and older children may accumulate smaller amounts of these agents in less mature infants.

Another major factor determining drug distribution is drug binding to plasma proteins. Albumin is the plasma protein with the greatest binding capacity. In general, protein binding of drugs is reduced in the neonate. This has been seen with local anesthetic drugs, diazepam, phenytoin, ampicillin, and phenobarbital. Therefore, the concentration of free (unbound) drug in plasma is

TABLE 59–3 Oral drug absorption (bioavailability) of various drugs in the neonate compared with older children and adults.

Drug	Oral Absorption
Acetaminophen	Decreased
Ampicillin	Increased
Diazepam	Normal
Digoxin	Normal
Penicillin G	Increased
Phenobarbital	Decreased
Phenytoin	Decreased
Sulfonamides	Normal

increased initially. Because the free drug exerts the pharmacologic effect, this can result in greater drug effect or toxicity despite a normal or even low plasma concentration of total drug (bound plus unbound). Consider a therapeutic dose of a drug (eg, diazepam) given to a patient. The concentration of total drug in the plasma is 300 mcg/L. If the drug is 98% protein-bound in an older child or adult, then 6 mcg/L is the concentration of free drug. Assume that this concentration of free drug produces the desired effect in the patient without producing toxicity. However, if this drug is given to a preterm infant in a dosage adjusted for body weight and it produces a total drug concentration of 300 mcg/L—and protein binding is only 90%—then the free drug concentration will be 30 mcg/L, or five times higher. Although the higher free concentration may result in faster elimination (see Chapter 3), this concentration may be quite toxic initially.

Some drugs compete with serum bilirubin for binding to albumin. Drugs given to a neonate with jaundice can displace bilirubin from albumin. Because of the greater permeability of the neonatal blood-brain barrier, substantial amounts of bilirubin may enter the brain and cause kernicterus. This was in fact observed when sulfonamide antibiotics were given to preterm neonates as prophylaxis against sepsis. Conversely, as the serum bilirubin rises for physiologic reasons or because of a blood group incompatibility, bilirubin can displace a drug from albumin and substantially raise the free drug concentration. This may occur without altering the total drug concentration and would result in greater therapeutic effect or toxicity at normal concentrations. This has been shown to happen with phenytoin.

Drug Metabolism

The metabolism of most drugs occurs in the liver (see Chapter 4). The drug-metabolizing activities of the cytochrome P450-dependent mixed-function oxidases and the conjugating enzymes are substantially lower (50–70% of adult values) in early neonatal life than later. The point in development at which enzymatic activity is maximal depends upon the specific enzyme system in question. Glucuronide formation reaches adult values (per kilogram body weight) between the third and fourth years of life. Because of the neonate's decreased ability to metabolize drugs, many drugs have slow clearance rates and prolonged elimination half-lives. If drug doses and dosing schedules are not altered appropriately, this immaturity predisposes the neonate to adverse effects from drugs that are metabolized by the liver. Table 59–4 demonstrates how neonatal and adult drug elimination half-lives can differ and how the half-lives of phenobarbital and phenytoin decrease as the neonate grows older. The process of maturation must be considered when administering drugs to this age group, especially in the case of drugs administered over long periods.

Another consideration for the neonate is whether or not the mother was receiving drugs (eg, phenobarbital) that can induce early maturation of fetal hepatic enzymes. In this case, the ability of the neonate to metabolize certain drugs will be greater than expected, and one may see less therapeutic effect and lower plasma drug concentrations when the usual neonatal dose is given. During toddlerhood (12–36 months), the metabolic rate of many

TABLE 59–4 Comparison of elimination half-lives of various drugs in neonates and adults.

Drug	Neonatal Age	Neonates $t_{1/2}$ (hours)	Adults $t_{1/2}$ (hours)
Acetaminophen		2.2–5	0.9–2.2
Diazepam		25–100	40–50
Digoxin		60–70	30–60
Phenobarbital	0–5 days	200	64–140
	5–15 days	100	
	1–30 months	50	
Phenytoin	0–2 days	80	12–18
	3–14 days	18	
	14–50 days	6	
Salicylate		4.5–11	10–15
Theophylline	Neonate	13–26	5–10
	Child	3–4	

drugs exceeds adult values, often necessitating larger doses per kilogram than later in life.

Drug Excretion

The glomerular filtration rate is much lower in newborns than in older infants, children, or adults, and this limitation persists during the first few days of life. Calculated on the basis of body surface area, glomerular filtration in the neonate is only 30–40% of the adult value. The glomerular filtration rate is even lower in neonates born before 34 weeks of gestation. Function improves substantially during the first week of life. At the end of the first week, the glomerular filtration rate and renal plasma flow have increased 50% from the first day. By the end of the third week, glomerular filtration is 50–60% of the adult value; by 6–12 months, it reaches adult values (per unit surface area). Therefore, drugs that depend on renal function for elimination are cleared from the body very slowly in the first weeks of life. Subsequently, during toddlerhood, it exceeds adult values, often necessitating larger doses per kilogram than in adults, as described previously for drug-metabolic rate.

Penicillins, for example, are cleared by preterm infants at 17% of the adult rate based on comparable surface area and 34% of the adult rate when adjusted for body weight. The dosage of ampicillin for a neonate less than 7 days old is 50–100 mg/kg/d in two doses at 12-hour intervals. The dosage for a neonate over 7 days old is 100–200 mg/kg/d in three doses at 8-hour intervals. A decreased rate of renal elimination in the neonate has also been observed with aminoglycoside antibiotics (kanamycin, gentamicin, neomycin, and streptomycin). The dosage of gentamicin for a neonate less than 7 days old is 5 mg/kg/d in two doses at 12-hour intervals. The dosage for a neonate over 7 days old is 7.5 mg/kg/d in three doses at 8-hour intervals. Total body clearance of digoxin is directly dependent upon adequate renal function, and accumulation of digoxin can occur when glomerular filtration is decreased. Since renal function in a sick infant may not improve at the predicted rate during the first weeks and months of life, appropriate adjustments in dosage and dosing schedules may be very difficult. In this situation, adjustments are best made on the basis of plasma drug concentrations determined at intervals throughout the course of therapy.

Although great focus is naturally concentrated on the neonate, it is important to remember that toddlers may have *shorter* elimination half-lives of drugs than older children and adults, due probably to *increased* renal elimination and metabolism. For example, the dose per kilogram of digoxin is much higher in toddlers than in adults. The mechanisms for these developmental changes are still poorly understood.

Special Pharmacodynamic Features in the Neonate

The appropriate use of drugs has made possible the survival of neonates with severe abnormalities who would otherwise die within days or weeks after birth. For example, administration of indomethacin (see Chapter 35) causes the rapid closure of a patent ductus arteriosus, which would otherwise require surgical closure in an infant with a normal heart. Infusion of prostaglandin E_1, on the other hand, causes the ductus to remain open, which can be lifesaving in an infant with transposition of the great vessels or tetralogy of Fallot (see Chapter 18). An unexpected effect of such infusion has been described. The drug caused antral hyperplasia with gastric outlet obstruction as a clinical manifestation in 6 of 74 infants who received it. This phenomenon appears to be dose-dependent. Neonates are also more sensitive to the central depressant effects of opioids than are older children and adults, necessitating extra caution when they are exposed to some narcotics (eg, codeine) through breast milk.

PEDIATRIC DOSAGE FORMS & COMPLIANCE

The form in which a drug is manufactured and the way in which the parent dispenses the drug to the child determine the actual dose administered. Many drugs prepared for children are in the form of elixirs or suspensions. **Elixirs** are alcoholic solutions in which the drug molecules are dissolved and evenly distributed. No shaking is required, and unless some of the vehicle has evaporated, the first dose from the bottle and the last dose should contain equivalent amounts of drug. **Suspensions** contain undissolved particles of drug that must be distributed throughout the vehicle by shaking. If shaking is not thorough each time a dose is given, the first doses from the bottle may contain less drug than the last doses, with the result that less than the expected plasma concentration or effect of the drug may be achieved early in the course of therapy. Conversely, toxicity may occur late in the course of therapy, when it is not expected. This uneven distribution is a potential cause of inefficacy or toxicity in children taking phenytoin suspensions. It is thus essential that the prescriber know the form in which the drug will be dispensed and provide proper instructions to the pharmacist and patient or parent.

Compliance may be more difficult to achieve in pediatric practice than otherwise, since it involves not only the parent's conscientious effort to follow directions but also such practical matters as measuring errors, spilling, and spitting out. For example, the measured volume of "teaspoons" ranges from 2.5 to 7.8 mL. The parents should obtain a calibrated medicine spoon or syringe from the pharmacy. These devices improve the accuracy of dose measurements and simplify administration of drugs to children.

When evaluating compliance, it is often helpful to ask if an attempt has been made to give a further dose after the child has spilled half of what was offered. The parents may not always be able to say with confidence how much of a dose the child actually received. The parents must be told whether or not to wake the infant for its every-6-hour dose day or night. These matters should be discussed and made clear, and no assumptions should be made about what the parents may or may not do. Noncompliance frequently occurs when antibiotics are prescribed to treat otitis media or urinary tract infections and the child feels well after 4 or 5 days of therapy. The parents may not feel there is any reason to continue giving the medicine even though it was prescribed for 10 or 14 days. This common situation should be anticipated so the parents can be told why it is important to continue giving the medicine for the prescribed period even if the child seems to be "cured."

Practical and convenient dosage forms and dosing schedules should be chosen to the extent possible. The easier it is to administer and take the medicine and the easier the dosing schedule is to follow, the more likely it is that compliance will be achieved.

Consistent with their ability to comprehend and cooperate, children should also be given some responsibility for their own health care and for taking medications. This should be discussed in appropriate terms both with the child and with the parents. Possible adverse effects and drug interactions with over-the-counter medicines or foods should also be discussed. Whenever a drug does not achieve its therapeutic effect, the possibility of noncompliance should be considered. There is ample evidence that in such cases parents' or children's reports may be grossly inaccurate. Random pill counts and measurement of serum concentrations may help disclose noncompliance. The use of computerized pill containers, which record each lid opening, has been shown to be very effective in measuring compliance.

Because many pediatric doses are calculated—eg, using body weight—rather than simply read from a list, major dosing errors may result from incorrect calculations. Typically, tenfold errors due to incorrect placement of the decimal point have been described. In the case of digoxin, for example, an intended dose of 0.1 mL containing 5 mcg of drug, when replaced by 1.0 mL—which is still a small volume—can result in fatal overdosage. A good rule for avoiding such "decimal point" errors is to use a leading "0" plus decimal point when dealing with doses less than "1" and to avoid using a zero after a decimal point (see Chapter 65).

DRUG USE DURING LACTATION

Despite the fact that most drugs are excreted into breast milk in amounts too small to adversely affect neonatal health, thousands of women taking medications do not breast-feed because of misperception of risk. Unfortunately, physicians contribute heavily to this bias. It is important to remember that formula feeding is associated with higher morbidity and mortality in all socioeconomic groups.

Most drugs administered to lactating women are detectable in breast milk. Fortunately, the concentration of drugs achieved in breast milk is usually low (Table 59–5). Therefore, the total amount the infant would receive in a day is substantially less than what would be considered a "therapeutic dose." If the nursing mother must take medications and the drug is a relatively safe one, she should optimally take it 30–60 minutes after nursing and 3–4 hours before the next feeding. This allows time for many drugs to be cleared from the mother's blood, and the concentrations in breast milk will be relatively low. Drugs for which no data are available on safety during lactation should be avoided or breast-feeding discontinued while they are being given.

Most antibiotics taken by nursing mothers can be detected in breast milk. Tetracycline concentrations in breast milk are approximately 70% of maternal serum concentrations and present a risk of permanent tooth staining in the infant. Isoniazid rapidly reaches equilibrium between breast milk and maternal blood. The concentrations achieved in breast milk are high enough so that signs of pyridoxine deficiency may occur in the infant if the mother is not given pyridoxine supplements.

Most sedatives and hypnotics achieve concentrations in breast milk sufficient to produce a pharmacologic effect in some infants. Barbiturates taken in hypnotic doses by the mother can produce lethargy, sedation, and poor suck reflexes in the infant. Chloral hydrate can produce sedation if the infant is fed at peak milk concentrations. Diazepam can have a sedative effect on the nursing infant, but, most importantly, its long half-life can result in significant drug accumulation.

Opioids such as heroin, methadone, and morphine enter breast milk in quantities potentially sufficient to prolong the state of neonatal narcotic dependence if the drug was taken chronically by the mother during pregnancy. If conditions are well controlled and there is a good relationship between the mother and the physician, an infant could be breast-fed while the mother is taking methadone. She should not, however, stop taking the drug abruptly; the infant can be tapered off the methadone as the mother's dose is tapered. The infant should be watched for signs of narcotic withdrawal. Although codeine has been believed to be safe, a recent case of neonatal death from opioid toxicity revealed that the mother was an ultra rapid metabolizer of cytochrome 2D6 substrates, producing substantially higher amounts of morphine. Hence, polymorphism in maternal drug metabolism may affect neonatal exposure and safety. A subsequent case control study has shown that this situation is not rare. The FDA has published a warning to lactating mothers to exert extra caution while using painkillers containing codeine.

Minimal use of alcohol by the mother has not been reported to harm nursing infants. Excessive amounts of alcohol, however, can produce alcohol effects in the infant. Nicotine concentrations in the breast milk of smoking mothers are low and do not produce effects in the infant. Very small amounts of caffeine are excreted in the breast milk of coffee-drinking mothers.

Lithium enters breast milk in concentrations equal to those in maternal serum. Clearance of this drug is almost completely dependent upon renal elimination, and women who are receiving lithium may expose the infant to relatively large amounts of the drug.

Radioactive substances such as iodinated ^{125}I albumin and other forms of radioiodine can cause thyroid suppression in infants and may increase the risk of subsequent thyroid cancer as much as tenfold. Breast-feeding is contraindicated after large doses and should be withheld for days to weeks after small doses. Similarly, breast-feeding should be avoided in mothers receiving cancer chemotherapy or being treated with cytotoxic or immunomodulating agents for collagen diseases such as lupus erythematosus or after organ transplantation.

PEDIATRIC DRUG DOSAGE

Because of differences in pharmacokinetics in infants and children, simple proportionate reduction in the adult dose may not be adequate to determine a safe and effective pediatric dose. The most reliable pediatric dose information is usually that provided by the manufacturer in the package insert. However, such information is not available for the majority of products, even when studies have been published in the medical literature, reflecting the reluctance of manufacturers to label their products for children. Recently, the FDA has moved toward more explicit expectations that manufacturers test their new products in infants and children. Still, most drugs in the common formularies, eg, *Physicians' Desk Reference*, are not specifically approved for children, in part because manufacturers often lack the economic incentive to evaluate drugs for use in the pediatric market.

Most drugs approved for use in children have recommended pediatric doses, generally stated as milligrams per kilogram or per pound. In the absence of explicit pediatric dose recommendations, an approximation can be made by any of several methods based on age, weight, or surface area. These rules are not precise and should not be used if the manufacturer provides a pediatric dose. When pediatric doses are calculated (either from one of the methods set forth below or from a manufacturer's dose), the pediatric dose should never exceed the adult dose.

With the current epidemic of child obesity, a fresh and careful look at pediatric drug dosing will be needed. Studies in adults indicate that dosing based on per kilogram of body weight may constitute overdosing, because most drugs are distributed based on lean body weight, rather than total (obese) weight.

Surface Area, Age, & Weight

Calculations of dosage based on age or weight (see below) are conservative and tend to underestimate the required dose. Doses based on surface area (Table 59–6) are more likely to be adequate.

Age (Young's rule):

$$Dose = \text{Adult dose} \times \frac{\text{Age (years)}}{\text{Age} + 12}$$

TABLE 59–5 Drugs often used during lactation and possible effects on the nursing infant.

Drug	Effect on Infant	Comments
Ampicillin	Minimal	No significant adverse effects; possible occurrence of diarrhea or allergic sensitization.
Aspirin	Minimal	Occasional doses probably safe; high doses may produce significant concentration in breast milk.
Caffeine	Minimal	Caffeine intake in moderation is safe; concentration in breast milk is low.
Chloral hydrate	Significant	May cause drowsiness if infant is fed at peak concentration in milk.
Chloramphenicol	Significant	Concentrations too low to cause gray baby syndrome; possibility of bone marrow suppression does exist; recommend not taking chloramphenicol while breast-feeding.
Chlorothiazide	Minimal	No adverse effects reported.
Chlorpromazine	Minimal	Appears insignificant.
Codeine	Variable, based on genetic polymorphism	Safe in most cases. Neonatal toxicity described when the mother is an ultra rapid 2D6 metabolizer, producing substantially more morphine from codeine.
Diazepam	Significant	Will cause sedation in breast-fed infants; accumulation can occur in newborns.
Dicumarol	Minimal	No adverse side effects reported; may wish to follow infant's prothrombin time.
Digoxin	Minimal	Insignificant quantities enter breast milk.
Ethanol	Moderate	Moderate ingestion by mother unlikely to produce effects in infant; large amounts consumed by mother can produce alcohol effects in infant.
Heroin	Significant	Enters breast milk and can prolong neonatal narcotic dependence.
Iodine (radioactive)	Significant	Enters milk in quantities sufficient to cause thyroid suppression in infant.
Isoniazid (INH)	Minimal	Milk concentrations equal maternal plasma concentrations. Possibility of pyridoxine deficiency developing in the infant.
Kanamycin	Minimal	No adverse effects reported.
Lithium	Variable	In some cases, large amounts in milk, but not in others.
Methadone	Significant	(See heroin.) Under close physician supervision, breast-feeding can be continued. Signs of opioid withdrawal in the infant may occur if mother stops taking methadone or stops breast-feeding abruptly.
Oral contraceptives	Minimal	May suppress lactation in high doses.
Penicillin	Minimal	Very low concentrations in breast milk.
Phenobarbital	Moderate	Hypnotic doses can cause sedation in the infant.
Phenytoin	Moderate	Amounts entering breast milk are not sufficient to cause adverse effects in infant.
Prednisone	Moderate	Low maternal doses (5 mg/d) probably safe. Doses 2 or more times physiologic amounts (> 15 mg/d) should probably be avoided.
Propranolol	Minimal	Very small amounts enter breast milk.
Propylthiouracil	Variable	Rarely may suppress thyroid function in infant.
Spironolactone	Minimal	Very small amounts enter breast milk.
Tetracycline	Moderate	Possibility of permanent staining of developing teeth in the infant. Should be avoided during lactation.
Theophylline	Moderate	Can enter breast milk in moderate quantities but not likely to produce significant effects.
Thyroxine	Minimal	No adverse effects in therapeutic doses.
Tolbutamide	Minimal	Low concentrations in breast milk.
Warfarin	Minimal	Very small quantities found in breast milk.

TABLE 59–6 Determination of drug dosage from surface area.[1]

Weight				
(kg)	(lb)	Approximate Age	Surface Area (m²)	Percent of Adult Dose
3	6.6	Newborn	0.2	12
6	13.2	3 months	0.3	18
10	22	1 year	0.45	28
20	44	5.5 years	0.8	48
30	66	9 years	1	60
40	88	12 years	1.3	78
50	110	14 years	1.5	90
60	132	Adult	1.7	102
70	154	Adult	1.76	103

[1]For example, if adult dose is 1 mg/kg, dose for 3-month-old infant would be 0.18 mg/kg or 1.1 mg total.

Reproduced, with permission, from Silver HK, Kempe CH, Bruyn HB: *Handbook of Pediatrics,* 14th ed. Originally published by Lange Medical Publications. Copyright © 1983 by the McGraw-Hill Companies, Inc.

Weight (somewhat more precise is Clark's rule):

$$Dose = Adult\ dose \times \frac{Weight\ (kg)}{70}$$

or

$$Dose = Adult\ dose \times \frac{Weight\ (lb)}{150}$$

In spite of these approximations, only by conducting studies in children can safe and effective doses for a given age group and condition be determined.

REFERENCES

American Heart Association (AHA) guidelines for cardiopulmonary resuscitation (CPR) and emergency cardiovascular care (ECC) of pediatric and neonatal patients: Pediatric basic life support. Circulation 2005;112(24 Suppl):IV1.

Benitz WE, Tatro DS: *The Pediatric Drug Handbook,* 3rd ed. Year Book, 1995.

Bennett PN: *Drugs and Human Lactation,* 2nd ed. Elsevier, 1996.

Berlin CM Jr: Advances in pediatric pharmacology and toxicology. Adv Pediatr 1997;44:545.

Besunder JB, Reed MD, Blumer JL: Principles of drug biodisposition in the neonate: A critical evaluation of the pharmacokinetic-pharmacodynamic interface. (Two parts.) Clin Pharmacokinet 1988;14:189, 261.

Briggs GG, Freeman RK, Yaffe SJ: Drugs in Pregnancy and Lactation. *A Reference Guide to Fetal and Neonatal Risk,* 6th ed. Williams & Wilkins, 2002.

Gavin PJ, Yogev R: The role of protease inhibitor therapy in children with HIV infection. Paediatr Drugs 2002;4:581.

Hansten PD, Horn JR: *Drug Interactions, Analysis and Management.* Facts & Comparisons. [Quarterly.]

Hendrick V et al: Birth outcomes after prenatal exposure to antidepressant medication. Am J Obstet Gynecol 2003;188:812.

Iqbal MM, Sohhan T, Mahmud SZ: The effects of lithium, valproic acid, and carbamazepine during pregnancy and lactation. J Toxicol Clin Toxicol 2001;39:381.

Ito S: Drug therapy for breast feeding women. N Engl J Med 2000;343:118.

Ito S, Koren G: Fetal drug therapy. Perinat Clin North Am 1994;21:1.

Kearns GL et al: Developmental pharmacology—drug disposition, action, and therapy in infants and children. N Engl J Med 2003;349:1157.

Koren G: *Medication Safety during Pregnancy and Breastfeeding; A Clinician's Guide,* 4th ed. McGraw-Hill, 2006.

Koren G, Klinger G, Ohlsson A: Fetal pharmacotherapy. Drugs 2002;62:757.

Koren G, Pastuszak A: Prevention of unnecessary pregnancy terminations by counseling women on drug, chemical, and radiation exposure during the first trimester. Teratology 1990;41:657.

Koren G, Pastuszak A, Ito E: Drugs in pregnancy. N Engl J Med 1998;338:1128.

Loebstein R, Koren G: Clinical pharmacology and therapeutic drug monitoring in neonates and children. Pediatr Rev 1998;19:423.

Madadi P et al: Pharmacogenetics of neonatal opioid toxicity following maternal use of codeine during breastfeeding: A case control study. Clin Pharmacol Ther 2009;85:31.

Neubert D: Reproductive toxicology: The science today. Teratog Carcinog Mutagen 2002;22:159.

Nottarianni LJ: Plasma protein binding of drugs in pregnancy and in neonates. Clin Pharmacokinet 1990;18:20.

Paap CM, Nahata MC: Clinical pharmacokinetics of antibacterial drugs in neonates. Clin Pharmacokinet 1990;19:280.

Peled N et al: Gastric-outlet obstruction induced by prostaglandin therapy in neonates. N Engl J Med 1992;327:505.

Rousseaux CG, Blakely PM: Fetus. In: Haschek WM, Rousseaux CG (editors). *Handbook of Toxicologic Pathology.* Academic Press, 1991.

Van Lingen RA et al: The effects of analgesia in the vulnerable infant during the perinatal period. Clin Perinatol 2002;29:511.

60

Special Aspects of Geriatric Pharmacology

Bertram G. Katzung, MD, PhD

CASE STUDY

A 77-year-old man comes to your office at his wife's insistence. He has had documented moderate hypertension for 10 years but does not like to take his medications. He says he has no real complaints, but his wife remarks that he has become much more forgetful lately and has almost stopped reading the newspaper and watching television. A Mini-Mental Examination reveals that he is oriented as to name and place but is unable to give the month or year. He cannot remember the names of his three adult children nor three random words (tree, flag, chair) for more than 2 minutes. No cataracts are visible, but he is unable to read standard newsprint without a powerful magnifier. Why doesn't he take his antihypertensive medications? What therapeutic measures are available for the treatment of Alzheimer's disease? How might macular degeneration be treated?

Society has traditionally classified everyone over 65 as "elderly," but most authorities consider the field of geriatrics to apply to persons over 75—even though this too is an arbitrary definition. Furthermore, chronologic age is only one determinant of the changes pertinent to drug therapy that occur in older people. In addition to the chronic diseases of adulthood, the elderly have an increased incidence of many conditions, including Alzheimer's disease, Parkinson's disease, and vascular dementia; stroke; visual impairment, especially cataracts and macular degeneration; atherosclerosis, coronary heart disease, and heart failure; diabetes; arthritis, osteoporosis, and fractures; cancer; and incontinence. As a result, the need for drug treatment is great in this age group.

Important changes in responses to some drugs occur with increasing age in many individuals. For other drugs, age-related changes are minimal, especially in the "healthy old." Drug usage patterns also change as a result of the increasing incidence of disease with age and the tendency to prescribe heavily for patients in nursing homes. General changes in the lives of older people have significant effects on the way drugs are used. Among these changes are the increased incidence with advancing age of several simultaneous diseases, nutritional problems, reduced financial resources, and—in some patients—decreased dosing adherence (also called compliance) for a variety of reasons. The health practitioner should be aware of the changes in pharmacologic responses that may occur in older people and should know how to deal with these changes.

PHARMACOLOGIC CHANGES ASSOCIATED WITH AGING

In the general population, measurements of functional capacity of most of the major organ systems show a decline beginning in young adulthood and continuing throughout life. As shown in Figure 60–1, there is no "middle-age plateau" but rather a linear decrease beginning no later than age 45. However, these data reflect the mean and do not apply to every person above a certain age; approximately one third of healthy subjects have no age-related decrease in, for example, creatinine clearance up to the age of 75. Thus, the elderly do not lose specific functions at an accelerated rate compared with young and middle-aged adults but rather accumulate more deficiencies with the passage of time. Some of these changes result in altered pharmacokinetics. For the pharmacologist and the clinician, the most important of these is the decrease in renal function. Other changes and concurrent diseases may alter the pharmacodynamic characteristics of particular drugs in certain patients.

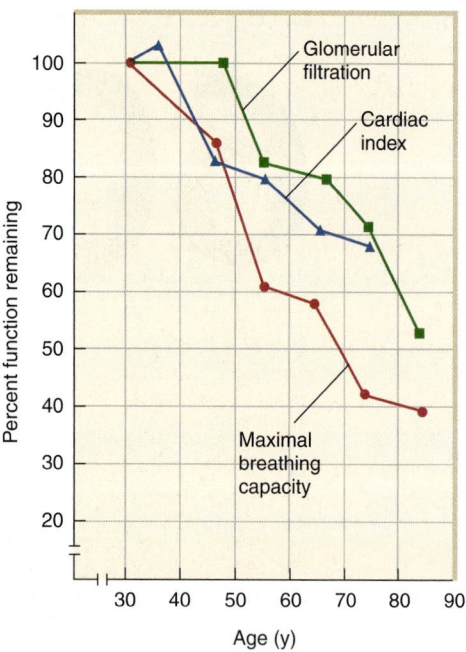

FIGURE 60–1 Effect of age on some physiologic functions. (Modified and reproduced, with permission, from Kohn RR: *Principles of Mammalian Aging.* Prentice-Hall, 1978.)

Pharmacokinetic Changes

A. Absorption

There is little evidence of any major alteration in drug absorption with age. However, conditions associated with age may alter the rate at which some drugs are absorbed. Such conditions include altered nutritional habits, greater consumption of nonprescription drugs (eg, antacids and laxatives), and changes in gastric emptying, which is often slower in older persons, especially in older diabetics.

B. Distribution

Compared with young adults, the elderly have reduced lean body mass, reduced body water, and increased fat as a percentage of body mass. Some of these changes are shown in Table 60–1. There is usually a decrease in serum albumin, which binds many drugs, especially weak acids. There may be a concurrent *increase* in serum orosomucoid (α-acid glycoprotein), a protein that binds many basic drugs. Thus, the ratio of bound to free drug may be significantly altered. As explained in Chapter 3, these changes may alter the appropriate loading dose of a drug. However since both the clearance and the effects of drugs are related to the free concentration, the steady-state effects of a maintenance dosage regimen should not be altered by these factors alone. For example, the loading dose of digoxin in an elderly patient with heart failure should be reduced (if used at all) because of the decreased apparent volume of distribution. The maintenance dose may have to be reduced because of reduced clearance of the drug.

C. Metabolism

The capacity of the liver to metabolize drugs does not appear to decline consistently with age for all drugs. Animal studies and some

TABLE 60–1 Some changes related to aging that affect pharmacokinetics of drugs.

Variable	Young Adults (20–30 years)	Older Adults (60–80 years)
Body water (% of body weight)	61	53
Lean body mass (% of body weight)	19	12
Body fat (% of body weight)	26–33 (women)	38–45
	18–20 (men)	36–38
Serum albumin (g/dL)	4.7	3.8
Kidney weight (% of young adult)	(100)	80
Hepatic blood flow (% of young adult)	(100)	55–60

clinical studies have suggested that certain drugs are metabolized more slowly; some of these drugs are listed in Table 60–2. The greatest changes are in phase I reactions, ie, those carried out by microsomal P450 systems. There are much smaller changes in the ability of the liver to carry out conjugation (phase II) reactions (see Chapter 4). Some of these changes may be caused by decreased liver blood flow (Table 60–1), an important variable in the clearance of drugs that have a high hepatic extraction ratio. In addition, there is

TABLE 60–2 Effects of age on hepatic clearance of some drugs.

Age-Related Decrease in Hepatic Clearance Found	No Age-Related Difference Found
Alprazolam	Ethanol
Barbiturates	Isoniazid
Carbenoxolone	Lidocaine
Chlordiazepoxide	Lorazepam
Chlormethiazole	Nitrazepam
Clobazam	Oxazepam
Desmethyldiazepam	Prazosin
Diazepam	Salicylate
Flurazepam	Warfarin
Imipramine	
Meperidine	
Nortriptyline	
Phenylbutazone	
Propranolol	
Quinidine, quinine	
Theophylline	
Tolbutamide	

a decline with age of the liver's ability to recover from injury, eg, that caused by alcohol or viral hepatitis. Therefore, a history of recent liver disease in an older person should lead to caution in dosing with drugs that are cleared primarily by the liver, even after apparently complete recovery from the hepatic insult. Finally, malnutrition and diseases that affect hepatic function—eg, heart failure—are more common in the elderly. Heart failure may dramatically alter the ability of the liver to metabolize drugs by reducing hepatic blood flow. Similarly, severe nutritional deficiencies, which occur more often in old age, may impair hepatic function.

D. Elimination

Because the kidney is the major organ for clearance of drugs from the body, the age-related decline of renal functional capacity is very important. The decline in creatinine clearance occurs in about two thirds of the population. It is important to note that this decline is not reflected in an equivalent rise in serum creatinine because the production of creatinine is also reduced as muscle mass declines with age; therefore, serum creatinine alone is not an adequate measure of renal function. The practical result of this change is marked prolongation of the half-life of many drugs, and the possibility of accumulation to toxic levels if dosage is not reduced in size or frequency. Dosing recommendations for the elderly often include an allowance for reduced renal clearance. If only the young adult dosage is known for a drug that requires renal clearance, a rough correction can be made by using the **Cockcroft-Gault** formula, which is applicable to patients from ages 40 through 80:

$$\text{Creatinine clearance (mL/min)} = \frac{(140 - \text{Age}) \times (\text{Weight in kg})}{72 \times \text{Serum creatinine in mg/dL}}$$

For women, the result should be multiplied by 0.85 (because of reduced muscle mass). It must be emphasized that this estimate is, at best, a *population* estimate and may not apply to a particular patient. If the patient has normal renal function (up to one third of elderly patients), a dose corrected on the basis of this estimate will be too low—but a low dose is initially desirable if one is uncertain of the renal function in any patient. If a precise measure is needed, a standard 12- or 24-hour creatinine clearance determination should be obtained. As indicated above, nutritional changes alter pharmacokinetic parameters. A patient who is severely dehydrated (not uncommon in patients with stroke or other motor impairment) may have an additional marked reduction in renal drug clearance that is completely reversible by rehydration.

The lungs are important for the excretion of volatile drugs. As a result of reduced respiratory capacity (Figure 60–1) and the increased incidence of active pulmonary disease in the elderly, the use of inhalation anesthesia is less common and parenteral agents more common in this age group. (See Chapter 25.)

Pharmacodynamic Changes

It was long believed that geriatric patients were much more "sensitive" to the action of many drugs, implying a change in the pharmacodynamic interaction of the drugs with their receptors. It is now recognized that many—perhaps most—of these apparent changes result from altered pharmacokinetics or diminished homeostatic responses. Clinical studies have supported the idea that the elderly are more sensitive to *some* sedative-hypnotics and analgesics. In addition, some data from animal studies suggest actual changes with age in the characteristics or numbers of a few receptors. The most extensive studies suggest a decrease in responsiveness to β-adrenoceptor agonists. Other examples are discussed below.

Certain homeostatic control mechanisms appear to be blunted in the elderly. Since homeostatic responses are often important components of the overall response to a drug, these physiologic alterations may change the pattern or intensity of drug response. In the cardiovascular system, the cardiac output increment required by mild or moderate exercise is successfully provided until at least age 75 (in individuals without obvious cardiac disease), but the increase is the result primarily of increased stroke volume in the elderly and not tachycardia, as in young adults. Average blood pressure goes up with age (in most Western countries), but the incidence of symptomatic orthostatic hypotension also increases markedly. It is thus particularly important to check for orthostatic hypotension on every visit. Similarly, the average 2-hour postprandial blood glucose level increases by about 1 mg/dL for each year of age above 50. Temperature regulation is also impaired, and hypothermia is poorly tolerated by the elderly.

Behavioral & Lifestyle Changes

Major changes in the conditions of daily life accompany the aging process and have an impact on health. Some of these (eg, forgetting to take one's pills) are the result of cognitive changes associated with vascular or other pathology. Others relate to economic stresses associated with greatly reduced income and, possibly, increased expenses due to illness. One of the most important changes is the loss of a spouse.

■ MAJOR DRUG GROUPS

CENTRAL NERVOUS SYSTEM DRUGS

Sedative-Hypnotics

The half-lives of many benzodiazepines and barbiturates increase by 50–150% between ages 30 and 70. Much of this change occurs during the decade from 60 to 70. For some of the benzodiazepines, both the parent molecule and its metabolites (produced in the liver) are pharmacologically active (see Chapter 22). The age-related decline in renal function and liver disease, if present, both contribute to the reduction in elimination of these compounds. In addition, an increased volume of distribution has been reported for some of these drugs. Lorazepam and oxazepam may be less affected by these changes than the other benzodiazepines. In addition to these pharmacokinetic factors, it is generally believed that the elderly vary more in their sensitivity to the sedative-hypnotic drugs on a pharmacodynamic basis as well. Among the toxicities of these drugs, ataxia and other signs of motor impairment should be particularly watched for in order to avoid accidents.

Analgesics

The opioid analgesics show variable changes in pharmacokinetics with age. However, the elderly are often markedly more sensitive to the respiratory effects of these agents because of age-related changes in respiratory function. Therefore, this group of drugs should be used with caution until the sensitivity of the particular patient has been evaluated, and the patient should then be dosed appropriately for full effect. Unfortunately, studies show that opioids are consistently *underutilized* in patients who require strong analgesics for chronic painful conditions such as cancer. There is no justification for underutilization of these drugs, especially in the care of the elderly, and good pain management plans are readily available (see Morrison, 2006; Rabow, 2011).

Antipsychotic & Antidepressant Drugs

The traditional antipsychotic agents (phenothiazines and haloperidol) have been very heavily used (and probably misused) in the management of a variety of psychiatric diseases in the elderly. There is no doubt that they are useful in the management of schizophrenia in old age, and also in the treatment of some symptoms associated with delirium, dementia, agitation, combativeness, and a paranoid syndrome that occurs in some geriatric patients (see Chapter 29). However, they are not fully satisfactory in these geriatric conditions, and dosage should not be increased on the assumption that full control is possible. There is no evidence that these drugs have any beneficial effects in Alzheimer's dementia, and on theoretical grounds the antimuscarinic effects of the phenothiazines might be expected to worsen memory impairment and intellectual dysfunction (see below).

Much of the apparent improvement in agitated and combative patients may simply reflect the sedative effects of the drugs. When a sedative antipsychotic is desired, a phenothiazine such as thioridazine is appropriate. If sedation is to be avoided, haloperidol or an atypical antipsychotic is more appropriate. Haloperidol has increased extrapyramidal toxicity, however, and should be avoided in patients with preexisting extrapyramidal disease. The phenothiazines, especially older drugs such as chlorpromazine, often induce orthostatic hypotension because of their α-adrenoceptor-blocking effects. They are even more prone to do so in the elderly. Dosage of these drugs should usually be started at a fraction of that used in young adults.

Lithium is often used in the treatment of mania in the aged. Because it is cleared by the kidneys, dosages must be adjusted appropriately and blood levels monitored. Concurrent use of thiazide diuretics reduces the clearance of lithium and should be accompanied by further reduction in dosage and more frequent measurement of lithium blood levels.

Psychiatric depression is thought to be underdiagnosed and undertreated in the elderly. The suicide rate in the over-65 age group (twice the national average) supports this view. Unfortunately,

the apathy, flat affect, and social withdrawal of major depression may be mistaken for senile dementia. Clinical evidence suggests that the elderly are as responsive to antidepressants (of all types) as younger patients but are more likely to experience toxic effects. This factor along with the reduced clearance of some of these drugs underlines the importance of careful dosing and strict attention to the appearance of toxic effects. If a tricyclic antidepressant is to be used, a drug with reduced antimuscarinic effects should be selected, eg, nortriptyline or desipramine (see Table 30–2). To minimize autonomic effects, a selective serotonin reuptake inhibitor (SSRI) may be chosen.

Drugs Used in Alzheimer's Disease

Alzheimer's disease is characterized by progressive impairment of memory and cognitive functions and may lead to a completely vegetative state, resulting in massive socioeconomic disruption, and early death. Prevalence increases with age and may be as high as 20% in individuals over 85. Both familial and sporadic forms have been identified. Early onset of Alzheimer's disease is associated with several gene defects, including trisomy 21 (chromosome 21), a mutation of the gene for presenilin-1 on chromosome 14, and an abnormal allele, ε4, for the lipid-associated protein, ApoE, on chromosome 19. Unlike the normal form, ApoE ε2, the ε4 form facilitates the formation of amyloid β deposits.

Pathologic changes include increased deposits of amyloid β peptide in the cerebral cortex, which eventually forms extracellular plaques and cerebral vascular lesions, and intraneuronal fibrillary tangles consisting of the tau protein (Figure 60–2). There is a progressive loss of neurons, especially cholinergic neurons, and thinning of the cortex. The loss of cholinergic neurons results in a marked decrease in choline acetyltransferase and other markers of cholinergic activity. Patients with Alzheimer's disease are often exquisitely sensitive to the central nervous system toxicities of drugs with antimuscarinic effects. Some evidence implicates excess excitation by glutamate as a contributor to neuronal death. In addition, abnormalities of mitochondrial function may contribute to neuronal death.

Many methods of treatment of Alzheimer's disease have been explored (Table 60–3). Most attention has been focused on the cholinomimetic drugs because of the evidence of loss of cholinergic neurons. Monoamine oxidase (MAO) type B inhibition with selegiline (L-deprenyl) has been suggested to have some beneficial effects. One drug that inhibits *N*-methyl-D-aspartate (NMDA) glutamate receptors is available (see below), and "ampakines," substances that facilitate synaptic activity at glutamate AMPA receptors, are under intense study. Some evidence suggests that lipid-lowering statins are beneficial. Rosiglitazone, a PPAR-γ (peroxisome proliferator-activated receptor-gamma) agent, has also been reported to have beneficial effects in a preliminary study. Unfortunately, this drug is associated with increased cardiovascular risk and its use has been restricted (see Chapter 41). So-called cerebral vasodilators are ineffective.

Tacrine (tetrahydroaminoacridine, THA), a long-acting cholinesterase inhibitor and muscarinic modulator, was the first drug

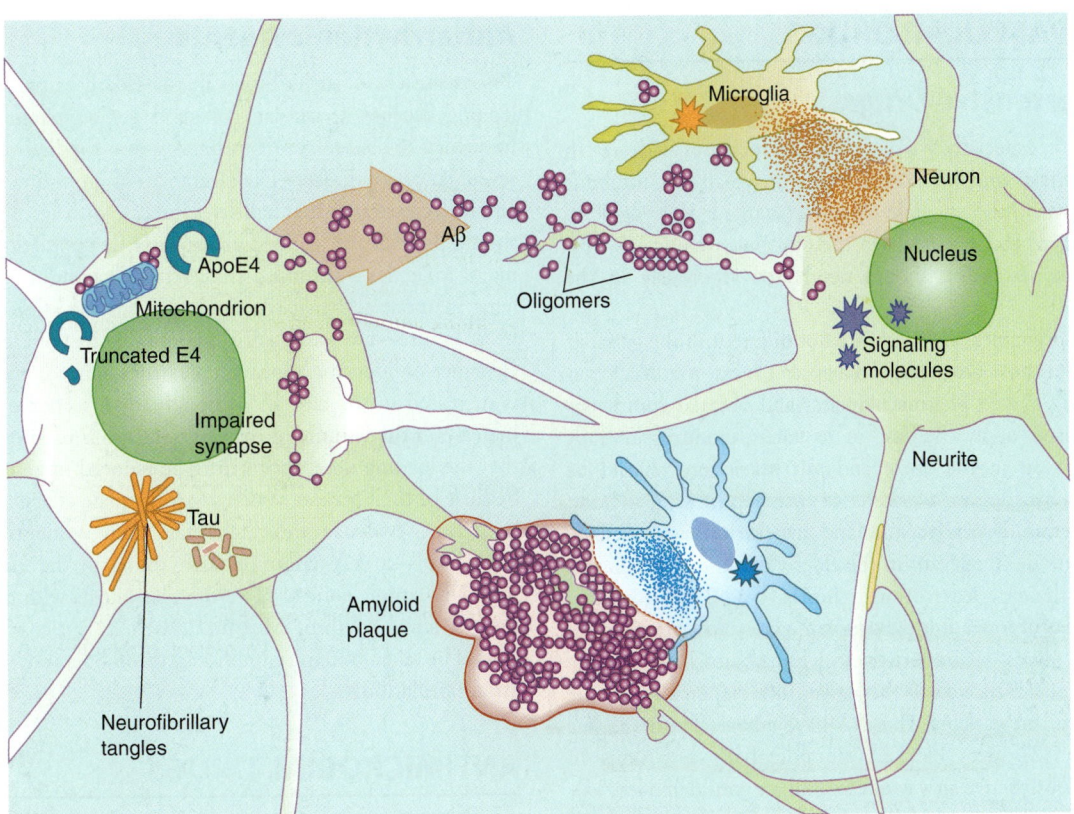

FIGURE 60–2 Some processes involved in Alzheimer's disease. From the left: mitochondrial dysfunction, possibly involving glucose utilization; synthesis of protein tau and aggregation in filamentous tangles; synthesis of amyloid β (Aβ) and secretion into the extracellular space, where it may interfere with synaptic signaling and accumulates in plaques. (Reproduced, with permission, from Robertson ED and Mucke L: 100 years and counting: Prospects for defeating Alzheimer's disease. Science 2006;314:781.)

shown to have any benefit in Alzheimer's disease. Because of its hepatic toxicity, tacrine has been almost completely replaced in clinical use by newer cholinesterase inhibitors: **donepezil, rivastigmine,** and **galantamine.** These agents are orally active, have adequate penetration into the central nervous system, and are much less toxic than tacrine. Although evidence for the benefit of cholinesterase inhibitors (and memantine; see below) is statistically significant, the clinical benefit from these drugs is modest and temporary.

The cholinesterase inhibitors cause significant adverse effects, including nausea and vomiting, and other peripheral cholinomimetic effects. These drugs should be used with caution in patients receiving other drugs that inhibit cytochrome P450 enzymes (eg, ketoconazole, quinidine; see Chapter 4). Preparations available are listed in Chapter 7.

Excitotoxic activation of glutamate transmission via NMDA receptors has been postulated to contribute to the pathophysiology of Alzheimer's disease. **Memantine** binds to NMDA receptor channels in a use-dependent manner and produces a noncompetitive blockade. This drug appears to be better tolerated and less toxic than the cholinesterase inhibitors. Memantine is available as Namenda in 5 and 10 mg oral tablets.

TABLE 60–3 Some potential strategies for the prevention or treatment of Alzheimer's disease.

Therapy	Comment
Cholinesterase inhibitors	Increase cholinergic activity; four drugs approved
N-methyl-D-aspartate glutamate antagonists	Inhibit glutamate excitotoxicity; 1 drug approved
Modifiers of glucose utilization	PPAR-γ agonists
Antilipid drugs	Statins (off-label use)
NSAIDs	Disappointing results with cyclooxygenase (COX)-2 inhibitors but interest continues
Anti-amyloid vaccines	In clinical trials
Anti-amyloid antibodies	Bapineuzumab in clinical trials
Inhibitors of amyloid β synthesis	γ-Secretase modulator studies in progress
Antioxidants	Disappointing results
Nerve growth factor	One very small trial

PPAR-γ, peroxisome proliferator-activated receptor-gamma.

CARDIOVASCULAR DRUGS

Antihypertensive Drugs

Blood pressure, especially systolic pressure, increases with age in Western countries and in most cultures in which salt intake is high. In women, the increase is more marked after age 50. Although treated conservatively in the past, most clinicians now believe that hypertension should be treated vigorously in the elderly.

The basic principles of therapy are not different in the geriatric age group from those described in Chapter 11, but the usual cautions regarding altered pharmacokinetics and blunted compensatory mechanisms apply. Because of its safety, nondrug therapy (weight reduction in the obese and salt restriction) should be encouraged. Thiazides are a reasonable first step in drug therapy. The hypokalemia, hyperglycemia, and hyperuricemia caused by these agents are more relevant in the elderly because of the higher incidence in these patients of arrhythmias, type 2 diabetes, and gout. Thus, use of low antihypertensive doses—rather than maximum diuretic doses—is important. Calcium channel blockers are effective and safe if titrated to the appropriate response. They are especially useful in patients who also have atherosclerotic angina (see Chapter 12). Beta blockers are potentially hazardous in patients with obstructive airway disease and are considered less useful than calcium channel blockers in older patients unless heart failure is present. Angiotensin-converting enzyme inhibitors are also considered less useful in the elderly unless heart failure or diabetes is present. The most powerful drugs, such as minoxidil, are rarely needed. Every patient receiving antihypertensive drugs should be checked regularly for orthostatic hypotension because of the danger of cerebral ischemia and falls.

Positive Inotropic Agents

Heart failure is a common and particularly lethal disease in the elderly. Fear of this condition may be one reason why physicians overuse cardiac glycosides in this age group. The toxic effects of digoxin are particularly dangerous in the geriatric population, since the elderly are more susceptible to arrhythmias. The clearance of digoxin is usually decreased in the older age group, and although the volume of distribution is often decreased as well, the half-life of this drug may be increased by 50% or more. Because the drug is cleared mostly by the kidneys, renal function must be considered in designing a dosage regimen. There is no evidence that there is any increase in pharmacodynamic sensitivity to the therapeutic effects of the cardiac glycosides; in fact, animal studies suggest a possible decrease in therapeutic sensitivity. On the other hand, there is probably an increase in sensitivity to the toxic arrhythmogenic actions. Hypokalemia, hypomagnesemia, hypoxemia (from pulmonary disease), and coronary atherosclerosis all contribute to the high incidence of digitalis-induced arrhythmias in geriatric patients. The less common toxicities of digitalis such as delirium, visual changes, and endocrine abnormalities (see Chapter 13) also occur more often in older than in younger patients.

Antiarrhythmic Agents

The treatment of arrhythmias in the elderly is particularly challenging because of the lack of good hemodynamic reserve, the frequency of electrolyte disturbances, and the high prevalence of severe coronary disease. The clearances of quinidine and procainamide decrease and their half-lives increase with age. Disopyramide should probably be avoided in the geriatric population because its major toxicities—antimuscarinic action, leading to voiding problems in men; and negative inotropic cardiac effects, leading to heart failure—are particularly undesirable in these patients. The clearance of lidocaine appears to be little changed, but the half-life is increased in the elderly. Although this observation implies an increase in the volume of distribution, it has been recommended that the loading dose of this drug be reduced in geriatric patients because of their greater sensitivity to its toxic effects.

Recent evidence indicates that many patients with atrial fibrillation—a very common arrhythmia in the elderly—do as well with simple control of ventricular rate as with conversion to normal sinus rhythm. Measures (such as anticoagulant drugs) should be taken to reduce the risk of thromboembolism in chronic atrial fibrillation.

ANTIMICROBIAL DRUGS

Several age-related changes contribute to the high incidence of infections in geriatric patients. There appears to be a reduction in host defenses in the elderly, manifested in the increase in both serious infections and cancer. This may reflect an alteration in T-lymphocyte function. In the lungs, a major age and tobacco-dependent decrease in mucociliary clearance significantly increases susceptibility to infection. In the urinary tract, the incidence of serious infection is greatly increased by urinary retention and catheterization in men.

Since 1940, the antimicrobial drugs have contributed more to the prolongation of life than any other drug group because they can compensate to some extent for this deterioration in natural defenses. The basic principles of therapy of the elderly with these agents are no different from those applicable in younger patients and have been presented in Chapter 51. The major pharmacokinetic changes relate to decreased renal function; because most of the β-lactam, aminoglycoside, and fluoroquinolone antibiotics are excreted by this route, important changes in half-life may be expected. This is particularly important in the case of the aminoglycosides, because they cause concentration- and time-dependent toxicity in the kidney and in other organs. The half-lives of gentamicin, kanamycin, and netilmicin are more than doubled. The increase may not be so marked for tobramycin.

ANTI-INFLAMMATORY DRUGS

Osteoarthritis is a very common disease of the elderly. Rheumatoid arthritis is less exclusively a geriatric problem, but the same drug therapy is usually applicable. The basic principles laid down in

Chapter 36 and the properties of the anti-inflammatory drugs described there apply fully here.

The nonsteroidal anti-inflammatory agents (NSAIDs) must be used with special care in geriatric patients because they cause toxicities to which the elderly are very susceptible. In the case of aspirin, the most important of these is gastrointestinal irritation and bleeding. In the case of the newer NSAIDs, the most important is renal damage, which may be irreversible. Because they are cleared primarily by the kidneys, these drugs accumulate more rapidly in the geriatric patient and especially in the patient whose renal function is already compromised beyond the average range for his or her age. A vicious circle is easily set up in which cumulation of the NSAID causes more renal damage, which causes more cumulation. There is no evidence that the cyclooxygenase (COX)-2 selective NSAIDs are safer with regard to renal function. Elderly patients receiving high doses of any NSAID should be carefully monitored for changes in renal function.

Corticosteroids are extremely useful in elderly patients who cannot tolerate full doses of NSAIDs. However, they consistently cause a dose- and duration-related increase in osteoporosis, an especially hazardous toxic effect in the elderly. It is not certain whether this drug-induced effect can be reduced by increased calcium and vitamin D intake, but it would be prudent to consider these agents (and bisphosphonates if osteoporosis is already present) and to encourage frequent exercise in any patient taking corticosteroids.

OPHTHALMIC DRUGS

Drugs Used in Glaucoma

Glaucoma is more common in the elderly, but its treatment does not differ from that of glaucoma of earlier onset. Management of glaucoma is discussed in Chapter 10.

Macular Degeneration

Age-related macular degeneration (AMD) is the most common cause of blindness in the elderly in the developed world. Two forms of advanced AMD are recognized: the neovascular "wet" form, which is associated with intrusion of new blood vessels in the subretinal space, and a more common "dry" form, which is not associated with abnormal vascularization. Although the cause of AMD is not known, smoking is a documented risk factor, and oxidative stress has long been thought to play a role. On this premise, antioxidants have been used to prevent or delay the onset of AMD. Proprietary oral formulations of vitamins C and E, β-carotene, zinc oxide, and cupric oxide are available. Evidence for the efficacy of these antioxidants is modest or absent. Oral drugs in clinical trials include the carotenoids lutein and zeaxanthin, and n-3 long-chain polyunsaturated fatty acids.

In advanced AMD, treatment has been moderately successful but only for the neovascular form. Neovascular AMD can now be treated with laser phototherapy or with antibodies against vascular endothelial growth factor (VEGF). Two antibodies are available: bevacizumab (Avastin, used off-label) and ranibizumab (Lucentis), as well as the oligopeptide pegaptanib (Macugen). The latter two are approved for neovascular AMD. These agents are injected into the vitreous for local effect. Ranibizumab is extremely expensive. Fusion proteins and RNA agents that bind VEGF are under study.

■ ADVERSE DRUG REACTIONS IN THE ELDERLY

The relation between the number of drugs taken and the incidence of adverse drug reactions has been well documented. In long-term care facilities, in which a high percentage of the population is elderly, the average number of prescriptions per patient varies between 6 and 8. Studies have shown that the percentage of patients with adverse reactions increases from about 10% when a single drug is being taken to nearly 100% when 10 drugs are taken. Thus, it may be expected that about half of patients in long-term care facilities will have recognized or unrecognized reactions at some time. Patients living at home may see several different practitioners for different conditions and accumulate multiple prescriptions for drugs with overlapping actions. It is useful to conduct a "brown bag" analysis in such patients. The brown bag analysis consists of asking the patient to bring to the practitioner a bag containing *all* the medications, supplements, vitamins, etc, that he or she is currently taking. Some prescriptions will be found to be duplicates, others unnecessary. The total number of medications taken can often be reduced by 30–50%.

The overall incidence of drug reactions in geriatric patients is estimated to be at least twice that in the younger population. Reasons for this high incidence undoubtedly include errors in prescribing on the part of the practitioner and errors in drug usage by the patient. Practitioner errors sometimes occur because the physician does not appreciate the importance of changes in pharmacokinetics with age and age-related diseases. Some errors occur because the practitioner is unaware of incompatible drugs prescribed by other practitioners for the same patient. For example, cimetidine, an H_2-blocking drug heavily prescribed (or recommended in its over-the-counter form) to the elderly, causes a much higher incidence of untoward effects (eg, confusion, slurred speech) in the geriatric population than in younger patients. It also inhibits the hepatic metabolism of many drugs, including phenytoin, warfarin, β blockers, and other agents. A patient who has been taking one of the latter agents without untoward effect may develop markedly elevated blood levels and severe toxicity if cimetidine is added to the regimen without adjustment of dosage of the other drugs. Additional examples of drugs that inhibit liver microsomal enzymes and lead to adverse reactions are described in Chapters 4 and 66.

Patient errors may result from nonadherence for reasons described below. In addition, they often result from use of nonprescription drugs taken without the knowledge of the physician. As noted in Chapters 63 and 64, many over-the-counter agents and herbal medications contain "hidden ingredients" with potent pharmacologic effects. For example, many antihistamines have significant sedative effects and are inherently more hazardous in patients with impaired cognitive function. Similarly, their antimuscarinic action may precipitate urinary retention in geriatric men or glaucoma in patients with a narrow anterior chamber angle. If the patient is also taking a metabolism inhibitor such as cimetidine, the probability of an adverse reaction is greatly increased. A patient taking an herbal medication containing gingko is more likely to experience bleeding while taking low doses of aspirin.

PRACTICAL ASPECTS OF GERIATRIC PHARMACOLOGY

The quality of life in elderly patients can be greatly improved and life span can be prolonged by the intelligent use of drugs. However, the prescriber must recognize several practical obstacles to compliance.

The expense of drugs can be a major disincentive in patients receiving marginal retirement incomes who are not covered or inadequately covered by health insurance. The prescriber must be aware of the cost of the prescription and of cheaper alternative therapies. For example, the monthly cost of arthritis therapy with newer NSAIDs may exceed $100, whereas that for generic aspirin is about $5 and for ibuprofen and naproxen, two older NSAIDs, about $20.

Nonadherence may result from forgetfulness or confusion, especially if the patient has several prescriptions and different dosing intervals. A survey carried out in 1986 showed that the population over 65 years of age accounted for 32% of drugs prescribed in the USA, although these patients represented only 11–12% of the population at that time. Since the prescriptions are often written by several different practitioners, there is usually no attempt to design "integrated" regimens that use drugs with similar dosing intervals for the conditions being treated. Patients may forget instructions regarding the need to complete a fixed duration of therapy when a course of anti-infective drug is being given. The disappearance of symptoms is often regarded as the best reason to halt drug taking, especially if the prescription was expensive.

Nonadherence may also be deliberate. A decision not to take a drug may be based on prior experience with it. There may be excellent reasons for such "intelligent" noncompliance, and the practitioner should try to elicit them. Such efforts may also improve compliance with alternative drug regimens, because enlisting the patient as a participant in therapeutic decisions increases the motivation to succeed.

Some errors in drug taking are caused by physical disabilities. Arthritis, tremor, and visual problems may all contribute. Liquid medications that are to be measured "by the spoonful" are especially inappropriate for patients with any type of tremor or motor disability. Use of a dosing syringe may be helpful in such cases. Because of decreased production of saliva, older patients often have difficulty swallowing large tablets. "Childproof" containers are often "elder-proof" if the patient has arthritis. Cataracts and macular degeneration occur in a large number of patients over 70.

Therefore, labels on prescription bottles should be large enough for the patient with diminished vision to read or should be color-coded if the patient can see but can no longer read.

Drug therapy has considerable potential for both helpful and harmful effects in the geriatric patient. The balance may be tipped in the right direction by adherence to a few principles:

1. Take a careful drug history. The disease to be treated may be drug-induced, or drugs being taken may lead to interactions with drugs to be prescribed.

2. Prescribe only for a specific and rational indication. Do not prescribe omeprazole for "dyspepsia." Expert guidelines are published regularly by national organizations and websites such as UpToDate.com.

3. Define the goal of drug therapy. Then start with small doses and titrate to the response desired. Wait at least three half-lives (adjusted for age) before increasing the dose. If the expected response does not occur at the normal adult dosage, check blood levels. If the expected response does not occur at the appropriate blood level, switch to a different drug.

4. Maintain a high index of suspicion regarding drug reactions and interactions. Know what other drugs the patient is taking, including over-the-counter and botanical (herbal) drugs.

5. Simplify the regimen as much as possible. When multiple drugs are prescribed, try to use drugs that can be taken at the same time of day. Whenever possible, reduce the number of drugs being taken.

REFERENCES

American College of Cardiology Foundation Task Force: ACCF/AHA 2011 Expert consensus document on hypertension in the elderly. J Am Coll Cardiol 2011;57:2037. http://content.onlinejacc.org/cgi/content/full/j.jacc.2011.01.008v1

Ancolli-Israel S, Ayalon L: Diagnosis and treatment of sleep disorders in older adults. Am J Geriatr Psychiatry 2006;14:95.

Aronow WS: Drug treatment of systolic and diastolic heart failure in elderly persons. J Gerontol A Biol Med Sci 2005;60:1597.

Birnbaum LS: Pharmacokinetic basis of age-related changes in sensitivity to toxicants. Annu Rev Pharmacol Toxicol 1991;31:101.

Calcado RT, Young NS: Telomere diseases. N Engl J Med 2009;361:2353.

Chatap G, Giraud K, Vincent JP: Atrial fibrillation in the elderly: Facts and management. Drugs Aging 2002;19:819.

Cockcroft DW, Gault MH: Prediction of creatinine clearance from serum creatinine. Nephron 1976;16:31.

Dergal JM et al: Potential interactions between herbal medicines and conventional drug therapies used by older adults attending a memory clinic. Drugs Aging 2002;19:879.

Docherty JR: Age-related changes in adrenergic neuroeffector transmission. Auton Neurosci 2002;96:8.

Drugs in the elderly. Med Lett Drugs Ther 2006;48:6.

Ferrari AU: Modifications of the cardiovascular system with aging. Am J Geriatr Cardiol 2002;11:30.

Goldberg TH, Finkelstein MS: Difficulties in estimating glomerular filtration rate in the elderly. Arch Intern Med 1987;147:1430.

Jager RD, Mieler WF, Miller JW: Age-related macular degeneration. N Engl J Med 2008;358:2606.

Karlsson I: Drugs that induce delirium. Dement Geriatr Cogn Disord 1999;10:412.

Kirby J et al: A systematic review of the clinical and cost-effectiveness of memantine in patients with moderately severe to severe Alzheimer's disease. Drugs Aging 2006;23:227.

Mangoni AA: Cardiovascular drug therapy in elderly patients: Specific age-related pharmacokinetic, pharmacodynamic and therapeutic considerations. Drugs Aging 2005;22:913.

McLean AJ, LeCouteur DG: Aging biology and geriatric clinical pharmacology. Pharmacol Rev 2004;56:163.

Morrison LJ, Morrison RS: Palliative care and pain management. Med Clin N Am 2006;90:983.

Palmer AM: Neuroprotective therapeutics for Alzheimer's disease: Progress and prospects. Trends Pharmacol Sci 2011;32:141.

Rabow MW, Pantilat SZ: Care at the end of life. *Current Medical Diagnosis & Treatment*, 50th ed., McPhee SJ, Papadakis MA, eds. McGraw-Hill, 2011.

Robertson ED, Mucke L: 100 Years and counting: Prospects for defeating Alzheimer's disease. Science 2006;314:781.

Rodriguez EG et al: Use of lipid-lowering drugs in older adults with and without dementia: A community-based epidemiological study. J Am Geriatr Soc 2002;50:1852.

Sawhney R, Sehl M, Naeim A: Physiologic aspects of aging: Impact on cancer management and decision making, part I. Cancer J 2005;11:449.

Staskin DR: Overactive bladder in the elderly: A guide to pharmacological management. Drugs Aging 2005;22:1013.

Steinman MA, Hanlon JT: Managing medications in clinically complex elders. JAMA 2010;304:1592.

Van Marum RJ: Current and future therapy in Alzheimer's disease. Fund Clin Pharmacol 2008;22:265.

Vik SA et al: Medication nonadherence and subsequent risk of hospitalisation and mortality among older adults. Drugs Aging 2006;23:345.

Wade PR: Aging and neural control of the GI tract. I. Age-related changes in the enteric nervous system. Am J Physiol Gastrointest Liver Physiol 2002;283:G489.

CASE STUDY ANSWER

This patient has several conditions that warrant careful treatment. Hypertension is eminently treatable; the steps described in Chapter 11 are appropriate and effective in the elderly as well as in young patients. Patient education is critical in combating his reluctance to take his medications. Alzheimer's disease may respond temporarily to one of the anticholinesterase agents (donepezil, rivastigmine, galantamine). Alternatively, memantine may be tried. Unfortunately, age-related macular degeneration (the most likely cause of his visual difficulties) is not readily treated, but the "wet" (neovascular) variety may respond well to one of the drugs currently available (bevacizumab, ranibizumab, pegaptanib). However, these therapies are expensive.

61

Dermatologic Pharmacology

Dirk B. Robertson, MD, & Howard I. Maibach, MD

CASE STUDY

A 22-year-old woman presents with a complaint of worsening psoriasis. She has a strong family history of the disease and has had lesions on her scalp and elbows for several years. She recently noted new lesions developing on her knees and the soles of her feet. She has been using topical over-the-counter hydrocortisone cream but admits that this treatment does not seem to help. What therapeutic options are available for the treatment of this chronic disease?

Diseases of the skin offer special opportunities to the clinician. In particular, the topical administration route is especially appropriate for skin diseases, although some dermatologic diseases respond as well or better to drugs administered systemically.

The general pharmacokinetic principles governing the use of drugs applied to the skin are the same as those involved in other routes of administration (see Chapters 1 and 3). Although often depicted as a simple three-layered structure (Figure 61–1), human skin is a complex series of diffusion barriers. Quantitation of the flux of drugs and drug vehicles through these barriers is the basis for pharmacokinetic analysis of dermatologic therapy, and techniques for making such measurements are rapidly increasing in number and sensitivity.

Major variables that determine pharmacologic response to drugs applied to the skin include the following:

1. **Regional variation in drug penetration:** For example, the scrotum, face, axilla, and scalp are far more permeable than the forearm and may require less drug for equivalent effect.

2. **Concentration gradient:** Increasing the concentration gradient increases the mass of drug transferred per unit time, just as in the case of diffusion across other barriers (see Chapter 1). Thus, resistance to topical corticosteroids can sometimes be overcome by use of higher concentrations of drug.

3. **Dosing schedule:** Because of its physical properties, the skin acts as a reservoir for many drugs. As a result, the "local half-life" may be long enough to permit once-daily application of drugs with short systemic half-lives. For example, once-daily application of corticosteroids appears to be just as effective as multiple applications in many conditions.

4. **Vehicles and occlusion:** An appropriate vehicle maximizes the ability of the drug to penetrate the outer layers of the skin. In addition, through their physical properties (moistening or drying effects), vehicles may themselves have important therapeutic effects. Occlusion (application of a plastic wrap to hold the drug and its vehicle in close contact with the skin) is extremely effective in maximizing efficacy.

■ REACTIONS TO DERMATOLOGIC MEDICATIONS

The skin reacts to many systemic medications with a variety of symptom-generating responses. In addition, some dermatologic medications themselves cause skin reactions. The major types of reactions are summarized in Table 61–1.

■ DERMATOLOGIC VEHICLES

Topical medications usually consist of active ingredients incorporated in a vehicle that facilitates cutaneous application. Important considerations in vehicle selection include the solubility of the active agent in the vehicle; the rate of release of the agent from the vehicle; the ability of the vehicle to hydrate the stratum corneum, thus enhancing penetration; the stability of the therapeutic agent in the vehicle; and interactions, chemical and physical, of the vehicle, stratum corneum, and active agent.

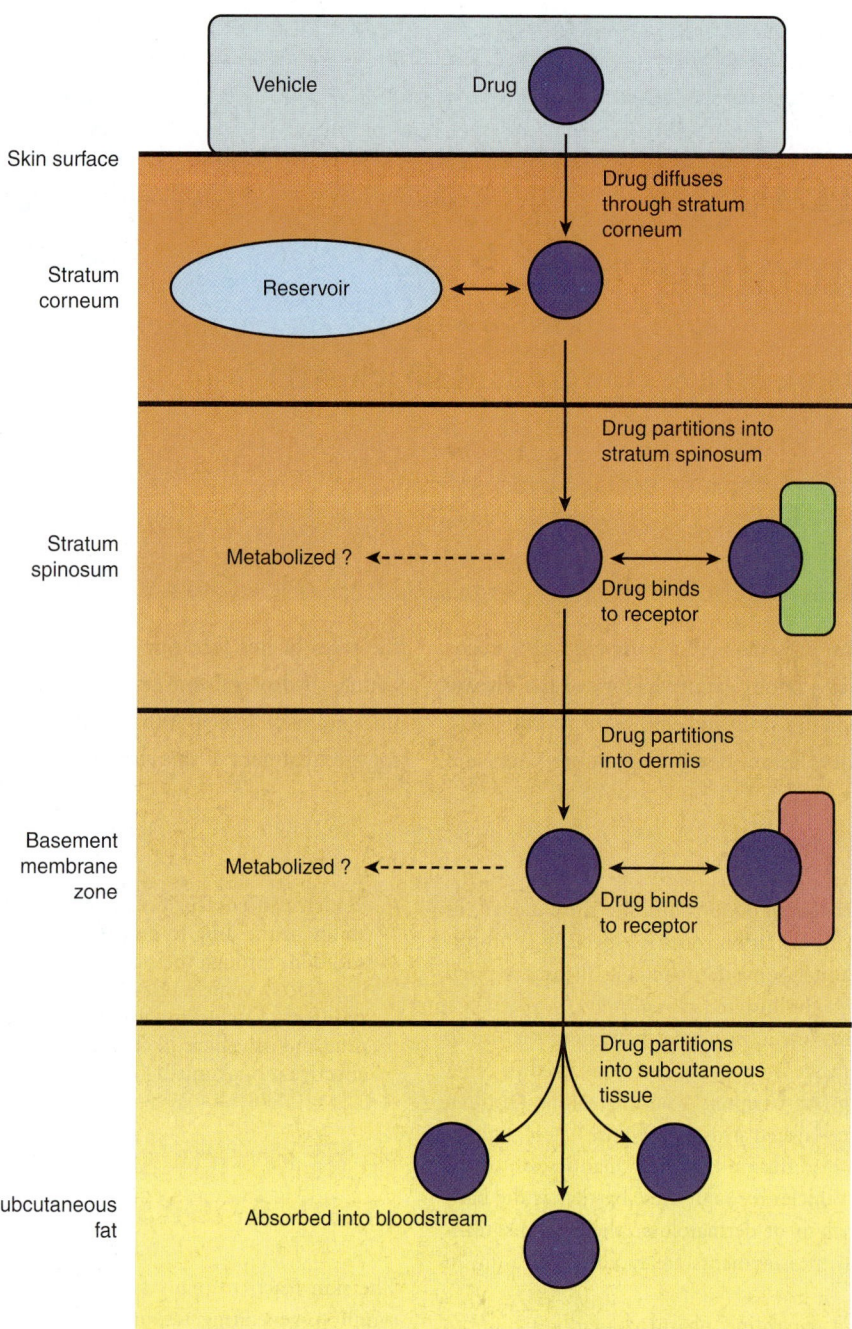

FIGURE 61–1 Schematic diagram of percutaneous absorption. (Redrawn from Orkin M, Maibach HI, Dahl MV: *Dermatology*. Appleton & Lange, 1991.)

Depending upon the vehicle, dermatologic formulations may be classified as tinctures, wet dressings, lotions, gels, aerosols, powders, pastes, creams, foams, and ointments. The ability of the vehicle to retard evaporation from the surface of the skin increases in this series, being least in tinctures and wet dressings and greatest in ointments. In general, acute inflammation with oozing, vesiculation, and crusting is best treated with drying preparations such as tinctures, wet dressings, and lotions, whereas chronic inflammation with xerosis, scaling, and lichenification is best treated with more lubricating preparations such as creams and ointments.

Tinctures, lotions, gels, foams, and aerosols are convenient for application to the scalp and hairy areas. Emulsified vanishing-type creams may be used in intertriginous areas without causing maceration.

Emulsifying agents provide homogeneous, stable preparations when mixtures of immiscible liquids such as oil-in-water creams are compounded. Some patients develop irritation from these agents. Substituting a preparation that does not contain them or using one containing a lower concentration may resolve the problem.

TABLE 61–1 Local cutaneous reactions to topical medications.

Reaction type	Mechanism	Comment
Irritation	Non-allergic	Most common local reaction
Photoirritation	Non-allergic	Phototoxicity; usually requires UVA exposure
Allergic contact dermatitis	Allergic	Type IV delayed hypersensitivity
Photoallergic contact dermatitis	Allergic	Type IV delayed hypersensitivity; usually requires UVA exposure
Immunologic contact urticaria	Allergic	IgE-mediated type I immediate hypersensitivity; may result in anaphylaxis
Non-immunologic contact urticaria	Non-allergic	Most common contact urticaria; occurs without prior sensitization

■ ANTIBACTERIAL AGENTS

TOPICAL ANTIBACTERIAL PREPARATIONS

Topical antibacterial agents may be useful in preventing infections in clean wounds, in the early treatment of infected dermatoses and wounds, in reducing colonization of the nares by staphylococci, in axillary deodorization, and in the management of acne vulgaris. The efficacy of antibiotics in these topical applications is not uniform. The general pharmacology of the antimicrobial drugs is discussed in Chapters 43–51.

Some topical anti-infectives contain corticosteroids in addition to antibiotics. There is no convincing evidence that topical corticosteroids inhibit the antibacterial effect of antibiotics when the two are incorporated in the same preparation. In the treatment of secondarily infected dermatoses, which are usually colonized with streptococci, staphylococci, or both, combination therapy may prove superior to corticosteroid therapy alone. Antibiotic-corticosteroid combinations may be useful in treating diaper dermatitis, otitis externa, and impetiginized eczema.

The selection of a particular antibiotic depends upon the diagnosis and, when appropriate, in vitro culture and sensitivity studies of clinical samples. The pathogens isolated from most infected dermatoses are group A β-hemolytic streptococci, *Staphylococcus aureus,* or both. The pathogens present in surgical wounds will be those resident in the environment. Information about regional patterns of drug resistance is therefore important in selecting a therapeutic agent. Prepackaged topical antibacterial preparations that contain multiple antibiotics are available in fixed dosages well above the therapeutic threshold. These formulations offer the advantages of efficacy in mixed infections, broader coverage for infections due to undetermined pathogens, and delayed microbial resistance to any single component antibiotic.

BACITRACIN & GRAMICIDIN

Bacitracin and gramicidin are peptide antibiotics, active against gram-positive organisms such as streptococci, pneumococci, and staphylococci. In addition, most anaerobic cocci, neisseriae, tetanus bacilli, and diphtheria bacilli are sensitive. Bacitracin is compounded in an ointment base alone or in combination with neomycin, polymyxin B, or both. The use of bacitracin in the anterior nares may temporarily decrease colonization by pathogenic staphylococci. Microbial resistance may develop following prolonged use. Bacitracin-induced contact urticaria syndrome, including anaphylaxis, occurs rarely. Allergic contact dermatitis occurs frequently, and immunologic allergic contact urticaria rarely. Bacitracin is poorly absorbed through the skin, so systemic toxicity is rare.

Gramicidin is available only for topical use, in combination with other antibiotics such as neomycin, polymyxin, bacitracin, and nystatin. Systemic toxicity limits this drug to topical use. The incidence of sensitization following topical application is exceedingly low in therapeutic concentrations.

MUPIROCIN

Mupirocin (pseudomonic acid A) is structurally unrelated to other currently available topical antibacterial agents. Most gram-positive aerobic bacteria, including methicillin-resistant *S aureus* (MRSA), are sensitive to mupirocin (see Chapter 50). It is effective in the treatment of impetigo caused by *S aureus* and group A β-hemolytic streptococci.

Intranasal mupirocin ointment for eliminating nasal carriage of *S aureus* may be associated with irritation of mucous membranes caused by the polyethylene glycol vehicle. Mupirocin is not appreciably absorbed systemically after topical application to intact skin.

RETAPAMULIN

Retapamulin is a semisynthetic pleromutilin derivative effective in the treatment of uncomplicated superficial skin infection caused by group A β-hemolytic streptococci and *S aureus*, excluding MRSA. Topical retapamulin 1% ointment is indicated for use in adult and pediatric patients, 9 months or older, for the treatment of impetigo. Recommended treatment regimen is twice-daily application for 5 days. Retapamulin is well tolerated with only occasional local irritation of the treatment site. To date only four cases of allergic contact dermatitis have been reported.

POLYMYXIN B SULFATE

Polymyxin B is a peptide antibiotic effective against gram-negative organisms, including *Pseudomonas aeruginosa, Escherichia coli,* enterobacter, and klebsiella. Most strains of proteus and serratia are resistant, as are all gram-positive organisms. Topical preparations may be compounded in either a solution or ointment base.

Numerous prepackaged antibiotic combinations containing polymyxin B are available. Detectable serum concentrations are difficult to achieve from topical application, but the total daily dose applied to denuded skin or open wounds should not exceed 200 mg in order to reduce the likelihood of neurotoxicity and nephrotoxicity. Allergic contact dermatitis to topically applied polymyxin B sulfate is uncommon.

NEOMYCIN & GENTAMICIN

Neomycin and gentamicin are aminoglycoside antibiotics active against gram-negative organisms, including *E coli*, proteus, klebsiella, and enterobacter. Gentamicin generally shows greater activity against *P aeruginosa* than neomycin. Gentamicin is also more active against staphylococci and group A β-hemolytic streptococci. Widespread topical use of gentamicin, especially in a hospital environment, should be avoided to slow the appearance of gentamicin-resistant organisms.

Neomycin is available in numerous topical formulations, both alone and in combination with polymyxin, bacitracin, and other antibiotics. It is also available as a sterile powder for topical use. Gentamicin is available as an ointment or cream.

Topical application of neomycin rarely results in detectable serum concentrations. However, in the case of gentamicin, serum concentrations of 1–18 mcg/mL are possible if the drug is applied in a water-miscible preparation to large areas of denuded skin, as in burned patients. Both drugs are water-soluble and are excreted primarily in the urine. Renal failure may permit the accumulation of these antibiotics, with possible nephrotoxicity, neurotoxicity, and ototoxicity.

Neomycin frequently causes allergic contact dermatitis, particularly if applied to eczematous dermatoses or if compounded in an ointment vehicle. When sensitization occurs, cross-sensitivity to streptomycin, kanamycin, paromomycin, and gentamicin is possible.

TOPICAL ANTIBIOTICS IN ACNE

Several systemic antibiotics that have traditionally been used in the treatment of acne vulgaris have been shown to be effective when applied topically. Currently, four antibiotics are so utilized: clindamycin phosphate, erythromycin base, metronidazole, and sulfacetamide. The effectiveness of topical therapy is less than that achieved by systemic administration of the same antibiotic. Therefore, topical therapy is generally suitable only in mild to moderate cases of inflammatory acne.

Clindamycin

Clindamycin has in vitro activity against *Propionibacterium acnes;* this has been postulated as the mechanism of its beneficial effect in acne therapy. Approximately 10% of an applied dose is absorbed, and rare cases of bloody diarrhea and pseudomembranous colitis have been reported following topical application. The hydroalcoholic vehicle and foam formulation (Evoclin) may cause drying and irritation of the skin, with complaints of burning and stinging. The water-based gel and lotion formulations are well tolerated and less likely to cause irritation. Allergic contact dermatitis is uncommon. Clindamycin is also available in fixed-combination topical gels with benzoyl peroxide (Acanya, BenzaClin, Duac), and with tretinoin (Ziana).

Erythromycin

In topical preparations, erythromycin base rather than a salt is used to facilitate penetration. The mechanism of action of topical erythromycin in inflammatory acne vulgaris is unknown but is presumed to be due to its inhibitory effects on *P acnes*. One of the possible complications of topical therapy is the development of antibiotic-resistant strains of organisms, including staphylococci. If this occurs in association with a clinical infection, topical erythromycin should be discontinued and appropriate systemic antibiotic therapy started. Adverse local reactions to erythromycin solution may include a burning sensation at the time of application and drying and irritation of the skin. The topical water-based gel is less drying and may be better tolerated. Allergic contact dermatitis is uncommon. Erythromycin is also available in a fixed combination preparation with benzoyl peroxide (Benzamycin) for topical treatment of acne vulgaris.

Metronidazole

Topical metronidazole is effective in the treatment of rosacea. The mechanism of action is unknown, but it may relate to the inhibitory effects of metronidazole on *Demodex brevis;* alternatively, the drug may act as an anti-inflammatory agent by direct effect on neutrophil cellular function. Oral metronidazole has been shown to be a carcinogen in susceptible rodent species, and topical use during pregnancy and by nursing mothers and children is therefore not recommended.

Adverse local effects of the water-based gel formulation (MetroGel) include dryness, burning, and stinging. Less drying formulations may be better tolerated (MetroCream, MetroLotion, and Noritate cream). Caution should be exercised when applying metronidazole near the eyes to avoid excessive tearing.

Sodium Sulfacetamide

Topical sulfacetamide is available alone as a 10% lotion (Klaron) and as a 10% wash (Ovace), and in several preparations in combination with sulfur for the treatment of acne vulgaris and acne rosacea. The mechanism of action is thought to be inhibition of *P acnes* by competitive inhibition of *p*-aminobenzoic acid utilization. Approximately 4% of topically applied sulfacetamide is absorbed percutaneously, and its use is therefore contraindicated in patients having a known hypersensitivity to sulfonamides.

Dapsone

Topical dapsone is available as a 5% gel (Aczone) for the treatment of acne vulgaris. The mechanism of action is unknown. Topical use in patients with glucose-6-phosphate dehydrogenase (G6PD) deficiency has not been shown to cause clinically relevant hemolysis or anemia. However, a slight decrease in hemoglobin concentration was noted in patients with G6PD deficiency, suggestive of mild hemolysis. To date, serious adverse reactions associated with oral dapsone use as delineated in Chapter 47 have not been reported with topical use. Adverse local side effects include mild dryness, redness, oiliness, and skin peeling. Application of dapsone gel followed by benzoyl peroxide may result in a temporary yellow discoloration of the skin and hair.

■ ANTIFUNGAL AGENTS

The treatment of superficial fungal infections caused by dermatophytic fungi may be accomplished (1) with topical antifungal agents, eg, clotrimazole, miconazole, econazole, ketoconazole, oxiconazole, sulconazole, sertaconazole, ciclopirox olamine, naftifine, terbinafine, butenafine, and tolnaftate; or (2) with orally administered agents, ie, griseofulvin, terbinafine, ketoconazole, fluconazole, and itraconazole. Superficial infections caused by candida species may be treated with topical applications of clotrimazole, miconazole, econazole, ketoconazole, oxiconazole, ciclopirox olamine, nystatin, or amphotericin B. Chronic generalized mucocutaneous candidiasis is responsive to long-term therapy with oral ketoconazole.

TOPICAL ANTIFUNGAL PREPARATIONS

TOPICAL AZOLE DERIVATIVES

The topical imidazoles, which currently include clotrimazole, econazole, ketoconazole, miconazole, oxiconazole, sulconazole, and sertaconazole, have a wide range of activity against dermatophytes (epidermophyton, microsporum, and trichophyton) and yeasts, including *Candida albicans* and *Pityrosporum orbiculare* (see Chapter 48).

Miconazole (Monistat, Micatin) is available for topical application as a cream or lotion and as vaginal cream or suppositories for use in vulvovaginal candidiasis. Clotrimazole (Lotrimin, Mycelex) is available for topical application to the skin as a cream or lotion and as vaginal cream and tablets for use in vulvovaginal candidiasis. Econazole (Spectazole) is available as a cream for topical application. Oxiconazole (Oxistat) is available as a cream and lotion for topical use. Ketoconazole (Nizoral) is available as a cream for topical treatment of dermatophytosis and candidiasis and as a shampoo or foam for the treatment of seborrheic dermatitis. Sulconazole (Exelderm) is available as a cream or solution. Sertaconazole (Ertaczo) is available as a cream. Topical antifungal-corticosteroid fixed combinations have been introduced on the basis of providing more rapid symptomatic improvement than an antifungal agent alone. Clotrimazole-betamethasone dipropionate cream (Lotrisone) is one such combination.

Once- or twice-daily application to the affected area will generally result in clearing of superficial dermatophyte infections in 2–3 weeks, although the medication should be continued until eradication of the organism is confirmed. Paronychial and intertriginous candidiasis can be treated effectively by any of these agents when applied three or four times daily. Seborrheic dermatitis should be treated with twice-daily applications of ketoconazole until clinical clearing is obtained.

Adverse local reactions to the imidazoles may include stinging, pruritus, erythema, and local irritation. Allergic contact dermatitis is uncommon.

CICLOPIROX OLAMINE

Ciclopirox olamine is a synthetic broad-spectrum antimycotic agent with inhibitory activity against dermatophytes, candida species, and *P orbiculare*. This agent appears to inhibit the uptake of precursors of macromolecular synthesis; the site of action is probably the fungal cell membrane.

Pharmacokinetic studies indicate that 1–2% of the dose is absorbed when applied as a solution on the back under an occlusive dressing. Ciclopirox olamine is available as a 1% cream and lotion (Loprox) for the topical treatment of dermatomycosis, candidiasis, and tinea versicolor. The incidence of adverse reactions has been low. Pruritus and worsening of clinical disease have been reported. The potential for allergic contact dermatitis is small.

Topical 8% ciclopirox olamine (Penlac nail lacquer) has been approved for the treatment of mild to moderate onychomycosis of fingernails and toenails. Although well tolerated with minimal side effects, the overall cure rates in clinical trials are less than 12%.

ALLYLAMINES: NAFTIFINE & TERBINAFINE

Naftifine hydrochloride and terbinafine (Lamisil) are allylamines that are highly active against dermatophytes but less active against yeasts. The antifungal activity derives from selective inhibition of squalene epoxidase, a key enzyme for the synthesis of ergosterol (see Figure 48–1).

They are available as 1% creams and other forms for the topical treatment of dermatophytosis, to be applied on a twice-daily dosing schedule. Adverse reactions include local irritation, burning sensation, and erythema. Contact with mucous membranes should be avoided.

BUTENAFINE

Butenafine hydrochloride (Mentax) is a benzylamine that is structurally related to the allylamines. As with the allylamines, butenafine inhibits the epoxidation of squalene, thus blocking the synthesis of ergosterol, an essential component of fungal cell membranes. Butenafine is available as a 1% cream to be applied once daily for the treatment of superficial dermatophytosis.

TOLNAFTATE

Tolnaftate is a synthetic antifungal compound that is effective topically against dermatophyte infections caused by epidermophyton, microsporum, and trichophyton. It is also active against *P orbiculare* but not against candida.

Tolnaftate (Aftate, Tinactin) is available as a cream, solution, powder, or powder aerosol for application twice daily to infected areas. Recurrences following cessation of therapy are common, and infections of the palms, soles, and nails are usually unresponsive to tolnaftate alone. The powder or powder aerosol may be used chronically following initial treatment in patients susceptible to tinea infections. Tolnaftate is generally well tolerated and rarely causes irritation or allergic contact dermatitis.

NYSTATIN & AMPHOTERICIN B

Nystatin and amphotericin B are useful in the topical therapy of *C albicans* infections but ineffective against dermatophytes. Nystatin is limited to topical treatment of cutaneous and mucosal candida infections because of its narrow spectrum and negligible absorption from the gastrointestinal tract following oral administration. Amphotericin B has a broader antifungal spectrum and is used intravenously in the treatment of many systemic mycoses (see Chapter 48) and to a lesser extent in the treatment of cutaneous candida infections.

The recommended dosage for topical preparations of nystatin in treating paronychial and intertriginous candidiasis is application two or three times a day. Oral candidiasis (thrush) is treated by holding 5 mL (infants, 2 mL) of nystatin oral suspension in the mouth for several minutes four times daily before swallowing. An alternative therapy for thrush is to retain a vaginal tablet in the mouth until dissolved four times daily. Recurrent or recalcitrant perianal, vaginal, vulvar, and diaper area candidiasis may respond to oral nystatin, 0.5–1 million units in adults (100,000 units in children) four times daily in addition to local therapy. Vulvovaginal candidiasis may be treated by insertion of 1 vaginal tablet twice daily for 14 days, then nightly for an additional 14–21 days.

Amphotericin B (Fungizone) is available for topical use in cream and lotion form. The recommended dosage in the treatment of paronychial and intertriginous candidiasis is application two to four times daily to the affected area.

Adverse effects associated with oral administration of nystatin include mild nausea, diarrhea, and occasional vomiting. Topical application is nonirritating, and allergic contact hypersensitivity is exceedingly uncommon. Topical amphotericin B is well tolerated and only occasionally locally irritating. The drug may cause a temporary yellow staining of the skin, especially when the cream vehicle is used.

ORAL ANTIFUNGAL AGENTS

ORAL AZOLE DERIVATIVES

Azole derivatives currently available for oral treatment of systemic mycosis include fluconazole (Diflucan), itraconazole (Sporanox), ketoconazole (Nizoral), and others. As discussed in Chapter 48,

imidazole derivatives act by affecting the permeability of the cell membrane of sensitive cells through alterations of the biosynthesis of lipids, especially sterols, in the fungal cell.

Patients with chronic mucocutaneous candidiasis respond well to a once-daily dose of 200 mg of ketoconazole, with a median clearing time of 16 weeks. Most patients require long-term maintenance therapy. Variable results have been reported in treatment of chromomycosis.

Ketoconazole is effective in the therapy of cutaneous infections caused by epidermophyton, microsporum, and trichophyton species. Infections of the glabrous skin often respond within 2–3 weeks to a once-daily oral dose of 200 mg. Palmar-plantar skin is slower to respond, often taking 4–6 weeks at a dosage of 200 mg twice daily. Infections of the hair and nails may take even longer before resolving, with low cure rates noted for tinea capitis. Tinea versicolor is responsive to short courses of a once-daily dose of 200 mg.

Nausea or pruritus occurs in approximately 3% of patients taking ketoconazole. More significant adverse effects include gynecomastia, elevations of hepatic enzyme levels, and hepatitis. Caution is advised when using ketoconazole in patients with a history of hepatitis. Routine evaluation of hepatic function is advisable for patients on prolonged therapy.

Fluconazole is well absorbed following oral administration, with a plasma half-life of 30 hours. In view of this long half-life, daily doses of 100 mg are sufficient to treat mucocutaneous candidiasis; alternate-day doses are sufficient for dermatophyte infections. The plasma half-life of itraconazole is similar to that of fluconazole, and detectable therapeutic concentrations remain in the stratum corneum for up to 28 days following termination of therapy. Itraconazole is effective for the treatment of onychomycosis in a dosage of 200 mg daily taken with food to ensure maximum absorption for 3 consecutive months. Recent reports of heart failure in patients receiving itraconazole for onychomycosis have resulted in recommendations that it not be given for treatment of onychomycosis in patients with ventricular dysfunction. Additionally, routine evaluation of hepatic function is recommended for patients receiving itraconazole for onychomycosis.

Administration of oral azoles with midazolam or triazolam has resulted in elevated plasma concentrations and may potentiate and prolong hypnotic and sedative effects of these agents. Administration with HMG-CoA reductase inhibitors has been shown to cause a significant risk of rhabdomyolysis. *Therefore, administration of the oral azoles with midazolam, triazolam, or HMG-CoA inhibitors is contraindicated.*

GRISEOFULVIN

Griseofulvin is effective orally against dermatophyte infections caused by epidermophyton, microsporum, and trichophyton. It is ineffective against candida and *P orbiculare*. Griseofulvin's mechanism of antifungal action is not fully understood, but it is active only against growing cells.

Following the oral administration of 1 g of micronized griseofulvin, drug can be detected in the stratum corneum 4–8 hours later. Reducing the particle size of the medication greatly increases absorption of the drug. Formulations that contain the smallest particle size are labeled "ultramicronized." Ultramicronized griseofulvin achieves bioequivalent plasma levels with half the dose of micronized drug. In addition, solubilizing griseofulvin in polyethylene glycol enhances absorption even further. Micronized griseofulvin is available as 250 mg and 500 mg tablets, and ultramicronized drug is available as 125 mg, 165 mg, 250 mg, and 330 mg tablets and as 250 mg capsules.

The usual adult dosage of the micronized ("microsize") form of the drug is 500 mg daily in single or divided doses with meals; occasionally, 1 g/d is indicated in the treatment of recalcitrant infections. The pediatric dosage is 10 mg/kg of body weight daily in single or divided doses with meals. An oral suspension is available for use in children.

Griseofulvin is most effective in treating tinea infections of the scalp and glabrous (nonhairy) skin. In general, infections of the scalp respond to treatment in 4–6 weeks, and infections of glabrous skin will respond in 3–4 weeks. Dermatophyte infections of the nails respond only to prolonged administration of griseofulvin. Fingernails may respond to 6 months of therapy, whereas toenails are quite recalcitrant to treatment and may require 8–18 months of therapy; relapse almost invariably occurs.

Adverse effects seen with griseofulvin therapy include headaches, nausea, vomiting, diarrhea, photosensitivity, peripheral neuritis, and occasionally mental confusion. Griseofulvin is derived from a penicillium mold, and cross-sensitivity with penicillin may occur. It is contraindicated in patients with porphyria or hepatic failure or those who have had hypersensitivity reactions to it in the past. Its safety in pregnant patients has not been established. Leukopenia and proteinuria have occasionally been reported. Therefore, in patients undergoing prolonged therapy, routine evaluation of the hepatic, renal, and hematopoietic systems is advisable. Coumarin anticoagulant activity may be altered by griseofulvin, and anticoagulant dosage may require adjustment.

TERBINAFINE

Terbinafine (described above) is quite effective given orally for the treatment of onychomycosis. Recommended oral dosage is 250 mg daily for 6 weeks for fingernail infections and 12 weeks for toenail infections. Patients receiving terbinafine for onychomycosis should be monitored closely with periodic laboratory evaluations for possible hepatic dysfunction.

■ TOPICAL ANTIVIRAL AGENTS

ACYCLOVIR, VALACYCLOVIR, PENCICLOVIR, & FAMCICLOVIR

Acyclovir, valacyclovir, penciclovir, and famciclovir are synthetic guanine analogs with inhibitory activity against members of the herpesvirus family, including herpes simplex types 1 and 2. Their mechanism of action, indications, and usage in the treatment of cutaneous infections are discussed in Chapter 49.

Topical acyclovir (Zovirax) is available as a 5% ointment; topical penciclovir (Denavir), as a 1% cream for the treatment of recurrent orolabial herpes simplex virus infection in immunocompetent adults. Adverse local reactions to acyclovir and penciclovir may include pruritus and mild pain with transient stinging or burning.

■ IMMUNOMODULATORS

IMIQUIMOD

Imiquimod is available as 5% cream (Aldara) for the treatment of external genital and perianal warts in adults, actinic keratoses on the face and scalp, and biopsy-proven primary basal cell carcinomas on the trunk, neck, and extremities. A lower 3.75% concentration cream (Zyclara) is available for the treatment of face and scalp actinic keratoses. The mechanism of its action is thought to be related to imiquimod's ability to stimulate peripheral mononuclear cells to release interferon-α and to stimulate macrophages to produce interleukins-1, -6, and -8, and tumor necrosis factor-α (TNF-α).

Imiquimod should be applied to the wart tissue three times per week and left on the skin for 6–10 hours prior to washing off with mild soap and water. Treatment should be continued until eradication of the warts is accomplished, but not for more than a total of 16 weeks. Recommended treatment of actinic keratoses consists of twice-weekly applications of the 5% cream on the contiguous area of involvement or nightly applications of the 3.75% cream. The cream is removed after approximately 8 hours with mild soap and water. Treatment of superficial basal cell carcinoma consists of five-times-per-week application to the tumor, including a 1-cm margin of surrounding skin, for a 6-week course of therapy.

Percutaneous absorption is minimal, with less than 0.9% absorbed following a single-dose application. Adverse side effects consist of local inflammatory reactions, including pruritus, erythema, and superficial erosion.

TACROLIMUS & PIMECROLIMUS

Tacrolimus (Protopic) and pimecrolimus (Elidel) are macrolide immunosuppressants that have been shown to be of significant benefit in the treatment of atopic dermatitis. Both agents inhibit T-lymphocyte activation and prevent the release of inflammatory cytokines and mediators from mast cells in vitro after stimulation by antigen-IgE complexes. Tacrolimus is available as 0.03% and 0.1% ointments, and pimecrolimus is available as a 1% cream. Both are indicated for short-term and intermittent long-term therapy for mild to moderate atopic dermatitis. Tacrolimus 0.03% ointment and pimecrolimus 1% cream are approved for use in children older than 2 years of age, although all strengths are approved for adult use. Recommended dosing of both agents is twice-daily application to affected skin until clearing is noted. Neither medication should be used with occlusive dressings. The most common side effect of both drugs is a burning sensation in the applied area that improves with continued use. The Food and Drug Administration has added a black box warning regarding the long-term safety of topical tacrolimus and pimecrolimus because of animal tumorigenicity data.

■ ECTOPARASITICIDES

PERMETHRIN

Permethrin is toxic to *Pediculus humanus, Pthirus pubis*, and *Sarcoptes scabiei*. Less than 2% of an applied dose is absorbed percutaneously. Residual drug persists up to 10 days following application.

It is recommended that permethrin 1% cream rinse (Nix) be applied undiluted to affected areas of pediculosis for 10 minutes and then rinsed off with warm water. For the treatment of scabies, a single application of 5% cream (Elimite, Acticin) is applied to the body from the neck down, left on for 8–14 hours, and then washed off. Adverse reactions to permethrin include transient burning, stinging, and pruritus. Cross-sensitization to pyrethrins or chrysanthemums has been alleged but inadequately documented.

LINDANE (HEXACHLOROCYCLOHEXANE)

The gamma isomer of hexachlorocyclohexane was commonly called gamma benzene hexachloride, a misnomer, since no benzene ring is present in this compound. Percutaneous absorption studies using a solution of lindane in acetone have shown that almost 10% of a dose applied to the forearm is absorbed, to be subsequently excreted in the urine over a 5-day period. After absorption, lindane is concentrated in fatty tissues, including the brain.

Lindane (Kwell, etc) is available as a shampoo or lotion. For pediculosis capitis or pubis, 30 mL of shampoo is applied to dry hair on the scalp or genital area for 4 minutes and then rinsed off. No additional application is indicated unless living lice are present 1 week after treatment. Then reapplication may be required.

Recent concerns about the toxicity of lindane have altered treatment guidelines for its use in scabies; the current recommendation calls for a single application to the entire body from the neck down, left on for 8–12 hours, and then washed off. Patients should be retreated only if active mites can be demonstrated, and never within 1 week of initial treatment.

Concerns about neurotoxicity and hematotoxicity have resulted in warnings that lindane should be used with caution in infants, children, and pregnant women. The current USA package insert recommends that it not be used as a scabicide in premature infants and in patients with known seizure disorders. California has prohibited the medical use of lindane following evaluation of its toxicologic profile. The risk of adverse systemic reactions to lindane appears to be minimal when it is used properly and according to directions in adult patients. However, local irritation may occur, and contact with the eyes and mucous membranes should be avoided.

CROTAMITON

Crotamiton, *N*-ethyl-*o*-crotonotoluidide, is a scabicide with some antipruritic properties. Its mechanism of action is not known. Studies on percutaneous absorption have revealed detectable levels of crotamiton in the urine following a single application on the forearm.

Crotamiton (Eurax) is available as a 10% cream or lotion. Suggested guidelines for scabies treatment call for two applications to the entire body from the chin down at 24-hour intervals, with a cleansing bath 48 hours after the last application. Crotamiton is an effective agent that can be used as an alternative to lindane. Allergic contact dermatitis and primary irritation may occur, necessitating discontinuance of therapy. Application to acutely inflamed skin or to the eyes or mucous membranes should be avoided.

SULFUR

Sulfur has a long history of use as a scabicide. Although it is non-irritating, it has an unpleasant odor, is staining, and is thus disagreeable to use. It has been replaced by more aesthetic and effective scabicides in recent years, but it remains a possible alternative drug for use in infants and pregnant women. The usual formulation is 5% precipitated sulfur in petrolatum.

MALATHION

Malathion is an organophosphate cholinesterase inhibitor that is hydrolyzed and inactivated by plasma carboxylesterases much faster in humans than in insects, thereby providing a therapeutic advantage in treating pediculosis (see Chapter 7). Malathion is available as a 0.5% lotion (Ovide) that should be applied to the hair when dry; 4–6 hours later, the hair is combed to remove nits and lice.

BENZYL ALCOHOL

Benzyl alcohol (Ulesfia) is available as a 5% lotion for the treatment of head lice in patients older than 6 months. The lotion is applied to dry hair and left on for 10 minutes prior to rinsing off with water. Because the drug is not ovacidal, the treatment must be repeated after 7 days. Eye irritation and allergic contact dermatitis have been reported.

■ AGENTS AFFECTING PIGMENTATION

HYDROQUINONE, MONOBENZONE, & MEQUINOL

Hydroquinone, monobenzone (Benoquin, the monobenzyl ether of hydroquinone), and mequinol (the monomethyl ether of hydroquinone) are used to reduce hyperpigmentation of the skin. Topical hydroquinone and mequinol usually result in temporary lightening, whereas monobenzone causes irreversible depigmentation.

The mechanism of action of these compounds appears to involve inhibition of the enzyme tyrosinase, thus interfering with the biosynthesis of melanin. In addition, monobenzone may be toxic to melanocytes, resulting in permanent loss of these cells. Some percutaneous absorption of these compounds takes place, because monobenzone may cause hypopigmentation at sites distant from the area of application. Both hydroquinone and monobenzone may cause local irritation. Allergic contact dermatitis to these compounds can occur. Prescription combinations of hydroquinone, fluocinolone acetonide, and retinoic acid (Tri-Luma) and mequinol and retinoic acid (Solagé) are more effective than their individual components.

TRIOXSALEN & METHOXSALEN

Trioxsalen and methoxsalen are psoralens used for the repigmentation of depigmented macules of vitiligo. With the recent development of high-intensity long-wave ultraviolet fluorescent lamps, photochemotherapy with oral methoxsalen for psoriasis and with oral trioxsalen for vitiligo has been under intensive investigation.

Psoralens must be photoactivated by long-wavelength ultraviolet light in the range of 320–400 nm (ultraviolet A [UVA]) to produce a beneficial effect. Psoralens intercalate with DNA and, with subsequent UVA irradiation, cyclobutane adducts are formed with pyrimidine bases. Both monofunctional and bifunctional adducts may be formed, the latter causing interstrand cross-links. These DNA photoproducts may inhibit DNA synthesis. The major long-term risks of psoralen photochemotherapy are cataracts and skin cancer.

■ SUNSCREENS

Topical medications useful in protecting against sunlight contain either chemical compounds that absorb ultraviolet light, called sunscreens, or opaque materials such as titanium dioxide that reflect light, called sunshades. The three classes of chemical compounds most commonly used in sunscreens are p-aminobenzoic acid (PABA) and its esters, the benzophenones, and the dibenzoylmethanes.

Most sunscreen preparations are designed to absorb ultraviolet light in the ultraviolet B (UVB) wavelength range from 280 to 320 nm, which is the range responsible for most of the erythema and sunburn associated with sun exposure and tanning. Chronic exposure to light in this range induces aging of the skin and photocarcinogenesis. Para-aminobenzoic acid and its esters are the most effective available absorbers in the B region. Ultraviolet in the longer UVA range, 320–400 nm, is also associated with skin aging and cancer.

The benzophenones include oxybenzone, dioxybenzone, and sulisobenzone. These compounds provide a broader spectrum of absorption from 250 to 360 nm, but their effectiveness in the UVB erythema range is less than that of PABA. The dibenzoylmethanes include Parasol and Eusolex. These compounds absorb wavelengths throughout the longer UVA range, with maximum absorption at 360 nm. Patients particularly sensitive to UVA wavelengths include individuals with polymorphous light eruption, cutaneous lupus erythematosus, and drug-induced photosensitivity. In these patients, dibenzoylmethane-containing sunscreen may provide improved photoprotection. Ecamsule (Mexoryl) appears to provide greater UVA protection than the dibenzoylmethanes and is less prone to photodegradation.

The sun protection factor (SPF) of a given sunscreen is a measure of its effectiveness in absorbing erythrogenic ultraviolet light. It is determined by measuring the minimal erythema dose with and without the sunscreen in a group of normal people. The ratio of the minimal erythema dose with sunscreen to the minimal erythema dose without sunscreen is the SPF.

Recently updated FDA regulations limit the claimed maximum SPF value on sunscreen labels to 50+ because there is not sufficient data to show that products with SPF values higher than 50 provide greater protection for users. These new FDA regulations require that sunscreens labeled as "broad spectrum" sunscreens will have to pass a standard test comparing the amount of UVA radiation protection in relation to the amount of UVB radiation. Broad spectrum sunscreens with SPF values of 15 or higher help protect against not only sunburn, but also skin cancer and early skin aging when used as directed. Sunscreens with an SPF value between 2 and 14 will only be allowed to claim to help prevent sunburn. In addition, products claiming to be water resistant must indicate whether they remain effective for 40 minutes or 80 minutes while swimming or sweating, based on standard testing.

■ ACNE PREPARATIONS

RETINOIC ACID & DERIVATIVES

Retinoic acid, also known as *tretinoin* or *all-trans*-retinoic acid, is the acid form of vitamin A. It is an effective topical treatment for acne vulgaris. Several analogs of vitamin A, eg, 13-*cis*-retinoic acid (isotretinoin), have been shown to be effective in various dermatologic diseases when given orally. Vitamin A alcohol is the physiologic form of vitamin A. The topical therapeutic agent, **retinoic acid,** is formed by the oxidation of the alcohol group, with all four double bonds in the side chain in the *trans* configuration as shown.

Retinoic acid

Retinoic acid is insoluble in water but soluble in many organic solvents. Topically applied retinoic acid remains chiefly in the epidermis, with less than 10% absorption into the circulation. The small quantities of retinoic acid absorbed following topical application are metabolized by the liver and excreted in bile and urine.

Retinoic acid has several effects on epithelial tissues. It stabilizes lysosomes, increases ribonucleic acid polymerase activity, increases prostaglandin E_2, cAMP, and cGMP levels, and increases the incorporation of thymidine into DNA. Its action in acne has been attributed to decreased cohesion between epidermal cells and increased epidermal cell turnover. This is thought to result in the expulsion of open comedones and the transformation of closed comedones into open ones.

Topical retinoic acid is applied initially in a concentration sufficient to induce slight erythema with mild peeling. The concentration or frequency of application may be decreased if too much irritation occurs. Topical retinoic acid should be applied to dry skin only, and care should be taken to avoid contact with the corners of the nose, eyes, mouth, and mucous membranes. During the first 4–6 weeks of therapy, comedones not previously evident may appear and give the impression that the acne has been aggravated by the retinoic acid. However, with continued therapy, the lesions will clear, and in 8–12 weeks optimal clinical improvement should occur. A timed-release formulation of tretinoin containing microspheres (Retin-A Micro) delivers the medication over time and may be less irritating for sensitive patients.

The effects of tretinoin on keratinization and desquamation offer benefits for patients with photo damaged skin. Prolonged use of tretinoin promotes dermal collagen synthesis, new blood vessel formation, and thickening of the epidermis, which helps diminish fine lines and wrinkles. Specially formulated moisturizing 0.05% cream (Renova, Refissa) is marketed for this purpose.

The most common adverse effects of topical retinoic acid are erythema and dryness that occur in the first few weeks of use, but these can be expected to resolve with continued therapy. Animal studies suggest that this drug may increase the tumorigenic potential of ultraviolet radiation. In light of this, patients using retinoic acid should be advised to avoid or minimize sun exposure and use a protective sunscreen. Allergic contact dermatitis to topical retinoic acid is rare.

Adapalene (Differin) is a derivative of naphthoic acid that resembles retinoic acid in structure and effects. It is available for daily application as a 0.1% gel, cream, or lotion and a 0.3% gel. Unlike tretinoin, adapalene is photochemically stable and shows little decrease in efficacy when used in combination with benzoyl peroxide. Adapalene is less irritating than tretinoin and is most effective in patients with mild to moderate acne vulgaris. Adapalene is also available in a fixed-dose combination gel with benzoyl peroxide (Epiduo).

Tazarotene (Tazorac) is an acetylenic retinoid that is available as a 0.1% gel and cream for the treatment of mild to moderately severe facial acne. Topical tazarotene should be used by women of childbearing age only after contraceptive counseling. It is recommended that tazarotene should not be used by pregnant women.

ISOTRETINOIN

Isotretinoin is a synthetic retinoid currently restricted to the oral treatment of severe cystic acne that is recalcitrant to standard therapies. The precise mechanism of action of isotretinoin in cystic acne is not known, although it appears to act by inhibiting sebaceous gland size and function. The drug is well absorbed, extensively bound to plasma albumin, and has an elimination half-life of 10–20 hours.

Most patients with cystic acne respond to 1–2 mg/kg, given in two divided doses daily for 4–5 months. If severe cystic acne persists following this initial treatment, after a period of 2 months, a second course of therapy may be initiated. Common adverse effects resemble hypervitaminosis A and include dryness and itching of the skin and mucous membranes. Less common side effects

are headache, corneal opacities, pseudotumor cerebri, inflammatory bowel disease, anorexia, alopecia, and muscle and joint pains. These effects are all reversible on discontinuance of therapy. Skeletal hyperostosis has been observed in patients receiving isotretinoin with premature closure of epiphyses noted in children treated with this medication. Lipid abnormalities (triglycerides, high-density lipoproteins) are frequent; their clinical relevance is unknown at present.

Teratogenicity is a significant risk in patients taking isotretinoin; therefore, women of childbearing potential *must* use an effective form of contraception for at least 1 month before, throughout isotretinoin therapy, and for one or more menstrual cycles following discontinuation of treatment. A negative serum pregnancy test *must* be obtained within 2 weeks before starting therapy in these patients, and therapy should be initiated only on the second or third day of the next normal menstrual period. In the USA, health care professionals, pharmacists, and patients must utilize the mandatory iPLEDGE registration and follow-up system.

BENZOYL PEROXIDE

Benzoyl peroxide is an effective topical agent in the treatment of acne vulgaris. It penetrates the stratum corneum or follicular openings unchanged and is converted metabolically to benzoic acid within the epidermis and dermis. Less than 5% of an applied dose is absorbed from the skin in an 8-hour period. It has been postulated that the mechanism of action of benzoyl peroxide in acne is related to its antimicrobial activity against *P acnes* and to its peeling and comedolytic effects.

To decrease the likelihood of irritation, application should be limited to a low concentration (2.5%) once daily for the first week of therapy and increased in frequency and strength if the preparation is well tolerated. Fixed-combination formulations of 5% benzoyl peroxide with 3% erythromycin base (Benzamycin) or 1% clindamycin (BenzaClin, Duac), and 2.5% benzoyl peroxide with 1.2% clindamycin (Acanya) or 0.1% adapalene (Epiduo) appear to be more effective than individual agents alone.

Benzoyl peroxide is a potent contact sensitizer in experimental studies, and this adverse effect may occur in up to 1% of acne patients. Care should be taken to avoid contact with the eyes and mucous membranes. Benzoyl peroxide is an oxidant and may rarely cause bleaching of the hair or colored fabrics.

AZELAIC ACID

Azelaic acid is a straight-chain saturated dicarboxylic acid that is effective in the treatment of acne vulgaris (in the form of Azelex) and acne rosacea (Finacea). Its mechanism of action has not been fully determined, but preliminary studies demonstrate antimicrobial activity against *P acnes* as well as in vitro inhibitory effects on the conversion of testosterone to dihydrotestosterone. Initial therapy is begun with once-daily applications of the 20% cream or 15% gel to the affected areas for 1 week and twice-daily applications thereafter. Most patients experience mild irritation with redness and dryness of the skin during the first week of treatment. Clinical improvement is noted in 6–8 weeks of continuous therapy.

DRUGS FOR PSORIASIS

ACITRETIN

Acitretin (Soriatane), a metabolite of the aromatic retinoid etretinate, is quite effective in the treatment of psoriasis, especially pustular forms. It is given orally at a dosage of 25–50 mg/d. Adverse effects attributable to acitretin therapy are similar to those seen with isotretinoin and resemble hypervitaminosis A. Elevations in cholesterol and triglycerides may be noted with acitretin, and hepatotoxicity with liver enzyme elevations has been reported. Acitretin is more teratogenic than isotretinoin in the animal species studied to date, which is of special concern in view of the drug's prolonged elimination time (more than 3 months) after chronic administration. In cases where etretinate is formed by concomitant administration of acitretin and ethanol, etretinate may be found in plasma and subcutaneous fat for many years.

Acitretin must not be used by women who are pregnant or may become pregnant while undergoing treatment or at any time for at least 3 years after treatment is discontinued. Ethanol must be strictly avoided during treatment with acitretin and for 2 months after discontinuing therapy. Patients must not donate blood during treatment and for 3 years after acitretin is stopped.

TAZAROTENE

Tazarotene (Tazorac) is a topical acetylenic retinoid prodrug that is hydrolyzed to its active form by an esterase. The active metabolite, tazarotenic acid, binds to retinoic acid receptors, resulting in modified gene expression. The precise mechanism of action in psoriasis is unknown but may relate to both anti-inflammatory and antiproliferative actions. Tazarotene is absorbed percutaneously, and teratogenic systemic concentrations may be achieved if applied to more than 20% of total body surface area. Women of childbearing potential must therefore be advised of the risk prior to initiating therapy, and adequate birth control measures must be utilized while on therapy.

Treatment of psoriasis should be limited to once-daily application of either 0.05% or 0.1% gel not to exceed 20% of total body surface area. Adverse local effects include a burning or stinging sensation (sensory irritation) and peeling, erythema, and localized edema of the skin (irritant dermatitis). Potentiation of photosensitizing medication may occur, and patients should be cautioned to minimize sunlight exposure and to use sunscreens and protective clothing.

CALCIPOTRIENE & CALCITRIOL

Calcipotriene (Dovonex) is a synthetic vitamin D_3 derivative (available as a 0.005% cream or scalp lotion) that is effective in the treatment of plaque-type psoriasis vulgaris of moderate severity.

Improvement of psoriasis was generally noted following 2 weeks of therapy, with continued improvement for up to 8 weeks of treatment. However, fewer than 10% of patients demonstrate total clearing while on calcipotriene as single-agent therapy. Adverse effects include burning, itching, and mild irritation, with dryness and erythema of the treatment area. Care should be taken to avoid facial contact, which may cause ocular irritation. A once-daily two-compound ointment containing calcipotriene and betamethasone dipropionate (Taclonex) is available. This combination is more effective than its individual ingredients and is well tolerated, with a safety profile similar to betamethasone dipropionate.

Calcitriol (Vectical) contains 1,25-dihydroxycholecalciferol, the hormonally active form of vitamin D_3. Calcitriol 3 mcg/g ointment is similar in efficacy to calcipotriene 0.005% ointment for the treatment of plaque-type psoriasis on the body and is better tolerated in intertriginous and sensitive areas of the skin. Clinical studies show comparable safety data regarding adverse cutaneous and systemic reactions between topical calcitriol and calcipotriene ointment.

BIOLOGIC AGENTS

Biologic agents useful in treating adult patients with moderate to severe chronic plaque psoriasis include the T-cell modulator alefacept, the TNF-α inhibitors etanercept, infliximab, and adalimumab, and the cytokine inhibitor ustekinumab. TNF-α inhibitors are also discussed in Chapters 36 and 55.

ALEFACEPT

Alefacept (Amevive) is an immunosuppressive dimeric fusion protein that consists of the extracellular CD2-binding portion of the human leukocyte function antigen-3 linked to the Fc portion of human IgG_1. Alefacept interferes with lymphocyte activation, which plays a role in the pathophysiology of psoriasis, and causes a reduction in subsets of CD2 T lymphocytes and circulating total CD4 and CD8 T-lymphocyte counts. The recommended dosage is 7.5 mg given once weekly as an intravenous bolus or 15 mg once weekly as an intramuscular injection for a 12-week course of treatment. Patients should have CD4 lymphocyte counts monitored weekly while taking alefacept, and dosing should be withheld if CD4 counts are below 250 cells/µL. The drug should be discontinued if the counts remain below 250 cells/µL for 1 month. Alefacept is an immunosuppressive agent and should not be administered to patients with clinically significant infection. Because of the possibility of an increased risk of malignancy, it should not be administered to patients with a history of systemic malignancy.

TNF INHIBITORS: ETANERCEPT, INFLIXIMAB, & ADALIMUMAB

Etanercept (Enbrel) is a dimeric fusion protein consisting of the extracellular ligand-binding portion of the human TNF receptor linked to the Fc portion of human IgG_1. Etanercept binds selectively to TNF-α and -β and blocks interaction with cell surface TNF receptors that play a role in the inflammatory process of plaque psoriasis. The recommended dosage of etanercept in psoriasis is a 50 mg subcutaneous injection given twice weekly for 3 months followed by a maintenance dose of 50 mg weekly.

Infliximab (Remicade) is a chimeric IgG_1 monoclonal antibody composed of human constant and murine variable regions. Infliximab binds to the soluble and transmembrane forms of TNF-α and inhibits binding of TNF-α with its receptors. The recommended dose of infliximab is 5 mg/kg given as an intravenous infusion followed by similar doses at 2 and 6 weeks after the first infusion and then every 8 weeks thereafter.

Adalimumab (Humira) is a recombinant $1gG_1$ monoclonal antibody that binds specifically to TNF-α and blocks its interaction with cell surface TNF receptors. The recommended dose for adalimumab in psoriasis is an initial dose of 80 mg administered subcutaneously followed by 40 mg given every other week starting 1 week after the initial dose.

Serious life-threatening infections, including sepsis and pneumonia, have been reported with the use of TNF inhibitors. Patients should be evaluated for tuberculosis risk factors and tested for latent tuberculosis infection prior to starting therapy. Concurrent use with other immunosuppressive therapy should be avoided. In clinical trials of all TNF-blocking agents more cases of lymphoma were observed compared with control patients. Patients with a prior history of prolonged phototherapy treatment should be monitored for nonmelanoma skin cancers.

USTEKINUMAB

Ustekinumab (Stelara) is a human $IgG_1\kappa$ monoclonal antibody that binds with high affinity and specificity to interleukin (IL)-12 and IL-23 cytokines inhibiting TH1 and TH17 cell-mediated responses, which are involved in the pathogenesis of psoriasis. The recommended treatment protocol is 45 mg for patients weighing less than 100 kg and 90 mg for patients weighing more than 100 kg given as a subcutaneous injection initially, followed by the same dose 4 weeks later, and then once every 12 weeks. Serious allergic reactions including angioedema and anaphylaxis have occurred and caution should be exercised in patients receiving allergy immunotherapy. Serious infections, especially from mycobacterial organisms, are possible and patients must be evaluated for tuberculosis prior to initiating therapy. Live vaccines, including Bacillus Calmette-Guérin (BCG), should not be given with ustekinumab. One case of reversible posterior leukoencephalopathy syndrome (RPLS) has been reported.

■ ANTI-INFLAMMATORY AGENTS

TOPICAL CORTICOSTEROIDS

The remarkable efficacy of topical corticosteroids in the treatment of inflammatory dermatoses was noted soon after the introduction of hydrocortisone in 1952. Numerous analogs are now available that offer extensive choices of potencies, concentrations, and vehicles. The therapeutic effectiveness of topical corticosteroids is based primarily on their anti-inflammatory activity. Definitive explanations of the effects of corticosteroids on endogenous mediators of inflammation await further experimental clarification. The antimitotic effects of corticosteroids on human epidermis may account for an additional mechanism of action in psoriasis and other dermatologic diseases associated with increased cell turnover. The general pharmacology of these endocrine agents is discussed in Chapter 39.

Chemistry & Pharmacokinetics

The original topical glucocorticosteroid was hydrocortisone, the natural glucocorticosteroid of the adrenal cortex. The 9α-fluoro derivative of hydrocortisone was active topically, but its salt-retaining properties made it undesirable even for topical use. Prednisolone and methylprednisolone are as active topically as hydrocortisone (Table 61–2). The 9α-fluorinated steroids dexamethasone and betamethasone did not have any advantage over hydrocortisone. However, triamcinolone and fluocinolone, the acetonide derivatives of the fluorinated steroids, do have a distinct efficacy advantage in topical therapy. Similarly, betamethasone is not very active topically, but attaching a 5-carbon valerate chain to the 17-hydroxyl position results in a compound over 300 times as active as hydrocortisone for topical use. Fluocinonide is the 21-acetate derivative of fluocinolone acetonide; the addition of the 21-acetate enhances the topical activity about five-fold. Fluorination of the corticoid is not required for high potency.

Corticosteroids are only minimally absorbed following application to normal skin; for example, approximately 1% of a dose of hydrocortisone solution applied to the ventral forearm is absorbed. Long-term occlusion with an impermeable film such as plastic wrap is an effective method of enhancing penetration, yielding a tenfold increase in absorption. There is a marked regional anatomic variation in corticosteroid penetration. Compared with the absorption from the forearm, hydrocortisone is absorbed 0.14 times as well through the plantar foot arch, 0.83 times as well through the palm, 3.5 times as well through the scalp, 6 times as well through the forehead, 9 times as well through vulvar skin, and 42 times as well through scrotal skin. Penetration is increased severalfold in the inflamed skin of atopic dermatitis; and in severe exfoliative diseases, such as erythrodermic psoriasis, there appears to be little barrier to penetration.

Experimental studies on the percutaneous absorption of hydrocortisone fail to reveal a significant increase in absorption when applied on a repetitive basis and a single daily application may be effective in most conditions. Ointment bases tend to give better activity to the corticosteroid than do cream or lotion vehicles. Increasing the concentration of a corticosteroid increases the penetration but not proportionately. For example, approximately 1% of a 0.25% hydrocortisone solution is absorbed from the forearm. A 10-fold increase in concentration causes only a fourfold increase in absorption. Solubility of the corticosteroid in the vehicle is a significant determinant of the percutaneous absorption of a topical steroid. Marked increases in efficacy are noted when optimized

TABLE 61–2 Relative efficacy of some topical corticosteroids in various formulations.

Concentration in Commonly Used Preparations	Drug	Concentration in Commonly Used Preparations	Drug
Lowest efficacy		**Intermediate efficacy (continued)**	
0.25–2.5%	Hydrocortisone	0.05%	Fluticasone propionate (Cutivate)
0.25%	Methylprednisolone acetate (Medrol)	0.05%	Desonide (Desowen)
0.1%	Dexamethasone[1] (Decaderm)	0.025%	Halcinonide[1] (Halog)
1.0%	Methylprednisolone acetate (Medrol)	0.05%	Desoximetasone[1] (Topicort L.P.)
0.5%	Prednisolone (MetiDerm)	0.05%	Flurandrenolide[1] (Cordran)
0.2%	Betamethasone[1] (Celestone)	0.1%	Triamcinolone acetonide[1]
Low efficacy		0.025%	Fluocinolone acetonide[1]
0.01%	Fluocinolone acetonide[1] (Fluonid, Synalar)	**High efficacy**	
0.01%	Betamethasone valerate[1] (Valisone)	0.05%	Fluocinonide[1] (Lidex)
0.025%	Fluorometholone[1] (Oxylone)	0.05%	Betamethasone dipropionate[1] (Diprosone, Maxivate)
0.05%	Alclometasone dipropionate (Aclovate)	0.1%	Amcinonide[1] (Cyclocort)
0.025%	Triamcinolone acetonide[1] (Aristocort, Kenalog, Triacet)	0.25%	Desoximetasone[1] (Topicort)
0.1%	Clocortolone pivalate[1] (Cloderm)	0.5%	Triamcinolone acetonide[1]
0.03%	Flumethasone pivalate[1] (Locorten)	0.2%	Fluocinolone acetonide[1] (Synalar-HP)
Intermediate efficacy		0.05%	Diflorasone diacetate[1] (Florone, Maxiflor)
0.2%	Hydrocortisone valerate (Westcort)	0.1%	Halcinonide[1] (Halog)
0.1%	Mometasone furoate (Elocon)	**Highest efficacy**	
0.1%	Hydrocortisone butyrate (Locoid)	0.05%	Betamethasone dipropionate in optimized vehicle (Diprolene)[1]
0.1%	Hydrocortisone probutate (Pandel)	0.05%	Diflorasone diacetate[1] in optimized vehicle (Psorcon)
0.025%	Betamethasone benzoate[1] (Uticort)		
0.025%	Flurandrenolide[1] (Cordran)	0.05%	Halobetasol propionate[1] (Ultravate)
0.1%	Betamethasone valerate[1] (Valisone)	0.05%	Clobetasol propionate[1] (Temovate)
0.1%	Prednicarbate (Dermatop)		

[1]Fluorinated steroids.

vehicles are used, as demonstrated by newer formulations of betamethasone dipropionate and diflorasone diacetate.

Table 61–2 groups topical corticosteroid formulations according to approximate relative efficacy. Table 61–3 lists major dermatologic diseases in order of their responsiveness to these drugs. In the first group of diseases, low- to medium-efficacy corticosteroid preparations often produce clinical remission. In the second group, it is often necessary to use high-efficacy preparations, occlusion therapy, or both. Once a remission has been achieved, every effort should be made to maintain the improvement with a low-efficacy corticosteroid.

The limited penetration of topical corticosteroids can be overcome in certain clinical circumstances by the intralesional injection of relatively insoluble corticosteroids, eg, triamcinolone acetonide, triamcinolone diacetate, triamcinolone hexacetonide, and betamethasone acetate-phosphate. When these agents are injected into the lesion, measurable amounts remain in place and are gradually released for 3–4 weeks. This form of therapy is often effective for the lesions listed in Table 61–3 that are generally unresponsive to topical corticosteroids. The dosage of the triamcinolone salts should be limited to 1 mg per treatment site, ie, 0.1 mL of 10 mg/mL suspension, to decrease the incidence of local atrophy (see below).

Adverse Effects

All absorbable topical corticosteroids possess the potential to suppress the pituitary-adrenal axis (see Chapter 39). Although most patients with pituitary-adrenal axis suppression demonstrate only a laboratory test abnormality, cases of severely impaired stress

TABLE 61–3 Dermatologic disorders responsive to topical corticosteroids ranked in order of sensitivity.

Very responsive
Atopic dermatitis
Seborrheic dermatitis
Lichen simplex chronicus
Pruritus ani
Later phase of allergic contact dermatitis
Later phase of irritant dermatitis
Nummular eczematous dermatitis
Stasis dermatitis
Psoriasis, especially of genitalia and face
Less responsive
Discoid lupus erythematosus
Psoriasis of palms and soles
Necrobiosis lipoidica diabeticorum
Sarcoidosis
Lichen striatus
Pemphigus
Familial benign pemphigus
Vitiligo
Granuloma annulare
Least responsive: Intralesional injection required
Keloids
Hypertrophic scars
Hypertrophic lichen planus
Alopecia areata
Acne cysts
Prurigo nodularis
Chondrodermatitis nodularis chronica helicis

response can occur. Iatrogenic Cushing's syndrome may occur as a result of protracted use of topical corticosteroids in large quantities. Applying potent corticosteroids to extensive areas of the body for prolonged periods, with or without occlusion, increases the likelihood of systemic effects. Fewer of these factors are required to produce adverse systemic effects in children, and growth retardation is of particular concern in the pediatric age group.

Adverse local effects of topical corticosteroids include the following: atrophy, which may present as depressed, shiny, often wrinkled "cigarette paper"-appearing skin with prominent telangiectases and a tendency to develop purpura and ecchymosis; corticoid rosacea, with persistent erythema, telangiectatic vessels, pustules, and papules in central facial distribution; perioral dermatitis, steroid acne, alterations of cutaneous infections, hypopigmentation, hypertrichosis; increased intraocular pressure; and allergic contact dermatitis. The latter may be confirmed by patch

testing with high concentrations of corticosteroids, ie, 1% in petrolatum, because topical corticosteroids are not irritating. Screening for allergic contact dermatitis potential is performed with tixocortol pivalate, budesonide, and hydrocortisone valerate or butyrate. Topical corticosteroids are contraindicated in individuals who demonstrate hypersensitivity to them. Some sensitized subjects develop a generalized flare when dosed with adrenocorticotropic hormone or oral prednisone.

TAR COMPOUNDS

Tar preparations are used mainly in the treatment of psoriasis, dermatitis, and lichen simplex chronicus. The phenolic constituents endow these compounds with antipruritic properties, making them particularly valuable in the treatment of chronic lichenified dermatitis. Acute dermatitis with vesiculation and oozing may be irritated by even weak tar preparations, which should be avoided. However, in the subacute and chronic stages of dermatitis and psoriasis, these preparations are quite useful and offer an alternative to the use of topical corticosteroids.

The most common adverse reaction to coal tar compounds is an irritant folliculitis, necessitating discontinuance of therapy to the affected areas for a period of 3–5 days. Photoirritation and allergic contact dermatitis may also occur. Tar preparations should be avoided in patients who have previously exhibited sensitivity to them.

■ KERATOLYTIC & DESTRUCTIVE AGENTS

SALICYLIC ACID

Salicylic acid has been extensively used in dermatologic therapy as a keratolytic agent. The mechanism by which it produces its keratolytic and other therapeutic effects is poorly understood. The drug may solubilize cell surface proteins that keep the stratum corneum intact, thereby resulting in desquamation of keratotic debris. Salicylic acid is keratolytic in concentrations of 3–6%. In concentrations greater than 6%, it can be destructive to tissues.

Salicylic acid

Salicylism and death have occurred following topical application. In an adult, 1 g of a topically applied 6% salicylic acid preparation will raise the serum salicylate level not more than 0.5 mg/dL of plasma; the threshold for toxicity is 30–50 mg/dL. Higher serum levels are possible in children, who are therefore at a greater risk for salicylism. In cases of severe intoxication, hemodialysis is the treatment of choice (see Chapter 58). It is advisable

to limit both the total amount of salicylic acid applied and the frequency of application. Urticarial, anaphylactic, and erythema multiforme reactions may occur in patients who are allergic to salicylates. Topical use may be associated with local irritation, acute inflammation, and even ulceration with the use of high concentrations of salicylic acid. Particular care must be exercised when using the drug on the extremities of patients with diabetes or peripheral vascular disease.

PROPYLENE GLYCOL

Propylene glycol is used extensively in topical preparations because it is an excellent vehicle for organic compounds. It has been used alone as a keratolytic agent in 40–70% concentrations, with plastic occlusion, or in gel with 6% salicylic acid.

Only minimal amounts of a topically applied dose are absorbed through normal stratum corneum. Percutaneously absorbed propylene glycol is oxidized by the liver to lactic acid and pyruvic acid, with subsequent utilization in general body metabolism. Approximately 12–45% of the absorbed agent is excreted unchanged in the urine.

Propylene glycol is an effective keratolytic agent for the removal of hyperkeratotic debris. It is also an effective humectant and increases the water content of the stratum corneum. The hygroscopic characteristics of propylene glycol may help it to develop an osmotic gradient through the stratum corneum, thereby increasing hydration of the outermost layers by drawing water out from the inner layers of the skin.

Propylene glycol is used under polyethylene occlusion or with 6% salicylic acid for the treatment of ichthyosis, palmar and plantar keratodermas, psoriasis, pityriasis rubra pilaris, keratosis pilaris, and hypertrophic lichen planus.

In concentrations greater than 10%, propylene glycol may act as an irritant in some patients; those with eczematous dermatitis may be more sensitive. Allergic contact dermatitis occurs with propylene glycol, and a 4% aqueous propylene glycol solution is recommended for the purpose of patch testing.

UREA

Urea in a compatible cream vehicle or ointment base has a softening and moisturizing effect on the stratum corneum. It has the ability to make creams and lotions feel less greasy, and this has been utilized in dermatologic preparations to decrease the oily feel of a preparation that otherwise might feel unpleasant. It is a white crystalline powder with a slight ammonia odor when moist.

Urea is absorbed percutaneously, although the amount absorbed is minimal. It is distributed predominantly in the extracellular space and excreted in urine. Urea is a natural product of metabolism, and systemic toxicities with topical application do not occur.

Urea increases the water content of the stratum corneum, presumably as a result of the hygroscopic characteristics of this naturally occurring molecule. Urea is also keratolytic. The mechanism of action appears to involve alterations in prekeratin and keratin, leading to increased solubilization. In addition, urea may break hydrogen bonds that keep the stratum corneum intact.

As a humectant, urea is used in concentrations of 2–20% in creams and lotions. As a keratolytic agent, it is used in 20% concentration in diseases such as ichthyosis vulgaris, hyperkeratosis of palms and soles, xerosis, and keratosis pilaris. Concentrations of 30–50% applied to the nail plate have been useful in softening the nail prior to avulsion.

PODOPHYLLUM RESIN & PODOFILOX

Podophyllum resin, an alcoholic extract of *Podophyllum peltatum*, commonly known as mandrake root or May apple, is used in the treatment of condyloma acuminatum and other verrucae. It is a mixture of podophyllotoxin, α and β peltatin, desoxypodophyllotoxin, dehydropodophyllotoxin, and other compounds. It is soluble in alcohol, ether, chloroform, and compound tincture of benzoin.

Percutaneous absorption of podophyllum resin occurs, particularly in intertriginous areas and from applications to large moist condylomas. It is soluble in lipids and therefore is distributed widely throughout the body, including the central nervous system.

The major use of podophyllum resin is in the treatment of condyloma acuminatum. Podophyllotoxin and its derivatives are active cytotoxic agents with specific affinity for the microtubule protein of the mitotic spindle. Normal assembly of the spindle is prevented, and epidermal mitoses are arrested in metaphase. A 25% concentration of podophyllum resin in compound tincture of benzoin is recommended for the treatment of condyloma acuminatum. Application should be restricted to wart tissue only, to limit the total amount of medication used and to prevent severe erosive changes in adjacent tissue. In treating cases of large condylomas, it is advisable to limit application to sections of the affected area to minimize systemic absorption. The patient is instructed to wash off the preparation 2–3 hours after the initial application, because the irritant reaction is variable. Depending on the individual patient's reaction, this period can be extended to 6–8 hours on subsequent applications. If three to five applications have not resulted in significant resolution, other methods of treatment should be considered.

Toxic symptoms associated with excessively large applications include nausea, vomiting, alterations in sensorium, muscle weakness, neuropathy with diminished tendon reflexes, coma, and even death. Local irritation is common, and inadvertent contact with the eye may cause severe conjunctivitis. Use during pregnancy is contraindicated in view of possible cytotoxic effects on the fetus.

Pure podophyllotoxin (podofilox) is approved for use as either a 0.5% solution or gel (Condylox) for application by the patient in the treatment of genital condylomas. The low concentration of podofilox significantly reduces the potential for systemic toxicity. Most men with penile warts may be treated with less than 70 μL per application. At this dose, podofilox is not routinely detected in the serum. Treatment is self-administered in treatment cycles of twice-daily application for 3 consecutive days followed by a 4-day drug-free period. Local adverse effects include inflammation, erosions, burning pain, and itching.

SINECATECHINS

Sinecatechins 15% ointment (Veregen) is a prescription botanical drug product of a partially purified fraction of the water extract of green tea leaves from *Camellia sinensis* containing a mixture of catechins. Sinecatechins ointment is indicated for the topical treatment of external genital and perianal warts in immunocompetent patients 18 years and older. The mechanism of action is unknown. Sinecatechins ointment should be applied three times daily to the warts until complete clearance, not to exceed 16 weeks of therapy.

FLUOROURACIL

Fluorouracil is a fluorinated pyrimidine antimetabolite that resembles uracil, with a fluorine atom substituted for the 5-methyl group. Its systemic pharmacology is described in Chapter 54. Fluorouracil is used topically for the treatment of multiple actinic keratoses.

Approximately 6% of a topically applied dose is absorbed—an amount insufficient to produce adverse systemic effects. Most of the absorbed drug is metabolized and excreted as carbon dioxide, urea, and α-fluoro-β-alanine. A small percentage is eliminated unchanged in the urine. Fluorouracil inhibits thymidylate synthetase activity, interfering with the synthesis of DNA and, to a lesser extent, RNA. These effects are most marked in atypical, rapidly proliferating cells.

Fluorouracil is available in multiple formulations containing 0.5%, 1%, 2%, and 5% concentrations. The response to treatment begins with erythema and progresses through vesiculation, erosion, superficial ulceration, necrosis, and finally reepithelialization. Fluorouracil should be continued until the inflammatory reaction reaches the stage of ulceration and necrosis, usually in 3–4 weeks, at which time treatment should be terminated. The healing process may continue for 1–2 months after therapy is discontinued. Local adverse reactions may include pain, pruritus, a burning sensation, tenderness, and residual postinflammatory hyperpigmentation. Excessive exposure to sunlight during treatment may increase the intensity of the reaction and should be avoided. Allergic contact dermatitis to fluorouracil has been reported, and its use is contraindicated in patients with known hypersensitivity.

NONSTEROIDAL ANTI-INFLAMMATORY DRUGS

A topical 3% gel formulation of the nonsteroidal anti-inflammatory drug diclofenac (Solaraze) has shown moderate effectiveness in the treatment of actinic keratoses. The mechanism of action is unknown. As with other NSAIDs, anaphylactoid reactions may occur with diclofenac, and it should be given with caution to patients with known aspirin hypersensitivity (see Chapter 36).

AMINOLEVULINIC ACIDS

Aminolevulinic acid (ALA) is an endogenous precursor of photosensitizing porphyrin metabolites. When exogenous ALA is provided to the cell through topical applications, protoporphyrin IX (PpIX) accumulates in the cell. When exposed to light of appropriate wavelength and energy, the accumulated PpIX produces a photodynamic reaction resulting in the formation of cytotoxic superoxide and hydroxyl radicals. Photosensitization of actinic keratoses using ALA (Levulan Kerastick) and illumination with a blue light photodynamic therapy illuminator (BLU-U) is the basis for ALA photodynamic therapy.

Treatment consists of applying ALA 20% topical solution to individual actinic keratoses followed by blue light photodynamic illumination 14–18 hours later. Transient stinging or burning at the treatment site occurs during the period of light exposure. Patients *must* avoid exposure to sunlight or bright indoor lights for at least 40 hours after ALA application. Redness, swelling, and crusting of the actinic keratoses will occur and gradually resolve over a 3- to 4-week time course. Allergic contact dermatitis to methyl ester may occur.

■ ANTIPRURITIC AGENTS

DOXEPIN

Topical doxepin hydrochloride 5% cream (Zonalon) may provide significant antipruritic activity when utilized in the treatment of pruritus associated with atopic dermatitis or lichen simplex chronicus. The precise mechanism of action is unknown but may relate to the potent H_1- and H_2-receptor antagonist properties of dibenzoxepin tricyclic compounds. Percutaneous absorption is variable and may result in significant drowsiness in some patients. In view of the anticholinergic effect of doxepin, topical use is contraindicated in patients with untreated narrow-angle glaucoma or a tendency to urinary retention.

Plasma levels of doxepin similar to those achieved during oral therapy may be obtained with topical application; the usual drug interactions associated with tricyclic antidepressants may occur. Therefore, monoamine oxidase inhibitors must be discontinued at least 2 weeks prior to the initiation of doxepin cream. Topical application of the cream should be performed four times daily for up to 8 days of therapy. The safety and efficacy of chronic dosing has not been established. Adverse local effects include marked burning and stinging of the treatment site which may necessitate discontinuation of the cream in some patients. Allergic contact dermatitis appears to be frequent, and patients should be monitored for symptoms of hypersensitivity.

PRAMOXINE

Pramoxine hydrochloride is a topical anesthetic that can provide temporary relief from pruritus associated with mild eczematous dermatoses. Pramoxine is available as a 1% cream, lotion, or gel and in combination with hydrocortisone acetate. Application to the affected area two to four times daily may provide short-term relief of pruritus. Local adverse effects include transient burning and stinging. Care should be exercised to avoid contact with the eyes.

■ TRICHOGENIC & ANTITRICHOGENIC AGENTS

MINOXIDIL

Topical minoxidil (Rogaine) is effective in reversing the progressive miniaturization of terminal scalp hairs associated with androgenic alopecia. Vertex balding is more responsive to therapy than frontal balding. The mechanism of action of minoxidil on hair follicles is unknown. Chronic dosing studies have demonstrated that the effect of minoxidil is not permanent, and cessation of treatment will lead to hair loss in 4–6 months. Percutaneous absorption of minoxidil in normal scalp is minimal, but possible systemic effects on blood pressure (see Chapter 11) should be monitored in patients with cardiac disease.

FINASTERIDE

Finasteride (Propecia) is a 5α-reductase inhibitor that blocks the conversion of testosterone to dihydrotestosterone (see Chapter 40), the androgen responsible for androgenic alopecia in genetically predisposed men. Oral finasteride, 1 mg/d, promotes hair growth and prevents further hair loss in a significant proportion of men with androgenic alopecia. Treatment for at least 3–6 months is necessary to see increased hair growth or prevent further hair loss. Continued treatment with finasteride is necessary to sustain benefit. Reported adverse effects include decreased libido, ejaculation disorders, and erectile dysfunction, which resolve in most men who remain on therapy and in all men who discontinue finasteride.

There are no data to support the use of finasteride in women with androgenic alopecia. Pregnant women should not be exposed to finasteride either by use or by handling crushed tablets because of the risk of hypospadias developing in a male fetus.

BIMATOPROST

Bimatoprost (Latisse) is a prostaglandin analog that is available as a 0.03% ophthalmic solution to treat hypotrichosis of the eyelashes. The mechanism of action is unknown. Treatment consists of nightly application to the skin of the upper eyelid margins at the base of the eyelashes using a separate disposable applicator for each eyelid. Contact lenses should be removed prior to bimatoprost application. Side effects include pruritus, conjunctival hyperemia, skin pigmentation, and erythema of the eyelids. Although iris darkening has not been reported with applications confined to the upper eyelid skin, increased brown iris pigmentation, which is likely to be permanent, has occurred when bimatoprost ophthalmic solution was instilled onto the eye.

EFLORNITHINE

Eflornithine (Vaniqa) is an irreversible inhibitor of ornithine decarboxylase, which catalyzes the rate-limiting step in the biosynthesis of polyamines. Polyamines are required for cell division and differentiation, and inhibition of ornithine decarboxylase affects the rate of hair growth. Topical eflornithine has been shown to be effective in reducing facial hair growth in approximately 30% of women when applied twice daily for 6 months of therapy. Hair growth was observed to return to pretreatment levels 8 weeks after discontinuation. Local adverse effects include stinging, burning, and folliculitis.

■ ANTINEOPLASTIC AGENTS

Alitretinoin (Panretin) is a topical formulation of 9-*cis*-retinoic acid which is approved for the treatment of cutaneous lesions in patients with AIDS-related Kaposi's sarcoma. Localized reactions may include intense erythema, edema, and vesiculation necessitating discontinuation of therapy. Patients who are applying alitretinoin should not concurrently use products containing DEET, a common component of insect repellant products.

Bexarotene (Targretin) is a member of a subclass of retinoids that selectively binds and activates retinoid X receptor subtypes. It is available both in an oral formulation and as a topical gel for the treatment of cutaneous T-cell lymphoma. Teratogenicity is a significant risk for both systemic and topical treatment with bexarotene, and women of childbearing potential must avoid becoming pregnant throughout therapy and for at least 1 month following discontinuation of the drug. Bexarotene may increase levels of triglycerides and cholesterol; therefore, lipid levels must be monitored during treatment.

Vorinostat (Zolinza) and **romidepsin** (Istodax) are histone deacetylase inhibitors that are approved for the treatment of cutaneous T-cell lymphoma in patients with progressive, persistent, or recurrent disease after prior systemic therapy. Adverse effects include thrombocytopenia, anemia, and gastrointestinal disturbances. Pulmonary embolism, which has occurred with vorinostat, has not been reported to date with romidepsin.

■ ANTISEBORRHEA AGENTS

Table 61–4 lists topical formulations for the treatment of seborrheic dermatitis. These are of variable efficacy and may

TABLE 61–4 Antiseborrhea agents.

Active Ingredient	Typical Trade Name
Betamethasone valerate foam	Luxiq
Chloroxine shampoo	Capitrol
Coal tar shampoo	Ionil-T, Pentrax, Theraplex-T, T-Gel
Fluocinolone acetonide shampoo	FS Shampoo
Ketoconazole shampoo and gel	Nizoral, Xolegel
Selenium sulfide shampoo	Selsun, Exsel
Zinc pyrithione shampoo	DHS-Zinc, Theraplex-Z

necessitate concomitant treatment with topical corticosteroids for severe cases.

■ MISCELLANEOUS MEDICATIONS

A number of drugs used primarily for other conditions also find use as oral therapeutic agents for dermatologic conditions. A few such preparations are listed in Table 61–5.

REFERENCES

General

Bronaugh R, Maibach HI: Percutaneous Penetration: *Principles and Practices*, 4th ed. Taylor & Francis, 2005.

Wakelin S, Maibach HI: *Systemic Drugs in Dermatology*. Manson, 2004.

Wolverton S: *Comprehensive Dermatologic Drug Therapy*, 2nd ed. Saunders, 2007.

Antibacterial, Antifungal, & Antiviral Drugs

Aly R, Beutner K, Maibach HI: *Cutaneous Microbiology*. Marcel Dekker, 1996.

James WD: Clinical practice. Acne. N Engl J Med 2005;352:1463.

McClellan KJ et al: Terbinafine. An update of its use in superficial mycoses. Drugs 1999;58:179.

Ectoparasiticides

Elgart ML: A risk-benefit assessment of agents used in the treatment of scabies. Drug Saf 1996;14:386.

Agents Affecting Pigmentation

Levitt J: The safety of hydroquinone. J Am Acad Dermatol 2007;57:854.

Stolk LML, Siddiqui AH: Biopharmaceutics, pharmacokinetics, and pharmacology of psoralens. Gen Pharmacol 1988;19:649.

Retinoids & Other Acne Preparations

Leyden JJ: Topical treatment of acne vulgaris: Retinoids and cutaneous irritation. J Am Acad Dermatol 1998;38:S1.

TABLE 61–5 Miscellaneous medications and the dermatologic conditions in which they are used.

Drug or Group	Conditions	Comment
Alitretinoin	AIDS-related Kaposi's sarcoma	See also Chapter 49.
Antihistamines	Pruritus (any cause), urticaria	See also Chapter 16.
Antimalarials	Lupus erythematosus, photosensitization	See also Chapter 36.
Antimetabolites	Psoriasis, pemphigus, pemphigoid	See also Chapter 54.
Becaplermin	Diabetic neuropathic ulcers	See also Chapter 41.
Bexarotene	Cutaneous T-cell lymphoma	See also Chapter 54.
Corticosteroids	Pemphigus, pemphigoid, lupus erythematosus, allergic contact dermatoses, and certain other dermatoses	See also Chapter 39.
Cyclosporine	Psoriasis	See also Chapter 55.
Dapsone	Dermatitis herpetiformis, erythema elevatum diutinum, pemphigus, pemphigoid, bullous lupus erythematosus	See also Chapter 47.
Denileukin diftitox	Cutaneous T-cell lymphoma	See also Chapter 54.
Drospirenone/ethinyl estradiol	Moderate female acne	See also Chapter 39.
Interferon	Melanoma, viral warts	See also Chapter 55.
Mycophenolate mofetil	Bullous disease	See also Chapter 55.
Romidepsin	Cutaneous T-cell lymphoma	See also Chapter 54.
Thalidomide	Erythema nodosum leprosum	See also Chapters 47 and 55.
Vorinostat	Cutaneous T-cell lymphoma	See also Chapter 54

Shalita AR et al: Tazarotene gel is safe and effective in the treatment of acne vulgaris. A multicenter, double-blind, vehicle-controlled study. Cutis 1999;63:349.

Thami GP, Sarkar R: Coal tar: Past, present and future. Clin Exp Dermatol 2002;27:99.

Weinstein GD et al: Topical tretinoin for treatment of photodamaged skin. Arch Dermatol 1991;127:659.

Anti-Inflammatory Agents

Brazzini B, Pimpinelli N: New and established topical corticosteroids in dermatology: Clinical pharmacology and therapeutic use. Am J Clin Dermatol 2002;3:47.

Surber C, Maibach HI: *Topical Corticosteroids*. Karger, 1994.

Williams JD, Griffiths CE: Cytokine blocking agents in dermatology. Clin Exp Dermatol 2002;27:585.

Keratolytic & Destructive Agents

Roenigk H, Maibach HI (editors): *Psoriasis*, 3rd ed. Marcel Dekker, 1998.

CASE STUDY ANSWER

Initial therapy consisting of twice-daily applications of a medium-strength topical corticosteroid combined with once-daily topical calcipotriene or calcitriol should provide adequate control for this patient's localized psoriasis. A coal tar shampoo should be initiated for her scalp psoriasis with nightly application of a corticosteroid solution to recalcitrant plaques.

Drugs Used in the Treatment of Gastrointestinal Diseases

Kenneth R. McQuaid, MD

CASE STUDY

A 21-year-old woman comes with her parents to discuss therapeutic options for her Crohn's disease. She was diagnosed with Crohn's disease 2 years ago, and it involves her terminal ileum and proximal colon, as confirmed by colonoscopy and small bowel radiography. She was initially treated with mesalamine and budesonide with good response, but over the last 2 months, she has had a relapse of her symptoms. She is experiencing fatigue, cramping, abdominal pains, and nonbloody diarrhea up to 10 times daily, and she has had a 15-lb weight loss.

She has no other significant medical or surgical history. Her current medications are mesalamine 2.4 g/d and budesonide 9 mg/d. She appears thin and tired. Abdominal examination reveals tenderness without guarding in the right lower quadrant; no masses are palpable. On perianal examination, there is no tenderness, fissure, or fistula. Her laboratory data are notable for anemia and elevated C-reactive protein. What are the options for immediate control of her symptoms and disease? What are the long-term management options?

INTRODUCTION

Many of the drug groups discussed elsewhere in this book have important applications in the treatment of diseases of the gastrointestinal tract and other organs. Other groups are used almost exclusively for their effects on the gut; these are discussed in the following text according to their therapeutic uses.

■ DRUGS USED IN ACID-PEPTIC DISEASES

Acid-peptic diseases include gastroesophageal reflux, peptic ulcer (gastric and duodenal), and stress-related mucosal injury. In all these conditions, mucosal erosions or ulceration arise when the caustic effects of aggressive factors (acid, pepsin, bile) overwhelm the defensive factors of the gastrointestinal mucosa (mucus and bicarbonate secretion, prostaglandins, blood flow, and the processes of restitution and regeneration after cellular injury). Over

90% of peptic ulcers are caused by infection with the bacterium *Helicobacter pylori* or by use of nonsteroidal anti-inflammatory drugs (NSAIDs). Drugs used in the treatment of acid-peptic disorders may be divided into two classes: agents that reduce intragastric acidity and agents that promote mucosal defense.

AGENTS THAT REDUCE INTRAGASTRIC ACIDITY

PHYSIOLOGY OF ACID SECRETION

The parietal cell contains receptors for gastrin (CCK-B), histamine (H_2), and acetylcholine (muscarinic, M_3) (Figure 62–1). When acetylcholine (from vagal postganglionic nerves) or gastrin (released from antral G cells into the blood) bind to the parietal cell receptors, they cause an increase in cytosolic calcium, which in turn stimulates protein kinases that stimulate acid secretion from a H^+/K^+-ATPase (the proton pump) on the canalicular surface.

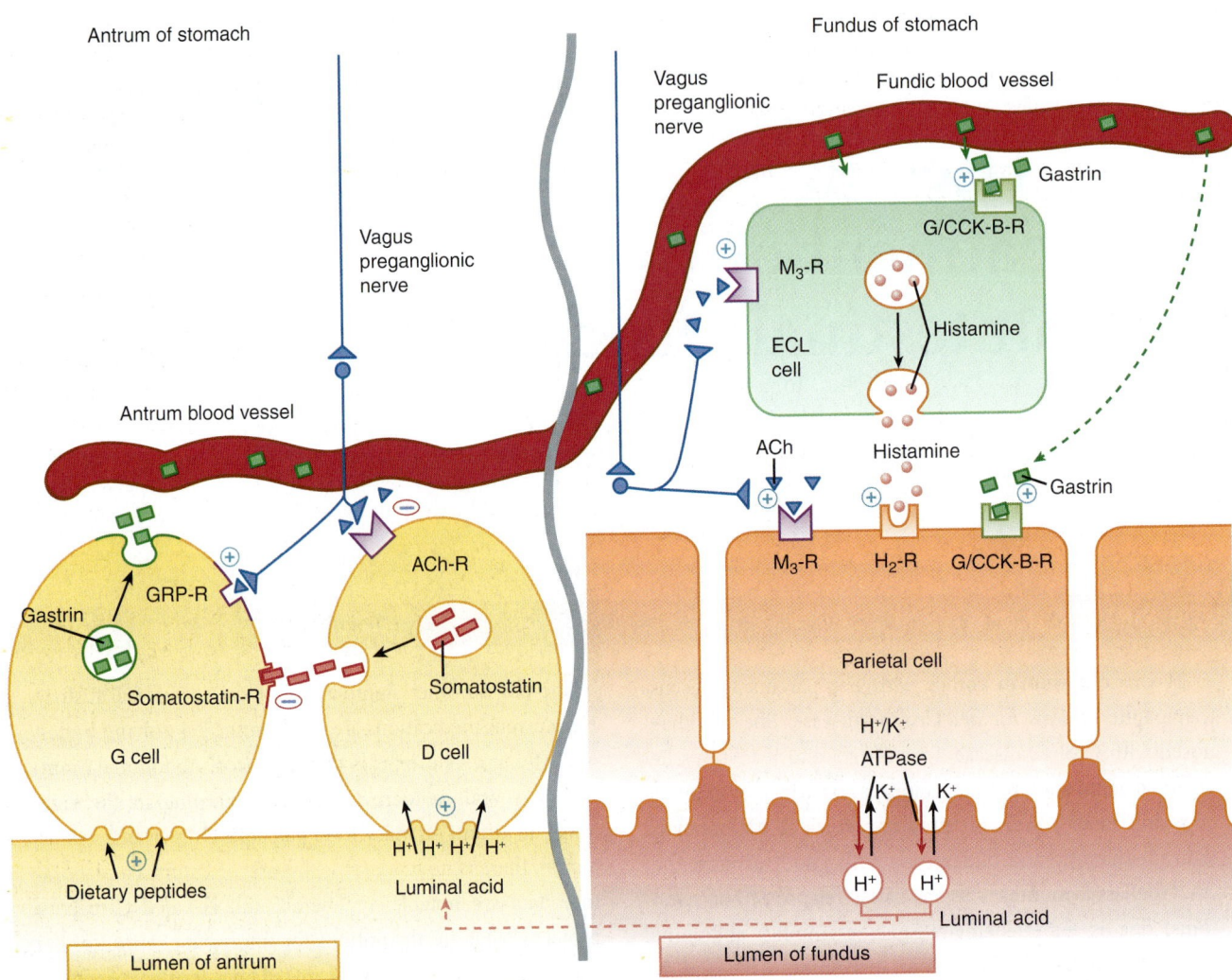

FIGURE 62–1 Schematic model for physiologic control of hydrogen ion (acid) secretion by the parietal cells of the gastric fundic glands. Parietal cells are stimulated to secrete acid (H^+) by gastrin (acting on gastrin/CCK-B receptor), acetylcholine (M_3 receptor), and histamine (H_2 receptor). Acid is secreted across the parietal cell canalicular membrane by the H^+/K^+-ATPase proton pump into the gastric lumen. Gastrin is secreted by antral G cells into blood vessels in response to intraluminal dietary peptides. Within the gastric body, gastrin passes from the blood vessels into the submucosal tissue of the fundic glands, where it binds to gastrin-CCK-B receptors on parietal cells and enterochromaffin-like (ECL) cells. The vagus nerve stimulates postganglionic neurons of the enteric nervous system to release acetylcholine (ACh), which binds to M_3 receptors on parietal cells and ECL cells. Stimulation of ECL cells by gastrin (CCK-B receptor) or acetylcholine (M_3 receptor) stimulates release of histamine. Within the gastric antrum, vagal stimulation of postganglionic enteric neurons enhances gastrin release directly by stimulation of antral G cells (through gastrin-releasing peptide, GRP) and indirectly by inhibition of somatostatin secretion from antral D cells. Acid secretion must eventually be turned off. Antral D cells are stimulated to release somatostatin by the rise in intraluminal H^+ concentration and by CCK that is released into the bloodstream by duodenal I cells in response to proteins and fats (not shown). Binding of somatostatin to receptors on adjacent antral G cells inhibits further gastrin release. ATPase, H^+/K^+-ATPase proton pump; CCK, cholecystokinin; M_3, muscarinic receptors.

In close proximity to the parietal cells are gut endocrine cells called *enterochromaffin-like (ECL) cells*. ECL cells also have receptors for gastrin and acetylcholine, which stimulate histamine release. Histamine binds to the H_2 receptor on the parietal cell, resulting in activation of adenylyl cyclase, which increases intracellular cyclic adenosine monophosphate (cAMP) and activates protein kinases that stimulate acid secretion by the H^+/K^+-ATPase. In humans, it is believed that the major effect of gastrin upon acid secretion is mediated indirectly through the release of histamine from ECL cells rather than through direct parietal cell stimulation. In contrast, acetylcholine provides potent direct parietal cell stimulation.

ANTACIDS

Antacids have been used for centuries in the treatment of patients with dyspepsia and acid-peptic disorders. They were the mainstay of treatment for acid-peptic disorders until the advent of H2–receptor antagonists and proton pump inhibitors. They continue to be used commonly by patients as nonprescription remedies for the treatment of intermittent heartburn and dyspepsia.

Antacids are weak bases that react with gastric hydrochloric acid to form a salt and water. Their principal mechanism of action is reduction of intragastric acidity. After a meal, approximately 45 mEq/h of hydrochloric acid is secreted. A single dose of 156 mEq of antacid given 1 hour after a meal effectively neutralizes gastric acid for up to 2 hours. However, the acid-neutralization capacity among different proprietary formulations of antacids is highly variable, depending on their rate of dissolution (tablet versus liquid), water solubility, rate of reaction with acid, and rate of gastric emptying.

Sodium bicarbonate (eg, baking soda, Alka Seltzer) reacts rapidly with hydrochloric acid (HCL) to produce carbon dioxide and sodium chloride. Formation of carbon dioxide results in gastric distention and belching. Unreacted alkali is readily absorbed, potentially causing metabolic alkalosis when given in high doses or to patients with renal insufficiency. Sodium chloride absorption may exacerbate fluid retention in patients with heart failure, hypertension, and renal insufficiency. **Calcium carbonate** (eg, Tums, Os-Cal) is less soluble and reacts more slowly than sodium bicarbonate with HCl to form carbon dioxide and calcium chloride ($CaCl_2$). Like sodium bicarbonate, calcium carbonate may cause belching or metabolic alkalosis. Calcium carbonate is used for a number of other indications apart from its antacid properties (see Chapter 42). Excessive doses of either sodium bicarbonate or calcium carbonate with calcium-containing dairy products can lead to hypercalcemia, renal insufficiency, and metabolic alkalosis (milk-alkali syndrome).

Formulations containing **magnesium hydroxide** or **aluminum hydroxide** react slowly with HCl to form magnesium chloride or aluminum chloride and water. Because no gas is generated, belching does not occur. Metabolic alkalosis is also uncommon because of the efficiency of the neutralization reaction. Because unabsorbed magnesium salts may cause an osmotic diarrhea and aluminum salts may cause constipation, these agents are commonly administered together in proprietary formulations (eg, Gelusil, Maalox, Mylanta) to minimize the impact on bowel function. Both magnesium and aluminum are absorbed and excreted by the kidneys. Hence, patients with renal insufficiency should not take these agents long-term.

All antacids may affect the absorption of other medications by binding the drug (reducing its absorption) or by increasing intragastric pH so that the drug's dissolution or solubility (especially weakly basic or acidic drugs) is altered. Therefore, antacids should not be given within 2 hours of doses of tetracyclines, fluoroquinolones, itraconazole, and iron.

H₂-RECEPTOR ANTAGONISTS

From their introduction in the 1970s until the early 1990s, H₂-receptor antagonists (commonly referred to as H₂ blockers) were the most commonly prescribed drugs in the world (see Clinical Uses). With the recognition of the role of *H pylori* in ulcer disease (which may be treated with appropriate antibacterial therapy) and the advent of proton pump inhibitors, the use of prescription H₂ blockers has declined markedly.

Chemistry & Pharmacokinetics

Four H₂ antagonists are in clinical use: cimetidine, ranitidine, famotidine, and nizatidine. All four agents are rapidly absorbed from the intestine. Cimetidine, ranitidine, and famotidine undergo first-pass hepatic metabolism resulting in a bioavailability of approximately 50%. Nizatidine has little first-pass metabolism. The serum half-lives of the four agents range from 1.1 to 4 hours; however, duration of action depends on the dose given (Table 62–1). H₂ antagonists are cleared by a combination of hepatic metabolism, glomerular filtration, and renal tubular secretion. Dose reduction is required in patients with moderate to severe renal (and possibly severe hepatic) insufficiency. In the elderly, there is a decline of up to 50% in drug clearance as well as a significant reduction in volume of distribution.

Cimetidine

TABLE 62–1 Clinical comparisons of H₂–receptor blockers.

Drug	Relative Potency	Dose to Achieve > 50% Acid Inhibition for 10 Hours	Usual Dose for Acute Duodenal or Gastric Ulcer	Usual Dose for Gastroesophageal Reflux Disease	Usual Dose for Prevention of Stress–Related Bleeding
Cimetidine	1	400–800 mg	800 mg HS or 400 mg bid	800 mg bid	50 mg/h continuous infusion
Ranitidine	4–10	150 mg	300 mg HS or 150 mg bid	150 mg bid	6.25 mg/h continuous infusion or 50 mg IV every 6–8 h
Nizatidine	4–10	150 mg	300 mg HS or 150 mg bid	150 mg bid	Not available
Famotidine	20–50	20 mg	40 mg HS or 20 mg bid	20 mg bid	20 mg IV every 12 h

BID, twice daily; HS, bedtime.

Pharmacodynamics

The H_2 antagonists exhibit competitive inhibition at the parietal cell H_2 receptor and suppress basal and meal-stimulated acid secretion (Figure 62–2) in a linear, dose-dependent manner. They are highly selective and do not affect H_1 or H_3 receptors (see Chapter 16). The volume of gastric secretion and the concentration of pepsin are also reduced.

H_2 antagonists reduce acid secretion stimulated by histamine as well as by gastrin and cholinomimetic agents through two mechanisms. First, histamine released from ECL cells by gastrin or vagal stimulation is blocked from binding to the parietal cell H_2 receptor. Second, direct stimulation of the parietal cell by gastrin or acetylcholine has a diminished effect on acid secretion in the presence of H_2-receptor blockade.

The potencies of the four H_2-receptor antagonists vary over a 50-fold range (Table 62–1). When given in usual prescription doses however, all inhibit 60–70% of total 24-hour acid secretion. H_2 antagonists are especially effective at inhibiting nocturnal acid secretion (which depends largely on histamine), but they have a modest impact on meal-stimulated acid secretion (which is stimulated by gastrin and acetylcholine as well as histamine). Therefore, nocturnal and fasting intragastric pH is raised to 4–5 but the impact on the daytime, meal-stimulated pH profile is less. Recommended prescription doses maintain greater than 50% acid inhibition for 10 hours; hence, these drugs are commonly given twice daily. At doses available in over-the-counter formulations, the duration of acid inhibition is less than 6 hours.

Clinical Uses

H_2-receptor antagonists continue to be prescribed but proton pump inhibitors (see below) are steadily replacing H_2 antagonists for most clinical indications. However, the over-the-counter preparations of the H_2 antagonists are heavily used by the public.

A. Gastroesophageal Reflux Disease (GERD)

Patients with infrequent heartburn or dyspepsia (fewer than 3 times per week) may take either antacids or intermittent H_2 antagonists. Because antacids provide rapid acid neutralization, they afford faster symptom relief than H_2 antagonists. However, the effect of antacids is short-lived (1–2 hours) compared with H_2 antagonists (6–10 hours). H_2 antagonists may be taken prophylactically before meals in an effort to reduce the likelihood of heartburn. Frequent heartburn is better treated with twice-daily H_2 antagonists (Table 62–1) or proton pump inhibitors. In patients with erosive esophagitis (approximately 50% of patients with GERD), H_2 antagonists afford healing in less than 50% of patients; hence proton pump inhibitors are preferred because of their superior acid inhibition.

B. Peptic Ulcer Disease

Proton pump inhibitors have largely replaced H_2 antagonists in the treatment of acute peptic ulcer disease. Nevertheless, H_2 antagonists are still sometimes used. Nocturnal acid suppression by H_2 antagonists affords effective ulcer healing in most patients

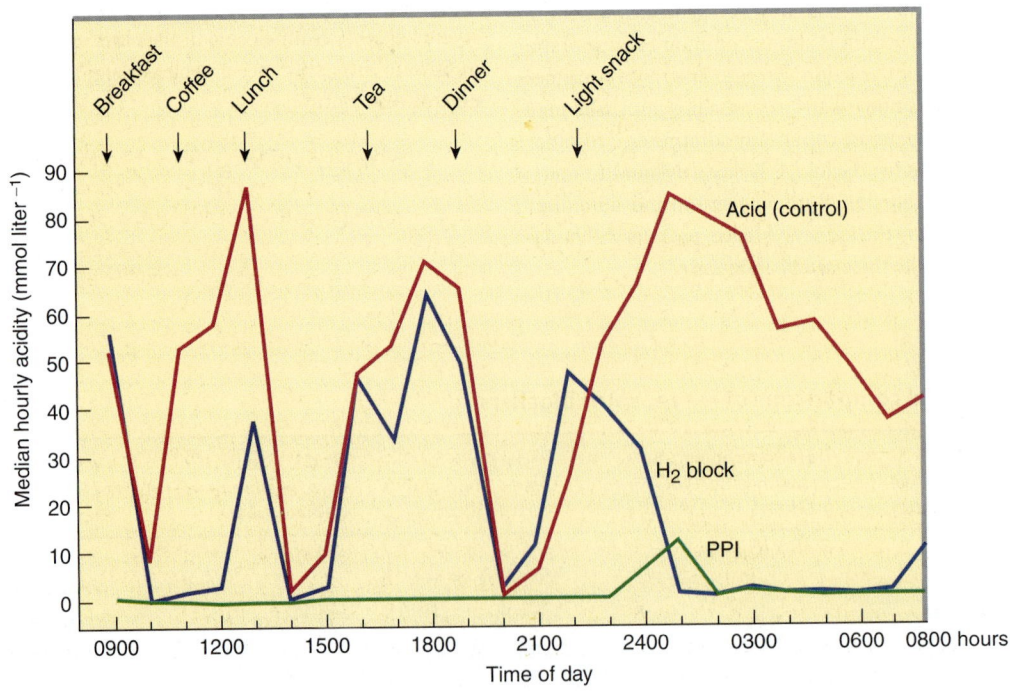

FIGURE 62–2 Twenty-four-hour median intragastric acidity pretreatment (red) and after 1 month of treatment with either ranitidine, 150 mg twice daily (blue, H_2 block), or omeprazole, 20 mg once daily (green, PPI). Note that H_2-receptor antagonists have a marked effect on nocturnal acid secretion but only a modest effect on meal-stimulated secretion. Proton pump inhibitors (PPIs) markedly suppress meal-stimulated and nocturnal acid secretion. (Redrawn from data in Lanzon-Miller S et al: Twenty-four-hour intragastric acidity and plasma gastrin concentration before and during treatment with either ranitidine or omeprazole. Aliment Pharmacol Ther 1987;1:239.)

with uncomplicated gastric and duodenal ulcers. Hence, all the agents may be administered once daily at bedtime, resulting in ulcer healing rates of more than 80–90% after 6–8 weeks of therapy. For patients with ulcers caused by aspirin or other NSAIDs, the NSAID should be discontinued. If the NSAID must be continued for clinical reasons despite active ulceration, a proton pump inhibitor should be given instead of an H_2 antagonist to more reliably promote ulcer healing. For patients with acute peptic ulcers caused by *H pylori*, H_2 antagonists no longer play a significant therapeutic role. *H pylori* should be treated with a 10- to 14-day course of therapy including a proton pump inhibitor and two antibiotics (see below). This regimen achieves ulcer healing and eradication of the infection in more than 90% of patients. For the minority of patients in whom *H pylori* cannot be successfully eradicated, H_2 antagonists may be given daily at bedtime in half of the usual ulcer therapeutic dose to prevent ulcer recurrence (eg, ranitidine, 150 mg; famotidine, 20 mg).

C. Nonulcer Dyspepsia

H_2 antagonists are commonly used as over-the-counter agents and prescription agents for treatment of intermittent dyspepsia not caused by peptic ulcer. However, benefit compared with placebo has never been convincingly demonstrated.

D. Prevention of Bleeding from Stress-Related Gastritis

Clinically important bleeding from upper gastrointestinal erosions or ulcers occurs in 1–5% of critically ill patients as a result of impaired mucosal defense mechanisms caused by poor perfusion. Although most critically ill patients have normal or decreased acid secretion, numerous studies have shown that agents that increase intragastric pH (H_2 antagonists or proton pump inhibitors) reduce the incidence of clinically significant bleeding. However, the optimal agent is uncertain at this time. For patients without a nasoenteric tube or with significant ileus, intravenous H_2 antagonists are preferable over intravenous proton pump inhibitors because of their proven efficacy and lower cost. Continuous infusions of H_2 antagonists are generally preferred to bolus infusions because they achieve more consistent, sustained elevation of intragastric pH.

Adverse Effects

H_2 antagonists are extremely safe drugs. Adverse effects occur in less than 3% of patients and include diarrhea, headache, fatigue, myalgias, and constipation. Some studies suggest that intravenous H_2 antagonists (or proton pump inhibitors) may increase the risk of nosocomial pneumonia in critically ill patients.

Mental status changes (confusion, hallucinations, agitation) may occur with administration of intravenous H_2 antagonists, especially in patients in the intensive care unit who are elderly or who have renal or hepatic dysfunction. These events may be more common with cimetidine. Mental status changes rarely occur in ambulatory patients.

Cimetidine inhibits binding of dihydrotestosterone to androgen receptors, inhibits metabolism of estradiol, and increases serum prolactin levels. When used long-term or in high doses, it may cause gynecomastia or impotence in men and galactorrhea in

women. These effects are specific to cimetidine and do not occur with the other H_2 antagonists.

Although there are no known harmful effects on the fetus, H_2 antagonists cross the placenta. Therefore, they should not be administered to pregnant women unless absolutely necessary. The H_2 antagonists are secreted into breast milk and may therefore affect nursing infants.

H_2 antagonists may rarely cause blood dyscrasias. Blockade of cardiac H_2 receptors may cause bradycardia, but this is rarely of clinical significance. Rapid intravenous infusion may cause bradycardia and hypotension through blockade of cardiac H_2 receptors; therefore, intravenous injections should be given over 30 minutes. H_2 antagonists rarely cause reversible abnormalities in liver chemistry.

Drug Interactions

Cimetidine interferes with several important hepatic cytochrome P450 drug metabolism pathways, including those catalyzed by CYP1A2, CYP2C9, CYP2D6, and CYP3A4 (see Chapter 4). Hence, the half-lives of drugs metabolized by these pathways may be prolonged. Ranitidine binds 4–10 times less avidly than cimetidine to cytochrome P450. Negligible interaction occurs with nizatidine and famotidine.

H_2 antagonists compete with creatinine and certain drugs (eg, procainamide) for renal tubular secretion. All of these agents except famotidine inhibit gastric first-pass metabolism of ethanol, especially in women. Although the importance of this is debated, increased bioavailability of ethanol could lead to increased blood ethanol levels.

PROTON PUMP INHIBITORS

Since their introduction in the late 1980s, these efficacious acid inhibitory agents have assumed the major role for the treatment of acid-peptic disorders. Proton pump inhibitors (PPIs) are now among the most widely prescribed drugs worldwide due to their outstanding efficacy and safety.

Chemistry & Pharmacokinetics

Six proton pump inhibitors are available for clinical use: **omeprazole, esomeprazole, lansoprazole, dexlansoprazole, rabeprazole,** and **pantoprazole.** All are substituted benzimidazoles that resemble H_2 antagonists in structure (Figure 62–3) but have a completely different mechanism of action. Omeprazole and lansoprazole are racemic mixtures of *R*- and *S*-isomers. Esomeprazole is the *S*-isomer of omeprazole and dexlansoprazole the *R*-isomer of lansoprazole. All are available in oral formulations. Esomeprazole and pantoprazole are also available in intravenous formulations (Table 62–2).

Proton pump inhibitors are administered as inactive prodrugs. To protect the acid-labile prodrug from rapid destruction within the gastric lumen, oral products are formulated for delayed release as acid-resistant, enteric-coated capsules or tablets. After passing through the stomach into the alkaline intestinal lumen, the enteric

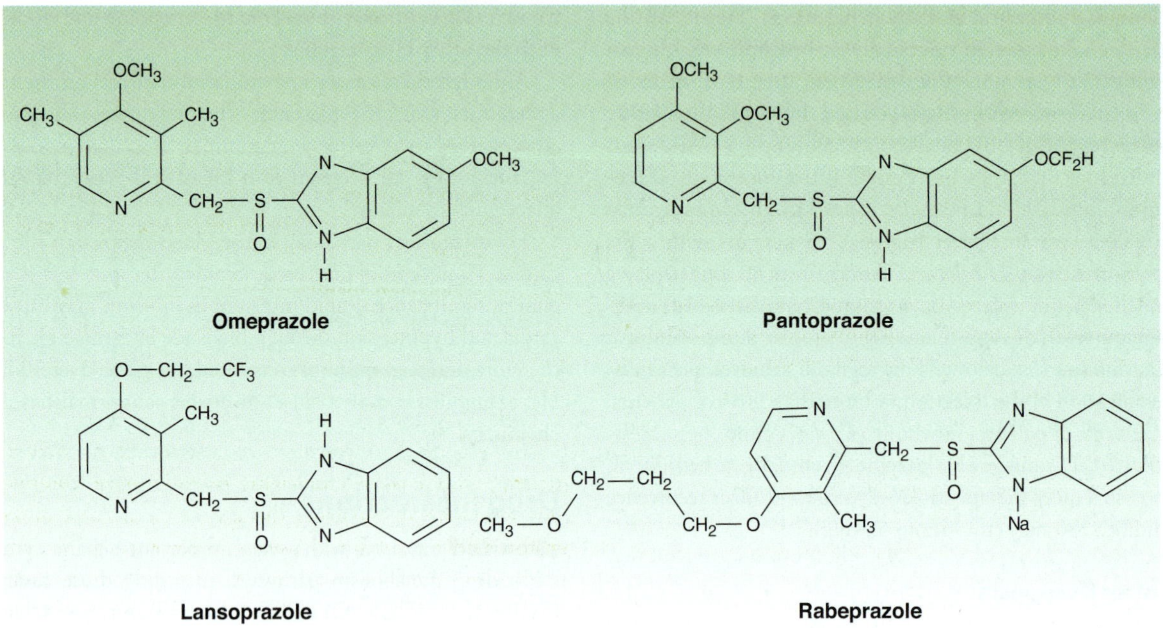

FIGURE 62–3 Molecular structure of the proton pump inhibitors: omeprazole, lansoprazole, pantoprazole, and the sodium salt of rabeprazole. Omeprazole and esomeprazole have the same chemical structure (see text).

coatings dissolve and the prodrug is absorbed. For children or patients with dysphagia or enteral feeding tubes, capsule formulations (but not tablets) may be opened and the microgranules mixed with apple or orange juice or mixed with soft foods (eg, applesauce). Lansoprazole is also available as a tablet formulation that disintegrates in the mouth, or it may be mixed with water and administered via oral syringe or enteral tube. Omeprazole is also available as a powder formulation (capsule or packet) that contains sodium bicarbonate (1100–1680 mg $NaHCO_3$; 304–460 mg of sodium) to protect the naked (non-enteric-coated) drug from acid degradation. When administered on an empty stomach by mouth or enteral tube, this "immediate-release" suspension results in rapid omeprazole absorption (T_{max} < 30 minutes) and onset of acid inhibition.

The proton pump inhibitors are lipophilic weak bases (pK$_a$ 4–5) and after intestinal absorption diffuse readily across lipid membranes into acidified compartments (eg, the parietal cell canaliculus). The prodrug rapidly becomes protonated within the canaliculus and is concentrated more than 1000-fold by Henderson-Hasselbalch trapping (see Chapter 1). There, it rapidly undergoes a molecular conversion to the active form, a reactive thiophilic sulfenamide cation, which forms a covalent disulfide bond with the H^+/K^+-ATPase, irreversibly inactivating the enzyme.

The pharmacokinetics of available proton pump inhibitors are shown in Table 62–2. Immediate-release omeprazole has a faster onset of acid inhibition than other oral formulations. Although differences in pharmacokinetic profiles may affect speed of onset and duration of acid inhibition in the first few days of therapy, they are of little clinical importance with continued daily administration. The bioavailability of all agents is decreased approximately 50% by food; hence, the drugs should be administered on

TABLE 62–2 Pharmacokinetics of proton pump inhibitors.

Drug	pK$_a$	Bioavailability (%)	$t_{1/2}$ (h)	T_{max} (h)	Usual Dosage for Peptic Ulcer or GERD
Omeprazole	4	40–65	0.5–1.0	1–3	20–40 mg qd
Esomeprazole	4	>80	1.5	1.6	20–40 mg qd
Lansoprazole	4	>80	1.0–2.0	1.7	30 mg qd
Dexlansoprazole	4	NA	1.0–2.0	5.0	30–60mg qd
Pantoprazole	3.9	77	1.0–1.9	2.5–4.0	40 mg qd
Rabeprazole	5	52	1.0–2.0	3.1	20 mg qd

GERD, gastroesophageal reflux disease; NA, data not available.

an empty stomach. In a fasting state, only 10% of proton pumps are actively secreting acid and susceptible to inhibition. Proton pump inhibitors should be administered approximately 1 hour before a meal (usually breakfast), so that the peak serum concentration coincides with the maximal activity of proton pump secretion. The drugs have a short serum half-life of about 1.5 hours, but acid inhibition lasts up to 24 hours owing to the irreversible inactivation of the proton pump. At least 18 hours are required for synthesis of new H^+/K^+-ATPase pump molecules. Because not all proton pumps are inactivated with the first dose of medication, up to 3–4 days of daily medication are required before the full acid-inhibiting potential is reached. Similarly, after stopping the drug, it takes 3–4 days for full acid secretion to return.

Proton pump inhibitors undergo rapid first-pass and systemic hepatic metabolism and have negligible renal clearance. Dose reduction is not needed for patients with renal insufficiency or mild to moderate liver disease but should be considered in patients with severe liver impairment. Although other proton pumps exist in the body, the H^+/K^+-ATPase appears to exist only in the parietal cell and is distinct structurally and functionally from other H^+-transporting enzymes.

The intravenous formulations of esomeprazole and pantoprazole have characteristics similar to those of the oral drugs. When given to a fasting patient, they inactivate acid pumps that are actively secreting, but they have no effect on pumps in quiescent, nonsecreting vesicles. Because the half-life of a single injection of the intravenous formulation is short, acid secretion returns several hours later as pumps move from the tubulovesicles to the canalicular surface. Thus, to provide maximal inhibition during the first 24–48 hours of treatment, the intravenous formulations must be given as a continuous infusion or as repeated bolus injections. The optimal dosing of intravenous proton pump inhibitors to achieve maximal blockade in fasting patients is not yet established.

From a pharmacokinetic perspective, proton pump inhibitors are ideal drugs: they have a short serum half-life, they are concentrated and activated near their site of action, and they have a long duration of action.

Pharmacodynamics

In contrast to H_2 antagonists, proton pump inhibitors inhibit both fasting and meal-stimulated secretion because they block the final common pathway of acid secretion, the proton pump. In standard doses, proton pump inhibitors inhibit 90–98% of 24-hour acid secretion (Figure 62–2). When administered at equivalent doses, the different agents show little difference in clinical efficacy. In a crossover study of patients receiving long-term therapy with five proton pump inhibitors, the mean 24-hour intragastric pH varied from 3.3 (pantoprazole, 40 mg) to 4.0 (esomeprazole, 40 mg) and the mean number of hours the pH was higher than 4 varied from 10.1 (pantoprazole, 40 mg) to 14.0 (esomeprazole, 40 mg). Although dexlansoprazole has a delayed-release formulation that results in a longer T_{max} and greater AUC than other proton pump inhibitors, it appears comparable to other agents in the ability to suppress acid secretion. This is because acid suppression is more dependent upon irreversible

inactivation of the proton pump than the pharmacokinetics of different agents.

Clinical Uses

A. Gastroesophageal Reflux Disease (GERD)

Proton pump inhibitors are the most effective agents for the treatment of nonerosive and erosive reflux disease, esophageal complications of reflux disease (peptic stricture or Barrett's esophagus), and extraesophageal manifestations of reflux disease. Once-daily dosing provides effective symptom relief and tissue healing in 85–90% of patients; up to 15% of patients require twice-daily dosing.

GERD symptoms recur in over 80% of patients within 6 months after discontinuation of a proton pump inhibitor. For patients with erosive esophagitis or esophageal complications, long-term daily maintenance therapy with a full-dose or half-dose proton pump inhibitor is usually needed. Many patients with nonerosive GERD may be treated successfully with intermittent courses of proton pump inhibitors or H_2 antagonists taken as needed ("on demand") for recurrent symptoms.

In current clinical practice, many patients with symptomatic GERD are treated empirically with medications without prior endoscopy, ie, without knowledge of whether the patient has erosive or nonerosive reflux disease. Empiric treatment with proton pump inhibitors provides sustained symptomatic relief in 70–80% of patients, compared with 50–60% with H_2 antagonists. Because of recent cost reductions, proton pump inhibitors are being used increasingly as first-line therapy for patients with symptomatic GERD.

Sustained acid suppression with twice-daily proton pump inhibitors for at least 3 months is used to treat extraesophageal complications of reflux disease (asthma, chronic cough, laryngitis, and noncardiac chest pain).

B. Peptic Ulcer Disease

Compared with H_2 antagonists, proton pump inhibitors afford more rapid symptom relief and faster ulcer healing for duodenal ulcers and, to a lesser extent, gastric ulcers. All the pump inhibitors heal more than 90% of duodenal ulcers within 4 weeks and a similar percentage of gastric ulcers within 6–8 weeks.

1. H pylori-associated ulcers—For *H pylori*-associated ulcers, there are two therapeutic goals: to heal the ulcer and to eradicate the organism. The most effective regimens for *H pylori* eradication are combinations of two antibiotics and a proton pump inhibitor. Proton pump inhibitors promote eradication of *H pylori* through several mechanisms: direct antimicrobial properties (minor) and—by raising intragastric pH—lowering the minimal inhibitory concentrations of antibiotics against *H pylori*. The best treatment regimen consists of a 14-day regimen of "triple therapy": a proton pump inhibitor twice daily; clarithromycin, 500 mg twice daily; and either amoxicillin, 1 g twice daily, or metronidazole, 500 mg twice daily. After completion of triple therapy, the proton pump inhibitor should be continued once daily for a total of 4–6 weeks to ensure complete ulcer healing. Alternatively, 10 days of "sequential treatment" consisting on days 1–5 of a proton pump inhibitor twice daily plus amoxicillin, 1 g twice daily, and followed on days 6–10 by five additional days of a proton pump inhibitor twice daily, plus clarithromycin, 500 mg twice daily, and tinidazole, 500 mg twice daily, has been shown to be a highly effective treatment regimen.

2. NSAID-associated ulcers—For patients with ulcers caused by aspirin or other NSAIDs, either H₂ antagonists or proton pump inhibitors provide rapid ulcer healing so long as the NSAID is discontinued; however continued use of the NSAID impairs ulcer healing. In patients with NSAID-induced ulcers who require continued NSAID therapy, treatment with a once- or twice-daily proton pump inhibitor more reliably promotes ulcer healing.

Asymptomatic peptic ulceration develops in 10–20% of people taking frequent NSAIDs, and ulcer-related complications (bleeding, perforation) develop in 1–2% of persons per year. Proton pump inhibitors taken once daily are effective in reducing the incidence of ulcers and ulcer complications in patients taking aspirin or other NSAIDs.

3. Prevention of rebleeding from peptic ulcers—In patients with acute gastrointestinal bleeding due to peptic ulcers, the risk of rebleeding from ulcers that have a visible vessel or adherent clot is increased. Rebleeding of this subset of high-risk ulcers is reduced significantly with proton pump inhibitors administered for 3–5 days either as high-dose oral therapy (eg, omeprazole, 40 mg orally twice daily) or as a continuous intravenous infusion. It is believed that an intragastric pH higher than 6 may enhance coagulation and platelet aggregation. The optimal dose of intravenous proton pump inhibitor needed to achieve and maintain this level of near-complete acid inhibition is unknown; however, initial bolus administration of esomeprazole or pantoprazole (80 mg) followed by constant infusion (8 mg/h) is commonly recommended.

C. Nonulcer Dyspepsia

Proton pump inhibitors have modest efficacy for treatment of non-ulcer dyspepsia, benefiting 10–20% more patients than placebo. Despite their use for this indication, superiority to H₂ antagonists (or even placebo) has not been conclusively demonstrated.

D. Prevention of Stress-Related Mucosal Bleeding

As discussed previously (see H₂-Receptor Antagonists) proton pump inhibitors (given orally, by nasogastric tube, or by intravenous infusions) may be administered to reduce the risk of clinically significant stress-related mucosal bleeding in critically ill patients. The only proton pump inhibitor approved by the Food and Drug Administration (FDA) for this indication is an oral immediate-release omeprazole formulation, which is administered by nasogastric tube twice daily on the first day, then once daily. For patients with nasoenteric tubes, immediate-release omeprazole may be preferred to intravenous H₂ antagonists or other proton pump inhibitors because of comparable efficacy, lower cost, and ease of administration.

For patients without a nasoenteric tube or with significant ileus, intravenous H₂ antagonists are preferred to intravenous proton pump inhibitors because of their proven efficacy and lower cost. Although proton pump inhibitors are increasingly used, there are no controlled trials demonstrating efficacy or optimal dosing.

E. Gastrinoma and Other Hypersecretory Conditions

Patients with isolated gastrinomas are best treated with surgical resection. In patients with metastatic or unresectable gastrinomas, massive acid hypersecretion results in peptic ulceration, erosive esophagitis, and malabsorption. Previously, these patients required vagotomy and extraordinarily high doses of H₂ antagonists, which still resulted in suboptimal acid suppression. With proton pump inhibitors, excellent acid suppression can be achieved in all patients. Dosage is titrated to reduce basal acid output to less than 5–10 mEq/h. Typical doses of omeprazole are 60–120 mg/d.

Adverse Effects

A. General

Proton pump inhibitors are extremely safe. Diarrhea, headache, and abdominal pain are reported in 1–5% of patients, although the frequency of these events is only slightly increased compared with placebo. Increasing cases of acute interstitial nephritis have been reported. Proton pump inhibitors do not have teratogenicity in animal models; however, safety during pregnancy has not been established.

B. Nutrition

Acid is important in releasing vitamin B₁₂ from food. A minor reduction in oral cyanocobalamin absorption occurs during proton pump inhibition, potentially leading to subnormal B₁₂ levels with prolonged therapy. Acid also promotes absorption of food-bound minerals (non-heme iron, insoluble calcium salts, magnesium). Several case-control studies have suggested a modest increase in the risk of hip fracture in patients taking proton pump inhibitors over a long term compared with matched controls. Although a causal relationship is unproven, proton pump inhibitors may reduce calcium absorption or inhibit osteoclast function. Pending further studies, patients who require long-term proton pump inhibitors—especially those with risk factors for osteoporosis—should have monitoring of bone density and should be provided calcium supplements. Cases of severe, life-threatening hypomagnesemia with secondary hypocalcemia due to proton pump inhibitors have been reported; however, the mechanism of action is unknown.

C. Respiratory and Enteric Infections

Gastric acid is an important barrier to colonization and infection of the stomach and intestine from ingested bacteria. Increases in gastric bacterial concentrations are detected in patients taking proton pump inhibitors, which is of unknown clinical significance. Some studies have reported an increased risk of both community-acquired respiratory infections and nosocomial pneumonia among patients taking proton pump inhibitors.

There is a 2- to 3-fold increased risk for hospital- and community-acquired *Clostridium difficile* infection in patients taking proton pump inhibitors. There also is a small increased risk of other enteric infections (eg, *Salmonella, Shigella, E coli, Campylobacter*), which should be considered particularly when traveling in under-developed countries.

D. Potential Problems Due to Increased Serum Gastrin

Gastrin levels are regulated by intragastric acidity. Acid suppression alters normal feedback inhibition so that median serum gastrin levels rise 1.5- to 2-fold in patients taking proton pump inhibitors. Although gastrin levels remain within normal limits in most patients, they exceed 500 pg/mL (normal, < 100 pg/mL) in 3%. Upon stopping the drug, the levels normalize within 4 weeks. The rise in serum gastrin levels may stimulate hyperplasia of ECL and parietal cells, which may cause transient rebound acid hypersecretion with increased dyspepsia or heartburn after drug discontinuation, which abate within 2–4 weeks after gastrin and acid secretion normalize. In female rats given proton pump inhibitors for prolonged periods, hypergastrinemia caused gastric carcinoid tumors that developed in areas of ECL hyperplasia. Although humans who take proton pump inhibitors for a long time also may exhibit ECL hyperplasia, carcinoid tumor formation has not been documented. At present, routine monitoring of serum gastrin levels is not recommended in patients receiving prolonged proton pump inhibitor therapy.

E. Other Potential Problems Due to Decreased Gastric Acidity

Among patients infected with *H pylori*, long-term acid suppression leads to increased chronic inflammation in the gastric body and decreased inflammation in the antrum. Concerns have been raised that increased gastric inflammation may accelerate gastric gland atrophy (atrophic gastritis) and intestinal metaplasia—known risk factors for gastric adenocarcinoma. A special FDA Gastrointestinal Advisory Committee concluded that there is no evidence that prolonged proton pump inhibitor therapy produces the kind of atrophic gastritis (multifocal atrophic gastritis) or intestinal metaplasia that is associated with increased risk of adenocarcinoma. Routine testing for *H pylori* is not recommended in patients who require long-term proton pump inhibitor therapy. Long-term proton pump inhibitor therapy is associated with the development of small benign gastric fundic-gland polyps in a small number of patients, which may disappear after stopping the drug and are of uncertain clinical significance.

Drug Interactions

Decreased gastric acidity may alter absorption of drugs for which intragastric acidity affects drug bioavailability, eg, ketoconazole, itraconazole, digoxin, and atazanavir. All proton pump inhibitors are metabolized by hepatic P450 cytochromes, including CYP2C19 and CYP3A4. Because of the short half-lives of proton pump inhibitors, clinically significant drug interactions are rare. Omeprazole may inhibit the metabolism of warfarin, diazepam, and phenytoin. Esomeprazole also may decrease metabolism of diazepam. Lansoprazole may enhance clearance of theophylline. Rabeprazole and pantoprazole have no significant drug interactions.

The FDA has issued a warning about a potentially important adverse interaction between clopidogrel and proton pump inhibitors. Clopidogrel is a prodrug that requires activation by the hepatic P450 CYP2C19 isoenzyme, which also is involved to varying degrees in the metabolism of proton pump inhibitors (especially omeprazole, esomeprazole, lansoprazole, and dexlansoprazole). Thus, proton pump inhibitors could reduce clopidogrel activation (and its antiplatelet action) in some patients. Several large retrospective studies have reported an increased incidence of serious cardiovascular events in patients taking clopidogrel and a proton pump inhibitor. In contrast, three smaller prospective randomized trials have not detected an increased risk. Pending further studies, proton pump inhibitors should be prescribed to patients taking clopidogrel only if they have an increased risk of gastrointestinal bleeding or require them for chronic gastroesophageal reflux or peptic ulcer disease, in which case agents with minimal CYP2C19 inhibition (pantoprazole or rabeprazole) are preferred.

MUCOSAL PROTECTIVE AGENTS

The gastroduodenal mucosa has evolved a number of defense mechanisms to protect itself against the noxious effects of acid and pepsin. Both mucus and epithelial cell-cell tight junctions restrict back diffusion of acid and pepsin. Epithelial bicarbonate secretion establishes a pH gradient within the mucous layer in which the pH ranges from 7 at the mucosal surface to 1–2 in the gastric lumen. Blood flow carries bicarbonate and vital nutrients to surface cells. Areas of injured epithelium are quickly repaired by restitution, a process in which migration of cells from gland neck cells seals small erosions to reestablish intact epithelium. Mucosal prostaglandins appear to be important in stimulating mucus and bicarbonate secretion and mucosal blood flow. A number of agents that potentiate these mucosal defense mechanisms are available for the prevention and treatment of acid-peptic disorders.

SUCRALFATE

Chemistry & Pharmacokinetics

Sucralfate is a salt of sucrose complexed to sulfated aluminum hydroxide. In water or acidic solutions it forms a viscous, tenacious paste that binds selectively to ulcers or erosions for up to 6 hours. Sucralfate has limited solubility, breaking down into sucrose sulfate (strongly negatively charged) and an aluminum salt. Less than 3% of intact drug and aluminum is absorbed from the intestinal tract; the remainder is excreted in the feces.

Pharmacodynamics

A variety of beneficial effects have been attributed to sucralfate, but the precise mechanism of action is unclear. It is believed that the negatively charged sucrose sulfate binds to positively charged proteins in the base of ulcers or erosion, forming a physical barrier that restricts further caustic damage and stimulates mucosal prostaglandin and bicarbonate secretion.

Clinical Uses

Sucralfate is administered in a dosage of 1 g four times daily on an empty stomach (at least 1 hour before meals). At present, its clinical uses are limited. Sucralfate (administered as a slurry through a nasogastric tube) reduces the incidence of clinically significant upper gastrointestinal bleeding in critically ill patients hospitalized in the intensive care unit, although it is slightly less effective than intravenous H_2 antagonists. Sucralfate is still used by many clinicians for prevention of stress-related bleeding because of concerns that acid inhibitory therapies (antacids, H_2 antagonists, and proton pump inhibitors) may increase the risk of nosocomial pneumonia.

Adverse Effects

Because it is not absorbed, sucralfate is virtually devoid of systemic adverse effects. Constipation occurs in 2% of patients due to the aluminum salt. Because a small amount of aluminum is absorbed, it should not be used for prolonged periods in patients with renal insufficiency.

Drug Interactions

Sucralfate may bind to other medications, impairing their absorption.

PROSTAGLANDIN ANALOGS

Chemistry & Pharmacokinetics

The human gastrointestinal mucosa synthesizes a number of prostaglandins (see Chapter 18); the primary ones are prostaglandins E and F. **Misoprostol,** a methyl analog of PGE_1, has been approved for gastrointestinal conditions. After oral administration, it is rapidly absorbed and metabolized to a metabolically active free acid. The serum half-life is less than 30 minutes; hence, it must be administered 3–4 times daily. It is excreted in the urine; however, dose reduction is not needed in patients with renal insufficiency.

Pharmacodynamics

Misoprostol has both acid inhibitory and mucosal protective properties. It is believed to stimulate mucus and bicarbonate secretion and enhance mucosal blood flow. In addition, it binds to a prostaglandin receptor on parietal cells, reducing histamine-stimulated cAMP production and causing modest acid inhibition. Prostaglandins have a variety of other actions, including stimulation of intestinal electrolyte and fluid secretion, intestinal motility, and uterine contractions.

Clinical Uses

Peptic ulcers develop in approximately 10–20% of patients who receive long-term NSAID therapy (see Proton Pump Inhibitors,

above). Misoprostol reduces the incidence of NSAID-induced ulcers to less than 3% and the incidence of ulcer complications by 50%. It is approved for prevention of NSAID-induced ulcers in high-risk patients; however, misoprostol has never achieved widespread use owing to its high adverse-effect profile and need for multiple daily dosing. As discussed, proton pump inhibitors may be as effective as and better tolerated than misoprostol for this indication. Cyclooxygenase-2-selective NSAIDs, which may have less gastrointestinal toxicity (see Chapter 36), offer another option for patients at high risk for NSAID-induced complications.

Adverse Effects & Drug Interactions

Diarrhea and cramping abdominal pain occur in 10–20% of patients. Because misoprostol stimulates uterine contractions (see Chapter 18), it should not be used during pregnancy or in women of childbearing potential unless they have a negative serum pregnancy test and are compliant with effective contraceptive measures. No significant drug interactions are reported.

BISMUTH COMPOUNDS

Chemistry & Pharmacokinetics

Two bismuth compounds are available: **bismuth subsalicylate,** a nonprescription formulation containing bismuth and salicylate, and **bismuth subcitrate potassium.** In the USA, bismuth subcitrate is available only as a combination prescription product that also contains metronidazole and tetracycline for the treatment of *H pylori.* Bismuth subsalicylate undergoes rapid dissociation within the stomach, allowing absorption of salicylate. Over 99% of the bismuth appears in the stool. Although minimal (< 1%), bismuth is absorbed; it is stored in many tissues and has slow renal excretion. Salicylate (like aspirin) is readily absorbed and excreted in the urine.

Pharmacodynamics

The precise mechanisms of action of bismuth are unknown. Bismuth coats ulcers and erosions, creating a protective layer against acid and pepsin. It may also stimulate prostaglandin, mucus, and bicarbonate secretion. Bismuth subsalicylate reduces stool frequency and liquidity in acute infectious diarrhea, due to salicylate inhibition of intestinal prostaglandin and chloride secretion. Bismuth has direct antimicrobial effects and binds enterotoxins, accounting for its benefit in preventing and treating traveler's diarrhea. Bismuth compounds have direct antimicrobial activity against *H pylori.*

Clinical Uses

In spite of the lack of comparative trials, nonprescription bismuth compounds (eg, Pepto-Bismol, Kaopectate) are widely used by patients for the nonspecific treatment of dyspepsia and acute diarrhea. Bismuth subsalicylate also is used for the prevention of traveler's diarrhea (30 mL or 2 tablets four times daily).

Bismuth compounds are used in 4-drug regimens for the eradication of *H pylori* infection. One regimen consists of a proton pump inhibitor twice daily combined with bismuth subsalicylate (2 tablets; 262 mg each), tetracycline (250–500 mg), and metronidazole (500 mg) four times daily for 10–14 days. Another regimen consists of a proton pump inhibitor twice daily combined with three capsules of a combination prescription formulation (each capsule containing bismuth subcitrate 140 mg, metronidazole 125 mg, and tetracycline 125 mg) taken four times daily for 10 days. Although these are effective, standard "triple therapy" regimens (ie, proton pump inhibitor, clarithromycin, and amoxicillin or metronidazole twice daily for 14 days) generally are preferred for first-line therapy because of twice-daily dosing and superior compliance. Bismuth-based quadruple therapies are commonly used as second-line therapies.

Adverse Effects

All bismuth formulations have excellent safety profiles. Bismuth causes harmless blackening of the stool, which may be confused with gastrointestinal bleeding. Liquid formulations may cause harmless darkening of the tongue. Bismuth agents should be used for short periods only and should be avoided in patients with renal insufficiency. Prolonged usage of some bismuth compounds may rarely lead to bismuth toxicity, resulting in encephalopathy (ataxia, headaches, confusion, seizures). However, such toxicity is not reported with bismuth subsalicylate or bismuth citrate. High dosages of bismuth subsalicylate may lead to salicylate toxicity.

■ DRUGS STIMULATING GASTROINTESTINAL MOTILITY

Drugs that can selectively stimulate gut motor function (**prokinetic** agents) have significant potential clinical usefulness. Agents that increase lower esophageal sphincter pressures may be useful for GERD. Drugs that improve gastric emptying may be helpful for gastroparesis and postsurgical gastric emptying delay. Agents that stimulate the small intestine may be beneficial for postoperative ileus or chronic intestinal pseudo-obstruction. Finally, agents that enhance colonic transit may be useful in the treatment of constipation. Unfortunately, only a limited number of agents in this group are available for clinical use at this time.

PHYSIOLOGY OF THE ENTERIC NERVOUS SYSTEM

The enteric nervous system (see also Chapter 6) is composed of interconnected networks of ganglion cells and nerve fibers mainly located in the submucosa (submucosal plexus) and between the circular and longitudinal muscle layers (myenteric plexus). These networks give rise to nerve fibers that connect with the mucosa and muscle. Although extrinsic sympathetic and parasympathetic nerves project onto the submucosal and myenteric plexuses, the enteric

nervous system can independently regulate gastrointestinal motility and secretion. Extrinsic primary afferent neurons project via the dorsal root ganglia or vagus nerve to the central nervous system (Figure 62–4). Release of serotonin (5-HT) from intestinal mucosa enterochromaffin (EC) cells stimulates 5-HT₃ receptors on the extrinsic afferent nerves, stimulating nausea, vomiting, or abdominal pain. Serotonin also stimulates submucosal 5-HT$_{1P}$ receptors of the intrinsic primary afferent nerves (IPANs), which contain calcitonin gene-related peptide (CGRP) and acetylcholine and project to myenteric plexus interneurons. 5-HT₄ receptors on the presynaptic terminals of the IPANs appear to enhance release of CGRP or acetylcholine. The myenteric interneurons are important in controlling the peristaltic reflex, promoting release of excitatory mediators proximally and inhibitory mediators distally. Motilin may stimulate excitatory neurons or muscle cells directly. Dopamine acts as an inhibitory neurotransmitter in the gastrointestinal tract, decreasing the intensity of esophageal and gastric contractions.

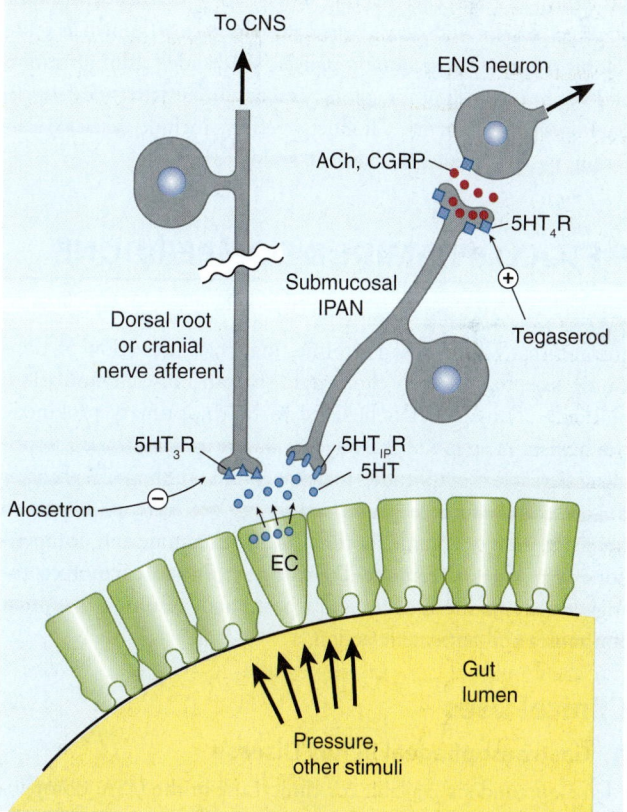

FIGURE 62–4 Release of serotonin (5-HT) by enterochromaffin (EC) cells from gut distention stimulates submucosal intrinsic primary afferent neurons (IPANs) via 5-HT$_{1P}$ receptors and extrinsic primary afferent neurons via 5-HT₃ receptors (5-HT$_{1P}$R, 5-HT₃R). Submucosal IPANs activate the enteric neurons responsible for peristaltic and secretory reflex activity. Stimulation of 5-HT₄ receptors (5-HT₄R) on presynaptic terminals of IPANs enhances release of acetylcholine (ACh) and calcitonin gene-related peptide (CGRP), promoting reflex activity. CNS, central nervous system; ENS, enteric nervous system. (Redrawn from Gershon MD: Serotonin and its implication for the management of irritable bowel syndrome. Rev Gastroenterol Dis 2003;3[Suppl 2]:S25.)

Although there are at least 14 serotonin receptor subtypes, 5-HT drug development for gastrointestinal applications to date has focused on **5-HT$_3$-receptor antagonists and 5-HT$_4$-receptor agonists.** These agents—which have effects on gastrointestinal motility and visceral afferent sensation—are discussed under Drugs Used for the Treatment of Irritable Bowel Syndrome and Antiemetic Agents. Other drugs acting on 5-HT receptors are discussed in Chapters 16, 29, and 30.

CHOLINOMIMETIC AGENTS

Cholinomimetic agonists such as bethanechol stimulate muscarinic M$_3$ receptors on muscle cells and at myenteric plexus synapses (see Chapter 7). Bethanechol was used in the past for the treatment of GERD and gastroparesis. Owing to multiple cholinergic effects and the advent of less toxic agents, it is now seldom used. The acetylcholinesterase inhibitor neostigmine can enhance gastric, small intestine, and colonic emptying. Intravenous neostigmine has enjoyed a resurgence in clinical usage for the treatment of hospitalized patients with acute large bowel distention (known as acute colonic pseudo-obstruction or Ogilvie's syndrome). Administration of 2 mg results in prompt colonic evacuation of flatus and feces in the majority of patients. Cholinergic effects include excessive salivation, nausea, vomiting, diarrhea, and bradycardia.

METOCLOPRAMIDE & DOMPERIDONE

Metoclopramide and domperidone are dopamine D$_2$-receptor antagonists. Within the gastrointestinal tract activation of dopamine receptors inhibits cholinergic smooth muscle stimulation; blockade of this effect is believed to be the primary prokinetic mechanism of action of these agents. These agents increase esophageal peristaltic amplitude, increase lower esophageal sphincter pressure, and enhance gastric emptying but have no effect on small intestine or colonic motility. Metoclopramide and domperidone also block dopamine D$_2$ receptors in the chemoreceptor trigger zone of the medulla (area postrema), resulting in potent antinausea and antiemetic action.

Clinical Uses

A. Gastroesophageal Reflux Disease

Metoclopramide is available for clinical use in the USA; domperidone is available in many other countries. These agents are sometimes used in the treatment of symptomatic GERD but are not effective in patients with erosive esophagitis. Because of the superior efficacy and safety of antisecretory agents in the treatment of heartburn, prokinetic agents are used mainly in combination with antisecretory agents in patients with regurgitation or refractory heartburn.

B. Impaired Gastric Emptying

These agents are widely used in the treatment of patients with delayed gastric emptying due to postsurgical disorders (vagotomy, antrectomy)

and diabetic gastroparesis. Metoclopramide is sometimes administered in hospitalized patients to promote advancement of nasoenteric feeding tubes from the stomach into the duodenum.

C. Nonulcer Dyspepsia

These agents lead to symptomatic improvement in a small number of patients with chronic dyspepsia.

D. Prevention of Vomiting

Because of their potent antiemetic action, metoclopramide and domperidone are used for the prevention and treatment of emesis.

E. Postpartum Lactation Stimulation

Domperidone is sometimes recommended to promote postpartum lactation (see also Adverse Effects).

Adverse Effects

The most common adverse effects of metoclopramide involve the central nervous system. Restlessness, drowsiness, insomnia, anxiety, and agitation occur in 10–20% of patients, especially the elderly. Extrapyramidal effects (dystonias, akathisia, parkinsonian features) due to central dopamine receptor blockade occur acutely in 25% of patients given high doses and in 5% of patients receiving long-term therapy. Tardive dyskinesia, sometimes irreversible, has developed in patients treated for a prolonged period with metoclopramide. For this reason, long-term use should be avoided unless absolutely necessary, especially in the elderly. Elevated prolactin levels (caused by both metoclopramide and domperidone) can cause galactorrhea, gynecomastia, impotence, and menstrual disorders.

Domperidone is extremely well tolerated. Because it does not cross the blood-brain barrier to a significant degree, neuropsychiatric and extrapyramidal effects are rare.

MACROLIDES

Macrolide antibiotics such as **erythromycin** directly stimulate motilin receptors on gastrointestinal smooth muscle and promote the onset of a migrating motor complex. Intravenous erythromycin (3 mg/kg) is beneficial in some patients with gastroparesis; however, tolerance rapidly develops. It may be used in patients with acute upper gastrointestinal hemorrhage to promote gastric emptying of blood before endoscopy.

■ LAXATIVES

The overwhelming majority of people do not need laxatives; yet they are self-prescribed by a large portion of the population. For most people, intermittent constipation is best prevented with a high-fiber diet, adequate fluid intake, regular exercise, and the heeding of nature's call. Patients not responding to dietary changes or fiber supplements should undergo medical evaluation before initiating long-term laxative treatment. Laxatives may be classified by their major mechanism of action, but many work through more than one mechanism.

BULK-FORMING LAXATIVES

Bulk-forming laxatives are indigestible, hydrophilic colloids that absorb water, forming a bulky, emollient gel that distends the colon and promotes peristalsis. Common preparations include natural plant products (**psyllium, methylcellulose**) and synthetic fibers (**polycarbophil**). Bacterial digestion of plant fibers within the colon may lead to increased bloating and flatus.

STOOL SURFACTANT AGENTS (SOFTENERS)

These agents soften stool material, permitting water and lipids to penetrate. They may be administered orally or rectally. Common agents include **docusate** (oral or enema) and **glycerin suppository**. In hospitalized patients, docusate is commonly prescribed to prevent constipation and minimize straining. **Mineral oil** is a clear, viscous oil that lubricates fecal material, retarding water absorption from the stool. It is used to prevent and treat fecal impaction in young children and debilitated adults. It is not palatable but may be mixed with juices. Aspiration can result in a severe lipid pneumonitis. Long-term use can impair absorption of fat-soluble vitamins (A, D, E, K).

OSMOTIC LAXATIVES

The colon can neither concentrate nor dilute fecal fluid: fecal water is isotonic throughout the colon. Osmotic laxatives are soluble but nonabsorbable compounds that result in increased stool liquidity due to an obligate increase in fecal fluid.

Nonabsorbable Sugars or Salts

These agents may be used for the treatment of acute constipation or the prevention of chronic constipation. **Magnesium hydroxide (milk of magnesia)** is a commonly used osmotic laxative. It should not be used for prolonged periods in patients with renal insufficiency due to the risk of hypermagnesemia. **Sorbitol** and **lactulose** are nonabsorbable sugars that can be used to prevent or treat chronic constipation. These sugars are metabolized by colonic bacteria, producing severe flatus and cramps.

High doses of osmotically active agents produce prompt bowel evacuation (purgation) within 1–3 hours. The rapid movement of water into the distal small bowel and colon leads to a high volume of liquid stool followed by rapid relief of constipation. The most commonly used purgatives are **magnesium citrate** and **sodium phosphate**. Sodium phosphate is available as a nonprescription liquid formulation and by prescription as a tablet formulation. When taking these agents, it is very important that patients maintain adequate hydration by taking increased oral liquids to compensate for fecal fluid loss. Sodium phosphate frequently causes hyperphosphatemia, hypocalcemia, hypernatremia, and hypokalemia. Although these electrolyte abnormalities are clinically insignificant in most patients, they may lead to cardiac arrhythmias or acute renal failure due to tubular deposition of calcium phosphate (nephrocalcinosis). Sodium phosphate preparations should not be used in patients who are frail or elderly, have renal insufficiency, have significant cardiac disease, or are unable to maintain adequate hydration during bowel preparation.

Balanced Polyethylene Glycol

Lavage solutions containing **polyethylene glycol (PEG)** are used for complete colonic cleansing before gastrointestinal endoscopic procedures. These balanced, isotonic solutions contain an inert, nonabsorbable, osmotically active sugar (PEG) with sodium sulfate, sodium chloride, sodium bicarbonate, and potassium chloride. The solution is designed so that no significant intravascular fluid or electrolyte shifts occur. Therefore, they are safe for all patients. The solution should be ingested rapidly (2–4 L over 2–4 hours) to promote bowel cleansing. For treatment or prevention of chronic constipation, smaller doses of PEG powder may be mixed with water or juices (17 g/8 oz) and ingested daily. In contrast to sorbitol or lactulose, PEG does not produce significant cramps or flatus.

STIMULANT LAXATIVES

Stimulant laxatives (cathartics) induce bowel movements through a number of poorly understood mechanisms. These include direct stimulation of the enteric nervous system and colonic electrolyte and fluid secretion. There has been concern that long-term use of cathartics could lead to dependence and destruction of the myenteric plexus, resulting in colonic atony and dilation. More recent research suggests that long-term use of these agents probably is safe in most patients. Cathartics may be required on a long-term basis, especially in patients who are neurologically impaired and in bed-bound patients in long-term care facilities.

Anthraquinone Derivatives

Aloe, senna, and **cascara** occur naturally in plants. These laxatives are poorly absorbed and after hydrolysis in the colon, produce a bowel movement in 6–12 hours when given orally and within 2 hours when given rectally. Chronic use leads to a characteristic brown pigmentation of the colon known as "melanosis coli." There has been some concern that these agents may be carcinogenic, but epidemiologic studies do not suggest a relation to colorectal cancer.

Diphenylmethane Derivatives

Bisacodyl is available in tablet and suppository formulations for the treatment of acute and chronic constipation. It also is used in conjunction with PEG solutions for colonic cleansing prior to colonoscopy. It induces a bowel movement within 6–10 hours when given orally and 30–60 minutes when taken rectally. It has minimal systemic absorption and appears to be safe for acute and long-term use. Phenolphthalein, another agent in this class, was removed from the market owing to concerns about possible cardiac toxicity.

CHLORIDE CHANNEL ACTIVATOR

Lubiprostone is a prostanoic acid derivative labeled for use in chronic constipation and irritable bowel syndrome (IBS) with predominant constipation. It acts by stimulating the type 2 chloride channel (ClC-2) in the small intestine. This increases chloride-rich fluid secretion into the intestine, which stimulates intestinal motility and shortens intestinal transit time. Over 50% of patients experience a bowel movement within 24 hours of taking one dose. There appears to be no loss of efficacy with long-term therapy. After discontinuation of the drug, constipation may return to its pretreatment severity. Lubiprostone has minimal systemic absorption but is designated category C for pregnancy because of increased fetal loss in guinea pigs. Lubiprostone may cause nausea in up to 30% of patients due to delayed gastric emptying.

OPIOID RECEPTOR ANTAGONISTS

Acute and chronic therapy with opioids may cause constipation by decreasing intestinal motility, which results in prolonged transit time and increased absorption of fecal water (see Chapter 31). Use of opioids after surgery for treatment of pain as well as endogenous opioids also may prolong the duration of postoperative ileus. These effects are mainly mediated through intestinal mu (μ)-opioid receptors. Two selective antagonists of the μ-opioid receptor are commercially available: **methylnaltrexone** bromide and **alvimopan.** Because these agents do not readily cross the blood-brain barrier, they inhibit peripheral μ-opioid receptors without impacting analgesic effects within the central nervous system. Methylnaltrexone is approved for the treatment of opioid-induced constipation in patients receiving palliative care for advanced illness who have had inadequate response to other agents. It is administered as a subcutaneous injection (0.15 mg/kg) every 2 days. Alvimopan is approved for short-term use to shorten the period of postoperative ileus in hospitalized patients who have undergone small or large bowel resection. Alvimopan (12 mg capsule) is administered orally within 5 hours before surgery and twice daily after surgery until bowel function has recovered, but for no more than 7 days. Because of possible cardiovascular toxicity, alvimopan currently is restricted to short-term use in hospitalized patients only.

SEROTONIN 5-HT₄-RECEPTOR AGONISTS

Stimulation of 5-HT$_4$ receptors on the presynaptic terminal of submucosal intrinsic primary afferent nerves enhances the release of their neurotransmitters, including calcitonin gene-related peptide, which stimulate second-order enteric neurons to promote the peristaltic reflex (Figure 62–4). These enteric neurons stimulate proximal bowel contraction (via acetylcholine and substance P) and distal bowel relaxation (via nitric oxide and vasoactive intestinal peptide).

Tegaserod is a serotonin 5-HT$_4$ partial agonist that has high affinity for 5-HT$_4$ receptors but no appreciable binding to 5-HT$_3$ or dopamine receptors. Tegaserod was approved for the treatment of patients with chronic constipation and IBS with predominant constipation. Although tegaserod initially appeared to be extremely safe, it was voluntarily removed from the general market in 2007 because of an increased incidence of serious cardiovascular events. These adverse events have been attributed to inhibition of the 5-HT$_{1B}$ receptor. Another partial 5-HT$_4$ agonist, **cisapride,** was also associated with an increased incidence of cardiovascular events that was attributed to inhibition of cardiac hERG (human ether-a-go-go-related gene) K$^+$ channels, which resulted in QT$_c$ prolongation in some patients.

Prucalopride is a high-affinity 5-HT$_4$ agonist that is available in Europe (but not in the USA) for the treatment of chronic constipation in women. In contrast to cisapride and tegaserod, it does not appear to have significant affinities for either hERG channels or 5-HT$_{1B}$. In three 12-week clinical trials of patients with severe chronic constipation, it resulted in a significant increase in bowel movements compared with placebo. The long-term efficacy and safety of this agent require further study.

GUANYLATE CYCLASE C AGONISTS

Linaclotide is a poorly absorbed 14-amino-acid peptide that binds to the guanylate cylase C receptor on the luminal surface of intestinal enterocytes, activating the cystic fibrosis transmembrane conductance channel and stimulating intestinal fluid secretion. Preliminary results of phase 3 clinical trials confirm its efficacy in patients with chronic constipation. Further studies are anticipated.

■ ANTIDIARRHEAL AGENTS

Antidiarrheal agents may be used safely in patients with mild to moderate acute diarrhea. However, these agents should not be used in patients with bloody diarrhea, high fever, or systemic toxicity because of the risk of worsening the underlying condition. They should be discontinued in patients whose diarrhea is worsening despite therapy. Antidiarrheals are also used to control chronic diarrhea caused by such conditions as irritable bowel syndrome (IBS) or inflammatory bowel disease (IBD).

OPIOID AGONISTS

As previously noted, opioids have significant constipating effects (see Chapter 31). They increase colonic phasic segmenting activity through inhibition of presynaptic cholinergic nerves in the submucosal and myenteric plexuses and lead to increased colonic transit time and fecal water absorption. They also decrease mass colonic movements and the gastrocolic reflex. Although all opioids have antidiarrheal effects, central nervous system effects and potential for addiction limit the usefulness of most.

Loperamide is a nonprescription opioid agonist that does not cross the blood-brain barrier and has no analgesic properties or potential for addiction. Tolerance to long-term use has not been reported. It is typically administered in doses of 2 mg taken one to four times daily. **Diphenoxylate** is a prescription opioid agonist that has no analgesic properties in standard doses; however, higher doses have central nervous system effects, and prolonged use can lead to opioid dependence. Commercial preparations commonly contain small amounts of atropine to discourage overdosage (2.5 mg diphenoxylate with 0.025 mg atropine). The anticholinergic properties of atropine may contribute to the antidiarrheal action.

COLLOIDAL BISMUTH COMPOUNDS

See the section under Mucosal Protective Agents in earlier text.

BILE SALT-BINDING RESINS

Conjugated bile salts are normally absorbed in the terminal ileum. Disease of the terminal ileum (eg, Crohn's disease) or surgical resection leads to malabsorption of bile salts, which may cause colonic secretory diarrhea. The bile salt-binding resins **cholestyramine, colestipol,** or **colesevelam,** may decrease diarrhea caused by excess fecal bile acids (see Chapter 35). These products come in a variety of powder and pill formulations that may be taken one to three times daily before meals. Adverse effects include bloating, flatulence, constipation, and fecal impaction. In patients with diminished circulating bile acid pools, further removal of bile acids may lead to an exacerbation of fat malabsorption. Cholestyramine and colestipol bind a number of drugs and reduce their absorption; hence, they should not be given within 2 hours of other drugs. Colesevelam does not appear to have significant effects on absorption of other drugs.

OCTREOTIDE

Somatostatin is a 14-amino-acid peptide that is released in the gastrointestinal tract and pancreas from paracrine cells, D cells, and enteric nerves as well as from the hypothalamus (see Chapter 37). Somatostatin is a key regulatory peptide that has many physiologic effects:

1. It inhibits the secretion of numerous hormones and transmitters, including gastrin, cholecystokinin, glucagon, growth hormone, insulin, secretin, pancreatic polypeptide, vasoactive intestinal peptide, and 5-HT.
2. It reduces intestinal fluid secretion and pancreatic secretion.
3. It slows gastrointestinal motility and inhibits gallbladder contraction.
4. It reduces portal and splanchnic blood flow.
5. It inhibits secretion of some anterior pituitary hormones.

The clinical usefulness of somatostatin is limited by its short half-life in the circulation (3 minutes) when it is administered by intravenous injection. **Octreotide** is a synthetic octapeptide with actions similar to somatostatin. When administered intravenously, it has a serum half-life of 1.5 hours. It also may be administered by subcutaneous injection, resulting in a 6- to 12-hour duration of action. A longer-acting formulation is available for once-monthly depot intramuscular injection.

Clinical Uses

A. Inhibition of Endocrine Tumor Effects

Two gastrointestinal neuroendocrine tumors (carcinoid, VIPoma) cause secretory diarrhea and systemic symptoms such as flushing and wheezing. For patients with advanced symptomatic tumors that cannot be completely removed by surgery, octreotide decreases secretory diarrhea and systemic symptoms through inhibition of hormonal secretion and may slow tumor progression.

B. Other Causes of Diarrhea

Octreotide inhibits intestinal secretion and has dose-related effects on bowel motility. In low doses (50 mcg subcutaneously), it stimulates motility, whereas at higher doses (eg, 100–250 mcg subcutaneously), it inhibits motility. Octreotide is effective in higher doses for the treatment of diarrhea due to vagotomy or dumping syndrome as well as for diarrhea caused by short bowel syndrome or AIDS. Octreotide has been used in low doses (50 mcg subcutaneously) to stimulate small bowel motility in patients with small bowel bacterial overgrowth or intestinal pseudo-obstruction secondary to scleroderma.

C. Other Uses

Because it inhibits pancreatic secretion, octreotide may be of value in patients with pancreatic fistula. The role of octreotide in the treatment of pituitary tumors (eg, acromegaly) is discussed in Chapter 37. Octreotide is sometimes used in gastrointestinal bleeding (see below).

Adverse Effects

Impaired pancreatic secretion may cause steatorrhea, which can lead to fat-soluble vitamin deficiency. Alterations in gastrointestinal motility cause nausea, abdominal pain, flatulence, and diarrhea. Because of inhibition of gallbladder contractility and alterations in fat absorption, long-term use of octreotide can cause formation of sludge or gallstones in over 50% of patients, which rarely results in the development of acute cholecystitis. Because octreotide alters the balance among insulin, glucagon, and growth hormone, hyperglycemia or, less frequently, hypoglycemia (usually mild) can occur. Prolonged treatment with octreotide may result in hypothyroidism. Octreotide also can cause bradycardia.

■ DRUGS USED IN THE TREATMENT OF IRRITABLE BOWEL SYNDROME

IBS is an idiopathic chronic, relapsing disorder characterized by abdominal discomfort (pain, bloating, distention, or cramps) in association with alterations in bowel habits (diarrhea, constipation, or both). With episodes of abdominal pain or discomfort, patients note a change in the frequency or consistency of their bowel movements.

Pharmacologic therapies for IBS are directed at relieving abdominal pain and discomfort and improving bowel function.

For patients with predominant diarrhea, antidiarrheal agents, especially loperamide, are helpful in reducing stool frequency and fecal urgency. For patients with predominant constipation, fiber supplements may lead to softening of stools and reduced straining; however, increased gas production may exacerbate bloating and abdominal discomfort. Consequently, osmotic laxatives, especially milk of magnesia, are commonly used to soften stools and promote increased stool frequency.

For chronic abdominal pain, low doses of tricyclic antidepressants (eg, amitriptyline or desipramine, 10–50 mg/d) appear to be helpful (see Chapter 30). At these doses, these agents have no effect on mood but may alter central processing of visceral afferent information. The anticholinergic properties of these agents also may have effects on gastrointestinal motility and secretion, reducing stool frequency and liquidity. Finally, tricyclic antidepressants may alter receptors for enteric neurotransmitters such as serotonin, affecting visceral afferent sensation.

Several other agents are available that are specifically intended for the treatment of IBS.

ANTISPASMODICS (ANTICHOLINERGICS)

Some agents are promoted as providing relief of abdominal pain or discomfort through antispasmodic actions. However, small or large bowel spasm has not been found to be an important cause of symptoms in patients with IBS. Antispasmodics work primarily through anticholinergic activities. Commonly used medications in this class include **dicyclomine** and **hyoscyamine** (see Chapter 8). These drugs inhibit muscarinic cholinergic receptors in the enteric plexus and on smooth muscle. The efficacy of antispasmodics for relief of abdominal symptoms has never been convincingly demonstrated. At low doses, they have minimal autonomic effects. However, at higher doses they exhibit significant additional anticholinergic effects, including dry mouth, visual disturbances, urinary retention, and constipation. For these reasons, antispasmodics are infrequently used.

SEROTONIN 5-HT$_3$-RECEPTOR ANTAGONISTS

5-HT$_3$ receptors in the gastrointestinal tract activate visceral afferent pain sensation via extrinsic sensory neurons from the gut to the spinal cord and central nervous system. Inhibition of afferent gastrointestinal 5-HT$_3$ receptors may reduce unpleasant visceral afferent sensation, including nausea, bloating, and pain. Blockade of central 5-HT$_3$ receptors also reduces the central response to visceral afferent stimulation. In addition, 5-HT$_3$-receptor blockade on the terminals of enteric cholinergic neurons inhibits colonic motility, especially in the left colon, increasing total colonic transit time.

Alosetron is a 5-HT$_3$ antagonist that has been approved for the treatment of patients with severe IBS with diarrhea (Figure 62–5). Four other 5-HT$_3$ antagonists (ondansetron, granisetron, dolasetron, and palonosetron) have been approved for the prevention and treatment of nausea and vomiting (see Antiemetics); however, their efficacy in the treatment of IBS has not been determined. The differences between these 5-HT$_3$ antagonists that determine their pharmacodynamic effects have not been well studied.

Pharmacokinetics & Pharmacodynamics

Alosetron is a highly potent and selective antagonist of the 5-HT$_3$ receptor. It is rapidly absorbed from the gastrointestinal tract with a bioavailability of 50–60% and has a plasma half-life of 1.5 hours but a much longer duration of effect. It undergoes extensive hepatic cytochrome P450 metabolism with renal excretion of most metabolites. Alosetron binds with higher affinity and dissociates more slowly from 5-HT$_3$ receptors than other 5-HT$_3$ antagonists, which may account for its long duration of action.

Clinical Uses

Alosetron is approved for the treatment of women with severe IBS in whom diarrhea is the predominant symptom ("diarrhea-predominant IBS"). Its efficacy in men has not been established. In a dosage of 1 mg once or twice daily, it reduces IBS-related lower abdominal pain, cramps, urgency, and diarrhea. Approximately 50–60% of patients report adequate relief of pain and discomfort with alosetron compared with 30–40% of patients treated with placebo. It also leads to a reduction in the mean number of bowel movements per day and improvement in stool consistency. Alosetron has not been evaluated for the treatment of other causes of diarrhea.

Adverse Events

In contrast to the excellent safety profile of other 5-HT$_3$-receptor antagonists, alosetron is associated with rare but serious gastrointestinal toxicity. Constipation occurs in up to 30% of patients with diarrhea-predominant IBS, requiring discontinuation of the drug in 10%. Serious complications of constipation requiring hospitalization or surgery have occurred in 1 of every 1000 patients. Episodes of ischemic colitis—some fatal—have been reported in up to 3 per 1000 patients. Given the seriousness of these adverse events, alosetron is restricted to women with severe diarrhea-predominant IBS who have not responded to conventional therapies and who have been educated about the relative risks and benefits.

Drug Interactions

Despite being metabolized by a number of CYP enzymes, alosetron does not appear to have clinically significant interactions with other drugs.

SEROTONIN 5-HT$_4$-RECEPTOR AGONISTS

The pharmacology of tegaserod was discussed previously under Laxatives. This agent was approved for the short-term treatment of women with IBS who had predominant constipation. Controlled studies demonstrated a modest improvement (approximately 15%)

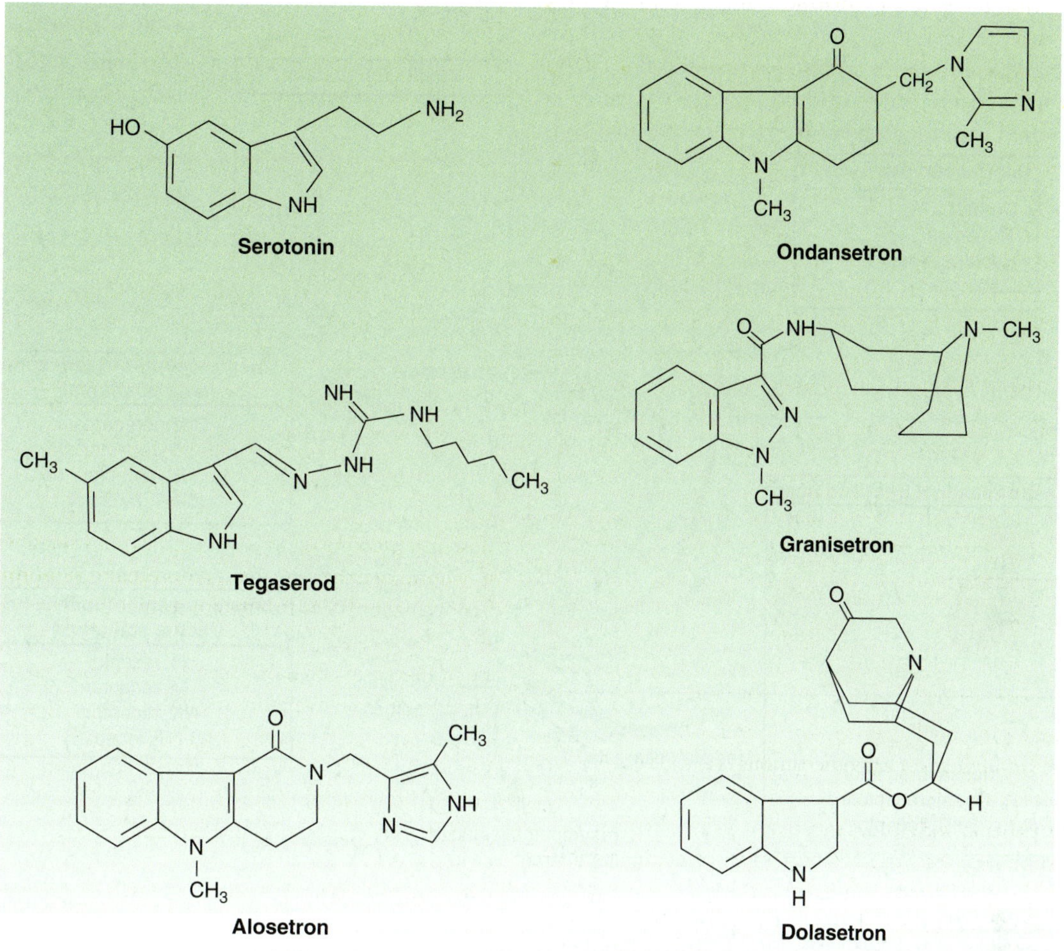

FIGURE 62–5 Chemical structure of serotonin; the 5-HT$_3$ antagonists ondansetron, granisetron, dolasetron, and alosetron; and the 5-HT$_4$ partial agonist tegaserod.

in patient global satisfaction and a reduction in severity of pain and bloating in patients treated with tegaserod, 6 mg twice daily, compared with placebo. Owing to an increased number of cardiovascular deaths observed in post-marketing studies in patients taking tegaserod, it was voluntarily removed from the market.

CHLORIDE CHANNEL ACTIVATOR

As discussed previously, lubiprostone is a prostanoic acid derivative that stimulates the type 2 chloride channel (ClC-2) in the small intestine and is used in the treatment of chronic constipation. Lubiprostone recently was approved for the treatment of women with IBS with predominant constipation. Its efficacy for men with IBS is unproven. The approved dose for IBS is 8 mcg twice daily (compared with 24 mcg twice daily for chronic constipation). Lubiprostone has not been compared with other less expensive laxatives (eg, milk of magnesia). Lubiprostone is listed as category C for pregnancy and should be avoided in women of child-bearing age.

■ ANTIEMETIC AGENTS

Nausea and vomiting may be manifestations of a wide variety of conditions, including adverse effects from medications; systemic disorders or infections; pregnancy; vestibular dysfunction; central nervous system infection or increased pressure; peritonitis; hepatobiliary disorders; radiation or chemotherapy; and gastrointestinal obstruction, dysmotility, or infections.

PATHOPHYSIOLOGY

The brainstem "vomiting center" is a loosely organized neuronal region within the lateral medullary reticular formation and coordinates the complex act of vomiting through interactions with cranial nerves VIII and X and neural networks in the nucleus tractus solitarius that control respiratory, salivatory, and vasomotor centers. High concentrations of muscarinic M$_1$, histamine H$_1$, neurokinin 1 (NK$_1$), and serotonin 5-HT$_3$ receptors have been identified in the vomiting center (Figure 62–6).

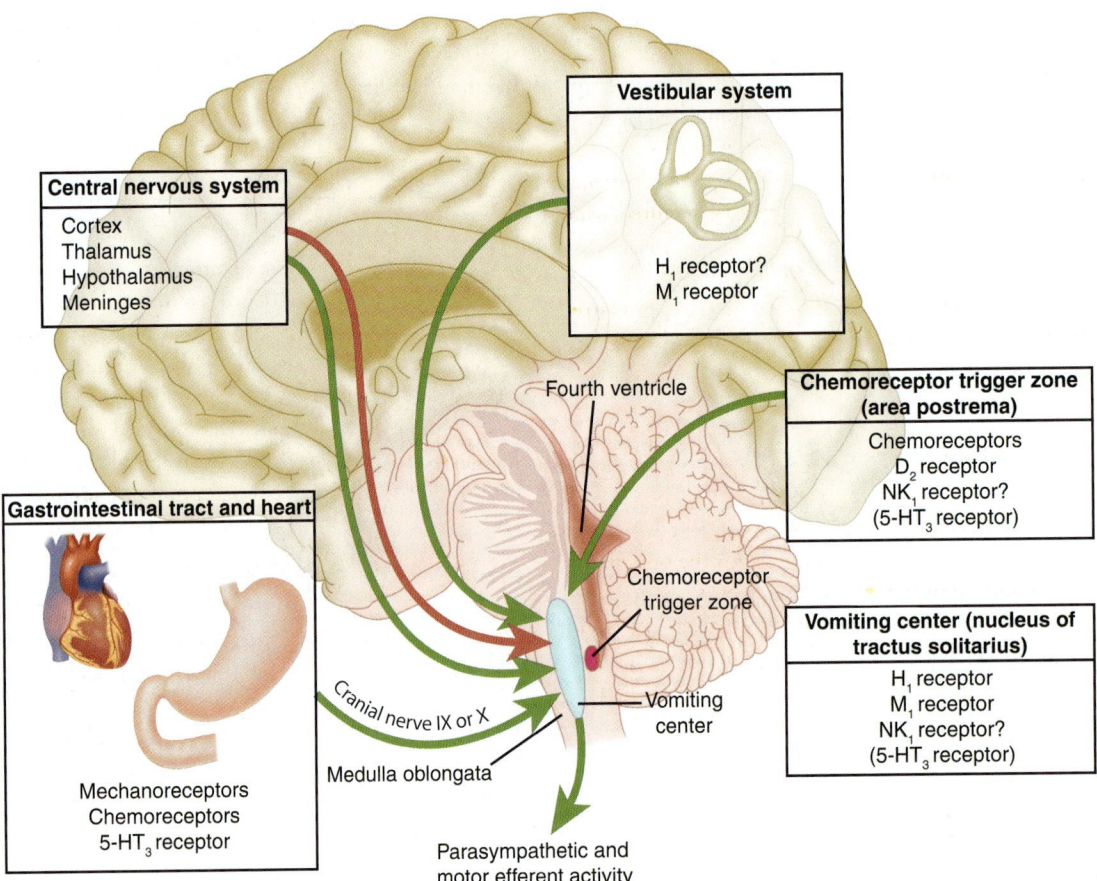

FIGURE 62–6 Neurologic pathways involved in pathogenesis of nausea and vomiting (see text). (Modified and reproduced, with permission, from Krakauer EL et al: Case records of the Massachusetts General Hospital. N Engl J Med 2005;352:817.)

There are four important sources of afferent input to the vomiting center:

1. The "chemoreceptor trigger zone" or area postrema is located at the caudal end of the fourth ventricle. This is outside the blood-brain barrier but is accessible to emetogenic stimuli in the blood or cerebrospinal fluid. The chemoreceptor trigger zone is rich in dopamine D_2 receptors and opioid receptors, and possibly serotonin 5-HT_3 receptors and NK_1 receptors.

2. The vestibular system is important in motion sickness via cranial nerve VIII. It is rich in muscarinic M_1 and histamine H_1 receptors.

3. Vagal and spinal afferent nerves from the gastrointestinal tract are rich in 5-HT_3 receptors. Irritation of the gastrointestinal mucosa by chemotherapy, radiation therapy, distention, or acute infectious gastroenteritis leads to release of mucosal serotonin and activation of these receptors, which stimulate vagal afferent input to the vomiting center and chemoreceptor trigger zone.

4. The central nervous system plays a role in vomiting due to psychiatric disorders, stress, and anticipatory vomiting prior to cancer chemotherapy.

Identification of the different neurotransmitters involved with emesis has allowed development of a diverse group of antiemetic agents that have affinity for various receptors. Combinations of antiemetic agents with different mechanisms of action are often used, especially in patients with vomiting due to chemotherapeutic agents.

SEROTONIN 5-HT_3 ANTAGONISTS

Pharmacokinetics & Pharmacodynamics

Selective 5-HT_3-receptor antagonists have potent antiemetic properties that are mediated in part through central 5-HT_3-receptor blockade in the vomiting center and chemoreceptor trigger zone but mainly through blockade of peripheral 5-HT_3 receptors on extrinsic intestinal vagal and spinal afferent nerves. The antiemetic action of these agents is restricted to emesis attributable to vagal stimulation (eg, postoperative) and chemotherapy; other emetic stimuli such as motion sickness are poorly controlled.

Four agents are available in the USA: **ondansetron, granisetron, dolasetron, and palonosetron.** (Tropisetron is another agent available outside the USA.) The first three agents (ondansetron, granisetron, and dolasetron, Figure 62–5) have a serum half-life of 4–9 hours and may be administered once daily by oral or intravenous routes. All three drugs have comparable efficacy and tolerability when administered at equipotent doses. Palonosetron is a newer intravenous agent that has greater affinity for the 5-HT$_3$ receptor and a long serum half-life of 40 hours. All four drugs undergo extensive hepatic metabolism and are eliminated by renal and hepatic excretion. However, dose reduction is not required in geriatric patients or patients with renal insufficiency. For patients with hepatic insufficiency, dose reduction may be required with ondansetron.

5-HT$_3$-receptor antagonists do not inhibit dopamine or muscarinic receptors. They do not have effects on esophageal or gastric motility but may slow colonic transit.

Clinical Uses

A. Chemotherapy-Induced Nausea and Vomiting

5-HT$_3$-receptor antagonists are the primary agents for the prevention of acute chemotherapy-induced nausea and emesis. When used alone, these drugs have little or no efficacy for the prevention of delayed nausea and vomiting (ie, occurring > 24 hours after chemotherapy). The drugs are most effective when given as a single dose by intravenous injection 30 minutes prior to administration of chemotherapy in the following doses: ondansetron, 8 mg; granisetron, 1 mg; dolasetron, 100 mg; or palonosetron, 0.25 mg. A single oral dose given 1 hour before chemotherapy may be equally effective in the following regimens: ondansetron 8 mg twice daily or 24 mg once; granisetron, 2 mg; dolasetron, 100 mg. Although 5-HT$_3$-receptor antagonists are effective as single agents for the prevention of chemotherapy-induced nausea and vomiting, their efficacy is enhanced by combination therapy with a corticosteroid (dexamethasone) and NK$_1$-receptor antagonist (see below).

B. Postoperative and Postradiation Nausea and Vomiting

5-HT$_3$-receptor antagonists are used to prevent or treat postoperative nausea and vomiting. Because of adverse effects and increased restrictions on the use of other antiemetic agents, 5-HT$_3$-receptor antagonists are increasingly used for this indication. They are also effective in the prevention and treatment of nausea and vomiting in patients undergoing radiation therapy to the whole body or abdomen.

Adverse Effects

The 5-HT$_3$-receptor antagonists are well-tolerated agents with excellent safety profiles. The most commonly reported adverse effects are headache, dizziness, and constipation. All four agents cause a small but statistically significant prolongation of the QT interval, but this is most pronounced with dolasetron. Although cardiac arrhythmias have not been linked to dolasetron, it should not be administered to patients with prolonged QT or in conjunction with other medications that may prolong the QT interval (see Chapter 14).

Drug Interactions

No significant drug interactions have been reported with 5-HT$_3$-receptor antagonists. All four agents undergo some metabolism by the hepatic cytochrome P450 system but they do not appear to affect the metabolism of other drugs. However, other drugs may reduce hepatic clearance of the 5-HT$_3$-receptor antagonists, altering their half-life.

CORTICOSTEROIDS

Corticosteroids (dexamethasone, methylprednisolone) have antiemetic properties, but the basis for these effects is unknown. The pharmacology of this class of drugs is discussed in Chapter 39. These agents appear to enhance the efficacy of 5-HT$_3$-receptor antagonists for prevention of acute and delayed nausea and vomiting in patients receiving moderately to highly emetogenic chemotherapy regimens. Although a number of corticosteroids have been used, dexamethasone, 8–20 mg intravenously before chemotherapy, followed by 8 mg/d orally for 2–4 days, is commonly administered.

NEUROKININ RECEPTOR ANTAGONISTS

Neurokinin 1 (NK$_1$)-receptor antagonists have antiemetic properties that are mediated through central blockade in the area postrema. **Aprepitant** (an oral formulation) is a highly selective NK$_1$-receptor antagonist that crosses the blood-brain barrier and occupies brain NK$_1$ receptors. It has no affinity for serotonin, dopamine, or corticosteroid receptors. **Fosaprepitant** is an intravenous formulation that is converted within 30 minutes after infusion to aprepitant.

Pharmacokinetics

The oral bioavailability of aprepitant is 65%, and the serum half-life is 12 hours. Aprepitant is metabolized by the liver, primarily by the CYP3A4 pathway.

Clinical Uses

Aprepitant is used in combination with 5-HT$_3$-receptor antagonists and corticosteroids for the prevention of acute and delayed nausea and vomiting from highly emetogenic chemotherapeutic regimens. Combined therapy with aprepitant, a 5-HT$_3$-receptor antagonist, and dexamethasone prevents acute emesis in 80–90% of patients compared with less than 70% treated without aprepitant. Prevention of delayed emesis occurs in more than 70% of patients receiving combined therapy versus 30–50% treated without aprepitant. NK$_1$-receptor antagonists may be administered for 3 days as follows: oral aprepitant 125 mg or intravenous fosaprepitant 115 mg given 1 hour before chemotherapy, followed by oral aprepitant 80 mg/d for 2 days after chemotherapy.

Adverse Effects & Drug Interactions

Aprepitant may be associated with fatigue, dizziness, and diarrhea. The drug is metabolized by CYP3A4 and may inhibit the metabolism of other drugs metabolized by the CYP3A4 pathway. Several chemotherapeutic agents are metabolized by CYP3A4, including docetaxel, paclitaxel, etoposide, irinotecan, imatinib, vinblastine, and vincristine. Drugs that inhibit CYP3A4 metabolism may significantly increase aprepitant plasma levels (eg, ketoconazole, ciprofloxacin, clarithromycin, nefazodone, ritonavir, nelfinavir, verapamil, and quinidine). Aprepitant decreases the international normalized ratio (INR) in patients taking warfarin.

PHENOTHIAZINES & BUTYROPHENONES

Phenothiazines are antipsychotic agents that can be used for their potent antiemetic and sedative properties (see Chapter 29). The antiemetic properties of phenothiazines are mediated through inhibition of dopamine and muscarinic receptors. Sedative properties are due to their antihistamine activity. The agents most commonly used as antiemetics are **prochlorperazine, promethazine,** and **thiethylperazine.**

Antipsychotic butyrophenones also possess antiemetic properties due to their central dopaminergic blockade (see Chapter 29). The main agent used is **droperidol,** which can be given by intramuscular or intravenous injection. In antiemetic doses, droperidol is extremely sedating. Previously, it was used extensively for postoperative nausea and vomiting, in conjunction with opiates and benzodiazepines for sedation for surgical and endoscopic procedures, for neuroleptanalgesia, and for induction and maintenance of general anesthesia. Extrapyramidal effects and hypotension may occur. Droperidol may prolong the QT interval, rarely resulting in fatal episodes of ventricular tachycardia including torsades de pointes. Therefore, droperidol should not be used in patients with QT prolongation and should be used only in patients who have not responded adequately to alternative agents.

SUBSTITUTED BENZAMIDES

Substituted benzamides include **metoclopramide** (discussed previously) and **trimethobenzamide.** Their primary mechanism of antiemetic action is believed to be dopamine-receptor blockade. Trimethobenzamide also has weak antihistaminic activity. For prevention and treatment of nausea and vomiting, metoclopramide may be given in the relatively high dosage of 10–20 mg orally or intravenously every 6 hours. The usual dose of trimethobenzamide is 300 mg orally, or 200 mg by intramuscular injection. The principal adverse effects of these central dopamine antagonists are extrapyramidal: restlessness, dystonias, and parkinsonian symptoms.

H₁ ANTIHISTAMINES & ANTICHOLINERGIC DRUGS

The pharmacology of anticholinergic agents is discussed in Chapter 8 and that of H₁ antihistaminic agents in Chapter 16. As single agents, these drugs have weak antiemetic activity, although they are particularly useful for the prevention or treatment of motion sickness. Their use may be limited by dizziness, sedation, confusion, dry mouth, cycloplegia, and urinary retention. **Diphenhydramine** and one of its salts, **dimenhydrinate,** are first-generation histamine H₁ antagonists that also have significant anticholinergic properties. Because of its sedating properties, diphenhydramine is commonly used in conjunction with other antiemetics for treatment of emesis due to chemotherapy. **Meclizine** is an H₁ antihistaminic agent with minimal anticholinergic properties that also causes less sedation. It is used for the prevention of motion sickness and the treatment of vertigo due to labyrinth dysfunction.

Hyoscine (scopolamine), a prototypic muscarinic receptor antagonist, is one of the best agents for the prevention of motion sickness. However, it has a very high incidence of anticholinergic effects when given orally or parenterally. It is better tolerated as a transdermal patch. Superiority to dimenhydrinate has not been proved.

BENZODIAZEPINES

Benzodiazepines such as lorazepam or diazepam are used before the initiation of chemotherapy to reduce anticipatory vomiting or vomiting caused by anxiety. The pharmacology of these agents is presented in Chapter 22.

CANNABINOIDS

Dronabinol is Δ⁹-tetrahydrocannabinol (THC), the major psychoactive chemical in marijuana (see Chapter 32). After oral ingestion, the drug is almost completely absorbed but undergoes significant first-pass hepatic metabolism. Its metabolites are excreted slowly over days to weeks in the feces and urine. Like crude marijuana, dronabinol is a psychoactive agent that is used medically as an appetite stimulant and as an antiemetic, but the mechanisms for these effects are not understood. Because of the availability of more effective agents, dronabinol now is uncommonly used for the prevention of chemotherapy-induced nausea and vomiting. Combination therapy with phenothiazines provides synergistic antiemetic action and appears to attenuate the adverse effects of both agents. Dronabinol is usually administered in a dosage of 5 mg/m² just prior to chemotherapy and every 2–4 hours as needed. Adverse effects include euphoria, dysphoria, sedation, hallucinations, dry mouth, and increased appetite. It has some autonomic effects that may result in tachycardia, conjunctival injection, and orthostatic hypotension. Dronabinol has no significant drug-drug interactions but may potentiate the clinical effects of other psychoactive agents.

Nabilone is a closely related THC analog that has been available in other countries and is now approved for use in the USA.

■ DRUGS USED TO TREAT INFLAMMATORY BOWEL DISEASE

Inflammatory bowel disease (IBD) comprises two distinct disorders: ulcerative colitis and Crohn's disease. The etiology and pathogenesis of these disorders remain unknown. For this reason, pharmacologic treatment of inflammatory bowel disorders often involves drugs that belong to different therapeutic classes and have different but non-specific mechanisms of anti-inflammatory action. Drugs used in inflammatory bowel disease are chosen on the basis of disease severity, responsiveness, and drug toxicity (Figure 62–7).

AMINOSALICYLATES

Chemistry & Formulations

Drugs that contain **5-aminosalicylic acid (5-ASA)** have been used successfully for decades in the treatment of inflammatory bowel diseases (Figure 62–8). 5-ASA differs from salicylic acid only by the addition of an amino group at the 5 (meta) position. Aminosalicylates are believed to work topically (not systemically) in areas of diseased gastrointestinal mucosa. Up to 80% of unformulated, aqueous 5-ASA is absorbed from the small intestine and does not reach the distal small bowel or colon in appreciable quantities. To overcome the rapid absorption of 5-ASA from the proximal small intestine, a number of formulations have been designed to deliver 5-ASA to various distal segments of the small bowel or the colon. These include **sulfasalazine, olsalazine, balsalazide,** and various forms of **mesalamine.**

A. Azo Compounds

Sulfasalazine, balsalazide, and olsalazine contain 5-ASA bound by an azo (N=N) bond to an inert compound or to another 5-ASA molecule (Figure 62–8). In sulfasalazine, 5-ASA is bound to sulfapyridine; in balsalazide, 5-ASA is bound to 4-aminobenzoyl-β-alanine; and in olsalazine, two 5-ASA molecules are bound together. The azo structure markedly reduces absorption of the parent drug from the small intestine. In the terminal ileum and colon, resident bacteria cleave the azo bond by means of an azoreductase enzyme, releasing the active 5-ASA. Consequently, high

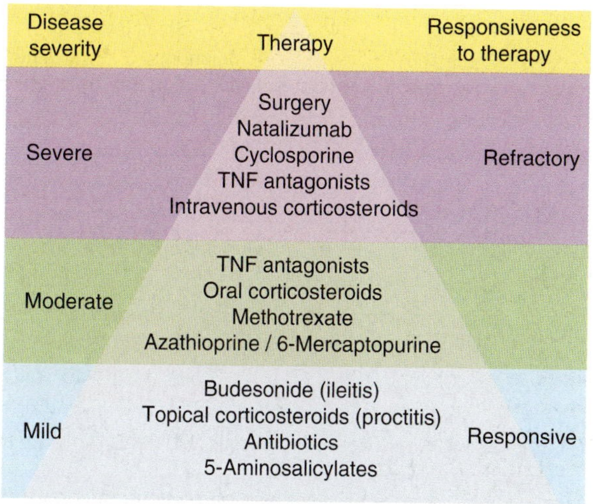

FIGURE 62–7 Therapeutic pyramid approach to inflammatory bowel diseases. Treatment choice is predicated on both the severity of the illness and the responsiveness to therapy. Agents at the bottom of the pyramid are less efficacious but carry a lower risk of serious adverse effects. Drugs may be used alone or in various combinations. Patients with mild disease may be treated with 5-aminosalicylates (with ulcerative colitis or Crohn's colitis), topical corticosteroids (ulcerative colitis), antibiotics (Crohn's colitis or Crohn's perianal disease), or budesonide (Crohn's ileitis). Patients with moderate disease or patients who fail initial therapy for mild disease may be treated with oral corticosteroids to promote disease remission; immunomodulators (azathioprine, mercaptopurine, methotrexate) to promote or maintain disease remission; or anti-TNF antibodies. Patients with moderate disease who fail other therapies or patients with severe disease may require intravenous corticosteroids, anti-TNF antibodies, or surgery. Natalizumab is reserved for patients with severe Crohn's disease who have failed immunomodulators and TNF antagonists. Cyclosporine is used primarily for patients with severe ulcerative colitis who have failed a course of intravenous corticosteroids. TNF, tumor necrosis factor.

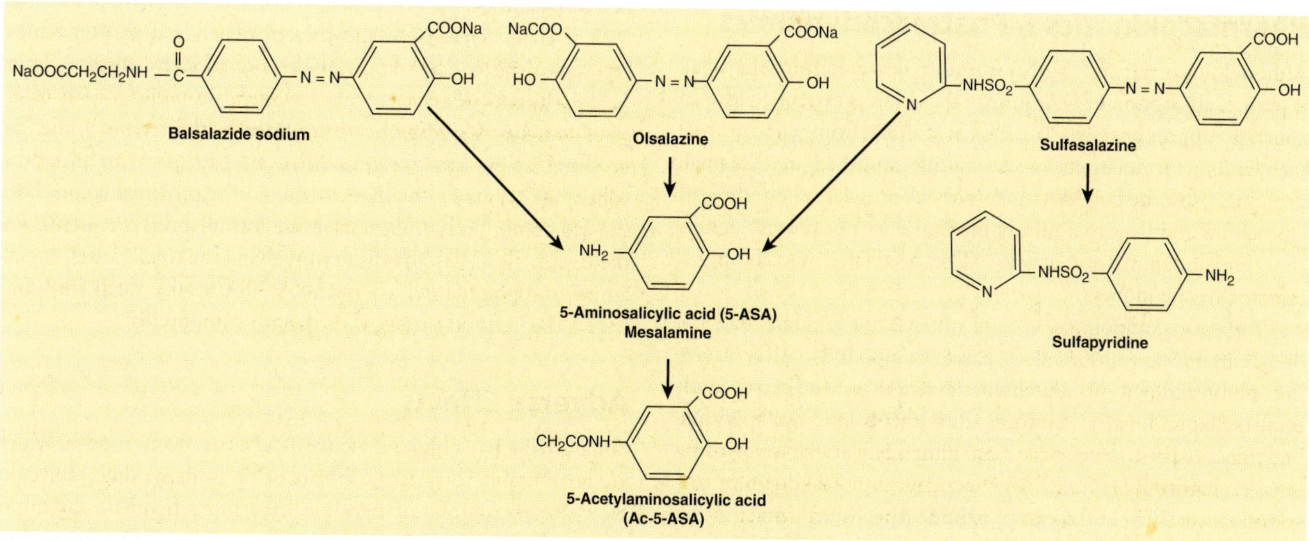

FIGURE 62–8 Chemical structures and metabolism of aminosalicylates. Azo compounds (balsalazide, olsalazine, sulfasalazine) are converted by bacterial azoreductase to 5-aminosalicylic acid (mesalamine), the active therapeutic moiety.

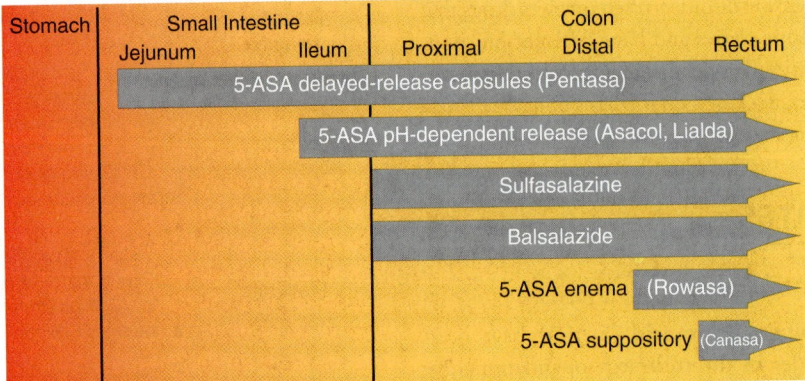

FIGURE 62–9 Sites of 5-aminosalicylic acid (5-ASA) release from different formulations in the small and large intestines.

concentrations of active drug are made available in the terminal ileum or colon.

B. Mesalamine Compounds

Other proprietary formulations have been designed that package 5-ASA itself in various ways to deliver it to different segments of the small or large bowel. These 5-ASA formulations are known generically as **mesalamine. Pentasa** is a mesalamine formulation that contains timed-release microgranules that release 5-ASA throughout the small intestine (Figure 62–9). **Asacol** and **Apriso** have 5-ASA coated in a pH-sensitive resin that dissolves at pH 6-7 (the pH of the distal ileum and proximal colon). **Lialda** also uses a pH-dependent resin that encases a multimatrix core. On dissolution of the pH-sensitive resin in the colon, water slowly penetrates its hydrophilic and lipophilic core, leading to slow release of mesalamine throughout the colon. 5-ASA also may be delivered in high concentrations to the rectum and sigmoid colon by means of enema formulations (**Rowasa**) or suppositories (**Canasa**).

Pharmacokinetics & Pharmacodynamics

Although unformulated 5-ASA is readily absorbed from the small intestine, absorption of 5-ASA from the colon is extremely low. In contrast, approximately 20–30% of 5-ASA from current oral mesalamine formulations is systemically absorbed in the small intestine. Absorbed 5-ASA undergoes *N*-acetylation in the gut epithelium and liver to a metabolite that does not possess significant anti-inflammatory activity. The acetylated metabolite is excreted by the kidneys.

Of the azo compounds, 10% of sulfasalazine and less than 1% of balsalazide are absorbed as native compounds. After azoreductase breakdown of sulfasalazine, over 85% of the carrier molecule sulfapyridine is absorbed from the colon. Sulfapyridine undergoes hepatic metabolism (including acetylation) followed by renal excretion. By contrast, after azoreductase breakdown of balsalazide, over 70% of the carrier peptide is recovered intact in the feces and only a small amount of systemic absorption occurs.

The mechanism of action of 5-ASA is not certain. The primary action of salicylate and other NSAIDs is due to blockade of prostaglandin synthesis by inhibition of cyclooxygenase. However, the aminosalicylates have variable effects on prostaglandin production. It is thought that 5-ASA modulates inflammatory mediators derived from both the cyclooxygenase and lipoxygenase pathways. Other potential mechanisms of action of the 5-ASA drugs relate to their ability to interfere with the production of inflammatory cytokines. 5-ASA inhibits the activity of nuclear factor-κB (NF-κB), an important transcription factor for proinflammatory cytokines. 5-ASA may also inhibit cellular functions of natural killer cells, mucosal lymphocytes, and macrophages, and it may scavenge reactive oxygen metabolites.

Clinical Uses

5-ASA drugs induce and maintain remission in ulcerative colitis and are considered to be the first-line agents for treatment of mild to moderate active ulcerative colitis. Their efficacy in Crohn's disease is unproven, although many clinicians use 5-ASA agents as first-line therapy for mild to moderate disease involving the colon or distal ileum.

The effectiveness of 5-ASA therapy depends in part on achieving high drug concentration at the site of active disease. Thus, 5-ASA suppositories or enemas are useful in patients with ulcerative colitis or Crohn's disease confined to the rectum (proctitis) or distal colon (proctosigmoiditis). In patients with ulcerative colitis or Crohn's colitis that extends to the proximal colon, both the azo compounds and mesalamine formulations are useful. For the treatment of Crohn's disease involving the small bowel, mesalamine compounds, which release 5-ASA in the small intestine, have a theoretic advantage over the azo compounds.

Adverse Effects

Sulfasalazine has a high incidence of adverse effects, most of which are attributable to systemic effects of the sulfapyridine molecule. Slow acetylators of sulfapyridine have more frequent and more severe adverse effects than fast acetylators. Up to 40% of patients cannot tolerate therapeutic doses of sulfasalazine. The most common problems are dose-related and include nausea, gastrointestinal upset, headaches, arthralgias, myalgias, bone marrow suppression, and malaise. Hypersensitivity to sulfapyridine (or, rarely, 5-ASA) can result in fever, exfoliative dermatitis, pancreatitis, pneumonitis, hemolytic anemia, pericarditis, or hepatitis. Sulfasalazine has also been associated with oligospermia, which reverses upon discontinuation of the drug. Sulfasalazine impairs folate absorption and processing; hence, dietary supplementation with 1 mg/d folic acid is recommended.

In contrast to sulfasalazine, other aminosalicylate formulations are well tolerated. In most clinical trials, the frequency of drug adverse events is similar to that in patients treated with placebo. For unclear reasons, olsalazine may stimulate a secretory diarrhea—which should not be confused with active inflammatory bowel disease—in 10% of patients. Rare hypersensitivity reactions may occur with all aminosalicylates but are much less common than with sulfasalazine. Careful studies have documented subtle changes indicative of renal tubular damage in patients receiving high doses of aminosalicylates. Rare cases of interstitial nephritis are reported, particularly in association with high doses of mesalamine formulations; this may be attributable to the higher serum 5-ASA levels attained with these drugs. Sulfasalazine and other aminosalicylates rarely cause worsening of colitis, which may be misinterpreted as refractory colitis.

GLUCOCORTICOIDS

Pharmacokinetics & Pharmacodynamics

In gastrointestinal practice, prednisone and prednisolone are the most commonly used oral glucocorticoids. These drugs have an intermediate duration of biologic activity allowing once-daily dosing.

Hydrocortisone enemas, foam, or suppositories are used to maximize colonic tissue effects and minimize systemic absorption via topical treatment of active inflammatory bowel disease in the rectum and sigmoid colon. Absorption of hydrocortisone is reduced with rectal administration, although 15–30% of the administered dosage is still absorbed.

Budesonide is a potent synthetic analog of prednisolone that has high affinity for the glucocorticoid receptor but is subject to rapid first-pass hepatic metabolism (in part by CYP3A4), resulting in low oral bioavailability. A controlled-release oral formulation of budesonide (Entocort) is available that releases the drug in the distal ileum and colon, where it is absorbed. The bioavailability of controlled-release budesonide capsules is approximately 10%.

As in other tissues, glucocorticoids inhibit production of inflammatory cytokines (TNF-α, IL-1) and chemokines (IL-8); reduce expression of inflammatory cell adhesion molecules; and inhibit gene transcription of nitric oxide synthase, phospholipase A_2, cyclooxygenase-2, and NF-κB.

Clinical Uses

Glucocorticoids are commonly used in the treatment of patients with moderate to severe active inflammatory bowel disease. Active disease is commonly treated with an initial oral dosage of 40–60 mg/d of prednisone or prednisolone. Higher doses have

not been shown to be more efficacious but have significantly greater adverse effects. Once a patient responds to initial therapy (usually within 1–2 weeks), the dosage is tapered to minimize development of adverse effects. In severely ill patients, the drugs are usually administered intravenously.

For the treatment of inflammatory bowel disease involving the rectum or sigmoid colon, rectally administered glucocorticoids are preferred because of their lower systemic absorption.

Oral controlled-release budesonide (9 mg/d) is commonly used in the treatment of mild to moderate Crohn's disease involving the ileum and proximal colon. It appears to be slightly less effective than prednisolone in achieving clinical remission, but has significantly less adverse systemic effects.

Corticosteroids are not useful for maintaining disease remission. Other medications such as aminosalicylates or immunosuppressive agents should be used for this purpose.

Adverse Effects

Adverse effects of glucocorticoids are reviewed in Chapter 39.

PURINE ANALOGS: AZATHIOPRINE & 6-MERCAPTOPURINE

Pharmacokinetics & Pharmacodynamics

Azathioprine and 6-mercaptopurine (6-MP) are purine antimetabolites that have immunosuppressive properties (see Chapters 54 and 55).

The bioavailability of azathioprine (80%) is superior to 6-MP (50%). After absorption azathioprine is rapidly converted by a nonenzymatic process to 6-MP. 6-Mercaptopurine subsequently undergoes a complex biotransformation via competing catabolic enzymes (xanthine oxidase and thiopurine methyltransferase) that produce inactive metabolites and anabolic pathways that produce active thioguanine nucleotides. Azathioprine and 6-MP have a serum half-life of less than 2 hours; however, the active 6-thioguanine nucleotides are concentrated in cells resulting in a prolonged half-life of days. The prolonged kinetics of 6-thioguanine nucleotide results in a median delay of 17 weeks before onset of therapeutic benefit from oral azathioprine or 6-MP is observed in patients with inflammatory bowel disease.

Clinical Uses

Azathioprine and 6-MP are important agents in the induction and maintenance of remission of ulcerative colitis and Crohn's disease. Although the optimal dose is uncertain, most patients with normal thiopurine-S-methyltransferase (TPMT) activity (see below) are treated with 6-MP, 1–1.5 mg/kg/d, or azathioprine, 2–2.5 mg/kg/d. After 3–6 months of treatment, 50–60% of patients with active disease achieve remission. These agents help maintain remission in up to 80% of patients. Among patients who depend on long-term glucocorticoid therapy to control active disease, purine analogs allow dose reduction or elimination of steroids in the majority.

Adverse Effects

Dose-related toxicities of azathioprine or 6-MP include nausea, vomiting, bone marrow depression (leading to leukopenia, macrocytosis, anemia, or thrombocytopenia), and hepatic toxicity. Routine laboratory monitoring with complete blood count and liver function tests is required in all patients. Leukopenia or elevations in liver chemistries usually respond to medication dose reduction. Severe leukopenia may predispose to opportunistic infections; leukopenia may respond to therapy with granulocyte stimulating factor. Catabolism of 6-MP by TPMT is low in 11% and absent in 0.3% of the population, leading to increased production of active 6-thioguanine metabolites and increased risk of bone marrow depression. TPMT levels can be measured before initiating therapy. These drugs should not be administered to patients with no TPMT activity and should be initiated at lower doses in patients with intermediate activity. Hypersensitivity reactions to azathioprine or 6-MP occur in 5% of patients. These include fever, rash, pancreatitis, diarrhea, and hepatitis.

As with transplant recipients receiving long-term 6-MP or azathioprine therapy, there appears to be an increased risk of lymphoma among patients with inflammatory bowel disease. These drugs cross the placenta; however, there are many reports of successful pregnancies in women taking these agents, and the risk of teratogenicity appears to be small.

Drug Interactions

Allopurinol markedly reduces xanthine oxide catabolism of the purine analogs, potentially increasing active 6-thioguanine nucleotides that may lead to severe leukopenia. Allopurinol should not be given to patients taking 6-MP or azathioprine except in carefully monitored situations.

METHOTREXATE

Pharmacokinetics & Pharmacodynamics

Methotrexate is another antimetabolite that has beneficial effects in a number of chronic inflammatory diseases, including Crohn's disease and rheumatoid arthritis (see Chapter 36), and in cancer (see Chapter 54). Methotrexate may be given orally, subcutaneously, or intramuscularly. Reported oral bioavailability is 50–90% at doses used in chronic inflammatory diseases. Intramuscular and subcutaneous methotrexate exhibit nearly complete bioavailability.

The principal mechanism of action is inhibition of dihydrofolate reductase, an enzyme important in the production of thymidine and purines. At the high doses used for chemotherapy, methotrexate inhibits cellular proliferation. However, at the low doses used in the treatment of inflammatory bowel disease (12–25 mg/wk), the antiproliferative effects may not be evident. Methotrexate may interfere with the inflammatory actions of interleukin-1. It may also stimulate increased release of adenosine, an endogenous anti-inflammatory autacoid. Methotrexate may also stimulate apoptosis and death of activated T lymphocytes.

Clinical Uses

Methotrexate is used to induce and maintain remission in patients with Crohn's disease. Its efficacy in ulcerative colitis is uncertain. To induce remission, patients are treated with 15–25 mg of methotrexate once weekly by subcutaneous injection. If a satisfactory response is achieved within 8–12 weeks, the dose is reduced to 15 mg/wk.

Adverse Effects

At higher dosage, methotrexate may cause bone marrow depression, megaloblastic anemia, alopecia, and mucositis. At the doses used in the treatment of inflammatory bowel disease, these events are uncommon but warrant dose reduction if they do occur. Folate supplementation reduces the risk of these events without impairing the anti-inflammatory action.

In patients with psoriasis treated with methotrexate, hepatic damage is common; however, among patients with inflammatory bowel disease and rheumatoid arthritis, the risk is significantly lower. Renal insufficiency may increase risk of hepatic accumulation and toxicity.

ANTI-TUMOR NECROSIS FACTOR THERAPY

Pharmacokinetics & Pharmacodynamics

A dysregulation of the helper T cell type 1 (TH1) response and regulatory T cells (Tregs) is present in inflammatory bowel disease, especially Crohn's disease. One of the key proinflammatory cytokines in inflammatory bowel disease is tumor necrosis factor (TNF). TNF is produced by the innate immune system (eg, dendritic cells, macrophages), the adaptive immune system (especially TH1 cells), and nonimmune cells (fibroblasts, smooth muscle cells). TNF exists in two biologically active forms: soluble TNF and membrane-bound TNF. The biologic activity of soluble and membrane-bound TNF is mediated by binding to TNF receptors (TNFR) that are present on some cells (especially TH1 cells, innate immune cells, and fibroblasts). Binding of TNF to TNFR initially activates components including NF-κB that stimulate transcription, growth, and expansion. Biologic actions ascribed to TNFR activation include release of proinflammatory cytokines from macrophages, T-cell activation and proliferation, fibroblast collagen production, up-regulation of endothelial adhesion molecules responsible for leukocyte migration, and stimulation of hepatic acute phase reactants. Activation of TNFR may later lead to apoptosis (programmed cell death) of activated cells.

Three monoclonal antibodies to human TNF are approved for the treatment of inflammatory bowel disease: infliximab, adalimumab, and certolizumab (Table 62–3). Infliximab and adalimumab are antibodies of the IgG$_1$ subclass. Certolizumab is a recombinant antibody that contains an Fab fragment that is conjugated to polyethylene glycol (PEG) but lacks an Fc portion. The Fab portions of infliximab and certolizumab are chimeric mouse-human antibodies but adalimumab is fully humanized. Infliximab

TABLE 62–3 Anti-TNF antibodies used in inflammatory bowel disease.

	Infliximab	Adalimumab	Certolizumab
Class	Monoclonal antibody	Monoclonal antibody	Monoclonal antibody
% Human	75%	100%	95%
Structure	IgG$_1$	IgG$_1$	Fab fragment attached to PEG (lacks Fc portion)
Route of administration	Intravenous	Subcutaneous	Subcutaneous
Half–life	8–10 days	10–20 days	14 days
Neutralizes soluble TNF	Yes	Yes	Yes
Neutralizes membrane-bound TNF	Yes	Yes	Yes
Induces apoptosis of cells expressing membrane-bound TNF	Yes	Yes	No
Complement-mediated cytotoxicity of cells expressing membrane–bound TNF	Yes	Yes	No
Induction dose	5 mg/kg at 0, 2, and 6 weeks	160 mg, 80 mg, and 40 mg at 0, 2, and 4 weeks	400 mg at 0, 2, and 4 weeks
Maintenance dose	5 mg/kg every 8 weeks	40 mg every 2 weeks	400 mg every 4 weeks

TNF, tumor necrosis factor.

is administered as an intravenous infusion. At therapeutic doses of 5–10 mg/kg, the half-life of infliximab is approximately 8–10 days, resulting in plasma disappearance of antibodies over 8–12 weeks. Adalimumab and certolizumab are administered by subcutaneous injection. The half-life for both is approximately 2 weeks.

All three agents bind to soluble and membrane-bound TNF with high affinity, preventing the cytokine from binding to its receptors. Binding of all three antibodies to membrane-bound TNF also causes reverse signaling that suppresses cytokine release. When infliximab or adalimumab bind to membrane-bound TNF, the Fc portion of the human IgG$_1$ region promotes antibody-mediated apoptosis, complement activation, and cellular cytotoxicity of activated T lymphocytes and macrophages. Certolizumab, without an Fc portion, lacks these properties.

Clinical Uses

All three agents are approved for the acute and chronic treatment of patients with moderate to severe Crohn's disease who have had an inadequate response to conventional therapies. Infliximab also is approved for the acute and chronic treatment of moderate to severe ulcerative colitis. With induction therapy, all three agents lead to symptomatic improvement in 60% and disease remission in 30% of patients with moderate to severe Crohn's disease, including patients who have been dependent on glucocorticoids or who have not responded to 6-MP or methotrexate. The median time to clinical response is 2 weeks. Induction therapy is generally given as follows: infliximab 5 mg/kg intravenous infusion at 0, 2, and 6 weeks; adalimumab 160 mg (in divided doses) initially and 80 mg subcutaneous injection at 2 weeks; and certolizumab 400 mg subcutaneous injection at 0, 2, and 4 weeks. Patients who

respond may be treated with chronic maintenance therapy, as follows: infliximab 5 mg/kg intravenous infusion every 8 weeks; adalimumab 40 mg subcutaneous injection every 2 weeks; certolizumab 400 mg subcutaneous injection every 4 weeks. With chronic, regularly scheduled therapy, clinical response is maintained in more than 60% of patients and disease remission in 40%. However, one-third of patients eventually lose response despite higher doses or more frequent injections. Loss of response in many patients may be due to the development of antibodies to the TNF antibody or to other mechanisms.

Infliximab is approved for the treatment of patients with moderate to severe ulcerative colitis who have had inadequate response to mesalamine or corticosteroids. After induction therapy of 5–10 mg/wk at 0, 2, and 6 weeks, 70% of patients have a clinical response and one third achieve a clinical remission. With continued maintenance infusions every 8 weeks, approximately 50% of patients have continued clinical response.

Adverse Effects

Serious adverse events occur in up to 6% of patients with anti-TNF therapy. The most important adverse effect of these drugs is infection due to suppression of the T$_H$1 inflammatory response. This may lead to serious infections such as bacterial sepsis, tuberculosis, invasive fungal organisms, reactivation of hepatitis B, listeriosis, and other opportunistic infections. Reactivation of latent tuberculosis, with dissemination, has occurred. Before administering anti-TNF therapy, all patients must undergo testing with tuberculin skin tests or interferon gamma release assays. Prophylactic therapy for tuberculosis is warranted for patients with positive test results before beginning anti-TNF therapy.

More common but usually less serious infections include upper respiratory infections (sinusitis, bronchitis, and pneumonia) and cellulitis. The risk of serious infections is increased markedly in patients taking concomitant corticosteroids.

Antibodies to the antibody (ATA) may develop with all three agents. These antibodies may attenuate or eliminate the clinical response and increase the likelihood of developing acute or delayed infusion or injection reactions. Antibody formation is much more likely in patients given episodic anti-TNF therapy than regular scheduled injections. In patients on chronic maintenance therapy, the prevalence of ATA with infliximab is 10%, certolizumab 8%, and adalimumab 3%. Antibody development also is less likely in patients who receive concomitant therapy with immunomodulators (ie, 6-MP or methotrexate). Concomitant treatment with anti-TNF agents and immunomodulators may increase the risk of lymphoma.

Infliximab intravenous infusions result in acute adverse infusion reactions in up to 10% of patients, but discontinuation of the infusion for severe reactions is required in less than 2%. Infusion reactions are more common with the second or subsequent infusions than with the first. Early mild reactions include fever, headache, dizziness, urticaria, or mild cardiopulmonary symptoms that include chest pain, dyspnea, or hemodynamic instability. Reactions to subsequent infusions may be reduced with prophylactic administration of acetaminophen, diphenhydramine, or corticosteroids. Severe acute reactions include significant hypotension, shortness of breath, muscle spasms, and chest discomfort; such reactions may require treatment with oxygen, epinephrine, and corticosteroids.

A delayed serum sickness-like reaction may occur 1–2 weeks after anti-TNF therapy in 1% of patients. These reactions consist of myalgia, arthralgia, jaw tightness, fever, rash, urticaria, and edema and usually require discontinuation of that agent. Positive antinuclear antibodies and anti-double-stranded DNA develop in a small number of patients. Development of a lupus-like syndrome is rare and resolves after discontinuation of the drug.

Rare but serious adverse effects of all anti-TNF agents also include severe hepatic reactions leading to acute hepatic failure, demyelinating disorders, hematologic reactions, and new or worsened congestive heart failure in patients with underlying heart disease. Anti-TNF agents may cause a variety of psoriatic skin rashes, which usually resolve after drug discontinuation.

Lymphoma appears to be increased in patients with untreated inflammatory bowel disease. Anti-TNF agents may further increase the risk of lymphoma in this population, although the relative risk is uncertain. An increased number of cases of hepatosplenic T-cell lymphoma, a rare but usually fatal disease, have been noted in children and young adults, virtually all of whom have been on combined therapy with immunomodulators, anti-TNF agents, or corticosteroids.

ANTI-INTEGRIN THERAPY

Integrins are a family of adhesion molecules on the surface of leukocytes that may interact with another class of adhesion molecules on the surface of the vascular endothelium known as selectins, allowing circulating leukocytes to adhere to the vascular endothelium and subsequently move through the vessel wall into the tissue. Integrins consist of heterodimers that contain two subunits, alpha and beta. **Natalizumab** is a humanized IgG_4 monoclonal antibody targeted against the $\alpha 4$ subunit, and thereby blocks several integrins on circulating inflammatory cells and thus prevents binding to the vascular adhesion molecules and subsequent migration into surrounding tissues.

Natalizumab has shown significant efficacy for a subset of patients with moderate to severe Crohn's disease. Unfortunately, in initial clinical trials of patients with Crohn's disease and multiple sclerosis, 3 of 3100 patients treated with natalizumab developed progressive multifocal leukoencephalopathy due to reactivation of a human polyomavirus (JC virus), which is present in latent form in over 80% of adults. All three patients were receiving concomitant therapy with other immunomodulators. After voluntary withdrawal and review of the drug by the manufacturer in 2005, it was approved by the FDA in 2008 for patients with moderate to severe Crohn's disease who have failed other therapies through a carefully restricted program. The approved dosage is 300 mg every 4 weeks by intravenous infusion, and patients should not be on other immune suppressant agents. Approximately 50% of patients respond to initial therapy with natalizumab. Of patients with an initial response, long-term response is maintained in 60% and remission in over 40%. Other adverse effects include acute infusion reactions and a small risk of opportunistic infections.

■ PANCREATIC ENZYME SUPPLEMENTS

Exocrine pancreatic insufficiency is most commonly caused by cystic fibrosis, chronic pancreatitis, or pancreatic resection. When secretion of pancreatic enzymes falls below 10% of normal, fat and protein digestion is impaired and can lead to steatorrhea, azotorrhea, vitamin malabsorption, and weight loss. Pancreatic enzyme supplements, which contain a mixture of amylase, lipase, and proteases, are the mainstay of treatment for pancreatic enzyme insufficiency. Two major types of preparations in use are **pancreatin** and **pancrelipase.** Pancreatin is an alcohol-derived extract of hog pancreas with relatively low concentrations of lipase and proteolytic enzymes, whereas pancrelipase is an enriched preparation. On a per-weight basis, pancrelipase has approximately 12 times the lipolytic activity and more than 4 times the proteolytic activity of pancreatin. Consequently, pancreatin is no longer in common clinical use. Only pancrelipase is discussed here.

Pancrelipase is available worldwide in both non-enteric-coated and enteric-coated preparations. Formulations are available in sizes containing varying amounts of lipase, amylase, and protease. However, manufacturers' listings of enzyme content do not always reflect true enzymatic activity. Pancrelipase enzymes are rapidly and permanently inactivated by gastric acids. Therefore, non-enteric-coated preparations (eg, Viokase tablets or powder) should be given concomitantly with acid suppression therapy (proton pump inhibitor or H$_2$ antagonist) to reduce acid-mediated destruction within the stomach. Enteric-coated formulations are more commonly used because they do not require concomitant acid suppression therapy. In 2006, the FDA announced that all products must undergo an approval process to demonstrate product quality, safety, and efficacy. At present, three formulations (all enteric-coated capsules) are approved for use (Creon, Pancreaze, Zenpep).

Pancrelipase preparations are administered with each meal and snack. Enzyme activity may be listed in international units (IU) or USP units. One IU is equal to 2–3 USP units. Dosing should be individualized according to the age and weight of the patient, the degree of pancreatic insufficiency, and the amount of dietary fat intake. Therapy is initiated at a dose that provides 60,000–90,000 USP units (20–30,000 IU) of lipase activity in the prandial and postprandial period—a level that is sufficient to reduce steatorrhea to a clinically insignificant level in most cases. Suboptimal response to enteric-coated formulations may be due to poor mixing of granules with food or slow dissolution and release of enzymes. Gradual increase of dose, change to a different formulation, or addition of acid suppression therapy may improve response. For patients with feeding tubes, microspheres may be mixed with enteral feeding prior to administration.

Pancreatic enzyme supplements are well tolerated. The capsules should be swallowed, not chewed, because pancreatic enzymes may cause oropharyngeal mucositis. Excessive doses may cause diarrhea and abdominal pain. The high purine content of pancreas extracts may lead to hyperuricosuria and renal stones. Several cases of colonic strictures were reported in patients with cystic fibrosis who received high doses of pancrelipase with high lipase activity. These high-dose formulations have since been removed from the market.

BILE ACID THERAPY FOR GALLSTONES

Ursodiol (ursodeoxycholic acid) is a naturally occurring bile acid that makes up less than 5% of the circulating bile salt pool in humans and a much higher percentage in bears. After oral administration, it is absorbed, conjugated in the liver with glycine or taurine, and excreted in the bile. Conjugated ursodiol undergoes extensive enterohepatic recirculation. The serum half-life is approximately 100 hours. With long-term daily administration, ursodiol constitutes 30–50% of the circulating bile acid pool. A small amount of unabsorbed conjugated or unconjugated ursodiol passes into the colon, where it is either excreted or undergoes dehydroxylation by colonic bacteria to lithocholic acid, a substance with potential hepatic toxicity.

Pharmacodynamics

The solubility of cholesterol in bile is determined by the relative proportions of bile acids, lecithin, and cholesterol. Although prolonged ursodiol therapy expands the bile acid pool, this does not

appear to be the principal mechanism of action for dissolution of gallstones. Ursodiol decreases the cholesterol content of bile by reducing hepatic cholesterol secretion. Ursodiol also appears to stabilize hepatocyte canalicular membranes, possibly through a reduction in the concentration of other endogenous bile acids or through inhibition of immune-mediated hepatocyte destruction.

Clinical Use

Ursodiol is used for dissolution of small cholesterol gallstones in patients with symptomatic gallbladder disease who refuse cholecystectomy or who are poor surgical candidates. At a dosage of 10 mg/kg/d for 12–24 months, dissolution occurs in up to 50% of patients with small (< 5–10 mm) noncalcified gallstones. It is also effective for the prevention of gallstones in obese patients undergoing rapid weight loss therapy. Several trials demonstrate that ursodiol 13–15 mg/kg/d is helpful for patients with early-stage primary biliary cirrhosis, reducing liver function abnormalities and improving liver histology.

Adverse Effects

Ursodiol is practically free of serious adverse effects. Bile salt–induced diarrhea is uncommon. Unlike its predecessor, chenodeoxycholate, ursodiol has not been associated with hepatotoxicity.

DRUGS USED TO TREAT VARICEAL HEMORRHAGE

Portal hypertension most commonly occurs as a consequence of chronic liver disease. Portal hypertension is caused by increased blood flow within the portal venous system and increased resistance to portal flow within the liver. Splanchnic blood flow is increased in patients with cirrhosis due to low arteriolar resistance that is mediated by increased circulating vasodilators and decreased vascular sensitivity to vasoconstrictors. Intrahepatic vascular resistance is increased in cirrhosis due to fixed fibrosis within the spaces of Disse and hepatic veins as well as reversible vasoconstriction of hepatic sinusoids and venules. Among the consequences of portal hypertension are ascites, hepatic encephalopathy, and the development of portosystemic collaterals—especially gastric or esophageal varices. Varices can rupture, leading to massive upper gastrointestinal bleeding.

Several drugs are available that reduce portal pressures. These may be used in the short term for the treatment of active variceal hemorrhage or long term to reduce the risk of hemorrhage.

SOMATOSTATIN & OCTREOTIDE

The pharmacology of octreotide is discussed above under Antidiarrheal Agents. In patients with cirrhosis and portal hypertension, intravenous somatostatin (250 mcg/h) or octreotide (50 mcg/h) reduces portal blood flow and variceal pressures; however, the mechanism by which they do so is poorly understood. They do not appear to induce direct contraction of vascular smooth muscle. Their activity may be mediated through inhibition of release of glucagon and other gut peptides that alter mesenteric blood flow. Although data from clinical trials are conflicting, these agents are probably effective in promoting initial hemostasis from bleeding esophageal varices. They are generally administered for 3–5 days.

VASOPRESSIN & TERLIPRESSIN

Vasopressin (antidiuretic hormone) is a polypeptide hormone secreted by the hypothalamus and stored in the posterior pituitary. Its pharmacology is discussed in Chapters 17 and 37. Although its primary physiologic role is to maintain serum osmolality, it is also a potent arterial vasoconstrictor. When administered intravenously by continuous infusion, vasopressin causes splanchnic arterial vasoconstriction that leads to reduced splanchnic perfusion and lowered portal venous pressures. Before the advent of octreotide, vasopressin was commonly used to treat acute variceal hemorrhage. However, because of its high adverse-effect profile, it is no longer used for this purpose. In contrast, for patients with acute gastrointestinal bleeding from small bowel or large bowel vascular ectasias or diverticulosis, vasopressin may be infused—to promote vasospasm—into one of the branches of the superior or inferior mesenteric artery through an angiographically placed catheter. Adverse effects with systemic vasopressin are common. Systemic and peripheral vasoconstriction can lead to hypertension, myocardial ischemia or infarction, or mesenteric infarction. These effects may be reduced by coadministration of nitroglycerin, which may further reduce portal venous pressures (by reducing portohepatic vascular resistance) and may also reduce the coronary and peripheral vascular vasospasm caused by vasopressin. Other common adverse effects are nausea, abdominal cramps, and diarrhea (due to intestinal hyperactivity). Furthermore, the antidiuretic effects of vasopressin promote retention of free water, which can lead to hyponatremia, fluid retention, and pulmonary edema.

Terlipressin is a vasopressin analog that appears to have similar efficacy to vasopressin with fewer adverse effects. Although this agent is available in other countries, it has never been approved for use in the USA.

BETA-RECEPTOR-BLOCKING DRUGS

The pharmacology of β-receptor-blocking agents is discussed in Chapter 10. Beta-receptor antagonists reduce portal venous pressures via a decrease in portal venous inflow. This decrease is due to a decrease in cardiac output (β_1 blockade) and to splanchnic vasoconstriction (β_2 blockade) caused by the unopposed effect of systemic catecholamines on α receptors. Thus, nonselective β blockers such as propranolol and nadolol are more effective than selective β_1 blockers in reducing portal pressures. Among patients with cirrhosis and esophageal varices who have not previously had an episode of variceal hemorrhage, the incidence of bleeding among patients treated with nonselective β blockers is 15% compared with 25% in control groups. Among patients with a history of variceal hemorrhage, the likelihood of recurrent hemorrhage is 80% within 2 years. Nonselective β blockers significantly reduce the rate of recurrent bleeding, although a reduction in mortality is unproved.

SUMMARY Drugs Used Primarily for Gastrointestinal Conditions

Subclass	Mechanism of Action	Effects	Clinical Applications	Pharmacokinetics, Toxicities, Interactions
DRUGS USED IN ACID-PEPTIC DISEASES				
• Proton pump inhibitors (PPIs), eg, omeprazole, lanso prazole	Irreversible blockade of H⁺, K⁺-ATPase pump in active parietal cells of stomach	Long-lasting reduction of stimulated and nocturnal acid secretion	Peptic ulcer, gastroesophageal reflux disease, erosive gastritis	Half-lives much shorter than duration of action • low toxicity • reduction of stomach acid may reduce absorption of some drugs and increase that of others

- *H₂-receptor blockers, eg, cimetidine: Effective reduction of nocturnal acid but less effective against stimulated secretion; very safe, available over the counter (OTC). Cimetidine, but not other H₂ blockers, is a weak antiandrogenic agent and a potent CYP enzyme inhibitor*
- *Sucralfate: Polymerizes at site of tissue damage (ulcer bed) and protects against further damage; very insoluble with no systemic effects; must be given four times daily*
- *Antacids: Popular OTC medication for symptomatic relief of heartburn; not as useful as PPI and H₂ blockers in peptic diseases*

DRUGS STIMULATING MOTILITY				
• Metoclopramide	D₂-receptor blocker • removes inhibition of acetylcholine neurons in enteric nervous system	Increases gastric emptying and intestinal motility	Gastric paresis (eg, in diabetes) • antiemetic (see below)	Parkinsonian symptoms due to block of central nervous system (CNS) D₂ receptors

- *Domperidone: Like metoclopramide, but less CNS effect; not available in USA*
- *Cholinomimetics: Neostigmine often used for colonic pseudo-obstruction in hospitalized patients*
- *Macrolides: Erythromycin useful in diabetic gastroparesis but tolerance develops*

LAXATIVES				
• Magnesium hydrox ide, other nonabsorb able salts and sugars	Osmotic agents increase water content of stool	Usually causes evacuation within 4–6 h, sooner in large doses	Simple constipation; bowel prep for endoscopy (especially PEG solutions)	Magnesium may be absorbed and cause toxicity in renal impairment

- *Bulk-forming laxatives: Methylcellulose, psyllium, etc: increase volume of colon, stimulate evacuation*
- *Stimulants: senna, cascara; stimulate activity; may cause cramping*
- *Stool surfactants: Docusate, mineral oil; lubricate stool, ease passage*
- *Chloride channel activator: Lubiprostone, prostanoic acid derivative, stimulates chloride secretion into intestine, increasing fluid content*
- *Opioid receptor antagonists: Alvimopan, methylnaltrexone; block intestinal μ-opioid receptors but do not enter CNS, so analgesia is maintained*
- *5-HT₄ agonists: Tegaserod; activates enteric 5-HT₄ receptors and increases intestinal motility*

ANTIDIARRHEAL DRUGS				
• Loperamide	Activates μ-opioid receptors in enteric nervous system	Slows motility in gut with negligible CNS effects	Nonspecific, noninfectious diarrhea	Mild cramping but little or no CNS toxicity

- *Diphenoxylate: Similar to loperamide, but high doses can cause CNS opioid effects and toxicity*
- *Colloidal bismuth compounds: Subsalicylate and citrate salts available. OTC preparations popular and have some value in travelers' diarrhea due to adsorption of toxins*
- *Kaolin + pectin: Adsorbent compounds available OTC in some countries*

DRUGS FOR IRRITABLE BOWEL SYNDROME (IBS)				
• Alosetron	5-HT₃ antagonist of high potency and duration of binding	Reduces smooth muscle activity in gut	Approved for severe diarrhea-predominant IBS in women	Rare but serious constipation • ischemic colitis • infarction

- *Anticholinergics: Nonselective action on gut activity, usually associated with typical antimuscarinic toxicity*
- *Chloride channel activator: Lubiprostone (see above); useful in constipation-predominant IBS in women*

(continued)

Subclass	Mechanism of Action	Effects	Clinical Applications	Pharmacokinetics, Toxicities, Interactions
ANTIEMETIC DRUGS				
• Ondansetron, other 5-HT$_3$ antagonists	5-HT$_3$ blockade in gut and CNS with shorter duration of binding than alosetron	Extremely effective in preventing chemotherapy-induced and postoperative nausea and vomiting	First-line agents in cancer chemotherapy; also useful for postop emesis	Usually given IV but orally active in prophylaxis • 4–9 h duration of action • very low toxicity but may slow colonic transit
• Aprepitant	NK$_1$-receptor blocker in CNS	Interferes with vomiting reflex • no effect on 5-HT, dopamine, or steroid receptors	Effective in reducing both early and delayed emesis in cancer chemotherapy	Given orally • IV fosaprepitant available • fatigue, dizziness, diarrhea • CYP interactions

- *Corticosteroids: Mechanism not known but useful in antiemetic IV cocktails*
- *Antimuscarinics (scopolamine): Effective in emesis due to motion sickness; not other types*
- *Antihistaminics: Moderate efficacy in motion sickness and chemotherapy-induced emesis*
- *Phenothiazines: Act primarily through block of D$_2$ and muscarinic receptors*
- *Cannabinoids: Dronabinol is available for use in chemotherapy-induced nausea and vomiting, but is associated with CNS marijuana effects*

Subclass	Mechanism of Action	Effects	Clinical Applications	Pharmacokinetics, Toxicities, Interactions
DRUGS USED IN INFLAMMATORY BOWEL DISEASE (IBD)				
• 5-Aminosalicylates, eg, mesalamine in many formulations • Sulfasalazine	Mechanism uncertain • may be inhibition of eicosanoid inflammatory mediators	Topical therapeutic action • systemic absorption may cause toxicity	Mild to moderately severe Crohn's disease and ulcerative colitis	Sulfasalazine causes sulfonamide toxicity and may cause GI upset, myalgias, arthralgias, myelosuppression • other aminosalicylates much less toxic
• Purine analogs and antimetabolites, eg, 6-mercaptopurine, methotrexate	Mechanism uncertain • may promote apoptosis of immune cells • Methotrexate blocks dihydrofolate reductase	Generalized suppression of immune processes	Moderately severe to severe Crohn's disease and ulcerative colitis	GI upset, mucositis • myelosuppression • purine analogs may cause hepatotoxicity, but rare with methotrexate at the low doses used
• Anti-TNF antibodies, eg, infliximab, others	Bind tumor necrosis factor and prevent it from binding to its receptors	Suppression of several aspects of immune function, especially T$_H$1 lymphocytes	Infliximab: Moderately severe to severe Crohn's disease and ulcerative colitis • others approved in Crohn's disease	Infusion reactions • reactivation of latent tuberculosis • increased risk of dangerous systemic fungal and bacterial infections

- *Corticosteroids: Generalized anti-inflammatory effect; see Chapter 39*

Subclass	Mechanism of Action	Effects	Clinical Applications	Pharmacokinetics, Toxicities, Interactions
PANCREATIC SUPPLEMENTS				
• Pancrelipase	Replacement enzymes from animal pancreatic extracts	Improves digestion of dietary fat, protein, and carbohydrate	Pancreatic insufficiency due to cystic fibrosis, pancreatitis, pancreatectomy	Taken with every meal • may increase incidence of gout

- *Pancreatin: Similar pancreatic extracts but much lower potency; rarely used*

Subclass	Mechanism of Action	Effects	Clinical Applications	Pharmacokinetics, Toxicities, Interactions
BILE ACID THERAPY FOR GALLSTONES				
• Ursodiol	Reduces cholesterol secretion into bile	Dissolves gallstones	Gallstones in patients refusing or not eligible for surgery	May cause diarrhea

Subclass	Mechanism of Action	Effects	Clinical Applications	Pharmacokinetics, Toxicities, Interactions
DRUGS USED TO TREAT VARICEAL HEMORRHAGE				
• Octreotide	Somatostatin analog • mechanism not certain	May alter portal blood flow and variceal pressures	Patients with bleeding varices or at high risk of repeat bleeding	Reduced endocrine and exocrine pancreatic activity • other endocrine abnormalities • GI upset

- *β Blockers: Reduce cardiac output and splanchnic blood flow; see Chapter 10*

PREPARATIONS AVAILABLE

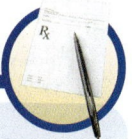

ANTACIDS

Aluminum hydroxide gel* (AlternaGEL, others)
Oral: 300, 500, 600 mg tablets; 400, 500 mg capsules; 320, 450, 675 mg/5 mL suspension

Calcium carbonate* (Tums, others)
Oral: 350, 420, 500, 600, 650, 750, 1000, 1250 mg chewable tablets; 1250 mg/5 mL suspension

Combination aluminum hydroxide and magnesium hydroxide preparations* (Maalox, Mylanta, Gaviscon, Gelusil, others)
Oral: 400 to 800 mg combined hydroxides per tablet, capsule, or 5 mL suspension

H₂ HISTAMINE RECEPTOR BLOCKERS

Cimetidine (generic, Tagamet, Tagamet HB*)
Oral: 200,* 300, 400, 800 mg tablets; 300 mg/5 mL liquid
Parenteral: 300 mg/2 mL, 300 mg/50 mL for injection

Famotidine (generic, Pepcid, Pepcid AC,* Pepcid Complete*)
Oral: 10, 20 mg tablets,* gelcaps*; powder to reconstitute for 40 mg/5 mL suspension
Parenteral: 10 mg/mL for injection

Nizatidine (generic, Axid, Axid AR*)
Oral: 75 mg tablets*; 150, 300 mg capsules

Ranitidine (generic, Zantac, Zantac 75*)
Oral: 75,* 150, 300 mg tablets
Parenteral: 1, 25 mg/mL for injection

SELECTED ANTICHOLINERGIC DRUGS

Atropine (generic)
Oral: 0.4 mg tablets
Parenteral: 0.05, 0.1, 0.3, 0.4, 0.5, 0.8, 1 mg/mL for injection

Belladonna alkaloids tincture (generic)
Oral: 0.27–0.33 mg/mL liquid

Dicyclomine (generic, Bentyl, others)
Oral: 10, 20 mg capsules; 20 mg tablets; 10 mg/5 mL syrup
Parenteral: 10 mg/mL for injection

Glycopyrrolate (generic, Robinul)
Oral: 1, 2 mg tablets
Parenteral: 0.2 mg/mL for injection

Hyoscyamine (Anaspaz, Levsin, others)
Oral: 0.125, 0.15 mg tablets; 0.375 mg timed-release capsules; 0.125 mg/5 mL oral elixir and solution
Parenteral: 0.5 mg/mL for injection

Scopolamine (generic, Transderm Scop)
Oral: 0.4 mg tablets
Transdermal patch: 1.5 mg/2.5 cm²
Parenteral: 0.4, 1 mg/mL for injection

PROTON PUMP INHIBITORS

Esomeprazole (Nexium)
Oral: 20, 40 mg delayed-release capsules
Parenteral: 20, 40 mg vial powder for IV injection

Omeprazole (Prilosec, Prilosec OTC,* Zegerid)
Oral: 10, 20, 40 mg delayed-release capsules; 20 mg delayed-release tablet*

Lansoprazole (Prevacid)
Oral: 15, 30 mg delayed-release capsules; 15, 30 mg orally disintegrating tablet containing delayed-release granules; 15, 30 mg delayed-release granules for oral suspension
Parenteral: 30 mg powder for injection

Dexlansoprazole (Dexilant)
Oral: 30, 60 mg delayed-release capsules

Pantoprazole (Protonix)
Oral: 20, 40 mg delayed-release tablets; 40 mg delayed-release granules for oral suspension
Parenteral: 40 mg/vial powder for IV injection

Rabeprazole (Aciphex)
Oral: 20 mg delayed-release tablets

MUCOSAL PROTECTIVE AGENTS

Misoprostol (Cytotec)
Oral: 100, 200 mcg tablets

Sucralfate (generic, Carafate)
Oral: 1 g tablets; 1 g/10 mL suspension

DIGESTIVE ENZYMES

Pancrelipase (Creon, Pancrease, Zenpep)
Oral: Delayed-release capsules containing varying amounts of lipase, protease, and amylase activity. See manufacturers' literature for details.

DRUGS FOR MOTILITY DISORDERS & SELECTED ANTIEMETICS

5-HT₃-RECEPTOR ANTAGONISTS
Alosetron (Lotronex)
Oral: 0.5, 1 mg tablets

Dolasetron (Anzemet)
Oral: 50, 100 mg tablets
Parenteral: 20 mg/mL for injection

Granisetron (generic, Kytril)
Oral: 1 mg tablets; 2 mg/10 mL oral solution
Parenteral: 0.1, 1 mg/mL for injection

Ondansetron (generic, Zofran)
Oral: 4, 8, 16, 24 mg tablets; 4, 8 mg orally disintegrating tablets; 4 mg/5 mL oral solution
Parenteral: 2 mg/mL, 32 mg/50 mL for IV injection

Palonosetron (Aloxi)
Oral: 0.5 mg capsules
Parenteral: 0.05 mg/mL for injection

OTHER MOTILITY AND ANTIEMETIC AGENTS

Aprepitant (Emend)
Oral: 80, 125 mg capsules

Dronabinol (Marinol)
Oral: 2.5, 5, 10 mg capsules

Fosaprepitant (Emend)
Parenteral: 115 mg/10 mL for IV injection

Metoclopramide (generic, Reglan, others)
Oral: 5, 10 mg tablets; 5 mg/5 mL syrup, 10 mg/mL concentrated solution
Parenteral: 5 mg/mL for injection

Nabilone (Cesamet)
Oral: 1 mg tablets

Prochlorperazine (Compazine)
Oral: 5, 10, 25 mg tablets; 10, 15, 30 mg capsules; 1 mg/mL solution
Rectal: 2.5, 5, 25 mg suppositories
Parenteral: 5 mg/mL for injection

Promethazine (generic, Phenergan, others)
Oral: 10, 13.2, 25, 50 mg tablets; 5, 6.25, 10 mg/5 mL syrup
Rectal: 10, 12.5, 25, 50 mg suppositories
Parenteral: 25, 50 mg/mL for IM or IV injection

Scopolamine (Transderm Scop)
Transdermal patch: 1.5 mg/2.5 cm^2

Tegaserod (Zelnorm)
Oral: 2, 6 mg tablets

Trimethobenzamide (generic, Tigan, others)
Oral: 250, 300 mg capsules
Parenteral: 100 mg/mL for injection

SELECTED ANTI–INFLAMMATORY DRUGS USED IN GASTROINTESTINAL DISEASE (SEE ALSO CHAPTER 55)

Adalimumab (Humira)
Parenteral: 40 mg/0.8 mL for subcutaneous injection by syringe or auto-pen

Balsalazide (Colazal)
Oral: 750 mg capsules

Budesonide (Entocort)
Oral: 3 mg capsules

Certolizumab (Cimzia)
Parenteral: 200 mg powder (reconstituted with 1 mL) for subcutaneous injection

Hydrocortisone (Cortenema, Cortifoam, Proctofoam–HC)
Rectal: 100 mg/60 mL unit retention enema; 90 mg/applicatorful intrarectal foam
Anal: 1% hydrocortisone/1% pramoxine as aerosol application

Infliximab (Remicade)
Parenteral: 100 mg powder for intravenous injection

Mesalamine (5–ASA)
Oral: Asacol: 400 mg, 800 mg delayed-release tablets; Pentasa: 250 mg controlled-release capsules; Lialda: 1.2 g delayed-release tablets; Apriso: 375 mg delayed-release capsules
Rectal: Rowasa: 4 g/60 mL suspension
Canasa: 1000 mg suppositories

Methylprednisolone (Medrol Enpack)
Rectal: 40 mg/bottle retention enema

Olsalazine (Dipentum)
Oral: 250 mg capsules

Sulfasalazine (generic, Azulfidine)
Oral: 500 mg tablets and delayed-release enteric-coated tablets

SELECTED ANTIDIARRHEAL DRUGS

Bismuth subsalicylate* (Pepto–Bismol, others)
Oral: 262 mg caplets, chewable tablets; 130, 262, 524 mg/15 mL suspension

Difenoxin (Motofen)
Oral: 1 mg (with 0.025 mg atropine sulfate) tablets

Diphenoxylate (generic, Lomotil, others)
Oral: 2.5 mg (with 0.025 mg atropine sulfate) tablets and liquid

Loperamide* (generic, Imodium)
Oral: 2 mg tablets, capsules; 1 mg/5 mL liquid

BULK-FORMING LAXATIVES*

Methylcellulose (generic, Citrucel)
Oral: bulk powder, capsules

Psyllium (generic, Serutan, Metamucil, others)
Oral: granules, bulk powder, wafer

OTHER SELECTED LAXATIVE DRUGS

Alvimopan (Entereg)
Oral: 12 mg capsules

Bisacodyl* (generic, Dulcolax, others)
Oral: 5 mg enteric-coated tablets
Rectal: 5 mg, 10 mg suppositories

Cascara sagrada* (generic)
Oral: 325 mg tablets; 5 mL per dose fluid extract (approximately 18% alcohol)

Docusate* (generic, Colace, others)
Oral: 50, 100, 250 mg capsules; 100 mg tablets; 20, 50, 60, 150 mg/15 mL syrup

Lactulose (Chronulac, Cephulac)
Oral: 10 g/15 mL syrup

Lubiprostone (Amitiza)
Oral: 8, 24 mcg capsules

Magnesium hydroxide [milk of magnesia, Epsom Salt]* (generic)
Oral: 400, 800 mg/5 mL aqueous suspension

Methylnaltrexone bromide (Relistor)
Parenteral: 12 mg/0.6 mL

Polycarbophil* (Equalactin, Mitrolan, FiberCon, Fiber–Lax)
Oral: 500, 625 mg tablets; 500 mg chewable tablets

Polyethylene glycol electrolyte solution (Co–Lyte, GoLYTELY, HalfLytely, Moviprep, others)
Oral: Powder for oral solution, makes 2L or 4L

Senna* (Senokot, ExoLax, others)
Oral: 8.6, 15, 17, 25 mg tablets; 8.8, 15 mg/mL liquid

Sodium Phosphate (Fleets Phospho-soda, OsmoPrep, Visicol)
Oral: 1.5 g tablets; 10 g/15 mL liquid

DRUGS THAT DISSOLVE GALLSTONES

Ursodiol (generic, Actigall, URSO)
Oral: 250, 500 mg tablets; 300 mg capsules

*Over-the-counter formulations.

REFERENCES

Acid-Peptic Diseases

Boparai V et al: Guide to the use of proton pump inhibitors in adult patients. Drugs 2008;68:925.

Kahrilas PJ: Gastroesophageal reflux disease. N Engl J Med 2008;359:1700.

Kahrilas PJ et al: American Gastroenterological Association Medical Position Statement on the management of gastroesophageal reflux disease. Gastroenterology 2008;135:1383.

Kwok CS et al: Meta-analysis: The effects of proton pump inhibitors on cardiovascular events and mortality in patients receiving clopidogrel. Aliment Pharmacol Ther 2010;31:810.

Lanza FL et al: Guidelines for the prevention of NSAID-related ulcer complications. Am J Gastronterol 2009;104:728.

McColl KE: *Helicobacter pylori* infection. N Engl J Med 2010;362:1597.

Schubert ML et al: Control of gastric acid secretion in health and disease. Gastroenterology 2008;134:1872.

Wu DC et al: Sequential and concomitant therapy with four drugs is equally effective for eradication of *H pylori* infection. Clin Gastroenterol Hepatol 2010;8:36.

Yang YX et al: Safety of proton pump inhibitor exposure. Gastroenterology 2010;139:1115.

Motility Disorders

DeMaeyer JH et al: 5-HT$_4$ receptor agonists: Similar but not the same. Neurogastroenterol Motil 2008;20:99.

Patrick A et al: Review article: Gastroparesis. Aliment Pharmacol Ther 2008;27:724.

Reddymasu SC et al: Severe gastroparesis: medical therapy or gastric electrical stimulation. Clin Gastroenterol Hepatol 2010;8:117.

Laxatives

American College of Gastroenterology Task Force: An evidence-based approach to the management of chronic constipation in North America. Am J Gastroenterol 2005;100(Suppl 1):S1.

Becker G et al: Novel opioid antagonists for opioid-induced bowel dysfunction and postoperative ileus. Lancet 2009;373:1198.

Bouras EP et al: Chronic constipation in the elderly. Gastroenterol Clin North Am 2009;38:463.

Camilleri M et al: Prucalopride for constipation. Expert Opin Pharmacother 2010;11:451.

Johanson JF et al: Multicenter, 4-week, double-blind, randomized, placebo-controlled trial of lubiprostone, a locally-active type-2 chloride channel activator, in patients with chronic constipation. Am J Gastroenterol 2008;103:170.

Lembo A et al: Efficacy of linaclotide for patients with chronic constipation. Gastroenterology 2010;138:886.

Rao SS: Constipation: Evaluation and treatment of colonic and anorectal motility disorders. Gastrointest Endosc Clin North Am 2009;19:117.

Thomas J et al: Methylnaltrexone for opioid-induced constipation in advanced illness. N Engl J Med 2008;358:2332.

Wald A: A 27-year old woman with constipation: Diagnosis and treatment. Clin Gastroenterol Hepatol 2010;8:838.

Antidiarrheal Agents

Baker DE: Loperamide: A pharmacologic review. Rev Gastroenterol Disord 2007;7(Suppl 3):S11.

Odunsi-Shiyanbade ST et al: Effects of chenodeoxycholate and a bile acid sequestrant, colesevelam, on intestinal transit and bowel function. Clin Gastroenterol Hepatol 2010;8:159.

Schiller LR: Diarrhea and malabsorption in the elderly. Gastroenterol Clin North Am 2009;38:481.

Drugs Used for Irritable Bowel Syndrome

Camilleri M: Review article: New receptor targets for medical therapy in irritable bowel syndrome. Aliment Pharmacol Ther 2010;31;35.

Grundman O et al: Irritable bowel syndrome: Epidemiology, diagnosis and treatment: an update for health-care practitioners. J Gastroenterol Hepatol 2010;25:691.

Mayer EA: Clinical practice. Irritable bowel syndrome. N Engl J Med 2008;358:1692.

Antiemetic Agents

Hasketh PJ: Chemotherapy-induced nausea and vomiting. N Engl J Med 2008;358:2482.

Le TP et al: Update on the management of postoperative nausea and vomiting and postdischarge nausea vomiting in ambulatory surgery. Anesthesiol Clin 2010;28:225.

Roila F et al; Guideline update for MASCC and ESMO in the prevention of chemotherapy- and radiotherapy-induced nausea and vomiting: Results of the Perugia consensus conference. Ann Oncol 2010;21(Suppl 5):v232.

Drugs Used for Inflammatory Bowel Disease

Abraham C et al: Inflammatory bowel disease. N Engl J Med 2009;361:2066.

Benchimol EI et al: Traditional corticosteroids for induction of remission in Crohn's disease. Cochrane Database Syst Rev 2008 Apr 16(2):CD006792.

Bernstein CN et al: World Gastroenterology Organization Practice Guidelines for the diagnosis and management of IBD in 2010. Inflamm Bowel Dis 2010;16:112.

Columbel JF et al: Infliximab, azathioprine, or combination therapy for Crohn's disease. N Engl J Med 2010;362:1383.

De Silva S et al: Optimizing the safety of biologic therapy for IBD. Nat Rev Gastroenterol Hepatol 2010;7:93.

Devlin SM et al: Evolving inflammatory bowel disease treatment paradigms: Top-down versus step-up. Gastroenterol Clin North Am 2009;38:577.

Etchevers MJ et al: Optimizing the use of tumor necrosis factor inhibitors in Crohn's disease: a practical approach. Drugs 2010;70:190.

Hanauer SB: Evolving concepts in treatment and disease modification in ulcerative colitis. Aliment Pharmacol Ther 2008;27(Suppl 1):15.

Kornbluth A et al: Ulcerative colitis guidelines in adults: American College of Gastroenterology, Practice Parameters Committee. Am J Gastroenterol 2010;105:501.

Patel V et al: Methotrexate for maintenance of remission in Crohn's disease. Cochrane Database Syst Rev 2009;7:CD006884.

Peyrin-Biroulet L et al: Efficacy and safety of tumor necrosis factor antagonists in Crohn's disease: Meta-analysis of placebo-controlled trials. Clin Gastroenterol Hepatol 2008;6:644.

Prefontaine E et al: Azathioprine or 6-mercaptopurine for induction of remission in Crohn's disease. Cochrane Database Syst Rev 2010;16:CD000545.

Rosenberg LN et al: Efficacy and safety of drugs in ulcerative colitis. Expert Opin Drug Saf 2010;9:573.

Sandborn WJ et al: Once-daily dosing of delayed-release oral mesalamine (400-mg tablet) is as effective as twice-daily dosing for maintenance of remission for ulcerative colitis. Gastroenterology 2010;138:1286.

Pancreatic Enzyme Supplements

Whitcomb DC et al: Pancrelipase delayed-release capsules (CREON) for exocrine pancreatic insufficiency due to chronic pancreatitis or pancreatic surgery: A double-blind randomized trial. Am J Gastroenterol 2010;105:2276.

Bile Acids for Gallstone Therapy

Hempfling W, Dilger K, Beuers U: Systematic review: Ursodeoxycholic acid—adverse effects and drug interactions. Aliment Pharmacol Ther 2003;18:963.

Drugs for Portal Hypertension

Dell'Era A et al: Acute variceal bleeding: Pharmacological treatment and primary/secondary prophylaxis. Best Pract Clin Gastronterol 2008;22:279.

Garcia-Tsao G et al: Management of varices and variceal hemorrhage in cirrhosis. N Engl J Med 2010;362:823.

CASE STUDY ANSWER

The immediate goals of therapy are to improve this young woman's symptoms of abdominal pain, diarrhea, weight loss, and fatigue. Equally important goals are to reduce the intestinal inflammation in hopes of preventing progression to intestinal stenosis, fistulization, and need for surgery. One option now is to "step up" her therapy by giving her a slow, tapering course of systemic corticosteroids (eg, prednisone) for 8–12 weeks in order to quickly bring her symptoms and inflammation under control while also initiating therapy with an immunomodulator (eg, azathioprine or mercaptopurine) in hopes of achieving long-term disease remission. If satisfactory disease control is not achieved within 3–6 months, therapy with an anti-TNF agent then would be recommended. Alternatively, patients with moderate-to-severe Crohn's disease who have failed mesalamine may be treated upfront with *both* an anti-TNF agent and immunomodulators, which achieves higher remission rates than either agent alone and may improve long-term outcomes.

Therapeutic & Toxic Potential of Over-the-Counter Agents

Robin L. Corelli, PharmD

CASE STUDY

A 66-year-old man presents to his primary care provider for worsening shortness of breath, chest congestion, and symptoms of a severe cold (cough, rhinorrhea, nasal congestion, drowsiness) over the past week. His past medical history is significant for heart failure, hypertension, and hyperlipidemia. His current medications include lisinopril 20 mg daily, simvastatin 40 mg daily, furosemide 40 mg daily, and potassium chloride 20 mEq daily. The patient reports sporadic compliance with his prescribed medications but admits to taking several over-the-counter (OTC) medications over the past 5 days for his recent cold symptoms, including Alka-Seltzer Plus Cold Formula (2 tablets every 4 hours during the day), Sudafed (60 mg every 6 hours), and Advil PM (2 tablets at bedtime). His social history is significant for alcohol use (3–4 beers/night). His vital signs include the following: afebrile, blood pressure 172/94 mm Hg, pulse 84 bpm, respiratory rate 16/min. On physical examination an S_3 gallop is heard; 3+ pitting edema is noted in his lower extremities, and a chest examination reveals inspiratory rales bilaterally. What drugs do OTC "cold" preparations typically contain? Which of the OTC medications might have contributed to the patient's current hypertension? Are any of these preparations implicated in the signs of heart failure?

In the USA, drugs are divided by law into two classes: those restricted to sale by prescription only and those for which directions for safe use by the public can be written. The latter category constitutes the nonprescription or over-the-counter (OTC) drugs. In 2010, the American public spent approximately $17 billion on over 100,000 OTC products to medicate themselves for ailments ranging from acne to warts. These products contain approximately 1000 active ingredients in various forms and combinations.

It is apparent that many OTC drugs are no more than "me too" products advertised to the public in ways that suggest significant differences between them. For example, there are over 100 different systemic analgesic products, almost all of which contain aspirin, acetaminophen, nonsteroidal anti-inflammatory drugs (NSAIDs) such as ibuprofen, or a combination of these agents as primary ingredients. They are made different from one another by the addition of questionable ingredients such as caffeine or antihistamines; by brand names chosen to suggest a specific use or strength ("women's," "migraine," "arthritis," "maximum"); or by special dosage formulations (enteric-coated tablets, geltabs, liquids, orally disintegrating strips and tablets, sustained-release products, powders, seltzers). There is a price attached to all of these features, and in most cases a less expensive generic product can be equally effective. It is probably safe to assume that the public is generally overwhelmed and confused by the wide array of products presented and will probably use those that are most heavily advertised.

Over the past four decades the Food and Drug Administration (FDA) has been engaged in a methodical review of OTC ingredients for both safety and efficacy. There have been two major outcomes of this review: (1) Ingredients designated as ineffective or unsafe for their claimed therapeutic use are being eliminated from OTC product formulations (eg, antimuscarinic agents have been eliminated from OTC sleep aids, attapulgite and polycarbophil can no longer be marketed as OTC antidiarrheal products); and (2) agents previously available by prescription only have been made available for OTC use because they were judged by the review panel to be generally safe and effective for consumer use without medical supervision (Table 63–1). The prescription-to-OTC

TABLE 63-1 Selected agents switched from prescription to OTC status by the Food and Drug Administration.

Ingredient	Indication	Year Ingredient First Switched	Single-Ingredient Product Examples
Systemic agents			
Cetirizine	Antihistamine	2007	Zyrtec
Cimetidine	Acid reducer (H_2 blocker)	1995	Tagamet HB
Clemastine	Antihistamine	1992	Tavist Allergy
Famotidine	Acid reducer (H_2 blocker)	1995	Pepcid AC
Fexofenadine	Antihistamine	2011	Allegra 12 Hour, Allegra 24 Hour
Ibuprofen	Analgesic, antipyretic (NSAID)	1984	Advil, Motrin IB
Lansoprazole	Acid reducer (proton pump inhibitor)	2009	Prevacid 24 HR
Levonorgestrel	Emergency contraceptive	2006	Plan B One-Step
Loratadine	Antihistamine	2002	Claritin, Alavert
Naproxen sodium	Analgesic, antipyretic (NSAID)	1994	Aleve
Nicotine transdermal system	Smoking cessation	1996	Nicoderm CQ
Nicotine polacrilex gum	Smoking cessation	1996	Nicorette
Nizatidine	Acid reducer (H_2 blocker)	1996	Axid AR
Omeprazole	Acid reducer (proton pump inhibitor)	2003	Prilosec OTC, Zegerid OTC
Orlistat	Weight loss aid	2007	Alli
Polyethylene glycol	Laxative	2006	MiraLax
Ranitidine	Acid reducer (H_2 blocker)	1995	Zantac 75, Zantac 150
Topical agents			
Butenafine	Antifungal (topical)	2001	Lotrimin Ultra
Butoconazole	Antifungal (vaginal)	1995	Femstat-3
Clotrimazole	Antifungal (vaginal)	1990	Gyne-Lotrimin-7, Gyne-Lotrimin-3
Cromolyn	Nasal antiallergy	1997	Nasalcrom
Ketoconazole	Dandruff shampoo	1997	Nizoral A-D
Ketotifen fumarate	Ophthalmic antihistamine	2006	Alaway, Zaditor
Miconazole	Antifungal (vaginal)	1991	Monistat-7, Monistat-3
Minoxidil	Hair growth stimulant	1996	Rogaine Regular and Extra Strength For Men, Rogaine For Women
Naphazoline/Pheniramine	Ophthalmic decongestant antihistamine	1994	Naphcon A, Opcon A, Visine-A
Terbinafine	Antifungal (topical)	1999	Lamisil AT
Tioconazole	Antifungal (vaginal)	1997	Monistat-1, Vagistat-1

switch process has significantly enhanced and expanded self-care options for US consumers. Indeed, more than 700 OTC products contain ingredients and dosages that were available only by prescription less than 30 years ago. Some agents such as docosanol and the nicotine polacrilex lozenge have bypassed the prescription route altogether and have been released directly to the OTC market. Other OTC ingredients previously available in low doses only are now available in higher-strength or original prescription strength formulations. Examples of other prescription drugs with the potential for future OTC reclassification include nicotine replacement therapy (oral inhaler, nasal spray) for smoking cessation, proton-pump inhibitors (pantoprazole) for heartburn, and second-generation nonsedating antihistamines (desloratadine, fexofenadine, levocetirizine) for relief of allergy and cold symptoms. The frequency of prescription-to-OTC switches, while commonplace in the mid-1990s, has largely declined over the past decade. The prescription-to-OTC reclassification process is both costly and rigorous and fewer prescription medications are appropriate candidates for a switch (eg, a consumer can self-diagnose and safely treat the condition). For example, the cholesterol-lowering agents cholestyramine, lovastatin, and pravastatin were denied OTC status on the basis that these agents could not be used safely and effectively in an OTC setting. The nonprescription drug advisory committee believed that diagnosis and ongoing management by a health care professional was necessary for the management of hyperlipidemia, a chronic, asymptomatic condition with potentially life-threatening consequences. In a similar recommendation, oral acyclovir for OTC use in the treatment of recurrent genital herpes was not approved because of concerns about misdiagnosis and inappropriate use leading to increased viral resistance.

There are three reasons why it is essential for clinicians to be familiar with the OTC class of products. First, many OTC medications are effective in treating common ailments, and it is important to be able to help the patient select a safe, effective product. Because managed-care practices encourage clinicians to limit the cost of drugs they prescribe, many will recommend effective OTC treatments to their patients, since these drugs are rarely paid for by the insurance plan (Table 63–2). Second, many of the active ingredients contained in OTC drugs may worsen existing medical conditions or interact with prescription medications. (See Chapter 66, Important Drug Interactions & Their Mechanisms.) Finally, the misuse or abuse of OTC products may actually produce significant medical complications. Phenylpropanolamine, for example, a sympathomimetic previously found in many cold, allergy, and weight control products, was withdrawn from the United States market by the FDA based on reports that the drug increased the risk of hemorrhagic stroke. Dextromethorphan, an antitussive found in many cough and cold preparations, has been increasingly abused in high doses (eg, > 5–10 times the recommended antitussive dose) by adolescents as a hallucinogen. Although severe complications associated with dextromethorphan as a single agent in overdose are uncommon, many dextromethorphan-containing products are formulated with other ingredients (acetaminophen, antihistamines, and sympathomimetics) that can be fatal in overdose. Additionally, pseudoephedrine, a decongestant contained in numerous OTC cold preparations, has been used in the illicit manufacture of methamphetamine. A general awareness of these products and their formulations will enable clinicians to more fully appreciate the potential for OTC drug-related problems in their patients.

Table 63–2 lists examples of OTC products that may be used effectively to treat common medical problems. The selection of one ingredient over another may be important in patients with certain medical conditions or in patients taking other medications. These are discussed in detail in other chapters. The recommendations listed in Table 63–2 are based on the efficacy of the ingredients and on the principles set forth in the following paragraphs.

1. Select the product that is simplest in formulation with regard to ingredients and dosage form. In general, single-ingredient products are preferred. Although some combination products contain effective doses of all ingredients, others contain therapeutic doses of some ingredients and subtherapeutic doses of others. Furthermore, there may be differing durations of action among the ingredients, and there is always a possibility that the clinician or patient is unaware of the presence of certain active ingredients in the product. Acetaminophen, for example, is in many cough and cold preparations; a patient unaware of this may take separate doses of analgesic in addition to that contained in the cold preparation, potentially leading to hepatotoxicity.
2. Select a product that contains a therapeutically effective dose.
3. Consumers and providers should carefully read the "Drug Facts" label to determine which ingredients are appropriate based on the patient's symptoms, underlying health conditions, and whatever is known about the medications the patient is already taking. This is critical because many products with the same brand name contain different ingredients that are labeled for different uses. For example, multiple laxative products (with different active ingredients) carry the Dulcolax name including Dulcolax Balance (polyethylene glycol), Dulcolax Laxative (bisacodyl), and Dulcolax Stool Softener (docusate sodium). This marketing practice of "extending a brand name" across product lines, while legal, is confusing and can lead to medication errors.
4. Recommend a generic product if one is available.
5. Be wary of "gimmicks" or advertising claims of specific superiority over similar products.
6. For children, the dose, dosage form, and palatability of the product are prime considerations.

Certain ingredients in OTC products should be avoided or used with caution in selected patients because they may exacerbate existing medical problems or interact with other medications the patient is taking. Many of the more potent OTC ingredients are hidden in products where their presence would not ordinarily be expected (Table 63–3). Although OTC medications have standardized label formatting and content requirements that specify the indications for use, dosage, warnings, and active and inactive ingredients contained in the product, many consumers do not carefully read or comprehend this information. Lack of awareness of the ingredients in OTC products and the belief by many providers that OTC products are ineffective and harmless may cause diagnostic confusion and perhaps interfere with therapy. For example, innumerable OTC products, including analgesics and allergy, cough, and cold preparations, contain sympathomimetics. These agents should be avoided or used cautiously by type 1 diabetics and patients with hypertension, angina, or hyperthyroidism. Aspirin should not be used in children and adolescents for viral infections (with or without fever) because of an increased risk of Reye's syndrome. Aspirin and other NSAIDs should be avoided by individuals with active peptic ulcer disease, certain platelet disorders, and patients taking oral anticoagulants. Cimetidine, an H$_2$-receptor antagonist, is a well-known inhibitor of hepatic drug metabolism and can increase the blood levels and toxicity of drugs such as phenytoin, theophylline, and warfarin.

Overuse or misuse of OTC products may induce significant medical problems. A prime example is rebound congestion from the regular use of decongestant nasal sprays for more than 3 days. The improper and long-term use of some antacids (eg, aluminum hydroxide) may cause constipation and even impaction in elderly people, as well as hypophosphatemia. Laxative abuse can result in abdominal cramping and fluid and electrolyte disturbances. Insomnia, nervousness, and restlessness can result from the use of sympathomimetics or caffeine hidden in many OTC products (Table 63–3). The long-term use of some analgesics containing large amounts of caffeine may produce rebound headaches, and long-term use of analgesics has been associated with interstitial nephritis. OTC products containing aspirin, other salicylates, acetaminophen, ibuprofen, or naproxen may increase the risk of hepatotoxicity and gastrointestinal hemorrhage in individuals who consume three or more alcoholic drinks daily. Recent evidence

TABLE 63–2 Ingredients of known efficacy for selected OTC classes.

OTC Category	Ingredient and Usual Adult Dosage	Product Examples	Comments
Acid reducers (H₂ antagonists)	Cimetidine, 200 mg once or twice daily	Tagamet HB, various generic	These products have been approved for the relief of "heartburn associated with acid indigestion, and sour stomach." They should not be taken for longer than 2 weeks and are not recommended for children < 12 years of age.
	Famotidine, 10–20 mg once or twice daily	Pepcid AC, Maximum Strength Pepcid AC, various generic	
	Nizatidine, 75 mg once or twice daily	Axid AR	
	Ranitidine, 75–150 mg once or twice daily	Zantac 75, Zantac 150, various generic	
Acid reducers (proton pump inhibitors)	Lansoprazole, 15 mg once daily for 14 days	Prevacid 24 HR	Proton pump inhibitors are approved for the treatment of frequent heartburn in adults (≥ 18 years of age) with symptoms of heartburn 2 or more days per week. These products are not intended for immediate relief of heartburn, as they may take 1–4 days for full effect. They should not be taken for more than 14 days or more often than every 4 months unless directed by a physician. Omeprazole magnesium 20.6 mg is equivalent to 20 mg of omeprazole (prescription strength).
	Omeprazole magnesium, 20.6 mg once daily for 14 days	Prilosec OTC, various generic	
	Omeprazole (20 mg) with sodium bicarbonate (1100 mg), once daily for 14 days	Zegerid OTC	
Acne preparations	Benzoyl peroxide, 5%, 10%	Clearasil, Oxy-10, various generic	One of the most effective acne preparations. Apply sparingly once or twice daily. Decrease concentration or frequency if excessive skin irritation occurs.
Allergy and "cold" preparations	Chlorpheniramine, 4 mg every 4–6 hours; 8 mg (extended-release) every 8–12 hours; 12 mg (extended-release) every 12 hours	Chlor-Trimeton Allergy, various generic	Antihistamines alone relieve most symptoms associated with allergic rhinitis or hay fever. Chlorpheniramine, brompheniramine, and clemastine may cause less drowsiness than diphenhydramine. Cetirizine, fexofenadine and loratadine (second generation antihistamines), are therapeutically comparable to first-generation agents; these agents have minimal anti-cholinergic effects and are therefore associated with a lower incidence of sedation. Occasionally, symptoms unrelieved by the antihistamine respond to the addition of a sympathomimetic decongestant. OTC sale of products containing pseudoephedrine is restricted (see comments under Decongestants, systemic).
	Clemastine, 1.34 mg every 12 hours	Tavist Allergy	
	Cetirizine, 10 mg every 24 hours	Zyrtec, various generic	
	Diphenhydramine, 25–50 mg every 4–6 hours	Benadryl Allergy, various generic	
	Fexofenadine 60 mg every 12 hours; 180 mg every 24 hours	Allegra 12 Hour, Allegra 24 Hour	
	Loratadine, 10 mg every 24 hours	Alavert, Claritin, various generic	
	Brompheniramine (4 mg) with phenylephrine (10 mg) every 4 hours	Dimetapp Cold & Allergy, various generic	
	Cetirizine (5 mg) with pseudoephedrine (120 mg) every 12 hours	Zyrtec-D	
	Chlorpheniramine (4 mg) with phenylephrine (10 mg) every 4 hours	Allerest PE, Sudafed PE Sinus & Allergy, various generic	
	Fexofenadine (60 mg) with pseudoephedrine (120 mg) every 12 hours	Allegra-D 12 Hour	
	Loratadine (5 mg) with pseudoephedrine (120 mg) every 12 hours	Claritin-D 12 Hour	
	Loratadine (10 mg) with pseudoephedrine (240 mg) every 24 hours	Claritin-D 24 Hour	
	Triprolidine (2.5 mg) with phenylephrine (10 mg) every 4 hours	Actifed Cold & Allergy, various generic	

(continued)

TABLE 63-2 Ingredients of known efficacy for selected OTC classes. (Continued)

OTC Category	Ingredient and Usual Adult Dosage	Product Examples	Comments
Analgesics and antipyretics	Acetaminophen, 325–650 mg every 4–6 hours; 650–1300 mg (extended-release) every 8 hours	Panadol, Tylenol, Extra Strength Tylenol, Tylenol 8-Hour, various generic	Acetaminophen lacks anti-inflammatory activity but is available as a liquid; this dosage form is used primarily for infants and children who cannot chew or swallow tablets. Use of products containing acetaminophen may increase the risk of severe liver damage in individuals who ingest more than 4 g in 24 hours, take with other drugs containing acetaminophen, or consume ≥ three alcoholic drinks daily. In January 2011, the FDA announced that manufacturers of prescription acetaminophen combination products must limit the maximum amount of acetaminophen in these formulations to 325 mg per dosage unit to reduce the risk of severe liver injury from acetaminophen overdosing. There are numerous product modifications, including the addition of antacids and caffeine; enteric-coated tablets and seltzers; long-acting or extra-strength formulations; and various mixtures of analgesics. None has any substantial advantage over a single-ingredient product. Aspirin should be used cautiously in certain individuals (see text). Use of products containing aspirin may increase the risk of severe gastrointestinal hemorrhage in individuals who consume ≥ 3 alcoholic drinks daily. Use of products containing NSAIDs may increase the risk of severe gastrointestinal hemorrhage in individuals who are age 60 or older, have had stomach ulcers or bleeding problems, take anticoagulant or steroid drugs, take other drugs containing prescription or nonprescription NSAIDs, consume 3 or more alcoholic drinks daily or take more or for a longer time than directed. Long-term continuous use of NSAIDs may increase the risk of heart attack or stroke.
	Aspirin, 325–650 mg every 4–6 hours	Bayer Aspirin, Ecotrin, Bufferin, various generic	
	Ibuprofen, 200–400 mg every 4–6 hours (not to exceed 1200 mg in a 24-hour period)	Advil, Motrin IB, various generic	
	Naproxen sodium, 220 mg every 8–12 hours (not to exceed 660 mg in a 24-hour period)	Aleve, various generic	
Antacids	Magnesium hydroxide and aluminum hydroxide alone or in combination; calcium carbonate, dosage varies; consult product labeling	Alternagel, Maalox, Milk of Magnesia, Mylanta, Tums, various generic	Combinations of magnesium and aluminum hydroxide are less likely to cause constipation or diarrhea and offer high neutralizing capacity. Some preparations include simethicone, an antiflatulent to relieve symptoms of bloating and pressure.
Antihelminthics (pinworm infection)	Pyrantel pamoate, 11 mg/kg (maximum: 1 g)	Pin-X, Reese's Pinworm	Treat all members of the household. Consult physician for children < 2 years of age or < 25 lb. Undergarments, pajamas, and linens should be washed daily until the infection is resolved. If symptoms persist beyond 2 weeks, contact a physician to determine if a repeat dose is indicated.
Antidiarrheal agents	Bismuth subsalicylate, 524 mg every 30–60 minutes as needed up to 8 doses daily	Kaopectate, Pepto-Bismol, various generics	Antidiarrheals should not be used if diarrhea is accompanied by fever > 101°F or if blood or mucus is present in stool. Bismuth salts can cause dark discoloration of the tongue and/or stools. Salicylates are absorbed and can cause tinnitus if coadministered with aspirin.
	Loperamide, 4 mg initially, then 2 mg after each loose stool, not to exceed 8 mg in 24 hours	Imodium A-D, various generic	Loperamide, a synthetic opioid, acts on intestinal smooth muscle to decrease motility allowing for absorption of water and electrolytes. Poorly penetrates the CNS and has a lower risk of side effects compared with diphenoxylate or opiates. Not considered a controlled substance.

(continued)

TABLE 63–2 Ingredients of known efficacy for selected OTC classes. (Continued)

OTC Category	Ingredient and Usual Adult Dosage	Product Examples	Comments
Antifungal topical preparations	Butenafine, 1% (cream) apply to affected areas once daily	Lotrimin Ultra	Effective for the treatment of tinea pedis (athlete's foot), tinea cruris (jock itch), and tinea corporis (ringworm). Clotrimazole and miconazole also effective against *Candida albicans*. Clinicians should be aware that products carrying the same brand name do not necessarily contain the same active ingredient.
	Clotrimazole, 1% (cream, powder, solution), apply to affected areas twice daily (morning and evening)	Lotrimin AF (various formulations), various generic	
	Miconazole, 2% (cream, powder, solution), apply to affected areas twice daily (morning and night)	Cruex, Desenex, Lotrimin AF (powder, spray), Zeasorb-AF	
	Terbinafine, 1% (cream, gel, solution), apply to affected areas once daily (ringworm/jock itch) or twice daily (athlete's foot)	Lamisil AT	
	Tolnaftate, 1% (cream, powder, spray, solution), apply to affected areas twice daily (morning and night)	Lamisil AF Defense (powder), Tinactin, Ting cream, various generic	
	Undecylenic acid, 12–25% (powder, solution) apply to affected areas twice daily	Blis-To-Sol, Elon Dual Defense Anti-Fungal	
Antifungal vaginal preparations	Clotrimazole (1%, 2% vaginal cream, 100 mg, 200 mg tablet); see comments for dosage	Gyne-Lotrimin-7, Gyne-Lotrimin-3, various generic	Topical vaginal antifungals should only be used for treatment of recurrent vulvovaginal candidiasis in otherwise healthy, nonpregnant women previously diagnosed by a clinician. Insert one applicatorful (1%) or one tablet (100 mg) intravaginally at bedtime for 7 consecutive days. Alternatively: Insert one applicatorful (2%) or one tablet (200 mg) intravaginally at bedtime for 3 consecutive days.
	Miconazole (2%, 4% vaginal cream; 100 mg, 200 mg, 1200 mg vaginal suppositories); see comments for dosage	Monistat-7, Monistat-3, Vagistat-3, various generic	Insert one applicatorful intravaginally at bedtime for 3 consecutive days (4%) or 7 consecutive days (2%). Alternatively: Insert one suppository intravaginally at bedtime for 1 day (1200 mg), 3 consecutive days (200 mg), or 7 consecutive days (100 mg).
	Tioconazole, 6.5% vaginal ointment, one applicatorful intravaginally at bedtime (single dose)	Monistat-1, Vagistat-1, various generic	
Anti-inflammatory topical preparations	Hydrocortisone, 0.5% (cream, ointment, lotion), 1% (cream, gel, ointment, lotion, spray)	Cortaid, Cortizone-10, Preparation H, Hydrocortisone, various generic	Used to temporarily relieve itching and inflammation associated with minor rashes due to contact or allergic dermatitides, insect bites, and hemorrhoids. Apply sparingly to affected areas two to four times daily.
Antiseborrheal agents	Coal tar, 0.5-5% shampoo, dosage varies; consult product labeling	Denorex Therapeutic, Ionil T Plus, various generic	Tar derivatives inhibit epidermal proliferation and may possess antipruritic and antimicrobial activity.
	Ketoconazole, 1% shampoo, apply every 3–4 days	Nizoral A-D	Synthetic azole antifungal agent with activity versus *Pityrosporum ovale*, a fungus that may cause seborrhea and dandruff. Massage over entire scalp for 3 minutes. Rinse thoroughly and repeat application.
	Pyrithione zinc, 1–2% shampoo, apply once or twice weekly	Head & Shoulders, Selsun Blue Salon, various generic	Both selenium sulfide and zinc pyrithione are cytostatic agents that decrease epidermal turnover rates. Massage into wet scalp for 2–3 minutes. Rinse thoroughly and repeat application. Selenium sulfide can be irritating to the eyes and skin.
	Selenium sulfide, 1% shampoo, apply once or twice weekly	Head & Shoulders Intensive Treatment, Selsun Blue Medicated, various generic	

(continued)

TABLE 63–2 Ingredients of known efficacy for selected OTC classes. (Continued)

OTC Category	Ingredient and Usual Adult Dosage	Product Examples	Comments
Antitussives	Codeine, 10–20 mg every 4–6 hours, not to exceed 120 mg in 24 hours (with guaifenesin)	Guiatuss AC, Mytussin AC, various generic	Acts centrally to increase the cough threshold. In doses required for cough suppression, the addiction liability associated with codeine is low. Codeine-containing antitussive combinations are schedule V narcotics, and OTC sale is restricted in some states.
	Dextromethorphan, 10–20 mg every 4 hours or 30 mg every 6–8 hours; 60 mg (extended-release suspension) every 12 hours	Delsym 12-Hour Cough, Hold DM, Robitussin Cough, Vicks 44 Dry Cough, various generic	Dextromethorphan is a nonopioid congener of levorphanol without analgesic or addictive properties. Often is used with antihistamines, decongestants, and expectorants in combination products. In high dosages (> 2 mg/kg) dextromethorphan can induce phencyclidine-like hallucinogenic effects.
Decongestants, topical	Oxymetazoline, 0.05% nasal solution, 2–3 sprays per nostril not more often than every 10–12 hours Phenylephrine (0.5%, 1%), nasal solution, 2–3 sprays per nostril no more often than every 4 hours	Afrin, Dristan, Neo-Synephrine Nighttime 12 Hour, Sudafed OM, Vicks Sinex, various generic Neo-Synephrine, various generic	Topical sympathomimetics are effective for the temporary acute management of rhinorrhea associated with common colds and allergies. Long-acting agents (oxymetazoline-containing products) are generally preferred, although phenylephrine is equally effective. Topical decongestants should not be used for longer than 3 days to prevent rebound nasal congestion.
Decongestants, systemic	Phenylephrine, 10 mg every 4 hours Pseudoephedrine, 60 mg every 4–6 hours or 120 mg (extended-release) every 12 hours, or 240 mg (extended-release) every 24 hours	Sudafed PE, various generic combination products Sudafed, various generic	Oral decongestants have a prolonged duration of action but may cause more systemic effects, including nervousness, excitability, restlessness, and insomnia. Also available in antihistamine, antitussive, expectorant, and analgesic combination products. Federal regulations established to discourage the illicit manufacture of methamphetamine specify that all drug products containing pseudoephedrine must be stored in locked cabinets or behind the pharmacy counter and can only be sold in limited quantities to consumers after they provide photo identification and sign a logbook.
Emergency contraceptive	Levonorgestrel, 1.5 mg tablet taken as soon as possible within 72 hours after unprotected intercourse	Plan B One-Step	Levonorgestrel prevents ovulation and may inhibit fertilization or implantation. Reduces the chance of pregnancy by up to 89% when taken as directed within 72 hours after unprotected intercourse. Plan B is available behind the counter at pharmacies and sold under the supervision of a licensed pharmacist. A prescription is needed for women ≤ 17 years of age.
Expectorants	Guaifenesin, 200–400 mg every 4 hours; 600–1200 mg (extended-release) every 12 hours	Mucinex, Robitussin, various generic	The only OTC expectorant recognized as safe and effective by the FDA. Often used with antihistamines, decongestants, and antitussives in combination products.
Hair growth stimulants	Minoxidil, 2% solution (for women), 5% foam, solution (for men), apply 1/2 capful (foam) or 1 mL (solution) to affected areas of scalp twice daily	Rogaine for Men, Rogaine for Women, Rogaine Extra Strength for Men	Minoxidil appears to directly stimulate hair follicles resulting in increased hair thickness and reduced hair loss. Treatment for 4 months or longer may be necessary to achieve visible results. If new hair growth is observed, continued treatment is necessary as hair density returns to pretreatment levels within months following drug discontinuation.

(continued)

TABLE 63–2 Ingredients of known efficacy for selected OTC classes. (Continued)

OTC Category	Ingredient and Usual Adult Dosage	Product Examples	Comments
Laxatives	Bulk formers: Polycarbophil, psyllium, and methylcellulose preparations. Dosage varies; consult product labeling	Citrucel, Fibercon, Konsyl, Metamucil, various generic	The safest laxatives for chronic use include the bulk formers and stool softeners. Saline laxatives and stimulants may be used acutely but not chronically (see text). Bulk formers hold water and expand in stool, promoting peristalsis.
	Hyperosmotics: Glycerin, 2–3 g suppository per rectum daily. Polyethylene glycol 3350 (powder), 17 g dissolved in 4–8 oz of beverage daily	Fleet Glycerin Suppository, various generic; Dulcolax Balance, MiraLax	Glycerin induces a local irritant effect in combination with an osmotic effect. Polyethylene glycol formulations are large, poorly absorbed molecules that induce an osmotic effect causing distention and catharsis.
	Stool softeners: Docusate sodium, 50–500 mg daily. Docusate calcium, 240 mg daily	Colace, Dulcolax, Surfak, various generic	Softens fecal material via detergent action that allows water to penetrate stool.
	Stimulant laxatives: Bisacodyl, 5–15 mg daily. Senna, dosage varies, consult product labeling	Dulcolax, Ex-Lax, Senokot, various generic	Stimulant laxative actions include direct irritation of intestinal mucosa or stimulation of the myenteric plexus, resulting in peristalsis. These agents may also cause alteration of fluid and electrolyte absorption, resulting in luminal fluid accumulation and bowel evacuation.
Pediculicides (head lice)	Permethrin 1%	Nix	Instructions for use vary; consult product labeling. Avoid contact with eyes. Comb out nits. Linens, pajamas, combs, and brushes should be washed daily until the infestation is eliminated. For pyrethrin products, retreat in 7–10 days to kill any newly hatched nits. Permethrin products have residual effects for up to 10 days; therefore, reapplication is not required unless live nits are visible 7 days or more after the initial treatment.
	Pyrethrins (0.3%) combined with piperonyl butoxide (3–4%)	A-200, RID	
Sleep aids	Diphenhydramine, 25–50 mg at bedtime	Nytol, Simply Sleep, Sominex, various generic	Diphenhydramine and doxylamine are antihistamines with well-documented CNS depressant effects. Because insomnia may be indicative of a serious underlying condition requiring medical attention, patients should consult a physician if insomnia persists continuously for longer than 2 weeks.
	Doxylamine, 25 mg 30 minutes before bedtime	Unisom, various generic	
Smoking cessation aids	Nicotine polacrilex gum; dosage varies; consult product labeling	Nicorette, various generic	Nicotine replacement products in combination with behavioral support approximately double long-term cessation rates compared with placebo. Review directions for use carefully, since product strengths vary and self-titration and tapering may be necessary.
	Nicotine polacrilex lozenge, dosage varies, consult product labeling	Nicorette, various generic	
	Nicotine (transdermal system), dosage varies; consult product labeling	Nicoderm CQ, various generic	
Weight loss aids	Orlistat, 60 mg with each meal containing fat (not to exceed 180 mg/d)	Alli	Approved for weight loss in overweight adults ≥ 18 years of age when used in combination with a reduced-calorie, low-fat diet and exercise program. Orlistat is a nonsystemically absorbed inhibitor of gastrointestinal lipase that blocks the absorption of dietary fat. OTC formulation is a half-strength version of the prescription product (Xenical).

TABLE 63–3 Hidden ingredients in OTC products.

Hidden Drug or Drug Class	OTC Class Containing Drug	Product Examples
Alcohol (percent ethanol)	Cough syrups, cold preparations	Theraflu Nighttime (10%); Vicks NyQuil Cold & Flu Liquid (10%); Vicks NyQuil Cough (10%)
	Mouthwashes	Listerine (27%); Scope (15%); Cepacol (14%)
Antihistamines	Analgesics	Advil PM; Alka-Seltzer PM; Excedrin PM; Bayer PM; Extra Strength Doan's PM; Goody's PM Pain Relief Powder; Tylenol PM
	Menstrual products	Midol Menstrual Complete; Pamprin Multi-Symptom
	Sleep aids	Nytol; Simply Sleep; Sominex; Unisom
Aspirin and other salicylates	Antidiarrheals	Pepto-Bismol (bismuth subsalicylate); Kaopectate (bismuth subsalicylate)
	Cold/allergy preparations	Alka-Seltzer Plus Flu
Caffeine (mg/tablets or as stated)	Analgesics	Anacin (32); Anacin Maximum Strength (32); Arthritis Strength BC (65/pre-measured packet); BC Powder (65/pre-measured packet); Excedrin Extra Strength (65); Excedrin Migraine (65); Excedrin Tension Headache (65); Goody's Extra Strength Headache Powder (33/pre-measured packet); Goody's Cool Orange (65/pre-measured packet)
	Menstrual products	Excedrin Menstrual Complete (65); Midol Menstrual Complete (60); Pamprin Max (65)
	Stimulants	NoDoz (200); Vivarin (200)
Local anesthetics (usually benzocaine)	Antitussives/lozenges	Cepacol Sore Throat Lozenges; Chloraseptic Sore Throat; Sucrets Sore Throat; Sucrets Complete
	Dermatologic preparations	Americaine; Bactine; Dermoplast; Lanacane; Solarcaine
	Hemorrhoidal products	Americaine Ointment; Nupercainal; Tronolane; Tucks Ointment
	Toothache, cold sore, and teething products	Anbesol; Kank-A; Orajel; Zilactin-B
Sodium (mg/tablet or as stated)	Analgesics	Alka-Seltzer Original Effervescent Tablet (567); Alka-Seltzer Extra Strength Effervescent Tablet (588); Bromo-Seltzer Granules (959/pre-measured packet)
	Antacids	Alka-Seltzer Original Effervescent Tablet (567); Alka-Seltzer Extra Strength Effervescent Tablet (588); Alka-Seltzer Gold (309); Alka-Seltzer Heartburn Relief (575); Brioschi (500/6 g dose); Bromo-Seltzer Granules (959/pre-measured packet)
	Cold/cough preparations	Alka-Seltzer Plus Formulations: Day Cold (416); Cold & Cough (415); Flu (387); Night Cold (474)
	Laxatives	Fleets Enema (4,439 mg, of which 275-400 mg/enema is absorbed)
Sympathomimetics	Analgesics	Excedrin Sinus Headache; Sine-Off; Sinutab; Tylenol Congestion & Pain; Tylenol Sinus Severe Congestion
	Asthma products	Bronkaid Dual Action; Primatene Mist; Primatene Tablets
	Cold/cough/allergy preparations	Advil Cold & Sinus; Alka-Seltzer Plus (many); Comtrex Severe Cold & Sinus; Congestac; Contac Cold+Flu; Dimetapp (many); Dristan Cold; PediaCare (many); Robitussin Cough, Cold & Flu; Robitussin Cough & Cold CF; Sudafed PE Cold & Cough; Theraflu (many); Triaminic (many); Tylenol Cold (many); Tylenol Sinus (many); Tylenol Allergy (many); Vicks (many)
	Hemorrhoidal products	Hemorid; Preparation H (cream, ointment, suppository)

suggests the long-term use of certain NSAIDs may increase the risk of heart attack or stroke. Furthermore, acute ingestion of large amounts of acetaminophen by adults or children can cause serious, and often fatal, hepatotoxicity. Antihistamines may cause sedation or drowsiness, especially when taken concurrently with sedative-hypnotics, tranquilizers, alcohol, or other central nervous system depressants. Antihistamines and other substances contained in OTC topical and vaginal products may induce allergic reactions.

Finally, use of OTC cough and cold preparations in the pediatric population has been under scrutiny by the FDA based on a lack of efficacy data in children less than 12 years of age and reports of serious toxicity in children. In 2008, the FDA issued an advisory alert recommending that OTC cough and cold agents (eg, products containing antitussives, expectorants, decongestants, and antihistamines) not be used in infants and children less than 2 years of age because of the potential for serious and possibly life-threatening adverse events. More recently, in October 2008, leading pharmaceutical manufacturers voluntarily modified product labels on OTC cough and cold preparations to state, "do not use" in children under 4 years of age. Further safety reviews by the FDA regarding the use of these agents in children between the ages of 2 and 11 are ongoing.

There are three major drug information sources for OTC products. *Handbook of Nonprescription Drugs* is the most comprehensive resource for OTC medications; it evaluates ingredients contained in major OTC drug classes and lists the ingredients included in many OTC products. *Nonprescription Drug* Therapy is an online reference that is updated monthly; it provides detailed OTC product information and patient counseling instructions. *Physicians' Desk Reference for Nonprescription Drugs, Dietary Supplements and Herbs*, a compendium of manufacturers' information regarding OTC products, is published annually but is somewhat incomplete with regard to the number of products included. Any health care provider who seeks more specific information regarding OTC products may find useful the references listed below.

REFERENCES

Consumer Healthcare Products Association website: http://www.chpa-info.org/

Handbook of Nonprescription Drugs, 17th ed. American Pharmacists Association, 2011.

Lessenger JE, Feinberg SD: Abuse of prescription and over-the-counter medications. J Am Board Fam Med 2008;21:45.

Nonprescription Drug Therapy. Facts and Comparisons 4.0 (online). Wolters Kluwer Health, 2011.

Physicians' Desk Reference for Nonprescription Drugs, Dietary Supplements and Herbs, 32nd ed. Thomson Healthcare, 2011.

Sharfstein JM, North M, Serwint JR: Over the counter but no longer under the radar—pediatric cough and cold medications. N Engl J Med 2007;357:232.

US Food and Drug Administration: Center for Drug Evaluation and Research. Office of Nonprescription Products website: http://www.fda.gov/cder/offices/otc/default.htm

CASE STUDY ANSWER

OTC cold medications typically contain antihistamines (eg, brompheniramine, chlorpheniramine, diphenhydramine), antitussives (eg, dextromethorphan), expectorants (eg, guaifenesin), and nasal decongestants (eg, phenylephrine, pseudoephedrine). Systemic nasal decongestants (contained in Alka-Seltzer and Sudafed) stimulate α_1-adrenoceptors and may raise blood pressure through direct vasoconstrictor effects. Additionally, NSAIDs (contained in Advil PM) increase blood pressure and may reduce the effectiveness of antihypertensive agents. NSAIDs may also exacerbate heart failure through increased fluid retention and elevated blood pressure. Alka-Seltzer cold preparations should be avoided in patients with heart failure due to the high sodium content, which can lead to fluid retention. The sodium content in one dose of Alka-Seltzer Plus cold medicine (948 mg/dose) provides approximately half of the maximum recommended sodium allowance for patients with heart failure.

64

Dietary Supplements & Herbal Medications[*]

Cathi E. Dennehy, PharmD, & Candy Tsourounis, PharmD

CASE STUDY

A 65-year-old man with a history of coronary artery disease, high cholesterol, type 2 diabetes, and hypertension presents with a question about a dietary supplement. He is in good health, exercises regularly, and eats a low-fat, low-salt diet. His most recent laboratory values show that his low-density lipoprotein (LDL) cholesterol is still slightly above goal at 120 mg/dL (goal < 100 mg/dL) and his hemoglobin A_{1C} is well controlled at 6%. His blood pressure is also well controlled. His medications include simvastatin, metformin, benazepril, and aspirin. He also regularly takes a vitamin B complex supplement and coenzyme Q10. He asks you if taking a garlic supplement could help to bring his LDL cholesterol down to less than 100 mg/dL. What are two rationales for why he might be using a coenzyme Q10 supplement? Are there any supplements that could increase bleeding risk if taken with aspirin?

The medical use of plants in their natural and unprocessed form undoubtedly began when the first intelligent animals noticed that certain food plants altered particular body functions. While there is a great deal of historical information about the use of plant-based supplements, there is also much unreliable information from poorly designed clinical studies that do not account for randomization errors, confounders, and—most importantly—a placebo effect that can contribute 30–50% of the observed response. Since the literature surrounding dietary supplements is evolving and much of it is not peer-reviewed, it is recommended that reputable evidence-based resources be used to help guide treatment decisions. An unbiased and regularly updated compendium of basic and clinical reports regarding botanicals is *Pharmacists Letter/Prescribers Letter Natural Medicines Comprehensive Database* (see references). Another evidence-based resource is *Natural Standard*, which includes an international, multi-disciplinary collaborative website, http://www.naturalstandard.com. Unfortunately, the evidence available to these objective and unbi-

ased evaluators is rarely adequate to permit clear conclusions. As a result, all statements regarding positive benefits should be regarded as preliminary and even conclusions regarding safety should be considered tentative at this time.

For legal purposes, "dietary supplements" are distinguished from "prescription drugs" derived from plants (morphine, digitalis, atropine, etc) by virtue of being available without a prescription and, unlike "over-the-counter medications," are legally considered dietary supplements rather than drugs. This distinction eliminates the need for proof of efficacy and safety prior to marketing and also places the burden of proof on the Food and Drug Administration (FDA) to prove that a supplement is harmful before its use can be restricted or removed from the market. Although manufacturers are prohibited from marketing unsafe or ineffective products, the FDA has met significant challenges from the supplement industry largely due to the strong lobbying effort by supplement manufacturers and the variability in interpretation of the Dietary Supplement Health and Education Act (DSHEA). DSHEA defines dietary supplements as vitamins, minerals, herbs or other botanicals, amino acids or dietary supplements used to supplement the diet by increasing dietary intake, or concentrates, metabolites, constituents, extracts, or any combination of these ingredients. For the purposes of this chapter, plant-based substances and synthetic purified

---

[*]The industry marketing these materials is replacing the terms "herbal medication" and "botanical medication" with the term "dietary supplement" in order to avoid legal liability and added governmental regulation. For the purposes of this chapter, they are identical.

chemicals will be referred to as dietary supplements. Among the purified chemicals, glucosamine, coenzyme Q10, and melatonin are of significant pharmacologic interest.

This chapter provides some historical perspective and describes the evidence provided by randomized, double-blind, placebo-controlled trials, meta-analyses, and systematic reviews involving several of the most commonly used agents in this class. Ephedrine, the active principle in Ma-huang, is discussed in Chapter 9.

HISTORICAL & REGULATORY FACTORS

Under the DSHEA, dietary supplements are not considered over-the-counter drugs in the USA but rather food supplements used for health maintenance. Although dietary supplements are regulated as food, consumers may use them in the same fashion as drugs and even use them in place of drugs or in combination with drugs.

In 1994, the United States Congress, influenced by growing "consumerism" as well as strong manufacturer lobbying efforts, passed the DSHEA. DSHEA required the establishment of Good Manufacturing Practice (GMP) standards for the supplement industry; however, it was not until 2007 that the FDA issued a final rule on the proposed GMP standards. This 13-year delay allowed supplement manufacturers to self-regulate the manufacturing process and resulted in many instances of adulteration, misbranding, and contamination. Therefore, much of the criticism regarding the dietary supplement industry involves a lack of product purity and variations in potency. Under the new GMP standards, large and small dietary supplement manufacturers should now be in compliance with this legislation. The FDA, however, has limited resources to adequately investigate and oversee compliance with manufacturing standards, particularly since many ingredient suppliers are based overseas. Furthermore, the dietary supplement ingredient supply chain is complex and federal regulators are not able to adequately inspect manufacturing facilities in a timely or efficient matter.

Because of the problems that resulted from self-regulation, another law, the Dietary Supplement and Non-Prescription Drug Consumer Protection Act, was approved in 2006. This law requires manufacturers, packers, or distributors of supplements to submit reports of serious adverse events to the FDA. Serious adverse events are defined as death, a life-threatening event, hospitalization, a persistent or significant disability or incapacity, congenital anomaly or birth defect, or an adverse event that requires medical or surgical intervention to prevent such outcomes based on reasonable medical judgment. These reports are intended to identify trends in adverse effects and would help to alert the public to safety issues.

CLINICAL ASPECTS OF THE USE OF BOTANICALS

Many United States consumers have embraced the use of dietary supplements as a "natural" approach to their health care. Unfortunately, misconceptions regarding safety and efficacy of the agents are common, and the fact that a substance can be called "natural" does not of course guarantee its safety. In fact, these products may be inherently inert, toxic, or may have been adulterated, misbranded, or contaminated either intentionally or unintentionally in a variety of ways.

Adverse effects have been documented for a variety of dietary supplements; however, under-reporting of adverse effects is likely since consumers do not routinely report, and do not know how to report an adverse effect if they suspect that the event was caused by consumption of a supplement. Furthermore, chemical analysis is rarely performed on the products involved, including those products that are described in the literature as being linked to an adverse event. This leads to confusion about whether the primary ingredient or an adulterant caused the adverse effect. In some cases, the chemical constituents of the herb can clearly lead to toxicity. Some of the herbs that should be used cautiously or not at all are listed in Table 64–1.

An important risk factor in the use of dietary supplements is the lack of adequate testing for drug interactions. Since botanicals may contain hundreds of active and inactive ingredients, it is very difficult and costly to study potential drug interactions when they are combined with other medications. This may present significant risks to patients.

■ BOTANICAL SUBSTANCES

ECHINACEA (*ECHINACEA PURPUREA*)

Chemistry

The three most widely used species of *Echinacea* are *Echinacea purpurea*, *E pallida*, and *E angustifolia*. The chemical constituents include flavonoids, lipophilic constituents (eg, alkamides, polyacetylenes), water-soluble polysaccharides, and water-soluble caffeoyl conjugates (eg, echinacoside, cichoric acid, caffeic acid). Within any marketed echinacea formulation, the relative amounts of these components are dependent upon the species used, the method of manufacture, and the plant parts used. *E purpurea* has been the most widely studied in clinical trials. Although the active constituents of echinacea are not completely known, cichoric acid from *E purpurea* and echinacoside from *E pallida and E angustifolia*, as well as alkamides and polysaccharides, are most often noted as having immune-modulating properties. Most commercial formulations, however, are not standardized for any particular constituent.

Pharmacologic Effects

A. Immune Modulation

The effect of echinacea on the immune system is controversial. In vivo human studies using commercially marketed formulations of *E purpurea* have shown increased phagocytosis, total circulating white blood cells, monocytes, neutrophils, and natural killer cells but not immunostimulation. In vitro, *E purpurea* juice increased production of interleukins-1, -6, and -10, and tumor necrosis factor-α by human macrophages. Enhanced natural killer cell activity and antibody-dependent cellular toxicity was also observed

TABLE 64–1 Various supplements and some associated risks.

Commercial Name, Scientific Name, Plant Parts	Intended Use	Toxic Agents, Effects	Comments
Aconite *Aconitum* species	Analgesic	Alkaloid, cardiac and central nervous system effects	Avoid
Aristolochic acid *Aristolochia* species	Traditional Chinese medicine; various uses	Carcinogen, nephrotoxicity	Avoid
Black cohosh *Cimicifuga racemosa*	Menopausal symptoms	Hepatotoxicity	Avoid[1]
Borage *Borago officinalis* Tops, leaves	Anti-inflammatory; diuretic	Pyrrolizidine alkaloids, hepatotoxicity	Avoid
Chaparral *Larrea tridentata* Twigs, leaves	Anti-infective; antioxidant; anticancer	Hepatotoxicity	Avoid
Coltsfoot *Tussilago farfara* Leaves, flower	Upper respiratory tract infections	Pyrrolizidine alkaloids, hepatotoxicity	Avoid ingestion of any parts of plant; leaves may be used topically for anti-inflammatory effects for up to 4–6 weeks
Comfrey *Symphytum* species Leaves and roots	Internal digestive aid; topical for wound healing	Pyrrolizidine alkaloids, hepatotoxicity	Avoid ingestion; topical use should be limited to 4–6 weeks
Ephedra, Ma-huang *Ephedra* species	Diet aid; stimulant; bronchodilator	Central nervous system toxicity, cardiac toxicity	Avoid in patients at risk for stroke, myocardial infarction, uncontrolled blood pressure, seizures, general anxiety disorder
Germander *Teucrium chamaedrys* Leaves, tops	Diet aid	Hepatotoxicity	Avoid
Gland-derived extracts (thymus, adrenal, thyroid)	Hormone replacement	Risk of bacterial, viral, or prion transmission; variable hormone content	Avoid
Human placenta derivatives	Antirheumatic; anti-inflammatory	Risk of bacterial, viral, or prion transmission	Avoid
Jin Bu Huan	Analgesic; sedative	Hepatotoxicity	Avoid
Kava-kava	Anxiety	Hepatotoxicity	Avoid
Pennyroyal *Mentha pulegium* or *Hedeoma pulegioides* Extract	Digestive aid; induction of menstrual flow; abortifacient	Pulegone and pulegone metabolite, liver failure, renal failure	Avoid
Poke root *Phytolacca americana*	Antirheumatic	Hemorrhagic gastritis	Avoid
Royal jelly *Apis mellifera* (honeybee)	Tonic	Bronchospasm, anaphylaxis	Avoid in patients with chronic allergies or respiratory diseases; asthma, chronic obstructive pulmonary disease, emphysema, atopy
Sassafras *Sassafras albidum* Root bark	Blood thinner	Safrole oil, hepatocarcinogen in animals	Avoid

[1]Cases of hepatotoxicity have occurred; these cases are rare given the widespread use of black cohosh

with *E purpurea* extract in cell lines from both healthy and immunocompromised patients. Studies using the isolated purified polysaccharides from *E purpurea* have also shown cytokine activation. Polysaccharides by themselves, however, are unlikely to accurately reproduce the activity of the entire extract.

B. Anti-Inflammatory Effects

Certain echinacea constituents have demonstrated anti-inflammatory properties in vitro. Inhibition of cyclooxygenase, 5-lipoxygenase, and hyaluronidase may be involved. In animals, application of *E purpurea* prior to application of a topical irritant reduced both paw and ear edema. Despite these laboratory findings, randomized, controlled clinical trials involving echinacea for wound healing have not been performed in humans.

C. Antibacterial, Antifungal, Antiviral, and Antioxidant Effects

In vitro studies have reported some antibacterial, anti-fungal, antiviral, and antioxidant activity with echinacea constituents. In vitro, a standardized extract of the aerial parts of *E purpurea* demonstrated potent virucidal ($MIC_{100} < 1$ µg/mL) against influenza and herpes simplex viruses and potent bactericidal activity against *Streptococcus pyogenes*, *Haemophilus influenzae*, and *Legionella pneumophila* in human bronchial cells. The pro-inflammatory cytokine release caused by these viruses and bacteria were also reversed by echinacea.

Clinical Trials

Echinacea is most often used to enhance immune function in individuals who have colds and other respiratory tract infections.

Two recent reviews have assessed the efficacy of echinacea for this primary indication. A review by the Cochrane Collaboration involved 16 randomized trials with 22 comparisons. Trials were included if they involved monopreparations of echinacea for cold treatment or prevention. Prevention trials involving rhinovirus inoculation versus natural cold development were excluded. Overall, the review concluded that there was some evidence of efficacy for the aerial (above-ground) parts of *E purpurea* plants in the early treatment of colds but that efficacy for prevention and for other species of echinacea was not clearly shown. Among the placebo-controlled comparisons for cold treatment, echinacea was superior in nine trials, showed a positive trend in one trial, and was insignificant in six trials.

A separate meta-analysis involving 14 randomized, placebo-controlled trials of echinacea for cold treatment or prevention was published in *Lancet*. In this review, echinacea decreased the odds of developing clear signs and symptoms of a cold by 58% and decreased symptom duration by 1.25 days. This review, however, was confounded by the inclusion of four clinical trials involving multi-ingredient echinacea preparations, as well as three studies using rhinovirus inoculation versus natural cold development.

Echinacea has been used investigationally to enhance hematologic recovery following chemotherapy. It has also been used as an adjunct in the treatment of urinary tract and vaginal fungal infections. These indications require further research before they can be accepted in clinical practice. *E purpurea* is ineffective in treating recurrent genital herpes.

Adverse Effects

Flu-like symptoms (eg, fever, shivering, headache, vomiting) have been reported following the intravenous use of echinacea extracts. Adverse effects with oral commercial formulations are minimal and most often include unpleasant taste, gastrointestinal upset, or rash. In one large clinical trial, pediatric patients using an oral echinacea product were significantly more likely to develop a rash (~ 5%) than those taking placebo.

Drug Interactions & Precautions

Until the role of echinacea in immune modulation is better defined, this agent should be avoided in patients with immune deficiency disorders (eg, AIDS, cancer), autoimmune disorders (eg, multiple sclerosis, rheumatoid arthritis), and patients with tuberculosis. While there are no reported drug interactions for echinacea, some preparations have a high alcohol content and should not be used with medications known to cause a disulfiram-like reaction. In theory, echinacea should also be avoided in persons taking immunosuppressant medications (eg, organ transplant recipients).

Dosage

It is recommended to follow the dosing on the package label, as there may be slight variations in dose based on the product manufacturer. Standardized preparations made from the above-ground parts of *E purpurea* (Echinaforce, Echinaguard) as an alcoholic extract or fresh pressed juice have some clinical support and may be taken within the first 24 hours of cold symptoms. It should not be used as a preventative agent or for longer than 10–14 days.

GARLIC (*ALLIUM SATIVUM*)

Chemistry

The pharmacologic activity of garlic involves a variety of organo-sulfur compounds. Dried and powdered formulations contain many of the organosulfur compounds found in raw garlic and will likely be standardized to allicin or alliin content. Allicin is responsible for the characteristic odor of garlic, and alliin is its chemical precursor. Dried powdered formulations are often enteric-coated to protect the enzyme allinase (the enzyme that converts alliin to allicin) from degradation by stomach acid. Aged garlic extract has also been studied in clinical trials, but to a lesser degree than dried, powdered garlic. Aged garlic extract contains no alliin or allicin and is odor-free. Its primary constituents are water-soluble organosulfur compounds, and packages may carry a standardization to the compound *S*-allylcysteine.

Pharmacologic Effects

A. Cardiovascular Effects

In vitro, allicin and related compounds inhibit HMG-CoA reductase, which is involved in cholesterol biosynthesis (see Chapter 35), and exhibit antioxidant properties. Several clinical trials have investigated the lipid-lowering potential of garlic. The most recent meta-analysis involved 29 randomized, double-blind, placebo-controlled trials and found a small but significant reduction in both total cholesterol (–0.19 mmol/L) and triglycerides (–0.011 mmol/L), but no effect on low- or high-density lipoproteins. These results echoed another review in patients with baseline hypercholesterolemia (total cholesterol > 200 mg/dL) that found a significant reduction in total cholesterol of 5.8% using garlic for

2–6 months. The effect of garlic became insignificant, however, when dietary controls were in place. Results of a study by the National Center of Complementary and Alternative Medicine (NCCAM) evaluating three different sources of garlic (fresh, powdered, and aged garlic extract) in adults with moderately elevated cholesterol contradicted the findings of these reviews and found no effect of any formulation of garlic versus placebo on LDL cholesterol. Cumulatively, these data indicate that garlic is unlikely to be effective in reducing cholesterol to a clinically significant extent. Clinical trials report antiplatelet effects (possibly through inhibition of thromboxane synthesis or stimulation of nitric oxide synthesis) following garlic ingestion. A majority of human studies also suggest enhancement of fibrinolytic activity. These effects in combination with antioxidant effects (eg, increased resistance to low-density lipoprotein oxidation) and reductions in total cholesterol might be beneficial in patients with atherosclerosis. A randomized, controlled trial among persons with advanced coronary artery disease who consumed dried powdered garlic for 4 years showed significant reductions in secondary markers (plaque accumulation in the carotid and femoral arteries) as compared with placebo, but primary endpoints (death, stroke, myocardial infarction) were not assessed.

Garlic constituents may affect blood vessel elasticity and blood pressure. A variety of mechanisms have been proposed. There have been a limited number of randomized, controlled trials in humans for this indication. Ten trials were included in a systematic review and meta-analysis that found no effect on systolic or diastolic pressure in patients without elevated systolic blood pressure but a significant reduction in systolic and diastolic pressure among the three trials involving patients with elevated systolic blood pressure.

B. Endocrine Effects

The effect of garlic on glucose homeostasis does not appear to be significant in persons with diabetes. Certain organosulfur constituents in garlic, however, have demonstrated hypoglycemic effects in nondiabetic animal models.

C. Antimicrobial Effects

The antimicrobial effect of garlic has not been extensively studied in clinical trials. Allicin has been reported to have in vitro activity against some gram-positive and gram-negative bacteria as well as fungi (*Candida albicans*), protozoa (*Entamoeba histolytica*), and certain viruses. The primary mechanism involves the inhibition of thiol-containing enzymes needed by these microbes. Given the availability of safe and effective prescription antimicrobials, the usefulness of garlic in this area appears limited.

D. Antineoplastic Effects

In rodent studies, garlic inhibits procarcinogens for colon, esophageal, lung, breast, and stomach cancer, possibly by detoxification of carcinogens and reduced carcinogen activation. Several epidemiologic case-control studies demonstrate a reduced incidence of stomach, esophageal, and colorectal cancers in persons with high dietary garlic consumption.

Adverse Effects

Following oral ingestion, adverse effects may include nausea (6%), hypotension (1.3%), allergy (1.1%), and bleeding (rare). Breath and body odor have been reported with an incidence of 20–40% at recommended doses using enteric-coated powdered garlic formulations. Contact dermatitis may occur with the handling of raw garlic.

Drug Interactions & Precautions

Because of reported antiplatelet effects, patients using anticlotting medications (eg, warfarin, aspirin, ibuprofen) should use garlic cautiously. Additional monitoring of blood pressure and signs and symptoms of bleeding is warranted. Garlic may reduce the bioavailability of saquinavir, an antiviral protease inhibitor, but it does not appear to affect the bioavailability of ritonavir.

Dosage

Dried, powdered garlic products should be standardized to contain 1.3% alliin (the allicin precursor) or have an allicin-generating potential of 0.6%. Enteric-coated formulations are recommended to minimize degradation of the active substances. A daily dose of 600–900 mg/d of powdered garlic is most common. This is equivalent to one clove of raw garlic (2–4 g) per day.

GINKGO (*GINKGO BILOBA*)

Chemistry

Ginkgo biloba extract is prepared from the leaves of the ginkgo tree. The most common formulation is prepared by concentrating 50 parts of the crude leaf to prepare one part of extract. The active constituents in ginkgo are flavone glycosides and terpenoids (ie, ginkgolides A, B, C, J, and bilobalide).

Pharmacologic Effects

A. Cardiovascular Effects

In animal models and some human studies, ginkgo has been shown to increase blood flow, reduce blood viscosity, and promote vasodilation, thus enhancing tissue perfusion. Enhancement of endogenous nitric oxide (see Chapter 19) and antagonism of platelet-activating factor have been observed in animal models.

Ginkgo biloba has been studied for its effects on mild to moderate occlusive peripheral arterial disease. Among 11 randomized, placebo-controlled studies involving 477 participants using standardized ginkgo leaf extract (EGb761) for up to 6 months, a nonsignificant trend toward improvements in pain-free walking distance (increase of 64.5 meters) was observed (p = .06).

The Ginkgo Evaluation of Memory (GEM) study evaluated cardiovascular outcomes associated with the long-term use of ginkgo for 6 years in 3069 patients over 75 years of age. Daily use of 240 mg/d EGb761 did not affect the incidence of hypertension or reduce blood pressure among persons with hypertension or prehypertension. No significant effects in cardiovascular disease mortality or events or hemorrhagic stroke were observed. There was, however, a significant reduction in peripheral vascular disease events in the ginkgo arm versus the placebo arm.

B. Metabolic Effects

Antioxidant and radical-scavenging properties have been observed for the flavonoid fraction of ginkgo as well as some of the terpene constituents. In vitro, ginkgo has been reported to have superoxide dismutase-like activity and superoxide anion- and hydroxyl radical-scavenging properties. The flavonoid fraction has also been observed to have anti-apoptotic properties. In some studies, it has also demonstrated a protective effect in limiting free radical formation in animal models of ischemic injury and in reducing markers of oxidative stress in patients undergoing coronary artery bypass surgery.

C. Central Nervous System Effects

In aged animal models, chronic administration of ginkgo for 3–4 weeks led to modifications in central nervous system receptors and neurotransmitters. Receptor densities increased for muscarinic, α_2, and 5-HT$_{1a}$ receptors and decreased for β adrenoceptors. Increased serum levels of acetylcholine and norepinephrine and enhanced synaptosomal reuptake of serotonin have also been reported. Additional effects include reduced corticosterone synthesis and inhibition of amyloid-beta fibril formation.

Ginkgo has been used to treat cerebral insufficiency and dementia of the Alzheimer type. The term *cerebral insufficiency*, however, includes a variety of manifestations ranging from poor concentration and confusion to anxiety and depression as well as physical complaints such as hearing loss and headache. For this reason, studies evaluating cerebral insufficiency tend to be more inclusive and difficult to assess than trials evaluating dementia. An updated meta-analysis of ginkgo for cognitive impairment or dementia was performed by the Cochrane Collaboration. They reviewed 36 randomized, double-blind, placebo-controlled trials ranging in length from 3 to 52 weeks. Significant improvements in cognition and activities of daily living were observed at 12 but not 24 weeks. Significant improvements in clinical global improvement, however, were observed at 24 but not 12 weeks. The authors concluded that the effects of ginkgo in the treatment of cognitive impairment and dementia were unpredictable and unlikely to be clinically relevant. In the GEM study, the effects of gingko as a prophylactic agent to prevent progression to dementia were assessed. No benefit was observed with 6 years of ginkgo treatment. To date, there is no known therapy that prevents progression to dementia.

D. Miscellaneous Effects

Ginkgo has been studied for its effects in allergic and asthmatic bronchoconstriction, short-term memory in healthy, non-demented adults, erectile dysfunction, tinnitus and hearing loss, and macular degeneration. For each of these conditions, there is insufficient evidence to warrant clinical use.

Adverse Effects

Adverse effects have been reported with a frequency comparable to that of placebo. These include nausea, headache, stomach upset, diarrhea, allergy, anxiety, and insomnia. A few case reports noted bleeding complications in patients using ginkgo. In a few of these cases, the patients were also using either aspirin or warfarin.

Drug Interactions & Precautions

Ginkgo may have antiplatelet properties and should not be used in combination with antiplatelet or anticoagulant medications. One case of an enhanced sedative effect was reported when ginkgo was combined with trazodone. Seizures have been reported as a toxic effect of ginkgo, most likely related to seed contamination in the leaf formulations. Uncooked ginkgo seeds are epileptogenic due to the presence of ginkgotoxin. Ginkgo formulations should be avoided in individuals with preexisting seizure disorders.

Dosage

Ginkgo biloba dried leaf extract is usually standardized to contain 24% flavone glycosides and 6% terpene lactones. The daily dose ranges from 120 to 240 mg of the dried extract in two or three divided doses.

GINSENG

Chemistry

Ginseng may be derived from any of several species of the genus *Panax*. Of these, crude preparations or extracts of *Panax ginseng*, the Chinese or Korean variety, and *P quinquefolium*, the American variety, are most often available to consumers in the United States. The active principles appear to be the triterpenoid saponin glycosides called ginsenosides or panaxosides, of which there are approximately 30 different types. It is recommended that commercial *P ginseng* formulations be standardized to contain 4–10% ginsenosides.

Other plant materials are commonly sold under the name ginseng but are not from *Panax* species. These include Siberian ginseng (*Eleutherococcus senticosus*) and Brazilian ginseng (*Pfaffia paniculata*). Of these, Siberian ginseng is more widely available in the USA. Siberian ginseng contains eleutherosides but no ginsenosides. Currently, there is no recommended standardization for eleutheroside content in Siberian ginseng products.

Pharmacology

An extensive literature exists on the potential pharmacologic effects of ginsenosides. Unfortunately, the studies differ widely in the species of *Panax* used, the ginsenosides studied, the degree of purification applied to the extracts, the animal species studied, and the measurements used to evaluate the responses. A remarkable list of reported beneficial pharmacologic effects include modulation of immune function (induced mRNA expression for interleukins-2 and -1α, interferon-γ, and granulocyte-macrophage colony-stimulating factor; activated B and T cells, natural killer cells, and macrophages); central nervous system effects (increased proliferating ability of neural progenitors; increased central levels of acetylcholine, serotonin, norepinephrine, and dopamine in the cerebral cortex); antioxidant activity; anti-inflammatory effects (inhibition of TNF-α, interleukin-1β, and vascular and intracellular cell adhesion molecules); antistress activity (ie, stimulation of pituitary-adreno-cortical system, agonist at glucocorticoid receptor); analgesia (inhibition of substance P); vasoregulatory effects (increased endothelial nitric oxide and inhibition of prostacyclin production); cardioprotective activity (reduced ventricular remodeling and cardiac hypertrophy in animal models of myocardial ischemia); antiplatelet activity; improved glucose homeostasis (increased insulin release, number of insulin receptors, and insulin sensitivity); and anticancer properties (reduced tumor angiogenesis, increased tumor cell apoptosis).

Clinical Trials

Ginseng is most often claimed to help improve physical and mental performance or to function as an "adaptogen," an agent that helps the body to return to normal when exposed to stressful or noxious stimuli. Unfortunately, the clinical trials evaluating ginseng for these indications have shown few if any benefits. Some randomized controlled trials evaluating "quality of life" have claimed significant benefits in some subscale measures of quality of life but rarely in overall composite scores using *P ginseng*. Better results have been observed with *P quinquefolium* and *P ginseng* in lowering postprandial glucose indices in subjects with and without diabetes. This was the subject of a recent systematic review in which 15 studies (13 randomized and 2 nonrandomized) were evaluated. Nine of the studies reported significant reductions in blood glucose. Newer randomized, placebo-controlled trials have reported some immunomodulating benefits of *P quinquefolium* (four trials) and *P ginseng* (one trial) in preventing upper respiratory tract infections. Use of ginseng for 2–4 months in healthy seniors may reduce the incidence of acquiring the common cold as well as the duration of symptoms. Because of heterogeneity in these trials, however, these findings are insufficient to warrant recommending the use of ginseng for this indication at this time. Two case-control studies, a cohort study and one randomized, double-blind, placebo-controlled study, also suggest a non-organ-specific cancer preventative effect with long-term administration of *P ginseng*. In summary, the strongest support for use of *P ginseng* or *P quinquefolium* currently relates to its effects in cold prevention, lowering postprandial glucose, and nonspecific cancer prevention.

Adverse Effects

Vaginal bleeding and mastalgia have been described in case reports. Central nervous system stimulation (eg, insomnia, nervousness) and hypertension have been reported in patients using high doses (more than 3 g/d) of *P ginseng*. Methylxanthines found in the ginseng plant may contribute to this effect. Vasoregulatory effects of ginseng are unlikely to be clinically significant.

Drug Interactions & Precautions

Irritability, sleeplessness, and manic behavior have been reported in psychiatric patients using ginseng in combination with other medications (phenelzine, lithium, neuroleptics). Ginseng should be used cautiously in patients taking any psychiatric, estrogenic, or hypoglycemic medications. Ginseng has antiplatelet properties and should not be used in combination with warfarin. Cytokine stimulation has been claimed for both *P ginseng* and *P quinquefolium* in vitro and in animal models. In a randomized, double-blind, placebo-controlled study, *P ginseng* significantly increased natural killer cell activity versus placebo with 8 and 12 weeks of use. Immunocompromised individuals, those taking immune stimulants, and those with autoimmune disorders should use ginseng products with caution.

Dosing

One to two grams of the crude *P ginseng* root or its equivalent is considered standard dosing. Two hundred milligrams of standardized *P ginseng* extract is equivalent to 1 g of the crude root. Ginsana has been used as a standardized extract in some clinical trials and is available in the USA.

MILK THISTLE (*SILYBUM MARIANUM*)

Chemistry

The fruit and seeds of the milk thistle plant contain a lipophilic mixture of flavonolignans known as silymarin. Silymarin comprises 2–3% of the dried herb and is composed of three primary isomers, silybin (also known as silybinin or silibinin), silychristin (silichristin), and silydianin (silidianin). Silybin is the most prevalent and potent of the three isomers and accounts for about 50% of the silymarin complex. Products should be standardized to contain 70–80% silymarin.

Pharmacologic Effects

A. Liver Disease

In animal models, milk thistle purportedly limits hepatic injury associated with a variety of toxins, including *Amanita* mushrooms, galactosamine, carbon tetrachloride, acetaminophen, radiation, cold ischemia, and ethanol. In vitro studies and some in vivo studies demonstrate that silymarin reduces lipid peroxidation, scavenges free radicals, and enhances glutathione and superoxide dismutase levels. This may contribute to membrane stabilization and reduce toxin entry.

Milk thistle appears to have anti-inflammatory properties. In vitro, silybin strongly and noncompetitively inhibits lipoxygenase activity and reduces leukotriene formation. Inhibition of leukocyte migration has been observed in vivo and may be a factor when acute inflammation is present. Silymarin also inhibits tumor necrosis factor-α–mediated activation of nuclear factor kappa B (NF-κB), which promotes inflammatory responses. One of the most unusual mechanisms claimed for milk thistle involves an increase in RNA polymerase I activity in nonmalignant hepatocytes but not in hepatoma or other malignant cell lines. By increasing this enzyme's activity, enhanced protein synthesis and cellular regeneration may occur in healthy but not malignant cells.

In an animal model of cirrhosis, it reduced collagen accumulation, and in an in vitro model it reduced expression of the fibrogenic cytokine transforming growth factor-β. If confirmed, milk thistle may have a role in the treatment of hepatic fibrosis.

In animal models, silymarin has a dose-dependent stimulatory effect on bile flow that could be beneficial in cases of cholestasis. To date, however, there is insufficient evidence to warrant the use of milk thistle for these indications.

B. Chemotherapeutic Effects

Preliminary in vitro and animal studies of the effects of silymarin and silybinin have been carried out with several cancer cell lines. In murine models of skin cancer, silybinin and silymarin were said to reduce tumor initiation and promotion. Induction of apoptosis has also been reported using silymarin in a variety of malignant human cell lines (eg, melanoma, prostate, leukemia cells, bladder transitional-cell papilloma cells, and hepatoma cells). Inhibition of cell growth and proliferation by inducing a G_1 cell cycle arrest has also been claimed in cultured human breast and prostate cancer cell lines. The use of milk thistle in the clinical treatment of cancer has not yet been adequately studied but preliminary trials are under way.

C. Lactation

Historically, milk thistle has been used by herbalists and midwives to induce lactation in pregnant or postpartum women. In female rats, milk thistle increases prolactin production. As such, it is possible that it could have an effect on human breast milk production. Clinical trial data are lacking, however, for this indication, as are safety data on nursing mothers and infants. Until further data become available, milk thistle should not be used for this indication.

Clinical Trials

Milk thistle has been used to treat acute and chronic viral hepatitis, alcoholic liver disease, and toxin-induced liver injury in human patients. A systematic review of 13 randomized trials involving 915 patients with alcoholic liver disease or hepatitis B or C found no significant reductions in all-cause mortality, liver histopathology, or complications of liver disease with 6 months of use. A significant reduction in liver-related mortality was claimed using the data from all the surveyed trials, but not when the data were limited to trials of better design and controls. It was concluded that the effects of milk thistle in improving liver function or mortality from liver disease are currently poorly substantiated. Until additional well-designed clinical trials (possibly exploring higher doses) can be performed, a clinical effect can be neither supported nor ruled out.

Although milk thistle has not been confirmed as an antidote following acute exposure to liver toxins in humans, parenteral silybin is nevertheless marketed and used in Europe as an antidote in *Amanita phalloides* mushroom poisoning. This use is based on favorable outcomes reported in case-control studies.

Adverse Effects

Milk thistle has rarely been reported to cause adverse effects when used at recommended doses. In clinical trials, the incidence of adverse effects (eg, gastrointestinal upset, dermatologic, headaches) was comparable to that of placebo. At high doses (> 1500 mg), it can have a laxative effect caused by stimulation of bile flow and secretion.

DRUG INTERACTIONS, PRECAUTIONS, & DOSING

There are no reported drug-drug interactions or precautions for milk thistle. Recommended dosage is 280–420 mg/d, calculated as silybin, in three divided doses.

ST. JOHN'S WORT (*HYPERICUM PERFORATUM*)

Chemistry

St. John's wort, also known as hypericum, contains a variety of constituents that might contribute to its claimed pharmacologic activity in the treatment of depression. Hypericin, a marker of standardization for currently marketed products, was thought to be the primary antidepressant constituent. Recent attention has focused on hyperforin, but a combination of several compounds is probably involved. Commercial formulations are usually prepared by soaking the dried chopped flowers in methanol to create a hydroalcoholic extract that is then dried.

Pharmacologic Effects

A. Antidepressant Action

The hypericin fraction was initially reported to have MAO-A and -B inhibitor properties. Later studies found that the concentration required for this inhibition was higher than that achieved with recommended dosages. In vitro studies using the commercially formulated hydroalcoholic extract have shown inhibition of nerve terminal reuptake of serotonin, norepinephrine, and dopamine. While the hypericin constituent did not show reuptake inhibition for any of these systems, the hyperforin constituent did. Chronic administration of the commercial extract has also been reported to significantly down-regulate the expression of cortical β adrenoceptors and up-regulate the expression of serotonin receptors (5-HT$_2$) in a rodent model.

Other effects observed in vitro include sigma receptor binding using the hypericin fraction and GABA receptor binding using the commercial extract. Interleukin-6 production is also reduced in the presence of the extract.

1. Clinical trials for depression—The most recent systematic review and meta-analysis involved 29 randomized, double-blind, controlled trials (18 compared St. John's wort to placebo, 5 to tricyclic antidepressants, and 12 to selective serotonin reuptake inhibitors [SSRIs]). Only studies meeting defined classification criteria for major depression were included. St. John's wort was reported to be more efficacious than placebo and equivalent to prescription reference treatments including the SSRIs for mild to moderate depression but with fewer side effects. Most trials used 900 mg/d of St. John's wort for 4–12 weeks. Depression severity was mild to moderate in 19 trials, moderate to severe in 9 trials, and not stated in one trial. These data support a role for St. John's wort in relieving symptoms of major depression.

St. John's wort has been studied for several other indications related to mood, including premenstrual dysphoric disorder, climacteric complaints, somatoform disorders, and anxiety. These studies are too few in number, however, to draw any firm conclusions regarding efficacy.

B. Antiviral and Anticarcinogenic Effects

The hypericin constituent of St. John's wort is photolabile and can be activated by exposure to certain wavelengths of visible or ultraviolet A light. Parenteral formulations of hypericin (photoactivated just before administration) have been used investigationally to treat HIV infection (given intravenously) and basal and squamous cell carcinoma (given by intralesional injection). In vitro, photoactivated hypericin inhibits a variety of enveloped and non-enveloped viruses as well as the growth of cells in some neoplastic tissues. Inhibition of protein kinase C and inhibition of singlet oxygen radical generation have been proposed as possible mechanisms. The latter could inhibit cell growth or cause cell apoptosis. These studies were carried out using the isolated hypericin constituent of St. John's wort; the usual hydroalcoholic extract of St. John's wort has not been studied for these indications and should not be recommended for patients with viral illness or cancer.

Adverse Effects

Photosensitization is related to the hypericin and pseudohypericin constituents in St. John's wort. Consumers should be instructed to wear sunscreen and eye protection while using this product when exposed to the sun. Hypomania, mania, and autonomic arousal have also been reported in patients using St. John's wort.

Drug Interactions & Precautions

Inhibition of reuptake of various amine transmitters has been highlighted as a potential mechanism of action for St. John's wort. Drugs with similar mechanisms (ie, antidepressants, stimulants) should be used cautiously or avoided in patients using St. John's wort due to the risk of serotonin syndrome (see Chapters 16 and 30). This herb may induce hepatic CYP enzymes (3A4, 2C9, 1A2) and the P-glycoprotein drug transporter. This has led to case reports of subtherapeutic levels of numerous drugs, including digoxin, birth control drugs (and subsequent pregnancy), cyclosporine, HIV protease and nonnucleoside reverse transcriptase inhibitors, warfarin, irinotecan, theophylline, and anticonvulsants.

Dosage

The most common commercial formulation of St. John's wort is the dried hydroalcoholic extract. Products should be standardized to 2–5% hyperforin, although most still bear the older standardized

marker of 0.3% hypericin. The recommended dosing for mild to moderate depression is 900 mg of the dried extract per day in three divided doses. Onset of effect may take 2–4 weeks. Long-term benefits beyond 12 weeks have not been sufficiently studied.

SAW PALMETTO (SERENOA REPENS OR SABAL SERRULATA)

Chemistry

The active constituents in saw palmetto berries are not well defined. Phytosterols (eg, β-sitosterol), aliphatic alcohols, polyprenic compounds, and flavonoids are all present. Marketed preparations are dried lipophilic extracts that are generally standardized to contain 85–95% fatty acids and sterols.

Pharmacologic Effects

Saw palmetto is most often promoted for the treatment of benign prostatic hyperplasia (BPH). Enzymatic conversion of testosterone to dihydrotestosterone (DHT) by 5α-reductase is inhibited by saw palmetto in vitro. Specifically, saw palmetto shows a noncompetitive inhibition of both isoforms (I and II) of this enzyme, thereby reducing DHT production. In vitro, saw palmetto also inhibits the binding of DHT to androgen receptors. Additional effects that have been observed in vitro include inhibition of prostatic growth factors, blockade of α_1 adrenoceptors, and inhibition of inflammatory mediators produced by the 5-lipoxygenase pathway.

The clinical pharmacology of saw palmetto in humans is not well defined. One week of treatment in healthy volunteers failed to influence 5α-reductase activity, DHT concentration, or testosterone concentration. Six months of treatment in patients with BPH also failed to affect prostate-specific antigen (PSA) levels, a marker that is typically reduced by enzymatic inhibition of 5α-reductase. In contrast, other researchers have reported a reduction in epidermal growth factor, DHT levels, and antagonist activity at the nuclear estrogen receptor in the prostate after 3 months of treatment with saw palmetto in patients with BPH.

Clinical Trials

The most recent review involved 30 randomized controlled trials in men with symptoms consistent with BPH. Fourteen trials used saw palmetto monotherapy compared to placebo and found no significant improvement in most urologic symptoms (eg, international prostate symptom scores, peak flow, prostate size). Although nocturia was significantly improved with saw palmetto compared to placebo, when studies were limited to those of higher quality and larger sample size, this significance was lost. In contrast, saw palmetto, 320 mg/d, was shown to have comparable efficacy to 5 mg/d of finasteride (a prescription 5α-reductase inhibitor) and 0.4 mg/d of tamsulosin (a prescription α blocker) in one randomized, double-blind, clinical trial each, lasting 6 months and 1 year, respectively. These two trials lacked placebo controls.

Adverse Effects

Adverse effects are reported with an incidence of 1–3%. The most common include abdominal pain, nausea, diarrhea, fatigue, headache, decreased libido, and rhinitis. Saw palmetto has been associated with a few rare case reports of pancreatitis, liver damage, and increased bleeding risk, but due to confounding factors, causality remains inconclusive. In comparison to tamsulosin and finasteride, saw palmetto was claimed to be less likely to affect sexual function (eg, ejaculation).

Drug Interactions, Precautions, & Dosing

No drug-drug interactions have been reported for saw palmetto. Because saw palmetto has no effect on the PSA marker, it will not interfere with prostate cancer screening using this test. Recommended dosing of a standardized dried extract (containing 85–95% fatty acids and sterols) is 160 mg orally twice daily. Patients should be instructed that it may take 4–6 weeks for onset of clinical effects.

■ PURIFIED NUTRITIONAL SUPPLEMENTS

COENZYME Q10

Coenzyme Q10, also known as CoQ, CoQ10, and ubiquinone, is found in the mitochondria of many organs, including the heart, kidney, liver, and skeletal muscle. After ingestion, the reduced form of coenzyme Q10, ubiquinol, predominates in the systemic circulation. Coenzyme Q10 is a potent antioxidant and may have a role in maintaining healthy muscle function, although the clinical significance of this effect is unknown. Reduced serum levels have been reported in Parkinson's disease.

Clinical Uses

A. Hypertension

In early clinical trials, small but significant reductions in systolic and diastolic blood pressure were reported after 8–10 weeks of coenzyme Q10 supplementation. The exact mechanism is unknown but, if correct, might be related to the antioxidant and vasodilating properties of coenzyme Q10. In three well-designed randomized, placebo-controlled trials, coenzyme Q10 was reported to significantly lower systolic blood pressure and diastolic blood pressure by 11 mm Hg and 7 mm Hg, respectively, as compared with no change in the placebo groups. Whether coenzyme Q10 can be used to lower blood pressure remains unclear. Since all three clinical trials have shown a benefit, it is possible that publication bias may be present. Furthermore, an exaggerated treatment effect may occur as adequate randomization, blinding, and concealment of allocation have been questioned for these studies.

B. Heart Failure

Low endogenous coenzyme Q10 levels have been associated with worse heart failure outcomes, but this association is likely because low levels are a marker for more advanced heart failure, rather than a predictor of disease. Despite these findings, coenzyme Q10 is often advocated to improve heart muscle function in patients with heart failure. According to the most recent meta-analysis, coenzyme Q10 was shown to improve ejection fraction by 3.7% with a more significant effect being observed in patients not receiving angiotensin-converting enzyme inhibitors. It is unclear whether the improvements in ejection fraction are applicable to all patients with heart failure, as more research is required to assess the role of coenzyme Q10 in heart failure and its impact on disease severity.

C. Ischemic Heart Disease

The effects of coenzyme Q10 on coronary artery disease and chronic stable angina are modest but appear promising. A theoretical basis for such benefit could be metabolic protection of the ischemic myocardium. Double-blind, placebo-controlled trials have demonstrated that coenzyme Q10 supplementation improved a number of clinical measures in patients with a history of acute myocardial infarction (AMI). Improvements have been observed in lipoprotein a, high-density lipoprotein cholesterol, exercise tolerance, and time to development of ischemic changes on the electrocardiogram during stress tests. In addition, very small reductions in cardiac deaths and rate of reinfarction in patients with previous AMI have been reported (absolute risk reduction 1.5%).

D. Prevention of Statin-Induced Myopathy

Statins reduce cholesterol by inhibiting the HMG-CoA reductase enzyme (see Chapter 35). This enzyme is also required for synthesis of coenzyme Q10. Initiating statin therapy has been shown to reduce endogenous coenzyme Q10 levels, which may block steps in muscle cell energy generation, possibly leading to statin-related myopathy. It is unknown whether a reduction in intramuscular coenzyme Q10 levels leads to statin myopathy or if the myopathy causes cellular damage that reduces intramuscular coenzyme Q10 levels. In one of the largest studies, when rosuvastatin was used in patients with heart failure, there was no association between statin-induced low coenzyme Q10 levels and a worse heart failure outcome. Furthermore, the study found no observable difference in the incidence of statin-induced myopathy regardless of endogenous coenzyme Q10 levels. More information is needed to determine which patients with statin-related myopathy might benefit most from coenzyme Q10 especially as it relates to the specific statin, the dose, and the duration of therapy.

Adverse Effects

Coenzyme Q10 is well tolerated, rarely leading to any adverse effects at doses as high as 3000 mg/d. In clinical trials, gastrointestinal upset, including diarrhea, nausea, heartburn, and anorexia, has been reported with an incidence of less than 1%. Cases of maculopapular rash and thrombocytopenia have very rarely been observed. Other rare adverse effects include irritability, dizziness, and headache.

Drug Interactions

Coenzyme Q10 shares a structural similarity with vitamin K, and an interaction has been observed between coenzyme Q10 and warfarin. Coenzyme Q10 supplements may decrease the effects of warfarin therapy. This combination should be avoided or very carefully monitored.

Dosage

As a dietary supplement, 30 mg of coenzyme Q10 is adequate to replace low endogenous levels. For cardiac effects, typical dosages are 100–600 mg/d given in two or three divided doses. These doses increase endogenous levels to 2–3 mcg/mL (normal for healthy adults, 0.7–1 mcg/mL).

GLUCOSAMINE

Glucosamine is found in human tissue, is a substrate for the production of articular cartilage, and serves as a cartilage nutrient. Glucosamine is commercially derived from crabs and other crustaceans. As a dietary supplement, glucosamine is primarily used for pain associated with knee osteoarthritis. Sulfate and hydrochloride forms are available, but recent research has shown the hydrochloride form to be ineffective.

Pharmacologic Effects & Clinical Uses

Endogenous glucosamine is used for the production of glycosaminoglycans and other proteoglycans in articular cartilage. In osteoarthritis, the rate of production of new cartilage is exceeded by the rate of degradation of existing cartilage. Supplementation with glucosamine is thought to increase the supply of the necessary glycosaminoglycan building blocks, leading to better maintenance and strengthening of existing cartilage.

Many clinical trials have been conducted on the effects of both oral and intra-articular administration of glucosamine. Early studies reported significant improvements in overall mobility, range of motion, and strength in patients with osteoarthritis. More recent studies have reported mixed results, with both positive and negative outcomes. One of the largest and well-designed clinical trials, which compared glucosamine, chondroitin sulfate, the combination, celecoxib, and placebo, found no benefit for glucosamine therapy in mild to moderate disease. Unfortunately the investigators studied the glucosamine hydrochloride formulation, which has been shown to be inferior to the sulfate formulation. The formulation of glucosamine appears to play an important role with regard to efficacy. More research is needed to better define the specific patient populations that stand to benefit from glucosamine sulfate.

Adverse Effects

Glucosamine sulfate is very well tolerated. In clinical trials, mild diarrhea and nausea were occasionally reported. Cross allergenicity in people with shellfish allergies is a potential concern; however, this is unlikely if the formulation has been properly manufactured and purified.

Drug Interactions & Precautions

Glucosamine sulfate may increase the international normalized ratio (INR) in patients taking warfarin, increasing the risk for bruising and bleeding. The mechanism is not well understood and may be dose-related as increases in INR have occurred when the glucosamine dose was increased. Until more is known, the combination should be avoided or very carefully monitored.

Dosage

The dosage used most often in clinical trials is 500 mg three times daily or 1500 mg once daily. Glucosamine does not have direct analgesic effects, and improvements in function, if any, may not be observed for 1–2 months.

MELATONIN

Melatonin, a serotonin derivative produced by the pineal gland and some other tissues (see also Chapter 16), is believed to be responsible for regulating sleep-wake cycles. Release coincides with darkness; it typically begins around 9 PM and lasts until about 4 AM. Melatonin release is suppressed by daylight. Melatonin has also been studied for a number of other functions, including contraception, protection against endogenous oxidants, prevention of aging, treatment of depression, HIV infection, and a variety of cancers. Currently, melatonin is most often used to prevent jet lag and to induce sleep.

Pharmacologic Effects & Clinical Uses

A. Jet Lag

Jet lag, a disturbance of the sleep-wake cycle, occurs when there is a disparity between the external time and the traveler's endogenous circadian clock (internal time). The internal time regulates not only daily sleep rhythms but also body temperature and many metabolic systems. The synchronization of the circadian clock relies on light as the most potent "zeitgeber" (time giver).

Jet lag is especially common among frequent travelers and airplane cabin crews. Typical symptoms of jet lag may include daytime drowsiness, insomnia, frequent awakenings, and gastrointestinal upset. Clinical studies with administration of melatonin have reported subjective reduction in daytime fatigue, improved mood, and a quicker recovery time (return to normal sleep patterns, energy, and alertness). Although taking melatonin has not been shown to adjust circadian patterns of melatonin release, it may have a role in helping people fall asleep once they arrive at their new destination. When traveling across five or more time zones, jet lag symptoms are reduced when taking melatonin close to the target bedtime (10 PM to midnight) at the new destination. The benefit of melatonin is thought to be greater as more time zones are crossed. In addition, melatonin appears more effective for eastbound travel than for westward travel. Finally, maximizing exposure to daylight on arrival at the new destination can also aid in resetting the internal clock.

B. Insomnia

Melatonin has been studied in the treatment of various sleep disorders, including insomnia and delayed sleep-phase syndrome. It has been reported to improve sleep onset, duration, and quality when administered to healthy volunteers, suggesting a pharmacologic hypnotic effect. Melatonin has also been shown to increase rapid-eye-movement (REM) sleep. These observations have been applied to the development of ramelteon, a prescription hypnotic, which is an agonist at melatonin receptors (see Chapter 22).

Clinical studies in patients with primary insomnia have shown that oral melatonin supplementation may alter sleep architecture. Subjective improvements in sleep quality and improvements in sleep onset and sleep duration have been reported. Specifically, melatonin taken at the desired bedtime, with bedroom lights off, has been shown to improve morning alertness and quality of sleep as compared to placebo. These effects have been observed in both young and older adults (18–80 years of age). Interestingly, baseline endogenous melatonin levels were not predictive of exogenous melatonin efficacy.

C. Female Reproductive Function

Melatonin receptors have been identified in granulosa cell membranes, and significant amounts of melatonin have been detected in ovarian follicular fluid. Melatonin has been associated with midcycle suppression of luteinizing hormone surge and secretion. This may result in partial inhibition of ovulation. Nightly doses of melatonin (75–300 mg) given with a progestin through days 1–21 of the menstrual cycle resulted in lower mean luteinizing hormone levels. Therefore, melatonin should not be used by women who are pregnant or attempting to conceive. Furthermore, melatonin supplementation may decrease prolactin release in women and therefore should be used cautiously or not at all while nursing.

D. Male Reproductive Function

In healthy men, chronic melatonin administration ($\geq$ 6 months) decreased sperm quality, possibly by aromatase inhibition in the testes. However, when endogenous melatonin levels were measured in healthy men, high endogenous melatonin concentrations were associated with enhanced sperm quality and short-term in vitro exposure to melatonin improved sperm motility. Until more is known, melatonin should not be used by couples who are actively trying to conceive.

Adverse Effects

Melatonin appears to be well tolerated and is often used in preference to over-the-counter "sleep-aid" drugs. Although melatonin is associated with few adverse effects, some next-day drowsiness has been reported as well as fatigue, dizziness, headache, and irritability. Melatonin may affect blood pressure as both increases and decreases in blood pressure have been observed. Careful monitoring is recommended, particularly in patients initiating melatonin therapy while taking antihypertensive medications.

Drug Interactions

Melatonin drug interactions have not been formally studied. Various studies, however, suggest that melatonin concentrations are altered by a variety of drugs, including nonsteroidal anti-inflammatory drugs, antidepressants, β-adrenoceptor agonists and antagonists, scopolamine, and sodium valproate. The relevance of these effects is unknown. Melatonin is metabolized by CYP450 1A2 and may interact with other drugs that either inhibit or induce the 1A2 isoenzyme, including fluvoxamine. Melatonin may decrease prothrombin time and may theoretically decrease the effects of warfarin therapy. A dose-response relationship between the plasma concentration of melatonin and coagulation activity has been suggested according to one in vitro analysis. If combination therapy is desired, careful monitoring is recommended especially if melatonin is being used on a short-term basis. Melatonin may interact with nifedipine, possibly leading to an increased blood pressure and heart rate. The exact mechanism is unknown.

Dosage

A. Jet Lag

Daily doses of 0.5–5 mg appear to be equally effective for jet lag; however, the 5-mg dose resulted in a faster onset of sleep and better sleep quality than lower doses. The immediate-release formulation is preferred and should be given at the desired sleep time (10 PM–midnight) upon arrival at the new destination and for 1–3 nights after arrival. The value of extended-release formulations remains unknown, as evidence suggests the short-acting, high-peak effect of the immediate-release formulation to be more effective. Exposure to daylight at the new time zone is also important to regulate the sleep-wake cycle.

B. Insomnia

Doses of 0.3–10 mg of the immediate-release formulation orally given once nightly have been tried. The lowest effective dose should be used first and may be repeated in 30 minutes up to a maximum of 10–20 mg. Sustained-release formulations are effective and may be used but currently do not appear to offer any advantages over the immediate-release formulations. Sustained-release formulations are also more costly.

REFERENCES

Abenavoli L et al: Milk thistle in liver diseases: Past, present, and future. Phytother Res 2010;24:1423.

Agbabiaka TB et al: Serenoa repens (saw palmetto): A systematic review of adverse events. Drug Saf 2009;32:637.

Alpers DH: Garlic and its potential for prevention of colorectal cancer and other conditions. Curr Opin Gastroenterol 2009;25:116.

Barnes J et al: Echinacea species (Echinacea angustifolia (DC.) Hell., Echinacea pallida (Nutt.) Nutt., Echinacea purpurea (L.) Moench): A review of their chemistry, pharmacology and clinical properties. Pharm Pharmacol 2005;57:929.

Bent S: Herbal medicine in the United States: Review of efficacy, safety, and regulation: Grand rounds at University of California, San Francisco Medical Center. J Gen Intern Med 2008;23:854.

Bent S et al: Saw palmetto for benign prostatic hyperplasia. N Engl J Med 2006;354:557.

Birks J et al: Ginkgo biloba for cognitive impairment and dementia. Cochrane Database Syst Rev 2009;(1):CD003120.

Brzezinski A et al: Effects of exogenous melatonin on sleep: A meta-analysis. Sleep Med Rev 2005;9:41.

Buck AC: Is there a scientific basis for the therapeutic effects of Serenoa repens in benign prostatic hyperplasia? Mechanisms of action. J Urol 2004;172:1792.

Butterweck V, Schmidt M: St John's wort: Role of active compounds for its mechanism of action and efficacy. Wien Med Wochenschr 2007;157:356.

DeKosky ST et al: *Gingko biloba* for prevention of dementia. A randomized controlled trial. JAMA 2008;300:2253.

De Smet PA: Herbal remedies. N Engl J Med 2002;347:2046.

Geng J et al: Ginseng for cognition. Cochrane Database of Systematic Reviews 2010, Issue 12. Art. No.: CD007769. DOI:10.1002/14651858.CD007769.pub2.

Goel V et al: A proprietary extract from the Echinacea plant (Echinacea purpurea) enhances systemic immune response during a common cold. Phytother Res 2005;19:689.

Herxheimer A, Petrie KJ. Melatonin for the prevention and treatment of jet lag. Cochrane Database Syst Rev 2002, issue 2:CD001520.

Ho MJ, Bellusci A, Wright JM: Blood pressure lowering efficacy of coenzyme Q10 for primary hypertension. Cochrane Database Syst Rev 2009, issue 4:CD007435.

Jellin JM et al: Pharmacist's Letter/Prescriber's Letter Natural Medicines Comprehensive Database, 14th ed. Therapeutic Research Faculty, 2010.

Krebs Seida J et al: North American (Panax quinquefolius) and Asian ginseng (Panax ginseng) preparations for prevention of the common cold in healthy adults: a systematic review. Evid Based Complement Alternat Med 2011, article ID 282151. DOI:10.1093/ecam/nep068.

Linde K et al: Echinacea for preventing and treating the common cold. Cochrane Database Syst Rev 2006;(1):CD000530.

Linde K et al: St. John's wort for major depression. Cochrane Database Syst Rev 2008, issue 4:CD000448.

Linde K: St John's wort—an overview. Forsch Komplementmed 2009;16:146.

McMurray JV, et al: Coenzyme Q10, rosuvastatin, and clinical outcomes in heart failure: A pre-specified substudy of CORONA (controlled rosuvastatin multinational study in heart failure). J Am Coll Cardiol 2010;56:1196.

Natural Standard: http://www.naturalstandard.com. (Evidence-based compendium authored by academics, available to institutions.)

Nicolai SP et al: From the Cochrane library: Ginkgo biloba for intermittent claudication. Vasa 2010;39:153.

Radad K et al: Ginsenosides and their CNS targets. CNS Neurosci Ther 2010;17. DOE:10.1111/j.1755-5949.2010.00208x.

Rambaldi A et al: Milk thistle for alcoholic and/or hepatitis B or C virus liver diseases. Cochrane Database Syst Rev 2007;(4):CD003620.

Reinhart KM et al: Effects of garlic on blood pressure in patients with and without systolic hypertension: A meta-analysis. Ann Pharmacother 2008;42:1766.

Reinhart KH et al: The impact of garlic on lipid parameters: a systematic review and meta-analysis. Nutr Res Rev 2009;22:39.

Saller R et al: An updated systematic review with meta-analysis for the clinical evidence of silymarin. Forsch Komplementarmed 2008;15:9.

Sharma M et al: Bactericidal and anti-inflammatory properties of a standardized Echinacea extract (Echinaforce): Dual actions against respiratory bacteria. Phytomed 2010;17:563.

Shi C et al: Ginkgo biloba extract in Alzheimer's disease: From action mechanisms to medical practice. Int J Mol Sci 2010;11:107.

Stevinson C, Pittler MH, Ernst E: Garlic for treating hypercholesterolemia. A meta-analysis of randomized clinical trials. Ann Intern Med 2000;133:420.

Tacklind J et al: Serenoa repens for benign prostatic hyperplasia. Cochrane Database Syst Rev 2009;(15):CD001423.

Towheed T et al: Glucosamine therapy for treating osteoarthritis. Cochrane Database Syst Rev 2005, issue 2:CD002946.

Yun TK: Non-organ specific preventative effect of long-term administration of Korean Red Ginseng extract on incidence of human cancers. J Med Food 2010;13:489.

CASE STUDY ANSWER

Garlic has not been shown to significantly lower LDL cholesterol. It has been shown to have a small but significant lowering effect on total cholesterol, but only when dietary controls were not in place. There is limited evidence to suggest that garlic may lower plaque burden in patients with coronary artery disease (CAD). It is advisable to monitor blood pressure for 2 weeks after initiating a garlic supplement since he is on prescription medications for hypertension. This patient might be using coenzyme Q10 for CAD or hypertension, or because he takes simvastatin. Current literature does not support a reduced risk of statin-related myopathy. The data supporting benefits of coenzyme Q10 in patients with CAD are preliminary and limited to studies in persons with a previous myocardial infarction. Several of the dietary supplements reviewed in this chapter (garlic, ginkgo, and ginseng) have antiplatelet effects that could be additive with aspirin. If this patient were also taking warfarin, additional interactions could occur with coenzyme Q10 (vitamin K-like structure), St. John's wort (cytochrome P450 1A2, 2C9, 3A4 inducer), and melatonin (in vitro decreased prothrombin time), leading to a decreased warfarin effect, or with glucosamine (increased international normalized ratio), leading to an increased warfarin effect.

Rational Prescribing & Prescription Writing

65

Paul W. Lofholm, PharmD, &
Bertram G. Katzung, MD, PhD

Once a patient with a clinical problem has been evaluated and a diagnosis has been reached, the practitioner can often select from a variety of therapeutic approaches. Medication, surgery, psychiatric treatment, radiation, physical therapy, health education, counseling, further consultation, and no therapy are some of the options available. Of these options, drug therapy is by far the one most frequently chosen. In most cases, this requires the writing of a prescription. A written prescription is the prescriber's order to prepare or dispense a specific treatment—usually medication—for a specific patient. When a patient comes for an office visit, the physician or other authorized health professional prescribes medications 67% of the time, and an average of one prescription per office visit is written because more than one prescription may be written at a single visit.

In this chapter, a plan for prescribing is presented. The physical form of the prescription, common prescribing errors, and legal requirements that govern various features of the prescribing process are then discussed. Finally, some of the social and economic factors involved in prescribing and drug use are described.

RATIONAL PRESCRIBING

Like any other process in health care, writing a prescription should be based on a series of rational steps.

1. **Make a specific diagnosis:** Prescriptions based merely on a desire to satisfy the patient's psychological need for some type of therapy are often unsatisfactory and may result in adverse effects. A specific diagnosis, even if it is tentative, is required to move to the next step. For example, in a patient with a probable diagnosis of rheumatoid arthritis, the diagnosis and the reasoning underlying it should be clear and should be shared with the patient.

2. **Consider the pathophysiologic implications of the diagnosis:** If the disorder is well understood, the prescriber is in a much better position to offer effective therapy. For example, increasing knowledge about the mediators of inflammation makes possible more

effective use of nonsteroidal anti-inflammatory drugs (NSAIDs) and other agents used in rheumatoid arthritis. The patient should be provided with the appropriate level and amount of information about the pathophysiology. Many pharmacies, websites, and disease-oriented public and private agencies (eg, American Heart Association, American Cancer Society, Arthritis Foundation) provide information sheets suitable for patients.

3. **Select a specific therapeutic objective:** A therapeutic objective should be chosen for each of the pathophysiologic processes defined in the preceding step. In a patient with rheumatoid arthritis, relief of pain by reduction of the inflammatory process is one of the major therapeutic goals that identifies the drug groups that will be considered. Arresting the course of the disease process in rheumatoid arthritis is a different therapeutic goal, which might lead to consideration of other drug groups and prescriptions.

4. **Select a drug of choice:** One or more drug groups will be suggested by each of the therapeutic goals specified in the preceding step. Selection of a drug of choice from among these groups follows from a consideration of the specific characteristics of the patient and the clinical presentation. For certain drugs, characteristics such as age, other diseases, and other drugs being taken are extremely important in determining the most suitable drug for management of the present complaint. In the example of the patient with probable rheumatoid arthritis, it would be important to know whether the patient has a history of aspirin intolerance or ulcer disease, whether the cost of medication is an especially important factor and the nature of the patient's insurance coverage, and whether there is a need for once-daily dosing. Based on this information, a drug would probably be selected from the NSAID group. If the patient is intolerant of aspirin and does not have ulcer disease but does have a need for low-cost treatment, ibuprofen or naproxen would be a rational choice.

5. **Determine the appropriate dosing regimen:** The dosing regimen is determined primarily by the pharmacokinetics of the drug in that patient. If the patient is known to have disease of the organs required for elimination of the drug selected, adjustment of the average regimen is needed. For a drug such as ibuprofen, which is eliminated mainly by the kidneys, renal function should be assessed. If renal function is normal, the

half-life of ibuprofen (about 2 hours) requires administration three or four times daily. The dose suggested in this book, drug handbooks, and the manufacturer's literature is 400–800 mg four times daily.

6. **Devise a plan for monitoring the drug's action and determine an end point for therapy:** The prescriber should be able to describe to the patient the kinds of drug effects that will be monitored and in what way, including laboratory tests (if necessary) and signs and symptoms that the patient should report. For conditions that call for a limited course of therapy (eg, most infections), the duration of therapy should be made clear so that the patient does not stop taking the drug prematurely and understands why the prescription probably need not be renewed. For the patient with rheumatoid arthritis, the need for prolonged—perhaps indefinite—therapy should be explained. The prescriber should also specify any changes in the patient's condition that would call for changes in therapy. For example, in the patient with rheumatoid arthritis, development of gastrointestinal bleeding would require an immediate change in drug therapy and a prompt workup of the bleeding. Major toxicities that require immediate attention should be explained clearly to the patient.

7. **Plan a program of patient education:** The prescriber and other members of the health team should be prepared to repeat, extend, and reinforce the information transmitted to the patient as often as necessary. The more toxic the drug prescribed, the greater the importance of this educational program. The importance of informing and involving the patient in each of the above steps must be recognized, as shown by experience with teratogenic drugs (see Chapter 59). Many pharmacies routinely provide this type of information with each prescription filled, but the prescriber must not assume that this will occur.

THE PRESCRIPTION

Although a prescription can be written on any piece of paper (as long as all of the legal elements are present), it usually takes a specific form. A typical printed prescription form for outpatients is shown in Figure 65–1.

In the hospital setting, drugs are prescribed on a particular page of the patient's hospital chart called the **physician's order sheet (POS)** or **chart order.** The contents of that prescription are specified in the medical staff rules by the hospital's Pharmacy and Therapeutics Committee. The patient's name is typed or written on the form; therefore, the orders consist of the name and strength of the medication, the dose, the route and frequency of administration, the date, other pertinent information, and the signature of the prescriber. If the duration of therapy or the number of doses is not specified (which is often the case), the medication is continued until the prescriber discontinues the order or until it is terminated as a matter of policy routine, eg, a stop-order policy.

A typical chart order might be as follows:

11/15/08

10:30 a.m.

    (1) **Ampicillin 500 mg IV q6h × 5 days**

    (2) **Aspirin 0.6 g per rectum q6h prn temp over 101**

                                          [Signed] Janet B. Doe, MD

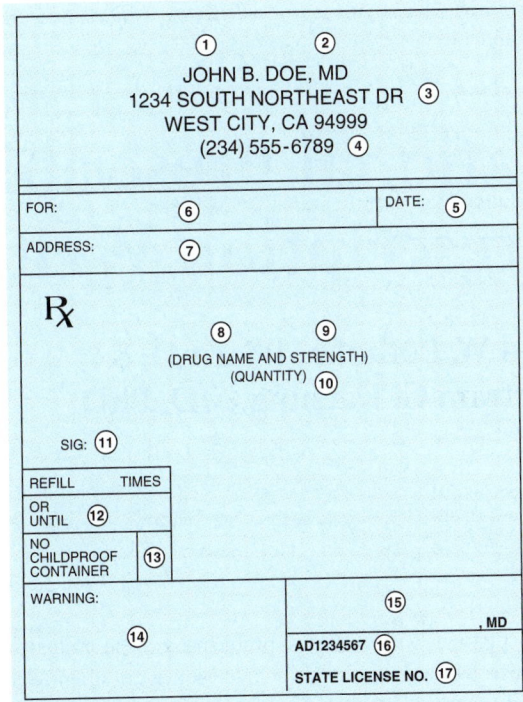

FIGURE 65–1 Common form of outpatient prescription. Circled numbers are explained in the text.

Thus, the elements of the hospital chart order are equivalent to the central elements (5, 8–11, 15) of the outpatient prescription.

Elements of the Prescription

The first four elements (see circled numerals in Figure 65–1) of the outpatient prescription establish the identity of the prescriber: name, license classification (ie, professional degree), address, and office telephone number. Before dispensing a prescription, the pharmacist must establish the prescriber's bona fides and should be able to contact the prescriber by telephone if any questions arise. Element [5] is the date on which the prescription was written. It should be near the top of the prescription form or at the beginning (left margin) of the chart order. Since the order has legal significance and usually has some temporal relationship to the date of the patient-prescriber interview, a pharmacist should refuse to fill a prescription without verification by telephone if too much time has elapsed since its writing.

Elements [6] and [7] identify the patient by name and address. The patient's name and full address should be clearly spelled out.

The body of the prescription contains the elements [8] to [11] that specify the medication, the strength and quantity to be dispensed, the dosage, and complete directions for use. When writing the drug name (element [8]), either the brand name (proprietary name) or the generic name (nonproprietary name) may be used. Reasons for using one or the other are discussed below. The strength of the medication [9] should be written in metric units. However, the prescriber should be familiar with both

systems now in use: metric and apothecary. For practical purposes, the following approximate conversions are useful:

> **1 grain (gr) = 0.065 grams (g), often rounded to 60 milligrams (mg)**
>
> **15 gr = 1 g**
>
> **1 ounce (oz) by volume = 30 milliliters (mL)**
>
> **1 teaspoonful (tsp) = 5 mL**
>
> **1 tablespoonful (tbsp) = 15 mL**
>
> **1 quart (qt) = 1000 mL**
>
> **1 minim = 1 drop (gtt)**
>
> **20 drops = 1 mL**
>
> **2.2 pounds (lb) = 1 kilogram (kg)**

The strength of a solution is usually expressed as the quantity of solute in sufficient solvent to make 100 mL; for instance, 20% potassium chloride solution is 20 grams of KCl per deciliter (g/dL) of final solution. Both the concentration and the volume should be explicitly written out.

The quantity of medication prescribed should reflect the anticipated duration of therapy, the cost, the need for continued contact with the clinic or physician, the potential for abuse, and the potential for toxicity or overdose. Consideration should be given also to the standard sizes in which the product is available and whether this is the initial prescription of the drug or a repeat prescription or refill. If 10 days of therapy are required to effectively cure a streptococcal infection, an appropriate quantity for the full course should be prescribed. Birth control pills are often prescribed for 1 year or until the next examination is due; however, some patients may not be able to afford a year's supply at one time; therefore, a 3-month supply might be ordered, with refill instructions to renew three times or for 1 year (element [12]). Some third-party (insurance) plans limit the amount of medicine that can be dispensed—often to only a month's supply. Finally, when first prescribing medications that are to be used for the treatment of a chronic disease, the initial quantity should be small, with refills for larger quantities. The purpose of beginning treatment with a small quantity of drug is to reduce the cost if the patient cannot tolerate it. Once it is determined that intolerance is not a problem, a larger quantity purchased less frequently is sometimes less expensive.

The directions for use (element [11]) must be both drug-specific and patient-specific. The simpler the directions, the better; and the fewer the number of doses (and drugs) per day, the better. Patient noncompliance (also known as nonadherence, failure to adhere to the drug regimen) is a major cause of treatment failure. To help patients remember to take their medications, prescribers often give an instruction that medications be taken at or around mealtimes and at bedtime. However, it is important to inquire about the patient's eating habits and other lifestyle patterns, because many patients do not eat three regularly spaced meals a day.

The instructions on how and when to take medications, the duration of therapy, and the purpose of the medication must be explained to each patient both by the prescriber and by the pharmacist. (Neither should assume that the other will do it.)

Furthermore, the drug name, the purpose for which it is given, and the duration of therapy should be written on each label so that the drug may be identified easily in case of overdose. An instruction to "take as directed" may save the time it takes to write the orders out but often leads to noncompliance, patient confusion, and medication error. The directions for use must be clear and concise to prevent toxicity and to obtain the greatest benefits from therapy.

Although directions for use are no longer written in Latin, many Latin apothecary abbreviations (and some others included below) are still in use. Knowledge of these abbreviations is essential for the dispensing pharmacist and often useful for the prescriber. Some of the abbreviations still used are listed in Table 65–1.

Note: It is always safer to write out the direction without abbreviating.

Elements [12] to [14] of the prescription include refill information, waiver of the requirement for childproof containers, and additional labeling instructions (eg, warnings such as "may cause drowsiness," "do not drink alcohol"). Pharmacists put the name of the medication on the label unless directed otherwise by the prescriber, and some medications have the name of the drug stamped or imprinted on the tablet or capsule. Pharmacists must place the expiration date for the drug on the label. If the patient or prescriber does not request waiver of childproof containers, the pharmacist or dispenser must place the medication in such a container. Pharmacists may not refill a prescription medication without authorization from the prescriber. Prescribers may grant authorization to renew prescriptions at the time of writing the prescription or over the telephone. Elements [15] to [17] are the prescriber's signature and other identification data.

PRESCRIBING ERRORS

All prescription orders should be legible, unambiguous, dated (and timed in the case of a chart order), and signed clearly for optimal communication between prescriber, pharmacist, and nurse. Furthermore, a good prescription or chart order should contain sufficient information to permit the pharmacist or nurse to discover possible errors before the drug is dispensed or administered.

Several types of prescribing errors are particularly common. These include errors involving omission of needed information; poor writing perhaps leading to errors of drug dose or timing; and prescription of drugs that are inappropriate for the specific situation.

Omission of Information

Errors of omission are common in hospital orders and may include instructions to "resume pre-op meds," which assumes that a full and accurate record of the "pre-op meds" is available; "continue present IV fluids," which fails to state exactly what fluids are to be given, in what volume, and over what time period; or "continue eye drops," which omits mention of which eye is to be treated as well as the drug, concentration, and frequency of administration. Chart orders may also fail to discontinue a prior medication when a new

TABLE 65–1 Abbreviations used in prescriptions and chart orders.

Abbreviation	Explanation	Abbreviation	Explanation
$\overline{a}$	before	PO	by mouth
ac	before meals	PR	per rectum
agit	shake, stir	prn	when needed
Aq	water	q	every
Aq dest	distilled water	qam, om	every morning
bid	twice a day	qd (do not use)	every day (write "daily")
$\overline{c}$	with	qh, q1h	every hour
cap	capsule	q2h, q3h, etc	every 2 hours, every 3 hours, etc
D5W, D_5W	dextrose 5% in water	qhs	every night at bedtime
dil	dissolve dilute	qid	four times a day
disp, dis	dispense	qod (do not use)	every other day
elix	elixir	qs	sufficient quantity
ext	extract	rept, repet	may be repeated
g	gram	Rx	take
gr	grain	$\overline{s}$	without
gtt	drops	SC, SQ	subcutaneous
h	hour	sid (veterinary)	once a day
hs	at bedtime	Sig, S	label
IA	intra-arterial	sos	if needed
IM	intramuscular	$\overline{ss}$, ss	one-half
IV	intravenous	stat	at once
IVPB	IV piggyback	sup, supp	suppository
kg	kilogram	susp	suspension
mcg, µg (do not use)	microgram (always write out "microgram")	tab	tablet
mEq, meq	milliequivalent	tbsp, T (do not use)	tablespoon (always write out "15 mL")
mg	milligram	tid	three times a day
no	number	Tr, tinct	tincture
non rep	do not repeat	tsp (do not use)	teaspoon (always write out "5 mL")
OD	right eye	U (do not use)	units (always write out "units")
OS, OL	left eye	vag	vaginal
OTC	over-the-counter	i, ii, iii, iv, etc	one, two, three, four, etc
OU	both eyes	ʒ (do not use)	dram (in fluid measure 3.7 mL)
$\overline{p}$	after	Ʒ (do not use)	ounce (in fluid measure 29.6 mL)
pc	after meals		

one is begun; may fail to state whether a regular or long-acting form is to be used; may fail to specify a strength or notation for long-acting forms; or may authorize "as needed" (prn) use that fails to state what conditions will justify the need.

Poor Prescription Writing

Poor prescription writing is traditionally exemplified by illegible handwriting. However, other types of poor writing are common and often more dangerous. One of the most important is the misplaced or ambiguous decimal point. Thus ".1" is easily misread as "1," a tenfold overdose, if the decimal point is not unmistakably clear. This danger is easily avoided by always preceding the decimal point with a zero. On the other hand, appending an unnecessary zero after a decimal point increases the risk of a tenfold overdose, because "1.0 mg" is easily misread as "10 mg," whereas "1 mg" is not. The slash or virgule ("/") was traditionally used as a substitute for a decimal point. This should be abandoned

because it is too easily misread as the numeral "1." Similarly, the abbreviation "U" for units should never be used because "10U" is easily misread as "100"; the word "units" should *always* be written out. Doses in micrograms should always have this unit written out because the abbreviated form ("μg") is very easily misread as "mg," a 1000-fold overdose! Orders for drugs specifying only the number of dosage units and not the total dose required should not be filled if more than one size dosage unit exists for that drug. For example, ordering "one ampule of furosemide" is unacceptable because furosemide is available in ampules that contain 20, 40, or 100 mg of the drug. The abbreviation "OD" should be used (if at all) only to mean "the right eye"; it has been used for "every day" and has caused inappropriate administration of drugs into the eye. Similarly, "Q.D." or "QD" should not be used because it is often read as "QID," resulting in four daily doses instead of one. Acronyms and abbreviations such as "ASA" (aspirin), "5-ASA" (5-aminosalicylic acid), "6MP" (6-mercaptopurine), etc, should not be used; drug names should be written out. Unclear handwriting can be lethal when drugs with similar names but very different effects are available, eg, acetazolamide and acetohexamide, methotrexate and metolazone. In this situation, errors are best avoided by noting the indication for the drug in the body of the prescription, eg, "acetazolamide, for glaucoma."

Inappropriate Drug Prescriptions

Prescribing an inappropriate drug for a particular patient results from failure to recognize contraindications imposed by other diseases the patient may have, failure to obtain information about other drugs the patient is taking (including over-the-counter drugs), or failure to recognize possible physicochemical incompatibilities between drugs that may react with each other. Contraindications to drugs in the presence of other diseases or pharmacokinetic characteristics are listed in the discussions of the drugs described in this book. The manufacturer's package insert usually contains similar information. Some of the important drug interactions are listed in Chapter 66 of this book as well as in package inserts.

Physicochemical incompatibilities are of particular concern when parenteral administration is planned. For example, certain insulin preparations should not be mixed. Similarly, the simultaneous administration of antacids or products high in metal content may compromise the absorption of many drugs in the intestine, eg, tetracyclines. The package insert and the *Handbook on Injectable Drugs* (see References) are good sources for this information.

E-PRESCRIBING

Electronic prescribing of prescriptions is gaining momentum in the USA. Congress has passed legislation to support this health care initiative. Essentially e-prescribing provides an electronic flow of information between the prescriber, intermediary, pharmacy, and health plan. The health plan can provide information on patient eligibility, formulary, benefits, costs, and sometimes, a medication history. The prescriber selects the medication, strength, dosage form, quantity, and directions for use and the prescription is transmitted to the pharmacy where the appropriate data fields are populated. The pharmacist reviews the order and, if appropriate, dispenses the prescription. The electronic system must be Health Insurance Portability and Accountability Act (HIPAA)-compliant, and there needs to be a business association agreement between the parties involved.

Prescribers can obtain decision support information such as disease-drug and drug-drug interaction information or cost information prior to prescribing as part of the health plan information. Prescriptions can be clear in their writing, but pull-down drug lists can create new errors. Prescription renewals can be processed electronically and drug misuse or abuse may be identifiable. Theoretically, time to process prescription orders should be reduced and patients would have their medication ready when they arrive at the pharmacy.

The Drug Enforcement Administration has begun to issue tentative rules for e-prescribing of controlled substances. Currently, only registered prescribers can e-prescribe, and there will be several independent identification proofing sources required: a unique pin number, or retinal scan, or a finger print. The objective is to prevent drug diversion. Pharmacies currently can order controlled drugs via computer using a specific form once they are certified.

COMPLIANCE

Compliance (sometimes called adherence) is the extent to which patients follow treatment instructions. There are four types of noncompliance leading to medication errors.

1. The patient fails to obtain the medication. Some studies suggest that one third of patients never have their prescriptions filled. Some patients leave the hospital without obtaining their discharge medications, whereas others leave the hospital without having their prehospitalization medications resumed. Some patients cannot afford the medications prescribed.

2. The patient fails to take the medication as prescribed. Examples include wrong dosage, wrong frequency of administration, improper timing or sequencing of administration, wrong route or technique of administration, or taking medication for the wrong purpose. This usually results from inadequate communication between the patient and the prescriber and the pharmacist.

3. The patient prematurely discontinues the medication. This can occur, for instance, if the patient incorrectly assumes that the medication is no longer needed because the bottle is empty or symptomatic improvement has occurred.

4. The patient (or another person) takes medication inappropriately. For example, the patient may share a medication with others for any of several reasons.

Several factors encourage noncompliance. Some diseases cause no symptoms (eg, hypertension); patients with these diseases therefore have no symptoms to remind them to take their medications. Patients with painful conditions such as arthritis may continually change medications in the hope of finding a better one.

Characteristics of the therapy itself can limit the degree of compliance; patients taking a drug once a day are much more likely to be compliant than those taking a drug four times a day. Various patient factors also play a role in compliance. Patients living alone are much less likely to be compliant than married patients of the same age. Packaging may also be a deterrent to compliance—elderly arthritic patients often have difficulty opening their medication containers. Lack of transportation as well as various social or personal beliefs about medications are likewise barriers to compliance.

Strategies for improving compliance include enhanced communication between the patient and health care team members; assessment of personal, social, and economic conditions (often reflected in the patient's lifestyle); development of a routine for taking medications (eg, at mealtimes if the patient has regular meals); provision of systems to assist taking medications (ie, containers that separate drug doses by day of the week, or medication alarm clocks that remind patients to take their medications); and mailing of refill reminders by the pharmacist to patients taking drugs chronically. The patient who is likely to discontinue a medication because of a perceived drug-related problem should receive instruction about how to monitor and understand the effects of the medication. Compliance can often be improved by enlisting the patient's active participation in the treatment.

LEGAL FACTORS (USA)

The United States government recognizes two classes of drugs: (1) over-the-counter (OTC) drugs and (2) those that require a prescription from a licensed prescriber (Rx Only). OTC drugs are those that can be safely self-administered by the layman for self-limiting conditions and for which appropriate labels can be written for lay comprehension (see Chapter 63). Half of all drug doses consumed by the American public are OTC drugs.

Physicians, dentists, podiatrists, and veterinarians—and, in some states, specialized pharmacists, nurses, physician's assistants, and optometrists—are granted authority to prescribe dangerous drugs (those bearing the federal legend statement, "Rx Only") on the basis of their training in diagnosis and treatment (see Box: Who May Prescribe?). Pharmacists are authorized to dispense prescriptions pursuant to a prescriber's order provided that the medication order is appropriate and rational for the patient. Nurses are authorized to administer medications to patients subject to a prescriber's order (Table 65–2).

Because of the multiplicity of third-party payers (health insurers) and Medicare and Medicaid claimants, the concept of electronic processing of prescriptions ("e-prescribing") has become urgent. (Further information about e-prescribing may be found at

TABLE 65–2 Prescribing authority of certain allied health professionals in selected states.

State	Pharmacists	Nurse Practitioners	Physician's Assistants	Optometrists
California	Yes, under protocol[1]; must be trained in clinical practice	Yes[2]	Yes, under protocol[1]	Yes; limited to certain drug classes
Florida	Yes, according to state formulary; protocol not required	Yes[2]	Yes[2]	Yes; limited to certain drug classes
Michigan	Yes, under protocol; must be specially qualified by education, training, or experience	Yes; do not need physician supervision	Yes[2]	Yes; limited to certain drug classes
Mississippi	Yes, under protocol in an institutional setting	Yes,[2] under narrowly specified conditions	No	Yes; limited to certain drug classes
Nevada	Yes, under protocol, within a licensed medical facility	Yes[2]	Yes[2]	Yes; limited to certain drug classes
New Mexico	Yes, under protocol, must be "pharmacist clinician"	Yes; do not need physician supervision	Yes[2]	Yes; limited to certain drug classes
North Dakota	Yes, under protocol in an institutional setting	Yes; do not need physician supervision	Yes	Yes; limited to certain drug classes
Oregon	Yes, under guidelines set by the state board	Yes; do not need physician supervision	Yes[2]	Yes; limited to certain drug classes
Texas	Yes, under protocol set for a particular patient in an institutional setting	Yes; do not need physician supervision	Yes	Yes; limited to certain drug classes
Washington	Yes, under guidelines set by the state board	Yes; do not need physician supervision	Yes[2]	Yes; limited to certain drug classes

[1]Under protocol; see Box: Who May Prescribe?

[2]In collaboration with or under the supervision of a physician.

Who May Prescribe?

The right to prescribe drugs has traditionally been the responsibility of the physician, dentist, podiatrist, or veterinarian. Prescribing now includes—in a number of states and in varying degrees—pharmacists, nurse practitioners, nurse midwives, physician's assistants, and optometrists (see Table 65–2). In the future, physical therapists may be licensed to prescribe drugs relevant to their practice. The development of large health maintenance organizations has greatly strengthened this expansion of prescribing rights because it offers these extremely powerful economic bodies a way to reduce their expenses.

The primary organizations controlling the privilege of prescribing in the USA are the state boards, under the powers delegated to them by the state legislatures. As indicated in Table 65–2, many state boards have attempted to reserve some measure of the primary responsibility for prescribing to physicians by requiring that the ancillary professional work with or under a physician according to a specific protocol. In the state of California, this protocol must include a statement of the training, supervision, and documentation requirements of the arrangement and must specify referral requirements, limitations to the list of drugs that may be prescribed (ie, a formulary), and a method of evaluation by the supervising physician. The protocol must be in writing and must be periodically updated (see reference: An Explanation of the Scope of RN Practice, 1994).

http://www.cms.hhs.gov/eprescribing/.) To further standardize electronic prescription transmission and billing, the Centers for Medicare and Medicaid (CMS) issued regulations effective in 2008 requiring all US health care providers to obtain a National Provider Identification (NPI) number. This 10-digit identifier is issued by the National Plan and Provider Enumeration System (NPPES) at https://NPPES.cms.hhs.gov. The purpose of the NPI is to identify all health care transactions (and associated costs) incurred by a particular practitioner with a single number.

In addition to a health care provider's unique identification number, some states require that prescriptions for controlled substances be written on tamper-resistant security prescription forms. The purpose of this legislation is to prevent forgeries and to tighten the control of prescription order forms.

The concept of a "secure" prescription form was expanded by the federal government in 2008 to all prescriptions written for Medicaid patients. Any prescription for a Medicaid patient must be written on a security form if the pharmacist is to be compensated for the prescription service. In turn, the use of "triplicate" prescription forms was eliminated and replaced with an online electronic transmission system whereby orders for Schedule II and Schedule III prescriptions are transmitted to a company that acts as a repository for these transactions. In California, it is called the CURES program (Controlled Substances Utilization Review and Evaluation System). Additional information about CURES may be found at http://ag.ca.gov/bne/trips.php.

Prescription drugs are controlled by the United States Food and Drug Administration as described in Chapter 5. The federal legend statement as well as the package insert is part of the packaging requirements for all prescription drugs. The package insert is the official brochure setting forth the indications, contraindications, warnings, and dosing for the drug.

The prescriber, by writing and signing a prescription order, controls who may obtain prescription drugs. The pharmacist may purchase these drugs, but they may be dispensed only on the order of a legally qualified prescriber. Thus, a **prescription** is actually three things: the **physician's order in the patient's chart,** the **written order to which the pharmacist refers** when dispensing, and the patient's **medication container with a label affixed.**

Whereas the federal government controls the drugs and their labeling and distribution, the state legislatures control who may prescribe drugs through their licensing boards, eg, the Board of Medical Examiners. Prescribers must pass examinations, pay fees, and—in the case of some states and some professions—meet other requirements for relicensure such as continuing education. If these requirements are met, the prescriber is licensed to order dispensing of drugs.

The federal government and the states further impose special restrictions on drugs according to their perceived potential for abuse (Table 65–3). Such drugs include opioids, hallucinogens, stimulants, depressants, and anabolic steroids. Special requirements

TABLE 65–3 Classification of controlled substances. (See Inside Front Cover for examples.)

Schedule	Potential for Abuse	Other Comments
I	High	No accepted medical use; lack of accepted safety as drug.
II	High	Current accepted medical use. Abuse may lead to psychological or physical dependence.
III	Less than I or II	Current accepted medical use. Moderate or low potential for physical dependence and high potential for psychological dependence.
IV	Less than III	Current accepted medical use. Limited potential for dependence.
V	Less than IV	Current accepted medical use. Limited dependence possible.

must be met when these drugs are to be prescribed. The Controlled Drug Act requires prescribers and dispensers to register with the Drug Enforcement Agency (DEA), pay a fee, receive a personal registration number, and keep records of all controlled drugs prescribed or dispensed. Every time a controlled drug is prescribed, a valid DEA number must appear on the prescription blank.

Prescriptions for substances with a high potential for abuse (Schedule II drugs) cannot be refilled. However, multiple prescriptions for the same drug may be written with instructions not to dispense before a certain date and up to a total of 90 days. Prescriptions for Schedules III, IV, and V can be refilled if ordered, but there is a five-refill maximum, and in no case may the prescription be refilled after 6 months from the date of writing. Schedule II drug orders may not be transmitted over the telephone, and some states require a tamper-resistant security prescription blank to reduce the chances for drug diversion.

These restrictive prescribing laws are intended to limit the amount of drugs of abuse that are made available to the public.

Unfortunately, the inconvenience occasioned by these laws— and an unwarranted fear by medical professionals themselves regarding the risk of patient tolerance and addiction—continues to hamper adequate treatment of patients with terminal conditions. This has been shown to be particularly true in children and elderly patients with cancer. *There is no excuse for inadequate treatment of pain in a terminal patient; not only is addiction irrelevant in such a patient, it is actually uncommon in patients who are being treated for pain* (see Chapter 31).

Some states have recognized the underutilization of pain medications in the treatment of pain associated with chronic and terminal conditions. California, for example, has enacted an "intractable pain treatment" act that reduces the difficulty of renewing prescriptions for opioids. Under the provisions of this act, upon receipt of a copy of the order from the prescriber, eg, by fax, a pharmacist may write a prescription for a Schedule II substance for a patient under hospice care or living in a skilled nursing facility or in cases in which the patient is expected to live less than 6 months, provided that the prescriber countersigns the order (by fax); the word "exemption" with regulatory code number is written on a typical prescription, thus providing easier access for the terminally ill.

Medication Therapy Management

The Medicare Modernization Act of 2003 established the requirement that Medicare Part D plan sponsors offer a Medication Therapy Management (MTM) program to their beneficiaries. The MTM program is targeted for patients who have at least two chronic diseases and have used multiple drugs at significant expense (initially a $4000 annual drug expense and now lowered to $3000/yr). The pharmacist collects the patient's drug information and analyzes the drug history and drug utilization information with the objective to optimize drug therapy,

lower costs, improve drug safety, and improve the patients' understanding of their medications. Pharmacists collaborate with physicians to address the drug therapy challenges in these high-use groups.

Labeled & Off-Labeled Uses of Drugs

In the USA, the FDA approves a drug only for the specific uses proposed and documented by the manufacturer in its New Drug Application (see Chapter 5). These approved (labeled) uses or indications are set forth in the package insert that accompanies the drug. For a variety of reasons, these labeled indications may not include all the conditions in which the drug might be useful. Therefore, a clinician may wish to prescribe the agent for some other, unapproved (off-label), clinical condition, often on the basis of adequate or even compelling scientific evidence. Federal laws governing FDA regulations and drug use place no restrictions on such unapproved use.*

Even if the patient suffers injury from the drug, its use for an unlabeled purpose does not in itself constitute "malpractice." However, the courts may consider the package insert labeling as a complete listing of the indications for which the drug is considered safe unless the clinician can show that other use is considered safe by competent expert testimony.

Drug Safety Surveillance

Governmental drug-regulating agencies have responsibility for monitoring drug safety. In the USA, the FDA-sponsored Med Watch program collects data on safety and adverse drug effects (ADEs) through mandatory reporting by drug manufacturers and voluntary reporting by health care practitioners. Practitioners may submit reports on any suspected adverse drug (or medical device) effect using a simple form obtainable from http://www.fda.gov/medwatch/index.html. The FDA is expected to use these data to establish an adverse effect rate. It is not clear that the FDA has sufficient resources at present to carry out this mandate, but they are empowered to take further regulatory actions if deemed necessary. A similar vaccine reporting program is in place to monitor vaccine safety.

The FDA has also increased requirements for labeling on drugs that carry special risks. Dispensers of medications are required to distribute "Med Guides" to patients when these medications are dispensed. These guides are provided by the manufacturers of the medications. In addition, pharmacists often provide patient educational materials that describe the drug, its

---

*"Once a product has been approved for marketing, a physician may prescribe it for uses or in treatment regimens or patient populations that are not included in the approved labeling. Such 'unapproved' or, more precisely, 'unlabeled' uses may be appropriate and rational in certain circumstances, and may, in fact, reflect approaches to drug therapy that have been extensively reported in medical literature."—FDA Drug Bull 1982;12:4.

use, adverse effects, storage requirements, methods of administration, what to do when a dose is missed, and the potential need for ongoing therapy.

SOCIOECONOMIC FACTORS

Generic Prescribing

Prescribing by generic name offers the pharmacist flexibility in selecting the particular drug product to fill the order and offers the patient a potential savings when there is price competition. For example, the brand name of a popular sedative is *Valium*, manufactured by Hoffmann-LaRoche. The generic (public nonproprietary) name of the same chemical substance adopted by United States Adopted Names (USAN) and approved by the FDA is *diazepam*. All diazepam drug products in the USA meet the pharmaceutical standards expressed in the *United States Pharmacopeia (USP)*. However, there are several manufacturers, and prices vary greatly. For drugs in common use, the difference in cost between the trade-named product and generic products varies from less than twofold to more than 100-fold.

In most states and in most hospitals, pharmacists have the option of supplying a generically equivalent drug product even if a proprietary name has been specified in the order. If the prescriber wants a particular brand of drug product dispensed, handwritten instructions to "dispense as written" or words of similar meaning are required. Some government-subsidized health care programs and many third-party insurance payers *require* that pharmacists dispense the cheapest generically equivalent product in the inventory (generic substitution). However, the principles of drug product selection by private pharmacists do not permit substituting one therapeutic agent for another (therapeutic substitution); that is, dispensing trichlormethiazide for hydrochlorothiazide would not be permitted without the prescriber's permission even though these two diuretics may be considered pharmacodynamically equivalent. Pharmacists within managed care organizations may follow different policies; see below.

It cannot be assumed that every generic drug product is as satisfactory as the trade-named product, although examples of unsatisfactory generics are rare. Bioavailability—the effective absorption of the drug product—varies between manufacturers and sometimes between different lots of a drug produced by the same manufacturer. In spite of the evidence, many practitioners avoid generic prescribing, thereby increasing medical costs. In the case of a very small number of drugs, which usually have a low therapeutic index, poor solubility, or a high ratio of inert ingredients to active drug content, a specific manufacturer's product may give more consistent results. In the case of life-threatening diseases, the advantages of generic substitution may be outweighed by the clinical urgency so that the prescription should be filled as written.

In an effort to codify bioequivalence information, the FDA publishes *Approved Drug Products with Therapeutic Equivalence Evaluations*, with monthly supplements, commonly called "the Orange Book." The book contains listings of multi-source products in one of two categories: Products given a code beginning with the letter "A" are considered bioequivalent to a reference standard formulation of the same drug and to all other versions of that product with a similar "A" coding. Products not considered bioequivalent are coded "B." Of the approximately 8000 products listed, 90% are coded "A." Additional code letters and numerals are appended to the initial "A" or "B" and indicate the approved route of administration and other variables.

Mandatory drug product selection on the basis of price is common practice in the USA because third-party payers (insurance companies, health maintenance organizations, etc) enforce money-saving regulations. If outside a managed care organization, the prescriber can sometimes override these controls by writing "dispense as written" on a prescription that calls for a brand-named product. However, in such cases, the patient may have to pay the difference between the dispensed product and the cheaper one.

Within most managed care organizations, formulary controls have been put in place that force the selection of less expensive medications whenever they are available. In a managed care environment, the prescriber often selects the drug group rather than a specific agent, and the pharmacist dispenses the formulary drug from that group. For example, if a prescriber in such an organization decides that a patient needs a thiazide diuretic, the pharmacist automatically dispenses the single thiazide diuretic carried on the organization's formulary. As noted below, the choice of drugs for the organization's formulary may change from time to time, depending on negotiation of prices and rebates with different manufacturers.

Other Cost Factors

The private pharmacy bases its charges on the cost of the drug plus a fee for providing a professional service. Each time a prescription is dispensed, there is a fee. The prescriber controls the frequency of filling prescriptions by authorizing refills and specifying the quantity to be dispensed. However, for medications used for chronic illnesses, the quantity covered by insurance may be limited to the amount used in 1 month. Thus, the prescriber can save the patient money by prescribing standard sizes (so that drugs do not have to be repackaged) and, when chronic treatment is involved, by ordering the largest quantity consistent with safety, expense, and third-party plan. Optimal prescribing for cost savings often involves consultation between the prescriber and the pharmacist. Because of continuing increases in the wholesale prices of drugs in the USA, prescription costs have risen dramatically over the past 3 decades; and from 1999 to 2009, the number of prescriptions purchased has increased 39% while the population grew 9% (see Box: The Cost of Prescriptions).

The Cost of Prescriptions

The cost of prescriptions has risen dramatically in the last several decades. The average price for a single prescription in the USA in 2004 was $55. By 2006, this average cost had risen to $75. In the California Medicaid Sector, the average charge was over $80, with generic products being under $40 per prescription and brand-name products over $140. This rise is occasioned by new technology, marketing costs, and stockholder expectations. The pharmaceutical industry typically posts profits of 10-15% annually, whereas the retail business sector shows a 3% profit. The cost to the patient for many new drugs such as statins exceeds $1000 per year. The cost of some therapeutic antibody products (eg, MABs) is more than $10,000 per year. Pharmaceuticals tend to be the highest out-of-pocket health-related cost because other health care services are covered by health insurance, whereas prescriptions often are not, although this is changing.

Because of public and political pressure resulting from this problem, the US Congress enacted the Medicare Modernization Act in 2003 establishing the Medicare Part D plan. This voluntary prescription plan provides for partial payment by private medical insurance companies for some prescriptions for patients who are Medicare-eligible. Unfortunately, the complexity of the legislation and the resulting confusing insurance plans with gaps in coverage, formulary and quantity limits, and the favored economic treatment given the pharmaceutical industry, prevent this plan from solving the high drug cost problem.

High drug costs have caused payers and consumers alike to do without or seek alternative sources. Because most other governments, eg, Canada, have done a better job in controlling drug prices, the prices for the same drug are usually less in other countries than those in the United States. This fact has caused a number of US citizens to purchase their drugs "off-shore" in a variety of countries for "personal use" in quantities up to a 3-month supply—at substantial savings, often as much as 50%. However, there is no assurance that these drugs are always what they are purported to be, or that they will be delivered in a timely manner, or that there is a traditional doctor-pharmacist-patient relationship and the safeguards that such a relationship offers.

Without a true universal health care program, the cost of drugs in the USA will continue to be subject to the negotiating power (or lack thereof) of the purchasing group-insurance company, hospital consortium, HMO, small retail pharmacy, etc, and will be driven primarily by the economic policies of the large manufacturers. In most companies, these policies favor executive compensation and stockholder dividends above the interests of consumers or employees. Thus far, only the US Veterans Administration system, the larger HMOs, and a few "big box" stores have proved strong enough to control costs through bulk purchases of drugs and serious negotiation of prices with manufacturers. Until new legislation gives other organizations the same power to negotiate, or pricing policies are made more equitable, no real solution to the drug cost problem can be expected.

REFERENCES

American Pharmacists Association and The National Association of Chain Drug Stores: MTM in Pharmacy Practice, Core Elements v. 2, 2008.

An explanation of the scope of RN practice including standardization procedures. Board of Registered Nursing, State of California, August 1994.

Avorn J: Part "D" for "defective"—The Medicare drug benefit chaos. N Engl J Med 2006;354:1339.

Bell, D: A toolset for e-prescribing implementation. Rand Health, US AHRQ, 2011.

California Business and Professions Code, Chapter 9, Division 2, Pharmacy Law. Department of Consumer Affairs, Sacramento, California, 2011.

Conroy S et al: Educational interventions to reduce prescribing errors. Arch Dis Child 2008;93:313.

Do we pay too much for prescriptions? Consumer Reports 1993;58:668.

Graber MA, Easton-Carr R: Poverty and pain: Ethics and the lack of opioid pain medications in fixed-price, low-cost prescription plans. Ann Pharmacother 2008;42:1913.

Hendrickson R (editor): *Remington's Practice and Science of Pharmacy.* Advanced Concepts Institute, 2005.

Jerome JB, Sagan P: The USAN nomenclature system. JAMA 1975;232:294.

Kesselheim AS et al: Clinical equivalence of generic and brand-name drugs used in cardiovascular disease. A systematic review and meta-analysis. JAMA 2008;300:2514.

Lesar TS, Briceland L, Stein DS: Factors related to errors in medication prescribing. JAMA 1997;277:312.

Prescription drug costs. http://www.kaiseredu.org/Issue-Modules/Prescription-Drug-Costs/Background-Brief.aspx

Schnipper JL et al: Role of pharmacist counseling in preventing adverse drug events after hospitalization. Arch Intern Med 2006;166:565.

Trissel LA: *Handbook on Injectable Drugs,* 13th ed. American Society of Hospital Pharmacists, 2005. (With supplements.)

Use of approved drugs for unlabeled indications. FDA Drug Bull 1982;12:4.

WHO Drug Action Committee: *Model Guide to Good Prescribing.* WHO, 1994.

66

Important Drug Interactions & Their Mechanisms

John R. Horn, PharmD, FCCP

One of the factors that can alter the response to drugs is the concurrent administration of other drugs. There are several mechanisms by which drugs may interact, but most can be categorized as pharmacokinetic (absorption, distribution, metabolism, excretion), pharmacodynamic (additive, synergistic, or antagonistic effects), or combined interactions. The general principles of pharmacokinetics are discussed in Chapters 3 and 4; the general principles of pharmacodynamics in Chapter 2.

Botanical medications ("herbals") may interact with each other or with conventional drugs. Unfortunately, botanicals are much less well studied than other drugs, so information about their interactions is scanty. Pharmacodynamic interactions are described in Chapter 64. Pharmacokinetic interactions that have been documented (eg, St. John's wort) are listed in Table 66–1.

Knowledge of the mechanism by which a given drug interaction occurs is often clinically useful, since the mechanism may influence both the time course and the methods of circumventing the interaction. Some important drug interactions occur as a result of two or more mechanisms.

PREDICTABILITY OF DRUG INTERACTIONS

The designations listed in Table 66–1 are used here to *estimate* the predictability of the drug interactions. These estimates are intended to indicate simply whether or not the interaction will occur, and they do not always mean that the interaction is likely to produce an adverse effect. Whether or not the interaction occurs (precipitant drug produces a measurable change in the object drug) and produces an adverse effect depends on both patient- and drug-specific factors. Patient factors can include intrinsic drug clearance, genetics, gender, concurrent diseases, and diet. Drug-specific factors include dose, route of administration, drug formulation, and the sequence of drug administration. The most important factor that can mitigate the risk of patient harm

is recognition by the prescriber of a potential interaction followed by appropriate action.

Pharmacokinetic Mechanisms

The gastrointestinal **absorption** of drugs may be affected by concurrent use of other agents that (1) have a large surface area upon which the drug can be adsorbed, (2) bind or chelate, (3) alter gastric pH, (4) alter gastrointestinal motility, or (5) affect transport proteins such as P-glycoprotein and organic anion transporters. One must distinguish between effects on absorption *rate* and effects on *extent* of absorption. A reduction in only the absorption rate of a drug is seldom clinically important, whereas a reduction in the extent of absorption is clinically important if it results in subtherapeutic serum concentrations.

The mechanisms by which drug interactions alter drug **distribution** include (1) competition for plasma protein binding, (2) displacement from tissue binding sites, and (3) alterations in local tissue barriers, eg, P-glycoprotein inhibition in the blood-brain barrier. Although competition for plasma protein binding can increase the free concentration (and thus the effect) of the displaced drug in plasma, the increase will be transient owing to a compensatory increase in drug disposition. The clinical importance of protein binding displacement has been overemphasized; current evidence suggests that such interactions are unlikely to result in adverse effects. Displacement from tissue binding sites would tend to transiently increase the blood concentration of the displaced drug.

The **metabolism** of drugs can be stimulated or inhibited by concurrent therapy, and the importance of the effect varies from negligible to dramatic. Drug metabolism primarily occurs in the liver and the wall of the small intestine, but other sites include plasma, lung, and kidney. Induction (stimulation) of cytochrome P450 isozymes in the liver and small intestine can be caused by drugs such as barbiturates, bosentan, carbamazepine, efavirenz, nevirapine, phenytoin, primidone, rifampin, rifabutin, and St. John's wort. Enzyme inducers can also increase the activity of phase II metabolism such as glucuronidation. Enzyme induction does not take place quickly; maximal effects usually occur after 7–10 days and require an equal or longer time to dissipate after the enzyme inducer is stopped. Rifampin, however, may produce enzyme induction after only a few doses. Inhibition of metabolism generally takes place more quickly than enzyme induction and may begin as soon as sufficient tissue concentration of the inhibitor is achieved. However, if the half-life of the affected (object) drug is long, it may take a week or more (three to four half-lives) to reach a new steady-state serum concentration. Drugs that may inhibit the cytochrome P450 metabolism of other drugs include amiodarone, androgens, atazanavir, chloramphenicol, cimetidine, ciprofloxacin, clarithromycin, cyclosporine, delavirdine, diltiazem, diphenhydramine, disulfiram, enoxacin, erythromycin, fluconazole, fluoxetine, fluvoxamine, furanocoumarins (substances in grapefruit juice), indinavir, isoniazid, itraconazole, ketoconazole, metronidazole, mexiletine, miconazole, nefazodone, omeprazole, paroxetine, propoxyphene, quinidine, ritonavir, sulfamethizole, verapamil, voriconazole, zafirlukast, and zileuton.

The **renal excretion** of active drug can also be affected by concurrent drug therapy. The renal excretion of certain drugs that are weak acids or weak bases may be influenced by other drugs that affect urinary pH. This is due to changes in ionization of the drug, as described in Chapter 1 under Ionization of Weak Acids and Weak Bases; the Henderson-Hasselbalch equation. For some drugs, active secretion into the renal tubules is an important elimination pathway. P-glycoprotein, organic anion transporters, and organic cation transporters are involved in active tubular secretion of some drugs, and inhibition of these transporters can inhibit renal elimination with attendant increase in serum drug concentrations.

Pharmacodynamic Mechanisms

When drugs with similar pharmacologic effects are administered concurrently, an additive or synergistic response is usually seen. The two drugs may or may not act on the same receptor to produce such effects. In theory, drugs acting on the same receptor or process are usually additive, eg, benzodiazepines plus barbiturates. Drugs acting on different receptors or sequential processes may be synergistic, eg, nitrates plus sildenafil or sulfonamides plus trimethoprim. Conversely, drugs with opposing pharmacologic effects may reduce the response to one or both drugs. Pharmacodynamic drug interactions are relatively common in clinical practice, but adverse effects can usually be minimized if one understands the pharmacology of the drugs involved. In this way, the interactions can be anticipated and appropriate countermeasures taken.

Combined Toxicity

The combined use of two or more drugs, each of which has toxic effects on the same organ, can greatly increase the likelihood of organ damage. For example, concurrent administration of two nephrotoxic drugs can produce kidney damage, even though the dose of either drug alone may have been insufficient to produce toxicity. Furthermore, some drugs can enhance the organ toxicity of another drug, even though the enhancing drug has no intrinsic toxic effect on that organ.

TABLE 66–1 Important drug interactions.

Drug or Drug Group	Properties Promoting Drug Interaction	Clinically Documented Interactions
Alcohol	Chronic alcoholism results in enzyme induction. Acute alcoholic intoxication tends to inhibit drug metabolism (whether person is alcoholic or not). Severe alcohol-induced hepatic dysfunction may inhibit ability to metabolize drugs. Disulfiram-like reaction in the presence of certain drugs. Additive central nervous system depression with other central nervous system depressants.	**Acetaminophen:** [NE] Increased formation of hepatotoxic acetaminophen metabolites (in chronic alcoholics). **Acitretin:** [P] Increased conversion of acitretin to etretinate (teratogenic). **Anticoagulants, oral:** [NE] Increased hypoprothrombinemic effect with acute alcohol intoxication. **Central nervous system depressants:** [HP] Additive or synergistic central nervous system depression. **Insulin:** [NE] Acute alcohol intake may increase hypoglycemic effect of insulin (especially in fasting patients). *Drugs that may produce a disulfiram-like reaction:* **Cephalosporins:** [NP] Disulfiram-like reactions are noted with cefamandole, cefoperazone, cefotetan, and moxalactam. **Chloral hydrate:** [NP] Mechanism not established. **Disulfiram:** [HP] Inhibited aldehyde dehydrogenase. **Metronidazole:** [NP] Mechanism not established. **Sulfonylureas:** [NE] Chlorpropamide is most likely to produce a disulfiram-like reaction; acute alcohol intake may increase hypoglycemic effect (especially in fasting patients).

HP, Highly predictable. Interaction occurs in almost all patients receiving the interacting combination; P, Predictable. Interaction occurs in most patients receiving the combination; NP, Not predictable. Interaction occurs only in some patients receiving the combination; NE, Not established. Insufficient data available on which to base estimate of predictability.

(continued)

TABLE 66–1 Important drug interactions. (Continued)

Drug or Drug Group	Properties Promoting Drug Interaction	Clinically Documented Interactions
Allopurinol	Inhibits hepatic drug-metabolizing enzymes. Febuxostat (another drug used in gout) will also inhibit the metabolism of azathioprine and mercaptopurine.	**Anticoagulants, oral:** [NP] Increased hypoprothrombinemic effect. **Azathioprine:** [P] Decreased azathioprine detoxification resulting in increased azathioprine toxicity. **Mercaptopurine:** [P] Decreased mercaptopurine metabolism resulting in increased mercaptopurine toxicity.
Antacids	Antacids may adsorb drugs in gastrointestinal tract, thus reducing absorption. Antacids tend to speed gastric emptying, thus delivering drugs to absorbing sites in the intestine more quickly. Some antacids (eg, magnesium hydroxide with aluminum hydroxide) alkalinize the urine somewhat, thus altering excretion of drugs sensitive to urinary pH.	**Atazanavir:** [NP] Decreased absorption of atazanavir (requires acid for absorption). **Digoxin:** [NP] Decreased gastrointestinal absorption of digoxin. **Indinavir:** [NP] Decreased absorption of indinavir (requires acid for absorption). **Iron:** [P] Decreased gastrointestinal absorption of iron with calcium-containing antacids. **Itraconazole:** [P] Reduced gastrointestinal absorption of itraconazole due to increased pH (itraconazole requires acid for dissolution). **Ketoconazole:** [P] Reduced gastrointestinal absorption of ketoconazole due to increased pH (ketoconazole requires acid for dissolution). **Quinolones:** [HP] Decreased gastrointestinal absorption of ciprofloxacin, norfloxacin, and enoxacin (and probably other quinolones). **Salicylates:** [P] Increased renal clearance of salicylates due to increased urine pH; occurs only with large doses of salicylates. **Sodium polystyrene sulfonate:** [NE] Binds antacid cation in gut, resulting in metabolic alkalosis. **Tetracyclines:** [HP] Decreased gastrointestinal absorption of tetracyclines. **Thyroxine:** [NP] Reduced gastrointestinal absorption of thyroxine.
Anticoagulants, oral	Metabolism inducible. Susceptible to inhibition of CYP2C9-mediated metabolism. Highly bound to plasma proteins. Anticoagulation response altered by drugs that affect clotting factor synthesis or catabolism.	*Drugs that may increase anticoagulant effect:* **Acetaminophen:** [NE] Impaired synthesis of clotting factors. **Amiodarone:** [P] Inhibited anticoagulant metabolism. **Anabolic steroids:** [P] Altered clotting factor disposition? **Chloramphenicol:** [NE] Decreased dicumarol metabolism (probably also warfarin). **Cimetidine:** [HP] Decreased warfarin metabolism. **Clofibrate:** [P] Mechanism not established. **Clopidogrel:** [NP] Decreased warfarin metabolism and inhibits platelet function. **Danazol:** [NE] Impaired synthesis of clotting factors? **Dextrothyroxine:** [P] Enhanced clotting factor catabolism? **Disulfiram:** [P] Decreased warfarin metabolism. **Erythromycin:** [NP] Probably inhibits anticoagulant metabolism. **Fluconazole:** [P] Decreased warfarin metabolism. **Fluoxetine:** [P] Decreased warfarin metabolism. **Gemfibrozil:** [NE] Mechanism not established. **Lovastatin:** [NP] Decreased warfarin metabolism. **Metronidazole:** [P] Decreased warfarin metabolism. **Miconazole:** [NE] Decreased warfarin metabolism.

HP, Highly predictable. Interaction occurs in almost all patients receiving the interacting combination; P, Predictable. Interaction occurs in most patients receiving the combination; NP, Not predictable. Interaction occurs only in some patients receiving the combination; NE, Not established. Insufficient data available on which to base estimate of predictability.

(continued)

TABLE 66–1 Important drug interactions. (Continued)

Drug or Drug Group	Properties Promoting Drug Interaction	Clinically Documented Interactions
Anticoagulants, oral (cont.)		**Nonsteroidal anti-inflammatory drugs:** [P] Inhibition of platelet function, gastric erosions; some agents increase hypoprothrombine-mic response (unlikely with diclofenac, ibuprofen, or naproxen).
		Propafenone: [NE] Probably decreases anticoagulant metabolism.
		Quinidine: [NP] Additive hypoprothrombinemia.
		Salicylates: [HP] Platelet inhibition with aspirin but not with other salicylates; [P] large doses have hypoprothrombinemic effect.
		Simvastatin: [NP] Decreased warfarin metabolism.
		Sulfinpyrazone: [NE] Inhibited warfarin metabolism.
		Sulfonamides: [NE] Inhibited warfarin metabolism.
		Thyroid hormones: [P] Enhanced clotting factor catabolism.
		Trimethoprim-sulfamethoxazole: [P] Inhibited warfarin metabolism; displaces from protein binding.
		Voriconazole: [NP] Decreased warfarin metabolism.
		See also Alcohol; Allopurinol.
		Drugs that may decrease anticoagulant effect:
		Aminoglutethimide: [P] Enzyme induction.
		Barbiturates: [P] Enzyme induction.
		Bosentan: [P] Enzyme induction.
		Carbamazepine: [P] Enzyme induction.
		Cholestyramine: [P] Reduced absorption of anticoagulant.
		Glutethimide: [P] Enzyme induction.
		Nafcillin: [NE] Enzyme induction.
		Phenytoin: [NE] Enzyme induction; anticoagulant effect may increase transiently at start of phenytoin therapy due to protein-binding displacement.
		Primidone: [P] Enzyme induction.
		Rifabutin: [P] Enzyme induction.
		Rifampin: [P] Enzyme induction.
		St. John's wort: [NE] Enzyme induction.
		Effects of anticoagulants on other drugs:
		Hypoglycemics, oral: [P] Dicumarol inhibits hepatic metabolism of tolbutamide and chlorpropamide.
		Phenytoin: [P] Dicumarol inhibits metabolism of phenytoin.
Antidepressants, tricyclic and heterocyclic	Inhibition of amine uptake into postganglionic adrenergic neuron. Antimuscarinic effects may be additive with other antimuscarinic drugs. Metabolism inducible. Susceptible to inhibition of metabolism via CYP2D6, CYP3A4, and other CYP450 enzymes.	**Amiodarone:** [P] Decreased antidepressant metabolism.
		Barbiturates: [P] Increased antidepressant metabolism.
		Bupropion: [NE] Decreased antidepressant metabolism.
		Carbamazepine: [NE] Enhanced metabolism of antidepressants.
		Cimetidine: [P] Decreased antidepressant metabolism.
		Clonidine: [P] Decreased clonidine antihypertensive effect.
		Guanadrel: [P] Decreased uptake of guanadrel into sites of action.
		Guanethidine: [P] Decreased uptake of guanethidine into sites of action.
		Haloperidol: [P] Decreased antidepressant metabolism.
		Monoamine oxidase inhibitors: [NP] Some cases of excitation, hyperpyrexia, mania, and convulsions, especially with serotonergic antidepressants such as clomipramine and imipramine, but many patients have received combination without ill effects.

HP, Highly predictable. Interaction occurs in almost all patients receiving the interacting combination; P, Predictable. Interaction occurs in most patients receiving the combination; NP, Not predictable. Interaction occurs only in some patients receiving the combination; NE, Not established. Insufficient data available on which to base estimate of predictability.

(continued)

TABLE 66–1   Important drug interactions. (Continued)

Drug or Drug Group	Properties Promoting Drug Interaction	Clinically Documented Interactions
Antidepressants, tricyclic and heterocyclic (cont.)		**Quinidine:** [NE] Decreased antidepressant metabolism.
		Rifampin: [P] Increased antidepressant metabolism.
		Selective serotonin reuptake inhibitors (SSRIs): [P] Fluoxetine and paroxetine inhibit CYP2D6 and decrease metabolism of antidepressants metabolized by this enzyme (eg, desipramine). Citalopram, sertraline, and fluvoxamine are only weak inhibitors of CYP2D6, but fluvoxamine inhibits CYP1A2 and CYP3A4 and thus can inhibit the metabolism of antidepressants metabolized by these enzymes.
		Sympathomimetics: [P] Increased pressor response to norepinephrine, epinephrine, and phenylephrine.
		Terbinafine: [P] Decreased antidepressant metabolism.
Azole antifungals	Inhibition of CYP3A4 (itraconazole = ketoconazole > posaconazole > voriconazole > fluconazole). Inhibition of CYP2C9 (fluconazole, voriconazole). Susceptible to enzyme inducers (itraconazole, ketoconazole, voriconazole). Gastrointestinal absorption pH-dependent (itraconazole, ketoconazole, posaconazole). Inhibition of P-glycoprotein (itraconazole, ketoconazole, posaconazole).	**Barbiturates:** [P] Increased metabolism of itraconazole, ketoconazole, voriconazole.
		Calcium channel blockers: [P] Decreased calcium channel blocker metabolism.
		Carbamazepine: [P] Decreased carbamazepine metabolism. Potential increased metabolism of azole antifungal.
		Cisapride: [NP] Decreased metabolism of cisapride; possible ventricular arrhythmias.
		Colchicine: [P] Decreased metabolism and transport of colchicine.
		Cyclosporine: [P] Decreased metabolism of cyclosporine.
		Digoxin: [NE] Increased plasma concentrations of digoxin with itraconazole, posaconazole, and ketoconazole.
		H₂-receptor antagonists: [NE] Decreased absorption of itraconazole, ketoconazole, and posaconazole.
		HMG-CoA reductase inhibitors: [HP] Decreased metabolism of lovastatin, simvastatin, and, to a lesser extent, atorvastatin.
		Phenytoin: [P] Decreased metabolism of phenytoin with fluconazole and probably voriconazole.
		Pimozide: [NE] Decreased pimozide metabolism.
		Proton pump inhibitors: [P] Decreased absorption of itraconazole, ketoconazole, and posaconazole.
		Rifabutin: [P] Decreased rifabutin metabolism. Increased metabolism of itraconazole, ketoconazole, and voriconazole.
		Rifampin: [P] Increased metabolism of itraconazole, ketoconazole, and voriconazole.
		See also Antacids; Anticoagulants, oral.
Barbiturates	Induction of hepatic microsomal drug metabolizing enzymes. Additive central nervous system depression with other central nervous system depressants.	**Beta-adrenoceptor blockers:** [P] Increased β-blocker metabolism.
		Calcium channel blockers: [P] Increased calcium channel blocker metabolism.
		Central nervous system depressants: [HP] Additive central nervous system depression.
		Corticosteroids: [P] Increased corticosteroid metabolism.
		Cyclosporine: [NE] Increased cyclosporine metabolism.
		Delavirdine: [P] Increased delavirdine metabolism.
		Doxycycline: [P] Increased doxycycline metabolism.
		Estrogens: [P] Increased estrogen metabolism.
		Methadone: [NE] Increased methadone metabolism.
		Phenothiazine: [P] Increased phenothiazine metabolism.
		Protease inhibitors: [NE] Increased protease inhibitor metabolism.
		Quinidine: [P] Increased quinidine metabolism.
		Sirolimus: [NE] Increased sirolimus metabolism.

HP, Highly predictable. Interaction occurs in almost all patients receiving the interacting combination; P, Predictable. Interaction occurs in most patients receiving the combination; NP, Not predictable. Interaction occurs only in some patients receiving the combination; NE, Not established. Insufficient data available on which to base estimate of predictability.

(continued)

TABLE 66–1 Important drug interactions. (Continued)

Drug or Drug Group	Properties Promoting Drug Interaction	Clinically Documented Interactions
Barbiturates (*cont.*)		**Tacrolimus:** [NE] Increased tacrolimus metabolism.
		Theophylline: [NE] Increased theophylline metabolism; reduced theophylline effect.
		Valproic acid: [P] Decreased phenobarbital metabolism.
		See also Anticoagulants, oral; Antidepressants, tricyclic.
Beta-adrenoceptor blockers	Beta-blockade (especially with nonselective agents such as propranolol) alters response to sympathomimetics with β-agonist activity (eg, epinephrine). Beta blockers that undergo extensive first-pass metabolism may be affected by drugs capable of altering this process. Beta blockers may reduce hepatic blood flow.	*Drugs that may increase β-blocker effect:*
		Cimetidine: [P] Decreased metabolism of β blockers that are cleared primarily by the liver, eg, propranolol. Less effect (if any) on those cleared by the kidneys, eg, atenolol, nadolol.
		Selective serotonin reuptake inhibitors (SSRIs): [P] Fluoxetine and paroxetine inhibit CYP2D6 and increase concentrations of timolol, propranolol, metoprolol, carvedilol, and labetalol.
		Drugs that may decrease β-blocker effect:
		Enzyme inducers: [P] Barbiturates, phenytoin, and rifampin may enhance β-blocker metabolism; other enzyme inducers may produce similar effects.
		Nonsteroidal anti-inflammatory drugs: [P] Indomethacin reduces antihypertensive response; other prostaglandin inhibitors probably also interact.
		Effects of β blockers on other drugs:
		Clonidine: [NE] Hypertensive reaction if clonidine is withdrawn while patient is taking propranolol.
		Insulin: [P] Inhibition of glucose recovery from hypoglycemia; inhibition of symptoms of hypoglycemia (except sweating); increased blood pressure during hypoglycemia.
		Prazosin: [P] Increased hypotensive response to first dose of prazosin.
		Sympathomimetics: [P] Increased pressor response to epinephrine (and possibly other sympathomimetics); this is more likely to occur with nonselective β blockers.
		See also Barbiturates; Theophylline.
Bile acid–binding resins	Resins may bind with orally administered drugs in gastrointestinal tract. Resins may bind in gastrointestinal tract with drugs that undergo enterohepatic circulation, even if the latter are given parenterally.	**Acetaminophen:** [NE] Decreased gastrointestinal absorption of acetaminophen.
		Digitalis glycosides: [NE] Decreased gastrointestinal absorption of digitoxin (possibly also digoxin).
		Furosemide: [P] Decreased gastrointestinal absorption of furosemide.
		Methotrexate: [NE] Reduced gastrointestinal absorption of methotrexate.
		Mycophenolate: [P] Reduced gastrointestinal absorption of mycophenolate.
		Thiazide diuretics: [P] Reduced gastrointestinal absorption of thiazides.
		Thyroid hormones: [P] Reduced thyroid absorption.
		See also Anticoagulants, oral.
Calcium channel blockers	Verapamil, diltiazem, and perhaps nicardipine (but not nifedipine) inhibit hepatic drug-metabolizing enzymes. Metabolism (via CYP3A4) of diltiazem, felodipine, nicardipine, nifedipine, verapamil, and probably other calcium channel blockers subject to induction and inhibition.	**Atazanavir:** [NE] Decreased metabolism of calcium channel blockers.
		Carbamazepine: [P] Decreased carbamazepine metabolism with diltiazem and verapamil; possible increase in calcium channel blocker metabolism.
		Cimetidine: [NP] Decreased metabolism of calcium channel blockers.
		Clarithromycin: [P] Decreased metabolism of calcium channel blockers.
		Colchicine: Decreased colchicine metabolism and transport with diltiazem and verapamil.
		Conivaptan: [NE] Decreased metabolism of calcium channel blockers.

HP, Highly predictable. Interaction occurs in almost all patients receiving the interacting combination; P, Predictable. Interaction occurs in most patients receiving the combination; NP, Not predictable. Interaction occurs only in some patients receiving the combination; NE, Not established. Insufficient data available on which to base estimate of predictability.

(continued)

TABLE 66–1 Important drug interactions. (Continued)

Drug or Drug Group	Properties Promoting Drug Interaction	Clinically Documented Interactions
Calcium channel blockers (*cont.*)		**Cyclosporine:** [P] Decreased cyclosporine metabolism with diltiazem, nicardipine, verapamil.
		Erythromycin: [P] Decreased metabolism of calcium channel blockers. **Phenytoin:** [NE] Increased metabolism of calcium channel blockers.
		Rifampin: [P] Increased metabolism of calcium channel blockers.
		Sirolimus: [P] Decreased sirolimus metabolism with diltiazem, nicardipine, verapamil.
		Tacrolimus: [P] Decreased tacrolimus metabolism with diltiazem, nicardipine, verapamil.
		See also Azole antifungals; Barbiturates; Theophylline; Digitalis glycosides.
Carbamazepine	Induction of hepatic microsomal drug-metabolizing enzymes. Susceptible to inhibition of metabolism, primarily by CYP3A4.	**Atazanavir:** [NE] Decreased metabolism of carbamazepine.
		Cimetidine: [P] Decreased carbamazepine metabolism.
		Clarithromycin: [P] Decreased carbamazepine metabolism.
		Corticosteroids: [P] Increased corticosteroid metabolism.
		Cyclosporine: [P] Increased cyclosporine metabolism and possible decreased carbamazepine metabolism.
		Danazol: [P] Decreased carbamazepine metabolism.
		Doxycycline: [P] Increased doxycycline metabolism.
		Erythromycin: [NE] Decreased carbamazepine metabolism.
		Fluvoxamine: [NE] Decreased carbamazepine metabolism.
		Estrogens: [P] Increased estrogen metabolism.
		Haloperidol: [P] Increased haloperidol metabolism.
		Isoniazid: [P] Decreased carbamazepine metabolism.
		Nefazodone: [NE] Decreased carbamazepine metabolism.
		Propoxyphene: [HP] Decreased carbamazepine metabolism and possible increased propoxyphene metabolism.
		Rifampin: [P] Increased carbamazepine metabolism.
		Selective serotonin reuptake inhibitors (SSRIs): [NE] Fluoxetine and fluvoxamine decrease carbamazepine metabolism.
		Sirolimus: [P] Increased sirolimus metabolism.
		St. John's wort: [P] Increased carbamazepine metabolism.
		Tacrolimus: [P] Increased tacrolimus metabolism.
		Theophylline: [NE] Increased theophylline metabolism.
		See also Anticoagulants, oral; Antidepressants, tricyclic; Azole antifungals; Calcium channel blockers.
Chloramphenicol	Inhibits hepatic drug-metabolizing enzymes.	**Phenytoin:** [P] Decreased phenytoin metabolism.
		Sulfonylurea hypoglycemics: [P] Decreased sulfonylurea metabolism.
		See also Anticoagulants, oral.

HP, Highly predictable. Interaction occurs in almost all patients receiving the interacting combination; P, Predictable. Interaction occurs in most patients receiving the combination; NP, Not predictable. Interaction occurs only in some patients receiving the combination; NE, Not established. Insufficient data available on which to base estimate of predictability.

(continued)

TABLE 66–1 Important drug interactions. (Continued)

Drug or Drug Group	Properties Promoting Drug Interaction	Clinically Documented Interactions
Cimetidine	Inhibits hepatic microsomal drug-metabolizing enzymes. (Ranitidine, famotidine, and nizatidine do not.) May inhibit the renal tubular secretion of weak bases.	**Atazanavir:** [NP] Decreased absorption of atazanavir (requires acid for absorption; other H₂ blockers and proton pump inhibitors would be expected to have the same effect). **Benzodiazepines:** [P] Decreased metabolism of alprazolam, chlordiazepoxide, diazepam, halazepam, prazepam, and clorazepate but not oxazepam, lorazepam, or temazepam. **Carmustine:** [NE] Increased bone marrow suppression. **Indinavir:** [NP] Decreased absorption of indinavir (requires acid for absorption; other H₂ blockers and proton pump inhibitors would be expected to have the same effect). **Lidocaine:** [P] Decreased metabolism of lidocaine; increased serum lidocaine concentrations. **Phenytoin:** [NE] Decreased phenytoin metabolism; increased serum phenytoin concentrations. **Procainamide:** [P] Decreased renal excretion of procainamide; increased serum procainamide concentrations. **Quinidine:** [P] Decreased metabolism of quinidine; increased serum quinidine concentrations. **Theophylline:** [P] Decreased theophylline metabolism; increased plasma theophylline concentrations. *See also* Anticoagulants, oral; Antidepressants, tricyclic; Azole antifungals; Beta-adrenoceptor blockers; Calcium channel blockers; Carbamazepine.
Cisapride	Susceptible to inhibition of metabolism by CYP3A4 inhibitors. High cisapride serum concentrations can result in ventricular arrhythmias.	**Atazanavir:** [NE] Decreased metabolism of cisapride; possible ventricular arrhythmia. **Clarithromycin:** [NP] Decreased metabolism of cisapride; possible ventricular arrhythmia. **Cyclosporine:** [NE] Decreased metabolism of cisapride; possible ventricular arrhythmia. **Erythromycin:** [NP] Decreased metabolism of cisapride; possible ventricular arrhythmia. **Nefazodone:** [NP] Possibly decreased metabolism of cisapride by CYP3A4; possible ventricular arrhythmia. **Ritonavir:** [NE] Decreased metabolism of cisapride; possible ventricular arrhythmia. **Selective serotonin reuptake inhibitors (SSRIs):** [NP] Fluvoxamine inhibits CYP3A4 and probably decreases cisapride metabolism; possible ventricular arrhythmia. *See also* Azole antifungals.
Colchicine	Susceptible to inhibition of CYP3A4 metabolism and P-glycoprotein transport.	**Amiodarone:** [NP] Decreased colchicine metabolism and transport. **Amprenavir:** [P] Decreased colchicine metabolism. **Carbamazepine:** [P] Increased metabolism of colchicine. **Clarithromycin:** [P] Decreased colchicine metabolism and transport. **Cyclosporine:** [P] Decreased colchicine metabolism and transport. **Dronedarone:** [NE] Decreased colchicine transport. **Erythromycin:** [P] Decreased colchicine metabolism and transport. **Nefazodone:** [NE] Decreased colchicine metabolism. **Rifampin:** [P] Increased colchicine metabolism. **Ritonavir:** [P] Decreased colchicine metabolism. *See also* Azole antifungals, Calcium channel blockers.

HP, Highly predictable. Interaction occurs in almost all patients receiving the interacting combination; P, Predictable. Interaction occurs in most patients receiving the combination; NP, Not predictable. Interaction occurs only in some patients receiving the combination; NE, Not established. Insufficient data available on which to base estimate of predictability.

(continued)

TABLE 66–1 Important drug interactions. (Continued)

Drug or Drug Group	Properties Promoting Drug Interaction	Clinically Documented Interactions
Cyclosporine	Metabolism inducible. Susceptible to inhibition of metabolism by CYP3A4. (Tacrolimus and sirolimus appear to have similar interactions.)	**Aminoglycosides:** [NE] Possible additive nephrotoxicity. **Amphotericin B:** [NE] Possible additive nephrotoxicity. **Amprenavir:** [P] Increased cyclosporine metabolism. **Androgens:** [NE] Increased serum cyclosporine. **Atazanavir:** [NE] Decreased metabolism of cyclosporine. **Barbiturates:** [P] Increased cyclosporine metabolism. **Carbamazepine:** [P] Increased cyclosporine metabolism. **Clarithromycin:** [P] Decreased cyclosporine metabolism. **Erythromycin:** [NP] Decreased cyclosporine metabolism. **Lovastatin:** [NP] Decreased metabolism of lovastatin. Myopathy and rhabdomyolysis noted in patients taking lovastatin and cyclosporine. **Nefazodone:** [P] Decreased cyclosporine metabolism. **Phenytoin:** [NE] Increased cyclosporine metabolism. **Pimozide:** [NE] Decreased pimozide metabolism. **Quinupristin:** [P] Increased cyclosporine metabolism. **Rifampin:** [P] Increased cyclosporine metabolism. **Ritonavir:** [P] Decreased cyclosporine metabolism. **Simvastatin:** [NP] Decreased metabolism of simvastatin. Myopathy and rhabdomyolysis noted in patients taking simvastatin and cyclosporine. **St. John's wort:** [NP] Increased cyclosporine metabolism. *See also* Azole antifungals; Barbiturates; Calcium channel blockers.
Digitalis glycosides	Digoxin susceptible to alteration of gastrointestinal absorption. Digitalis toxicity may be increased by drug-induced electrolyte imbalance (eg, hypokalemia). Digitoxin metabolism inducible. Renal and nonrenal excretion of digoxin susceptible to inhibition.	*Drugs that may increase digitalis effect:* **Amiodarone:** [P] Increased plasma digoxin concentrations. **Azithromycin:** [NP] Increased plasma concentration of digoxin. **Clarithromycin:** [P] Increased plasma concentration of digoxin. **Diltiazem:** [P] Increased plasma digoxin and additive AV conduction effects. **Erythromycin:** [NP] Increased plasma concentration of digoxin. **Potassium-depleting drugs:** [P] Increases likelihood of digitalis toxicity. **Propafenone:** [P] Increases plasma digoxin levels. **Quinidine:** [HP] Increased digoxin plasma concentrations; displaces digoxin from tissue binding sites. **Spironolactone:** [NE] Decreased renal digoxin excretion and interferes with some serum digoxin assays. **Verapamil:** [P] Increased plasma digoxin levels and additive AV conduction effects. *See also* Azole antifungals. *Drugs that may decrease digitalis effect:* **Kaolin-pectin:** [P] Decreased gastrointestinal digoxin absorption. **Rifampin:** [NE] Increased metabolism of digitoxin and elimination digoxin. **Sulfasalazine:** [NE] Decreased gastrointestinal digoxin absorption. *See also* Antacids; Bile acid–binding resins.

HP, Highly predictable. Interaction occurs in almost all patients receiving the interacting combination; P, Predictable. Interaction occurs in most patients receiving the combination; NP, Not predictable. Interaction occurs only in some patients receiving the combination; NE, Not established. Insufficient data available on which to base estimate of predictability.

(continued)

TABLE 66–1 Important drug interactions. (Continued)

Drug or Drug Group	Properties Promoting Drug Interaction	Clinically Documented Interactions
Disulfiram	Inhibits hepatic microsomal drug-metabolizing enzymes. Inhibits aldehyde dehydrogenase.	**Benzodiazepines:** [P] Decreased metabolism of chlordiazepoxide and diazepam but not lorazepam and oxazepam. **Metronidazole:** [NE] Confusion and psychoses reported in patients receiving this combination; mechanisms unknown. **Phenytoin:** [P] Decreased phenytoin metabolism. *See also* Alcohol; Anticoagulants, oral.
Estrogens	Metabolism inducible. Enterohepatic circulation of estrogen may be interrupted by alteration in bowel flora (eg, due to antibiotics).	**Ampicillin:** [NP] Interruption of enterohepatic circulation of estrogen; possible reduction in oral contraceptive efficacy. Some other oral antibiotics may have a similar effect. **Bosentan:** [NP] Enzyme induction leading to reduced estrogen effect. **Corticosteroids:** [P] Decreased metabolism of corticosteroids leading to increased corticosteroid effect. **Griseofulvin:** [NE] Possible inhibition of oral contraceptive efficacy; mechanism unknown. **Phenytoin:** [NP] Increased estrogen metabolism; possible reduction in oral contraceptive efficacy. **Primidone:** [NP] Increased estrogen metabolism; possible reduction in oral contraceptive efficacy. **Rifabutin:** [NP] Increased estrogen metabolism; possible reduction in oral contraceptive efficacy. **Rifampin:** [NP] Increased estrogen metabolism; possible reduction in oral contraceptive efficacy. **St. John's wort:** [NE] Increased estrogen metabolism; possible reduction in oral contraceptive efficacy. *See also* Barbiturates; Carbamazepine.
HMG-CoA reductase inhibitors	Lovastatin, simvastatin, and, to a lesser extent, atorvastatin are susceptible to CYP3A4 inhibitors; lovastatin, simvastatin, and, to a lesser extent, atorvastatin are susceptible to CYP3A4 inducers; increased risk of additive myopathy risk with other drugs that can cause myopathy.	**Amiodarone:** [NP] Decreased statin metabolism. **Atazanavir:** [NP] Decreased statin metabolism. **Carbamazepine:** [P] Increased statin metabolism. **Clarithromycin:** [P] Decreased statin metabolism. **Clofibrate:** [NP] Increased risk of myopathy. **Cyclosporine:** [P] Decreased statin metabolism. **Diltiazem:** [NE] Decreased statin metabolism. **Erythromycin:** [P] Decreased statin metabolism. **Gemfibrozil:** [NP] Increased plasma lovastatin and simvastatin and increase the risk of myopathy. **Indinavir:** [NE] Decreased statin metabolism. **Nefazodone:** [NE] Decreased statin metabolism. **Rifampin:** [P] Increased statin metabolism. **Ritonavir:** [NE] Decreased statin metabolism. **St. John's wort:** [NP] Increased statin metabolism. **Verapamil:** [NE] Decreased statin metabolism. *See also* Azole antifungals; Cyclosporine.
Iron	Binds with drugs in gastrointestinal tract, reducing absorption.	**Methyldopa:** [NE] Decreased methyldopa absorption. **Mycophenolate:** [P] Decreased absorption of mycophenolate. **Quinolones:** [P] Decreased absorption of ciprofloxacin and other quinolones. **Tetracyclines:** [P] Decreased absorption of tetracyclines; decreased efficacy of iron. **Thyroid hormones:** [P] Decreased thyroxine absorption. *See also* Antacids.

HP, Highly predictable. Interaction occurs in almost all patients receiving the interacting combination; P, Predictable. Interaction occurs in most patients receiving the combination; NP, Not predictable. Interaction occurs only in some patients receiving the combination; NE, Not established. Insufficient data available on which to base estimate of predictability.

(continued)

TABLE 66–1 Important drug interactions. (Continued)

Drug or Drug Group	Properties Promoting Drug Interaction	Clinically Documented Interactions
Levodopa	Levodopa degraded in gut prior to reaching sites of absorption. Agents that alter gastrointestinal motility may alter degree of intraluminal degradation. Anti-parkinsonism effect of levodopa susceptible to inhibition by other drugs.	**Clonidine:** [NE] Inhibited antiparkinsonism effect. **Monoamine oxidase inhibitors:** [P] Hypertensive reaction (carbidopa prevents the interaction). **Papaverine:** [NE] Inhibited antiparkinsonism effect. **Phenothiazines:** [P] Inhibited antiparkinsonism effect. **Phenytoin:** [NE] Inhibited antiparkinsonism effect. **Pyridoxine:** [P] Inhibited antiparkinsonism effect (carbidopa prevents the interaction). *See also* Antimuscarinics.
Lithium	Renal lithium excretion sensitive to changes in sodium balance. (Sodium depletion tends to cause lithium retention.) Susceptible to drugs enhancing central nervous system lithium toxicity.	**ACE inhibitors:** [NE] Probably reduce renal clearance of lithium; increase lithium effect. **Angiotensin II receptor blockers:** [NE] Probably reduce renal clearance of lithium; increase lithium effect. **Diuretics (especially thiazides):** [P] Decreased excretion of lithium; furosemide may be less likely to produce this effect than thiazide diuretics. **Haloperidol:** [NP] Occasional cases of neurotoxicity in manic patients, especially with large doses of one or both drugs. **Methyldopa:** [NE] Increased likelihood of central nervous system lithium toxicity. **Nonsteroidal anti-inflammatory drugs:** [NE] Reduced renal lithium excretion (except sulindac and salicylates). **Theophylline:** [P] Increased renal excretion of lithium; reduced lithium effect.
Macrolides	The macrolides clarithromycin and erythromycin are known to inhibit CYP3A4 and P-glycoprotein. Azithromycin does not appear to inhibit CYP3A4 but is a modest inhibitor of P-glycoprotein.	**Pimozide:** [NE] Increased pimozide concentrations. **Quinidine:** [P] Increased serum quinidine concentrations. **Theophylline:** [P] Decreased metabolism of theophylline. *See also* Anticoagulants, oral; Calcium channel blockers; Carbamazepine; Cisapride; Colchicine; Cyclosporine; Digitalis glycosides; HMG-CoA reductase inhibitors.
Monoamine oxidase inhibitors (MAOIs)	Increased norepinephrine stored in adrenergic neuron. Displacement of these stores by other drugs may produce acute hypertensive response. MAOIs have intrinsic hypoglycemic activity.	**Anorexiants:** [P] Hypertensive episodes due to release of stored norepinephrine (benzphetamine, diethylpropion, mazindol, phendimetrazine, phentermine). **Antidiabetic agents:** [P] Additive hypoglycemic effect. **Buspirone:** [NE] Possible serotonin syndrome; *avoid* concurrent use. **Dextromethorphan:** [NE] Severe reactions (hyperpyrexia, coma, death) have been reported. **Guanethidine:** [P] Reversal of the hypotensive action of guanethidine. **Mirtazapine:** [NE] Possible serotonin syndrome; *avoid* concurrent use. **Narcotic analgesics:** [NP] Some patients develop hypertension, rigidity, excitation; meperidine may be more likely to interact than morphine. **Nefazodone:** [NE] Possible serotonin syndrome; *avoid* concurrent use. **Phenylephrine:** [P] Hypertensive episode, since phenylephrine is metabolized by monoamine oxidase. **Selective serotonin reuptake inhibitors (SSRIs):** [P] Fatalities have occurred due to serotonin syndrome; contraindicated in patients taking MAOIs. **Sibutramine:** [NE] Possible serotonin syndrome; *avoid* concurrent use.

HP, Highly predictable. Interaction occurs in almost all patients receiving the interacting combination; P, Predictable. Interaction occurs in most patients receiving the combination; NP, Not predictable. Interaction occurs only in some patients receiving the combination; NE, Not established. Insufficient data available on which to base estimate of predictability.

(continued)

TABLE 66–1 Important drug interactions. (Continued)

Drug or Drug Group	Properties Promoting Drug Interaction	Clinically Documented Interactions
Monoamine oxidase inhibitors (MAOIs) (cont.)		**Sympathomimetics (indirect-acting):** [HP] Hypertensive episode due to release of stored norepinephrine (amphetamines, ephedrine, isometheptene, phenylpropanolamine, pseudoephedrine).
		Tramadol: [NE] Possible serotonin syndrome; *avoid* concurrent use.
		Venlafaxine: [NE] Possible serotonin syndrome; *avoid* concurrent use.
		See also Antidepressants, tricyclic and heterocyclic; Levodopa.
Nonsteroidal anti-inflammatory drugs (NSAIDs)	Prostaglandin inhibition may result in reduced renal sodium excretion, impaired resistance to hypertensive stimuli, and reduced renal lithium excretion. Most NSAIDs inhibit platelet function; may increase likelihood of bleeding due to other drugs that impair hemostasis.	**ACE inhibitors:** [P] Decreased antihypertensive response.
		Angiotensin II receptor blockers: [P] Decreased antihypertensive response.
		Furosemide: [P] Decreased diuretic, natriuretic, and antihypertensive response to furosemide.
		Hydralazine: [NE] Decreased antihypertensive response to hydralazine.
		Methotrexate: [NE] Possibly increased methotrexate toxicity (especially with anticancer doses of methotrexate).
		Selective serotonin reuptake inhibitors (SSRIs): Increased risk of bleeding due to platelet inhibition.
		Thiazide diuretics: [P] Decreased diuretic, natriuretic, and antihypertensive response.
		Triamterene: [NE] Decreased renal function noted with triamterene plus indomethacin in both healthy subjects and patients.
		See also Anticoagulants, oral; Beta-adrenoceptor blockers; Lithium.
Phenytoin	Induces hepatic microsomal drug metabolism. Susceptible to inhibition of metabolism by CYP2C9 and, to a lesser extent, CYP2C19.	*Drugs whose metabolism is stimulated by phenytoin:*
		Corticosteroids: [P] Decreased serum corticosteroid levels.
		Doxycycline: [P] Decreased serum doxycycline levels.
		Methadone: [P] Decreased serum methadone levels; watch for withdrawal symptoms.
		Mexiletine: [NE] Decreased serum mexiletine levels.
		Quinidine: [P] Decreased serum quinidine levels.
		Theophylline: [NE] Decreased serum theophylline levels.
		See also Calcium channel blockers; Cyclosporine; Estrogens.
		Drugs that inhibit phenytoin metabolism:
		Amiodarone: [P] Increased serum phenytoin; possible reduction in serum amiodarone.
		Capecitabine: [NE] Increased serum phenytoin.
		Chloramphenicol: [P] Increased serum phenytoin.
		Felbamate: [P] Increased serum phenytoin.
		Fluorouracil: [NE] Increased serum phenytoin.
		Fluvoxamine: [NE] Increased serum phenytoin.
		Isoniazid: [NP] Increased serum phenytoin; problem primarily with slow acetylators of isoniazid.
		Metronidazole: [NP] Increased serum phenytoin.
		Ticlopidine: [NP] Increased serum phenytoin.
		See also Azole antifungals; Cimetidine; Disulfiram.
		Drugs that enhance phenytoin metabolism:
		Carbamazepine: [P] Decreased serum phenytoin levels.
		Rifampin: [P] Decreased serum phenytoin levels.

HP, Highly predictable. Interaction occurs in almost all patients receiving the interacting combination; P, Predictable. Interaction occurs in most patients receiving the combination; NP, Not predictable. Interaction occurs only in some patients receiving the combination; NE, Not established. Insufficient data available on which to base estimate of predictability.

(continued)

TABLE 66–1 Important drug interactions.

Drug or Drug Group	Properties Promoting Drug Interaction	Clinically Documented Interactions
Pimozide	Susceptible to CYP3A4 inhibitors; may exhibit additive effects with other agents that prolong QT_c interval.	**Nefazodone:** [NE] Decreased pimozide metabolism. *See also* Azole antifungals; Cyclosporine; Macrolides.
Potassium-sparing diuretics (amiloride, eplerenone, spironolactone, triamterene)	Additive effects with other agents increasing serum potassium concentration. May alter renal excretion of substances other than potassium (eg, digoxin, hydrogen ions).	**ACE inhibitors:** [NP] Additive hyperkalemic effect. **Angiotensin II receptor blockers:** [NP] Additive hyperkalemic effect. **Potassium-sparing diuretics:** [P] Additive hyperkalemic effect. **Potassium supplements:** [P] Additive hyperkalemic effect; especially a problem in presence of renal impairment. *See also* Digitalis glycosides; Nonsteroidal anti-inflammatory drugs.
Probenecid	Interference with renal excretion of drugs that undergo active tubular secretion, especially weak acids. Inhibition of glucuronide conjugation of other drugs.	**Clofibrate:** [P] Reduced glucuronide conjugation of clofibric acid. **Methotrexate:** [P] Decreased renal methotrexate excretion; possible methotrexate toxicity. **Palatrexate:** [P] Decreased renal palatrexate excretion; possible palatrexate toxicity. **Penicillin:** [P] Decreased renal penicillin excretion. **Salicylates:** [P] Decreased uricosuric effect of probenecid (interaction unlikely with less than 1.5 g of salicylate daily).
Quinidine	Substrate of CYP3A4. Inhibits CYP2D6. Renal excretion susceptible to changes in urine pH. Additive effects with other agents that prolong the QT_c interval.	**Acetazolamide:** [P] Decreased renal quinidine excretion due to increased urinary pH; elevated serum quinidine. **Amiodarone:** [NP] Increased serum quinidine levels. **Kaolin-pectin:** [NE] Decreased gastrointestinal absorption of quinidine. **Rifampin:** [P] Increased hepatic quinidine metabolism. **Thioridazine:** [NE] Decreased thioridazine metabolism; additive prolongation of QT_c interval. *See also* Anticoagulants, oral; Antidepressants, tricyclic; Barbiturates; Cimetidine; Digitalis glycosides; Macrolides; Phenytoin.
Quinolone antibiotics	Susceptible to inhibition of gastrointestinal absorption. Some quinolones inhibit CYP1A2.	**Caffeine:** [P] Ciprofloxacin, enoxacin, pipedemic acid, and, to a lesser extent, norfloxacin inhibit caffeine metabolism. **Sucralfate:** [HP] Reduced gastrointestinal absorption of ciprofloxacin, norfloxacin, and probably other quinolones. **Theophylline:** [P] Ciprofloxacin, enoxacin, and, to a lesser extent, norfloxacin inhibit theophylline metabolism; gatifloxacin, levofloxacin, lomefloxacin, ofloxacin, and sparfloxacin appear to have little effect. *See also* Antacids; Anticoagulants, oral; Iron.
Rifampin	Inducer (strong) of hepatic microsomal drug-metabolizing enzymes.	**Corticosteroids:** [P] Increased corticosteroid hepatic metabolism; reduced corticosteroid effect. **Mexiletine:** [NE] Increased mexiletine metabolism; reduced mexiletine effect. **Sulfonylurea hypoglycemics:** [P] Increased hepatic metabolism of tolbutamide and probably other sulfonylureas metabolized by the liver (including chlorpropamide). **Theophylline:** [P] Increased theophylline metabolism; reduced theophylline effect. *See also* Anticoagulants, oral; Azole antifungals; Beta-adrenoceptor blockers; Calcium channel blockers; Cyclosporine; Digitalis glycosides; Estrogens.

HP, Highly predictable. Interaction occurs in almost all patients receiving the interacting combination; P, Predictable. Interaction occurs in most patients receiving the combination; NP, Not predictable. Interaction occurs only in some patients receiving the combination; NE, Not established. Insufficient data available on which to base estimate of predictability.

(continued)

TABLE 66–1 Important drug interactions.

Drug or Drug Group	Properties Promoting Drug Interaction	Clinically Documented Interactions
Salicylates	Interference with renal excretion of drugs that undergo active tubular secretion. Salicylate renal excretion dependent on urinary pH when large doses of salicylate used. Aspirin (but not other salicylates) interferes with platelet function. Large doses of salicylates have intrinsic hypoglycemic activity.	**Carbonic anhydrase inhibitors:** [NE] Increased acetazolamide serum concentrations; increase salicylate toxicity due to decreased blood pH. **Corticosteroids:** [P] Increased salicylate elimination; possible additive toxic effect on gastric mucosa. **Heparin:** [NE] Increased bleeding tendency with aspirin, but probably not with other salicylates. **Methotrexate:** [P] Decreased renal methotrexate clearance; increases methotrexate toxicity (primarily at anticancer doses). **Sulfinpyrazone:** [HP] Decreased uricosuric effect of sulfinpyrazone (interaction unlikely with less than 1.5 g of salicylate daily). *See also* Antacids; Anticoagulants, oral; Probenecid.
Selective serotonin reuptake inhibitors	Selective serotonin reuptake inhibitors (SSRIs) can lead to excessive serotonin response when administered with other serotonergic drugs (eg, MAOIs). Some SSRIs inhibit various cytochrome P450s including CYP2D6, CYP1A2, CYP3A4, and CYP2C19.	**Theophylline:** [P] Decreased metabolism by fluvoxamine-induced inhibition of CYP. *See also* Anticoagulants, oral; Antidepressants, tricyclic and heterocyclic; Beta-adrenoceptor blockers; Carbamazepine; Cisapride; Colchicine; Cyclosporine; HMG-CoA reductase inhibitors; Monoamine oxidase inhibitors; Nonsteroidal anti-inflammatory drugs; Phenytoin; Pimozide.
Theophylline	Susceptible to inhibition of hepatic metabolism by CYP1A2. Metabolism inducible.	**Benzodiazepines:** [NE] Inhibition of benzodiazepine sedation. **Beta-adrenoceptor blockers:** [NP] Decreased theophylline bronchodilation especially with nonselective β blockers. **Diltiazem:** [NP] Decreased theophylline metabolism. **Smoking:** [HP] Increased theophylline metabolism. **Tacrine:** [NP] Decreased theophylline metabolism. **Ticlopidine:** [NE] Decreased theophylline metabolism. **Verapamil:** [NP] Decreased theophylline metabolism. **Zileuton:** [NP] Decreased theophylline metabolism. *See also* Barbiturates; Carbamazepine; Cimetidine; Lithium; Macrolides; Phenytoin; Quinolones; Rifampin.

HP, Highly predictable. Interaction occurs in almost all patients receiving the interacting combination; P, Predictable. Interaction occurs in most patients receiving the combination; NP, Not predictable. Interaction occurs only in some patients receiving the combination; NE, Not established. Insufficient data available on which to base estimate of predictability.

REFERENCES

Asberg A: Interactions between cyclosporin and lipid-lowering drugs: Implications for organ transplant recipients. Drugs 2003;63:367.

Blanchard N et al: Qualitative and quantitative assessment of drug-drug interaction potential in man, based on Ki, IC50 and inhibitor concentration. Curr Drug Metab 2004;5:147.

deMaat MM et al: Drug interactions between antiretroviral drugs and comedicated agents. Clin Pharmacokinet 2003;42:223.

DuBuske LM: The role of P-glycoprotein and organic anion-transporting polypeptides in drug interactions. Drug Saf 2005;28:789.

Egger SS et al: Potential drug-drug interactions in the medication of medical patients at hospital discharge. Eur J Clin Pharmacol 2003;58:773.

Hansten PD: Understanding drug interactions. Sci Med 1998;5:16.

Hansten PD, Horn JR: *Drug Interactions Analysis and Management.* Facts & Comparisons. 2011. [Quarterly.]

Hansten PD, Horn JR: *The Top 100 Drug Interactions. A Guide to Patient Management.* H&H Publications, 2011.

Juurlink DN et al: Drug-drug interactions among elderly patients hospitalized for drug toxicity. JAMA 2003;289:1652.

Kim RB (editor): *The Medical Letter Handbook of Adverse Interactions. Medical Letter,* 2003.

Leucuta SE, Vlase L: Pharmacokinetics and metabolic drug interactions. Curr Clin Pharmacol 2006;1:5.

Levy RH et al (editors): *Metabolic Drug Interactions.* Lippincott Williams & Wilkins, 2000.

Lin JH, Yamazaki M: Role of P-glycoprotein in pharmacokinetics: Clinical implications. Clin Pharmacokinet 2003;42:59.

Tatro DS (editor): *Drug Interaction Facts.* Facts & Comparisons. 2011. [Quarterly.]

Thelen K, Dressman JB: Cytochrome P540-mediated metabolism in the human gut wall. J Pharm Pharmacol 2009;61:541.

Williamson EM: Drug interactions between herbal and prescription medicines. Drug Saf 2003;26:1075.

Appendix: Vaccines, Immune Globulins, & Other Complex Biologic Products

Harry W. Lampiris, MD, & Daniel S. Maddix, PharmD

Vaccines and related biologic products constitute an important group of agents that bridge the disciplines of microbiology, infectious diseases, immunology, and immunopharmacology. A list of the most important preparations is provided here. The reader who requires more complete information is referred to the sources listed at the end of this appendix.

ACTIVE IMMUNIZATION

Active immunization consists of the administration of antigen to the host to induce formation of antibodies and cell-mediated immunity. Immunization is practiced to induce protection against many infectious agents and may utilize either inactivated (killed) materials or live attenuated agents (Table A–1). Desirable features of the ideal immunogen include complete prevention of disease, prevention of the carrier state, production of prolonged immunity with a minimum of immunizations, absence of toxicity, and suitability for mass immunization (eg, cheap and easy to administer). Active immunization is generally preferable to passive immunization—in most cases because higher antibody levels are sustained for longer periods of time, requiring less frequent immunization, and in some cases because of the development of concurrent cell-mediated immunity. However, active immunization requires time to develop and is therefore generally inactive at the time of a specific exposure (eg, for parenteral exposure to hepatitis B, concurrent hepatitis B IgG [passive antibodies] and active immunization are given to prevent illness).

Current recommendations for routine active immunization of children are given in Table A–2.

PASSIVE IMMUNIZATION

Passive immunization consists of transfer of immunity to a host using preformed immunologic products. From a practical standpoint, only immunoglobulins have been used for passive immunization, because passive administration of cellular components of the immune system has been technically difficult and associated with graft-versus-host reactions. Products of the cellular immune system (eg, interferons) have also been used in the therapy of a wide variety of hematologic and infectious diseases (see Chapter 55).

Passive immunization with antibodies may be accomplished with either animal or human immunoglobulins in varying degrees of purity. These may contain relatively high titers of antibodies directed against a specific antigen or, as is true for pooled immune globulin, may simply contain antibodies found in most of the population. Passive immunization is useful for (1) individuals unable to form antibodies (eg, congenital agammaglobulinemia); (2) prevention of disease when time does not permit active immunization (eg, postexposure); (3) for treatment of certain diseases normally prevented by immunization (eg, tetanus); and (4) for treatment of conditions for which active immunization is unavailable or impractical (eg, snakebite).

Complications from administration of *human* immunoglobulins are rare. The injections may be moderately painful and rarely a sterile abscess may occur at the injection site. Transient hypotension and pruritus occasionally occur with the administration of intravenous immune globulin (IVIG) products, but generally are mild. Individuals with certain immunoglobulin deficiency states (IgA deficiency, etc) may occasionally develop hypersensitivity reactions to immune globulin that may limit therapy.

TABLE A–1 Materials commonly used for active immunization in the United States.[1]

Vaccine	Type of Agent	Route of Administration	Primary Immunization	Booster[2]	Indications
Diphtheria tetanus acellular pertussis (DTaP)	Toxoids and inactivated bacterial components	Intramuscular	See Table A–2	None	For all children
Haemophilus influenzae type b conjugate (Hib)[3]	Bacterial polysaccharide conjugated to protein	Intramuscular	One dose (see Table A–2 for childhood schedule)	Not recommended	1. For all children 2. Asplenia and other at-risk conditions
Hepatitis A	Inactivated virus	Intramuscular	One dose (see Table A–2 for childhood schedule) (administer at least 2–4 weeks before travel to endemic areas)	At 6–12 months for long-term immunity	1. Travelers to hepatitis A endemic areas 2. Homosexual and bisexual men 3. Injection drug users 4. Chronic liver disease or clotting factor disorders 5. Persons with occupational risk for infection 6. Persons living in, or relocating to, endemic areas 7. Household and sexual contacts of individuals with acute hepatitis A (with additional gamma globulin in select patients) 8. For all children
Hepatitis B	Inactive viral antigen, recombinant	Intramuscular (subcutaneous injection is acceptable in individuals with bleeding disorders)	Three doses at 0, 1, and 6 months (see Table A–2 for childhood schedule)	Not routinely recommended	1. For all infants 2. Preadolescents, adolescents, and young adults 3. Persons with occupational, lifestyle, or environmental risk 4. Hemophiliacs 5. Persons with end-stage renal disease, HIV, or chronic liver disease 6. Postexposure prophylaxis 7. Household and sexual contacts of individuals with acute and chronic hepatitis B
Human papillomavirus (HPV)[4]	Virus-like particles of the major capsid protein	Intramuscular	Three doses at 0, 2, and 6 months (HPV4) or 0, 1, and 6 months (HPV2)[4]	None	HPV2 or HPV4 for females between 9 and 26 years of age; HPV4 for males aged 9–26 years
Influenza, inactivated	Inactivated virus or viral components	Intramuscular	One dose (Children < 9 years who are receiving influenza vaccine for the first time should receive two doses administered at least 1 month apart.)	Yearly with current vaccine	1. Adults > 18 years 2. Persons with high-risk conditions (eg, asthma) 3. Health care workers and others in contact with high-risk groups 4. Residents of nursing homes and other residential chronic care facilities 5. All children aged 6 months to 18 years 6. Women who will be pregnant during the influenza season

1164

Vaccine	Type	Route of Administration	Primary Immunization	Booster	Indications
Influenza, live attenuated	Live virus	Intranasal	Split dose in each nostril. Children age 5–8 who are receiving influenza vaccine for the first time should receive two doses administered 6–10 weeks apart	Yearly with current vaccine	Healthy persons aged 19–49 years who desire protection against influenza. May be substituted for inactivated vaccine in healthy children 2–18 years
Measles-mumps-rubella (MMR)	Live virus	Subcutaneous	See Table A–2	None	1. For all children 2. Adults born after 1956
Meningococcal conjugate vaccine	Bacterial polysaccharides conjugated to diphtheria toxoid	Intramuscular	One dose	Unknown	1. All adolescents 2. Preferred over polysaccharide vaccine in persons aged 11–55 years
Meningococcal polysaccharide vaccine	Bacterial polysaccharides of serotypes A/C/Y/W-135	Subcutaneous	One dose	Every 5 years if there is continuing high risk of exposure	1. Military recruits 2. Travelers to areas with hyperendemic or epidemic meningococcal disease 3. Individuals with asplenia, complement deficiency, or properdin deficiency 4. Control of outbreaks in closed or semiclosed populations 5. College freshmen who live in dormitories 6. Microbiologists who are routinely exposed to isolates of *Neisseria meningitidis*
Pneumococcal conjugate vaccine	Bacterial polysaccharides conjugated to protein	Intramuscular or subcutaneous	See Table A–2	None	For all children
Pneumococcal polysaccharide vaccine	Bacterial polysaccharides of 23 serotypes	Intramuscular or subcutaneous	One dose	Repeat after 5 years in patients at high risk	1. Adults ≥ 65 years 2. Persons at increased risk for pneumococcal disease or its complications
Poliovirus vaccine, inactivated (IPV)	Inactivated viruses of all three serotypes	Subcutaneous	See Table A–2 for childhood schedule. Adults: Two doses 4–8 weeks apart, and a third dose 6–12 months after the second	One-time booster dose for adults at increased risk of exposure	1. For all children 2. Previously unvaccinated adults at increased risk for occupational or travel exposure to polioviruses
Rabies	Inactivated virus	Intramuscular	**Preexposure:** Three doses at days 0, 7, and 21 or 28 **Postexposure:** Four doses at days 0, 3, 7, and 14	Serologic testing every 6 months to 2 years in persons at high risk	1. **Preexposure** prophylaxis in persons at risk for contact with rabies virus 2. **Postexposure** prophylaxis (administer with rabies immune globulin)
Rotavirus	Live virus	Oral	See Table A–2	None	For all infants. The series of 3 doses should be initiated by age 14 weeks and completed by age 32 weeks
Tetanus-diphtheria (Td or DT)[5]	Toxoids	Intramuscular	Two doses 4–8 weeks apart, and a third dose 6–12 months after the second	Every 10 years or a single booster at age 50	1. All adults 2. Postexposure prophylaxis if > 5 years has passed since last dose

(continued)

TABLE A–1 Materials commonly used for active immunization in the United States.[1] (Continued)

Vaccine	Type of Agent	Route of Administration	Primary Immunization	Booster[2]	Indications
Tetanus, diphtheria, pertussis (Tdap)	Toxoids and inactivated bacterial components	Intramuscular	Substitute 1 dose of Tdap for Td in patients 19–64 years of age	None	All adults < 65 years
Typhoid, Ty21a oral	Live bacteria	Oral	Four doses administered every other day	Four doses every 5 years	Risk of exposure to typhoid fever
Typhoid, Vi capsular polysaccharide	Bacterial polysaccharide	Intramuscular	One dose	Every 2 years	Risk of exposure to typhoid fever
Varicella	Live virus	Subcutaneous	Two doses 4–8 weeks apart in persons past their 13th birthday (see Table A–2 for childhood schedule)	Unknown	1. For all children 2. Persons past their 13th birthday without a history of varicella infection or immunization 3. Postexposure prophylaxis in susceptible persons
Yellow fever	Live virus	Subcutaneous	One dose 10 years to 10 days before travel	Every 10 years	1. Laboratory personnel who may be exposed to yellow fever virus 2. Travelers to areas where yellow fever occurs
Zoster	Live virus	Subcutaneous	One dose	None	All adults ≥ 60 years of age

[1]Dosages for the specific product, including variations for age, are best obtained from the manufacturer's package insert.

[2]One dose unless otherwise indicated.

[3]Three Hib conjugate vaccines are available for use: (1) oligosaccharide conjugate Hib vaccine (HbOC), (2) polyribosylribitol phosphate-tetanus toxoid conjugate (PRP-T), and (3) *Haemophilus influenzae* type b conjugate vaccine (meningococcal protein conjugate) (PRP-OMP).

[4]Two HPV vaccines are available for use: (1) quadrivalent vaccine (HPV4) for the prevention of cervical, vaginal, and vulvar cancers (in females) and genital warts (in males and females), and (2) bivalent vaccine (HPV2) for the prevention of cervical cancers in females.

[5]Td is tetanus and diphtheria toxoids for use in persons ≥ 7 years of age (contains less diphtheria toxoid than DPT and DT). DT is tetanus and diphtheria toxoids for use in persons < 7 years of age (contains the same amount of diphtheria toxoid as DPT).

TABLE A–2 Recommended routine childhood immunization schedule.

Age	Immunization	Comments
Birth to 2 months	Hepatitis B vaccine (HBV)	**Infants born to seronegative mothers:** Administration should begin at birth, with the second dose administered at least 4 weeks after the first dose. **Infants born to seropositive mothers:** Should receive the first dose within 12 hours after birth (with hepatitis B immune globulin), the second dose at 1–2 months of age, and the third dose at 6–18 months of age.
2 months	Diphtheria and tetanus toxoids and acellular pertussis vaccine (DTaP), inactivated poliovirus vaccine (IPV), *Haemophilus influenzae* type b conjugate vaccine (Hib),[1] pneumococcal conjugate vaccine (PCV), rotavirus vaccine (RV)	
1–2 months	HBV	The second dose should be given at least 4 weeks after the first dose.
4 months	DTaP, Hib,[1] IPV, PCV, RV	
6 months	DTaP, Hib,[1] PCV, RV	
6–18 months	HBV, IPV, influenza	The third dose of HBV should be given at least 16 weeks after the first dose and at least 8 weeks after the second dose, but not before age 6 months. Influenza vaccine should be administered annually to children aged 6 months to 18 years.
12–15 months	Measles-mumps-rubella vaccine (MMR), Hib,[1] PCV, varicella vaccine	The second dose of varicella vaccine should be administered at age 4–6 years
12–18 months	DTaP at 15–18 months	DTaP may be given as early as age 12 months.
12–23 months	Hepatitis A vaccine	Two doses ≥ 6 months apart.
4–6 years	DTaP IPV, MMR, varicella vaccine	The second dose of MMR should be routinely administered at age 4–6 years but may be given during any visit if at least 4 weeks have elapsed since administration of the first dose. The second dose should be given no later than age 11–12 years.
11–12 years	Tetanus, diphtheria, pertussis (Tdap) vaccine, human papillomavirus vaccine (HPV),[2] meningococcal conjugate vaccine	Three doses of HPV should be administered to females at 0, 1–2, and 6 months. HPV4 may be administered to males aged 9–18 years to reduce the likelihood of developing genital warts.

[1]Three Hib conjugate vaccines are available for use: (1) oligosaccharide conjugate Hib vaccine (HbOC), (2) polyribosylribitol phosphate-tetanus toxoid conjugate (PRP-T), and (3) *Haemophilus influenzae* type b conjugate vaccine (meningococcal protein conjugate) (PRP-OMP). Children immunized with PRP-OMP at 2 and 4 months of age do not require a dose at 6 months of age.

[2]Two HPV vaccines are available for use: (1) quadrivalent vaccine (HPV4) for the prevention of cervical, vaginal, and vulvar cancers (in females) and genital warts (in males and females), and (2) bivalent vaccine (HPV2) for the prevention of cervical cancers in females.

Adapted from MMWR Morb Mortal Wkly Rep 2010;58:(51&52).

Conventional immune globulin contains aggregates of IgG; it will cause severe reactions if given intravenously. However, if the passively administered antibodies are derived from *animal* sera, hypersensitivity reactions ranging from anaphylaxis to serum sickness may occur. Highly purified immunoglobulins, especially from rodents or lagomorphs, are the least likely to cause reactions. To avoid anaphylactic reactions, tests for hypersensitivity to the animal serum must be performed. If an alternative preparation is not available and administration of the specific antibody is deemed essential, desensitization can be carried out.

Antibodies derived from human serum not only avoid the risk of hypersensitivity reactions but also have a much longer half-life in humans (about 23 days for IgG antibodies) than those from animal sources (5–7 days or less). Consequently, much smaller doses of human antibody can be administered to provide therapeutic concentrations for several weeks. These advantages point to the desirability of using human antibodies for passive protection whenever possible. Materials available for passive immunization are summarized in Table A–3.

LEGAL LIABILITY FOR UNTOWARD REACTIONS

It is the physician's responsibility to inform the patient of the risk of immunization and to use vaccines and antisera in an appropriate manner. This may require skin testing to assess the risk of an untoward reaction. Some of the risks previously described are,

TABLE A–3 Materials available for passive immunization.[1]

Indication	Product	Dosage	Comments
Black widow spider bite	Aontivenin (*Latrodectus mactans*), equine	One vial (6000 units) IV or IM.	For persons with hypertensive cardiovascular disease or age < 16 or > 60 years.
Bone marrow transplantation	Immune globulin (intravenous [IV])[2]	500 mg/kg IV on days 7 and 2 prior to transplantation and then once weekly through day 90 after transplantation.	Prophylaxis to decrease the risk of infection, interstitial pneumonia, and acute graft-versus-host disease in adults undergoing bone marrow transplantation.
Botulism	Botulism antitoxin, equine	Consult the CDC.[3]	Treatment and prophylaxis of botulism. Available from the CDC.[3] Incidence of serum reactions is 10–20%.
	Botulism immune globulin (IV)	50 mg/kg IV.	For the treatment of patients < 1 year of age with infant botulism caused by toxin type A or B.
Chronic lymphocytic leukemia (CLL)	Immune globulin (IV)[2]	400 mg/kg IV every 3–4 weeks. Dosage should be adjusted upward if bacterial infections occur.	CLL patients with hypogammaglobulinemia and a history of at least one serious bacterial infection.
Cytomegalovirus (CMV)	Cytomegalovirus immune globulin (IV)	Consult the manufacturer's dosing recommendations.	Prophylaxis of CMV infection in bone marrow, kidney, liver, lung, pancreas, and heart transplant recipients.
Diphtheria	Diphtheria antitoxin, equine	20,000–120,000 units IV or IM depending on the severity and duration of illness.	Early treatment of respiratory diphtheria. Available from the CDC.[3] Anaphylactic reactions in ≥ 7% of adults and serum reactions in ≥ 5–10% of adults.
Hepatitis A	Immune globulin (intramuscular [IM])	**Preexposure prophylaxis:** 0.02 mL/kg IM for anticipated risk of ≤ 3 months, 0.06 mL/kg for anticipated risk of > 3 months, repeated every 4–6 months for continued exposure. **Postexposure:** 0.02 mL/kg IM as soon as possible after exposure up to 2 weeks.	Preexposure and postexposure hepatitis A prophylaxis. The availability of hepatitis A vaccine has greatly reduced the need for preexposure prophylaxis. Patients > 40 years should receive hepatitis A vaccine in addition to immune globulin for postexposure prophylaxis
Hepatitis B	Hepatitis B immune globulin (HBIG)	0.06 mL/kg IM as soon as possible after exposure up to 1 week for percutaneous exposure or 2 weeks for sexual exposure. 0.5 mL IM within 12 hours after birth for perinatal exposure.	Postexposure prophylaxis in nonimmune persons following percutaneous, mucosal, sexual, or perinatal exposure. Hepatitis B vaccine should also be administered.
HIV-infected children	Immune globulin (IV)[2]	400 mg/kg IV every 28 days.	HIV-infected children with recurrent serious bacterial infections or hypogammaglobulinemia.
Idiopathic thrombocytopenic purpura (ITP)	Immune globulin (IV)[2]	Consult the manufacturer's dosing recommendations for the specific product being used.	Response in children with ITP is greater than in adults. Corticosteroids are the treatment of choice in adults, except for severe pregnancy-associated ITP.
Kawasaki disease	Immune globulin (IV)[2]	400 mg/kg IV daily for 4 consecutive days within 4 days after the onset of illness. A single dose of 2 g/kg IV over 10 hours is also effective.	Effective in the prevention of coronary aneurysms. For use in patients who meet strict criteria for Kawasaki disease.
Measles	Immune globulin (IM)	**Normal hosts:** 0.25 mL/kg IM. **Immunocompromised hosts:** 0.5 mL/kg IM (maximum 15 mL for all patients).	Postexposure prophylaxis (within 6 days after exposure) in nonimmune contacts of acute cases.
Primary immunodeficiency disorders	Immune globulin (IV)[2]	Consult the manufacturer's dosing recommendations for the specific product being used.	Primary immunodeficiency disorders include specific antibody deficiencies (eg, X-linked agammaglobulinemia) and combined deficiencies (eg, severe combined immunodeficiencies).

(continued)

TABLE A–3 Materials available for passive immunization.[1] (Continued)

Indication	Product	Dosage	Comments
Rabies	Rabies immune globulin	20 IU/kg. The full dose should be infiltrated around the wound and any remaining volume should be given IM at an anatomic site distant from vaccine administration.	Postexposure rabies prophylaxis in persons not previously immunized with rabies vaccine. Must be combined with rabies vaccine.
Respiratory syncytial virus (RSV)	Palivizumab	15 mg/kg IM once prior to the beginning of the RSV season and once monthly until the end of the season.	For use in infants and children < 24 months with chronic lung disease or a history of premature birth (≤ 35 weeks' gestation).
Rubella	Immune globulin (IM)	0.55 mL/kg IM.	Nonimmune pregnant women exposed to rubella who will not consider therapeutic abortion. Administration does not prevent rubella in the fetus of an exposed mother.
Snake bite (coral snake)	Antivenom (*Micrurus fulvius*), equine	At least 3–5 vials (30–50 mL) IV initially within 4 hours after the bite. Additional doses may be required.	Neutralizes venom of eastern coral snake and Texas coral snake. Serum sickness occurs in almost all patients who receive > 7 vials.
Snake bite (pit vipers)	Antivenom (Crotalidae) polyvalent immune Fab, ovine	An initial dose of 4–6 vials should be infused intravenously over 1 hour. The dose should be repeated if initial control is not achieved. After initial control, 2 vials should be given every 6 hours for up to 3 doses.	For the management of minimal to moderate North American crotalid envenomation.
Tetanus	Tetanus immune globulin	**Postexposure prophylaxis:** 250 units IM. For severe wounds or when there has been a delay in administration, 500 units is recommended. **Treatment:** 3000–6000 units IM.	Treatment of tetanus and postexposure prophylaxis of nonclean, nonminor wounds in inadequately immunized persons (less than two doses of tetanus toxoid or less than three doses if wound is > 24 hours old).
Vaccinia	Vaccinia immune globulin	Consult the CDC.[3]	Treatment of severe reactions to vaccinia vaccination, including eczema vaccinatum, vaccinia necrosum, and ocular vaccinia. Available from the CDC.[3]
Varicella	Varicella-zoster immune globulin	**Weight (kg)** — **Dose (units)** ≤ 10 — 125 IM 10.1–20 — 250 IM 20.1–30 — 375 IM 30.1–40 — 500 IM ≥ 40 — 625 IM	**Postexposure prophylaxis** (preferably within 48 hours but no later than within 96 hours after exposure) in susceptible immunocompromised hosts, selected pregnant women, and perinatally exposed newborns.

[1]Passive immunotherapy or immunoprophylaxis should always be administered as soon as possible after exposure. Prior to the administration of animal sera, patients should be questioned and tested for hypersensitivity.

[2]See the following references for an analysis of additional uses of intravenously administered immune globulin: Ratko TA et al: Recommendations for off-label use of intravenously administered immunoglobulin preparations. JAMA 1995;273:1865; and Feasby T et al: Guidelines on the use of intravenous immune globulin for neurologic conditions. Transfus Med Rev 2007;21(2 Suppl 1)S57.

[3]Centers for Disease Control and Prevention, 404-639-3670 during weekday business hours; 770-488-7100 during nights, weekends, and holidays (emergency requests only).

however, currently unavoidable; on balance, the patient and society are clearly better off accepting the risks for routinely administered immunogens (eg, influenza and tetanus vaccines).

Manufacturers should be held legally accountable for failure to adhere to existing standards for production of biologicals. However, in the present litigious atmosphere of the USA, the filing of large liability claims by the statistically inevitable victims of good public health practice has caused many manufacturers to abandon efforts to develop and produce low-profit but medically valuable therapeutic agents such as vaccines. Since the use and sale of these products are subject to careful review and approval by government bodies such as the Surgeon General's Advisory Committee on Immunization Practices and the Food and Drug Administration, "strict product liability" (liability without fault) may be an inappropriate legal standard to apply when rare reactions to biologicals, produced and administered according to government guidelines, are involved.

RECOMMENDED IMMUNIZATION OF ADULTS FOR TRAVEL

Every adult, whether traveling or not, should be immunized with tetanus toxoid and should also be fully immunized against poliomyelitis, measles (for those born after 1956), and diphtheria. In addition, every traveler must fulfill the immunization requirements of the health authorities of the countries to be visited. These are listed in *Health Information for International Travel*, available from the Superintendent of Documents, United States Government Printing Office, Washington, DC 20402. A useful website is http://wwwnc.cdc.gov/travel/page/vaccinations.aspx. *The Medical Letter on Drugs and Therapeutics* also offers periodically updated recommendations for international travelers (see *Treatment Guidelines from The Medical Letter,* 2006;4:25). Immunizations received in preparation for travel should be recorded on the International Certificate of Immunization. ***Note:*** Smallpox vaccination is not recommended or required for travel in any country.

REFERENCES

Ada G: Vaccines and vaccination. N Engl J Med 2001;345:1042.

Advice for travelers. Treat Guidel Med Lett 2009;7:83.

Avery RK: Immunizations in adult immunocompromised patients: Which to use and which to avoid. Cleve Clin J Med 2001;68:337.

CDC Website: http://www.cdc.gov/vaccines/

Dennehy PH: Active immunization in the United States: Developments over the past decade. Clin Micro Rev 2001;14:872.

Gardner P, Peter G: Vaccine recommendations: Challenges and controversies. Infect Dis Clin North Am 2001;15:1.

Gardner P et al: Guidelines for quality standards for immunization. Clin Infect Dis 2002;35:503.

General recommendations on immunization. Recommendations of the Advisory Committee on Immunization Practices (ACIP). MMWR Morb Mortal Wkly Rep 2011;60(2):1.

Hill DR et al: The practice of travel medicine: Guidelines by the Infectious Diseases Society of America. Clin Infect Dis 2006;43:1499.

Keller MA, Stiehm ER: Passive immunity in prevention and treatment of infectious diseases. Clin Microbiol Rev 2000;13:602.

Pickering LK et al: Immunization programs for infants, children, adolescents, and adults: Clinical practice guidelines by the Infectious Diseases Society of America. Clin Infect Dis 2009;49:817.

Recommended adult immunization schedule—United States, 2010. MMWR Morb Mortal Wkly Rep 2010;59:1.

Recommended immunization schedules for persons aged 0 through 18 years—United States, 2010. MMWR Morb Mortal Wkly Rep 2007;58(51&52).

Index

Note: Page numbers in boldface type indicate major discussions. A *t* following a page number indicates tabular material, and an *f* following a page number indicates a figure.